Vascular *and* Endovascular Surgery

A Comprehensive Review

Editor:
Wesley S. Moore, MD
Professor and Chief Emeritus
Division of Vascular and Endovascular Surgery
University of California, Los Angeles
Los Angeles, California

Associate Editors:
Peter F. Lawrence, MD
Wiley Barker Professor of Surgery
Chief of the Division of Vascular and Endovascular Surgery
Department of Surgery
University of California, Los Angeles
Los Angeles, California

Gustavo S. Oderich, MD
Professor of Surgery
Director of Aortic Center
Director of Vascular Surgery Training Programs
Division of Vascular and Endovascular Surgery
Mayo Clinic
Rochester, Minnesota

Ninth Edition

ELSEVIER

ELSEVIER

1600 John F. Kennedy Blvd.
Ste 1800
Philadelphia, PA 19103-2899

VASCULAR AND ENDOVASCULAR SURGERY:
A COMPREHENSIVE REVIEW, NINTH EDITION

ISBN: 978-0-323-48011-6

Notices

Practitioners and researchers must always rely on their own experience and knowledge in evaluating and using any information, methods, compounds or experiments described herein. Because of rapid advances in the medical sciences, in particular, independent verification of diagnoses and drug dosages should be made. To the fullest extent of the law, no responsibility is assumed by Elsevier, authors, editors or contributors for any injury and/or damage to persons or property as a matter of products liability, negligence or otherwise, or from any use or operation of any methods, products, instructions, or ideas contained in the material herein.

Library of Congress Control Number: 2018942663

Publisher: Russell Gabbedy
Senior Content Development Specialist: Deidre Simpson
Publishing Services Manager: Catherine Jackson
Project Manager: Kate Mannix
Design Direction: Margaret Reid
Illustrations Manager: Nichole Beard

Printed in China

Last digit is the print number: 9 8 7 6 5 4 3 2 1

CONTRIBUTORS

Christopher J. Abularrage, MD
Associate Professor
Division of Vascular Surgery and Endovascular Therapy
The Johns Hopkins Hospital
Baltimore, Maryland
59: Prosthetic Graft Infection

Olamide Alabi, MD
Assistant Professor of Surgery
Division of Vascular Surgery and Endovascular Therapy
Department of Surgery
Emory University School of Medicine
Atlanta, Georgia
34: Natural History and Nonoperative Treatment of Chronic Lower Extremity Ischemia

Mark M. Archie, MD
Division of Vascular Surgery
University of California, Los Angeles
Los Angeles, California
53: Etiology and Management of Varicose Veins: Surgery, Endovenous Ablation, and Sclerotherapy

Dean J. Arnaoutakis, MD, MBA
Assistant Professor of Surgery
Division of Vascular Surgery and Endovascular Therapy
University of Florida
Gainesville, Florida
23: Surgical Management of Aortoiliac Occlusive Disease

Margaret W. Arnold, MD
Assistant Professor of Surgery
Division of Vascular Surgery and Endovascular Therapy
Johns Hopkins University School of Medicine
Baltimore, Maryland
61: Management of Complications After Endovascular Abdominal Aortic Aneurysm Repair

Enrico Ascher, MD
Vascular Institute of New York;
Division of Vascular Surgery
NYU Lutheran Medical Center
New York, New York
28: Surgical Management of Femoral, Popliteal, and Tibial Arterial Occlusive Disease

Gener Augustin, MD
Vascular Surgery and Endovascular Therapy
University Hospitals Cleveland Medical Center
Cleveland, Ohio
35: Thrombolysis for Arterial and Graft Occlusions: Technique and Results

Micheal Toma Ayad, MD
Southcoast Physicians Group Vascular and Endovascular Surgery
Dartmouth, Massachusetts
48: Surgical and Endovascular Management of Vascular Trauma, Including Aortic Transection

Amir F. Azarbal, MD
Assistant Professor of Surgery
Division of Vascular Surgery
Oregon Health and Science University
Portland, Oregon

Ali Azizzadeh, MD, FACS
Professor
Department of Cardiothoracic and Vascular Surgery
McGovern Medical School
University of Texas Health Science Center at Houston
Houston, Texas
36: Descending Thoracic and Thoracoabdominal Aortic Aneurysms: General Principles and Open Surgical Repair

John T. Baber, Jr., MD, MBA
Fellow, Vascular and Endovascular Surgery
Department of Surgery
New York-Presbyterian Hospital
Weill Cornell/Columbia University Medical Centers
New York, New York
13: Medical Management of Vascular Disease, Including Pharmacology of Drugs used in Vascular Disease Management

J. Dennis Baker, MD
Emeritus Professor of Surgery
Division of Vascular Surgery
UCLA School of Medicine
Los Angeles, California
14: The Noninvasive Vascular Diagnostic Laboratory

Donald T. Baril, MD
Associate Professor of Surgery
Division of Vascular Surgery
University of California, Los Angeles
Los Angeles, California
18: Atherectomy and Arterial Closure Devices: Selection, Technique, and Results

Wiley F. Barker, MD
Professor Emeritus of Surgery and Vascular Surgery
University of California, Los Angeles
Los Angeles, California
1: A History of Vascular Surgery

Neal R. Barshes, MD, MPH
Associate Professor of Surgery
Michael E. DeBakey Department of Surgery
Baylor College of Medicine
Houston, Texas
62: Diabetic Foot Complications: A Primer for Vascular Surgeons

Michael Belkin, MD
Chief, Division of Vascular Surgery
Brigham & Women's Hospital
Harvard University
Boston, Massachusetts
23: Surgical Management of Aortoiliac Occlusive Disease

John D. Bisognano, MD, PhD
Professor of Medicine/Cardiology
Internal Medicine
University of Rochester Medical Center
Rochester, New York
66: Carotid Sinus Stimulation: Background, Technique, and Future Directions

Ruth L. Bush, MD, JD, MPH
Professor of Surgery and Medicine
Michael E. DeBakey VA Medical Center
Baylor College of Medicine
Houston, Texas
24: Angioplasty and Stenting for Aorto-Iliac Occlusive Disease: Technique and Results

Danielle E. Cafasso, DO, MPH
Fellow of Vascular & Endovascular Surgery
Vascular & Endovascular Surgery
New York Presbyterian Hospital
New York, New York
21: Endovascular Repair of Extracranial Cerebrovascular Lesions

Catherine Cagiannos, MD
Division of Vascular Surgery and Endovascular Therapy
Michael E. DeBakey Department of Surgery
Baylor College of Medicine
Houston, Texas

John George Carson, MD
Assistant Professor of Surgery
Department of Surgery
University of California–Davis
Sacramento, California
59: Prosthetic Graft Infection

Neal S. Cayne, MD
Director of Endovascular Surgery
Professor of Surgery
Division of Vascular Surgery
New York University Medical Center
New York, New York
28: Surgical Management of Femoral, Popliteal, and Tibial Arterial Occlusive Disease; 43: Open Surgical and Endovascular Management of Ruptured Abdominal Aortic Aneurysm

Ankur Chandra, MD, RPVI
Director of Quality
VQI Southern California VOICe;
Co-Director, Vascular Diagnostic Laboratory
Division of Vascular and Endovascular Surgery
Scripps Clinic/Scripps Green Hospital
La Jolla, California
14: The Noninvasive Vascular Diagnostic Laboratory

Kristofer M. Charlton-Ouw, MD
Associate Professor
Department of Cardiothoracic and Vascular Surgery
McGovern Medical School
University of Texas Health Science Center at Houston
Houston, Texas
36: Descending Thoracic and Thoracoabdominal Aortic Aneurysms: General Principles and Open Surgical Repair

Jayer Chung, MD, MSc
Assistant Professor
Division of Vascular Surgery and Endovascular Therapy
Michael E DeBakey Department of Surgery
Baylor College of Medicine
Houston, Texas
12: Patterns of Diabetic Vascular Disease

Dawn M. Coleman, MD
Handleman Research Professor
Associate Professor of Surgery and Pediatrics & Communicable Disease
Section of Vascular Surgery
University of Michigan
Ann Arbor, Michigan
46: Splanchnic and Renal Artery Aneurysms; 49: Venous Thromboembolic Disease

Anthony J. Comerota, MD
Director
Jobst Vascular Center
The Toledo Hospital
Toledo, Ohio;
Adjunct Professor of Surgery
Vascular Surgery
University of Michigan
Ann Arbor, Michigan
50: Thrombolysis and Mechanical Thrombectomy for Deep Venous Thrombosis and Pulmonary Embolism

Enrique Criado, MD, FACS
MidMichigan Health
Midland, Michigan
20: Surgical Reconstruction of the Supraaortic Trunks and Vertebral Arteries

Thomas G. DeLoughery, MD
Professor of Hematology/Oncology and Laboratory Medicine
Knight Cancer Institute
Oregon Health & Science University
Portland, Oregon
6: Hemostasis and Thrombosis

Ralph G. DePalma, MD, FACS
Special Operattions Officer
Office of Research and Development
Department of Veterans Affairs
Washington, DC;
Professor of Surgery
Norman Rich Department of Surgery
Uniformed Services University of the Health Sciences
Bethesda, Maryland
7: Atherosclerosis: Pathology, Pathogenesis, and Medical Management

Brian G. DeRubertis, MD
Associate Professor of Surgery
Division of Vascular Surgery
UCLA School of Medicine
Los Angeles, California
30: Infrainguinal Endovascular Reconstruction: Technique and Results

Jeffrey B. Edwards, MD
Resident, Division of Vascular Surgery
University of South Florida College of Medicine
Tampa, Florida
66: Carotid Sinus Stimulation: Background, Technique, and Future Directions

Christian Eisenring, MSN, ACNP-c
Division of Cardiothoracic Surgery
Department of Cardiothoracic Surgery
David Geffen School of Medicine
University of California–Los Angeles
Los Angeles, California
29: Endoscopic Harvesting of the Saphenous Vein

Jonathan L. Eliason, MD
Eliason Lindenauer Professor of Surgery
Department of Vascular Surgery
University of Michigan
Ann Arbor, Michigan
46: Splanchnic and Renal Artery Aneurysms

Sharif H. Ellozy, MD
Division of Vascular and Endovascular Surgery
Weil Cornell Medicine
New York, New York
61: Management of Complications After Endovascular Abdominal Aortic Aneurysm Repair

Anthony L. Estrera, MD
Department of Cardiothoracic and Vascular Surgery
McGovern Medical School
University of Texas Health Science Center at Houston
Houston, Texas
36: Descending Thoracic and Thoracoabdominal Aortic Aneurysms: General Principles and Open Surgical Repair

Ronald M. Fairman, MD
The Clyde F. Barker–William Maul Measey Professor in Surgery
Chief, Division of Vascular Surgery and Endovascular Therapy
Vice-Chairman for Clinical Affairs, Department of Surgery
Professor of Surgery in Radiology
Hospital of the University of Pennsylvania
Philadelphia, Pennsylvania
42: Endovascular Repair of Juxtarenal (Chimney), Infrarenal, and Iliac Artery Aneurysms

Alik Farber, MD, FACS
Professor of Surgery and Radiology
Associate Chair of Surgery
Division of Vascular and Endovascular Surgery
Boston University School of Medicine
Boston Medical Center
Boston, Massachusetts
16: Vascular Grafts: Characteristics and Rational Selection

Steven M. Farley, MD
Associate Professor of Surgery
Division of Vascular and Endovascular Surgery
University of California, Los Angeles
Los Angeles, California
54: Management of Venous Leg Ulcers; 63: The Wound Care Center and Limb Salvage

Julie Ann Freischlag, MD
Chief Executive Officer and Dean
Wake Forest Medical Center
Winston Salem, North Carolina
59: Prosthetic Graft Infection

Nicholas J. Gargiulo III, MD, FACS
Vascular Surgeon
Department of Surgery
Division of Vascular Surgery
The Brookdale University Hospital and Medical Center
New York, New York
28: Surgical Management of Femoral, Popliteal, and Tibial Arterial Occlusive Disease

Hugh A. Gelabert, MD
Professor of Surgery
UCLA School of Medicine
Los Angeles, California
11: Antibiotic Prophylaxis in Vascular Disease Management; 33: Thoracic Outlet Syndrome and Vascular Disease of the Upper Extremity; 55: Portal Hypertension

Bruce L. Gewertz, MD
Chair and Vice-President of Interventional Services
Department of Surgery
Cedars-Sinai Medical Center
Los Angeles, California
25: Diagnosis and Surgical Management of the Visceral Ischemic Syndromes

David L. Gillespie, MD, RVT, FACS
Chief, Department of Vascular and Endovascular Surgery
Southcoast Health System
Fall River, Massachusetts;
Affiliated Professor of Surgery
Uniformed Services University
Bethesda, Maryland
48: Surgical and Endovascular Management of Vascular Trauma Including Aortic Transection

Peter Gloviczki, MD
Joe M. and Ruth Roberts Professor of Surgery, Emeritus
Chair Emeritus
Division of Vascular and Endovascular Surgery
Mayo Clinic
Rochester, Minnesota
9: Venous Vascular Malformations; 32: Thoracic and Lumbar Sympathectomy: Indications, Technique, and Results; 51: Surgical Management of Chronic Venous Obstruction

Jerry Goldstone, MD
Professor Emeritus
Department of Surgery
Case Western Reserve University School of Medicine
Cleveland, Ohio;
Consulting Professor
Department of Vascular Surgery
Stanford University School of Medicine,
Stanford, California
41: Aneurysms of the Aorta and Iliac Arteries

Antoinette S. Gomes, MD
Professor of Radiological Sciences & Medicine
Department of Radiological Sciences
David Geffen School of Medicine at UCLA
Los Angeles, California
15: Principles of Imaging in Vascular Disease

Ryan A. Haqq, MD
Resident Physician
University of Alabama
Birmingham, Alabama
26: Diagnosis and Management of Renal Vascular Occlusive Disease

Peter K. Henke, MD
Leland Ira Doan Professor of Surgery
Section of Vascular Surgery
University of Michigan
Ann Arbor, Michigan
49: Venous Thromboembolic Disease

Ying Huang, MD, PhD
Assistant Professor of Surgery
Division of Vascular and Endovascular Surgery
Mayo Clinic
Rochester, Minnesota
51: Surgical Management of Chronic Venous Obstruction

Glenn C. Hunter, MD, FRCSC, FRCSED
Professor of Surgery Emeritus
Department of Surgery
University of Arizona
Tucson, Arizona
60: Noninfectious Complications in Vascular Surgery

Karl A. Illig, MD
Professor of Surgery
Division of Vascular Surgery
University of South Florida Morsani School of Medicine
Tampa, Florida
66: Carotid Sinus Stimulation: Background, Technique, and Future Directions

Benjamin Jacobs, MD
House Officer
General Surgery
University of Michigan
Ann Arbor, Michigan
49: Venous Thromboembolic Disease

Krishna Mohan Jain, MD
Clinical Professor of Surgery
Western Michgan University
Homer Stryker MD School of Medicine
Kalamazoo, Michigan
67: Building an Outpatient Interventional Suite

Arjun Jayaraj, MD, FACS
Vascular Surgeon
RANE Center for Venous and Lymphatic Diseases at St. Dominic Hospital
Jackson, Mississippi
52: Endovascular Repair of Chronic Venous Obstruction

Juan Carlos Jimenez, MD, FACS
Associate Clinical Professor of Surgery
Gonda (Goldschmied) Vascular Center
UCLA Center for Wound Healing and Limb Preservation
UCLA Hyperbaric Medicine
David Geffen School of Medicine at UCLA;
Attending Surgeon
Ronald Reagan-UCLA Medical Center
ULCA-Santa Monica Hospital
Santa Monica, California
29: Endoscopic Harvesting of the Saphenous Vein; 60: Noninfectious Complications in Vascular Surgery; 64: Lower Extremity Amputation

Daniel J. Johnston, MD
Clinical Assistant Professor of Surgery
Western Michigan University
Homer Stryker MD School of Medicine
Kalamazoo, Michigan
67: Building an Outpatient Interventional Suite

William D. Jordan, Jr., MD
Professor of Surgery
Chief, Division of Vascular Surgery and Endovascular Therapy
Department of Surgery
Emory University School of Medicine
Atlanta, Georgia
24: Angioplasty and Stenting for Aortoiliac Occlusive Disease: Technique and Results

Vikram Kashyap, MD, FACS
Chief, Division of Vascular Surgery and Endovascular Surgery
Alan H. Markowitze MD Master Clinician for Cardiac and Vascular Surgery
Director, Vascular Center
Harrington Heart and Vascular Institute
University Hospitals Cleveland Medical Center;
Professor of Surgery
Case Western Reserve University
Cleveland, Ohio
35: Thrombolysis for Arterial and Graft Occlusions: Technique and Results

Ahmed Kayssi, MD, MSc, MPH
Vascular Surgery and Wound Care
Department of Surgery
University of Toronto
Toronto, Ontario, Canada
57: Hemodialysis and Vascular Access

Melina R. Kibbe, MD
Colin G. Thomas Professor of Surgery
Chair, Department of Surgery
University of North Carolina
Chapel Hill, North Carolina
58: Neointimal Hyperplasia

Andrew Kimball, MD
House Officer
General Surgery
University of Michigan
Ann Arbor, Michigan
49: Venous Thromboembolic Disease

Jordan Knepper, MD
Henry Ford Allegiance
Vascular Health
Jackson, Mississippi
49: Venous Thromboembolic Disease

Ted R. Kohler, MD
Professor Emeritus
Department of Surgery
University of Washington
Seattle, Washington
3: Anatomy, Physiology, and Pharmacology of the Vascular Wall

Ralf R. Kolvenbach, MD
Professor
Department of Vascular Surgery and Endovascular Therapy
Augusta Hospital
Duesseldorf, Germany
44: Laparoscopic Aortic Surgery for Aneurysm and Occlusive Disease: Technique and Results

Andrew K. Kurklinsky, MD, MACP
Department of Cardiovascular Medicine
Mayo Clinic
Jacksonville, Florida
56: Lymphedema

Mimmie Kwong, MD
Resident (PGY-4)
Vascular Surgery
University of California–Davis
Sacramento, California
59: Prosthetic Graft Infection

Mario Lachat, MD, FEBVS, FECTS
Professor, Head of Vascular Surgery
Clinic for Cardiovascular Surgery
University Hospital Zurich
Zurich, Switzerland
43: Open Surgical and Endovascular Management of Ruptured Abdominal Aortic Aneurysm

Gregg S. Landis, MD
Chief of Vascular Surgery
Division of Vascular Surgery
Northwell Health
New York, New York
28: Surgical Management of Femoral, Popliteal, and Tibial Arterial Occlusive Disease

Gregory J. Landry, MD
Professor of Surgery
Chief, Division of Vascular Surgery
Knight Cardiovascular Institute
Oregon Health & Science University
Portland, Oregon
8: Nonatherosclerotic Vascular Disease; 34: Natural History and Nonoperative Treatment of Chronic Lower Extremity Ischemia

Peter F. Lawrence, MD
Wiley Barker Professor of Surgery
Chief of the Division of Vascular and Endovascular Surgery
Department of Surgery
University of California, Los Angeles
Los Angeles, California
22: Carotid Body Tumors: Diagnosis and Surgical Management; 54: Management of Venous Leg Ulcers; 63: The Wound Care Center and Limb Salvage

Wesley Kwan Lew, MD
Vascular Surgeon
Kaiser Sunset
Los Angeles, California
38: Combined Endovascular and Surgical (Hybrid) Approach to Aortic Arch and Thoracoabdominal Aortic Pathology

Timothy K. Liem, MD, MBA
Professor of Surgery
Knight Cardiovascular Institute
Oregon Health & Science University
Portland, Oregon
6: Hemostasis and Thrombosis

Evan C. Lipsitz, MD, MBA
Chief, Division of Vascular and Endovascular Surgery
Cardiothoracic and Vascular Surgery
Montefiore Medical Center
Albert Einstein College of Medicine
New York, New York
28: Surgical Management of Femoral, Popliteal, and Tibial Arterial Occlusive Disease

Chris Longton, RN
Business Manager
Advanced Vascular Surgery
Kalamazoo, Michigan
67: Building an Outpatient Interventional Suite

Alan B. Lumsden, MD
Professor and Chairman
Department of Cardiovascular Surgery
Houston Methodist DeBakey Heart & Vascular Center
Houston Methodist Hospital
Houston, Texas
17: Introduction to Endovascular Surgery: Arterial Access, Guide Wires, Catheters, Sheaths, Angioplasty Catheters, and Stents; 45: Building a Hybrid Operating Suite, Including Robotic Capability

Michel S. Makaroun, MD
Professor of Surgery
University of Pittsburgh
Pittsburgh, Pennsylvania
37: Endovascular Repair of Thoracic Aortic Aneurysm

Neel A. Mansukhani, MD
Vascular Surgery Resident
Deparment of Surgery
Northwestern University
Chicago, Illinois
58: Neointimal Hyperplasia

David S. Maxwell, MD[†]
2: Embryology of the Vascular System

Dieter Mayer, MD, FEBVS
Director of Vascular Surgery
Department of Surgery
Canton Hospital of Fribourg
Fribourg, Switzerland
43: Open Surgical and Endovascular Management of Ruptured Abdominal Aortic Aneurysm

James F. McKinsey, MD
Chief of Vascular Surgery and Endovascular Interventions
Department of Surgery
New York Presbyterian/Columbia University
New York, New York
25: Diagnosis and Surgical Management of the Visceral Ischemic Syndromes

Charles C. Miller III, MD
Professor and Vice Chair, Research
Department of Cardiothoracic and Vascular Surgery
McGovern Medical School
University of Texas Health Science Center at Houston
Houston, Texas
36: Descending Thoracic and Thoracoabdominal Aortic Aneurysms: General Principles and Open Surgical Repair

[†]Deceased

Joseph L. Mills, MD
Professor and Chief of Vascular Surgery and Endovascular Therapy
Michael E. DeBakey Department of Surgery
Baylor College of Medicine
Houston, Texas
12: Patterns of Diabetic Vascular Disease; 31: Endovascular Repair of Infrapopliteal Arterial Occlusive Disease; 62: Diabetic Foot Complications: A Primer for Vascular Surgeons

Erica L. Mitchell, MD
Professor of Surgery
Medical Director Salem Health Medical Group Vascular Surgery
Division of Vascular Surgery
Oregon Health and Science University
Portland, Oregon
34: Natural History and Nonoperative Treatment of Chronic Lower Extremity Ischemia

Gregory L. Moneta, MD
Professor
Division of Vascular Surgery
Oregon Health and Science University
Portland, Oregon
34: Natural History and Nonoperative Treatment of Chronic Lower Extremity Ischemia

Miguel Montero-Baker, MD
Associate Chief of Vascular Surgery
Division of Vascular and Endovascular Surgery
Michael E. DeBakey Department of Surgery
Baylor College of Medicine
Houston, Texas
31: Endovascular Repair of Infrapopliteal Arterial Occlusive Disease

Wesley S. Moore, MD
Professor and Chief Emeritus
Division of Vascular and Endovascular Surgery
University of California, Los Angeles
Los Angeles, California
19: Extracranial Cerebrovascular Disease: The Carotid Artery

Rameen S. Moridzadeh, MD
Division of Vascular and Endovascular Surgery
University of California, Los Angeles
Los Angeles, California
22: Carotid Body Tumors: Diagnosis and Surgical Management; 55: Portal Hypertension

John S. Munn, MD
Clinical Assistant Professor of Surgery
Western Michigan University
Homer Stryker MD School of Medicine
Kalamazoo, Michigan
67: Building an Outpatient Interventional Suite

Daiva Nevidomskyte, MD
Assistant Professor
Department of Vascular and Endovascular Surgery
Duke University
Durham, North Carolina
10: Congenital Arterial Malformations

Richard F. Neville, MD
Associate Director, Heart and Vascular Institute
Director, Vascular Services
INOVA Health System;
Vice Chairmanm Surgical Subspecialties
Department of Surgery
INOVA Fairfax
Falls Church, Virginia
57: Hemodialysis and Vascular Access

Andrea Obi, MD
Assistant Professor of Surgery
Section of Vascular Surgery
University of Michigan
Ann Arbor, Michigan
49: Venous Thromboembolic Disease

Jessica Beth O'Connell, MD, FACS
Deputy Director, Surgical & Perioperative Careline
Co-Chief, Vascular Surgery Service
Department of Veterans Affairs
VA Greater Los Angeles Healthcare System;
Associate Clinical Professor
Gonda (Goldschmied) Vascular Center
ULCA Department of Surgery
Los Angeles, California
7: Atherosclerosis: Pathology, Pathogenesis, and Medical Management; 13: Medical Management of Vascular Disease, Including Pharmacology of Drugs Used in Vascular Disease Management

Gustavo S. Oderich, MD
Professor of Surgery
Director of Aortic Center
Director of Vascular Surgery Training Programs
Division of Vascular and Endovascular Surgery
Mayo Clinic
Rochester, Minnesota
27: Angioplasty and Stenting for Mesenteric and Renal Artery Disease; 39: Fenestrated-Branched and Parallel Stent-Grafts for Endovascular Repair of Aortic Arch and Thoracoabdominal Aortic Aneurysms

Jigar A. Patel, MD
Vascular Surgery Fellow
Assistant Professor of Surgery
Uniformed Services University of the Health Sciences
Walter Reed National Military Medical Center
Bethesda, Maryland
4: Anatomy and Surgical Exposure of the Vascular System

Benjamin J. Pearce, MD, FACS
Associate Professor and Program Director
Division of Vascular Surgery and Endovascular Therapy
University of Alabama-Birmingham
Birmingham, Alabama
26: Diagnosis and Management of Renal Vascular Occlusive Disease

Wande B. Pratt, MD, MPH
Staff Vascular Surgeon
Department of Surgery
Christian Hospital
St. Louis, Missouri
36: Descending Thoracic and Thoracoabdominal Aortic Aneurysms: General Principles and Open Surgical Repair

William J. Quiñones-Baldrich, MD
Professor of Surgery
Department of Vascular Surgery
David Geffen School of Medicine at UCLA;
Director, UCLA Aortic Center
UCLA Medical Center
Los Angeles, California
35: Thrombolysis for Arterial and Graft Occlusions: Technique and Results; 38: Combined Endovascular and Surgical (Hybrid) Approach to Aortic Arch and Thoracoabdominal Aortic Pathology; 65: Anterior Spine Exposure: Operative Techniques for the Vascular Surgeon

Seshadri Raju, MD
Professor Emeritus of Surgery
Director, the RANE Center
River Oaks Hospital
Jackson, Mississippi
52: Endovascular Repair of Chronic Venous Obstruction

Todd E. Rasmussen, MD
Shumacker Professor of Surgery
Associate Dean for Clinical Research
F. Edward Herbert School of Medicine
Uniformed Services University of the Health Sciences
Bethesda, Maryland
4: Anatomy and Surgical Exposure of the Vascular System

David A. Rigberg, MD
Professor
Deparment of Vascular Surgery
David Geffen School of Medicine at UCLA
Los Angeles, California
33: Thoracic Outlet Syndrome and Vascular Disease of the Upper Extremity; 53: Etiology and Management of Varicose Veins: Surgery, Endovenous Ablation, and Sclerotherapy; 55: Portal Hypertension

Scott T. Robinson, MD, PhD
House Officer
Vascular Surgery
University of Michigan
Ann Arbor, Michigan
49: Venous Thromboembolic Disease

Johnathon Rollo, MD
Assistant Professor
Division of Vascular Surgery
University of Washington
Seattle, Washington
18: Atherectomy and Arterial Closure Devices: Selection, Technique, and Results; 30: Infrainguinal Endovascular Reconstruction: Technique and Results

Thom W. Rooke, MD
Krehbiel Professor of Vascular Medicine
Vascular Center
Mayo Clinic
Rochester, Minnesota
56: Lymphedema

Mark C. Rummel, MD
Clinical Assistant Professor of Surgery
Western Michigan University
Homer Stryker MD School of Medicine
Kalamazoo, Michigan
67: Building an Outpatient Interventional Suite

Hazim J. Safi, MD, FACS, FRCS
Professor and Chairman
Department of Cardiothoracic and Vascular Surgery
McGovern Medical School
University of Texas Health Science Center at Houston
Houston, Texas
36: Descending Thoracic and Thoracoabdominal Aortic Aneurysms: General Principles and Open Surgical Repair

Taimur Saleem, MD
Vascular Surgery Fellow
UCLA Department of Surgery
Division of Vascular Surgery
David Geffen School of Medicine
University of California, Los Angeles
Los Angeles, California
7: Atherosclerosis: Pathology, Pathogenesis, and Medical Management; 11: Antibiotic Prophylaxis in Vascular Disease Management

Giuliano de A. Sandri, MD
Aortic Research Fellow
Division of Vascular and Endovascular Surgery
Mayo Clinic
Rochester, Minnesota
27: Angioplasty and Stenting for Mesenteric and Renal Artery Disease; 39: Fenestrated-Branched and Parallel Stent-Grafts for Endovascular Repair of Aortic Arch and Thoracoabdominal Aortic Aneurysms

Peter A. Schneider, MD
Chief
Division of Vascular Therapy
Kaiser Foundation Hospital
Honolulu, Hawaii
21: Endovascular Repair of Extracranial Cerebrovascular Lesions; 30: Infrainguinal Endovascular Reconstruction: Technique and Results

Lewis B. Schwartz, MD
Vascular Surgery
Department of Surgery
Advocate Lutheran General Hospital
Park Ridge, Illinois
25: Diagnosis and Surgical Management of the Visceral Ischemic Syndromes

Aamir S. Shah, MD
Associate Director of Aortic Program
Cardiothoracic and Vascular Surgery
Cedars-Sinai Medical Center
Los Angeles, California
25: Diagnosis and Surgical Management of the Visceral Ischemic Syndromes

Sherene Shalhub, MD, MPH, FACS
Assistant Professor of Surgery
Division of Vascular Surgery
University of Washington
Seattle, Washington
40: Acute and Chronic Aortic Dissection: Medical Management, Surgical Management, Endovascular Management, and Results

Palma M. Shaw, MD
Associate Professor of Surgery
General Surgery
Upstate Medical Center
Syracuse, New York
65: Anterior Spine Exposure: Operative Techniques for the Vascular Surgeon

Maxim E. Shaydakov, MD, PhD
General Surgery Resident
Department of Surgery
UT Health San Antonio
San Antonio, Texas
50: Thrombolysis and Mechanical Thrombectomy for Deep Venous Thrombosis and Pulmonary Embolism

Cynthia K. Shortell, MD
Professor and Chief of Vascular Surgery
Department of Vascular and Endovascular Surgery
Duke University
Durham, North Carolina
10: Congenital Arterial Malformations

Daniel Silverberg, MD
Senior Consultant
Department of Vascular Surgery
The Chaim Sheba Medical Center
Tel Hashomer, Israel
61: Management of Complications After Endovascular Abdominal Aortic Aneurysm Repair

Michael J. Singh, MD, FACS, RPVI
Co-Director of Aortic Center
UPMC Heart and Vascular Institute
Associate Professor of Surgery
Division of Vascular Surgery
University of Pittsburgh Medical Center
Pittsburgh, Pennsylvania
37: Endovascular Repair of Thoracic Aortic Aneurysm

Jeffrey J. Siracuse, MD, RPVI, FACS
Associate Professor of Surgery and Radiology
Division of Vascular and Endovascular Surgery
Boston University School of Medicine
Boston Medical Center
Boston, Massachusetts
16: Vascular Grafts: Characteristics and Rational Selection

James C. Stanley, MD
Professor Emeritus of Surgery
Department of Vascular Surgery
University of Michigan
Ann Arbor, Michigan
46: Splanchnic and Renal Artery Aneurysms

Benjamin W. Starnes, MD
The Alexander W. Clowes Endowed Chair
Professor of Surgery
Chief, Vascular Surgery Division
University of Washington
Seattle, Washington
40: Acute and Chronic Aortic Dissection: Medical Management, Surgical Management, Endovascular Management, and Results

Gale L. Tang, MD
Associate Professor
Department of Surgery
University of Washington
VA Puget Sound Health Care System
Seattle, Washington
3: Anatomy, Physiology, and Pharmacology of the Vascular Wall

Emanuel Junio R. Tenorio, MD, PhD
Aortic Research Fellow
Division of Vascular and Endovascular Surgery
Mayo Clinic
Rochester, Minnesota
27: Angioplasty and Stenting for Mesenteric and Renal Artery Disease

Frank J. Veith, MD
Professor of Surgery
New York University
New York, New York;
Professor of Surgery
The William J. von Liebig Chair in Vascular Surgery
The Cleveland Clinic
Cleveland, Ohio
28: Surgical Management of Femoral, Popliteal, and Tibial Arterial Occlusive Disease; 43: Open Surgical and Endovascular Management of Ruptured Abdominal Aortic Aneurysm

Thomas Wakefield, MD
Department of Surgery
Section of Vascular Surgery
University of Michigan
Ann Arbor, Michigan
49: Venous Thromboembolic Disease

Grace J. Wang, MD, MSCE
Assistant Professor of Surgery
Division of Vascular Surgery and Endovascular Therapy
Hospital of the University of Pennsylvania
Philadelphia, Pennsylvania
42: Endovascular Repair of Juxtarenal (Chimney), Infrarenal, and Iliac Artery Aneurysms

Sarah Michelle Wartman, MD
Fellow, Vascular Surgery
University of Southern California
Los Angeles, California
47: Aneurysms of the Peripheral Arteries

Fred A. Weaver, MD, MMM
Professor and Chief
Vascular Surgery and Endovascular Therapy
Keck Medical Center of the University of Southern California
Los Angeles, California
47: Aneurysms of the Peripheral Arteries

Paul W. White, MD
Program Director, Vascular Surgery Fellowship
Associate Professor of Surgery
Walter Reed National Military Medical Center;
Associate Professor of Surgery
Uniformed Services University of the Health Sciences
Bethesda, Maryland
Consultant to the Surgeon General for Vascular Surgery
United States
4: Anatomy and Surgical Exposure of the Vascular System

R. Eugene Zierler, MD
Medical Director
D. E. Strandness Jr. Vascular Laboratory
University of Washington Medical Center
Harborview Medical Center;
Professor
Department of Surgery
University of Washington School of Medicine
Seattle, Washington
5: Hemodynamics for the Vascular Surgeon

PREFACE TO THE NINTH EDITION

The ninth edition has been completely revised and the chapters have been organized under sections. These sections include general principles, arterial occlusive disease, arterial aneurysm disease, venous disease, complications, and miscellaneous topics. The signature chapters, organized under sections, remain. The signature chapter authors have fully updated their material. In recognition of the continuing expansion of endovascular technology as well as medical management, new chapters have been added. These include Chapter 10, Congenital Arterial Malformations; Chapter 18, Atherectomy and Arterial Closure Devices: Selection, Technique, and Results; Chapter 22, Carotid Body Tumors: Diagnosis and Surgical Management; Chapter 45, Building a Hybrid Operating Suite Including Robotic Capability; and Chapter 54, Management of Venous Leg Ulcers.

This textbook serves as a comprehensive treatise and reference for those managing patients with vascular disease, particularly the vascular surgeon. It is also the companion text for the annual UCLA/SVS vascular review course.

In summary, we have a completely revised and up-to-date volume directed to the comprehensive management of patients with vascular disorders.

Wesley S. Moore, MD

PREFACE TO THE FIRST EDITION

During the past 20 years of rapid growth and development in vascular surgery, many graduates of general surgery programs found that their training in vascular surgery represented a valuable new resource for their hospital and practice communities. That training in vascular surgery often provided an important edge in establishing a new practice and led to the widespread use of the term general and vascular surgery on the community announcements and business cards of new surgeons.

Yet in 1969, a survey conducted by a committee composed of James A. DeWeese, F. William Blaisdell, and John H. Foster discovered that among the 83 residents graduating from the 22 general surgery training programs surveyed, only 19 had performed more than 40 arterial reconstructive procedures during the course of their training, and more than half of the graduating residents had performed fewer than 20 arterial reconstructive procedures. The DeWeese committee, which had been established in 1969 to develop a document on optimal resources in vascular surgery, thus concluded that there was considerable suboptimal vascular surgery being performed in the United States, owing to a combination of both inadequate training and continued deficiencies in vascular surgery experience following training. A survey of the frequency of vascular operations in 1143 hospitals across the United States had revealed that in over 75% of these hospitals, fewer than 10 aneurysm resections and 10 femoropopliteal arterial reconstructions were conducted annually. This discovery led to the unfortunate conclusion that many surgeons were performing only occasional vascular operations, often leading to poor results.

The substance of the DeWeese report was reviewed by the two national vascular societies and their responsible leadership. This paved the way for, among other things, the definition of adequate training in vascular surgery and the recommendation that physicians who wish to practice vascular surgery spend an additional year of training to guarantee adequate experience in the speciality. To ensure prospective candidates that a given fellowship program in vascular surgery would provide a broad and responsible experience, the vascular societies established a committee for program evaluation and endorsements from which program directors could request review. Programs reviewed and found to meet the criteria of appropriate education as established by the committee would be announced annually.

Program evaluation by the joint council of the two national vascular societies was taken on as a temporary responsibility because the role would ultimately become the purview of the Residency Review Committee and the Liaison Committee for Graduate Medical Education. It was recognized that once adequate training programs were developed, the certification of candidates successfully completing training rested with the American Board of Surgery.

After approximately 10 years of experience, debate, and review, the American Board of Medical Specialties approved an application by the American Board of Surgery to grant "Certification of Special Competence in General Vascular Surgery." The first examination for certification was given to qualified members of the American Board of Surgery and Thoracic Surgery in June 1982. The second written examination was held in November 1983 in several centers across the United States.

The intent of this textbook is to provide a comprehensive review of vascular surgery, together with the related medical and basic science disciplines. This edition of the text has been developed to accompany a postgraduate course designed to help candidates prepare for the examination leading to certification in general vascular surgery. Accordingly, a list of questions designed to aid the reader in self-examination completes each chapter. All question sets simply represent the authors" opinion, a fair and adequate survey of the material covered, as none of the chapter authors is a member of the American Board of Surgery (this would be a conflict of interest).

Although chapter outlines were suggested by an editorial committee, the final chapter test represents, in the opinion of its authors, core material in each subject. Particular effort to identify and separate generally accepted concepts from new or controversial material was made. Although this book was designed as a comprehensive review to prepare for an examination, it is also in view of its organization and content, a comprehensive text of vascular surgery.

Wesley S. Moore, MD

†Deceased

A History of Vascular Surgery

Wiley F. Barker

History is not a precise record, for it is only that which has been remembered or written down. Inevitably, there is much personal interpretation of that original material. In addition, interpreting events from the past is often difficult, and history sometimes changes as new information becomes available. It is often hard for an observer to see recent events in proper perspective, especially when the observer is close to or involved with those events.

In the last few years, there have been immense developments in molecular biology and in the techniques of minimally invasive surgery and interventional endovascular procedures. The value of these developments remains difficult to assess, despite their incalculable promise for the future. As Mao Zedong reportedly replied when asked about the effect of the French Revolution on the revolution in China, "It is much too soon to tell."

This chapter is presented in sections that can be considered as a series of scenes and acts. As with many modern stage plays, different actors appear in different scenes in different roles, and many scenes take place concurrently and must be observed from different points of view, depending on the subject at hand. Ultimately, the whole fits together.

PROLOGUE

Although some might argue that Guy de Chauliac or Ambroise Paré should properly be called the sires of surgery, John Hunter is the prototype of the modern vascular surgeon. He was an unbelievably productive and tireless worker, cut from the same Scottish mold as his brother William, who was 10 years older. John was largely unlettered, whereas William had become sophisticated through his education at Glasgow, yet they shared a frenetic capacity for work and an incurable curiosity.

To place the Hunters in a clear perspective in regard to nonmedical history, one should note that they were contemporaries of George Washington and Benjamin Franklin. William Hunter was born in Scotland in 1718, his brother John was born 10 years later; William died in 1783, and John died in 1793.[1,2] John was even made a member of the American Philosophical Society, although he never attended a meeting.

William Hunter preceded John to London, where he soon established a busy medical practice and interested himself in many subjects, including aneurysms. In fact, William proposed the concept that a lancet used carelessly during bloodletting might enter both artery and vein, and after healing, the two channels might be connected. He thus imagined an arteriovenous fistula. He soon found just such a patient and described the clinical manifestations with great accuracy.[3] William's primary activity, however, was focused on obstetrics and on the teaching of anatomy. John became his assistant in this latter project.

John Hunter is remembered for many things, but especially for his studies of the dynamics and efficiency of collateral arterial circulation, which he described in the vessels feeding the antlers of a stag after he had interrupted the major arteries in its neck. More renown came from his ligation of the femoral artery in its subsartorial course at a distance above a popliteal aneurysm—in Hunter's canal.[1,2]

To be sure, others had preceded him in performing proximal ligation of arteries to treat aneurysms. In the third century, a Roman surgeon named Antyllus had described proximal and distal ligation of the artery, followed by incision of the aneurysm and removal of its contents—a formidable operation without either anesthesia or asepsis.[4] In 1680, Purmann, faced with a large aneurysm in the antecubital space, performed ligation of the vessels and excision of the aneurysmal mass.[5] In 1714, Anel described an operation in which he placed one ligature on the artery at the proximal extent of the aneurysm. Hunter, however, had found that the ligature would sometimes cut through the artery when it was placed too close to the popliteal aneurysm; therefore he chose a site that was more remote, but was easily reached by the surgeon and would preserve collaterals. Most of Anel's patients suffered from false aneurysms caused by bloodletting in otherwise healthy arteries. The femoropopliteal aneurysms treated by Hunter were due to degenerative processes, probably a mixture of syphilis and trauma.[1,6]

Many other surgeons were ligating aneurysms in various anatomic sites at this time. Cooper, one of John Hunter's students, was soon established as one of the early vascular surgeons when he ligated the carotid artery for an aneurysm in 1805,[7] as well as the aorta for an iliac artery aneurysm.[8] Only these few important events occurred before the latter part of the nineteenth century.

At the time, ligation was virtually the only procedure available to surgeons for the management of arterial problems, and those problems were limited to the control of hemorrhage and the treatment of aneurysms. Hallowell in Newcastle-on-Tyne performed one arterial repair of an artery torn during bloodletting. The laceration was a short one, and at the suggestion of Lambert, he placed a short (¼ inch) steel pin through the edges of the wound and looped a ligature around it in a figure-of-eight pattern, approximating the edges of the wound with apparent success. Hallowell wrote to William Hunter concerning this operation in 1761, foreseeing that if this were a successful technique, "we might be able to cure wounds of some arteries that would otherwise require amputation, or be altogether incurable."[9] That Hallowell wrote to William instead of John is probably due to William's published work on arteriovenous fistulas secondary to inept bloodletting. Twelve years later in 1773, Asman reviewed the Newcastle repair, attempted some experiments of his own that were disastrous, and concluded that such a procedure could not work and that Lambert and Hallowell's efforts had probably failed as well.[10] After Asman's criticism, the matter of arterial repair rested quietly for nearly another 100 years.

John Hunter's less widely known contributions are scattered throughout the immense museum he left to the Royal College of Surgeons of England, and they hint at an understanding of arterial pathology that would not be general knowledge for half a century. They include dissections of several atherosclerotic aortic bifurcations (specimens P.1177 and P.1178), showing the atheromatous lesion at the aortic bifurcation that Leriche would describe 150 years later; a carotid bifurcation with an ulcerated atheroma from a patient who died of a ruptured syphilitic thoracic aneurysm (specimen P.1171); and an extracranial internal carotid aneurysm (specimen P.282) in a patient whose neatly described symptoms are almost typical of what today are recognized as classic transient ischemic episodes.[11] Regrettably, most of Hunter's notes did not survive to provide more than this fragmentary view of his understanding of vascular disease. To cap it all, in a postmortem specimen, Hunter had dissected the atheromatous layers (although the term atheroma had not yet come into use) from the remaining intact wall of an atherosclerotic terminal aorta (specimen P.1176), foreshadowing dos Santos by 150 years.

Both Hunter and Cooper seemed to hold with the teleologic belief of the times that when senile or spontaneous gangrene occurred in older persons, thrombosis of the major vessels supervened so that the patient would not bleed to death when the gangrenous part separated.[12] It was Cruveilhier who first clearly stated that the phrase "gangrene due to obstruction of the arteries" by thickening and by thrombosis should replace the terms spontaneous and senile gangrene,[13] but he attributed the concept to Dupuytren.

The recognition that arterial obstruction causes functional disability that limits the use of the affected part may have arisen in the veterinary world. Bouley described the clinical picture in a horse in 1831.[14]

Four years later in 1835, a nearly anonymous physician on the ward of a Professor Louis provided the first clear description of human claudication. Barth's patient was a 51-year-old woman who died of heart failure resulting from mitral valvular disease. His report described her incidental history of claudication in terms that we would recognize today.[15] In the postmortem report, he noted thrombosis of the terminal aorta and included a sketch suggesting that the lesion was a thrombosed hypoplastic terminal aorta, a contracted atherosclerotic lesion, or a combination of both. Barth also repeated Hunter's observation that the obstructing material could be separated easily from the residual intact arterial wall. Barth was never identified further, not even by an initial.

Charcot is often erroneously given credit for recognizing the syndrome of intermittent claudication caused by arterial insufficiency in humans.[16] Charcot described, just as Bouley had done, the vanishing pulses, the cold extremity, and what is now recognized as the loss of sympathetic tone in a horse in the throes of a spasm of severe claudication; he reported a human case as well. Homans liked to joke that Charcot observed the former because he spent so much time at the horse races.

As a neurologist, Charcot was familiar with intermittent claudication in humans caused by various neurologic processes. The patient Charcot described, however, suffered claudication in one leg secondary to an old gunshot wound that resulted in occlusion of the iliac artery and an aneurysm proximal to the occlusion. The aneurysm, which was adherent to and in communication with the jejunum, gave rise to a series of small gastrointestinal hemorrhages before the final fatal episode. Charcot thus deserves credit for identifying the herald hemorrhages that often presage major bleeding from an aortoenteric fistula. (Charcot credited both Bouley and Barth with their prior observations regarding claudication.)

SUCCESSFUL ARTERIAL SUTURE

Such information was of little utility to surgeons, however, until arterial repair became a reality. Consistent with the observations of Asman, several German masters had deemed arterial repair (as opposed to ligation) to be impossible. Langenbeck stated in 1825 that, because the primary requirement for healing is perfect rest, an arterial incision could never heal as long as the pulsatile movements of the arterial wall continued.[17] Heinecke was certain that the patient would bleed to death through the suture holes and the apposed edges of the arterial wall.[18]

Repair of small injuries to veins, however, was becoming an established procedure. The lateral ligature, in which a clamp is placed on the defect in the venous wall and a ligature is tied around the puckered wall, had been performed in 1816.[19] The first lateral suture of a venous defect (an erosion of the common jugular vein from an infected neck wound) was undertaken by Czerny in 1881, but the patient died of sepsis and hemorrhage.[20] Jassinowsky[19] credits Schede[21] with the first successful repair of a large venous injury (to the common femoral vein) by lateral sutures.

Going beyond the stage of venous repair, Eck reported the experimental creation of a portocaval fistula in dogs.[22] The original description hints that he had little to confirm his success. Among a series of eight dogs, one died within 24 hours, six lived 2 to 6 days, and the one survivor "tired of life in the laboratory and ran away after 2 months." The doctoral dissertation of Jassinowsky, written in 1889 and based purely on library research, reviewed the published information on arterial suture and concluded that it could not be successful at that time, but that there might be hope in the future.[19]

Only 2 years later, however, Jassinowsky himself succeeded. In 1891, he reported his successful animal experiments involving arterial suture.[23] The suture he described was passed carefully only two-thirds of the way through the media; he tried to avoid penetrating the intima, except in very thin-walled vessels. This effort should be recognized for its intrinsic difficulty using even the finest milliner's needles, because without sutures swaged onto needles, two pieces of suture have to be dragged through the arterial wall. Dörfler modified Jassinowsky's method and passed the suture through all thicknesses of the arterial wall.[24] He also recognized that the arterial suture exposed in the lumen of the vessel did no harm if uninfected. He observed that it soon became covered with a glistening membrane. Shortly thereafter in 1896, Jaboulay and Briau described successful end-to-end carotid arterial anastomoses in animals using an everting U-shaped suture.[25]

Jaboulay was one of the surgeons in Lyon, France, under whom Carrel studied. When Sadi Carnot, the president of the Republic of France, was wounded by an assassin and died because no one dared to try to repair his portal vein, Carrel was highly critical, because he believed that blood vessels could be sutured as well as any other tissue.[26] He soon undertook experimental arterial anastomoses; some of the earliest of these were arteriovenous communications in which the high-flow system ensured patency. Carrel's contributions to technical arterial surgery included methods that vascular surgeons routinely use today.[27,28] He devised the triangulation suture to facilitate end-to-end anastomosis, described the patch technique to anastomose a small vessel to the side of a larger one (as in replantation of an inferior mesenteric artery), and pioneered the use of vessel grafts and organ transplantation. His work, however, was not fully accepted in the United States for many years. In part, this stemmed from disputes that arose between him and Guthrie, who was his coworker for 1 year.[29]

In contrast, European surgeons not only accepted Carrel's work but also began to follow his lead. In 1906, Goyanes of Madrid, Spain, resected a popliteal aneurysm, then restored arterial continuity with an in situ venous graft using the popliteal vein, which was probably the first successful clinical vascular replacement.[30]

Surgeons in the United States were beginning to perform vascular surgery in their own way. In New Orleans in 1888, Matas described a landmark operation.[31] He stumbled onto the surgical procedure for which he is commonly remembered, endoaneurysmorrhaphy, when an aneurysm for which he had ligated only the proximal brachial artery, with apparent initial success, began to pulsate again 10 days later. Reportedly, it was a medical student who called this to the professor's attention. He chose to reoperate and to ligate the brachial artery distally. Even after this distal ligation, the aneurysm continued to pulsate, and he was forced to open the aneurysm, clean out the sac (the operation performed by Antyllus), and oversew the other arteries feeding the aneurysm from inside the sac. This foreshadowed the problems with endoleaks that confound vascular surgeons who place endovascular aortic prostheses today.

Matas's operation differed from that of Antyllus, in that Matas used a suture within the aneurysmal sac to obliterate the feeding vessels instead of ligating them outside the sac. The extensive dissection that would have been required outside might have damaged the collateral circulation and other adherent anatomic structures. It was many years before Matas performed another endoaneurysmorrhaphy, because most patients were treated successfully by simple proximal ligation.[32] Matas ultimately expanded the descriptions of his technique to include "restorative" and "reconstructive" modifications, and he reported an approach to the arteriovenous fistula through the venous component,[33] as had been proposed by Bickham.[34]

Murphy, of Chicago, performed a series of experiments on animals in which he successfully restored continuity by invagination of the proximal into the distal vessel. In 1897, he presented a successful human case.[35] Edwards briefly revived this anastomotic technique of invagination when he recommended the use of the first braided nylon grafts.[36]

Murphy's invagination techniques were reflected in other nonsuture methods of anastomosis: Nitze[37] and Payr[38] used small metal or ivory rings through which the vessel was drawn, everted, and tied in place; this unit was then inserted into the mouth of the distal vessel, and another ligature secured it there. This is substantially the Blakemore tube,[39] used during World War II, albeit without signal success.[40]

During his tenure at Johns Hopkins Hospital, W.S. Halsted had an abundance of traumatic and syphilitic aneurysms commanding his attention. In the early 1900s, Carrel visited Halsted and described his own technical experiments, including his early arteriovenous anastomoses. As a result, Halsted almost made history in 1907 when he faced the dilemma of a patient whose popliteal artery and vein had been sacrificed during an en bloc dissection of a sarcoma of the popliteal space.[41] Halsted went to the other leg, took the saphenous vein, reversed it, and anastomosed the distal saphenous vein to the proximal femoral artery. For his distal anastomosis, however, he chose the popliteal vein. Although the graft pulsated for 40 minutes, it soon thrombosed. It is possible that Halsted was pursuing the chimera of reversal of arterial flow through the venous bed. One can only imagine what a dramatic leap forward vascular surgery would have made if Halsted, with his superb supporting cast of talented surgeons, had chosen the popliteal artery for the distal anastomosis and had achieved a truly successful arterial reconstruction in the pattern of the modern vascular surgeon.

There is considerable literature on attempts to revascularize ischemic extremities via arteriovenous anastomoses. San Martín[42] and A. E. Halsted[43] attempted to improve the distal circulation using arteriovenous anastomoses.

Meanwhile, German surgeons such as Höpfner,[44] Lexer,[45,46] and Jeger[47] had become familiar with the use of short (<10 cm) vein grafts. Höpfner described the bypass procedure, which was illustrated in an encyclopedic book by Jeger. Jeger's book, republished posthumously in 1937, included a foreword that described Jeger's replantation of the completely severed arm of a German soldier, which he had performed in 1914. One year later, Jeger came to an untimely death from typhus while on the Russian front.

Lexer collected and reported on 65 vein transplants, 13 of which were his personal cases.[45] In 8 of these 13 cases, Lexer had obtained a distal pulse. This report prompted a Polish surgeon, Weglowski, to present his own personal series of 51 vein grafts, mostly for trauma, operated on between 1914 and 1921; in 40 patients he could document good distal pulses and normal arterial tracings.[48] Yet all this seemed to be forgotten for the next 25 years as Germany suffered the agonies of the interbellum years, and as the forceful and charismatic personality of Leriche appeared on the scene (Leriche's role is described in a later section).

ABDOMINAL AORTIC ANEURYSMS

Beyond the management of trauma to the arteries, the aneurysm is clearly one of the great surgical challenges. The previous section detailed early attempts to treat peripheral aneurysms, but these were sporadic and lacked a continuing series.

Vesalius is said to have been the first to describe an abdominal aneurysm.[49] The successful management of the abdominal aneurysm is certainly one of vascular surgery's major accomplishments. The technical maneuvers described previously concerning the ligation of aneurysms in various anatomic sites usually involved aneurysms of the peripheral vessels; aneurysms of the trunk were sacrosanct, because proximal control was not feasible. Cooper had continued many of Hunter's studies, including evaluation of collateral arterial supplies. In 1805, he had ligated the common carotid artery for an aneurysm,[7] but he opened the door for even wider surgical applications when, in 1818, he ligated the abdominal aorta to control external hemorrhage from an aneurysm of the external iliac artery that had eroded to the surface of the skin of the flank, bleeding openly at that site.[9]

Interest in the treatment of major vessel aneurysms lagged for almost a century. Eventually Colt, at the end of the nineteenth century, used wire to pack an aneurysm and then heated the wire.[50] Blakemore and King revived interest in this technique in 1938,[51] and many surgeons undertook modifications of the wiring technique, largely without success. Meanwhile, more direct attempts were being made by the major actors in the next scene: Matas of New Orleans and Halsted of Baltimore. Their interest in the management of vessel trauma, and in the management of late sequelae of such trauma, provided material for the fertile imaginations of the many surgeons who were emboldened to follow in their footsteps. Reid reported the experience of the Johns Hopkins Hospital (headed by Halsted) with aneurysms in 1926.[52] The aneurysms treated included many varieties, both anatomic and etiologic, but treatment of abdominal aneurysms was substantially a failure. These operations were only preparation for the end of ligation as a treatment for aneurysms of the abdominal aorta.

Matas finally accomplished a successful aortic ligation (just below the renal arteries) for an aneurysm at the bifurcation of the aorta. He reported it first in 1925 and then again in 1940.[53,54] In the issue of *Annals of Surgery* that contained Matas's second report was a similar paper by Elkin,[55] as well as a hint of the coming era of vascular reconstruction in a report by Bigger of Virginia.[56] Bigger had ligated the neck of an abdominal aneurysm using fascia that he expected to loosen gradually and allow restoration of flow. With the protection of this temporary control, he performed a plication of the aneurysm, restoring the aorta to its proper caliber. The patient had a protracted survival without recurrence of the aneurysm and also with restoration of femoral pulses.

About this time, however, cardiac surgery began to emerge. During the first decade of the twentieth century, Jeger had proposed valved venous grafts between the left pulmonary veins and the left ventricle to bypass mitral stenosis, and a valved venous graft from the left ventricle to the innominate artery to bypass aortic stenosis.[47] In the mid 1920s, Cutler and colleagues[57] had attempted to treat mitral stenosis surgically, but with minimal success. A valvulotome was used through a ventricular approach.

Nonetheless, the influence of these attempts led Gross to the successful ligation and, 5 years later, division of the patent ductus arteriosus.[58,59] In Baltimore, Blalock and Taussig[60] began their series of pioneering surgical procedures for various cardiac anomalies, the first and most dramatic of which was the "blue baby" operation—the creation of a systemic shunt from the subclavian artery to the pulmonary artery in patients with congenital pulmonic stenosis.

Crafoord and Nylin[61] reported the successful end-to-end anastomosis of the aorta after resection of an aortic coarctation at the same time that Gross and Hufnagel[62] carried out their first case. This last operation demonstrated that lesions of the thoracic and abdominal segments of the aorta were amenable to a surgical approach.

Development of Vascular Prostheses

Although arterial homografts functioned fairly well in the aorta (discussed later), they were difficult to obtain, harvest, sterilize, and store. Grafts other than those of the aorta fared poorly. Homografts of smaller vessels containing a higher proportion of smooth muscle were even less satisfactory. The development of an artificial arterial substitute would allow the expansion of arterial reconstruction.

Following the experience in the laboratory reported by Abbe,[63] Tuffier had used rigid tubes of metal and of paraffined glass to try to replace small- to medium-size arteries during World War I, without success.[64] Similar tubes were used in World War II, but the results were no better than those obtained by immediate ligation of the artery.[40] Hufnagel chose a more inert surface, methylmethacrylate, as well as a tube with a better hemodynamic design.[65] Hufnagel's tubes functioned remarkably well in animal experiments, except for the difficulty in securing them within a major artery such as the aorta without the risk of ultimate erosion. Eventually the use of pliable plastic fabrics virtually eliminated the rigid tube.

In 1947, Hufnagel reported on the use of rapid freezing for the preservation of arterial homografts and suggested their utility in the repair of long aortic coarctations.[66] Gross, who at first feared that frozen vessels could not survive, published a laboratory and clinical report on his experiences with homografts preserved in electrolyte solutions for use in various cardiac operations, but particularly for the management of coarctation of the aorta.[67] Swan soon used a homograft for a thoracic aneurysm associated with a coarctation.[68]

The arterial homograft initially seemed to be a good substitute for the thoracic or abdominal aorta. At first, fresh grafts were used; then they were preserved in Tyrode's solution. Improvements in the preservation of grafts by freezing[69] and then lyophilization[70] facilitated the development of arterial graft banks. Early successes were soon erased by late failures of the homografts, however, and a truly satisfactory aortic substitute was sorely needed.

In 1952, Voorhees and colleagues observed that fabric threads in a chamber of the heart soon became covered with endothelium.[71] Dörfler had made a similar gross observation 60 years earlier, but had not carried the observation to its conclusion.[64] Voorhees and associates at Columbia pursued experiments not only with Vinyon-N but also with parachute silk and other materials. Many fabrics were tried, and most were quickly discarded. Braided and crimped nylon tubes were introduced by Edwards and Tapp,[36] but it was soon discovered that nylon rapidly lost strength and was unsatisfactory.[72] Both Orlon[73] and Teflon[74] were used. Szilagyi and colleagues[75] and Julian and colleagues[76] introduced various fabrications of Dacron. The transcripts of the vascular surgery meetings of the late 1950s might be mistaken for a textile journal, as various weaves, deniers, calenderizing, and the advantages of braid versus knit versus taffeta weaves were discussed. The summation of the principles of vascular grafting by Wesolowski and coworkers had enunciated the importance of porosity,[77,78] but the substantially nonporous Teflon undercut that thesis.

The knitted Dacron introduced by DeBakey and colleagues placed a generally successful graft in the hands of every surgeon.[79] Subsequent modifications by the addition of velour to the surface by Sauvage[80] and also by Cooley[81] refined this outstanding contribution. Wesolowski and colleagues' concept[78] that the fabric tube would become "encapsulated" and might develop a firm new endothelial surface has been pursued as a goal but has not been achieved in humans.

The immediate porosity of the grafts has been troublesome on occasion, especially in patients who require heparinization or in whom even minor blood loss from a weeping graft is intolerable. Impregnation with either collagen[82] or albumin[83] was a useful advance. Teflon in the form of an extruded tube (Gore-Tex) rather than as a woven or knitted fabric was introduced clinically by Soyer,[84] and it has achieved great popularity. Introduced first for use as a venous substitute, it came to be used extensively in arterial reconstructions as a second choice after autologous vein,[85] although Quiñones-Baldrich and colleagues[86] expressed a preference for Gore-Tex in femoral anastomoses above the knee, preserving the vein for more distal reconstructions if such become necessary.

Biological substitutes other than the arterial homograft have also been suggested. Rosenberg and associates used bovine carotid arteries that had been subjected to enzymatic treatment to remove all the tissue-specific protein, except the basic structural collagen of the bovine artery.[87] Sawyer and colleagues[88] attempted to modify the bovine heterograft by inducing a negatively charged lining in an effort to inhibit thrombosis. Dardik and coworkers[89] used treated umbilical vein grafts supported with a mesh of Dacron as a peripheral arterial substitute.

The world turns, however, and there is currently renewed interest in the use of cryopreserved (frozen but not lyophilized) arterial homografts, especially in infected aortic sites. Experience is limited, and this topic deserves to be in a clinical area rather than a historic one.

Modern Management of Aortic Aneurysms

The grave risk posed by abdominal aneurysms was exposed in a timely paper by Estes in 1951.[90] Other experiences with the aorta were preparing the way for present-day management of abdominal aneurysms. Alexander and Byron[91,92] had resected a thoracic aneurysm associated with coarctation of the aorta and successfully oversewn the ends of the vessel, although the patient ultimately died of renovascular hypertension. Swan had used a homograft to replace a thoracic aneurysm.[68]

Various attempts were made to use either reactive cellophane[93] or the tissue-irritating plasticizer dicetyl phosphate[94] as a means of inducing sclerosis that might restrain the dilatation of the aneurysm. These attempts to control the growth of the aneurysm were not rewarding.

Oudot[95] set the stage for other forms of aortic replacement when he used a homograft to restore circulation in a patient with Leriche syndrome. Dubost is recognized as the pioneer who first successfully replaced an abdominal aneurysm with a homograft on March 19, 1951.[96] Schaffer and Hardin[97] actually preceded Dubost by 4 weeks, but their publication appeared considerably later and focused on the use of a polythene shunt to maintain distal circulation during the operation rather than on the priority of resecting the aneurysm itself. It appears that Wylie actually accomplished a successful endarterectomy of an abdominal aneurysm on January 13, 1951. Similarly, Freeman and Leeds treated three patients, two successfully, with inlay grafts of the patient's own iliac veins beginning on February 12, 1951. Wylie's and Freeman's operations were not graft replacements, however, but rather modifications of Bigger's procedure.[56]

Dubost's operation was soon followed by those of Julian,[98] Brock,[99] DeBakey,[100] and Bahnson.[101] It is a curious twist of fate to find that Dubost had left the practice of colorectal surgery to become a cardiac surgeon after he saw Blalock and Bahnson perform dramatic cardiac operations while they were visiting France in the late 1940s. Szilagyi's[102] classic study of the benefits of the operation in 1966 provided confirmation and justification of the thesis Estes had presented in 1950.

The complicated abdominal aneurysm still posed a major problem. Ellis was one of the first to implant the renal arteries into the graft when the aneurysm was found to include their orifices.[103] Etheredge[104] extended this operation to resect a major thoracoabdominal aortic aneurysm. He used a heparinized plastic shunt of the type described in Schaffer's resection and replacement of an abdominal aneurysm with a homograft in March

1951. Etheredge established the shunt, divided the aorta, and performed the proximal anastomosis; he then moved the clamp down the graft after each successive visceral anastomosis was completed and finished with the lower aortic anastomosis to the graft.

DeBakey and colleagues[105] reported in 1956 a series of complicated abdominal and thoracoabdominal aneurysms that were resected with a technique similar to that later used by Shumacker.[106] In 1973, Stoney and Wylie[107] popularized the long thoracoabdominal incision for the approach to this lesion. The great advance in the management of these complicated lesions was made by Crawford,[108] who introduced a direct approach to the aneurysm in which the aorta is clamped above and below and then opened throughout the length of the aneurysm. A fabric graft is sewn into the proximal aorta; the major groups of arteries, including the lower intercostals when possible, are sewn into the wall of the fabric tube using the expeditious Carrel patch method of anastomosis; then the distal anastomosis is completed. This direct method has greatly simplified the approach to these challenging lesions.

The placement of a graft within the lumen of an aneurysm—whether abdominal, thoracic, or peripheral—was logically extended by a technique that allows one to place the graft within the aneurysm from a distance through a short arteriotomy in either the femoral or the external iliac artery. The evolution of this method stems circuitously from Dotter and coworkers.[109] In 1983, they attempted to improve the results of simple arterial dilatation or to maintain the patency of a graft with small end-arterial spiral coils. After several generations of devices that did not gain wide acceptance, Palmaz and associates[110] introduced a metal mesh stent that can be expanded by balloon dilatation, which secures the stent in place. Introduced originally to maintain the patency of a segment of artery that had undergone percutaneous dilatation, this method was at first used in occlusive disease, but Parodi and colleagues[111] modified the technique to secure a fabric graft that had been placed within an aneurysm. Although initially used as a tube graft, modifications soon allowed the placement of bifurcation grafts.[112,113] The anticipated decrease in morbidity and mortality accompanying this method led to its widespread use, although not all aneurysms are amenable. The need for prolonged follow-up versus the security of a one-time operation has raised the clinical question of the ultimate role of the endovascular repair of aneurysms. Here the narrative becomes so contemporaneous as to require clinical rather than historical description.

PERIPHERAL ARTERIAL ANEURYSMS

The peripheral arterial aneurysm was one of the first arterial lesions treated by surgeons, but its importance paled beside the advances made in the management of the aortic aneurysm. The early history of treatment by ligation was described earlier.

In 1949, Linton used Leriche's concept of arteriectomy and sympathectomy for the management of 14 patients who had popliteal aneurysms—an ingenious approach that resulted in no amputations in his series.[114] The patients received a preliminary sympathectomy; shortly afterward, or sometimes at the same operation, the aneurysm was resected, with ligation of the artery above and below it.

The ability to replace vessels of the size of the popliteal artery brought to the fore the concept that the popliteal aneurysm had a risk-benefit pattern similar to that of the abdominal aneurysm. If operations were done electively, the results were excellent, but once thrombosis occurred, the risk to the limb was grave, as Wychulis and associates demonstrated.[115] Wylie (in the discussion of Wychulis[115]) and Edwards[116] introduced the procedure of excluding the aneurysm and restoring flow through a bypass technique.

OCCLUSIVE ARTERIAL DISEASE

As mentioned earlier in this chapter, it was not until the middle of the nineteenth century that the relationship between arterial occlusion and gangrene was clearly established. Repair of acute injuries had been accomplished, but management of more chronic arterial obstructions had hardly been considered a surgical problem. Recognition of the clinical symptoms of less severe ischemia came to surgery by way of veterinary medicine.[14] The association between the sympathetic nervous system and the arteries was recognized in the early twentieth century, especially during World War I.

Leriche, born in 1879, had been educated and trained at Lyon, where he had known Jaboulay and Carrel. Shortly after Leriche completed his training, World War I broke out, and Leriche acquired considerable experience with wounds of the extremities. After he was demobilized, Leriche continued to work in a trauma hospital in Lyon for several years. There he saw many patients with posttraumatic neuralgias, and he developed his concepts of the role of the sympathetic nervous system and the possible treatment by periarterial sympathectomy, about which he had first written in 1917.[117] Then, seeing patients with arterial thrombosis caused by artérite (a nonspecific term used by French surgeons to describe arterial disease and occlusion in general), Leriche concluded that if the patient was seen before the occluding thrombosis was too widespread, local resection of the thrombosed artery provided relief. Because many patients did well after this simple procedure and soon developed relatively warm feet, he concluded that the collateral circulation in these patients must have been satisfactory and that the coldness of the extremity was due to vasospasm rather than insufficient arterial flow. He therefore applied the principle of sympathectomy, first as a periarterial operation, then as an arteriectomy (excising the obstructed segment), and then as a division of the sympathetic rami.[118]

Diez,[119] dissatisfied with the results of periarterial sympathectomy, modified that operation into the lumbar ganglionectomy. At nearly the same time, Royle[120] and Hunter[121] introduced the same fruitless operation for the management of spasm in striated muscle. Use of this operation for the management of pain syndromes and ischemic extremities remains controversial.

It seems likely that the forcefulness of Leriche's personality led European surgical thought to diverge from the known techniques of vascular grafting. This is not to say that Leriche actively spoke against the use of grafts; in fact, it was noted by some of his former trainees that he often said that it would be ideal to connect the two ends of a severed artery by a graft, but the risk of infection and the distance to be bridged always seemed too great. Instead, he offered arterial excision and sympathectomy, an approach that seemed to be beneficial and posed less risk.

One of Leriche's most important early observations was the definition of the syndrome that now bears his name, the atherosclerotic obliteration of the terminal aorta and the iliac arteries. He described this in 1923, during the period when he was beginning to evaluate arteriectomy.[122] It would be 17 years, however, before he found a suitable case in which he could perform resection of the aortic bifurcation and lumbar sympathectomy.[123] Leriche's surgical clinic became famous, and he attracted a long line of surgeons who came to learn: DeBakey, Learmonth, dos Santos, and Kunlin, to name a few.

The possibility of effective arterial suture anastomosis had been developed through the ideas of Jaboulay[25] and Carrel[27] at Lyon. After World War I, another surgeon from Lyon assumed a major role in vascular surgery.

In 1909, Murphy removed an embolus from the common iliac artery and restored flow into the femoral system. Although locally successful, distal thrombosis required a distal amputation.[124] Two years later, Labey (as cited by Mosny and Dumont[125]) removed an embolus from the artery of a patient, with complete success. Embolectomy was thereafter performed with occasional success worldwide, but it did not become a fully satisfactory procedure because of the need to operate hastily, before extensive distal thrombosis supervened. After the clinical introduction of heparin by Murray,[126] it became possible to extend the indications for embolectomy and to extend the time limit for undertaking the procedure and thus improve the results.

Surgeons such as João Cid dos Santos and his father, Reynaldo, used heparin to prevent thrombosis after performing the nearly forgotten Matas endoaneurysmorrhaphy.[127] The younger dos Santos believed that with the protection of heparin, he might be able to remove chronically adherent arterial emboli and their associated thrombus and achieve healing without rethrombosis. After finding such a patient with advanced renal disease and a seriously ischemic extremity, dos Santos removed the clot and reestablished flow. He was chided by the pathologist for having removed the intima as well. After another successful case, in which he removed a chronic thrombosis of the subclavian, axillary, and brachial arteries secondary to scalenus anticus syndrome, he sent his report to Leriche. Leriche presented the work in the name of dos Santos to the French Academy of Surgery[128] and introduced endarterectomy to the surgical world. It is interesting to note that neither of these patients suffered primarily from the usual forms of atherosclerotic thrombosis.

Subsequently, Freeman and colleagues,[129,130] Wylie and associates,[131] and others adopted the operation, using the open technique that was championed primarily by Bazy and coworkers.[132] In September 1951, Wylie described endoaneurysmectomy and endarterectomy of the aorta. At the time, my colleagues and I had undertaken six procedures without success, but in the summer of 1951, Wylie had visited us, and in October 1951 we performed the first successful endarterectomy in our series.[133] The operation consisted of a combination of the Matas endoaneurysmorrhaphy and the dos Santos endarterectomy (or the technique as revised by Reboul): an abdominal aneurysm was endarterectomized, tailored to a proper size, and wrapped with fascia lata, and an endarterectomy in continuity was performed throughout the length of the left iliofemoropopliteal system. In fact, these operations were only extensions of the aneurysm repair performed by Bigger in 1940.[56]

Cannon and Barker later introduced the long, closed endarterectomy using intraluminal strippers,[134] which was a modification of the original method of dos Santos. Several similar varieties of endarterectomy loops were devised by Butcher[135] and by Vollmar and Laubaeh,[136] among others. A period of early success was followed by disenchantment owing to the difficulty of the operation in comparison with the increasingly popular grafting procedures.

Leriche and his close associate Kunlin had not had great technical success with endarterectomy, especially in the femoral artery system. Kunlin revived the use of the vein graft in the form of a long venous bypass.[137] His first patient had already undergone arteriectomy and sympathectomy, thus justifying the then-unorthodox procedure.

Veins had been used for short (4 to 8 cm) replacements on rare occasions during the prior 40 years. This technique has persisted as the basic method of arterial reconstruction ever since.

Saphenous vein grafting was useful only in the femoral and iliofemoral systems, however, and it remained for Oudot to perform a comparable reconstructive operation on the aorta using an aortic homograft,[95] which thoracic and cardiac surgeons were already using to replace segments of the thoracic aorta. Oudot was presented with a 51-year-old patient with claudication as a result of proximal iliac and distal aortic occlusion. Oudot's operation is commonly described as a simple bifurcation graft, common iliac to common iliac, but it was actually a much more complicated procedure. He approached the bifurcation extraperitoneally through a left flank incision and resected the bifurcation. The patient's internal iliacs were found to be thrombosed and were ligated. The external iliac arteries of the graft were very small, but the graft's internal iliacs were large; Oudot therefore anastomosed the graft's internal iliacs to the patient's external iliacs. However, he did the left-sided anastomosis first and then found that the repaired vessel obstructed his view and hindered manipulations of the right-sided anastomosis. This difficult anastomosis thrombosed promptly. Oudot made the best of a bad situation and pointed out that he had done a perfect experiment, as there was still some discussion from Leriche's camp about whether grafting at this level would be worthwhile. On the right side, Oudot had performed substantially nothing more than an arteriectomy; on the left, he had reconstituted the lumen. The right side was warm but pulseless and still fatigued easily, whereas the left side had a pulse and did not tire. Six months later, Oudot reoperated on the patient, who was still complaining of right-sided claudication; he performed an iliac-to-iliac "extraanatomic" bypass, as had been suggested by Kunlin in 1951.

A few months later, Oudot climbed Annapurna with the French team. Shortly after his return to France, he was killed in an automobile crash at the age of 40.

The saga of the treatment of arterial disease continues with the development and then the failure of artery banks and the introduction of the plastic prosthesis, but by 1952 the stage was set for nearly everything that is done today. Linton's espousal of the reversed saphenous vein in 1952 confirmed the approach of Kunlin and established the procedure of choice for peripheral reconstruction for many years.[138]

Endarterectomy did not die out completely; it persists in carotid operations, but only occasionally is it used in the aorta and as part of local tailoring procedures elsewhere. Edwards made one important attempt to use it in the femoral artery by means of a long patch; the procedure worked well unless the patch was so wide that it created a stagnant column of blood in the femoral artery.[139] Femoropopliteal endarterectomy fell from favor because of its limited applicability to reconstructions that ended proximal to the distal portion of the popliteal artery. The full open repair was tedious, and most surgeons had limited success in restoring flow.

In recent years, however, closed endarterial procedures have become commonplace. Dotter and Judkins began in 1956 by using a stiff dilator,[140] a procedure that was not widely accepted. Gruntzig and Hopff modified this method by using a balloon that could distend and fracture the stenotic plaque.[141]

Endarterial procedures have been extended to include not only dilatation and placement of emboli of several kinds in bleeding arteries but also removal of atherosclerotic lesions by endarterial manipulations through a percutaneous route. A major requirement for endarterial procedures was believed to be endarterial visualization, beyond that provided by contrast radiography. Visualization began effectively with the work of Greenstone and others.[142]

Actual removal of plaque by several mechanical means followed: Simpson and associates[143] used a side-biting forceps in a catheter, Kensey and coworkers[144] used a catheter through which a rapidly rotating auger-like tip was passed, and Ahn and colleagues[145] advocated a high-speed rotary bur. Others have used various forms of laser energy to destroy plaque.[146] In one procedure, the laser recognizes the difference between plaque and normal arterial wall.[147] In another, the laser-heated probe "melts" the atheroma.[148] Further mechanical dilatation often accompanies these initial coring methods. Appraisal of these methods, however, belongs in the clinical rather than the historical section of this volume; they appear to achieve only limited removal of the atheromatous material and much less satisfactory results than the classic techniques of endarterectomy, albeit without requiring a major operative procedure.

Dotter and others[109] proposed the addition of intraluminal stents to maintain graft patency, as well as the patency of vessels that had been dilated. In the surgical literature, this maneuver was largely ignored until Palmaz and associates[110] introduced balloon-expandable stents, which were first used to maintain patency in dilated arteries. The use of percutaneous arterial dilatation and endarterectomy has suffered from inadequate and inconstant reporting standards in the hands of many nonsurgeons, but the technique appears to have reached a level of acceptance that requires the definition of its historical role.

Parodi and coworkers[111] hybridized the technique of endarterial placement of these stents and added the placement of fabric grafts, a technique described previously in the section on aneurysms.

Two other important extensions of distal femoral reconstruction came on the scene. The first was introduction of the graft to the infrapopliteal artery. In 1960, Palma[149] published descriptions of vein graft insertions into the tibial arteries. Later information from Palma (personal communication, 1990) indicates that these were performed as early as 1956. McCaughan described the exposure of the "distal popliteal artery" (more commonly known as the *tibioperoneal trunk*) and anastomoses to it in 1958,[150] but his work went unrecognized because of his unconventional terminology. In that article, McCaughan[151] described a successful graft into the tibial vessels in July 1957, using an exposure in the upper third of the calf. He presented six additional patients with grafts into the tibial segment in 1960. In 1966, McCaughan[152] went one step further when he reported four grafts in which the distal insertion of the graft was into the posterior tibial artery at the ankle. Morris and coworkers[153] and Tyson and DeLaurentis[154] were other contemporary pioneers in the development of various configurations of infrapopliteal procedures.

The second extension of distal femoral reconstruction was application of the in situ vein graft, with destruction of valvular competence within the vein, by Hall.[155] The procedure did not receive much attention until it was revitalized by Leather and associates in 1981.[156] Many variations on the theme of the distal bypass have been introduced, combining free grafts and in situ methods.

Dardik and associates introduced the use of tanned human umbilical vein and then added a distal arteriovenous fistula.[157] The fistula was not a revival of earlier attempts by Carrel and others to revascularize an extremity through the veins, rather it was an attempt to provide sufficient outflow for a long graft to ensure its patency, with some of the graft flow still directed through the distal arterial tree. DeLaurentis and Friedman introduced a method of sequential multiple bypasses in the extremity,[158] and Veith and associates[159] carried this to extremes with bypasses from one tibial artery to another, and even with bypasses beginning and ending below the malleolus. Nehler's group[160] applied this small vessel bypass technique to the management of small vessel disease in the distal upper extremity.

A different approach to the ischemic lower limb was advocated by Oudot and Cormier[161] when they observed how frequently the superficial femoral artery was occluded, but the profunda femoris remained patent. Martin and coworkers described an extended form of profundaplasty, particularly as the site of insertion of a graft from above.[162]

None of these advances in reconstructive surgery has been helpful in the management of the frustrating syndrome of thromboangiitis obliterans, or Buerger's disease. It is likely that von Winiwarter[163] was describing the pathologic process of thromboangiitis obliterans, but his description and clinical correlation are ambiguous. Certainly, Buerger described the clinical picture,[164] although neither he nor von Winiwarter noted the association with tobacco or the involvement of the upper extremities.

One other major contribution rounds out this section. In 1963, Fogarty and coworkers devised one of the most useful methods for managing occlusive arterial disease—the balloon embolectomy catheter for the extraction of clot in the treatment of embolization.[165] This technique has been modified for use in many other arterial and venous operations and has even been adapted to many general surgical uses.

The development of endarterial stenting and grafting has already been mentioned. These methods have undoubtedly improved the results of arterial dilatation, but the lack of standardized methods of reporting in the nonvascular literature and the overenthusiastic promotion of the method still cloud its value. Furthermore, the application of these techniques has become a point of conflict among radiologists, cardiologists, and surgeons over whose "turf" it should be. Some areas are obviously suitable for treatment by an interventional radiologist or cardiologist, but in many instances the presence and active participation of a surgeon in the operating room are mandatory. In any event, comparison of methods and results should be made possible by accurate and standardized methods of analysis. Here again, current clinical choices supersede historical interpretation.

ARTERIAL TRAUMA

Arterial injuries have always been a challenge to surgeons. Trauma was the source of Hallowell's first arterial repair. During the years after the Civil War, Mitchell described the syndrome of burning pain ("causalgia") that followed many arterial injuries[166]; it was this lesion that had intrigued Leriche and led to his interest in the sympathetic nervous system.[118] Halsted had remarked on surgeons' fascination with arterial injuries. During World War I, Makins[167] surveyed the injuries to blood vessels incurred by the British forces. DeBakey and Simeone[168] provided a similar service for U.S. forces after World War II and noted almost no benefit from the vascular surgical techniques then available because of the incidental and associated surgical complications and the problem of delay.

Few arterial injuries were treated definitively, except for ligation of the artery, until the Korean War. Before that time, the main interest in arterial injuries seemed to be estimating the likelihood of survival of the limb and selecting the appropriate level for ligation of the artery. Generations of anatomy students learned the "site of election" for ligation of various arteries.

During the Korean War, however, Jahnke and Howard,[169] Hughes,[170] and Spencer and Grewe[171] participated in a program in which acute vascular injuries were treated with fresh vein grafts. Whelan and coworkers[172] and Rich and Hughes[173] continued using these techniques of arterial repair in Vietnam. The Registry of Vascular Injuries from Vietnam, as maintained at the Walter Reed Army Medical Center under the direction of Rich, has continued to yield a monumental body of information concerning acute vascular repair. Civilian medical centers have continued to apply these techniques to the everyday patterns of vessel injuries.

The arteriovenous fistula is one sequela of trauma to the major vessels that poses a special challenge to surgeons. Its acute effects on the distal circulation, its systemic effects as a major left-to-right shunt, and its local changes, which result in increased blood flow through the feeding arterial supply, are all intriguing examples of the body's adaptability—or lack thereof.

The arteriovenous fistula was first described by Hunter.[3] The lesion did not become common until the end of the nineteenth century, as weapons (i.e., high-speed projectiles) and the injuries they caused changed. Volumes have been written in an attempt to interpret the diverse physiologic parameters involved in this lesion, but as early as 1913, Soubbotitich[174] noted that simple ligation of the proximal artery should never be done. Not long after, Lexer introduced the "ideal" operation,[45] consisting of resection of the aneurysmal sac and restoration of flow through the artery with a short venous graft if the ends of the artery could not be brought back together. Reconstruction of the vein was desirable but not mandatory. Bickham suggested approaching the arterial repair through the venous component of the sac, with repair of the vein if possible[34]—a modification of the Matas endoaneurysmorrhaphy.

For the most part, however, until the Korean War era in the 1950s and later, the most common form of surgical management was quadruple ligation and excision of the sac and fistula. Such an operation depended on the development of sufficient collateral circulation to the distal limb to allow the limb to survive after arterial interruption, but it had to be done before the extra load placed on the heart by a left-to-right shunt caused serious cardiac disability; timing was thus a matter of delicate clinical judgment. Holman,[175] whose lifelong interest in the arteriovenous fistula began during his training at Johns Hopkins, was the most eminent contributor to the understanding of the physiology of the arteriovenous fistula. With the advent of prompt exploration and repair of acute arterial injuries, it was anticipated that the number of late arteriovenous fistulas would be greatly reduced, but this has not been the case. The current ability to reconstruct the artery diminishes the need to delay to allow the development of collateral circulation, as was once necessary.

EXTRACRANIAL CEREBROVASCULAR ARTERIAL OCCLUSIONS

The critical nature of the blood flow to the brain through the great arteries of the neck was recognized by the ancient Greeks, who named the carotid artery after the symptoms that followed its occlusion—asphyxia, or stupor. The clinical importance of carotid artery stenosis and obstruction was only slowly accepted by the neurologic community in general, however, despite the fact that eminent neurologists such as Savory,[176] Hunt,[177] and Fisher[178,179] had observed the relationship between arterial lesions and atheroembolic phenomena many years before surgical treatment became accepted.

The first elective attempt to restore flow to the ischemic brain was made by Carrea and associates in 1951 but not reported until 1955.[180] The proximal portion of the diseased internal carotid artery was excised, and flow was restored by an anastomosis of the unusually large proximal external carotid artery to the cut end of the distal internal carotid. A slightly different reconstruction of the carotid bifurcation, necessitated by a gunshot wound, was accomplished by Lefèvre in 1918.[181] He resected the carotid bulb, ligated the common trunk, and anastomosed the distal ends of the internal and external carotid arteries to provide the brain with the arterial supply from the rich anastomoses of the external carotid artery.

The most widely acclaimed early carotid reconstruction and the one that truly began the modern reconstructive era was the resection of the carotid bifurcation and restoration of carotid flow by anastomosis of the common carotid to the internal carotid by Eastcott and colleagues in 1954.[182] It now appears that others, including Cooley and colleagues,[183] Roe,[184] and DeBakey,[185] were among the first to successfully perform true carotid endarterectomies. As was the case with Estes[90] and his paper justifying the approach to abdominal aneurysms, so the report to the National Research Council of Great Britain by Yates and Hutchinson[186] indicated the importance of occlusive disease of the carotid and vertebral arteries.

Whisnant and associates[187] in Rochester, Minnesota, identified the risk of stroke in the presence of transient ischemic attacks and provided the solid basis for operation on the carotid artery to prevent major strokes. Hollenhorst[188] called attention to the bright cholesterol emboli seen in the eye grounds that are pathognomonic of atherosclerotic embolization, but Julian and associates[189] and Moore and Hall[190] clearly demonstrated that embolization was the major cause of transient cerebral ischemic symptoms, rather than simple hemodynamics. Further landmark studies of the morphology of carotid plaque and its evolution were presented by Imparato and coworkers[191] and Lusby and associates.[192] Moore and Hall[193] and others among Wylie's group called attention to the role of carotid back-pressure in identifying patients whose brains needed protection from ischemia during the period of operative occlusion.

Operation for symptomatic patients was soon relatively well accepted, but operation to prevent stroke in asymptomatic patients whose carotid stenosis manifests as a bruit or a measurable change in retinal artery pressure or some other noninvasive laboratory test remains controversial. Work by Thompson and colleagues[194] is the predominant authoritative source, despite criticism concerning its lack of perfect controls. Dixon and associates[195] provided further evidence of the role of large, asymptomatic ulcerations of the carotid bifurcation. Berguer and coworkers[196] showed that many "asymptomatic" patients with carotid lesions actually demonstrate multiple small cerebral infarcts that are not clearly reflected in the patient's symptoms.

In 1992, Moore summarized several early multicenter, randomized trials that were performed to compare carotid endarterectomy with nonsurgical methods.[197] These trials revealed carotid endarterectomy to be so highly effective that many early criticisms of the operation were quieted. An immense body of controversial literature exists concerning the role of anticoagulant or antiplatelet agents to prevent thrombosis or thromboembolization, but these modalities remain an adjunct to carotid endarterectomy performed by trained surgeons. Continuing comparisons of several different modalities continue to define appropriate clinical measures.

The surgeon's inability to clear the totally occluded bifurcation safely and effectively has been addressed by the use of microsurgical techniques. Yasargil and associates[198] first popularized this technique. Many neurosurgeons have become skillful in the performance of extracranial-to-intracranial bypass. A randomized study cast serious doubts about the value of this technique in preventing strokes,[199] and its true role remains to be clarified.

VISCERAL VASCULAR OCCLUSIONS

One of the most important lesions in relatively small arteries is the occlusive lesion in the coronary arteries. Longmire and colleagues[200] performed a few successful coronary endarterectomies in 1958. The difficulties associated with endarterectomy in small vessels led others to use the vein graft, first as a replacement by Favoloro[201] in 1968 and then as a bypass by Johnson and associates[202] in 1969.

Renal arterial insufficiency has been treated successfully for many years. Goldblatt and coworkers[203] recognized the importance of renal ischemia as a cause of arterial hypertension, and others explained the details of the deranged physiology. Freeman and associates[129] were among the first to treat this lesion successfully, leading to the surgical management of renovascular hypertension. DeCamp and coworkers,[204] Poutasse,[205] and Foster and associates[206] were leaders in the perfection of these techniques.

Recognition of several forms of fibromuscular hyperplasia in the renal artery was followed by its identification in the internal carotid artery by Connett and Lansche.[207] Ehrenfeld and associates put the surgical management of this lesion on a firm footing.[208]

Occlusive disease is much less common in the mesenteric vessels than in most other visceral beds, but it is frequently lethal when it does occur. It was commonly recognized only when it had reached an advanced stage and caused extensive intestinal necrosis. Dunphy[209] in 1936 related the progression of symptoms of mesenteric ischemia to frank intestinal infarction. Fifteen years later, Klass[210] removed an embolus from the superior mesenteric artery successfully, although the patient died of his primary cardiovascular disease. Barker and Cannon[133] included in their first endarterectomy series a patient who underwent a superior mesenteric endarterectomy at the same time as an aortoiliac procedure. In 1957, Shaw and Rutledge[211] performed an embolectomy of the superior mesenteric artery without concomitant bowel resection. The following year, Shaw and Maynard[212] identified two patients with both malabsorption and mesenteric ischemia who were treated successfully by endarterectomy. In the meantime, Mikkelsen and Zaro[213] reported similar experiences from California, and they clarified the useful term intestinal angina.

The meandering mesenteric collaterals so well described by Kountz and associates[214] provided a radiographic sign suggesting the presence of serious stenosis of the celiac axis and superior mesenteric vessels. Recognition of this sign has become cause for careful evaluation of the mesenteric vessels, whether found in the radiology suite or the operating room.

One of the important nonsurgical lesions that mimics obstructive mesenteric vascular disease is the nonocclusive form of mesenteric vascular insufficiency identified by Heer and associates.[215] This condition occurs in forms of cardiogenic shock in which the cardiac output is low and the mesenteric vascular resistance is high.

The extrinsic compression syndrome of the celiac axis is a subject capable of generating considerable discussion. Marable and associates first described this as compression by the arcuate ligament of the diaphragm.[216] Some authors believe that other anatomic structures, such as the neural components of the celiac ganglion, may also be involved. Many support the existence of this lesion, whatever its anatomic cause, as a source of serious symptoms; others forcefully deny its existence.[217]

EXTRAANATOMIC BYPASS AND VASCULAR INFECTIONS

There are many technical and mechanical advances that cannot properly be placed in any of the previously described compartments of the history of vascular surgery. One of these is the concept of extraanatomic bypass. The term itself is controversial. It has been suggested that the term implies a bypass outside the body instead of outside the classic anatomic routes, but its usage is so well established that it is retained here. It was proposed as a possibility by Kunlin[137] and actually carried out as an ilioiliac bypass by way of the prevesical space by Oudot in 1951. Although rerouting of flow through short shunts had been done by many surgeons for various reasons, the first dramatic step was taken by Blaisdell and colleagues,[218] who led a graft from the thoracic aorta extraperitoneally to the femoral artery. Shortly thereafter, this anatomic arrangement was modified as the axillofemoral and then the axillobifemoral graft in 1963 by Blaisdell and Hall.[219]

The axillofemoral bypass was first advised as a means of establishing flow to the extremity in the presence of an infected aortic reconstruction that had to be removed. Similarly, in 1966, Mahoney and Whelan[220] introduced the obturator bypass to avoid an established infection in the groin. Vetto[221] introduced a slightly different anatomic variant—the femorofemoral bypass—in 1962, 11 years after Oudot's ilioiliac operation. Today the pattern of unusual anatomic configurations seems limited only by the patient's needs and the surgeon's ingenuity.

One of the important indications for replacement of the classic aortic prosthesis is the development of an aortoenteric fistula. These lesions have plagued surgeons since the first aortic grafts were performed. Elliott and coauthors[222] contributed one of the first important papers toward the understanding of this problem. Later, Busuttil and associates[223] defined the common primary role played by the false aneurysm at the aortic suture line and clarified the management.

VENOUS SURGERY

The history of venous surgery is in one sense older and in another sense newer than that of arterial surgery. Venous repairs were undertaken before arterial repairs were generally successful. Most of the first generation of arterial surgeons learned about the vagaries of the venous system as their first experiences in vascular surgery. Varicose veins, venous thrombosis, pulmonary embolism, and the postphlebitic extremity were the four major topics.

Although operations on the veins were the major procedures that vascular surgeons were called on to perform in the first half of the twentieth century, venous surgery was overshadowed by the more glamorous arterial reconstructions until recently, when the American Venous Forum was established to study the management of problems involving the veins. Phlebology never lost its major role in Europe, and the Venous Forum has returned venous surgery to prominent status in the United States.

The earliest modern operations for varicosities consisted of little more than local excision of the varix, and it was probably Trendelenburg who introduced the physiologically useful ligation of the long saphenous vein in the upper leg.[224,225] Trendelenburg's interruption of the saphenous vein was carried out in the midthigh. Although Trendelenburg's operation introduced and was directed at the concept of reversal of flow in the diseased saphenous system, the collaterals at the saphenous bulb allowed prompt return to a pattern of saphenous flow toward the foot. Homans[226] is generally credited with defining the importance of interrupting the saphenous vein flush with the femoral vein and dividing its major collateral trunks in the first few centimeters below that junction.

Babcock devised techniques to strip or avulse veins by means of extraluminal strippers,[227] and for many years the Mayo external stripper has been a useful instrument to facilitate dissection of the vein.[228]

Radical stripping of the major saphenous trunks has become less common in the last quarter century, once the importance of preserving a nonvaricose vein for possible later use as an arterial conduit became an important consideration.

Pulmonary embolism has long been a major problem for physicians in all areas of medical practice. In 1908, Trendelenburg introduced the operation of pulmonary embolectomy.[229] This operation was undertaken infrequently and was usually unsuccessful, but its rare successes have continued to challenge surgeons. It is an operation that can be applied more frequently today because of the ability to support the patient's cardiovascular system until the operation can be performed. The role of direct operation may be lessened by the ability to place catheters in the pulmonary artery and dissolve the clot with thrombolytic agents.[230]

In 1934, the true relationship between deep venous thrombosis of the leg veins and pulmonary embolism was clarified by Homans,[231,232] who matched the ends of a thrombus taken from the pulmonary artery at autopsy with a residual clot in the popliteal vein, showing that this must have been the source of the embolus. Homans recognized that the great venous sinuses in the soleal veins were capable of returning large quantities of blood during exercise, but at rest, blood might be stagnant there. Thus, given the other factors of Virchow's triad (stagnant flow, endothelial injury, and increased coagulability), one might anticipate spontaneous thrombosis at that site. In fact, subsequent studies with radioiodinated fibrinogen showed an alarming rate of thrombosis there. Fortunately, only a small proportion of these thromboses yields thrombi that propagate into the mainline channels and produce serious clinical problems.

The next step in the management of patients with venous thrombosis was also made by Homans,[233] who introduced ligation of the superficial femoral vein where it joins the deep femoral system in the groin. The introduction of this procedure must be viewed in the context of the times, when there was no practical anticoagulant commonly in use. Allen,[234] Veal,[235] and others quickly took up this operation.

Homans experienced disappointment over the outcome of a patient whose superficial femoral vein he and I had ligated. A clot propagated through the deep femoral system and into the common femoral vein, causing an embolism and the patient's death, despite the interruption of the superficial femoral vein.

The preferred level of venous ligation was moved upward because of other similar failures of superficial femoral vein interruption. First, the common femoral and then the iliac veins were ligated bilaterally. These operations could be performed under local anesthesia through groin incisions, but it was soon recognized that bilateral ligation of the iliac veins was preferred to the common femoral site. Vena caval interruption soon became the procedure of choice. It is hard to identify who first ligated the vena cava for pulmonary embolism, but Northway and Buxton,[236] O'Neill,[237] and Collins and coworkers[238] are all credited with early reports.

It seems unfortunate that once anticoagulants became readily available—first warfarin (Coumadin) and then heparin—their combination with ligation was not common; ligation and anticoagulation were used on an either-or basis by most physicians. Simple ligation without anticoagulant therapy was often associated with extension of thrombosis in the stagnant systems below the ligature, which led to severe postphlebitic symptoms. Anlyan and colleagues,[239] Bowers and Leb,[240] and others seriously criticized interruption, giving rise to a school that treated venous thrombosis primarily with increasingly large doses of heparin.[241] The extent of postphlebitic syndrome, however, seems to be more clearly related to the extent of the inflammatory thrombophlebitic process and its destruction of the valves in the leg than to ligation or the level of ligation.[242] The successful use of large doses of heparin has greatly diminished the need for venous interruption.

Spencer[243] introduced another approach to caval interruption, however, to maintain some flow through the cava but still prevent the passage of emboli to the lungs by plication of the cava with sutures. Other extraluminal occlusive devices were suggested by Moretz and associates,[244] Miles and colleagues,[245] and Adams and DeWeese.[246] Mobin-Uddin's invention of a transvenous umbrella[247] and Greenfield's transvenous wire trap[248] reduced the need for major venous interruption by open surgical methods even further.

The problems of the postphlebitic extremity remain. This syndrome was well described by Homans,[249] but his contributions to its treatment were not particularly fruitful, except that they represent the culmination of the best forms of nonoperative management. Trout,[250] Linton,[251] and Dodd and Cockett[252] separately advocated methods that accomplish subfascial interruption of the communicating veins in the lower leg; this procedure remains a surgical standard.

The re-creation of a venous drainage channel that is protected from regurgitant flow offered a new approach to this old problem. Kistner demonstrated a technique of converting an incompetent valve into a competent one.[253] Venous transposition, redirecting flow through a competent vein and around an area of venous incompetence, is another approach used by Dale[254] and Palma and Esperoti.[255]

Taheri and coworkers[256] published the results of a free graft of a valved segment of the axillary vein into the diseased femoral system. Taheri and others[257] went even farther, attempting to develop prosthetic venous valves.

HIGHLIGHTS IN DIAGNOSTIC MODALITIES

The diagnosis of both arterial and venous diseases has long depended on the use of contrast radiography. One of the first to use this technique successfully in a living patient was Brooks,[258] who injected sodium iodide to demonstrate the lesions of Buerger's disease in digital vessels. Moniz described "arterial encephalography" for neurologic lesions in 1927.[259] His presentation was not only a seminal paper; it also defined the technical needs of the radiographer in terms that are pertinent nearly 80 years later.

In the audience at Moniz's presentation was dos Santos (the elder). He and his colleagues soon published the basic technical approach to arteriography of the vessels of the abdomen and their branches.[260] Each of these authors foresaw the great advances that would accompany the development of rapid cassette changers and less toxic contrast media, but the techniques of image enhancement and subtraction by electronic means are recent and highly effective contributions.

One of the major technical advances for the angiographer was Seldinger's technique,[261] which, instead of using a single needle to inject contrast material, used a catheter that was passed over a wire that had been introduced through the primary vessel puncture. The guidewire was first advanced to the desired site, then the appropriate catheter was advanced over the wire. Wire and catheter could be alternated so that injections could be made at different sites and at different rates. With this method, a catheter can be placed and injection can be achieved at almost any intravascular site in the body. The culmination of these technical advances is the clarification and modification of the radiographic image by subtraction, digitization, enhancement, and various electronic manipulations.

A totally different field of radiology was signaled by the work of Dotter and Judkins,[140] who used a rigid dilator passed through a large needle under fluoroscopic guidance to dilate narrowed arteries in 1956. Dotter's contributions were followed by those of Gruntzig.[141] This percutaneous intravascular technique evolved into the burgeoning field of interventional rather than purely diagnostic radiology.

The growth of vascular surgery in recent years has been almost synonymous with the development of methods of noninvasive diagnosis of peripheral vascular disease. This is an outgrowth of those methods commonly taken for granted, which had their humble beginnings in the stethoscope, the sphygmomanometer,[262] and the ophthalmoscope.

The measurement of many physiologic parameters in the laboratory was extended to the patient by such physicians as Winsor,[263] whose definition of pressure gradients remains a critical basis for the clinical estimation of the severity of arterial obstruction. Combined with a sphygmomanometer and a Doppler sensor, evaluation of segmental arterial pressures became a useful means of evaluating peripheral arterial disease and identifying segmental pressure differences, just as Winsor had done with less accurate sensing methods.

Other common measurements performed in the early vascular diagnostic laboratories included digital and segmental plethysmography and skin temperature and resistance, both before and after sympathetic blockade.

Pachon[264] introduced a modification of the sphygmomanometer and the segmental plethysmograph; the oscillometer provided a rough measure of the volume of the distensile arterial pulse wave. The values obtained bore no physiologic definition, but comparisons at different levels in one extremity, of comparable levels in opposite extremities, or at one site on successive occasions provided the surgeon with some objective evidence of change. Although the stethoscope is used by all physicians, its role in the evaluation of murmurs over the peripheral arteries was clarified and codified by Edwards and Levine[265] and then by Wylie and McGuiness[266] at a surprisingly late date. The usefulness of inexpensive auscultation has diminished as electronic assessment has become readily available.

One of the interesting early techniques was that of Baillart,[267] who used the ophthalmoscope and concurrent ophthalmodynamometry to evaluate lesions of the eye and thus estimate retinal arterial pressures, which were assumed to reflect pressure and hence flow through the internal carotid artery. Operator sensitivity and reproducibility, critical aspects of many such techniques, were such that the method's utility was not great. Kartchner[268] and Gee[269] and their respective colleagues introduced a recording device to reproduce relative pressure curves within the ocular globe or to compare the peak time of the retinal artery pulse wave, which is reflected in the globe's pressure, with the arrival of the pulse wave in the earlobe; this enabled estimation of the severity of obstruction in the carotid system. Gee and associates developed a method to evaluate the back-pressure in the stenotic carotid artery to predict the necessity of a shunt during operative carotid occlusion. Their method, however, is actually of greater value in evaluating the forward pressure beyond the stenotic carotid artery; it provides more precise measurement of the pressures but does not provide time relationships, as Kartchner's system does. These subtle physiologic evaluations of the intraocular arterial pressure as an indirect reflection of the intracranial carotid flow have been supplanted by more direct physiologic studies of the extracranial arteries in the neck.

Ultrasonography has become one of the most popular modalities in its many ramifications. Leopold and associates[270] used classic ultrasonic imaging (B-mode) techniques to outline the aorta and identify aneurysmal changes there.

Use of the ultrasonic flow detector was soon modified by Brockenbrough to determine the direction of flow through the supraorbital artery,[271] which is reversed in the presence of high-grade obstruction of the ipsilateral carotid artery. Machleder and Barker dramatized the technique,[272] but extreme operator sensitivity limits its use.

Imaging of the crude Doppler signal was introduced by Thomas and coworkers,[273] who simply mounted a Doppler probe on a scanning device. Increased sophistication of these scanning methods ultimately led to duplex scanning techniques.

Ultrasonography in another form (i.e., either the continuous or the gated Doppler mode that measures the shift in frequency of the ultrasonic signal reflected from moving red blood cells) was introduced by Strandness and colleagues[274] and by Sumner and Strandness.[275] Here, ultrasonic B-mode scanning defines the anatomy and obtains a reference point to be combined with pulsed, "gated" Doppler reflections to show blood flow patterns and velocities at the designated site within the lumen. Use of these studies is limited to vessels that can be "reached" by the Doppler signal.[276] This method became widely used to evaluate the carotid bifurcation, but its application has now been extended as a monitor in peripheral arterial sites, vertebral arteries,[277] mesenteric vessels,[278] and at the operating table.[279] Evaluation of the circle of Willis is also possible, but is not consistently reliable.[280]

Carotid angiography has been shown to contribute a major proportion of the morbidity and mortality associated with carotid surgery in many randomized trials. As a result, duplex imaging has rapidly replaced it as the primary diagnostic tool for carotid artery disease. It provides highly accurate anatomic as well as physiologic data, although arteriography is still necessary in some patients.

A new twist on computed tomography was introduced by Kalender and associates.[281] Use of this form of spiral computed tomography has become more common, and although its images may lose some of the detail obtained by other methods, it provides a superb overall picture of the course and collaterals of an arterial segment, and its software allows manipulation so that the three-dimensional image can be visualized from many different angles. Magnetic resonance imaging has become a useful evaluation tool, especially of the aorta, and magnetic resonance angiography also shows promise,[282] but these techniques are at the stage of clinical rather than historical evaluation at the moment.

Evaluation of the venous side of the circulation beyond classic physical examination has not yielded such exact information. Cranley and coworkers[283] introduced "phleborheography," which evaluates changes in venous pulse, outflow, and respiratory excursions to diagnose deep venous disease of the legs. Wheeler's impedance plethysmography[284] is less sophisticated and easier to handle, but perhaps less informative.

The Doppler velocity probe, despite some drawbacks related to operator sensitivity, remains a useful method for identifying lesions in the major superficial veins, such as in the groin, the popliteal space, and the axilla. It can also be used in the post-phlebitic extremity to identify both regurgitant flow in superficial channels and flow from communicating veins. It can be used even in the presence of brawny edema, which otherwise obscures much of the venous system from sight and palpation.

Just as the duplex scan in carotid surgery has become popular, color-assisted duplex imaging is an important part of the evaluation of the venous system,[285] where its use was first popularized.

VASCULAR ACCESS SURGERY

Kolff's introduction of hemodialysis in the mid 1950s revolutionized nephrology,[286] but it also added to the number of difficult procedures that vascular surgeons are asked to perform, including providing and maintaining access to the vascular system, often on an emergency basis. Vascular access surgery lacks the glamour of much of the rest of vascular surgery, but it constitutes a significant portion of vascular surgical practice. The construction and maintenance of a well-functioning access site demand both surgical skill and judgment.

The first approaches involved the use of silicone tubing as an external shunt between the arterial and venous systems in the arm.[287] The natural progression by Brescia and his team was to use a direct arteriovenous fistula, usually in the arm.[288] The fistula results in dilated veins suitable for recurrent punctures. The addition of an autologous vein graft to allow a better fistula and better access to the vein[289] was soon followed by the use of other materials as shunts, both biologic and plastic.[290]

THORACIC OUTLET SYNDROMES

The problems and care of the varied thoracic outlet syndromes are shared by vascular surgeons, orthopedists, neurosurgeons, and physiotherapists. Although first treated surgically as an exostosis of the first rib in 1861,[291] clear anatomic understanding was achieved through the works of Murphy,[292] Adson and Coffey,[293] and Ochsner and coworkers.[294] It appeared to early authors that a cervical rib was the offending anatomic structure, but Adson and Coffey introduced the concept of entrapment of the brachial plexus and accompanying artery by the anterior scalene muscle and the highest rib. Naffziger and Grant confirmed the mechanical origins of the syndrome and demonstrated the anterior supraclavicular approach.[295] One of the illustrations, however, taking an anatomist's point of view from inside the chest, showed the anatomy that Roos would subsequently use in his transaxillary approach.[296] Falconer and Li[297] proposed resection of the first rib to relieve the costoclavicular compression of the vessels. Edwards offered a thesis that consolidated the anatomic and evolutionary origins of these syndromes, pointing out that the human is one of the few animals in which there is a descent of the heart and great vessels in relation to the shoulder girdle, which leads to draping of the great vessels over the highest rib, whatever its number might be.[298]

The surgical approaches to this area have been varied: paraspinal and anterior supraclavicular and transaxillary. The latter involves no major muscle division and provides a better cosmetic result. It is especially helpful in muscular athletes, who are prone to symptoms from compression.

The most common form involves pressure on the nerves and arteries, but a slightly different anatomic arrangement is responsible for the variations in Paget-Schroetter syndrome, in which obstruction of the venous system is the major problem. McLeery and coworkers[299] defined the anatomic basis of intermittent venous obstruction from the subclavian and anterior scalene muscles.

QUESTIONS

1. Implantation of a small artery into the side of a larger one by the patch technique was described by whom?
   a. Linton
   b. W. Hunter
   c. DeBakey
   d. Carrel
   e. Hufnagel
2. The first treatment of arterial obstruction in the leg by an endarterial approach was reported by whom?
   a. Homans
   b. Cannon
   c. Wylie
   d. Dotter
   e. Leriche
3. The chronic burning pain described by Mitchell is known as what?
   a. Artérite
   b. Thromboangiitis
   c. Causalgia
   d. Peripheral neuritis
   e. Postherpetic neuralgia
4. The first successful coronary artery reconstruction for angina was performed by whom?
   a. May
   b. DeBakey and Cooley
   c. Cooley and Morris
   d. Edwards and Lyons
   e. Longmire and Cannon
5. Who is commonly credited with interrupting major draining veins in the leg to treat deep venous thrombosis?
   a. Holman
   b. Hall
   c. Homans
   d. Allen
   e. Trendelenburg
6. The duplex scan was introduced to evaluate what?
   a. Flow in the venous system
   b. Carotid stenosis
   c. Size and progression of abdominal aneurysms
   d. Raynaud's syndrome
   e. Pulmonary embolism
7. The possibility of an extraanatomic bypass of an obstructed artery was first proposed by ____________ and carried out by ____________.
   a. J. Hunter and Cooper
   b. Wylie and Moore
   c. DeBakey and Morris
   d. Kunlin and Oudot
   e. Linton and Darling
8. John Hunter's famous operation to cure popliteal aneurysm consisted of what?
   a. Ligation of the popliteal artery above and below the aneurysm
   b. Sympathectomy and excision of the aneurysm
   c. Sympathectomy and ligation of the common femoral artery

d. Sympathectomy and external compression (using the Massachusetts General compressor) of the popliteal artery
e. Ligation of the "superficial" femoral artery in the subsartorial region

9. Murray's introduction of heparin to clinical use led which surgeon to attempt delayed arterial embolectomy?
   a. Homans
   b. Osler
   c. Kunlin
   d. J. dos Santos
   e. Matas

10. Although not described in the exact words, the principle behind the concept of endoleaks following operation for aneurysm was described by whom?
   a. Vesalius
   b. J. Hunter
   c. Holman
   d. Matas
   e. Parodi

BIBLIOGRAPHY

Bigger IA. Surgical treatment of aneurysm of the aorta: Review of the literature and report of two cases, one apparently successful. *Ann Surg*. 1940;112:879–894.

Blaisdell FW, Hall AD. Axillary-femoral artery bypass for lower extremity ischemia. *Surgery*. 1963;54:563–568.

Blalock A, Taussig HB. The surgical treatment of malformations of the heart in which there is pulmonary stenosis or pulmonary atresia. *JAMA*. 1945;128:189–202.

Buerger L. Thromboangiitis obliterans: A study of the vascular lesions leading to presenile spontaneous gangrene. *Am J Med Sci*. 1908;136:567–580.

Carrel A. The surgery of blood vessels, etc. *Johns Hopkins Hosp Bull*. 1907;190:18–28.

Charcot JM. Obstruction artérielle et claudication intermittente dans le cheval et dans l'homme. *Mem Soc Biol*. 1858;1:225–238.

Crafoord C, Nylin G. Congenital coarctation of the aorta and its surgical treatment. *J Thorac Surg*. 1945;14:347–361.

DeBakey ME, Cooley SA, Crawford ES, et al. Clinical application of a new flexible knitted Dacron arterial substitute. *Arch Surg*. 1958;77:713–724.

DeCamp P, Snyder CH, Bost RB. Severe hypertension due to congenital stenosis of artery to solitary kidney: Correction by splenorenal anastomosis. *Arch Surg*. 1957;75:1026–1030.

Dobson J. *John Hunter*. Edinburgh: E & S Livingstone; 1969.

dos Santos JC. Sur la désobstruction des thromboses artérielles anciennes. *Mem Acad Chir*. 1947;73:409–411.

dos Santos R, Lamas A, Caldas P. L'artériographie des membres, de l'aorte et des ses branches abdominales. *Bull Mem Soc Natl Chir*. 1929;55:587–601.

Dubost C, Allary M, Oeconomos N. Resection of an aneurysm of the abdominal aorta: Reestablishment of the continuity by a preserved human arterial graft, with result after five months. *Arch Surg*. 1952;64:405–408.

Dunphy JE. Abdominal pain of vascular origin. *Am J Med Sci*. 1936;92:109–113.

Eastcott HHG, Pickering GW, Rob C. Reconstruction of internal carotid artery in a patient with intermittent attacks of hemiplegia. *Lancet*. 1954;2:994–996.

Edwards WS, Tapp JS. Chemically treated nylon tubes as arterial grafts. *Surgery*. 1955;38:61–76.

Fogarty TJ, Cranley JJ, Krause RJ, et al. A method of extraction of arterial emboli and thrombi. *Surg Gynecol Obstet*. 1963;116: 241–244.

Gross RE. Complete surgical division of the patent ductus arteriosus. *Surg Gynecol Obstet*. 1944;78:36–43.

Holman E. Clinical and experimental observations on arteriovenous fistulae. *Ann Surg*. 1940;112:840–878.

Homans J. Thrombosis of the deep veins of the lower leg causing pulmonary embolism. *N Engl J Med*. 1934;211: 993–997.

Homans J. The late results of femoral thrombophlebitis and their treatment. *N Engl J Med*. 1946;235:249–253.

Jaboulay M, Briau E. Recherches expérimentales sur la suture et la greffe artérielles. *Bull Lyon Med*. 1896;81:97–99.

Jahnke EJ Jr, Howard JM. Primary repair of major arterial injuries. *Arch Surg*. 1953;66:646–649.

Jassinowsky A. Die Arteriennaht: Eine experimentelle Studie [dissertation]; 1889. Dorpat, Estonia, University of Tartu.

Julian OC, Dye WS, Javid H, et al. Ulcerative lesions of the carotid artery bifurcation. *Arch Surg*. 1963;86:803–809.

Kistner RL. Surgical repair of the incompetent vein valve. *Arch Surg*. 1975;110:1336–1342.

Kolff WJ. The first clinical experience with the artificial kidney. *Ann Intern Med*. 1965;62:608–619.

Kunlin J. Le traitement de l'ischemie artéritique par la greffe veineuse longue. *Rev Chir*. 1951;70:207–235.

Leriche R. Des oblitérations artérielles hautes (oblitération de la terminasion de l'aorte) comme causes des insuffisances circulatoires des membres inférieures. *Bull Mem Soc Chir Paris*. 1923;49:1404–1406.

Longmire WP Jr, Cannon JA, Kattus HA. Direct-vision coronary endarterectomy for angina pectoris. *N Engl J Med*. 1958;259: 993–999.

Marrangoni AC, Cecchini LP. Homotransplantation of arterial segments by the freeze-drying method. *Ann Surg*. 1951;134: 977–983.

Matas R. Traumatic aneurism of the brachial artery. *Med News*. 1888;53:462–466.

Moore WS, Hall AD. Carotid artery back pressure: A test of cerebral tolerance to temporary carotid artery occlusion. *Arch Surg*. 1969;99:702–710.

Murphy JB. Resection of arteries and veins injured in continuity … end to end suture … experimental and clinical research. *Med Rec*. 1897;51:73–88.

Murray GDW. Heparin in thrombosis and embolism. *Br J Surg*. 1940;27:567–576.

Ochsner A, Gage M, DeBakey ME. Scalenus anticus (Naffziger) syndrome. *Am J Surg*. 1935;28:669–693.

Parodi J, Palmaz JC, Barone HD. Transfemoral intraluminal graft implantation for abdominal aortic aneurysms. *Ann Vasc Surg*. 1991;5:491–499.

Strandness DE, Schultz RD, Sumner DS, et al. Ultrasonic flow detection: A useful technique in the evaluation of peripheral vascular disease. *Am J Surg*. 1967;113:311–320.

Thompson JE, Patman RD, Talkington CM. Asymptomatic carotid bruit. *Ann Surg*. 1978;188:308–316.

Voorhees AB Jr, Jaretzki A III, Blakemore AH. Use of tubes constructed of Vinyon-"N" cloth in bridging arterial defects. *Ann Surg*. 1952;135:332–336.

Winsor T. Pressure gradients: Influence of arterial disease on the systolic blood pressure gradients of the extremity. *Am J Med Sci*. 1950;220:117–126.

References available online at ExpertConsult.com.

CHAPTER 2

Embryology of the Vascular System

David S. Maxwell[†]

It is quite evident that the vascular apparatus does not independently and by itself "unfold" into the adult pattern. On the contrary, it reacts continuously in a most sensitive way to the factors of its environment, the pattern in the adult being the result of the sum of the environmental influences that have played upon it throughout the embryonic period. We thus find that this apparatus is continuously adequate and complete for the structures as they exist at any particular stage as the environmental structures progressively change; the vascular apparatus also changes and thereby is always adapted to the newer conditions. Furthermore, there are no apparent ulterior preparations at any time for the supply and drainage of other structures which have not yet made their appearance. For each stage it is an efficient and complete going-mechanism, apparently uninfluenced by the nature of its subsequent morphology.

George L. Streeter (1918)

This observation made more than 80 years ago exemplifies the finest tradition of the working scientist: years of attention to the most minute details of a subject, which eventuate in the broadest and most comprehensive view of the fundamental issues. In this statement, Streeter summarizes all that needs to be said and virtually all that can be said about the development of the vascular system, save for some specific details that would only embellish the theme he has laid out.

The story of the development of the vascular system encompasses the life span of the organism. This system retains the ability to grow, change, regenerate, and add on in response to the changing needs of the tissues, from the earliest stages of embryonic life to the final breath. Thus, it supports normal growth, wound healing, and revascularization of tissues endangered by restricted flow in existing vessels, just as it supports the new growth of tumors and transiently develops a highly efficient transport and exchange system through the uteroplacental circulation during pregnancy. All this is accomplished by the opening and enlarging of preexisting vessels and the budding of new vascular growth from preexisting stem vessels. That it may eventually fail to respond to adequately supply the myocardium or the central nervous system is not as remarkable as the fact that it responds so well for so long. It seems likely that, in the embryonic and fetal history of the vascular system, there would be clues to the mysteries that surround this responsiveness throughout life. Furthermore, in the prenatal unfolding of the vascular system lie the origins of the various cardiovascular malformations to which the human organism is subject. We do not yet know whether the mechanisms of growth and the stimuli to vascularization of the embryo and fetus are the same as those that encourage and sustain the responsiveness of the vasculature in the postnatal organism.

This chapter does not attempt to review the enormous literature on the subject, and many exciting details are omitted in the interest of providing a simple narrative exposition of the high points. The organizational scheme first discusses a short history of the heart, which is simply a greatly modified blood vessel, followed by descriptions of the development of the large arteries and veins. The chapter concludes with some comments on the growth of small vessels, which, like acorns, must appear and flourish first to produce the mighty trunk and branches of the vascular tree.

EARLY HISTORY

An organism of a cubic millimeter or so in volume (depending on the surface area and other factors related to the effectiveness of diffusion) may thrive without a vascular system. The human embryo enjoys the elaboration of a vascular system from its earliest stages, almost as if it can anticipate that its bulk will soon require a highly sophisticated transport system. As the embryonic disk becomes recognizable, blood islands rapidly accumulate around the periphery of the disk. These isolated "puddles" begin to coalesce and communicate with one another until the embryo resembles a bloody sponge. Most prominent is the precephalic region, where the seemingly random coalescence of blood islands forms a network in the region soon to be identified as the cardiogenic plate (Fig. 2.1*A*).

[†]Deceased

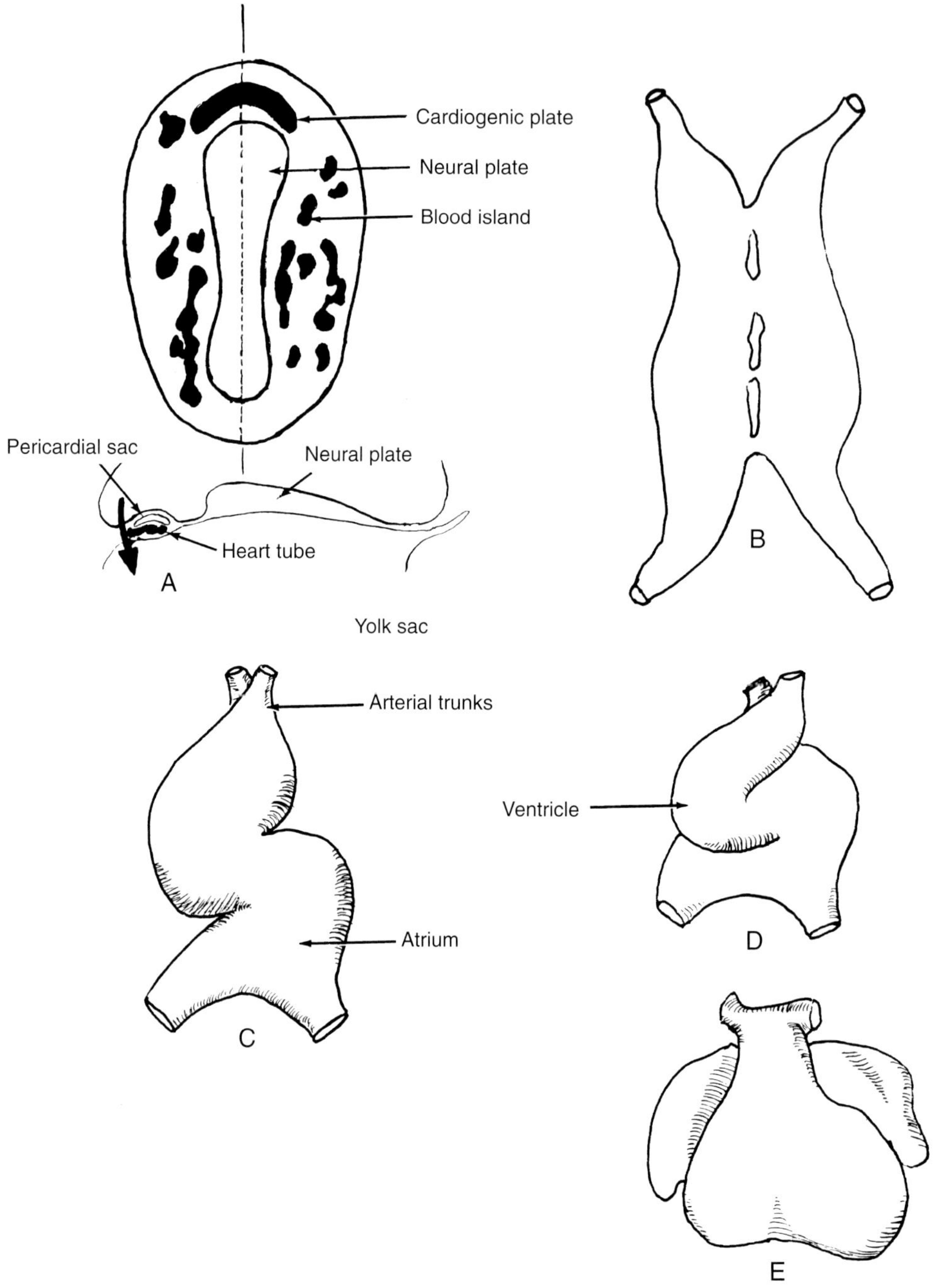

FIG 2.1 **A,** Embryonic disk from above, with the head of the embryo facing upward. The *dotted line* indicates the plane of the longitudinal section below, with the cranial end to the left. In the section, the pericardial sac is above the heart tube, but as the head folds under the forebrain (direction of the *large arrow*), the positions of the heart and sac will be reversed, with the heart invaginating from above the pericardial sac. **B,** The two parallel primitive heart tubes (dorsal view) fuse in the midline to form a single heart tube and a single-chambered heart. **C-E,** Successive stages of the folding of the heart tube, viewed from the front. The venous end of the tube swings posteriorly to form the atria, whereas the arterial end (ventricles) remains anterior. This represents the loop stage. (Adapted from Moore KL: *The developing human,* ed 3, Philadelphia, 1982, WB Saunders, 1982; and Rushmer RF: *Cardiovascular dynamics,* ed 2, Philadelphia, 1961, WB Saunders.)

In these earliest stages of development, the vascular system manifests some of its greatest mysteries: to what extent is the developmental pattern dictated by tissue needs and demands (possibly through the release of angiogenic factors or through stimuli provided by metabolic products), and to what extent is it dictated by factors such as extravascular pressures restricting flow in one set of possible blood channels and forcing the enlargement of adjacent alternative routes of blood flow? To what extent is the overall pattern dictated genetically? The similarity of the vascular tree from one individual to another favors the speculation that there is a detailed genetic code. The variability from one to another—each pattern seemingly equally efficient in supporting tissues and organs—argues for development according to need and use and based on mechanical and other adventitious factors.

In the case of the heart, a detailed genetic code is surely the guiding factor. Here, curiously, we begin with a parallel pair of cardiac tubes that fuse into one large tube; the latter then divides internally into the right and left hearts. At first glance, this seems inefficient. Why not simply have each original tube of the pair form a right or left heart? The reason is clear when examining the details of internal division of the heart, in which the single outflow tract is divided in such a way as to connect the right heart to the primitive vessels supplying the pulmonary circuit and to connect the remaining members of the branchial arch arteries to the left heart.

HEART

Our interest in the development of the heart in this chapter is restricted to its bearing on the origins of the great vessels. The heart is simply a highly modified artery from both histologic and embryologic viewpoints. Histologically, it resembles a muscular artery because it has three layers to its walls: adventitia (epicardium), tunica media (myocardium), and tunica intima (endocardium). At the beginning, the heart tubes are simply a parallel pair of vessels, seemingly little different from the other components of the random network of primitive blood vessels. Nonetheless, the fusion of these two tubes and the development of a feeble myocardial investment around the endothelium quickly lead to irregular contractions of the musculature, with feeble and inefficient ejection of blood. Subsequent events include the development of septa, dividing the single-chambered heart into right and left halves, and the appearance of valves that dictate unidirectional flow. The heart is beating with increasing regularity and with an efficiency-improving peristalsis and force as the myocardial element thickens and cytodifferentiates. Presumably from these first feeble, sporadic beats there is a stirring of the blood contents of the primitive vessels, perhaps providing some benefit to the growing tissues around them and perhaps beginning to stimulate the enlargement of those channels that will survive into later embryonic stages. Beginning to channel blood through preferred pathways leads to closure and disappearance of less satisfactory routes and enlargement of the more successful channels into definitive blood vessels that are soon worthy of names recognizable in terms of the adult circulatory pattern. Channel formation from blood islands might be influenced simply by the choice of the lowest resistance among the available pathways.

The now-fused heart tube (see Fig. 2.1*B*) begins to invaginate the presumptive pericardial cavity, acquiring its visceral and parietal layers of pericardium while still a single-chambered heart configured as a simple, relatively straight tube. As the somites begin to appear in the neck and trunk region, the heart tube begins to fold on itself, first bulging ventrally, further invaginating the pericardial sac. The heart that is now swinging ventrocaudally comes to lie in front of the head and will continue its descent down the front of the neck and into the anterior chest. The ventrally directed bulge created by the U-shaped fold of the heart characterizes the loop stage.[1] The ventral limb of the U is the arterial outflow path, and the dorsal limb of the U will become the venous inflow tract (see Fig. 2.1*C* to *E*). By the 10-somite stage, approximately 3 weeks' ovulation age, the heart has begun to fold in a coronal plane as well, directing the ventricular region to the left and forming a recognizable outflow tract, now termed the *bulbus cordis,* whose distal part is called the *truncus arteriosus* (see Fig. 2.1*C*). At this stage, the heart is still a single-chambered structure innocent of valves but completely enclosed in a pericardial sac and demonstrably beating, albeit irregularly. There is no single primordium, no segment of the primitive heart tube, that can be identified as leading to a specific cardiac cavity in the early postloop stage. Instead, there are microscopically and experimentally identifiable zones, each of which gives rise to a specific anatomic region of a definitive cardiac cavity. These primordia are most accurately termed *primitive cardiac regions;* therefore referring to segments of the heart tube as forerunners of the chambers of the fully formed heart is misleading.[1] The folds in the heart tube and the peristaltic nature of myocardial contraction lead to a predetermined direction of flow out through the bulbus cordis, the folds acting as inefficient valves to direct the flow. Such early vitality is not surprising, because the cardiovascular system is the earliest to attain form and function among the organ systems of the body. The heart is disproportionately large for the size of the embryo at this stage, and this disproportion remains until birth, with only a modest decline in heart-to-body ratio toward birth. Obviously, this occurs because the heart must support not only the growing tissue of the organism but also the embryo's share of the enormous placental circulation.

It is worth digressing here to emphasize the functional problems faced by the developing heart. It is required to form and to function in such a way as to maintain and support the growth of the developing organism in an intrauterine (aquatic) environment; that is, it must support an organism incapable of independent gas exchange and dependent on the placenta for oxygen and nutriments and for other metabolic exchange. The lungs are developed rather late and require only to be supplied with enough blood to support their growth. To perfuse the embryonic lungs with a rate of blood flow commensurate with an air-breathing existence would be energetically inefficient and perhaps an impediment to their growth and development, but during the early stages of development of the cardiovascular system, the lungs are simply not sufficiently developed to be called anything other than *buds,* volumetrically incapable of containing any significant quantity of blood. As a result, the heart must develop a mechanism whereby it can support the organism in an aquatic environment with extensive exchange across the placenta and provide adequate distribution of blood throughout the growing body of the embryo; however, it must simultaneously develop a configuration that will enable it to shift its mode of function instantly at birth to support the organism by way of pulmonary gas exchange. Simply put, in fetal and embryonic life, the two sides of the heart function as two pumps operating in parallel, with the output of both ventricles distributed to the placenta and to the growing tissues of the body, and with no interdependence of the output. However, the two hearts must have the means to shift from functioning in parallel to functioning in tandem at birth, wherein the outflow of one heart becomes the inflow of the other, and blood is obligated to perfuse the pulmonary circuit, return to the heart, and then perfuse the systemic circuit, and so on. One emphasis of this chapter is to focus on the development of features that render the heart capable of these sequential and different modes of function.

ARTERIES

During the early folding of the heart, and with identification of a bulbus cordis and truncus arteriosus as an outflow tract, the aortic arches are beginning to form. The truncus arteriosus is continuous with a ventral aorta. This large, single-channeled artery is connected to a pair of dorsal aortas through a series of branchial (pharyngeal) arch arteries. The developing pharynx passes through a period in its development when it is said to mimic the development of the gill apparatus of fish. Outpouchings of the pharyngeal wall grow as pockets toward the surface, where they are met or at least approached by corresponding infoldings of the ectodermal surface. Normally these outpouchings and infoldings neither meet nor coalesce to form gill slits or fistulas. The supporting tissue on both sides of the pouches is endowed with a cartilaginous supporting bar, a nerve, and a blood vessel, respectively known as the *branchial arch (pharyngeal) cartilage, branchial arch nerve,* and *branchial arch artery*. The first such cartilaginous bar is Meckel's cartilage, in front of the first pharyngeal pouch; the second, Reichert's cartilage, lies between the first and second pouches. The pharynx is supported by six arch complexes, surrounding and intervening between the pharyngeal pouches. The arteries of these arches are the connectives from the ventral aorta to the dorsal aortas, and they appear in sequence from cranial to caudal. Rarely are more than three such arch arteries identifiable at one time; in this case, as elsewhere in the embryo, the cranial development leads or precedes that occurring more caudally. As the fourth arch artery appears, the first is being transformed into its successor structures and ceases to be identifiable as an arch artery. In humans, there are five such arch arteries, numbered 1, 2, 3, 4, and 6, in recognition of the dropping out in phylogeny of the fifth arch artery, which has no significant role in human development (the fifth pharyngeal pouch fuses with the fourth at its opening into the pharynx; its rudimentary arch between the fourth and fifth pouches contributes to the formation of the larynx). In contrast to the constancy of innervation of the derivatives of the pharyngeal arches, the vascular supply to the arches is subject to later, often extensive modification. The motor nerve to an arch persists throughout phylogeny and throughout ontogenetic development in supplying the derivatives of that arch (first arch, mandibular nerve; second arch, facial nerve; third arch, glossopharyngeal nerve; fourth through sixth arches, recurrent and superior laryngeal nerves and vagal pharyngeal nerve). The geometric representation of the arch artery pattern and the fate of those arteries are summarized in Fig. 2.2. The paired dorsal aortas sweep posteriorly and fuse in the midline to form a single dorsal aorta (see Fig. 2.2, *inset*) posterior to entry points of the arch arteries.

The lungs begin their development as a ventrally directed outgrowth from the pharynx, and the single tube that will become the trachea descends into the presumptive chest cavity, where it branches into a pair of lung buds. These buds receive a small blood supply from branches of the sixth aortic arch arteries (see Fig. 2.2*A*). Clearly the sixth arch arteries will have a role in the development of the pulmonary arterial tree. The developmental problem posed here is that the sixth arch arteries are initially part of the systemic circulation, simply representing the most caudal of the branchial arch arteries springing from the truncus arteriosus and uniting with the dorsal aortas. In the division of the heart tube into right and left hearts, some provision must be made for joining the right ventricular outflow tract to the sixth arch arteries and joining the remainder of the great branchial arch system and aortas with the left ventricle. The rationale for fusion of the primitive heart tubes into a single channel and subsequent division is now clarified by this need to divide the bulbus cordis and truncus arteriosus into a pulmonary artery and an aortic artery. The manner of that division solves the problem of connecting the right ventricle and the developing pulmonary artery to the lungs and connecting the remainder of the arch arteries to the systemic circulation and the left ventricle. The interested reader is encouraged to examine the article by Congdon[2] for further clarification of this point.

The heart is divided into four chambers that compose two separate hearts, with provision for a parallel mode of function before birth and a tandem mode after birth. The umbilical veins (after the sixth week, a single left umbilical vein) return blood to the fetal heart by their union with the inferior vena cava. This return route sees the umbilical vein enter the liver, where a shunt, the ductus venosus, bypasses the complex hepatic circulation and shunts the blood directly into the inferior vena cava. Thus, the right atrium receives a supply of freshly oxygenated blood, in contrast to the adult condition. Before separation of the right and left atria, that placental return is into the single atrial chamber, which is diagrammatically depicted in Fig. 2.3*A*. The single chamber undergoes a constriction in the plane of the atrioventricular orifices and the atrioventricular sulcus on the exterior of the heart. From the margins of this constriction, endocardial cushions grow inward to begin the formation of the tricuspid and mitral valves. The single atrium begins its separation into halves by downgrowth from the dorsocranial wall of a filmy crescentic curtain—the septum primum (see Fig. 2.3*B*). The leading invaginated edge of the crescent grows down toward the floor of the single atrium; that floor forms by virtue of the

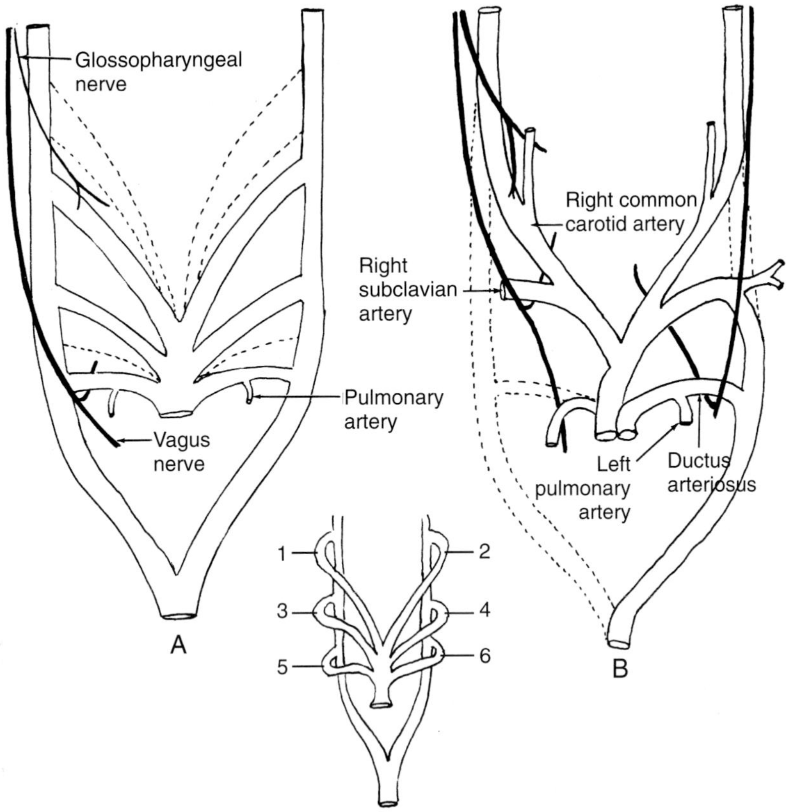

FIG 2.2 Fate of the branchial arch arteries. **A,** Primitive arrangement of six arch arteries. Arches 1 and 2 have formed and have been accommodated into the vessels of the head (dotted lines indicate arteries that are no longer arches—that is, 1, 2, and 5). Arches 3, 4, and 6 connect the ventral aorta (aortic sac and truncus arteriosus) with the paired dorsal aortas. The latter fuse posteriorly to form a single dorsal aorta. **B,** Subsequent disposition of these vessels. The *dotted lines* indicate vessels that normally disappear, including the right sixth arch beyond the right pulmonary artery. The glossopharyngeal nerve (motor to the third arch) and the recurrent laryngeal nerve (motor to the sixth arch derivatives) are shown. The recurrent laryngeal nerve is a branch of the vagus "recurring" around the sixth arch in **A;** in **B,** these nerves recur around the ductus arteriosus and around the right subclavian. **Inset,** The first three aortic arch arteries from the front (ventral) view during the branchial period. At no time are all arch arteries evident at the same time. The paired dorsal aortas unite into a single dorsal aorta posterior to the entry of the arch arteries. The postbranchial period, when the heart descends from the branchial region into the chest, is characterized by modification of the arch system into the adult disposition of the derived arteries.

growth of the atrioventricular valve primordia. Fig. 2.3*B* shows the septum primum from the right side as it progresses toward complete closure of the single atrial chamber in its midline. In addition, just before the foramen primum closes, a group of perforations forms in the dorsocranial part of the partition (see Fig. 2.3*B*) and then coalesces into a foramen secundum (see Fig. 2.3*C*). This process is necessary because throughout this developmental sequence, the heart is pumping blood to and returning it from the placenta, and the returning blood must be shunted from the right side of the heart into the left atrium in large volume to sustain the systemic circulation. Therefore at no point in fetal life may the right and left atria be functionally separate. During the time that the placental circulation is intact, the pressure in the right atrium exceeds that in the left atrium, and a right-to-left shunt will be operative. As a result, the foramen secundum opens just in time to continue that shunt as the foramen primum closes. Next, on the right side of the septum primum, a much more robust and rigid septum secundum begins its downgrowth, following the same pattern as that of the septum primum (see Fig. 2.3*C*); a crescent-shaped leading edge grows down from above toward the endocardial cushions that will finally separate the atria from the ventricles. This downgrowth of the septum secundum comes to overlie the orifice of the foramen secundum. Fortunately, the septum secundum is sturdy and relatively unyielding, whereas the septum primum is thin and curtainlike. As long as the free lower edge of the septum secundum fails to reach the floor of the atrium, thus forming the foramen ovale, the elevated pressure in the right atrium pushes blood through the ovale, deflecting the septum primum and allowing blood to pass through the foramen secundum into

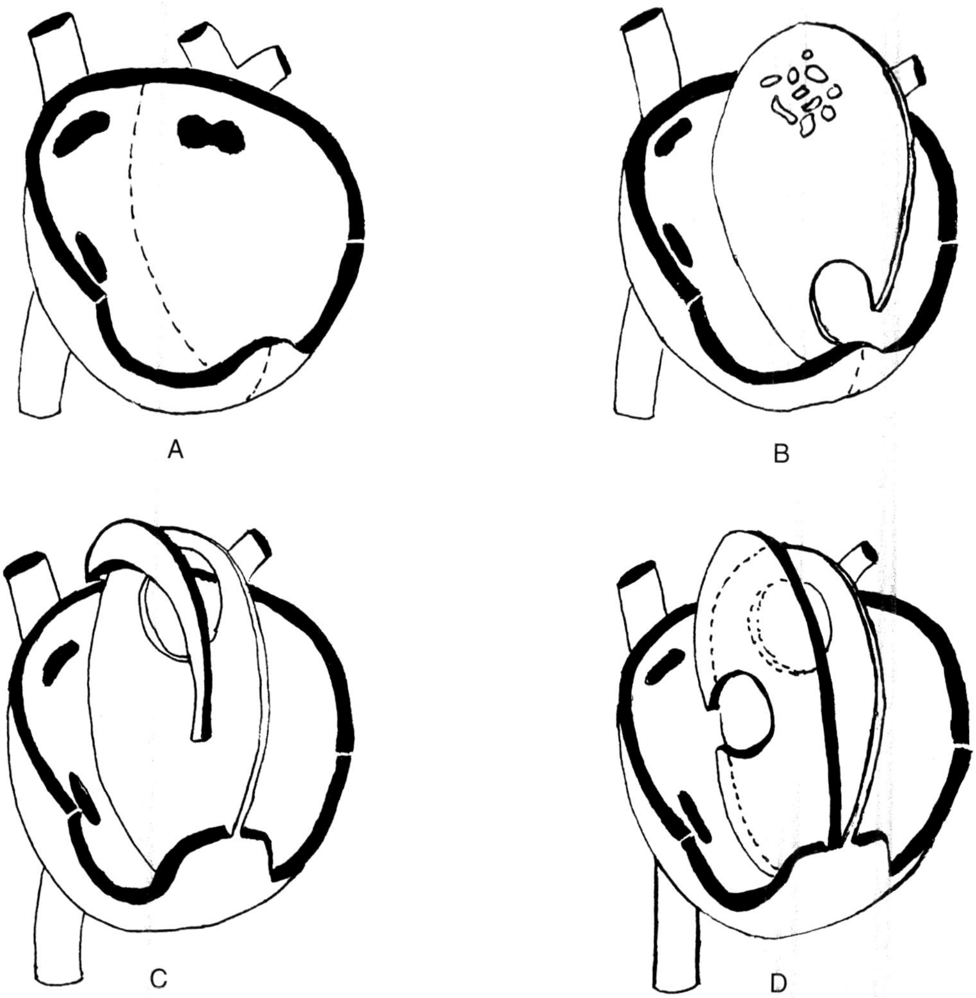

FIG 2.3 The single early atrium is represented as a hollow sphere, from an anterolateral view. The atrioventricular canals are the lower part of the cutaway sphere. **A,** The *dotted line* indicates the plane of division into right and left atria. The entry of the superior and inferior venae cavae (right atrial segment of the sphere) and the pulmonary arteries (left segment of the sphere) is indicated by entering tubes. **B-D,** Successive stages in development of the interatrial septum. In **B,** the septum primum grows downward, leaving a free margin as the ostium primum. As this ostium prepares to close, holes appear in the upper posterior part of the septum, which in **C** have coalesced into an ostium secundum. In **C,** the septum secundum begins to grow downward to the right of the septum primum, covering the ostium secundum on that side. The free margin of the septum secundum does not close over in **D,** leaving the foramen ovale open. The right atrial contents flow into the left atrium via the foramen ovale and ostium secundum. (Adapted from Tuchmann-Duplessis H, David HG, Haegel P: *Illustrated human embryology,* New York, 1972, Springer-Verlag.)

the left atrium and permitting continuation of the obligatory right-to-left shunt. Inasmuch as the downgrowth of the septum secundum is arrested, leaving a fixed foramen ovale, such a shunt operates throughout the intrauterine life of the organism. The orifice of the foramen ovale is just above and medial to the orifice of the inferior vena cava (see Fig. 2.3*D*), so that inferior caval (i.e., placental) blood is preferentially directed into that foramen, and then into the left atrium, with remarkably little mixing of this oxygenated blood with the oxygen-poor blood returning via the superior vena cava.

The division of the ventricles and the single aortic outflow path are both simpler to understand and more critically complex. The ventricle begins to divide by the upward growth of a muscular partition of myocardium from the cardiac apex toward the truncus arteriosus (Fig. 2.4*A*); this will form the muscular part of the interventricular septum. At the same time, a pair of ridges (the spiral ridges) grow toward each other as outgrowths of the walls of the truncus arteriosus. These ridges will fuse to form a spiral septum, dividing the septum from above downward. The lower ends of the spiral ridges contribute to the formation of the final septal closure (see Fig. 2.4*B*). This phenomenon is extraordinarily complex, involves early histologic changes, and is probably initiated by hemodynamic influences and is subsequently controlled by genetic factors (see the analysis by Fanapazir

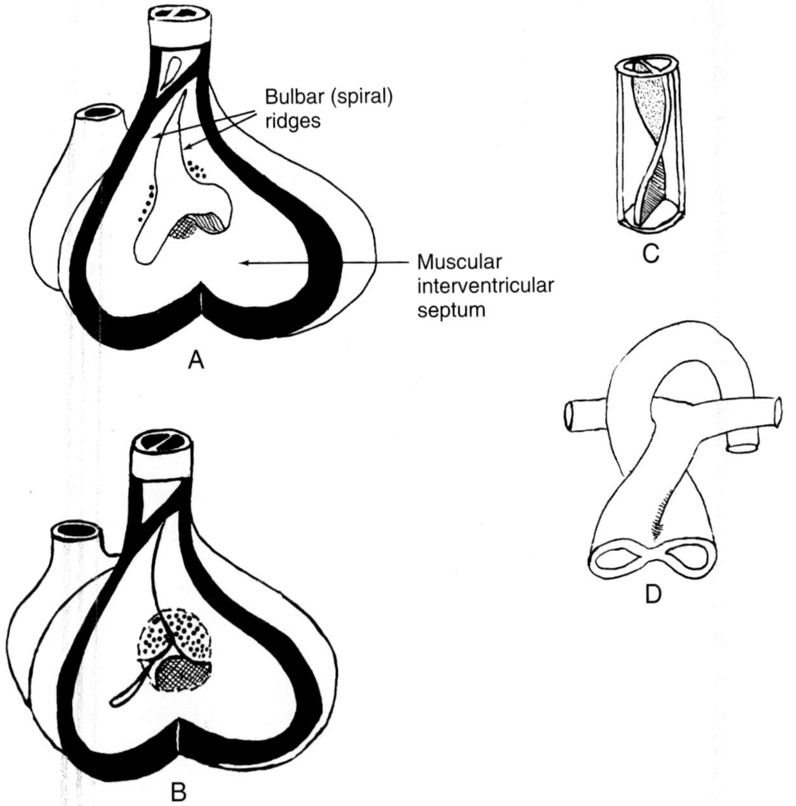

FIG 2.4 Stages in the division of the ventricle and formation of the great arteries from the truncus arteriosus and bulbus cordis. **A,** The ventricle has begun to divide, with formation of the muscular part of the interventricular septum by means of growth of the ventricular wall musculature. The bulbus cordis is dividing into two vessels, beginning with the growing together of two spiral ridges. **B,** The two spiral ridges meet and fuse to divide the bulbus cordis into two outflow tracts: the pulmonary artery and the ascending aorta. The ridges at their lower extremities *(stippled cushions)* meet a muscular cushion derived from the muscular interventricular septum *(hatched)* to form the membranous part of the interventricular septum (outlined by *dotted lines*). The spiral character of the arterial division connects the sixth arch arteries to the right ventricle and connects the left ventricle to the other arch arteries and their derivatives. **C,** Spiral septum shown diagrammatically, in a cutaway cylinder representing the single bulbus cordis. The hatched surface of the septum represents the aortic side of the division, and the stippled side represents the pulmonary surface of the septum. The two resulting arteries must spiral around each other, as in **D.** Derived from a single tube, they are constrained to remain wrapped in a single pericardial sleeve. (Adapted from Tuchmann-Duplessis H, David HG, Haegel P: *Illustrated human embryology,* New York, 1972, Springer-Verlag; and Moore KL: *The developing human,* Philadelphia, 1982, WB Saunders.)

and Kaufman[3]). The membranous interventricular septum is formed where the three cushions meet. Fig. 2.4*C* and 2.4*D* schematically depict the spiral arrangement of the division of the truncus arteriosus whereby the single outflow tract is divided into pulmonary and aortic tubes, each connected to its corresponding ventricular cavity. The complexity of the closure lies in the precise pitch of the spiral septum; its lower end must be aligned with the upthrusting muscular cushion so as to meet accurately in a single plane. Interference in the fusion of these cushions into a complete membranous septum will lead to a membranous interventricular septal defect. Misalignment of the spiral ridges may result in failure of the great arteries to form and function independently through the accident of a pulmonary aortic fistula. Misalignment of the lower end of the dividing arteries and asymmetry in the positioning of the spiral ridges could lead to such errors as an overriding aorta, with the right ventricular contents partially ejected into the aorta. The features of the tetralogy of Fallot can be readily interpreted as a result of such misalignment in the truncus division. The tetralogy consists of an overriding aorta, pulmonary stenosis, membranous septal defect (presumably due to asymmetrical division of the proximal truncus arteriosus), and right ventricular hypertrophy (secondary to the right-to-left shunt through the overriding aorta and to the stenotic pulmonary artery).

A superbly illustrated and classic account of early experimental findings, as well as an excellent historical review of the anatomy and physiology of fetal circulation, can be found in the book by Barclay and associates.[4] More recent summaries can be obtained in standard works by Arey,[5] Clemente,[6] Hamilton and Mossman,[7] Moore,[8] Sabin,[9] and Tuchmann-Duplessis and associates.[10]

The original plan of five pairs of aortic arch arteries (see Fig. 2.2) becomes modified by incorporation of the first two arch arteries into the internal carotid system, dropping out of the paired dorsal aortas between the third and fourth arches, and participation in the formation of the common carotid arteries by the third arches. Caudal to the lost segments of dorsal aortas, the fourth arches become the roots of the subclavian arteries; the right sixth arch is lost distal to its pulmonary branch, and the left sixth arch becomes the left pulmonary artery, with the segment distal to the pulmonary "branch" serving as the ductus arteriosus (see Fig. 2.2*B*). This arterial shunt vessel develops specialized muscle in its tunica media, which is stimulated to contract and shut down the shunt vessel after birth. It is believed that abnormal migration of some of this specialized smooth muscle into the aortic wall accounts for aortic stenosis, the stricture developing in the aorta at the site of this ectopic ductus muscle after birth.

The closure of this right-to-left shunt on the arterial side at birth results in a great increase in pulmonary blood flow (the resistance of pulmonary vessels drops dramatically with inflation of the lungs and elongation of helicine arteries). On the venous side, the rise in left atrial pressure and loss of umbilical venous return arrest the interatrial right-to-left shunt. Elevated left atrial pressure results in the two interatrial septa operating as a flap valve, closing the foramen ovale by applying the curtainlike septum primum against the left one (see Fig. 2.3*D*).

Certainty in the derivation of the arteries of the head is not easy to achieve. The arteries form from a loose network of interconnected vessels in which it is often impossible to distinguish between arteries and veins.[11] The artery of the first arch becomes a part of the internal carotid artery, which also forms in part from persistence of the rostral parts of the dorsal aortas. The second arch artery appears in the form of the stapedial artery. This artery of the tympanic cavity passes through the annulus (obturator foramen) in the stapes, and in some mammals it persists in this form. In humans, this form of stapedial artery may remain into adulthood as a surgically troublesome vascular anomaly. This artery of the second arch for a time supplies three branches (supraorbital, infraorbital, and mandibular), distributed with the divisions of the trigeminal nerve. An anastomosis between the infraorbital and mandibular branches of the stapedial artery and the external carotid artery is said to give rise to the maxillary artery and its middle meningeal branch. It is further argued that the orbital anastomotic branch of the middle meningeal artery is the remnant of the original supraorbital branch of the stapedial artery. Some information is indicated in the phylogenetic history of the artery. In most mammals, the originally small external carotid artery, as it grows forward, taps the origin of the stapedial artery and appropriates its branches, which at one stroke reduces the size and causes the disappearance of the original stapedial artery and extends the distribution of the external carotid. As Romer said, "the process is analogous to 'stream piracy,' whereby one river taps the headwaters of another."[12] Padget offers a detailed discussion and critical appraisal of the literature of the general mammalian stapedial artery and of the human artery, and her discussion is recommended to the interested reader.[13]

The third arch artery forms the common carotid arteries and the first segments of the internal carotid arteries. Thus, it is probable that portions of the first three arches all contribute to the external carotid arteries. The left fourth arch forms the arch of the aorta, and the left dorsal aorta distal to the point of union of this arch forms the descending aorta, along with the single dorsal aorta more caudally (see Fig. 2.2*B*). The entirety of the right dorsal aorta is lost. The right horn of the aortic sac forms the brachiocephalic artery, from which the right common carotid and subclavian arteries spring.

The sixth arches are associated with the pulmonary blood supply, first as the source of the small twigs to the lung buds. Those twigs and their parent stems from the truncus arteriosus become the definitive pulmonary arteries. At this point it should be clear why the complex twist of the spiral septum dividing the truncus arteriosus is necessary. In dividing the truncus, it is essential to connect the right ventricle to the origins of the sixth arches from the truncus, leaving the more rostral arch arteries connected to the part of the truncus connected to the left ventricle. The arch arteries spring from a single vessel, the truncus, and must end as arteries arising from separate arteries—the sixth arising from the pulmonary artery, and the first through fourth from the aortic component of the truncus. The twisting division of the truncus also accounts for the intertwined course of the pulmonary artery and the ascending aorta; their derivation from a single vessel, the truncus, accounts for these great arteries being wrapped in a single pericardial sleeve (see Fig. 2.4*D*).

The branchial arches develop nerve supplies along with their vascular supplies, and it is an axiom of anatomy that nerve supply is never lost once it is established. The motor nerves of the branchial arches supply the structures derived from those arches, no matter what developmental events ensue. In Fig. 2.2, the position of the glossopharyngeal nerve as the motor nerve of the third arch, and the recurrent laryngeal branch of the vagus as the motor nerve of the sixth arch, can be seen as these nerves are drawn caudally by the descent of the heart and growth of the branchial arch system. The recurrent branch of the vagus is in fact the motor nerve derived from the nucleus ambiguus of the brainstem, which happens to distribute by way of the vagus, having emerged from the brainstem as the cranial root of the spinal accessory nerve (cranial nerve XI). The recurring course of the nerve is accounted for by its inherited requirement of lying caudal to the sixth arch artery. The distal part of the left sixth arch artery becomes the ductus arteriosus (the ligamentum arteriosum after birth); thus arises the asymmetry in the courses of the two recurrent laryngeal nerves. The left nerve is constrained to maintain its original relationship to its arch artery as that artery is drawn down into the chest by the descent of the heart. The right nerve loses that constraint as the sixth arch drops out distal to the origin of the pulmonary artery. The only persisting arch to prevent the nerve's remaining in the neck as the heart descends is the fourth arch on the right side (the right subclavian artery), around which the nerve recurring in the adult human is found (see Fig. 2.2*B*). If, during thyroid surgery, the surgeon finds that the right recurrent nerve does not come up around the subclavian artery, he or she should take that as a warning that a developmental abnormality in the formation of the right subclavian artery might be expected (e.g., a retroesophageal right subclavian). In that event, the right subclavian forms from the right seventh intersegmental artery and part of the right dorsal aorta, the right fourth arch artery, and right dorsal aorta having involuted cranial to the origin of the seventh intersegmental artery.[8]

The developing embryo in its earliest stages is supported by a yolk sac of nutriment, sustaining growth until the placenta is sufficiently developed to assume those duties. The embryo lies on the surface of the yolk sac, with the interior of the latter in continuity with the developing gastrointestinal tract. The digestive tract cranial to the yolk sac is termed the *foregut,* that caudal to the yolk sac is termed the *hindgut,* and that directly connected to the yolk sac is termed the *midgut.* Three aortic branches, midline and unpaired, arise to supply each of these segments of the digestive tract, and these arteries remain the source of arterial blood for those portions of the tract and their derivatives. Thus, the celiac artery is the artery of the foregut and the derivatives of the foregut, including the liver and spleen. The artery of the midgut is the superior mesenteric artery; the artery of the hindgut is the inferior mesenteric artery. During development, the digestive tract outgrows the room available for it in the abdominal cavity and temporarily herniates out into the umbilical cord. Its return from this extraabdominal sojourn is accompanied by a rotation that accounts for the disposition of the stomach, the duodenum, and the bowel in the adult. The axis of rotation around which this reentry into the abdomen occurs is the superior mesenteric artery.[14]

The kidneys begin their development in the pelvis and migrate cranially to their final position on the posterior abdominal wall. The pelvic kidneys derive their arterial blood supply from the iliac system; as they ascend, the previous arterial supply drops out and new vessels from the aorta are established. The ascent and the history of the previous blood supply can be seen in the sources of small vessels supplying the ureter, their origins indicating the stems of vessels formerly supplying the kidney. Should the ascent of the kidney be arrested, the blood supply at the time remains the supply into adulthood. Thus, the ascent of the horseshoe kidney is arrested by the overhanging inferior mesenteric artery, and the horseshoe kidney has arterial blood supplied from common iliac vessels or the aorta at a level lower than the origin of the normal renal arteries. In addition, accessory renal arteries usually arise below the renal arteries and enter the inferior pole of the kidney, attesting to a previous source of blood that did not entirely disappear with ascent to the final renal destination.

The limbs seem to be organized around a central arterial stem, so that from the beginning an axial artery is identifiable. Fig. 2.5 depicts the changes in circulatory pattern for the two limbs. Generally, the axial artery in large part disappears and certainly ceases to be the principal source of limb blood.

In the upper limb, the axial artery passes down the core of the limb to the hand plexus. It is a continuation of the subclavian and axillary systems, already established in the 5-mm embryo, and is the forerunner of the brachial artery and, more distally, the interosseous artery. The upper limb axial artery sprouts a median branch and an ulnar arterial branch on the medial side of the stem artery. The median branch temporarily joins with the ulnar branch in the volar arch. A radial sprout follows on the preaxial side of the limb, and this new branch usurps the median's connection with the volar arch. The distal axial artery persists as the anterior interosseous artery. This pattern is completed before the end of the second month, and the early dominance of the axial and median arteries is permanently lost. The median artery persists as a branch of the anterior interosseous artery, serving as the nutrient artery of the median nerve. It may persist in an enlarged form as an anomaly, accompanying the median nerve into the palm and retaining its connection with and contribution to the palmar arterial arches.

Fig. 2.5 shows the steps by which the adult pattern of arterial supply to the lower limb is derived from the axial artery of the limb bud. The axial vessel is the sciatic artery, a direct branch of the umbilical; it is the primary source of the blood for the limb bud in the 9-mm embryo. The major stem artery for the limb becomes the femoral artery, as the latter continues the course of the external iliac. The femoral artery annexes the foot plexus of the sciatic artery and the origin of this axial vessel. The remaining proximal "stump" of the once-dominant sciatic artery persists as the inferior gluteal artery. A branch of the latter, the artery of the sciatic nerve, is all that remains of the former glory of the sciatic artery. The distal parts of the sciatic stem, appropriated by the femoral artery near its origin from the external iliac, give rise to the anterior tibial artery, which connects with the plantar arch distally. The newer, more distal femoral artery establishes a new connection to the distal sciatic so that it and the plantar arch come to branch from the sciatic. The most distal segment of the sciatic shifts its origin to the posterior tibial as the peroneal, and the adult pattern is established. The remnants of the sciatic persist (from above downward) as the inferior gluteal with its small artery of the sciatic nerve, the popliteal artery, and the peroneal artery. In the adult arterial plan, these persisting segments of the original sciatic artery no longer have continuity with one another in any significant way.

The umbilical arteries, carrying blood to the placenta for gas and metabolite exchange, appear as large branches of the internal iliac arteries and persist unmodified throughout gestation. These arteries develop robust branches to the upper surface of the urinary bladder. At birth, the segments of the umbilical arteries distal to the origin of the arteries to the bladder are obliterated and remain as fibrous cords—the medial umbilical ligaments. The stem of these arteries and the branches to the bladder are henceforth known as the *superior vesicle arteries.*

VEINS

As the arterial distribution system develops, appropriate return pathways arise simultaneously. The venous system is extensively interconnected, with a great capacity for collateral routes of venous return, and arteries are generally accompanied by corresponding veins. The short review of the venous system in this section focuses only on the great systems of veins that arise early

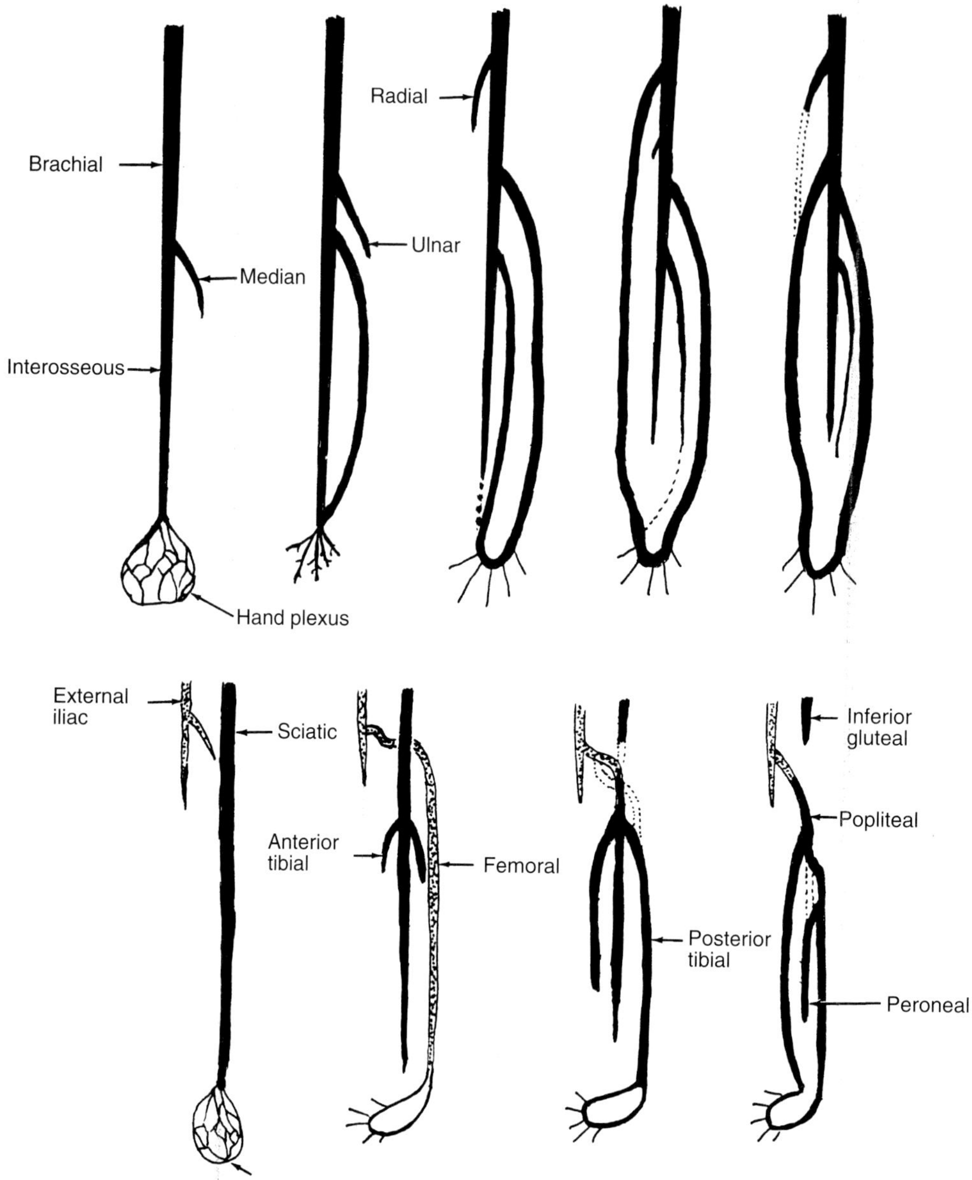

FIG 2.5 Development of the arterial pattern of the limbs. **Top row,** Upper limb. The upper limb is initially organized around a single axial artery—the brachial and its interosseous continuation—terminating in a hand plexus. The hand plexus will develop into the palmar arches. The stem artery gives rise in succession to the median, ulnar, and radial arteries. The median artery normally has an evanescent existence as a major vessel, losing its connection with the hand plexus, which it usurped from the axial vessel. **Bottom row,** Lower limb. The axial vessel for the lower limb is the sciatic, which remains in the adult as the inferior gluteal, and portions of the popliteal and peroneal arteries. The femoral artery arises from the external iliac and appropriates the distal part of the sciatic to dominate the vascular distribution of the limb. The anterior tibial artery arises as a branch of the popliteal; the posterior tibial is developed from the union of the femoral and the popliteal. Notice in the third figure from the left that an upper segment of the femoral artery is lost, allowing the popliteal to become interposed. (Adapted from Arey LB: *Developmental anatomy,* ed 7, Philadelphia, 1965, WB Saunders.)

in embryonic life and give rise to the major collecting pathways recognizable in the normal adult. As a result, even such important but developmentally simple systems as the pulmonary venous system are not discussed here.

A passing comment on venous valves is appropriate here, to draw attention to a provocative analysis and comparative study of superficial veins in the limbs of primates.[15] The number and spacing of venous valves are dictated genetically and are relevant to the need to maintain optimum pressures within capillary beds to ensure a balanced fluid exchange in tissues. The distance between venous valves in the limbs is sufficient to provide the transcapillary pressure gradients required for an equilibrium in fluid efflux and return to the vascular bed; it is not, as previously supposed, an adaptation to counter the effects of gravity in the bipedal posture.

The veins of the embryo fall into three major groups: vitelline (omphalomesenteric) veins, umbilical veins, and the cardinal system of veins. The coalesced blood islands that give rise to undifferentiated blood networks develop a venous side, as they do an arterial side, as directions of blood flow become established through them. Preferential pathways emerge on the venous side, giving rise to larger and more dominant veins that undergo modification as regional or organ-specific changes occur. Many of the venous channels developed in support of fetal life disappear as the need for them vanishes through subsequent development.

The vitelline veins are the veins of the yolk sac. They pass through the intestinal portal of the umbilical cord, alongside the (at first) wide channel of communication between the sac and the midgut region of the alimentary canal. A vitelline plexus is formed of communicating venous channels between the vitelline veins in the septum transversum. As the liver develops in the septum, it infringes on the vitelline plexus, separating it into hepatic sinusoids. Despite this encroachment, the vitelline pathway from the septum transversum into the heart persists as hepaticocardiac channels. The right channel of this return persists as the terminal segment of the inferior vena cava (Fig. 2.6). The vitelline plexus also surrounds the duodenum during the stage of hepatic growth, and the plexus is further distorted when the herniated midgut returns in a spiraling motion into the abdominal cavity. It is this rotation during the return that brings the duodenum into its transverse position and fixes this position by peritonealization. This position forces the blood in the surrounding plexus to shunt from the right to the left vitelline vein, which is the segment of the vitelline system lying just caudal to the transversely oriented duodenum. The left vitelline vein then sends its blood directly across to the liver by way of its dorsal anastomosis with the persistent cranial end of the right vitelline vein.

The portal vein thus formed does not spiral around the duodenum, as commonly described and illustrated; instead, it is short and straight, with the duodenum spiraling around it. The ease with which these changes occur can be understood if two basic facts are appreciated: (1) the essentially plexiform nature of the embryonic vascular system, and (2) the natural tendency for blood to seek the most direct route of flow because of hydrodynamic factors. (Refer to the clear sequence of illustrations of this development in Hamilton and Mossman,[7] page 274.)

The umbilical veins, entering the abdominal cavity by way of the umbilicus, must also traverse the septum transversum to arrive at the heart, and their septal segments within the septum also become enmeshed with the vitelline veins in the hepatic plexus of sinusoids. In the 5-mm embryo, the umbilical veins communicate extensively with the vitelline plexus in the liver. Two days later, the right umbilical vein undergoes atrophy, and all placental blood returns to the fetal heart via the left vein. The left vein's channel through the liver enlarges to accommodate this enhanced flow and forms the ductus venosus, a direct channel through the liver between the left umbilical vein and the inferior vena cava. This channel obliterates at birth with cessation of flow through the umbilical system, and the intrahepatic shunt is replaced by the ligamentum venosum. There is a sphincter in this shunt that regulates umbilical flow, which is a particularly important feature to prevent overloading of the fetal heart during uterine contractions. This sphincter's closure at birth contributes to the prompt obliteration of the shunt. The course of the left umbilical vein caudal to the liver is in the free margin of the ventral mesentery. The obliterated umbilical vein between the umbilicus and liver is the ligamentum teres hepatis of the adult, lying in the free margin of the falciform ligament; the latter is the adult counterpart of the ventral mesentery between the liver and the anterior abdominal wall.

The cardinal veins are the body wall veins of the embryo and fetus. There are several sets designated by distinguishing names. The anterior cardinal veins (also termed *precardinal veins*) drain the cranial region of the early embryo. The posterior cardinal veins drain the caudal portion and arise slightly later than the anterior cardinals. The subcardinal veins appear shortly after the posterior cardinal veins and are derived in conjunction with the rapidly growing progenitor of the kidney, the mesonephros. The term *supracardinal veins* is sometimes used to designate lateral sympathetic or thoracolumbar line veins or paraureteric veins. To limit the number of cardinal veins requiring attention, in discussing the veins of the posterior body wall anterior to the segmental vessels, the term *lateral sympathetic veins* is used instead.

The primary head vein of the embryo evolves into the complex system of dural sinuses and venous pathways of the head, and the reader is referred to the classic accounts of Streeter[16] and Padget,[11,13] whose illustrations amply clarify the changes leading to the adult pattern. The anterior and posterior cardinal veins unite behind the heart to form the common cardinal veins, or ducts of Cuvier (right and left). The union of the ducts of Cuvier is the ductus venosus at the venous end of the heart. Part of the ductus venosus becomes incorporated into the walls of the atria, most notably the right atrium.

The posterior cardinal veins are the first of a series of caudal longitudinal body wall veins, which form an interconnected system (see Fig. 2.6), giving rise to the caudal body wall venous drainage and to the inferior vena cava and azygos system of veins.

The subcardinal veins appear soon after the posterior cardinal veins as a pair of veins along the medial side of the urogenital folds. They are associated with the mesonephros and probably arise as a series of longitudinal anastomoses for the plexuses of the mesonephroi. They drain the mesonephroi and the germinal epithelium and terminate cranially and caudally by connecting with the posterior cardinal veins (see Fig. 2.6). The subcardinal veins unite with each other and, along their lengths, with the posterior cardinal veins through anastomoses; the multiple transverse anastomoses of these veins are probably their most distinctive feature. One of these anastomoses is the intersubcardinal anastomosis between the two veins ventral to the aorta. The right subcardinal vein establishes a communication with the liver sinusoids, and that segment becomes the hepatic segment of the inferior vena cava (see Fig. 2.6). The preaortic anastomosis comes into play in the establishment of the vena cava inferior to that segment.

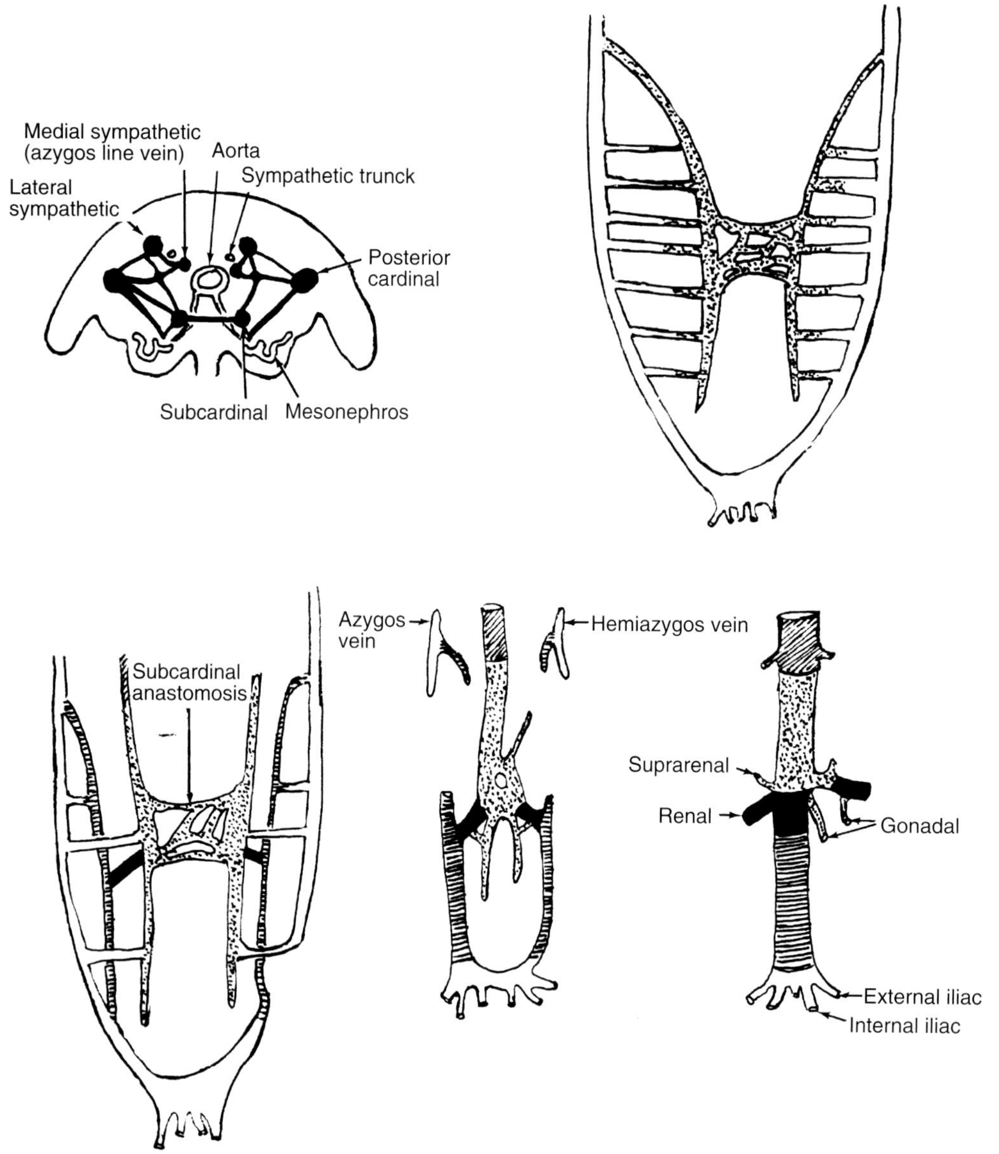

FIG 2.6 Development of the large veins. **Upper left,** Schematic cross-section of the embryo shows the relative positions and extensive interconnections of the major body wall veins. **Upper right** and **lower row** (left to right), Succession of stages in the development of the inferior vena cava and the related body wall veins. The key in the lower row identifies the component veins making up the inferior vena cava (lower right). For simplicity, the azygos and hemiazygos veins are depicted as if they arise from the lateral sympathetic veins, but in fact they arise as derivatives from the parallel medial sympathetic (azygos line) veins. (Adapted from Williams PL, Wendell-Smith CP, Treadgold S: *Basic human embryology,* ed 2, Philadelphia, 1969, JB Lippincott; and Hollinshead WH, Rosse L: *Textbook of anatomy,* ed 4, Philadelphia, 1985, Harper and Row.)

The lateral sympathetic veins appear soon after the hepatic segment of the inferior vena cava, anterior to the segmental vessels. They appear first as a plexus but quickly become a longitudinal trunk, ending cranially in the posterior cardinal vein and anastomosing posteriorly with the subcardinal vein, especially strongly on the right side. The part caudal to that latter anastomosis persists, and most of the remainder of the lateral sympathetic veins regresses; the persisting right caudal segment survives as the infrarenal part of the inferior vena cava (see Fig. 2.6). As the lateral sympathetic veins appear, a medial pair (medial sympathetic or azygos line veins) also arises, but medial to the sympathetic trunk in the abdominal wall. These veins link across the midline and, with the loss of an intermediate segment on the left side, form the azygos system of veins.

The adult pattern is completed by the emerging dominance of the right common cardinal vein. The left upper intercostal spaces drain into the remainder of the left common cardinal vein, which connects with the left brachiocephalic vein after the lateral part of the left common cardinal is lost. The left superior intercostal vein is formed in part by the left posterior and anterior cardinal veins. The potential communication between the two may persist as a left superior vena cava; the latter's position may be identified in the normal adult as the oblique cardiac vein (of Marshall), which can be traced to the left superior intercostal vein as a reminder of that origin.

The inferior vena cava has a complex origin. The hepatic segment, as noted previously, is derived from the cranial segment of the right vitelline vein and the hepatic sinusoids. A prerenal segment forms distal to this as an anastomosis between the hepatic segment and the right subcardinal vein. This latter vein forms the prerenal segment (down to the junction of the renal veins). A renal segment is formed from a renal collar (note the preaortic anastomosis between the subcardinals described previously). The renal collar is an anastomosis involving this preaortic anastomosis and anastomoses between the right subcardinal and lateral sympathetic veins. A postrenal segment forms from the lumbar part of the right lateral sympathetic vein down to the level of the common iliac veins. The common iliacs join with the lower part of the inferior vena cava as the postcardinal veins degenerate, forcing the iliacs to find this secondary route of venous return to the heart. As the kidneys come to rest in the adult position, the definitive renal veins are formed as connections to the inferior vena cava through anastomoses between the subcardinal and lateral lumbar veins. On the left side, the longer path to the inferior vena cava is accomplished through recruitment of this anastomosis between the subcardinal veins. On the right, this anastomosis is incorporated into the formation of the renal segment of the inferior vena cava, and the situation is less complex.

The multiple sources incorporated into the inferior vena cava, including anastomoses across the midline, can lead to some bizarre malformations. Most dramatic of these is the rare retrocaval ureter, which is clearly not a malformation of the ureter or a misguided path of ascent of the kidney; rather, it must be interpreted as incorporation of unusual components of the renal collar into the inferior vena cava. Accounts in the literature agree on this interpretation of a caval rather than a ureteric malformation.[17-19]

GROWTH OF NEW VESSELS

It would be helpful to know whether the development of new blood vessels in the fetus and during postnatal growth is a model for vascular proliferation under other circumstances. It is likely that this is so, although the factors that stimulate and direct such growth might be quite different. The central nervous system (CNS) provides a model that has been studied by a variety of means. The relative maturity of the brain at birth provides an existing and fully functional vascular tree that can be used as a model of a relatively mature vascular system. The further growth and development of the CNS dictate the need for postnatal neovascularization to support further maturation of the tissue.

Examination of the vascularization of the CNS addresses a fundamental issue in vascular growth during development: To what extent is development of a vascular bed a permissive condition for the subsequent onset of function; that is, to what extent is it anticipatory of and necessary for function? Or, conversely, to what extent is the development of a vasculature the response to the greater metabolic demands of a tissue as it increases or begins to achieve the functional levels expected of it at full maturation?

Studying CNS regions at the time of onset of measurable function (e.g., the auditory system) reveals that vascular sprouting parallels such events in their time courses (Skolnik and Maxwell, unpublished observations). Such observations cannot distinguish cause and effect, and perhaps they must go hand in hand—functional and vascular maturation identically timed or responsive to some common signal from yet another source. Greater temporal resolution would have to be applied than we have been able to achieve to date.

It is possible to describe the manner of new vessel growth in the CNS and to derive some quantitative information. Rowan and Maxwell[20] studied the postnatal rat cerebral cortex, which is structurally and cytologically quite immature at birth and undergoes a remarkable degree of maturation in the first 3 weeks after birth. CNS blood vessels are the only CNS tissue elements to display alkaline phosphatase activity. Using a simple histochemical procedure, it is possible to visualize small vessels by light and electron microscopy, relying on the enzyme reaction to label vessels—and those cells in the process of becoming vessels through cytodifferentiation—with no ambiguity whatsoever.[21] It has been widely accepted that new vessels in the CNS and perhaps elsewhere begin as a proliferation of solid cords of cells that later canalize (i.e., develop lumens). Yet such a mechanism seems improbable on purely mechanistic grounds, and this does not seem to be the case in the CNS. In this tissue, postnatal growth of new vessels seems to occur by budding from preexisting vessels; the buds are recognizable by their enzyme content and by the presence of lumens, although they are collapsed and empty. The lumens are not identifiable by light microscopy; therefore the interpretation of solid cords of cells is understandable. The buds or sprouts have characteristic cytoplasmic protuberances, or fingers, that "explore" in advance of growth of the sprout, seeming to seek the most appropriate path or perhaps sensing the direction where vessel growth will best satisfy the perceived need. Figs. 2.7 through 2.10 show a series of such sprouts from the rat cerebral cortex. These sprouts presumably link with a venous channel, establishing hemodynamics, which should serve to open the lumen as a capillary link. Fig. 2.11 is an electron micrograph of such a sprout, in which the unopened state of the lumen is evident. Because CNS arteries prominently display alkaline phosphatase activity, and because sprouts at their earliest detectable stages also display this enzyme, it is likely that postnatal vascularization proceeds by arteriolar sprouting, with subsequent linkage to the venous bed. An excellent historical review of the study of growth and differentiation of blood vessels and a statement of the status of the field can be found in Eriksson and Zarem's chapter in *Microcirculation*.[22]

The factors that induce an arteriole to sprout may be multiple, and possibly legion. An enormous literature on angiogenic factors is available for the CNS and other tissues, including tumors. Attention must be drawn, however, to a series of papers announcing a major achievement by Vallee's group at Harvard.[23-25] These investigators isolated and analyzed an angiogenic factor from human carcinoma cells, marking the first time that an

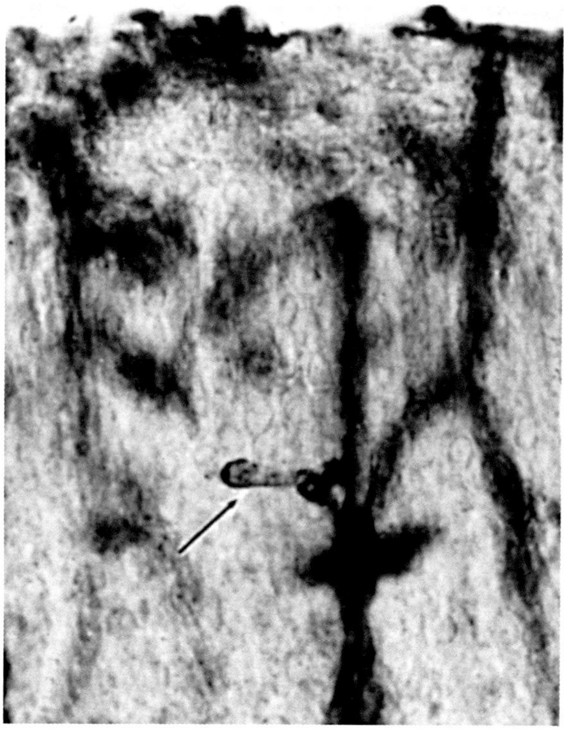

FIG 2.7 Light micrograph of rat cerebral cortex, reacted for alkaline phosphatase. A vascular sprout *(arrow)* is seen in the superficial cortex 2 days after birth. The cortical surface is at the top (∞1548). (Courtesy Dr. R. Rowan.)

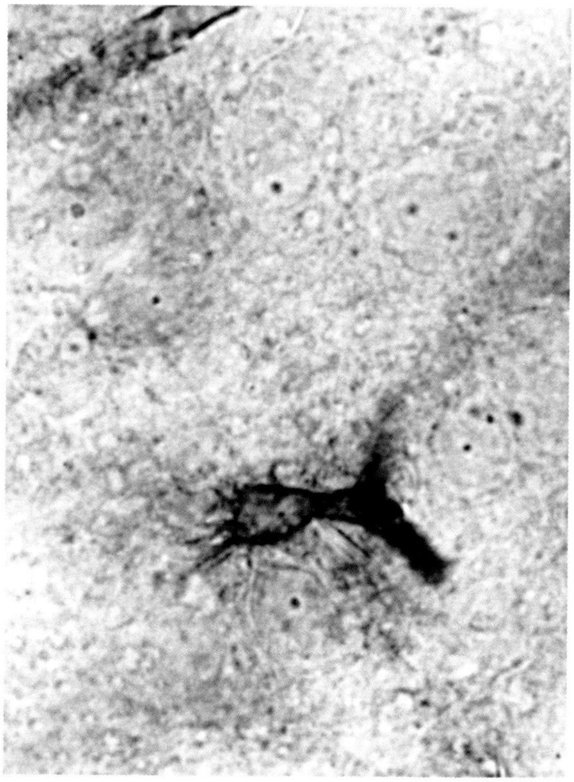

FIG 2.9 Light micrograph of rat cerebral cortex, reacted for alkaline phosphatase. A vascular sprout is seen in the middle third of the cortex 8 days after birth. Pseudopodia are evident at the tip (∞3148). (Courtesy Dr. R. Rowan.)

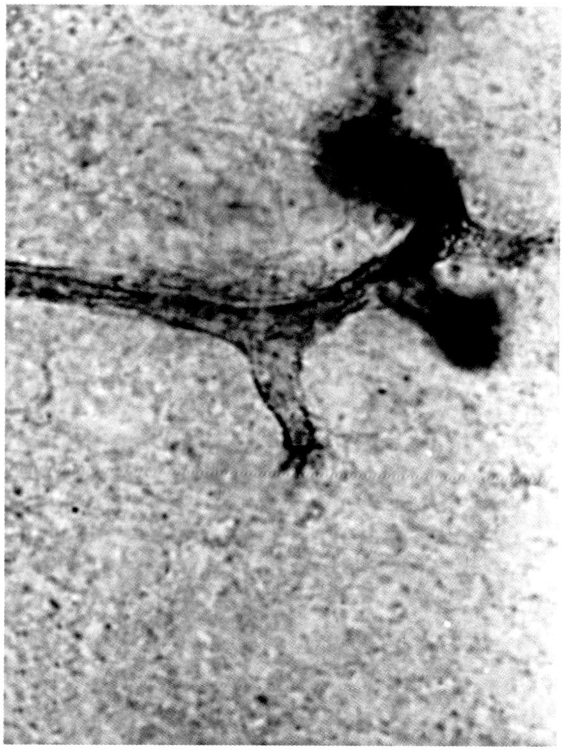

FIG 2.8 Light micrograph of rat cerebral cortex, reacted for alkaline phosphatase. A vascular sprout is seen in the middle third of the rat cortex 7 days after birth. Delicate exploratory fingers, or pseudopodia, are seen at the tip of the sprout (∞3148). (Courtesy Dr. R. Rowan.)

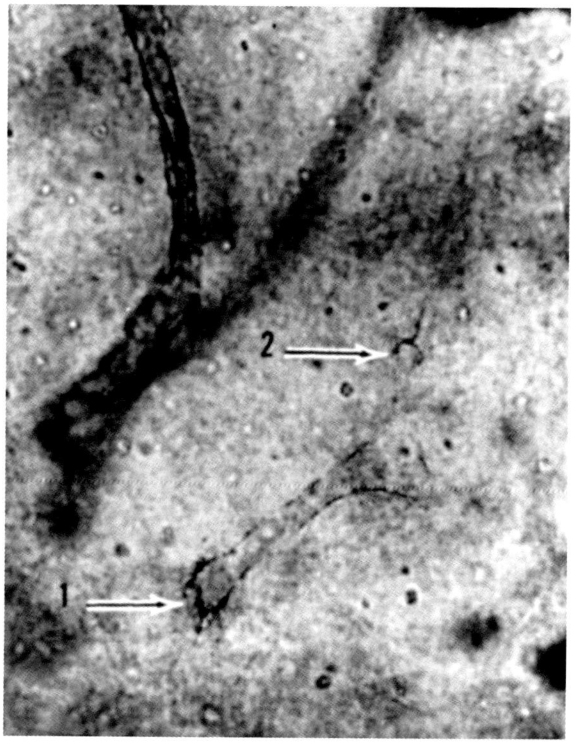

FIG 2.10 Light micrograph of rat cerebral cortex, reacted for alkaline phosphatase. A branched sprout with two tips *(arrows)* is evident. The larger tip (*1*) extends down and to the left of the stem vessel; the smaller tip (*2*) extends upward. The parent sprout and the two sprout tips are much less intensely stained than are the mature vessels dominating the upper and left parts of the micrograph (∞3148). (Courtesy Dr. R. Rowan.)

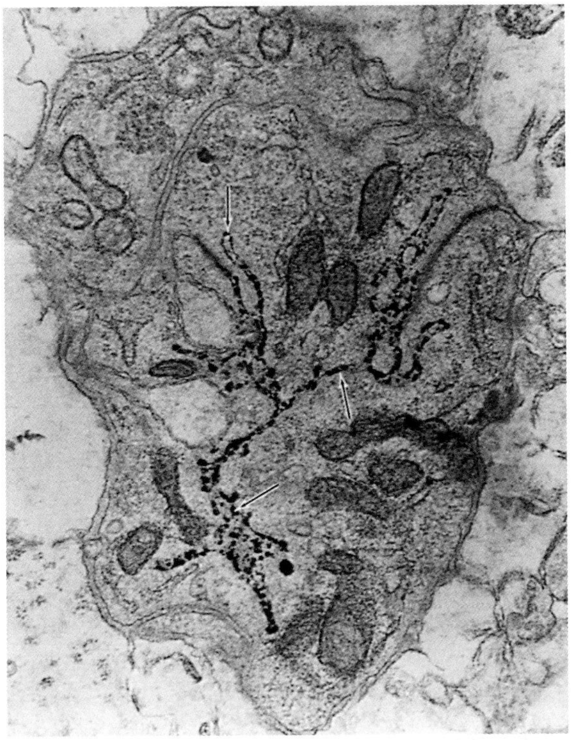

FIG 2.11 Electron micrograph of a sprout in the middle third of the rat cortex 8 days after birth. The unopened lumen *(arrows)* is delicately outlined by the deposition of enzyme (alkaline phosphatase) reaction product (∞42,200). (Courtesy Dr. R. Rowan.)

angiogenic factor was isolated, its amino acid sequence determined, and its genetic code identified. Curiously, this factor (angiogenin) is remarkably similar in its amino acid sequence to a ribonuclease, and the unraveling of the biologic meaning of this similarity and possible relationship will be fascinating to watch in the literature. This is not to say that only one angiogenic protein is the cause of neovascularization. There may be many, perhaps different ones, operating in the embryo and fetus, in the adult during wound healing, and in neoplasms. There is abundant evidence that tissue metabolites are capable of stimulating vascular development (e.g., high carbon dioxide and low oxygen content in tissue fluids). A complex list of possibilities will have to be sorted to determine which factors act to stimulate the production or release of specific angiogenic factors from cells (and which cells) and which are sufficient factors in their own right, acting directly on preexisting vessels.

It might not be satisfying to conclude with a dismaying array of unanswered questions. It is compelling evidence, however, that the questions are there and that the vigorous activity taking place in laboratories around the world will eventually yield some answers. The control of neovascularization, of which the embryo is such a master, may allow us to apply these concepts to a wide spectrum of problems afflicting adults in our clinics and hospitals.

References available online at expertconsult.com.

3 CHAPTER

Anatomy, Physiology, and Pharmacology of the Vascular Wall

Gale L. Tang, Ted R. Kohler

NORMAL ANATOMY

The primary purpose of the vascular system is to serve as a nonthrombogenic conduit for blood flow, which is necessary for the delivery of oxygen, nutrients, hormonal signals, and cellular components throughout the body. The cellular elements of blood vessels, (endothelial cells, smooth muscle cells, fibroblasts, and niche progenitor cells) are similar throughout the vasculature. However, structure and function varies throughout the vascular tree to allow for the dynamic regulation of blood flow, primarily regulated by changes in arteriolar resistance and venous capacitance. In addition, the vasculature regulates the cellular and molecular trafficking between the intravascular and extravascular space, as well as into and out of the vessel wall. As discussed later in this chapter, the normal adaptive responses of the endothelium and smooth muscle cells to inflammation and injury account for some of the atherosclerotic changes or vessel wall thickening after transplantation.

The organization of the cellular elements and extracellular matrix components varies dramatically throughout the vasculature, accounting for its distinctive anatomic and physiologic features at various sites. Vessels larger than capillaries possess three distinct layers or tunics, called the *intima, media,* and *adventitia*. These layers are generally thicker and better defined in arteries than in veins. In arteries, the intima is composed of a sheet of endothelial cells lining the luminal surface and a subendothelial extracellular matrix basement membrane. It is divided from the media by an internal elastic lamina. Rare inflammatory cells and smooth muscle cells may be found within the normal intima, although larger populations are seen as a reaction to injury or as a result of atherosclerotic disease. The media contains circular smooth muscle fibers embedded in a matrix of collagen, elastin, and proteoglycans and is divided from the adventitia by an external elastic lamina. Although the media is composed mostly of smooth muscle cells, there is increasing evidence that smooth muscle cell progenitors reside in niche populations within the media.[1] Both the internal and external elastic laminae are visualized as bright white lines using B-mode ultrasonography, allowing a measurement of intima-media thickness, which can be used as a surrogate marker for atherosclerosis.[2] The adventitia, which serves as the strength layer after endarterectomy, is composed primarily of loose connective tissue and fibroblasts. Inflammatory cells, nerve fibers, niche progenitor cells,[1,3] a nutrient microcirculation (known as the *vasa vasorum*),[4,5] and a lymphatic network[6] also reside within the adventitia.

Arterial Anatomy

The arterial tree can be divided into three separate categories: large elastic arteries, medium muscular arteries, and small arteries. The aorta and its major branches are classified as large elastic arteries, while the distributing arteries to major organs comprise the muscular arteries, and the arteries within organs comprise the small arteries. From small arteries, blood flow travels through arterioles to capillary beds, then to postcapillary venules and small veins, and blood flow then returns to the heart via larger veins. Collateral arteries are a special class of muscular arteries that traverse from one artery to another, rather than feeding into arterioles.[7] Normally there is little flow through collateral arteries and they have low shear stress. However, when the main conduit artery is obstructed, collateral artery flow and shear stress increase substantially, as a compensatory mechanism, which after adaption eventually can restore up to one-third of the normal conduit artery blood flow (Fig. 3.1).

The aortic media is composed of well-defined lamellar units; each unit consists of a concentric plate of elastin and a circumferentially oriented layer of smooth muscle cells, surrounded by a network of type III collagen fibrils embedded in a matrix of basal lamina. Finer elastin fibers compose a network between lamellae, as do bundles of interstitial type I collagen.[8] As the aorta becomes more distant from the heart, the percentage of collagen increases and the elastin decreases, so that the thoracic aorta and its major branches have more elastin than collagen and the abdominal aorta has more collagen than elastin.

The tangential tension on an artery wall can be approximately estimated with Laplace's law (tension is proportional to the product of the radius and the pressure). Because blood pressure is similar in animals of all sizes, the average wall tangential tension per lamellar unit is remarkably constant across different species.[9] The upper two-thirds of the thoracic aorta, which is thicker than 28 lamellar units, also contains a medial vasa vasorum.[4,5] The

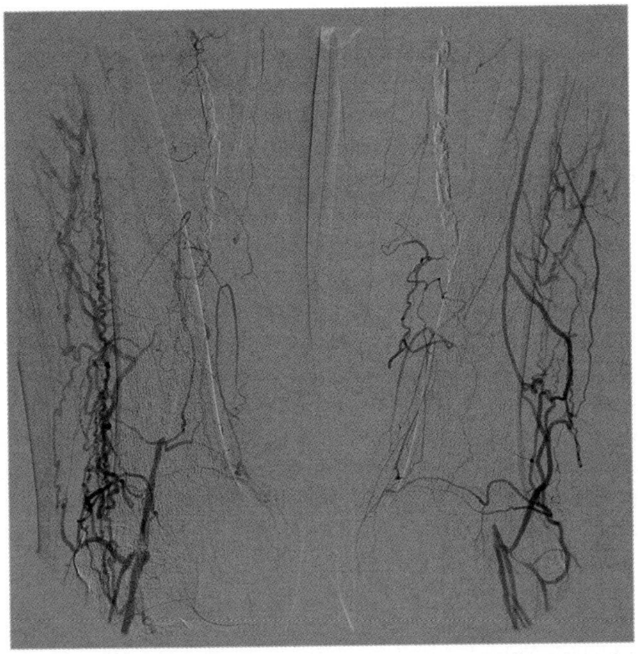

FIG 3.1 Digital subtraction angiogram demonstrating abundant collaterals from the bilateral profunda femoris arteries reconstituting the above-knee popliteal arteries. Note that the collaterals traverse between two muscular arteries and that they have both dilated and elongated, resulting in a characteristic corkscrew appearance.

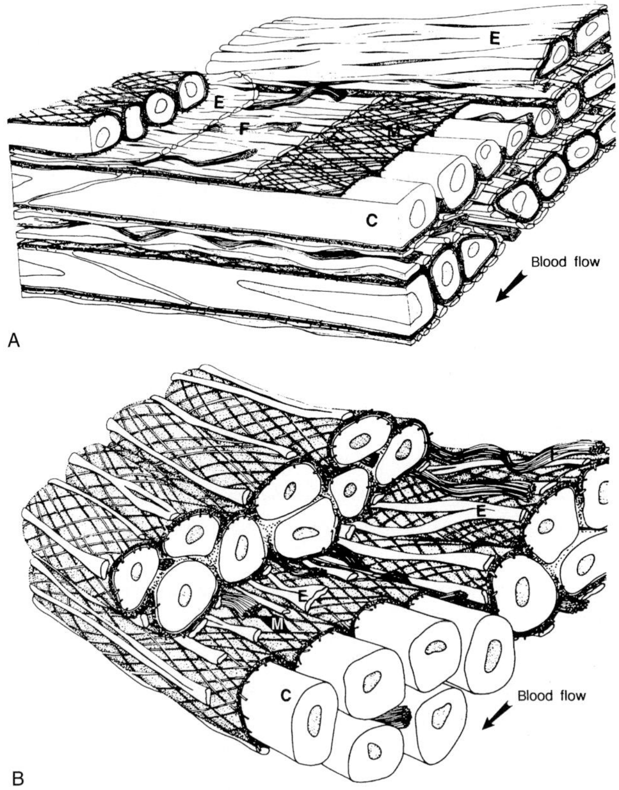

FIG 3.2 Schematic representation of the lamellar organization of elastic (A) and muscular (B) arteries. Each unit is composed of a group of commonly oriented smooth muscle cells *(C)* surrounded by matrix *(M)* consisting of basal lamina and a fine meshwork of collagen and surrounded by elastic fibers *(E)* oriented in the same direction as the long axes of the cells. Wavy collagen bundles *(F)* lie between the elastic fibers. The elastic lamellae are much better defined in the elastic arteries (A) than in the muscular arteries (B). (From Clark JM, Glagov S: Transmural organization of the arterial media: the lamellar unit revisited. *Arteriosclerosis* 5:19, 1985.)

dependence of the abdominal aortic wall on luminal nutrition, because of the lack of a medial vasa vasorum, may explain its increased propensity to aneurysm formation.

In contrast to elastic arteries, where collagen and elastin comprise approximately 60% of the dry weight of the media, muscular arteries contain proportionally more smooth muscle cells and less collagen and elastin, allowing them to alter their diameter rapidly through vasodilation or vasoconstriction. In addition, their ratio of media to lumen is higher, contributing to their function as resistive arteries (Fig. 3.2). Elastin is diminished as arteries become smaller, and the internal and external elastic lamellae become discontinuous and fragmented. The smallest arteries (arterioles) consist of only an endothelium, a layer of smooth muscle cells, and a filamentous collagenous adventitia. At the capillary level, only the endothelium remains, supported by an occasional contractile connective tissue cell known as a *pericyte*.[10]

The differentiation of these three types of arteries has significance because each class of vessel is subject to different pathology and diseases.[11] Atherosclerosis affects the elastic and muscular arteries, whereas medial calcific sclerosis is limited to muscular arteries, and small arteries are subject to diffuse fibromuscular thickening and hyalinization.

Venous Anatomy

Veins, as befitting their role as capacitance vessels under low-pressure conditions,[12] are larger and thinner walled than arteries. Despite this, the vasa vasorum in veins is denser than in arteries and has increased medial wall flow, suggesting that luminal blood flow is less capable of providing nutritional support to the vein wall.[13] Disruption of the vasa vasorum in veins, during vein graft harvest, may lead to wall damage and worse patency rates.[14] The subendothelial layer of the intima is missing entirely in veins, and an internal elastic lamina is present only in larger veins. The medial layer contains few smooth muscle cells, collagen, and elastin. Thin bicuspid valves, consisting of two layers of endothelium sandwiched around a layer of connective tissue, support unidirectional flow to the heart. They are present in larger numbers in peripheral extremity veins and are rarely present in central veins. The contractile state of both venules and veins is largely controlled by sympathetic adrenergic activity.

Veins can be divided into three systems: deep (located below the muscular fascia, paralleling arteries and providing approximately 90% to 95% of the extremity drainage), superficial (providing the remaining 5% to 10% of drainage), and perforating (connecting the deep and superficial systems). The usual direction of flow is from the superficial to the deep system. There is substantially more variation in venous anatomy than arterial anatomy.[15] The function of venous valves is to decrease the hydrostatic pressure from the weight of blood within each segment of the venous system when standing and to prevent retrograde flow. Entrapment of venous valves from fibrotic scarring resulting from incomplete resolution of deep venous thrombosis can cause venous obstruction, estimated to contribute to approximately 80% of chronic venous insufficiency. The other 20% results from primary valvular incompetence. Evidence suggests that the increased collagen with decreased smooth muscle and elastin found in varicose veins may occur prior to the development of incompetent valves, leading to reflux.[15a]

ACUTE REGULATION OF BLOOD FLOW AND VESSEL DIAMETER

The basic structural components described previously combine to allow the vasculature to dynamically regulate blood flow by changing luminal area and wall thickness, both in an acute reaction (e.g., increased blood flow induced by exercise, vascular injury, temperature, and pain) and in chronic structural changes to the structural wall, induced by ongoing stimuli (hypertension, increased or decreased inflow or outflow, and pathologic inflammation). These alterations require changes within the individual cellular elements, as well as cell-cell interactions, which allow the fully formed vessel to function as an integrated organ.

Blood flow within the vasculature creates unique biomechanical forces on the vessel walls at different levels throughout the vascular tree—these biomechanical forces are pressure and shear stress. Pressure is created by the hydrostatic force of cardiac contraction, with the addition of the hydrostatic pressure created by gravity. Gravity is a compressive force that also creates wall tension. The greatest wall tension occurs in the large elastic vessels. Wall tension is distributed across all three layers of the vessel wall and determines wall thickness. Shear stress primarily affects the endothelium and is a result of drag caused by the tangential flow of viscous blood over the intimal surface. This force causes endothelial cells to align with the direction of flow. In laminar conditions, the magnitude of shear stress is directly proportional to blood flow and fluid viscosity and inversely related to the cube of the radius.[16] Shear stress is normally maintained in mammals at a constant between 10 and 20 dynes/cm^2 at all levels of the arterial tree.[17] Both developing and mature vessels respond to changes in hemodynamic forces by adjusting their diameters to maintain a constant level of shear stress. Acutely, this occurs by altering vasomotor tone.[18] The reaction of arteries and arterioles to vasoactive substances is dependent on the stage in development, the species, and the particular vascular bed.[19]

Vasodilators

Pharmacologic vasodilators can be classified as endothelial dependent or endothelial independent.[20] Relaxation of the isolated rabbit aorta and other arteries induced by acetylcholine and other muscarinic receptor agonists was initially demonstrated to be dependent on the presence of endothelial cells, by Furchgott and Zawadzki in 1980.[21] In the absence of endothelial cells, acetylcholine causes contraction of the arterial wall instead of relaxation. There are three main families of endothelial-dependent vasodilators that trigger separate mechanisms, leading to vasodilation.[19] The first and most potent is the soluble gas nitric oxide (NO, previously known as *endothelial-derived relaxation factor*), produced by endothelial nitric oxide synthase (eNOS) from L-arginine, which was identified in 1987.[20] NO stimulates guanylate cyclase in vascular smooth muscle cells, leading to an increase in cyclic guanosine monophosphate (cGMP) and activation of cGMP-dependent protein kinase and vasodilation. The second family is the prostaglandins, with prostacyclin as the classic example. Prostacyclin is produced by cyclooxygenase (COX) enzymes from arachidonic acid and causes a cyclic adenosine monophosphate–dependent hyperpolarization of vascular smooth muscle cells leading to vasodilation. The last family is the endothelial-derived hyperpolarizing factors (EDHFs). They cause vasodilation by stimulating Ca^{2+}-activated K^+ channels or Na^+/K^+-ATPase, leading to hyperpolarization of vascular smooth muscle cells. EDHF family members include hydrogen peroxide, carbon monoxide, hydrogen sulfide, C-natriuretic peptide, K^+, and epoxyeicosatrienoic acids (EETs).[19] In contrast, other pharmacologic agents such as adenosine, papaverine, isoproterenol, and nitrovasodilators (e.g., sodium nitroprusside, which acts as a direct NO donor) can cause vasodilation, even in the absence of endothelial cells.

Vasoconstrictors

Vasoconstriction results from increased intracellular Ca^{2+} within vascular smooth muscle cells. This commonly occurs from activation of the sympathetic nervous system or increased circulating epinephrine interacting with cell surface adrenergic receptors. The endothelium can also produce vasoconstricting factors in response to arachidonic acid, hypoxia, and in some isolated cerebral vessels by stretch.[20,22] Arachidonic acid is metabolized by COX into endoperoxides, which are vasoconstrictors, and further metabolized by other enzymes to thromboxanes, which are potent vasoconstrictors. Reactive oxygen species, formed as by-products of COX generation of prostanoids, also stimulate vasoconstriction at least partially through uncoupling of eNOS to produce superoxide anion instead of NO.[22,23] Endothelin and angiotensin II are both peptide vasoconstrictors that have been isolated from cultured endothelial cells. Increases in shear stress suppress endothelin gene expression and increase the production of eNOS by endothelial cells; endothelin promotes smooth muscle growth, whereas NO suppresses it.

It is likely that these endothelium-derived relaxing and constricting factors contribute to long-term vascular adaptation in response to changes in blood flow. Flow patterns also affect the expression of receptors and chemoattractants involved in leukocyte recruitment, including intercellular adhesion molecule-1, vascular cell adhesion molecule-1, and monocyte chemoattractant protein-1.[24] Missing or abnormal endothelium can contribute to certain pathologic conditions associated with acute and chronic vasospasm, such as atypical angina from coronary vasospasm and cerebrovasospasm after cerebral hemorrhage. In addition, endothelial dysfunction, as measured by abnormal flow-mediated vasodilation of the brachial or radial artery in response to reactive hyperemia, can be detected in the presence of most major cardiovascular risk factors, including hypertension, tobacco exposure (either active or passive), dyslipidemia, aging, diabetes mellitus, obesity, hyperhomocysteinemia, and chronic inflammation.[25]

LONG-TERM ADAPTATIONS OF THE ARTERIAL WALL

Vessels subjected to chronic changes in blood flow remodel by altering their structure to regain an appropriate level of shear stress and return vasomotor tone to normal.[18] For example, during embryonic development, higher-volume flow leads to vessel enlargement, whereas lower-volume flow leads to vessel regression. Similarly, in adult vessels, an artery proximal to an arteriovenous fistula will enlarge and can eventually become aneurysmal.[26] Conversely, an artery carrying less flow, either from proximal obstruction or a decrease in outflow (e.g., following amputation or paralysis), will adapt by decreasing its diameter.[18,27,28]

Diseased vessel segments also adapt to alterations in blood flow. A coronary artery with an enlarging atherosclerotic plaque is subject to increased blood flow velocity in the area of luminal stenosis. The coronary artery acutely responds by vasodilating and chronically undergoes a process known as outward remodeling to preserve luminal diameter (Glagov phenomenon). This adaptive process works to preserve a normal luminal diameter as long as the intimal lesion does not exceed 40% of the area within the internal elastic lamina, at which point pathologic narrowing begins.[29] This process is dependent on an intact endothelium to translate the biomechanical information from shear stress to biochemical signals that regulate vessel diameter. Vessels denuded of endothelium in general do not respond to changes in flow.[30]

Regulation of Medial and Intimal Thickening

As described previously, arterial wall thickness is initially determined by tangential tension. Wall thickening is a prominent feature of most pathologic processes. Hypertension causes arterial medial thickening in both humans and animals. Atherosclerosis, hypercholesterolemia, and reaction to injury, such as endothelial denudation, cause intimal thickening.[31-33] Exactly how these responses are regulated is not clear, although it is certain that in each instance smooth muscle cells proliferate and drive accumulation of extracellular matrix.[33,34] In addition, hypercholesterolemia promotes the accumulation of lipids and lipoproteins, followed by lipid-filled macrophages into the intimal lesion.[32]

Because smooth muscle accumulation is a central feature of most forms of vascular wall thickening, it is worth discussing the currently understood mechanisms of smooth muscle growth control.[34,35] Although smooth muscle cell proliferation is required during growth and development, these cells are predominantly quiescent in adult vessels. In the adult rat, smooth muscle cells turn over at a rate of 0.06% per day, which is barely detectable by available methods.[36] Vascular smooth muscle cells can be stimulated by various pathologic conditions to undergo a phenotypic switch to a synthetic phenotype. In this state, they undergo high levels of proliferation, migration into the intimal layer, and generation of significant amounts of extracellular matrix components. A recent theory suggests that resident or perhaps bone marrow–derived progenitor cells, rather than quiescent mature smooth muscle cells, are the primary cells contributing to vascular remodeling in response to arterial injury or disease.[1,35] Regulation of the contractile and synthetic phenotypic states is incompletely understood but appears to occur at the transcriptional level; this regulation clearly is critical to the problems of arterial wall remodeling in reaction to primary hypertension, as well as local susceptibility to atherosclerotic change.

Because of the importance of vascular smooth muscle cells in pathologic processes, including atherosclerosis and restenosis in response to arterial and vein grafts, as well as balloon angioplasty and stenting, many in vivo models of smooth muscle cell growth and proliferation have been developed.[37-40] Perhaps increasingly relevant is a model using angioplasty balloon dilation in the rat carotid artery, with or without stent implantation. In this model, significant intimal hyperplasia is observed only when the internal elastic lamina is ruptured.[39,40] However, the best characterized model is the balloon injury model, in which smooth muscle cell proliferation is stimulated by the passage of an inflated balloon catheter along an artery.[41,42] The passage of the inflated balloon both stretches the arterial wall and denudes the endothelium. Immediately following balloon passage, platelets adhere to the denuded wall, spread, and degranulate, releasing numerous growth factors, chemotactic factors, and vasoactive substances.

Endothelial denudation and platelet adherence are followed 1 to 2 days later by the stimulation of medial smooth muscle proliferation and migration across the internal elastic lamina to form a neointima.[36] This response can be dramatic, as illustrated by the marked increase in thymidine incorporation index (a measure of DNA replication, and therefore proliferation) in the ballooned rat carotid artery (Fig. 3.3). Smooth muscle cells commit to proliferation early after injury; this response can be blocked by giving heparin during the first few days after injury. Heparin blocks entry in the cell cycle, significantly reducing

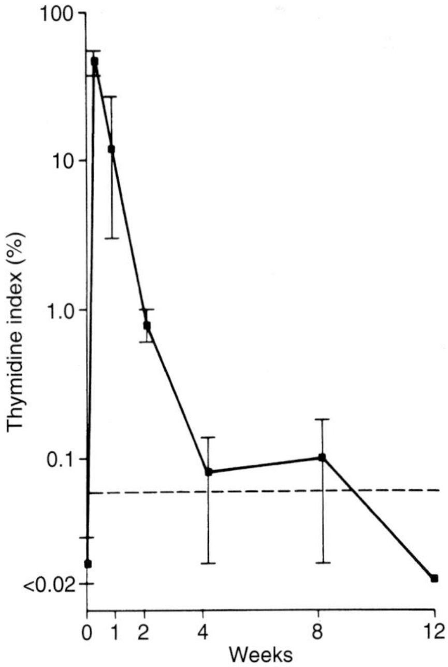

FIG 3.3 Smooth muscle cell proliferation rates following balloon catheter injury of the rat carotid artery, as measured by the percentage of cells that incorporate thymidine. Proliferation is greatest at 48 hours and falls rapidly thereafter. (Modified from Clowes AW, Reidy MA, Clowes MM: Kinetics of cellular proliferation after arterial injury. I. Smooth muscle growth in the absence of endothelium, *Lab Invest* 49:327, 1983.)

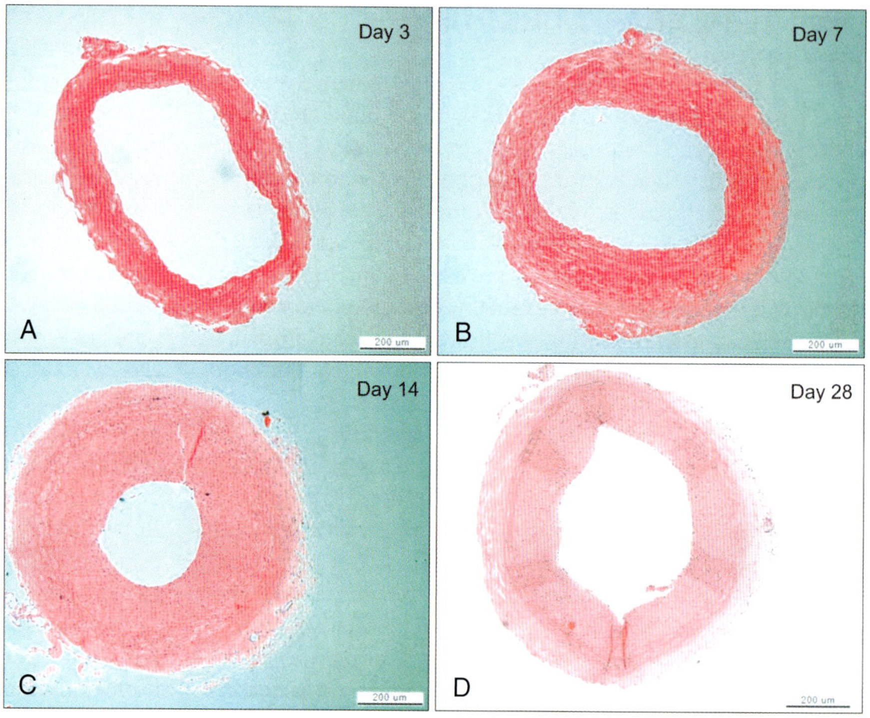

FIG 3.4 Histologic Cross-sections of the Region Lacking Endothelium in Injured Rat Carotid Arteries Stained With Hematoxylin and Eosin. (A) Denuded vessel at 3 days. Note the loss of endothelium. (B and C) Denuded vessel at 7 days. The neointima is now thickened because of smooth muscle proliferation. (C) Denuded vessel at 2 weeks. Further intimal thickening has occurred. (D) Denuded vessel at 4 weeks with increased extracellular matrix and decreased nuclear content within the neointima. (From Park YJ, Min SI, Jung IM, et al: Different responses of neointimal cells to imatinib mesylate and rapamycin compared with normal vascular smooth muscle cells, *Vasc Specialist Int* 30:5–10, 2014.)

both the number of dividing cells and the eventual mass of neointima.[43] Not all smooth muscle cells respond equally to mitogenic stimuli, probably because of the differing phenotypes of smooth muscle cells that can be derived from either the mesoderm or the ectoderm, as well as the presence or absence of progenitor cells.[35]

The initial proliferative response of smooth muscle cells occurs in the media of the injured artery and does not lead to an increase in wall thickness. Rather, the wall thickens only after the smooth muscle cells migrate into the intima and proliferate. This process persists for approximately 2 weeks and spontaneously subsides regardless of whether endothelium reappears at the luminal surface. Intimal thickness is further increased by the accumulation of extracellular matrix synthesized by the smooth muscle cells (Fig. 3.4).[44]

Several lines of evidence suggest that platelet degranulation stimulates smooth muscle cell proliferation and migration.[45-47] Many growth factors, including platelet-derived growth factor (PDGF), transforming growth factor-β, and an epidermal growth factor–like protein, are found within platelet granules.[48,49] Of these, PDGF appears to be the dominant growth factor affecting vascular smooth muscle cells after injury, as evidenced by work using anti-PDGF antibodies or infusion of PDGF after balloon injury.[47,50] Injured arteries in thrombocytopenic animals show little intimal thickening.[51] This effect occurs despite no measurable change in smooth muscle cell proliferation, suggesting that platelets are more important in stimulating migration rather than cell proliferation.[46] However, it remains unknown where soluble growth factors and other platelet-derived granular proteins go after being released from the platelet. An attractive hypothesis is that they accumulate within the arterial wall and stimulate subsequent smooth muscle growth and migration.

Despite intensive study, the mechanisms that start or stop the intimal thickening process are still poorly understood. Several interesting and potentially important observations about the process have been made. First, the surface of the injured artery will only accumulate a single layer of platelets. Fibrin and microthrombi are seen at the luminal surface only when an artery that has already undergone intimal thickening is injured again or when small craters have been formed in the luminal surface in association with adherent macrophages in hypercholesterolemic animals.[52] Therefore active fulminant thrombosis is not a usual reaction to injury; when it occurs, it must represent a major aberration of vessel function.

In models in which reendothelialization occurs early or partial deendothelialization occurs without medial injury, intimal thickening does not develop, although one or two rounds of medial smooth muscle cell proliferation may occur. This observation suggests that the endothelium normally suppresses smooth muscle proliferation and migration from the media into the intima. This suggestion is supported by the isolation of smooth muscle growth inhibitors from the vessel wall. In addition, the endothelium can synthesize a heparin-like molecule that inhibits in vitro smooth muscle cell growth; heparin suppresses both proliferation and migration of smooth muscle cells in vitro and in vivo.[53] The endothelium also releases NO in a flow-dependent manner; NO is a growth inhibitor for smooth muscle cells.[54,55] These findings suggest that an intact, functional endothelium actively maintains the medial smooth muscle cells and smooth muscle progenitor cells in a quiescent state, as opposed to the quiescent state resulting from a lack of growth factors. These findings also support the more general concept that the cells of the vascular wall communicate with each other and regulate each other's function.

In 1973, Ross and Glomset proposed that atherosclerosis is initiated by endothelial injury.[56] This theory has been modified and refined over the past 30 years, with a more recent recognition of the importance of the role of inflammation and inflammatory cells.[32,33] In its current state the theory proposes that injury leads to endothelial cell dysfunction, which changes endothelial permeability, adhesive characteristics, and responses to various growth factors. The changes in endothelial permeability allow inflammatory cells, such as activated platelets, monocytes, and T lymphocytes, to infiltrate into the arterial wall. The subsequent cell-cell interaction between endothelial cells, smooth muscle cells, and inflammatory cells create a fibroproliferative response, which eventually leads to the formation of atherosclerotic plaque.

Arterial Stiffening

Increased arterial thickness is also associated with loss of arterial elasticity frequently seen in aging. There is gradual fragmentation of elastin within the aorta and accumulation of stiffer collagen fibers within the media, decreasing aortic compliance. This causes an increase in pulse wave velocity and a decrease in the reservoir function of the aorta, leading to increased systolic and pulse pressure. This process is independent of atherosclerosis.[57] In animal models, inhibition of matrix metalloproteinases blunts this effect and the associated systolic hypertension.[58] Likely mechanisms include inflammatory cell infiltration into the aorta, endothelial dysfunction with decreased NO production, and increased oxidative stress with aging.[57]

CELL-CELL COMMUNICATION WITHIN THE VASCULAR WALL

The importance of cell-cell communication within the vascular wall has now been introduced 3 times, once in regard to chronic vasodilation in response to increased flow, second in regard to control of vascular smooth muscle cell proliferation and migration, and third in regard to the initiation of the atherosclerotic plaque. The following section will explore the participants and kinds of messages in more detail, especially as they pertain to growth control and maintenance of the antithrombotic state. Cell-cell communication can be direct by means of intercellular junctions or can occur at a distance through paracrine and hormonal communication by molecules secreted into the extracellular space.

Direct cell-cell communication across gap junctions has been demonstrated in monolayers of endothelium[59] and in mixed cell populations between endothelial and smooth muscle cells.[60,61] Gap junctions have been demonstrated morphologically between endothelial cells as well as between endothelial and smooth muscle cells in vitro and in vivo. The significance of these direct links has not been well defined, although in culture, pericytes and smooth muscle cells can inhibit endothelial cell growth when the cells are in contact with one another.[61] Plasma membrane preparations from confluent large vessel endothelium also actively inhibit growing endothelial cells.[59,62] In vivo, endothelial proliferation occurs in the absence of pericytes; this growth ceases when pericytes become associated with the endothelium.[63] Some aspects of vasodilation are likely translated from the endothelium to smooth muscle cells by gap junctions.[60] In addition, direct intercellular links may help to regulate endothelial proliferation and endothelial-mediated vascular relation in collateral vessels by propagating signals from one cell to the next upstream from a large vessel occlusion to a downstream vessel.[64,65] These intercellular links provide a mechanism for a local response by the vessel wall in the absence of release and wide dissemination of potent vasoactive or growth-regulating substances.

Cell-cell communication over distances is mediated by secreted soluble factors. As previously mentioned, platelets, which are non-nucleated fragments of megakaryocytes, carry granules bearing an array of potent mitogens. Platelets are clearly involved in wound healing, atherogenesis, angiogenesis, and vascular remodeling.[66] This is evidenced by the observation that whole blood serum contains much more growth-promoting activity than does serum lacking platelets (plasma-derived serum); this observation led to the isolation of PDGF from platelet alpha granules and more recently has led to work demonstrating platelet-progenitor cell interactions.[66,67] PDGF is a basic dimeric protein with a molecular weight of approximately 30 kD and acts as a potent smooth muscle cell mitogen at active concentrations of nanograms per milliliter.[68,69] In addition, its mitogenic activity, it also stimulates smooth muscle cell migration, contraction, and extracellular matrix synthesis and serves as a chemotactic factor for other inflammatory cells. This last activity is likely responsible for its in vivo activity of stimulation of granulation tissue when placed in a subcutaneously implanted wound chamber[70] and has been exploited as the topical agent Regranex (becaplermin or recombinant human PDGF-BB) for use in assisting wound healing.

In 1983 the structure of the oncogene *v-sis*, a gene associated with cellular transformation by the simian sarcoma virus, was found to be almost identical to the *PDGF* gene structure.[71,72] This discovery, coupled with the finding that a variety of both normal and oncogenic cells synthesize and secrete active PDGF, raised the possibility that only subtle changes in gene regulation separate normal wound healing from malignant, unregulated growth of tumor cells. In terms of vascular wall components, endothelium, smooth muscle cells, and leukocytes, including macrophages, have been demonstrated to express the *PDGF* gene (c-sis) both in vitro and in vivo.[69] All the activities of PDGF within the vascular wall are incompletely characterized; however, as previously discussed, its primary role in animals undergoing balloon-catheter carotid injury appears to be to stimulate smooth muscle cell migration rather than proliferation.[47,50] Recently, PDGF also has been found to be upregulated—along with acidic fibroblast growth factor, basic fibroblast growth factor (bFGF), and vascular endothelial growth factor—within developing collateral arteries.[73]

In contrast, smooth muscle cell proliferation is likely to be primarily stimulated by intracellular mitogens released from injured medial smooth muscle cells. Hydrostatic distention models of arterial injury that do not cause significant endothelial injury lead to significant smooth muscle cell proliferation without migration, presumably because of a lack of platelet degranulation in this model.[74] In addition, when the endothelium is injured using a fine nylon loop that does not damage the media, very little smooth muscle cell proliferation is observed.[75,76] The principal mitogen responsible for smooth muscle cell proliferation after injury appears to be bFGF.[77] Both bFGF messenger RNA and protein are found in the uninjured vessel wall.[78] Infusion or local administration of bFGF after arterial injury causes a marked increase in smooth muscle cell proliferation and intimal thickening, whereas infusion of antibodies against bFGF causes a significant reduction in smooth muscle cell proliferation.[78-80] Interestingly, bFGF is not mitogenic for smooth muscle cells in uninjured vessels, suggesting that other products of injury are required to induce mitogenesis. When smooth muscle cells are cultured from injured media, they produce up to fivefold more PDGF than do cells cultured from uninjured arteries.[81] Smooth muscle cells derived from injured media also express messenger RNA for insulin-like growth factor[82,83] and transforming growth factor-β,[83] both of which are mitogenic for smooth muscle cells in vitro. Thus injury to smooth muscle cells may stimulate cell growth in a paracrine fashion by releasing a number of mitogens.

The rate of blood flow, which as previously discussed affects the diameter of developing and mature arteries, also influences intimal hyperplasia in injured vessels and vascular grafts. Wall thickening of vein and synthetic grafts is increased in areas of reduced flow[84,85] and is reduced by high flow (Fig. 3.5).[86,87] Increased flow causes regression of intima in endothelialized expanded polytetrafluoroethylene grafts implanted into baboons.[88] These changes are presumably the result of the endothelial response to changes in shear stress, resulting in the release of factors that regulate the arterial diameter and wall structure. For example, reduced flow causes an increase in PDGF expression in rat carotid arteries.[75] High flow upregulates NOS in synthetic grafts; this effect can be blocked by the local infusion of a NOS inhibitor.[76] Interestingly, flow also appears to affect intimal hyperplasia in balloon-injured rat carotid arteries, even though the endothelium is denuded in this model.[77] This finding implies that surface smooth muscle cells can respond to flow in a manner similar to that of endothelium. Finally, restoration of eNOS activity by gene transfer into the denuded wall of injured rat carotid arteries suppresses intimal hyperplasia and increases vessel reactivity.[78]

Growth control of the vascular wall must involve a complex interaction between endothelial cells, vascular smooth muscle cells, inflammatory cells, progenitor cells, and the extracellular matrix. In addition to growth factors, platelets also release chemotactic factors for progenitor and inflammatory cells (e.g., stromal-cell derived factor-1),[89] whereas endothelial cells can upregulate adhesion molecules and chemotactic factors that also attract inflammatory cells.[90] Activated vascular wall cells can amplify the initial stimulus (perhaps an influx of platelet-derived factors) by producing PDGF, PDGF-like proteins, and other growth-promoting factors that further act on vascular wall cells. These and other factors likely also act to regulate the traffic of leukocytes and progenitor cells in and out of the wall; the activated leukocytes and progenitors could then reciprocate by producing additional factors to affect the function of the vascular wall cells. These findings support the theory that there is a great deal of crosstalk between the cells within the vascular wall and those within the blood, with many complex feedback loops.[91,92]

POSSIBLE THERAPIES FOR PREVENTION OF RESTENOSIS

New therapeutic possibilities for preventing restenosis are emerging from the increasing understanding of the cellular and

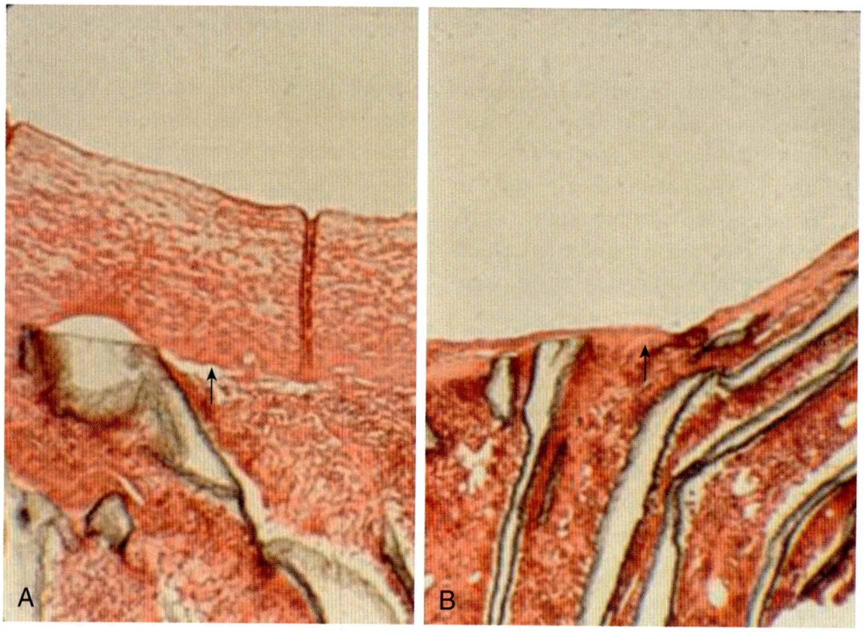

FIG 3.5 Cross-sections of Polytetrafluoroethylene Grafts 3 Months After Placement in the Aortoiliac Circulation in Baboons. (A) Control side with normal flow. (B) Experimental side with a distal arteriovenous fistula causing increased flow. The *arrows* indicate the junction of the graft and neointima. Scale bar, 100 μm. (Modified from Kohler TR, Kirkman TR, Kraiss LW, et al: Increased blood flow inhibits neointimal hyperplasia in endothelialized vascular grafts, *Circ Res* 69:1557, 1991.)

molecular events surrounding the formation of intimal hyperplasia.[92] A complete listing of therapeutic strategies is beyond the scope of this chapter, but therapies that are already in clinical practice are worth noting. We have previously emphasized the importance of the platelet in triggering activation of the vascular cell wall in response to injury. Multiple antiplatelet drugs are commonly used in clinical practice, including aspirin (irreversible COX inhibitor); dipyridamole (phosphodiesterase and thromboxane synthase inhibitor); cilostazol (phosphodiesterase-3 inhibitor); thienopyridines such as ticlopidine, clopidogrel, and prasugrel (adenosine diphosphate receptor inhibitors); and abciximab (chimeric human-murine monoclonal antibody blocking the glycoprotein IIb/IIIa receptor). Interestingly, although vein graft patency was not improved by the addition of clopidogrel to aspirin in a randomized trial, prosthetic bypass patency was improved.[93] Although cilostazol is more commonly used for its vasodilatory properties in improving symptoms of intermittent claudication, recent evidence suggests it also has a role in suppressing intimal hyperplasia after angioplasty and stenting procedures.[94,95] Lastly, abciximab reduces the incidence of repeated procedures, death, and myocardial infarction after coronary angioplasty.[96] A single dose was able to improve clinical results 3 years out from the procedure, suggesting either that platelet blockade can abort the initiation of the intimal hyperplastic response or that the drug affects smooth muscle cell proliferation and migration.[97]

Of the various strategies for local control of smooth muscle cell proliferation following vascular injury, drug-eluting stents have had the most success, primarily in the coronary circulation,[98] whereas local delivery of radiation and antisense oligonucleotides to inhibit cell cycle regulatory proteins lacked clinical efficacy.[99,100] The first generation of drug-eluting stents provides local delivery of the potent cell cycle inhibitors sirolimus and paclitaxel via a permanent polymer coating.[98] However, there have been several reports of delayed stent thrombosis (up to 5 years after implantation), generally after cessation of dual antiplatelet therapy.[101] When examined histologically, drug-eluting stents show delayed endothelialization,[102] which has been theorized to result from inflammation and hypersensitivity to the permanent polymers used to coat the stent and allow drug delivery. Second-generation drug-eluting stents elute zotarolimus and everolimus and are coated with new polymers that cause less inflammation. Third-generation drug-eluting stents—which feature biodegradable polymers, are polymer-free, or are completely biodegradable, thus avoiding the problems incited by late stent fracture—are under development and starting to enter clinical use.[103,104] Paclitaxel drug-eluting stents[105,106] and balloons[107-109] have demonstrated efficacy in the peripheral arterial system as well. The ideal device would inhibit intimal hyperplasia while encouraging positive outward remodeling and early reendothelialization.

REGULATION OF HEMOSTASIS

Normal arteries are resistant to thrombosis, even with complete cessation of blood flow for a prolonged period. However, blood within a damaged vessel clots readily. This empirical observation led to the theory that the endothelium must produce one or more antithrombotic or anticoagulant molecules, which has been borne out by the isolation of these molecules. The endothelium must also be capable of expressing an extensive array of procoagulant functions; these molecules have also been isolated and determined to be regulated by messages from the blood or from neighboring cells.[110]

On the anticoagulation side of the balance, the endothelium synthesizes several membrane-associated proteins that have extracellular heparan sulfate moieties, which, like heparin, increase the affinity of antithrombin III for thrombin.[111] This interaction occurs at the level of the endothelial surface and causes rapid inactivation of circulating thrombin and other activated serine proteases in the clotting cascade, including factors VII, IX, and X. As previously observed, heparan sulfate also impedes smooth muscle cell proliferation; this in conjunction with its anticoagulant properties helps to impede two aspects of the response to injury.[53] In addition, endothelial cells synthesize and secrete thrombomodulin, which acts as a cell surface receptor for thrombin. Thrombin bound to thrombomodulin loses it proteolytic activity for fibrinogen and activates protein C instead. Activated protein C binds protein S on the endothelial surface and, as a complex, degrades factors Va and VIIIa to inhibit the clotting cascade. The importance of this pathway is amply demonstrated by the prothrombotic tendencies of patients with genetic protein C and S deficiencies and patients with factor V Leiden, in which a point mutation renders factor V resistant to activated protein C cleavage. Endothelial cells synthesize tissue factor pathway inhibitor. Heparin increases its release into the plasma, where it quenches the activity of tissue factor–bound factor VII. Lastly, endothelial cells synthesize and secrete tissue plasminogen activator, as well as binding sites to colocalize tissue plasminogen activator and plasminogen on the endothelial surface and enhance fibrinolytic activity at the blood vessel wall.[110,112]

On the procoagulation side, endothelial cells synthesize and secrete von Willebrand factor, which supports platelet adhesion, fibronectin, which stabilizes fibrin clot by cross-linking fibrin monomers, and thrombospondin, which promotes platelet aggregate stabilization and depresses fibrinolysis. In addition, under certain pathologic conditions, such as exposure to inflammatory mediators (e.g., endotoxin, interleukin-1, tumor necrosis factor) from the blood or possibly also from resident macrophages, the endothelium downregulates its antithrombotic properties by internalizing thrombomodulin and decreasing production of heparan sulfate proteoglycans. The endothelium also upregulates several prothrombotic pathways, including expression of tissue factor, release of P-selectin, generation of platelet-activating factor, secretion of plasminogen activator inhibitor, and exposure of factor IX/Xa binding sites.[110,112] In addition, endothelial cells also synthesize and express interleukin-1, which could affect the underlying smooth muscle cells.[113]

Only 0.2% of the total thrombin released during the process of thrombosis is generated during the initiation phase. The vast majority of thrombus-associated thrombin is formed after clotting is complete and continues to be released by the mural thrombus. After endothelial injury, thrombin can come into contact with the subendothelial smooth muscle cells. Thrombin is a mitogen for vascular smooth cells in vitro. Furthermore, antithrombin agents can block the increase in PDGF gene expression that is the normal response to injury; it can also limit the smooth muscle cell proliferation following injury. In addition to thrombomodulin, thrombin also binds to a class of protease activated receptors. In normal vessels, thrombin receptors are primarily expressed in the endothelium; however, significant expression is found both in smooth muscle cells in atherosclerotic plaques as well as those reacting to vascular injury. Likewise, thrombomodulin production by smooth muscle cells is rapidly upregulated in response to endothelial denudation or damage; this appears to reduce the mitogenic effect of thrombin on smooth muscle cells. Vasodilatory prostaglandins negatively regulate the expression of thrombin protease activated receptors and upregulate the transcription of thrombomodulin.[114] The derangements of the normal antithrombotic endothelial surface associated with atherosclerotic plaques, as well as the significant inflammatory component within the plaque, presumably have a direct bearing on the thrombotic complications associated with end-stage atherosclerosis.

SUMMARY

The vasculature should not be regarded as a passive conduit for blood flow, but as an organ with integrated endothelial, smooth muscle, fibroblasts, and progenitor cells that can respond to physical and chemical stimuli in the blood by adjusting vascular diameter and thickness acutely and over time. Vascular wall cells participate in local and systemic inflammatory reactions and communicate among themselves to express factors regulating cell proliferation, inflammatory cell trafficking, and coagulation.

REVIEW QUESTIONS

1. In normal arteries, most of the smooth muscle cells are found in which area?
   a. Intima
   b. Media
   c. Adventitia
   d. None of the above
2. Arteries respond to an increase in blood flow by doing which of the following?
   a. Contracting
   b. Dilating
   c. Intermittently contracting
   d. Intermittently dilating
3. Endothelial cells synthesize and secrete substances that cause what?
   a. Vasodilatation
   b. Vasoconstriction
   c. Both vasodilatation and vasoconstriction
   d. None of the above
4. What causes injured arteries to thicken?
   a. Medial smooth muscle hyperplasia
   b. Intimal smooth muscle hyperplasia
   c. Intimal endothelial hyperplasia
   d. None of the above
5. Atherogenesis begins with endothelial dysfunction, which includes all of the following except which of the following?
   a. Increased permeability.
   b. Increase in adhesion receptors for inflammatory cells.
   c. Increased responsiveness to growth factors.
   d. Increased uptake of cholesterol by regenerating endothelium.
6. Smooth muscle cells respond to PDGF by doing which of the following?
   a. Proliferating
   b. Synthesizing matrix
   c. Migrating
   d. All of the above
7. What is not a proven anti-restenosis therapy?
   a. Drug-eluting stents
   b. Drug-eluting balloons
   c. Radiation therapy
   d. Antiplatelet drugs
8. Based on in vitro studies, endothelial cells appear to express molecules that regulate the behavior of the blood at the luminal surface. Which of the following endothelium-derived molecules act to sustain the anticoagulant state? (There may be more than one correct answer.)
   a. Heparan sulfate
   b. Von Willebrand factor
   c. Plasminogen activator inhibitor
   d. Thrombomodulin
   e. Prostacyclin
9. Which of the following molecules are procoagulants? (There may be more than one correct answer.)
   a. Heparan sulfate
   b. Von Willebrand factor
   c. Plasminogen activator inhibitor
   d. Thrombomodulin
   e. Prostacyclin
10. In general, inflammatory mediators (e.g., interleukin-1) cause endothelial cells to express which of the following?
   a. Increased procoagulant activities
   b. Increased anticoagulant activities
   c. Increased endothelium-derived relaxing factor
   d. None of the above

References available online at ExpertConsult.com.

CHAPTER 4

Anatomy and Surgical Exposure of the Vascular System

Jigar A. Patel, Paul W. White, Todd E. Rasmussen

GENERAL PRINCIPLES

Knowledge of vascular anatomy and surgical exposures are foundational components of vascular surgery. A detailed understanding of the location of blood vessels, surrounding structures, and the methods to obtain a safe and effective working space around a vessel are critical for any vascular operation. Careful preoperative planning of the approach to any vessel facilitates the performance of the actual operation. Proximal and distal control of vessels is as important as exposure of the actual operative field. On occasion, using a separate incision or exposure for control can be very helpful. As endovascular techniques mature and newer technology emerges, open exposure will remain an essential and basic skill. We will follow a systematic head-to-toe discussion of the anatomy and common exposures of the major blood vessels. Because the major veins usually run in close proximity to major arteries, we will focus on arterial exposures in this chapter for the most part.

EXPOSURE OF THE CAROTID ARTERY

The carotid artery is divided into three zones corresponding to the three zones of the neck described for penetrating neck trauma (Fig. 4.1).[1] The left common carotid artery originates directly off the aortic arch, and the right common carotid artery is a branch of the innominate artery. The exposure of the proximal common carotid arteries and other supra-aortic trunks within zone 1 is primarily through a thoracic incision and will be discussed in the exposure of the aortic arch.

The common carotid artery ascends through the neck without any branches within the carotid sheath, medial to the internal jugular vein and anterior to the vagus nerve, and bifurcates typically at the level of the fourth cervical vertebrae, 2.5 cm below the angle of the mandible, deep to the common facial vein as it enters the internal jugular vein. The bifurcation lies within the carotid triangle, which is bound by the anterior border of the sternocleidomastoid muscle (SCM) laterally, the posterior belly of the digastric muscle and stylohyoid muscle superiorly, and the superior belly of the omohyoid muscle inferiorly.[2] The internal carotid artery is a direct continuation of the common carotid artery into the skull. Rising almost straight vertically from the bifurcation, it enters the skull through the carotid canal in the petrous portion of the temporal bone. The XII cranial nerve passes anteriorly from lateral to medial over the internal carotid artery within a few centimeters superior to the carotid bifurcation. As it passes over the artery, it gives off a small branch, the superior root of the ansa cervicalis.[3]

An incision along the anterior border of the SCM allows access to almost the entire cervical carotid artery, with the cranial aspect of the incision angled behind the earlobe if access to the distal internal carotid artery is required. This incision is easily extended into a median sternotomy for access to the supra-aortic trunks in zone 1 of the neck. Alternatively, a transverse incision along a patient's skin crease can be made for better cosmetic outcomes. This incision typically is best for carotid bifurcation exposure and should be used with caution as more cephalic or caudal exposure through this incision is difficult. In transcervical, penetrating trauma, a transverse cervical collar incision extending to each side of the SCM may provide access to both sides of the neck, with posterior extension for more cephalad exposure.[4]

Extending the neck slightly, using a shoulder roll and turning the head toward the contralateral side, facilitates exposure, but in trauma patients the cervical spine must be cleared before performing these maneuvers. The platysma is the first muscular layer, followed by the deep cervical fascia. The dissection is carried down along the anterior border of the SCM. The muscle is elevated away from the deep carotid sheath and retracted laterally. The common facial vein lies over the carotid bifurcation and should be ligated to expose the carotid arteries. The common carotid artery is isolated and controlled first. Avoiding excessive manipulation may prevent embolism. After the common carotid artery is encircled by a vessel loop, the internal carotid artery can be exposed lateral and deep to the external carotid artery. Retraction of the internal jugular vein facilitates exposure of the internal carotid artery as it lies anterior to the artery.

Cranial and somatic nerve injury is the most common neurologic complication of carotid endarterectomy with the potential of causing significant morbidity, with an incidence of injury ranging between 5% and 20%.[5] Understanding the anatomy of the neck and relations to the carotid artery helps to understand the location and course of important cranial nerves, particularly cranial nerves IX, X, and XII, but also the mandibular branch of VII, and XI (Table 4.1).

The most frequently injured cranial nerve is the hypoglossal nerve.[6] The nerve courses between the internal carotid artery and internal jugular vein and travels anterior to the artery as it descends, about 2 cm above the carotid bifurcation. The

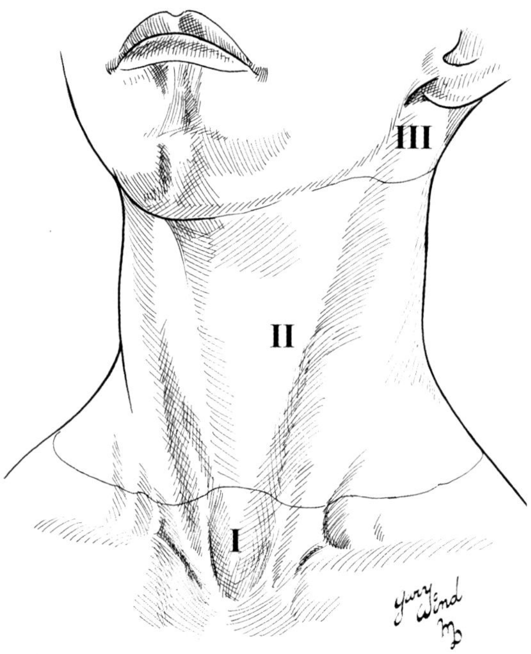

FIG 4.1 Division of the Neck into Three Zones Zone I extends from the clavicle to the cricoid cartilage, zone II from the cricoid cartilage to the angle of the mandible, and zone III from the angle of the mandible to the base of the skull. (Reproduced with permission from Valentine RJ, Wind GG: Carotid arteries. In *Anatomic exposures in vascular surgery*, Philadelphia, 2003, Lippincott Williams & Wilkins, p 41, © by RJ Valentine and GG Wind.)

descending branch of the hypoglossal nerve, also known as the ansa cervicalis, comes off the hypoglossal trunk and is typically anterior and parallel to the carotid arteries. It can be traced back to the hypoglossal trunk and can be helpful in identifying the hypoglossal nerve. The ansa cervicalis may be sacrificed, which will allow additional exposure of the distal internal carotid artery, with care taken to avoid excessive traction on the hypoglossal nerve. The hypoglossal nerve and its descending branch also travel along with the sternocleidomastoid artery and vein. This artery can be ligated to allow for additional hypoglossal nerve mobilization, but injury to the hypoglossal nerve must be avoided.[2]

The recurrent laryngeal nerve is the second most commonly injured nerve.[6] Originating within the mediastinum, the branch ascends into the neck and is typically away from the internal carotid artery; however, traction on the vagus nerve can result in injury.[2] Rarely, the recurrent laryngeal nerve can arise off the vagus at the level of the carotid bifurcation as a nonrecurrent laryngeal nerve. This occurs more frequently on the right, with an incidence of 0.3% to 0.8%, and can be seen when dissecting medial or posterior to the carotid bulb.[7]

The superior laryngeal nerve arises from the vagus near the distal internal carotid artery and courses posterior to the artery and descends obliquely with the superior thyroid artery, where it branches into an internal and external branch. It is subject to injury during carotid artery clamping.[2]

The mandibular branch of the facial nerve descends from the parotid gland, deep to the platysma along the angle of the mandible. Its course may be variable, traveling more inferiorly,

TABLE 4.1 Regional Nerves Encountered During Exposure of the Carotid Bifurcation

Nerve Branch	Location Encountered	Test for Function	Remarks
Mandibular ramus of facial nerve (cranial nerve VII)	Deep to platysma muscle; can be 5–10 mm below inferior margin of mandible	Ask patient to show teeth; check for paralysis of lower lip	Use gentle retraction of mandible; nerve is pulled down when head is rotated to opposite side
Great auricular nerve (C2, C3)	Anteromedial surface of SCM muscle anterior to and below ear	Anesthesia of ear and adjacent scalp	May cause ipsilateral occipital headache when damaged
Cutaneous cervical nerve (C2, C3)	Subcutaneous on deep fascia	Anesthesia of skin below mandible	Warn patient preoperatively about possible sensory loss
Glossopharyngeal nerve (cranial nerve IX)	Between external and internal carotid arteries; branch is the carotid sinus nerve, also known as the *nerve of Hering*	Loss of ability to swallow	Manipulation of branch nerve may cause bradycardia or hypotension; IV atropine or local infiltration of the nerve with lidocaine relieves circulatory changes
Vagus nerve (cranial nerve X)	Within carotid sheath; between IJV and CCA; directly behind proximal ICA	Indirect laryngoscopy for vocal cord function	Dissect "right on" distal CCA and ICA to avoid injury, avoid past-pointing with occluding clamp tips
External branch of superior laryngeal nerve (branch of cranial nerve X)	Adjacent and medial to superior thyroid artery	Loss of function of cricothyroid muscle	Inability to produce high tones
Hypoglossal nerve (cranial nerve XII)	Main nerve trunk crosses ICA and ECA 1–2 cm above bifurcation, SCM artery and vein branches sling around nerve, dividing these branches improves distal ICA exposure	Extended tongue deviates to side of injured nerve	Visualize descending branch first and follow it to main nerve trunk; carefully ligate "sling" vessels to maintain dry operative field

CCA, Common carotid artery; *ECA*, external carotid artery; *ICA*, internal carotid artery; *IJV*, internal jugular vein; *IV*, intravenous; *SCM*, sternocleidomastoid.

causing it to be prone to traction injury during exposure of the distal internal carotid artery.[2,6]

The glossopharyngeal and spinal accessory nerves are structures in the cephalad portion of the neck that are prone to injury during retraction. The glossopharyngeal nerve courses in close proximity to the stylopharyngeus and stylohyoid muscles, and the spinal accessory nerve pierces the SCM and courses posteriorly to the trapezius muscle. The risk of injury to these nerves and the other cranial nerves increases as more maneuvers are performed to expose the distal internal carotid artery.

The greater auricular nerve, supplying the skin around the angle of the mandible and lower ear, courses high along the base of the skull, typically around the superior extent of a longitudinal incision, and the transverse cervical cutaneous nerves travel along the inferior aspect of the incision supplying the skin of the ipsilateral anterior neck.

Access to the internal jugular vein can be obtained with the same exposure of the carotid artery within the carotid sheath, except with gentle medial retraction of the carotid artery.

The external carotid artery courses medially and cephalad, behind the neck of the mandible, where it divides into multiple branches. For management of external carotid arterial injury, the external carotid artery may be ligated without consequence because of the rich collateral flow.[8]

The exposure of the carotid artery becomes more complex as it rises to the skull base with many structures closely adjacent. Exposure of the distal internal carotid artery within zone III of the neck poses significant challenges for optimal visualization and for performing a safe distal anastomosis. Five steps can be performed to optimize exposure of the distal internal carotid artery (Fig. 4.2).

The first step is to divide the arterial branches from the external carotid, often off the occipital branch of the artery, to the cephalad portion of the sternocleidomastoid. Any lymph nodes in this area can be carefully excised as well. Second, the ansa cervicalis can be divided and the hypoglossal nerve gently retracted medially and superiorly. Third, the posterior belly of the digastric muscle and the occipital branch of the external carotid artery can be divided. Fourth, the styloid process can be resected with a rongeur after division of the stylohyoid, styloglossus, and stylopharyngeus muscles, which insert onto the styloid process. This allows for an additional 0.5 cm of exposure.[9] Extreme care must be taken during division and retraction as the hypoglossal and glossopharyngeal nerves both run deep to these muscles, the facial nerve crosses anterior to the styloid process, the spinal accessory nerve crosses posterior to the styloid process, and the spinal accessory nerve crosses posterior to the digastric muscle near its origin on the mastoid process. Mock and colleagues demonstrated in human cadavers that division of these structures can allow exposure of the internal carotid artery to the level of the first cervical vertebrae.[9]

Lastly, anterior subluxation of the mandible with temporary intermaxillary fixation by intraoral wires and penetrating towel clamps on interdental Steinmann pin wiring would allow for an additional 1 to 2 cm of exposure to reach the base of the skull (Figs. 4.3 and 4.4).[10-12] These maneuvers require extensive interdisciplinary planning with an oromaxillofacial or plastic and

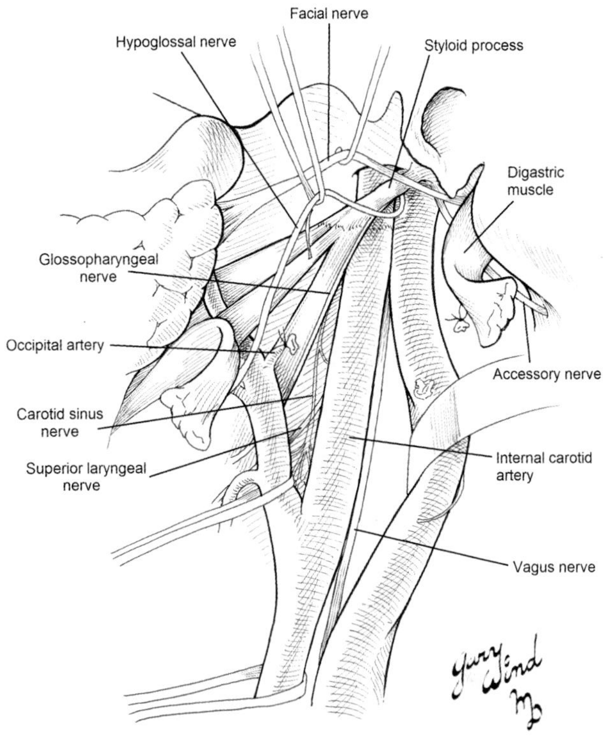

FIG 4.2 Exposure of the Distal Carotid Artery Note the relationship of the styloid process to the artery. The posterior belly of the digastric muscle and the occipital artery are divided. (Reproduced with permission from Valentine RJ, Wind GG: Carotid arteries. In *Anatomic exposures in vascular surgery*, Philadelphia, 2003, Lippincott Williams & Wilkins, p 48, © by RJ Valentine and GG Wind.)

reconstructive surgeon with nasotracheal intubation. It is important to differentiate mandibular subluxation with dislocation because, with dislocation, there is a higher risk for joint capsular or ligamentous injury.

The most aggressive but greatest exposure comes with the complete vertical mandibular ramus osteotomy with translocation or removal of the ramus segment with plated reimplantation.[13]

EXPOSURE OF THE VERTEBRAL ARTERY

Exposure of the vertebral arteries is becoming less frequent with the increasing use of endovascular techniques in treating vertebral artery stenosis and hemorrhage.[14,15] The vertebral arteries lie deep within the neck, coursing within the transverse processes of the cervical vertebra for much of their length. They arise from the first part of the subclavian artery bilaterally approximately at the level of the C6 or C7 vertebrae. The vertebral veins form a dense plexus adjacent to the artery as it enters the sixth transverse process and ascends the neck. On the left, the thoracic duct enters the subclavian vein between the internal jugular vein and vertebral vein and should be identified when exposing the proximal left vertebral artery.

The vertebral artery is divided into four segments (Fig. 4.5). V1, the most proximal or ostial segment, extends from the origin

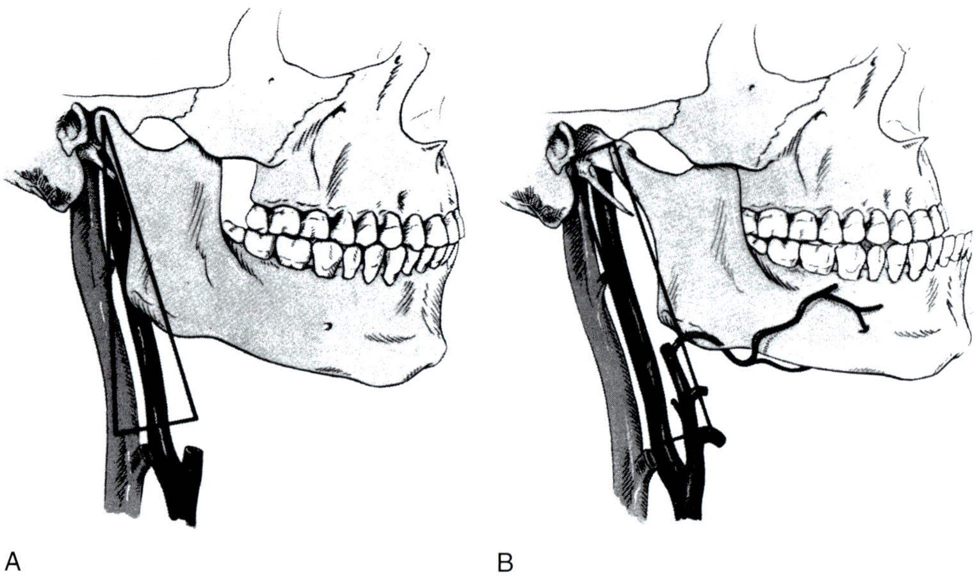

FIG 4.3 With anterior subluxation of the condyle of the mandible, the narrow angle (A) between the carotid artery and the mandible is widened (B) to increase exposure of the distal internal carotid artery. (From Fisher DF, Jr, Clagett GP, Parker JI, et al: Mandibular subluxation for high carotid exposure, *J Vasc Surg* 1:727, 1984.)

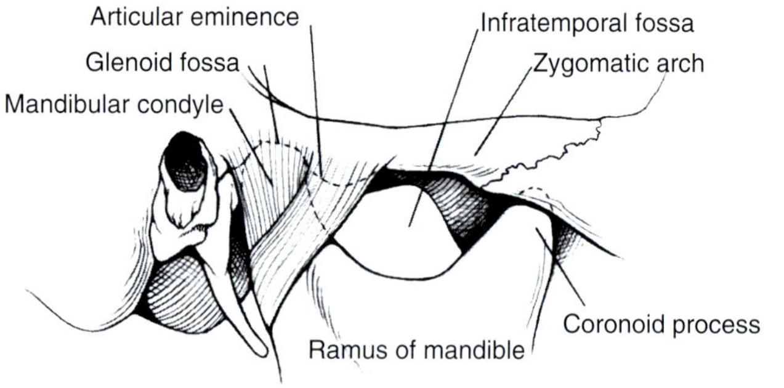

FIG 4.4 Anterior subluxation moves the condyle of the mandible to the articular eminence but not to the infratemporal fossa, as would occur with dislocation of the mandible, risking injury. (From Fisher DF, Jr, Clagett GP, Parker JI, et al: Mandibular subluxation for high carotid exposure, *J Vasc Surg* 1:727, 1984.)

of the artery off the subclavian artery to the C6 transverse foramen, anatomically marked by the convergence of the longitudinal longus colli muscle and anterior scalene muscle inserting on the C6 process tubercle. V2, the interosseous or transversary segment, travels through the anterior aspect of C6 transverse process foramen up to the axis (C2). V3 is the extracranial, suboccipital segment spanning from the artery's emergence from C2, through the atlas' transverse (C1) process to the base of the skull, where it penetrates the atlantooccipital membrane and dura. V4 is the intradural, intracranial segment of the artery to the convergence with the contralateral vertebral artery to form the basilar artery. It is noteworthy that in approximately 40% of patients the vertebral arteries are of different sizes. One artery may be dominant, while the other is minor or hypoplastic. In approximately 10% of cases the vertebral artery enters the cervical transverse foramen at a level higher than C6, in which the artery will course anterior to the longus colli muscle.[16]

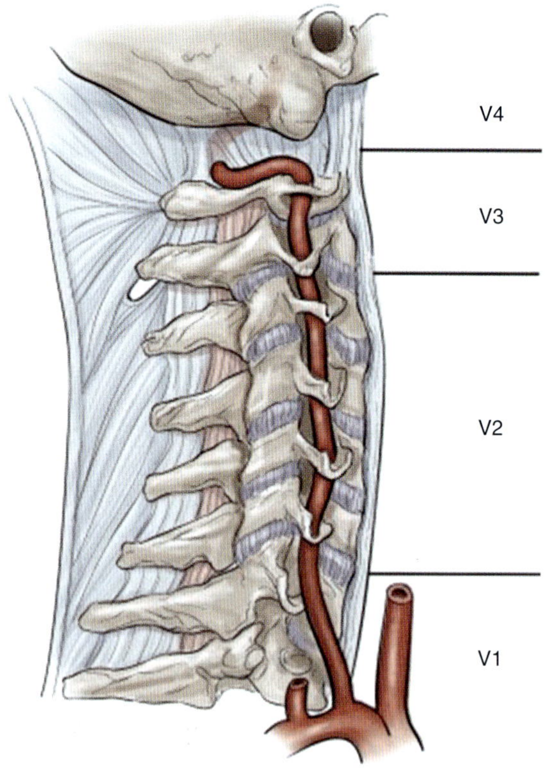

FIG 4.5 The four anatomic segments of the vertebral artery. (From Weaver FA, Herscu G: Neck and Thoracic Outlet. In Rasmussen TE, Tai NRM, editors: *Rich's Vascular Trauma*, ed. 3, Philadelphia, 2016, Elsevier, p. 141.)

Careful preoperative planning based on computed tomographic or digitally subtracted angiographic imaging allows the surgeon to choose the exposure technique. Two approaches used to expose V1 are the transverse supraclavicular approach and the vertical anterior cervical approach.[17]

In the supraclavicular approach, an 8-cm transverse incision is made 1 cm above the clavicle. The external jugular vein is ligated, and the clavicular head of the SCM is transected. The sternal head can usually be retracted medially but can be transected if necessary. The omohyoid muscle crosses the carotid sheath at this level and is divided to expose the carotid sheath. The sheath is opened vertically, the carotid artery is retracted medially, and the jugular vein, vagus nerve, and cervical sympathetic chain are retracted laterally with the sternal head of the SCM. Lateral to the carotid sheath lies the scalene fat pad containing the thoracic duct on the left side. It should be ligated as proximal to the subclavian vein as possible to void injuries that can cause a leak postoperatively.[17] Deep to the fat pad on the anterior aspect of the anterior scalene muscle is the phrenic nerve running superior-laterally to inferior-medially. The inferior thyroid artery crosses diagonally over the vertebral artery at V1. On the medial side, the prevertebral aponeurosis over the longus colli muscle is incised, exposing the sympathetic chain that should be protected. At this point, an inverted V can be seen created by the longus colli muscle medially, the anterior scalene muscle and phrenic nerve laterally, and the apex pointing to the vertebral artery. Arising lateral to the vertebral artery is the second branch of the subclavian artery, the thyrocervical trunk, which can be differentiated from the vertebral artery by its multiple branches. The inferior thyroid artery and vertebral veins are then ligated, and the dissection can be carried cephalad to the C6 transverse process and caudal to the subclavian artery to fully expose the V1 segment. The longus colli muscle can be cut along the lateral aspect of the vertebral body to expose the foramen. The transverse approach allows for a faster but more limited exposure, whereas the cervical approach is useful for extended exposure of other segments at the expense of a more difficult and time-consuming dissection.[18]

The vertical anterior cervical approach uses the same incision as a longitudinal incision for a carotid endarterectomy. The SCM is retracted laterally, the omohyoid muscle divided, and the carotid sheath with its contents retracted medially and the scalene fat pad retracted laterally with the phrenic nerve. Similarly, the inferior thyroid artery and vertebral veins are ligated, and dissection is carried in both directions for complete exposure. This approach is useful if the distal vertebral artery may need to be exposed, as in a common carotid-vertebral artery bypass or vertebral artery transposition.[19]

Exposure of the V2 segment begins similarly to the anterior cervical exposure of V1 with extension of the incision cephalad to the mastoid process, angling posteriorly toward the ear. With the SCM retracted laterally, the carotid sheath and pharynx are retracted as medially as possible to expose the prevertebral fascia. This fascia is vertically incised medial to the sympathetic chain, and the fascia is retracted laterally to maintain the branches from the chain to the nerve roots posterolaterally. Again, the distal exposure of V1 exposes the longus colli and anterior scalene muscles converging to the C6 anterior tubercle of the transverse process. The anterior longitudinal ligament is incised vertically against the vertebral column and swept off with a periosteal elevator en bloc with the longus colli and longus capitus muscles. Bleeding may be encountered here with the extensive venous plexus that runs with the vertebral artery, and dissection lateral or posterior to the anterior transverse process tubercle risks injury to the cervical nerve roots as they emerge.[20] Using a small rongeur, the anterior arch of the transverse process can be removed to open the bony canal, exposing the vertebral artery. At the level of C3, the vertebral artery begins to course laterally as the C2 transverse foramen is more lateral than the rest. At this level, dissection over the anterolateral aspect of the vertebral body is preferred to visualize and feel the angle of C2 safely.

The V3 segment has a more intricate course between C2 and the skull base. C1 and C2 are the most mobile vertebrae of the entire spine and have the most intervertebral space. At this level, the vertebral artery contains redundant length as it traverses from the atlas to the foramen magnum at the base of the skull. It takes a sharp posterior turn after emerging from the atlas foramen, travels in a posterior groove, and then turns anterior to penetrate through the atlantooccipital ligament and dura within the foramen magnum.[21] During this course, multiple small branches are given off that create collaterals with the external carotid artery and supply the cervical vertebrae and meninges.

The most commonly described approach is the anterolateral approach, which begins again similar to the exposure of V1 and V2 with a longitudinal incisional along the medial border of the SCM, extending posteriorly toward the mastoid process behind the ear. The carotid sheath structures are retracted medially. The SCM can be completely transected, partially transected, or preserved, with care taken to preserve the spinal accessory nerve that enters the muscle within a few centimeters of its insertion point on the mastoid process. The splenius capitis and longissimus capitis muscles are also transected off the mastoid process with a 5- to 10-mm cuff for reattachment. This exposes the levator scapulae and splenius cervicis muscles that can be detached from the C1 transverse process to expose the vertebral artery between C1 and C2.[22]

Exposure of the V3 segment to the base of the skull and V4 segment is best accomplished through the suboccipital approach described extensively by Berguer.[22,23] The patient is positioned in the prone, "park bench" position in which the head is tilted and resting over an extended contralateral forearm. The incision is curvilinear, transverse from the posterior midline to the mastoid process and extending downward along the posterior border of the SCM. From superficial to deep, the following structures are sequentially identified and divided: the medial trapezius toward its insertion, the semispinalis capitis, the splenius capitis, the longissimus capitis, and SCMs. The spinal accessory nerve is exposed by the division and reflection of the sternocleidomastoid. The transverse process of C1 is palpated. Lastly, the obliquus capitis superior muscle and the lateral half of the rectus capitus posterior major muscle are cut to fully expose the base of the skull. The vertebral artery surrounded by its venous plexus is then visible. Berguer describes a technique to ligate these bridging veins by using an 8-0 Prolene suture passed on the needle backward. Bipolar cautery can also be used. Upon completion, the splenius capitis and semispinalis muscles are reapproximated and the SCM reinserted.[22,23]

EXPOSURE OF THE AORTIC ARCH

Exposure of the aortic arch can be achieved through two primary approaches: a median sternotomy for the ascending aorta, the brachiocephalic artery, the proximal right subclavian artery, and the right and left common carotid arteries (Fig. 4.6). The most accepted approach to the proximal left subclavian artery is with a left anterolateral thoracotomy.[24] Both of these exposures may require supraclavicular extension or counterincisions, which will be described in this section. The ultimate goal is to allow for proximal and distal control with maximal visualization and working space and minimal morbidity (Fig. 4.7).

EXPOSURE OF THE BRACHIOCEPHALIC ARTERY

Exposure of the first two trunks of the aortic arch begins with a median sternotomy. There must be coordination with the anesthesia team to deflate the lungs to avoid injury to the pleural space or lung parenchyma during the division of the sternum. A well-placed sternal retractor provides wide access to the anterior mediastinum. The first structure encountered is the thymus gland, which should be divided vertically in the midline, ligating its blood supply coming from the internal thoracic arteries and draining into the brachiocephalic and internal thoracic veins. The internal jugular veins course anteriorly to the subclavian arteries and are joined by the subclavian veins to form the brachiocephalic veins. The left brachiocephalic vein courses obliquely across the midline anterior to the aortic arch to unite with the right brachiocephalic vein around the level of the first sternocostal joint. The internal thyroid and thymic veins drain into the left brachiocephalic vein and should be ligated to provide wide mobilization of the venous trunk to retract it superiorly. The left brachiocephalic trunk can be ligated in instances necessitating urgent proximal control of the innominate artery.[25] Once the left brachiocephalic vein has been retracted superiorly or ligated and divided, the aortic arch can now be visualized (Fig. 4.8). If access to the ascending aortic arch is required, the pericardial sac is opened.

The apex of the aortic arch runs obliquely from the right anterior aspect of the mediastinum to the left posterior aspect. As a result, the brachiocephalic artery is the anterior-most aortic branch, followed by the left common carotid, with the left subclavian artery posterior. Therefore the proximal left subclavian artery has very limited exposure through a median sternotomy.

The trachea and apical lung parenchyma and pleura lie just deep to the brachiocephalic or innominate artery, with the right vagus nerve passing inferiorly just distal and anterior to origin of the right subclavian artery. The right recurrent laryngeal nerve passes under and medial to the proximal right subclavian artery as it ascends back up the neck. The confluence of the right subclavian and internal jugular veins creating the right brachiocephalic vein lies anterior to the subclavian artery. The veins must be retracted laterally to expose the innominate and proximal right subclavian arteries.

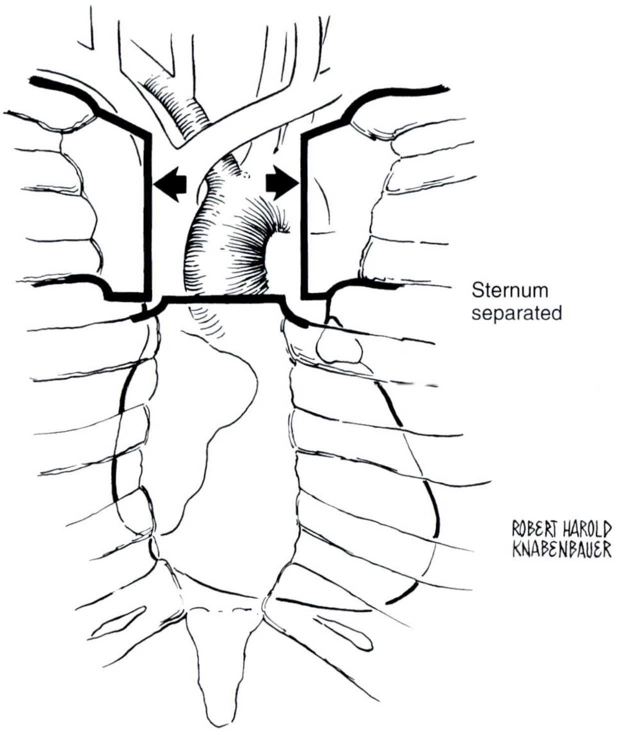

FIG 4.6 A median sternotomy, exposing the ascending aorta and arch vessels. (From Sakopoulos AG, Ballard JL, Gundry SR: Minimally invasive approach for aortic branch vessel reconstruction, *J Vasc Surg* 31:200, 2000.)

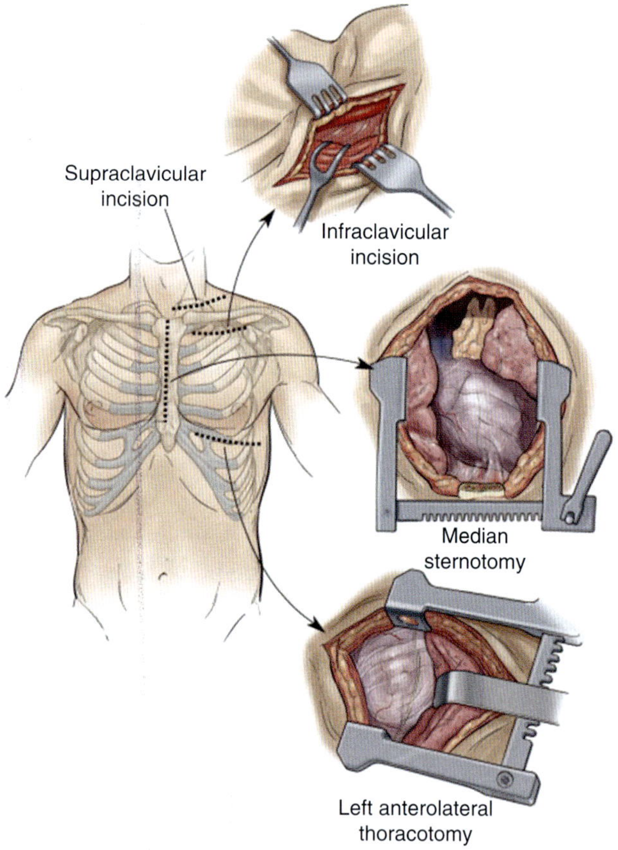

FIG 4.7 Incisions for the different aortic arch branches may vary to provide the greatest exposure. (From Baker A, Clouse WD: Upper Extremity and Junctional Zone Injuries. In Rasmussen TE, Tai NRM, editors: *Rich's Vascular Trauma,* ed. 3, Philadelphia, 2016 Elsevier, p. 159.)

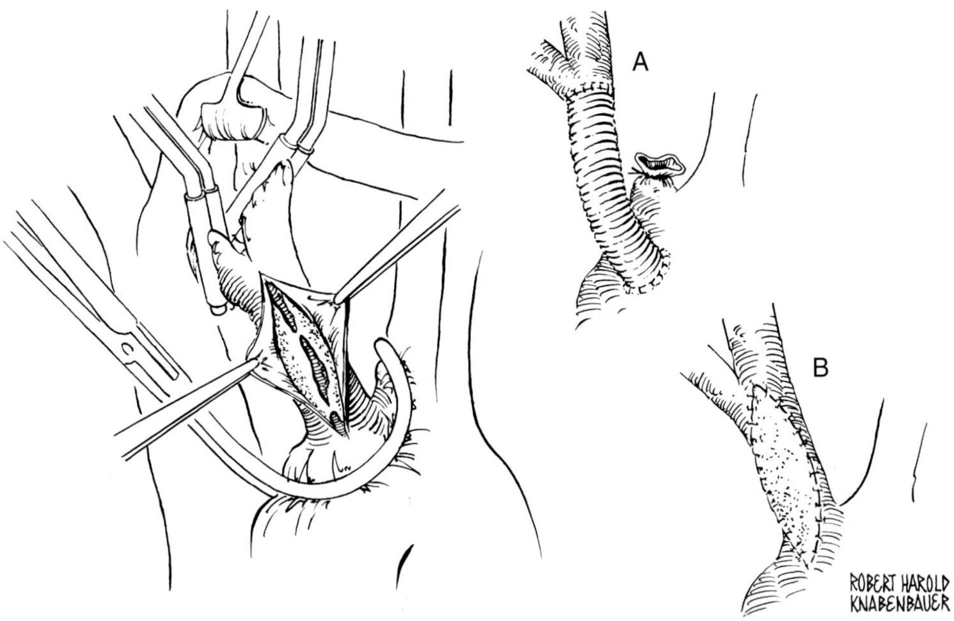

FIG 4.8 Surgical Exposure of an Innominate Artery With Visible Atherosclerotic Stenosis (A) Repair by proximal exclusion and ascending aorta–to–innominate artery bypass. (B) Repair by endarterectomy and patch angioplasty. (From Sakopoulos AG, Ballard JL, Gundry SR: Minimally invasive approach for aortic branch vessel reconstruction, *J Vasc Surg* 31:200, 2000.)

The full median sternotomy is considered the standard approach for aortic arch exposure; however, a minimally invasive approach with a partial upper sternotomy to the level of the third rib has been described in a series of patients with promising results. It requires transection of the sternum at the third rib, forming an inverted "T" on the sternum.[26] During the transection, the internal thoracic arteries run close to the sternal edge and can be injured, risking vascular compromise to the sternum. Another technique, by Tominaga and colleagues, approached exposure of the entire aortic arch with an L-incision, described as a left anterolateral thoracotomy and upper partial median sternotomy.[27]

EXPOSURE OF THE RIGHT SUBCLAVIAN ARTERY

The subclavian arteries are divided into three segments, proximal, middle, and distal, based on the relation to the anterior scalene muscle. The proximal segment spans from the origin of the artery to the medial border of the anterior scalene muscle. The middle segment is the portion directly posterior to the anterior scalene muscle. Lastly, the distal segment is the portion from the lateral margin of the anterior scalene muscle to the outer border of the first rib, where it becomes the axillary artery.

The proximal right subclavian artery is exposed through a median sternotomy. The incision can be extended superiorly along the anterior border of the respective SCM or along a supraclavicular, transverse line to expose the middle segment of the subclavian artery as it crosses into the thoracic outlet (Fig. 4.9). The dissection will require division of the sternothyroid and sternothyroid muscles attaching to the manubrium, and the sternal and clavicular heads of the SCM.

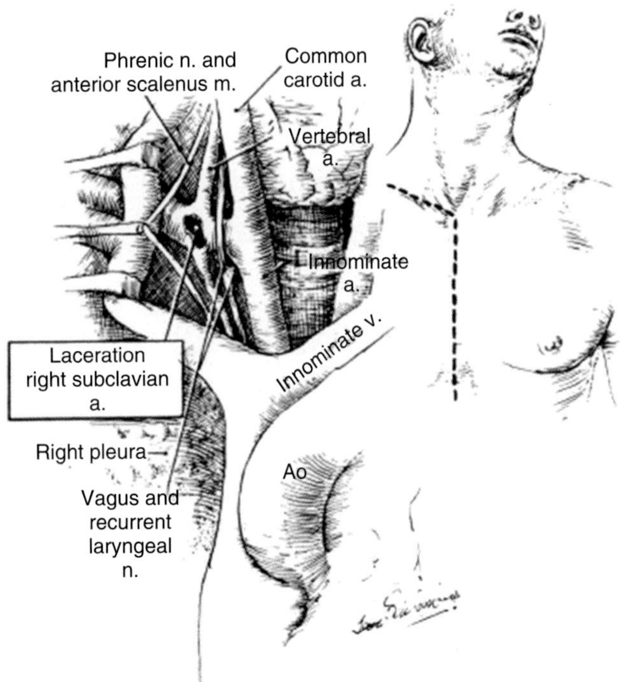

FIG 4.9 Exposure of the right subclavian artery through a median sternotomy and supraclavicular incision. Note the location of the phrenic, vagus, and recurrent laryngeal nerves, which must be identified and protected. *Ao*, Aorta. (From Ernst C: Exposure of the subclavian arteries, *Semin Vasc Surg* 2:202, 1989.)

The second and third portions of both the right and left subclavian arteries are exposed through a supraclavicular approach. An 8- to 10-cm transverse incision approximately 1 to 2 cm above the clavicle is deepened through the platysma muscle. Subplatysmal flaps are developed superiorly and inferiorly. The external jugular vein is typically ligated, and the clavicular head of the SCM is resected. The sternal head can be retracted medially or divided as needed. The omohyoid muscle is divided. The scalene fat pad is then encountered. The internal jugular vein composes the medial border of the fat pad and the subclavian vein its inferior border. The fat pad is mobilized along these veins at its medial and inferior borders and reflected. The phrenic nerve lies just below the fat pad on the anterior surface of the anterior scalene muscle, and the nerve should be identified and preserved as the fat pad is mobilized. The phrenic nerve can be carefully mobilized off the anterior scalene muscle. The subclavian artery lies just posterior to the anterior scalene, and careful sharp division of the muscle will expose the middle and distal portions of the artery. The brachial plexus lies just posterior to the artery. Sharp dissection will prevent thermal injury to the brachial plexus, thoracic duct, and vagus and phrenic nerves, all of which travel in the vicinity.[28] Resection of the middle of the clavicle can also provide exposure for the middle and distal segments of the subclavian artery, particularly in cases of trauma.[28] As the subclavian artery is dissected, the vertebral, internal thoracic, and thyrocervical arteries are encountered on the proximal segment of the subclavian artery, medial to the anterior scalene muscle. Of these vessels, the thyrocervical trunk can be ligated, whereas the vertebral and internal thoracic arteries should be preserved.

EXPOSURE OF THE PROXIMAL COMMON CAROTID ARTERIES

The right common carotid artery is exposed in the same manner as the brachiocephalic artery, with a median sternotomy with extension of the incision along the right anterior SCM. The cervical incision can be made in continuity with the sternotomy incision or separately if a more distal common carotid artery dissection is needed. A similar maneuver is performed for the left common carotid artery, except its course begins slightly posterior on the aortic arch. The vagus nerve can be identified running between the left common carotid and left subclavian arteries as it crosses the aortic arch and gives off the left recurrent laryngeal nerve that moves behind the ligamentum arteriosum and back into the neck.

Through the cervical extension of the sternotomy, the platysma is divided, and the investing fascia, also known as the deep cervical fascia, is incised to lateralize the SCM. The sternothyroid and sternothyroid muscles are divided, exposing the internal jugular vein that is retracted laterally to fully expose the proximal common carotid artery.[2]

EXPOSURE OF THE LEFT SUBCLAVIAN ARTERY

As the aorta curves to the left and posteriorly to the left side of the trachea, the left subclavian artery is the third and most posterior branch. It is relatively inaccessible through a median sternotomy. The most common means for exposure is through a left anterolateral thoracotomy in the fourth intercostal space. For access to the middle segment of the subclavian artery or the proximal common carotid artery, a separate left supraclavicular incision can be made. A third approach combines both the anterolateral thoracotomy and supraclavicular incision with a connecting sternotomy, sometimes called the "trap-door," or "book-flap" thoracotomies.[28,29] Because separate incisions for adequate proximal exposure are accomplished with reduced morbidity, the trap-door incision is not usually recommended and typically performed only in cases of penetrating trauma for emergent control.[29,30]

To perform the anterolateral thoracotomy, the patient's shoulder should be elevated behind the scapula and the arm adducted to 90 degrees, with single lung ventilation. A curvilinear incision is made in the fourth intercostal space from the medial border of the sternum to the anterior axillary line. Dissection through the pectoralis fascia and muscle to the intercostal space is followed by entry into the pleural space to reduce the lung to allow the incision to be opened completely without parenchymal injury. The internal thoracic vascular bundle may require ligation to avoid traction avulsion after the rib spreader is placed. The lung is retracted inferiorly, exposing the lateral aspect of the aortic arch, and the mediastinal pleura is incised. The surgeon must be cognizant to identify the left vagus, recurrent laryngeal and phrenic nerves, and the thoracic duct, which comes up posterolateral to the left subclavian artery to drain into the junction of the left subclavian and internal jugular veins. The thoracic duct should be ligated unless it can be confidently protected during the entire operation to prevent a chyle leak or chylothorax. At this point, vascular control can be obtained at the origin of the left subclavian artery, and the proximal segment of the subclavian artery can be fully exposed (Fig. 4.10).

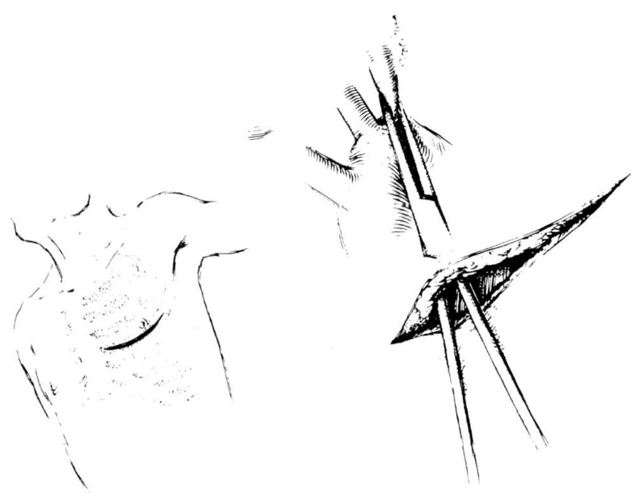

FIG 4.10 Anterior thoracotomy with placement of a vascular clamp for control of bleeding from the proximal left subclavian artery. (From Trunkey D: Great vessel injury. In Blaisdell F, Trunkey D, editors: *Trauma management*, vol 3, *Cervicothoracic trauma*, New York, 1986, Thieme, p 255.)

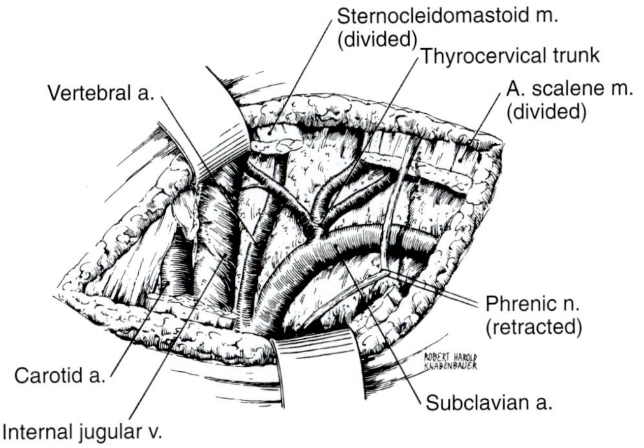

FIG 4.11 Exposure of the second portion of the left subclavian artery via a supraclavicular incision. In this depiction, the lateral head of the sternocleidomastoid muscle and the anterior scalene muscle are divided.

To gain access to the middle and distal segment of left subclavian artery as it courses over the first rib, a supraclavicular incision similar to the one described for the right subclavian artery is used. When mobilizing the scalene fat pad on the left, the thoracic duct should be identified and preserved or ligated as it enters the subclavian vein posteriorly near the junction with the jugular vein (Fig. 4.11).

EXPOSURE OF THE DESCENDING THORACIC AORTA

Distal to the takeoff of the left subclavian artery at the ligamentum arteriosum, the aorta courses to the abdomen anterior and to the left of the vertebral bodies and posterolateral to the esophagus. As it descends, the aorta migrates toward the midline, where it pierces the diaphragm around T12 through the aortic hiatus to become the abdominal aorta. The hemiazygos vein runs posterior to the aorta, and the thoracic duct runs to the right over the vertebrae. The descending thoracic aorta gives off many paired branches that must be attended to during dissection of the thoracic aorta, and these include the bronchial, mediastinal, esophageal, intercostal, and superior phrenic arteries.

Exposure of the descending thoracic aorta is best achieved by a left posterolateral thoracotomy. If extension into the abdominal aorta is warranted, then a left thoracoabdominal incision will provide the additional exposure. In the posterolateral approach the patient is positioned in the right lateral decubitus position with all four extremities padded to avoid iatrogenic neuropathy. Double-lumen endotracheal intubation is performed to provide single-lung ventilation. An incision is made in any space between the fourth and seventh intercostal space, dependent on the level of the thoracic aorta to be exposed, with or without the resection of the rib. The incision is oriented along the rib space, starting anterior to the midaxillary line and extended cephalad toward the tip of the scapula. Once the subcutaneous tissue is dissected, the latissimus dorsi muscle is divided, and the serratus anterior can be either divided or retracted posteriorly with a self-retraining retractor. Upward retraction of the scapula allows access to the chest wall to count the ribs to ensure the correct rib space is entered.

With the lung deflated, the intercostal muscles are divided just above the lower rib to avoid injury to the intercostal neurovascular bundle. With the lung retracted anteriorly, the aorta is seen invested in the mediastinal pleura that is then incised to obtain vascular control at any level. Incision of the pleura should be against the aorta as the hemiazygos vein runs posterolaterally to the aorta within 1 cm. The esophagus must be dissected off the aorta, which can be done bluntly. Dissection should also occur at the level of a rib at the costovertebral junction to avoid injury to an intercostal artery branch. For dissection proximally near the aortic arch, the vagus and phrenic nerves must be protected. The ligamentum arteriosum can be divided to provide access to the inner aspect of the aortic arch, but the left recurrent laryngeal nerve should be preserved. The pulmonary artery abuts the proximal thoracic aorta and should be retracted with care. For visualization of the distal thoracic aorta, the inferior pulmonary ligament is divided.[31]

If the planned operation requires intraabdominal aorta to be exposed, it is best performed with a thoracoabdominal incision. The patient should be positioned in a modified, "lazy" right lateral decubitus position with the hips rotated approximately 45 degrees to the right or the shoulder elevated approximately 60 degrees with the support of a bean bag. This allows widening of the left thorax, as well as exposure of the groin.[32] The superior aspect of the incision is the same as a posterolateral thoracotomy with the rib space chosen preoperatively based on the extent of the thoracic aorta to be exposed. For exposure of the visceral segment of the aorta, the thoracic incision is continued inferomedially, across the costal margin to a point along the ipsilateral rectus muscle or a point off the midline (Fig. 4.12). For further abdominal aortic exposure, the incision is extended in a paramedian incision or along the midline on the linea alba as in a laparotomy (Fig. 4.13).[33]

Entry in to the chest is the same as with any thoracotomy and with clear communication with the anesthesia team. A rib retractor is placed, and the costal margin is divided to connect the thoracic wound with the abdominal incision. The diaphragm can be divided in multiple ways. With a partial division of the diaphragm to the level of the central tendon, there tends to be minimal pulmonary compromise but at the expense of requiring additional dissection to open the aortic hiatus.[34] Other approaches are to circumferentially incise the diaphragm muscle approximately 2 to 3 cm from the costal margin and chest wall, or to completely incise the diaphragm radially. The latter two techniques provide the best exposure; however, reconstruction is more difficult with similar pulmonary outcomes. The circumferential incision may reduce the risk of a phrenic nerve injury.[35]

EXPOSURE OF THE SUPERIOR VENA CAVA

The superior vena cava is best approached through a median sternotomy. Once the right brachiocephalic vein is exposed as in the exposure of the right subclavian artery, the junction of the two brachiocephalic veins can be seen lateral to the ascending aorta. The pericardial sac may need to be incised carefully, paying

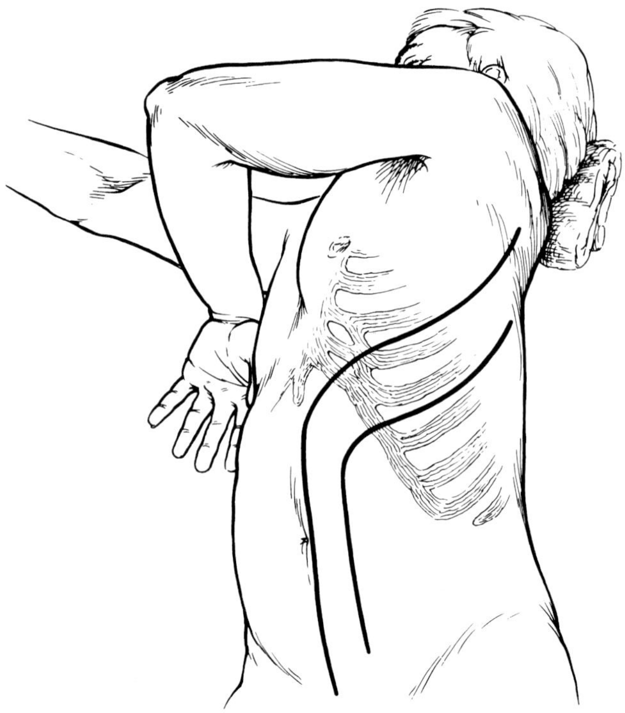

FIG 4.12 Incision options for thoracoabdominal aortic procedures are based on the extent of thoracic aorta to be exposed and the desire to stay in an extraperitoneal plane. (From Rutherford RB: Thoracoabdominal aortic exposures. In Rutherford RB, editor: *Atlas of vascular surgery: basic techniques and exposures*, Philadelphia, 1993, WB Saunders, p 223.)

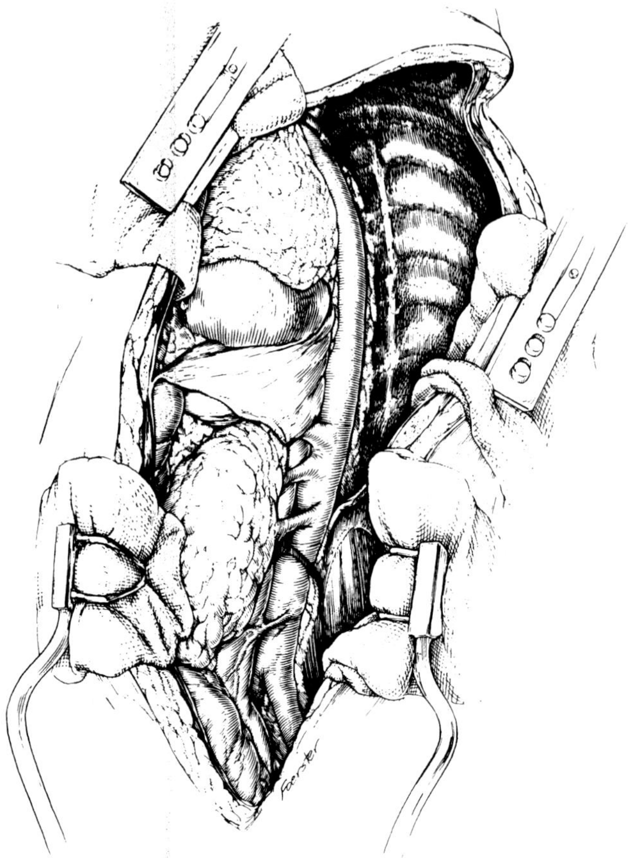

FIG 4.13 Thoracoabdominal aortic exposure from the origin of the left subclavian artery to the common iliac arteries. (From Rutherford RB: Thoracoabdominal aortic exposures. In Rutherford RB, editor: *Atlas of vascular surgery: basic techniques and exposures*, Philadelphia, 1993, WB Saunders, p 233.)

attention to the phrenic nerve passing more posteriorly, to expose the portions of the superior vena cava closest to the heart.[31]

EXPOSURE OF THE AXILLARY ARTERY

The axillary artery is divided into three parts defined by their relative location to the pectoralis minor muscle. The first part begins as the subclavian artery exits the thoracic outlet at the first rib and is medial to the pectoralis minor. The second part is posterior to the muscle, and the third part is lateral to the pectoralis minor. The axillary artery gives off multiple branches throughout its course, and these can be ligated. The axillary vein courses anteromedial to the artery and thus is exposed and retracted first before encountering the artery. The brachial plexus closely invests and intertwines with the artery and must be meticulously protected.

The approach is dependent on which portion and how much artery is to be exposed. Access to the first part of the axillary artery is achieved through a lateral infraclavicular incision, whereas exposure of the second and third part requires lateral extension into the upper arm or an axillary incision (Fig. 4.14).

For the infraclavicular approach, the arm is abducted to 90 degrees, and an incision is made approximately 2 to 3 cm parallel and below the lateral half of the clavicle. The pectoralis major muscle is separated along the course of its fibers or divided to expose the posterior fascia and clavipectoral fascia, which are then opened. A fat pad is seen and contains the axillary neurovascular

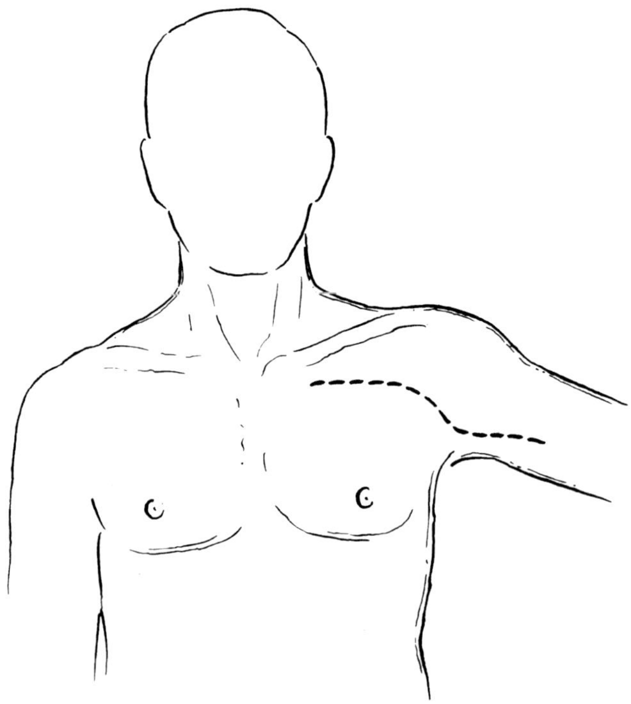

FIG 4.14 Incision for exposure of the axillary artery.

structures, with the pectoralis minor muscle defining the lateral extent of the dissection. The first vessel encountered is the axillary vein anteromedial to the artery, and the brachial plexus is invested closely posterior to the vessels at this portion of the artery. The lateral pectoral nerve typically crosses over the axillary vessels near pectoralis minor to innervate the pectoralis major. The lateral pectoral nerve arises off the lateral cord of the brachial plexus, and the medial pectoral nerve arises off the medial chord. They are named for their parental chord, not their relative position to each other, because the lateral pectoral nerve is actually medial to the medial pectoral nerve. The axillary vein can be retracted caudally, and any tributaries can be ligated as needed. The axillary artery is then isolated. For better mobilization and exposure, branches coming off the artery, including the supreme thoracic or thoracoacrominal arteries, can be ligated.

For distal exposure of the axillary artery, the infraclavicular incision is extended on to the proximal arm over the deltoid muscle in the deltopectoral groove, across the pectoralis major muscle, and toward the medial aspect of the arm. This approach will allow for exposure of the entire course of the axillary artery with minimal mobility or range of motion restrictions. After dissection through the subcutaneous tissue, the superior border of pectoralis major muscle can be identified and retracted inferomedially, exposing the clavipectoral fascia with the pectoralis minor muscle deep to it. Once the fascia is incised, the third part of the axillary artery can be isolated. It is at this portion that the brachial plexus can wrap around the artery. Particularly, the formation of the median nerve is usually anterior to the artery. Division of the pectoralis minor muscle at its insertion on the coracoid process exposes the second part of the artery, and care must be taken to avoid injury to the pectoral nerves innervating both pectoralis muscles.

In the case of more proximal arterial exposure including the distal subclavian artery, a separate supraclavicular incision can be made for proximal arterial control. In a penetrating trauma scenario the clavicle can be resected with extension of the incision toward the axilla to expose both the distal subclavian artery and entire axillary artery.[36] The second and third portions of the axillary artery can also be exposed through an incision in the axilla. Care should be taken to preserve the long thoracic nerve and thoracodorsal nerve as they course along the chest wall. The pectoralis major is retracted medial, and the pectoralis minor can be divided to expose the neurovascular bundle. The median nerve runs anteriorly to the distal axillary artery and the ulnar nerve and axillary vein run medially to the artery.

EXPOSURE OF THE BRACHIAL ARTERY

The brachial artery is the continuation of the axillary artery as it passes the teres major muscle and courses to its bifurcation in the antecubital fossa. The brachial artery has only a few branches: the profunda brachii artery, the superior ulnar collateral artery, and the inferior ulnar collateral artery. These branches typically provide collateral flow and can be ligated as needed for optimal exposure.

Exposure of the brachial artery in the upper medial arm is based on its anatomic course between the triceps and biceps muscles. A straight incision is made longitudinally over the segment of brachial artery to be exposed (Fig. 4.15). Segmental incisions or a continuous incision can be made for proximal and distal access. When crossing the elbow crease distally, the incision in the antecubital fossa should be made in an S shape to reduce the risk for skin contractures. In the antecubital fossa, the basilic vein and medial antebrachial cutaneous nerve lie superficial to the bicipital aponeurosis and should be retracted. The bicipital aponeurosis can be divided, but the biceps tendon proper must be preserved.

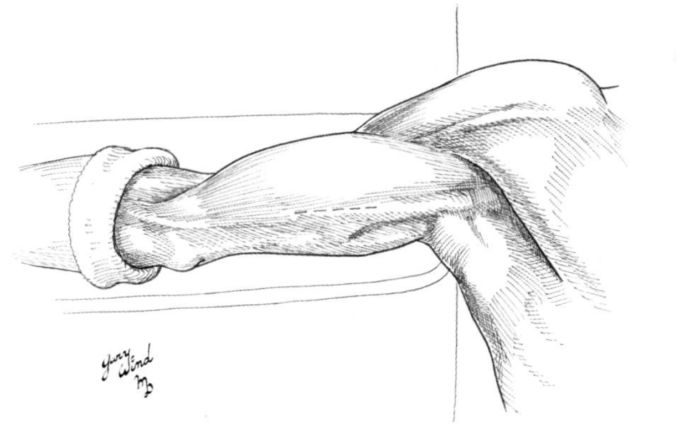

FIG 4.15 A longitudinal incision is made between the biceps and triceps muscles with the arm abducted. (Reproduced with permission from Valentine RJ, Wind GG: Brachial artery. In *Anatomic exposures in vascular surgery*, Philadelphia, 2003, Lippincott Williams & Wilkins, p 185, © by RJ Valentine and GG Wind.)

Incising the deep brachial fascia along the medial aspect of the biceps muscle exposes the basilic vein, median nerve, and brachial artery. The vein typically runs 1 to 2 cm inferior to the artery and may penetrate the deep fascia to course more superficially. The median nerve lies directly superficial to the artery and must be gently retracted away from the artery. In the antecubital fossa the bicipital aponeurosis is opened to expose the artery, where its bifurcation can be seen just distal to the antecubital fossa near the radial tuberosity near the intersection of the brachioradialis and pronator teres muscles.

EXPOSURE OF THE RADIAL ARTERY

The radial artery continues into the forearm from the brachial artery and travels with the radial nerve, along a path from the antecubital fossa to the styloid process laterally. Preoperative planning is needed to determine which aspect of the artery needs to be exposed. Incisions are oriented longitudinally with the course of the artery primarily on the lateral aspect of the volar forearm.[37] Identification of the proximal radial artery is easiest just below the antecubital fossa at the bifurcation of the brachial artery. The antebrachial fascia surrounds the entire forearm and is a continuation of the brachial fascia of the upper arm. The radial artery can be found coursing just deep to and along medial border of the brachioradialis muscle (Fig. 4.16). The medial border of the brachioradialis can be used as a landmark for incisions to expose the length of the radial artery in the forearm. After dividing the subcutaneous tissues and fascia, the radial

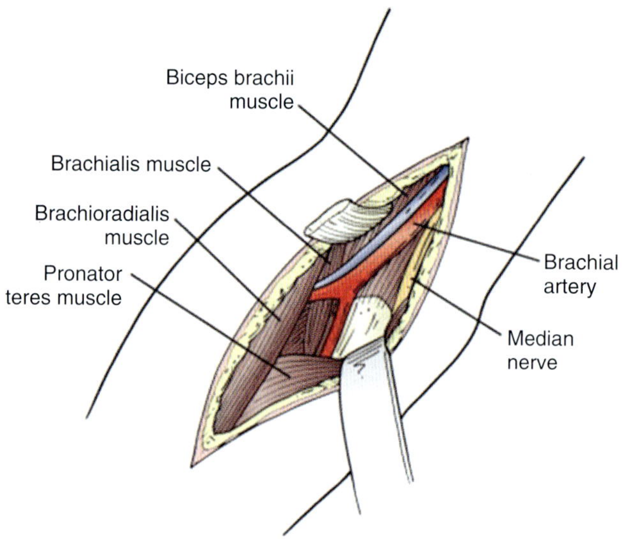

FIG 4.16 Exposure of the distal brachial artery and proximal radial artery with a longitudinal incision along the course of the artery, with an S-shaped curve across the antecubital fossa. (From Baker A, Clouse WD: Upper Extremity and Junctional Zone Injuries. In Rasmussen TE, Tai NRM, editors: *Rich's Vascular Trauma*, ed. 3, Philadelphia, 2016 Elsevier, p. 162.)

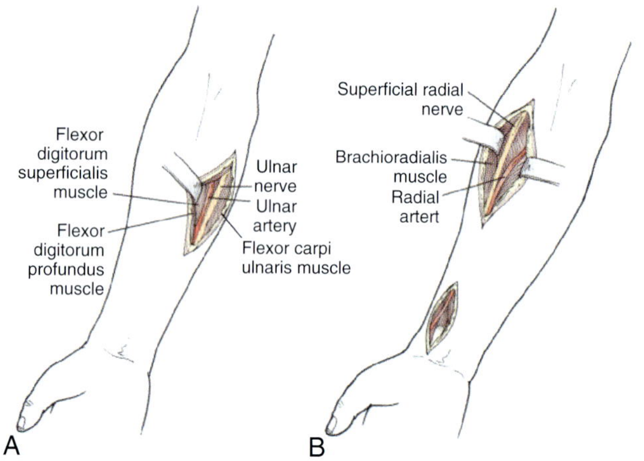

FIG 4.17 (A) Exposure of the ulnar artery on the medial aspect of the volar forearm. (B) Exposure of the middle and distal radial artery as it courses along the medial border of the brachioradialis muscle. (From Baker A, Clouse WD: Upper Extremity and Junctional Zone Injuries. In Rasmussen TE, Tai NRM, editors: *Rich's Vascular Trauma,* ed. 3, Philadelphia, 2016 Elsevier, p. 163.)

artery can be exposed by retracting the brachioradialis laterally and the pronator teres medially (Fig. 4.17B).

A longitudinal incision near the radial pulse proximal to the wrist allows distal exposure (see Fig. 4.17B). Again, the antebrachial fascia must be incised to expose the artery. At this level, the radial artery lies just below the fascia between the flexor carpi radialis tendon medially and the brachioradialis tendon laterally, with the superficial radial nerve accompanying the artery.

EXPOSURE OF THE ULNAR ARTERY

The ulnar artery's course differs significantly from the radial artery's. At the bifurcation, the ulnar artery sharply courses medially and immediately dives under the pronator teres muscle. It courses deep to the flexor muscles to approximately halfway down the forearm where it becomes superficial. This deep proximal course makes identification and exposure difficult with the added need to protect the ulnar nerve running with the artery.

To expose the ulnar artery in the forearm, slight flexion of the hand helps to relax the flexor muscles. An incision over the medial forearm is made approximately 10 cm below the elbow. The fascia is incised. The flexor digitorum superficialis is reflected laterally. As the artery courses more distally, it travels under the flexor carpi ulnaris, which can be retracted medially (see Fig. 4.17A). The ulnar nerve joins the ulnar artery approximately a third of the way down the forearm and must be protected along its course to the hand. Near the wrist, toward the hypothenar eminence, a longitudinal incision medial to the flexor carpi ulnaris tendon will expose the artery. At the wrist, a superficial palmar branch of the ulnar nerve runs above the fascia and should be protected.

EXPOSURE OF THE ABDOMINAL AORTA

The abdominal aorta can be divided four segments: supraceliac, visceral, juxtarenal, and infrarenal. The supraceliac aorta spans from the aortic hiatus at the diaphragm to the celiac trunk. The visceral segment of the abdominal aorta spans from the celiac trunk to the renal arteries and includes the origin of the superior mesenteric artery. The juxtarenal aorta includes only the origins of the renal arteries. The infrarenal aorta includes the distal portion of the aorta below the origin of the renal arteries to its bifurcation and includes the origin of inferior mesenteric artery. Each of the segments of the abdominal aorta can be accessed through either the transperitoneal or retroperitoneal approach, although certain segments are more easily reached by one or the other. Consideration should also be given to the extent any of the visceral arteries need to be exposed. The vascular surgeon should be familiar with both techniques. Prior surgical history, location of stomas, body habitus, and involvement of the iliac arteries are a few of the factors to consider when choosing an incision. Inflammatory aneurysms and aneurysms in the presence of a horseshoe kidney are best approached from the retroperitoneum.

TRANSPERITONEAL APPROACHES

Most transperitoneal approaches begin with a long midline laparotomy from the xiphoid process to the pubis, although a transverse incision above the umbilicus also provides wide access to the peritoneal cavity. A brief examination of the peritoneum and intraperitoneal organs should be performed. A large self-retaining retractor system is a necessity. Transperitoneal access to the supraceliac aorta can be carried out through the lesser sac. Through an upper midline laparotomy incision, the left triangular ligament of the liver is taken down and the left liver lobe is retracted superolaterally to the right to expose the proximal stomach. The gastrohepatic ligament is incised vertically along its middle portion to spare the hepatic branch of the right vagus nerve or a replaced or accessory left hepatic artery, which

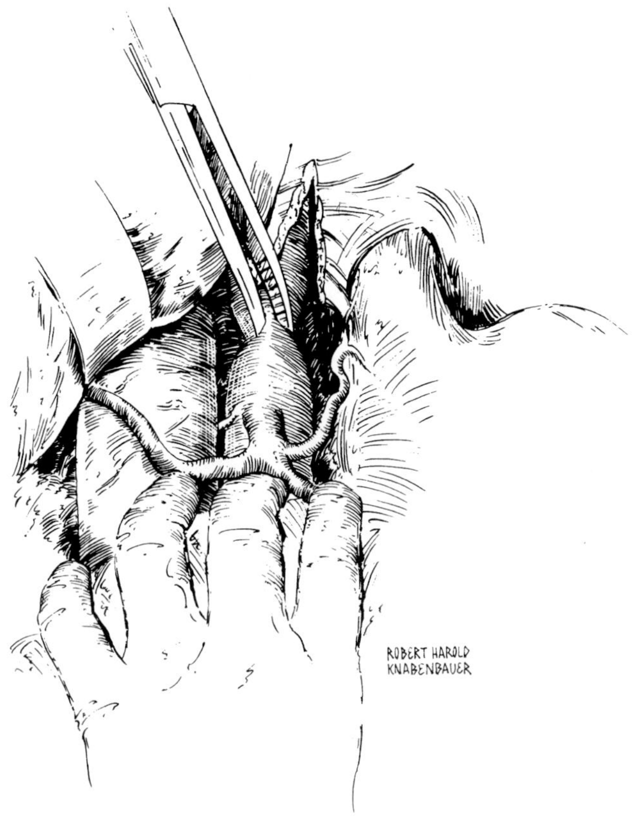

FIG 4.18 Exposure of the abdominal aorta at the diaphragm.

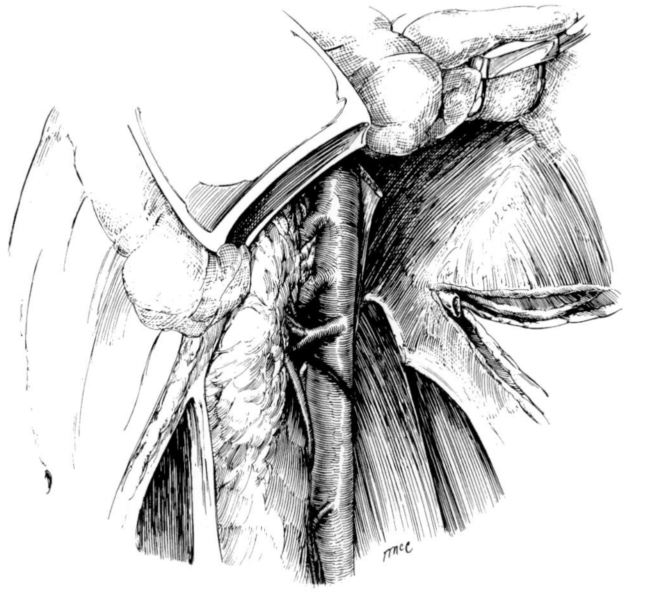

FIG 4.19 Division of the median arcuate ligament and left diaphragmatic crus facilitates suprarenal and supraceliac exposure. (From Rutherford RB: Thoracoabdominal aortic exposures. In Rutherford RB, editor: *Atlas of vascular surgery: basic techniques and exposures*, Philadelphia, 1993, WB Saunders, p 207.)

occurs in approximately 10% of the population arising from the left gastric artery, as these structures travel along the cephalad portion of the ligament.

Once in the lesser sac, the esophagus and gastric cardia are retracted to the left to expose the right crus of the diaphragm. Dividing the right crus of the diaphragm will expose the aorta anterior to the spine (Fig. 4.18). The periaortic fascia can be cleared bluntly but should not be circumferentially cleaned because intercostal or lumbar arteries and the lumbar venous plexus are posterior and exceedingly difficult to control if they bleed. Additional proximal exposure is facilitated with division of the median arcuate ligament which forms across the right and left crura over the aorta (Fig. 4.19). Any further proximal extension above the median arcuate ligament is within the posterior mediastinum, and entry into the pleura to cause a pneumothorax should be considered should a patient become difficult to ventilate or hypotensive.

To expose the visceral segment of the aorta or as an alternative exposure of the supraceliac aorta, a left medial visceral rotation can be performed (Fig. 4.20). The descending colon is mobilized by dividing the avascular white line of Toldt from the splenic flexure to the sigmoid colon, followed by dividing the splenophrenic and splenocolic ligaments. The spleen and the pancreatic body and tail are rotated anteriorly as this dissection is developed. The left kidney is mobilized and the gonadal and lumbar veins off the left renal vein are ligated to free the left renal vein. At this point the left colon, spleen, pancreas, stomach, left kidney, left adrenal gland, and small bowel are

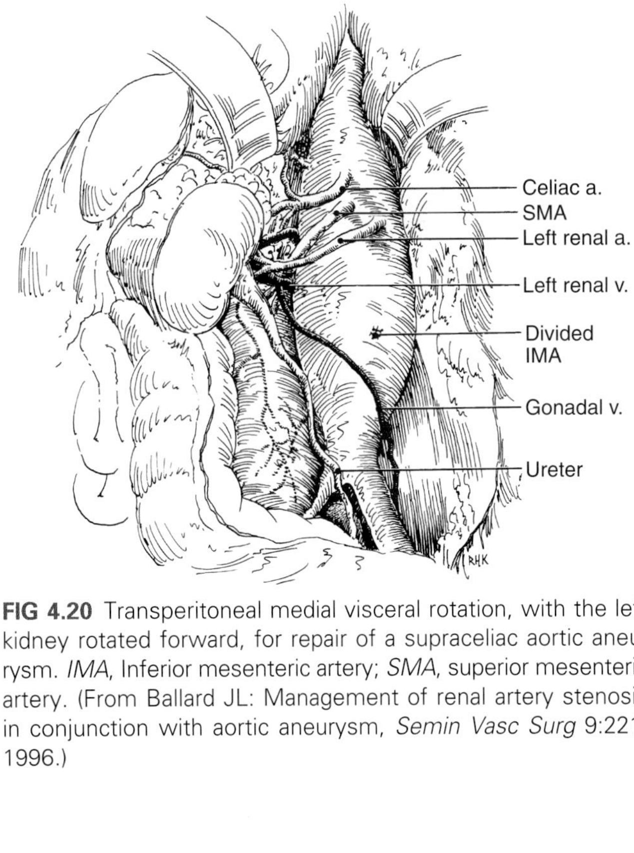

FIG 4.20 Transperitoneal medial visceral rotation, with the left kidney rotated forward, for repair of a supraceliac aortic aneurysm. *IMA*, Inferior mesenteric artery; *SMA*, superior mesenteric artery. (From Ballard JL: Management of renal artery stenosis in conjunction with aortic aneurysm, *Semin Vasc Surg* 9:221, 1996.)

retracted medially to expose the entire abdominal aorta from the diaphragm to the aortic bifurcation. The left crus be divided for additional proximal exposure. Alternatively, the left kidney can be left in place and the aorta approached anterior to the renal artery and vein.

The juxtarenal and infrarenal aorta can also be approached through the peritoneum. After a laparotomy or a transverse abdominal incision, the small bowel is packed into the right side of the abdomen or eviscerated. The retroperitoneum is incised just to the left of the duodenum. The duodenum is then mobilized and retracted to the right. The renal vein should be identified, mobilized, and controlled at the cephalad portion of the field. Careful dissection can expose the aorta to the origin of the superior mesenteric artery, but the visceral segment cannot be exposed through this approach. The vena cava can be identified to the right of the aorta, but extensive dissection and mobilization of the vena cava is contraindicated. The remainder of the infrarenal aorta can be exposed by dissecting through the retroperitoneum. The plane of dissection should pass to the right of the inferior mesenteric artery origin. At the level of the aortic bifurcation, circumferential isolation or control at this level should be avoided. The iliac veins run posterior to the bifurcation and are usually inseparable from the aorta without significant injury and bleeding; therefore, distal aortic control should be performed at the level of the common iliac arteries. Dissection of the fibrous tissue over the origin of the left common iliac artery should be avoided to preserve the nervi erigentes and prevent postoperative retrograde ejaculation and sexual dysfunction.

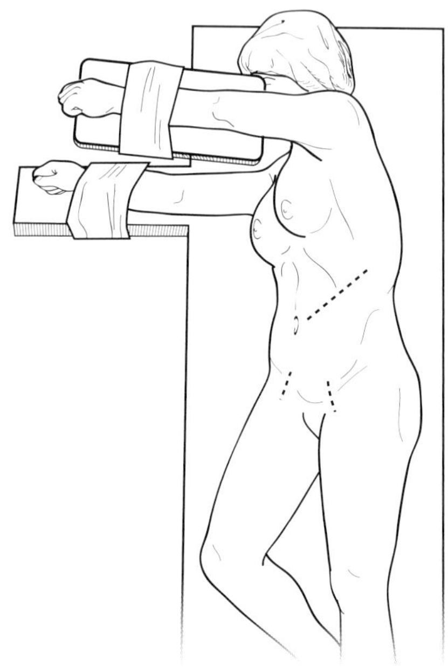

FIG 4.21 Positioning for Exposure of the Retroperitoneal Aorta The patient is positioned right lateral decubitus with the hips rotated open, which will unwind the torso allowing for greater exposure of bilateral groins as well as the left flank.

RETROPERITONEAL APPROACHES

A retroperitoneal approach should be used when access to multiple segments of the aorta is required, for additional exposure of the distal thoracic aorta, and in cases of inflammatory aortic aneurysms, but it can also be used electively for infrarenal aortic exposure. The difficult access to the distal right common iliac artery from this approach should be kept in mind. A left oblique incision extending from the tip of the 12th rib, or near the axillary line, toward the umbilicus is made and can be extended caudally as needed for infrarenal aortic exposure (Fig. 4.21). If more proximal exposure of the aorta is required, the incision can be based off of a higher rib. The external and internal oblique muscles are divided in the direction of their fibers, and the transversalis fascia is incised exposing the peritoneum. Medially, toward the lateral aspect of the rectus sheath, the peritoneum and transversalis fascia may be fused and therefore division of the transversalis fascia should be carefully extended to this point. Blunt dissection facilitates separation of the peritoneum from the abdominal wall and should be extended over the psoas muscle. The fascia over the psoas should be left in place to avoid injury to the genitofemoral nerve. The left kidney can be rotated anteriorly with the peritoneal contents or allowed to remain posteriorly. In either case the ureter should be identified and preserved. If rotating the left kidney, Gerota fascia is incised and blunt dissection posterior to the left kidney will medialize the kidney and displace it anteriorly. This will medialize the left ureter from the field and expose small renal and lumbar venous branches that can be ligated to expose the anterolateral aorta. It is prudent to identify the left renal artery at its origin to ensure that it is protected from any retractors or excessive tension.

Dissection along the proximal aorta is similar to the transperitoneal approach with left medial visceral rotation in that the left crus can be divided. Combined with the thoracic aspect of dissection and division of the diaphragm as previously described, the supraceliac aorta, aortic hiatus, and the descending thoracic aorta can be widely exposed.

EXPOSURE OF THE CELIAC TRUNK

The usual anatomy of celiac trunk consists of three branches: the common hepatic and the left gastric and splenic arteries, arising from a short 1- to 2-cm trunk that comes off the aorta at a 90-degree angle 2 to 3 cm below the aortic hiatus.

Exposure of the branches of the celiac trunk is best approached through the peritoneum. Similar to the supraceliac aortic exposure, the celiac trunk is seen within the cephalad portion of the lesser sac, covered in posterior peritoneum. Additional proximal aorta is uncovered for proximal control by incising the median arcuate ligament and right and left crura. The celiac ganglion is invested within a fibrous sheath surrounding the celiac trunk and must be divided vertically, exposing the branches and the segment of aorta between the celiac trunk and superior mesenteric artery, which can be as short as 3 mm. Isolation of the common hepatic artery is best performed just over the pylorus or first portion of the duodenum. It is important to note that the common bile duct will ascend just lateral to the artery as it courses into the hepatoduodenal ligament. The splenic artery can be approached from the left after mobilizing the splenic flexure and descending colon by incising the white line of Toldt and medializing the spleen and body and tail of the pancreas en bloc. The kidney should remain posterior in its investing fascia. The artery can be seen taking a tortuous path along the superior border of the pancreas, at times being embedded within its parenchyma and abutting the splenic vein. It can also be approached through the lesser sac by dividing the gastrocolic ligament and dissecting along the superior border of the pancreas.

EXPOSURE OF THE SUPERIOR MESENTERIC ARTERY

The superior mesenteric artery comes off the aorta descends behind the neck of the pancreas, medial to the bordering superior mesenteric vein. The artery courses over the third portion of the duodenum and gives off its first major branch, the middle colic artery. It then branches to supply the right colon and small bowel.

Exposure of the superior mesenteric artery varies according to the portion of the artery to be exposed. The origin is best approached through the gastrohepatic ligament, similar to the exposure of the celiac trunk, followed by caudal retraction of the pancreas or through a left medial visceral rotation. The left renal vein runs transversely posterior to the superior mesenteric artery, between the artery and the aorta. Exposure of the retropancreatic portion of the superior mesenteric artery is best achieved by a left medial visceral rotation to include the distal pancreas.

More distal exposure of the superior mesenteric artery is obtained by approaching the superior mesenteric anteriorly through the peritoneum. The anterior approach requires elevation of the transverse mesocolon to trace the middle colic artery proximally to its origin in the superior mesentery artery. The visceral peritoneum is cut at the base of the mesocolon and medial to the Ligament of Treitz to expose the superior mesenteric artery in the root of the small bowel mesentery (Fig. 4.22).

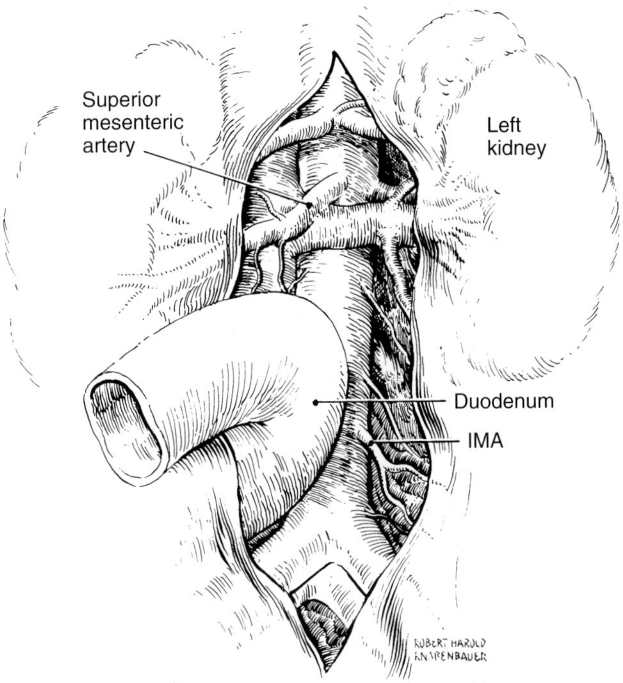

FIG 4.22 Infracolic Exposure of the Superior Mesenteric Artery The pancreas and transverse colon are not shown but are retracted upward and forward. *IMA*, Inferior mesenteric artery.

EXPOSURE OF THE RENAL ARTERIES

The renal arteries originate off the aorta around the L1 and L2 vertebrae, just inferior to the Ligament of Treitz, and they are slightly posterolateral as the kidneys. The left renal artery and vein are typically slightly cephalad compared with the right, and the arteries typically lay posterior the vein on both sides. The renal artery is a terminal artery, which explains why disruptions in their flow cause immediate ischemia.

Exposure of the renal arteries on either side can be approached transperitoneally or retroperitoneally, with techniques similar to exposure of the abdominal aorta, described earlier.

Transperitoneal exposure is accomplished with one of three types of incisions: midline, flank, or transverse.[38] A midline abdominal incision or a supraumbilical transverse incision can be used for bilateral arterial exposure with or without an aortic component to a repair. An ipsilateral flank incision allows for exposure of the blood supply of one kidney. In the midline approach, similar to exposure of the abdominal aorta, the transverse colon is reflected superiorly, and the small bowel is retracted to the right or eviscerated to expose the retroperitoneum. The ligament of Treitz is taken down, and the posterior peritoneum is incised. The left renal vein should come into view and should be dissected out toward the renal hilum and across the midline to the right. Exposure of either renal artery origin requires mobilization of the left renal vein and usually requires ligation and division of the left gonadal, adrenal, and lumbar veins to provide optimal, safe retraction. At this point the vein can be retracted cranially or caudally to expose the juxtarenal aorta and the left renal artery origin. The medial wall of the inferior vena cava must be separated and retracted slightly to the right, whereas the left renal vein is retracted cranially, to identify the origin of the right renal artery. The right renal artery passes posteriorly to the inferior vena cava (Fig. 4.23). The left renal vein can be ligated if the left adrenal and gonadal veins have not been already ligated, but ligation can lead to renal compromise. To allow development of these collaterals, the left renal vein is ligated as close to the vena cava as possible.[39]

The left renal artery can also be exposed by a left medial visceral rotation as described previously (Fig. 4.24).

The right renal artery can also be approached through a right visceral medial rotation. The right colon is mobilized and retracted to the left. A Kocher maneuver frees the duodenum and exposes the vena cava, left renal vein, and aorta (Fig. 4.25). Dissection along the right edge of the inferior vena cava brings the right renal vein into view. The right renal artery passes directly behind the inferior vena cava, so the inferior vena cava must be cleared and mobilized above and below the renal artery. Ligating lumbar venous branches is helpful in avoiding venous bleeding around the cava. The vena cava is then retracted medially, and the renal vein retracted cranially or caudally to expose the right renal artery from its origin to the renal pelvis (Fig. 4.26).

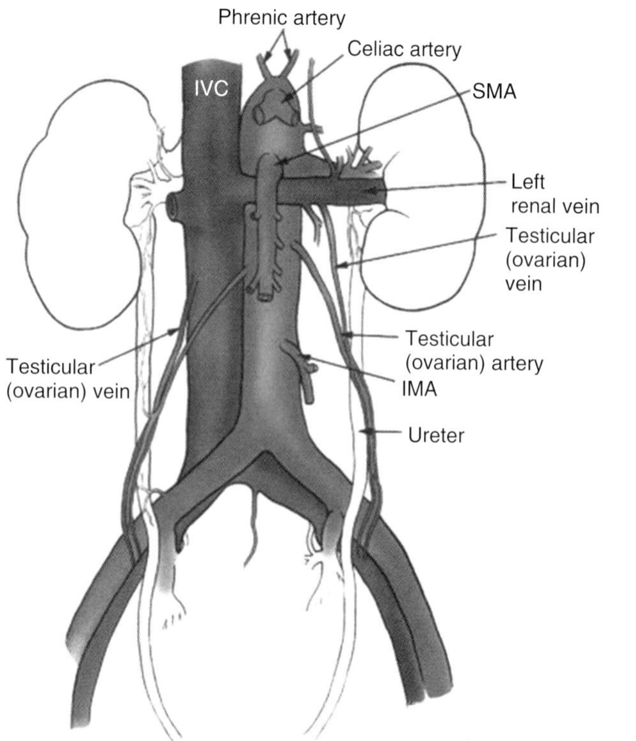

FIG 4.23 Relationship of the renal artery and vein. *IVC,* Inferior vena cava; *IMA,* Inferior mesenteric artery; *SMA,* superior mesenteric artery. (From Kumar NG, Knipp BS, Gillespie DL: Lower Extremity Vascular Trauma. In Rasmussen TE, Tai NRM, editors: *Rich's Vascular Trauma,* ed. 3, Philadelphia, 2016 Elsevier, p. 176.)

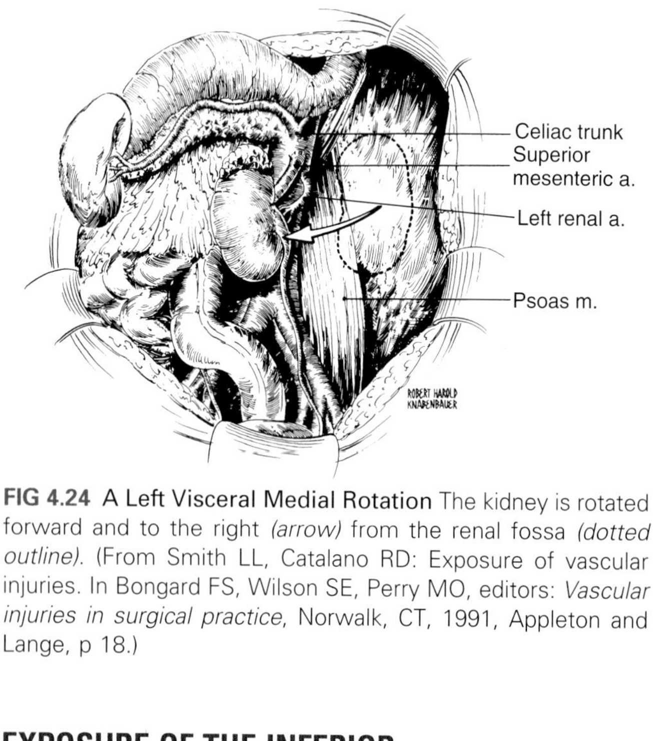

FIG 4.24 A Left Visceral Medial Rotation The kidney is rotated forward and to the right *(arrow)* from the renal fossa *(dotted outline).* (From Smith LL, Catalano RD: Exposure of vascular injuries. In Bongard FS, Wilson SE, Perry MO, editors: *Vascular injuries in surgical practice,* Norwalk, CT, 1991, Appleton and Lange, p 18.)

EXPOSURE OF THE INFERIOR MESENTERIC ARTERY

The inferior mesenteric artery is the lowest of the visceral arteries. It usually supplies the left colon, but robust collaterals with the superior mesenteric artery through the marginal artery of

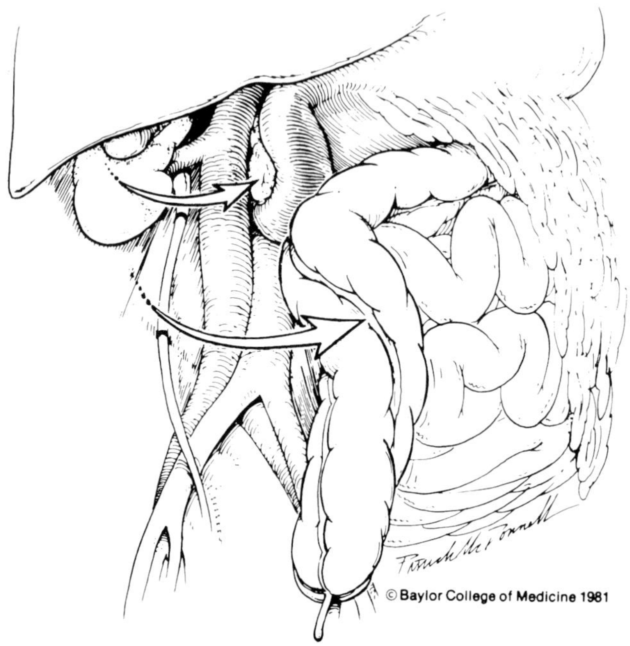

FIG 4.25 A right visceral medial rotation with mobilization of the right colon and kocherization of the duodenum. The right kidney can also be mobilized to inspect the posterior surface of the vena cava, if necessary. (Courtesy M. Dohrmann, the original illustrator.)

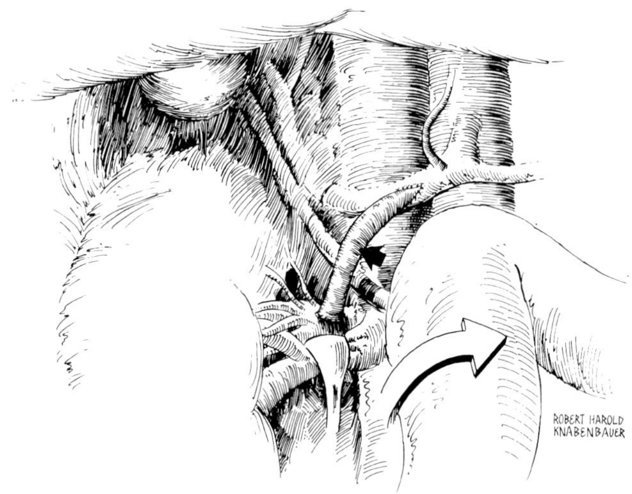

FIG 4.26 Hepatic-to–Right Renal Artery Bypass The duodenum is kocherized *(open arrow)* for exposure. The reverse saphenous vein bypass is identified *(solid arrow).* Note the retraction of the right renal vein for exposure.

Drummond, and meandering mesenteric artery or the arc of Riolan usually ensure that the inferior mesenteric artery can be ligated or covered by an endograft. Exposure of the inferior mesenteric artery typically is performed transperitoneally. The approach is identical to the exposure of the infrarenal aorta.

EXPOSURE OF THE ILIAC ARTERIES

The common iliac arteries descend along posterior abdominal wall from the level of the umbilicus or L4 to the sacral promontory. They lie anterior and lateral to the ipsilateral iliac vein. The right common iliac artery passes anterior to the left common iliac vein and can compress it, leading to May-Thurner Syndrome. At the level of the sacral promontory, the common iliac arteries bifurcate. The internal iliac arteries wrap over and medial to the common iliac veins and dive posteriorly as they give off multiple branches, and the external iliac arteries sweep laterally around the pelvic sidewall just medial to the psoas muscle exiting the abdomen posterior to the inguinal ligaments.

Exposure of the common iliac vessels is essentially a caudal extension of the dissection of the infrarenal aorta. In the transperitoneal approach through a low midline abdominal incision, after mobilization of the bowel and mesentery cranially, the posterior peritoneum is incised vertically over the right common iliac artery, not over the aortic bifurcation or left common iliac artery, where the sympathetic nerves are most dense. Lateral retraction with blunt dissection will expose the right common iliac artery with the common iliac vein confluence intimately associated with the artery posterolaterally. The ureter must be identified as it courses over the iliac artery bifurcation on both sides and dissected out to be lateralized to avoid injury. The cecal mesentery and the inferior portions of the root of the small bowel mesentery can be divided to allow more cephalad exposure of the right common iliac artery and distal aorta.

The left common iliac artery can be approached through the peritoneum either medial or lateral to the sigmoid colon. If medial, the approach is similar to the approach to the right common iliac, although again care should be taken to avoid the origin of the left common iliac to avoid the nervi erigentes. The lateral approach is completed by mobilizing the sigmoid colon from its peritoneal attachments. The ureter should be identified and preserved as it crosses over the common iliac artery bifurcation or external iliac artery.

For the retroperitoneal approach, an ipsilateral oblique curvilinear incision from 2 to 3 cm above the pubis to 2 to 3 cm from the anterior superior iliac spine is made. The external and internal oblique muscles and their aponeuroses are opened, and the transversus abdominus and transversalis fascia are opened to expose the peritoneum. The peritoneum is swept away from the anterior abdominal wall as it courses posteriorly to the psoas muscle. Attention should be paid to identifying the ilioinguinal and genitofemoral nerves traveling over psoas and iliacus muscles. The external iliac artery will be encountered first. Again, the ureter should be identified and preserved as it crosses the iliac bifurcation or external iliac artery. It is best to leave the ureter attached to and reflected with the peritoneum as the peritoneum retracted medially. Exposure from this approach can reach the aortic bifurcation and to the distal external iliac artery at the inguinal ligament. More distal exposure should be completed with a separate vertical groin incision with division of the inguinal ligament (Fig. 4.27).

The internal iliac arteries track deeper into the pelvis and are accessed through the transperitoneal iliac arterial exposure, except with more medial and inferior extension. The veins abut and course posteromedial to their corresponding artery, and one must be cognizant of their location during the entire exposure. Mobilization of the iliac veins typically requires ligation of multiple iliosacral veins that drain into the iliac veins to avoid avulsion or traction injury that can be difficult to control.

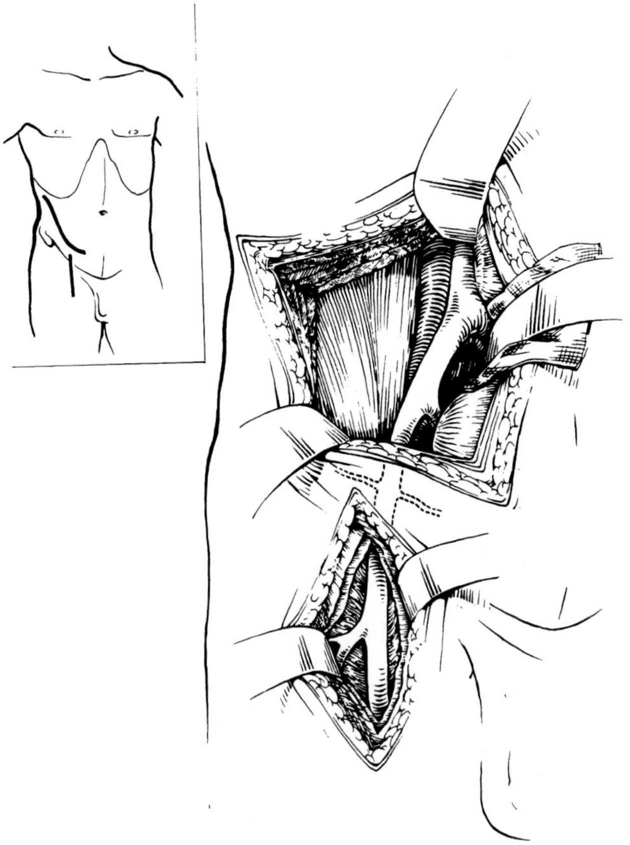

FIG 4.27 Extraperitoneal exposure of the distal common and external iliac arteries. Counterincision at the groin facilitates iliofemoral reconstruction.

EXPOSURE OF THE INFERIOR VENA CAVA

The inferior vena cava, formed by confluence of the common iliac veins around L5 and under the right common iliac artery, ascends on the right of the aorta anterior to the vertebral column. Retroperitoneal exposure is performed through a right flank incision, mirroring the left-sided approach to exposing the intraabdominal aorta. Lumbar veins will be draining into the vena cava posteriorly at every level and may need to be ligated or protected to ensure that they will not bleed after avulsion or traction injury.

Transperitoneal exposure requires a right medial visceral rotation of the cecum and ascending colon and a Kocher maneuver to mobilize the duodenum and head of the pancreas. The retrohepatic inferior vena cava is accessed with a subcostal extension of the midline abdominal incision, or a chevron incision, as alternatives to a midline incision. The right triangular ligament of the liver is incised to expose the bare area of the liver. Small hepatic vein draining directly into the vena cava can be ligated. The liver can then be retracted to the left (Fig. 4.28).

Suprahepatic and supradiaphragmatic vena cava exposure can be very difficult because of the small space between the heart and hepatic veins and is best accomplished through the chest. A median sternotomy with or without extension into the abdomen provides access to the pericardium which should be opened. The vena cava can be controlled as it drains into the right atrium.

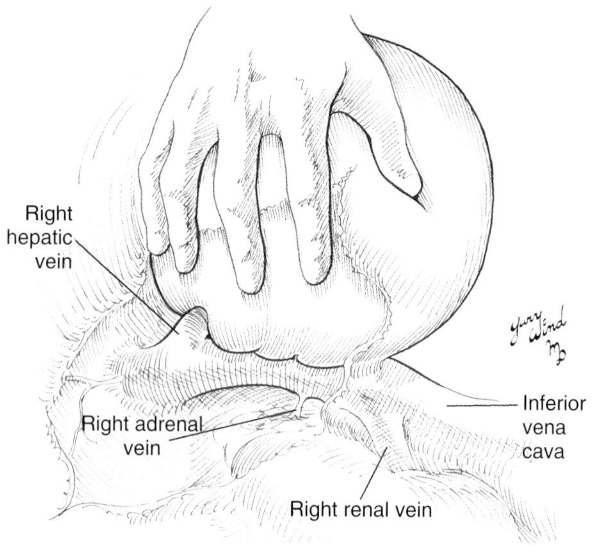

FIG 4.28 Exposure of the retrohepatic inferior vena cava after division of the right coronary and triangular ligaments. (Reproduced with permission from Valentine RJ, Wind GG: Inferior vena cava. In Brown B, McAvery M: *Anatomic exposures in vascular surgery*, Philadelphia, 2003, Lippincott Williams & Wilkins, p 344, © by RJ Valentine and GG Wind.)

For the portion of the vena cava below the pericardial sac, the central tendon of the diaphragm can be incised and retracted if needed.[40,41]

EXPOSURE OF THE PORTAL, SUPERIOR MESENTERIC, AND SPLENIC VEINS

The portal vein can be exposed in the porta hepatis through a transperitoneal approach. A subcostal or chevron incision is usually used. The hepatic flexure of the colon and the first and second portions of the duodenum are retracted caudally, whereas the liver is retracted cephalad. Usually, within the hepaticoduodenal ligament, the bile duct runs anterior to the portal vein and hepatic artery with the hepatic artery to the left of the portal vein. A replaced right hepatic artery will travel just to the right of the portal vein. The hepaticoduodenal ligament should be opened on its right, posterior side to directly expose the portal vein.

The superior mesenteric vein is exposed in a similar manner as the distal superior mesenteric artery. The transverse mesocolon is elevated, and the middle colic vessels are traced to their origins off the superior mesenteric vessels through and incision in the peritoneum at the base of the mesocolon.

The splenic vein runs along the posterior surface of the pancreas, with multiple small branches directly draining the pancreas. Using a midline or left subcostal incision, one approaches the splenic vein through the lesser sac by developing a plane along the inferior edge of the pancreas. As the body of the pancreas is rotated superiorly, the small pancreatic veins must be carefully ligated. The splenic vein can then be mobilized off the posterior surface of the pancreas.

EXPOSURE OF COMMON FEMORAL ARTERY

The common femoral artery is the extension of the external iliac artery below the inguinal ligament. The artery exits the abdomen just medial to the midpoint of the inguinal ligament, with the common femoral vein medial and the femoral nerve lateral to the artery. The artery and vein cross under the inguinal ligament deep to the fascia lata, with the greater saphenous vein and small branches of the artery piercing through the fascia at the foramen ovale. The common femoral artery varies in length between 1 and 10 cm and is between usually between 8 and 10 mm in diameter.

Exposure of the common femoral artery is usually carried out with a vertical groin incision just medial to the midpoint of the inguinal ligament or two fingerbreadths lateral to the pubic tubercle. An oblique incision parallel to and a fingerbreadth below the inguinal ligament can also be used if a limited section of the artery needs to be exposed. Multiple small arteries, including the superficial epigastric and external pudendal arteries, and branches of the saphenous vein may be encountered in variable positions and number and may be ligated. The fascia lata is opened, and the sartorius muscle is retracted laterally to expose the femoral sheath containing the common femoral artery and vein. Cephalad exposure can be obtained by retracting the inguinal ligament or dividing it for 1 to 2 cm. The deep circumflex iliac vein, which often crosses the external iliac artery just above the inguinal ligament, should be carefully identified and ligated if necessary. The ligament should be reconstructed if divided. Caudally, the common femoral artery divides into the superficial femoral artery and deep (profunda) femoral artery. The location of the bifurcation can often be identified by the change in diameter between the common and superficial femoral arteries.

EXPOSURE OF DEEP FEMORAL ARTERY

The deep profunda artery dives deeper into the thigh between the pectineus and adductor longus and brevis muscles approximately 3 to 8 cm from the inguinal ligament and runs closely along the medial femur. The artery arises from the common femoral artery posterolaterally. As it descends along the femur, it gives off a first major branch, the lateral circumflex femoral artery, and multiple perforating branches. The sartorius muscle acts as an important landmark to identify the zone of the deep femoral artery, similar to that of the pectoralis muscle to the axillary artery. The deep femoral artery is usually divided into three parts.[42] The deep femoral artery can be used as an outflow site in cases where the common femoral artery cannot be used due to scarring or infection in the groin. The first portion of the artery is exposed through the same incision and with a similar dissection as that described for the common femoral artery.[43]

A lateral approach to the midportion of the deep femoral has also been described. The incision is made along the lateral border of the sartorius muscle. Once through the fascia lata, the sartorius muscle is retracted medially, and the rectus femoris is identified. The fascia overlying the rectus femoris muscle is incised

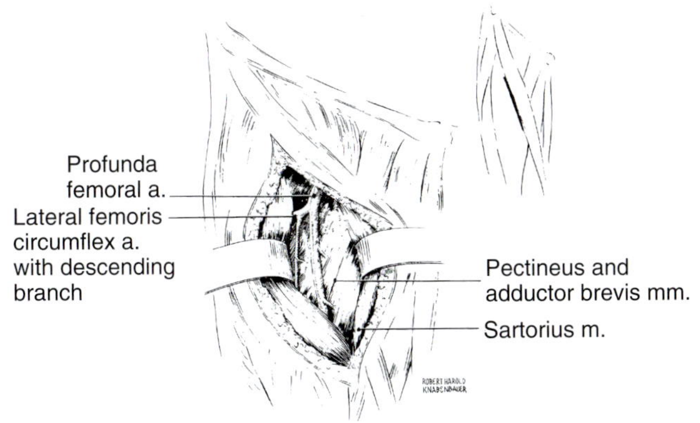

FIG 4.29 Lateral Approach to the Deep Femoral Artery *Upper right,* The incision is lateral to the sartorius muscle. *Lower left,* Exposure of the deep femoral vessel.

to allow lateral retraction of this muscle, which will expose the deep artery (Fig. 4.29). To fully expose the trunk, the lateral femoral circumflex vein traverses over the artery's origin and must be ligated.

The more distal deep femoral artery exposure can shorten the distance between inflow and outflow vessels, which reduces the length of conduit required. An alternative posteromedial approach has been developed to access the deep femoral artery through a more medially placed incision. Dissection is performed between the adductor longus muscle anteriorly and the adductor brevis, adductor magnus, and gracilis muscles posteriorly. Once these muscles are retracted, the deep femoral artery and accompanying vein are exposed against the femur and vastus medialis, which has a raphe attaching to the adductor longus muscle that must be divided.[44]

EXPOSURE OF SUPERFICIAL FEMORAL ARTERY

The superficial femoral artery courses in a more or less straight line caudally from the common femoral artery once the deep profunda femoral artery branches off. It runs along the undersurface of the sartorius muscle and crosses over the adductor longus at the midthigh (Fig. 4.30). This passage through the thigh is called the adductor or Hunter canal and is bound by the sartorius muscle anteriorly, the vastus medialis muscle laterally, and the adductor longus and magnus muscles posteromedially, with the latter muscle's aponeurosis splitting to form the adductor hiatus. As the artery passes medially with the rest of the neurovascular bundle, it becomes the popliteal artery. Exposure of the any part of the length of the superficial femoral artery (and vein) is best accomplished by a longitudinal incision along the lateral border of the sartorius muscle. Similar to the exposure of the common femoral artery, the fascia lata is incised proximally and the sartorius muscle is retracted laterally in the proximal thigh or medially in the distal thigh. The superficial femoral vein twists around the artery and receives multiple branches as it ascends to its confluence in the groin. The saphenous nerve must be protected during dissection as it also passes through Hunter canal.

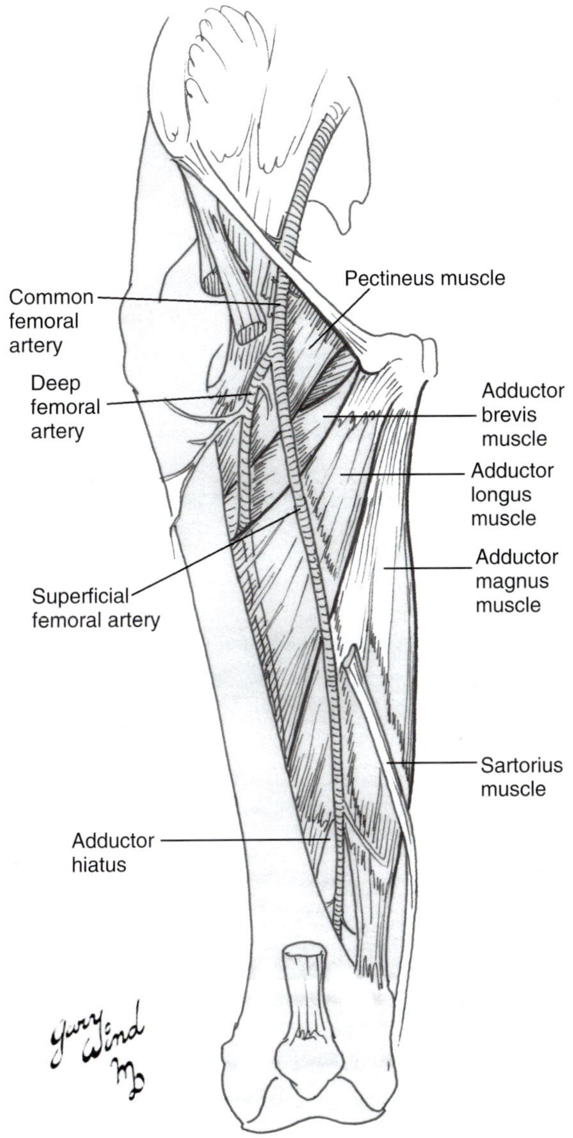

FIG 4.30 The Course of the Superficial and Deep Femoral Arteries Note the sartorius muscle has been removed better visualization. (Reproduced with permission from Valentine RJ, Wind GG: Vessels of the thigh. In Brown B, McAvery M: *Anatomic exposures in vascular surgery*, Philadelphia, 2003, Lippincott Williams & Wilkins, p 418, © by RJ Valentine and GG Wind.)

EXPOSURE OF POPLITEAL ARTERY

The popliteal artery spans from the adductor canal to the tibioperoneal trunk behind the tibial tuberosity and is invested in a fibrous sheath and cushioned by a small fat pad within the popliteal fascia. Multiple branches are given off in the proximal and middle popliteal artery that supplies the surrounding muscles and knee joint. Three of these important collateral vessels, the superior, middle, and inferior genicular arteries, divide the popliteal artery into three segments to aid in choosing the optimal exposure.[45]

The suprageniculate and infrageniculate segments of the popliteal artery can be approached from the medial aspect or

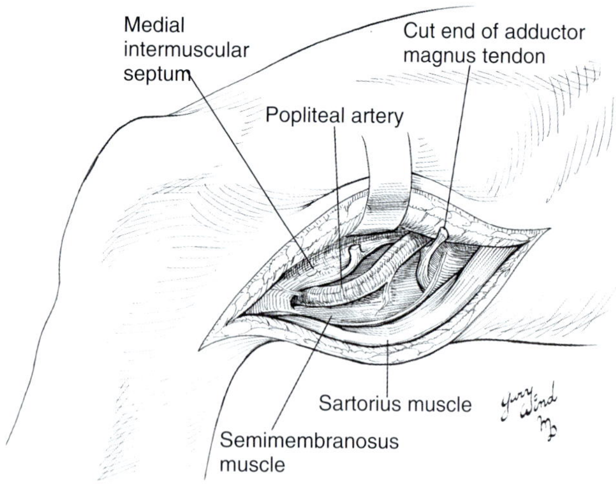

FIG 4.31 Medial Exposure of the Suprageniculate Popliteal Artery The fascia between the adductor magnus and intermuscular septum must be divided, and the adductor magnus tendon can be divided. (Reproduced with permission from Valentine RJ, Wind GG: Popliteal artery. In Brown B, McAvery M: *Anatomic exposures in vascular surgery*, Philadelphia, 2003, Lippincott Williams & Wilkins, p 446, © by RJ Valentine and GG Wind.)

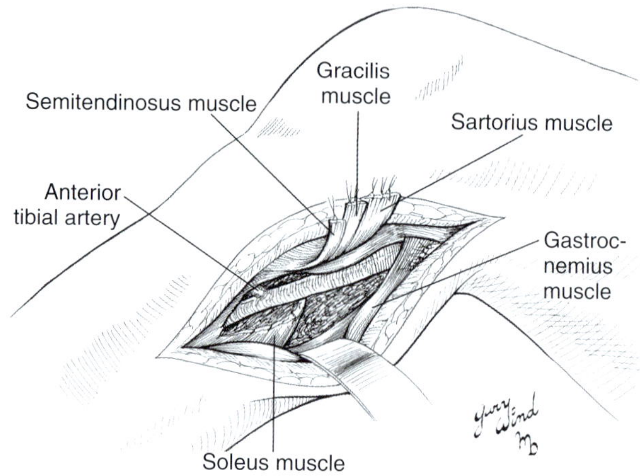

FIG 4.32 The tendons of the semitendinosus, gracilis, and sartorius muscles are divided, as well as the soleus muscle attachments to the tibia, to expose the infragenicular popliteal artery in the medial approach. (Reproduced with permission from Valentine RJ, Wind GG: Popliteal artery. In Brown B, McAvery M: *Anatomic exposures in vascular surgery*, Philadelphia, 2003, Lippincott Williams & Wilkins, p 453, © by RJ Valentine and GG Wind.)

less commonly from the lateral aspect, and the midpopliteal segment is typically approached from posteriorly through the popliteal fossa.

To isolate the proximal popliteal artery medially, an incision is made along the anterior border of the sartorius muscle. The sartorius muscle is retracted posterior and the vastus medialis muscle is the retracted anteriorly to expose a fascia to connect the adductor magnus and semimembranosus muscles together. Care must be taken to avoid injury to the saphenous vein during the skin incision and the saphenous nerve that overlies the deep fascia. The artery within the neurovascular bundle lies just posterior to the femur itself (Fig. 4.31).

Medial exposure of the distal popliteal artery is accomplished through an incision 1 to 2 cm behind the posteromedial aspect of the proximal tibia, with care taken to avoid the saphenous vein, which should be posterior to the incision. The fascia is incised and the gastrocnemius muscle is retracted posteriorly, and the semitendinosus, gracilis muscles in the proximal part of the exposure, and sartorius muscle in the distal part can be retracted anteriorly. If additional or wider exposure is required, the tendons of these muscles can be divided (Fig. 4.32). Within the popliteal neurovascular sheath, the vein is usually medial and encountered first. It can be retracted posteriorly to expose the artery.

Less commonly, the popliteal artery can be reached from the lateral approach, particularly in the setting of reoperation.[46] To expose the above-knee popliteal segment, an incision is made along the edge of the biceps femoris muscle and vastus muscles. The fascia lata is incised, and the biceps femoris muscle is retracted posteriorly, whereas the vastus muscle contained by the lateral intermuscular septum is retracted anteriorly. A thin layer of fascia connecting the hamstring to the femur must be divided, and the neurovascular bundle is just medial to this fascial layer. Of

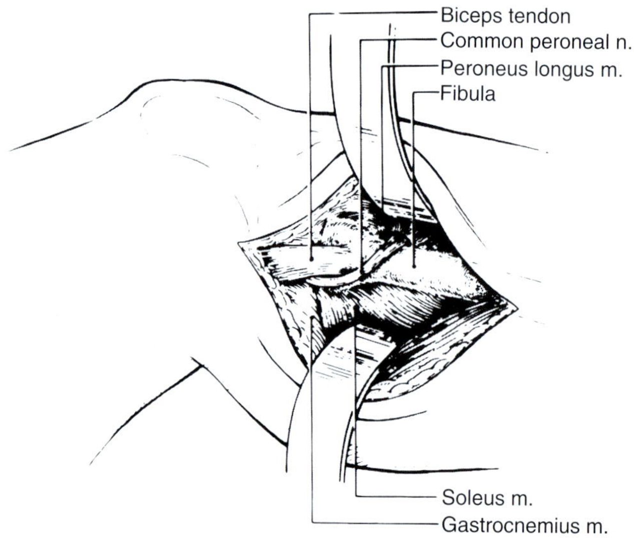

FIG 4.33 Lateral Approach to the Distal Popliteal Artery Note the common peroneal nerve coursing around the neck of the fibula. (From Veith F, Ascer E, Gupta S: Lateral approach to the popliteal artery, *J Vasc Surg* 6:119, 1987.)

note, the tibial and peroneal nerves are avoided because they are retracted posteriorly between the biceps femoral heads. To expose the below-knee segment, an incision is made over the fibular head and the biceps femoris muscle insertion is identified. The tendon is divided, protecting the common peroneal nerve as it courses over the fibular head (Fig. 4.33). The upper third of the fibula is cleared with periosteal elevators, and the bone shaft is resected. Once the bone is removed, the distal popliteal artery and tibioperoneal trunk can be seen and isolated (Fig. 4.34).[46]

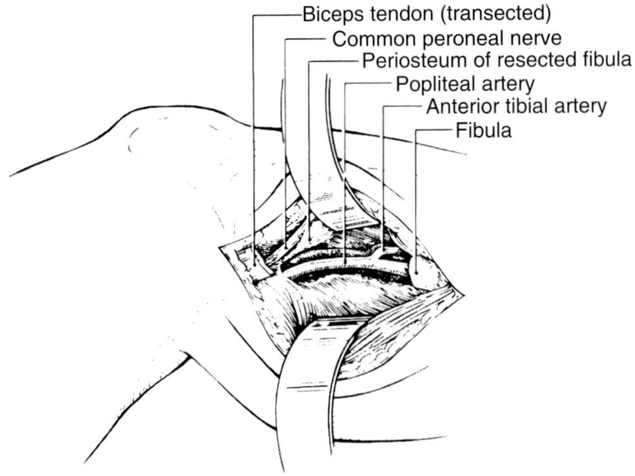

FIG 4.34 Lateral approach to the distal popliteal artery and tibioperoneal trunk after removal of the proximal fibula. Note the transected tendon of the biceps muscle and the intact common peroneal nerve. (From Veith F, Ascer E, Gupta S: Lateral approach to the popliteal artery, *J Vasc Surg* 6:119, 1987.)

Lastly, the posterior approach to the midpopliteal artery can be used for isolated exposure of this middle segment of the artery with limited ability to expose the proximal and distal aspects. This approach is particularly useful in entrapment syndromes, aneurysms, reoperations, or other focal pathology.[47] Patients are placed in the prone position with an S-shaped incision across the popliteal fossa, starting from the posteromedial thigh. The small saphenous vein lies above the deep fascia and is ligated. Once the deep fascia is entered, the sural nerve is retracted laterally. The tibial nerve is the first major structure of the neurovascular bundle which is encountered. The peroneal nerve can be found superiorly within the field but runs laterally along the biceps femoris insertion. Both nerves can be retracted laterally. Deep to the tibial nerve, the popliteal artery and vein are seen within its sheath, with the artery typically medial and deep to the vein (Fig. 4.35).

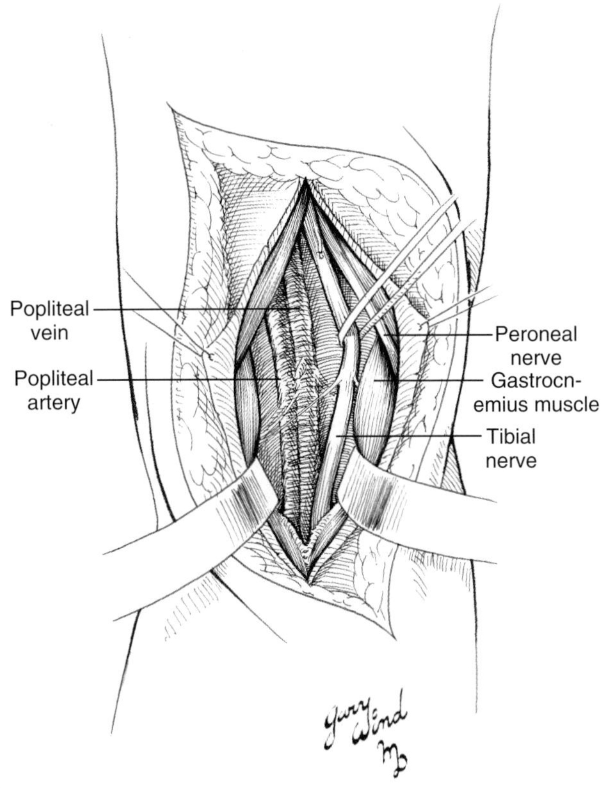

FIG 4.35 Through an S-shaped incision in the popliteal fossa, the tibial nerve is the first structure encountered and retracted laterally to expose the popliteal artery. (Reproduced with permission from Valentine RJ, Wind GG: Popliteal artery. In Brown B, McAvery M: *Anatomic exposures in vascular surgery*, Philadelphia, 2003, Lippincott Williams & Wilkins, p 465, © by RJ Valentine and GG Wind.)

EXPOSURE OF THE ANTERIOR TIBIAL ARTERY

The anterior tibial artery runs at the deep apex of the anterior compartment over the interosseous membrane (Fig. 4.36). Exposure is performed by making a longitudinal incision in the anterolateral aspect of the proximal leg, approximately 2 cm lateral to the tibia. The muscles encountered are the anterior tibial muscle anteriorly, and the extensor hallicus longus and extensor digitorum longus muscles laterally. As the plane between these muscles is developed, the anterior tibial neurovascular bundle is exposed, containing two accompanying veins, the deep peroneal nerve and the anterior tibial artery.

Distally the artery and deep peroneal nerve will run between the medial anterior tibial tendon and the lateral extensor hallicus longus tendon. At the ankle the artery and nerve pass medially to laterally deep to the extensor hallucis tendon and emerge between the extensor digitorum and hallicus tendons. The superior extensor retinaculum can be divided to provide additional mobility of the tendons. As the artery passes beneath the inferior extensor retinaculum, it becomes the dorsalis pedis artery.

EXPOSURE OF THE POSTERIOR TIBIAL ARTERY

The posterior tibial artery comes off of the tibioperoneal trunk approximately 2 cm distal to the takeoff of the anterior tibial artery from the popliteal artery.[48] The posterior tibial artery runs in the deep compartment behind the tibia alongside the tibial nerve and a host of venous tributaries (see Fig. 4.36). The same incision for exposure of the distal popliteal artery can be used to expose the tibioperoneal trunk and the proximal posterior tibial artery. Once the deep fascia has been incised, the gastrocnemius muscle is retracted posteriorly and the soleus muscle is released off the posterior tibia to expose the neurovascular bundle. The artery will run between the posterior tibial and flexor digitorum longus muscles, with the tibial nerve deep to the artery.

Exposure of more distal posterior tibial artery is similar with the soleus muscle released and retracted and the artery against the flexor digitorum longus muscle. In the distal third of the leg, an incision medial to the calcaneal tendon exposes the posterior tibial neurovascular bundle with the posterior tibial artery and tibial nerve between the flexor digitorum longus and flexor hallicus longus muscles.

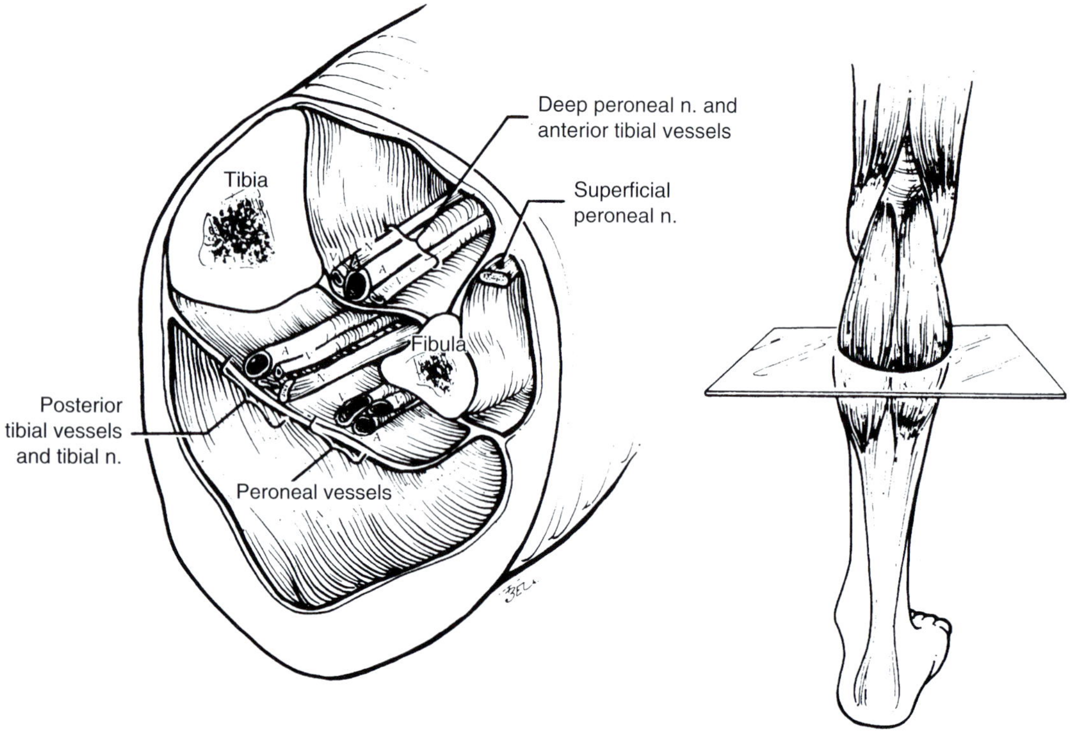

FIG 4.36 Cross-section of the leg showing the location of the anterior tibial artery in the anterior compartment of the leg and the posterior tibial and peroneal arteries in the deep posterior compartment. (From Briggs S, Seligson D: Management of extremity trauma. In Richardson D, Polk H, Flint M, editors: *Trauma: clinical care and pathophysiology*, Chicago, 1987, Year Book Medical, p 544.)

EXPOSURE OF THE PERONEAL ARTERY

The peroneal artery also runs in the deep compartment of the leg, along the medial aspect of the fibula, and it courses deeper into the leg along the interosseous membrane (see Fig. 4.36). Using the same exposure for the posterior tibial artery, the peroneal artery is situated deeper along the intermuscular septum. The soleus is taken down and retracted posteriorly along with the posterior tibial neurovascular bundle. The plane of dissection is carried deeper with the peroneal artery running on the anterior surface of the flexor hallicus longus muscle, posterior to the septum.

From the lateral aspect, similar to the lateral exposure of the popliteal artery, the fibula can be resected to expose the peroneal artery.[49]

REVIEW QUESTIONS

1. Which of the following nerves has the highest incidence of injury during carotid endarterectomy?
   a. Recurrent laryngeal nerve
   b. Hypoglossal nerve
   c. Superior laryngeal nerve
   d. Glossopharyngeal nerve
2. Regarding carotid artery exposure, all of the following are true except:
   a. The distal internal carotid artery is crossed anteriorly by the hypoglossal nerve.
   b. The vagus nerve passes posterolateral to the carotid bifurcation.
   c. Distal exposure is safely facilitated by anterior dislocation of the mandible.
   d. Distal exposure may be facilitated by division of the posterior belly of the digastric muscle and the stylohyoid muscle.
3. Exposure of the origin of the left subclavian artery is best achieved through a:
   a. Median sternotomy
   b. Left posterolateral thoracotomy
   c. Left anterolateral thoracotomy
   d. Left infraclavicular incision
4. During repair of an infrarenal abdominal aortic aneurysm, all of the following statements are true except:
   a. Autonomic nerve fibers crossing the left common iliac artery should be protected to preserve erectile function.

   b. A large anastomotic artery appearing on arteriography between the superior and inferior mesenteric arteries indicates satisfactory perfusion of the left colon with little risk of ischemia if the inferior mesenteric artery is ligated.
   c. A large lumbar artery near the renal arteries should be preserved, if possible, because this may represent a significant contribution to the anterior spinal artery.
   d. Skeletonization of the left common iliac artery increases the risk of retrograde ejaculation and/or sexual dysfunction.
5. During the dissection of the popliteal artery from the posterior approach, which of the following anatomic relationships is usually correct?
   a. The peroneal nerve runs medial to the popliteal artery.
   b. The tibial nerve is superficial to the popliteal artery.
   c. The popliteal artery is superficial to the popliteal vein.
   d. The tibial nerve runs deep to the popliteus muscle.
6. Which of the following nerves are at risk of injury during exposure of the brachial artery at the antecubital fossa?
   a. Radial nerve
   b. Ulnar nerve
   c. Musculocutaneous nerve
   d. Median nerve
7. Which of the following anatomic relationships is incorrect?
   a. The anterior tibial artery runs in the anterior compartment of the leg.
   b. The peroneal artery runs in the deep posterior compartment of the leg.
   c. The popliteal artery begins as it emerges from the inguinal ligament.
   d. The deep femoral artery travels along the medial aspect of the femur.
8. All of the following vascular relationships are usually correct except:
   a. The right renal artery passes posterior to the inferior vena cava.
   b. The left renal vein runs anterior to the superior mesenteric artery.
   c. The common facial vein typically runs superficial to the carotid artery bifurcation.
   d. The right common iliac artery passes anterior to the left common iliac vein.
9. Which of the following anatomic segments is correct?
   a. Zone 3 of the carotid artery is between the sternal notch and hyoid bone.
   b. V2 of the vertebral artery runs within the transverse foramen.
   c. The first part of the axillary artery is posterior to the pectoralis minor muscle.
   d. Zone 3 of the carotid artery is best approached through a supraclavicular incision.
10. In general, in the extremities, incisions should be made:
   a. Along the lines of Langerhans to reduce scarring
   b. Transversely
   c. Parallel to the course of the artery so they can be easily extended
   d. They should not be made. Modern vascular surgery can accomplish all therapies through endovascular means.

BIBLIOGRAPHY

Ballard JL. Anatomy and surgical exposure of the vascular system. In: Moore WS, ed. *Vascular and Endovascular Surgery: A Comprehensive Review*. 8th ed. Philadelphia: Elsevier; 2013.

Cronenwett JL, Johnston KW. *Rutherford's Vascular Surgery*. 7th ed. Philadelphia: Elsevier, Society of Vascular Surgery; 2010.

Rasmussen T, Tai N. *Rich's Vascular Trauma*. 3rd ed. Philadelphia: Elsevier, Society of Vascular Surgery; 2016.

Wind GG, Valentine RJ. *Anatomic Exposures in Vascular Surgery*. 3rd ed. Philadelphia: Wolters Kluwer; 2013.

References available online at ExpertConsult.com.

5 CHAPTER

Hemodynamics for the Vascular Surgeon

R. Eugene Zierler

Blood flow in human arteries and veins can be described in terms of hemodynamic principles that provide the theoretical foundation for the treatment of vascular disease. The major mechanisms of arterial disease are obstruction of the lumen and disruption of the vessel wall. The clinical significance of an obstructive arterial lesion depends on its location, severity, and duration, as well as on the ability of the circulation to compensate by increasing cardiac output and developing collateral pathways. Open surgical or endovascular treatment requires the identification and correction of arterial lesions associated with significant hemodynamic disturbances. Disruption of the arterial wall occurs with ruptured aneurysms or trauma. The tendency of aneurysms to rupture is determined by characteristics of the arterial wall, intraluminal pressure, and size. In this situation, the role of surgical intervention is to prevent rupture or to control hemorrhage and reestablish arterial continuity.

On the venous side of the circulation, the major hemodynamic mechanisms of disease are obstruction and valvular incompetence. These are generally the sequelae of thrombosis in the deep venous system, and they produce venous hypertension distal to the involved venous segment. The clinical consequences of venous hypertension are the signs and symptoms of the postthrombotic syndrome: pain, edema, subcutaneous fibrosis, pigmentation, stasis dermatitis, and ulceration. Treatment of this condition involves elevation, external compression, venous interruption, and, rarely, direct venous interventions.

This chapter begins with a discussion of the hemodynamic principles and vessel wall properties that govern arterial flow. The hemodynamic alterations produced by arterial stenoses and their effect on flow patterns in human limbs are considered next. These principles are then related to the treatment of arterial obstruction. Finally, the hemodynamics of the venous system are briefly reviewed and related to the pathophysiology and treatment of venous disease.

BASIC PRINCIPLES OF ARTERIAL HEMODYNAMICS

Fluid Pressure

The pressure in a fluid system is defined as force per unit area and expressed in units such as dynes per square centimeter (dyn/cm^2) or millimeters of mercury (mm Hg). Intravascular arterial pressure *(P)* has three components: (1) the dynamic pressure produced by contraction of the heart, (2) the hydrostatic pressure, and (3) the static filling pressure. Hydrostatic pressure is determined by the specific gravity of blood and the height of the point of measurement above a specific reference level. The reference level in the human body is considered to be the right atrium. The hydrostatic pressure is given by the following equation:

$$P(\text{hydrostatic}) = -\rho g h \qquad \textbf{[Equation 5.1]}$$

where ρ is the specific gravity of blood (approximately 1.056 g/cm^3), g is the acceleration due to gravity (980 cm/s^2), and h is the distance in centimeters above or below the right atrium. The magnitude of hydrostatic pressure may be large. In a man 5 feet 8 inches tall, this pressure at ankle level is around 89 mm Hg.[1] The static filling pressure represents the residual pressure that exists in the absence of arterial flow. This pressure is determined by the volume of blood and the elastic properties of the vessel wall, and it is typically in the range of 5 to 10 mm Hg.

Fluid Energy

Blood flows through the arterial system in response to differences in total fluid energy. Although pressure gradients are the most obvious forces involved, other forms of energy drive the circulation.[2] Total fluid energy *(E)* can be divided into potential energy (E_p) and kinetic energy (E_k). The components of potential energy are intravascular pressure *(P)* and gravitational potential energy.

The factors contributing to intravascular pressure are described in the preceding text. Gravitational potential energy represents the ability of a volume of blood to do work because of its height above a specific reference level. The formula for gravitational potential energy is the same as that for hydrostatic pressure (see Eq. 5.1) but with an opposite sign: $+\rho gh$. Because the gravitational potential energy and hydrostatic pressure usually cancel each other out and the static filling pressure is relatively low, the predominant component of potential energy is the dynamic pressure produced by cardiac contraction. Potential energy can be expressed as follows:

$$E_p = P + (\rho g h) \qquad \textbf{[Equation 5.2]}$$

Kinetic energy represents the ability of blood to do work on the basis of its motion. It is proportional to the specific gravity of blood and the square of blood velocity *(v)*, in centimeters per second:

$$E_k = \tfrac{1}{2}\rho v^2 \qquad \textbf{[Equation 5.3]}$$

By combining Eqs. 5.2 and 5.3, an expression for the total fluid energy per unit volume of blood (in ergs per cubic centimeter) can be obtained:

$$E = P + \rho gh + \tfrac{1}{2}\rho v^2 \quad \textbf{[Equation 5.4]}$$

Fluid Energy Losses

Bernoulli's Principle

When fluid flows from one point to another, its total energy *(E)* along any given streamline is constant provided that flow is steady and there are no frictional energy losses. This is in accordance with the law of conservation of energy and constitutes Bernoulli's principle:

$$P_1 + \rho gh_1 + \tfrac{1}{2}\rho v_1^2 = P_2 + \rho gh_2 + \tfrac{1}{2}\rho v_2^2 \quad \textbf{[Equation 5.5]}$$

This equation expresses the relationships among pressure, gravitational potential energy, and kinetic energy in an idealized fluid system. In the horizontal diverging tube shown in Fig. 5.1, steady flow between point 1 and point 2 is accompanied by an increase in cross-sectional area and a decrease in flow velocity. Although the fluid moves against a pressure gradient of 2.5 mm Hg and therefore gains potential energy, the total fluid energy remains constant because of the lower velocity and a proportional loss of kinetic energy. In other words, the widening of the tube results in the conversion of kinetic energy to potential energy in the form of pressure. In a converging tube, the opposite would occur; a pressure drop and increase in velocity would result in potential energy being converted to kinetic energy.

The situation depicted in the preceding example is not observed in human arteries because the ideal flow conditions specified in the Bernoulli relationship are not present. The fluid energy lost in moving blood through the arterial circulation is dissipated mainly in the form of heat. When this source of energy loss is accounted for, Eq. 5.5 becomes the following:

$$P_1 + \rho gh_1 + \tfrac{1}{2}\rho v_1^2 = P_2 + \rho gh_2 + \tfrac{1}{2}\rho v_2^2 + \text{heat} \quad \textbf{[Equation 5.6]}$$

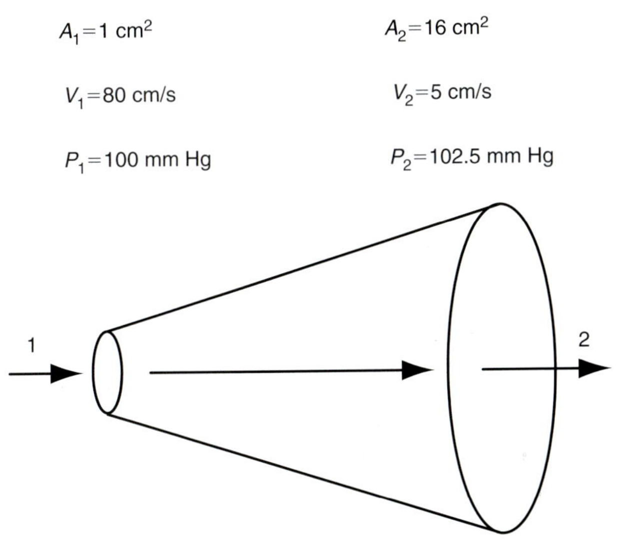

FIG 5.1 Effect of Increasing Cross-sectional Area on Pressure in a Frictionless Fluid System. While pressure increases, total fluid energy remains constant as a result of a decrease in velocity. (Redrawn from Sumner DS: The hemodynamics and pathophysiology of arterial disease. In Rutherford RB, editor: *Vascular Surgery*, Philadelphia, 1977, WB Saunders.)

Viscous Energy Losses and Poiseuille's Law

Energy losses in flowing blood occur either as viscous losses resulting from friction or as inertial losses related to changes in the velocity or direction of flow. The term *viscosity* describes the resistance to flow that arises because of the intermolecular attractions between fluid layers. The coefficient of viscosity (η) is defined as the ratio of shear stress (τ) to shear rate (D):

$$\eta = \frac{\tau}{D} \quad \textbf{[Equation 5.7]}$$

Shear stress is proportional to the energy loss resulting from friction between adjacent fluid layers, whereas shear rate is the relative velocity of adjacent fluid layers. Fluids with particularly strong intermolecular attractions offer a high resistance to flow and have high coefficients of viscosity. For example, motor oil has a higher coefficient of viscosity than water.[3] The unit of viscosity is the poise, which equals 1 dyne-s/cm². Because it is difficult to measure viscosity directly, relative viscosity is often used to relate the viscosity of a fluid to that of water. The relative viscosity of plasma is approximately 1.8, whereas the relative viscosity of whole blood is in the range of 3 to 4.

Because viscosity increases exponentially with increases in hematocrit, the concentration of red blood cells is the most important factor affecting the viscosity of whole blood. The viscosity of plasma is determined largely by the concentration of plasma proteins. These constituents of blood are also responsible for its non-Newtonian character. In a Newtonian fluid, viscosity is independent of shear rate or flow velocity. Because blood is a suspension of cells and large protein molecules, its viscosity can vary greatly with shear rate (Fig. 5.2). Blood viscosity increases rapidly at low shear rates but approaches a constant value at higher shear rates. In most of the arterial circulation, the prevailing shear rates place the blood viscosity on the asymptotic portion of the curve. Thus, for arteries with diameters greater than approximately 1 mm, human blood resembles a constant-viscosity or Newtonian fluid.

Poiseuille's law describes the viscous energy losses that occur in an idealized flow model. This law states that the pressure gradient along a tube ($P_1 - P_2$, in dynes per square centimeter) is directly proportional to the mean flow velocity ($\overline{V}$, in centimeters per second) or volume flow (*Q*, in cubic centimeters per second), the tube length (*L*, in centimeters), and the fluid viscosity (η, in poise) and is inversely proportional to either the second or fourth power of the radius (*r*, in centimeters):

$$P_1 - P_2 = \overline{V}\frac{8L\eta}{r^2} = Q\frac{8L\eta}{\pi r^4} \quad \textbf{[Equation 5.8]}$$

When this equation is simplified to Pressure = flow × resistance, it is analogous to Ohm's law of electrical circuits.

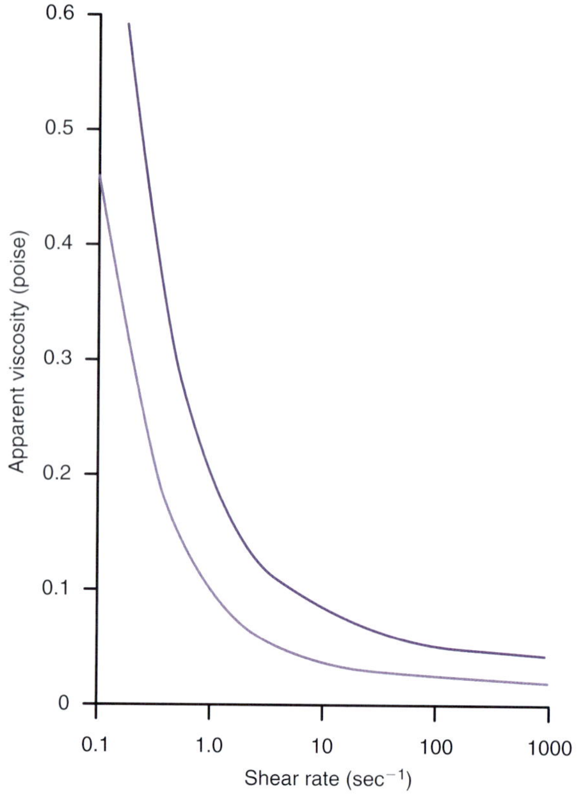

FIG 5.2 Viscosity of Human Blood as a Function of Shear Rate. Values range between the two lines. (From Strandness DE, Sumner DS: *Hemodynamics for Surgeons*, New York, 1975, Grune and Stratton.)

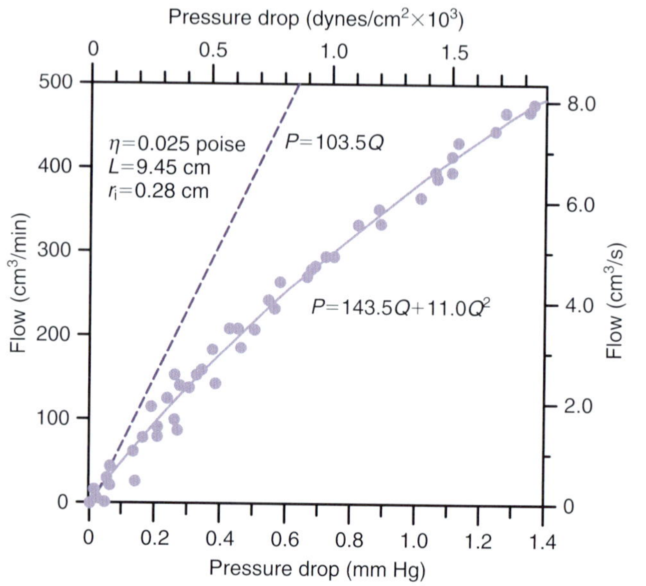

FIG 5.3 Pressure Drop Across a 9.45-cm Length of Canine Femoral Artery at Varying Flow Rates. The experimental data line *(solid)* has both linear and squared terms, corresponding to viscous and inertial energy losses. The pressure-flow curve predicted by Poiseuille's law *(dashed line)* depicts much lower energy losses than those actually observed. (From Sumner DS: The hemodynamics and pathophysiology of arterial disease. In Rutherford RB, editor: *Vascular Surgery*, Philadelphia, 1977, WB Saunders.)

The strict application of Poiseuille's law requires the steady, laminar flow of a Newtonian fluid in a straight, rigid, cylindrical tube. Because these conditions seldom exist in the arterial circulation, Poiseuille's law can only estimate the minimum pressure gradient or viscous energy losses that may be expected in arterial flow. Energy losses owing to inertial effects often exceed viscous energy losses, particularly in the presence of arterial disease.

Inertial Energy Losses

Energy losses related to inertia (ΔE) are proportional to a constant (K), the specific gravity of blood, and the square of blood velocity:

$$\Delta E = K \tfrac{1}{2} \rho v^2 \qquad \textbf{[Equation 5.9]}$$

Because velocity is the only independent variable in this equation, inertial energy losses result from the acceleration and deceleration of pulsatile flow, variations in lumen diameter, and changes in the direction of flow at points of curvature and branching. The combined effects of viscous and inertial energy losses are illustrated in Fig. 5.3. When the pressure drop across an arterial segment is measured at varying flow rates, the experimental data fit a line with both linear (viscous) and squared (inertial) terms. The viscous energy losses predicted by Poiseuille's law are considerably less than the total energy loss actually observed.

Vascular Resistance

Hemodynamic resistance (R) can be defined as the ratio of the energy drop between two points along an artery $(E_1 - E_2)$ to the mean blood flow (Q):

$$R = \frac{E_1 - E_2}{Q} \cong \frac{P_1 - P_2}{Q} \qquad \textbf{[Equation 5.10]}$$

Because the kinetic energy term $(\tfrac{1}{2}\rho v^2)$ is typically a small component of the total fluid energy and the artery is usually assumed to be horizontal so that the gravitational potential energy terms $(\rho g h)$ cancel, Eq. 5.4 can be used to express resistance as the simple ratio of pressure drop $(P_1 - P_2)$ to flow. Thus Eq. 5.10 becomes a rearranged version of Poiseuille's law (see Eq. 5.8), and the minimum resistance or viscous energy losses are given by the resistance term

$$R = \frac{8L\eta}{\pi r^4} \qquad \textbf{[Equation 5.11]}$$

The hemodynamic resistance of an arterial segment increases as the flow velocity increases, provided that the lumen size remains constant (Fig. 5.4). These additional energy losses are related to inertial effects and are proportional to $\tfrac{1}{2}\rho v^2$.

According to Eq. 5.11, the predominant factor influencing hemodynamic resistance is the fourth power of the radius. The relationship between radius and pressure drop for various flow rates along a 10-cm vessel segment is shown in Fig. 5.5. For a

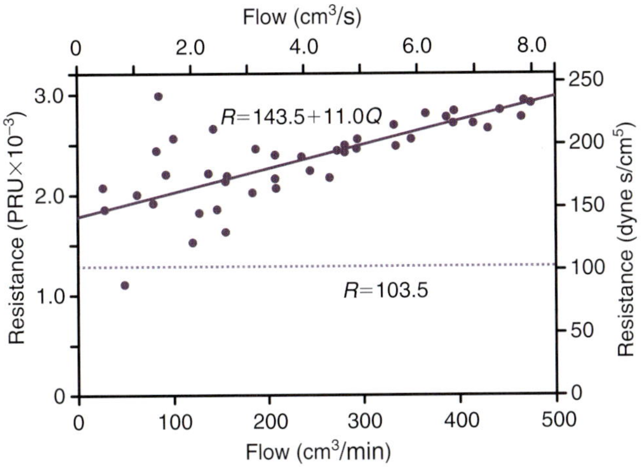

FIG 5.4 Resistance Derived from the Pressure-Flow Curve in Fig. 5.3. The resistance increases with increasing flow. Constant resistance predicted by Poiseuille's law is shown by the dotted line. *PRU,* Peripheral resistance unit. (From Sumner DS: The hemodynamics and pathophysiology of arterial disease. In Rutherford RB, editor: *Vascular Surgery*, Philadelphia, 1977, WB Saunders.)

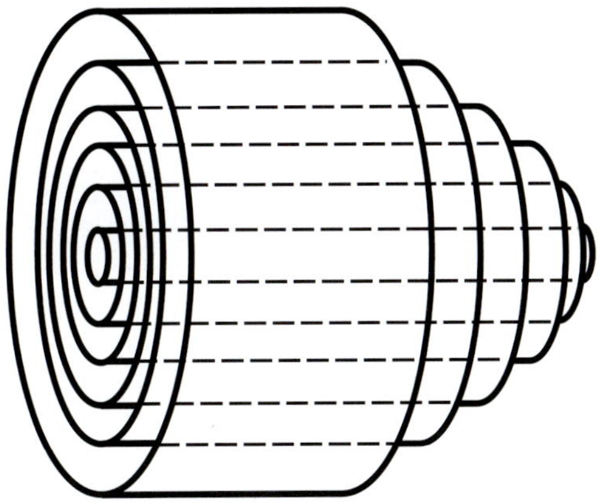

FIG 5.6 Concentric Laminae of Fluid in a Cylindrical Tube. Flow is from *left* to *right*. The *center* laminae move more rapidly than those near the periphery, and the flow profile is parabolic. (From Strandness DE, Sumner DS: *Hemodynamics for Surgeons*, New York, 1975, Grune and Stratton.)

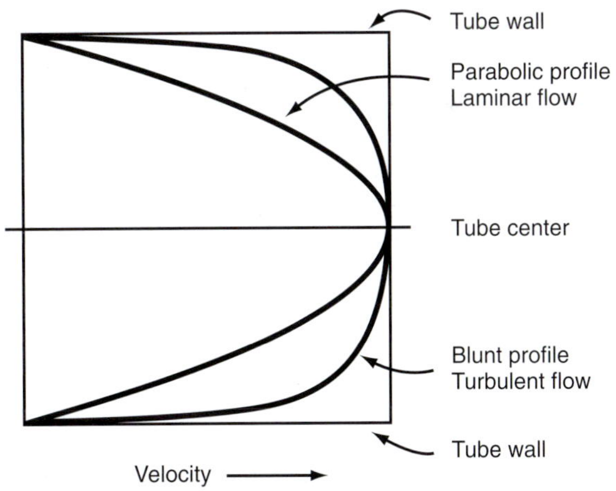

FIG 5.7 Velocity Profiles of Steady Laminar and Turbulent Flow. Velocity is lowest adjacent to the tube wall and maximal in the center. (From Sumner DS: The hemodynamics and pathophysiology of arterial disease. In Rutherford RB, editor: *Vascular Surgery*, Philadelphia, 1977, WB Saunders.)

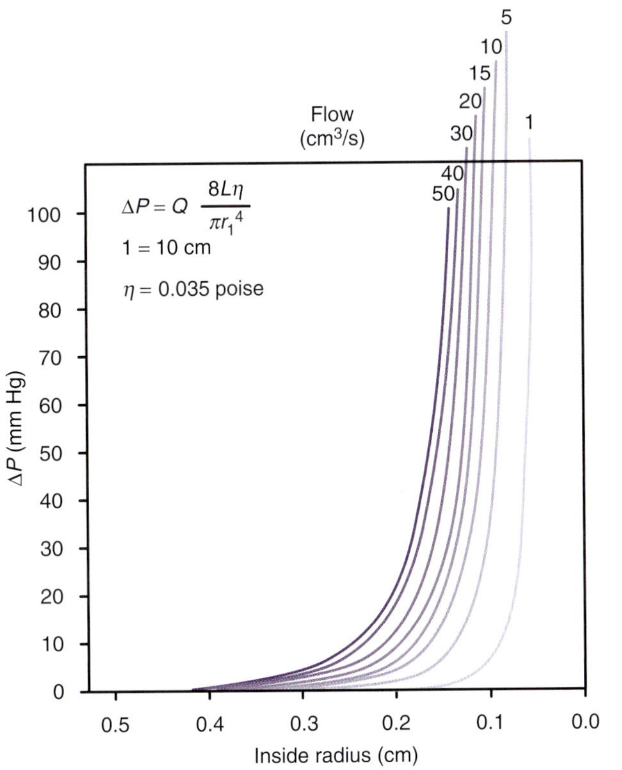

FIG 5.5 Relationship of Pressure Drop to the Inside Radius of a Cylindrical Tube 10 cm in Length at Various Rates of Steady Laminar Flow. Flow rates are comparable to those in the human iliac artery. (From Strandness DE, Sumner DS: *Hemodynamics for Surgeons*, New York, 1975, Grune and Stratton.)

wide range of flow rates, the pressure drop is negligible until the radius is reduced to approximately 0.3 cm; for radii less than 0.2 cm, the pressure drop increases rapidly. These observations may explain the frequent failure of femoropopliteal autogenous vein bypass grafts less than 4 mm in diameter.[4]

In the human circulation, approximately 90% of the total vascular resistance results from flow through the arteries and capillaries, whereas the remaining 10% results from venous flow. The arterioles and capillaries are responsible for more than 60% of the total resistance, whereas the large- and medium-sized arteries account for only about 15%.[2] Thus, the arteries that are most commonly affected by atherosclerotic occlusive disease are normally vessels with low resistance.

Blood Flow Patterns

Laminar Flow

In the steady-state conditions specified by Poiseuille's law, the flow pattern is laminar. All motion is parallel to the walls of the tube, and the fluid is arranged in a series of concentric layers, or laminae, like those shown in Fig. 5.6. While the velocity within each lamina remains constant, the velocity is lowest adjacent to the tube wall and increases toward the center of the tube. This results in a velocity profile that is parabolic in shape (Fig. 5.7).

As discussed previously, the energy expended in moving one lamina of fluid over another is proportional to viscosity.

Turbulent Flow

In contrast to the linear streamlines of laminar flow, turbulence is an irregular flow state in which velocity varies rapidly with respect to space and time. These random velocity changes result in the dissipation of fluid energy as heat. Although turbulent flow is uncommon in normal arteries, the arterial flow pattern is often disturbed.[5] The condition of disturbed flow is an intermediate state between stable laminar flow and fully developed turbulence. It is a transient perturbation in the laminar streamlines that disappears as the flow proceeds downstream. Arterial flow may become disturbed at points of branching and curvature.

When turbulence is the result of a stenotic arterial lesion, it generally occurs immediately downstream from the stenosis and may be present only over the systolic portion of the cardiac cycle when the velocities are highest. Under conditions of turbulent flow, the velocity profile changes from the parabolic shape of laminar flow to a rectangular or blunt shape (see Fig. 5.7). Because of the random velocity changes, energy losses are greater for a turbulent or disturbed flow state than for a laminar flow state. Consequently the linear relationship between pressure and flow expressed by Poiseuille's law cannot be applied. This deviation from Poiseuille's law in arterial flow is shown in Fig. 5.3.

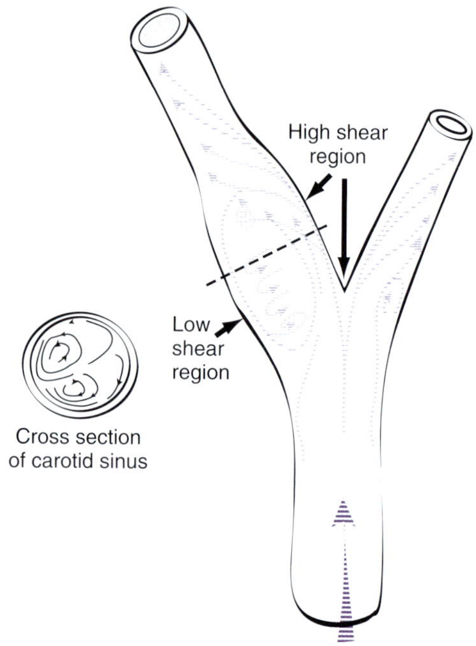

FIG 5.8 **Carotid Artery Bifurcation Showing an Area of Flow Separation Adjacent to the Outer Wall of the Bulb.** Rapid flow is associated with high shear stress, whereas the slower flow of the separation zone produces a region of low shear. (From Zarins CK, Giddens DP, Glagov S: Atherosclerotic plaque distribution and flow velocity profiles in the carotid bifurcation. In Bergan JJ, Yao JST, editors: *Cerebrovascular Insufficiency*, New York, 1983, Grune and Stratton.)

Boundary Layer Separation

In fluid flowing through a tube, the portion of fluid adjacent to the tube wall is referred to as the *boundary layer*. This layer is subject to both frictional interactions with the tube wall and viscous forces generated by the more rapidly moving fluid toward the center of the tube. When the tube geometry changes suddenly, as at points of curvature, branching, or variations in lumen diameter, small pressure gradients are created that cause the boundary layer to stop or reverse direction. This change results in a complex, localized flow pattern known as an area of *boundary layer separation* or *flow separation*.[6]

Areas of boundary layer separation have been observed in models of arterial anastomoses and bifurcations.[7,8] In the carotid artery bifurcation shown in Fig. 5.8, the central rapid flow stream of the common carotid artery is compressed along the inner wall of the carotid bulb, producing a region of high shear stress. An area of flow separation has formed along the outer wall of the carotid bulb that includes helical flow patterns and flow reversal. The region of the carotid bulb adjacent to the separation zone is subject to relatively low shear stresses. Distal to the bulb, in the internal carotid artery, flow reattachment occurs and a more laminar flow pattern is present.

The complex flow patterns described in models of the carotid bifurcation have also been documented in human subjects by pulsed Doppler studies.[9,10] As shown in Fig. 5.9, the Doppler spectral waveform obtained near the inner wall of the carotid bulb is typical of the forward flow pattern found in the internal carotid artery. However, sampling of flow along the outer wall of the bulb demonstrates lower velocities with periods of both forward and reverse flow. These spectral characteristics are consistent with the presence of flow separation and are considered to be a normal finding, particularly in young individuals.[10] Alterations in arterial distensibility with increasing age make flow separation less prominent in older individuals.[11]

The clinical importance of boundary layer separation is that these localized flow disturbances may contribute to the formation of atherosclerotic plaques.[12] Examination of human carotid bifurcations, both at autopsy and during surgery, indicates that intimal thickening and atherosclerosis tend to occur along the outer wall of the carotid bulb, whereas the inner wall is relatively spared.[8] These findings suggest that atherosclerotic lesions form near areas of flow separation and low shear stress.

Pulsatile Flow

In a pulsatile system, pressure and flow vary continuously with time and the velocity profile changes throughout the cardiac cycle. The hemodynamic principles already discussed are based on steady flow, and they are not adequate for a precise description of pulsatile flow in the arterial circulation; however, as previously stated, they can be used to determine the minimum energy losses occurring in a specific flow system. The resistance term of Poiseuille's law (see Eq. 5.11) estimates viscous energy losses in steady flow, but it does not account for the inertial effects, arterial wall elasticity, and wave reflections that influence pulsatile flow. The term *vascular impedance* is used to describe the resistance or opposition offered by a peripheral vascular bed to pulsatile blood flow.[3]

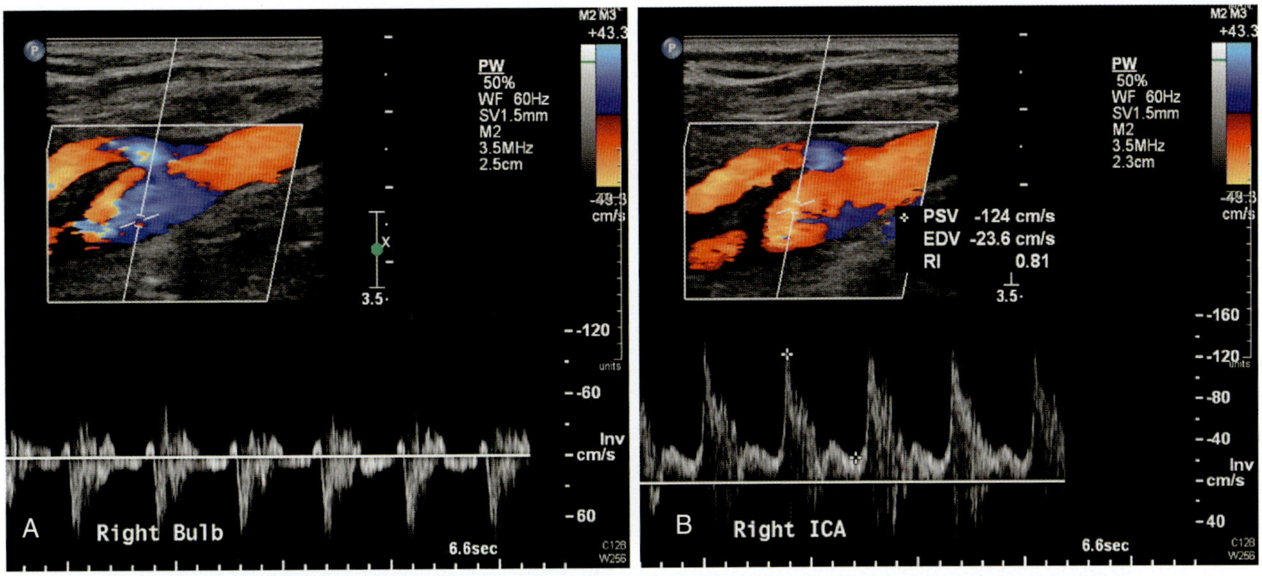

FIG 5.9 Flow Separation in the Normal Carotid Bulb as Shown by Duplex Scanning With Spectral Waveform Analysis. (A) The waveform obtained with the pulsed Doppler sample volume positioned near the outer wall the bulb includes both forward and reverse flow components and relatively low velocities, indicating an area of flow separation. (B) When the sample volume is placed near the inner wall of the internal carotid artery *(ICA)*, the waveform shows predominantly forward flow and higher velocities.

Pulsatile flow appears to be important for optimal organ function. For example, when a kidney is perfused by steady flow instead of pulsatile flow, a reduction in urine volume and sodium excretion occurs.[13] The critical effect of pulsatile flow is probably exerted on the microcirculation. Although the exact mechanism is unknown, transcapillary exchange, arteriolar tone, and lymphatic flow are all influenced by the pulsatile nature of blood flow.

Bifurcations and Branches

The branches of the arterial system produce sudden changes in the flow pattern that are potential sources of energy loss. However, the effect of branching on the total pressure drop in normal arterial flow is relatively small. Arterial branches commonly take the form of bifurcations. Flow patterns in a bifurcation are determined mainly by the area ratio and the branch angle. The area ratio is defined as the combined area of the secondary branches divided by the area of the primary artery.

Bifurcation flow can be analyzed in terms of pressure gradient, velocity, and transmission of pulsatile energy. According to Poiseuille's law, an area ratio of 1.41 would allow the pressure gradient to remain constant along a bifurcation. If the combined area of the branches equals the area of the primary artery, the area ratio is 1.0, and there is no change in the velocity of flow.[14] For efficient transmission of pulsatile energy across a bifurcation, the vascular impedance of the primary artery should equal that of the branches, a situation that occurs with an area ratio of 1.15 for larger arteries and 1.35 for smaller arteries.[15] Human infants have a favorable area ratio of 1.11 at the aortic bifurcation, but there is a gradual decrease in the ratio with age. In the teenage years, the average area ratio is less than 1.0; in the 20s, it is less than 0.9; and by the 40s, it drops below 0.8.[16] This decline in the area ratio of the aortic bifurcation leads to an increase in both the velocity of flow in the secondary branches and the amount of reflected pulsatile energy. For example, with an area ratio of 0.8, approximately 22% of the incident pulsatile energy is reflected in the infrarenal aorta. This mechanism may play a role in the localization of atherosclerosis and aneurysms in this arterial segment.[17]

The curvature and angulation of an arterial bifurcation can also contribute to the development of flow disturbances. As blood flows around a curve, the high-velocity portion of the stream is subjected to the greatest centrifugal force; rapidly moving fluid in the center of the vessel tends to flow outward and be replaced by the slower fluid originally located near the arterial wall. This can result in complex helical flow patterns, such as those observed in the carotid bifurcation.[9] As the angle between the secondary branches of a bifurcation is increased, the tendency to develop turbulent or disturbed flow also increases. The average angle between the human iliac arteries is 54 degrees; however, with diseased or tortuous iliac arteries, this angle can approach 180 degrees.[3] In the latter situation, flow disturbances are particularly likely to develop.

Tangential Stress and Tension

The tangential stress (τ) within the wall of a fluid-filled cylindrical tube can be expressed as follows:

$$\tau = P\frac{r}{\delta} \qquad \text{[Equation 5.12]}$$

where P is the pressure exerted by the fluid (in dynes per square centimeter), r is the internal radius (in centimeters), and δ is the thickness of the tube wall (in centimeters). Stress (τ) has the dimensions of force per unit area of tube wall (dynes per square centimeter). Thus tangential stress is directly proportional to pressure and radius but inversely proportional to wall thickness.

Eq. 5.12 is similar to Laplace's law, which defines tangential tension (T) as the product of pressure and radius:

$$T = Pr \qquad \textbf{[Equation 5.13]}$$

Tension is given in units of force per tube length (dynes per centimeter). The terms *stress* and *tension* have different dimensions and describe the forces acting on the tube wall in different ways. Laplace's law can be used to characterize thin-walled structures such as soap bubbles; however, it is not suitable for describing the stresses in arterial walls.

The Properties of Arterial Walls in Specific Conditions

Aging and atherosclerosis. Arterial walls become less distensible with age. This increase in stiffness cannot be explained on the basis of atherosclerosis alone.[3] Alterations in the elastin fibers and elastic lamellae, together with an increase in wall thickness, probably account for this increase in arterial stiffness. Changes associated with aging include fragmentation of elastic lamellae and deposition of collagen between the elastin layers. This tends to maintain the elastin fibers in the extended state. Calcium is also deposited near the elastin fibers and contributes to the increased thickness of the arterial wall.

The effects of atherosclerosis on the mechanical properties of the arterial wall are complex and difficult to distinguish from those caused by aging. In the early stages, arterial distensibility can actually increase as elastin fibers are disrupted; however, as the disease progresses, fibrosis and calcification tend to make the arterial wall less distensible.

Endarterectomy. During an endarterectomy the atherosclerotic plaque is removed, along with the intima and a portion of the media, leaving behind a tube consisting of the outer media and adventitia. This reduces the wall thickness to approximately one-third of its original value and, according to Eq. 5.12, should result in an increase in tangential stress. As would be expected, endarterectomy decreases the stiffness of an artery to circumferential expansion.[18] Still, the endarterectomized artery remains stiffer and less distensible than a normal artery; this indicates that the components responsible for strength and stiffness are concentrated in the outer layers of the arterial wall. It is because of this anatomic arrangement that endarterectomy is possible.

Aneurysms. When the structural components of the arterial wall are weakened, aneurysms can form. Rupture occurs when the tangential stress within the arterial wall becomes greater than the tensile strength. Fig. 5.10 shows a tube with an outside diameter of 2 cm and a wall thickness of 0.2 cm, dimensions similar to those of atherosclerotic aortas.[1] If the internal pressure is 150 mm Hg, the tangential wall stress is 8.0×10^5 dynes/cm^2. Expansion of the tube to form an aneurysm with a diameter of 6 cm results in a decrease in wall thickness to 0.06 cm. The increased radius and decreased wall thickness increase the wall

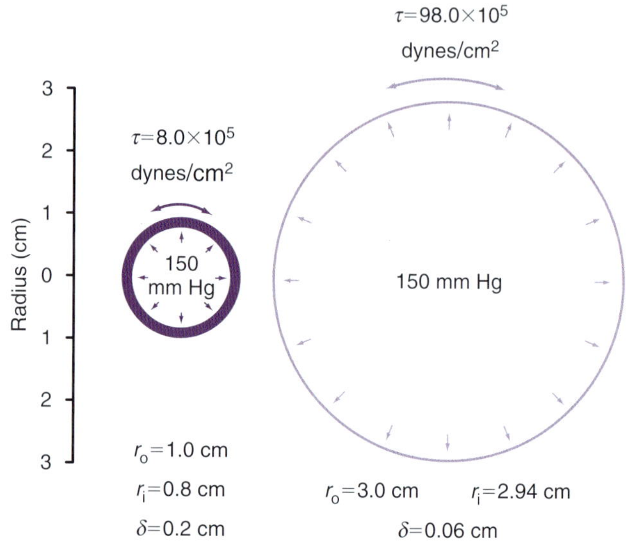

FIG 5.10 End-on view of a cylinder 2 cm in diameter that is expanded to 6 cm in diameter while the wall area remains constant. δ, Wall thickness; r_i, inside radius; r_o, outside radius; τ, tangential wall stress. (From Sumner DS: The hemodynamics and pathophysiology of arterial disease. In Rutherford RB, editor: *Vascular Surgery*, Philadelphia, 1977, WB Saunders.)

stress to 98.0×10^5 dynes/cm^2, assuming that the pressure remains constant. In this example, the diameter has been enlarged by a factor of 3, and the wall stress has increased by a factor of 12.

Although the tensile strength of collagen is extremely high, it constitutes only approximately 15% of the aneurysm wall.[19] Furthermore, the collagen fibers in an aneurysm are sparsely distributed and subject to fragmentation. The tendency of larger aneurysms to rupture is readily explained by the effect of increased radius on tangential stress (see Eq. 5.12) and the degenerative changes in the arterial wall. The relationship between tangential stress and blood pressure accounts for the contribution of hypertension to the risk of rupture.

The diverging and converging geometry of aneurysms can result in complex flow patterns that include areas of boundary layer separation and flow reversal.[20] These patterns explain the frequent accumulation of thrombus in aneurysms, which often confines the flow stream to an area not much larger than that of the native artery. Because this thrombus increases the effective thickness of the vessel wall, it may reduce tangential stress and provide some protection against rupture. However, the tensile strength of thrombus and arterial wall are different, and the contribution of thrombus to the integrity of an aneurysm is impossible to predict.[3] Furthermore, the thrombus within an aneurysm is often not circumferential. In this situation, Eq. 5.12 can be applied to the wall segment without thrombus, and the tangential stress at that site depends on the maximum internal radius.

Another factor to consider is that in approximately 55% of ruptured abdominal aortic aneurysms, the site of rupture is in the posterolateral aspect of the aneurysm wall.[21] The posterior wall of the aorta is relatively fixed against the spine, and repeated flexion of the wall in that area can result in structural fatigue. Such fatigue would produce a localized area of weakness that might predispose to rupture.

HEMODYNAMICS OF ARTERIAL STENOSIS

Energy Losses

According to Poiseuille's law (see Eq. 5.8), the radius of a stenotic segment has a much greater effect on viscous energy losses than its length. Inertial energy losses, which occur at the entrance (contraction effects) and exit (expansion effects) of a stenosis, are proportional to the square of blood velocity (see Eq. 5.9). Energy losses are also influenced by the geometry of a stenosis; a gradual tapering results in less energy loss than an irregular or abrupt change in luminal size. A converging vessel geometry tends to stabilize laminar flow and flatten the velocity profile, whereas a diverging vessel produces an elongated velocity profile and a less stable flow pattern.

Fig. 5.11 illustrates the energy losses related to a stenosis 1 cm long. The viscous losses are relatively small and occur within the stenotic segment. Inertial losses resulting from contraction and expansion are much greater. The energy lost at the exit of a stenosis can be significant because of the sudden expansion of the flow stream and dissipation of kinetic energy in a zone of turbulence. Because most of the energy loss in this example results from inertial effects, the length of the stenosis is relatively unimportant.[1]

Bruits and Poststenotic Dilatation

The presence of an audible sound or bruit over an artery is usually regarded as a clinical sign of arterial disease. Stenoses or irregularities of the vessel lumen produce turbulent flow patterns that set up vibrations in the arterial wall. These vibrations generate displacement waves that radiate through the surrounding tissues and can be detected as audible sounds. Such vibrations are probably the main source of sound in the arterial system.[3] Generally, a soft, midsystolic bruit is associated with a relatively minor lesion that does not significantly reduce flow or pressure. A bruit with a loud diastolic component suggests a stenosis severe enough to reduce flow and produce a pressure drop. A bruit may be absent when an artery is nearly occluded or when the flow rate is extremely low.

A dilated area distal to a stenosis is a common clinical finding. Poststenotic dilation has been observed in the thoracic aorta below coarctations, distal to arterial stenoses at the thoracic outlet, and distal to atherosclerotic lesions. The most likely explanation for this phenomenon is that arterial wall vibrations result in structural fatigue of elastin fibers. In a series of animal model studies, poststenotic dilatations did not develop unless a bruit was present distal to the stenosis.[22] It appears that vibrations in the audible range may weaken elastin fibers and break down links between collagen fibers. When this occurs, the arterial wall distal to the stenosis becomes more distensible and subject to localized dilatation.

Critical Arterial Stenosis

The degree of arterial narrowing required to produce a significant reduction in blood pressure or flow is called a *critical stenosis*. Because the energy losses associated with a stenosis are inversely proportional to the fourth power of the radius at that site (see Eq. 5.8), there is an exponential relationship between energy loss (pressure drop) and reduction in lumen size. When this relationship is illustrated graphically, the curves have a single sharp bend (Fig. 5.12; also see Fig. 5.5). These

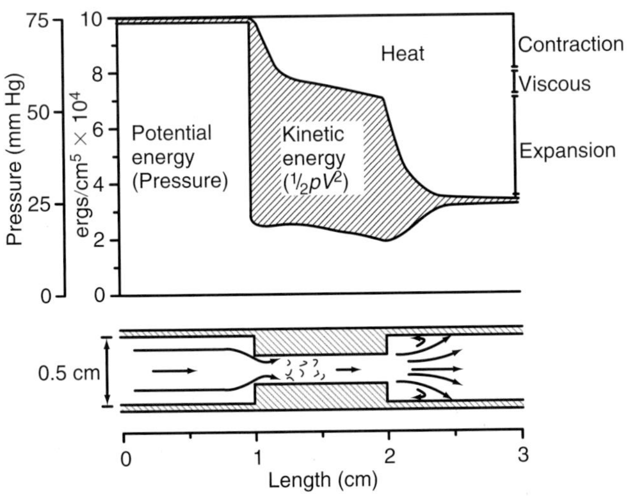

FIG 5.11 Energy losses resulting when blood flows steadily through a stenosis 1 cm in length. Inertial losses (contraction and expansion) are much larger than viscous losses. (From Sumner DS: The hemodynamics and pathophysiology of arterial disease. In Rutherford RB, editor: *Vascular Surgery*, Philadelphia, 1977, WB Saunders.)

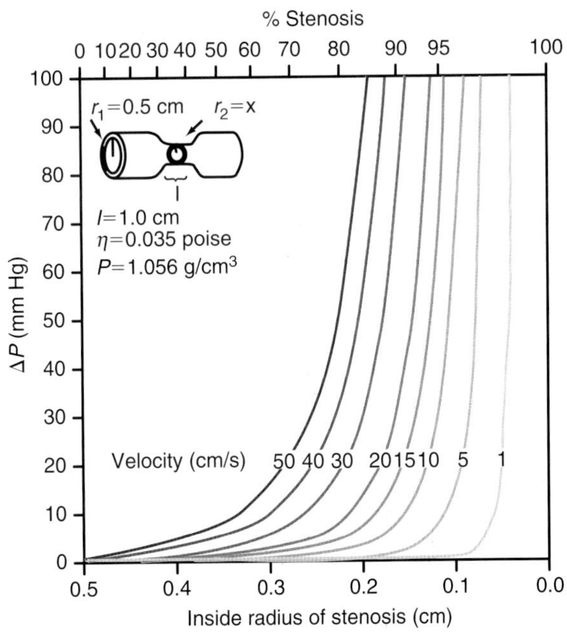

FIG 5.12 Relationship of pressure drop across a stenosis (ΔP) to the radius of the stenotic segment (or % stenosis) for various flow velocities. (From Strandness DE, Sumner DS: *Hemodynamics for Surgeons*, New York, 1975, Grune and Stratton.)

observations provide theoretical support for the concept of critical stenosis.[23,24]

As previously noted, blood flow velocity is a major determinant of fluid energy losses (see Eqs. 5.8 and 5.9). Thus the pressure drop across a stenosis varies with the flow rate. Because flow velocity depends on the distal hemodynamic resistance, the critical stenosis value also varies with the resistance of the runoff bed. In Fig. 5.12, a system with a high flow velocity (low resistance) shows a reduction in pressure with less narrowing than a system with low flow velocity (high resistance). The higher flow velocities produce curves that are less sharply bent, making the point of critical stenosis less distinct.

Another observation related to critical stenosis is that the decrease in flow is linearly related to the increase in pressure gradient as long as the peripheral resistance remains constant (Fig. 5.13).[24] In this situation, the curves for pressure drop and flow reduction are mirror images of each other, and the critical stenosis value is the same for both. Many vascular beds are able to maintain a constant level of blood flow over a wide range of perfusion pressures by the mechanism of autoregulation. This is achieved by constriction of resistance vessels in response to an increase in blood pressure and dilation of resistance vessels when blood pressure decreases. For example, autoregulation permits the brain to maintain normal flow rates down to perfusion pressures in the range of 50 to 60 mm Hg.[25]

In general, significant changes in pressure and flow begin to occur when the arterial lumen has been reduced by approximately 50% of its diameter or 75% of its cross-sectional area; however, the concept of critical stenosis is strictly valid only when the flow conditions are specified. Consequently, a stenosis that is not significant at resting flow rates can become critical when flow rates are increased by reactive hyperemia or exercise. For example, iliac stenoses that do not appear severe by arteriography may be associated with significant pressure gradients during exercise.[26] Because of the complex geometry of atherosclerotic lesions and the wide variation in arterial flow rates, it is often difficult to predict the hemodynamic significance of a lesion based on the apparent reduction in lumen size. Therefore physiologic testing by blood pressure measurement must be used to document the clinical severity of arterial lesions.[27,28]

Effect of Stenosis Length and Multiple Stenoses

Poiseuille's law predicts that the radius of a stenosis will have a much greater effect on viscous energy losses than its length (see Eq. 5.8). If the length of a stenosis is doubled, the viscous energy losses are also doubled; however, reducing the radius by half increases energy losses by a factor of 16. Furthermore, inertial energy losses are independent of stenosis length and are especially prominent at the exit of a stenosis (see Fig. 5.11). Because energy losses are primarily due to entrance and exit effects, separate short stenoses tend to be more significant than a single longer stenosis. It has been shown experimentally that when stenoses that are not significant individually are arranged in series, large reductions in pressure and flow can occur.[29] Thus multiple

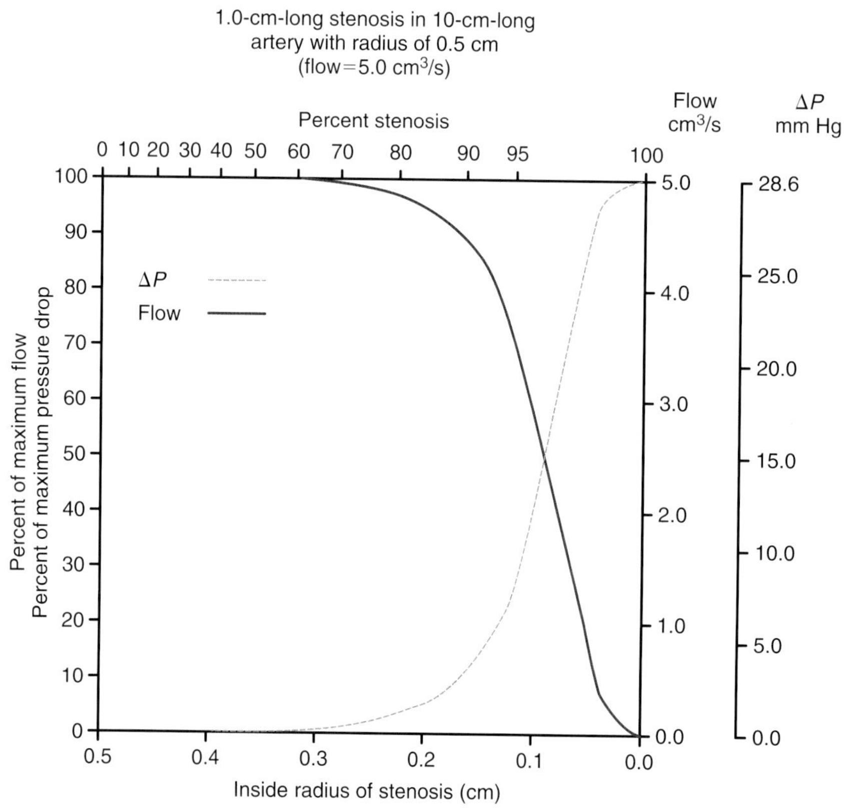

FIG 5.13 Effect of Increasing Stenosis on Blood Flow and Pressure Drop Across the Stenotic Segment. Collateral and peripheral resistances are considered to be fixed. (From Strandness DE, Sumner DS: *Hemodynamics for Surgeons*, New York, 1975, Grune and Stratton.)

subcritical stenoses may have the same effect as a single critical stenosis. Based on the preceding discussion, several points can be made about stenoses in series. When two stenoses are of similar diameter, removal of one provides only a modest increase in blood flow. If the stenoses have different diameters, removal of the least severe has little effect, whereas removal of the most severe can improve blood flow significantly.

ARTERIAL FLOW PATTERNS IN HUMAN LIMBS

Collateral Circulation

When arterial obstruction occurs, blood must pass through a network of collateral vessels to bypass the diseased segment. The functional capacity of the collateral circulation varies according to the level and extent of occlusive lesions. For example, the profunda-geniculate system can compensate to a large degree for an isolated superficial femoral artery occlusion; however, the addition of an iliac lesion severely limits collateral flow.

A typical hemodynamic circuit includes the diseased major artery, a parallel system of collateral vessels, and the peripheral runoff bed (Fig. 5.14). The collateral system consists of stem arteries, which are large distributing branches; a midzone of smaller intramuscular channels; and reentry vessels that join the major artery distal to the point of obstruction.[30] These vessels are preexisting pathways that enlarge when flow through the parallel major artery is reduced. The main stimuli for collateral development are an abnormal pressure gradient across the collateral system and increased velocity of flow through the midzone vessels.[31] This mechanism is consistent with the gradual improvement in collateral circulation that results from a regular exercise program in patients with lower extremity arterial occlusive disease.[32]

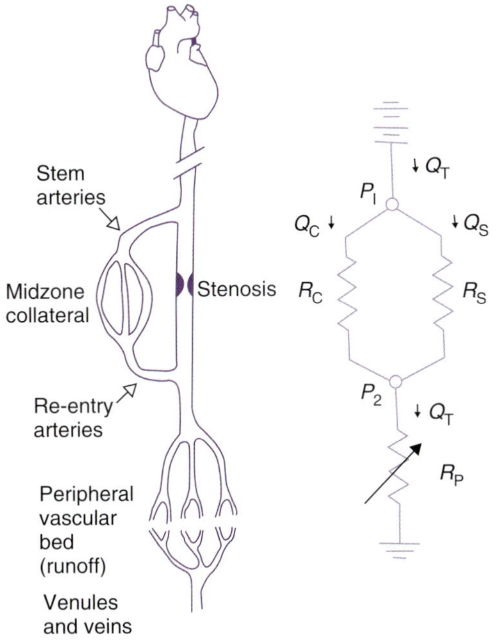

FIG 5.14 Major Components of a Hemodynamic Circuit Containing a Stenotic Artery. The analogous electrical circuit is shown on the right, with the heart represented as a battery and the central veins as a ground. Flows are represented by Q_T (total), Q_C (collateral), and Q_S (stenosis). Resistances are represented by R_C (collateral), R_S (stenosis), and R_P (peripheral runoff); R_C and R_S are fixed and R_P is variable. (From Sumner DS: The hemodynamics and pathophysiology of arterial disease. In Rutherford RB, editor: *Vascular Surgery*, Philadelphia, 1977, WB Saunders.)

Collateral vessels are smaller, longer, and more numerous than the major arteries they replace. Although considerable enlargement can occur in the midzone vessels, collateral resistance is always greater than that of the original unobstructed artery. In addition, the acute changes in collateral resistance during exercise are minimal.[33] Therefore the resistance of a collateral system is, for practical purposes, fixed.

Distribution of Vascular Resistance and Blood Flow

Unlike collateral resistance, the resistance of a peripheral runoff bed is highly variable. The muscular arterioles are primarily responsible for regulating peripheral resistance and controlling the distribution of blood flow to various capillary beds. Arteriolar tone is mainly determined by the sympathetic nervous system, but it is also subject to the influence of locally produced metabolites.

When discussing blood flow in the lower limb, it is useful to separate vascular resistance into segmental and peripheral components. Segmental resistance consists of the relatively fixed parallel resistances of the major normal or diseased artery and the bypassing collateral vessels, such as the superficial femoral artery and the profunda-geniculate system. Peripheral resistance includes the highly variable resistances of the distal calf muscle arterioles and cutaneous circulation. Normally the resting segmental resistance is low and the peripheral resistance is relatively high; therefore, the pressure drop across the femoropopliteal segment is minimal. With exercise, the peripheral resistance falls, and flow through the segmental arteries increases by a factor of up to 10, with little or no pressure drop.

With moderate arterial disease, such as an isolated superficial femoral artery occlusion, the segmental resistance is increased as a result of collateral flow and an abnormal pressure drop is present across the thigh. Because of a compensatory decrease in peripheral resistance, the total resistance of the limb and the resting blood flow often remain in the normal range.[34] During exercise, the segmental resistance remains high and fixed, whereas the peripheral resistance decreases further. However, the capacity of the peripheral circulation to compensate for a high segmental resistance is limited, and exercise flow is less than normal. In this situation, exercise is associated with a still larger pressure drop across the diseased arterial segment. The clinical result is calf muscle ischemia and claudication.

When arterial disease becomes severe, as in combined iliofemoral and tibioperoneal occlusive disease, the compensatory decrease in peripheral resistance may be unable to provide normal blood flow at rest. In this case, there is a marked pressure drop across the involved arterial segments and little or no increase in blood flow with exercise. Claudication is severe, and ischemic rest pain or ulceration may develop.

Arterial Pulses and Waveforms

The heart generates a complex pressure pulse that is modified by arterial wall properties and changes in vascular resistance as it progresses distally. Normally the peak systolic pressure is amplified as it passes down the lower limb due to a progressive decrease in arterial compliance and reflections originating from the relatively high peripheral resistance.[3] Consequently the systolic pressure at the ankle is higher than that in the upper arm and the ankle-brachial pressure ratio is greater than 1; however, the diastolic and mean pressures gradually decrease as the blood moves distally.

When blood flows through an arterial stenosis or a high-resistance collateral bed, the distal pulse pressure is reduced to a greater extent than the mean pressure.[35] This indicates that the systolic pressure beyond a lesion is a more sensitive indicator of hemodynamic significance than the mean pressure. It is well known that palpable pedal pulses in patients with superficial femoral artery stenosis can disappear after leg exercise. This occurs when increased flow through high-resistance vessels causes a reduction in pulse pressure. The contour of the pressure pulse also reflects the presence of proximal arterial disease. These changes can be demonstrated plethysmographically and include a delayed upslope, rounded peak, and bowing of the downslope away from the baseline.[36]

Changes in the flow or velocity pulse are also useful to characterize the state of the arterial system. Although the peak pressure increases, the peak of the flow pulse decreases as the periphery is approached.[3] The flow pattern in the major arteries of the leg is normally triphasic (Fig. 5.15). An initial large, forward-velocity phase resulting from cardiac systole is followed by a brief phase of flow reversal in early diastole and a third smaller phase of forward flow in late diastole. This triphasic pattern is modified by a variety of factors, including proximal arterial disease and changes in peripheral resistance. For example, body heating, which causes vasodilation and decreased resistance, abolishes the second phase of flow reversal; on exposure to cold, resistance increases and the reverse-flow phase becomes more prominent. Because a stenotic lesion is accompanied by a compensatory decrease in peripheral resistance, one of the earliest changes noted distal to a stenosis is the disappearance of the reverse-flow phase (see Fig. 5.15). As a stenosis becomes more severe, the distal flow pattern becomes monophasic, with a slow rise, a rounded peak, and a gradual decline toward the baseline in diastole. The character of the flow pulse proximal to an arterial obstruction is variable and depends on the capacity of the collateral circulation.

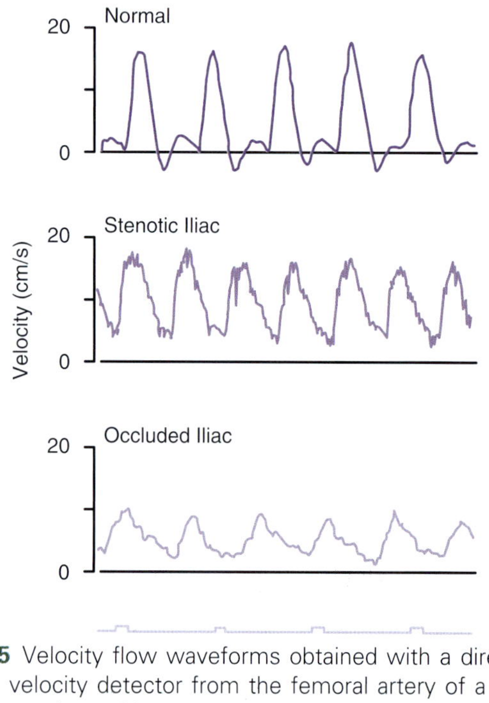

FIG 5.15 Velocity flow waveforms obtained with a directional Doppler velocity detector from the femoral artery of a normal subject, a patient with external iliac stenosis, and a patient with common iliac occlusion. (From Strandness DE, Sumner DS: *Hemodynamics for Surgeons,* New York, 1975, Grune and Stratton.)

Pressure and Flow in Normal Limbs

As the pressure pulse moves distally, the systolic pressure rises, the diastolic pressure falls, and the pulse pressure becomes wider. The fall in mean arterial pressure between the heart and ankle is normally less than 10 mm Hg. In normal individuals at rest, the ratio of ankle systolic pressure to brachial systolic pressure (ankle-brachial index) has a mean value of 1.11 ± 0.10.[37] Moderate exercise in normal extremities produces little or no drop in ankle systolic pressure. Strenuous effort may be associated with a drop of several millimeters of mercury; however, pressures return rapidly to resting levels after cessation of exercise.

The average blood flow in the normal human leg is in the range of 300 to 500 mL/min under resting conditions.[3] Blood flow to the muscles of the lower leg is approximately 2.0 mL/100 g/min. With moderate exercise, total leg blood flow increases by a factor of 5 to 10, and muscle blood flow rises to approximately 30 mL/100 g/min. During strenuous exercise, muscle blood flow can reach 70 mL/100 g/min. After cessation of exercise, blood flow decreases rapidly and returns to resting values within 1 to 5 minutes.

Pressure and Flow in Limbs With Arterial Obstruction

If an arterial lesion is hemodynamically significant at rest, there is a measurable reduction in distal blood pressure. Generally limbs with a lesion at one anatomic level have an ankle-brachial index between 0.9 and 0.5, whereas limbs with occlusions at multiple anatomic levels have an index less than 0.5.[28] The ankle-brachial index also correlates with the clinical severity of disease: in limbs with intermittent claudication, the index has a mean value of 0.59 ± 0.15; in limbs with ischemic rest pain, 0.26 ± 0.13; and in limbs with impending gangrene, 0.05 ± 0.08.[37] Because of the increased segmental vascular resistance in limbs with arterial occlusive disease, the ankle systolic blood pressure falls dramatically during leg exercise. As indicated in Figs. 5.16 to 5.18, the extent and duration of the pressure drop are proportional to the severity of the arterial lesions. By monitoring the ankle systolic pressure before and after treadmill exercise, two components of the physiologic response can be evaluated: (1) the

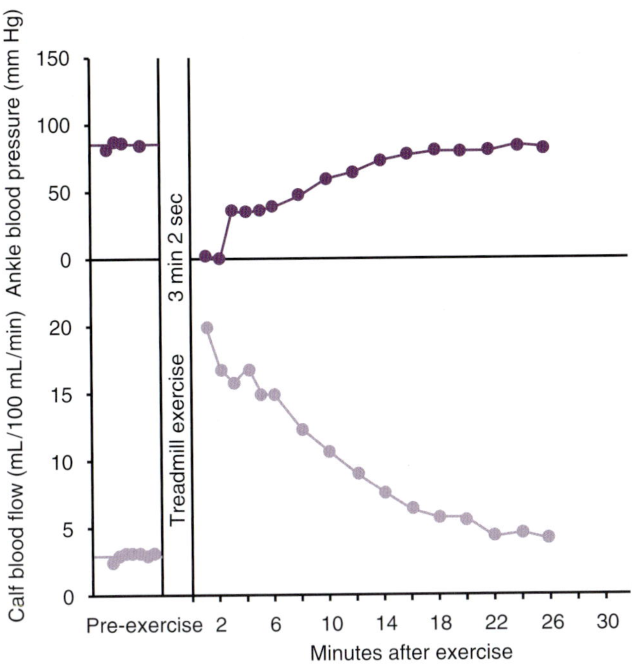

FIG 5.16 Pre- and post-exercise ankle blood pressure and calf blood flow in a patient with severe stenosis of the superficial femoral artery. (From Sumner DS, Strandness DE: The relationship between calf blood flow and ankle blood pressure in patients with intermittent claudication, *Surgery* 65:763–771, 1969.)

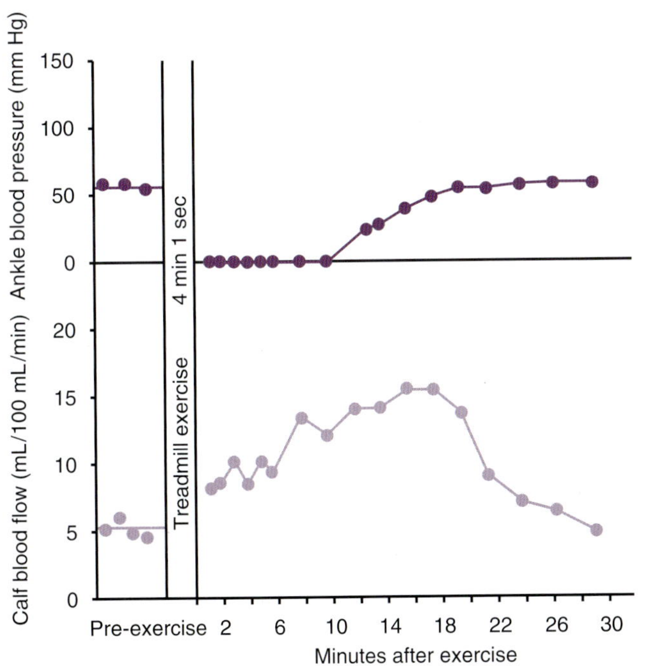

FIG 5.17 Pre- and post-exercise ankle blood pressure and calf blood flow in a patient with iliac stenosis and superficial femoral artery occlusion. (From Sumner DS, Strandness DE: The relationship between calf blood flow and ankle blood pressure in patients with intermittent claudication, *Surgery* 65:763–771, 1969.)

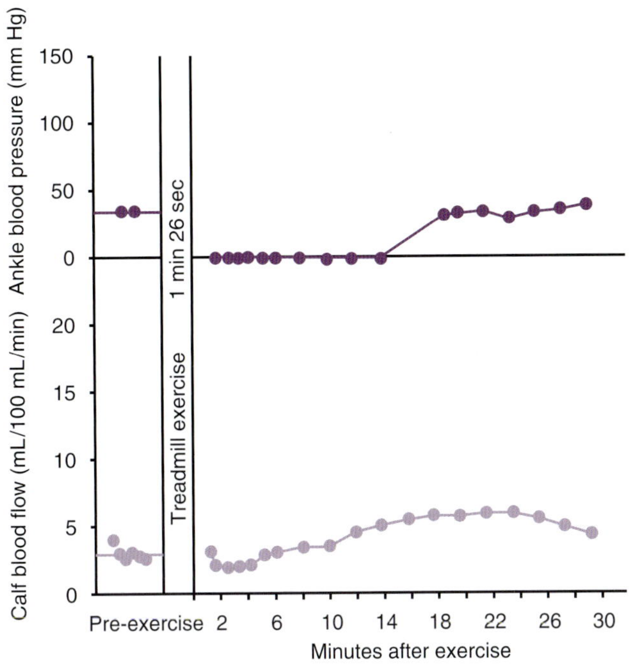

FIG 5.18 Pre- and post-exercise ankle blood pressure and calf blood flow in a patient with occlusion of the iliac, common femoral, and superficial femoral arteries. This patient had moderate rest pain and severe claudication. (From Sumner DS, Strandness DE: The relationship between calf blood flow and ankle blood pressure in patients with intermittent claudication, *Surgery* 65:763–771, 1969.)

magnitude of the immediate pressure drop and (2) the time for recovery to resting pressure. The changes in both of these parameters are proportional to the severity of arterial disease.[38]

Resting leg or calf blood flow in patients with intermittent claudication is often not significantly different from values obtained in normal individuals. However, the capacity to increase limb blood flow during exercise is quite limited, and pain occurs in the muscles that have been rendered ischemic. As the occlusive process becomes more severe, the decrease in peripheral vascular resistance can no longer compensate, and resting flow may be less than normal. When this occurs, ischemic rest pain or ulceration may appear.

Vascular Steal

Hemodynamic arrangements in which one vascular bed draws blood away or "steals" from another can occur in a variety of situations. A vascular steal can arise when two runoff beds with different resistances must be supplied by a limited source of arterial inflow.

Multiple-Level Occlusive Disease

One example of the steal phenomenon involves a limb with lesions in both the iliac and superficial femoral arteries.[1] The orifice of the profunda femoris artery, which supplies the variable resistance of the thigh, is between the fixed resistances of these two arterial lesions. The resistance of the distal calf runoff bed is also variable. Under resting conditions, normal leg blood flow can be maintained by a nearly maximal decrease in calf resistance and a moderate decrease in thigh resistance. In this situation the ankle systolic pressure will be abnormally decreased. With the increased metabolic demands of exercise, the thigh resistance can decrease further, but the calf resistance has already reached its lower limit; this results in a further pressure drop across the proximal iliac lesion, which reduces the pressure perfusing the calf. Blood flow to the calf is decreased until the thigh resistance rises and thigh blood flow begins to fall. In this situation, the effect of exercise is to increase thigh blood flow, decrease calf blood flow, and decrease distal blood pressure. The thigh steals blood from the calf because the proximal iliac lesion restricts inflow to both runoff beds.

Subclavian Steal Syndrome

In the subclavian steal syndrome, reversal of flow in the vertebral artery is associated with subclavian artery occlusion and symptoms of brainstem ischemia.[39] When occlusion is present in the proximal subclavian artery on the left or the innominate artery on the right, the pressure at the origin of the ipsilateral vertebral artery is reduced. This can result in reversal of flow in the vertebral artery, which then serves as a source of collateral circulation to the arm. The increased demands of arm exercise tend to augment the reversed flow, and the patient may experience ischemia of the brainstem. The hemodynamic effect is more severe with innominate artery occlusion than with isolated subclavian occlusion. With innominate occlusion, the origin of the right common carotid is also subject to reduced pressure, and the patterns of collateral circulation to the arm and brain become quite complicated. Blood passing down the vertebral artery on the side of the occlusion may be recovered in part by the right common carotid artery; however, during arm exercise, flow in the right common carotid may be reduced.

It is important to distinguish between symptomatic and asymptomatic subclavian steal. The presence of reversed vertebral artery flow, as demonstrated by arteriography, may be a normal variant without clinical significance.[40] In true subclavian steal syndrome, there is often a definite relationship between arm exercise and symptoms of brainstem ischemia. There will also be objective evidence of decreased blood flow to the involved arm, such as a diminished radial pulse and lowered brachial blood pressure relative to the contralateral arm.[41]

Extraanatomic Bypass Grafts

When an extraanatomic bypass is performed, a single donor artery must supply several vascular beds. In the case of a femorofemoral crossover graft, one iliac is the donor artery, the leg ipsilateral to the donor artery is the donor limb, and the contralateral leg is the recipient limb. Studies of crossover grafts in animal models have shown that the immediate effect of the graft is to double the flow in the donor artery.[42,43] When an arteriovenous fistula is created in the recipient limb, graft flows may increase by a factor of 10 without any evidence of a steal from the donor limb.

These experimental observations are consistent with hemodynamic data from patients with femorofemoral grafts.[44] Improvement in the ankle-brachial index on the recipient side can be achieved even in the presence of significant occlusive disease in both the donor and recipient limbs. Although the ankle-brachial index may decrease slightly on the donor side, a symptomatic steal is extremely uncommon. The most important factor contributing to vascular steal with a femorofemoral graft is stenosis of the donor iliac artery, and in that setting, a steal is most likely to occur during exercise, when flow rates are increased. A mildly stenotic iliac can be used as a donor artery when high flow rates are not needed, as in the treatment of ischemic rest pain. However, when increased flow rates are required to improve the walking distance of a patient with claudication, stenosis of the donor iliac artery may result in a steal from the donor limb. Occlusive disease in the arteries of the donor limb distal to the origin of the femorofemoral graft does not result in a steal, provided that the donor iliac artery is normal. These principles also apply to other types of extraanatomic bypass grafts, including axillary-axillary, carotid-subclavian, and axillofemoral grafts.[42,45]

HEMODYNAMIC PRINCIPLES AND THE TREATMENT OF ARTERIAL DISEASE

It should be apparent from the preceding discussion that the high fixed segmental resistance of the diseased major arteries and collaterals is responsible for decreased peripheral blood flow. Therefore, to be most effective in improving peripheral blood flow and relieving ischemic symptoms, therapy must be directed toward lowering this abnormally high segmental resistance. Because the peripheral resistance has already been lowered to compensate for the increased segmental resistance, attempts to further reduce the peripheral resistance are seldom beneficial.[46] Although walking exercise therapy has been shown to improve collateral function, the degree of clinical improvement is usually modest, and there is usually little change in the ankle pressure.[32,47] In general, exercise therapy is best suited for patients with mild, stable claudication who are not candidates for direct intervention.

Direct Arterial Intervention

The most satisfactory approach to reducing the fixed segmental resistance is direct intervention by open surgical or catheter-based techniques. In patients with occlusive disease involving a single anatomic level, a successful procedure should return all hemodynamic parameters to normal or near normal. This should be evident as an increase in the ankle-brachial index and an improvement in the ankle pressure response to leg exercise.[48] However, because it is seldom possible to perform a perfect arterial reconstruction, it is common to detect a minor degree of residual hemodynamic impairment. When occlusions involve multiple levels, the treatment of one level should result in significant improvement, and the persisting hemodynamic abnormality should then reflect the remaining untreated disease. In such cases, the improvement is usually sufficient to increase claudication distance or relieve ischemic rest pain. The relative severity of lesions at different levels is often difficult to determine clinically; however, the basic principle is to initially treat the most proximal level of hemodynamically significant occlusive disease.

The factors required for optimal function of arterial grafts can be analyzed in terms of hemodynamic principles. As noted previously, vessel diameter is the main determinant of hemodynamic resistance, so the diameter of a graft is considerably more important than its length. All prosthetic grafts develop a pseudointimal layer of variable thickness that further reduces the effective diameter.[3] Therefore, whenever the situation permits, a graft with a relatively large diameter should be used. Graft diameter is often limited by arterial size. To minimize energy losses associated with entrance and exit effects, the diameter of a graft should approximate that of the adjacent artery. When arteries of unequal size must be joined, a gradual transition is preferable. Thus the graft should be slightly smaller than the proximal artery and slightly larger than the distal artery.

Theoretically, end-to-end anastomoses are preferable to those done end-to-side, because the end-to-end configuration eliminates energy losses resulting from curvature and angulation. However, these losses appear to be minimal under physiologic conditions, and in most clinical situations the anastomotic angle is determined by technical factors. For example, reversed angulation has been used successfully in the construction of aortorenal and femorofemoral bypass grafts. Nevertheless, as a general rule, the smallest anastomotic angle that is technically feasible should be used. The width of an end-to-side anastomosis should be approximately equal to the diameter of the graft; the length of an anastomosis is less important but does serve as the main determinant of anastomotic angle.

Bifurcation grafts, such as those used for aortofemoral bypass, are subject to the same general hemodynamic considerations as arterial bifurcations and branches. Most commercially available grafts have secondary limbs with diameters that are half that of the primary tube, resulting in an area ratio of 0.5. In this configuration, each of the secondary limbs has 16 times the resistance of the primary tube, and in parallel they offer eight times the primary tube resistance. The flow velocity in the secondary limbs is doubled, and almost 50% of the incident pulsatile energy is reflected at the graft bifurcation.[3] As discussed previously, the area ratio determines the hemodynamic characteristics of a bifurcation with regard to pressure gradient, flow velocity, and transmission of pulsatile energy. However, the optimal area ratio for grafts has not been established, and the geometry of bifurcation grafts has received relatively little attention. Instead, the development of prosthetic grafts has emphasized features such as graft material, porosity, and surface characteristics. Despite theoretical disadvantages, commercially available grafts have functioned extremely well in a variety of clinical applications.

Vasodilators

The rationale for the use of vasodilators is that they lower peripheral vascular resistance and improve limb blood flow. Although this may occur in normal limbs, it is unlikely to be beneficial in limbs in which peripheral resistance is already decreased as a result of arterial disease. There is even a theoretical possibility that dilating vessels in relatively normal areas could divert blood away from the areas of ischemia. Most clinical studies of vasodilator therapy have failed to show a significant effect.[49,50] There is no conclusive evidence that vasodilators can increase flow in either collateral vessels or severely ischemic tissues. Consequently there is no theoretical or clinical support for vasodilator therapy.

Sympathectomy

Because the purpose of sympathectomy is to reduce peripheral resistance by release of vasomotor tone, it is subject to the same general criticisms as vasodilator therapy. Because sympathectomy has little, if any, influence on collateral resistance, there is no rational basis for its use in the treatment of intermittent claudication.[51] Furthermore, exercise-induced muscle ischemia alone is a potent stimulus for peripheral vasodilatation. The use of sympathectomy for cutaneous ischemia has some physiologic basis because the predominant effect is dilation of cutaneous arterioles. However, clinical improvement can occur only if the ischemic tissues are capable of further vasodilatation, as demonstrated by reactive hyperemia testing.[36] Beneficial results have been obtained in patients with mild rest pain and superficial ischemic ulcers; patients with severe rest pain and extensive tissue loss are not likely to respond.[51]

Rheologic Agents

According to Poiseuille's law, hemodynamic resistance is directly proportional to blood viscosity (see Eqs. 5.8 and 5.11). If the pressure remains constant and viscosity is reduced, flow increases in proportion to the fall in viscosity. Procedures for lowering blood viscosity are most often used in the immediate postoperative period to increase flow through a reconstructed arterial segment. Low-molecular-weight dextran (average molecular weight 40,000) is the most commonly used agent for reducing blood viscosity. The increased peripheral blood flow observed after intravenous administration of low-molecular-weight dextran is the result of both peripheral vasodilatation secondary to blood volume expansion and changes in viscosity due to hemodilution.[3] Dextran solutions also influence red blood cell aggregation and platelet function.[52]

HEMODYNAMICS OF THE VENOUS SYSTEM

The venous system of the lower extremities includes the deep veins beneath the muscular fascia, the superficial veins above the muscular fascia, and the perforating veins that penetrate the muscular fascia and connect the superficial and deep veins. The structure of the vein wall is considerably different from that of the arteries. For example: (1) the vein wall is much thinner, being anywhere from one-third to one-tenth as thick as that of the systemic arteries; (2) there is little elastic tissue in the wall of the vein; (3) the venous media is almost exclusively a muscular layer; (4) venules have no media and no smooth muscle; and (5) a major part of the walls of the larger veins is composed of adventitia. An important characteristic of the veins is the presence of valves, which are essential for proper function and have a bicuspid structure with a fine connective tissue skeleton covered by endothelium on both surfaces. The major function of venous valves is to ensure antegrade flow and prevent reflux from the deep to the superficial veins. The distribution of valves in the lower extremity corresponds to those regions where the effects of gravity are greatest, with the number increasing from proximal to distal.

From a clinical standpoint, the area of greatest interest in the lower extremity venous system is below the knee. This is the most common site for the development of venous thrombosis, and it is also the region of the leg where the complications of postthrombotic syndrome are evident. The veins of the soleus muscle are referred to as the *soleal sinuses* because of their capacious size and lack of venous valves. These sinuses are the most common site for the development of venous thrombosis.

The perforating veins that normally carry blood from the superficial to the deep veins are key elements in venous function. These short channels have the following features: (1) they penetrate the deep or muscular fascia, (2) they contain valves, (3) they are found predominantly below the knee, and (4) they vary in number from 90 to 200.[53] Although not commonly thought of as such, the great and small saphenous veins have all the characteristics of perforating veins. One relatively constant large perforator can be found on the medial aspect of the distal thigh, and this is one of the few that establishes a direct communication between the great saphenous vein and the deep venous system. A common misconception is that the perforating veins along the medial aspect of the lower leg communicate directly with the great saphenous vein. In fact, they communicate most commonly with its major tributary, the posterior arch vein. Normally there are four relatively constant perforators that join the posterior arch vein, and when these are diseased, they contribute to the pathogenesis of the postthrombotic syndrome. The region in the vicinity of the lowest two perforating veins is often referred to as the *gaiter area*.[53] As discussed later in this chapter, the function of the venous wall and its associated valves becomes evident when the effects of gravity and the calf muscle pump are considered.

Normal Pressure and Flow Relationships

A major factor in venous physiology that explains the capacitance function of these vessels is that they can undergo large changes in volume with very little change in transmural pressure. This is not due to the elastic properties of the vein walls but rather to the fact that they tend to collapse under the influence of a low transmural pressure.[54] Veins are actually stiffer than arteries when they are compared at the same distending pressure. This results from the paucity of elastic tissue and the prominent adventitia, which consists largely of collagen.

One of the remarkable features of the venous system is the wide range of flow rates that can be found—from high flows to nearly complete stasis. Flow rates depend on a variety of complex interactive factors, such as body position, level of activity, vascular fluid volume, and ambient temperature. Because it is virtually impossible to measure instantaneous venous flow in either the superficial or the deep veins, it is necessary to look at measurements of venous pressure and relate these to specific conditions or disease states.

Resting Venous Pressure

The venous pressures that exist in the absence of pulsatile flow are shown in Fig. 5.19 which shows the hydrostatic model of a 6-foot-tall "dead man." If the case of an open rigid tube is considered, pressure at the top would be zero (atmospheric). In the body, the arteries and veins can be represented as a series of parallel tubes, with the veins being collapsible and the arteries rigid. When the system is filled with fluid but not enough to entirely distend the collapsible venous tube, the pressure in the collapsed portion of the tube is atmospheric. Pressures in the rigid arterial tube must be equal to those in the collapsible tube up to the zero point. Above the zero pressure point, the pressures in the rigid tube are negative because the collapsed tube representing the veins prevents free communication between the two segments.

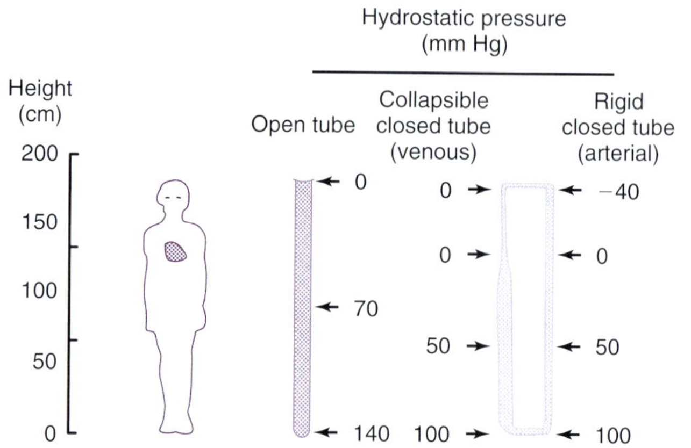

FIG 5.19 Hydrostatic Pressures Measured in the Upright "dead man." The pressures in the open tube are those expected in a rigid tube of equal height. The pressures in the closed tubes are those expected in a system of closed, connected parallel tubes. (From Strandness DE, Sumner DS: *Hemodynamics for Surgeons*, New York, 1975, Grune and Stratton.)

When we examine the venous pressure relationships in a "living man"—in the supine and erect positions—some important facts can be noted (Fig. 5.20).[55] There is a point just below the diaphragm where the pressures in the arteries and veins remain constant regardless of position. This has been termed the *hydrostatic indifferent point* (HIP). This point changes only when the subject is placed head down, and then it is located at the level of the right atrium. The zero pressure level is in the region of the right atrium, usually at the level of the fourth intercostal space. The effect of gravity is the same throughout the vascular system in a supine subject. Raising an arm above the head in the erect position produces some dramatic changes. The arteriovenous pressure gradient in the foot remains the same (83 mm Hg), but in the hand it falls to a level of 31 mm Hg.[56]

Although there is no difference in the pressure gradient across the capillaries in the feet between the supine and the standing positions, some important changes do occur. On assuming the standing position, there is a translocation of blood into the veins of the legs (approximately 500 mL).[57] There is also a marked increase in the transmural venous pressure at the foot as a result of the effect of gravity. With this increase in pressure, fluid is forced out of the capillaries into the tissues. Although some of this fluid may be picked up by the lymphatics, other factors must come into play if edema is to be prevented. The single most important element in preventing the continued accumulation of interstitial fluid is the calf muscle pump. This can dramatically

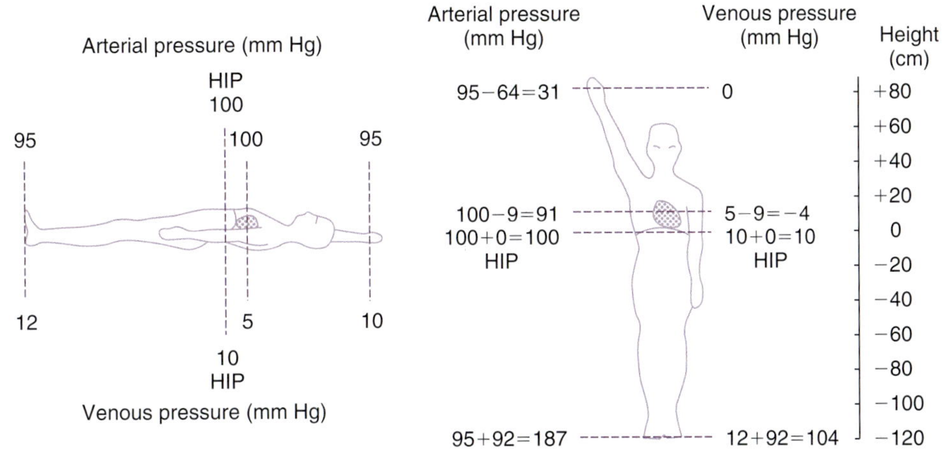

FIG 5.20 Intravascular Pressures Present in the Normal Supine and Erect Human. The hydrostatic indifferent point *(HIP)* is located just below the diaphragm. (From Strandness DE, Sumner DS: *Hemodynamics for Surgeons*, New York, 1975, Grune and Stratton.)

lower the pressure in the veins and capillaries, thus promoting the return of interstitial fluid to the circulation.

Pressure Changes During Exercise

Features that distinguish normal individuals from patients with venous disease are best understood by examining the pressure changes that occur with leg exercise. Although patients with chronic arterial disease can usually be distinguished from normal subjects under resting conditions by measurement of distal arterial blood pressure, this is not the case with venous disease. For patients with venous problems, it is only when the calf muscle pump is activated that the abnormality is apparent. The calf muscle pump produces important changes in venous volume, flow rate, and flow direction: (1) it lowers the venous pressure in the dependent limb; (2) it reduces venous volume in the exercising limb; and (3) it increases venous return.

With quiet standing, the venous pressure at the level of the foot remains constant, but this is dramatically altered with even a single step. As noted in Fig. 5.21, at the completion of a single step, the venous pressure is low and requires several seconds to return to the pre-step level.[58] When a normal individual walks, the venous pressure remains at a low and steady level throughout the period of exercise. Calf volume initially falls but gradually increases during exercise as the arterial inflow rises (Fig. 5.22). It should be emphasized that the observed pressure changes at the level of the foot are entirely dependent on intact and functioning venous valves in the distal limb. The calf muscle pump essentially empties the local venous system during contraction. With relaxation, the veins are nearly empty and the venous pressure is very low. These changes are vital to maintaining normal venous return and protecting the limb from edema.

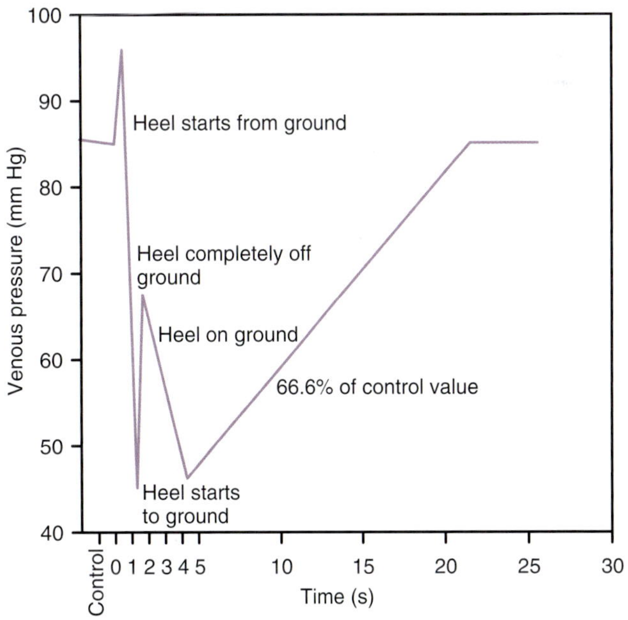

FIG 5.21 Changes in the mean saphenous vein pressure measured at the level of the ankle that occur with a single step. (Redrawn from Pollack AA, Wood EH: Human venous pressure in the saphenous vein at the ankle during exercise and changes in posture, *J Appl Physiol* 1:649–662, 1949.)

Venous Flow Patterns

Flow on the venous side of the circulation is influenced by a variety of factors, including respiration, the filling pressure of the right heart, body position, the activity of the calf muscle pump, and the amount of arterial inflow. The patterns of blood flow in the femoral artery and vein are shown in Fig. 5.23. Flow velocity in the normal femoral vein is lowest at peak inspiration, when the intraabdominal pressure resulting from descent of the diaphragm is at its maximum. In theory, the changes in velocity of venous flow in the subclavian vein should be opposite to those in the femoral vein—that is, highest at peak inspiration, when intrathoracic pressure is at its minimum.

As noted earlier, the presence of competent valves prevents reflux of blood and an increase in venous pressure. This can be shown when the pressure is suddenly increased above a competent iliofemoral valve (Fig. 5.24). A cough and a Valsalva maneuver result in a sharp increase in pressure above the valve but not

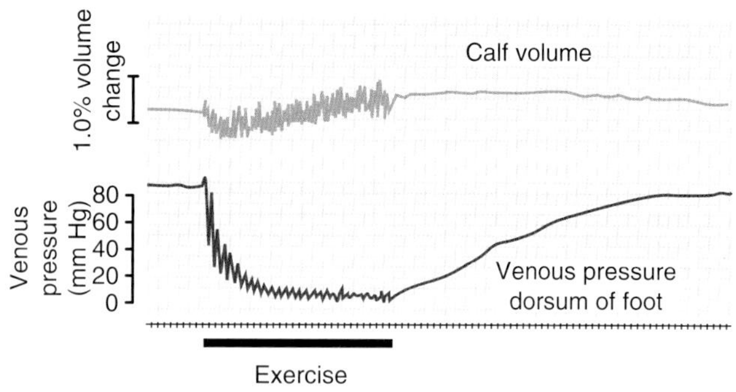

FIG 5.22 **Normal Calf Volume and Venous Pressure Response to Calf Muscle Exercise.** Pressure changes were measured in a dorsal foot vein. Venous pressure falls rapidly, remains low throughout the period of exercise, and returns slowly to baseline after calf muscle contraction ceases. (From Strandness DE, Sumner DS: *Hemodynamics for Surgeons*, New York, 1975, Grune and Stratton.)

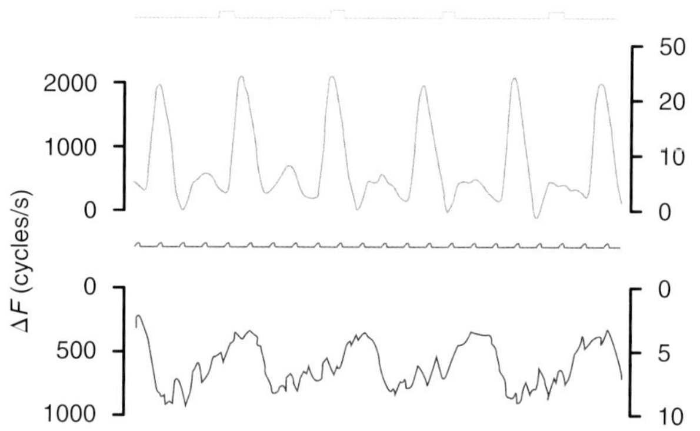

FIG 5.23 Comparison of the flow velocity patterns in the common femoral artery *(top)* and common femoral vein *(bottom)* in the supine position with normal respiration. The venous velocity patterns are dominated by the pressure changes that occur with respiration. ΔF, Doppler shift frequency, which is proportional to velocity. (From Strandness DE, Sumner DS: *Hemodynamics for Surgeons*, New York, 1975, Grune and Stratton.)

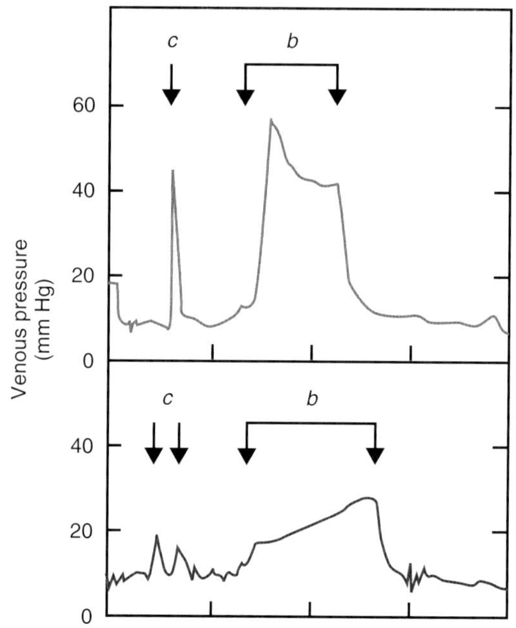

FIG 5.24 Effect of a cough *(c)* and a Valsalva maneuver *(b)* on the venous pressure in a patient with a competent valve at the iliofemoral level. *Upper panel,* Pressure changes above the valve. *Lower panel,* Pressure changes below the valve. (From Ludbrook J, Beale G: Femoral venous valves in relation to varicose veins, *Lancet* 1:79–81, 1962.)

below it. There is no reflux of blood flow through the valve during either of these maneuvers.

Abnormal Pressure and Flow Relationships

The most common manifestations of abnormal venous function are primary varicose veins and the postthrombotic syndrome. Current evidence suggests that primary varicose veins are often familial. The initial abnormality in this condition appears to be incompetence of the terminal valves of the great and small saphenous veins, which permits reflux of blood. With the passage of time, progressive dilation and incompetence of the other valves occurs. Dodd and Cockett[59] also include patients with idiopathic perforator vein incompetence in the primary varicose vein group. Although this may be valid, it is likely that many of these incompetent perforators occur secondary to episodes of deep vein thrombosis that result in destruction of the valves.

The flow abnormality produced by loss of valvular competence at any level of the venous system is easily demonstrated with a Doppler velocity detector. The flow patterns shown in Fig. 5.25

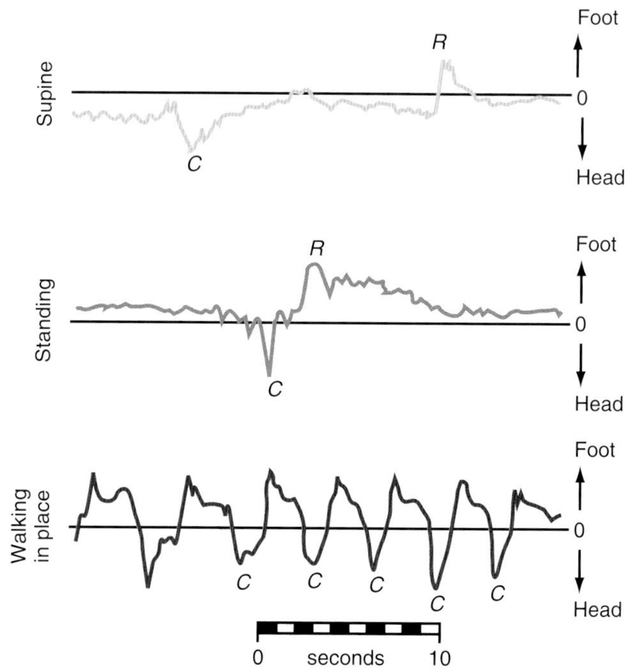

FIG 5.25 Changes in venous velocity recorded from an incompetent great saphenous vein in a patient with primary varicose veins. The effects of muscular contraction *(C)* and relaxation *(R)* are indicated for the supine and standing positions. The bidirectional flow that occurs with walking is also shown. (From Strandness DE, Sumner DS: *Hemodynamics for Surgeons*, New York, 1975, Grune and Stratton.)

are from the great saphenous vein of a patient with primary varicose veins. In the supine position, flow with calf contraction is antegrade, with a slight and transient period of reflux during relaxation; however, with standing, the opposite is noted, with flow being toward the foot. Walking in place clearly illustrates the rapid changes in direction that occur with each step as a result of loss of valvular competence. When the pressure in the veins on the dorsum of the foot is measured during exercise in a patient with primary varicose veins, the deviations from normal are evident (Fig. 5.26). The pressure does not fall to normally low levels, and it returns to the preexercise level much faster when walking is stopped. If a tourniquet is placed around the upper calf, this pattern is normalized as long as the valves in the deep system are competent.

With the development of acute deep vein thrombosis, two major factors determine the long-term outcome: (1) the location and extent of the residual venous obstruction and (2) the condition of the valves below the knee in the area of the calf muscle pump.[60-63] Because these vary greatly from one patient to another, it is not surprising that the pressure responses also show a wide variation. Four examples of the types of patterns that can be observed are shown in Fig. 5.27. It is clear that even with primary varicose veins, the pressure changes at the level of the foot are abnormal with exercise (see Figs. 5.26 and 5.27). However, patients

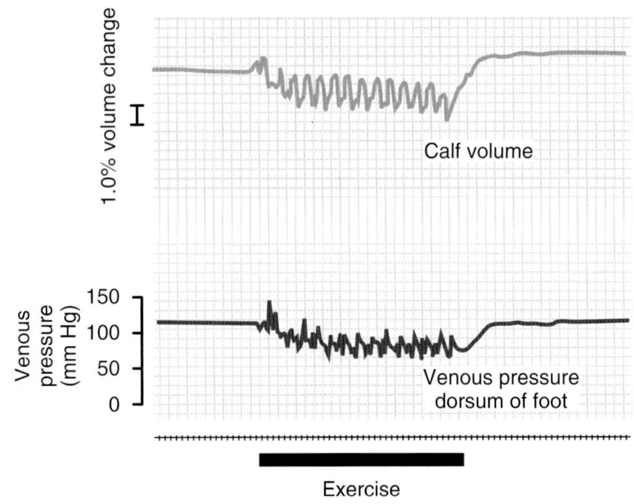

FIG 5.26 Calf volume and venous pressure changes recorded from a dorsal foot vein of a patient with primary varicose veins. The pressure does not fall to the low levels seen in normal subjects (see Fig. 5.22), and it returns to baseline much faster. (From Strandness DE, Sumner DS: *Hemodynamics for surgeons*, New York, 1975, Grune and Stratton.)

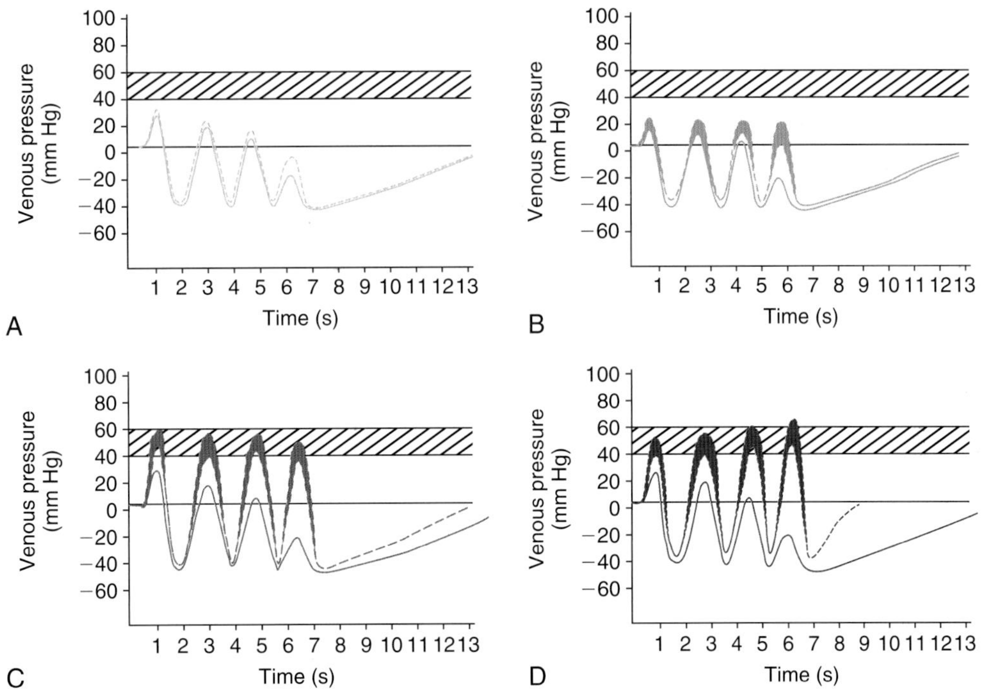

FIG 5.27 Pressure Changes in the Great Saphenous Vein at the Ankle During Four Steps. In each panel, the normal response is noted by the solid line. (A) Primary varicose veins and no leg ulcers. (B) Varicose veins, incompetent ankle perforators, normal deep veins, and no leg ulcers. (C) Varicose veins, incompetent ankle perforators, normal deep veins, and leg ulcers present. (D) Varicose veins, incompetent ankle perforators, abnormal deep veins, and leg ulcers present. (From Arnoldi CC, Linderholm H: On the pathogenesis of the venous leg ulcer, *Acta Chir Scand* 134:427–440, 1968.)

with this very common condition generally complain of minimal edema and rarely develop ulceration. The factors that appear to be responsible for development of the postthrombotic syndrome relate primarily to the status of the deep veins below the knee and the perforating veins. The most abnormal venous pressures and flows occur in the area where ulceration develops and are due to valvular incompetence in both the distal deep veins and their connections with the superficial venous system. With this combination, the high pressures that can be generated by activation of the calf muscle pump result in ambulatory venous hypertension in the lower leg.

In 1978, Browse and Burnand[64] offered a reassessment of the factors responsible for development of the postthrombotic syndrome. They recognized that the clinical condition could occur only with damage to the deep venous system and postulated that the abnormally high venous pressures would lead to the development of multiple new capillaries in the dermis, with large pores in the venular side. As a result, there would be extravasation of large molecules such as fibrinogen and coagulation factors. These factors, in conjunction with tissue factors, would lead to the conversion of fibrinogen to fibrin. If this were combined with inadequate fibrinolysis, fibrin would accumulate in the tissues and produce a barrier to the diffusion of both oxygen and nutrients. The end result would be tissue anoxia and death of the skin in the affected region.

Hemodynamic Principles and the Treatment of Venous Disease

In contrast to the arterial side of the circulation, there are few direct therapeutic approaches that can correct the underlying hemodynamic abnormalities of venous disease. Although obstruction of inflow to a limb is the most commonly treated arterial abnormality, mechanical interference with venous outflow is a rare cause of chronic venous insufficiency.

One uncommon exception to this observation is the patient with venous claudication. This entity occurs in the specific clinical setting of chronic iliofemoral venous occlusion, and in most cases, the major deep veins distal to the groin are patent and competent. With vigorous lower extremity exercise, the patient is unable to adequately empty and decompress the deep venous system, and the thigh becomes tense and very painful. After the patient stops exercising, it often requires 15 to 30 minutes for the pain and tightness to resolve. It is important to recognize that this syndrome rarely occurs with ordinary exercise and thus tends to be seen in relatively young patients who indulge in vigorous activities such as jogging, skiing, or tennis. The underlying mechanism of venous claudication involves the collateral veins that bypass the obstructed segment and have a relatively high, fixed resistance.[65] This high outflow resistance results in a marked increase in venous volume during exercise. In some circumstances, it may be feasible to provide therapeutic relief with a crossover saphenous vein graft using the proximal saphenous vein from the opposite limb; however, this is rarely done because the symptoms in most patients produce only minimal disability. Recanalization of occluded iliofemoral venous segments may also be possible with endovascular techniques.[66]

Other surgical procedures designed to treat chronic venous insufficiency, particularly in the superficial veins, consist of either removing or ablating the offending veins or interrupting them at some point along their course. These procedures are done to eliminate sites of reflux and restore the pressure-flow relationship to normal. The value of these techniques when the abnormalities involve the distal deep veins in the lower extremity is limited, since those venous segments are not currently amenable to direct intervention. There has been some interest in promoting valvular competence in the proximal femoral vein in the thigh, either by a direct surgical approach through a longitudinal venotomy or by transposition of a competent venous valve.[67,68] However, the effectiveness of these procedures is questionable because there is no evidence to support the concept of the so-called critical valve, and the alterations of pressure and flow are nearly always secondary to abnormalities in the distal deep veins.

The most common form of therapy for chronic venous insufficiency is the use of support stockings that provide external compression and thus minimize the amount of edema that occurs during ambulation.[69] The exact mechanism of compression therapy remains poorly understood.[70] In theory, the stocking should reduce the transmural venous pressure gradient in a graduated fashion, with the highest compression pressures in the ankle area and diminishing pressures proximally up the limb. The amount of pressure exerted by a stocking depends on the elastic tension in the garment and the radius of the limb. Compression pressure should be in the range of 80 to 90 mm Hg while standing, 50 to 60 mm Hg while sitting, and 0 mm Hg in the recumbent position. This is obviously not possible with any single stocking; therefore a compromise must be accepted.

Elevation of the legs above the level of the heart is also a standard method for relieving the symptoms of chronic venous insufficiency. The physiologic basis for the use of elevation depends on three major effects: (1) it reduces venous pressure by decreasing the hydrostatic component related to gravity; (2) it promotes the reabsorption of edema fluid; and (3) it prevents ambulatory venous hypertension. Periodic elevation and external compression therapy are essential for the treatment of chronic venous insufficiency. When strictly adhered to, a regimen of elevation and compression minimizes edema, improves skin nutrition, and avoids ulceration in the majority of patients.

CONCLUSION

The fundamental principles of hemodynamics often seem remote from the routine clinical problems faced by vascular surgeons. The purpose of this chapter has been to show how these mathematical and physical concepts provide the basis for a rational approach to the pathophysiology, diagnosis, and treatment of vascular disease. These principles are also important for understanding the noninvasive diagnostic techniques discussed elsewhere in this book. The use of objective hemodynamic data is an essential step in the initial clinical evaluation and follow-up of patients with vascular disease.

REVIEW QUESTIONS

1. Viscous energy losses in flowing blood result from which of the following?
   a. Changes in the velocity and direction of flow
   b. Friction between adjacent layers of moving blood
   c. Turbulent flow in areas of stenosis
   d. Disturbed flow at points of branching
   e. Areas of boundary layer separation
2. Poiseuille's law states that pressure gradients in an idealized flow model are inversely proportional to which of the following?
   a. Mean flow velocity
   b. Tube or stenosis length
   c. Blood viscosity
   d. Tube or stenosis radius
   e. Volume flow rate
3. Inertial energy losses in blood flow are related primarily to which of the following?
   a. Changes in the velocity and direction of flow
   b. Blood viscosity
   c. Specific gravity of blood
   d. Friction between adjacent layers of moving blood
   e. Mean blood pressure
4. The critical stenosis value for a particular artery depends on which of the following?
   a. Length of the arterial segment
   b. Tangential wall stress
   c. Blood viscosity
   d. Compliance of the arterial wall
   e. Flow rate and peripheral vascular resistance
5. Which of the following statements about the collateral circulation is false?
   a. Collateral vessels are preexisting pathways that enlarge when the parallel major artery is occluded.
   b. The vascular resistance of the collateral bed is relatively fixed.
   c. Collateral artery resistance is usually less than that of the original unobstructed parallel artery.
   d. An abnormal pressure gradient across the collateral bed may stimulate the further development of collateral pathways.
   e. The midzone of the collateral bed consists of small intramuscular vessels.
6. Which of the following is not related to tangential stress and rupture of arterial aneurysms?
   a. Volume flow rate through the aneurysm
   b. Arterial blood pressure
   c. Internal radius of the aneurysm
   d. Tensile strength of collagen
   e. Thickness of the aneurysm wall
7. With an extraanatomic bypass, such as a femorofemoral crossover graft, a vascular steal from the donor limb is most likely to occur in which of the following circumstances?
   a. There is occlusive disease in both the donor and the recipient limbs.
   b. There is an occlusive lesion in the donor artery.
   c. Severe occlusive disease is present in the donor limb.
   d. The recipient limb has only mild occlusive disease.
   e. The donor limb is hemodynamically normal.
8. Venous claudication is characterized by all of the following except:
   a. Chronic iliofemoral venous occlusion
   b. Thigh pain with vigorous exercise
   c. High-resistance venous collaterals
   d. Minimal disability with ordinary activities
   e. Valvular incompetence in the tibial veins
9. Which of the following is not a function of the calf muscle pump?
   a. It lowers venous pressure in the dependent limb.
   b. It reduces venous volume in the exercising limb.
   c. It improves arterial blood flow to the exercising muscle.
   d. It increases venous return to the right heart.
   e. It minimizes the accumulation of interstitial fluid in the distal limb.
10. All of the following contribute to the pathogenesis of the postthrombotic syndrome except
   a. Deep vein thrombosis with chronic obstruction of the deep veins
   b. Extravasation of blood components into the subcutaneous tissues
   c. Incompetence of the venous valves in the deep veins below the knee
   d. The presence of primary varicose veins
   e. Ambulatory venous hypertension

BIBLIOGRAPHY

Berguer R, Hwang NHC. Critical arterial stenosis—a theoretical and experimental solution. *Ann Surg.* 1974;180:39–50.

Carter SA. Response of ankle systolic pressure to leg exercise in mild or questionable arterial disease. *N Engl J Med.* 1972;287:578–582.

Flanigan DP, Tullis JP, Streeter VL, et al. Multiple subcritical arterial stenosis: effect on poststenotic pressure and flow. *Ann Surg.* 1977;186:663–668.

Killewich LA, Martin R, Cramer M, et al. Pathophysiology of venous claudication. *J Vasc Surg.* 1984;1:507–511.

Ku DN, Giddens DP, Phillips DJ, et al. Hemodynamics of the normal human carotid bifurcation—in vitro and in vivo studies. *Ultrasound Med Biol.* 1985;1:13–26.

Lee BB, Nicolaides AN, Myers K, et al. Venous hemodynamic changes in lower limb venous disease: The UIP consensus according to scientific evidence. *Int Angiol.* 2016;35:236–352.

May AG, Van de Berg L, DeWeese JA, et al. Critical arterial stenosis. *Surgery*. 1963;54:250–259.

Phillips DJ, Greene FM Jr, Langlois Y, et al. Flow velocity patterns in the carotid bifurcations of young, presumed normal subjects. *Ultrasound Med Biol*. 1983;1:39–49.

Sumner DS, Strandness DE Jr. The relationship between calf blood flow and ankle blood pressure in patients with intermittent claudication. *Surgery*. 1969;65:763–771.

Sumner DS, Strandness DE Jr. The hemodynamics of the femoro-femoral shunt. *Surg Gynecol Obstet*. 1972;134: 629–636.

References available online at expertconsult.com.

CHAPTER 6

Hemostasis and Thrombosis

Timothy K. Liem, Thomas G. DeLoughery

INTRODUCTION

Most of the bleeding that occurs during surgery or in association with trauma is mechanical and usually can be controlled. In contrast, nonsurgical bleeding most commonly is caused by the concomitant administration of antithrombotic medications, and less commonly by congenital or acquired defects of the hemostatic system. The vascular surgeon must understand the hemostatic pathways and the characteristics of the various antithrombotic agents in sufficient depth to prevent or arrest bleeding and restore hemostasis. In addition, vascular surgeons play an integral role in the surgical and medical management of patients who develop arterial and venous thromboembolism (VTE). This requires an in-depth knowledge of the myriad demographic; situational, inherited, and acquired risk factors for thrombosis, as well as a solid understanding of the various medical options available to alter the balance between thrombosis and hemostasis.

HEMOSTASIS

Components of Hemostasis

Hemostasis is the process by which bleeding from injured tissue is controlled. Although hemostasis is a dynamic process, it can be divided into several components: vessel response to injury, platelet activation, fibrin formation, fibrinolysis, and coagulation inhibition. Each component has numerous modulatory mechanisms.

Vessel Response

When a vessel is injured, the interaction of humoral, neurogenic, and myogenic systems leads to temporary vasoconstriction in the muscular arteries and arterioles. Mechanisms for vasoconstriction may include the release of thromboxane A_2 (TXA_2) by activated platelets, endothelin by endothelial cells, bradykinin, and fibrinopeptide B. Vasoconstriction has less of a role in obtaining hemostasis in veins and venules.

In normal vessels, endothelial cells cover the luminal surface, forming a monolayer with tight cell-cell interaction.[1] In their quiescent state, endothelial cells are actively antithrombotic. They synthesize and secrete several modulators that lead to vasodilation, decreased platelet aggregation, decreased levels of thrombin, factors Va and VIIIa, and factors IXa and Xa, by which an antithrombotic state is promoted. Specifically, prostacyclin and nitric oxide are potent vasodilators and inhibitors of platelet aggregation. Heparan sulfates accelerate the activity of antithrombin (AT), thereby inactivating thrombin. Thrombomodulin (TM) also inactivates thrombin[2] by forming the thrombomodulin-thrombin complex, a potent activator of the natural anticoagulant protein C[3], which with the help of cofactor protein S, inactivates factors Va and VIIIa, leading to decreased thrombin and factor Xa levels. Tissue factor pathway inhibitor (TFPI), which is bound to the endothelial surface, strongly inhibits the extrinsic coagulation pathway after heparin administration.[4,5] Tissue-type plasminogen activator (t-PA) and urokinase are synthesized, which bind fibrinogen and fibrin, increase plasmin, and promote fibrinolysis.

The endothelium also possesses substantial procoagulant activity and acts as a scaffold for hemostasis when stimulated after vessel injury. Tissue factor (thromboplastin, factor III) is a protein that is constitutively expressed by most cells; however, endothelial cells only express tissue factor when stimulated by agonists such as thrombin or endotoxin. Vessel injury causes endothelial denudation and activation, which results in the exposure of tissue factor to low circulating levels of activated factor VII in blood to form complexes that catalyze the conversion of factor IX to IXa and factor X to Xa, leading to thrombin formation.

Endothelial cells also synthesize and secrete von Willebrand factor (vWF), which is necessary for platelet adhesion to the vessel wall. This factor has binding sites for collagen, platelet glycoproteins (GPs) Ib and IIb/IIIa, and factor VIII. Factor VIII and vWF circulate together as a complex. Endothelial cells, in addition to the liver, synthesize factor V. Factors V and VIII are cleaved by thrombin into their activated states (Va and VIIIa) and then become integral components of membrane-bound complexes that accelerate the formation of thrombin and factor Xa (Fig. 6.1). Endothelial cells also synthesize plasminogen activator inhibitor (PAI-1), which rapidly inactivates circulating t-PA.

Platelet Activation

Platelets are small, discoid-shaped, anuclear cells with an average circulatory life span of 8 to 12 days. There are usually 150,000 to 300,000 platelets/mL in human blood. Platelets are released as cytoplasmic fragments of megakaryocytes within bone marrow.

The platelet membrane is composed of a phospholipid bilayer, GPs, and proteins. Circulating proteins interact with the carbohydrate moieties of the GPs. Several surface receptors are known

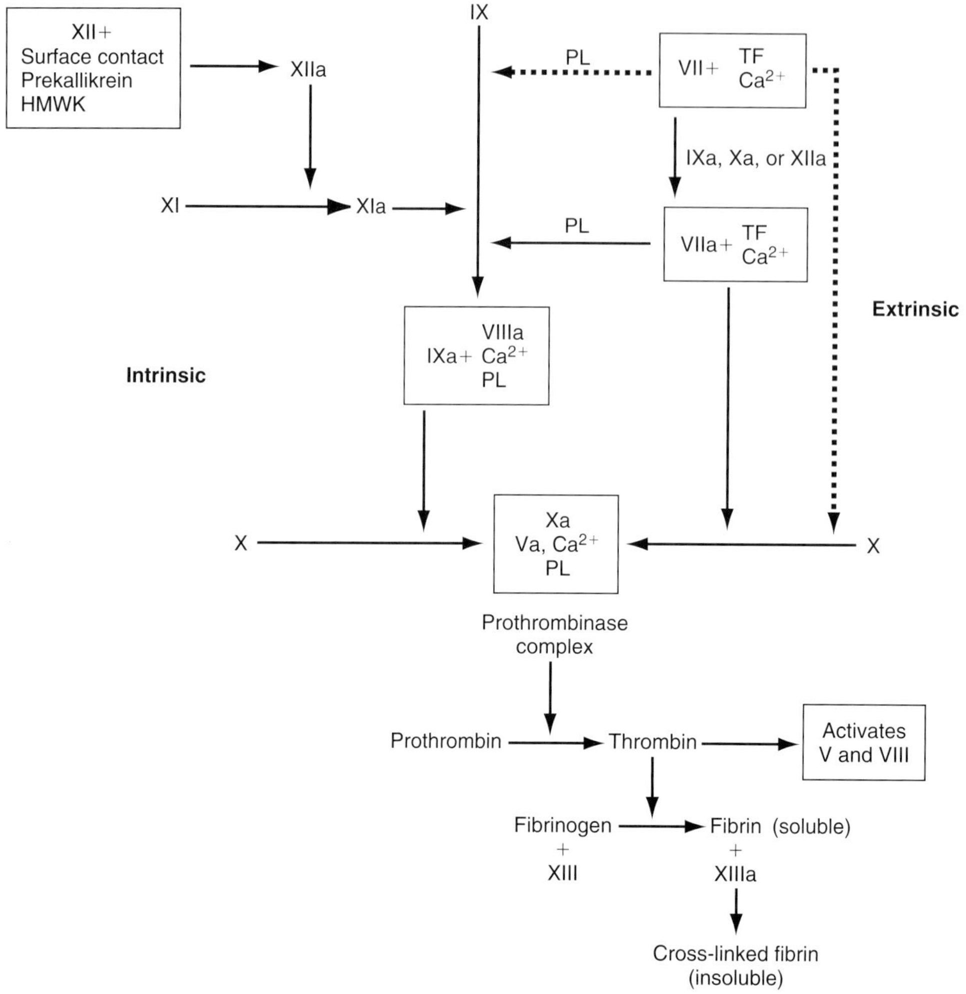

FIG 6.1 The Intrinsic and Extrinsic Pathways of Coagulation. The intrinsic pathway is initiated by surface contact; the extrinsic pathway is initiated by the release of tissue factor *(TF)* from tissues injured during surgery or trauma. Factor VIIa possesses an activity 100-fold greater than that of factor VII. The pathways are interrelated and operate in tandem to achieve hemostasis. *HMWK*, High-molecular-weight kininogen; *PL*, phospholipid from activated platelet or endothelial membranes.

to exist. Some of the more common receptors bind thrombin, adenosine diphosphate (ADP), TXA_2, fibrinogen, collagen, and vWF.[6] Platelets contain three types of storage granules: (1) dense granules, which contain serotonin, ADP, adenosine triphosphate (ATP), and calcium; (2) α-granules, which contain coagulation proteins (high-molecular-weight kininogen [HMWK], fibrinogen, fibronectin, factor V, vWF, platelet factor 4), growth factors, and adhesion proteins (fibronectin, thrombospondin, P-selectin); and (3) lysosomes.

The initial stage of hemostasis, consisting of vasoconstriction and platelet plug formation, is termed *primary hemostasis*. Immediately after vascular injury, platelets adhere to the subendothelial matrix via proteins, such as collagen and vWF. vWF binds primarily to the GP Ib-IX-V complex and the GP IIb-IIIa complex, whereas collagen binds via the GP Ia-IIa complex and GP IV. Collagen-induced platelet activation results in platelet shape change and release of prothrombotic α- and dense granule contents. Granule release reactions further amplify platelet activation and aggregation via several proteins, including vWF, fibrinogen, and ADP.

Platelet activation is associated with numerous downstream signals, including protein kinase C activation, inositol triphosphate formation, intracellular calcium mobilization, and the generation of arachidonic acid. Arachidonic acid is then converted by cyclooxygenase-1 (COX-1) to prostaglandin endoperoxides (PGG_2, PGH_2). PGG_2 is converted to TXA_2 by thromboxane synthetase. PGG_2, PGH_2, and TXA_2 stimulate further aggregation and platelet granule release.[7]

Regardless of the agonist, the final common pathway for platelet aggregation involves a conformational change in the GP IIb-IIIa complex that leads to the reversible exposure of binding sites for fibrinogen, which allows fibrinogen to form bridges between adjacent platelets, forming the platelet aggregate.[8]

Numerous medications inhibit platelet function at several steps in the pathway described previously. Aspirin irreversibly inhibits platelet COX-1, inhibiting TXA_2-mediated platelet aggregation for the life of the platelet. Clopidogrel, ticagrelor, and prasugrel inhibit ADP-mediated platelet activation and aggregation.[9,10] Novel GP IIb-IIIa inhibitors prevent platelet aggregation by blocking the binding of fibrinogen.[11]

Fibrin Formation

The platelet plug, which is required for normal hemostasis, deaggregates unless thrombin is generated and fibrin stabilization of the plug occurs; this is known as *secondary hemostasis*. The formation of fibrin requires the interaction of platelet aggregates, endothelial cells, and plasma coagulation proteins.

Plasma coagulation proteins have been designated by the Roman numerals I through XIII (the letter "a" follows the Roman numeral when the factor has been activated), and all of these factors are synthesized in the liver. The hepatic synthesis of factors II, VII, IX, and X is vitamin K dependent. When vitamin K is not available, these factors are synthesized and released but are not biologically active.

The sequence of enzymatic events leading to thrombin formation is the coagulation cascade (see Fig. 6.1). The intrinsic pathway is activated when plasma is exposed to a negatively charged surface such as subendothelium, collagen, or endotoxin. Factor XII is activated to XIIa by the interaction of HMWK, prekallikrein, and the negatively charged surface; however, the physiologic significance of factor XII activation is unclear because deficiencies in factor XII, HMWK, and prekallikrein are not associated with any clinical bleeding diatheses.

The extrinsic pathway is the more physiologic route for the generation of thrombin and fibrin. It is initiated by the exposure of tissue factor, which binds to low levels of circulating factor VIIa in the presence of calcium (TF-VIIa).[12,13] This complex activates factor X and factor IX.[14] Factor Xa alone does not generate thrombin efficiently; however, factors Xa and thrombin together can activate factors VII, V, and VIII. Factors Va and VIIIa are critical components of the prothrombinase and tenase complexes (see Fig. 6.1), respectively, which are 10^5-fold to 10^6-fold more active at generating thrombin than their serine protease factors acting independently.[13]

Thrombin proteolytically cleaves peptides from the fibrinogen molecule, resulting in the polymerization of fibrin monomers to form a gel. Thrombin also activates factor XIII in a reaction that is greatly accelerated (>80-fold) by the presence of fibrin.[15] Factor XIIIa covalently cross-links adjacent fibrin monomers, forming a stable clot that is more resistant to lysis by plasmin.

Coagulation Inhibition

Several mechanisms have evolved to control the rate of thrombin and fibrin formation (Fig. 6.2). AT is a serine protease inhibitor that is synthesized in the liver and endothelial cells. AT inhibits numerous coagulation factors, but its most important targets are thrombin and factor Xa. AT activity is enhanced at least 1000-fold whenever it binds to circulating heparin or endothelial-bound heparin-like molecules. After the AT–heparin complex binds to an activated coagulation factor, the heparin dissociates and continues to act as a catalyst for the formation of other AT–serine enzyme complexes.

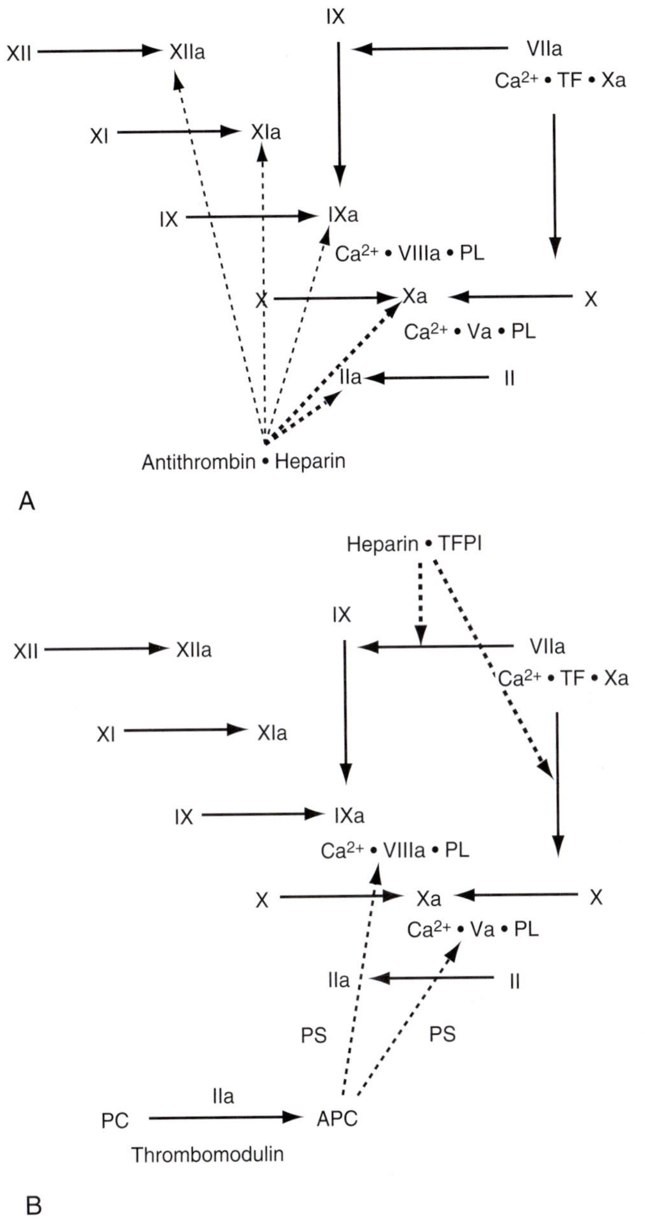

FIG 6.2 Sites of Activity for Natural Anticoagulants. *Dotted lines* indicated inhibitory activity. *APC*, Activated protein C; *PC*, protein C; *PL*, phospholipid; *PS*, protein S; *TF*, tissue factor; *TFPI*, tissue factor pathway inhibitor.

TFPI is an enzyme inhibitor synthesized by the endothelium and megakaryocytes.[16,17] It binds to the TF-VIIa-Xa complex and inhibits the further activation of factors X and IX.[18] TFPI is constitutively expressed on the endothelium, and its activity and antigen levels increase dramatically after the administration of heparin.

TM is a proteoglycan expressed on the surface of most endothelial cells[2] that binds thrombin, causes a conformational change in the substrate binding site, and renders the thrombin molecule incapable of binding active coagulation factors. TM also accelerates the inactivation of thrombin by AT.[19,20]

Protein C and protein S are synthesized by the liver, but protein S has also been found in endothelium and platelets.[21,22] Activated protein C (APC) binds to protein S on the endothelial or platelet surface and cleaves several peptide bonds in factors Va and VIIIa, resulting in decreased formation of the prothrombinase and tenase complexes.

Heparin cofactor II is another specific thrombin inhibitor that forms a stable 1 : 1 complex with thrombin. Heparin, heparan-like molecules, and dermatan sulfate accelerate the activity of heparin cofactor II. Unlike AT, heparin cofactor II cannot inhibit other coagulation factors. The plasma concentration of heparin cofactor II (70 µg/L) is much lower than that of AT (150 mg/L), and it is unlikely that heparin cofactor II has a major role in the regulation of hemostasis.

Fibrinolysis. Plasminogen, an inactive precursor synthesized in the liver, can be converted to plasmin by several plasminogen activators. Circulating t-PA does not activate plasminogen efficiently; however, both t-PA and plasminogen have high affinity for fibrin, which acts as a template for accelerated plasminogen activation (>1000-fold).[23,24] Thus the primary role for t-PA–activated plasmin is the lysis of preexisting formed fibrin clots. Alternatively, exogenously administered t-PA may activate non-bound plasminogen, resulting in the release of free plasmin, leading to the limited breakdown of fibrinogen, platelet receptors, factor V, and factor VIII, leading to a systemic fibrinolytic state.

t-PA is commercially available in several forms. Recombinant human t-PA is the most widely used agent for peripheral vascular applications, and it is Food and Drug Administration (FDA) indicated for acute ischemic stroke, acute myocardial infarction, and massive pulmonary embolism. Tenecteplase is a recombinant variant of t-PA with amino acid substitutions at three sites, resulting in a longer half-life and a higher affinity for thrombus-bound plasminogen. Each step within the plasminogen activation system has a known inhibitor. PAI-1 is released by endothelial cells, platelets, and hepatocytes. This inhibitor efficiently inactivates t-PA and two-chain u-PA and performs other functions, including the inhibition of thrombin and smooth muscle cell migration. α_2-Antiplasmin inactivates circulating plasmin more readily than it does fibrin-bound plasmin, thus decreasing overall systemic fibrinolysis.

Preoperative Evaluation

Clinical Evaluation

A thorough history and physical examination will detect the majority of bleeding disorders preoperatively. Laboratory testing is warranted if a bleeding disorder is present or suspected. Careful questioning should distinguish a congenital bleeding disorder from an acquired one. Determining the pattern of inheritance can further aid in identifying a congenital deficiency. A history of bleeding problems beginning in childhood or at the beginning of menses implies an inherited bleeding disorder. A history of postoperative or spontaneous bleeding in a family member is important, because many patients with inherited disorders do not experience serious bleeding until challenged by an operative procedure or trauma. All patients should be asked about bleeding after tooth extraction, minor trauma, circumcision, and other surgical procedures.

An acquired hemostatic disorder should be suspected in adults who bleed during or after surgery or trauma, but who have no previous history of bleeding disorders; however, some patients with congenital disorders, such as von Willebrand disease, may not demonstrate a bleeding diathesis until challenged. Patients with liver disease are at increased risk for developing a coagulopathy during surgery, after trauma, and after massive transfusion. A detailed history of drug use is also important, because many drugs alter platelet function and predispose patients to bleeding complications.

Physical examination should include a thorough inspection for ecchymoses, petechiae, purpura, hemangiomas, jaundice, hematomas, and hemarthroses. Petechiae, ecchymoses, and mucocutaneous bleeding (epistaxis, gastrointestinal or genitourinary bleeding, menorrhagia) are more commonly associated with defects in primary hemostasis. Bleeding into deep tissues (hemarthroses, muscle, and retroperitoneal hematomas) tends to occur with defects in coagulation. Signs of hepatic insufficiency should be noted, because these patients may have decreased production of coagulation proteins. Patients with myeloproliferative disorders, some malignant neoplasms, collagen disorders, or renal insufficiency are at increased risk for bleeding complications.

Laboratory Screening

Screening laboratory tests include the prothrombin time (PT; often reported as the international normalized ratio [INR]), activated partial thromboplastin time (aPTT), platelet count, and occasionally, platelet functional analyzer and mixing tests. Thromboelastography (TEG) and rotational thromboelastometry (ROTEM) may be useful in the resuscitation of patients who develop trauma-induced coagulopathy.[25] However, these latter tests have no established role in the preoperative screening for coagulopathy.

The PT assesses the extrinsic pathway and is prolonged by deficiencies of prothrombin, fibrinogen, and factors V, VII, and X. The INR is also useful for monitoring patients who are prescribed vitamin-K antagonists (VKA). The aPTT is prolonged by deficiencies of factors in the intrinsic pathway, including VIII, IX, XI, and XII. To a lesser extent, aPTT detects factor deficiencies in the common pathway: V, X, prothrombin, and fibrinogen. The aPTT is also prolonged by heparin and is used to monitor patients receiving heparin anticoagulation therapy.

Platelet count is a key component in evaluating the patient with suspected thrombocytopenia; however, this test does not offer information regarding platelet function. Platelet function analyzers (PFA-100) are used to quantify congenital and acquired platelet dysfunction and von Willebrand disease. They are also helpful when preoperatively screening those with a positive family history of bleeding disorders, or those with liver or renal disease. The PFA-100 can be used to identify possible causes for intraoperative or postoperative bleeding, monitor treatment for von Willebrand disease, and identify those high-risk patients who are resistant to aspirin therapy. Essentially the PFA-100 measures how fast platelets adhere, activate, and aggregate into a platelet plug onto a collagen coated membrane in the presence of either epinephrine or ADP. In the presence of epinephrine, the PFA-100 allows for the detection of aspirin-induced defects, and in the presence of ADP, more severe platelet defects may be detected.[26]

TABLE 6.1 **Common Causes of Elevated Prothrombin Time and Activated Partial Thromboplastin Time in the Presence and Absence of Bleeding**

BLEEDING				NO BLEEDING
Increased aPTT/ Increased PT	**Increased aPTT/ Normal PT**	**Normal aPTT/ Increased PT**	**Normal aPTT/ Normal PT**	**Increased aPTT/ Increased PT**
Heritable Causes				
Deficient factors I, II, V, X Dysfibrinogenemia	Deficient factors VIII, IX, XI von Willebrand disease	Factor VII deficiency Dysfibrinogenemia von Willebrand disease	Platelet function disorders Dysfibrinogenemia Factor XIII deficiency α_2-antiplasmin deficiency PAI-1 deficiency	Deficient factors XI, XII, kininogen, prekallikrein Factor VII deficiency
Acquired Causes				
Factor inhibitors against II, V, X DIC Liver disease Vitamin K deficiency Paraproteinemia Amyloidosis Heparin therapy	Factor inhibitors against VIII, IX, XI Heparin therapy	Warfarin therapy Liver disease Vitamin K deficiency DIC Paraproteinemia Specific inhibitors of Factor VII	Platelet inhibitors Thrombolytic agents von Willebrand syndrome	Lupus anticoagulant Heparin therapy Warfarin therapy or vitamin K deficiency Liver disease Dysfibrinogenemia Specific inhibitor of Factor V

aPTT, Activated partial thromboplastin time; *DIC*, disseminated intravascular coagulation; *PT*, prothrombin time.

In those patients with elevated aPTT, the presence of factor inhibitors may be suspected. A useful test in determining the presence of factor inhibitors is the mixing study. In a mixing study, normal plasma is added in a 1:1 ratio to a patient's plasma. If the aPTT corrects to normal, a specific factor deficiency (factors VIII, IX) is suspected. If the aPTT does not correct with the addition of normal plasma to the sample, the test is suggestive of the presence of a specific or nonspecific factor inhibitor in the patient's sample. The abnormal mix then can be incubated at 37°C for 30 to 60 minutes and reassessed. If there is no change in the aPTT, the patient likely has a nonspecific inhibitor such as lupus anticoagulant. If the aPTT increases after incubation, the patient likely has a specific factor inhibitor such as anti–factor VIII antibodies. Mixing studies are sensitive but not specific and should be used only as a screening test. If lupus anticoagulant or other factor inhibitors are suspected, further testing is required to confirm the diagnosis.[26] The common causes of elevated PT/INR and aPTT are shown in Table 6.1.

Platelet Disorders

Hemorrhagic complications can occur because of quantitative or qualitative platelet disorders that are acquired or congenital in origin. Thrombocytopenia and qualitative platelet defects are among the most common causes of bleeding in surgical patients. Spontaneous bleeding may occur when platelet counts fall to <20,000/mm^3. Platelet counts between 30,000 and 50,000/mm^3 are adequate to ensure hemostasis, provided that there are no associated functional platelet or coagulation disorders. Platelet counts of 50,000 to 100,000/mm^3 are required to restore hemostasis during bleeding.

Thrombocytopenia can occur from increased platelet destruction, abnormal production, dilution, or temporary sequestration (usually in the spleen). Increased destruction can occur via nonimmune or immune mechanisms. Non–immune-mediated thrombocytopenia occurs in hemolytic-uremic syndrome, thrombotic thrombocytopenic purpura, disseminated intravascular coagulation (DIC), and some vasculitides. In these syndromes, platelets are stimulated to aggregate within the microcirculation, often affecting the brain, kidneys, heart, lungs, and adrenal glands.[27] Early plasmapheresis and plasma transfusion (platelet-poor fresh frozen plasma [FFP], cryoprecipitate-poor plasma), along with high-dose glucocorticoid administration, can reverse most cases of thrombotic thrombocytopenic purpura.[28,29] Platelet transfusions should be used only for intracerebral or other life-threatening hemorrhagic complications. The treatment for hemolytic-uremic syndrome varies considerably but may include hemodialysis, heparin therapy, and plasma exchange, depending on the duration and severity of the illness. GP IIb-IIIa inhibitors may become a useful adjunct in the hemolytic-uremic syndrome.[30]

Immune-mediated platelet destruction (immune thrombocytopenia) can occur with certain collagen vascular diseases (lupus erythematosus) and lymphoproliferative disorders (chronic lymphocytic leukemia, non-Hodgkin lymphoma), or it may be drug induced. Acute ITP is a postinfectious thrombocytopenia that occurs predominantly in children and is usually self-limited. Chronic ITP is idiopathic and results when autoimmune antibodies are generated against the platelet membrane. Initial therapy for the chronic form consists of corticosteroids followed by more definitive therapy (e.g., rituximab, splenectomy, or platelet growth factors) in nonresponders. Severely thrombocytopenic patients with major hemorrhagic complications and patients requiring urgent surgery can be treated with platelet transfusions or intravenous (IV) gamma globulin.

Some drugs (e.g., vancomycin, quinidine, quinine, sulfonamides, penicillins, valproic acid, heparin) can induce thrombocytopenia via the formation of antigen-antibody complexes on the platelet surface, increasing platelet destruction. In general, discontinuation of the drug reverses the thrombocytopenia within

2 to 5 days. Adjuvant therapy for active bleeding may include corticosteroids, platelet transfusions, and in some cases, IV gamma globulin. These are often ineffective until the medication is no longer in circulation. Heparin-induced thrombocytopenia (HIT) is a prothrombotic condition, as discussed later in the section on thrombosis.

Impaired platelet production may be caused by aplastic anemia, radiation, myelosuppressive drugs, viral infections, vitamin B_{12} and folate deficiencies, and several other drugs (ethanol, estrogens, interferon, thiazides). Thrombocytopenia also has been described in association with numerous congenital disorders (Fanconi aplastic anemia, sex-linked recessive thrombocytopenia, Alport syndrome).

Thrombocytopenia commonly occurs after massive transfusions of banked blood. In general, the replacement of one blood volume decreases the platelet count by one-third to half.[31] Nevertheless, abnormal bleeding is uncommon, and the routine administration of platelets following massive transfusion is not warranted unless hemorrhage is ongoing.[32] Hypothermia (body temperature less than 32°C) also may cause thrombocytopenia. Each unit of single-donor platelet should increase the patient platelet count by 5000 to 10,000/mL, whereas a single unit of platelets via pheresis should increase the recipient's platelet count by 30,000 to 60,000/mL.

Qualitative Disorders of Platelet Function

Disturbances of platelet adherence and aggregation rarely cause spontaneous bleeding, but certainly may exacerbate bleeding after surgery and trauma. These disorders should be suspected when bleeding occurs in patients with normal coagulation studies and platelet counts. The most common *congenital* qualitative disorder of platelet function is von Willebrand disease. Bernard-Soulier syndrome, Glanzmann thrombasthenia, storage pool diseases, and diseases of platelet activation are rare qualitative platelet disorders, and they will not be covered further in this chapter.

Von Willebrand disease is the most common inherited bleeding disorder, characterized by a deficiency or defect in vWF. It has been classified into six subtypes (1, 2A, 2B, 2M, 2N, 3), with type 1 being the most common (70%).[33] Type 1 von Willebrand disease is usually inherited as an autosomal dominant trait with incomplete penetrance. In general, patients manifest epistaxis, ecchymoses, menorrhagia, and posttraumatic or postsurgical bleeding. Decreased platelet adherence causes prolongation of the bleeding time. The aPTT also may be elevated because most patients with this disease have concomitant decreases in factor VIII coagulation activity (VIII:C). Although much less common, subtypes 2 and 3 are associated with more severe bleeding complications, with subtypes 2N and 3 also demonstrating hemophilia-like symptoms (due to either poor factor VIII binding or markedly diminished vWF and factor VIII).

Treatment of von Willebrand disease can consist of replacement (cryoprecipitate and von Willebrand factor concentrates) or medical therapy (vasopressin, antifibrinolytic agents). Approximately 80% of patients with type 1 disease respond to desmopressin acetate (1-deamino-8-D-arginine vasopressin [DDAVP]) with increased vWF:Ag and VIII:C (within 60 minutes) that can last for 4 to 6 hours. Unfortunately, response to therapy cannot be predicted without trial administration. Repeated administration of DDAVP (every 12 hours) may be required for patients with type 1 disease who undergo surgical procedures. Most type 2 and type 3 patients do not respond to DDAVP. Antifibrinolytic agents (ε-aminocaproic acid, tranexamic acid) have been used for the treatment of mucocutaneous bleeding and for prophylaxis during oral surgical procedures.[34] Patients who are unresponsive to DDAVP may require replacement therapy during the perioperative period. Until recently, cryoprecipitate (rich in vWF, factors VIII and XIII, and fibronectin) was the treatment of choice. More recently, purified von Willebrand concentrates have been used successfully.[35] For major procedures, factor is given to achieve vWf levels of >80%. Specific levels of factor VIII or less commonly vWf levels are used to monitor response to replacement therapy.

Acquired qualitative platelet abnormalities may be caused by certain drugs, uremia, cirrhosis, myeloproliferative disorders, and dysproteinemias. As noted previously, aspirin and ADP-receptor inhibitors inhibit platelet function. Aspirin acetylates platelet COX-1 and -2, inhibiting thromboxane-mediated platelet activation and prostaglandin production for the life of the platelet. Clopidogrel, cangrelor, prasugrel, and ticagrelor are various classes of ADP-receptor inhibitors that inhibit ADP-mediated GP IIb-IIIa receptor expression. Clopidogrel binds irreversibly, whereas the newer agents demonstrate reversible binding to the $P2Y_{12}$ component of the platelet ADP receptor. Nonsteroidal antiinflammatory drugs (e.g., indomethacin, ibuprofen) reversibly inhibit cyclooxygenase. Numerous antibiotics, including some β-lactams, cephalosporins, and nitrofurantoin, impair platelet aggregation and prolong the bleeding time. Mechanisms can include the inhibition of agonist binding to the membrane receptor and inhibition of intracellular signal transduction. Platelet GP IIb-IIIa inhibitors (e.g., abciximab, eptifibatide, tirofiban) block the binding of fibrinogen to the GP IIb-IIIa receptor and effectively prevent platelet aggregation in a dose-dependent fashion. The correction of bleeding can be accomplished with platelet transfusions.

Uremia causes defective platelet adherence and aggregation, resulting in a prolonged PFA-100 as well. Clinical manifestations can include petechiae, ecchymoses, and mucocutaneous bleeding. The pathophysiology remains unclear, but may involve impaired thromboxane and calcium metabolism or defective platelet-subendothelial adhesion (via vWF). DDAVP has been shown to shorten bleeding times preoperatively in uremic patients.[36] IV DDAVP, 0.3 to 0.4 µg/kg over 15 to 30 minutes, shortens the bleeding time in most patients within 1 hour. Hemodialysis, peritoneal dialysis, and rarely the use of conjugated estrogens have been implemented with some success.

Coagulation factor deficiencies, DIC, dysfibrinogenemias, impaired thrombopoiesis, platelet sequestration, and impaired platelet aggregation all contribute to the hemostatic defects associated with liver failure. Therapy is nonspecific but can include DDAVP and platelet transfusions for severe thrombocytopenia.

Disorders of Secondary Hemostasis

Congenital Disorders

Congenital disorders of coagulation usually involve a single factor. Preoperative transfusion of the appropriate factor is necessary and may be required during surgery and postoperatively as well. Deficiencies of factor XII, HMWK, and prekallikrein cause prolongation of the aPTT but do not cause significant bleeding diatheses. Deficiencies of the remaining factors can result in serious bleeding after surgery or trauma.

Hemophilia A (factor VIII deficiency) is the most common of the inherited coagulation defects, with a prevalence of 1 in 10,000 males. Hemophilia B (Christmas disease, factor IX deficiency) has a prevalence of approximately 1 in 50,000 males. Both are X-linked recessive disorders that are clinically indistinguishable. The severity of these disorders depends on the levels of factor VIII or IX that are present. Severely affected individuals (factor levels <1%) manifest spontaneous hemarthroses and deep tissue hematomas during infancy or early childhood. Patients with mild to moderate hemophilia (factor levels >5%) may develop hemorrhagic complications only after surgery or trauma.

Patients with hemophilia A who require major surgery should receive factor VIII replacement to achieve 100% of normal activity just before the procedure. For each unit per kilogram of body weight infused, the factor VIII level is increased by approximately 0.02 U/mL (normal activity is 1 U/mL).[37] Levels should be monitored postoperatively, and replacement therapy should be repeated every 12 hours to maintain at least 50% of normal activity until all wounds are healed.[38] Factor VIII levels can be restored using virus-inactivated factor VIII concentrate, or recombinant factor VIII. DDAVP (which increases factor VIII levels) and tranexamic acid may be used as adjunctive therapies in patients with mild hemophilia to reduce or avoid the need for replacement therapy during oral or minor surgical procedures.

Patients with hemophilia B should have at least 100% of normal activity before major surgery and for the first 7 to 10 days postoperatively. Factor IX can be replaced with purified factor IX or recombinant factor IX. However, replacement therapy for hemophilia A and B is complicated by the development of inhibitors to factors VIII and IX in approximately 20% of patients. Alternative strategies include the use of high-dose factor VIII or recombinant factor VIIa (rVIIa) and attempts to induce immune tolerance.

Rare coagulation factor deficiencies of factors II, V, VII, and X occur with a prevalence of 1:500,000 to 1:1,000,000. They are usually transmitted with an autosomal recessive pattern. The most severe complications occur with deficiencies of factors II and X.[39] In general, only low levels of factor activity (10% to 20% of normal) are required for normal hemostasis. Replacement therapy for factors II and X can be accomplished with FFP or factor concentrates. Factor IX concentrates contain significant amounts of factors II and X and can be used for their replacement. The short half-life of factor VII requires a more frequent replacement schedule using factor VII concentrates. rVIIa also can be used for factor VII deficiencies. Factor V deficiencies can be treated with FFP, because factor V concentrates are not yet commercially available.

Abnormalities of fibrinogen and fibrinolysis are also heritable. Afibrinogenemia is a rare disorder transmitted as an autosomal recessive trait; hypofibrinogenemia can occur in heterozygous individuals. Clinical manifestations include gastrointestinal and mucous membrane bleeding, hemarthroses, intracranial hemorrhage, and recurrent fetal loss. The PT and aPTT, which are markedly prolonged, usually correct when mixed with normal plasma. Replacement therapy with cryoprecipitate or fibrinogen concentrates is usually reserved for active bleeding, the perioperative period, and prophylaxis during pregnancy. The goal of fibrinogen therapy for hemostasis should be >150 mg/dL. Each unit of cryoprecipitate usually increases the fibrinogen level by approximately 10 mg/dL.[40]

Dysfibrinogenemias are a heterogeneous group of disorders that can cause defective fibrin formation, polymerization, cross-linkage, or impaired fibrinolysis. Patients may manifest mild to moderate bleeding diatheses (30%) or recurrent thromboses (20%).[41] The PT and aPTT usually are normal, but functional assays for fibrinogen (thrombin time) are abnormal. Cryoprecipitate or fibrinogen concentrates are indicated for hemorrhage, but contraindicated for acute thrombotic episodes.

Congenital hyperfibrinolytic states can result in delayed bleeding. The congenital hyperfibrinolytic states include heterozygous and homozygous α_2-antiplasmin deficiencies and functionally abnormal or deficient PAI-1.[42] The whole blood clot lysis time and the euglobulin clot lysis time are characteristically shortened. Antifibrinolytic agents (ε-aminocaproic acid or tranexamic acid) are recommended for the management of active bleeding.[43]

Acquired Disorders

Patients develop coagulation disorders because of deficiencies of coagulation proteins, synthesis of nonfunctioning factors, and consumption or inadequate replacement of coagulation proteins.

Hepatic insufficiency can cause decreased plasma levels of several coagulation factors (including factors II, V, VII, IX, X, XIII, and fibrinogen) because of a decreased synthetic capacity, defective posttranslational modification (γ-carboxylation), and an increased breakdown of activated factors (with subclinical DIC). Although liver disease is a risk factor for bleeding, paradoxically, it is also a risk factor for thrombosis, perhaps due to decreased synthesis of protein C, S, and AT. Thrombocytopenia can also occur because of increased splenic sequestration and decreased production of growth factors by the liver (thrombopoietin); however, levels of factor VIII and vWF may be elevated because they are synthesized in extrahepatic locations. The correction of coagulation factor deficits and thrombocytopenia is accomplished with FFP and platelet transfusions, respectively. Vitamin K administration alone does not completely reverse the coagulopathy.

Vitamin K deficiency can cause a bleeding diathesis as a result of the synthesis of nonfunctional forms of the vitamin K–dependent coagulation factors II, VII, IX, and X. Normal sources of vitamin K include dietary intake (e.g., leafy green vegetables, soybean oil) and vitamin K synthesis by normal intestinal flora. Vitamin K deficiency can be caused by poor dietary intake, decreased intestinal absorption of vitamin K, decreased production by the gut flora, and liver failure. This situation more commonly arises in patients receiving antibiotic bowel preparations or long-term parenteral nutrition (without vitamin K supplementation). Vitamin K deficiency also occurs in patients who have a prolonged recovery after intestinal surgery and in those with intrinsic bowel diseases (e.g., Crohn disease, celiac sprue, ulcerative colitis), as well as in patients with obstructive jaundice. Vitamin K should be administered preoperatively to patients with hepatic insufficiency, obstructive jaundice, malabsorption states, or malnutrition. Patients with an intact enterohepatic circulation can receive vitamin K orally (2.5 to 5 mg), with normalization of the PT within 24 to 48 hours. Slow IV administration (over 30 minutes) should be used in patients with biliary obstruction or malabsorption. Patients who require urgent correction of the PT should receive slow IV vitamin K and replacement therapy (4-factor prothrombin complex concentrates [PCC]).

DIC is characterized by the systemic generation of fibrin, often resulting in the thrombosis of small- and medium-sized blood vessels. The consumption of clotting factors, increased fibrinolysis, and thrombocytopenia also results in impaired coagulation and hemorrhagic complications. DIC is mediated by several cytokines (including tumor necrosis factor-α and interleukin-6), which result in the excess generation of thrombin. Fibrinolytic activity, which is initially increased via the release of t-PA, can become depressed in some patients due to elevated PAI-1. DIC can develop in association with bacterial infections (gram-positive and gram-negative infections), trauma, malignancy, obstetric complications, hemolytic transfusion reactions, giant hemangiomas (Kasabach-Merritt syndrome), and aortic aneurysms. A compensated DIC, in which coagulation factors and platelets are replaced as they are consumed, may be asymptomatic or may appear with ecchymoses and petechiae. Surgery, trauma, hypotension, or transfusion reactions can exacerbate the coagulopathy and hypofibrinolysis, leading to excessive bleeding and intravascular thrombosis.

A combination of laboratory tests may help to confirm the clinical diagnosis of DIC. These tests include detection of thrombocytopenia or a rapidly decreasing platelet count, prolongation of the PT and aPTT, and the presence of fibrin degradation products (D-dimer assay, latex agglutination for fibrous degradation products). Extrinsic pathway coagulation proteins (factors II, V, VII, and X) and physiologic coagulation inhibitors (AT, protein C) usually are depressed, whereas vWF and factor VIII levels may be increased.[44] The fibrinogen level is variably affected by DIC.

The first goal of management is eliminating the cause of DIC. When this is possible, the intravascular coagulation ceases with the return of normal hemostasis. In severe DIC, with ongoing blood loss, patients are best managed by replacing deficient blood elements using FFP (up to 6 units per 24 hours) and platelets while the precipitating cause of DIC is eliminated.[44] Administration of AT and protein C concentrates may retard the consumption of coagulation factors, although this remains to be proven. Some trials have demonstrated a benefit with the administration of heparin or low-molecular-weight heparin (LMWH).[45,46] Given that patients with DIC already have a coagulopathy, heparin should be used cautiously (lower IV doses of 300 to 500 units/h) and with careful clinical observation and laboratory monitoring. Direct thrombin inhibitors (hirudin, recombinant TM), APC, and extrinsic pathway inhibitors (recombinant TFPI) are under investigation as well.

Management of Anticoagulation

More than 30 million prescriptions for VKA are written in the United States every year, for indications such as therapy for acute arterial and VTE and prophylaxis against thromboembolism in patients with chronic atrial fibrillation and mechanical heart valves.[47] As a result, VKA-associated bleeding has become the most frequent cause of emergency room visits for medication-associated complications.[48]

Over the past few years, several direct oral anticoagulants (DOAC) received FDA approval for the treatment and prevention of VTE and for prophylaxis against thromboembolism in chronic atrial fibrillation. The use of these medications has risen rapidly, rivaling the volume of prescriptions written for VKAs. Although the overall risk for major bleeding is lower with the DOACs, the risk for gastrointestinal bleeding may be higher. Treatment strategies for the reversal of VKAs and DOACs will be discussed in this section.

Treatment Strategies for Vitamin K Antagonist–Associated Bleeding

Vitamin K antagonists require periodic monitoring of the INR, and this is commonly performed by specialized anticoagulation clinics and primary care and specialist physicians, with some protocols allowing for patient self-management. For most indications, an INR range of 2.0 to 3.0 is suggested, with the exception of patients with mechanical mitral heart valves and patients with antiphospholipid antibody (APA) syndrome who have had prior episodes of arterial thrombosis. In these latter instances, the typical INR goal range is 3.0 to 4.0.

Controlled clinical studies have shown that treatment with VKAs increases the risk of major bleeding by 0.5% per year and the risk of intracranial hemorrhage by 0.2% per year.[49] Risk factors associated with hemorrhage in patients treated with VKAs include target INR greater than three,[50] patient age, cytochrome P450 CYP2C9 polymorphisms that decrease VKA metabolism,[51] and renal and hepatic insufficiency. The addition of antiplatelet therapy and nonsteroidal antiinflammatory medications in the setting of VKA therapy also increases the risk of major bleeding and gastrointestinal bleeding by 2.5-fold and 11-fold, respectively.[52-54]

In the presence of bleeding, patients should be assessed for hemodynamic stability and a potential bleeding source. Treatment algorithms suggest stratification into those with clinically relevant nonmajor bleeding and those with major bleeding.[55] In either situation, the VKA should be discontinued, volume replacement should be administered, and local hemostasis should be applied (if possible). Red blood cells may be indicated for symptomatic anemia, and platelets for patients with recent usage of antiplatelet medications. In the setting of nonmajor bleeding, lower doses of vitamin K should be administered (1 mg to 2 mg slow IV), with an expected normalization of the INR within 12 to 16 hours. In patients with major bleeding, higher doses of vitamin K should be administered (5 to 10 mg slow IV). Regardless of vitamin K dosage, VKA reversal will not be immediate.

Immediate reversal may be achieved with the IV administration of 4-factor prothrombin complex concentrate (4-factor

PCC). PCCs are lyophilized concentrates of a standardized amount of factor IX and differing amounts of factors II, VII, and X that vary by manufacturer. They are virally inactivated, undergo prion reducing processes, and are administered in small volumes (40 to 80 mL). The dosing should be guided by the patient INR, as shown here:

	4-Factor PCC dosing
INR 2–4	25 Units/kg IV
INR 4–6	35 Units/kg IV
INR >6	50 Units/kg IV

INR, International normalized ratio; *IV*, intravenous.

PCCs are indicated for the urgent reversal of VKA in those patients exhibiting major bleeding or those requiring urgent surgical or other invasive procedures (<6 hours). PCCs are *not* recommended for VKA reversal in the elective setting, for elevated INR without bleeding or an urgent need for surgery, for use in massive transfusions, coagulopathy of liver disease, patients with a recent history of thrombosis, ischemic stroke or DIC, or patients with a history of HIT. Complications of PCC use include thrombosis, DIC, hemorrhage, and viral transmission.[56]

Although commonly used to reverse the INR in patients taking warfarin, factor replacement using FFP has several disadvantages. FFP elicits only a 2% to 4% rise in factor activity per unit infused, and large volumes of FFP often are required to correct an elevated INR. In addition, there is an associated risk of transfusion-related acute lung injury (TRALI), anaphylaxis, and transmission of viral infections. FFP must be thawed before infusion and needs to be cross-matched to ensure ABO compatibility, limiting the rapidity of INR correction and hemorrhage cessation. Because of the variability of vitamin K–dependent clotting factors in FFP, others have studied the effect of clotting factor concentrates on the INRs of anticoagulated patients who require rapid correction. Makris and colleagues[57] found that patients given FFP did not normalize their INR, whereas those treated with clotting factor concentrates did, largely due to increased factor IX levels in the clotting factor concentrate compared with the factor IX levels found in FFP.

rVIIa replacement also has been used to correct INR and halt hemorrhage in patients taking VKAs. rVIIa forms complexes with tissue factor to activate factors IX and X, initiating the clotting cascade while bypassing the activation of factors VIII and IX. A typical dose of rVIIa is 5 to 16 μg/kg IV.[58] However, a comparison of rVIIa with 4-factor PCC (Octaplex, Octapharma AG, Lachen, Switzerland) showed that although both rVIIa and PCC corrected the INR, only PCC restored endogenous thrombin generation, which is the key end point in restoring hemostasis.[59]

Treatment Strategies for Direct Oral Anticoagulant-Associated Bleeding

Several DOAC have received FDA approval for the treatment and prevention of VTE, and for thromboembolism prophylaxis in patients with chronic atrial fibrillation. These include dabigatran (direct thrombin inhibitor), rivaroxaban, apixaban, and edoxaban (factor Xa inhibitors). Despite their lower overall risk for clinically relevant bleeding when compared with VKA, many clinicians had early reservations about DOACs, due to the inability to monitor or effectively reverse these agents.

None of the commonly available coagulation assays will accurately monitor serum levels of dabigatran. The aPTT and activated clotting time will give an approximation of dabigatran activity, but the relationship is nonlinear. Of all the common coagulation assays, the dilute thrombin time is the most sensitive and has the greatest potential utility. For factor Xa inhibitors, only the aPTT provides an approximation of activity, more so for rivaroxaban than for apixaban. Assays for anti–factor Xa activity (as used for LMWH) have some potential, but will require further development, specific for each of these DOAC agents.

Patients with DOAC-associated bleeding also should be stratified into those with minor, moderate-to-severe, and life-threatening bleeding.[60] Given the shorter half-lives of the DOACs, mild bleeding may only require temporary discontinuation or a delay in the next dosage of medication. Moderate-to-severe bleeding is treated with mechanical compression or surgical intervention, if applicable, and blood product transfusion/fluid replacement for symptomatic anemia. Dabigatran-associated major bleeding may be treated with oral charcoal administration (if <2 hours since ingestion) or hemodialysis (>60% removal with dialysis). However, the specific dabigatran reversal agent, idarucizumab (FDA approved in 2015), is likely to be more effective. With life-threatening bleeding, prothrombin complex concentrates, or rVIIa, may be administered as well, especially for bleeding associated with the direct factor Xa inhibitors (rivaroxaban, apixaban, edoxaban), at least until factor Xa–specific reversal agents become FDA approved. The most promising reversal agent (andexanet alpha) normalizes factor Xa activity within 15 minutes of IV bolus administration.[61]

Perioperative Management

Patients who receive antithrombotic therapy and subsequently require surgical or other invasive procedures must be assessed to determine the best method of anticoagulation management to minimize the risk of periprocedural bleeding and thrombosis. Detailed recommendations are available in the 2012 American College of Chest Physicians (ACCP) Evidence-Based Clinical Practice Guidelines, with updated recommendations regarding the perioperative management of DOACs published in 2016.[62,63] Several factors should be considered when developing an optimal management strategy. These include the risk for perioperative thromboembolism, risk for perioperative bleeding, and the pharmacokinetic profile of the anticoagulant medication in question. Table 6.2 shows an ACCP thromboembolism risk stratification for patients receiving anticoagulation for three common indications: mechanical heart valves, atrial fibrillation, and VTE. For patients with mechanical valves, perioperative thromboembolism risk is influenced by the position of the valve, valve design, and the presence of recent stroke or transient ischemic attack. Perioperative risk for patients with atrial fibrillation and VTE is primarily guided by the classification system: congestive heart failure, hypertension, age ≥75 years, diabetes, stroke ($CHADS_2$) score, and time interval since the most recent VTE, respectively.

These perioperative thromboembolism risks should be weighed against the risk for bleeding. Patients undergoing *minimal*

TABLE 6.2 Risk Stratification and Recommendations for Perioperative Arterial or Venous Thromboembolism

	INDICATION FOR ANTITHROMBOTIC THERAPY		
Risk	**Mechanical Heart Valve**	**Atrial Fibrillation**	**VTE**
High	Any MVR, older aortic valve, recent CVA or TIA (<6 months)	$CHADS_2$ score, 5–6; recent CVA or TIA (<3 months); rheumatic valve disease	VTE within 3 months; severe thrombophilia; Prot C, Prot S, AT deficiency; antiphospholipid antibody; multiple abnormalities
Moderate	Bileaflet AVR plus one of: atrial fibrillation, prior CVA or TIA, HTN, DM, CHF, or age >75 y	$CHADS_2$, score 3–4	VTE 3–12 months ago; nonsevere thrombophilia (heterozygous factor V Leiden or prothrombin mutation); recurrent VTE; active cancer (<6 months)
Low	Bileaflet AVR without other CVA risk factors	$CHADS_2$, score 0–2	VTE >12 months ago and no other risk factors

AT, Antithrombin; *AVR*, aortic valve replacement; *$CHADS_2$*, classification system: congestive heart failure, hypertension, age ≥75 years, diabetes, stroke; *CHF*, congestive heart failure; *CVA*, cerebrovascular accident; *DM*, diabetes mellitus; *HTN*, hypertension; *IV*, intravenous; *LMWH*, low-molecular weight heparin; *MVR*, mitral valve replacement; *ProtC*, protein C; *ProtS*, protein S; *SC*, subcutaneous; *TIA*, transient ischemic attack; *VTE*, venous thromboembolism.

From Douketis JD, Berger PB, Dunn AS, et al: Perioperative management of antithrombotic therapy: American College of Chest Physicians Evidence-Based Clinical Practice Guidelines (9th edition). *Chest* 141:326S–350S, 2012.

TABLE 6.3 Recommended Perioperative Management for Patients Receiving Anticoagulation

Thromboembolic Risk	Nonminimal Bleeding-Risk Procedures	Minimal Bleeding-Risk Procedures
High	DOAC: Interrupt DOAC therapy, LMWH bridging not suggested Warfarin: Interrupt warfarin therapy with LMWH bridging suggested based on clinician judgment[a]	No interruption of anticoagulant therapy suggested
Moderate	DOAC: Interrupt DOAC therapy, LMWH bridging not suggested Warfarin: Consider interrupting warfarin therapy without LMWH bridging on the basis of clinician judgment[a]	No interruption of anticoagulant therapy suggested
Low	DOAC: Interrupt DOAC therapy, LMWH bridging not suggested Warfarin: Interrupt warfarin therapy, LMWH bridging not necessary[a]	No interruption of anticoagulant therapy suggested

[a]Consider administering prophylactic dose LMWH for VTE prevention in patients undergoing high bleeding-risk procedures or those at high risk of VTE.

DOAC, Direct oral anticoagulation; *LMWH*, low–molecular–weight heparin.

Modified from Spyropoulos AC, Al-Badri A, Sherwood MW, Douketis JD: Periprocedural management of patients receiving a vitamin K antagonist or a direct oral anticoagulant requiring an elective procedure or surgery. *J Thromb Haemost* 14:875–885, 2016.

bleeding-risk procedures (minor dental or dermatologic procedures, cataract surgery, pacemaker, or defibrillator implantation) generally do not require interruption of their anticoagulant therapy, with the caveat that DOAC medications should be withheld on the day of the procedure. In patients who are to undergo a higher bleeding-risk procedure, Table 6.3 lists some anticoagulation management strategies. These recommendations have evolved in recent years, with a trend away from bridging anticoagulation. Recent meta-analyses and a large randomized clinical trial of patients receiving chronic anticoagulation for atrial fibrillation (BRIDGE) have demonstrated that bridging anticoagulation was consistently associated with a three- to fourfold increased risk for perioperative major bleeding, *without* a reduction in the rate of acute thromboembolic episodes.[64,65]

The meta-analyses data regarding perioperative warfarin bridging are limited by the heterogeneity of the studies included, with varying bridging protocols or indications for anticoagulation. In addition, the recent BRIDGE trial was limited by the relatively low inclusion rate of patients who were deemed to be at the highest risk for thromboembolism (approximately 3% had $CHADS_2$ scores or 5 to 6). In addition, only 11% of patients underwent major or high bleeding-risk procedures. In combination, these data do suggest that patients with warfarin-treated chronic atrial fibrillation, who are at low to moderate risk for thromboembolism, may withhold bridging around the time of surgery or other invasive procedures. Patients at high risk of thromboembolism (prosthetic heart valves, higher $CHADS_2$ score) are still being evaluated in an ongoing clinical trial (NCT 00432796). Until further data is available, warfarin-treated patients at high risk for thromboembolism should still receive bridging anticoagulation (see Table 6.3).

Given the more recent approval of DOAC medications, there are less data to guide perioperative management. In general, bridging with parenteral anticoagulants is likely unnecessary, due to the shorter half-lives of these newer oral anticoagulants. Spyropoulos and colleagues suggest that these medications should be withheld to allow 2 to 3 half-lives between the last dose and a low bleeding-risk surgery, and 4 to 5 half-lives between the last DOAC dose and a high bleeding-risk surgery.[63] In patients with a creatinine clearance >30 to 50 mL/min, the last dose should be taken 2 days prior to a low bleeding-risk procedure, and 3 days prior to a high bleeding-risk procedure. In patients with significantly impaired renal function, these authors recommend a longer interruption interval.

Resumption of DOAC or warfarin anticoagulation during the postoperative period is dependent upon the patient's ability to absorb these medications adequately, timing until peak onset of activity, risk for arterial or VTE, and risk for bleeding. Warfarin usually may be restarted within 12 to 24 hours, since its therapeutic effect usually is delayed for several days. The therapeutic effect of DOACs occurs much more rapidly, in the range of 2 to 4 hours after ingestion. Therefore, these latter medications should be withheld for at least 24 hours for low bleeding-risk procedures, and 48 to 72 hours for high bleeding-risk procedures. During this time interval, surgeons usually should consider the option to administer prophylactic dose parenteral anticoagulation as well.

THROMBOSIS

In 1856, Virchow suggested that thrombus formation was the result of an interaction among an injured surface, stasis, and the hypercoagulability of blood.[66] One or more components of Virchow triad can be invoked when determining the cause of in vivo thrombosis. Hypofibrinolysis is the only major process not recognized by Virchow that contributes to intravascular thrombosis.

The heritable thrombophilic conditions (with the exception of congenital hyperhomocysteinemia), and most of the acquired ones as well, are more closely associated with VTE (Table 6.4). Some acquired conditions such as APA syndrome, HIT, and some malignancies have a recognized association with both arterial and venous thromboses. The more common heritable and acquired hypercoagulable states are discussed later, as are the indications for testing and the optimal timing for the performance of these assays. A detailed description of the various antithrombotic medications that are used for the management of established arterial and venous thromboses, and prophylaxis against thromboembolism, are discussed in other chapters. This chapter will discuss anticoagulation management with specific regard to the management of specific hypercoagulable conditions.

TABLE 6.4 Acquired and Heritable Risk Factors for Venous Thrombosis

Acquired	Heritable	Mixed Etiology
Immobilization	Antithrombin deficiency	High factor VIII
Plaster cast	Protein C deficiency	High factor IX
Trauma	Protein S deficiency	High factor XI
Major surgery	Factor V Leiden	High levels of fibrinogen
Orthopedic surgery	Prothombin 20210A	High levels of TAFI
Malignancy	Dysfibrinogenemia	Low levels of TFPI
Oral contraceptives	Factor XIII 34val	APC-resistance in absence of F V Leiden
Hormonal replacement therapy	Fibrinogen (G) 10034T	Hyperhomocysteinemia
Antiphospholipid antibodies	Non-O blood group	High PAI-3
Myeloproliferative disorders		
Central venous catheters		
Age		
Obesity		

APC, Activated protein C; *PAI-3*, plasminogen activator inhibitor-3; *TAFI*, thrombin-activatable fibrinolysis inhibitor; *TFPI*, tissue factor pathway inhibitor.

Modified from Rosendaal FR and Reitsma PH: Genetics of venous thrombosis. *J Thromb Haemost* 7(S1):301–304, 2009.

Prothrombotic Conditions

Inherited Prothrombotic Conditions

APC resistance is most commonly caused by a mutation in the factor V gene, during which Arg506 is replaced with Gln (factor V Leiden), making activated factor V resistant to degradation by APC.[67] It is the most common inherited hypercoagulable condition, occurring in approximately 12% to 33% of patients with VTE.[68-71] In contrast, it has a prevalence of 3% to 6% in control populations.[69-71] The white population is affected more commonly than black, Asian, or Native American populations. Individuals who are heterozygous for the factor V mutation have a 2.7-fold to sevenfold increased risk for VTE, whereas homozygous patients may have an 80-fold increased risk.[70,71] A small percentage of patients with APC resistance do not have the Leiden mutation. Other factor V mutations (factor V Cambridge, factor V HR2 haplotype) can also cause APC resistance.[72,73]

Functional APC resistance can be detected by performing the aPTT in the presence and absence of purified APC. In general, an aPTT ratio (aPTT with APC/aPTT without APC) of less than 2 is considered a positive study (normal is 2.4 to 4.0). Numerous factors can affect the accuracy of the aPTT ratio, including protein C deficiency, the presence of anticoagulants, and antiphospholipid antibodies. Modifications to this functional assay have improved its sensitivity and specificity.[74] DNA testing using the polymerase chain reaction to amplify the factor V Leiden mutation is standard. The optimal management of patients with APC resistance remains to be defined. APC-resistant individuals in high-risk situations (e.g., pregnancy, surgery) should receive thrombosis prophylaxis. Patients with prior thrombotic episodes may benefit from long-term warfarin therapy. This is especially true for patients with multiple prior episodes, thromboses in unusual locations, and multiple inherited thrombophilic mutations.

Prothrombin 20210A is a mutation (G to A substitution) in the prothrombin gene at nucleotide 20210, resulting in increased levels of plasma prothrombin.[75] The prothrombin 20210A mutation is present in 18% of selected patients with strong family histories of VTE, 6.2% of unselected patients with a first episode of thrombosis, and 2.3% of healthy controls. The prevalence is even higher in southern European whites.[76] A significant number of patients have more than one congenital thrombophilic condition, further increasing their risk for VTE.[75,77]

AT deficiency was the first reported congenital thrombophilic condition.[78] It is transmitted with an autosomal dominant pattern and has a prevalence of 1 : 5000 in the population.[79] AT deficiency has been detected in approximately 1% of patients with venous thromboses, conferring a risk that may be as high as 50-fold greater than normal.[80,81] The lifetime risk for developing a thrombotic episode ranges between 17% and 50%.[82] Although thromboembolism may occur spontaneously, it is usually associated with a precipitating event such as surgery, trauma, or pregnancy. Arterial thromboses, although less common than venous thromboses, also occur. AT levels may be reduced to less than 80% of normal in other conditions, including hepatic insufficiency, DIC, acute venous thrombosis, sepsis, and nephrotic syndrome, and in patients receiving heparin or estrogen supplementation.

The mainstay of therapy in AT-deficient patients with VTE is still heparin anticoagulation, although supranormal dosages may be required.[83] AT concentrates may be appropriate in patients who do not achieve adequate anticoagulation with heparin alone. The minimum level of AT necessary to prevent thrombosis is unknown; however, it is suggested that levels be adjusted to greater than 80% of normal activity. AT can be replaced with AT concentrate (1 U/kg increases the AT activity by 1% to 2%) or FFP. Asymptomatic patients should receive thrombosis prophylaxis during high-risk situations such as prolonged immobilization, surgery, or pregnancy; however, long-term warfarin therapy is usually reserved for AT-deficient patients who have experienced thrombotic events.

Protein C and protein S deficiencies account for a number of disorders. Congenital protein C deficiency may be transmitted as an autosomal dominant or recessive trait and has a prevalence of 1:200 to 1:500.[84,85] The incidence of thrombosis varies, depending on the population in question. Studies identifying protein C deficiency in healthy blood donors demonstrate a low prevalence of venous thrombosis, whereas studies that screen patients with VTE find a higher prevalence of protein C deficiency compared with controls.[80,84-86] Overall, inherited protein C deficiency is associated with an approximately sevenfold increased risk for developing a first venous thromboembolic event.[86] Common sites for venous thromboses include the lower extremities, mesenteric veins, and cerebral venous sinuses. Functional and immunologic assays are available to establish the diagnosis of protein C deficiency. Healthy adults have protein C antigen levels ranging from 70% to 140% of normal. Patients with antigen levels less than 55% are likely to have heterozygous protein C deficiency.

Approximately 60% of the total protein S circulates bound to C4b complement-binding protein.[87] Deficiency states can occur with decreased total protein S, decreased free protein S, and decreased functional protein S activity (with total and free protein S concentrations in the normal range). Histories of patients with congenital protein S deficiencies are similar to those of patients with protein C deficiency, although arterial thromboses also have been described in patients with protein S deficiency. Protein S can be measured with functional assays, which assess the ability to catalyze the inhibition of factor Va by APC, or immunologic assays.

Both protein C and protein S are vitamin K–dependent proteins synthesized in the liver. Consequently, plasma levels may be decreased in patients with hepatic insufficiency. Acquired protein C and protein S deficiencies can also occur with warfarin administration, vitamin K deficiency (malabsorption, biliary obstruction), sepsis, DIC, and acute thromboses, and in patients receiving some chemotherapeutic medications. Because C4b is also an acute-phase reactant, inflammatory conditions can increase C4b levels, causing a decrease in free protein S and an increased tendency toward thrombosis.[88]

Heparin is the first line of therapy in the management of acute thromboembolic episodes in patients with known protein C and S deficiencies. Because warfarin-induced skin necrosis is more likely to occur in patients with protein C deficiency, heparin therapy should overlap with the first 4 or 5 days of warfarin therapy, and large loading dosages of warfarin should be avoided. Longer-term treatment with warfarin is effective in the prevention of recurrent venous thromboembolic episodes in patients with protein C and protein S deficiencies. FFP occasionally may be required to restore functional levels of protein C and protein S.

Abnormalities of fibrinogen and fibrinolysis include *dysfibrinogenemias*, which may impair any of the steps involved in the generation and cross-linkage of fibrin. These anomalies have been reported in association with bleeding diatheses (30%) and VTE (20%). Therapeutic alternatives have been described earlier.

Elevated factor XI is a mild risk factor for the development of venous thrombosis.[89,90] Factor XI levels in the 90th percentile or greater confer a 2.2-fold relative risk for the development of venous thrombosis. Even lower factor XI levels demonstrate a linear dose-response relationship with thrombotic risk. The underlying cause for elevated factor XI levels remains to be determined.

Acquired Prothrombotic Conditions

Many clinical disorders predispose to thrombosis by activating the coagulation system or causing platelet aggregation. Soft tissue trauma, thermal injuries, and operative dissection all predispose to thrombosis through the release of tissue factor and activation of the extrinsic coagulation pathway.

Sepsis predisposes to thrombosis via multiple mechanisms. Gram-positive bacteria may directly cause platelet aggregation and subsequent thrombosis. Gram-negative bacterial endotoxin may stimulate platelet aggregation but may also, through interaction with leukocytes and endothelial cells, cause TF-like activation of the coagulation system. Endotoxin is known to be a major stimulus for the development of DIC.

As many as 11% of patients with *malignancies* have venous thromboembolic complications.[91] Pancreatic, prostate, gastrointestinal, and lung cancers have a particularly strong association with thrombosis. Conversely, patients with unprovoked VTE are more likely to be diagnosed with cancer (up to 7.6%).[92] However, aggressive screening for occult malignancies in patients with VTE has not been shown to be cost-effective or to result in improved long-term survival.

Pregnancy is associated with a fourfold increased risk for VTE.[81,93] The risk may be threefold to fivefold greater in the immediate postpartum period. *Oral contraceptives and hormonal replacement therapy* are also associated with an approximately threefold increased risk, which is conferred immediately and is reversible.[94] Dinger and colleagues performed a case-control study evaluating newer preparations with lower doses of ethinylestradiol, but found similar rates of VTE between patients using low-dose and standard-dose combined oral contraceptives.[95]

Although the exact mechanism is unclear, women taking oral contraceptives demonstrate increased levels of thrombin and fibrinogen, with decreased levels of protein S and plasminogen activators.

Antiphospholipid antibodies (ApL), including lupus anticoagulants and anticardiolipin antibodies, are immunoglobulin (Ig) G, IgM, or IgA, which are directed against phospholipid-binding proteins (prothrombin and β_2-GP I). These antibodies interfere with in vitro phospholipid-dependent clotting assays, such as aPTT, kaolin clotting time, and the dilute Russell viper venom time. In vivo, antiphospholipid antibodies may promote thrombosis by interfering with the activation of protein C.[96] The presence of antiphospholipid antibodies is associated with a ninefold increased risk for venous thrombosis. Clinical manifestations of the antiphospholipid syndrome may include venous and arterial thromboses (coronary, cerebral) and recurrent fetal loss. Lupus anticoagulants are also associated with arterial thrombosis. As many as 50% of patients who are positive for lupus anticoagulants and undergo vascular surgical procedures develop thrombotic complications.[97] Patients with thrombotic episodes should receive heparin (usually LMWH) and warfarin anticoagulation, since evidence regarding use of the DOACs is preliminary. Long-term warfarin therapy (at higher intensity, INR greater than three) has been shown to reduce the recurrence of thrombosis.[98] The optimal duration of anticoagulation is unclear.

Heparin-associated antibodies (HAAbs) and *HIT* are important considerations for patients receiving anticoagulation therapy. HAAbs IgG and IgM target the heparin–platelet factor 4 complex. These immune complexes bind to the Fcγ-RII platelet receptor, causing pathophysiologic platelet activation, aggregation, and thrombocytopenia. The incidence of HAAb formation varies widely, depending on the indications for heparin, the type of heparin used, and the tests used to detect HAAbs. LMWHs are associated with a significantly decreased incidence of HAAb formation and HIT.[99] Up to 20% of patients who undergo vascular surgical procedures develop HAAbs, which are associated with a greater than twofold increased risk for thrombotic complications.[100] Overall, the incidence of HIT ranges between 2% and 9%, depending on the type of heparin used, the route of administration, and the definition of thrombocytopenia used.[101,102] Most authors use a platelet count of less than 100,000/mm^3 to define HIT-associated thrombocytopenia. However, thrombocytopenia is not a prerequisite for the development of thrombotic complications.

The diagnosis of HIT may be made according to the following criteria:

1. The development of thrombocytopenia or a significantly decreased platelet count while receiving heparin
2. Resolution of thrombocytopenia after cessation of heparin
3. Exclusion of other causes for thrombocytopenia
4. A positive HAAb assay (two-point platelet aggregation assay, serotonin release assay, enzyme-linked immunosorbent assay)

However, obtaining a prompt diagnosis may be problematic, since HAAb assays are time-consuming and may not be readily available at every institution. As a result, some patients with a low probability of HIT may undergo unnecessary interruption of anticoagulation in the presence of acute arterial or VTE. Instead, a validated clinical scoring system (4Ts Scoring System) recently has been developed to essentially exclude the diagnosis in patients with a low clinical probability of having HIT (Table 6.5).[103] Patients with a low probability 4Ts score have a 0.998 negative predictive value for HIT. Patients with a 4Ts score ≤3 may continue heparin, and alternative diagnoses should be considered. If the 4Ts score is ≥4, patients should discontinue heparin, start an alternative anticoagulant, and receive confirmatory HAAb lab testing.

In the short term, most HAAb-positive patients require continued anticoagulation, but there are a limited number of agents that have FDA approval in this setting (argatroban and bivalirudin). Warfarin has been the standard of care for long-term anticoagulation in HIT, but typically should not be initiated until after the platelet count returns to normal. In this setting, patients had been treated as inpatients with IV argatroban and frequent platelet counts. Low-molecular-weight heparin (LMWH)

TABLE 6.5 The 4Ts Scoring System

4Ts Category	2 Points	1 Point	0 Points
Thrombocytopenia	Platelet counts fall >50% and platelet nadir ≥20	Platelet count 30%–50% or platelet nadir 10–19	Platelet counts fall <30% or platelet nadir <10
Timing of platelet counts fall	Clear onset days 5–10 or platelet fall ≤1 day (prior heparin exposure within 30 days)	Consistent with days 5–10, but unclear (missing platelet counts); Onset after date 10; Or fall ≤1 day (prior heparin exposure 30–100 days ago)	Platelet count ≤4 days without recent exposure
Thrombosis or other sequela	New thrombosis (confirmed); Skin necrosis; Acute systemic reaction post intravenous unfractionated heparin bolus	Progressive or recurrent thromboses; Non-necrotizing (erythematosus) skin lesions; suspected thrombosis (not proven)	None
Other causes of thrombocytopenia	None apparent	Possible	Definite

4Ts score is the some of the values in each of the categories. 1–3 low probability, 4–5 intermediate probability, and 6–8 high probability of HIT. Modified from Cuker A, Gimotty PA, Crowther M, Warkentin TE: Predictive value of the 4Ts scoring system for heparin-induced thrombocytopenia: a systematic review and meta-analysis, *Blood* 120(20):4160–4167, 2012.

should *not* be used to treat patients with acute HIT due to significant antibody cross-reactivity, persistence of thrombocytopenia, and potential for new thromboembolism. Fondaparinux and rivaroxaban are direct factor Xa inhibitors that are subcutaneously and orally administered, respectively. Although not FDA approved in the setting of HIT, there is accumulating evidence that these agents may be safe and effective in the setting of HIT.[104-106]

However, the problem remains for patients with HIT or HAAbs who require vascular or cardiac surgery, when intraoperative administration of anticoagulation prior to arterial or venous clamping is needed. In this situation, we have treated HIT-positive patients with argatroban at a dose of 300 mcg/kg prior to arterial clamping (not an FDA approved dosing), and replaced heparin flushes with argatroban flushes at 10 mg/1000 mL normal saline.[107] Alternatively, patients who undergo peripheral intervention also may receive bivalirudin with an IV bolus of 0.75 mg/kg, followed by an IV infusion at 1.75 mg/kg/h.[108]

Hyperhomocysteinemia can be caused by inborn errors of metabolism (cystathionine β-synthase deficiency, methylene tetrahydrofolate reductase variant) or, more commonly, by acquired deficiencies in vitamin B_6, vitamin B_{12}, and folic acid. Elevated homocysteine is an independent risk factor for myocardial infarction, stroke, and peripheral arterial atherothrombosis[109]; it is also an independent risk factor for venous thrombosis, with an odds ratio of approximately 2 to 2.5.[110-112] The risk may be much higher in patients with combined hyperhomocysteinemia and other thrombophilic conditions.[113,114] Homocystinemia can be detected using fasting plasma levels or after methionine loading (100 mg/kg). Elevated homocysteine levels can be effectively reduced with folate, vitamin B_6, and vitamin B_{12} supplementation.[115] Despite this association, two randomized placebo-controlled trials have failed to show a reduction in VTE after correction of hyperhomocysteinemia.[116,117] The underlying link between hyperhomocysteinemia and increased VTE risk has yet to be elucidated.

Surgery and trauma are strong risk factors for the development of venous thrombosis. VTE occurs in up to 25% of patients undergoing general surgical procedures without thrombosis prophylaxis. Orthopedic procedures (hip and knee replacement, hip fracture repair) are associated with an even greater risk for VTE (45% to 61%). The incidence of VTE in trauma patients depends on the severity of injury. Multisystem trauma is associated with a greater than 50% incidence.[118]

Myeloproliferative diseases (polycythemia vera, chronic myelogenous leukemia, myeloid metaplasia, essential thrombocytosis), hypergammaglobulinemia, and hyperfibrinogenemia may predispose to thrombosis by causing a hyperviscous state. At clinical presentation, patients manifest cerebral (arterial and venous), coronary, pulmonary, and peripheral arterial and venous thromboemboli. Hemolytic-uremic syndrome and thrombotic thrombocytopenic purpura cause microvascular thromboses and thrombocytopenia.

Indications and Timing for Thrombophilia Screening

Venous Thromboembolism

Before 1993, heritable prothrombotic conditions were detected in less than 5% of patients with VTE. Since the discovery of Factor V Leiden and the prothrombin 20210A mutation, the number of VTE patients with a detectable thrombophilia has increased significantly. Despite this significant prevalence of thrombophilia, there has been a significant move *away* from routine testing for several reasons.

First, the more frequently identifiable thrombophilias (especially factor V Leiden and prothrombin gene mutation) are moderate risk factors for a first-time VTE, but they are weak risk factors for recurrent VTE (Table 6.6)[119]. Thus, the presence or absence of the more common thrombophilias does not significantly affect the recommended duration of anticoagulation in most circumstances. In patients with a proximal DVT or PE provoked by surgery or a nonsurgical transient risk factor, the ACCP guidelines recommend 3 months of anticoagulation, given the relatively low rate of recurrent VTE.[120] In addition, the American Society of Hematology recommends against thrombophilia testing in this population, with the caveat that testing decisions are more complex when VTE occurs in association with pregnancy, hormonal therapy, or a strong family history for thrombophilia or thrombosis.[121] In patients with a first unprovoked VTE, and those with multiple unprovoked VTEs, the ACCP guidelines recommend at least 3 months of anticoagulation, and for patients at low or moderate risk of bleeding, they suggest extended anticoagulation with no predetermined stop date. Again, the more common thrombophilias do not factor into the recommended duration of therapy. Lastly, the risk for postthrombotic syndrome and long-term mortality are unaffected by the presence of a heritable thrombophilia.[122,123]

TABLE 6.6 Prevalence of Thrombophilia and Relative Risk Estimates for Thrombosis

	Antithrombin Deficiency	Protein C Deficiency	Protein S Deficiency	Factor V Leiden	Prothrombin 20210A
Prevalence in general population	0.02%	0.2%	0.03%–0.13%	3%–7%	0.7%–4%
Prevalence in consecutive VTE patients	1%	3%	2%	20%	5%
Relative risk for 1st VTE	5–10	4–6.5	1–10	3–5	2–3
Relative risk for recurrent VTE	1.9–2.6	1.4–1.8	1.0–1.4	1.4	1.4
Relative risk for arterial thrombosis	No association	No consistent association	No consistent association	1.3	0.9

VTE, Venous thromboembolism.
Modified from Middeldorp S: Inherited thrombophilia: a double-edged sword. *Hematology Am Soc Hematol Educ Program* 2016(1):1–9, 2016.

Consensus guidelines recently have been published that summarize recommendations for patients with provoked and unprovoked VTE, as well as common circumstances in which family members of those with VTE might seek additional thrombophilia testing, and these are summarized in Box 6.1.[124]

For patients who do undergo a thrombophilia evaluation, testing usually includes genotype assays for factor V Leiden and prothrombin 20210A variant; testing for AT, protein C, and protein S deficiency; factor VIII activity; fasting homocysteine; and testing for anticardiolipin antibodies and lupus anticoagulant. In patients with visceral vein thrombosis, testing for paroxysmal nocturnal hemoglobinuria (PNH) and myeloproliferative syndrome should be performed. PNH is screened for with a flow cytometry assay, and myeloproliferative syndromes are detected with DNA testing for the *JAK2* mutation. In addition, patients who develop thrombocytopenia or arterial/venous thrombosis while receiving heparin or LMWH should be evaluated with the 4Ts test, and those with a score of ≥4 should undergo testing for HAAbs.

BOX 6.1 Anticoagulation Forum Guidance Regarding the Evaluation of Hereditary and Acquired Thrombophilia

1. Do not perform thrombophilia testing following a provoked VTE. Note: A positive thrombophilia evaluation is not a sufficient basis to offer extended anticoagulation.
2. Do not perform thrombophilia testing following an unprovoked VTE, unless a patient at low risk of bleeding planned to stop anticoagulation, and a positive test would influence this decision. Note: A negative thrombophilia evaluation is not a sufficient basis to stop anticoagulation in a patient with an unprovoked VTE, low bleeding risk, and willingness to continue therapy.
3. Do not test for thrombophilia in asymptomatic family members of patient with VTE or heritable thrombophilia. Note: Family history of VTE already confers an elevated risk, and a negative thrombophilia evaluation does not eliminate this risk. These relatives should receive prophylaxis in high-risk situations regardless of test results.
4. Do not perform thrombophilia testing in asymptomatic family members of patients with VTE or heritable thrombophilia who are contemplating estrogen. Note: Women contemplating estrogen use who have a first-degree relative with VTE and a known heritable thrombophilia should test for that thrombophilia if it would alter the decision. Family history of VTE itself confers an elevated risk of estrogen-associated VTE, but the absolute risk remains very low, especially in younger women considering oral contraceptive use.
5. Do not perform thrombophilia testing in asymptomatic family members of patients with VTE or heritable thrombophilia who are contemplating pregnancy. Note: Women contemplating pregnancy who have a first-degree relative with VTE and known heritable thrombophilia should test for that thrombophilia if it would alter VTE prophylaxis. If multiple family members are affected by VTE, a more potent thrombophilia (AT deficiency) may be present, potentially altering VTE prophylaxis.
6. Do not perform thrombophilia testing at the time of VTE diagnosis or during the initial 3 months of anticoagulation.

AT, Antithrombin; *VTE*, venous thromboembolism.
Modified from Stevens SM, Willer SC, Bauer KA, et al: Guidance for the evaluation and treatment of hereditary and acquired thrombophilia, *J Thromb Thrombolysis* 41(1):154–164, 2016.

Acute thrombosis, inflammation, a large thrombus burden, pregnancy, and estrogen use may cause transient depression of AT, protein C, and protein S levels. Concomitant administration of oral vitamin K antagonists also decreases protein C and protein S activity. If abnormal results are obtained under these conditions, then repeated testing should be performed once the acute thrombosis has resolved and after discontinuation of the vitamin K antagonist. To avoid the need and expense of repeated testing, many clinicians do not perform the thrombophilia testing until after 3 months of anticoagulation, waiting 2 to 4 weeks after the anticoagulation has been discontinued. It is also important to remember that many antiphospholipid antibodies are transient, and the official criteria for APA syndrome require two positive test results at least 12 weeks apart.

Arterial Thromboembolism

The relationship between thrombophilia and arterial thrombosis is not as well established. A 2008 large systematic review suggested that several of the heritable and acquired hypercoagulable conditions have a probable association with coronary artery disease, myocardial infarction, and stroke, but there was no identifiable association with peripheral artery disease or thrombosis (Table 6.7).[125] More recently, smaller observational studies and meta-analyses have recognized an association between various heritable and acquired hypercoagulable conditions (AT, protein C, and protein S deficiency; lupus anticoagulant, APA, factor V Leiden, and prothrombin 20210A mutation; PNH; hyperfibrinogenemia; elevated homocysteine) and peripheral artery disease, lower extremity ischemia, and lower extremity graft thrombosis.[126-129] However, given that most of these are retrospective single center studies, the overall quality of evidence for a significant association is still low.

The available clinical data is unable to provide clear guidance regarding indications for thrombophilia testing in patients with

TABLE 6.7 Heritable and Acquired Hypercoagulable States That Have a Probable Association With Arterial Disease

Hypercoagulable State	Arterial Disease
Fibrinogen level	CAD, stroke
Prothrombin G20210A	CAD, stroke
Factor V Leiden	stroke
PAI -1 level	CAD
Platelet GP IIIa Leu33Pro	CAD
Hyperhomocysteinemia	CAD, stroke
MTHFR C677T	CAD, stroke
C-reactive protein	MI
Oral contraceptives	MI, stroke
Hormone replacement	Stroke

CAD, Coronary artery disease; *GP*, glycoprotein; *MI*, myocardial infarction; *MTHFR*, methylenetetrahydrofolate reductase; *PAI*, plasminogen activator inhibitor.
Modified from Chan MY, Andreotti F, Becker RC: Hypercoagulable states in cardiovascular disease. *Circulation* 118:2286–2297, 2008.

peripheral artery disease and acute arterial thrombosis. In part, this may be due to the complex pathophysiology that results in acute limb or organ ischemia. For example, patients with peripheral artery disease often have multiple other risk factors such as diabetes, hypertension, hyperlipidemia, and tobacco use that contribute to the development of atherosclerosis and atherothrombosis. Many patients with these risk factors will present with acute limb ischemia in the absence of any detectable thrombophilia. Another confounding factor is that patients with acute arterial thromboembolism often have concomitant cardiogenic sources of embolism (atrial fibrillation, aortic or mitral valvular disease, intracardiac thrombus).[130] Chan and colleagues suggested that younger patients who develop arterial thrombosis in the absence of traditional atherosclerotic risk factors should be screened for a thrombophilia, as shown in Box 6.2.[125]

We reviewed the prevalence and spectrum of thrombophilia in 112 patients at our institution who presented with acute peripheral artery thrombosis or thromboembolism over a 7-year period, excluding patients with known atherosclerotic occlusive disease and trauma-associated arterial thrombosis.[131] Fifty percent of patients had an identifiable cardiogenic source alone, 25% had an identifiable thrombophilia alone, 14% had cardiogenic and thrombophilic etiologies, and 11% had neither. The more common thrombophilias identified in our patients matched those shown in Box 6.2, with antiphospholipid antibodies (40%) and malignancy (30%) being two more common conditions. Patients with arterial thrombosis and thrombophilia were younger, had fewer comorbidities, and were more likely to have a family history of thrombosis, yet they had a higher rate of limb amputation and mortality when compared with nonthrombophilic patients. Given these results, we test all patients who present with idiopathic peripheral artery thrombosis for antiphospholipid antibodies and myeloproliferative disorders, and make sure they receive age-appropriate screening for malignancy. Practically speaking, however, many patients also receive a computerized tomography angiogram (CTA) of the chest, abdomen, and pelvis, not as an evaluation for malignancy, but rather as part of the workup for a proximal source of thromboembolism.

BOX 6.2 Clinical Features Suggesting Underlying Thrombophilia in Patients With Arterial Thrombosis

Arterial thrombosis with any of the following clinical features:	Screen for:
1. Previous arterial thrombosis and age ≤50 (male) or ≤55 (female) 2. Age ≤55 (male) or ≤60 (female) with no other atherosclerosis risk factors 3. No significant coronary stenosis on angiography	Antiphospholipid antibodies Essential thrombocythemia Polycythemia vera Malignancy Cocaine metabolites
1. Age ≤55 (male) or ≤60 (female) and strong family history	Homocysteinemia Factor V Leiden Prothrombin 20210

Modified from Chan MY, Andreotti F, Becker RC: Hypercoagulable states in cardiovascular disease. *Circulation* 118:2286-2297, 2008.

Caveats in Management of Thrombosis and Thrombophilia

Until several years ago, unfractionated heparin, LMWH, and warfarin were the more commonly used antithrombotic agents. Now, physicians and patients have several other options available, including orally or intravenously administered direct thrombin inhibitors and orally administered factor Xa inhibitors. Numerous other drugs have become FDA approved for limited indications, including argatroban, bivalirudin, and fondaparinux. The basic pharmacokinetic properties of each of these anticoagulants are shown in Tables 6.8 and 6.9. Numerous other agents are in development or in clinical trials (e.g., recombinant TFPI, GP Ib inhibitors, other factor IIA inhibitors), but they are not discussed further in this chapter.

Patients with VTE who require anticoagulation may receive unfractionated heparin, LMWH, or fondaparinux, as an initial

TABLE 6.8 Direct Thrombin Inhibitors

	Desirudin	Bivalrudin	Argatroban	Dabigatran
FDA approved indications	• DVT prophylaxis THR	• UA/NSTEMI undergoing early invasive strategy • PCTA/PCI with or without HIT/HITTS	• HIT • PCI	• Non-valvular a fib • Treatment of DVT/PE
Route of administration	IV or SC	IV or SC	IV	Oral
Peak effect (h)	1–3	1–3	1–3	1–3
Half-life (h)	2–3	0.42	0.5–0.85	14–17
Renal clearance	Primary route of elimination: 40%–50% as unchanged drug	Primary route of elimination: 20% as unchanged drug	22%–24% excreted in urine, 16% as unchanged drug	80% excreted in urine
Dialyzable	Yes	Yes. 25% removed	Yes. 20% removed	Yes. 65% removed but concentrations rebound as drug re-equilibrates

DVT, Deep vein thrombosis; *FDA*, Food and Drug Administration; *HIT*, heparin-induced thrombocytopenia; *IV*, intravenous.

TABLE 6.9 Factor Xa Inhibitors

	Fondaparinux (Indirect)	Rivaroxaban	Apixaban	Edoxaban
FDA approved indications	• DVT prophylaxis following THR/TKR/HFS (including extended prophylaxis) and • Abdominal surgery • Treatment of DVT/PE	• DVT prophylaxis THR/TKR • Nonvalvular a fib • Treatment and extended treatment of DVT/PE	• DVT prophylaxis following THR/TKR • Treatment and extended treatment of DVT/PE • Nonvalvular a fib	• Treatment of DVT/PE following 5–10 days parenteral AC • Nonvalvular a fib
Route of administration	Subcutaneous	Oral	Oral	Oral
Peak effect (h)	2–3	2–4	1–3	1–3
Half-life (h)	17–21	5–9	8–15	9–11
Renal clearance	Primary route: 77% as unchanged drug	33%	25%	50%
Dialyzable	Yes, 20% removed. Due to risk of accumulation, use is contraindicated.	No. Not FDA approved, risk of accumulation, use not recommended.	No. Dosing recommendations in package insert. Due to risk of accumulation, use not recommended.	No. Not FDA approved, risk of accumulation, use not recommended.

DVT, Deep vein thrombosis; *FDA*, Food and Drug Administration.

parenteral agent, allowing a transition to warfarin or other vitamin-K antagonist. Alternatively, most patients with VTE may receive one of the FDA-approved DOAC medications. Some require an initial parenteral bridge as in the case with dabigatran and edoxaban, while other DOACs are FDA approved as monotherapy, as in the case with rivaroxaban or apixaban.

The choice of antithrombotic agents generally is not affected by the presence of a thrombophilia, except in a few select circumstances. In patients with cancer-associated VTE, the 2016 ACCP guidelines suggest at least 3 months of therapeutic LMWH.[120] This is based on earlier studies showing that LMWH was associated with a lower rate of VTE recurrence or mortality (with some tumors), while later studies showed only a lower rate of nonmajor bleeding.[132-134] Limited recent data show that the DOACs also may be a safe and effective alternative to long-term LMWH in cancer-associated VTE.[135] In the setting of pregnancy-associated VTE, LMWH is likely the safest option since many of the other agents have the potential to cross the placenta.

In patients who are deemed to be at high likelihood of having HAAbs or HIT, the options for alternative anticoagulation in the acute setting include argatroban, bivalirudin, or fondaparinux (fondaparinux is not FDA approved in HIT). When transitioning to longer-term therapy, patients either may continue with therapeutic fondaparinux, or they may transition to one of the DOACs (also not FDA-approved), given the increasing evidence for their effectiveness in the setting of HIT. Typically these decisions should be made in collaboration between the vascular surgery and hematology teams.

Patients who are diagnosed with APA syndrome may represent a particular challenge with regard to the most appropriate choice of antithrombotic therapy. First, patients should be classified based on clinical presentation: vascular thrombosis versus pregnancy morbidity.[136] Patients with vascular thrombosis may develop one or more episodes of arterial, venous, or small vessel thrombosis in any tissue or organ. Those with pregnancy morbidity may present with:

1. Greater than or equal to one unexplained deaths of a morphologically healthy fetus at or beyond the 10th week gestation
2. Greater than or equal to one premature births of a morphologically healthy newborn before the 34th week of gestation due to eclampsia or severe preeclampsia
3. Greater than or equal to three unexplained consecutive spontaneous abortions before the 10th week of gestation

In order to meet laboratory criteria for antiphospholipid syndrome, patients should be test-positive for lupus anticoagulant, anticardiolipin antibodies (IgG or IgM medium or high titers), or anti-β2-glycoprotein 1 antibody (IgG or IgM) on at least two occasions (≥12 weeks apart).

Antithrombotic prophylaxis or therapy in this population may be classified as primary (no prior thrombosis) versus secondary (established arterial or venous thrombosis). Primary thromboprophylaxis in patients with systemic lupus and positive lab titers should include hydroxychloroquine and low-dose aspirin. Titer-positive patients without systemic lupus may receive long-term prophylaxis with aspirin alone. Patients with APA syndrome and a first *venous thrombosis* should receive indefinite warfarin (goal INR 2.0 to 3.0), whereas those with *arterial thrombosis* should receive warfarin with an INR goal range ≥3.0 or a combination of warfarin (goal INR 2.0 to 3.0) and antiplatelet therapy. Those patients who are refractory to these regimens can be considered for long-term LMWH, hydroxychloroquine, and statin therapy.[137] The prophylaxis and treatment options for patients with strongly positive lab titers and recurrent pregnancy loss are even more complex, and a full description is beyond the scope of this chapter. However, the regimen usually includes low-dose aspirin plus unfractionated heparin or LMWH, with the dosing dependent on the patient's clinical presentation.[137]

REVIEW QUESTIONS

1. A patient with atrial fibrillation (classification system: congestive heart failure, hypertension, age ≥75 years, diabetes, stroke [$CHADS_2$] score of 3) is receiving chronic oral anticoagulation, and needs a femoral popliteal bypass. Which of the following statements is true regarding perioperative low-molecular-weight heparin bridging?
   a. Patients taking warfarin should receive bridging anticoagulation with therapeutic low-molecular-weight heparin (LMWH).
   b. Patients taking a direct oral anticoagulant (e.g., Rivaroxaban) should receive bridging anticoagulation with therapeutic LMWH.
   c. When compared with no bridging, perioperative LMWH bridging is associated with a similar risk of major bleeding.
   d. When compared with no bridging, perioperative LMWH bridging is associated a similar risk of acute thromboembolism.
2. Regarding the management of heparin-induced thrombocytopenia (HIT), which of the following is true?
   a. Unfractionated heparin and low-molecular-weight heparin have a similar incidence of heparin-associated antibody formation.
   b. If the clinical scoring system demonstrates a low probability of HIT, laboratory testing for HIT is unnecessary.
   c. Low-molecular-weight heparin can be administered safely in patients with established HIT.
   d. The platelet count must be less than 100,000/mm^3 to be diagnosed with HIT.
3. Which of the following statements regarding von Willebrand disease is false?
   a. Defects of primary hemostasis commonly cause petechiae and ecchymoses.
   b. Hemophilic disorders commonly cause hemarthroses and deep tissue hematomas.
   c. Von Willebrand disease is the most common inherited bleeding disorder.
   d. Type 1 von Willebrand disease is usually unresponsive to DDAVP.
   e. Cryoprecipitate and some factor VIII concentrates are rich in von Willebrand factor (vWF).
4. Which of the following statements regarding thrombophilia testing and treatment for patients with venous thromboembolism (VTE) is true?
   a. Thrombophilia testing is not indicated for most patients with *unprovoked* VTE.
   b. Thrombophilia testing is indicated for most patients with *provoked* VTE.
   c. Thrombophilia testing is indicated for asymptomatic family members of patients with known heritable thrombophilias.
   d. Warfarin is ineffective in patients with antiphospholipid syndrome.
5. Following major surgical procedures in patients with hemophilia A, factor VIII plasma activity should be at least:
   a. 5% of normal
   b. 25% of normal
   c. 50% of normal
   d. 75% of normal
   e. 100% of normal
6. A 52-year-old male develops acute left lower extremity ischemia due to superficial femoral artery thrombosis. He has no atherosclerosis risk factors. Which of the following thrombophilias is the most likely contributor?
   a. Prothrombin gene mutation
   b. Factor V Leiden
   c. Antiphospholipid antibodies
   d. Hyperhomocysteinemia
7. A 78-year-old patient with heart failure is on chronic warfarin for a left iliofemoral deep vein thrombosis (DVT). His international normalized ratio (INR) is 4.2, and he develops a spontaneous large retroperitoneal hemorrhage causing hypotension. Which of the following statements regarding anticoagulation management is true?
   a. Warfarin and direct oral anticoagulants (DOAC) have a similar rate of major hemorrhage.
   b. Intravenous (IV) vitamin K should result in normalization of the INR within 2 to 3 hours.
   c. 4-factor prothrombin complex concentrates normalize the INR within 30 minutes.
   d. Each unit of fresh frozen plasma elicits approximately a 15% to 20% increase in factor activity, normalizing the INR after 3 to 4 units.
8. Which of the following statements regarding the risk associated with pregnancy and hormonal therapy is false?
   a. The risk of venous thrombosis decreases after delivery.
   b. The thrombosis risks associated with oral contraceptives are immediate and reversible.
   c. Oral contraceptives are associated with a two- to fourfold increased risk for venous thrombosis.
   d. LMWHs have been shown to be safe and effective in pregnant patients with venous thromboembolism.
9. Which of the following is not a vitamin K–dependent coagulation factor?
   a. Factor II
   b. Factor V
   c. Factor VII
   d. Factor IX
   e. Factor X
10. Which of the following is not a major regulator of the coagulation cascade?
   a. Antithrombin
   b. Protein C
   c. Protein S
   d. Tissue factor pathway inhibitor
   e. Heparin cofactor II

BIBLIOGRAPHY

Chan MY, Andreotti F, Becker RC. Hypercoagulable states in cardiovascular disease. *Circulation*. 2008;118:2286–2297.

Cuker A, Gimotty PA, Crowther M, Warkentin TE. Predictive value of the 4Ts scoring system for heparin–induced thrombocytopenia: a systematic review and meta–analysis. *Blood*. 2012;120(20): 4160–4167.

Kearon C, Akl EA, Ornelas J, et al. Antithrombotic therapy for VTE disease: chest guideline and expert panel report. *Chest*. 2016; 149(2):315–352.

Levy JH, Faraoni D, Spring JL, et al. Managing new oral anticoagulants in the perioperative and intensive care unit setting. *Anesthesiology*. 2013;118:1466–1474.

Middeldorp S. Inherited thrombophilia: a double-edged sword. *ASH Education Book*. 2016;2016(1):1–9.

Ruiz-Irastorza G, Crowther M, Branch W, Khamashta MA. Antiphospholipid syndrome. *Lancet*. 2010;376(9751):1498–1509.

Ruiz-Irastorza G, Cuadrado MJ, Ruiz-Arruza I, et al. Evidence-based recommendations for the prevention and long-term management of thrombosis in antiphospholipid antibody-positive patients: report of a task force at the 13th International Congress on Antiphospholipid Antibodies. *Lupus*. 2011;20(2):206–218.

Schulman S, Beyth RJ, Clive K, et al. Hemorrahagic complications of anticoagulant and thrombolytic treatment. *Chest*. 2008;133: 257S–298S.

Scully M, Gates C, Neave L. How we manage patients with heparin-induced thrombocytopenia. *Br J Haematol*. 2016; 174(1):9–15.

Spyropoulos AC, Al-Badri A, Sherwood MW, Douketis JD. Periprocedural management of patients receiving a vitamin K antagonist or a direct oral anticoagulant requiring an elective procedure or surgery. *J Thromb Haemost*. 2016;14:875–885.

Stevens SM, Willer SC, Bauer KA, et al. Guidance for the evaluation and treatment of hereditary and acquired thrombophilia. *J Thromb Thrombolysis*. 2016;41(1):154–164.

Yates SG, Sarod R. New strategies for effective treatment of vitamin K antagonist-associated bleeding. *J Thromb Haemost*. 2015; 13(suppl 1):S180–S186.

References available online at ExpertConsult.com.

7 CHAPTER

Atherosclerosis: Pathology, Pathogenesis, and Medical Management

Taimur Saleem, Ralph G. DePalma, Jessica Beth O'Connell

Vascular surgeons commonly treat patients with the manifestations of atherosclerosis. An improved understanding of atherosclerosis and advances in its treatment now provide scientifically based prevention and management strategies. Precise lesion classification, accurate imaging, a better understanding of atherogenesis, and increasingly effective medical treatment before and after vascular interventions all promise to result in improved long-term results. The pivotal role of lipids in the pathogenesis of atherosclerosis and the impact of lipid reduction on atherosclerotic plaque has long been known, as well as more recent information on the crucial roles of inflammatory and immune responses that affect arterial plaques. Novel risk factors, such as elevated blood levels of biomarkers, including inflammatory cytokines, metalloproteinases, and smooth muscle growth factors, including glucose and insulin for late progression, all contribute to our understanding of atherosclerosis and its progression. Advanced imaging can now also detect unstable plaques prone to rupture, thrombosis, and downstream embolization. Prospective randomized trials using drugs, micronutrients, and other interventions continue to provide therapeutic guidelines. Coronary thrombosis or stroke, the main causes of death in patients with peripheral arterial disease,[1] have improved management strategies to increase overall survival and enhance long-term results of atherosclerosis management in other vascular beds.

Vascular surgeons must be familiar with the location and natural history of individual lesions and, in considering various interventions, distinguish primary prevention from secondary treatment. When active intervention is required, vascular surgeons must use strategies geared toward the specific pathology of lesions in particular arterial sites. For example, a stenotic lesion composed of smooth muscle and well-organized collagen, although capable of causing distal ischemia, is a much safer lesion than a plaque containing an unstable core of atheromatous debris beneath a tenuous cap. The smooth stenosis of an adductor hiatus plaque in the femoral artery, causing stable claudication, is clearly not as threatening as unstable symptomatic carotid or coronary plaques characterized by soft cores beneath friable caps. These lesions have differing vulnerabilities based on differing composition and morphology.[2]

We now recognize that operative or endovascular treatment of segmental lesions does not prevent the progression of systemic atherosclerosis elsewhere and ensuring long-term results requires both medical treatment and lifestyle interventions.

Variations in patterns and rates of progression of atherosclerosis also have significant implications for the timing and choice of treatment.[3,4] Considering the atherosclerotic process as a single disease leads to oversimplification; with considerable lesion diversity and clinical presentation, atherosclerosis also can be viewed as a polypathogenic process comprising a group of closely related vascular disorders.[5,6] Multiple risk factors promoting atherosclerosis and its complications include dyslipidemia, smoking, diabetes, hypertension, and proinflammatory factors. The multiplicity of disease-promoting factors makes a single-disease–single-etiology view difficult to reconcile. This chapter discusses atherosclerosis as a single entity, while recognizing its heterogeneous pathologic characteristics and differing clinical presentations, which will be discussed in subsequent chapters. Despite the complexity and heterogeneity of the atherosclerotic process, new treatment strategies have resulted in increasingly successful treatment outcomes. More effective medical therapy and advances in endovascular and surgical approaches, based on a better understanding of the pathology and pathogenesis of atherosclerotic disease, have been fruitful in improving the survival and quality of life of patients with atherosclerotic disease in multiple vascular beds.

PATHOLOGY

General Concepts

The term *atheroma* derives from the Greek *athere,* meaning "porridge" or "gruel" and *sclerosis,* meaning "induration" or "hardening." A gruel-like color and consistency and induration or hardening exists to various degrees in different plaques, different disease stages, and different individuals. In 1755, von Haller[7] first applied the term *atheroma* to a common type of plaque that, on sectioning, exuded a yellow, soft content from its core.[7] Fig. 7.1 illustrates a typical fibrous plaque containing a central atheromatous core with a fibrous or fibromuscular cap, macrophage accumulation, and round cell adventitial infiltration. A previous generic definition of atherosclerotic plaque as "a variable combination of changes in the intima of arteries consisting of focal accumulation of lipids, complex carbohydrates, blood and blood products, fibrous tissue and calcium deposits"[8] failed to encompass the full spectrum of atherosclerotic lesions. Advanced plaques invade the media, and at certain stages produce bulging or even enlarged arteries. Round cell infiltration, medial changes,

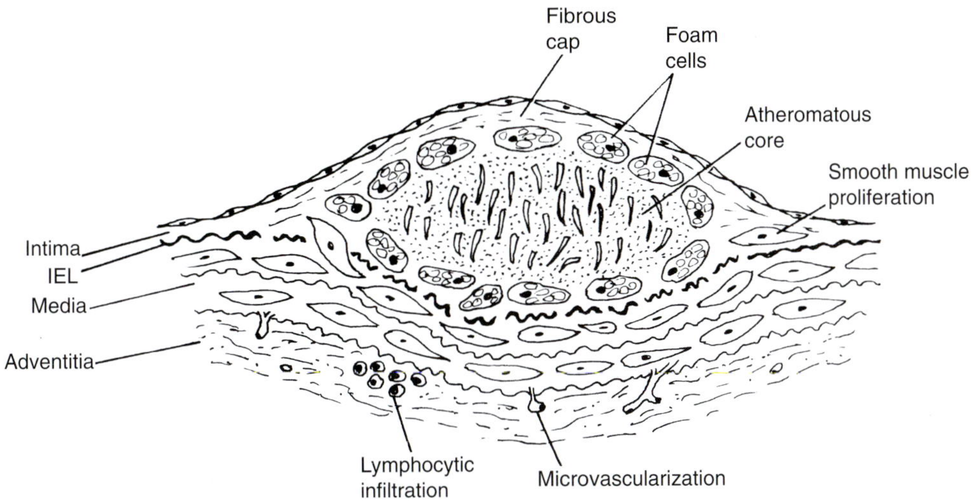

FIG 7.1 Typical Atheroma or Type IV Lesion. Note the central lipid core, fibrous cap, macrophage accumulation, and zone of synthetically active smooth muscle at the "shoulders" of the core. Note too the tendency of the lesion to bulge outward, neovascularization, and adventitial lymphocyte infiltration. *IEL,* Internal elastic lamina. (Modified from DePalma RG: Pathology of atheromas. In Bell PRF, Jamieson CW, Ruckley CV, editors: *Surgical Management of Vascular Disease*, London, 1992, WB Saunders, p 21.)

and neovascularization characterize advanced atherosclerotic lesions. The atherosclerotic process ultimately involves the entire arterial wall. The process is complex and variable and, although not all atherosclerotic lesions evolve in the same way, certain progression patterns are more common than others.

The development of the lipid atherosclerotic core and its relationship to an overlying cap relate directly to plaque complications. The lipid "core" develops early in atherosclerosis and accumulates in the deep aspects of early lesions, before actual fibrous plaque formation begins.[9] Another important principle is recognition of the role of inflammation and immune reactions in the early and late stages of atherogenesis.[10,11] The inflammatory cascade includes appearance of proinflammatory cytokines such as interleukin-6 (IL-6), tumor necrosis factor (TNF)-α, and antiinflammatory cytokines such as IL-10 within arterial tissue and arising from the bloodstream. Lipid accumulation appears to attract inflammatory cells that produce cytokines locally, whereas cytokines or biomarkers derived from a variety of tissues appear systemically in atherosclerotic subjects. For example, in atherosclerotic patients with claudication, plasma levels of inflammatory cytokines TNF-α and IL-6 are elevated, whereas antiinflammatory IL-10 levels are reduced.[12] Elevated levels of cytokines such as TNF-α and its receptors also affect the arterial wall.[13-15] The atherosclerotic plaque contains leukocytes, of which approximately 80% are monocytes or monocyte-derived macrophages. Lymphocytes, predominantly memory T cells,[16] constitute 5% to 20% of this cell population. Inflammation, size, and composition of the lipid core determine plaque instability or "vulnerability," which may result in sudden expansion, rupture, release of distal emboli, and vascular occlusion.

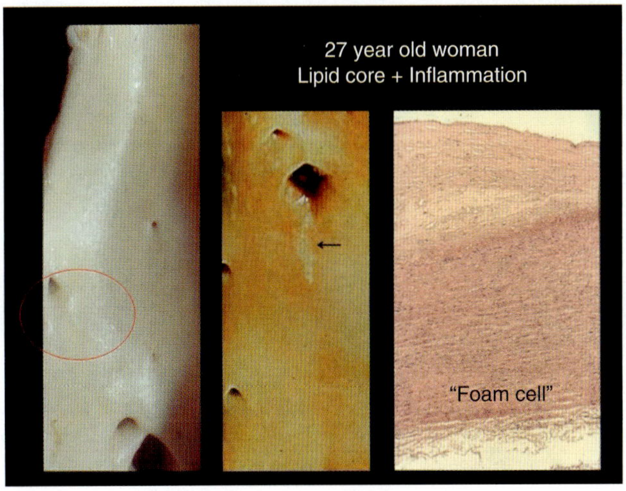

FIG 7.2 Early atherosclerotic plaque in thoracic aorta; note lipid core and inflammation.

Fatty Streaks

The first stages of atherosclerosis, fatty streaks (minimally raised yellow lesions), develop in vulnerable segments of the arterial tree. These lesions contain lipids deposited intracellularly in macrophages and smooth muscle cells. Stary and colleagues[17] defined initial fatty streaks and intermediate lesions of atherosclerosis as follows: type I lesions in children are early microscopic lesions, consisting of an increase in intimal macrophages and the appearance of foam cells. Type II fatty streak lesions are grossly visible (Fig. 7.2); in contrast to type I lesions, type II lesions stain with Sudan III or IV. Foam cells and lipid droplets appear in intimal smooth muscle cells and heterogeneous droplets of extracellular lipids characterize type II fatty streaks. Type III lesions are intermediate lesions, considered to be the bridge between the fatty streak (Fig. 7.3) and the prototypical type IV atheromatous fibrous plaque (see Fig. 7.1).[18] Type III lesions occur in plaque-prone locations in the arterial tree[19] at sites

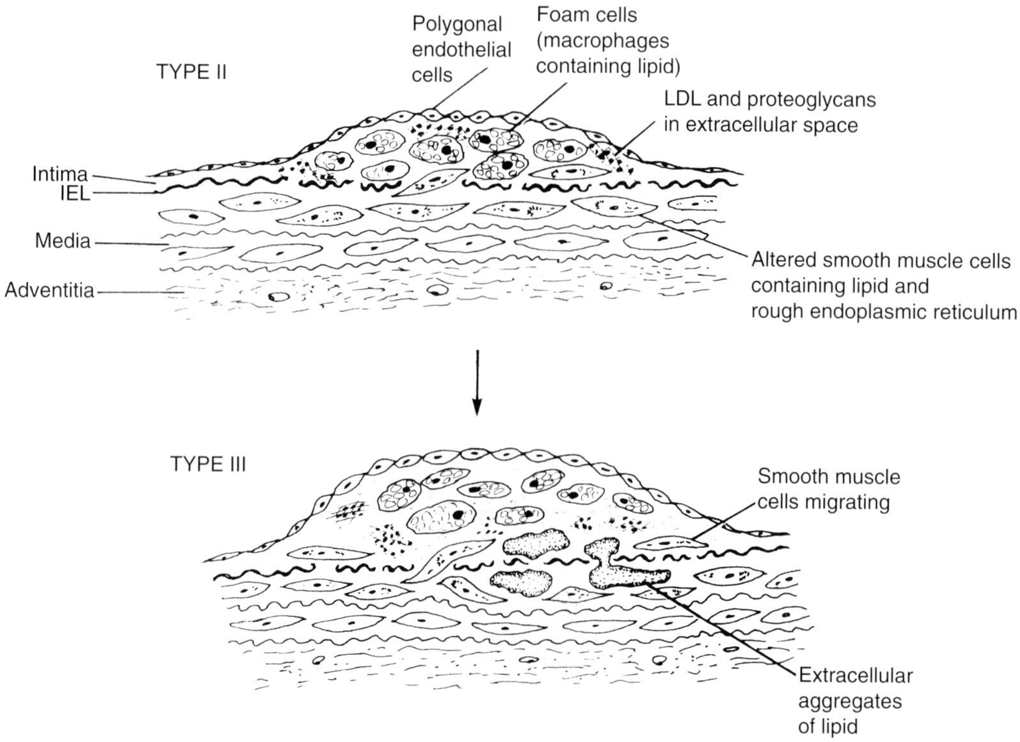

FIG 7.3 Type II fatty streak lesions with foam cells. Note the low-density lipoprotein *(LDL)* particles in the matrix and altered smooth muscle cells, with developed rough endoplasmic reticulum also containing lipid particles. Note too the evolution to an intermediate, more advanced lesion (type III) containing extracellular aggregates or pools of lipid deep in the intima and extending into the media. *IEL,* Internal elastic lamina. (From DePalma RG: Atherosclerosis: theories of etiology and pathogenesis. In Sidawy AN, Sumpio BE, DePalma RG, editors: *Basic Science of Vascular Disease*, Armonk, NY, 1997, Futura Publishing, pp 319–332.)

exposed to forces (particularly low-shear stress), promoting increased low-density lipoprotein (LDL) influx.[20]

The fatty streak type II lipids are chemically similar to those of plasma.[21] Plasma lipids may enter the arterial wall in several ways. As described in a review of pathogenesis,[22] LDL accumulation can occur because of (1) alterations in the permeability of the intima; (2) increases in the intimal interstitial space; (3) poor metabolism of LDL by vascular cells; (4) impeded transport of LDL from the intima to the media; (5) increased plasma LDL concentrations; or (6) specific binding of LDL to connective tissue components, particularly proteoglycans in the arterial intima. Experimental studies show that LDL cholesterol accumulates in the intima even before lesions develop and in the presence of intact endothelium. These observations support the classic descriptions of lesion formation by Aschoff[23] in the early 20th century and Virchow[24] in the mid-19th century.

A second event in early atherogenesis, as shown in animal experiments, is binding of monocytes to the endothelial lining, with their subsequent diapedesis into the subintimal layer, to become tissue macrophages.[25-27] Fatty streaks are populated mainly by monocyte-derived macrophages. These lipid-engorged scavenger cells mainly become the foam cells characterizing fatty streaks and more advanced lesions. LDL, altered by oxidation or acetylation, is taken up by the macrophages to form foam cells.[28] Oxidized LDL itself is a powerful chemoattractant for monocytes. Another component of this theory suggests that the endothelium modifies LDL to promote foam cell formation. In either case, oxidative reactions are seen as enhancing atheroma development.

The initial interactions of plasma LDL with the arterial wall and macrophages form the basis for the earliest lesion formation. LDL traverses the endothelium mostly through receptor-independent transport, possibly also through cell breaks.[29] Endothelial cells,[30] smooth muscle cells,[31] and macrophages[32] are all capable of promoting oxidation of LDL. The oxidized LDL, in turn, further attracts monocytes into the intima to promote their transformation into macrophages. Macrophages produce cytokines, thus initiating the inflammatory cascade. Oxidized LDL also induces genes and their products, which are not ordinarily expressed in normal vascular tissue. A notable example is tissue factor, the cellular initiator of the coagulation cascade, abundantly expressed by atheroma monocytes and foam cells.[33] Expression of tissue factor requires the presence of bacterial lipopolysaccharide, suggesting that hypercoagulability in atherosclerosis is enhanced by infectious factors.

Large numbers of macrophages and T lymphocytes in the plaques suggest cellular immune responses; oxidized lipoproteins, heat shock proteins, and microorganisms are all possible antigens. A study analyzing endarterectomy specimens by immunohistochemistry and reverse transcription polymerase chain reaction showed proinflammatory T cell cytokines, IL-2, and interferon-7 in a large proportion of plaques, indicating that a helper T cell 1–type cellular immune response likely occurs in the atherosclerotic plaque.[34]

Endothelium

Animal studies reveal that endothelial cells tend to be oriented parallel to the direction of flow; these cells show increased stigmata or stomata, increased proliferation, and a decrease in microfilament bundles.[25,26] In humans and animals, endothelial cells become polyhedral or rounded; in humans, there is also increased formation of multinucleated cells and cilia. Animal studies reveal increased proliferation and cell death, with retraction and exposure of subendothelial foam cells. The endothelium becomes more permeable to macromolecules in experimental models; in humans, it exhibits increased tissue factor expression and mural thrombus formation. Leukocyte adherence increases with the expression of a monocyte adhesion molecule (vascular cell adhesion molecule 1 [VCAM-1]). Endothelium-derived relaxing factor and prostacyclin release are decreased and vasoconstriction is enhanced.

Media

The smooth muscle shows increased proliferation, with increased rough endoplasmic reticulum, phenotypic changes, and increased production of altered intracellular and extracellular matrices. In humans, these matrices include increased expression of type I and type III collagen, dermatan sulfate, proteoglycan, and stromelysin. Smooth muscle cells also produce cytokines, including macrophage colony-stimulating factor, TNF, and monocyte chemoattractant protein-1. Myocytes accumulate native and modified lipoproteins by both native receptor pathways and nonspecific phagocytosis. These cells also express increased lipoprotein lipase activity; experimentally, they display a scavenger receptor similar to that of foam cells.

Macrophages

Macrophages proliferate and express monocyte chemoattractant protein-1, macrophage colony-stimulating factor, TNF, IL-1 and other interleukins, and platelet-derived growth factor (PDGF), along with cluster of differentiation (CD) immune antigens and, as previously described, tissue factor.[33] Plaque macrophages contain increased free and esterified cholesterol, increased acetyl coenzyme A, cholesterol acyltransferase, and acid cholesterol ester hydrolase. Neutral cholesterol ester hydrolase is decreased. These altered cells also express the scavenger receptor 15-lipoxygenase and exhibit increased lipoprotein oxidation products in humans and in animal models. These extensive changes indicate the complexity of the morphologic, functional, biochemical, and genetic expressions of the arterial wall in early atherosclerosis. The reader is referred to an original report for comprehensive details,[17] with references for the cellular alterations given.

Gelatinous Plaques

Intimal gelatinous lesions may sometimes be considered as precursors of atheromas. Haust described these lesions in 1971,[35] first noted in 1856 by Virchow[24] as potential progenitors of advanced atherosclerosis. Smith later described their identification and composition.[36] Gelatinous plaques are translucent and neutral in color, with central grayish opaque areas. Most plaques are characterized by finely dispersed, perifibrous lipid along with collagen strands around the lesions. Grossly, gelatinous lesions feel soft. With gentle lateral pressure, these plaques "wobble." The gelatinous material separates easily from the underlying arterial wall without entering a conventional endarterectomy plane. Gelatinous plaques appear in the aorta as extensive areas of flat, translucent thickenings, particularly in its lower abdominal segment. These lesions have a low lipid and high fluid content. In some plaques, numerous smooth muscle cells are present **and** the lesions contain substantial amounts of cross-linked fibrin.

Fibrous Plaques

Fig. 7.1 typifies a common prototypical atherosclerotic lesion: fibrous or type IV plaque. These lesions are composed of large numbers of smooth muscle cells and connective tissue, which form a fibrous cap over an inner yellow (atheromatous) core. This soft core contains cholesterol esters, mainly cholesteryl oleate, likely derived from disrupted foam cells. A second type of particle contains both free cholesterol and cholesterol linoleates. The early core is associated with vesicular lipids that are rich in free cholesterol.[9] These particles likely are derived directly from LDL, possibly by modification of LDL by specific lipolytic enzymes capable of hydrolyzing LDL cholesterol esters. Lipoprotein aggregation and fusion are thought to be the chief pathway of cholesterol ester accumulation. Fibrous plaques contain large numbers of smooth muscle cells, connective tissue cells, and macrophages. Over 2 decades ago, the importance of the composition and integrity of the atheromatous cap were emphasized, as this structure stabilizes the atheroma to prevent intraluminal rupture of its soft core.[37]

Fibrous plaques appear later than fatty streaks and often in similar locations. Fibrous plaques generally evolve from fatty streaks or from areas of fatty streak involvement. Gelatinous plaques, injured arterial areas, or thrombi less commonly may lead to fibrous plaque formation. Mural thrombi sometimes are converted into atheromas, as demonstrated by experimental intraarterial catheter implantation.[38]

Fibrous plaques protrude into the arterial lumen in fixed cut sections; however, when arteries are fixed at arterial pressure, they produce an external bulge. For example, coronary plaques in vivo must occupy at least 40% of the arterial wall before angiographic detection is possible.[39] Within certain limits, atheromatous luminal intrusion is compensated by arterial enlargement.[40] Compensatory remodeling of coronary arteries in subhuman primates and humans has been stressed as a protective response.[41] However, with lesion progression, ulceration, rupture, or overlying thrombosis, the arterial lumen may become suddenly compromised, a sequence characterizing coronary atheromas. A unique adaptive response involving dilation, with atheromatous involvement of the entire arterial wall and participation of inflammatory cells, immunologically active T lymphocytes, and elastolysis may predispose to aneurysm formation.

During the early stages of evolution from fatty streak to fibrous plaque, cholesterol esters appear in ordered arrays of intracellular lipid crystals. In intermediate type III and fibrous plaques, the lipids assume isotropic forms and occur extracellularly.[42] Cholesterol esters and oxysterols are highly irritating, causing severe inflammatory reactions in the connective tissue[43]; they probably behave similarly within the arterial wall to promote inflammation, fibrosis, and lymphocytic infiltration. Advancing neovascularization from the adventitia characterizes intermediate fibrofatty and fibrous plaque lesions. Atherosclerotic lesions contain immunoglobulin (Ig) G in large quantities, as well as other immunoglobulins and complement components. The IgG recognizes epitopes characteristic of oxidized LDL, indicating that immunologic processes characterize more advanced atherosclerotic plaques.[44] This process is associated with systemic effects; for example, patients with carotid atherosclerosis have higher antibody ratios of oxidized LDL and IgM than do comparable non-atherosclerotic controls.[45]

Experiments in complement-deficient rabbits suggest that the chronic inflammation of atherosclerosis is driven mainly by activation of the complement and monocyte-macrophage systems.[46] In this sequence, enzymatic degradation, not oxidation, is considered to be the central predisposing process.

Complicated Plaques

Fibrous plaques become complicated by calcification, ulceration, intraplaque hemorrhage, or necrosis. These later developments cause the clinical complications of myocardial infarction, stroke, and arterial occlusion causing gangrene. Aneurysm formation also may represent unique interactions with the atherosclerotic process. Alternatively, aneurysms have been viewed as nonspecific, inflammatory, degenerative, or purely mechanical arterial responses. Patients harboring aortic aneurysms have a higher prevalence of risk factors for atherosclerosis and concurrent atherosclerotic involvement of other arteries, suggesting a unique response to atherosclerosis involving a specific arterial segment in certain individuals.[47]

As with early plaque evolution,[17] advanced atherosclerotic lesions have been described and classified.[18] The type IV lesion has extracellular lipid as the precursor of the core. Lesions that contain a thick layer of fibrous connective tissue are characterized as type V lesions, whereas those with fissures, hematoma, or thrombus are characterized as type VI lesions. Type V lesions have been further described as largely calcified (type Vc) or consisting mainly of connective tissue with little or no lipid or calcium (type Vb). This definition of advanced disease includes atherosclerotic aneurysms, although aneurysm formation may follow other distinct sequences.

THEORIES OF ATHEROGENESIS

Lipid Hypothesis

Virchow believed that the cellular changes characterizing atherosclerosis were simply reactive responses to lipid infiltration.[24] Later, Aschoff remarked, "From plasma of low cholesterin content no deposition of lipids will occur even though mechanical conditions are favorable."[24] As can be seen from fatty streak to fibrous plaque evolution, lipids, particularly LDL cholesterol, have a pivotal role in lesion morphology, composition, and evolution. Early experiments by Anitschkow with cholesterol-fed rabbits appeared to validate a simple "lipid filtration hypothesis."[48] However, the atherosclerotic process was soon appreciated to be much more complex. Atherosclerosis develops in various species in proportion to the ease with which an experimental regimen displaces the normal lipid pattern toward hypercholesterolemia, particularly hyperbetalipoproteinemia. At the same time, arterial susceptibility and inflammatory responses vary among locations, species, and individuals. Enhanced inflammatory responses, genetically determined by toll-like receptors, influence atherogenesis.[49,50]

Canine and subhuman primate (rhesus and cynomolgus monkey) models develop atherosclerosis in response to dietary manipulation[50-60] and demonstrate plaque regression in response to serum cholesterol lowering. However, lesion production in susceptible species is not a result of simple dietary cholesterol overload. Any diet that causes hypercholesterolemia induces atherosclerosis. The presence of excess cholesterol is not necessary in atherogenic diets. In developmental subhuman primate feeding experiments, reduction of cholesterol content to 0.5% combined with sugar and eggs produced rapidly progressive plaques, whereas high cholesterol addition (up to 7% by weight) did not.[53,54] In rabbits, a variety of purified cholesterol-free diets with various amino acid compositions induces hypercholesterolemia and atherosclerosis.[60] Epidemiologic observations provide important circumstantial evidence linking hyperlipidemia to atherosclerosis.[61] Genetically determined hyperlipidemias provide compelling evidence that elevated LDL cholesterol is a prime etiologic factor in atherosclerosis, despite objections that highly cellular lipid-laden atheromas in these individuals might be atypical lesions.[62]

This important observation earned Brown and Goldstein a Nobel Prize.[63] Serum cholesterol levels are markedly elevated early in life; individuals with the homozygous condition die prematurely from atherosclerosis, rarely living beyond the age of 26 years. Unfortunately, the heterozygous condition is not uncommon, with total cholesterol levels ranging up to 350 mg/dL. These individuals account for 1 in 500 live births[64] and develop atherosclerosis during early middle age. The atheromas of these patients are similar in morphology to those seen in individuals with acquired hyperlipidemia or premature atherosclerosis associated with heavy smoking.

This unfortunate natural experiment is powerful evidence that elevated LDL cholesterol is a relentless factor in plaque formation and the rapid progression of atherosclerosis to lethal consequences. Liver transplantation has been successful in retarding the progress of this type of atherosclerosis.[65] Familial hypercholesterolemias are autosomal-dominant disorders produced by at least 12 different molecular defects of the LDL receptors. Familial abnormalities of high-density lipoprotein (HDL), a negative risk factor for atherosclerosis, also exist. In addition to LDL and HDL metabolism, surface proteins of the lipoprotein complex or apoproteins also appear to be relevant to pathogenesis. With the availability of effective therapy, a need for childhood screening for these disorders has been endorsed recently.[66]

Thrombogenic Hypothesis

In the mid-19th century, von Rokitansky postulated that fibrinous substances deposited on the arterial intimal surface because of abnormal hemostatic elements in the blood and could undergo metamorphosis into atheromatous masses containing cholesterol crystals and globules.[67] This theory posited that atheromatous lesions resulted mainly from degeneration of blood proteins (i.e., fibrin deposited in the arterial intima). Duguid[68] resurrected this theory in 1946 with the observation that in rabbits, indwelling arterial catheters or arterial injury caused cholesterol accumulation and arterial lesions in the absence of dietary cholesterol.

Mesenchymal Hypothesis: Hemodynamic Effects

Active smooth muscle cells with connective tissue production by these cells have been considered as primary, even crucial steps, in atherogenesis.[69-71] Proteoglycan, a ubiquitous arterial wall element, can trap infiltrated LDL, even when LDL is not elevated in the blood. Collagen is the other space-filling component of advanced atherosclerotic lesions. Hauss and colleagues[72] viewed the migration of smooth muscle cells from the media to the intima, with proliferation and production of connective tissue, as a nonspecific arterial reaction to any injury; atherosclerosis simply reflects a generic arterial response. Chisolm and colleagues[22] called this the "nonspecific" mesenchymal hypothesis. These scenarios are similar to wound-healing responses to injury. In part, this theory attempts to explain why physical factors such as shear stress, vasoactive agents, and repetitive injuries eventually lead to atheroma formation.

In one view, "Atherosclerosis constitutes the degenerative and reparative process consequent upon the hemodynamically induced engineering fatigue of the blood vessel wall."[63] This theory postulates "vibrations consisting of the pulsations associated with cardiac contractions and the vortex shedding generated in the blood vessels at branchings, unions, curvatures, and fusiform dilations (carotid sinus) over a lifetime are responsible for fatigue failure after a certain, but individually variable, number of vibrations."[63] Atherosclerosis, a process of wear and tear, therefore becomes an inexorable (and unavoidable) process associated with aging. In support of this concept, hypertension[73] and tachycardia induced in experimental animals receiving atherogenic feeding caused accelerated plaque development, whereas bradycardia induced by sinoatrial node ablation in monkeys reduced coronary and carotid atherosclerosis.[74,75]

Monoclonal Hypothesis: Smooth Muscle Proliferation

The morphologic similarity of smooth muscle proliferation in some atherosclerotic lesions to uterine smooth muscle myomas led to the suggestion that atherosclerotic lesions are derived from a singular or, at most, a few mutated smooth muscle cells that, like tumor cells, proliferate in an unregulated fashion.[70] This theory is based on the finding of only one allele for glucose-6-phosphate dehydrogenase in lesions from heterozygotes. A homology exists between the β chain of human PDGF and the protein product of the *v-sis* oncogene, which is a tumor-causing gene derived from simian sarcoma virus. Tumor-forming cells in culture express the genes for one or both of the PDGF chains and secrete PDGF into a culture medium. This hypothesis considers events causing smooth muscle cell proliferation to be a critical atherogenic factor. Actions of other growth factors, which might either stimulate or inhibit cell proliferation, depend on circumstances as well as on macrophage-derived cytokine activity. For example, the finding of transforming growth factor (TGF)-β receptors in human atherosclerosis provides evidence of an acquired resistance to apoptosis.[76] Resistance to apoptosis can lead to proliferation of resistant cell subsets associated with progression of lesions.

Response-to-Injury Hypothesis

Ross and Glomset[77] postulated two pathways for the promotion of atheroma formation. In the first pathway (e.g., in hypercholesterolemia), monocyte and macrophage migration occurs without endothelial denudation. In some instances, endothelial loss occurs, with platelets carpeting bare areas. In this event, platelets would stimulate proliferation of smooth muscle by releasing PDGF.

In the second pathway, the endothelium itself was postulated to release growth factors, stimulating smooth muscle proliferation. Experimental rabbit arterial balloon injury shows that regrowing endothelium induces myointimal proliferation beneath its advancing edges, stimulating accumulation of collagen[78] and glycosaminoglycans.[79] Stimulated smooth muscle itself then releases growth factors, leading to a continued autocrine proliferative response. In the initial iteration of this theory, the second pathway was thought to be relevant to atheroma stimulated by diabetes, possibly in relation to insulin-derived growth factors, cigarette smoking, or hypertension. Hypertension causes endothelial injury, but striking differences exist between the behavior of smooth muscle cells in atherosclerosis and hypertension. Atherosclerosis stimulates an overt smooth muscle proliferative response. In most instances, pure hypertension causes thickening of the arterial wall by virtue of increased protein synthesis, without an increase in cell number.[80]

Arterial trauma, such as clamping or balloon injury, produces stenoses and vascular injuries (ranging from minor to severe) and initiates both myointimal hyperplasia and atheromas. This mode of atherogenesis invokes the response to injury hypothesis. In this scenario, physical or chemical agents cause endothelial denudation, followed by platelet adherence and subsequent release of PDGF,[81] triggering smooth muscle migration proliferation and lipid accumulation. This sequence applies to specific arterial wall injuries, particularly when the internal elastic lamina is disrupted.

Injury as a global theory of atherogenesis is unsupported by subsequent observations of early atherogenesis. Arterial denudation is a rare finding in early atherogenesis in humans and animals, although endothelial cells may be injured or dysfunctional while remaining in place.[82] It is known that systemic endothelial dysfunction exists in atherosclerosis.[83] Endothelial dysfunction exerts profound effects on systemic vasodilatation and the upregulation of endothelial receptors, facilitating entry of cells and blood components through an apparently intact endothelium. Because all arterial wall cells secrete growth factors that are similar if not identical to PDGF and its derivatives, postulating physical endothelial disruption and platelet deposition is unnecessary.

The responses of the arterial wall after injury remain of considerable practical interest in both atherogenesis and intimal hyperplasia. With injury, early medial smooth muscle proliferation is the first step, influenced primarily by basic fibroblast growth factor.[84] Migration and production of an extracellular matrix are the second and third stages of injury. These mechanisms are relevant to trauma-provoked atheromas, which occur as a result of clamping or balloon injuries in the presence of modestly elevated levels of LDL cholesterol.[85] Angiotensin II also causes smooth muscle to proliferate and induces expression of growth factors.[86,87] One of these growth factors, TGF-β, exerts either stimulatory or inhibitory effects, depending on circumstances. Injury also induces medial angiotensinogen gene expression and angiotensin receptor expression.[88] Other smooth muscle antigens include thrombin, catecholamine, and possibly endothelin. As a result, atheromas developing in a setting of injury (mechanical, immunologic, or infectious) are influenced by trauma-induced growth factors in varying degrees and sequences. However, plasma LDL elevation accentuates neointimal hyperplasia[89,90] without actual atheroma formation.

Lesion Arrest or Regression

The potential for plaque regression and stabilization of vulnerable plaques is key in the consideration of prevention and treatment of atherosclerosis. Regression of atherosclerosis in response to lowered serum cholesterol has been demonstrated in autopsy studies of starved humans dating back to World War I,[23] in many animal models,[91] and in pioneering clinical angiographic trials combining cessation of smoking with lipid reduction.[92] In humans, trials of vascular end points have shown some impressive examples of regression in coronary arteries; more commonly, minimal anatomic regression is seen, along with slowing of progression, but with drastic reductions in coronary events.[93] Importantly, magnetic resonance imaging has documented favorable longitudinal changes in carotid plaque composition, with reduction of the lipid core and increased fibrous tissue.[94] As atherosclerotic plaques in experimental animals regress, plaque bulk is reduced, mainly by lipid egress. This regressive process has been shown convincingly in experiments using hypercholesterolemic dogs[52,53] and monkeys.[54-57] The exact mechanisms of lesion regression, particularly the roles of inflammatory and immune responses, are incompletely understood. Regression has been demonstrated using serial observations of decreased bulk of individual plaques; reduced luminal encroachment, as shown by edge defects on sequential angiography; and decreased plaque lipid and altered fibrous protein content measured histologically and chemically.[57] An important technical aspect of this research was the confirmation of regressive changes using immediate autopsy or surgical observation and biopsy. Grossly or histopathologically, plaque change correlated with observed regressive angiographic changes.[58,59] Stary[95] described regression of advanced lesions in atherosclerotic rhesus monkeys, clearly documenting disappearance of macrophages, macrophage-derived foam cells, lymphocytes, and extracellular lipids, as a result of drastic reduction of blood cholesterol for 42 months. Arterial wall calcium deposits, however, did not regress, and as might be expected, calcification is a definite limiting factor in regression as well as being important in the planning of endovascular interventions.

Sequential measurement of plaque content and composition are not readily obtained in humans, but angiography and ultrasonography are currently used to assess treatment effects. Experimentally, decreased luminal intrusion on sequential angiography coincided with decreased plaque size and reduced lipid content. In some instances, we found that plaque fibrous protein increased during regression.[57] Although residual fibrosis potentially limits plaque bulk reduction, fibrosis also converts a soft atheromatous plaque into a more stable lesion. Active lesions, particularly in the coronary arteries, are not necessarily the most occlusive ones. Although angiographic edge changes may be minimal, reduction in coronary events in response to lipid-lowering treatment likely relates more to plaque stabilization than to bulk reduction. To produce regression consistently, total serum cholesterol must be reduced to approximately 150 mg/dL. Modest serum cholesterol elevations exist, above which experimental lesions progress.[59] Antiplatelet treatment does not appear to retard plaque progression; combinations of antiplatelet agents, high-dose aspirin, and dipyridamole in the rhesus model caused rapid, dramatic plaque progression during hypercholesterolemia.[60] Favorable lipid thresholds for human regressive responses approximate a total serum cholesterol level of 150 to 170 mg/dL and an LDL level of 100 mg/dL or less, levels that Roberts cited in populations in which atherosclerosis is virtually absent.[96] This epidemiologic observation led him to conclude that elevated lipid levels are the single etiologic risk factor in atherogenesis. However, in extrapolating this concept to secondary treatment, inflammatory responses need to be considered. These responses likely contribute to plaque instability, leading to atherosclerotic complications, as often occurs in the late stages of atherosclerosis in the absence of hyperlipidemia.

In recent years, plaque morphology has garnered increasing interest. More research is in progress to elucidate high-risk features in plaques and their behaviors, including progression and specific complications, as well as the possibility of regression or arrest. Thus, particular plaque characteristics might better predict overt complications of atherosclerosis. This information in turn can improve our understanding about which plaques are likely to remain asymptomatic or potentially respond to medical therapy, versus which plaques have a higher likelihood of rupture. Such detailed understanding has important implications for medical and surgical management of atherosclerosis in specific sites. For instance, in carotid artery disease, the mechanism of stroke is most often related to the release of emboli from carotid plaques. However, carotid plaques exhibit wide morphologic variations (Fig. 7.4A and B). Unstable carotid plaques are associated with cerebral features of ischemic vascular injury including higher volumes of white matter lesions as possible markers for global cerebrovascular disease.[97] The results of the ongoing Plaque At risk (PARISK) study also may help us better diagnose and predict the behavior of particular carotid plaques.[98] Current noninvasive diagnostic modalities promise more precise information about plaque morphology. Lukanova and colleagues showed that the three commonly employed noninvasive imaging techniques (ultrasound, CT, and MRI) were all complementary to each other for optimal evaluation of carotid plaque morphology.[99] Biomechanical measurements such as shear stress and oscillatory shear

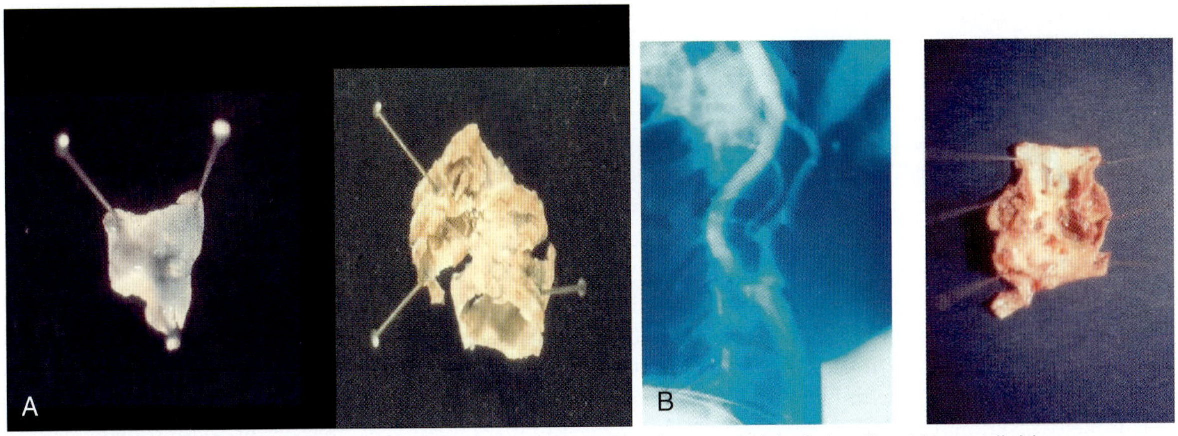

FIG 7.4 Heterogeneity of symptomatic carotid artery plaques. (A) *Left*: localized fibrous lipid poor carotid plaque; *right*: complex 32 mm ulcerated Council on Atherosclerosis, American Heart Association Class 6 atheroma. (B) Complex carotid plaque with ulceration and hemorrhage.

stress computed from MRI flow data may also help predict plaque rupture risk.[100]

MEDICAL MANAGEMENT

General Considerations

Populations free of coronary disease generally exhibit total cholesterol levels less than 150 mg/dL and LDL cholesterol levels less than 100 mg/dL. This observation questions the primacy of other atherosclerotic risk factors that commonly manifest in these relatively disease-free populations.[96] In examining the usefulness of the lipid hypothesis for treatment, rather than prevention, considerable positive evidence has accumulated to support an energetic approach to overall lipid reduction. The Heart Protection Study, a randomized, placebo-controlled trial using simvastatin in more than 20,000 individuals, showed a reduction of adverse cardiovascular events and prolongation of life when this agent was used for primary and secondary prevention, even in individuals without elevated lipid levels.[101] Statins have anti-inflammatory effects, as shown by decreased C-reactive protein levels.[102] These effects occur independent of LDL reduction.[103,104]

The National Cholesterol Education Program (NCEPIII) recommends a target LDL level of <100 mg/mL. For high-risk individuals, an optimal goal of <70 mg/mL is recommended. In contrast, the American College of Cardiology/American Heart Association (ACC/AHA) formulated guidelines in 2013 that endorsed cholesterol lowering treatment without specific targets; instead, an individual's absolute risk is used as a guide when choosing the optimal therapy.[105,106] Stringent lipid target levels can seldom be achieved with diet alone. The Heart Protection Study has recently addressed the issue of baseline C-reactive protein (CRP) in statin therapy. According to this study, allocation to simvastatin therapy proved effective, regardless of baseline levels of CRP and even in participants with normal lipid levels.[107] Currently, a statin, along with low-dose aspirin, clopidogrel (an antiplatelet agent), and angiotensin-converting enzyme (ACE) inhibitors are recommended for patients with peripheral arterial disease.[108]

Complications and deleterious clinical events associated with atherosclerosis are multiple and interactive. In the late stages, the instability of the fibrous plaques involves more than lipid dynamics. More than 4 decades ago, Holman and colleagues[109] pointed out "*a sharp line of distinction existing between atherogenesis and the subsequent evolution of lesions that may or may not precipitate clinical disease, for the factors involved in the evolution of lesions beyond the stage of fatty streaks may be entirely different from the factors that initiate fatty streaks.*" These factors include inflammatory and immune mechanisms, altered fibrous proteins, accumulation of blood elements, and cap rupture. Among interventions intended to produce plaque stabilization or regression, decreasing LDL cholesterol promotes favorable changes in atheromas and improved outcomes. Antiinflammatory effects of statins, as judged by biomarkers, are an important pleiotropic characteristic of these agents. The effect of cigarette smoking, a crucial promoter of complications of atherosclerosis, might be viewed as a contributor to inflammation, which cannot be overcome solely by lipid reduction.

In angiographic regression trials, the most favorable plaque changes in terms of arrest or regression relate to the degree and duration of blood lipid reduction. In peripheral arteries, regression and stabilization were 1.5- to 2.0-fold more common in treated subjects than in those receiving placebos.[92] Although angiographic studies show plaque regression trends, wall change or plaque reduction is usually quite modest compared to stabilization of vulnerable lesions. Intravascular ultrasound is an important tool in visualizing plaque relationships within the arterial wall in response to treatment. Serial angiography, which can only detect lesion encroachment, has detected favorable clinical results among patients randomly assigned to an experimental group consuming a 10% fat, 12-mg cholesterol diet and undergoing smoking cessation, stress management training, and exercise.[109] After 1 year, 82% of the treated group showed regressive changes in coronary artery plaques that depended, in some degree, on the amount of initial lesion encroachment. Importantly, a number of recent intravascular ultrasound studies in humans convincingly demonstrate regression of coronary atheroma in response to statin therapy.[110]

Treatment aims to improve the arterial lesions and improve complication-free patient survival. Increased fibrous protein synthesis produces a stable, fibrotic plaque as opposed to a soft, friable plaque containing an unstable, atheromatous core covered by a tenuous cap. However, a densely sclerotic, highly occlusive lesion can also cause distal ischemia. In evaluating these hypotheses with a view toward better prediction and control, ameliorating the atheroma itself and providing quantifiable evidence of favorable changes has correlated mostly with blood lipid reduction along with complete cessation of smoking.

Atherosclerosis is often segmental; bypassing or removing symptomatic arterial lesions in selected arterial segments minimizes the deleterious effects of dangerous lesions. These observations, made more than 40 years ago, were uniquely surgical insights and brought life- and limb-saving interventions to many patients.[3] Arterial interventions, which include endovascular approaches, evolved as highly effective means of treating patients with advanced, symptomatic atheromas, including specific patterns of coronary involvement, high-grade carotid lesions, and aortic disease. However, effective surgical or endovascular treatment of one arterial segment does not prevent disease progression in other segments—life expectancy remains shortened. Continued smoking after reconstruction makes matters worse, particularly after ill-advised infrainguinal or aortic reconstruction for stable claudicants. Aspirin, thrombolytics, and anticoagulants can prevent or minimize superimposed embolic phenomena and clotting, but underlying plaques continue to progress. Modification of inflammatory responses provoked by cytokine-derived or immune-modulating factors has potential and may now be practical, given the current ability to monitor blood levels for biomarkers such as inflammatory cytokines (IL-6) and high specificity C reactive protein (CRP), which predict cardiovascular complications and mortality.[111,112]

Insignificant or small plaques, particularly in coronary or cerebral arteries, can provoke arterial spasm. Atherosclerotic involvement impairs the normal action of endothelium-derived relaxing factor,[113-115] impairing vasodilator responses in coronary and cerebral arteries.[114] Dietary treatment of experimental atherosclerosis restores endothelium-dependent relaxation responses,[116] whereas long-term inhibition of nitric oxide synthesis by feeding promotes experimental atherosclerosis.[117]

Clinical Management

All individuals with two or more risk factors or any form of vascular disease require a lipid profile and an HbA1c blood sample. Fasting blood samples measure HDL cholesterol levels. The LDL cholesterol level is calculated as follows: LDL cholesterol = Total cholesterol – HDL cholesterol + (Triglycerides/5). This formula holds for fasting patients with triglycerides less than 400 mg/dL. Serum cholesterol levels must be obtained with patients on a regular diet outside the hospital. Acute illnesses cause sudden, inexplicable decrements in total serum cholesterol.

The National Cholesterol Education Program recommends dietary approaches as a first step for patients with hyperlipidemia.[118] The patient's age and sex are considered when choosing treatment. The initial emphasis is on physical activity and weight loss. It recommended that clinicians offer modestly hyperlipidemic patients information on diet and exercise in the form of walking. Drug treatment is delayed in patients with a low risk of coronary heart disease (e.g., no smoking, diabetes, or hypertension), in men younger than 45 years, and women younger than 55 years. Emphasis has been placed on high levels of HDL cholesterol, a powerful negative risk factor, but selectively increasing HDL levels is difficult to accomplish. Although these guidelines apply to primary prevention, virtually all patients with known vascular disease (i.e., presence of asymptomatic plaques or claudication) are candidates for drug therapy, usually with statins, cessation of smoking, and other lifestyle interventions.

Drug Therapy for Hyperlipidemia

Currently available drugs include cholestyramine and colestipol (bile acid sequestrants), nicotinic acid (a B-complex vitamin), and the widely used statin drugs. Statins are 3-hydroxy-3-methylglutaryl coenzyme A–reducing agents that include pravastatin, lovastatin, simvastatin, atorvastatin, and fluvastatin. These agents inhibit hepatic cholesterol biosynthesis. Gemfibrozil, a fibric acid derivative, is used to treat hypertriglyceridemia. Recent trials have shown that vitamin C and E supplements have no effect in preventing coronary heart disease events or in improving outcomes in established coronary heart disease.[119,120] Treatment that both lowers LDL cholesterol and raises HDL cholesterol is considered desirable. The dramatic results of intensive LDL lowering in the 2004 REVERSAL trial support the concept of "the lower the better" for treatment of patients with coronary artery disease.[121,122] A higher dose of atorvastatin (80 mg) was more effective than a lower dose of pravastatin (40 mg) in reducing LDL to 79 mg/dL, significantly reducing C-reactive protein while producing a significant reduction in atheroma volume and preventing the progression of coronary lesions. Statin drugs, combined with niacin in nondiabetics, have achieved dramatic reductions in coronary events, possibly related to nonlipid actions affecting endothelial function, inflammatory response, plaque stability, and thrombus formation.[123] The side effects of niacin, such as flushing, can be difficult to tolerate, and raising HDL levels remains less practical than lowering LDL levels. However, statin therapy may be associated with certain side effects, including liver disorders, neuromuscular disorders, new onset diabetes, cognitive dysfunction, cataracts, and rarely with immune-mediated necrotizing myopathy.[124,125] While an increased cancer risk was seen with the use of ezetimibe-simvastatin therapy in the Simvastatin and Ezetimibe in Aortic Stenosis (SEAS) study[126] in patients with aortic stenosis, this increased propensity was not confirmed in the 21-month follow-up of SEAS patients after the conclusion of the trial.[127]

Control of Associated Risk Factors

Cigarette Smoking

Cigarette smoking is a powerful risk factor for atherosclerotic disease, promoting its clinical complications even when lipids are normal. This addiction relates directly to limb amputation, high mortality owing to ischemic heart disease, and failure of aortic and femoropopliteal grafts.[128-130] The mechanisms by which cigarette smoking promotes atherosclerosis and graft thrombosis are incompletely understood. Carbon monoxidemia can predispose to endothelial injury, producing increased plasma flux and entry of LDL and other proteins. Cigarette smoking is associated with increased platelet reactivity, peripheral vasoconstriction, and lowered HDL levels.[131] From the standpoint of pathogenesis, lipid abnormalities are clearly important, but from the standpoint of clinical interventions for established disease, smoking cessation is critical in preventing amputation, myocardial infarction, and stroke.

At a minimum, clinical practice guidelines include routine institutional identification of and intervention with all tobacco users at every visit. Clinicians should ask about and record the tobacco use status of every patient. All smokers should be offered smoking cessation treatment at every office visit—nicotine replacement therapy short term, and bupropion long term to treat depression.[132] The latter drug offers prosexual benefits over other antidepressants. Cessation advice, even as brief as 3 minutes, is useful. Formal clinician-delivered support and life skills training are important treatment components for smoking cessation. The more intense the treatment, the more effective it will be in achieving long-term abstinence. Importantly, elective interventions in smokers for claudication alone should be avoided. Graft occlusion often occurs in chronic smokers and makes eventual amputation quite likely.

Hypertension

Control of hypertension prolongs life and reduces coronary mortality.[133] Chronic hypertension accelerates atherosclerosis in experimental hyperlipidemic animals.[134] Paradoxically, as with cigarette smoking, Asian and Caribbean populations exhibit hypertension with a low incidence of atherosclerotic disease in the absence of hyperlipidemia. In affluent societies, however, prospective studies show that hypertension is related to the risk of premature atherosclerotic disease, independent of the risk factors of hyperlipidemia and cigarette smoking.[135] Hypertension may be linked with risk factor clustering, including glucose intolerance, hyperinsulinemia, and dyslipidemia promoted by abdominal obesity,[136] comprising the metabolic syndrome, or syndrome X. Weight loss, exercise, and combined drug treatment for hypertriglyceridemia should be instituted. Treatment of hypertension with thiazide diuretics alone was not advantageous in terms of coronary outcome in a subgroup of men in the Multiple Risk Factor Intervention Trial,[137] likely owing to inadequate control of lipid levels when total cholesterol in the intervention group remained greater than 200 mg/dL, before the availability of statins. The current goal for blood pressure is 120/80 mm Hg using lifestyle changes, weight loss, and blood pressure medications based on patient age, race, and presence or absence of diabetes. Antihypertensive drugs with specific benefits include ACE inhibitors, diuretics, and β-blockers. Lifestyle alterations include weight reduction, reduced dietary sodium intake, reduced alcohol intake, increased physical activity, and possibly increased calcium intake.[138]

Exercise

Regular exercise decreases total serum cholesterol, LDL, and fasting triglycerides and has variable effects on HDL.[139] The preventive effects of exercise have been amply documented; a sedentary lifestyle is an important risk factor for coronary disease.[140] No study, however, has shown that exercise has a direct effect on established atherosclerotic plaques; experimental and clinical data have demonstrated arrest or regression of plaques with lipid reduction. Strenuous unsupervised exercise can be dangerous in the presence of preexisting coronary disease.[141] Exercise does not compensate for persistent uncorrected hyperlipidemia or continued cigarette smoking. This is an important message for patients with vascular disease. Exercise will not offset the effects of elevated total cholesterol and LDL or substitute for effective control of hypertension, where weight loss and drugs are prime requirements.[142]

Beneficial effects of exercise in peripheral vascular disease (i.e., increased walking distance) relate to improved skeletal muscle oxidative metabolism.[143] Exercise is important secondary therapy. Exercise programs can be more effective for claudication over the long term than surgical or endovascular intervention, particularly in infrainguinal atherosclerosis. In patients with coronary atherosclerosis, exercise prescriptions must be carefully structured. Before prescribing strenuous exercise, stress testing or monitoring to detect silent ischemic heart disease is recommended, and strenuous intermittent exercise is unadvisable. Recently, exercise has been shown to reduce CRP levels, demonstrating a favorable effect on this biomarker of inflammation.[144]

Diabetes

Diabetes, an increasingly prevalent risk factor, promotes atherosclerosis. Most patients with peripheral arterial disease who are nonsmokers are diabetic. In its singular form, diabetes is associated with severe infracrural and coronary atherosclerosis. One diabetes control trial showed a reduction in microvascular complications with "tight control" using insulin; unfortunately, this trial was not designed to study end points of macrovascular atherosclerotic complications.[145] Causes of enhanced atherogenesis in diabetes include abnormalities in apoproteins and lipoprotein particle distribution, particularly elevated levels of lipoprotein(a),[146] an independent thromboatherosclerotic risk factor. In poorly controlled diabetes, a procoagulant state exists. Increased glucose levels are associated with accelerated platelet aggregation in vitro, and accompanying hypertriglyceridemia enhances thrombogenic factors V, II, and X. Glycooxidation and oxidation contribute to LDL entry into macrophages, and glycation of proteins and plasma in the arterial wall contributes to accelerated atherosclerosis. Hormones, growth factors, cytokine-enhanced smooth muscle cell proliferation, and increased foam cell formation may relate to the pathogenesis of atherogenesis in diabetes mellitus.[147]

Both hyperinsulinemia and insulin resistance are associated with atherosclerosis,[148] and both occur in type 2 diabetes. Both insulin and glucose stimulate the growth of diabetic infragenicular smooth muscle cells.[149] A possible mechanism accounting for atherogenesis in diabetes is impaired vasoactivity;

troglitazone, an insulin-action enhancer, corrects impaired brachial artery vasoactivity in patients with occult impaired glucose tolerance.[150]

Consistent control of blood glucose is advisable, as described in Chapter 12 in this volume. A recent trial studying the effectiveness of intensive versus standard blood glucose control on cardiovascular events showed no significant effects upon cardiovascular events, death, or microvascular complications except for the progression of albuminuria.[151] For any given level of LDL, coronary heart disease risk is increased threefold to fivefold in diabetics compared with nondiabetics.[152] Other studies have shown an association of perioperative hyperglycemia with an increased risk of postoperative infections, longer length of stay, increased incidence of pneumonia, bacteremia, urinary tract infections, acute renal failure, and acute myocardial infarction. While HbA1c <7% correlates with good longer-term control of glucose in diabetics, moderately tight perioperative control (glucose <200 mg/dL) appears to prevent cardiac and infectious complications in cardiac surgery patients. However, "too tight" glucose control (target glucose 81 to 108 mg/dL) may result in increased hypoglycemic events and even increased mortality.[153]

Elevated triglyceride levels most commonly accompany severely elevated cholesterol levels in diabetics; this particular combination greatly increases the risk of adverse coronary events. Diabetics exhibit particular lipid abnormalities, including chylomicronemia, increased very-low-density lipoprotein (VLDL) levels, increased VLDL and chylomicron remnants, and triglyceride-rich LDL and HDL concentrations. Mamo and Proctor[154] emphasized the pathogenicity of these remnants. Glycosylation of lipoproteins and collagen relates directly to levels of glucose, contributing to increased binding of LDL by collagen, and glycosylated lipoproteins are taken up avidly by macrophages to transform them into foam cells. Extensive clinical experience documents the efficacy of bariatric surgery in diabetics with body mass index exceeding 35.[155] Target goals for treatment of diabetics include fasting glucose less than 110 mg/dL, hemoglobin A1c less than 7%, blood pressure less than 130/80 mm Hg, LDL less than 70 mg/dL, and triglycerides less than 150 mg/dL. The use of an ACE inhibitor with a statin should be considered in all cases.

Metformin monotherapy is recommended as an initial treatment in type 2 diabetics by the American Diabetes Association and has been confirmed by other authors. In a recent meta-analysis of more than 300 clinical trials, several glucose-lowering agents were compared concerning safety and relative efficacy in cardiovascular disease (CVD) outcomes. No significant differences were found between nine available classes of glucose-lowering drugs (including metformin) in cardiovascular or all-cause mortality outcomes. However, it appears that these agents do not have a significant effect on preventing morbidity or mortality from cardiovascular disease either.[156]

Antioxidants and Oxidative Stress

Treatment with antioxidants is based on the concept that oxidative stress related to reactive oxygen species promotes oxidized LDL to form foam cells and activate macrophages, which release inflammatory cytokines and growth factors that stimulate smooth muscle proliferation. Not all cytokines provoke the inflammatory response; IL-10, an anti-inflammatory cytokine, prevents atherosclerotic events in vitro and in vivo.[157] Conversely, plaque components such as metalloproteinases, inflammatory cytokines, and high-sensitivity CRP appear in the systemic circulation, presumably as markers of disease severity.[11,158] Biomarkers can be measured and evaluated as indicators of normal or pathogenic responses as well as pharmacologic responses to treatment. Determination of the exact relationships between biomarkers and plaque change requires both observational and outcome studies. Ideally, improved plaque morphology linked to improved outcomes provides the strongest evidence of validity of a particular biomarker. While oxidation is recognized as an important disease-promoting mechanism,[159,160] results of randomized trials with antioxidant vitamins have proved disappointing.[120] Vitamins C and E, at a molecular level, theoretically might function as pro-oxidants promoting formation of reactive oxidative species.

Elevated blood levels of homocysteine, earlier proposed as a thromboatherosclerotic risk factor,[161] have not shown promise. Elevated levels can be reduced by folic acid intake, but recent trial data from a 5-year study demonstrated no effect on cardiovascular outcomes, although homocysteine levels were effectively reduced.[162]

Iron Hypothesis

Sullivan first postulated the delay in heart risk in women after menopause related to total body iron stores, with iron accumulating particularly in men and in women after menopause.[163] Iron in its ferrous form is a powerful inflammatory and oxidizing agent believed to promote progressive inflammatory diseases.[164] Studies show that iron balance is regulated by the hormone hepcidin. Its action is relevant in that high hepcidin levels promote iron retention in macrophages, in turn relating to increased intralesional iron content and inflammation.[164,165] According to the "iron hypothesis," iron promotes atherosclerosis through its impact on multiple processes that culminate in the generation of reactive oxygen species (ROS), lipid peroxidation, endothelial activation and proliferation of smooth muscle cells and macrophages. According to the "refined iron hypothesis," hepcidin binds ferroportin (FPN) resulting in increased intracellular ROS and cholesterol levels, thus causing detrimental effects on atherosclerotic plaques.[166] Macrophages are pivotal in iron homeostasis and potentially play a role in the prevention of the toxic effects of iron that is released whenever intraplaque hemorrhage occurs.[166,167] The effect of deliberate reduction of iron stores was investigated in a single blinded clinical trial, the Iron and Atherosclerosis Study (FeAST).[168] Overall results did not show a difference in outcomes related to phlebotomy, but the study did demonstrate strikingly significant, age-related favorable outcomes, with improvement related to iron reduction occurring in younger participants (age 43 to 61 years).[169] Substudies carried out in FeAST participants at the Veterans' Administration (VA) Sierra Nevada Health Care System in Reno, Nevada, demonstrated inflammatory cytokine signatures in atherosclerotic participants compared with individuals apparently free of disease,[12] determined biomarker relationships to statin administration at baseline[170] and, upon completion of the 6-year study, demonstrated significant correlations between mortality, ferritin levels, and inflammatory biomarkers, particularly IL-6 and CRP.[171] Another line of evidence supporting the unfavorable health consequences of iron accumulation relates to regular blood donors, some of whom maintain protective ferritin levels characteristic of premenopausal women.[172]

Studies of blood donors in the United States and Finland[173-175] showed reduced risk of myocardial infarction in regular blood donors; however, a 2001 report[176] did not support this effect. Divergent outcomes could relate to the need to achieve significantly lowered ferritin levels that range from 17–25 ng/mL in premenopausal women. A later study of frequent blood donors achieving an average ferritin level of 17 ng/mL demonstrated that significantly improved flow mediated brachial artery dilation and reduced oxidative stress markers compared with infrequent blood donors' levels of average ferritin of 52 ng/mL.[177] Blood donation was initially reported to improve glucose control and insulin sensitivity in type 2 diabetics.[178] An additional set of observations, ultrasound longitudinal observation of carotid plaques, provided plaque observations relating changes to iron stores (ferritin levels) and to favorable outcomes in the study group.[179] These investigators concluded that the iron effect on carotid plaques related synergistically with elevated lipid levels, suggesting that iron excess promoted higher levels of oxidized LDL. An epidemiologic study compared iron parameters and oxidative markers in older men living in Crete and exhibiting lower disease risk compared with men of similar age living in Zutphen, the Netherlands.[180] Markers of oxidative stress were significantly lower in the healthier Cretan men together with a twofold lower mean ferritin level (mean 69.8 ng/mL) in Crete compared with men from Zutphen ($p < 0.0001$). The Mediterranean diet is low in iron content[181]; combined with other favorable characteristics, this diet might contribute to the difference between the two populations.

Racial disparity in outcomes of peripheral vascular disease exists among Black and White individuals. Amputation rates are higher in Black individuals compared to White individuals.[182] While reasons for these disparities remain elusive, one possible mechanism might be linked to the iron hypothesis. Improved clinical outcomes with lower ferritin and higher percent transferrin saturation in White but not Black individuals have previously been documented in literature. Additionally, lower hemoglobin and higher ferritin levels have been found in Black compared with White adults. These underlying metabolic differences may form the basis of protective mechanisms in White individuals against iron toxicity when compared to their Black counterparts. Differences in iron content of cells such as macrophages may translate into differences in the various inflammatory reactions involved in CVD.[183]

Antiplatelet and Anticoagulant Therapy

Antiplatelet therapy does not produce regressive effects on established lesions, although anti-inflammatory effects may occur. Favorable therapeutic effects relate mainly to the prevention of superimposed thrombosis on advanced plaques, as described in detail later. Generally, smaller rather than larger doses of aspirin are advantageous. The Physicians' Health Study showed that 325 mg of aspirin on alternate days reduced subsequent need for peripheral vascular surgery.[184] Aspirin doses ranging from 74 to 159 mg daily have been found to be as effective as larger doses. Aspirin is recommended as an adjunct, not an alternative, to managing accompanying cardiovascular risk factors.[185] Reports concerning the possible promotion of intraplaque hemorrhage in carotid lesions in patients receiving aspirin are conflicting.

Results of a long-term study of the effects of clopidogrel indicate a statistical advantage of this therapy over aspirin therapy alone. This population included patients with recent myocardial infarction, recent stroke, or established peripheral arterial disease.[184] The largest relative risk reduction for clopidogrel, compared with aspirin, was in fatal and nonfatal myocardial infarction—19.2%.[186,187] Antiplatelet therapy and oral anticoagulants appear to reduce the risk of graft occlusion and ischemic events after infrainguinal bypass surgery.[188] Oral anticoagulant therapy is the more effective treatment in high-risk patients. Evidence of the beneficial effects of antiplatelet and oral anticoagulant therapy was based on a small number of trials; there is no proof as to which modality is most effective in preventing graft occlusion and ischemic events.

The end point of epidemiologic and clinical studies of atherosclerosis usually involves a thrombotic episode.[189] A prospective study of hemostatic function and cardiovascular death showed that elevated levels of factors VIIc and VIIIc and fibrinogen, in addition to elevated plasma cholesterol levels, appeared to be important predisposing factors.[190,191] Elevated fibrinogen, a major risk factor for coronary artery disease, is associated with peripheral arterial disease in men[189]; leukocyte levels may be elevated in both disease states.[192] Continued low-dose aspirin therapy, as described previously, is the therapeutic mainstay of antiplatelet therapy,[184] although resistance to its antithrombotic effects might be present in a significant proportion of individuals.[193]

The use of low-dose daily aspirin is endorsed by the US Preventive Service Task Force (USPSTF) for the primary prevention of CVD in individuals 50 to 59 years of age, having a 10% or greater 10-year CVD risk and in whom bleeding risk is not increased. However, such individuals should also have a life expectancy of at least 10 years and they should take aspirin daily for a minimum of 10 years. For adults aged 60 years and above, the decision to start aspirin therapy should be individualized. In adults younger than 50 years of age, the use of daily aspirin for the primary prevention of CVD remains contentious due to current lack of evidence.[194]

However, the USPSTF recommendations have invited controversy. Between 1988 and 2005, six randomized controlled trials (British Doctors Trial, Thrombosis Prevention Trial, Women's Health Study, Primary Prevention Project, Physician's Health Study, and Hypertension Optimal Treat Trial) studied the impact of aspirin on reduction of CVD in adults without known CVD. Overall, these trials showed a net benefit of aspirin in reduction of cardiovascular events. Between 2008 and 2014, four other randomized controlled trials (Japanese Primary Prevention of Atherosclerosis With Aspirin for Diabetes, The Japanese

Primary Prevention Project, The Prevention of Progression of Arterial Disease and Diabetes) were conducted to study the benefit of aspirin for primary prevention of CVD in adults with high risk of CVD. In contrast to the earlier trials, these later trials have not demonstrated a significant benefit of aspirin therapy in primary prevention of CVD. As further robust studies on the subject progress, current findings underscore the importance of approaching each patient individually and tailoring their management according to their specific risk profile.[195,196] Younger age groups may derive more benefit from initiation of aspirin therapy compared those of more advanced age.

Vasoactive Drugs

Nonlipid strategies, beyond cholesterol reduction, include the use of β-adrenergic receptor blocking agents to reduce catecholamine release, calcium channel blockers to reduce wall stress and inhibit lipid intake, nitrates to relax vascular smooth muscle by nitric oxide release, and ACE inhibitors to block atherogenic effects on angiotensin II. The Heart Outcome Prevention Evaluation (HOPE) study showed that ACE inhibitors improved the primary end points of myocardial infarction, stroke, and death from cardiovascular causes.[197] The use of perioperative β-blockade for patients undergoing non-cardiac procedures has been brought into question as a result of the Perioperative Ischemic Evaluation (POISE) trial, demonstrating increased postoperative risks of perioperative metoprolol administration.[198] Current Surgical Complications Improvement Project (SCIP) guidelines recommend that patients receiving preoperative β-blockers continue to receive β-blockade postoperatively. When a clear indication for β-blockade exists, it appears best to begin this step well before operative intervention. In another separate issue concerning vasodilators, the drug cilostazol has been reported to be effective in improving walking distance.[199]

Future Directions and Perspectives

Atherosclerosis and Infection

Cytomegalovirus (CMV) and *Chlamydia pneumoniae* infections have been associated with atherosclerosis. Comprehensive reviews, summarizing biologic evidence supporting relationships between infection and atherosclerosis included CMV, which is a ubiquitous virus.[200,201] Seropositivity was reported to be associated with a high rate of restenosis after coronary bypass.[202]

The organism *C. pneumoniae* and its DNA have been detected in atherosclerotic plaques with some frequency.[203] Chlamydial heat shock protein co-localizes in plaques with *C. pneumoniae*–specific antigen,[201,204] leading to the hypothesis that *C. pneumoniae*–infected macrophages, upon entering the intima, mediate inflammatory and autoimmune responses by producing chlamydial heat shock proteins.[205,206] In addition to *C. pneumoniae* and CMV, *Helicobacter pylori* and herpesvirus have been suggested in the pathogenesis of atherosclerotic plaques. The deleterious effects of infection presumably relate to inflammation and bacterial heat shock proteins, inciting arterial inflammatory and autoimmune reactions. While the molecular mechanisms inciting arterial wall reactions are of pathogenic interest, the results of recent large, randomized prospective trials assessing the efficacy of antibiotics to prevent cardiovascular events have been negative.[207]

Observations linking periodontal disease epidemiologically to atherosclerosis[208] might be related to atherogenesis by increasing circulating inflammatory cytokine levels, possibly promoting a proatherogenic endothelial cell phenotype with loss of antithrombotic, growth inhibitory, and vasodilator properties.[209] Subjects with periodontal disease, along with diabetics, show impaired brachial artery dilation.[210] Oral infection in an experimental model with the periodontal pathogen *Porphyromonas gingivalis* has been shown to increase IL-6 levels and accelerate atherosclerosis.[211] Recently a protocol for a single randomized trial of periodontal treatment examining brachial flow measurements, inflammatory biomarkers, and other surrogates in individuals with periodontal disease and atherosclerosis has been registered.[212] As mentioned previously, the results of interventional trials serve as gold standards, but substantive results of the periodontal trials have yet to be reported at this time.

Proteinomics

There is currently an increasing interest to better characterize each individual's risk for CVD with a greater precision. Such characterization of "cardiovascular risk phenotype," based on proteinomic arrays, may in turn better guide clinicians in the choice of therapies. In a recent prospective cohort study, a 9-protein risk score was validated and utilized in the prediction of cardiovascular events. The 9 proteins included angiopoietin-2, matrix metalloproteinase-12, chemokine ligand 18, complement 7, α-1 antichymotrypsin complex, angiopoietin related protein 4, troponin I, growth differentiation factor 11/8, and α-2 antiplasmin. Overall, the risk score based on 9 proteins provided better discrimination when compared to the Framingham secondary event model (this model was refit to the cohorts in the study).[213] It is not unreasonable to predict that in the future, a combination of various factors based on clinical, genomic, and proteinomics data will probably provide the best prediction of an individual's risk for cardiovascular disease and events.

Iron Metabolism

In its ferrous form, iron is a powerful inflammatory and oxidizing agent as previously described. Ferritin levels may influence the levels of certain inflammatory cytokines.[171] As mentioned earlier, differences in iron metabolism between different groups potentially affect inflammatory responses and cascades seen in cardiovascular disease. Disease risk might relate to differential iron homeostasis between individuals, as well as genetic susceptibility in lipid and inflammatory responses among different groups. Further research into these areas includes revision of "normal range" for iron biomarkers among different populations, and reduction of heme dietary iron intake along with measures to correct dysmetabolic ferritin level elevation. In time, these efforts might lead to more targeted and precise strategies for primary and secondary prevention of cardiovascular disease.[214]

Comprehensive Risk Reduction Programs

Atherosclerosis remains a multifactorial disease with global involvement and manifestations within the cardiovascular system.

The risk of under-treatment of patients with atherosclerosis remains, as compared to standard primary risk reduction management guidelines. Comprehensive programs, based on guideline recommended risk reduction in patients with peripheral arterial disease, can reduce cardiovascular events as well as limb events. Targeted programs for these individuals need wider clinical application. An observational cohort study from Canada compared patients with peripheral arterial disease enrolled in the Systematic Assessment of Vascular Risk (SAVR) program with patients with peripheral arterial disease who were not enrolled in SAVR. The program included engagement of vascular surgeons, family physicians, and patients with PAD, and promoted the use of antiplatelet agents, statins, angiotensin-converting enzyme inhibitors, and close monitoring of blood pressure control, lipid control, diabetic glycemic control, smoking cessation, and reduction of body mass index. The former group had a significantly lower incidence of primary outcome measures (a composite risk ratio of death, acute myocardial infarction, or ischemic stroke) with an adjusted hazards ratio of 0.63. The SAVR group also fared better for most of the measures of secondary outcome (major and minor lower limb amputations and bypass surgeries). Engaged cooperation of specialists with a thorough understanding of vascular disease as part of a comprehensive risk reduction program can result in a significant improvement in overall outcomes of cardiovascular disease.[215]

Gut Microbiome

CVD risk maybe influenced by dietary nutrients with trimethylamine (TMA) moiety, including choline, L-carnitine, and phospatidylcholine. Gut microbes maybe involved in the process because of their role in the production of TMA. TMA is further metabolized by liver Flavin monoxygenases (FMO3 and FMO1) to form trimethylamine-N-oxide (TMAO). This in turn may lead to macrophage cholesterol accumulation and foam cell formation. High TMAO levels have been found to be associated with CVD. Therefore, modification of dietary practices or the gut microbiome represents an interesting future area of research in CVD prevention.[216-218]

New Pharmacologic Agents

Proprotein convertase subtilisin/kexin type 9 (PCSK9) represents a novel target for reduction of LDL-C. PCSK9 is a serine protease enzyme involved with degradation of hepatocyte LDL receptors.[219] It binds to the epidermal growth factor-like repeat A (EGF-A) domain of the low-density lipoprotein receptors (LDL-Rs). This in turn leads to fewer surface LDL receptors and reduces clearance of LDL from blood. PCSK9 inhibitors include drugs such as evolocumab, alirocumab, and bococizumab—agents that are monoclonal antibodies.[220] In 2015, the US Food and Drug Administration (FDA) approved Praluent (alirocumab) injection for use in addition to diet and maximally tolerated statin therapy in adult patients with heterozygous familial hypercholesterolemia (HeFH) or in patients with symptomatic CVD—this was the first drug of its class to get this approval. Repatha (evolocumab) is also now FDA-approved for use. Additionally, trials are underway to evaluate additional PCSK9 inhibitors including siRNA and adnectin. In various studies, PCSK9 inhibitors have shown a reduction of up to 57% in the levels of LDL-C as monotherapy and up to 73% when combined with statins. A PCSK9 vaccine is also being researched.[221] Also, PCSK9 genetic polymorphisms maybe linked to blood pressure among African Americans.[222,223]

SUMMARY

Effective medical therapy for atherosclerosis ideally induces plaque stabilization or regression and reduces adverse clinical events, and prolongs life. Recommendations derive from a broad base of pathologic evidence, imaging observations, and randomized trials. For stable claudicants with infrainguinal atherosclerosis and patients after vascular reconstruction, secondary prevention methods include cessation of smoking; aspirin (preferably 81 mg daily), clopidogrel, or both; lipid reduction of total cholesterol to less than 150 mg/dL and LDL less than 100 mg, best achieved with statins, which also offer antiinflammatory benefits; walking briskly for 30 to 60 minutes daily; and addition of ACE inhibitors for diabetics, even with normal blood pressure. These medical measures should not delay direct arterial interventions in the presence of life- or limb-threatening lesions. The provocative question in medical rather than surgical treatment of specific lesions (e.g., asymptomatic, stable carotid plaques)[224] requires highly reliable imaging and outcome studies to identify truly stable lesions and the best choices for individuals. Comparative effectiveness research, focusing on evidence to provide the best decisions for all stakeholders, will likely inform future treatment choices for aging patients with atherosclerotic disease.[225] A good example of the case in question is carotid artery disease and how the paradigm for its management continues to evolve. Best Medical Therapy (BMT), encompassing various combinations of proper diet, exercise, blood pressure control, use of statin and aspirin, is considered the cornerstone of management of asymptomatic carotid artery disease. Additionally, BMT has a significant role in prevention of recurrent cardiovascular events in individuals with symptomatic carotid artery disease.[226] In one study, BMT was associated with regression of the carotid artery plaque in up to 26% of the patients studied, while 15% of the patients had no change in the carotid plaque area.[227] More intensive versions of BMT have been associated with more significant reductions in plaque progression.[226] Vascular specialists, intervening at crucial times and in specific ways during the course of a complex chronic disease entity, atherosclerosis, need to understand opportunities and challenges implicit in assessing comparative effectiveness of selected treatments for individual patients with variable disease patterns.

REVIEW QUESTIONS

1. Type IV (fibrous plaques) usually evolve:
   a. In areas of fatty streak involvement
   b. From thrombotic clots
   c. In areas of endothelial shedding
   d. From gelatinous plaque progression
   e. From hypertrophic smooth muscle cells
2. Atherosclerotic plaque regression or stabilization is characterized by:
   a. Decreased fibrosis
   b. Lipid egress
   c. Less calcification
   d. Thrombolysis
   e. Activated macrophages
3. In atherosclerosis, macrophages in plaques produce all of the following except:
   a. Lipoproteins
   b. Interleukin (IL)1
   c. Metalloproteinases
   d. Growth factors
   e. Interleukin-10
4. Examples of inflammatory cytokines include all except:
   a. Interleukin (IL)-1
   b. IL-2
   c. IL-6
   d. Tumor necrosis factor (TNF)-α
   e. IL-10
5. Evidence-based medical management for patients with peripheral arterial disease usually includes:
   a. Folic acid supplements
   b. Statin administration
   c. Antioxidant vitamin C and E supplements
   d. Aspirin and dipyridamole
   e. β-blockade
6. Characteristics of unstable or vulnerable plaques include:
   a. A thin fibrous cap
   b. A prominent lipid core
   c. Intense round cell infiltration
   d. Variable degrees of luminal intrusion
   e. All of the above
7. Which of the following statements about genetic disorders promoting increased levels of low-density lipoprotein cholesterol and atherosclerosis is true?
   a. They are exceedingly rare.
   b. They are associated with type 1 diabetes.
   c. They occur in about 1 in 500 live births.
   d. They relate to surface defects in a high-density lipoprotein protein moiety.
   e. They can be treated with diet in most cases.
8. In stable patients, low ferritin levels are most commonly seen in:
   a. Hemochromatosis
   b. Middle-aged men
   c. Menstruating women
   d. Northern Europeans
   e. Postmenopausal women
9. Immediate preoperative management for patients undergoing vascular intervention may include all except:
   a. Aspirin administration
   b. Initiating β-blockade
   c. Prophylactic antibiotic administration
   d. Reinforcing smoking cessation advice
   e. Central line placement
10. Most recently accepted concepts of atherogenesis include:
    a. Intimal lipid infiltration
    b. Endothelial denudation
    c. Excess platelet derived growth factor
    d. Core lipid accumulation and inflammation
    e. Smooth muscle hypertrophy
11. The strongest recommendation to begin aspirin therapy from US Preventive Service Task Force (USPSTF) exists for which of the following age groups:
    a. 30 to 39 years
    b. 40 to 49 years
    c. 50 to 59 years
    d. 60 to 69 years
    e. 70 to 79 years
12. In high-risk individuals, the National Cholesterol Education Program (NCEPIII) recommends an optimal target LDL level of less than:
    a. 200 mg/mL
    b. 100 mg/mL
    c. 70 mg/mL
    d. 50 mg/mL
    e. 150 mg/mL
13. Mhem/M(Hb) macrophages are activated by:
    a. Antigen:antibody complexes
    b. Toll-like receptors
    c. Hemoglobin:haptoglobin complexes
    d. IL-10
    e. CXCL-4
14. Proprotein convertase subtilisin/kexin type 9 (PCSK9) is involved in the reduction of:
    a. HDL
    b. LDL–C
    c. Apo B–100
    d. Apo A–IV
    e. Apo B–48

References available online at ExpertConsult.com.

CHAPTER 8

Nonatherosclerotic Vascular Disease

Gregory J. Landry

Although the majority of arterial abnormalities of interest to vascular surgeons are caused by atherosclerosis, a significant number result from inflammatory, acquired, congenital, and developmental abnormalities. This chapter briefly describes the pathogenesis, symptoms, diagnosis, and treatment of a variety of nonatherosclerotic vascular diseases. Topics covered include vasospastic disorders, the vasculitides, heritable arteriopathies, anatomic anomalies, and a variety of other uncommon disease processes that may be encountered by vascular surgeons.

VASOSPASTIC DISORDERS

Raynaud syndrome (RS), variant angina, and migraine headache are the most frequent vasospastic disorders seen in clinical practice, with RS being the most common vasospastic condition referred to vascular surgeons.

Episodic digital ischemia (or RS) was first described by Maurice Raynaud in 1862. The digital ischemia in patients with this condition traditionally manifests as tricolor changes—white, blue, and red—although one or more of these color changes may be absent. The affected digits return to normal 10 to 15 minutes after removal of the precipitating stimulus (usually environmental cold or emotional stress), and the fingers remain normal between attacks.

The prevalence of RS in the general population varies with climate and, probably, ethnic origin. In cool, damp climates such as the Pacific Northwest, Scandinavia, and Great Britain, the prevalence approaches 20% to 25%.[1] It is not known whether the lower prevalence in warm, dry climates is due to a decreased occurrence of the syndrome or merely lack of patient complaints. RS occurs most frequently in young women.[2] The median age of onset of RS is 14 years, with only 27% of cases beginning after age 40.[3] Approximately one-quarter of patients have a family history of RS in a first-degree relative.[4]

The mechanism of vasoconstriction in RS remains a subject of debate. Raynaud speculated that sympathetic nervous system hyperactivity was responsible, a proposition disproved by Lewis in the 1920s when he demonstrated that blockade of digital nerve conduction did not prevent vasospasm.[5] Lewis then proposed the theory of a local vascular fault, the nature of which remains undefined.

In recent years, the focus in RS pathophysiology has been on alterations in peripheral adrenoceptor activity. Increased finger blood flow was noted in patients following α-adrenergic blockade with drugs such as reserpine. Oral and intraarterial reserpine were the cornerstones of medical management of RS for several years, but are no longer available Fig. 8.1.[6]

Research in human vessel models demonstrated increased α_2 receptor sensitivity to cold exposure.[7] α_2 Adrenoceptors appear to have a major role in the production of the symptoms of RS. Possible mechanisms of α_2-adrenergic–induced RS include an elevation in the number of α_2 receptor sites, receptor hypersensitivity, and alterations in the number of receptors exposed at any one time.[8,9]

The response of subcutaneous resistance vessels to acetylcholine has been shown to be diminished in patients with RS compared with controls, indicating a possible endothelium-dependent mechanism.[10] The possible roles of the vasoactive peptide endothelin, a potent vasoconstrictor, and calcitonin gene-related peptide (CGRP), a vasodilator, have also been investigated. Serum endothelin levels increased significantly with cold exposure in patients with RS compared with controls.[11,12] Depletion of endogenous CGRP may also contribute, because increased skin blood flow in response to CGRP infusion has been demonstrated in patients with RS compared with that in controls.[13]

Based on observations at the Mayo Clinic 70 years ago by Allen and Brown,[14] patients with Raynaud symptoms have traditionally been classified as having either Raynaud disease or Raynaud phenomenon, depending on the absence or presence of an associated systemic disease process. However, Raynaud disease may precede the development of an associated disease by years. In addition, this system does not address the underlying palmar and digital artery disease that may be present. Patients with cold- or stress-induced digital ischemia are referred to as having RS, thus avoiding the semantic conflict of *disease* versus *phenomenon*.

It is useful to subdivide patients with RS into two distinct pathophysiologic groups: obstructive and vasospastic, based on the presence or absence of arterial occlusive disease. Patients with vasospastic RS have patent digital arteries and normal digital artery pressures at room temperature. These patients have an abnormally forceful vasoconstrictive response to cold exposure or emotional stress, leading to digital arterial closure and episodic digital ischemic symptoms. Patients with obstructive RS have significant obstruction of either the palmar and digital arteries or the proximal arm arteries, with a concomitant reduction in

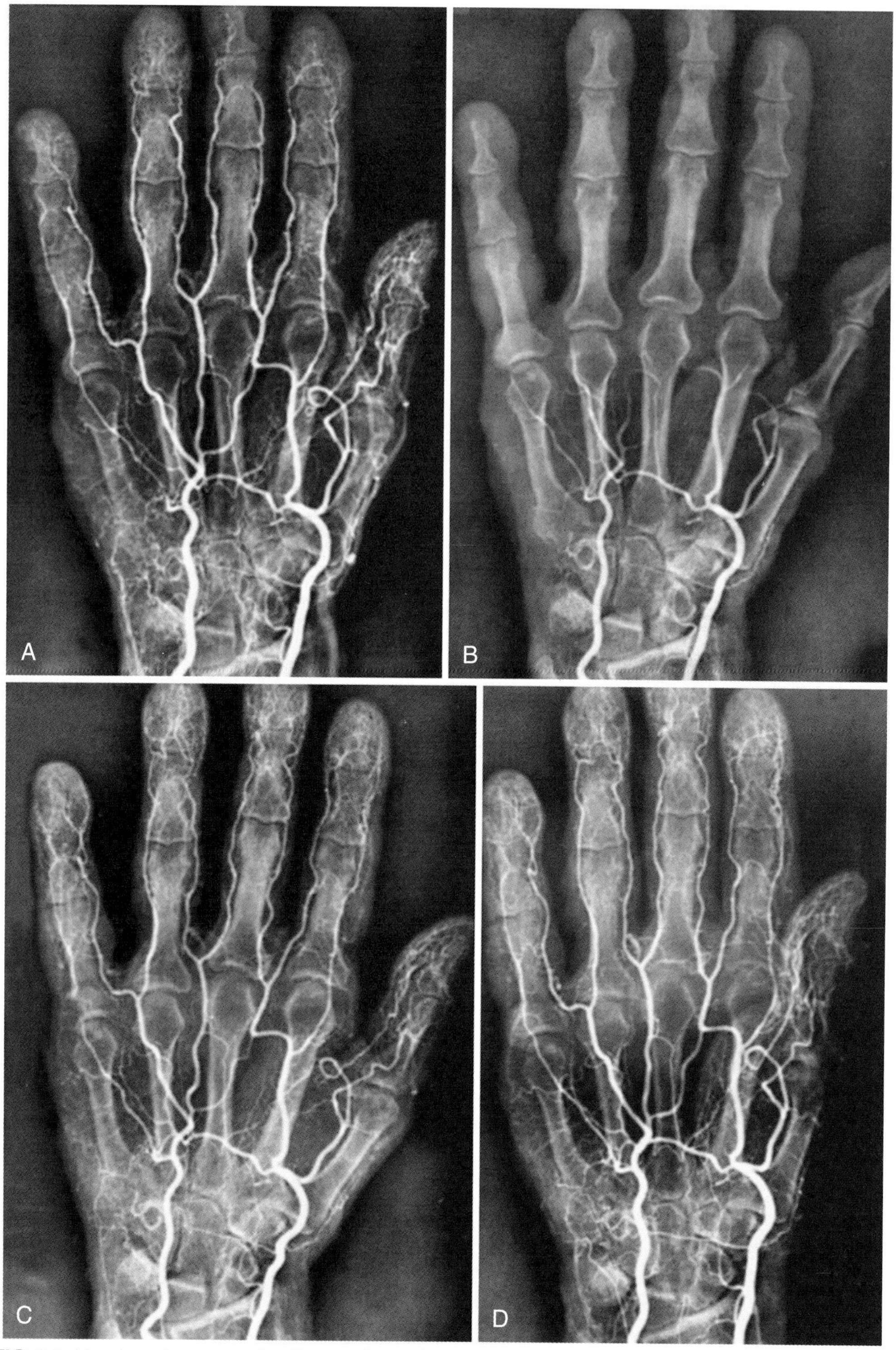

FIG 8.1 Hand angiograms of a Raynaud syndrome patient before and after cold exposure and before and after administration of intraarterial reserpine. A marked vasospastic response to cold exposure, which is blocked by reserpine administration, is demonstrated. (A) Before cold, before reserpine. (B) After cold, before reserpine. (C) Before cold, after reserpine. (D) After cold, after reserpine.

resting digital arterial pressure. In these patients, a normal vasoconstrictive response to cold appears to be sufficient to cause digital arterial closure with resultant episodic digital ischemia.

In patients with obstructive RS, the mechanism of the obstructive process is variable. Patients with connective tissue disease typically have an autoimmune vasculitis, which is probably the mechanism underlying the widespread digital and palmar artery occlusions. Patients who work with vibrating tools have a similar process and frequently develop a fibrotic form of palmar and digital artery obstruction, presumably associated with injury from repeated shear stress.[15] Hypercoagulable states may appear with digital artery occlusions, as can emboli from various sources, including valvular heart disease and subclavian, axillary, and ulnar aneurysms. Atherosclerosis involving the upper extremities is rarely seen in the younger age group but is occasionally observed in older patients.

A number of diseases have been recognized in association with RS, among which the connective tissue diseases are the most frequent; scleroderma is the most common. Associated diseases recognized in patients with RS are shown in Table 8.1.[16] Estimates of the percentage of patients with RS and an associated disease range from 30% to 80%.[1,17-19] It is important to note that the data from most series come from tertiary-care referral centers; therefore, they might not reflect the actual incidence in the general population and may overestimate the actual prevalence of associated diseases. The diagnosis of RS is made by history and physical examination. Noninvasive vascular laboratory testing is used to differentiate obstructive from vasospastic RS. Symptoms are typically described as coldness, numbness, or mild discomfort. Significant pain during attacks is conspicuously absent. Classically, both hands are involved, with frequent sparing of the thumbs. The lower extremities are infrequently involved. Most episodes are induced by cold; however, the cold threshold varies from patient to patient. Emotional stimuli can induce attacks in some patients. Episodes typically commence with blanching of one or several fingers extending as far as the metacarpophalangeal joint, rarely involving the palm or extending proximally to the wrist. This phase corresponds to vasoconstriction with the absence of blood in digital arteries. After rewarming, the first blood to reach the skin is desaturated, leading to finger cyanosis. Finally, reactive hyperemia leads to digital rubor. Episodes usually last as long as the cold stimulus is present and resolve within 10 to 15 minutes of rewarming. The hands and fingers are normal between attacks.

TABLE 8.1 Associated Diseases in Raynaud Syndrome Patients: Oregon Health Sciences University Series

Disease	No. of Patients
Autoimmune disease	**290**
Scleroderma	95
Undifferentiated connective tissue disease	24
Mixed connective tissue disease	23
Systemic lupus erythematosus	17
Sjögren syndrome	16
Rheumatoid arthritis	9
Positive serology	106
Other diseases or conditions	**300**
Atherosclerosis	46
Trauma	44
Hematologic abnormalities	42
Carpal tunnel syndrome	35
Frostbite	32
Buerger disease	28
Vibration	21
Hypersensitivity angiitis	18
Hypothyroidism	13
Cancer	13
Erythromelalgia	8
No associated disease	**498**
Total	**1088**

From Landry G, Edwards JM, McLafferty RM, et al: Long-term outcome of Raynaud's syndrome in a prospective analyzed cohort. *J Vasc Surg* 23:76–86, 1996.

A history suggestive of an associated connective tissue disease should be sought, including arthralgias, dysphagia, sclerodactyly, xerophthalmia, or xerostomia, as well as any prior history of large vessel occlusive disease, malignancy, hypothyroidism, frostbite, trauma, use of vibrating tools, and drug use. More than half of patients with carpal tunnel syndrome can have coexistent RS.[20] The examiner should carefully evaluate the pulses and assess the digits for evidence of active or healed ulceration, sclerodactyly, telangiectasia, and calcinosis. The optimal serologic evaluation has not been defined. It is common to obtain a complete blood cell count, erythrocyte sedimentation rate, antinuclear antibody titer, and rheumatoid factor. Patients who exhibit sudden-onset digital ischemia should be evaluated for hypercoagulable states. Tests for specific connective tissue diseases are obtained based on clinical suspicion. Importantly, the physical examination in patients with RS is frequently normal, and the diagnosis relies on history and noninvasive tests.

Routine vascular laboratory testing consists of digital photoplethysmography and digital blood pressures. The digital photoplethysmographic recording provides qualitative information on the character of the arterial waveform.[21] Normal digital blood pressure is within 30 mm Hg of brachial pressure. Patients with obstructive RS have blunted waveforms, whereas patients with vasospastic RS have either normal waveforms or a "peaked pulse." The peaked pulse pattern, first described by Sumner and Strandness,[22] appears to reflect increased vasospastic arterial resistance.

The utility of cold provocation testing remains controversial. Tests involving immersion of patients' hands in ice water are not clinically useful because of low specificity and reproducibility.[23,24] Of greater clinical utility is a digital hypothermic cold challenge test described by Nielson and Lassen.[25] This test is performed with a liquid-perfused cuff placed on the proximal phalanx of the target finger. The cuff is inflated to suprasystolic pressure for 5 minutes while it is perfused with cold water. The pressure at which blood flow is detected on deflation of the cuff is recorded. A control finger on the same hand is tested at room temperature. The test is repeated at several temperatures, and the result is expressed as the percentage drop in finger systolic pressure with cooling. This test has an overall sensitivity and accuracy of approximately 90%,[26] but is limited due to lack of widespread availability.

Duplex scanning does not appear to have a major role in the diagnosis of RS, although it can be used to search for proximal arterial obstructive or aneurysmal disease. Laser Doppler imaging quantifies digital microvascular blood flow and may have future diagnostic applications in RS.[27,28] Angiography was used extensively in the past, particularly in the evaluation of patients with obstructive RS. Patients with an underlying systemic disease process and bilateral palmar and digital arterial obstructive disease documented by vascular laboratory testing do not require angiography to confirm digital artery occlusive disease. Patients with unilateral disease, particularly those who have only one or two digits of one arm involved, should be considered for angiography to determine both the presence of bilateral disease and the presence of any proximal arterial disease.

Avoidance of triggering stimuli, such as cold or emotional stress, is the hallmark of conservative treatment.[29] We advise all patients with RS to avoid tobacco use, although a multicenter epidemiologic study suggested that RS is not strongly influenced by tobacco consumption.[30] Medications that have been associated with the causation of RS symptoms, such as ergot alkaloids and β-blockers, should be avoided if appropriate alternative therapies exist. More than 90% of patients with RS respond adequately to these simple conservative measures and require no additional treatment. The small number of patients who develop digital ulcers in association with obstructive RS can also be managed conservatively. A healing rate of 85% has been achieved with simple treatment consisting of soap and water scrubs, antibiotics as selected by culture, and conservative debridement.[31]

Calcium channel blockers are the most widely used pharmacologic agent for the treatment of RS. As a rule, patients with vasospastic RS respond more favorably to medical therapy than do those with occlusive RS. The dihydropyridine calcium channel blockers are most effective, and nifedipine has been the most studied, with a significant decrease in attack frequency and severity in numerous trials.[32] Potential side effects include headache, ankle swelling, pruritus, and, rarely, severe fatigue. Other calcium channel blockers include nicardipine, amlodipine, and felodipine.[33] Second-line medications with proven efficacy include α-blockers (prazosin),[34] angiotensin II receptor blockers (losartan),[35] serotonin reuptake inhibitors (fluoxetine),[36] phosphodiesterase 5 inhibitors (sildenafil, tadalafil),[37,38] and topical nitrates.[39] Intravenous prostaglandins, such as Iloprost, an analog of prostacyclin, have been shown to be effective in treating RS associated with systemic sclerosis[40,41] but have not been shown to be effective in oral form.[42,43] Endothelin receptor antagonists (bosentan) have also shown benefit in preventing and treating digital ulcers,[44] but have a high rate of liver toxicity and are approved by US Food and Drug Administration only for treatment of pulmonary hypertension. Temperature biofeedback, in which patients are taught hand warming through behavioral techniques, was initially believed to reduce symptom frequency in patients with vasospastic RS.[45] However, a randomized trial showed no improvement in symptoms after 1 year compared with a control technique.[46] Transcutaneous electrical nerve stimulation, which has been described as causing vasodilatation, resulted in only mild increases in skin temperature; it caused no improvements in digital plethysmography or transcutaneous partial pressure of oxygen in test hands and had a negligible effect on symptoms.[47] Anecdotal reports of the use of spinal cord stimulators report reduced pain and improved ulcer healing in refractory RS.[48] Acupuncture has also been suggested as a possible treatment alternative, with a significant reduction in frequency and severity of attacks.[49]

Several small case series have demonstrated decreased frequency of attacks and improved ulcer healing with chemical sympathectomy using an interdigital injection of botulinum toxin.[50,51] Surgical cervicothoracic sympathectomy has not been shown to have a lasting benefit in most series, with recurrence rates as high as 82% at 16 months of follow-up.[52] In a large series of patients undergoing thoracoscopic sympathectomy, increased digital artery perfusion was maintained out to 5 years of follow-up, although symptom recurrence occurred in 28% of patients.[53] Lumbar sympathectomy remains a viable option in patients with severely symptomatic lower extremity vasospasm and is amenable to minimally invasive laparoscopic techniques.[54] Periarterial neurectomy is performed by removing the adventitia of the radial, ulnar, palmar, or common digital arteries. Results have been mixed, with some series reporting improved quality of life and ulcer healing, although complication rates are as high as 37%[55]; therefore, widespread use is generally discouraged. Another recently described surgical technique involves autogenous fat grafting, in which fat harvested from the abdomen is injected at multiple sites in the hand. In small case series, improvements in pain and hand perfusion have been reported.[56] The mechanism is unknown but may involve generation of vascular growth factors from adipose-derived stem cells.

The long-term outcome of patients with RS is not known with certainty, although epidemiologic studies have shown that up to one-third of patients with RS can experience symptom resolution over time.[57] We reviewed our experience with more than 1000 RS patients followed for up to 23 years and found RS to be a relatively benign condition in the majority of patients.[16] We divided the patients into four groups at presentation to determine whether this classification scheme provided prognostic information: vasospastic RS with negative serologies, vasospastic RS with positive serologies, obstructive RS with negative serologies, and obstructive RS with positive serologies. Patients with no evidence of an associated disease or arterial obstruction did extremely well, with minimal risk of severe finger ischemia or development of an associated disease; those with obstruction and positive serologies were most likely to develop worsening finger ischemia and ulceration. A summary is presented in Table 8.2. Patients without a diagnosable connective tissue disorder, but with one or more clinical signs or laboratory tests suggesting such a disease, are much more likely to receive a diagnosis of connective tissue disorder at a later date. Current estimates of disease progression range from 2% to 6% in patients with initially negative serologic tests, and 30% to 75% in patients with positive serologic tests at presentation.[58]

SYSTEMIC VASCULITIS

Vasculitis has a deceptively simple definition—inflammation, often with necrosis and occlusive changes of the blood vessels—but its clinical manifestations are diverse and complex. The term *arteritis* has been used to describe many of these syndromes, but *vasculitis* is a more precise term, because many of the entities involve veins as well as arteries. Vasculitis can be generalized or

TABLE 8.2 Long-Term Outcome of Raynaud Syndrome Patients Based on Classification at Initial Presentation: Oregon Health Sciences University Series

Initial Classification	Initial Presence of Connective Tissue Disease (%)	Final Presence of Connective Tissue Disease (%)	Presence of Digital Ulceration (%)	Requirement for Digital or Phalangeal Amputation (%)
Spastic, negative serology	0.0	2.0	5.2	1.6
Spastic, positive serology	48.6	57.0	15.5	1.4
Obstructive, negative serology	0.0	8.5	48.2	19.0
Obstructive, positive serology	72.9	81.2	55.6	11.6

From Landry G, Edwards JM, McLafferty RM, et al: Long-term outcome of Raynaud's syndrome in a prospective analyzed cohort. *J Vasc Surg* 23:76–86, 1996.

BOX 8.1 Vasculitides With Potential Vascular Surgical Importance

Large Vessel Vasculitis
- Giant cell (temporal) arteritis
- Takayasu disease
- Radiation-induced arterial damage

Medium Vessel Vasculitis
- Polyarteritis nodosa (classic)
- Kawasaki disease
- Drug abuse arteritis
- Behçet disease
- Cogan syndrome
- Vasculitis associated with malignancy

Small Vessel Vasculitis
- Hypersensitivity vasculitis
- Henoch-Schönlein purpura
- Essential cryoglobulinemic vasculitis
- Vasculitis of connective tissue diseases

TABLE 8.3 Clinical Patterns in Giant Cell Arteritis

	Temporal Arteritis	Takayasu Disease
Age, sex	Elderly, white women	Young females
Pathology	Inflammatory cellular infiltrates giant cells	Same
Area of involvement	Usually branches of carotid; may involve any artery	Aortic arch and branches; pulmonary artery
Complications	Blindness	Hypertension, stroke
Response to steroids	Excellent	Unpredictable, unproved

localized. Knowledge of this condition is incomplete, and the currently used classification systems are filled with exceptions and overlapping syndromes. The most frequently used classification system is based on the size of the vessels (small, medium, large) involved in the vasculitic process (Box 8.1).[59] Medium and small vessel vasculitis is further subdivided by the presence or absence of antineutrophil cytoplasmic antibodies (ANCAs), a group of autoantibodies formed against enzymes found in primary granules of neutrophils. The most common ANCA-positive vasculitides include Wegener granulomatosis, microscopic polyangiitis, and Churg-Strauss syndrome, which are rarely encountered by vascular surgeons.[60]

The cause and pathogenesis of most vasculitides are complex and are currently either unknown or incompletely understood. The basic pathologic mechanism of vasculitis implicates immune-mediated injury, which can include recognition of a vascular structure as antigen, deposition of immune complexes in a vessel wall with complement activation and injury, direct deposition of antigen in a vessel wall, or a delayed hypersensitivity reaction.

The majority of vasculitides are associated with a cellular immunoreaction involving the production of soluble mediators including cytokines, arachidonic acid metabolites, and fibrinolytic and coagulation by-products. The production of cytokines results in neutrophilic, eosinophilic, monocytic, and lymphocytic interactions at the inflammatory site. Endothelial cells express cell membrane receptors specific for many of these inflammatory cells. Binding of inflammatory cells to the endothelial cell triggers intracellular production of additional endothelial cytokines that affect the local inflammatory environment. Complement binding is thought to aid the attachment of leukocytes to endothelial cells. Platelet interactions with both intact and injured endothelium can contribute to the inflammatory process through activation of coagulation pathways and release of cytokines capable of stimulating and modifying immune responses. The vascular surgeon attends to the sequelae of vasculitic injury in these diseases. Thrombosis, aneurysm formation, hemorrhage, or arterial occlusion may all follow or accompany transmural damage created by inflammatory reactions on the vascular wall. An abbreviated list of the vasculitides that have potential significance to vascular surgeons is presented in Box 8.1 and is considered in this section.

Large Vessel Vasculitis

Giant Cell Arteritis Group

The two conditions included in the giant cell arteritis (GCA) group are systemic giant cell, or temporal, arteritis and Takayasu disease. Although they have fairly distinctive clinical patterns (Table 8.3), the two entities likely represent different manifestations of the same disease process and are histologically similar with pathognomonic giant cells.[61] Glucocorticoids constitute the hallmark of therapy for each, although a variety of nonsteroidal immunosuppressants have also been employed with mixed results. Surgical and endovascular therapy are less frequently used but have a role in selective refractory patients.

Systemic giant cell arteritis (temporal arteritis). Systemic GCA occurs mainly in patients older than 50 years, is two- to sixfold more frequent in women, and is more prominent in whites. The annual incidence in white women older than 50 years is 15 to 25 cases per 100,000.[62]

GCA can involve any large artery of the body, although it has a propensity to affect branches of the carotid artery. The clinical history usually begins with a febrile myalgic process involving primarily the back, shoulder, and pelvic regions. Headache, malaise, anorexia, weight loss, and jaw claudication are common. Polymyalgia rheumatica, a clinical syndrome of aching and stiffness of the hip and shoulder girdle muscles lasting 4 weeks or longer and associated with an elevated erythrocyte sedimentation rate, is present in 50% to 75% of patients with temporal arteritis.[63]

The most characteristic complaint is severe pain along the course of the temporal artery, accompanied by tenderness and nodularity of the artery and overlying skin erythema. The involvement is frequently bilateral. Visual disturbances occur in more than 50% of patients. The mechanism of the visual alterations may be ischemic optic neuritis, retrobulbar neuritis, or occlusion of the central retinal artery. Unilateral blindness occurs in as many as 17% of patients with GCA, followed by contralateral, usually permanent, blindness in one-third of these patients within 1 week.[64] Amaurosis fugax is an important warning sign that precedes visual loss in 44% of patients.[65]

GCA can cause aneurysms or stenoses of the aorta or its main branches. Classic arteriographic findings of GCA include smooth, tapering stenoses of subclavian, axillary, and brachial arteries (Fig. 8.2). Both true thoracic aortic aneurysms and dissecting aneurysms can occur. Patients with GCA have a 17-fold increased risk of thoracic aortic aneurysms and a 2.4-fold increased risk of abdominal aortic aneurysms compared with age-matched controls.[66] Aortic involvement is best visualized with computed tomography (CT) or magnetic resonance angiography (MRA), in which aortic wall thickening is demonstrated.[67] Although rare, lower extremity involvement has also been described.[68] Laboratory findings supporting a diagnosis of GCA include an elevated erythrocyte sedimentation rate. The diagnostic criteria of the American College of Rheumatology include an erythrocyte sedimentation rate of at least 50 mm/h.[69] However, up to 25% of patients with GCA have a normal sedimentation rate at the time of diagnosis,[70] and this finding should not preclude treatment if clinical suspicion is high. C-reactive protein may be a more sensitive indicator of disease activity than the sedimentation rate.[71]

Temporal artery biopsy remains the gold standard of diagnosis in patients suspected of having GCA. Because of skip lesions, a specimen at least 2 cm long should be obtained. When possible, temporal artery biopsy should be performed before corticosteroid treatment; however, histologic evidence of arteritis may be found after up to 2 weeks of treatment.[72] Bilateral sequential temporal artery biopsies are frequently performed if the results of unilateral biopsy are inconclusive, but in 97% of cases, the two specimens show the same findings.[73] Characteristic findings on color-flow duplex scans have been described, typically a hypoechoic halo

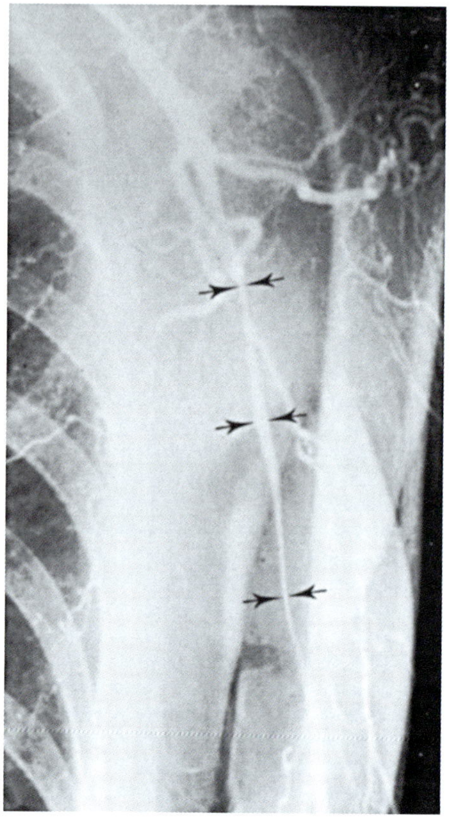

FIG 8.2 (A) Typical giant cell arteritis with smooth tapering of the axillary artery *(arrows)*. (B) Photomicrograph of an axillary artery involved with giant cell arteritis showing transmural inflammation *(large arrow)* and an inner zone of fibrosis *(small arrow)*. (From Rivers SP, Baur GM, Inahara T, et al: Arm ischemia secondary to giant cell arteritis. *Am J Surg* 143:554–558, 1982.)

around the artery corresponding with associated periarterial inflammation, with a sensitivity of 75% and specificity of 83% compared with temporal artery biopsies.[74]

The importance of a precise and early diagnosis lies in the early initiation of steroid therapy. Prompt steroid therapy frequently results in restoration of pulses and prevention of lasting visual disturbances. Typical treatment consists of initial high-dose intravenous steroids followed by a gradual oral taper. Most patients require at least 1 year of treatment, although some require lifelong therapy.[75,76] Although corticosteroids remain the cornerstone of medical therapy, cytotoxic agents (e.g., methotrexate),[77] immunosuppressants (e.g., azathioprine, cyclosporin), tumor necrosis factor (TNF) inhibitors (infliximab, etanercept),[78,79] and pyrimidine synthesis inhibitors (leflunomide)[80] are used occasionally. However, trials of steroid-sparing drugs have had mixed results. Surgical and endovascular therapy for GCA is rare due to overall good results with medical therapy. With the exception of those with aortic dissections, the life expectancy of patients with GCA is the same as that of the general population.[81]

Takayasu disease. Takayasu disease frequently affects the aorta and its major branches and, in contrast to GCA, the pulmonary artery. The majority of patients are Asian, about 85% are female, and the median age at onset is between 25 and 41 years.[82] The disease has two recognized stages. The first stage is

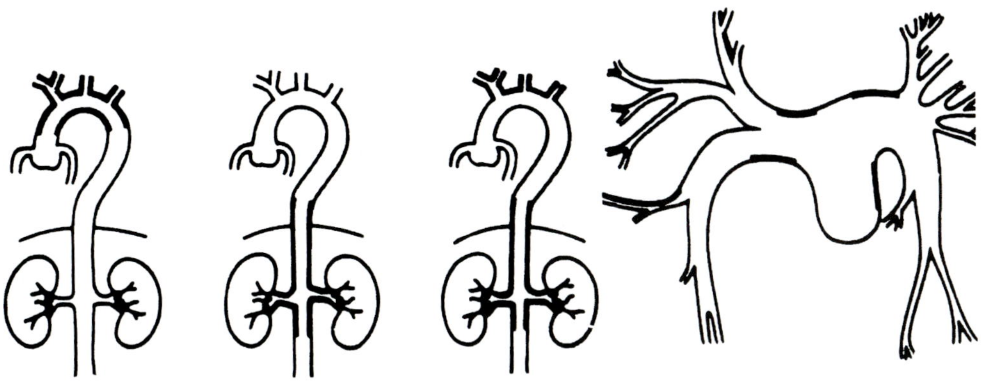

FIG 8.3 Diagrammatic representation of the recognized types of Takayasu arteritis. The areas of arterial involvement are shown in heavy lines. (From Lupi-Herrera E, Sanchez-Torres G, Marcustiamer J, et al: Takayasu arteritis: clinical study of 107 cases. *Am Heart J* 93:94–103, 1977.)

characterized by fever, myalgia, and anorexia in approximately two-thirds of patients. In the second stage, these symptoms may be followed by multiple arterial occlusive symptoms, with manifestations dependent on disease location.

The cardiovascular areas of involvement have been characterized as types I, II, III, and IV and are shown in Fig. 8.3. Type I is limited to involvement of the arch and arch vessels and occurs in 8.4% of patients. Type II involves the descending thoracic and abdominal aorta and accounts for 11.2% of cases. Type III involves the arch vessels and the abdominal aorta and its branches and accounts for 65.4% of cases. Type IV consists primarily of pulmonary artery involvement, with or without other vessels, and accounts for 15% of patients.[83] Most of the lesions are stenotic, although localized aneurysms have been reported. Arteriography has traditionally been the imaging modality of choice.[84] However, color-flow duplex scanning,[85] CT,[86] magnetic resonance imaging (MRI),[87] and positron emission tomography (PET) scanning[88] have emerged as important alternatives, providing information about both luminal and mural involvement in affected vessels.

Cardiovascular findings include diminished peripheral arterial pulsations and hypertension. The hypertension may be due to aortic coarctation or renal artery stenosis. Neurologic symptoms can result from hypertension or central nervous system ischemia associated with large artery occlusion or stenosis. Coronary artery involvement in Takayasu disease is rare. The cardiac pathologic feature most frequently found is nonspecific and appears to result from heart failure associated with systemic and pulmonary hypertension.

Available information suggests that a conservative surgical approach is best for these patients. The same spectrum of pharmacologic agents used to treat GCA is used in patients with Takayasu arteritis, with corticosteroids again being the primary agent used. Results of medical therapy, in general, are less consistent in patients with Takayasu arteritis. A poor long-term outcome is predicted by the presence of major complications (retinopathy, hypertension, aortic insufficiency, aneurysm formation) and a progressive disease course.[89]

Surgical intervention is generally reserved to treat symptomatic stenotic or, less commonly, aneurysmal lesions resulting from chronic Takayasu arteritis. Surgical intervention is best performed with the disease in a quiescent state. Restenosis rates in the presence of active disease are approximately 45%, compared with 12% restenosis rates with quiescent disease.[90] Acute phase reactants, such as erythrocyte sedimentation rate (ESR) and C-reactive protein (CRP), are often used to determine disease activity; however, these markers are not consistent. PET-CT may play an important role in defining metabolic activity associated with acute and quiescent states.[91] Successful surgical management requires bypass graft implantation into disease-free arterial segments and continuation of corticosteroid therapy.[92] Excellent long-term survival rates of up to 75% at 20 years have been reported in large operative series.[93] Owing to its inflammatory nature, endarterectomy has resulted in early failure and is generally not recommended.

Percutaneous transluminal angioplasty and stenting has had mixed success, with high early success rates of up to 90%[94]; however, high rates of in-stent restenosis have been reported.[95] In general, surgical intervention remains a more durable option.[96]

Radiation-Induced Arterial Damage

Radiation given for the treatment of regional malignancy causes well-recognized changes in arteries within the irradiated field. The primary changes consist of intimal thickening and proliferation, medial hyalinization, proteoglycan deposition, and cellular infiltration of the adventitia. Normal endothelium has a slow rate of turnover, and following irradiation, endothelial cells do not proliferate. Pleomorphic endothelial cells can develop as a result of irradiation, with exposure of the basement membrane leading to thrombosis of small vessels.[97] Postirradiation changes in large arteries often resemble atherosclerosis (Fig. 8.4).

Arteries in an irradiated area may develop stenosis years after exposure, thought to be due to chronic oxidative stress with upregulation of matrix metalloproteinases, proinflammatory cytokines, smooth muscle cell proliferation and apoptosis, with downregulation of nitric oxide.[98] There is an high incidence of carotid artery stenosis in patients years after neck irradiation, along with an increased likelihood of stroke.[99] The lesions vary from diffuse scarring to areas of typical atheromatous narrowing, with a preponderance of the latter. Patients who have had regional

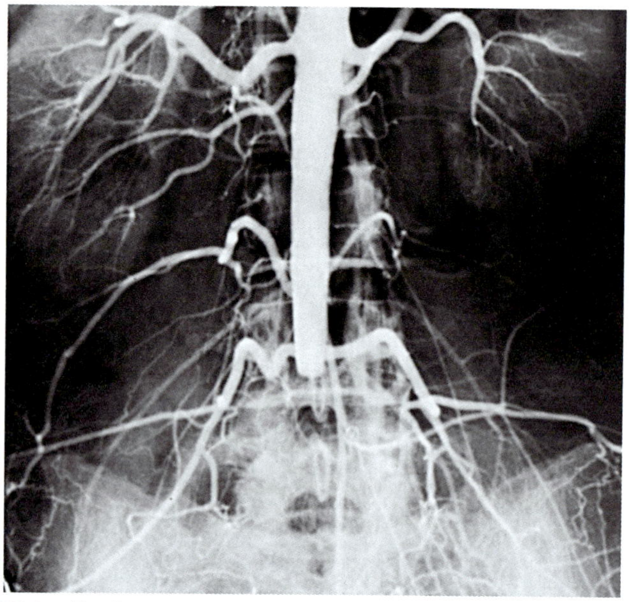

FIG 8.4 **Radiation Arteritis.** Arteriogram in a 40-year-old woman who received extensive internal and external irradiation for treatment of carcinoma of the cervix. There is a typical absence of atherosclerotic disease of the infrarenal aorta.

irradiation, especially of the cervical region, should have careful vascular follow-up, including noninvasive vascular laboratory examinations. Stenoses of the subclavian and axillary arteries have been demonstrated in patients undergoing radiation therapy for breast cancer and Hodgkin lymphoma, and aortoiliac involvement has been noted in patients undergoing abdominal or pelvic radiation therapy.

Vascular surgery on irradiated arteries can be performed using standard techniques. Prosthetic and autogenous bypass grafts, as well as endarterectomy, have all been performed satisfactorily.[100] Prudence suggests avoidance of a prosthetic graft in a field in which infection may be expected, such as a radical neck dissection after irradiation, and autologous vein reconstruction is preferred. Late graft infections occurring 2 to 5 years after surgery have been described.[101] The treatment of carotid artery stenosis in irradiated areas with percutaneous angioplasty and stenting has been reported, with excellent results,[102] although rates of restenosis and reintervention are significantly higher than in nonirradiated arteries and historical surgical controls. Although data are limited, endovascular treatment of other arterial beds appears to be safe and effective in selected cases.[103]

Medium Vessel Vasculitis

Polyarteritis Nodosa

Polyarteritis nodosa (PAN) is a disseminated disease characterized by focal necrotizing lesions involving primarily medium-sized muscular arteries. This is a rare disorder with a prevalence of 2 to 16 per 1 million, a male-female preponderance of 2-4:1, and a peak incidence in patients in their 40s.[104] The clinical manifestations of PAN are varied. It can involve only one organ or multiple organs simultaneously or sequentially over time. The most frequent manifestations of PAN include a characteristic crescent-forming glomerulonephritis, polyarteritis, polymyositis, and abdominal pain. A cutaneous form also exists, presenting with subcutaneous nodules, livedo reticularis, and cutaneous ulcers.[105]

The essential pathologic feature of PAN is focal transmural arterial inflammatory necrosis. The process begins with medial destruction, followed by a sequential acute inflammatory response, fibroblastic proliferation, and endothelial damage. The vascular injury is resolved by intimal proliferation, thrombosis, or aneurysm formation, all of which may culminate in luminal occlusion, with consequent organ ischemia and infarction.[106]

The ESR, CRP, and factor XIII–related protein, all nonspecific serologic markers of inflammation, are elevated in PAN. Positive hepatitis B serologies are common in adults with PAN.[107] This is also the most common vasculitis associated with hepatitis C and the human immunodeficiency virus (HIV).[108]

The hallmark of PAN is the formation of multiple saccular aneurysms associated with inflammatory destruction of the media, with the most frequently involved organs being the kidney, heart, liver, and gastrointestinal tract. Rupture of intraabdominal PAN aneurysms has been well described and may represent a surgical emergency.[109] Coil embolization of ruptured visceral aneurysms in PAN has also been described and represents an alternative to surgical intervention.[110] These aneurysms have been documented to regress on occasion after vigorous steroid and cyclophosphamide therapy, which should be recommended for all asymptomatic visceral aneurysms.[111] An arteriogram of a patient with PAN showing the typical visceral and renal artery aneurysms is shown in Fig. 8.5. Visceral PAN lesions can also lead to visceral artery narrowing incident to the inflammatory process, which can progress to occlusion. The visceral ischemia can manifest as cholecystitis, appendicitis, enteric perforation, gastrointestinal hemorrhage, or ischemic stricture formation with bowel obstruction.[112]

The routine use of steroid therapy has improved 5-year survival from 15% to the current 50% to 80%.[113] Cyclophosphamide can be added to the steroid regimen in acute, severe cases.[114] Antiviral agents can be used in hepatitis B virus (HBV)-induced PAN. Prognosis is influenced by the absence or presence of creatinemia, proteinuria, cardiomyopathy, and gastrointestinal or central nervous system involvement at the time of presentation. Five-year mortality with zero, one, or two or more of these signs was 12%, 26%, and 46%, respectively.[115] During the acute phase of PAN, renal and gastrointestinal lesions account for the majority of deaths, whereas cardiovascular and cerebral events account for mortality in chronic cases.

Kawasaki Disease

In the 1960s, Kawasaki observed 50 cases of a febrile exanthematous illness in Japan and coined the term *mucocutaneous lymph node syndrome*.[116] Over the next decade, the spread of the disease was noted worldwide, and it became known as Kawasaki disease. The disease occurs in all ethnic groups, although children of Japanese ancestry appear to be most susceptible. The annual incidence in Japan is 140 cases per 100,000 children younger than 5 years,[117] compared with the incidence in the United States of approximately 17 cases per 100,000 children.[118] The vasculitis associated with Kawasaki disease has a propensity to affect the

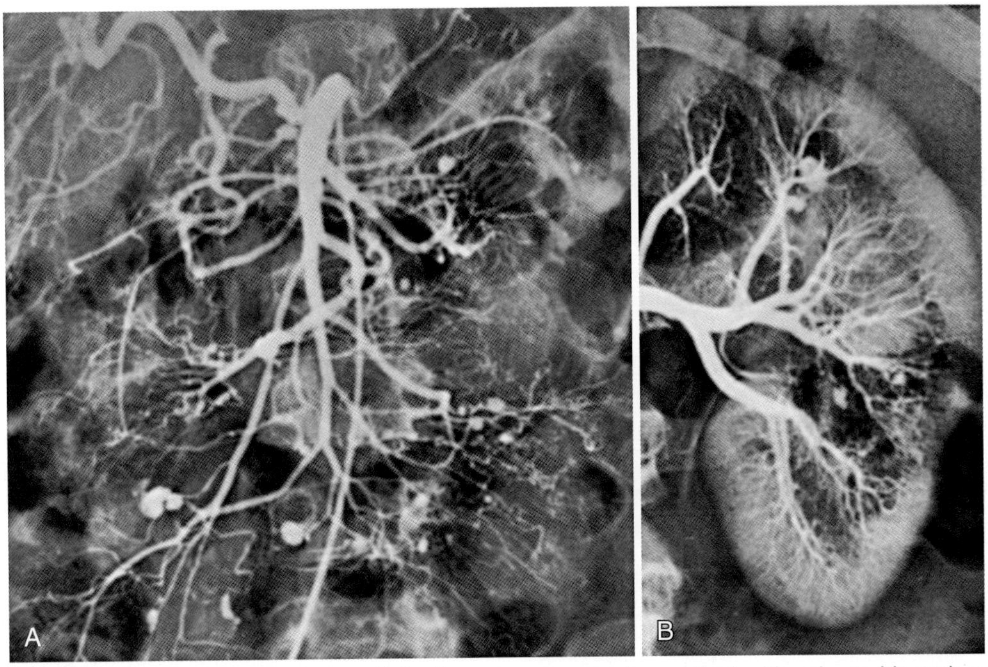

FIG 8.5 (A) Arteriogram showing multiple visceral aneurysms in a patient with polyarteritis nodosa. (B) Multiple renal artery aneurysms in the same patient.

coronary arteries, making it the most common cause of acquired heart disease in children in the developed world.[119]

The clinical criteria for diagnosis include: (1) high fever present for 5 days or more, (2) conjunctival congestion, (3) changes in the mucous membranes of the oral cavity, (4) peripheral edema or desquamation, (5) polymorphous exanthem, and (6) acute nonsuppurative swelling of the cervical lymph nodes. The presence of a prolonged high fever and any four of the five remaining criteria, in the absence of concurrent evidence of bacterial or viral infection, establishes the diagnosis.[120]

Kawasaki disease has a unimodal peak incidence at 1 year of age; it has not been described in neonates and is rarely observed for the first time in those older than 5 years. The acute symptoms can persist for 7 to 14 days before improvement occurs as the fever subsides. Notable laboratory features include elevation of the ESR and CRP, thrombocythemia, and elevated levels of von Willebrand factor.[121]

The etiology of Kawasaki disease is likely multifactorial. An infectious cause has long been assumed, given the self-limited nature of the disease, its seasonal incidence, and geographic outbreaks. However, no single infectious agent has been demonstrated. An immunologic defect has also been postulated, because there appears to be an altered immunoregulatory state in these patients, with decreased numbers of T cells and an increased proportion of activated helper T4 cells. Genetic susceptibility also appears to have a role in pathogenesis.[122] The most serious disease manifestation is coronary arteritis. The spectrum of documented coronary artery pathologic changes consists of active arteritis, thrombosis, calcification, and stenosis, although the distinguishing feature of Kawasaki disease is the formation of diffuse fusiform and saccular coronary artery aneurysms.

Routine echocardiography in patients with Kawasaki disease has demonstrated coronary artery dilation or aneurysms in 25% to 50%, with the aneurysms typically appearing in the second week of illness and reaching a maximum size from the third to eighth week after the onset of fever.[123] Echocardiography may show dilation of the right, left, or anterior descending coronary arteries, whereas the circumflex coronary artery is rarely involved.[124]

Systemic arteritis also occurs in Kawasaki disease, with iliac arteritis as prevalent as coronary arteritis. Aneurysm formation is far less frequent in the systemic arteries than in the coronary arteries, with one report identifying systemic arterial aneurysms (axillary and iliac) in 3.3% of 662 patients with Kawasaki disease and coronary artery aneurysms.[125] The healing process in the systemic arterial lesions can lead to focal arterial stenosis or aneurysm formation, just as in the coronary arteries. The coexistence of peripheral arterial involvement (subclavian and axillary arteries) and coronary artery aneurysms is shown in Fig. 8.6.

Thrombosis of coronary artery aneurysms is the overwhelming cause of death in the early stages of Kawasaki disease, causing acute myocardial infarction or arrhythmia. Coronary aneurysm rupture has also been described. With the initiation of aspirin and immune globulin therapy in the acute phase, the mortality from Kawasaki disease has decreased to 1.1%, and among patients with no cardiac sequelae does not differ from the general population.[126] Intravenous gamma globulin is typically given as a single-infusion high dose of 2 g/kg. Aspirin is given orally at a dose of 80 mg/kg per day until the child is afebrile, then continued in low-dose form (3 to 5 mg/kg per day) for an additional 6 to 8 weeks.[127] Approximately 10% to 15% of patients are refractory to standard therapy,[128] and corticosteroids or other immunosuppressant agents (e.g., infliximab, cyclosporin) are considered

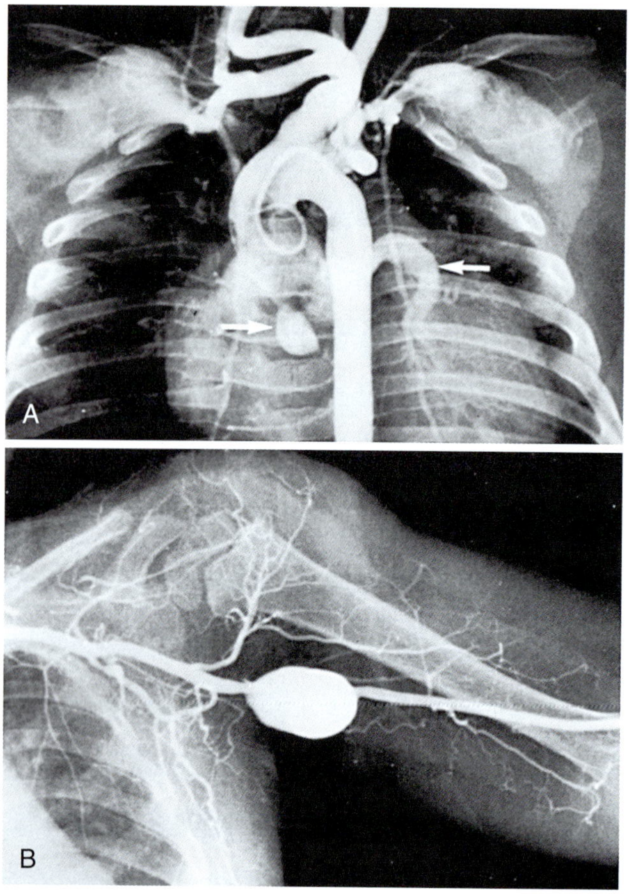

FIG 8.6 (A) Arteriogram of an infant with Kawasaki disease showing coronary artery aneurysms *(white arrows)* and massive subclavian artery aneurysms. (B) Arteriogram of a 2-year-old child showing a large axillary artery aneurysm resulting from Kawasaki disease.

in these patients.[129] Appropriate medical therapy during the acute phase can lead to aneurysm regression, with arteries less than 4 mm in diameter universally regressing, and those greater than 8 mm unlikely to regress.

Coronary artery bypass grafting was first used in Kawasaki disease in 1976.[130] The first procedure used the saphenous vein as a conduit; however, concerns over its potential to grow with the child have been raised. This concern led to the use of the internal mammary artery (unilateral or bilateral)[131] and the right gastroepiploic artery[132] for coronary revascularization in patients with Kawasaki disease. Five- and 15-year patency rates of internal mammary grafts are 91% in children older than 12 years of age, but only 73% and 65%, respectively, in patients younger than 12.[133] Percutaneous angioplasty of anastomotic lesions, however, has improved 10-year patency rates in this group to 94%.[134] Primary catheter-based interventions, such as stent implantation[135] and coronary rotational ablation,[136] have also had excellent results in selected cases of focal coronary artery stenosis. Cardiac transplantation for severe ischemic heart disease as a sequela of Kawasaki disease is considered in patients who are not candidates for revascularization because of distal coronary stenosis or aneurysms and those with severe irreversible myocardial dysfunction.[137] Overall survival of surgically treated patients is up to 95% at 25 years, although approximately one-third require reintervention during this time interval.[138]

Drug Abuse Arteritis

Intravenous drug abuse, particularly the use of methamphetamines or cocaine, is associated with a panarteritis similar in presentation and appearance to PAN,[139] with combinations of renal failure, central nervous system dysfunction, and localized intestinal necrosis and perforation. Isolated cerebral angiitis has also been reported in the setting of methamphetamine and cocaine abuse.[140,141] No medical therapy has proved effective for this condition. Necrotizing renal vasculitis secondary to oral methamphetamines ("ecstasy") has also been described.[142]

A second type of arterial obstruction has been reported in drug abuse patients following the accidental intraarterial injection of drugs during attempted intravenous injection. Parenteral agents can cause arterial injury and thrombosis due to chemical damage, perhaps related to the low pH of the injectant.[143] Another pattern of arterial damage results from the accidental injection of drug preparations intended for oral use. The practice of dissolving tablets for intravenous injection is harmful because of the large number of substances (e.g., silica, tragacanth) present. When this material is accidentally injected intraarterially, significant distal ischemia can result from obstruction of the small arteries by the inert materials (Fig. 8.7).[144]

No convincing evidence has demonstrated the value of any specific treatment in these patients. A number of therapeutic efforts have been tried, including anticoagulation, regional sympathetic block, and the administration of vasodilators, without proof of efficacy. The outcome appears to be determined at the time of injection by the quantity and concentration of injectant reaching the distal arterial bed. Nonetheless, heparin anticoagulation is favored if the patient is seen acutely and has no contraindications to this treatment. Compartment syndrome requiring fasciotomy is an infrequent but reported sequela.[145]

Behçet Disease

In 1937, Behçet described three patients with iritis and associated oral and genital mucocutaneous ulcerations, an association subsequently termed *Behçet disease*.[146] The associated vasculitis can cause both venous thromboses and specific arterial lesions. Venous thrombosis is the most frequent vascular disorder in Behçet disease, representing approximately 70% of vascular lesions and affecting up to one-third of patients.[147] Arterial lesions are less frequent, occurring in 1% to 7% of patients, and include occlusive and aneurysmal disease.[147] This systemic disease largely affects individuals from the Mediterranean area and East Asia and is more common in men.

The pathogenesis of vascular damage in Behçet disease appears to be an immune-mediated process. A humorally mediated cause has been suggested by the identification of enhanced neutrophil activity and circulating immune complexes in affected patients.[148] Specific T cell subsets have also been identified in high concentrations at the sites of vascular involvement, indicating a cellular-mediated process.[149] Activation of complement within the vessel wall can lead to destruction of the media and subsequent aneurysm formation. Vasa vasorum occlusion can then lead to

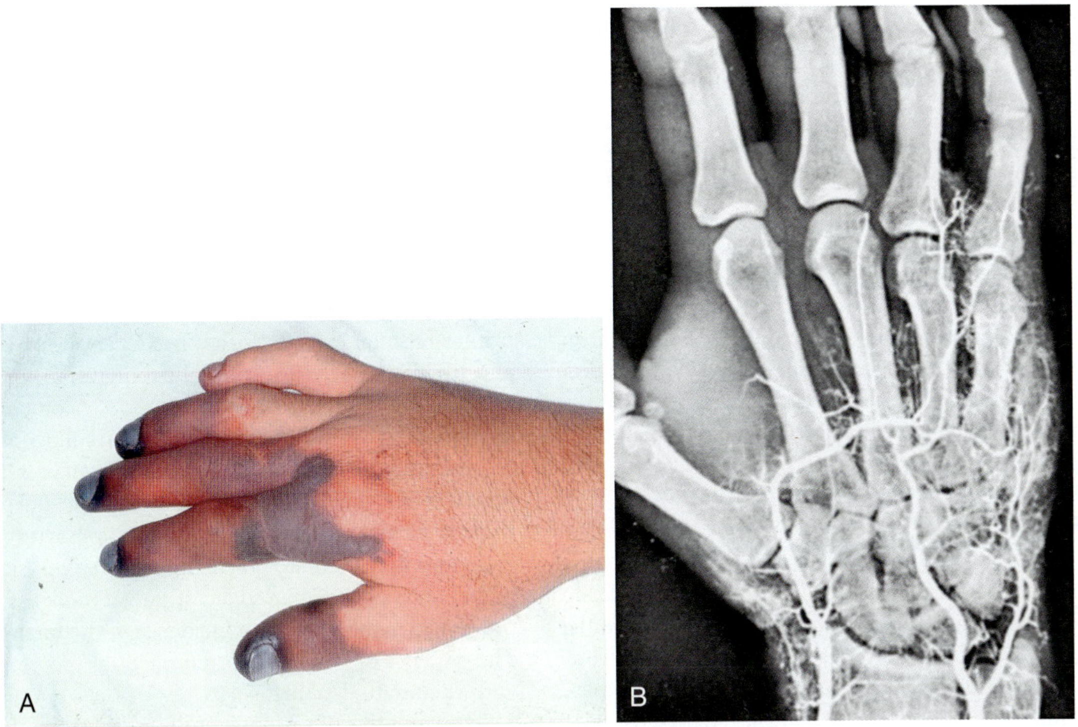

FIG 8.7 (A) Photograph of the hand of a 22-year-old man who injected a pentazocine tablet dissolved in tap water into his radial artery. The hand was severely ischemic, with gangrenous changes of the radial side. (B) Arteriogram showing massive arterial obstruction of the common and proper digital arteries to the thumb, index, and long fingers.

transmural necrosis of the large muscular arterial walls, with perforation and pseudoaneurysm formation.[150]

Behçet disease may have a genetic component because there is an increased incidence of the human leukocyte antigen (HLA)-B51 allele among patients with the disease, with resultant abnormalities in TNF-α expression.[151] Both viral and bacterial causes have been proposed, although definitive evidence is lacking.[152]

Large artery involvement is an uncommon but serious complication of Behçet disease. Arterial aneurysms, although distinctly less common than the mucocutaneous, ophthalmic, or arthritic lesions, are the most frequent cause of death in patients with Behçet disease.[153] Aneurysms have been described in numerous arteries, including the carotid, popliteal, femoral, iliac, pulmonary, and subclavian, but the aorta is the most frequent site of aneurysm formation in this disease.[147] The aneurysms frequently appear phlegmonous, suggesting acute bacterial infection, although cultures are typically negative. The arterial aneurysms are frequently multiple and may be metachronous. Unfortunately, interposition bypass grafts have a high incidence of thrombosis, in addition to the propensity to develop anastomotic pseudoaneurysms, which tend to occur within the first 18 months in up to 13% of cases.[154] Owing to the recognized difficulties of surgical aneurysm repair in Behçet disease, endovascular repair is emerging as the treatment of choice. The focal, saccular nature of these lesions makes them ideally suited to endovascular treatment. Excellent patency rates of endovascular treatment have been reported, but the fragile nature of the arteries puts patients at risk for pseudoaneurysm formation at seal zones, and aggressive stent oversizing is discouraged. Long-term immunosuppressive therapy is recommended after endovascular repair to limit pseudoaneurysm formation.[155]

Venous involvement is prominent, and lower extremity superficial or deep vein thrombosis occurs in 12% to 34% of patients, frequently alone or in association with arterial disease.[147] Thrombosis of the superior or inferior vena cava or of intracerebral veins occurs less frequently but can be fatal. Lifelong anticoagulation is often recommended in patients with Behçet disease who develop venous thrombosis, however, recent data suggests that immunosuppression is more important because the thrombosis is more likely due to vessel wall inflammation than hypercoagulability.[156]

Immunosuppressive agents, including azathioprine, corticosteroids, TNF-α antagonists (infliximab), and interferon-α, have been used with some success for nonarterial symptoms.[157] Although corticosteroids may prevent blindness and limit discomfort associated with the mucocutaneous disease, they do not appear to alter the progression or course of the underlying vascular disease. Currently, no uniformly satisfactory therapy exists for Behçet disease; however, early diagnosis and meticulous reconstructive management of identified arterial aneurysms have provided long-term limb salvage in some patients, despite the well-recognized propensity for arterial graft complications.[158] Vigilant follow-up is required once large artery disease is recognized.

Cogan Syndrome

Cogan syndrome is a rare condition consisting of interstitial keratitis and vestibuloauditory symptoms. It is a disease primarily of young adults, with the mean age of onset in the third decade. It is occasionally associated with a systemic vasculitis similar to PAN. Aortitis with subsequent development of clinically significant aortic insufficiency occurs in 10% of patients with Cogan syndrome.[159] Mesenteric vasculitis and thoracoabdominal aneurysms have also been described in association with Cogan syndrome.[160,161]

Daily administration of high-dose corticosteroids has been successful in reversing the visual and auditory components of Cogan syndrome, although deafness may be irreversible. The response of the aortitic component to steroids used singly or in combination with cyclosporine is less well established.[162] Surgical therapy, including aortic valve replacement, mesenteric revascularization, and thoracoabdominal aortic aneurysm repair, is occasionally indicated and can be performed safely.

Small Vessel Vasculitis

Hypersensitivity Vasculitis Group

The entities in the hypersensitivity vasculitis group include classic hypersensitivity vasculitis, mixed cryoglobulinemic vasculitis, and Henoch-Schönlein purpura. These conditions result from antigen exposure followed by antigen-antibody immune complex deposition in small arteries and arterial damage. Hypersensitivity vasculitis usually has prominent skin involvement. In some conditions, a drug, an environmental chemical, or the HBV may be implicated as the inciting antigen, but no causative agent is identified in more than half of cases. Henoch-Schönlein purpura is a self-limiting disease that occurs primarily in children and affects the skin, gastrointestinal tract, and kidneys. The disease course and findings are similar in cryoglobulinemic vasculitis, which may be associated with a hematologic malignancy or hepatitis B or C infection.[163]

The clinical syndromes typically associated with this group of diseases include skin rash, fever, and evidence of organ dysfunction, none of which specifically concerns vascular surgeons. It is clear, however, that some of these syndromes can manifest with arteritic involvement substantially limited to the hands and fingers. In these patients, the clinical picture is typically that of severe and widespread palmar and digital arterial occlusions and digital ischemia. The vasculitis can be treated with steroids, with the occasional use of immunosuppressive agents or plasmapheresis. The treatment of hand lesions can otherwise follow the approach outlined later in this chapter for Buerger disease.[164]

Vasculitis of Connective Tissue Diseases

The connective tissue diseases are often complicated by vasculitis. These diseases have associated immunologic abnormalities, and the occurrence of vasculitis in these patients likely results from immune-mediated damage, as described for other vasculitides.[165] Vasculitis frequently accompanies scleroderma, rheumatoid arthritis, and systemic lupus erythematosus.

Scleroderma is a generalized disorder of connective tissue, microvasculature, and small arteries. It is characterized by progressive scarring and small vessel occlusion in the skin, gastrointestinal tract, kidneys, lungs, and heart. CREST syndrome (calcinosis, RS, esophageal dysmotility, sclerodactyly, and telangiectases) describes a variant of scleroderma with limited cutaneous involvement. The vasculitis associated with scleroderma results in fibrinoid necrosis and concentric thickening of the intima, with deposition of layers of mucopolysaccharide.

Scleroderma is the most frequent connective tissue disease recognized in our patients with RS, as well as those with digital ulceration (Fig. 8.8).[16] Approximately 80% to 97% of patients with scleroderma have symptoms of RS. In our experience, the RS usually begins as vasospastic and progresses to the obstructive type.

The vasculitis associated with rheumatoid arthritis involves primarily small arteries with a predilection for vasa nervorum and the digital arteries. Intimal proliferation, medial necrosis, and progression to fibrosis with vessel occlusion occur. Symptoms of mononeuritis multiplex are common following involvement of small arteries. Cutaneous lesions are often present and include digital ulcers, nail fold infarcts, and palpable purpura.[166] Rarely, there is coronary, mesenteric, or cerebral artery involvement. Patients with rheumatoid arthritis who have positive ANCAs or higher titers of rheumatoid factor have a more aggressive disease course with a more frequent incidence of rheumatoid vasculitis.[167] The presence of vasculitis portends a poor prognosis for patients with rheumatoid arthritis.

The vasculitis of systemic lupus erythematosus is believed to be due to deposition of immune complexes.[168] The most frequent clinical vascular problem in lupus is RS, which can affect 80% of patients. Other vasculitic manifestations include palpable purpura and mononeuritis multiplex. Thrombotic disorders of the arterial and venous system occur in patients with lupus and appear to be related to the lupus anticoagulant, not vasculitis. IgA anti–double-stranded deoxyribonucleic acid (DNA) antibodies and anti–endothelial cell antibodies are markers of more virulent vasculitic involvement.[169] In addition to small vessel vasculitis, patients with systemic lupus erythematosus are clearly prone to premature large vessel atherosclerosis.[170]

Management of the vasculitides associated with the connective tissue diseases consists primarily of steroid therapy.[168] Steroids appear to have little or no role in the treatment of the occlusive vascular lesions of scleroderma. Immunosuppressive therapy with cyclophosphamide has also been shown to have modest

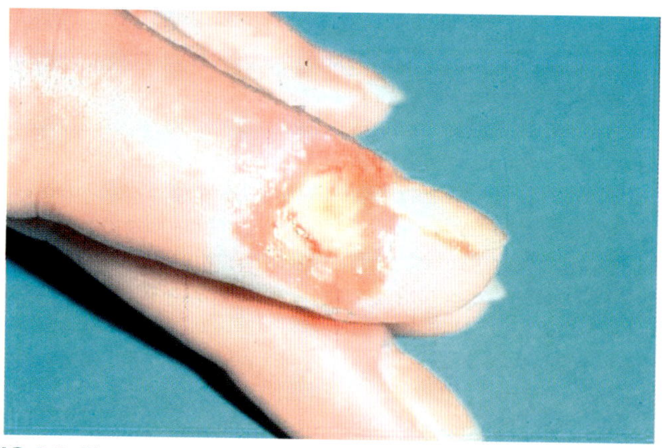

FIG 8.8 Photographs of a patient with scleroderma and a digital ulcer.

benefit in selected patients.[171] The treatment of RS associated with lupus or scleroderma is as described earlier.

Vasculitis Associated With Malignancy

Vasculitis associated with malignancy is infrequent. A strong association has been made between a systemic necrotizing vasculitis resembling PAN and hairy cell leukemia. The vasculitis in this situation presents after the diagnosis of leukemia and is indistinguishable from classic PAN. An immune-mediated mechanism is postulated. More frequently, vasculitides involving small vessels have been described in association with lymphoproliferative disorders. These have primarily cutaneous manifestations and minimal visceral involvement and are often referred to as *paraneoplastic vasculitides.*[172]

Vasculitis associated with solid tumors is rare, but resolution with tumor excision has been reported.[173] RS has been reported in association with carcinoma and lymphoproliferative malignancies. These cases were characterized by cold-induced ischemia, which frequently led to digital artery occlusion and ischemic ulcerations. The symptoms of finger ischemia preceded the diagnosis of malignancy, and several of these patients experienced marked improvement of their hand lesions after removal of the tumor.

BUERGER DISEASE

Buerger disease, also known as *thromboangiitis obliterans,* is a clinical syndrome characterized by the occurrence of segmental thrombotic occlusions of small- and medium-sized arteries in the lower and frequently the upper extremities, accompanied by a prominent arterial wall inflammatory cell infiltration.[174] Buerger disease is a discrete pathologic entity and is clinically distinct from atherosclerosis or immune arteritis. Affected patients are predominantly young male smokers (mean age, 34 years); they usually exhibit distal limb ischemia, frequently accompanied by localized digital gangrene.

Buerger disease appears to be on the decline in North America, although there has been an increase in the incidence in women. Women currently constitute up to 20% of patients in certain series.[175] It is unclear whether there is a true decline in incidence or simply more uniform application of strict diagnostic criteria. A large volume of patients continue to be reported from East and Southwest Asia. In patients with peripheral vascular disease, the reported incidence of Buerger disease is 0.75% in North America, 3.3% in Eastern Europe, and 16.6% in Japan.[176]

Approximately 40% to 50% of patients with Buerger disease have a history of superficial migratory thrombophlebitis, RS, or both.[175] The arterial lesions of Buerger disease usually occur in the distal portions of both the upper and the lower extremities and may be accompanied by digital gangrene, especially of the toes. Although there have been rare, well-documented reports, both arteriographically and pathologically, of iliac[177] and visceral artery involvement,[178] in the overwhelming majority of patients with thromboangiitis obliterans, disease is limited to the arteries distal to the elbow and knee. In North America, approximately 50% of patients with Buerger disease have isolated lower extremity involvement, 30% to 40% have upper and lower extremity involvement, and approximately 10% have isolated upper extremity involvement.[175]

The cause of Buerger disease remains unknown. Although a strong association with tobacco use has been recognized clinically, a causal relationship has not been conclusively demonstrated.[175] Most patients are heavy cigarette smokers, although cases of Buerger disease in users of smokeless tobacco[179] and cannabis[180] have also been reported. An increased cellular response to tobacco antigen has been noted in patients with Buerger disease, as well as in healthy smokers compared with nonsmokers. Tobacco is currently considered at least a permissive factor and likely a causative factor.

The major histocompatibility complex, specifically HLA-A9, -B5, -DR4, and -DRw6, has been implicated in Buerger disease, but its role is unclear.[175,181] Considerable evidence indicates that an autoimmune process is central to the illness. Several independent investigators have identified elevated levels of anticollagen antibodies[182] and antiendothelial antibodies[183] in patients with Buerger disease. Immunohistochemical analysis of the arterial wall of patients with Buerger disease demonstrates accumulation of immunoglobulins and complement in the intimal layer, with sparing of the medial and adventitial layers.[184]

The acute lesion of Buerger disease is a nonnecrotizing inflammation of the vascular wall with a prominent component of intraluminal thrombosis. In contrast to both atherosclerosis and immune arteritis, the internal elastic lamina remains intact in Buerger disease; therefore, Buerger disease is not a true vasculitis because it lacks vascular wall necrosis. Both T and B cell–mediated activation of macrophages or dendritic cells in the intima have been implicated in the pathogenesis of Buerger disease.[185] The chronic phase of Buerger disease includes a decline in hypercellularity, with the production of perivascular fibrosis and frequent recanalization of the luminal thrombus. Adjacent veins and nerves are frequently involved in the perivascular inflammatory process.

Currently, well-established diagnostic criteria exist to make the diagnosis of Buerger disease (Box 8.2).[175] The major criteria are essential for diagnosis, whereas the minor criteria are supportive. Central to the diagnosis is the onset of symptoms before the age of 45 years, a uniform exposure to tobacco, and absence of arterial lesions proximal to the knee or elbow. It is essential to exclude other frequent causes of limb ischemia in young adults. In North America, atherosclerosis is much more prevalent than Buerger disease, and major atherosclerotic risk factors such as hyperlipidemia, diabetes, and hypertension must be absent. Proximal sources of emboli (cardiac, proximal arterial occlusive, or aneurysmal disease), underlying autoimmune disease, hypercoagulable states, trauma, and local lesions (popliteal entrapment, adventitial cystic disease) must also be excluded. Serologic tests for autoimmune disease and hypercoagulable states are typically negative. Similar clinical diagnostic criteria were reported by Shionoya from Japan: (1) smoking history, (2) onset before the age of 50 years, (3) infrapopliteal arterial occlusion, (4) either upper limb involvement or phlebitis migrans, and (5) absence of other atherosclerotic risk factors.[186]

After the clinical criteria have been met, objective confirmation of distal occlusive disease limited to small- and medium-sized

BOX 8.2 Criteria for the Diagnosis of Buerger Disease

Major Criteria

- Onset of distal extremity ischemic symptoms before age 45 years
- Tobacco use
- Exclusion of the following:
  - Proximal embolic source (cardiac, thoracic outlet syndrome, arteriosclerosis obliterans, aneurysms)
  - Trauma and local lesions (entrapment, adventitial cyst)
  - Autoimmune disease
  - Hypercoagulable states
  - Atherosclerosis
  - Atherosclerotic risk factors (diabetes, hypertension, hyperlipidemia)
- No evidence of arterial disease proximal to popliteal or distal brachial arteries
- Objective documentation of distal occlusive disease by one of the following: plethysmography, histopathology, or arteriography

Minor Criteria

- Migratory superficial phlebitis
- Raynaud syndrome
- Upper extremity involvement
- Instep claudication

From Mills JL, Porter JM: Buerger disease: a review and update. *Semin Vasc Surg* 6:14–23, 1993.

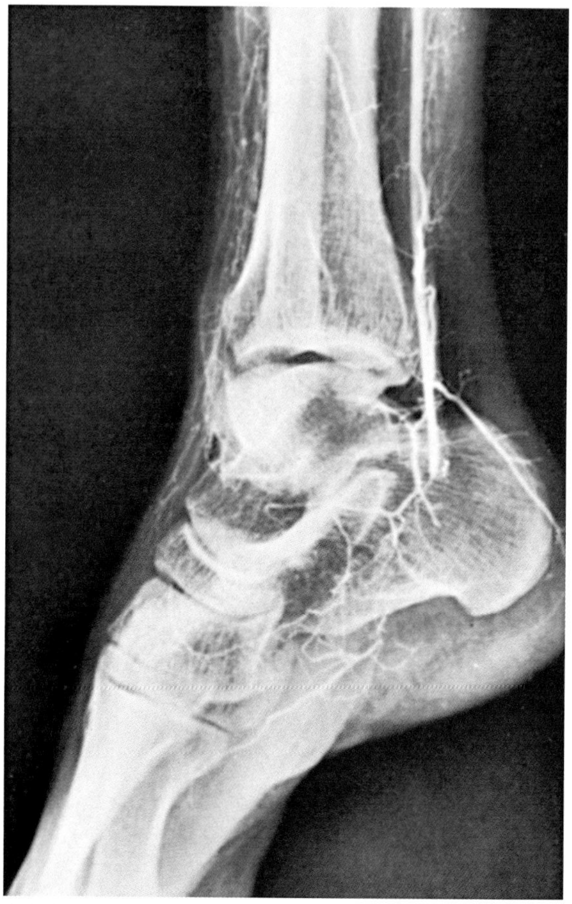

FIG 8.9 Arteriogram of patient with Buerger disease showing occlusion of the posterior tibial artery at the ankle, total occlusion of the anterior tibial artery, and numerous small collateral vessels.

vessels is required. This confirmation can be done with four-limb digital plethysmography, distinct histopathologic findings when available, or arteriography. The arteriographic findings reveal that the extremity arteries proximal to the popliteal and distal brachial levels are normal, proximal atherosclerosis and vascular calcification are absent, and there is an abrupt transition from a normal, smooth proximal vessel to an area of occlusion.[175] Involvement tends to be segmental rather than diffuse and is commonly symmetrical. In the upper extremity, the ulnar or radial artery is frequently occluded, and extensive digital and palmar arterial occlusion is uniformly present. In the lower extremity, the infrageniculate vessels are extensively diseased, with diffuse plantar arterial occlusion. Tortuous "corkscrew" collaterals frequently reconstitute patent distal arterial segments and, although not pathognomonic, are suggestive of Buerger disease (Fig. 8.9).

Digital plethysmography frequently provides especially important diagnostic information. In the typical patient with Buerger disease, obstructive arterial waveforms are present in all digits, providing objective evidence of widespread digital arterial occlusion or stenosis. Patients with unilateral digital plethysmographic abnormalities should undergo arteriography to rule out a proximal, potentially correctable arterial lesion causing the digital ischemia. In addition, patients with symptoms and objective findings localizing their disease to the distal feet and toes and who have normal hand and finger plethysmography should undergo arteriography to rule out a proximal embolic source for the ischemia.

The cornerstone of treatment for Buerger disease is complete tobacco abstinence. All other forms of treatment are palliative. The disease typically undergoes remissions and relapses that correlate closely with the cessation and resumption of cigarette smoking with patients sustaining no further tissue loss following cessation of smoking.[175] Conservative local treatment is appropriate for areas of finger ulceration and gangrene, with the primary goal being a clean, dry digit.[187] Debridement of ischemic ulcers, often including nail removal, is used frequently, accompanied by minimal rongeur removal of exposed phalangeal bone as needed. Any associated infection is treated with antibiotics. Proximal finger amputations are rarely required, and wrist or forearm amputations are rare. We have found thoracic sympathectomy ineffective, and we find no convincing evidence that this procedure is of any significant benefit in these patients.

The course of lower extremity Buerger disease stands in marked contrast to that observed with upper extremity involvement. Ischemic rest pain can be severe, and narcotic analgesics are frequently required. Several large series reported a 12% to 31% incidence of major leg amputation over a 5- to 10-year period.[188,189] Lumbar sympathectomy for refractory Buerger disease has been advocated by some, but results have been equivocal, with 50% ulcer healing rates at 6 months.[190] Anecdotal reports of improved lower extremity symptoms with the use of an implantable spinal cord stimulator are encouraging,[191] but the device has not yet been subjected to clinical trials.

Arteriography should be performed in all patients with threatened limb loss. If arteriography reveals a patent distal vessel and if autogenous vein is available, a distal arterial bypass may be considered. The use of autogenous vein is mandatory. Distal bypass is seldom feasible because of the diffuse nature of the arterial occlusive disease process. In our experience and that of others, the long-term results of reconstruction are mediocre. However, published data suggest that acceptable primary (30% to 49%) and secondary (47% to 63%) 5-year patency rates can be achieved in lower extremity bypasses, including inframalleolar bypasses, in patients with Buerger disease.[192,193] A novel operative approach developed in India involves a pedicled omental transfer to the lower extremity for limb-threatening ischemia.[194] In 62 patients treated, 94% experienced relief of pain, and none required amputation.

Many medications have been recommended for the treatment of Buerger disease, including corticosteroids, prostaglandin E1 (PGE1), vasodilators, hemorheologic agents, antiplatelet agents, and anticoagulants. There is no evidence that any are effective. A randomized European trial comparing the oral prostacyclin analog iloprost with placebo demonstrated improved pain control with iloprost, but no improvement in wound healing.[195] Preliminary results of gene therapy with intramuscular injection of vascular endothelial growth factor have been promising in promoting ulcer healing and limb salvage, but they remain investigational.[196,197]

Although lower-extremity Buerger disease portends a significantly worse prognosis for limb salvage than does atherosclerotic occlusive disease, life expectancy for patients with Buerger disease approaches that of an age-matched population. This is likely due to a lack of coronary artery involvement in the disease process. Reported survival is 97% at 5 years, 94% at 10 years, and 85% at 25 years.[188,189,198]

HERITABLE ARTERIOPATHIES

Hereditary disorders of the arterial wall typically affect the structure or stability of collagen or elastin, resulting in weakness of the arterial wall. These patients may possess characteristic phenotypic features, but they are often not recognized until the patient exhibits a catastrophic vascular complication. The heritable arteriopathies discussed in this chapter include Marfan syndrome, Ehlers-Danlos syndrome, Loeys-Dietz syndrome, cystic medial necrosis, and pseudoxanthoma elasticum. Arteriomegaly is also included in this section, although it is not strictly a heritable disease and there are no distinguishing phenotypic features.

Marfan Syndrome

Marfan syndrome is an inherited disorder of connective tissue characterized by abnormalities of the skeletal, ocular, and cardiovascular systems, with variable phenotypic expression.

Classic Marfan syndrome is caused by mutations in the fibrillin gene on chromosome 15.[199] Fibrillin, a large glycoprotein (350 kDa), is one of the structural components of the elastin-associated microfibrils. Both a reduction in fibrillin formation and abnormalities in the fibrillin molecule have been identified.[200]

The incidence of Marfan syndrome is estimated to be 1 in 5000, and there has been no identified race or sex preference.[201] Inheritance is by an autosomal dominant pattern, although nearly 25% of all cases are the result of spontaneous genetic mutations. In its classic form, the syndrome is easily recognizable and consists of abnormalities of the eye (subluxation of the lens), skeleton (arachnodactyly, extreme limb length, pectus excavatum or carinatum, and joint laxity), and cardiovascular system (aortic dilation and aortic valvular incompetence). The diagnosis is established on the basis of clinical manifestations in most cases. However, some patients have only one or a few of the characteristic features. Prenatal diagnosis can be accomplished using chorionic villus sampling.[202]

Patients with Marfan syndrome develop progressive dilation of the aortic root, with a resultant ascending aortic aneurysm and aortic valve incompetence (Fig. 8.10). A significant number have mitral valve prolapse and mitral insufficiency. Mild aortic isthmus coarctation may be associated with this syndrome, predisposing the patient to ascending aortic dissection. Less frequently, aneurysmal dilation and dissection involve the pulmonary, coronary, carotid, and splenic arteries and the infrarenal aorta.

If Marfan syndrome is untreated, life expectancy is approximately 40 years, with 95% of deaths related to cardiovascular causes. Progressive aortic root dilation leading to aortic dissection or aortic valvular insufficiency accounts for 80% of fatal complications. The remainder of deaths are due to congestive heart failure.[203]

Histopathologic evaluation of aortic segments from patients with Marfan syndrome has revealed cystic medial necrosis, with disruption of collagen fibers and fibrosis of the media.[204] Immunohistochemical analysis has revealed an upregulation of matrix

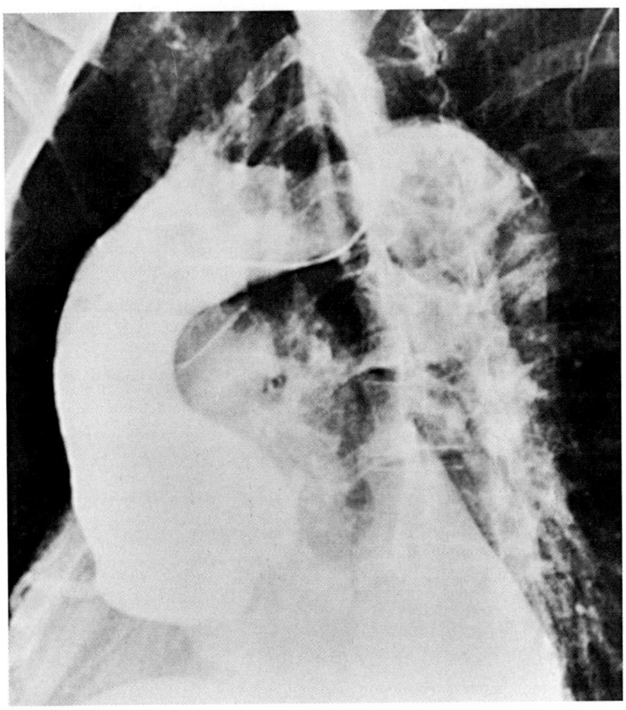

FIG 8.10 Thoracic aortogram of a patient with Marfan syndrome showing massive aortic dilation and associated aortic insufficiency.

metalloproteinases and abnormalities in elastin synthesis, leading to increased susceptibility to degradation by matrix metalloproteinases.[205] Compared with normal subjects, Marfan syndrome patients have decreased aortic distensibility and increased aortic stiffness indices in both the ascending and abdominal aortic regions, regardless of the aortic diameter.[206]

In view of the predictably progressive nature of the aortic dilation, all patients with Marfan syndrome should be followed from childhood with annual echocardiograms to detect aortic dilation.[207] There is evidence that β-blocker therapy initiated before the development of aortic incompetence can retard the onset of incompetence and perhaps retard aneurysmal degeneration,[203,208,209] and this remains the current standard of care with the goal of a resting heart rate less than 60 beats/min. Other potential medical therapies include angiotensin converting enzyme inhibitors and angiotensin II receptor blockers, which block transforming growth factor beta, the dysregulation of which is felt to contribute to the pathogenesis of Marfan syndrome.[210]

Elective repair of the aortic valve and ascending aorta should be accomplished prophylactically before severe aortic insufficiency compromises left ventricular function or the ascending aorta exceeds 6 cm in diameter, at which point the risk of dissection and rupture increases. Surgical intervention typically includes graft replacement of the ascending aorta, with concomitant aortic valve replacement, with 30-day mortality as low as 1.5% and 20-year survival of 59%.[211] Equally good results have been achieved with valve sparing aortic root reconstruction.[212]

As endovascular technology continues to improve, less invasive options for treatment of aortic arch pathology will surely emerge. The current consensus is still that endovascular repair be reserved for high-risk patients, as a bridge to open repair, or as part of a hybrid procedure.[213,214] Up to one-third of Marfan patients treated with stents will require reintervention, and Marfan syndrome was the strongest predictor of reintervention in the Talent registry.[215] Technical recommendations for stents placed in Marfan patients include landing in a graft whenever possible, oversizing less than 10% the native normal aortic diameter, and avoiding ballooning at the fixation sites.

Ehlers-Danlos Syndrome

Ehlers-Danlos syndrome includes a group of diseases described separately by Ehlers in 1899 and Danlos in 1908, characterized by hyperextensible skin, hypermobile joints, fragile tissues, and a bleeding diathesis primarily related to fragile vessels.[216,217] Ehlers-Danlos syndrome is the most frequent of the heritable connective tissue disorders and occurs in autosomal dominant, autosomal recessive, and sex-linked patterns, with an incidence of approximately 1 in 5000 births.[218] The most recent accepted classification system (Villefranche) recognizes six main types, including the vascular type (previously type IV).[219] Although the vascular type has the most severe vascular abnormalities, all types are associated with some degree of vascular fragility. The extreme fragility of tissues in many patients with Ehlers-Danlos syndrome leads to problems of surgical importance. The skin and soft tissues are easily disrupted, tend to fragment and tear with manipulation, and hold sutures and heal poorly. Wound dehiscence is common when surgery is required. The vascular type is caused by mutation of the *COLA31* gene and represents only about 5% of all cases of Ehlers-Danlos syndrome but causes the most severe arterial complications. These patients produce little or no type III collagen, which is of major structural importance in vessels, viscera, and skin. Patients are prone to spontaneous rupture of major vessels, aneurysm formation, and acute aortic dissections.[220] Other complications include spontaneous lacerations, false aneurysms, and arteriovenous fistulas. Hemorrhage can be life threatening despite normal platelet function and coagulation proteins. Defective type III collagen appears to facilitate bleeding by failing to stimulate platelets exposed to subendothelial connective tissue. The media of the arterial wall is thin and disorganized, with fragmented elastic fibers on microscopic examination. Treatment of spontaneous arterial rupture in patients with Ehlers-Danlos syndrome should be nonoperative, consisting of compression and transfusion whenever possible. If operation for major arterial disruption is required, the therapeutic objective should be ligation to control bleeding if this procedure can be accomplished without tissue loss. Arteriography carries special risks of vessel laceration and hemorrhage in these patients and should be avoided if possible. When necessary, open exposure with pledgeted repair of access sites is recommended.[221]

Despite the many pitfalls, major arterial reconstruction can be accomplished in patients with Ehlers-Danlos syndrome. In a Mayo Clinic series, perioperative mortality was low, but the morbidity was 46% and delayed graft complications occurred in 40% of arterial reconstructions, with only 68% of patients surviving to age 50.[222] Slightly better results were noted in a recent series from Johns Hopkins, in which survival free of any complications at 5 years was 85% and 54% following endovascular and open repairs respectively, although not all patients in this series had vascular Ehlers-Danlos syndrome.[221]

Medical therapy of vascular Ehlers-Danlos syndrome is not well established. Patients with vascular Ehlers-Danlos syndrome have been shown to have elevated levels of transforming growth factor beta (TGF-β). Celiprolol is a selective beta blocker, which has been shown to suppress TGF-β activity. In a small randomized controlled trial, patients with vascular Ehlers-Danlos syndrome treated with celiprolol had a decreased rate of arterial rupture compared to placebo.[223] Treatment with this and similar beta blockers, as well as the angiotensin receptor blockers, remain an area of research.

Cystic Medial Necrosis

Cystic medial necrosis is a condition associated with aortic dissection. It manifests pathologically with uniform hyaline degeneration of the media and replacement by a mucoid-appearing basophilic substance. Pathologic changes include a variety of metabolic conditions and syndromes affecting the composition and structure of collagen, elastin, and mucopolysaccharide ground substance. Thus, Marfan syndrome, Ehlers-Danlos syndrome, any of the mucopolysaccharidoses, and occasionally neurofibromatosis can all manifest with the typical arterial lesions and pathologic changes identified as cystic medial necrosis.

Although most patients with cystic medial necrosis have an identifiable clinical syndrome, most commonly Marfan syndrome

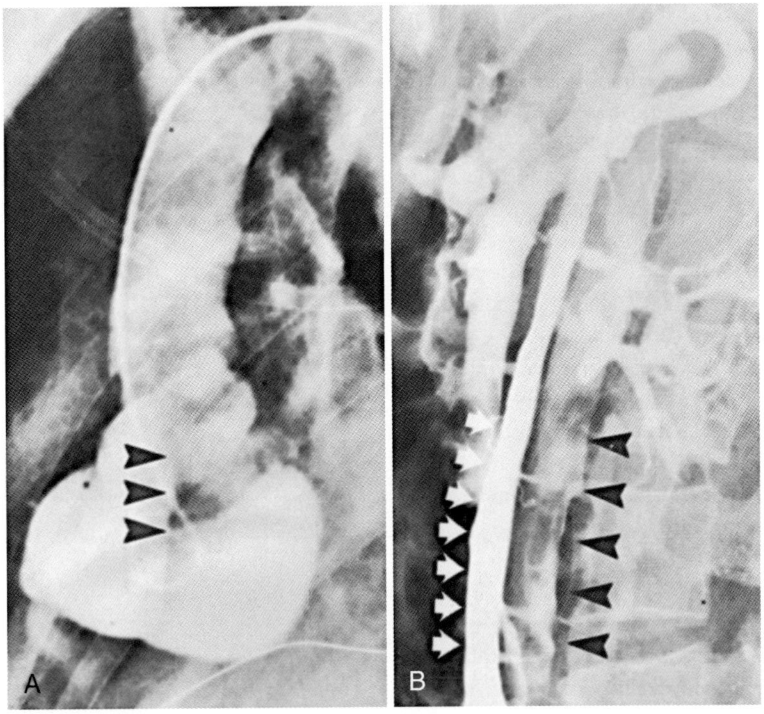

FIG 8.11 (A) Cystic medial necrosis with aortic root dissection. The junction of the true and false lumen is outlined *(black arrows)*. (B) Lateral aortogram of the same patient showing the outline of a double-lumen abdominal aorta (*white* and *black arrows*).

or Ehlers-Danlos syndrome, a distinct subpopulation of patients with aortic root disease and histologic findings consistent with cystic medial necrosis fail to show the classic phenotypes of either syndrome. These patients often seek treatment at an older age and with more advanced vascular disease. Ninety-four percent of the deaths in this patient group are related to cardiovascular disease, with the majority owing to aortic dissection, rupture, or sudden death (Fig. 8.11).[224]

Loeys-Dietz Syndrome

Initially described in 2005, the Loeys-Dietz syndrome is an autosomal dominant connective tissue disorder caused by a defect in the *TGF-β* gene.[225] Features of the clinical syndrome include hypertelorism, blue sclerae, bifid uvula, cleft palate, and arterial tortuosity and aortic aneurysm formation. Patients are particularly prone to ascending aorta dilation and dissection, the main source of death in affected individuals.[226] Aneurysm formation occurs at a younger age than Marfan and Ehlers-Danlos syndrome, and in general surgical results are better. Current recommendations for surgery include an aortic root diameter greater than 4 cm, descending thoracic aorta greater than 5 cm, and infrarenal aortic diameter greater than 4 cm. Women are susceptible to pregnancy complications and uterine rupture. Preventive therapy with β-blockers and angiotensin receptor blockers may slow the progression of disease.[227]

Neurofibromatosis

Neurofibromatosis, first described by von Recklinghausen in 1882, is an autosomal dominant mutation of chromosome 17 with variable clinical expression, including café-au-lait spots, neurofibromas, axillary or inguinal freckling, bone lesions, optic gliomas and iris lesions (Lisch nodules). Vascular lesions are also common, but likely underreported. Up to 25% of patients have hypertension related to renal artery stenosis or middle aortic syndrome.[228] Arterial aneurysms involving multiple arteries have also been reported, including renal, aortic, iliac, subclavian, visceral, popliteal, and radial. Surgical treatment of symptomatic lesions is indicated, although operations can be difficult because of associated vessel fragility and arteriovenous malformations.

Pseudoxanthoma Elasticum

Pseudoxanthoma elasticum is an inherited disorder of elastic tissue manifested clinically by loose, baggy skin with multiple creases and small, yellow-orange cutaneous papules in intertriginous areas (pseudoxanthomas). These patients also have changes in the eye (angioid streaks) and distinct vascular abnormalities. The prevalence of pseudoxanthoma elasticum is 1 in 70,000 to 160,000.[229] Studies have demonstrated an autosomal recessive inheritance in the majority, although there is also an autosomal dominant form.[230]

The basic pathologic change is degeneration of medial elastic fibers, with calcification, fragmentation, and secondary proliferation of the intima leading to luminal narrowing and obstruction. This change results in a markedly abnormal pulse contour owing to loss of the elastic recoil and distensibility of vessels and may be demonstrated plethysmographically. Arterial stenoses, occlusions, or both are the end results of this pathologic process and may involve the intracerebral and peripheral arteries.[231] Radiography frequently reveals extensive arterial calcification in a young patient without obvious risk factors for atherosclerosis. Arterial occlusive disease occurs at an early age, usually presenting in the 20s or 30s.[232] Decreased peripheral pulses and evidence of peripheral arterial occlusive disease can be found in 24% to 80% of these patients.[233] Symptoms include intermittent claudication, periodic abdominal pain, and angina.[234] Gastrointestinal hemorrhage is frequent and is believed to originate from the widespread arterial degeneration. Hypertension is common in these patients and is usually ascribed to extensive vascular calcification, although renovascular hypertension has been reported.

Standard techniques of vascular surgery, including autogenous vein bypass and endarterectomy, have been used with success in patients with pseudoxanthoma elasticum.[233] Anecdotal benefit from pentoxifylline for the relief of ischemic pain has been reported.[235] The indications for surgery in these patients are the same as for patients with arteriosclerotic occlusive disease.

Arteria Magna Syndrome

Leriche was the first to describe patients with arteria magna syndrome, which is characterized by extreme arterial dilation, elongation, and tortuosity, which he termed *dolicho et méga-artère*.[236] Since then, many such patients have been recognized, and the terms *arteria magna, arteria dolicho et magna,* and *arteriomegaly* have all been used to describe this condition. Pathologic study reveals that the arterial media of these patients has a striking loss of elastic tissue.[237]

Angiography in patients with this syndrome reveals characteristic changes. They have arterial widening and tortuosity (100% of patients), extremely slow arterial flow velocity (100% of patients), and multiple aneurysms (66% of patients; Fig. 8.12).[238] The slow arterial flow present in patients with this condition makes arteriography difficult. Large amounts of contrast must be used, and visualization of distal vessels may require multiple injections and special timing sequences with delayed filming.

The propensity to form arterial aneurysms at multiple sites results in the frequent need for surgical correction. Because of the generalized arterial dilation in these patients, standard criteria for determining the size of aneurysms to be repaired may not be useful. All patients with arteria magna should undergo annual examinations of all pertinent sites (aorta and iliac, femoral, and popliteal arteries), together with ultrasound imaging of nonpalpable or questionable areas. Any aneurysm that reaches twofold to 2.5-fold the size of the parent vessel or becomes symptomatic should be repaired. Arterial occlusions in these patients are almost always thrombotic or embolic complications of aneurysmal disease.

The relationship of arteria magna to typical atherosclerosis is uncertain. The syndrome occurs, albeit rarely, in young people with no evidence of atherosclerosis, and it has been reported in children. Lawrence and colleagues[239] reported a 36% familial incidence among first-degree relatives. Clinical experience suggests that most patients in the United States with arteria magna have significant associated atherosclerosis along with the usual risk factors, including tobacco use. In these patients, however, the atherosclerosis is typically nonocclusive, and dilation predominates.

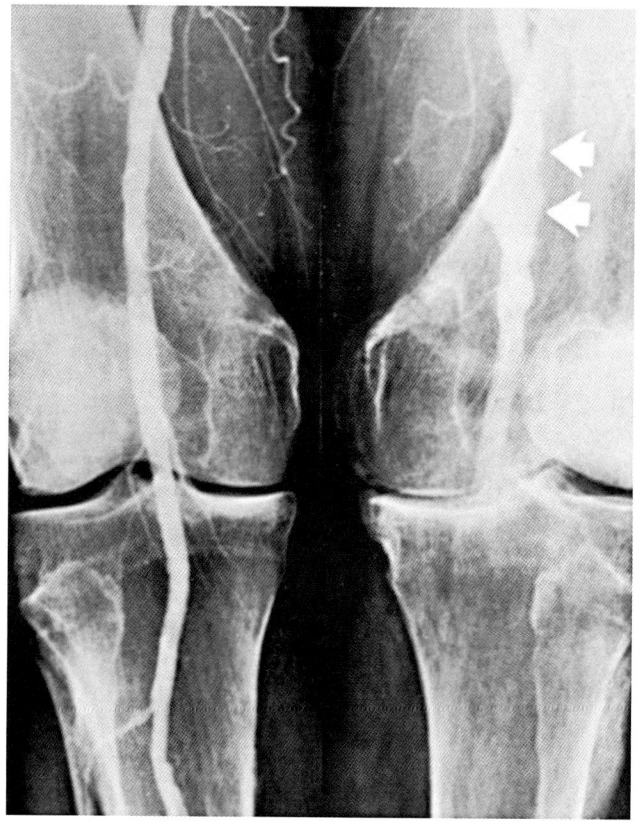

FIG 8.12 Arteriogram of a 68-year-old man showing very dilated popliteal arteries and a left popliteal aneurysm *(arrows)*. This patient's arterial dilatation extended throughout his body, a condition termed *arteria magna syndrome*.

CONGENITAL CONDITIONS AFFECTING THE ARTERIES

Abdominal Coarctation

Coarctation of the aorta below the diaphragm is a rare but well-recognized condition. Quain[240] described a stricture of the abdominal aorta in 1847 that he believed to be congenital in origin. In 1952, Glenn and coworkers[241] reported the first successful surgical repair, which consisted of bypassing the coarctation with a splenic artery graft. Since that time, the surgical treatment and clinical courses of a large number of patients have been reported.[242] Abdominal coarctation is usually discovered during an evaluation for hypertension. Most patients with abdominal coarctation become symptomatic during their teens, with complaints associated with hypertension, including headache, fatigue, shortness of breath, and palpitations. The hypertension is mediated through the renin-angiotensin system.[243] Severe leg ischemia is unusual,[244] but moderate claudication is often present. Involvement of the superior mesenteric artery occurs frequently, although symptoms of visceral ischemia are rare.

Physical findings in these patients include reduced or absent lower extremity pulses, with a noticeable femoral pulse delay. All patients have prominent abdominal systolic bruits, and many have systolic bruits in the lumbar region or lower posterior thoracic area. The natural history of untreated abdominal coarctation is severe hypertension, with death from renal or cardiac failure within a few years of the onset of symptoms.[245]

Multiple variants of abdominal coarctation have been described, with the variable factors being the precise location and length of the aortic involvement and the number of visceral branches affected. The origins of the visceral arteries may be involved even when they originate from an area of relatively uninvolved aorta. Stenosis or occlusion of the visceral arteries usually does not extend beyond a few millimeters from the origin, implicating a process that is primarily aortic.[242]

Two primary pathogenetic theories have been presented. The first proposes a congenital anomaly representing a failure of normal fusion of the two dorsal aortas of the embryo, resulting in aortic narrowing. The existence of multiple renal arteries in a number of these patients supports this theory because the formation of a single renal artery is a developmental step that coincides in both location and timing with fusion of the dorsal aortas. The congenital origin of abdominal coarctation in some of these patients may be related to intrauterine injury because the anomaly has been reported in association with the maternal rubella syndrome.[246] In patients in whom the lesion is congenital, the involved vessels are hypoplastic, without gross or microscopic inflammatory reaction.

The second proposed cause of abdominal coarctation is inflammation. In this group of patients, microscopic examination of involved arteries reveals pronounced inflammatory changes. This lesion is sometimes referred to as the *middle aortic syndrome* to emphasize its acquired rather than congenital nature.[247] This inflammatory middle aortic narrowing is probably a variant of Takayasu arteritis and appears to occur with a frequency reflecting the primarily Asian distribution of that disease.[248] Although this arteritis can be treated successfully with corticosteroids during the acute stage, the diagnosis is usually made later, when the chronic fibrotic and stenotic lesions are amenable only to surgical treatment.

Arteriography is necessary to define the extent of the lesion and to plan treatment (Fig. 8.13). Lateral and oblique views are helpful in detecting the extent of visceral vessel involvement. Renovascular hypertension is assumed, and renin studies or split renal function studies are not necessary unless the potential viability of a poorly visualized kidney is questionable (to determine the need for nephrectomy vs. revascularization).

Many authors have reported successful surgical treatment of abdominal coarctation by a variety of methods, including aortoaortic bypass, iliac or femoral bypass, prosthetic patch aortoplasty, and splenoaortic anastomosis.[242,249,250] In contrast to thoracic coarctation, prosthetic bypass grafting from the descending thoracic aorta to an uninvolved area of the infrarenal aorta or the iliac or femoral arteries has traditionally been the procedure of choice, although autologous repair with extensive aortic patching is often preferred if feasible.[242] When possible, a single abdominal operative incision is preferable, using medial visceral rotation to allow optimal exposure of the supraceliac aorta. Alternatively, this operation can be performed through a thoracoabdominal incision or through separate laparotomy and thoracotomy incisions. Complete revascularization has been reported as a staged procedure.[250] However, single-stage repair is recommended because most of these patients are young and tolerate extensive procedures well.[251] Results of surgical treatment of abdominal coarctation have been good. Stanley and associates[242] reviewed the results of 53 cases and found no operative mortality with either primary or secondary interventions, and overall graft patency of 97% at 5 years and 76% at 10 years.[242] In very small children, operation may be delayed until age 5 to 6 years, at which time increased vessel size allows a greater chance of successful repair, as long as cardiac and renal function can be preserved by medical management of hypertension. Successful repair of middle aortic coarctation with stent implantation has been reported, although long-term durability is unknown.[252,253]

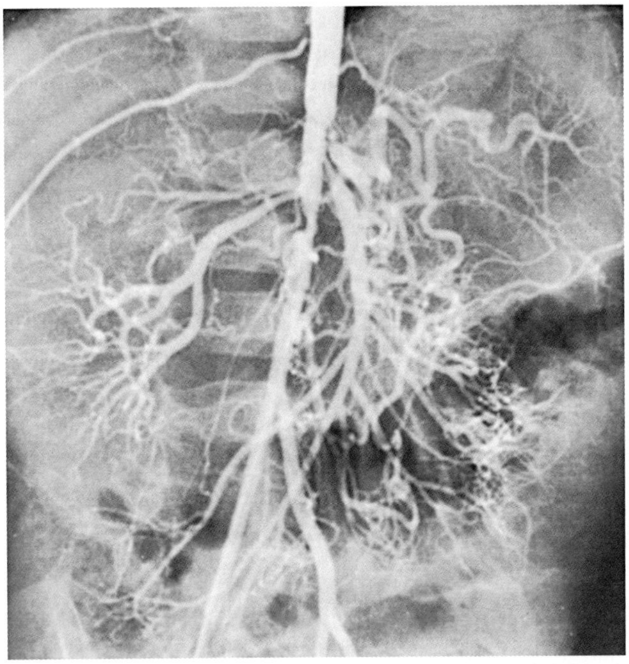

FIG 8.13 Abdominal aortic coarctation in a 2-year-old child with infrarenal aortic narrowing and high-grade stenoses at the origins of the celiac, superior mesenteric, and right renal arteries and nearly total occlusion of the left renal artery.

Persistent Sciatic Artery

In the embryo, the axial sciatic artery arises from the umbilical artery and supplies blood to the lower limb, following a dorsal course to the popliteal area and then proceeding through the midcalf to the ankle. As development proceeds, this artery is replaced in its upper part by the femoral artery developing from the external iliac artery. By the third month of gestation, the femoral artery predominates, and the vestiges of the sciatic artery remain only as the inferior gluteal artery, the distal popliteal artery, and the peroneal artery.[254]

Rarely, all or part of the sciatic artery persists into postnatal life as a large artery originating from the internal iliac artery, exiting the pelvis through the sciatic notch near the sciatic nerve, and following a course through the buttock and posterior thigh to join the popliteal artery in the popliteal fossa. The artery may coexist with a normal superficial femoral artery, or the superficial femoral artery may be hypoplastic. In some patients, the entire superficial femoral artery is absent, with the sciatic artery being the only vessel in the limb in continuity with the popliteal artery. The incidence of persistent sciatic artery is reportedly 0.03% to 0.06% in large series of femoral arteriograms, with one-third of all cases being bilateral.[255]

The anomalous lower extremity blood supply usually remains undetected until later life (mean age of detection, 51 years). Patients present with claudication or more severe lower extremity ischemic symptoms, pulsatile buttock masses,[256] or, rarely, sciatic neuropathy.[257] The anomalous artery has a proclivity for aneurysmal degeneration; up to 50% of detected sciatic arteries have been found to be aneurysmal.[258] Vascular surgeons are involved in treating both the aneurysmal and the ischemic manifestations. Although the traditional treatment is surgical ligation, endovascular coiling or covered stent placement is emerging as the procedure of choice.[259] Arterial reconstruction for lower extremity ischemia is typically performed with either femoropopliteal or iliopopliteal bypass.[260]

Popliteal Entrapment Syndromes

Stuart in 1879 was the first to describe the anatomic abnormality associated with popliteal entrapment,[261] and Hamming in 1959 reported the first successful treatment of the condition.[262] Love and Whelan[263] coined the term *popliteal artery entrapment syndrome* in 1965. The anatomic basis of this syndrome lies in the anomalous embryonic development of two independent structures, the popliteal artery and the gastrocnemius muscle.[264] Below the knee, the embryonic sciatic artery gives rise to the popliteal and tibial vessels. The femoral artery arises later as the amalgamation of a capillary plexus connecting branches of the external iliac artery proximally and branches of the sciatic artery distally. Both the femoral and sciatic arteries contribute to the popliteal artery. The femoral artery becomes dominant as the proximal sciatic artery regresses.

During this period of femoral maturation and sciatic regression, the heads of the gastrocnemius muscles develop. The anlage of the gastrocnemius muscle develops as a single muscle migrating cephalad from its origin on the calcaneus. As the gastrocnemius matures, it divides into larger medial and smaller lateral heads that gain their final attachments on the femoral epicondyles. The medial head of the gastrocnemius migrates from its lateral origin toward the medial epicondyle at the same developmental stage at which the mature popliteal artery is developing from the femoral and sciatic arteries.

A simplified classification system of popliteal entrapment recognizes four main variants based on the anomalous relationship of the popliteal artery and surrounding musculature (Fig. 8.14).[265,266] In type 1, accounting for approximately 50% of cases, the popliteal artery deviates medial to the normally placed medial head of the gastrocnemius muscle. Type 2 lesions (25% of cases) involve an abnormal attachment of the medial head of the gastrocnemius, with the popliteal artery passing medially but with less deviation than in type 1. In type 3 (6% of cases), the normally situated popliteal artery is compressed by muscle slips of the

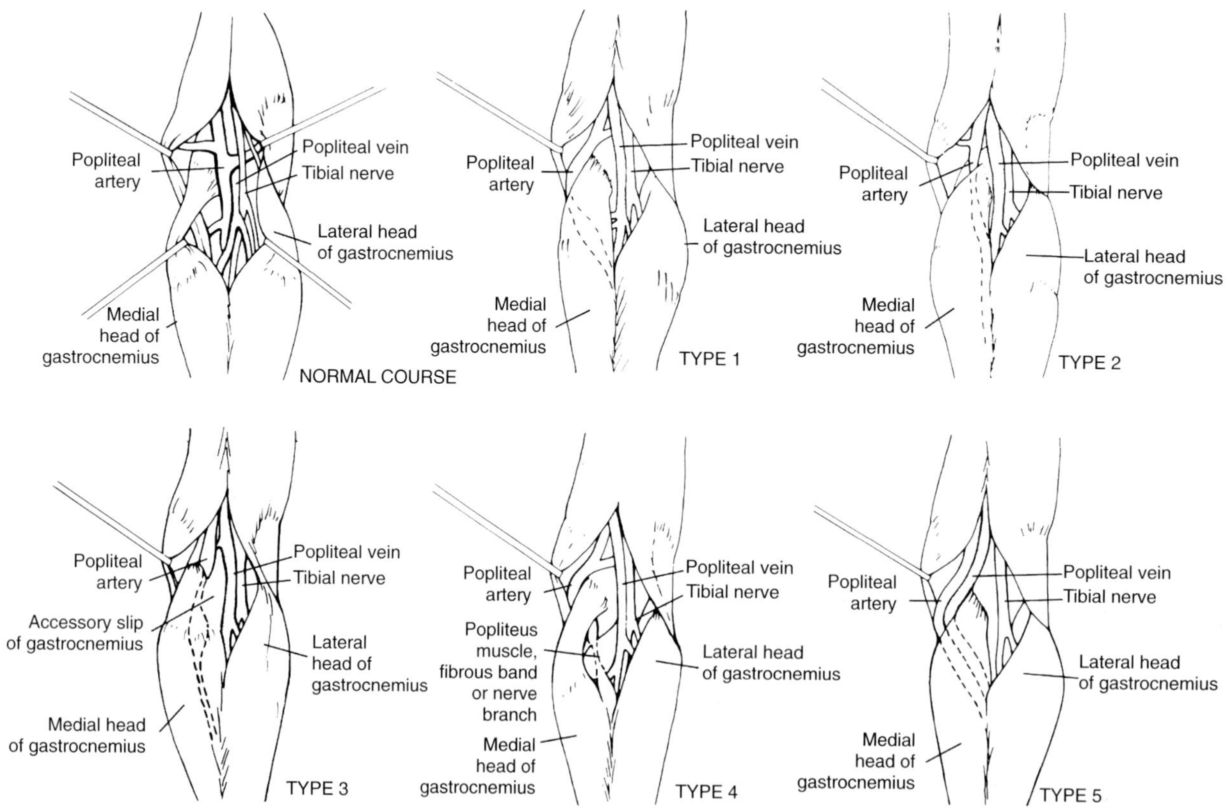

FIG 8.14 Diagram of the types of popliteal artery entrapment. (From Rich NM, Collins G, Jr, McDonald PT, et al: Popliteal vascular entrapment: its increasing interest. *Arch Surg* 114: 1377–1384, 1979.)

medial head of the gastrocnemius. Type 4 lesions have associated fibrous bands of the popliteus or plantar muscles compressing the popliteal artery. Type 5 lesions, in which the popliteal vein accompanies the artery in its abnormal course, and type 6 or functional entrapment, which occurs in symptomatic patients without identifiable anatomic abnormalities, have also been described.[267] The true incidence of popliteal artery entrapment syndrome is unknown. The reported incidence is increasing coincidentally with the development of more sophisticated diagnostic tests. A review of 20,000 patients screened with routine vascular laboratory testing identified verifiable popliteal artery entrapment syndrome in less than 1% of patients.[265] However, in an autopsy series, Gibson and colleagues[268] found an incidence of 3.5% in 86 postmortem examinations. Interestingly, all the patients were older than 60 years when they died, and the popliteal arteries showed no histologic abnormalities. Clearly, not all entrapped popliteal arteries become symptomatic. Approximately 90% of reported cases have occurred in men; more than half of these patients became symptomatic before age 30 years. The defect is bilateral in 20% of patients.[264]

Symptoms are due to obstruction of the popliteal artery with gastrocnemius contraction. Histopathologic changes distinct from typical atherosclerosis have been identified.[269] Repeated microtrauma leads to inflammatory cell infiltration and vessel wall disruption, which ultimately causes fibrosis and collagen scar formation. Thrombosis, embolism, or aneurysm formation may ensue. Symptomatic patients may have acute ischemia owing to popliteal artery occlusion (10%) or progressive intermittent claudication. Calf claudication in patients younger than 40 years is sufficiently infrequent that its presence should suggest the possibility of popliteal artery entrapment.

Most patients with popliteal entrapment are asymptomatic at rest. Symptomatic patients may have normal, reduced, or absent pulses of the lower leg. Ankle dorsiflexion or plantar flexion or knee extension may diminish or occlude distal pulses. Continuous-wave Doppler, photoplethysmography, and arterial duplex scanning have been used with these leg maneuvers to provide objective confirmation of popliteal artery entrapment.[270] However, these noninvasive tests and physical findings are nonspecific, as maneuver-induced pulse diminution can occur in normal individuals.

Arteriography demonstrating midpopliteal artery compression or medial deviation with the leg in a position of stress had been the gold standard for the diagnosis of popliteal artery entrapment syndrome during plantar flexion. The current gold standard for defining the popliteal anatomy at rest is MRI, which provides superior soft tissue definition and does not require the use of intravenous contrast to localize the vascular structures or define their patency status (Fig. 8.15).[271]

Treatment of this condition is surgical. If the syndrome is diagnosed early and minimal arterial changes are present, myotomy of the medial gastrocnemius head may be sufficient. Bypass grafting is required in patients with significant arterial stenosis, occlusion, or aneurysm formation.[272] Autogenous vein is the favored conduit for grafts across the knee. Both posterior and medial approaches have been described with similar results obtained with both techniques. Almost all patients are able to return to normal activity and have excellent long-term graft patency.[273,274]

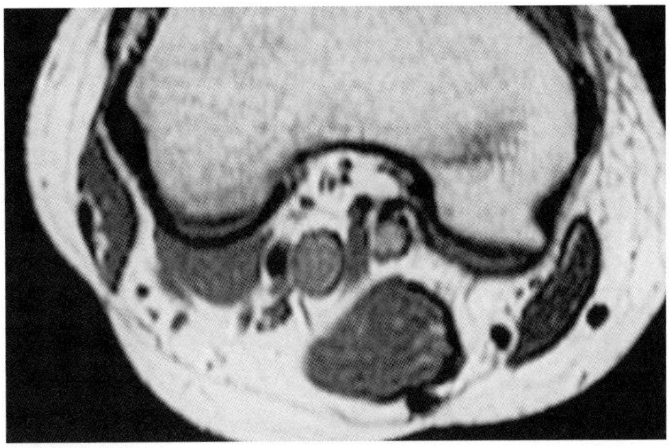

FIG 8.15 Magnetic resonance imaging scan showing the abnormal insertion of the medial head of the gastrocnemius muscle between the popliteal artery and vein. The popliteal artery ends up medial to the medial head of the gastrocnemius muscle.

Functional popliteal entrapment remains a controversial clinical entity. These patients have clinical findings of popliteal entrapment with normal popliteal fossa musculotendinous anatomy. Proposed mechanisms include popliteal artery compression due to gastrocnemius muscle hypertrophy, plantaris muscle hypertrophy or tendon compression, compression by the soleal sling, or against the lateral condyle of the tibia. Dynamic duplex and cross-sectional imaging demonstrating popliteal artery compression with plantar flexion can be used to support the diagnosis (Fig. 8.16). Surgical gastrocnemius debulking and release of the soleal sling have been performed with successful relief of symptoms.[275] Intraoperative duplex with provocative maneuvers has been used to determine adequacy of surgical debulking.[276]

Fibromuscular Dysplasia

Fibromuscular dysplasia (FMD) is a nonatherosclerotic, noninflammatory vascular disease most frequently involving the renal arteries of young white women. Detailed histologic studies have resulted in the recognition of at least four distinct pathologic types: intimal fibroplasia, medial fibroplasia, medial hyperplasia, and perimedial dysplasia.[277]

The first report of FMD by Leadbetter and Burkland[278] in 1938 described a patient with renal artery involvement. Approximately 75% of cases involve the renal artery, with the carotid and iliac arteries representing the second and third most common areas of involvement.[279] Rarely, femoral, popliteal, mesenteric, subclavian, axillary, forearm, vertebral, and coronary arteries may be involved. Multifocal disease is common with involvement of two vascular beds in 35%, three vascular beds in 22%, and four vascular beds in 9% in the US FMD registry.[280] Ten percent to 51% of patients with FMD of the internal carotid artery harbor intracranial aneurysms.[281] Ninety percent of adult patients with FMD are women. With renal involvement, 70% of patients display bilateral disease. The more severe disease almost always occurs on the right side. Lesions affecting the left renal artery alone occur in less than 10% of these patients. The prevalence of FMD

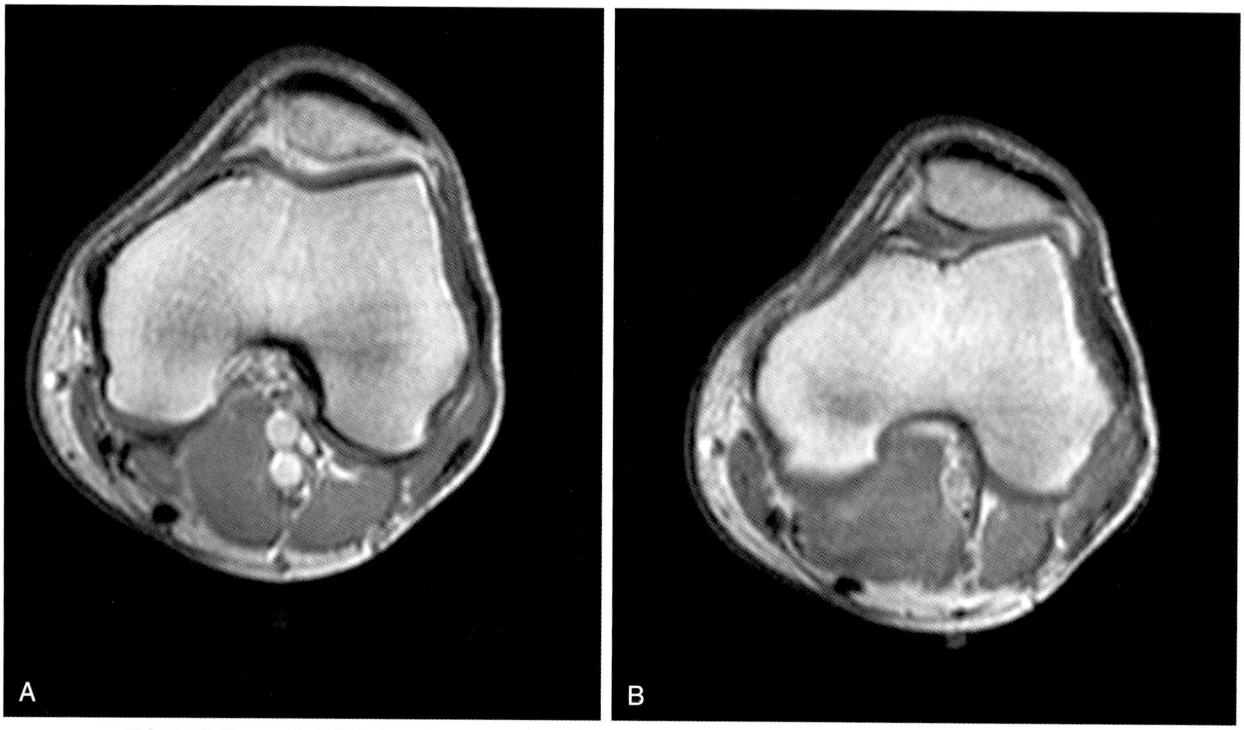

FIG 8.16 Dynamic MRI showing normal popliteal anatomy rest (A) with popliteal artery compression with plantar flexion (B). This patient went on to have gastrocnemius debulking with relief of claudication symptoms.

is unknown; however, renal FMD was identified in 3% to 6% of patients based on angiographic studies of kidney donors[282] and in the CORAL trial.[283] Carotid FMD prevalence is typically felt to be less frequent in the range of 0.3% to 3%, however in the US FMD registry it was only slightly less common than renal FMD.[280]

Medial fibroplasia accounts for 85% of FMD, perimedial dysplasia for 10%, and intimal fibroplasia for 5%.[277] The lesions of medial fibroplasia have the classic "string of beads" morphology on angiography (Fig. 8.17). The types are distinguished from one another by which vessel wall layer is primarily affected and by the tissue components that predominate. An increase of fibrous connective tissue, collagen, and ground substance within the media is characteristic of medial fibroplasia. The smooth muscle cell is multipotential and appears to be the source of the proliferative changes in FMD. Because histologic diagnoses are rarely obtained, the current recommendation is to classify lesions based on angiography as multifocal or unifocal.[284,285]

The cause of FMD is unknown. Several theories have been advanced, including (1) arterial stretching, (2) mural ischemia secondary to an abnormal distribution of vasa vasorum, (3) estrogenic (or other hormonal) effects on the arterial wall, (4) immunologic insult, and (5) anomalous embryologic development. A familial prevalence of 7% has been noted.[280] Symptoms produced by FMD are generally secondary to the associated arterial stenoses and are indistinguishable from those caused by atherosclerosis. Hypertension is the most frequent manifestation of renal artery FMD. For carotid FMD, transient ischemic attacks are rare, with most symptomatic patients having more nonspecific symptoms such as headache, pulsatile tinnitus, or dizziness.[280]

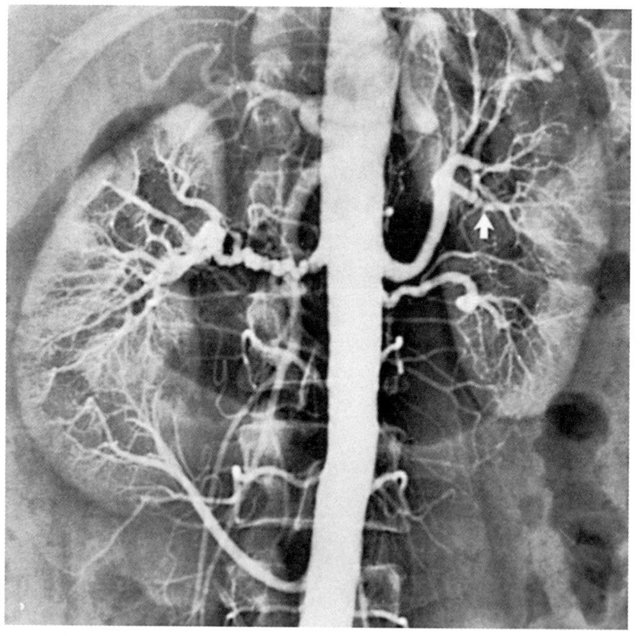

FIG 8.17 Fibromuscular Dysplasia (FMD). The superior right renal artery shows typical involvement extending beyond the primary branching. Moderate left kidney segmental artery FMD is present *(white arrow)*.

Duplex scanning of the renal arteries has proved useful in the diagnosis of renovascular FMD. As opposed to atherosclerotic renal artery stenosis, which typically involves the orifice or proximal renal artery, FMD lesions have a predilection for the middle and distal renal artery.[286] MRA and CT angiography are also frequently used imaging modalities, although they have not been systematically compared with contrast arteriography, which remains the gold standard for diagnosis.[287]

Treatment is recommended for arterial stenotic lesions only when they produce significant symptoms. Renovascular hypertension caused by FMD has responded more favorably to surgery than has that caused by atherosclerosis.[288-290] Technical success of surgical procedures ranges from 89% to 97%, with cured or improved hypertension in 67% to 93%.[288-290] Results of surgical management of children with renovascular FMD have been particularly encouraging, with cured or improved hypertension in 96% after up to 16 years of follow-up.[291] Percutaneous transluminal angioplasty has emerged as the primary treatment modality, with technical success rates of 94% to 100% and cured or improved hypertension in 74% to 88%,[292-294] although the duration of follow-up has not been as long as that of surgical series. FMD of the renal artery may be associated with the formation of renal artery aneurysms and renal artery dissection.

Treatment of cerebrovascular FMD is generally reserved for symptomatic patients. Unlike atherosclerotic disease, fibromuscular disease typically involves the distal extracranial internal carotid artery and stops before the internal carotid artery enters the base of the skull. Before the widespread application of percutaneous revascularization, surgical repair was the favored approach. Multiple techniques have been described, including open graduated internal dilation, patch angioplasty, and interposition grafting, depending on the location and extent of involvement.[295] However, percutaneous angioplasty has become the preferred treatment.

Cystic Adventitial Disease

Cystic adventitial disease is a rare condition that must always be considered in the differential diagnosis of claudication in a young patient. Single or multiple synovial-like cysts in the subadventitial layer of the arterial wall compressing the arterial lumen cause arterial stenosis. The cysts typically contain mucinous degenerative debris or clear, gelatinous material similar to that found in ganglia. Eighty percent of patients with this condition are men, and the median age at presentation is 42 years.[296] The first case report describing operative management was in 1954.[297] The popliteal artery is by far the most commonly involved artery, with the femoral and iliac arteries being the next most frequent areas of involvement. Femoral vein involvement has also been reported.[298]

The cause of cystic adventitial disease is unknown. The once-popular theory that it was caused by repeated arterial microtrauma has largely been abandoned. A direct communication with the adjacent knee joint, similar to a true ganglion, has been demonstrated in selected cases.[299,300] Currently, the most widely accepted theory is that the cysts result from the presence within the arterial wall of mucin-secreting cell rests derived embryologically from the synovial anlage of the knee joint.[301] On examination, the finding of a popliteal bruit and the absence of palpable pulses with knee flexion have been noted in a number of patients with cystic adventitial disease involving the popliteal artery. Diagnosis is possible using duplex or intravascular ultrasonography, CT, and MRI.[302] Arteriography may demonstrate segmental popliteal arterial occlusion or may show a "scimitar" sign of luminal encroachment by the cyst in a normally placed vessel that has no other signs of occlusive disease.[303]

Several methods of treatment have been described. Although spontaneous resolution has been reported,[304] for most patients, percutaneous or surgical treatment is required. Arteries with a small cyst have been successfully treated with CT- or ultrasound-guided needle aspiration or cyst enucleation,[305] although approximately 10% recur following this treatment. In more severely affected patients, segmental arterial replacement may be required. Patients with popliteal occlusion require bypass grafting with an autogenous conduit. Treatment has been successful in more than 90% of reported cases.[296,306]

External Iliac Endofibrosis

In the 1980s, thigh claudication symptoms in competitive cyclists was initially described, and the term *external iliac endofibrosis* was proposed.[307] Although this disorder is likely related to repetitive shear stress, it is not clear why specific individuals are affected, while the vast majority of competitive athletes are not at risk. Histologically, the process is distinctly different from atherosclerosis, with loosely packed collagen, no calcification, and minimal cellularity.[308] Primarily competitive cyclists are affected, but rare cases in other athletes, such as long-distance runners, have also been reported.[309]

Duplex ultrasound of the external iliac artery is often used as a diagnostic test, although a postexertional evaluation is often more illuminating because patients are often normal at rest (Fig. 8.18). MRI and contrast arteriography are also useful; however, findings are often subtle, with mild luminal narrowing over the length of the external iliac artery without focal stenoses (Fig. 8.19). Conservative therapy should be the initial therapeutic recommendation, because patients are typically only symptomatic with extreme levels of activity. For patients who wish to continue with competitive athletics, surgical options are available. Endofibrosectomy with saphenous vein patching is most frequently performed.[310] Often, the entire length of the external iliac artery needs to be treated because of the diffuse nature of the disease. Prosthetic bypass and endovascular interventions should be avoided because of the typically young age of affected individuals.[311] The majority of patients are eventually able to return to competitive athletic activities.

COMPARTMENT SYNDROME

Compartment syndrome occurs whenever tissue pressure within a confined space becomes sufficiently elevated to impair perfusion. If untreated, diminished nutritive blood flow results in limb dysfunction secondary to ischemic muscle contracture. The first clinical description of this syndrome was by von Volkmann more than a century ago in a report on contracture involving the arm following trauma. He attributed the deformity to a prolonged interruption of the vascular supply to the muscle.[312] In 1926, Jepson[313] reported successful experimental reproduction of the syndrome and demonstrated that early compartment decompression may prevent ischemic muscle paralysis and contracture.

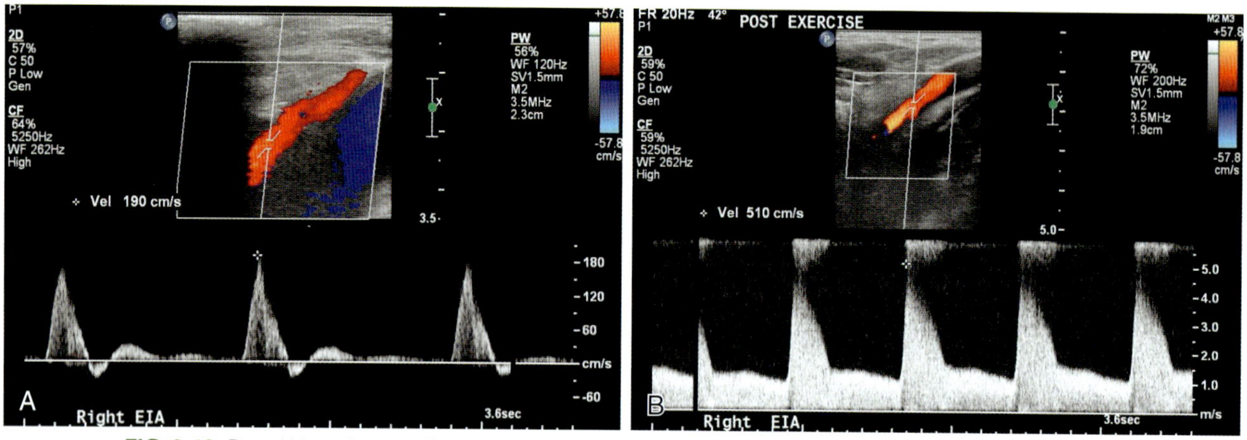

FIG 8.18 Pre- (A) and post- (B) exercise iliac artery duplex in young cyclist with right external iliac endofibrosis. Examination is normal at rest, with marked increase in peak systolic velocity and corresponding drop in ankle:brachial index with exercise.

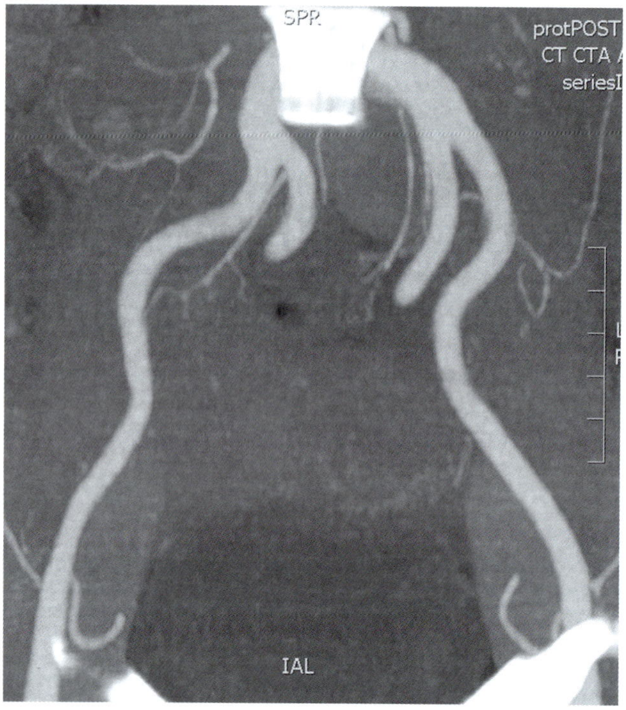

FIG 8.19 Computed tomography image of a patient with right external iliac endofibrosis. Note the subtle narrowing of the right external iliac artery in comparison with the left.

The multiple clinical causes of compartment syndrome have been well documented.[314] Any loss of vascular integrity, such as occurs following prolonged ischemia or reperfusion injury, leads to increased edema within a compartment. This edema then compromises venous outflow and increases venous and capillary pressures, leading to increased compartment pressure and decreased perfusion pressure. Pivotal to the development of the syndrome, whether from external compression or internal tissue swelling, is the production of sufficient intracompartment pressure to impair blood flow to the tissues.

The capillary leak following ischemia and reperfusion is believed to be mediated through inflammatory mediators and oxygen-derived free radicals.[315] The return of oxygenated blood to the microcirculation of ischemic tissue causes activation of inflammatory mediators locally and systemically. Neutrophil adherence to endothelium leads to oxidant release (H_2O_2, O_2, and OH^-), which damages the endothelium. Animal models suggest that treatment with free radical scavengers may mitigate the damage in compartment syndrome.[316] Experimentally blocking neutrophil adherence has also been shown to decrease reperfusion injury.[317]

There is no absolute pressure above which compartment syndrome invariably occurs, although tissue blood flow diminishes rapidly as intracompartment pressure approaches the level of the diastolic blood pressure. In addition, conditions such as hypotension or vasoconstriction may lead to the syndrome's occurrence at lower intracompartment pressures. In addition to the absolute and relative intracompartment pressures, the duration of ischemia is an important factor. Nerve tissue appears to be most susceptible to ischemia, with symptoms occurring within minutes and permanent damage at 2 hours or less. Muscle death begins at approximately 4 hours. Maximal muscle contracture appears to require approximately 12 hours of ischemia.[314] Skin and subcutaneous tissues are capable of tolerating periods of ischemia that are not tolerated by skeletal muscle or peripheral nerves.[318]

In patients with acute interruption of arterial blood flow, the incidence of compartment syndrome averages 8%.[319] The need for fasciotomy following revascularization is increased if the duration of ischemia was more than 6 hours or if there was a substantial period of shock in association with the arterial injury. Other circumstances increasing the need for fasciotomy include the occurrence of a tight swelling of the extremity preoperatively or intraoperatively, the combination of arterial and venous injury, and the presence of concomitant soft tissue crush injury. Compartment syndrome can develop in up to 30% of all extremities after combined fracture and arterial injury. Thrombolytic therapy for acute arterial occlusion must be recognized as a possible mode of reperfusion injury.[320]

In the lower leg, compartment syndrome most frequently occurs in the anterior compartment, followed by the lateral, deep posterior, and superficial posterior compartments. The quadriceps compartment in the thigh and the gluteal compartment in the buttock may be involved. In the upper extremity, the volar forearm compartment is most frequently involved, but involvement of the dorsal forearm, biceps, deltoid, and hand interosseous muscle compartments has also been reported.

The accurate diagnosis of compartment syndrome leading to successful treatment is based on recognition of the early signs and symptoms of increased compartment pressure. Diminished function of the extremity precedes nerve and muscle necrosis by several hours. Clinical signs include fullness and tenderness of the compartment, pain disproportionate to the physical findings, paresthesias of the compartment nerves, and weakness of the involved muscles. The palpable pulse status and Doppler pressures are unreliable reflections of intracompartment pressure. With compression of postcapillary venules and a continued fall in the arteriovenous perfusion gradient, tissue damage can occur despite continued arterial inflow and palpable pulses.[321]

In questionable clinical situations or when the patient is unable to communicate adequately, objective data reflecting either intracompartment pressure or nerve function may be monitored. Continuous or intermittent pressure determinations may be made by the Wick catheter technique, in which a plastic catheter is placed percutaneously into the compartment and connected to a pressure transducer.[322] A solid-state transducer that fits within a catheter tip in a hand-held unit, the "solid-state transducer in catheter" monitor, eliminates the artifacts inherent in pressure lines.[323] Surgical decompression is generally recommended for patients who have a compartment pressure of 40 mm Hg or greater or for those whose compartment pressure is greater than 30 mm Hg for 4 hours. Others argue that intervention based on fixed pressure is inappropriate and that critical intracompartment pressures occur within 30 mm Hg of the mean arterial pressure or 20 mm Hg of the diastolic pressure.[324]

Once compartment syndrome occurs, the time delay before treatment becomes the critical factor in determining outcome. Twelve hours appears to be the point beyond which significant residual dysfunction will likely occur despite adequate surgical decompression.[325] All circumferential bandages or casts should be removed at the first suspicion of increased compartment pressure to allow a complete examination of the extremity. The extremity should be placed at the level of the heart and not elevated, because elevation may further jeopardize ischemic compartment components. If physical examination, pressure measurements, or nerve conduction studies suggest a compartment syndrome, immediate surgical decompression is indicated. A frequently used decompressive technique is shown in Fig. 8.20.

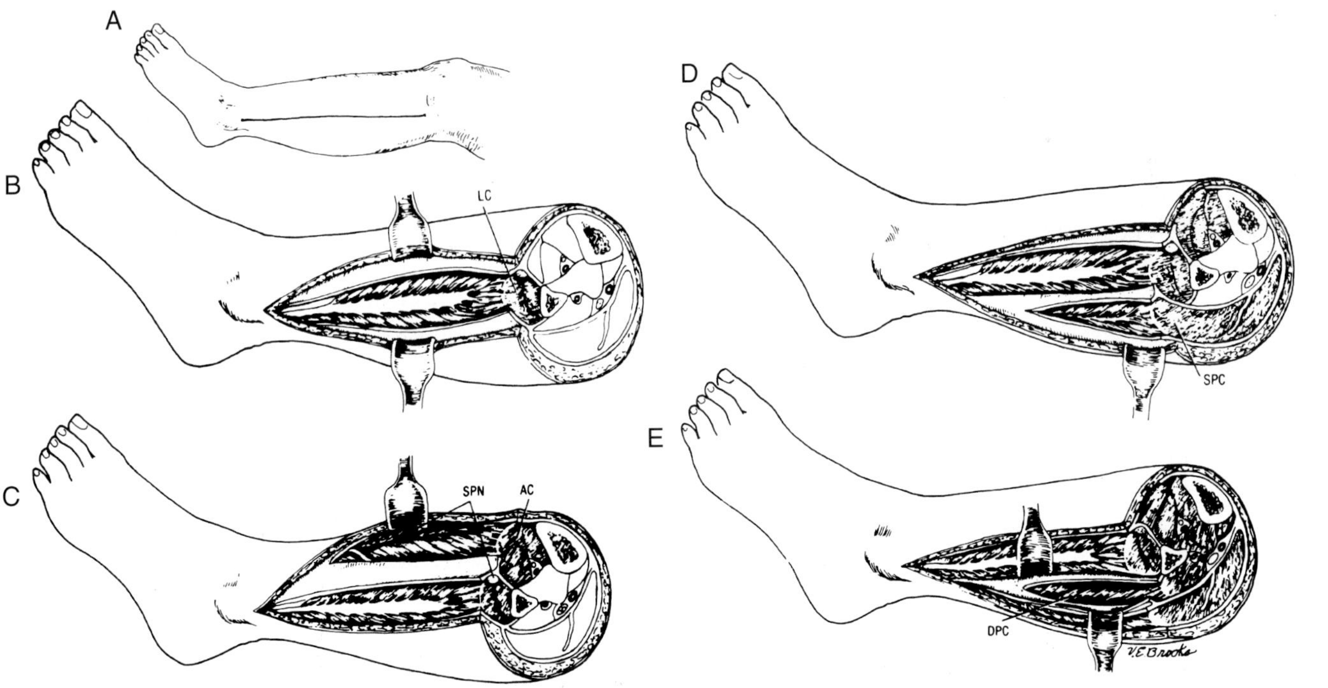

FIG 8.20 Parafibular decompression of all four compartments of the leg. (A) The skin incision runs the length of the fibula. (B) The lateral compartment *(LC)* is opened directly beneath the skin incision. (C) The anterior compartment *(AC)* is exposed by retracting the anterior skin flap and is opened over the entire length. Care is taken to preserve the superficial peroneal nerve *(SPN)*. (D) The superficial posterior compartment *(SPC)* is exposed by retracting the posterior skin flap and is opened over its entire length. (E) The lateral compartment is retracted anteriorly, and the superficial posterior compartment is retracted posteriorly after the fibular origin of the soleus muscle is released (not shown). This exposes the deep posterior compartment *(DPC)*, which is opened over its entire length. (From Matsen FA, Winquist RA, Krugmire RB: Diagnosis and management of compartmental syndromes. *J Bone Joint Surg* 62:286–291, 1980.)

Untreated compartment syndrome results in direct neurologic dysfunction or the development of contractures following fibrous replacement of myonecrosis. Symptomatic severity ranges from mild to critical, and amputation may be required. Frequent examination of the blood from patients with compartment syndrome may reveal elevated levels of creatinine phosphokinase as well as hyperkalemia. Subsequently, there may be myoglobinuria and renal failure.[326] In such patients, restoration of normal hemodynamics, the administration of mannitol to enhance urine flow and improve intrarenal blood distribution, and alkalinization of the urine to prevent precipitation of myoglobin within the renal tubules are specific therapeutic measures.[326] Prevention of the reperfusion syndrome has been shown in selected patients after the administration of hypertonic mannitol, presumably as a result of its free radical scavenging.[327] Deep muscle infections are uncommon but potentially life-threatening sequelae.

A rare but well-described form of compartment syndrome is exertional compartment syndrome seen in highly trained athletes.[328] As with other forms, the anterolateral compartments are most frequently affected. The diagnosis can be made by measuring compartment pressures at the point of exertional pain in affected individuals. Normal resting compartment pressures are less than 15 mm Hg. Compartment pressures are normally elevated following exercise but return to normal within 3 minutes.[329] The Pedowitz criteria for the diagnosis of chronic exertional compartment syndrome include pressures greater than 15 mm Hg at rest, greater than 30 mm Hg 1 minute after exercise, and greater than 20 mm Hg 5 minutes after exercise.[330] Turnipseed[329] described his experience of 276 patients with documented exertional compartment syndrome undergoing surgical treatment with open fasciectomy. Ninety-two percent of patients had complete relief of symptoms and return to normal activities.

REVIEW QUESTIONS

1. Which group with RS has the lowest risk of developing a connective tissue disease?
   a. Vasospastic, negative serologies
   b. Vasospastic, positive serologies
   c. Obstructive, negative serologies
   d. Obstructive, positive serologies
   e. Obstructive, unknown serologies
2. Vasculitis is a central feature in all of the following syndromes except:
   a. Kawasaki disease
   b. Cogan syndrome
   c. Behçet disease
   d. Takayasu disease
   e. Gilbert disease
3. The majority of patients with temporal arteritis are encompassed in which of the following groups?
   a. 50 years, male, white
   b. 50 years, female, nonwhite
   c. 50 years, male, nonwhite
   d. 50 years, male and female, nonwhite
   e. 50 years, female, white
4. What is the optimal initial treatment for subacute upper extremity ischemia caused by temporal arteritis?
   a. Steroids
   b. Endarterectomy
   c. Saphenous vein bypass
   d. Thrombolytic therapy
   e. Warfarin anticoagulation
5. Which of the following is of greatest benefit in the treatment of patients with Buerger disease?
   a. Sympathectomy
   b. Oral vasodilators
   c. Arterial reconstructive surgery
   d. Warfarin anticoagulation
   e. Cessation of tobacco use
6. Extensive vascular calcification in a young patient with normal parathyroid function suggests which of the following?
   a. Hyperlipidemia
   b. Hurler syndrome
   c. Pseudoxanthoma elasticum
   d. Marfan syndrome
   e. Ehlers-Danlos syndrome
7. Abdominal coarctation is most frequently discovered during evaluation for which symptom?
   a. Claudication
   b. Blue toe syndrome
   c. Weight loss
   d. Hypertension
   e. Abdominal pain
8. Calf claudication in a nonsmoker younger than 30 years is most commonly caused by which disorder?
   a. Popliteal entrapment syndrome
   b. Atherosclerosis
   c. Polyarteritis nodosa
   d. Takayasu disease
   e. Homocysteinemia
9. The early objective diagnosis of anterior compartment syndrome is best made by which finding?
   a. Absent dorsal pedal pulse
   b. Foot drop
   c. Tense swelling
   d. Localized compartment pain
   e. Compartment pressure measurement with Wick or the "solid-state transducer in catheter" monitor
10. Which of the following regarding popliteal artery entrapment is true?
    a. Usually associated with an abnormal relationship between the popliteal artery and the lateral head of gastrocnemius muscle
    b. Frequently seen in association with persistent sciatic artery
    c. Equally affects males and females
    d. Can occur with normal popliteal anatomy
    e. Predisposes affected individuals to anterior collateral ligament injury

BIBLIOGRAPHY

Espinosa G, Font J, Tassies D, et al. Vascular involvement in Behçet's disease. *Am J Med.* 2002;112:37–43.

Gio HVL, Greene PS, Alejo DE, et al. Replacement of the aortic root in patients with Marfan's syndrome. *N Engl J Med.* 1999;340:1307–1313.

Miyata T, Sato O, Koyama H, et al. Long-term survival after surgical treatment of patients with Takayasu's arteritis. *Circulation.* 2003;108:1474–1480.

Olin JW. Current concepts: thromboangiitis obliterans (Buerger's disease). *N Engl J Med.* 2000;343:864–869.

Salvarani C, Cantini F, Boiardi L, et al. Polymyalgia rheumatica and giant-cell arteritis. *N Engl J Med.* 2002;347:261–271.

Slovut DP, Olin JW. Current concepts: fibromuscular dysplasia. *N Engl J Med.* 2004;350:1862–1871.

Turnipseed WD. Popliteal entrapment syndromes. *J Vasc Surg.* 2002;35:910–915.

Wigley F. Raynaud's phenomenon. *N Engl J Med.* 2002;347:1001–1008.

SELECTED REFERENCES

1. Carpentier PH, Satger B, Poensin D, et al. Incidence and natural history of Raynaud phenomenon: a long-term follow-up (14 years) of a random sample from the general population. *J Vasc Surg.* 2006;44:1023–1028.
2. Kitamura S, Tsuda E, Kobayashi J, et al. Twenty-five-year outcome of pediatric coronary artery bypass surgery for Kawasaki disease. *Circulation.* 2009;120:60–68.
3. Saadoun D, Lambert M, Mirault T, et al. Retrospective analysis of surgery versus endovascular intervention in Takayasu arteritis a multicenter experience. *Circulation.* 2012;125:813–819.
4. Olin JW. Current concepts: thromboangiitis obliterans (Buerger's disease). *N Engl J Med.* 2000;343:864–869.
5. Waterman AL, Feezor RJ, Lee WA, et al. Endovascular treatment of acute and chronic aortic pathology in patients with Marfan syndrome. *J Vasc Surg.* 2012;55:1234–1241.
6. Brooke BS, Arnaoutakis G, McDonnell NB, et al. Contemporary management of vascular complications associated with Ehlers-Danlos syndrome. *J Vasc Surg.* 2010;51:131–139.
7. Loeys BL, Schwarze U, Holm T, et al. Aneurysm syndromes caused by mutations in the TGF-beta receptor. *N Engl J Med.* 2006;355:788–798.
8. Kranenburg G, de Jong PA, Mali WP, et al. Prevalence and severity of arterial calcifications in pseudoxanthoma elasticum (PXE) compared to hospital controls. Novel insights in the vascular phenotype of PXE. *Atherosclerosis.* 2017;256:7–14.
9. Olin JW, Froehlich J, Gu X, et al. The United States Registry for Fibromuscular Dysplasia: results in the first 447 patients. *Circulation.* 2012;125:3182–3190.
10. Collaborators IN. Diagnosis and management of iliac artery endofibrosis: results of a Delphi Consensus Study. *Eur J Vasc Endovasc Surg.* 2016;52:90–98.

References available online at ExpertConsult.com.

9 CHAPTER

Venous Vascular Malformations

Peter Gloviczki

Vascular malformations (VMs) are developmental abnormalities of the vascular system. They should be differentiated from vascular tumors or hemangiomas because they have different etiologies, growth patterns, treatments, and outcomes. Malformations can involve any segment of the vascular tree: arteries, capillaries, veins, or lymphatics. High-flow arteriovenous malformations are associated with the shunting of large amount of arterial blood into the venous system. These lesions can have significant hemodynamic manifestations, such as venous engorgement, distal limb ischemia, and high-output cardiac failure. High-flow malformations are discussed in detail in Chapter 10. This chapter focuses on low-flow venous vascular malformations (VVMs), which are seen most commonly in vascular clinics; many have a benign clinical course and require no special treatment. Many VMs are mixed, and some complex VVMs, like Klippel-Trenaunay syndrome (KTS), are associated with developmental abnormalities of other tissues, such as bone and soft tissue overgrowth or digital abnormalities.[1]

HISTORICAL NOTES

Birthmarks and congenital deformities afflicting humanity have been described by historians and depicted by painters for centuries. Malan and Puglionisi[2] were the first to attempt a classification of VMs (angiodysplasia), although the first practical guidelines for clinical classification and treatment were given by Szilagyi and colleagues.[3,4] Rutherford[5] also summarized the state of the art of VMs; of the multiple classifications published on these disorders, the Hamburg classification, in a revised form, is used most frequently.[6] Although surgical excision has been recommended for local lesions, selective catheterization and embolotherapy as well as percutaneous sclerotherapy that have changed the multidisciplinary management of VMs over the last decades.[6]

DEFINITION OF VASCULAR MALFORMATIONS AND VASCULAR TUMORS

VMs are localized errors of angiogenic development, whereas hemangiomas are vascular tumors. Mulliken and Glowacki[7,8] defined the endothelial characteristics and cell biology of VMs and vascular tumors. The term *hemangioma* should be reserved for vascular tumors alone; during the proliferative phase, they undergo growth and then usually resolution. The proliferative phase occurs during the first year, and spontaneous involution of hemangiomas is observed in 95% of cases by the age of 7 years. The female-to-male ratio is 5 to 1. Thirty percent of the hemangiomas are present at birth; the rest develop within the first 3 months of life. Endothelial hyperplasia is evident on biopsy specimens obtained from hemangiomas; these cells grow in tissue culture. In the proliferative phase, they incorporate [^{3}H]-thymidine and have an increased number of mast cells. Many patients with hemangiomas require no treatment at all.

In contrast, VMs are developmental, congenital abnormalities. There is increasing evidence that aberrant signaling at the molecular level results in dysfunction of normal proliferation, differentiation, maturation, and apoptosis of the vascular cells.[9] Localized, superficial VVMs or capillary VMs ("birthmarks" of the skin and the mucosa) are the most frequent, but VMs also occur in the skeletal muscles, pelvis, chest, visceral organs such as the lungs, gastrointestinal system, and brain. The abnormal vascular channels are lined by a continuous endothelium and surrounded by an abnormal complement of mural cells. Ninety percent of these cells are present at birth, and the male-to-female ratio is 1 to 1. VMs show no endothelial proliferation, no cell growth is observed in tissue culture, the cells do not incorporate [^{3}H]-thymidine, and no mast cells have been observed in biopsy specimens.[8] Clinically, no proliferation or spontaneous involution has been observed in VMs. The growth of the malformation is usually commensurate with the growth of the child, although hemodynamic factors (arteriovenous shunting, venous stasis) can accelerate growth and morbidity. Most low-flow VMs have a benign course, although complications such as bleeding, thrombophlebitis, skin changes, or infection may require treatment. High-flow arteriovenous malformations usually have a more ominous course and a worse prognosis. Treatment of these lesions, as discussed in Chapter 10, is often required.

DEVELOPMENT OF THE VASCULAR SYSTEM

The classification, clinical presentation, and prognosis of VMs are largely dependent on the point at which there is an arrest or abnormality in the development of the vascular system; therefore, it is worthwhile to review briefly the normal development of the vascular tree of the limbs. Primitive vascular channels first appear in the third week of gestation. During its development, the vascular system undergoes differentiation through multiple stages.[10] Stage 1 is the undifferentiated stage, with only a capillary network being present. Stage 2 is the retiform stage, when large plexiform structures can be seen. Stage 3, the maturation stage, includes development of large channels, arteries, and veins.

Vascular endothelial growth factor (VEGF) secreted by keratinocytes has been found to be responsible for inducing the penetration of capillary vessels into the avascular epidermis.[11] This invasion and the subsequent arterial differentiation are also guided by VEGF originating from sensory nerves.[12] A defective migratory response of endothelial cells to VEGF is the consequence of abnormal signaling of VEGF receptors. Malformations develop if the differentiation is abnormal and there is an arrest in the development of normal vascular tissue. It is indeed the persistence of the normal embryonic vascular system and any additional abnormal development that result in VMs.

CLASSIFICATION

Classification has been difficult because of the complex presentation and frequently mixed nature of VMs. The classification by Szilagyi and colleagues[3,4] was based primarily on Woollard's stages of embryologic development: capillary malformations develop when there is an arrest in stage 1 (Fig. 9.1). Although Szilagyi named them hemangiomas, these are not tumors but capillary or cavernous VM's. Microfistulous or macrofistulous arteriovenous malformations develop if there is an arrest in stage 2 (see Fig. 9.1). Persistence of large embryonic veins that develop in stage 3 is seen in patients with a persistent sciatic vein (Fig. 9.2) or in those with large lateral veins of the leg (Fig. 9.3). There are many mixed VMs owing to the involvement of several segments of the vascular system (capillaries, veins, lymphatics).

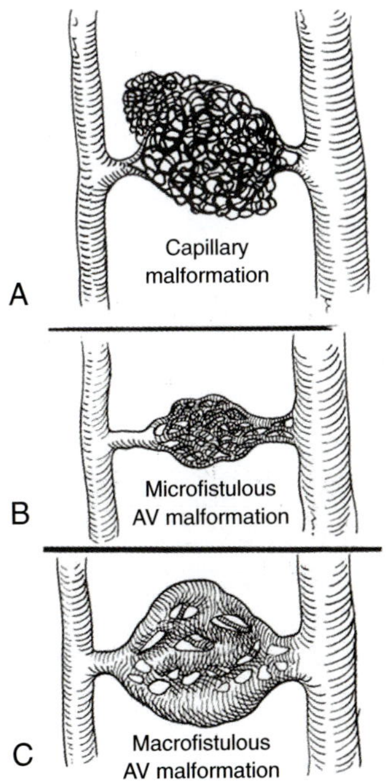

FIG 9.1 (A) Capillary malformation. (B) Microfistulous arteriovenous *(AV)* malformation. (C) Macrofistulous AV malformation.

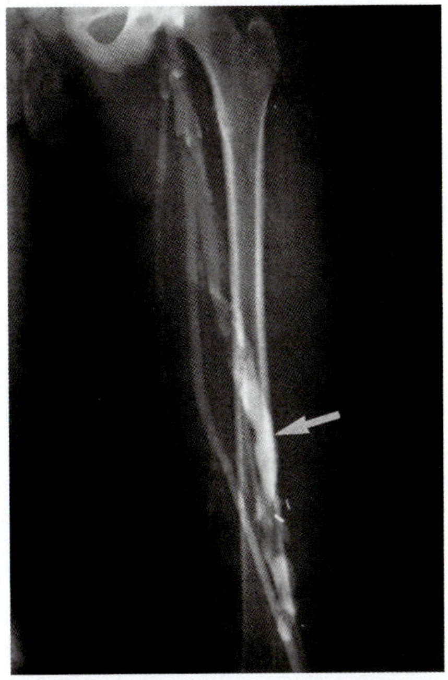

FIG 9.2 Persistent sciatic vein *(arrow)* in a 12-year-old girl. Surgical resection of the painful vein through a posterior approach resulted in an excellent clinical result at 7 years. The dilated vein contained no valves. (From Cherry KJ, Gloviczki P, Stanson AW: Persistent sciatic vein: diagnosis and treatment of a rare condition. *J Vasc Surg 23*:490–497, 1996.)

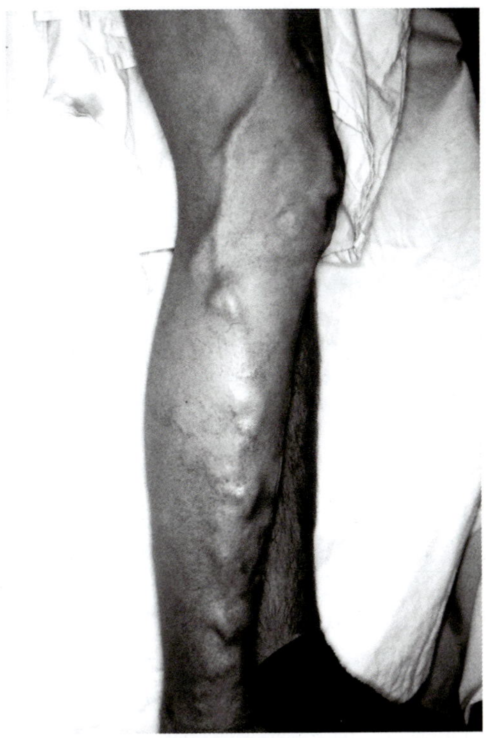

FIG 9.3 Persistent lateral embryonic veins in a 19-year-old male with Klippel-Trenaunay syndrome. (From Noel AA, Gloviczki P, Cherry KJ, Jr, et al: Surgical treatment of venous malformations in Klippel-Trenaunay syndrome. *J Vasc Surg 32*:840–847, 2000.)

The International Society for the Study for Vascular Anomalies (ISSVA) classification[13] distinguishes fast- and slow-flow VMs. A whole spectrum of malformations can be found between these two extremes.

The most recent recommendation is a combination of the modified Hamburg classification and the ISSVA classification, which divides the VMs into two major groups, low- and high-flow malformations (Table 9.1).[6] Low-flow malformation include VVMs as well as capillary, lymphatic, and combined lesions; high-flow VMs include arterial and arteriovenous malformations. Each malformation is then further classified for most categories into truncular or extratruncular forms, depending on the involvement of major axial vessels or branches of major arteries or veins.

VVMs may be truncular; these include aplasia or obstruction, stenosis or hypoplasia, dilations, and aneurysms. Many patients with KTS have persistence of large embryonic veins or hypoplasia, dilation, or aneurysmal dilation of the deep veins of the limb (Fig. 9.4).[1,14,15] The estimated prevalence of deep venous anomalies in patients with predominantly venous malformations was 47% in one study.[16] Phlebectasia, defined as dilated or aneurysmal deep veins, was the most frequent (36%), followed by aplasia or hypoplasia of the deep venous trunks (8%) and venous aneurysms (8%).

Extratruncular VVMs are the most frequent malformations; they can be diffuse (Fig. 9.5) or localized. Most venous malformations are localized defects of vascular morphogenesis that manifest as single or multiple bluish-purple lesions, mainly in the skin and mucosa.[17] Biopsy specimens show enlarged endothelial-lined vein-like channels with abnormal smooth muscle cells.

Capillary malformations, or port-wine stains, are frequent. These cutaneous lesions appear as red macular stains that darken over years (Fig. 9.6). Capillary malformations are typical in patients with Sturge-Weber syndrome, KTS, and Parkes Weber syndrome.[6]

Lymphatic malformations have been found frequently in some series. The truncular form includes obstruction or hypoplasia causing congenital lymphedema,[18,19] or dilation leading to valvular incompetence and rupture of lymphatics, causing chylous effusions or chylocutaneous fistulas owing to reflux of the chyle.[20,21] Most lymphatic cysts and lymphangiomas are lymphatic malformations, and many venous malformations contain lymphatic tissue.

TABLE 9.1 Classification of Vascular Malformations Based on Anatomy and Blood Flow

Malformation	Blood Flow
Arterial[a] Arteriovenous[a]	High flow
Venous[a] Lymphatic[a] Capillary	Low flow
Combined[a]	High flow or low flow

[a]Each can be extratruncular (diffuse or localized) or truncular (with obstruction or dilation).

Modified from Lee BB, Baumgartner I, Berlien P, et al: Diagnosis and treatment of venous malformations. Consensus document of the International Union of Phlebology (IUP): updated 2013. *Int Angiol* *34*:97–149, 2015. and Dasgupta R, Fishman SJ. ISSVA classification. *Semin Pediatr Surg* *23*:158–161, 2014.

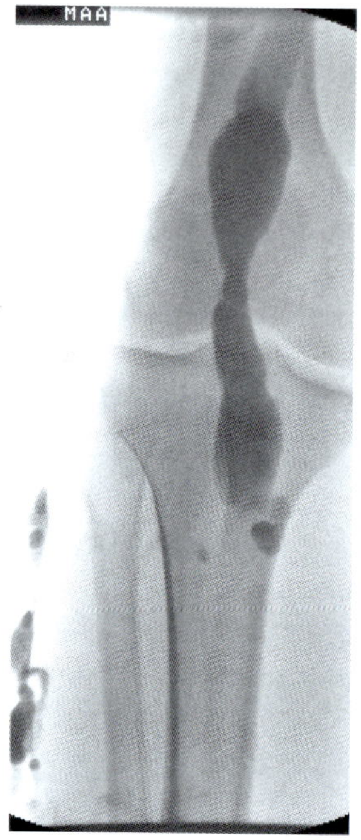

FIG 9.4 Aneurysmal dilation of the popliteal vein with a band-like narrowing associated with an atypical lateral varicosity in a 19-year-old male with Klippel-Trenaunay syndrome. (From Noel AA, Gloviczki P, Cherry KJ, Jr, et al: Surgical treatment of venous malformations in Klippel-Trenaunay syndrome. *J Vasc Surg* *32*: 840–847, 2000.)

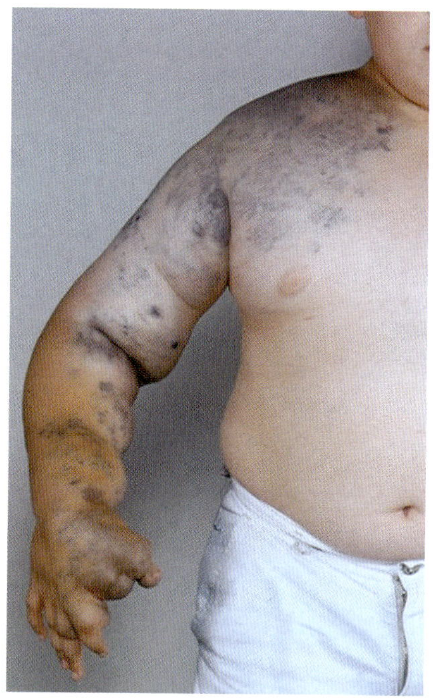

FIG 9.5 Diffuse extratruncular venous malformation involving the right arm. (Courtesy David J. Driscoll, MD, Mayo Foundation.)

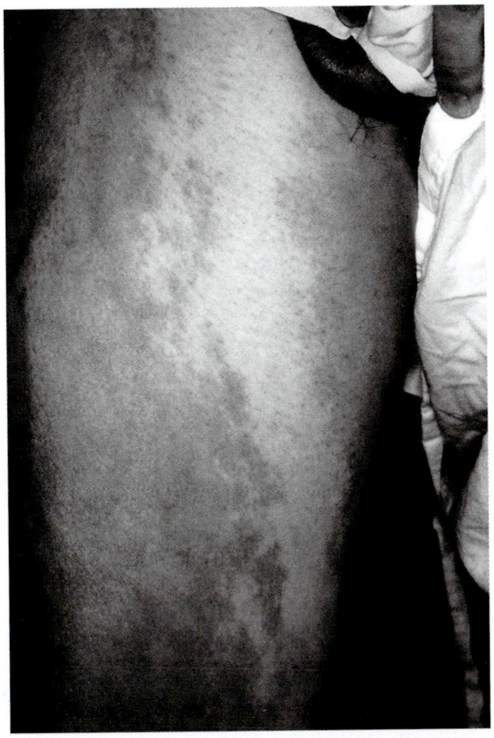

FIG 9.6 Port-wine stain (capillary malformation) on affected extremity of patient with Klippel-Trenaunay syndrome. Note also large lateral embryonic vein of the thigh. (From Noel AA, Gloviczki P, Cherry KJ, Jr, et al: Surgical treatment of venous malformations in Klippel-Trenaunay syndrome. *J Vasc Surg 32*: 840–847, 2000.)

More than 70% of the VMs are mixed, and these frequently complex abnormalities can include arterial, capillary, venous, or lymphatic elements as well. Although the Hamburg classification discourages the use of eponyms, some terms are named after physicians who first described the conditions; these have been widely accepted and used. The list of clinical syndromes of VM includes Parkes Weber, Klippel-Trenaunay, Servelle-Martorell (Fig. 9.7), Sturge-Weber, Rendu-Osler-Weber, von Hippel-Lindau, Kasabach-Merritt, Proteus (Fig. 9.8), and Maffucci syndromes (Table 9.2.)[1,12,22-24]

GENETICS

Genetic information on VMs has greatly increased in recent years.[25-27] Most VMs are sporadic, but autosomal dominant inheritance has also been described. Genetic studies of families have resulted in the identification of mutated genes[9,18,28,29] that have an important role in angiogenesis. These mutated genes in some patients encode tyrosine kinase receptors and intracellular signaling molecules. Vikkula and colleagues[30] identified the endothelial-specific angiopoietin receptor TIE2/TEK, located on 9p21, as the cause of familial mucocutaneous VMs. Glomuvenous malformations (venous malformations with glomus cells, or glomangiomas) are similar to VMs; most of these lesions are inherited, and Boon and colleagues[31] have identified the gene glomulin, a novel locus on the short arm of chromosome 1. Somatic mosaicism[32] with gene mutations was identified in Proteus syndrome *(AKT1)*, KTS *(AGGF1)*, Mafucci syndrome *(IDH1*

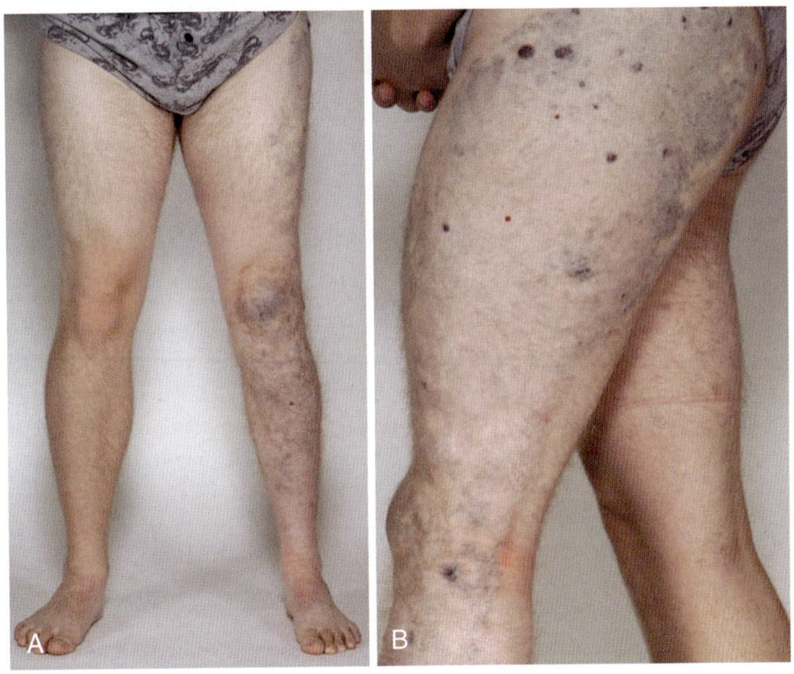

FIG 9.7 In Servelle-Martorell syndrome (A, anterior view, B, lateral view) the typical venous malformation is extratruncular and diffuse. The affected extremity is shorter, there are phleboliths present on plain radiographs, and there is no arteriovenous shunting. Spontaneous bone fracture and osteopenia are frequent. There are usually no port-wine stains. (Courtesy David J. Driscoll, MD, Mayo Foundation.)

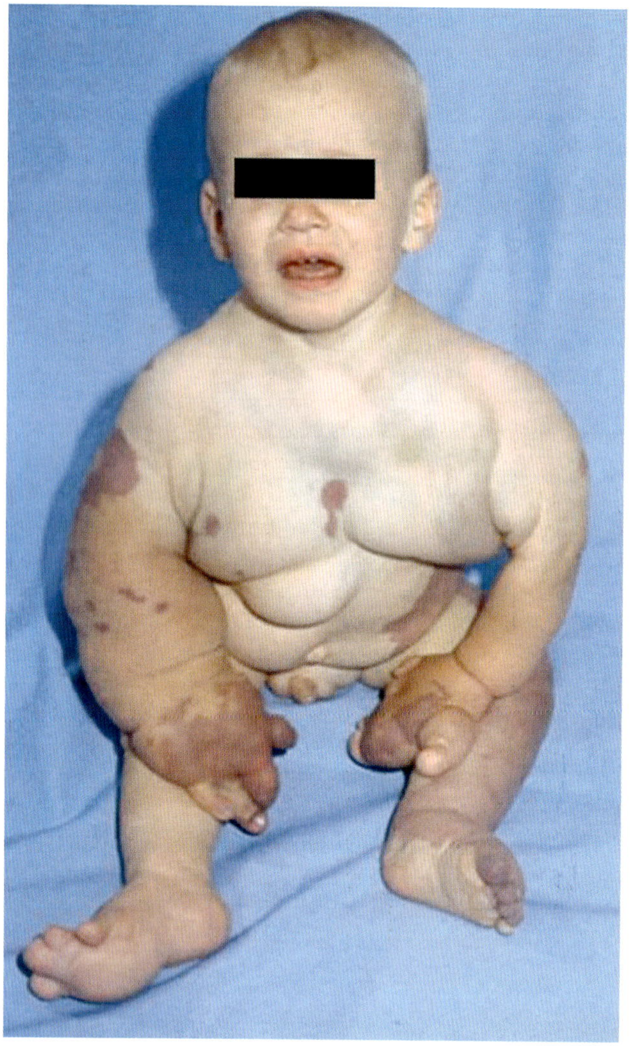

FIG 9.8 Patient with Proteus syndrome consisting of disproportionate overgrowth of multiple tissues, vascular malformations, and connective tissue or linear epidermal nevi. The patient had multiple lipomas and hyperostosis. (Courtesy David J. Driscoll, MD, Mayo Foundation.)

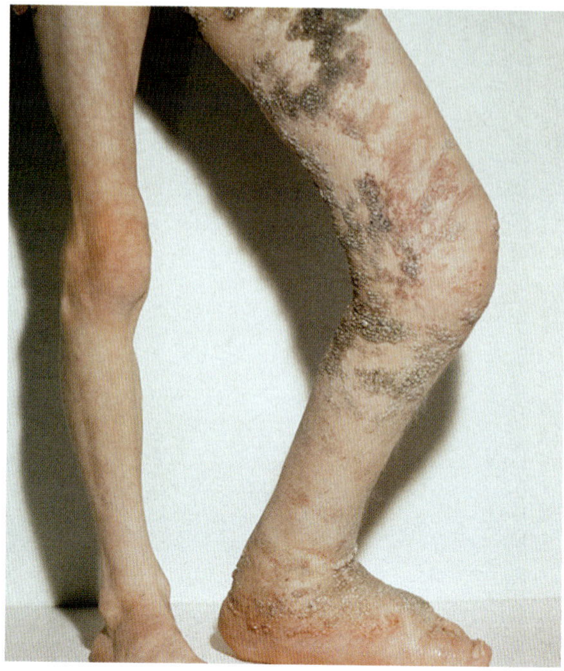

FIG 9.9 Klippel-Trenaunay syndrome with overgrowth of the left lower extremity by 12 cm.

and *IDH2*), Sturge–Weber syndrome *(GNAQ)*, and CLOVES syndrome *(PIK3CA)* (see Table 9.2).[33]

Port-wine stains have also been observed in families, and a genetic susceptibility for these capillary malformations has been suggested. Eerola and colleagues[28] identified a large locus, CMC1, on chromosome 5q. These authors used genetic mapping to identify a positional candidate gene, *RASA1*; heterozygous inactivating *RASA1* mutations were detected in families manifesting capillary malformations. Of interest, arteriovenous malformation, arteriovenous fistula, or Parkes Weber syndrome were also documented in all the families with this mutation.

Primary congenital lymphedema can be hereditary (Milroy disease), whereas late-onset primary lymphedema was also observed in multiple members of the same families (Meige disease).[34] Congenital lymphedema has been linked to chromosome 5q35.3, where the *VEGFR3* gene (VEGF receptor 3) is located. It is likely that congenital lymphedema is caused by a lack of sufficient signaling via the VEGFR3 receptor.[30]

INCIDENCE

VMs occur in approximately 1.5% of the population.[16] Published series of VMs seen at referral centers suggest that predominantly VVMs are the most common vascular anomalies; they are estimated to occur in between 1 of 5000 and 1 of 10,000 childbirths.[30] VVMs are certainly the most frequent that require medical attention.[6] Still, it is likely that capillary malformations or port-wine stains of the skin and mucosa are the most frequent VMs, occurring in 0.3% of childbirths.[28] Among 797 patients with VMs reported by Lee and colleagues,[35] 40% had predominantly lymphatic malformations.

CLINICAL PRESENTATION AND PHYSICAL EXAM

Patients with VVMs are frequently asymptomatic, and a birthmark of the skin or the mucosa is a cosmetic deformity only. However, patients who seek consultations by vascular surgeons may have a complex presentation or juvenile varicosity, and the limbs or pelvis may have extensive involvement by the malformation. Clinical presentations include varicose veins (see Fig. 9.3), limb edema or overgrowth (Fig. 9.9), port-wine stain, or digital anomalies (Figs. 9.10 and 9.11). The varicose veins are usually atypical, lateral, or suprapubic, although occasionally a varicosity may involve the great saphenous vein and its tributaries. Bleeding or leakage of lymph fluid from VVMs is not infrequent. Thrombophlebitis, cellulitis and lymphangitis, skin lesions, induration, pigmentation, and ulcerations can be signs of chronic venous insufficiency. Many of the patients with mixed lesions have associated lymphedema. Patients with pelvic involvement may exhibit hematuria and rectal bleeding. Any patient with

TABLE 9.2 **Clinical Syndromes Associated With Vascular Malformations**

Syndrome	Inheritance (Gene)	Type	Location	Characteristic Features	Treatment	Prognosis
Parkes Weber	Somatic mutations (RASA1)	AVM (intraosseal or close to epiphyseal plate), port-wine stain	Extremities, pelvis	Soft tissue and bony hypertrophy; varicosity (atypical); capillary and high-flow, high-shunt AVM	Observation, elastic support, embolization ± excision (localized lesions only)	Deep diffuse lesions have a poor prognosis
Klippel-Trenaunay	Somatic mutations (AGGF1)	Hemolymphatic malformation (VVM, lymphatic, and capillary malformation)	Extremities, pelvis, trunk	Soft tissue and bone hypertrophy; varicosities (lateral lumbar to foot pattern); capillary or venous vascular malformation, lymphatic malformation	Elastic support; Selective invasive Tx: epiphyseal stapling or selective excision or ablation of varicose veins, sclerotherapy	Usually good
Rendu-Osler-Weber (hereditary hemorrhagic telangiectasia)	Autosomal dominant (ENG, ACVRL1, MADH4)	Punctate angioma, telangiectasia, GI tract AVM	Skin, mucous membranes, liver, lungs, kidneys, brain, spinal cord	Epistaxis, hematemesis, melena, hematuria, hepatomegaly, neurologic symptoms	Transfusions; embolization vs. laser treatment ± excision	Good if bleeding can be controlled and no CNS manifestations
Sturge-Weber (encephalotrigeminal angiomatosis)	No (GNAQ)	CM	Trigeminal area, leptomeninges, choroid, oral mucosa	Convulsions, hemiplegia, ocular deformities, mental retardation, glaucoma, intracerebral calcification	Anticonvulsants, neurosurgical procedure	Guarded; depends on intracranial lesion
von Hippel-Lindau (oculo cerebellar hemangioblastomatosis)	Autosomal dominant (VHL)	Hemangioma	Retina, cerebellum	Cysts in cerebellum, pancreas, liver, adrenals, kidneys	Excision of cysts	Depends on intracranial lesion
Blue rubber bleb nevus	Autosomal dominant (TEK)	Cavernous venous malformation	Skin, GI tract, spleen, liver, CNS	Bluish, compressible rubbery lesions; GI bleeding; anemia	Transfusions, electrocoagulation, excision	Depends on CNS and GI involvement
Kasabach-Merritt	Autosomal dominant	Larger cavernous malformation	Trunk, extremities	Thrombocytopenia, hemorrhage, anemia, ecchymosis, purpura	Compression; transfusion of blood, platelets	Death from hemorrhage or infection
Maffucci (dyschondroplasia with vascular hamartoma)	Probably autosomal dominant (IDH1, IDH2)	AVM, cavernous lymphangioma	Fingers, toes, extremities, viscera	Enchondromas; spontaneous fractures; deformed, shorter extremity; vitiligo	Orthopedic management	Chance of malignancy 20%

AVM, Arteriovenous malformation; *CM*, capillary malformation; *CNS*, central nervous system; *GI*, gastrointestinal; *LM*, lymphatic malformation; *VVM*, venous vascular malformation; *VM*, vascular malformation.

varicose veins or port-wine stains with a longer or shorter limb could also have an underlying VM. Patients with primary or secondary lymphedema have limbs of identical length.

Low-flow VVMs should be differentiated from high-flow arteriovenous malformations based on the physical exam alone. If an arteriovenous malformation is present, the affected limb or pelvis may harbor a mass that is pulsatile; it may have a systolic-diastolic bruit and a palpable thrill that can be easily appreciated when the hand is placed over the affected area. The distal pulses are usually diminished and evidence of venous congestion distal to the fistula is frequent.

Diagnostic tests should focus on evaluation of the type and extent of the malformation. The presence or absence of any arteriovenous shunting must also be established. Physical examination of limb and pelvic lesions should be complemented by segmental systolic limb pressure measurement and establishment of the ankle-brachial index. Pulse volume recording is helpful in patients with arteriovenous malformations Placement of a tourniquet on a limb with a high-flow, high-shunt arteriovenous malformation and occlusion of the fistula will increase systolic blood pressure, which is followed by slowing of the heart rate because of a vagal response in the baroreceptors in the aorta and carotid arteries (bradycardia, or Branham sign). Duplex scanning will confirm other hemodynamic consequences of an arteriovenous shunt, such as low-resistance waveform in the arteries and pulsatile flow in the veins. Duplex scanning will also establish patency of the superficial and deep veins and other abnormalities, including an aneurysm or arterial dilation,

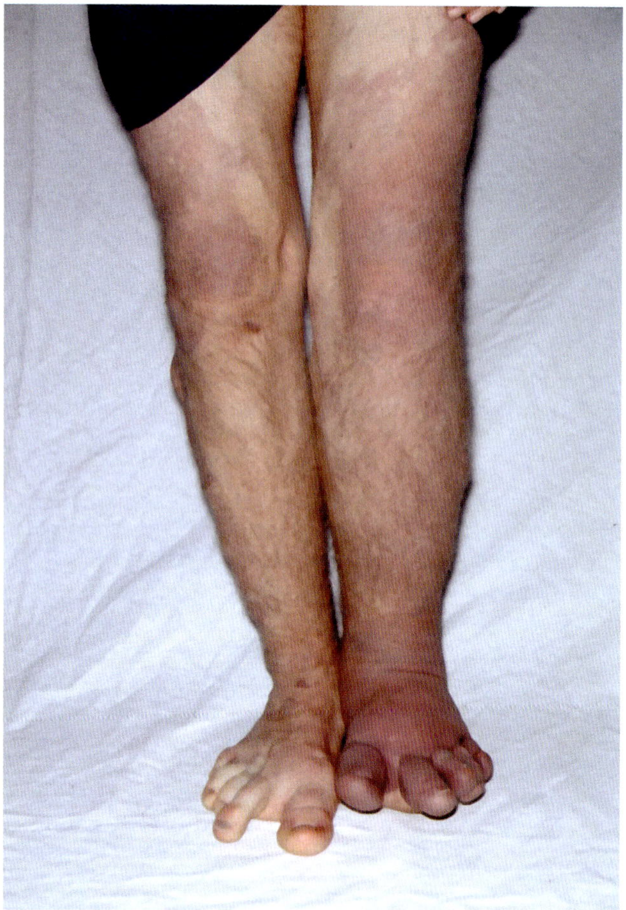

FIG 9.10 Klippel-Trenaunay syndrome with involvement of both lower extremities. Note the port-wine stain and digital anomalies.

hypoplasia, or valvular incompetence of the superficial or deep veins.

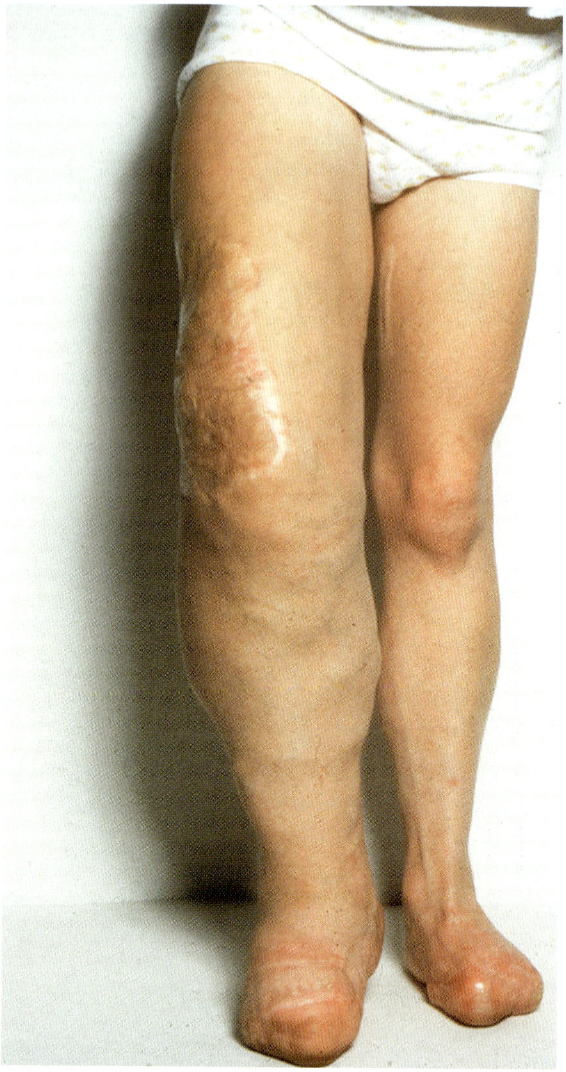

FIG 9.11 Bilateral leg involvement in Klippel-Trenaunay syndrome. Bilateral transmetatarsal amputations were needed because of digital anomalies.

IMAGING STUDIES

Scanograms are performed to document any length discrepancy between the limbs. Scanograms are long-bone radiographs that provide the most accurate measurement of the length of the long bones of the upper and lower limbs (Fig. 9.12).

Computed tomography angiography (CTA) and venography (CTV) have progressed rapidly in recent years; they provide excellent images of the malformations. A CTA will show the extent of involvement, but arteriovenous malformations might not always be distinguished from VVMs. Because intravenous contrast is required, appropriate timing of the imaging is needed, depending on the amount of blood shunted in the VM.

Magnetic resonance imaging (MRI), magnetic resonance arteriography (MRA) and magnetic resonance venography (MRV) have multiple advantages. MR can differentiate between muscle, bone, fat, and vascular tissue without the need for radiation or intravenous contrast, which can be deleterious to the kidneys. Axial, coronal, and sagittal images (Fig. 9.13) can be generated, and gadolinium enhancement provides high-quality angiography. High-flow and low-flow fistulas can be distinguished, as discussed in more detail in Chapter 10. Dynamic contrast-enhanced MRI has also emerged as an excellent imaging technique for VMs.[36,37]

Contrast arteriography is reserved for patients who are potential candidates for arterial embolization and have high-flow shunts. Contrast venography is reserved for patients who are potential candidates for venous intervention (see Fig. 9.5). Contrast venography is frequently done through multiple injections in the limb, with the use of a tourniquet or Esmarque bandage to visualize the deep system and with direct injection into the malformation before or after ethanol sclerotherapy or embolotherapy.

TREATMENT

Indications

There are absolute and relative indications for the treatment of low-flow VVMs. The absolute indication is hemorrhage. Bleeding from malformations can occur through defects in the skin or

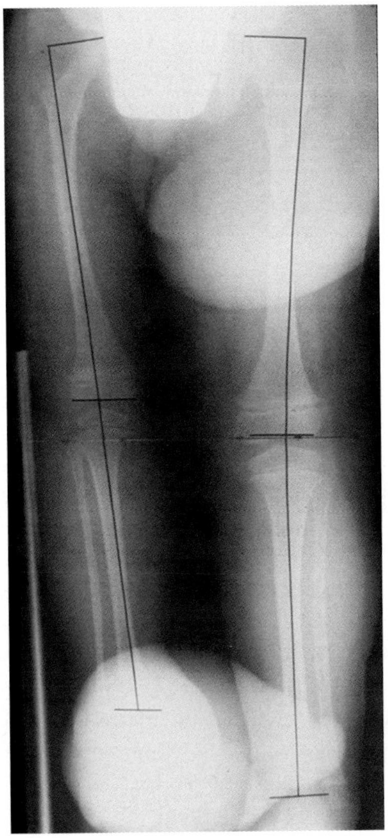

FIG 9.12 Long bone films (scanogram) confirm leg length discrepancy in bilateral Klippel-Trenaunay syndrome.

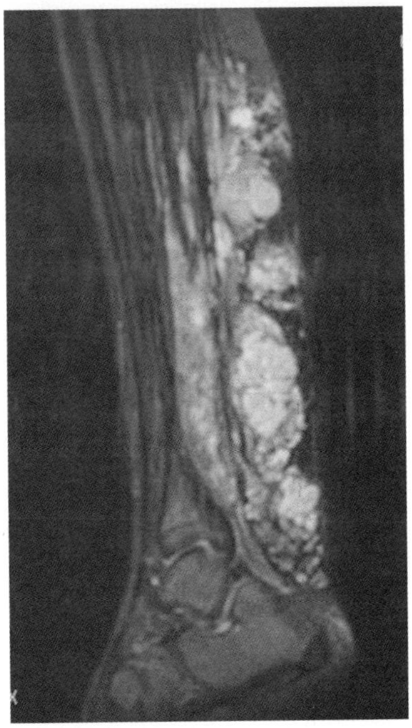

FIG 9.13 Magnetic resonance image of a predominantly venous malformation involving the superficial and deep compartments of the distal calf.

mucosa, or the patient can have an intramuscular or retroperitoneal hematoma, hematuria, rectal bleeding, hematemesis, hemoptysis, or intracerebral or intraspinal bleeding. Relative indications for treatment include pain, large varicosities, venous ulcers or skin changes, severe swelling, venous claudication, functional impairment, limb asymmetry, and cosmetic reasons. A multidisciplinary approach in the evaluation and treatment of VVMs provides the best chance for the patient. The team may include a pediatrician; pediatric, orthopedic, plastic, and vascular surgeons; an interventional radiologist; a cardiologist or vascular internist; and a physiatrist. Conservative treatment is used for most patients. Laser therapy has been used effectively for capillary malformations (port-wine stains). Effective and minimally invasive percutaneous techniques include transcatheter embolization and percutaneous or transcatheter sclerotherapy. Surgical excision is reserved for the minority of patients with localized superficial lesions or for those patients who have symptomatic juvenile varicose veins or localized venous malformations.

Conservative Treatment

Treatment of VVMs is most frequently conservative. Elastic garments or bandages, local wound care, compression dressings, special orthopedic footwear, and lifestyle modification may be required to manage daily life and improve limb function. Lymphedema is frequently managed using elastic garments, intermittent compression treatment, or lymphatic massage treatment by physical therapists. The psychological problem caused by a visible deformity should not be underestimated. Long-term antibiotic therapy may be needed for recurrent cellulitis, and patients who have had recurrent deep venous thrombosis are treated lifelong with anticoagulants.

Many patients with VVMs have thrombophilia. Baseline D-dimer and fibrinogen levels as part of the initial laboratory evaluations for patients with diffuse extratruncular VVMs are recommended.[6] In patients with thrombophilia, thrombosis prophylaxis before interventions is recommended, using low-molecular-weight heparin.[6] In those with repeated episodes of deep venous thrombosis, lifelong anticoagulation is often required.

Embolization

Embolization with selective catheterization has emerged as the primary therapy for arteriovenous malformations; it is rarely used for low-flow VVMs unless a main draining vein has to be occluded with embolotherapy for a more effective sclerotherapy of the distal VVM. Materials for embolization include polyvinyl alcohol particles (100 to 500 μm); absolute ethanol; stainless steel coils, usually with tufted Dacron, absorbable gelatin pledglets, powder coils, and cyanoacrylate adhesives. Coils are equivalent to surgical ligation, although the tufted Dacron and the addition of thrombin will generate more extensive thrombosis than ligation alone.

Detachable coils permit a double catheter technique to deliver the first coil as a filter to ensure accurate location of the others, while final detachment of the first coil is done at the end of the procedure. Size selection is important to avoid embolization through large veins. For very large veins, the use of vascular plugs can be considered. Particulate agents used for embolotherapy include gel foam, polyvinyl alcohol particles (100 to 500 μm), spherical embolics, or absorbable gelatin pledglets.

Sclerotherapy

Liquid and foam sclerosing agents permanently occlude or destroy the endothelium of the VVMs.[38] Sclerosing agents can cause endothelial damage due to their osmotic effect; they include hypertonic saline or detergents such as sodium morrhuate, sodium tetradecyl sulfate (STS), or polidocanol. The foam detergents are now used preferentially for sclerotherapy of VVMs, but absolute alcohol is also used frequently.[6,14,39]

Sclerosing agents cause shrinkage of the VVM due to thrombosis, inflammation, and scarring. Absolute ethanol induces denaturation of tissue protein, precipitating protoplasm, and destruction of the endothelial cells. For VVMs, it is delivered directly by percutaneous injection into lesions. Unfortunately alcohol sclerotherapy causes significant pain; therefore general anesthesia and pain control are frequently required. Absolute ethanol can also cause significant side effects. Treatment should be performed selectively and by a physician with expertise and knowledge of the dose- and toxicity-related complications.[40,41] For large VVMs, a pulmonary artery catheter and arterial pressure line monitoring is suggested, as well as giving dexamethasone sodium phosphate (3 to 10 mg) intravenously before the procedure. The maximal dose should not exceed 1 mL/kg body weight (maximum 30 to 60 mL).[39] Pulmonary hypertension should be monitored when large doses are given, and nitroglycerin can be used to treat pulmonary vasospasm. Yakes and colleagues[42] reported on a complication rate ranging from 10% to 30%, depending on their years of experience. Tissue necrosis, sloughing of the skin, and pulmonary hypertension are the most frequent side effects, followed by deep venous thrombosis, motor nerve injury, and sensory nerve injury.

One of the largest experiences using ethanol sclerotherapy of venous or arteriovenous malformations was compiled by Lee and colleagues.[43] In 87 patients who underwent 399 sessions of sclerotherapy for VVMs, the initial success rate was 95%. The mean follow-up was 24 months, and 71 of the 87 patients (82%) showed no recurrence of the treated lesion. Minor to major complications, mostly skin damage, developed after 47 sessions (12%) in 24 patients (28%). There was one permanent facial nerve palsy and one peroneal nerve palsy. The authors concluded that absolute ethanol sclerotherapy can deliver excellent results to patients with diffuse venous malformations, with a 25% rate of early and 3% rate of permanent complications. The low complication rate in this series was remarkable; most authors report complication rates between 10% and 30%. Complication rates in predominantly venous malformations are significantly lower than in patients who have arteriovenous shunting. The benefits and potential major complications of absolute alcohol sclerotherapy was emphasized by Villavicencio[44] and by Burrows and Mason.[40] According to recent guidelines, ethanol sclerotherapy has a high rate of complications and morbidity; therefore, its use should be restricted.[6]

Other materials that have been used for sclerotherapy include sotradecol and polidocanol liquid[45] or foam.[6,39] The advantage of foam detergent solutions is that smaller amounts can be used to achieve thrombosis. Sotradecol (STS) is used most frequently in the United States; one way to prepare the solution is to mix 10 mL of 3% STS (maximum dose of 0.5 mL/kg) with 2 mL of ethiodized oil (Ethiodol, a lipid-soluble contrast agent) and 10 mL of room air and prepare the foam using two syringes attached to each other with a three-way stopcock.[39] Polidocanol is less allergenic and produces less pain and a lower inflammatory response than other sclerosing solutions. Tessari and colleagues[46] use 1% polidocanol for duplex-guided foam sclerotherapy: two syringes were attached by a three-way stopcock; one was filled with polidocanol and the other with air. The foam is obtained by mixing the contents of the two syringes. Five to 10 mL of the foam is injected under duplex and venographic guidance into the venous malformation. Foam has been used with increasing frequency and with good results for VVMs.[6,14] Although longer follow-up is required, early complications are less than with ethanol sclerotherapy; foam has improved treatment and decreased complications in patients with VVMs.

Lidsky and colleagues[47] recently reported on results of treatment of 105 low-flow VVMs. Twenty-three (21.9%) patients were managed conservatively, and 38 (36.2%) were treated with sclerotherapy (STS, polidocanol, and/or ethanol). Another 18 (17.1%) were surgically resected, and 8 (7.6%) were managed with a combination of modalities. Response to sclerotherapy resulted in improvement in 32 (84.2%) patients, surgical resection resulted in improvement in 16 (88.9%), and combination therapy resulted in improvement in 8 (100%). Complications were observed in 6 (6.8%) patients (4 with ethanol sclerotherapy and 2 with resection). Since microfoam, a commercially prepared low-nitrogen gas mixture, is claimed to be safe, even in patients with patent foramen ovale, it has been approved in the United States and can be expected to be used more frequently for the treatment of VMs.[48]

Laser Treatment

Cutaneous capillary malformations (port-wine stains) were initially treated with argon lasers, with good results in many patients but with scarring that has been reported to occur in 5% to 24% of the cases.[49] The best results were obtained in adults with purple, well-vascularized lesions. Scarring has become less frequent with the introduction of yellow-light lasers.[50,51] The best results are achieved with the flash lamp-pumped pulsed dye laser. The 585-nm wavelength achieves deep tissue penetration while maintaining vascular specificity.[50] Both light- and dark-skinned patients can be treated with minimal intraoperative discomfort and a low chance of postoperative epidermal damage or pigmentary change. Lasers have revolutionized the treatment of superficial vascular lesions, especially port-wine stains and facial telangiectesias.[50,52] In a series of 56 patients with venous malformations, the success rate of laser treatment was 93%; 4% had minimal scarring and deformity, and no long-term complications were noted.[53]

Surgical Excision

Surgical excision of VVMs can be challenging and can result in significant blood loss. However, if such lesions are localized, they can be excised with a high rate of success. Exsanguination of the limb with an elastic (Esmarque) bandage and the use of a proximal tourniquet will greatly decrease blood loss and make the operation technically easier.[54] If excision is required, preoperative sclerotherapy or embolization should be considered to minimize bleeding. The use of a rapid cell saver is helpful and mandatory for extensive malformations. For extensive VVMs, which occur rarely, the only operation that serve to treat the patient is amputation. For these patients, amputation may mean cure, and a prosthesis can bring hope of functional recovery.

Recommendation of Invasive Treatment of Venous Vascular Malformations

A recent consensus document of the International Union of Phlebology[6] made the following recommendation on invasive therapy of VVMs: "for treatment of symptomatic VVMs, including the treatment of the lateral marginal vein, we recommend sclerotherapy, laser therapy, heat ablation with laser or radiofrequency, or surgical removal, depending on the expertise that is available, if evaluation confirms suitable anatomy and assured residual venous drainage." (Strength of recommendation: 1 [strong], Quality of evidence: C [low])

COMPLEX MALFORMATIONS

For vascular surgeons, management of complex clinical syndromes with VVMs deserves a separate discussion. The most frequently encountered problem of these rare malformations is the KTS.

KLIPPEL–TRENAUNAY SYNDROME

First described by Klippel and Trenaunay at the turn of the century, the clinical triad of this mixed malformation includes capillary malformations (port-wine stain), soft tissue and bone hypertrophy, atypical, usually lateral varicosity, and venous and lymphatic malformations (see Figs. 9.3, 9.5, 9.10, and 9.11).[1,6,15,55] The deep veins are frequently affected. The most frequent deep venous anomalies include ectasia or aneurysm, external compression, hypoplasia, aplasia, or persistent sciatic veins.[56] KTS is clearly a mesenchymal malformation that includes bone, soft tissue, and a mixed vascular, hemolymphatic malformation comprising predominantly venous, lymphatic, and capillary elements but no arteriovenous shunting. Many patients have lymphedema and some have cavernous lymphatic malformations. Although eponyms are discouraged by many experts, the term *KTS*, just like *Marfan* or *Down syndrome*, has been widely accepted and used by the public and the patients.

In a review of 252 patients with KTS, 246 (98%) had capillary malformations, 236 (94%) had soft tissue or bone hypertrophy, and 182 (72%) had varicosities or venous malformations.[57] The lower extremities were involved in 70%, and the malformation was bilateral in 19%. The upper extremity was involved in 74 of the 252 patients (29%). Symptoms of patients with KTS included swelling (70%), pain (7%), and bleeding (43 of 252; 17%). Thirty-nine patients (15%) had a history of superficial phlebitis, 4% had a history of deep venous thrombosis, and 4% had pulmonary embolism (PE), which was fatal in one case. Lateral varicose veins were frequent (56%). One percent had suprapubic varicosities owing to iliac vein agenesis or aplasia, and 19% of the patients had medial varicosities.

The management of KTS has been largely conservative, using elastic garments and treatment of any cellulitis or lymphangitis. Most patients who undergo surgical treatment do so because of overgrowth of one limb: these patients are managed with epiphiseodesis, with good results.[57]

Vascular interventions must be preceded by careful evaluation of the patency of the deep venous system. Ablation of the symptomatic incompetent superficial veins can be performed if the deep venous system is patent. Symptomatic, predominantly venous malformations can be managed by percutaneous sclerotherapy,[48,58,59] while localized capillary malformations of the skin respond to laser therapy. Large subcutaneous lateral embryonic veins can be treated well with invagination stripping or occasionally with endovenous thermal ablation or ambulatory miniphlebectomy. In a series of 49 patients with congenital varicose veins in 53 limbs, high ligation and stripping of the GSV as well as small and accessory saphenous and lateral embryonic veins was performed in 17 (32%), 10 (19%), 9 (17%), and 15 (28%) limbs, respectively. Two patients developed deep venous thrombosis, one had a PE, and one had peroneal nerve palsy. Freedom from disabling pain at 1, 3, and 5 years was 95%, 77%, and 59%, respectively, and freedom from secondary procedures was 78% at 3 years, and 74% at 5 years. Improvement in the venous clinical severity score at last follow-up was significant. In patients with a history of deep venous thrombosis or recurrent thrombophlebitis, preoperative placement of a vena cava filter should be considered.

Venous malformations and varicose veins can also be treated effectively, in multiple sessions using ethanol sclerotherapy or foam. In addition, endovenous thermal ablations with radiofrequency or laser have been used selectively for patients with KTS.[60] Long-term results with endothermal ablations are not well known because of the small number of VVM patients treated in single centers. Because of the rarity of this disorder and the presence of a mixed malformation, the multidisciplinary management of patients with KTS, just like with other complex VMs, is clearly warranted.

CONCLUSIONS

Improved imaging of the vascular system with duplex ultrasound scanning and MRI or CTA has changed the evaluation and treatment of patients with VVMs in recent years. Most venous VMs are still managed conservatively, but treatment options have increased for symptomatic patients, and they are less invasive. Treatment should be individualized, offering a combination of sclerotherapy, embolization, open surgery, and laser or radiofrequency ablation, depending on the expertise available and ensuring that venous drainage of the affected region or limb will not be compromised. Complex VVMs should be treated in specialized multidisciplinary centers.

REVIEW QUESTIONS

1. Which of the following lesion is not a VM?
   - **a.** Juvenile hemangioma
   - **b.** Port wine stain
   - **c.** Persistent sciatic vein
   - **d.** Congenital arteriovenous fistula
   - **e.** Venous VM
2. What type of VM is seen most frequently at vascular clinics?
   - **a.** Capillary
   - **b.** Arterial
   - **c.** Venous
   - **d.** Arteriovenous
   - **e.** Lymphatic
3. Which of the following statements is not true for VMs?
   - **a.** They have a proliferative phase and then undergo resolution.
   - **b.** The male to female ratio is 1 : 1.
   - **c.** They are developmental anomalies.
   - **d.** There is no cell growth in tissue culture.
   - **e.** They do not contain mast cells in biopsy specimen.
4. Which of the following classes are not part of the modified Hamburg classification used currently for VMs?
   - **a.** Arterial
   - **b.** Hemangiomatous
   - **c.** Venous
   - **d.** Arteriovenous
   - **e.** Lymphatic
5. In young patients with lateral varicose veins, preoperative evaluation must establish
   - **a.** Incompetence of the superficial veins
   - **b.** Incompetence in the deep veins
   - **c.** A normal saphenous system
   - **d.** A patent deep venous system
   - **e.** Leg length discrepancy
6. Which of the following findings are not typical for Klippel-Trenaunay syndrome?
   - **a.** Port wine stain
   - **b.** Lateral varicosity
   - **c.** Thrill with machinery murmur
   - **d.** Deep venous anomalies
   - **e.** Limb length discrepancy
7. A large cavernous low-flow venous malformation involves the left thigh and buttock in a 22-year-old woman. What is the most useful imaging study in this patient?
   - **a.** CT venogram
   - **b.** Duplex scan to exclude deep venous thrombosis
   - **c.** Intravascular ultrasound
   - **d.** MR imaging and MR venogram
   - **e.** Plethysmography
8. The best treatment for this patient, with symptoms of pain and frequent bleeding from a diffuse VVM of the thigh and buttock, is:
   - **a.** Surgical excision with skin graft
   - **b.** Radiofrequency ablation
   - **c.** Staged sclerotherapy
   - **d.** Transcatheter embolization with coils
   - **e.** Conservative management
9. Which of the following statements is true for the sclerotherapy of venous malformations?
   - **a.** Absolute alcohol injection is not painful.
   - **b.** The advantage of foam over liquid sclerotherapy is that smaller amounts of the detergent can be used to achieve venous thrombosis.
   - **c.** Ethanol sclerotherapy has significantly lower complication rates than foam sclerotherapy.
   - **d.** Venous malformations are best managed by transfemoral embolization of the feeding arteries.
   - **e.** Skin necrosis with ethanol sclerotherapy is very rare.
10. Patients with VVMs may have all of the following findings except
    - **a.** a machinery murmur over the lesion
    - **b.** a longer extremity
    - **c.** a shorter extremity
    - **d.** palpable phleboliths
    - **e.** a history of deep vein thrombosis

BIBLIOGRAPHY

Greene AK, Alomari AI. Management of venous malformations. *Clin Plast Surg*. 2011;38:83–93.

Lee BB, Baumgartner I, Berlien P, et al. Diagnosis and Treatment of Venous Malformations. Consensus Document of the International Union of Phlebology (IUP): updated 2013. *Int Angiol*. 2015;34:97–149.

Lee BB, Kim I, Huh S, et al. New experiences with absolute ethanol sclerotherapy in the management of a complex form of congenital venous malformation. *J Vasc Surg*. 2002;33:764–772.

Lidsky ME, Markovic JN, Miller MJ Jr, Shortell CK. Analysis of the treatment of congenital vascular malformations using a multidisciplinary approach. *J Vasc Surg*. 2012;56:1355–1362, discussion 62.

Malgor RD, Gloviczki P, Fahrni J, et al. Surgical treatment of varicose veins and venous malformations in Klippel-Trenaunay syndrome. *Phlebology*. 2016;31:209–215.

References available online at ExpertConsult.com.

CHAPTER 10

Congenital Arterial Malformations

Cynthia K. Shortell, Daiva Nevidomskyte

DEFINITION, INCIDENCE, AND CLINICAL SIGNIFICANCE

Congenital vascular malformations (CVMs) are rare developmental abnormalities of the vascular system that include a broad spectrum of arterial, venous, lymphatic, and capillary lesions. The overall incidence is estimated at 1.2% to 1.5%.[1-4] Congenital arterial malformations (AMs) without arteriovenous (AV) shunting are lesions that include abnormally formed arteries or anomalous anatomy due to persistence of the fetal arterial remnants. These pure AMs are extremely rare and represent only approximately 8% of all CVMs.[5] Arteriovenous malformations (AVMs) and combined lesions that involve venous, lymphatic, and high-flow (HF) arterial components, comprise the majority of congenital AMs. The prevalence of both intracranial and extracranial AVMs ranges from 5 to 613 per 1000,000 population.[6] Despite their relative rarity (10% to 20% of all CVMs), AVMs are the most challenging diagnostic and therapeutic pathology among all malformations[7]; therefore, the majority of this chapter is dedicated to discussing them.

DEVELOPMENT OF THE VASCULAR SYSTEM

The classification, clinical presentation, treatment, and outcomes of CVMs are dependent on the timing of developmental errors in the vascular system. Extratruncular CVMs arise before the formation of mature vascular trunks in the 4th to 6th weeks of gestation.[7-10] They possess mesenchymal cell characteristics that lead to progression and aggressive recurrence. Truncular CVMs originate in the final stage of angiogenesis in the 6th to 7th week of development and manifest as abnormal major axial vessels or persistence of embryonic vasculature.[2,8-10] They have lost embryonic characteristics and therefore, unlike extratruncular lesions, do not possess the potential to proliferate.[2,10-12]

Blood vessels and blood elements arise from the common mesenchymal precursor cells (hemangioblasts), which differentiate into blood cell and vascular precursors (angioblasts).[13-16] During vasculogenesis, angioblasts differentiate into endothelial cells that aggregate into small vessel cords and eventually form vessels.[9,13-16] After endothelial cells are established as vascular elements, under the influence of vascular endothelial growth factor (VEGF), they begin to sprout and form the primitive capillary retiform plexus.[8,15,16] As the vasculature matures, changes in hemodynamic requirements, growing metabolic demands, and growth factor secretion induce pruning and vessel remodeling.[13,15]

Extratruncular CVMs are thought to arise due to failure of the fetal capillary networks to undergo appropriate regression. Interestingly, AVMs are 20 times more common in the central nervous system, where apoptosis is rare.[17] These fetal nonfunctional AV channels later recanalize to form small AV connections that dilate, cause local ischemia, and subsequently enter a cycle of collateralization and recruitment.[16-18] As such, AVMs are characterized by direct flow from an artery to a vein in the absence of a normal capillary bed.[7,9-12] A central core or nidus forms as a network of densely packed, tortuous, poorly differentiated blood vessels with low resistance and vascular tone. The nidus with enlarged feeding arteries and draining veins is found in the majority of extratruncular AVMs.[7,17-21]

Truncular CVMs arise during later stages of vascular development and originate from fetal vessel trunks.[2,7-11] During early embryonic development the precursors of the heart, bulbus cordis and truncus arteriosus, are connected to the pair of dorsal aortas via a series of six pairs of pharyngeal arch arteries that develop in conjunction with the branchial pouches. In humans the five arch arteries are numbered 1, 2, 3, 4, and 6. The fifth arch eventually fuses with the fourth arch and carries no significance in later development. The paired dorsal aortas fuse in the midline to form a single dorsal aorta. The third and fourth dorsal arches, the seventh intersegmental artery, and the left dorsal aorta are the primary contributors to the normal aortic arch and its major thoracic branches. The segments of the bilateral aortic arch system that normally regress include the distal portion of the right sixth arch and the right-sided dorsal aorta. The distal part of the left sixth arch artery becomes ductus arteriosus or ligamentum arteriosum after birth. The right and left pulmonary arteries are formed from respective portions of sixth proximal arch segments. The left fourth arch becomes the aortic arch; the right fourth arch contributes to the innominate and proximal portion of the right subclavian artery. The third arches become the common carotid arteries and first segments of the internal carotid arteries. The seventh intersegmental arteries bilaterally become the subclavian and vertebral arteries. The left dorsal aorta becomes the descending thoracic aorta, as the entirety of the right dorsal aorta is lost.[8,22,23] Abnormal regression of aortic arches results in truncular anomalies associated with abnormal site and course of adult arterial anatomy.

Clinically, truncular lesions are defects in fully formed and often named vessels. A majority of the truncular lesions affecting arterial circulation are pure AMs. They are divided into obstructive (aplasia, hypoplasia, or stenosis) and dilated (localized and diffuse) forms.[7,9-11] Such anomalies present with hemodynamic and structural abnormalities that are treated with standard vascular or endovascular techniques.[10] Selected examples of truncular AMs are discussed at the end of the chapter. The truncular AMVs are extremely rare and will not be discussed in greater detail. They present with a fistulous connection between the artery and vein with no nidus. Examples include a patent ductus arteriosus, pulmonary arteriovenous fistula (AVF), direct communication between pelvic vessels, or femoral artery/vein.[7]

HISTORICAL BACKGROUND AND CLASSIFICATION

The history of CVMs has been plagued by incorrect descriptive terminology, eponymous nomenclature, and classification systems that are not based on clinical, anatomic, or flow characteristics. This historical lack of adequate classification has been an important factor obscuring the optimal approaches to diagnosis, treatment, and prognosis of these complex lesions.[19,24-26] The term "hemangioma" was used to describe a variety of vascular lesions with different etiologies and natural histories.[26,27] Terms such as "capillary or cavernous hemangioma" were used to describe both infantile hemangioma and CVMs.

The seminal study by Mulliken and Glowacki in 1982, which later formed the basis of International Society for the Study of Vascular Anomalies (ISSVA) classification system,[19] provided the first distinction between hemangiomas and CVMs.[27] Hemangiomas (vascular tumors) were classified as neoplastic disorders that histopathologically demonstrate rapid neonatal growth and increased endothelial cell turnover during their proliferative phase; during their involution phase, they then undergo slow fibrosis and exhibit diminished cellularity.[26-29] Vascular malformations were classified as embryologically developed, inborn errors of vascular morphogenesis, leading to structural anomalies present at birth and associated with normal endothelial proliferation.[27,30]

The Hamburg classification system, first proposed by Dr. S. Belov in 1988, placed the emphasis on embryogenesis of CVMs and their anatomic relationship to the major vascular trunks.[10,31] Initially, four major groups were identified: arterial, venous, arteriovenous (AV), and combined defects. Later, capillary and lymphatic malformations were added. Truncular and extratruncular categories subdivided lesions based on the predominant vessels present in the malformations—either peripheral vascular branches/tributaries or major axial trunks. Truncular and extratruncular lesions were separated based on the stage at which developmental defect occurred.[2,7,9-12] Truncular CVMs were divided into those with obstruction or stenosis (aplasia, hypoplasia, coarctation) and those with dilations (localized aneurysm, diffuse ectasia). Extratruncular malformations were localized or they were diffuse and infiltrating.[10] Occasionally both forms were combined and include capillary, arterial, venous, or lymphatic components. The distinction between truncular and extratruncular lesions is critical for successful treatment. Truncular lesions are treated to improve hemodynamics or eliminate physiologic burden with no risk of provocation. Extratruncular lesions are more challenging to manage due to their mesenchymal origin and proliferative potential that can be stimulated by interventions ("recruitment").

In 1992 the ISSVA was founded and in 1996 proposed an updated classification system based on histopathologic and flow characteristics, in addition to the clinical appearance of the lesions.[7,10,30,32,33] Vascular anomalies were divided into two categories: vascular tumors and vascular malformations (Table 10.1). This classification emphasized that CVMs, in contrast to vascular tumors, histologically and physiologically were not a proliferative neoplastic lesions. Vascular malformations were further subdivided into low-flow (LF) and HF groups, as well as mixed syndromes with various histopathologic features and flow components.[33,34] The latest version of ISSVA classification system was expanded in 2014 to include a section on malformations of individually named vessels ("truncular" malformations), as well as newly named anomalies and gene mutations involved in various subtypes of CVMs.[25] This classification system was meant to reflect the state of the art in vascular anomalies classification and reflect recent advances in knowledge and clinical associations.

In 2013 the International Union of Angiology (IUA) created a comprehensive classification system informed by both the ISSVA and Hamburg classification systems.[10,35] The new Integrated Classification System for the management of CVMs (Table 10.2) includes flow and vessel characteristics, as well as embryologic derivation (truncular vs. extratruncular). In the future this classification system should facilitate effective diagnosis and treatment of CVMs.[35]

EXTRATRUNCULAR ARTERIOVENOUS MALFORMATIONS

Extratruncular lesions result from defective development during the earlier stages of embryogenesis, when the vascular structures are still in the state of plexiform primordial vessels. As such, they possess mesenchymal cell characteristics to grow when stimulated externally (e.g., trauma, surgery, intervention) or internally (e.g., menarche, pregnancy, hormones).[10-17] Clinically, these lesions are masses of abnormal small/mid-sized vessels diffusely infiltrating various tissues and organ systems. The embryologic characteristics, combined with inappropriate treatment strategies, can provoke dormant, asymptomatic lesions to grow rapidly. Therefore, in addition to the hemodynamic impact on the affected vascular system, all extratruncular lesions, regardless of the type and location, carry the risk of progression and recurrence.[12]

Natural History and Clinical Presentation

Most AVMs are present at birth but may not become evident until later in childhood or adolescence, after the lesion has enlarged or become symptomatic.[20,21,30,32,33] AVMs are most common in the central nervous system[2,6,7]; however, intracranial lesions will not be discussed in this chapter. Extracranial AVMs are most commonly observed in the head and neck (50% to 70%), extremity

TABLE 10.1 International Society for the Study of Vascular Anomalies 2014 Classification of Vascular Anomalies Based on Etiology and Flow Characteristic

VASCULAR ANOMALIES				
	VASCULAR MALFORMATIONS			
Vascular Tumors	**Simple**	**Combined[b]**	**Of Major Named Vessels**	**Overgrowth Syndromes/ Other Anomalies**
Benign: • Infantile Hemangioma • Congenital Hemangioma (rapidly involuting, partially involuting, non-involuting,) • Pyogenic granuloma • Epithelioid hemangioma • Spindle cell hemangioma • Tufted angioma **Locally aggressive:** • Kaposiform hemangioendothelioma • Composite hemangioendothelioma • Kaposi sarcoma • Retiform hemangioendothelioma **Malignant:** • Angiosarcoma • Epithelioid hemangioendothelioma	**Arteriovenous Malformations (AVM)[a]:** • Sporadic • In CM-AVM • In HHT **Arteriovenous Fistula (AV)[a] (congenital):** • Sporadic • In CM-AVM • In HHT **Capillary Malformations (CM):** • Cutaneous and/or mucosal CM • Cutis Marmorata • Telangiectasia • Nevus simplex **Lymphatic Malformations (LM):** • Common LM (macro/micro/mixed cystic) • Generalized lymphatic anomaly • Primary lymphedema (various subtypes) **Venous Malformations (VM):** • Common VM • Blue rubber bleb nevus (Bean) syndrome • Glomuvenous • Cerebral cavernous • Familial VN cutaneo-mucosal	CVM CLM LVM CLVM CAVM[a] CLAVM[a] CVAVM[a] CLVAVM[a]	**Truncular, aka channel type:** Affect: • Lymphatics • Veins • Arteries[a] Anomalies of: • Origin • Course • Number • Length • Diameter (aplasia, hypoplasia, stenosis, ectasia, aneurysm) • Valves • Communication (AVF) • Persistence of embryonic vessel	CLOVES[a] Klippel-Trénaunay Maffuci Proteus Parkes Weber[a] Sturge-Weber[a] Bannayan-Riley-Ruvalcaba[a] PTEN hamartoma[a] Servelle-Martorell Limb CM + nonprogressive hypertrophy Macrocephaly-CM Microcephaly-CM

[a]Lesions with high-flow arterial component.
[b]Defined as two or more types of vascular malformations found in one lesion.
CAVM, Capillary arteriovenous malformation; *CLAVM*, capillary lymphatic arteriovenous malformation; *CLM*, capillary lymphatic malformation; *CLVM*, capillary lymphatic venous malformation; *CVAVM*, capillary venous arteriovenous malformation; *CVM*, capillary venous malformation; *HHT*, hereditary hemorrhagic telangiectasia; *LVM*, lymphatic venous malformation; *PTEN*, phosphatase and tensin homolog gene.
Modified from 20th ISSVA Workshop, Melbourne, April 2014 and Green AK: Arteriovenous malformations. In *Vascular anomalies. Classification, diagnosis & management.* St. Louis, MO, 2013, Quality Medical Publishing, p 160.

TABLE 10.2 Integrated Classification System for Congenital Vascular Malformations Combines Features of ISSVA and Modified Hamburg Classification Systems

CONGENITAL VASCULAR MALFORMATIONS					
Low Flow			**High Flow**		
Venous (VM)	Truncular	• Obstruction/narrowing • Dilation	**Arterial (AM)**	Truncular	• Obstruction/narrowing • Dilation
	Extratruncular	• Diffuse/infiltrating • Limited/localized		Extratruncular	• Diffuse/infiltrating • Limited/localized
Lymphatic (LM)	Truncular	• Obstruction/narrowing • Dilation	**Arteriovenous (AVM)**	Truncular	• Obstruction/narrowing • Dilation
	Extratruncular	• Diffuse/infiltrating • Limited/localized		Extratruncular	• Diffuse/infiltrating • Limited/localized
Capillary/microvascular					
Combined					
Syndrome associated			**Syndrome associated**		

ISSAV, International Society for the Study of Vascular Anomalies.

TABLE 10.3 Schobinger Severity Scoring System for Arteriovenous Malformations

Stage	Clinical Description
I (quiescence)	Warm, pink-bluish stain, arteriovenous shunting on Doppler, resembles capillary malformation or involuting hemangioma
II (expansion)	Same as stage I, plus enlargement, pulsatility, thrill/bruit and tortuous/tense veins
III (destruction)	Same as stage II, plus ulceration, bleeding, pain, steal, soft tissue necrosis. Osteolytic lesions may develop
IV (decompensation)	Same as stage III, plus progression to high-output congestive heart failure and left ventricular hypertrophy.

Modified from Green AK: Arteriovenous malformations. In *Vascular anomalies. Classification, diagnosis & management.* St. Louis, MO, 2013, Quality Medical Publishing, Inc., p 160.

(20% to 30%), trunk (5% to 10%), and visceral locations (1% to 5%).[3,7,9-12,30-39] Unlike vascular tumors, AVMs do not regress and their growth occurs simultaneously with the patient's physical development.[17-21,30] Lesions may progress more rapidly due to trauma, puberty, pregnancy, embolization, or resection-mediated ischemic injury. The mechanisms by which AVMs progress and recur following treatment include: collateralization and arterialization due to AV shunt, opening of latent AV shunts, aneurysm formation in arteries and veins, and angiogenesis and vasculogenesis.[30,36-41] Hormonal changes during adolescence and pregnancy also stimulate progression.[10,36,42-44] Estrogen, testosterone, and progesterone have been found to stimulate VEGF production, endothelial proliferation, and angiogenesis. During puberty, patients are at least a twofold risk of AVM progression.[36,37,39,43] Although pregnancy is not contraindicated in women with AVMs, patients should be warned of the potential of an aggressive lesion behavior during pregnancy.[17,30,36,37,43-45]

Extratruncular AVMs are classified according to the Schobinger severity scoring system (Table 10.3).[10,17,30,32,39] Stage I is quiescence: the AVM resembles a capillary malformation or involuting hemangioma (Fig. 10.1A). Stage II is expansion: the lesion becomes warmer and bigger and develops a throbbing sensation with a thrill and a bruit (see Fig. 10.1B). Stage III is that of tissue destruction: the aforementioned symptoms are accompanied by ulcers, hemorrhage, pain, and bony lytic lesions (see Fig. 10.1C). Stage IV is rare and signifies progression of all the previously mentioned symptoms to congestive failure with increased cardiac output, volume-pressure overload, and left ventricular hypertrophy. A high-output cardiac state occurs in 1% to 2% of peripheral AVMs.[20,30,36,39]

Genetic Basis

Most extratruncular AVMs are sporadic in nature and are caused by somatic (post)zygotic mutations with various penetrance patterns.[9,13,46] The precise genetic basis is unknown, but molecules that participate in AV differentiation and the angiogenesis pathway, such as Notch signaling proteins, are likely involved.[15,16,23,46,47] The genetic basis of several CVMs that occur as part of complex syndromes have been recently identified, and further studies will contribute to a better understanding of defective vascular morphogenesis. Newly discovered biomolecular pathways will serve as potential therapeutic targets for treatment of sporadic and syndromic CVMs.[20]

Hereditary hemorrhagic telangiectasia (HHT, also known as Rendu-Osler-Weber disease) is an autosomal dominant disorder characterized by multiple telangiectasias of the skin and gastrointestinal tract, as well as AVMs in the liver, lungs, and brain.[13,39,48,49] Spontaneous recurrent nosebleeds from telangiectasias of the nasal mucosa are the presenting sign in more than 90% of HHT patients.[49] The two major types of disease, HHT1 and HHT2, are caused by mutations in the endoglin *(ENG)* and activin receptor kinase *(ACVRL1)* genes, respectively. Both genes belong to the transforming growth factor-β (TGF-β) signaling pathway that regulates cell proliferation, migration, and differentiation. TGF-β is also responsible for maintaining extracellular vascular matrix. HHT1 has earlier onset and is more likely to have cerebral and pulmonary AVMs, whereas HHT2 has a later onset, lower penetrance, and more common hepatic AVMs.[3,39,48,49] Bevacizumab, a monoclonal antibody against VEGF, has been found to directly inhibit the VEGF proteins that can be elevated as a result of the HHT mutations and reduce epistaxis, telangiectasias, and iron-deficiency anemia.[50]

RASA1 is another autosomal dominant mutation responsible for capillary arteriovenous malformation (CAVM) syndrome.[10,39,46] Affected family members manifest small, multifocal capillary malformations, often with a pale halo. Approximately a third of the patients have AVMs, AVFs, or Parkes-Weber syndrome (PWS), which is characterized by soft tissue and skeletal overgrowth with or without lymphatic lesions, large cutaneous stains, and AV-microfistulas. Individuals with PWS who do not have multiple capillary lesions have a sporadic form of this syndrome without the *RASA1* mutation. The *RASA1* mutation leads to loss of inhibitory function on the Ras protein that takes part in endothelial cell proliferation, survival, and function, likely resulting in CAVM phenotype.[39,46]

Phosphatase and tensin homolog gene *(PTEN)* is an autosomal dominant mutation of a tumor suppressor gene involved in Cowden and Bannayan-Riley-Ruvalcaba syndromes.[10,39,46] *PTEN* hamartoma refers to the focal tissue overgrowth frequently containing AVMs. These syndromes share common features of macrocephaly, penile freckling, hamartomatous intestinal polyposis, asymmetrical overgrowth, and ectopic fat deposits (lipomas).[7,39,46,51] Patients usually have multiple intramuscular, paraspinal, or intracranial AVMs that are aggressive and difficult to control with embolization.[7,51-53]

Evaluation and Diagnostic Imaging

Distinguishing vascular tumors from vascular malformations and HF from LF lesions are essential steps in proper evaluation and treatment selection. The presence of arterial flow is the hemodynamic characteristic used to differentiate between HF and LF CVMs. Failure to identify arterial flow can have detrimental consequences in treatment outcomes if the patient with

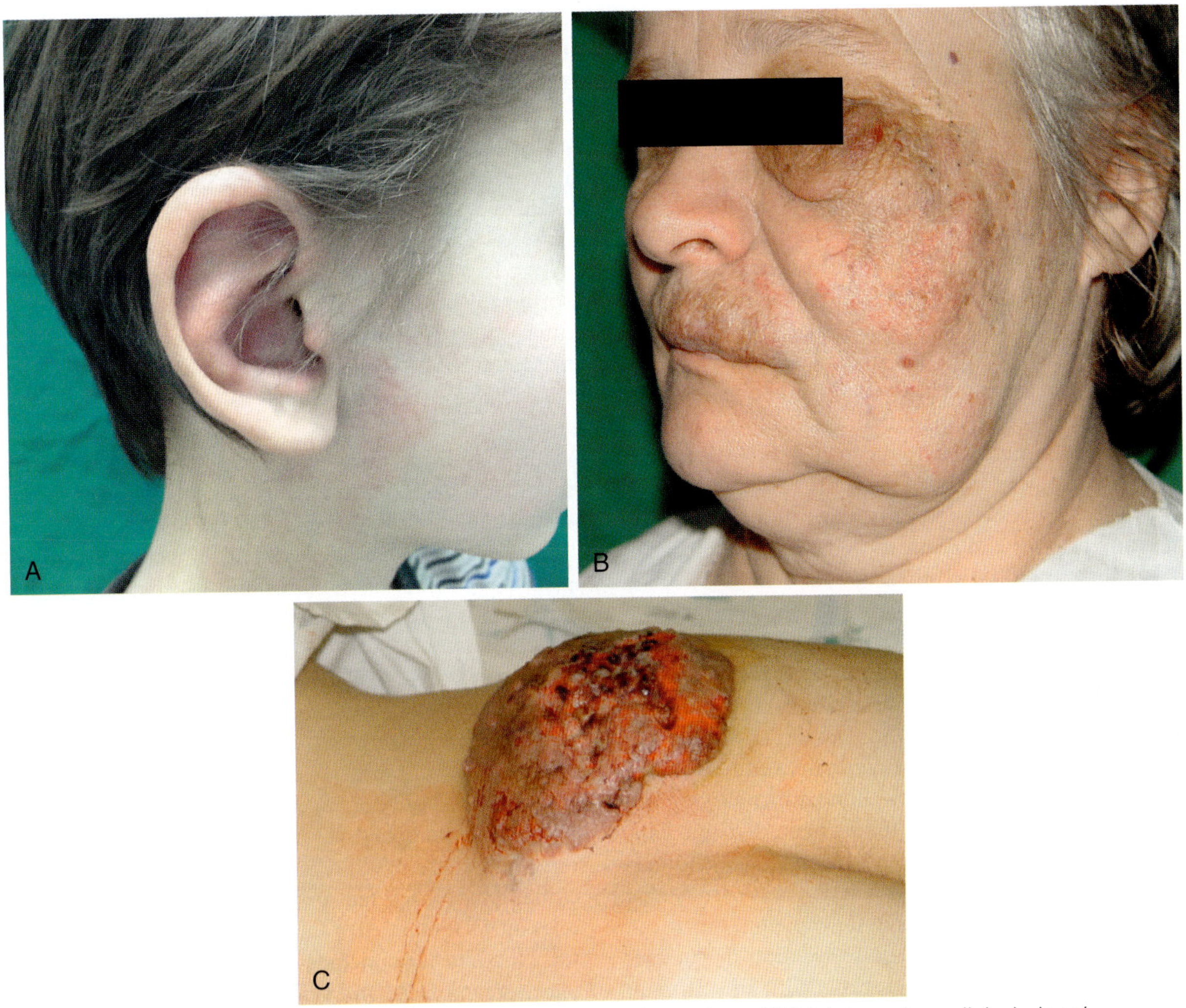

FIG 10.1 Schobinger staging of arteriovenous malformations (AVMs), based on clinical signs/symptoms. (A) Stage I AVM with blush, hyperpigmented stain and local warmth involving an ear and posterior cheek. (B) Stage II AVM of the left face with gradual expansion in size, increased discoloration, thickening, and soft tissue overgrowth. (C) Stage III AVM of the gluteal region had undergone dramatic expansion during pregnancy with progression to ulceration, necrosis, and hemorrhage. (Courtesy of Birute Vaisnyte, MD, PhD, Vilnius University, Vilnius University Hospital Santaros Klinikos.)

HF lesion is erroneously treated with techniques appropriate for LF CVM and vice versa.[25,54]

History and physical examination alone can differentiate 90% of AVMs.[10,17-21,30,32,33,37] It is important to note the timing of lesion appearance, progression, and any treatment attempts. The most important clinical characteristic used to differentiate between vascular tumors and CVMs is the absence of clinical regression among true malformations.[24,25,29] Infantile hemangiomas are neoplastic lesions that have an increased rate of cellular proliferation during the first year of life (proliferative phase) followed by slow, spontaneous regression (involution phase).[7,10,11,13,25] Therefore, by definition an adult presenting with a vascular lesion does not have a hemangioma,[25] despite the frequent use of this term by nonexperts.

Bedside Doppler examination with typical flow characteristics can help to distinguish HF from LF (such as capillary, lymphatic or venous) lesions.[10] Further imaging should be used to confirm the type of malformation, define anatomic extent and involvement of adjacent structures, and facilitate treatment planning.

Duplex ultrasound (US) is the best initial diagnostic study, especially for more focal, superficial lesions, and indeed should be considered part of the bedside physical exam to confirm diagnosis.[10,17-21] An HF AVM exhibits low-resistance high-velocity arterial flow with high diastolic flux and pulsatile venous outflow. Color Doppler shows a poorly defined hypervascular lesion with tortuous feeding arteries and dilated draining veins that can undergo aneurysmal degeneration as a result of long-standing arterialization. US can provide initial information about the lesion extent, proximity to the adjacent structures, relationship to normal anatomy, and patterns of drainage and reflux. On US the AVM can be differentiated from hemangioma because, in contrast to AVM, vascular tumors contain homogenous parenchymal tissue.[10,17-21,28,30]

Magnetic resonance imaging (MRI) has become the most important contemporary diagnostic modality. This study allows the clinician to define the anatomic extent and lesion relationship to the surrounding structures.[10,17-21,54-56] It also helps to distinguish among the HF and LF malformations. A typical CVM imaging protocol consists of spin echo (SE) or fast spin echo (FSE) T1-weighted sequences axial to the lesion with fat suppression in order to define the anatomy, tissue planes, and neurovascular structures. T2-weighted images in at least two planes (coronal, sagittal, or axial) have been found to be most sensitive and specific for detection of the extent and depth of the lesion because of a generally bright lesion signal intensity over a low signal intensity of surrounding fat, muscle, and bone.[10,57] These sequences demonstrate the content of the malformation. SE sequences with gadolinium help to distinguish HF AVMs from LF VMs or LMs because the signal voids on T2 sequences represent arterial feeding vessels and early filling of draining veins. Dilated feeding arteries and draining veins with a paucity of venous lakes are also indicative of HF lesions.[54] LF CVMs have increased intraluminal signal on T2-weighted images.[7,10,28,30,56,57] AVMs also exhibit a characteristic lack of soft tissue mass.

Dynamic contrast-enhanced MRI (dceMRI) has been reported to have increased specificity and sensitivity in differentiating between HF and LF CVMs.[54,56,58] Using multiple rapid bolus contrast injections over a period of time enables better demonstration of an enhanced lumen by eliminating background signal.[54,59] In addition to providing robust hemodynamic data, it also delineates feeding vessels, nidus morphology, and surrounding structures. Overall, MRI is a noninvasive study that provides anatomic and hemodynamic information, but it can be lengthy and noisy and might require sedation in younger children.[10] MRI is the preferred imaging modality for treatment follow-up.

Computed tomography (CT) is rarely used for the initial lesion evaluation because MRI is preferred; however, CT can complement MRI in demonstrating bony involvement, as well as provide some additional structural information.[7,10] Intravenous contrast and appropriate timing protocol (contrast bolus tracking technique) is needed to better distinguish the type of CVM and associated structures. Asymptomatic AVMs on CT angiogram should have no soft tissue component. Soft tissue enhancement suggests either a tumor (sarcoma) or inflammation due to infection, ischemia, or bleeding.[61] CT angiography is also reserved for patients who are unable to undergo MRI or for more rapid evaluation of acute symptoms, such as bleeding or airway compromise.[10,56]

Catheter-based angiography can be obtained if the diagnosis and/or flow characteristics remain equivocal following noninvasive imaging techniques and is essential in defining the lesion type. Angiographic classification system has been proposed by Yakes and is used to evaluate the feasibility of embolization treatment (Table 10.4).[25,60-66] Similar to the appearance on MRI or CT angiography, on angiography the AVM lesion appears as tortuous vessels with enlarged feeding arteries that rapidly shunt into dilated draining veins via a nidus. Catheter-based angiography allows for real-time evaluation of flow dynamics, main feeding arteries, collateral vessels, nidus, and draining veins.[20,31,56,67]

Conventional radiography is used to demonstrate erosive and intraosseous changes of adjacent bone and is recommended for evaluation of limb length discrepancy.[7,10,31,67]

Whole body blood pool scintigraphy (WBBPS) and transarterial lung perfusion scintigraphy (TLPS) are nuclear imaging techniques that have been recently introduced to quantitatively evaluate AVMs.[68-70] Using technetium 99m–tagged erythrocytes to detect abnormal blood pooling throughout the body, WBBPS allows localizing hidden lesions. Increased radiotracer pooling within the vascular lesions can be quantified before and after intervention to evaluate treatment efficacy.[10,19,21,28,69] TLPS uses technetium 99m–labeled microsphere albumin. Measuring radiotracer activity reaching the lungs that has passed unfiltered though the AVM shunt provides quantitative information on blood volume shunting through the AVM and allows calculation of shunt percentage. It can identify hidden micro-AV shunting that is difficult to detect on other modalities.[10,21,68-70] These two modalities are unique because they can document quantitative AV shut percentage through the nidus and can be used to objectively follow treatment response.[17,19,21,68-70]

General Treatment Principles

Compared with other CVMs, extratruncular AVMs are considered the most symptomatic and difficult to treat. Treatment goals are to manage symptoms, preserve function, prevent progression, and improve quality of life. Because such lesions are often diffuse and involve multiple tissue planes, a cure is rare. The best patient outcomes are achieved when treatment is based on a multidisciplinary approach that provides expertise from all disciplines relevant to the patient's lesion, and includes a patient navigator.[5,10,19,20] The team includes pediatricians; pediatric, orthopedic, plastic, craniofacial and vascular surgeons; interventional radiologists and cardiologists; ophthalmologists; hematologists; and dermatologists, as well as physical and occupational therapy specialists.[7-10,25,28] Patients with complex and diffuse AVMs need to be informed that multiple sessions and multimodal approach might be required. Treatment of extensive lesions is often palliative rather than curative.[25]

The selection of treatment modalities depends on the lesion type, size, location, patients' age, and Schobinger stage. The most important general principles are aggressive nidus control and absolute avoidance of proximal inflow vessel ligation or embolization because resultant ischemia and collateralization will stimulate enlargement and recurrence and prevent access for future embolizations.[9-13,17-21,30,37] Currently, there is no single uniformly effective medical/pharmacologic agent for AVM treatment. Some promising antiangiogenic agents include thalidomide, bevacizumab, sirolimus, interferon, and matrix metalloproteinase inhibitors.[50,72,73] Propranolol accelerates involution of hemangiomas but is not effective in treatment for AVMs.[18] In the future, better understanding of angiogenesis, vasculogenesis, and vascular remodeling will allow for development of patient- and lesion-specific therapeutic agents.

Treatment Indications and Timing

The absolute treatment indications for AVMs include hemorrhage (major or recurrent minor), gangrene or ulcer, distal steal

TABLE 10.4 Angiographic Classification of Arteriovenous Malformations on the Basis of Nidus Morphology Is Used for Preoperative Planning

AVM Type	Nidus Structure	Description		Treatment
I	Arteriovenous fistula	Less than three arteries shunted into single vein	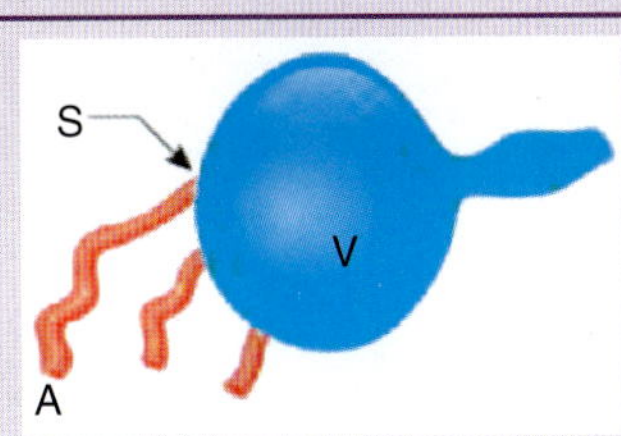	Unknown (rare)
II	Arteriolovenous fistula	Multiple arterioles shunted into single vein	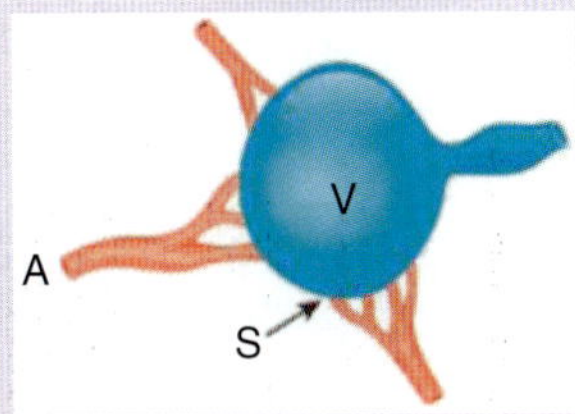	Transvenous approach or direct puncture
IIIA	Arteriolovenulous fistula without dilatation	Multiple shunts between arterioles and venules	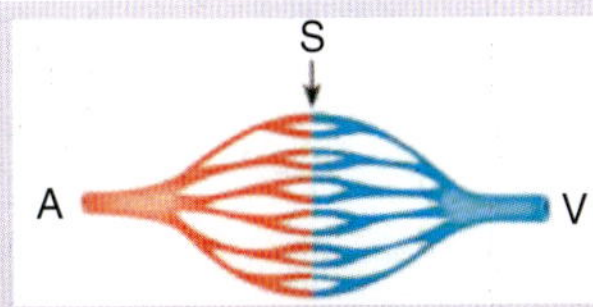	Transarterial approach
III B	Arteriolovenulous fistula with dilatation	Same as III A, but shunts are dilated	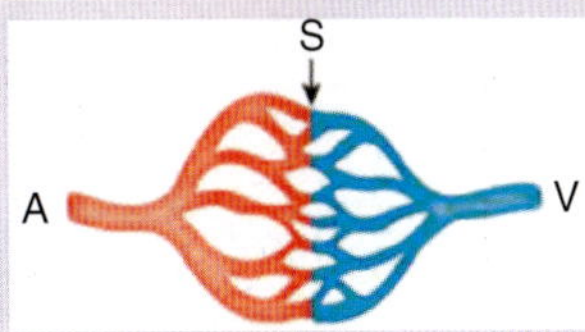	Transarterial approach or direct puncture

A, Artery; AVM, arteriovenous malformations; *S*, shunt; *V*, vein.
Modified from Lee BB, Antignani PL, Baraldini V, et al: ISVI-IUA consensus document diagnostic guidelines of vascular anomalies: vascular malformations and hemangiomas. *Int Angiol* 34:333–374, 2015.

with ischemic complications (acute or chronic arterial insufficiency, rest pain), high-output cardiac failure, and lesions located in vital areas that compromise daily function.[19] Relative indications include various signs and symptoms affecting quality of life and function, disabling pain, limb length discrepancy, cosmetic deformity, and lesions with a potentially high risk of future complications.[19,39] Treatment is usually not indicated for asymptomatic lesions in quiescent stage I. They should be observed, except in cases when complete cure can be achieved with minimal cosmetic damage and morbidity.[30,36-38,71] Some studies suggest that intervention on stage I lesions results in higher success and lower progression rates[36]; however, up to 17% of childhood AVMs remain asymptomatic until adulthood and do not require treatment.[17,19,21,37] Therefore, not all early AVMs require immediate attention. Embolization and incomplete resection of an asymptomatic lesion may actually stimulate further progression; therefore, treatment of asymptomatic lesions remains controversial.[37-39] Treatment of stage II lesions depends on symptoms and location. Stage III and IV lesions require treatment due to pain, bleeding, ulceration, or heart failure. Less favorable outcomes are achieved in more advanced AVMs, and recurrence is less likely when lower staged lesions are treated.[36-38,43]

Surgical Treatment

Surgical excision with complete eradication of the nidus is thought to offer the best opportunity for a "cure."[19] A compete surgical resection of the nidus is only possible in limited extratruncular and well-localized AVMs.[36,37,43,74] Various studies reported that 5% to 30% of AVMs are amendable to radical surgical treatment alone.[18,21,35,38,60-64,74-77] Most of these lesions are small or medium sized with minimal extension into adjacent structures (Fig. 10.2). Solitary intrapulmonary lesions in HHT or AVMs of the gastrointestinal (GI) tract can be managed with focal resection.[5,78] Due to potential hemorrhage, large residual deformities, injuries to adjacent structures, and high recurrence rates, a wide extirpation of large extratruncular infiltrating AVMs is dangerous and not recommended.[10,19,21] The role of surgical treatment has evolved over the past decade from "demolishing" operations described by Malan in 1974 to limited resections used in combination with endovascular therapy, as discussed later.[79]

Embolization

Embolization alone or in conjunction with surgical resection has developed as a primary treatment strategy for AVMs. Embolization

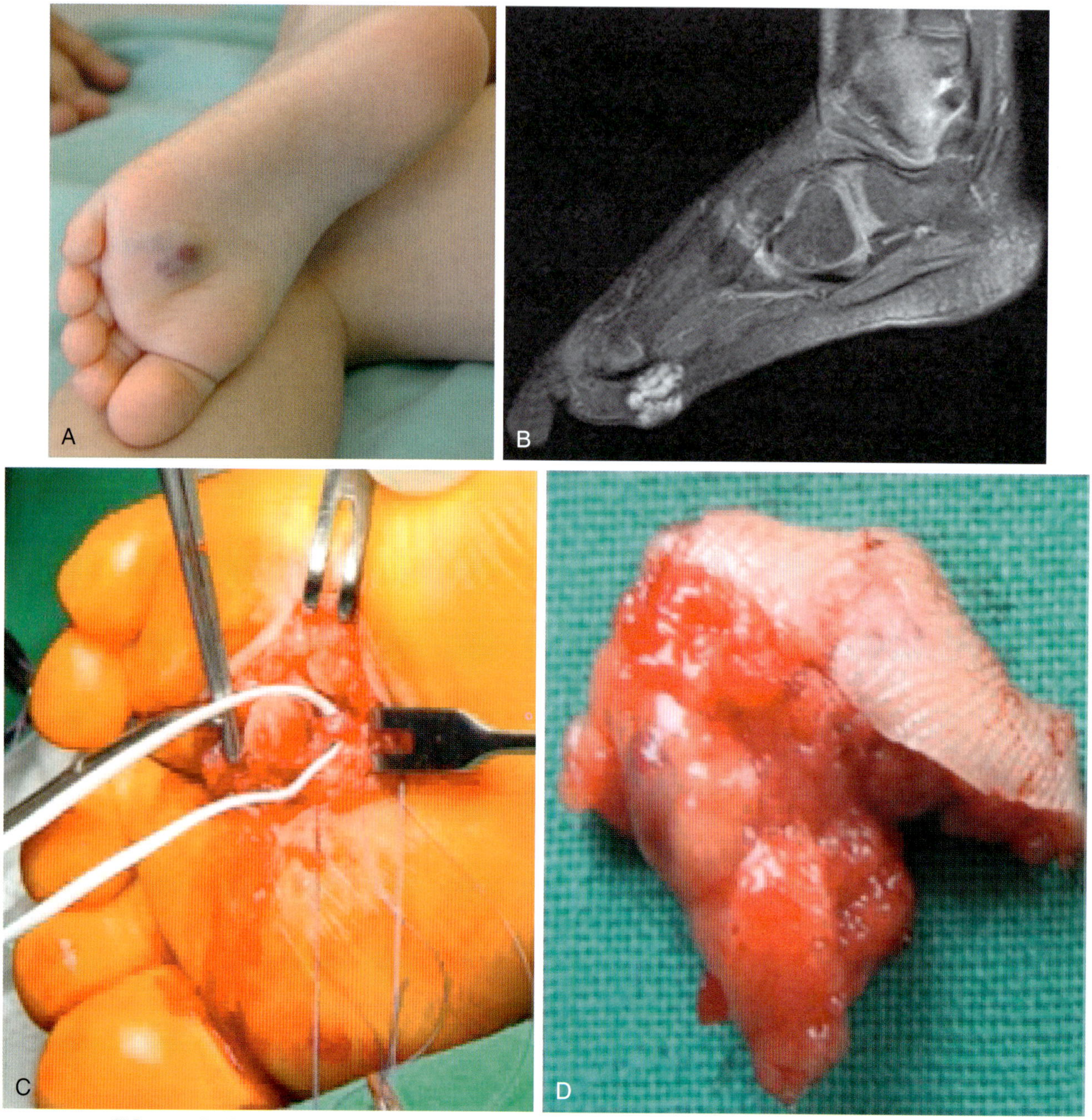

FIG 10.2 Radical surgical resection of a localized foot arteriovenous malformation (AVM) involving subcutaneous tissues of the plantar surface. (A) Initial clinical presentation. (B) Magnetic resonance angiography showing abnormal early venous filling of the AVM lesion. (C and D) Successful surgical resection with complete removal of AVM lesion. (Courtesy of Birute Vaisnyte, MD, PhD, Vilnius University, Vilnius University Hospital Santaros Klinikos.)

via transarterial, transvenous, or direct puncture approaches aims at eradicating the nidus, obliterating the most distal feeding arteries and immediate draining veins.[10] On the basis of the morphology of the nidus, an angiographic classification system has been developed (see Table 10.4).[10,60-67] It has been used as a predictive tool to guide therapeutic interventions and has prognostic value. In a study by Cho and colleagues (2006), the preferred approach for type II lesions is transvenous or direct puncture with or without coil embolization of the venous component of the nidus.[65] In this subtype of AVM, occlusion of the venous outflow with coils can be very effective and has been used to reduce the risk of tissue injury from arterial embolization with alcohol.[7,10] Type II lesions had the best therapeutic outcomes and highest cure rates with ethanol embolization.[65,80] Embolization via a transvenous approach is contraindicated in type III lesions because embolic material will not reach the nidus but rather block venous outflow, causing venous hypertension, hemorrhage, and progression if the arterial component of the nidus if not eradicated.[65] Type IIIA and IIIB lesions are best treated by direct puncture of the nidus or superselective embolization via an arterial approach.[25] Treatment of type IIIA lesions is challenging, due to lesion morphology, because transarterial embolization via small feeding vessels is often not feasible.[65]

Common embolic materials include liquid (dehydrated ethanol), semiliquid (*N*-butyl cyanoacrylate [nBCA] glue, ethylene vinyl alcohol copolymer [Onyx]), and solid embolic agents (coils, particles, and microvascular plugs).[10,32,56,81]

Transarterial embolization with ethanol has been reported to have cure rates up to 40% to 80%.[60-64] It can also be delivered through direct percutaneous injection to the lesion. Ethanol is a powerful sclerosant that causes endothelial cell damage due to protein denaturation and vascular wall destruction to the internal elastic lamina, promoting thrombosis. It permanently damages the AVM nidus. Yet this agent is associated with 10% to 30% complication rates for peripheral AVMs.[60-65,82] Most common complications are local tissue injuries such as skin blistering, necrosis, and neuropathy due to nontarget embolization and ethanol leakage into the peripheral system. Motor and sensory nerve injuries may occur. Therefore, superselective catheter positioning is essential. Ethanol-induced pulmonary hypertension is a life-threatening complication that can result in cardiac arrhythmia and cardiopulmonary collapse, so intraoperative monitoring of pulmonary and systemic pressure is essential to minimize potential complications. The total dose of ethanol should be limited to 0.5 to 1 mL/kg to avoid toxicity.[60-65] Serial embolizations of large AVMs increase the likelihood of cure and reduce the risk of tissue necrosis and postprocedure edema.[10,12,82]

nBCA and Onyx are safer alternatives to ethanol, with lower complication rates of approximately 4.8% to 17%.[31] nBCA is adhesive liquid glue that polymerizes when in contact with any ionic solution, such as blood within the nidus. It generates a mechanical vessel occlusion and an inflammatory reaction responsible for its action. Rapid nBCA delivery can be difficult to control and might result in proximal feeder occlusion, or the mixture might travel through the shunt to the lungs. Onyx is a less adhesive liquid polymerizing agent that can be injected at a slower, therefore more controlled, rate. This allows for more successful penetration of the nidus with less risk for nontarget embolization and pulmonary embolism (PE). Onyx leaves a more "spongy" mass, compared with the glues, and can be more easily resected later.[28] The drawbacks of both nBCA and Onyx are that late recanalization (11% to 18%) can occur and these agents might not be effective when used alone.[7,10,28,32,82] Therefore, rather than curative, they are palliative measures often used in preoperative staged embolization.

Mechanical occlusive devices such as coils and plugs are designed to focally occlude larger vessels and can be used in AV truncular lesions with direct connection between the artery and the vein.[20] Coils do not adequately penetrate the nidus. It is not appropriate to coil embolize primary arterial inflow to the AMV due to effects mentioned earlier. Coils are typically used as secondary devices to create a scaffold and facilitate further embolization with liquid agents. This allows limiting the volume of liquid agent.[19] Coil embolization via a transvenous approach has also been reported in several studies as an effective measure to decrease blood flow velocity through the nidus and hence decrease the amount of ethanol used.[19,24,60-64,80,82,83] Occlusion of the venous outflow with coils promotes thrombus formation and prevents potential PE.

There is no consensus regarding the most effective agent because each has its pros and cons in certain locations and lesion types. Combination of several agents and techniques may be used for optimal results.[12,20,35] Lidsky and colleagues[35] reported on the multidisciplinary treatment of 31 AVMs: eight (25.8%) were managed conservatively, eight (25.8%) were treated with transcatheter arterial embolization, six (19.4%) required embolization followed by ethanol sclerotherapy for a residual superficial component, and five (16.1%) were primarily resected. Symptom improvement was achieved in seven (87.5%) patients who underwent embolization, in four (80.0%) following surgical resection, and six (100%) following combination therapy.

Combined Treatment

Regardless of which embolic agent is used, AVMs have high recurrence rates. Embolization alone has been reported to have a 98% recurrence rates, compared with 81% following surgical or combined treatment (Fig. 10.3).[36] Patients treated with embolization alone had 14 times greater recurrence risk compared with patients treated with resection (with or without embolization). Higher recurrence rates are generally seen with the embolization-only approach because the nidus is not obliterated. Therefore, if anatomically feasible, optimal treatment should involve surgery or combined approach.[21] Combined treatment involves preoperative embolization followed by surgical lesion resection within 24 to 72 hours. It is a useful and effective measure for intraoperative hemorrhage control.[19]

Goldenberg and colleagues[84] described the impact of multiple embolizations on the outcomes of surgical resection in 31 patients with craniofacial AVMs. The number of preoperative embolization sessions was proportional to the lesion complexity and allowed for better surgical lesion identification. Twenty-two patients underwent total excision and nine subtotal resections. Recurrence rates were 15.8% in cases with precise limits versus 58.3% with imprecise limits and 18.2% after total resection versus 66.7% after subtotal resection during the follow-up period of 42.6 months. Large AVMs often require staged embolizations followed by several operative resections to fully remove the lesion or promote healing.[38]

Primary closure following resection of a large lesion is not always possible. Some of the adjunctive surgical techniques include skin grafts or free, local, or regional tissue flaps.[74,84] Where immediate primary closure or reconstruction is not feasible, vacuum-assisted closure devices can be used.[18]

Finally, amputation should not be excluded as a realistic treatment option, especially when the AVM is in an extremity with functional loss and/or is causing debilitating pain.[10,19] In fact, in patients with significant AV shunting and cardiac complications, amputation of the limb can expedite recovery and return the patient to a functional life.

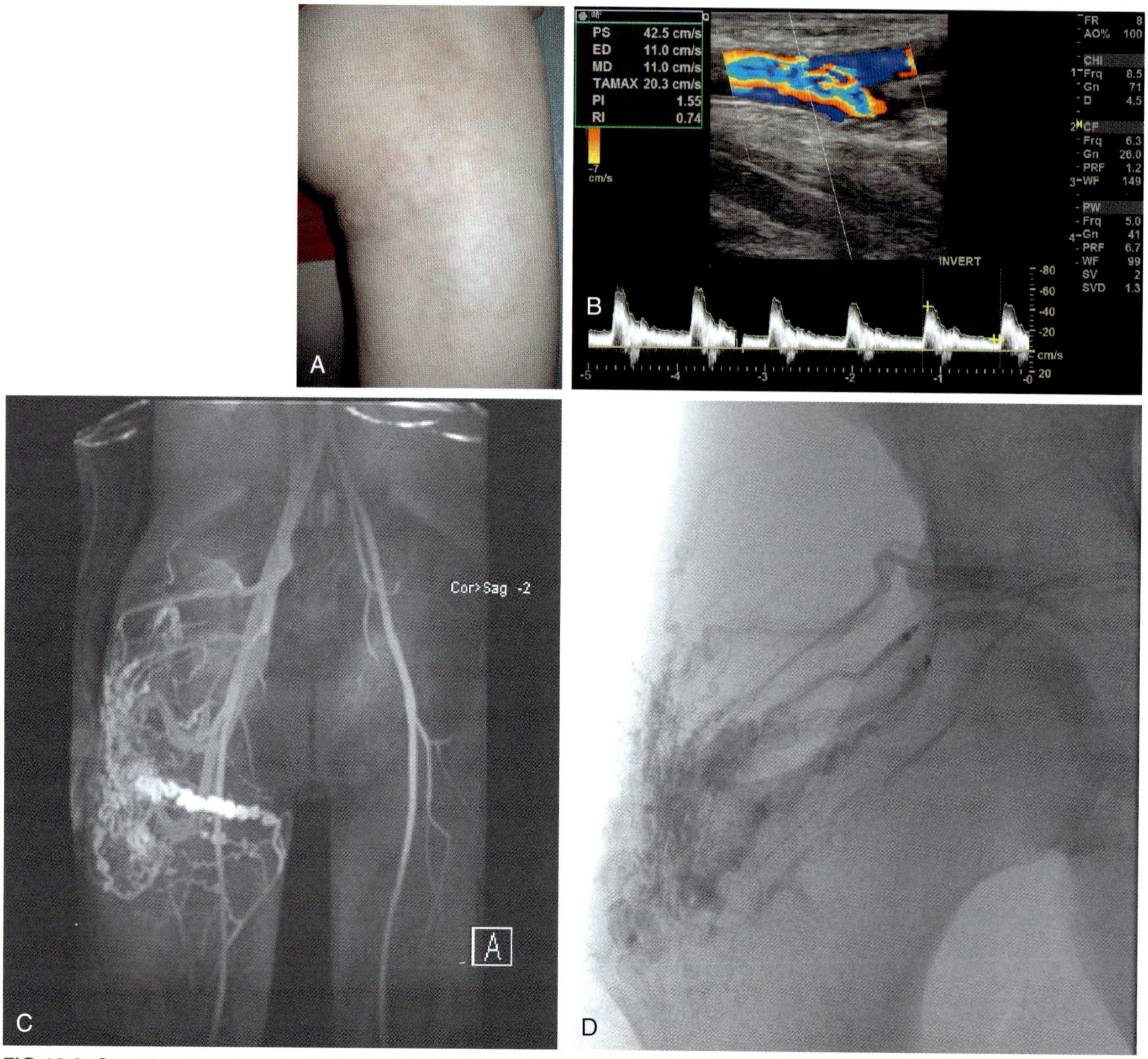

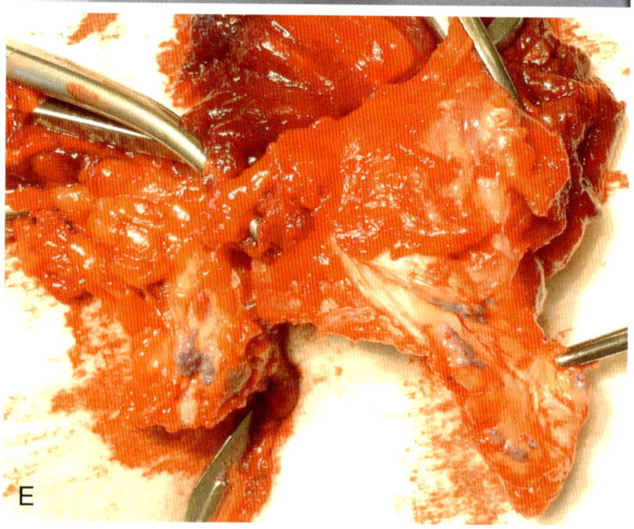

FIG 10.3 Combined treatment of a large right hip/buttock arteriovenous malformation (AVM) in an 18-year-old man with progressive development of hyperpigmentation, skin changes, and pain during puberty. This patient underwent six staged embolizations over the course of 4 years, followed by three staged surgical resections of the AVM lesion with removal of gluteus maximus and posterior thigh muscles. (A) Clinical presentation before lesion progression. (B) Duplex ultrasound finding of hemodynamically high-flow lesion with high diastolic flux along the feeding artery. (C) Magnetic resonance imaging findings confirming diffuse infiltrating extratruncular AVM within the gluteus muscle of the right buttock. (D) Arteriographic demonstration of the AVM lesion with the nidus during preoperative embolization of the lesion. (E) Surgical resection of gluteus maximus and posterior thigh muscles infiltrated by diffuse AVM. (Courtesy of Birute Vaisnyte, MD, PhD, Vilnius University, Vilnius University Hospital Santaros Klinikos.)

TRUNCULAR ARTERIAL MALFORMATIONS

Truncular AMs affect the aorta and major arteries of the limbs. As mentioned earlier, such defects include aplasia or obstruction, stenosis or hypoplasia, coarctation, and dilations or aneurysms. Anomalies of site and course of arteries are also possible. Many are asymptomatic, but some require treatment due to severe or even life-threatening hemodynamic or pathophysiologic disturbances. Compared with extratruncular lesions, diagnosis and treatment is more straightforward and in accordance with the principles of general vascular or endovascular surgery.[10]

Aberrant Right Subclavian Artery

Aberrant right subclavian artery (ARSA) is one of the most common congenital variants of the aortic arch, occurring in 0.5% to 2% of the population.[2,8,22,85] The ARSA originates in the proximal descending thoracic aorta and runs behind the esophagus. The aberrant origin of the RSA is caused by the involution of the right fourth vascular arch and proximal right dorsal aorta and the persistence of the seventh intersegmental artery originating from the proximal descending thoracic aorta, forming the abnormal course of the ARSA. A British surgeon, Bayford, first described the term "dysphagia lusoria" in 1794.[5] He described the autopsy findings in a 62-year-old woman who died of emaciation after years of dysphagia. This condition, in his own words, "may be called lusoria, from lusus naturae (Latin for 'freak of nature') that gives rise to it."[86] Most symptoms are related to development of dilation or aneurysm at the origin of RSA, occurring in nearly 60% of cases, known as Kommerell diverticulum.[85,86] It bears the name of a German radiologist who in 1936 reported the first clinical case of ARSA in the left-sided aortic arch.[88,89] The diverticulum at the origin of the ARSA artery is a remnant of the primitive right dorsal aorta.

Kommerell diverticulum can occur in a number of the aortic arch anomalies associated with aberrant course of subclavian arteries and be asymptomatic when discovered incidentally. When symptomatic, it causes tracheal or esophageal compression.[5] In the pediatric population, the symptoms frequently manifest as persistent cough, stridor, or respiratory compromise. The pathology can be misdiagnosed as a primary pulmonary or esophageal disorder. Dysphagia and thoracic pain are more commonly encountered in adults. The appearance of symptoms later in life may be due to development atherosclerotic arterial changes that make the artery wall stiffer and cause esophageal compression. Rarely, it can present as an emergency from aneurysm rupture or dissection of the native aorta.[5,85,90]

An accurate diagnosis is made noninvasively with computed tomography angiography (CTA) or magnetic resonance angiography (MRA). Catheter angiography is used as a confirmatory study. Esophageal compression due to ARSA can also be demonstrated on barium-contrast examination of the esophagus. A characteristic diagonal compression defect of the esophagus at the level of the third and fourth vertebrae is seen. Treatment is indicated in symptomatic patients or those with very large aneurysms because an embryologically abnormal vessels are prone to dissection or rupture.[85,90] Open surgical treatment with ARSA division and anastomosis to the ascending aorta or translocation to the right common carotid artery directly or via a short interposition bypass has been mainstay therapy for symptomatic lesions.[5,90] Excellent long-term patency is reported. A hybrid repair with coiling of the anomalous artery origin, combined with a carotid-subclavian bypass via right supraclavicular approach has been reported. In a recent review of 39 endovascular or hybrid published cases of ARSA, Yang and colleagues[87] reported that the hybrid approach, including thoracic stent grafting with distal subclavian ligation and reconstruction, was the most frequently used technique.

Right-Sided Aortic Arch

The right-sided aortic arch (RAA) is another common truncular anomaly of the aortic arch, reported in 0.05% of the population.[8,22,91] It results from inappropriate regression of the aortic arches with regression of the left instead of the right dorsal aorta. RAA is further subdivided into three types, according to the branching pattern of the arch vessels. In its simplest and most benign form the abnormality is a mirror-image dextrocardia with normal aortic branch anatomy. The other two types of RAA are RAA with aberrant left subclavian artery (ALSA) and RAA with isolation of the left subclavian artery (LSA).[91]

The RAA with ALSA is the most common subtype. In this anatomy, the left carotid artery is the first branch arising from the aorta, followed by the right carotid artery, right subclavian, and then ALSA. This anatomy forms due to the interruption of the dorsal segment of the left arch between the left common carotid and left subclavian arteries, with regression of the right ductus arteriosus in the hypothetical double arch.[22,23] The descending aorta appears either midline or to the right side. The ALSA may arise from the remnant of the left dorsal aortic root. In fact, Kommerell diverticulum is most frequently encountered in cases of the RAA with an ALSA.[89]

An RAA with isolation of the LSA is most rare and results from interruption of the left arch at two levels, with one level between the left common carotid and LSA and the other level distal to the attachment of the left ductus. The left carotid artery arises as the first branch of the right arch, followed by the right carotid artery and right subclavian arteries. The LSA does not have a connection with the aorta and receives retrograde flow via the left vertebral artery.[8,22,23] Despite it being a congenital anomaly, this pathology usually presents in the 4th to 5th decade of life, due to the lack of compensation for subclavian steal syndrome and vertebrobasilar insufficiency.[92,93]

Aortic Ring

Congenital anomalies of the aortic arch are usually incidental radiologic findings in asymptomatic patients, except when the anomaly constitutes a vascular ring that is formed when the abnormally developed arch vessels encircle the tracheobronchial tree and/or esophagus.[8,22,23] Depending on the origin of ligamentum arteriosum, the ring can be complete or incomplete. In the complete type of ring, both the trachea and the esophagus are fully encircled by the vascular anomaly. In the incomplete ring, the trachea and esophagus are not fully encircled. Patients with incomplete ring are usually asymptomatic.

Double aortic arch is the most common cause of a complete aortic ring. In this anomaly the ascending aorta divides into two separate arches. The left or anterior arch follows the course of the normal left-sided aorta and the right or posterior arch has a course to the left, behind the esophagus, before it joins the left arch.[91] The descending aorta is usually to the left side. Double aortic arch has various forms. Both arches may be patent, or an atretic (but persistent) segment may be present at one of the several locations in either arch. When both arches are patent, the right or left arch may be larger, or they may be similar in size. A cervical arch on either side, variable laterality of the descending thoracic aorta, coarctation of the major arch, and/or discontinuity of the central pulmonary arteries may be present. In more than 75% of patients the right arch is dominant, extends more cephalad, and is more posterior than the left.[91] Clinically, the onset and severity of symptoms of esophageal and tracheal obstruction are variable and depend on the tightness of the ring. Most patients present with stridor, recurrent respiratory infections, or dysphagia within the first 6 months of life.

CT angiography and MRI are the most effective imaging methods. Barium-contrast esophagogram and bronchoscopy are supplemental studies that help to prove the presence of the vascular ring. Surgical division of the complete aortic ring was first described by Gross in 1945.[94] In patients with complete vascular rings, surgical division releases the complete circle formed by the vascular and ligamentous structures around the trachea and esophagus. Video-assisted thoracoscopic surgical (VATS) techniques and endoscopic robotic-assisted techniques have been recently introduced to vascular ring ligation and division. These techniques have become more popular due to improved safety; low complication rates such as decreased surgical trauma and reduced intensive care unit and hospital stay, an enhanced recovery, and improved cosmetic results.[95,96] VATS was found to have excellent clinical outcomes, similar to those of the open thoracotomy approach.[96]

Persistent Sciatic Artery

Truncular AMs of lower extremities that are associated with aneurysm development include a fetal internal iliac artery and persistent sciatic artery (PSA).[2,5,97] The sciatic artery is an embryonic continuation of the internal iliac artery and functions as the earliest fetal axial blood supply to the lower extremity. Normally, it involutes by the third gestational month as the femoral artery develops. In adults, remnants of the sciatic artery persist as portions of the internal iliac, popliteal. and peroneal arteries.[8] In 0.03% to 0.06% of the population the sciatic artery does not regress in utero and is associated with a high incidence of complications, which include aneurysm formation (25% to 48%), aneurysm rupture, embolism, and sciatic nerve compression.[2,10,98] It has been reported that 30% to 60% of the PSAs cases present with lower extremity ischemia and up to 25% of patients have critical limb ischemia due to aneurysm thrombosis or distal embolization.[99]

In 75% of the cases the PSA is complete: it follows the course of the sciatic nerve and provides the major inflow to the thigh and lower extremity via the popliteal artery, and the superficial femoral artery (SFA) is absent or hypoplastic. In 25% of the cases the PSA is incomplete: the sciatic artery becomes hypoplastic in the thigh and the SFA is the major inflow vessel to the leg. Most incidental cases of a PSA do not require treatment, and 50% are partially asymptomatic.[2,22,98]

The classic physical exam finding of palpable pedal pulse in setting of absent femoral pulse is observed only in complete type PSA.[5,97] Duplex US is useful in confirming an absent SFA.[10] However, MRA, CTA, or catheter arteriography are more accurate in diagnosing the PSA and in identifying the type. Although asymptomatic PSAs should be observed, symptomatic patients should be treated based on the classification of the PSA, and presence or absence of aneurysmal degeneration, as well as distal embolization. In cases of incomplete type of PSA, aneurysm exclusion is sufficient because the SFA provides adequate lower extremity perfusion. When PSA is the dominant inflow vessel to the lower leg, exclusion of the aneurysm and revascularization with an interposition bypass graft are required. In patients with ischemia due to thrombosis or embolization from aneurysmal PSA, thrombolytic therapy may be useful before definitive revascularization. Endovascular techniques with embolization of incomplete PSA aneurysm or endovascular stent-graft exclusion of the complete form have been described. The endovascular approach avoids the morbidity of open operation and carries a decreased risk of sciatic nerve damage; however, long-term durability due to potential aneurysmal degeneration and stent fracture in gluteal region remains an issue.[99,100] A review described the intermediate and long-term outcomes in 29 symptomatic PSAs and found that regardless of the method of arterial reconstruction or PSA repair, the outcomes of different treatments for lower limb ischemia and PSAs were satisfactory. The patients remained asymptomatic during the follow-up period, which ranged from 2 months to 10 years.[101]

Aortic Coarctation

Aortic coarctations or hypoplasias are among the best-known and most commonly treated truncular AMs. Coarctation occurs in 5.1% to 8.1% of patients with congenital heart defects.[2,5] Aortic coarctation typically occurs in the proximal descending thoracic aorta, distal to the left SCA, as a stenosis in the juxtaductal region. Atypical coarctation or hypoplasia can occur anywhere along thoracic or abdominal aorta. Long segment thoracic and abdominal aortic coarctation is extremely rare, reported in approximately 0.5% to 2% of all coarctation cases.[5] Symptoms occur within the first 3 decades of life and include hypertension, lower extremity claudication, and mesenteric ischemia. Although open surgical repair continues to be the mainstay of treatment for aortic coarctation, endovascular techniques have emerged. Successful dilations and aortic stenting have been reported to delay or replace open surgical corrections. Balloon angioplasty, bare metal stents, and stent-grafts have been used for typical coarctation with increasing frequency, in spite of the need for close observation and repeat treatment of recurrences, which are more frequent than after open repairs.[2] A meta-analysis by Carr and colleagues[102] compared endovascular with surgical therapy for typical coarctation and concluded that primary angioplasty or stenting of adult aortic coarctation had similar morbidity to open repair; however, recurrence and reintervention rates were higher following endovascular interventions. Both therapies in the short term provided similar relief from hypertension. Primary stenting had the lowest risk and isolated angioplasty had the highest risk for complications. Although surgical complications were minor (bleeding, recurrent laryngeal nerve injury), endovascular interventions included more serious complications such as dissection, traumatic aneurysm, or stroke.[102] Long-term follow-up is needed to establish clinical equipoise between these two approaches.

Mid-Aortic Syndrome

Mid-aortic syndrome (MAS) is a rare congenital truncular AM or acquired condition with a total of approximately 200 cases described in literature.[103] The modern description of MAS was first published by Sen in 1963, who described 16 cases in young patients and named the syndrome.[104] It is characterized by segmental narrowing of the distal descending thoracic or abdominal aorta and frequently is accompanied by concomitant stenosis of renal (60% to 90%) and visceral aortic branches (20% to 40%) (Fig. 10.4).[103,105] The male-to-female ratio is 3:1. Congenital MAS is found in very young patients and is thought to occur due to incomplete fusion or and maturation of the paired embryonic dorsal aortas during the 4th week of gestation.[103] Another hypothesis suggests that acquired insults in utero or in early life (such as rubella infection) result in developmental disorders and hypoplasia of the growing aorta.[8] Acquired MAS is associated with neurofibromatosis, fibromuscular dysplasia, retroperitoneal fibrosis, Williams syndrome, mucopolysaccharidosis, and giant cell arteritis, including temporal and Takayasu arteritis. Young patients usually present with medically unresponsive hypertension, headache, and early fatigue with exertion. Rarely, it presents as bilateral lower extremity claudication or abdominal angina due to proximal stenosis and mesenteric hypoperfusion. In acquired MAS, signs and symptoms are associated with the underlying disease etiology. Diagnostic CTA or angiography usually shows robust collateral circulation due to narrowing of the abdominal aorta. Open surgical reconstructions include aortoaortic, aortorenal, and aortovisceral bypasses; reconstruction of narrowed renal/visceral branches with bypass grafting, or patch aortoplasty, are thought to offer the greatest durability. Seventy percent of patients have been reported to have normalized or improved blood pressure control.[103] However, these procedures are more challenging in children, and graft replacement may be required as the patient develops. Some studies suggest surgery as a definitive option but ideally not until later in life. Others advocate early surgical management with later revision as needed.[106,107] An endovascular approach is feasible for discrete stenoses that do not involve mesenteric or renal arteries. Few

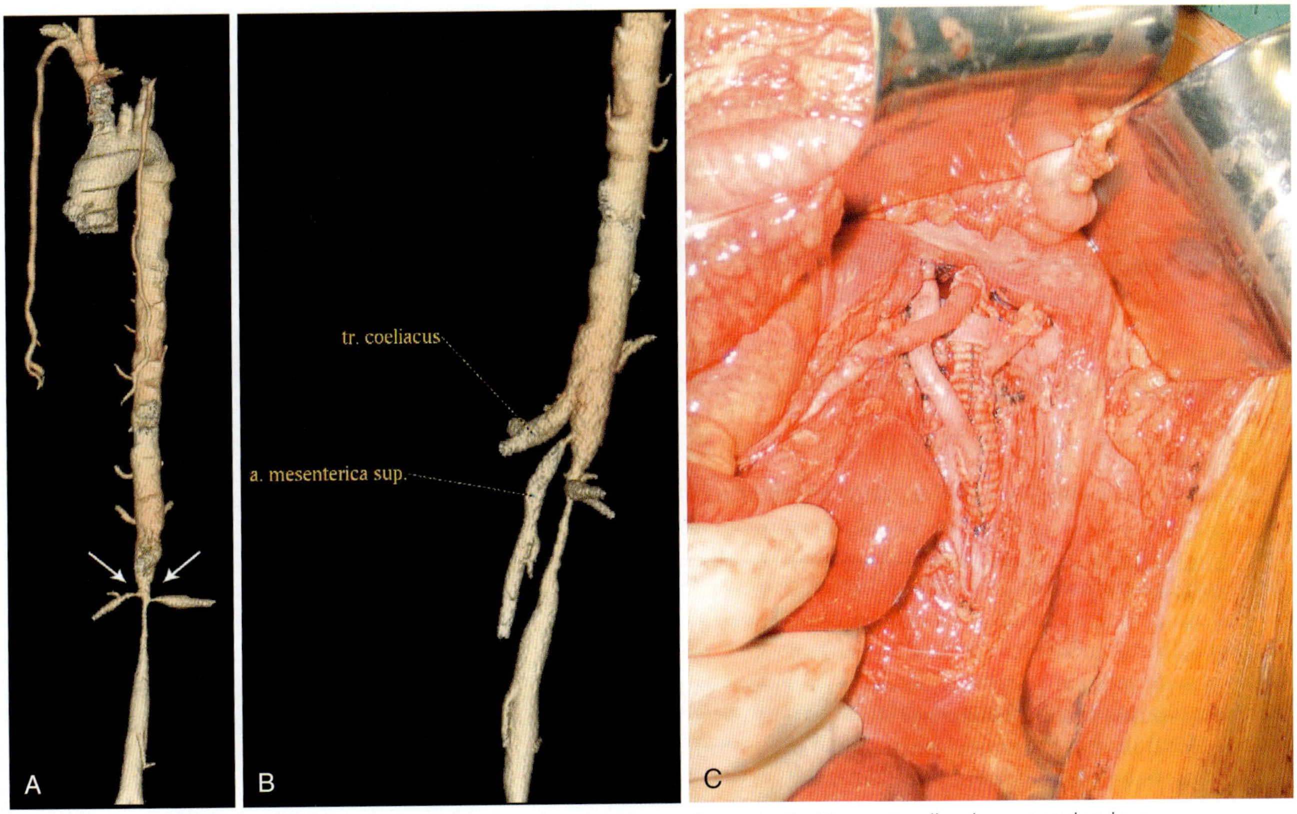

FIG 10.4 Mid-aortic syndrome associated with poorly controlled long-standing hypertension in a 21-year-old female. (A) Three-dimensional computed tomography reconstruction of the entire aorta demonstrates abdominal aortic coarctation and bilateral renal artery stenoses *(arrows)*. (B) Celiac and superior mesenteric artery stenoses with poststenotic dilation are seen in lateral projection. (C) The patient underwent surgical reconstruction with aortoaortic bypass using 8-mm Dacron graft and bilateral renal and mesenteric artery bypasses using saphenous vein. (Courtesy of Birute Vaisnyte, MD, PhD, Vilnius University, Vilnius University Hospital Santaros Klinikos.)

studies exist on stenting and percutaneous transluminal angioplasty (PTA) in children, but endovascular proponents argue that percutaneous interventions are less invasive, can be performed earlier, and reintervened upon as needed.

CONCLUSIONS

During recent decades, there have been significant advances in our understanding of CVM pathophysiology, which has led to improved diagnosis and management of patients with congenital AMs. Extratruncular AMs, and specifically AVMs, are challenging lesions that require an individualized approach and are best treated in centers of excellence under the management of multidisciplinary team. Accurate recognition of the correct pathology is essential in choosing appropriate treatment strategies. Even with the new treatment strategies, combined approaches, and multiple treatment sessions, most AVMs cannot be cured and remain lifelong medical issues. The primary treatment goal for patients with AVMs is to control lesion size and symptoms while optimizing the quality of life. Truncular AMs are encountered by a wider range of surgical specialists, and their diagnosis and treatment are more straightforward, so long-term outcomes are excellent.

REVIEW QUESTIONS

1. Which of the following is true regarding extratruncular CVMs?
   a. Extratruncular CVMs originate between 4th and 7th weeks of gestation
   b. They arise before the formation of mature vascular trunks and possess the ability to proliferate
   c. They manifest as abnormal major axial vessels or persistent embryonic vessels
   d. They can be differentiated from truncular CVMs by their location, distribution, and size
2. True or false: Extracranial AVMs are more common than intracranial AVMs.
3. The Integrated Classification System for CVMs includes all of the following components except:
   a. Flow characteristics
   b. Truncular versus extratruncular distinction
   c. Vessel characteristics
   d. Arteriovenous and combined anomalies
   e. Differentiation between benign and malignant hemangiomas
4. What is the most common location for extracranial AVMs?
   a. Head and neck region
   b. Pelvis
   c. Extremities
   d. Chest
   e. Genitalia
5. What is the most important clinical characteristic used to distinguish hemangiomas from true vascular malformations?
   a. Presence of arterial blood flow component
   b. The age of the patient
   c. Lesion appearance and distribution on physical exam
   d. Rapid growth in infancy, followed by gradual regression
6. A 25-year-old woman presents at 36 weeks' gestation with necrotic ulceration and hemorrhage from a right gluteal region AVM. She has a normal electrocardiogram and subsequent cardiac evaluation reveals no abnormalities. Which Schobinger stage does this patient fall into?
   a. Stage I
   b. Stage IIA
   c. Stage IIB
   d. Stage III
   e. Stage IV
7. According to the angiographic classification of AVMs, AVM lesions with multiple shunts between arterioles and venules are best treated with:
   a. Embolization of the nidus via transvenous approach
   b. Embolization of the nidus via transarterial approach
   c. Ligation or coil embolization of the proximal arterial inflow vessel
   d. Direct puncture
   e. Resection of extensive lesions
8. Which of the following statements regarding Kommerell diverticulum is false:
   a. It can cause symptoms of tracheal or esophageal compression in both children and adults
   b. It can be asymptomatic and discovered incidentally
   c. It is a dilation or aneurysm at the origin of the subclavian artery that occurs only in association with aberrant origin of the right subclavian artery
   d. Rarely it can present as an emergency from rupture or dissection of the native aorta
9. True or false: Patients with incidentally discovered persistent sciatic artery do not require immediate treatment.
10. Which of the following presentations is the most common for patients with mid-aortic syndrome?
    a. Bilateral lower extremity claudication
    b. Chronic mesenteric ischemia
    c. Poorly controlled hypertension
    d. Progressive kidney dysfunction

SELECTED REFERENCES

1. Charmeliet P. Angiogenesis in health and disease. *Nat Med.* 2003;9:653–660.
2. Markovic JV, Shortell CEK. Multidisciplinary treatment of extremity arteriovenous malformations. *J Vasc Surg: Venous and Lym Dis.* 2015;3:2009–2018.
3. Mulliken JB, Glowacki J. Hemangiomas and vascular malformations in infants and children: A classification system based on endothelial characteristics. *Plast Reconstr Surg.* 1982;69:412–422.
4. Lee BB, Antignani PL, Baraldini V, et al. ISVI-IUA consensus document. Diagnostic guidelines of vascular anomalies: vascular malformations and hemangiomas. *Int Angiol.* 2015;34: 333–374.
5. Liu AS, Mulliken JB, Zurakowski D, et al. Extracranial arteriovenous malformations: natural progression and recurrence after treatment. *Plast Reconstr Surg.* 2010;125: 1185–1194.
6. Greene AK, Orbach DB. Management of arteriovenous malformations. *Clin Plast Surg.* 2011;38:95–106.
7. Visser A, Fitzjohn T, Swee TT. Surgical management of arteriovenous malformation. *J Plast Reconstr Aesthet Surg.* 2011;64:283–291.
8. Skandalakis JE, Gray SW, Symbas P. The thoracic and abdominal aorta. In: Skandalakis JE, Gray SW, eds. *Embryology for Surgeons: The Embryological Basis for the Treatment of Congenital Anomalies.* 2nd ed. Baltimore: Williams & Wilkins; 1994: 976–1030.
9. van Hooft IM, Zeebregts CJ, van Sterkenburg SMM, et al. The persistent sciatic artery. *Eur J Vasc Endovasc Surg.* 2009;37: 585–591.
10. Yang C, Shu C, Li M, Li Q, Kopp R. Aberrant subclavian artery pathologies and Kommerell's diverticulum: a review and analysis of published endovascular/hybrid treatment options. *J Endovasc Ther.* 2012;19:373–382.

References available online at ExpertConsult.com.

11 CHAPTER

Antibiotic Prophylaxis in Vascular Disease Management

Hugh A. Gelabert, Taimur Saleem

INTRODUCTION

The use of antibiotics in vascular surgery has undergone significant change in the course of the past half-century. Initial experience with devastating arterial graft infections and significant data supporting antibiotic use led to overuse of antibiotics. More recent experience with restricted use of antibiotics has resulted in a more balanced approach. Our goal in this chapter is to review the use of antibiotics in vascular surgery both as prophylaxis and as therapeutic intervention. Specific instances of arterial infections and use of antibiotics in the management of them will also be addressed.

PROPHYLACTIC ANTIBIOTIC THERAPY

Although infections of implanted vascular prostheses are relatively uncommon, when they do occur, they are associated with significant morbidity and mortality. Complications of graft infection include pseudoaneurysm, anastomotic disruption, hemorrhage, fistula formation, and sepsis. Infection of a vascular graft almost always requires partial or complete graft removal, which is associated with a high incidence of amputation. Vascular graft infection leads to the patient's death in one-quarter to one-half of cases in contemporary series. These dire consequences have prompted laboratory and clinical investigation into the role of antibiotics in the prevention of vascular graft infection. The widespread use of prophylactic antibiotics in vascular surgery has significantly altered the microbiology and clinical presentation of graft infections. New insights have been gained into the pathogenesis of this process, and alternative methods of antibiotic delivery have been developed in animal models. This section presents the bacteriology and current understanding of the pathogenesis of graft infection, a historical overview of the development of antibiotic prophylaxis in vascular surgery, current recommendations for prophylaxis, and new directions in antibiotic delivery.

Clinical Significance of Graft Infection

The reported incidence of infection after the placement of vascular prostheses ranges from 1% to 6%. This relatively low rate of infection has remained stable over time, despite improvements in technique and the introduction of routine preoperative antibiotic prophylaxis. Two early series, from Hoffert and colleagues[1] in 1965 and Fry and Lindenauer[2] in 1967, reported graft infection rates of 6.0% (12 of 201) and 1.34% (12 of 890), respectively. In 1972, Szilagyi and colleagues[3] reported a large series of 3397 cases in which the graft infection rate was 1.9%. Later reports detailed similar findings. The series of Lorentzen and coauthors[4] from 1985 described graft infections in 62 of 2411 patients, a rate of 2.6%. Although the overall incidence of infection has not changed significantly, the use of antibiotic prophylaxis has clearly changed the clinical presentation of most vascular graft infections. Suppurative infections appearing in the first few weeks after graft implantation have given way to more insidious, low-grade, chronic infections.[5,6]

Infection in prosthetic grafts remains a critical issue in vascular surgery. Reported mortality rates from graft infection range from 25% to 75% (Table 11.1).[1,2,5,12-14] Mortality is greatest for proximal grafts, with almost uniform lethality reported in aortic stump sepsis.[2,3,9,12] Despite attempts to reduce mortality in aortic graft infection, it remains relatively high at 24% to 43%.[15-19] Peripheral graft infections are generally associated with lower mortality rates (as low as 6%).[19] Amputation rates are similar for survivors of aortic and peripheral graft infections, ranging from 22.5% to 43%.[3,8,11] In more recent series, reported amputation rates range from 24% to 27%.[18-20]

Principles of Antibiotic Prophylaxis

The goal of prophylactic antibiotic therapy is to prevent infection after surgery. The most important indication for antibiotic prophylaxis in vascular reconstructive surgery is the use of prosthetic materials. Synthetic materials provide a protective substrate for bacterial colonization and proliferation. Experimental studies have demonstrated that the presence of a foreign body increases the infectivity of *Staphylococcus aureus* 10,000-fold.[21] In light of the potentially catastrophic consequences of vascular graft infection, prophylactic antibiotics are recommended in patients undergoing procedures in which prosthetic materials are used.

The ideal prophylactic antibiotic should be bactericidal for the most common pathogens causing postoperative infection and adequately concentrated in serum and at the site of surgery. It should be present in adequate concentrations throughout the surgical procedure and nontoxic to the patient. In addition, its cost should be reasonable enough to justify its routine use.

Most vascular graft infections are caused by relatively few specific bacteria; therefore, broad-spectrum antibiotic prophylaxis is unnecessary. Selecting an antibiotic with the narrowest spectrum of activity that includes the most common pathogens

TABLE 11.1 Influence of Graft Site on Incidence and Outcome of Graft Infection

Author	Year	Type of Graft	Patients	Rate (%)[a]	Rate (%)[b]	Rate (%)
Hoffert and colleagues[1]	1965	Aortoiliac	84	0	NA	NA
		Aortofemoral	30	0	NA	NA
		Iliofemoropopliteal	83	13.0	75	25
Szilagyi and colleagues[3]	1972	Aortoiliac	418	0.7	0	66
		Aortofemoral	1244	1.6	21	53
		Iliofemoropopliteal	270	3.0	40	7
Bouhoutsos and colleagues[7]	1974	Aortoiliac/aortofemoral	412	1.5	0	50
		Iliofemoropopliteal	108	7.4	25	0
Liekweg and Greenfield[8]	1977	Aortoiliac	NR	NR	3	8
		Aortofemoral	NR	NR	11	47
		Iliofemoropopliteal	NR	NR	30	13
Yashar and colleagues[9]	1978	Aortoiliac	300	1.0	0	33
		Aortofemoral	210	2.9	33	50
		Iliofemoropopliteal	65	4.6	67	0
Casali and colleagues[10]	1980	Aortoiliac	NR	NR	0	50
		Aortofemoral	NR	NR	25	67
		Iliofemoropopliteal	NR	NR	33	33
Lorentzen and colleagues[4]	1985	Aortoiliac	515	0.0	NA	NA
		Aortofemoral	1497	3.0	22	29
		Iliofemoropopliteal	489	3.5	53	18
Edwards and colleagues[11]	1987	Aortic/aortoiliac	769	0.0	NA	NA
		Aortofemoral	1060	0.47	20	40
		Iliofemoropopliteal	583	2.9	12	18

[a]Primary graft infections only; excludes aortoenteric fistulas.
[b]Amputation rate among survivors.
NA, Not applicable; *NR*, not reported.

involved in graft infection will limit the emergence of resistant organisms. Antibiotics that are the principal line of therapy in difficult infections (such as vancomycin in the treatment of *Staphylococcus epidermidis* infections) should generally be reserved for that indication and not used in prophylaxis. Generally, the threshold for using prophylactic antibiotics in procedures without insertion of prosthetic material is high. This is particularly true in those instances where the consequence of an infection would present a low risk of serious sequelae. An example of this would be venous ablation or sclerotherapy. Less certainty arises in cases that involve open surgery with suture repair of the arteries. In such instances some hematoma is common, and infection would have the potential of resulting in an arterial disruption and hemorrhage. Although this may be a "clean" operation, the potential consequence of an infection could be devastating. For this reason, some would advise use of antibiotic prophylaxis.

Efforts have been made to identify risk factors that would predispose to infectious complications in vascular surgery. Basetti and colleagues noted that longer surgical times (>2 hours), reintervention on the same site within the first week, vascular stent placement in the inguinal canal, immunosuppression, and history of prosthetic surgery were identified as situations where antibiotic prophylaxis should be considered. Also, procedures including endograft placement, embolization and chemoembolization, and central venous access in immunocompromised individuals may merit antibiotic prophylaxis.[22] Ott and associates performed a retrospective analysis of cases to identify independent risk factors for surgical site infection. They specifically noted Fontaine stages III–IV, femoral grafting, postoperative drainage for more than 5 days, duration of operation greater than 214 minutes, and body mass index (BMI) greater than 29 as being significant risk factors for vascular infection.[23]

Bacteriology of Graft Infection

Gram-positive cocci, the predominant flora of the skin and dermal appendages, are most often responsible for vascular graft infections. Although the bacteriology of graft infection varies somewhat by anatomic site, when all sites are considered together, approximately 60% to 65% of reported cases are currently due to gram-positive organisms. The remaining 35% to 40% are largely due to gram-negative rods, which account for approximately half of all infections in intraabdominal (aortic, aortoiliac) grafts. Although *S. aureus* has historically been the most frequently cultured pathogen, the introduction of routine antibiotic prophylaxis and improved culture techniques have led to the emergence of *S. epidermidis* and other coagulase-negative staphylococci as the most frequent cause of vascular graft infection (Table 11.2). The most commonly cultured gram-negative rod is *Escherichia coli,* followed by *Proteus* species, *Pseudomonas* species, and *Klebsiella* species.

In early reports from the 1960s and 1970s, *S. aureus* was identified as the predominant pathogen in vascular graft infections. In 1965, Hoffert and colleagues[1] reported that *S. aureus* was cultured in 67% (8 of 12) of aortic, femoral, and popliteal

TABLE 11.2 Effect of Antibiotic Prophylaxis on the Microbiology of Graft Infection

Author	Year	Type of Graft	Antibiotics	CULTURED ORGANISMS (%)[a] *Staphylococcus aureus*	*Staphylococcus epidermidis*	*Escherichia coli*	Other GNRs	Culture Negative (%)
Hoffert and colleagues[1]	1965	Aortic and distal	No	67	17	8	25	17
Fry and Lindenauer[2]	1967	Aortic	No	67	0	25	8	8
Goldstone and Moore[5]	1974	Aortic and distal	In some cases[b]	41	26	15	11	7
Liekweg and Greenfield[8]	1977	Aortic and distal	No	50	4	13	18	NR
Bandyk and colleagues[6]	1984	Aortofemoral	Yes	10	60	13	23	10
Yeager and colleagues[19]	1985	Aortic	Yes	0	50	0	0	33
		Distal	Yes	14	14	0	29	43
Quiñones-Baldrich and colleagues[24]	1991	Aortic	Yes	13	21	18	45	21

[a]Expressed as the percentage of cases from which each organism was cultured.
[b]Prophylaxis administered in 10 of 27 cases of graft infection.
GNR, Gram-negative rod; *NR*, not reported.

reconstructions. Likewise, in a series of 890 aortic grafts from Fry and Lindenauer,[2] *S. aureus* was cultured in 67% (8 of 12) of cases. In 1967, Smith and colleagues[25] reported on nine cases of femoropopliteal graft infection, eight of which were due to *S. aureus*. In a review of 108 published cases of vascular graft infection reported between 1959 and 1974, Liekweg and Greenfield[8] noted that *S. aureus* was responsible for 50% of cases. The next most common pathogens were gram-negative rods (30.5%) and streptococci (8.5%); only 3.6% of cases were due to *S. epidermidis*.

Goldstone and Moore[5] were among the first to note the effects of antibiotic prophylaxis on the presentation and bacteriology of graft infection. They retrospectively reviewed the incidence of graft infection before and after the initiation of routine antibiotic prophylaxis. During the preantibiotic prophylaxis period (1959–1966), the vascular graft infection rate was 4.1% (9 of 222). From 1966 to 1973, when prophylactic antibiotic use became routine, the graft infection rate dropped to 1.5% (5 of 344). Of all staphylococcal infections treated at the author's institution between 1959 and 1973, 14 of 18 (78%) occurred before the routine use of prophylactic antibiotics.

Reviews of graft infection since the advent of routine antibiotic prophylaxis demonstrate an increasing incidence of late infections resulting from fastidious organisms such as *S. epidermidis* and other coagulase-negative staphylococci. Bandyk and colleagues[6] presented a report of 30 patients treated for aortofemoral graft infections from 1972 to 1982; 60% of these infections were due to *S. epidermidis*. The time of presentation influenced the microbiology of graft infection. Four of five early (<4 months) infections were due to gram-negative rods. Late infections (>4 months) were much more common, totaling 25; of these, 15 (60%) were due to *S. epidermidis*.

In 1985, Yeager and associates[19] reported a 9-year experience in which they managed 14 aortic and 11 peripheral graft infections. Whereas peripheral graft infections appeared an average of 8 months after surgery, aortic graft infections appeared an average of 5 years afterward. Of five primarily infected aortic grafts (not graft-enteric fistulas or erosions) with positive cultures, four were due to *S. epidermidis*. A wide range of organisms was cultured from peripheral grafts, including coagulase-positive and -negative staphylococci, gram-negative rods, anaerobic streptococci, and diphtheroids.

Edwards and associates[26] reported on 24 infections from a series of 2614 aortofemoropopliteal grafts over a 10-year period from 1975 to 1986; the majority (29%) were due to *S. aureus*. The authors noted, however, that prophylactic antibiotics were administered according to the departmental protocol in only 7 of 24 cases. This observation was supported by the fact that 63% of these infections appeared within 3 months of implantation. In addition, cultures were negative in 21% of patients, suggesting that the presence of fastidious organisms such as *S. epidermidis* may have been underestimated. In 1991, Quiñones-Baldrich and colleagues[24] reported an 18-year experience (1970–1988) with 45 aortic graft infections. Culture results were available for 38 of 45 patients. Gram-negative organisms, most commonly *Pseudomonas* species (21%) and *E. coli* (18%), were cultured from 24 patients (63%). Gram-positive cocci, most frequently *S. epidermidis* (21%), were cultured from 21 patients (55%). Of note is the fact that cultures grew multiple organisms in 39% of cases. There were eight (21%) negative cultures, again suggesting that the incidence of infection owing to fastidious organisms may have been underestimated.

Pathogenesis of Graft Infection

Although there is no definitive explanation of how graft infection occurs, the two principal routes of infection are thought to be direct contamination (bacteria present in the surgical wound) and hematogenous or lymphatogenous seeding. It is generally thought that most graft infections are caused by direct intraoperative contamination of the prosthesis. Potential sources of infecting organisms include the patient's skin, breaks in aseptic technique, adjacent active infections, transudation of bowel flora into the peritoneal space, and the diseased arterial tree itself, which may become colonized with pathogenic bacteria.

Skin Flora

The normal skin flora is the most important source of bacteria. Accordingly, preoperative skin preparation influences subsequent infection rates. Kaiser and coworkers[27] noted a higher rate of infection with a hexachlorophene-ethanol preparation compared with povidone-iodine. Close and colleagues[28] reported that hexachlorophene is more effective alone than when used in combination with ethanol. In a prospective study, Cruse demonstrated that preoperative hexachlorophene showering can be effective in reducing wound infection rates, and overzealous shaving may actually increase the risk of infection.[29] Wooster and colleagues[30] demonstrated that vascular grafts routinely become contaminated with skin organisms intraoperatively and suggested that careful attention to aseptic technique can significantly reduce this occurrence.

Groin incisions appear to have special significance in the development of vascular graft infections. Grafts involving an inguinal wound have a higher incidence of infection than do those that avoid this region.[3,5,7] Jamieson and colleagues[12] reported that the presence of a groin incision increased the risk of graft infection 3.5-fold; the presence of a groin complication such as a seroma or hematoma increased the risk of infection ninefold over patients without groin complications. Up to 33% of groin incisions with hematomas may develop infections.[9] Lorentzen and associates[4] reported that the highest incidence of infection was in patients who underwent aortobifemoral grafting for abdominal aortic aneurysms (5.9%), whereas there were no infections in 425 patients who underwent aortoiliac bypass for aneurysms (213) and occlusive atherosclerosis (212).

Gastrointestinal Flora

The gastrointestinal tract is a potential source of contamination during aortic reconstruction. Cultures of intestinal bag fluid have been reported by some investigators to yield enteric bacteria[8] and skin organisms such as coagulase-negative staphylococci.[31] In a report of 109 bowel bag cultures from abdominal aortic reconstructions, Scobie and colleagues[32] found positive cultures in 14% of patients. *S. epidermidis* was the single most common organism isolated ($n = 11$), whereas enteric flora were cultured in 12.

The impact of concomitant gastrointestinal surgery in the development of vascular graft infection is unclear. In separate series, DeBakey and colleagues,[33] Stoll,[34] and Hardy and colleagues[35] reported a total of 670 patients who underwent aortic graft placement and simultaneous gastrointestinal procedures, with no episodes of graft infection. These authors concluded that such coincident procedures can be undertaken safely. Other investigators, however, described the development of graft infection in patients undergoing simultaneous appendectomy,[5] cholecystectomy and gastrostomy,[36] and anterior resection.[30]

Arterial Colonization

The native arterial tree may harbor bacteria. The presence of pathogenic bacteria, particularly coagulase-negative staphylococci, in vascular tissues not previously operated on has been widely documented (Table 11.3). Lalka and colleagues[45] postulated that transient bacteremias resulting from breaks in the skin or mucous membranes may lead to arterial colonization. Bacterial contamination of vascular prostheses may therefore be inevitable in some cases. It is not yet clear, however, to what extent the presence of positive arterial wall cultures influences the likelihood of subsequent graft infection.

The 1977 report by Ernst and associates[31] of abdominal aortic aneurysmal wall cultures was one of the first to highlight the presence of pathogenic organisms in the native aorta. The overall incidence of positive cultures was 15%, and cultures were more likely to be positive when atherosclerotic disease was more advanced. Asymptomatic aneurysms were less likely to be culture positive (9%) than were symptomatic (13%) or ruptured aneurysms (35%). *S. epidermidis* was the most frequently isolated organism. The late graft sepsis rate was 10% in the culture-positive group versus 2% in the culture-negative group. In a similar report, Buckels and coauthors[39] described an 8% (22 of

TABLE 11.3 Positive Arterial Wall Cultures: Incidence and Significance

Author	Year	Culture Source	Positive Cultures (%)	Associated With Subsequent Infection?	Frequency of *Staphylococcus epidermidis* Among Positive Cultures (%)
Ernst and colleagues[31]	1977	Aortic aneurysms	15	Yes	53
Scobie and colleagues[32]	1979	Aortic aneurysms	23	No	71
Macbeth and colleagues[37]	1984	Femoropopliteal specimens	43	Yes	71
McAuley and colleagues[38]	1984	Aortic thrombus	14	No	NR
Buckels and colleagues[39]	1985	Aortic aneurysms	8	Yes	30
Durham and colleagues[40]	1987	Aortofemoropopliteal specimens	44	Yes	56
Schwartz and colleagues[41]	1987	Aortic aneurysms	10	No	54
Ilgenfritz and Jordan[42]	1988	Aortic aneurysms and atrial septal defects	20	No	55
Brandimarte and colleagues[43]	1989	Aortic aneurysms	31	No	NR
Wakefield and colleagues[44]	1990	Aortofemoropopliteal specimens	12	No	60

NR, Not reported.

275) incidence of positive cultures from aortic aneurysm contents. The incidence of graft sepsis was 32% (7 of 22) in patients with positive cultures, compared with 2.4% (6 of 253) in the culture-negative group.

Similar data suggest that lower extremity arteries can also become infected. In 1984, Macbeth and colleagues[37] reported on cultures of arterial wall specimens from 88 clean, elective, lower extremity revascularization procedures. Control cultures were taken from adjacent adipose or lymphatic tissue. Although all control cultures were negative, arterial wall cultures were positive in 43% of cases (38 of 88). Of these, 71% (27 of 38) grew *S. epidermidis*. The authors described three graft infections in 335 cases (0.9% infection rate), all of which had positive arterial wall cultures. Also included in this report was a retrospective review of 22 cases of graft infection for which arterial and graft culture data were available. Of the patients with positive arterial cultures, 57% (8 of 14) had suture line disruption, whereas there were no disruptions in the culture-negative group. Durham and colleagues[40] reported a series of 102 patients undergoing vascular reconstruction with a 74% (75 of 102) incidence of positive arterial wall cultures. *S. epidermidis* accounted for 56% of the cultured organisms. Six infections (3.5%) occurred over 18 months; all these patients had prior positive arterial cultures. No patients with negative arterial cultures developed graft infection. The greatest risk for graft infection appeared to be in patients with positive arterial wall cultures undergoing reoperation.

Hematogenous and Lymphatogenous Seeding

Hematogenous seeding of vascular prostheses is another potential source of graft infection. Anecdotal reports implicate urinary tract infection,[4,5] abdominal sepsis,[5,9,32] and other infections[3] in the development of vascular graft infections. Laboratory models demonstrate that bacteremia reliably produces prosthetic graft infections.[46-48]

Other Local and Systemic Factors

Open wounds on the distal lower extremities can be a source of contaminating bacteria. Hoffert and colleagues[1] noted that 75% of patients with graft infections (9 of 12) had open, infected lesions on the distal lower extremity at the time of graft implantation. Liekweg and Greenfield[8] reported that 33% of inguinal infections (20 of 60) occurred proximal to open foot infections. Bunt and Mohr[49] described the presence of bacteria cultured from a distally infected extremity in the inguinal lymph nodes of two patients undergoing lower extremity revascularization; both patients developed graft infection.

Prior vascular surgery has been implicated as a risk factor for vascular graft infection. Dense scar tissue, increased bleeding, and lymphatic leak may all contribute to this phenomenon. Goldstone and Moore[5] noted that 45% of patients (12 of 27) with graft infections had undergone one or more revisions of the original graft before developing an infection in the same region. In 8 of the 12 patients, the infection was in the groin. In the series by Edwards and coworkers,[26] 9 of 18 patients (50%) had undergone a previous vascular surgery at the site of the graft infection. Similarly, a report from Reilly and colleagues[17] described a history of multiple previous vascular procedures at the site of graft infection in 40% of cases. Johnson and associates[50] found that prior vascular procedures were not a significant risk factor for graft infection; however, only 12 of 135 patients in this series had prior operations at the site of infection.

The immunologic status of patients with vascular disease may also have an impact on the development of graft infection. Systemic disease, malnutrition, and medical debility may suppress the host response to invading microorganisms. Kwaan and colleagues[51] reported on 12 patients with advanced, fulminating graft infections, all of whom had critical deficiencies in immune status as determined by serum albumin, hemoglobin, immunoglobulin, and lymphocyte assays and by response to standard skin test antigens. Eight of 12 patients who received total parenteral nutrition had significant enhancement of immune response and accelerated recovery from the graft infection. Of the four patients who did not receive nutritional support, two had a prolonged convalescence, and two subsequently died from complications of graft infection.

Experimental Investigations

The suggestion that prophylactic antibiotic therapy may be effective in the prevention of surgical infections was first made 50 years ago.[52-56] In the early 1960s, Alexander and colleagues[57,58] demonstrated the efficacy of penicillin prophylaxis in experimental wound infections.

Lindenauer and associates[13] reported an experimental demonstration of the importance of antibiotics in preventing graft infection. Three groups of dogs underwent femoral arteriotomy with primary, Teflon patch, or vein patch closure. A fourth group received a sham operation alone. Wounds were contaminated with 10,000 to 100,000 *S. aureus* organisms. All subjects, except controls, received intramuscular procaine penicillin. Among control animals, the infection rate was 94% (8 of 9 shams, 3 of 3 arteriotomies, 3 of 3 Teflon patches, 3 of 3 vein patches). In animals treated with penicillin, the infection rate was 0% (15 shams, 5 arteriotomies, 5 Teflon patches, 5 vein patches). As a result, antibiotic therapy may sterilize a contaminated wound even in the presence of a prosthetic arterial patch.

Moore and colleagues[59] tested the utility of antibiotic prophylaxis in a canine model of hematogenous aortic graft contamination. Thirty minutes before laparotomy, dogs were infused intravenously with 10 million *S. aureus* organisms and then underwent placement of a Dacron infrarenal aortic graft. The experimental group received an IV dose of cephalothin (25 mg/kg), which was started just before the skin incision and continued for 30 minutes after the procedure. Experimental animals then received intramuscular cephalothin three times a day for 5 days; control animals received no antibiotics. Control animals experienced a significantly increased rate of positive cultures (72%) compared with animals that received perioperative cephalothin (24%).

Clinical Investigations

Early Experience

Until the mid-1970s, the use of antibiotics in vascular reconstruction with synthetic materials was largely based on personal preference. It is notable that in the series of Szilagyi and colleagues,[3] the graft infection rate among 2145 cases in which prophylactic antibiotics were not administered was 1.5%. Fry and Lindenauer[2] reported an incidence of 1.34% in 890 cases in which no antibiotics were used. These infection rates were comparable with, and often lower than, those reported in series in which prophylactic antibiotics were used.[12] Noting the preponderance of *S. aureus* in vascular graft infections, particularly in cases involving an inguinal incision, Szilagyi and colleagues[3] suggested a clinical trial of an antibiotic directed at this organism in reconstructions that required an inguinal anastomosis.

In 1974, Goldstone and Moore[5] published a review of the San Francisco Veterans Administration Hospital experience with vascular prosthetic infection. This series of 566 aortofemoropopliteal reconstructions was divided into two time periods: 1959 to 1965, when antibiotics were administered only postoperatively; and 1966 to 1973, when prophylaxis included preoperative, intraoperative, and postoperative antibiotics. The incidence of graft infection in the former group was 4.1% (9 of 222), compared with 1.5% (5 of 344) in the latter. Although the investigators conceded that greater experience and skill might have contributed to the lower incidence of infection, they maintained that the major factor responsible was the more appropriate use of antibiotics in the second group of patients. The following year, Perdue[60] published a similar retrospective review that suggested that the institution of routine antibiotic prophylaxis reduced the incidence of wound infections and other nosocomial infections in patients undergoing major arterial reconstructive procedures.

Prospective Trials

The first large, prospective, randomized, blinded clinical study of antibiotic prophylaxis in vascular reconstructive surgery was published by Kaiser and colleagues in 1978.[27] In that series, 462 patients undergoing aortofemoropopliteal reconstruction were randomized to receive either 1 g of cefazolin or a saline placebo. There were no graft infections among 225 patients who received cefazolin, compared with 4 of 237 placebo recipients (1.7%). When superficial skin infections and subcutaneous skin infections were considered in the analysis (Szilagyi classes I and II), the overall infection rates were 0.9% in the cefazolin group and 6.8% in the placebo group. Given no adverse drug reactions and no noted cefazolin resistance, the authors strongly recommended a short course of cefazolin prophylaxis in patients undergoing arterial reconstructive surgery.

The benefit of a short course of systemic cephalosporin prophylaxis in vascular reconstructive surgery was subsequently confirmed in a number of other prospective, randomized trials. In 1983, Salzmann[61] reported a trial of cefuroxime (a second-generation agent) and later cefotaxime (a third-generation agent) versus placebo in 300 patients undergoing aortofemoropopliteal reconstruction. The prophylaxis regimen was changed from cefuroxime to cefotaxime midway through the study because the latter was found to be more effective in vitro against the most common graft infection pathogens at the author's institution. Graft infection rates were 2.4% for the placebo group and 0.8% for the prophylaxis group. The incidence of wound infection was 15.1% in the placebo group and 3.0% in the prophylaxis group. No differences in infection rate were noted between the two antibiotics, and the author concluded that either agent could be used effectively in the prophylaxis of postoperative infection.

Addressing the question of duration of treatment for antibiotic prophylaxis, Hasselgren and colleagues[62] compared 1- and 3-day courses of cefuroxime versus placebo in lower extremity arterial reconstruction. There was only one graft infection in this small cohort of 110 patients, and it occurred in the placebo group. The wound infection rate was 16.7% for patients receiving placebo, compared with 3.8% in the 1-day and 4.3% in the 3-day prophylaxis groups. The investigators recommended that prophylactic antibiotic therapy be limited to a short-term course.

Robbs and associates reported a trial of cloxacillin plus gentamicin versus cefotaxime in infrainguinal arterial reconstruction.[63] This group had adopted a 48-hour course of cloxacillin plus gentamicin as their routine prophylaxis as a result of the predominance of *S. aureus* and gram-negative infections at their institution. Length of follow-up ranged from 6 to 20 months. The wound infection and graft infection rates for patients receiving cloxacillin plus gentamicin were 5.4% (7 of 129 wounds) and 1.5% (1 of 63 grafts), respectively. The rates for patients receiving cefotaxime were 6.3% (8 of 127 wounds) and 3.3% (2 of 61 grafts). The differences were not statistically significant. The authors concluded that the multiagent 2-day regimen conferred no advantage over the shorter, single-agent regimen.

Local Therapies

In 1980, Pitt and colleagues reported the results of a controlled study of cephradine prophylaxis in vascular procedures involving groin incisions in which topical, systemic, and topical plus systemic administration were compared.[64] Of 205 patients, 52 had prosthetic grafts placed, whereas the remainder received vein grafts. Infection rates were equivalent in these two groups. Wound infection rates were 0% for those receiving topical administration alone and systemic administration alone, 5.9% for patients receiving both, and 24.5% for controls. No distinction was made between graft (Szilagyi class III) and isolated wound (Szilagyi classes I and II) infections. Minimum follow-up was 4 weeks, but the mean length of follow-up was not indicated. Patients in whom synthetic graft material was used did not experience a higher incidence of wound infection. The authors concluded that topical and systemic prophylaxes were equally efficacious and that combined prophylaxis was unnecessary. The follow-up interval in this study, however, was not long enough to make conclusive statements.

Mohammed and colleagues compared the effect of prophylactic intraoperative wound irrigation with vancomycin (along with systemic antibiotics) to use of systemic antibiotics alone in a retrospective analysis of 454 patients undergoing aortofemoral or infrainguinal vascular surgery. They noted that use of vancomycin irrigation resulted in reduced incidence of superficial infections, but did not reduce inguinal wound dehiscence or deep infections.[65]

Use of a collagen implant impregnated with gentamicin sulfate for prophylaxis was studied retrospectively in 60 nondiabetic and nonobese patients undergoing infrainguinal prosthetic bypass procedures by Costa Almeida and colleagues. The results were promising in that the incidence of surgical site infection and the number of in-hospital days were reduced by the application of this implant when compared to the control group (0% vs. 20% for surgical site infection and mean of 5.66 days vs. 8.10 days for in-hospital days).[66] In another review of current literature, the potential role of a gentamicin-containing collagen implant for prophylaxis was discussed. This approach may have a beneficial effect in prevention of infection in patients who are at a high risk for infection or who are undergoing high-risk procedures.[67] Additional therapies described include the use of antibiotic-impregnated polymethyl methacrylate (PMMA; bone cement) beads with daptomycin, with or without the addition of tobramycin powder.[68,69]

Pretreatment of vascular grafts with antibiotics and fibrin sealant has also been investigated in in vitro experiments. Use of antibiotics with fibrin allows delayed release of antibiotic and a potentially longer period of resistance to infection.[70] In animal models using a vascular prosthesis, daptomycin has been seen to prevent staphylococcal biofilm formation. In the presence of rifampicin, the minimum inhibitory concentration (MIC) and the minimum bactericidal concentration of daptomycin are lower.[71] Some authors have cautioned against relying solely on systemic antibiotic prophylaxis for vascular grafts because of emergence of resistant microbial strains. Consideration for antimicrobial silver grafts has been highlighted in this regard.[72]

Hemodialysis Access

For hemodialysis access, the risk of infectious complications increases from arteriovenous fistulae (AVF) to arteriovenous grafts (AVGs) and central dialysis catheters.[73] In patients with AVGs, most infections arise from inoculation due to skin flora or seeding from distant sites. Infections due to *Staphylococcus* have been noted to occur more commonly in carriers than noncarriers. With regard to reduction of AVG infections, two prophylactic measures may have some merit for consideration including reduction of nasal carriage of the pathogen in carriers and use of cryopreserved human femoral vein as an alternative to prosthetic graft.[74]

Bennion and colleagues[75] examined the utility of antibiotic prophylaxis in patients with chronic renal insufficiency undergoing placement of a prosthetic arteriovenous shunt for hemodialysis. Patients were randomized to receive cefamandole or placebo just before placement of a polytetrafluoroethylene (PTFE) graft, followed by two subsequent doses. The wound infection rate for the cefamandole group was 10.5% (2 of 19), with one graft (Szilagyi class III) infection. The wound infection rate in the placebo group was 42.1% (8 of 19), with three graft infections. This high rate of infection is not uncommon in renal failure patients, and the study emphasized the importance of perioperative antibiotic prophylaxis.

A significant number of patients undergo minimally invasive percutaneous interventions aimed at maintenance of their dialysis access. Salman and colleagues recommended antibiotic prophylaxis in two particular situations in such patients: (1) peritoneal dialysis (PD) catheter placement and (2) insertion of an accidentally extruded tunneled hemodialysis catheter (TDC). In their experience, patients who developed clinical infection after percutaneous interventions had other comorbidities such as diabetes or advanced HIV. For prophylaxis, they used cefazolin for extruded TDC patients and vancomycin for PD catheter insertion. Overall, the rates of infection were low with no patients developing infection after PD catheter placement, one after angioplasty (0.04%), and one after tunneled catheter placement (0.3%).[76]

Tunneled central venous catheters can contribute to significant morbidity and mortality in patients with end-stage renal disease (ESRD) due to catheter-related infections. The question of consideration of prophylactic antibiotics in these patients is therefore an important one. In a prospective study, 60 patients were randomized between two groups. The group that received prophylactic antibiotics (1 gram cefazolin) prior to catheter insertion had a lower incidence of catheter loss due to infection ($P < .05$), catheter exit-site infections ($P < .05$), and tunnel infections ($P < .05$).[77] In oncology patients, a Cochrane review in 2013 did not find any benefit to the administration of routine prophylactic antibiotics to prevent Gram-positive catheter-related infections for long-term central venous catheters.[78]

Major Limb Amputation

McIntosh and colleagues conducted a review of literature to study the role of antibiotic prophylaxis in patients undergoing major limb amputations. They concluded that use of prophylactic antibiotics reduced rates of stump infection and even reamputation. The agent used for prophylaxis did not appear to affect outcomes.[79] Sadat and colleagues evaluated outcomes after major lower limb amputation in relation to the duration of antibiotic prophylaxis received. Their results showed lower wound infection, hospital length of stay, and revision rate for the amputation in patients who received 5 days of antibiotic prophylaxis.[80]

Arterial Closure Devices

Very low infection rates have been reported in the literature for patients undergoing angiography and angioplasty followed by deployment of arterial closure devices. A meta-analysis reviewed the incidence of infection in patients undergoing endovascular aortic repair involving use of vascular closure devices at access sites. Jaffan and colleagues reported a meta-analysis of closure device–related infections. They found no statistical difference in the rate of infection between patients who received antibiotic prophylaxis and those who did not. Based on these findings, the use of prophylactic antibiotics is not recommended.[81] Conditions that increase the risk of infectious complications after arterial closure device use include obesity, diabetes, and use of a closure device within the last 6 months.[82]

Angiography, Inferior Vena Cava Filter

In general, aseptic technique appears to be more important than antibiotic prophylaxis in angiographic procedures. Factors that increase the risk of infection in such procedures include repeated puncture or repeated catheterization of a sheath that is already in place or repeated intervention within 7 days if an endovascular stent is involved. Routine use of antibiotic prophylaxis before placement of an inferior vena cava (IVC) filter is currently not recommended. A fresh venous access site instead of a pre-existing conduit such as a central venous catheter is, however, recommended for the placement of IVC filters.[82]

Lower Extremity Superficial Venous Insufficiency Treatment

There is currently insufficient evidence in the literature to support the routine use of prophylactic antibiotics in procedures for lower extremity superficial venous insufficiency treatment such as varicose vein phlebectomy, endovascular thermal ablation, and sclerotherapy. Again, more emphasis is placed on use of aseptic technique.[82]

Autologous Vein Graft Reconstruction of Lower Extremity

A recent retrospective study from the Netherlands specifically included patients undergoing lower extremity arterial bypass using vein grafts between 2004 and 2012. One group received single-dose antibiotic prophylaxis, whereas the second group did not receive prophylaxis. The incidence of surgical site infections between the two groups was greater than 20% and not statistically significant.[83]

Comparisons of Antibiotic Regimens

Because it has become evident that a short course of a cephalosporin antibiotic is the ideal prophylaxis for vascular reconstructive procedures, several studies have focused on whether the most widely used cephalosporin, cefazolin, is the best choice. A large number of graft infections, particularly in abdominal grafts, are due to gram-negative rods. A theoretical disadvantage of first-generation cephalosporins such as cefazolin is that they are more vulnerable to gram-negative beta-lactamase than are second- and third-generation agents. Gram-negative activity is thus limited to *E. coli*, *Proteus* species, and *Klebsiella* species, and many hospital-acquired strains of these organisms are cefazolin resistant. It has also been demonstrated that other cephalosporins, such as the second-generation agent cefamandole, have greater in vitro activity against coagulase-negative staphylococci, which have been found to colonize the native arterial wall in a large number of patients. It is clear from previous studies by Salzmann,[61] Hasselgren and colleagues,[62] and Robbs and colleagues[63] that second- and third-generation cephalosporins can be used effectively in vascular surgery prophylaxis.

In 1989, Lalka and colleagues examined this issue in a prospective study of arterial wall microbiology and antibiotic penetration.[45] Forty-seven patients undergoing aortofemoropopliteal reconstruction were randomized to receive perioperative cefazolin or cefamandole, 1 g every 6 hours for nine doses. Serial samples of serum, subcutaneous fat, thrombus, atheroma, and arterial wall were obtained for culture and assay of drug levels by high-performance liquid chromatography. Serum and tissue levels of cefazolin were significantly higher than those of cefamandole at almost all time points. Positive arterial wall cultures were obtained in 41.4% of patients, and 68.8% of bacterial isolates were coagulase-negative staphylococci (half of these were slime producers). At times, the arterial wall concentration of both antibiotics fell below the geometric mean minimal inhibitory concentration for all organisms combined, but this occurred significantly more often with cefamandole. The investigators concluded that both antibiotics needed to be administered in larger doses (cefazolin, 1.5 g every 4 hours; cefamandole, 2 g every 3 hours) and that the antibiotics were essentially equal in efficacy if administered appropriately. This study corroborated the findings of Mutch and colleagues,[84] who noted that serum antibiotic levels did not correlate well with aortic tissue concentrations of bioactive antibiotic, and it suggested that arterial tissue levels rather than serum levels should be the standard for comparison of antibiotic efficacy.

Edwards and colleagues[85] reported a prospective trial of cefazolin versus the more β-lactamase–stable second-generation cephalosporin cefuroxime in patients undergoing aortic and peripheral vascular reconstruction. Prior studies had suggested that some failures of cefazolin prophylaxis were due to this agent's susceptibility to staphylococcal β-lactamase and that other cephalosporins might provide better protection in cardiac surgery.[27,86,87] Antibiotics were administered just before surgery, redosed intraoperatively, and continued every 6 hours postoperatively for 24 hours. Dosage and administration schedules were based on a prior pharmacokinetic study. The infection rate in the cefazolin group was 1% (3 of 287), versus 2.6% (7 of 272) in the cefuroxime group. This difference was not statistically significant. Cefuroxime exhibited lower trough concentrations than did cefazolin, and the length of the operative procedure was found to be a risk factor for infection only in the cefuroxime group. The investigators concluded that despite its lower resistance to β-lactamase, cefazolin provides better perioperative prophylaxis because of its greater antistaphylococcal potency and superior pharmacokinetic profile.[85] Data from this and other studies[27] suggest that intraoperative redosing of cefazolin should be more frequent in prolonged procedures than in routine therapeutic administration—that is, every 4 hours rather than every 6 hours.

A study done in Sweden[88] evaluated an antibiotic regimen for prophylaxis in patients undergoing vascular surgery involving groin incisions (n = 219). One group received cloxacillin for antimicrobial prophylaxis, whereas the second group received trimethoprim/sulfamethoxazole (TMP-SMX). This study failed to show a difference in the incidence of surgical site infections between the two groups.

Current Status of Antibiotic Prophylaxis

Antibiotic Selection

Cefazolin is currently the antibiotic of choice for routine vascular surgery prophylaxis. It is relatively inexpensive, has negligible toxicity and a low incidence of severe allergic reactions, and is active against many of the bacteria commonly implicated in graft infection (Tables 11.4 and 11.5). This is supported by current guidelines from the Agency of Healthcare Research and Quality.[89] Its pharmacokinetic profile is ideal for this indication, with reliably high peak serum concentrations and a long half-life of elimination compared with other cephalosporins.[85,90] It penetrates arterial tissue well, with drug concentrations exceeding the minimal inhibitory concentration of common graft infection pathogens in most instances.[45] Cefazolin is active against *S. aureus* (including penicillinase-producing strains), some strains of *S. epidermidis*, and the more commonly encountered gram-negative rods *E. coli*, *Proteus* species, and *Klebsiella* species. Most other gram-negative rods are resistant, including indole-positive *Proteus vulgaris*. Cephalothin, the other first-generation agent in common

TABLE 11.4 Wound Infections Among Patients Receiving Cefazolin or Placebo Prophylaxis

Prophylaxis	No. of Infections	No. of Patients	Infected (%)	Class I Infections (%)	Class II Infections (%)	Class III Infections (%)
Cefazolin	2	225	0.9[a]	0	2	0
Placebo	16	237	6.8[a]	4	8	4
Total	18	462	3.9	4	10	4

[a]Difference is significant at $P < .001$. Brachiocephalic procedures are not included.
From Kaiser AB, Clayson KR, Mulherin JL, et al: Antibiotic prophylaxis in vascular surgery. *Ann Surg* 188:283, 1978.

TABLE 11.5 Antibacterial Spectrum of Selected Antibiotics

	ANTIBACTERIAL ACTIVITY (MIC-90 IN µG/ML)[a]				
Antibiotic	***Staphylococcus aureus***	***Staphylococcus epidermidis***	***Escherichia coli***	***Klebsiella* spp.**	***Pseudomonas* spp.**
Cefazolin	1.0	0.8	5.0	6.0	R
Cephalothin	1.0	0.5	5.0	32.0	R
Cefamandole	1.0	2.0	4.0	8.0	R
Cefuroxime	2.0	1.0	4.0	R	R
Cefotaxime	2.0	8.0	0.25	0.25	32.0
Vancomycin	1.0	3.0	R	R	R
Penicillin V	ALP+: >25.0 ALP–: 0.03	0.02[b]	R	R	R
Oxacillin	0.25	0.2[b]	R	R	R
Gentamicin	0.6	2.0[b]	4.0	1.0	2.0
Ciprofloxacin	0.5	0.25	0.03	0.125	0.5
Rifampin	0.015	0.015	16.0	32.0	64.0

[a]MIC-90 is the minimal inhibitory concentration for 90% of strains. MIC >64 µg/mL is considered resistant. Values are approximate and may vary among institutions.
[b]Many strains are resistant.
ALP, Alkaline phosphatase; *R,* resistant.
Data from Mandell RGD, editor: *Principles and practice of infectious diseases*, ed 3, New York, 1989, Churchill Livingstone.

clinical use, is somewhat more resistant to staphylococcal β-lactamase, but it is less active against gram-negative organisms. More important, it is cleared from plasma fourfold to fivefold as rapidly as cefazolin.[90]

Later-generation cephalosporins have greater gram-negative activity and the potential benefit of increased resistance to staphylococcal β-lactamase; however, in vitro and in vivo activity against gram-positive cocci is reduced. Many investigators have tailored their choice of antibiotic to the predominant organisms responsible for graft infection at their particular institutions. Cefamandole,[45] cefuroxime,[91] and cefotaxime[63] have all been used effectively as prophylactic agents in prospective trials. However, cefamandole has fallen out of favor for routine use because of an association with hypoprothrombinemia and bleeding, particularly in elderly patients and those with renal insufficiency. Cefuroxime has been shown to have antistaphylococcal potency and pharmacokinetic properties inferior to those of cefazolin.[85] Third-generation agents such as cefotaxime have broad anti–gram-negative activity but are generally less active against staphylococci. Moreover, the later-generation cephalosporins are, in most instances, significantly more expensive than the first-generation agents. As a result, cefazolin remains the antibiotic of choice, except in specific instances when in vitro testing has revealed that another agent more adequately covers the principal pathogens of graft infection.

A potential disadvantage of cefazolin prophylaxis is the inconsistent activity of this agent against the organism that is currently responsible for the greatest number of graft infections, *S. epidermidis*. It has been shown that during hospitalization, patients acquire multiply resistant strains of this bacterium.[92,93] Up to 75% of *S. epidermidis* isolates at some institutions are now cefazolin resistant. Vancomycin is highly active against both *S. epidermidis* and *S. aureus;* resistance in these organisms is rarely encountered. Vancomycin, however, provides no gram-negative coverage. It is the drug of choice for prophylaxis in patients with a history of anaphylaxis to β-lactam antibiotics, often in combination with an aminoglycoside in procedures in which there is significant risk of gram-negative infection, such as aortic reconstruction. Vancomycin is also considered the antibiotic of choice for the prophylaxis of prosthetic hemodialysis access grafts and for patients known to be colonized with methicillin-resistant *S. aureus*. It is excreted primarily by glomerular filtration and therefore persists in high serum concentrations in patients with ESRD. Clindamycin is another alternative in patients with a history of anaphylaxis to β-lactam antibiotics.

The broad antibacterial spectrum, excellent tissue penetration, and low toxicity of the fluoroquinolones make them potentially ideal agents for the prophylaxis of surgical infections. Limited data are available concerning the use of fluoroquinolones for this indication, but there are reports of efficacy equal or superior to that of cephalosporin antibiotics in the prophylaxis of colorectal,[94,95] biliary,[94,96] and urologic surgery.[97-99] Auger and coauthors[100] reported a randomized study of pefloxacin, a nalidixic acid analog, and cefazolin in patients undergoing cardiac surgery. Of 111 patients, 14 receiving pefloxacin developed bacterial colonization at culture sites, compared with 11 in the cefazolin group. One patient who received cefazolin developed mediastinitis from a cefazolin-resistant strain of *S. epidermidis.* As yet, there are no published clinical trials of a fluoroquinolone versus a cephalosporin in the prophylaxis of peripheral vascular surgery procedures.

Resistant Bacteria

The contemporary use of antibiotics has resulted in further progression of bacterial resistance so that methicillin-resistant species of *Staphylococcus* are encountered more frequently. Institutional bacteriologic analysis may reveal an increased incidence of resistant species such as methicillin-resistant *Staphylococcus aureus* (MRSA). In recent reports, as many as 20% to 30% of vascular surgical site infections may be MRSA related.[101,102]

Measures that have been proposed to help address the risk of MRSA infections include surveillance of patients by nasal swab screening to identify high-risk patients, decolonization of carriers, and attention to host factors (nutritional support, control of hypothermia, and blood glucose regulation). Intranasal mupirocin may be considered for staphylococcal nasal decolonization.[22] The Centers for Disease Control and Prevention has offered guidelines that are directed at reducing surgical site infections. Attention to patient preparation, skin cleansing, hand disinfection, surgical site care, and sterile technique are emphasized. In addition, recommendations for the selection and use of antibiotics are proposed.[103]

In keeping with these recommendations, antibiotic prophylactic regimens must be adapted to these conditions to include agents directed at MRAS in high-risk populations. The use of daptomycin (a bactericidal cyclic lipopeptide) with cefazolin has been advocated. An alternative regimen is the use of vancomycin and cefazolin.[104] Other authors have reported the use of vancomycin alone for prophylaxis. In a report of 6465 patients undergoing cardiac procedures, Garey and colleagues[105] noted that the use of vancomycin resulted in reduction of the incidence of surgical site infections and a reduction in the incidence of coagulase-negative *Staphylococcus* species and MRSA infections. In another prospective study, low-risk patients undergoing elective vascular interventions were randomized to receive cefazolin, cefazolin and vancomycin, or cefazolin and daptomycin for prophylaxis. Patients in the cefazolin and daptomycin group had fewer infections compared to the other two groups. However, high-risk patients were not included in this study.[106] Recommendations for the first-line use of vancomycin or daptomycin should be tailored to local institutional patterns of incidence of methicillin-resistant *Staphylococcus* bacteria. Daptomycin has a favorable side-effect profile compared to vancomycin as well as short infusion time but higher cost.[106] Some authors have recommended daptomycin prophylaxis for up to 48 hours in patients who are colonized with MRSA and who are undergoing vascular procedures with a high risk for infection.[68]

A study by Payne and colleagues evaluated perioperative vancomycin administration as antibiotic prophylaxis in 34 consecutive patients (data from 21 patients were used for analysis) undergoing vascular procedures involving prosthetic material. Patients received a loading dose of vancomycin 12 hours prior to the surgery followed by a 24-hour infusion. It was seen that vancomycin achieved adequate serum concentrations in these patients. No adverse effects to vancomycin were reported in any patients.[107] Payne and colleagues also demonstrated that this modus operandi of antibiotic prophylaxis attains serum and vascular tissue concentrations above the MICs for pathogens involved in vascular graft infections.[108]

Antibiotic Administration

Prophylactic antibiotics are administered just before surgery and again intraoperatively during long procedures. Pharmacokinetic studies suggest that prophylactic antibiotics should be administered more frequently and in higher doses during surgery than is recommended for routine therapeutic indications (e.g., cefazolin 1.5 g every 4 hours).[27,86,109] Prophylaxis is usually continued postoperatively for up to 24 hours, and possibly longer when there is a theoretical risk of postoperative bacteremia from indwelling venous catheters, arterial lines, bladder catheters, and endotracheal tubes. The advantage of continuing coverage beyond the operating room, however, has not been clearly demonstrated. In the absence of these risk factors, there is clearly no advantage in extending antibiotic prophylaxis for longer than 24 hours.

Regimens of prophylaxis should be tailored to the type of vascular reconstruction undertaken. Cefazolin prophylaxis is recommended in all procedures involving the placement of prosthetic materials. It is probably not necessary in "clean" vascular procedures of the neck and upper extremities that do not involve the use of synthetic grafts. In contrast, the marked colonization and favorable bacterial environment of the lower abdomen and groin necessitate the use of antibiotic prophylaxis in all aortofemoropopliteal vascular procedures. The risk of gram-negative infection in aortic reconstruction may necessitate the addition of an aminoglycoside, particularly in institutions with a high degree of cefazolin resistance among gram-negative isolates. Alternatively, a second- or third-generation cephalosporin with broader anti–gram-negative activity may be substituted because this obviates the risk of aminoglycoside-associated nephrotoxicity.

Cephalosporins should be avoided in patients with a history of anaphylaxis to β-lactam antibiotics. Patients with a history of minor allergic reactions to penicillin antibiotics can be given a cephalosporin test dose to determine whether cross-reactivity is present. Reduced dosing of cefazolin and most other cephalosporins is recommended in renal insufficiency, based on the calculated creatinine clearance.

There is evidence that remote bacteremia may be implicated in vascular graft infection. Accordingly, oral prophylaxis is recommended for procedures that are highly associated with bacteremia, such as tooth extraction, cystoscopy, and colonoscopy. Wooster and colleagues[30] demonstrated in 200 vascular surgery patients undergoing cystoscopy that the incidence of bacteremia was 64% among inpatients and 8% among outpatients. For procedures such as tooth extraction and colonoscopy, prophylaxis must be tailored to the most common normal flora of the traumatized site. Penicillins are appropriate choices for major dental procedures, whereas broader gram-negative and anaerobic coverage may be warranted in colonoscopy. It should be emphasized, however, that the true risk of graft infection after procedures associated with bacteremia is unclear, and there is currently no consensus on the role of antibiotic prophylaxis in this setting.

PRIMARY ARTERIAL INFECTIONS

A primary arterial infection is a condition in which an infectious agent invades and destroys the wall of an artery, resulting in disruption of the normal arterial architecture and pseudoaneurysm formation. Ultimately these lesions can result in symptoms resulting from sepsis, compression, erosion, embolization, thrombosis, or hemorrhage. The essential features include the destruction of the arterial wall by an infectious process, septic illness, and rapid onset of pseudoaneurysm formation. The presentation varies from indolent to cataclysmic. Successful management requires familiarity with the processes involved and the ability to make prompt decisions at the time of surgery. The goal of this chapter is to review primary arterial infections in terms of their pathophysiology, diagnosis, and treatment.

Historical Perspective

In the 19th century, Rokitansky[110] and Koch[111] recognized an association between arterial infection and aneurysm formation. In 1885, Osler[112] presented the first comprehensive description of this relationship. In addressing the Royal College of Physicians, he described a 30-year-old man who had died from fever, chills, and pneumonia. At autopsy, the patient was found to have endocarditis involving the aortic valve, as well as multiple aneurysms of the thoracic aorta. Based on carefully described pathologic findings, Osler proposed a causal relationship between infection of the aortic wall and subsequent aneurysm formation. Because of a similarity between the beaded appearance of these aneurysms and fungal vegetations, he introduced the term *mycotic aneurysm* and thus the concept of primary arterial infection.

Definitions

There is no universally accepted definition of primary arterial infection. Moreover, there continues to be confusion regarding the general classification of infections that involve the native arterial tree. Although the term *mycotic aneurysm* initially signified an infected aneurysm found in association with bacterial endocarditis, it has come to denote an infected aneurysm of any type. Another problem is that there is considerable disparity among the several definitions that have been proposed. Finally, it should be recognized that, with the exception of a secondarily infected arterial aneurysm, most of these lesions are actually infected pseudoaneurysms. Most lesions arise by means of the local destruction of the arterial wall and the fibrous encapsulation of an expanding hematoma; therefore, these lesions do not have the histologic components of an arterial wall.

For practical purposes, *primary arterial infection* can be defined as the direct invasion of a pathogen into the wall of a native artery, irrespective of the preexisting state of the underlying artery or source of the pathogen. The term *mycotic aneurysm* is used to denote both true aneurysms and false aneurysms that are associated with infection of the arterial wall.

Pathogenesis

Five basic mechanisms have been implicated in the development of primary arterial infections. They can be grouped broadly as (1) oslerian mycotic aneurysms, (2) microbial arteritis with aneurysm formation, (3) infected aneurysms, (4) arterial injury with contamination, and (5) arteritis from contiguous spread.

Oslerian Mycotic Aneurysms: Embolization of Infected Cardiac Vegetations

Osler, in coining the term *mycotic aneurysm*, both named the condition and described what would be the most prevalent cause of primary arterial infection in the preantibiotic era. As he described it, a mycotic aneurysm is limited to the unique clinical condition characterized by bacterial endocarditis with septic embolization from valvular vegetations. These septic emboli lodge within the arterial wall, where a suppurative infection develops. The arterial wall is destroyed by the infection, and the resultant pseudoaneurysm is recognized as a mycotic aneurysm.

Considerable confusion has arisen because the term *mycotic aneurysm* has been expanded and applied to various types of infected aneurysms. Crane[113] attempted to classify mycotic aneurysms as primary and secondary types. He introduced the term *primary mycotic aneurysm* to refer to infected aortic aneurysms not associated with endocarditis or an infectious focus; secondary types were those that formed as a result of preceding endocarditis. Ponfick[114] and Eppinger[115] were among the first to characterize the anatomic features of these aneurysms pathologically. Ponfick[114] proposed that the initial insult to the arterial wall was a mechanical injury inflicted by the embolization of septic material. Eppinger in 1887 provided further support for the theory of septic emboli by culturing the same strain of bacteria from both vegetative lesions and the wall of an aneurysm in a patient with endocarditis. He applied the term *embolomycotic* to describe the combination of infectious and embolic components that led to the formation of mycotic aneurysms.[115]

Microbial Arteritis With Aneurysm Formation: Hematogenous Seeding

The second mechanism of arterial infection involves hematogenous microbial seeding of arteries during an episode of bacteremia. Microbial arteritis with aneurysm formation occurs when a normal or atherosclerotic artery becomes infected and the weakened artery becomes aneurysmal.

In 1906, the German pathologist Weisel[116] described distinctive pathologic changes in arterial walls that occurred during the course of an infectious disease, but were not related to cardiac valve vegetation emboli.[116] Lewis and Schrager[117] and Cathcart[118] presented case reports of infected peripheral aneurysms that developed in normal arteries of patients with osteomyelitis and typhoid fever, respectively. Despite these reports, nearly 30 years passed before consideration was given to the mechanism by which bacteremia led to arterial infection. Crane[113] described an infected aneurysm in a patient with hypoplasia of the aorta, but no associated bacterial endocarditis or other identifiable source of infection.[113] He proposed that the combination of the "force of the blood stream" and abnormal development of the aorta allowed bacteria to invade that portion of the aorta. This resulted in an arterial infection, disruption of the aortic wall, and an infected pseudoaneurysm. Revell extended the concept of aortic bacterial seeding one step further and proposed that the route of infection was through the aortic vasa vasorum.[119] Hawkins and Yeager,[120] acknowledging the resistance of arterial intima to infection, suggested that an intimal defect such as that produced by arteriosclerosis allowed bacterial localization and infection.

Infected Aneurysms

The term *infected aneurysm* refers to an infection of a preexisting aneurysm, most often by hematogenous microbiologic seeding of the aneurysm. The original aneurysm is most commonly atherosclerotic; however, it may also be the result of trauma or arteritis. The diseased artery becomes host to bacterial pathogens when these lodge within the intramural thrombus and arteriosclerotic intima.

Arterial Injury With Contamination

Another cause of arterial infections is mechanical arterial injury by contaminated instruments. This type of infection can occur after an inadvertent arterial puncture with a contaminated needle in a drug abuser, as an accidental contamination during radiologic procedures, during placement of hemodynamic monitoring catheters, or as a result of traumatic injury. The combination of mechanical disruption of the intima and seeding of the arterial lesion with pathogenic bacteria leads to the formation of suppurative arteritis and destroys a portion of the arterial wall. This subsequently becomes an infected arterial pseudoaneurysm.

Arteritis From Contiguous Spread

Arterial infections can also develop through the spread of infection from a contiguous focus. Contiguous infections that have been recognized as potential sources of bacteria include lesions such as osteomyelitis, infected lymph nodes, tuberculous lymph nodes, and abscesses from narcotic injection.[121] Bacteria, and less commonly mycobacteria or fungi, invade the artery either by direct extension or via lymphatics. They subsequently produce a necrotizing invasive infection of the arterial wall, with eventual destruction of the wall.

Other Forms of Arterial Infection

There are three other, less common forms of infected aneurysms: syphilitic aortitis, true fungal aneurysms, and primary (spontaneous) aortoenteric fistulas (AEFs). Because of significant differences in the pathogens and pathogenesis of these lesions, they merit separate discussion.

Syphilitic aneurysms are a rarely encountered complication of advanced syphilis. These lesions occur in approximately 10% of patients with the tertiary form of the disease.[122] These aneurysms commonly arise in the ascending aorta, frequently involve the aortic valve, and are secondary to treponemal invasion of the vasa vasorum. The reasons why *Treponema* species prefer this portion of the aorta remain unclear. After spirochete penetration, an infiltrate develops within the vessel wall consisting of plasma cells, epidermal cells, and giant cells. This infiltrate results in destruction of the elastic and muscular components of the tunica media, replacement of the normal wall with fibrous tissue, and dilation and subsequent formation of saccular aneurysms.

Fungal arterial infections are also extremely rare and occur most often in patients who are immunosuppressed. Common risk factors include diabetes, immunosuppressive medications, and chronic hematologic disorders such as leukemia or lymphoma. The species most often implicated are *Histoplasma capsulatum, Aspergillus fumigatus, Candida albicans,* and *Penicillium* species. These lesions most commonly result from colonization of a preexisting aneurysm or infection of a damaged artery.

HIV-related vasculitis can result in aneurysmal degeneration of the arterial wall. Radiologic appearance may be identical to that which results from a bacterial arterial infection. The distinction is noted in the pathologic evaluation of the affected arterial wall, which demonstrates acute and chronic adventitial inflammatory changes. Secondary bacterial infections may be present, and cultures may be positive in a minority of these patients. There appears to be a predilection toward carotid and femoral arteries; however, the aorta may also be involved.[123-125]

Spontaneous or "primary" AEFs arise as a consequence of progressive aneurysmal enlargement, with gradual erosion into an adjacent segment of the gastrointestinal tract. The erosion is thought to be facilitated by the indurated, atherosclerotic artery pressing against a tethered portion of bowel. The most common location for this erosion is the third portion of the duodenum. In their 1951 review of a series of 16,633 autopsies, Hirst and Affeldt[126] reported the incidence of this type of fistula to be 0.05%. Because the majority of patients with aortic aneurysms now undergo elective operation before they can progress to develop a primary AEF, the incidence of these lesions is thought to be considerably lower today. Patients with spontaneous AEFs may have an initial or "herald" bleed, which represents the initial hemorrhage of blood into the duodenum. In this presentation, the initial hemorrhage may abate then later resume in a more prolonged and dramatic manner. Presumably, a clot within the AEF is responsible for the intermittent nature of the bleeding episodes. This condition is considerably different from that associated with aortic graft infection, or secondary AEF. Secondary AEF is more common, more dangerous, and more difficult to manage.

Graft excision and remote reconstruction are the standard management of secondary AEF. In contrast, significant evidence exists that primary AEF can be managed by closure of the duodenal rent, debridement of the aorta, and in situ reconstruction with an arterial prosthesis. The prerequisites of this approach are the absence of purulence at the fistula site, a small defect in the duodenum, and a relatively healthy patient. It should be noted that the management of primary aortic infections (mycotic aneurysms) is similar to that of primary AEF, in that the absence of gross infection along with adequate debridement may allow in situ graft rcconstruction of the aorta.[127]

Causative Organisms

The organism most commonly associated with microbial aortitis is *Salmonella*. This is followed, in order of frequency, by *Streptococcus* species, *Bacteroides* species, *Arizona hinshawii, E. coli,* and *S. aureus*.[127] Studies that focus on subpopulations such as intravenous (IV) drug abusers or those with femoral mycotic aneurysms tend to identify a predominance of gram-positive bacteria such as staphylococci and streptococci, along with gram-negative organisms such as *E. coli* and *Pseudomonas* species.

The bacteriology of primary arterial infections has undergone considerable transformation since its original description in the mid-1800s (Fig. 11.1). Brown and colleagues[128] suggested that the reason for this change is antibiotic selective pressure leading to bacterial adaptation. There has also been a change in the relative incidence of pathogenic mechanisms with the more common use of invasive diagnostic modalities and the increased illicit use of IV drugs. The majority of arterial infections during the preantibiotic era were oslerian mycotic aneurysms; that is, they were related to bacterial endocarditis. The bacteriology of arterial infections during this period therefore was similar to that of endocarditis. Stengal and Wolferth[129] in the 1920s and Revell[119] in the 1940s reported that the predominant organisms were nonhemolytic streptococci, staphylococci, and pneumococci. Magilligan and Quinn,[130] in a 1986 review, subdivided 91 patients with bacterial endocarditis into two groups: those known to be IV drug abusers (36 patients) and those who were not (55 patients). Of the first group, the most common organisms were *S. aureus* (36%), *Pseudomonas* species (16%), polymicrobial organisms (15%), *Streptococcus faecalis* (13%), and *Streptococcus viridans* (11%). Organisms in the second group (non-IV drug abusers) were *S. viridans* (22%), *S. aureus* (20%), *S. faecalis* (14%), and *S. epidermidis* (11%). The declining incidence of rheumatic fever and the adoption of early, appropriate antibiotic treatment have resulted in a significant decrease in bacterial endocarditis. This in turn has resulted in a decline in the incidence of oslerian mycotic aneurysms in recent decades.

Concurrent with the declining incidence of oslerian mycotic aneurysms has been an increase in various other types of primary arterial infections. Principal among these are microbial arteritis and infected aneurysms. This may be due, in part, to the increasing age of the population and the simultaneous increase in the prevalence of atherosclerosis. The bacteriology of these arterial infections is different from that of oslerian mycotic aneurysms. The microorganisms most commonly associated with microbial arteritis are *Salmonella* species, *Staphylococcus* species, and *E. coli*. *Salmonella* species, in particular, have a striking propensity for invading diseased (atherosclerotic) aortas. In selected series, the involvement of *Salmonella* species has been reported to be as high as 50%. The most virulent species, *Salmonella choleraesuis* and *Salmonella typhimurium*, account for more than 60% of the reported cases of *Salmonella arteritis*.[131] Less commonly reported organisms associated with microbial arteritis include fungi and anaerobic organisms. Among the latter, *Bacteroides fragilis* has been reported in association with supraceliac aortic aneurysms.

The bacteriology of infected aneurysms is similar to that of both mycotic aneurysms and microbial arteritis. Despite this, some variation exists among reported series. Although Bennett and Cherry[132] reported a 66% incidence of *Salmonella* infections, Jarrett and associates[23] described a predominance of gram-positive cocci (59%), with *S. aureus* representing 41%. In two prospective studies of patients undergoing aneurysmectomy, cultures obtained from both the aneurysm wall and the bowel bag revealed a predominance of gram-positive organisms.[31,133] Both of these series are thought to represent cases of bacterial colonization. Despite the relative infrequency of gram-negative organisms observed in Jarrett's series, the distinction between gram-negative and gram-positive cultures proved clinically important. Patients with gram-negative bacteria demonstrated a greater likelihood of

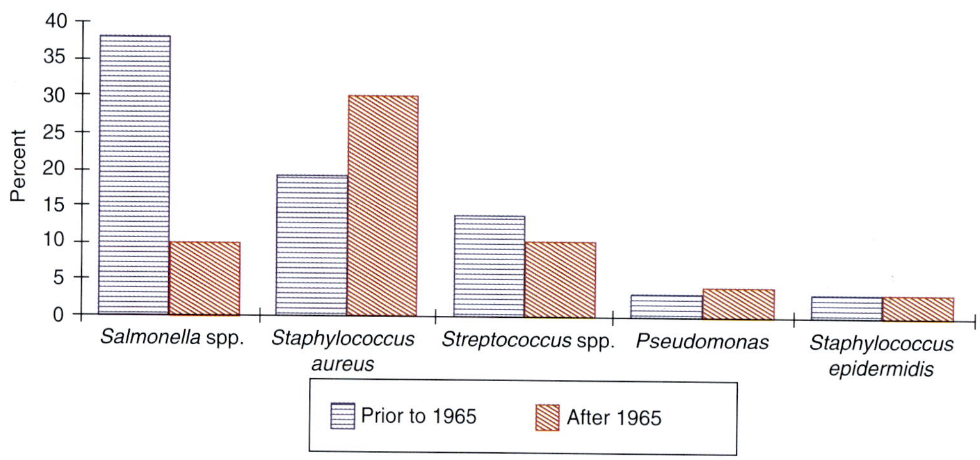

FIG 11.1 Organisms cultured from mycotic aneurysms. (From Brown SL, Busuttil RW, Baker JD, et al: Bacteriologic and surgical determinants of survival in patients with mycotic aneurysms. *J Vasc Surg* 1:541, 1984.)

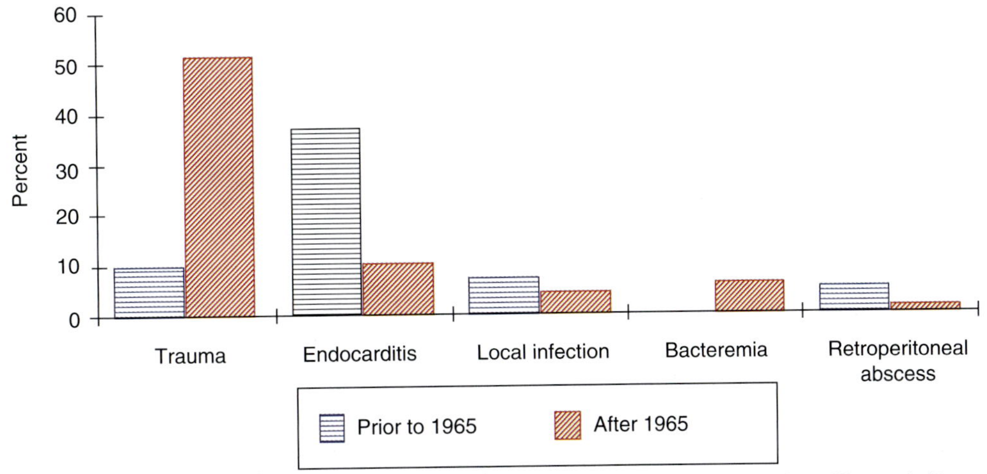

FIG 11.2 Causes of mycotic aneurysms. (From Brown SL, Busuttil RW, Baker JD, et al: Bacteriologic and surgical determinants of survival in patients with mycotic aneurysms. *J Vasc Surg* 1:541, 1984.)

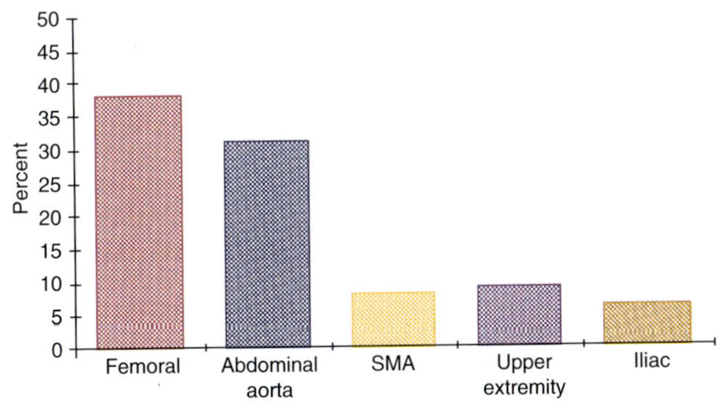

FIG 11.3 Distribution of mycotic aneurysms. *SMA*, Superior mesenteric artery. (From Brown SL, Busuttil RW, Baker JD, et al: Bacteriologic and surgical determinants of survival in patients with mycotic aneurysms. *J Vasc Surg* 1:541, 1984.)

aortic rupture than did those with gram-positive organisms. Specifically, the rupture rate associated with gram-negative bacterial isolates was 84%, whereas that associated with gram-positive bacterial cultures was 10%.

According to Brown and associates,[128] the most common infected aneurysms since 1965 are those that occur as a result of mechanical arterial injury with contamination of the vessel wall. The organism most frequently implicated in this type of arterial infection is *S. aureus*, which Brown's group cultured in as many as 30% of cases. Reddy and associates,[134] in a series of infected femoral false aneurysms, reported a 65% incidence of *S. aureus* and a 33% rate of polymicrobial infection. Although arterial infections secondary to contiguous spread are most commonly bacterial, mycobacterial and fungal infections may also occur in these lesions. As with microbial arteritis, *Salmonella* organisms are the predominant pathogen, and *Staphylococcus* organisms are second in frequency (Fig. 11.2).

The increased number of immunosuppressed patients in certain settings has resulted in an increase of reports indicating opportunistic infections. Patients with cancer, prolonged steroid use, transplantation, and other immunosuppressive conditions may present with infections. In these populations, infections from opportunistic agents are more prominent. Specifically noted are infections from *Campylobacter* species, *Listeria* species, and *Mycobacterium tuberculosis*.[135]

Anatomic Distribution

The anatomic distribution of primary arterial infections varies somewhat, depending on the pathologic type. True oslerian mycotic aneurysms most often involve the larger muscular and elastic arteries. In retrospective reviews, both Lewis and Schrager[117] and Brown and colleagues[128] found the most common sites of infection to be the abdominal aorta and the femoral and superior mesenteric arteries (Fig. 11.3). The predisposition for aortic involvement is thought to be related to the higher incidence of underlying atherosclerotic aneurysms in this location compared with other anatomic sites.

Microbial arteritis with aneurysm formation occurs when a pathogen localizes at the site of an arterial lesion such as an atherosclerotic plaque. As one would anticipate, the arteries most commonly involved are the ones that demonstrate advanced atherosclerotic changes—namely, the distal aorta and the femoral, iliac, and popliteal vessels. In theory, infected aneurysms can occur at any site within the arterial tree where there is a preexisting aneurysm. It is curious that all series in the literature demonstrate a strong propensity for involvement of the abdominal aorta. Involvement of this artery has been reported in up to 79% of cases. Whether this represents a tendency of the bacteria to infect aortic aneurysms or a study bias toward aortic aneurysms is not clear. Certainly, aortic aneurysms have been subjected to closer scrutiny than have other peripheral arterial aneurysms. This may account, in part, for this reported predilection.

Arterial infections due to mechanical injury with contamination most commonly involve arteries that have minimal soft tissue coverage. There are three main causes: accidental drug injection, vascular access, and trauma. Because these causes are related to the accessibility of the arteries and their superficial locations, these infections most commonly involve the femoral or brachial arteries. These locations also have an important effect on the presentation of these lesions, because femoral and brachial artery aneurysms are usually identified by the pulsatile mass, erythema, and tenderness of the aneurysm itself rather than by symptoms of arterial sepsis.

Clinical Presentation

The most common clinical presentation in patients with primary arterial infection is fever, leukocytosis, and tenderness over the affected artery. Patients may have a wide range of signs and symptoms, depending on the pathophysiology, bacteriology, and location of the infected artery or arteries. Most components of the clinical presentation can be assigned to one of two general groups: signs and symptoms resulting from infection or bacteremia, and signs and symptoms occurring secondary to local arterial involvement or aneurysm formation. Night sweats, general malaise, arthralgias, and increased fatigability in conjunction with fever and leukocytosis occur as a consequence of the recurrent bacteremias associated with sepsis from the arterial infections. In patients with oslerian mycotic aneurysms, the clinical signs and symptoms of bacterial endocarditis may be difficult to distinguish from those associated with the arterial infection. Similarly, symptoms in patients with arterial lesions that developed by spread from a contiguous suppurative source may derive from either infectious focus.

The second group of signs and symptoms occurs as a result of inflammation and aneurysmal dilatation of the infected artery. Localized tenderness is the most readily recognized symptom related to the inflammatory destruction of the arterial wall. Characteristics such as abdominal or peripheral bruits, neurologic defects from nerve compression, or pulsatile masses may also be present.

Thrombosis and thromboembolization are common sequelae of such arterial aneurysms. When they appear, they elicit associated symptoms such as ischemic digital or limb pain. Initially, these embolic presentations may be indistinguishable from similar events in uninfected aneurysms. If the embolic material is infected and causes a secondary arterial infection, the mycotic nature of the lesion may be revealed. Other findings of arterial infection include petechial skin lesions and septic arthritis.

Arterial rupture is common in cases of infected arterial aneurysms. This presentation is identical to that of any arterial rupture. If the damaged artery is contained and supported by a capsule of fibrous connective tissue, it may progress to form a pseudoaneurysm, and the principal symptom would be pain. If the rupture is uncontrolled, the presentation is that of hypotensive shock. If the rupture is in a superficial artery that erodes through the skin, the presentation is that of evident life-threatening hemorrhage.

Periarterial gas formation signals the presence of a gas-producing organism and should be a clear signal that urgent treatment is needed. Although this is not a common presentation, it should be considered in any patient who has unexplained periaortic gas and symptoms suggestive of sepsis.

Diagnostic Testing

The diagnosis of a primary arterial infection is based on elements of the clinical presentation, along with appropriate testing. The primary factor in making such a diagnosis is a high clinical suspicion, followed by a search for evidence to support the diagnosis of a primary arterial infection. The choice and use of diagnostic tests are of singular importance in identifying and substantiating the presence of an arterial infection. Because of the potentially fulminant course of these infections and the fatal outcome of improperly managed cases, diagnostic speed and accuracy are crucial. The basic elements of diagnostic testing include bacteriologic sampling and radiologic imaging.

Blood Cultures

The demonstration of bacterial organisms in association with an arterial lesion is central to the diagnosis of an arterial infection. The bacteria may be detected by either blood cultures or cultures of the arterial wall itself. Blood cultures, by virtue of their availability, are frequently one of the first tests done in patients suspected of having a significant infection. If the patient is floridly bacteremic, the blood culture may detect the circulating bacteria. However, several problems limit the usefulness of blood cultures. The incidence of negative blood cultures testifies to the fact that they are helpful in only a fraction of symptomatic patients; many patients with arterial infections never have positive blood cultures. In the review by Brown and associates,[128] only 60% of patients had positive preoperative blood cultures. In addition, blood cultures might not detect the infectious organism until several days or weeks have elapsed, limiting the test's effect on clinical management.

The presence of bacteria in the blood may be an important early clue to an arterial infection, but the information from such tests must be evaluated in the proper clinical context. Most bacteremic patients have an evident source of bacteremia that should be identified and treated. Patients with positive blood cultures and no clinical evidence of a concurrent infection should be examined for possible arterial lesions. The significance of a positive blood culture in an otherwise asymptomatic patient is difficult to determine without considering the patient's underlying problems and risk factors. It should also be noted that patients who are relatively asymptomatic (no systemic manifestations of sepsis) tend to have fewer positive blood cultures. As a result, in a study of patients undergoing clean arterial procedures, only 2% of blood cultures were positive, whereas 12% of arteries and 14% of periarterial adipose tissues harbored bacteria.[44] Obvious clues, such as a recently noted aneurysm or a history of drug abuse, may promote further investigation.

The type of organism identified in blood cultures may suggest a source of the infection. If a blood culture reveals *Salmonella* species in a patient with an aneurysm, an arterial infection should be seriously considered. Although *Staphylococcus* organisms are a common pathogen in arterial infections, their ubiquitous presence on skin often confuses the diagnosis and calls into question the results of the blood culture.

The importance of the preoperative blood culture is difficult to understate. It represents the earliest reliable clue to the presence of an arterial infection. Even in the event of a delayed result, such as when several days are required before the blood culture can identify the bacteria, the information provided may be invaluable in managing the patient.

Arterial Cultures

Arterial wall cultures may also help secure the diagnosis of an arterial infection. In any circumstance in which the diagnosis of an infectious aneurysm is entertained, arterial cultures should be attempted. The principal drawback to arterial wall cultures is the time required before any information about the infection is available. Patient management must therefore depend on other factors, such as the clinical setting, the index of suspicion, the presence of prior blood culture data, and the results of angiographic studies.

Because clinical decisions cannot always be based on arterial culture results, other techniques such as intraoperative Gram staining and frozen section of the arterial tissue are often considered. Unfortunately, these methods might not provide significant improvement in the detection of bacteria. In the study by Brown and associates,[128] although 60% of patients had positive preoperative blood cultures, only 20% of intraoperative Gram stains were positive. Arterial wall frozen sections have not seen widespread use, but they may prove helpful. Histologic findings of inflammation and bacterial invasion are strong evidence supporting the diagnosis of arterial infection.

When obtaining blood or arterial wall cultures, it should be noted that the type of organism can affect the yield of the tests. Brown and associates[128] noted that 60% of arterial wall cultures were negative. Approximately 25% of their cultures failed to detect any organism at all. Presumably, these were difficult organisms to collect and culture. *S. epidermidis* may be difficult to culture without sonicating the specimen. *Treponema pallidum* may require dark-field examination for identification. *M. tuberculosis* is a fastidious organism that is difficult to grow. These considerations should prompt the special attention of the pathology laboratory and the collection of adequate specimens.

Molecular Diagnosis of Arterial Infection

The molecular biology technique allows the evaluation of biological specimens for the detection of bacterial nucleic acids. This has been applied to the detection of bacteria within arterial samples. The application of techniques such as polymerase chain reaction (PCR) may allow the detection and amplification of genetic material from the bacteria within the arterial wall. These techniques diagnose the presence of microbiological organisms, identify the organism, and may identify the presence of resistant strains allowing for direction of antimicrobial therapy.

Da Silva and colleagues reported use of PCR for detection of bacterial ribosomal nucleic acid (RNA) in specimens of normal aortic tissue removed at the time of surgical repair.[136] Using universal eubacteria primers to amply 16SrRMA, they were able to identify the RNA from a wide variety of bacteria in the arterial specimen, thus demonstrating the potential of the technique. Their report is striking in its ability to detect bacteria that are ordinarily difficult to culture. Dickinson and colleagues[137] reported the application of this technique in the case of a 72-year-old man with a suspected mycotic femoral artery aneurysm and blood cultures that showed *S. pneumoniae*. Arterial wall samples subjected to routine culture techniques yielded no microorganisms. The same samples analyzed with pneumococcal primers for PCR were able to identify the presence of *S. pneumoniae*.

Dickinson used PCR to confirm the presence of a suspected pathogen, whereas da Silva used PCR to identify a wide spectrum of bacteria that were present in arterial tissue. Although widely available, these molecular techniques are not commonly used; they are costly, and interpretation of the test results might not be intuitive because they can detect both pathogenic and symbiotic bacteria. Still, these techniques could prove beneficial in the diagnosis of organisms that are notoriously difficult to culture, such as slow-growing organisms (e.g., mycobacteria) or those that produce biofilms (e.g., *S. epidermidis*). These techniques would likely allow improved diagnosis of bacteria present in the approximately 20% to 60% of suspected mycotic aneurysms that fail to yield bacterial growth on culture examination.

Nuclear Imaging: Tagged White Blood Cell Scans

Nuclear imaging has become an important tool in the identification of arterial graft infections, but it has not played as important a role in identifying primary arterial infections. The technique is based on the ability of various radioisotope markers to be linked to white blood cells, which then become involved in an inflammatory process. The advantages of these tests are their relatively low risk to the patient and the facility of their application. The principal drawback is that the tests may detect many inflammatory lesions, not just those that are the result of an arterial infection. The interpretation of the results of a nuclear scan must account for many clinical issues. Although the usefulness of these tests has been debated, in the absence of recent trauma or infection, the use of radiolabeled indium or gallium as markers may allow localization of an arterial infection.

Computed Tomography and Magnetic Resonance Imaging

The success of techniques such as computed tomography (CT) and magnetic resonance imaging (MRI) in identifying primary arterial infections depends largely on their ability to resolve the characteristic anatomic features of the lesions. Because of the detailed anatomic data these scans present, they have become popular in the evaluation of intraabdominal vascular lesions. There are some significant limitations, however, in regard to their ability to secure the diagnosis of an arterial infection.

The essential diagnostic characteristics of arterial infections include the presence of a focal defect in the wall of the aorta, the saccular shape of the aneurysm, and the tissue edema that accompanies the inflammatory reaction. Routine two-dimensional reconstruction of CT images does not readily allow recognition of the diagnostic features of mycotic aneurysms. A three-dimensional reconstruction does allow their recognition, but such reconstruction is not routinely performed and must be specifically requested.

MRI represents an improvement over CT scanning because current computer analysis allows a more flexible assemblage of the data and facilitates the recognition of essential diagnostic characteristics. MRI may not require intravascular contrast agents, which are frequently needed with CT. Finally, MRI is able to detect tissue differences with regard to certain molecular constituents. Another advantage of MRI is its ability to detect the accumulation of water in tissues; this tissue edema is frequently the hallmark of an inflammatory process and may identify an arterial infection.

Angiography

Angiography is the most widely used technique for the investigation and definition of arterial infections (Fig. 11.4). Historically it was the first method by which the characteristics of primary arterial infections were identified. Angiography served to define the characteristics of these lesions. Angiography is clearly superior in areas such as the intestinal mesentery and the visceral vessels, where the size of the arterial lesion may be less than the resolution of computed techniques. In the case of aortic mycotic aneurysms, the angiogram usually provides excellent definition of the defect in the aortic wall, the saccular pseudoaneurysm, and the contiguous arterial anatomy. Finally, the arteriogram offers the best definition of the relationship between the visceral vessels and the arterial defect—an essential step in planning patient management.

The role of arteriography in the management of a peripheral arterial infection has been questioned. Because some peripheral arterial infections can be managed with ligation and debridement without reconstruction, an angiogram might not be necessary. However, there is a benefit to assessing the native circulation before attempting arterial ligation. Should the limb require urgent revascularization after arterial ligation, an angiogram obtained before the ligation would be helpful in planning the revascularization. For this reason, an arteriogram of the involved vessels is strongly advised in all but emergent cases.

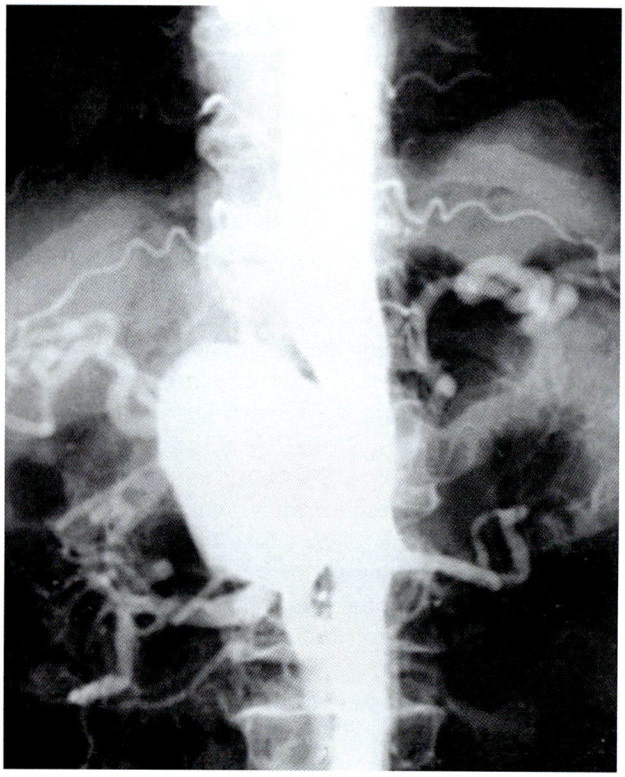

FIG 11.4 Angiogram of mycotic aortic aneurysm.

Hybrid Positron Emission Tomography and Computed Tomographic Scan

Positron emission tomography (PET) is a technique in which positron emissions from a biomarker are detected and displayed in an image. The PET scan relies on the ability of fludeoxyglucose, a glucose analog that has a positron-emitting radioactive isotope, to be taken up by high–glucose-using cells. In the setting of infections, these cells are macrophages, leucocytes, granulocytes, and inflammatory cells. The positron emission may then be detected by the PET scanner.

New "fusion technology" allows the images acquired from both a CT scanner and a PET scanner to be taken sequentially in the same session and combined into a single superposed or co-registered image. This allows combining the metabolic information of the PET scan with the spatial information of the CT scan. The technique may provide greater sensitivity and specificity in the detection and localization of an infection. Fukuchi and colleagues[138] described their initial experience with this technique when applied to suspected vascular graft infections in 2005. They observed that this technique might be of particular benefit in patients who might have an infection; however, the presentation is not clinically evident or severe. Their experience indicated that the PET/CT had a high sensitivity and that in several instances this resulted in false-positive scans. In addition, the PET techniques suffer the general limitation of requiring the production of radiopharmaceuticals for the scan—a process that is highly specialized, requires significant infrastructure, and is expensive. This technique is still far from general clinical application.

Timing of Diagnosis

The diagnosis of a primary arterial infection may be made preoperatively, intraoperatively, or postoperatively. Should the diagnosis be suspected before surgery, preoperative antibiotics may be commenced, and the patient can be better informed about potential problems. Plans can also be drawn for contingencies that might require alternative reconstructions. The diagnosis may be established or confirmed by the findings at surgery. The presence of gross purulence, engorged lymph nodes, and inflamed tissues helps to establish the diagnosis conclusively. Adjunctive tests such as the Gram stain and bacterial cultures may be performed. The intraoperative findings help determine the mode of arterial reconstruction. Gross infection, abscess, and pus should be taken as indications for debridement and remote reconstruction, whereas minimal evidence of infection may suggest reasonably good results from in situ reconstruction. If the diagnosis is confirmed in the postoperative period by positive bacterial cultures, a prolonged course of antibiotics and graft surveillance is advisable.

Natural History

Given the pathogenesis of a primary arterial infection—bacterial invasion, colonization, and destruction of an artery—the sequence of events after this initial insult is predictable and inexorable.

Destruction of the arterial wall leads to either the development of an arterial pseudoaneurysm or life-threatening hemorrhage. Which of these two events occurs is probably related to the rate of progression of the infection, its location, and the subsequent development of an inflammatory response. If the destruction of the arterial wall is gradual and accompanied by a vigorous inflammatory response, the arterial infection may produce a pseudoaneurysm. If the process of arterial infection leads to a rapid loss of arterial integrity, the arterial infection can result in hemorrhage.

Complications of arterial infections include those common to all aneurysms: embolization, thrombosis, and rupture. The high rupture rate is reflected in both the virulent course (rapid expansion and progression to rupture) and the high mortality of these lesions. For these reasons, mycotic aneurysms are urgent cases that should be repaired as soon as possible. One final complication, which is significantly increased in cases of primary arterial infection, is the rate of infection of the vascular reconstruction. Although the anticipated incidence of graft infection in "clean" cases is less than 1% or 2%, the incidence of graft infection after remote (extraanatomic) reconstruction in cases of primary arterial infection may be as high as 15%. In older series, when in situ reconstruction was performed in the face of a purulent infection and without concurrent antibiotics, the reinfection rate approached 100%.

Principles of Management

Two elemental principles form the basis of therapy in primary arterial infections: control of sepsis and arterial reconstruction.

Control of Sepsis

Antibiotic therapy and surgical debridement represent the primary treatment modalities for the control of sepsis in arterial infections. All infected arterial tissue must be debrided. It is important that the arterial resection encompass all inflamed tissues and continue to the point where the arterial tissue is normal and healthy. This helps to prevent recurrence of the infection and disruption of the arterial suture line.

Soft tissues adjacent to the infected artery that appear to be involved are also debrided. Major structures such as the vena cava and ureters are left intact. Retroperitoneal tissues that appear to be involved are resected as well. Once all infected tissues have been removed, the wound is thoroughly irrigated with an antibiotic solution—ideally, one that contains antibiotic directed toward the suspected pathogens (as detected by preoperative blood cultures). Surgical drains are useful when there is clear evidence of purulence or abscess. When collateral circulation allows, the excision may be accompanied by proximal and distal ligation and no effort to reconstruct the artery.

The use of antibiotics is mandatory in these situations. Broad-spectrum antibiotics must be initiated as soon as a strong clinical suspicion of arterial infection has been established. Blood cultures should be obtained before the initiation of antibiotics. When positive, these cultures are then used to select an antibiotic regimen with the highest therapeutic value and the fewest side effects. Negative cultures should not preclude the institution of broad-spectrum antibiotics when arterial infection is suspected. The use of high-dose preoperative antibiotics is directed toward sterilizing the aneurysm and adjacent tissues to minimize bacteremia and local contamination during surgical manipulation of infected tissues. Antibiotics must be continued until the source of the bacteremia has been corrected surgically or medically. Similarly, the primary source of bacteremia or local bacterial invasion must be controlled as a mainstay of therapy in all types of primary arterial infections. In patients with subacute bacterial endocarditis (SBE)-related mycotic aneurysms, specific consideration must be given to sterilization of cardiac valvular vegetations. When possible, a period of preoperative antibiotic administration is associated with improved outcome.

The duration of antibiotic treatment is somewhat controversial, and several competing regimens have been proposed. Several authors suggest that IV antibiotics be initiated before surgery and extended for no less than 6 weeks postoperatively.[139-141] In addition, these authors recommend that patients with prosthetic reconstructions, especially in situ prosthetic reconstructions, be prescribed lifelong oral regimens of suppressive antibiotics. Typically, oral TMP-SMX (Bactrim), a sulfa drug, or a first-generation cephalosporin or penicillin is the agent of choice.

Important technical points include the use of monofilament suture material in ligation and oversewing of the arteries. This recommendation is based on the superiority of monofilament over braided suture in resisting recurrent infection. Whenever possible, the resected arterial stump should be covered with a pedicle of healthy, viable tissue to further reduce the possibility of a recurrent infection and to accelerate healing of the arterial segment. In the abdomen, this tissue pedicle is frequently the omentum. A flap of fascia from the prevertebral fascia and ligaments can be used to reinforce the aortic suture line. In the periphery, muscle transposition is the preferred means of obtaining tissue coverage. In the femoral region, this is most readily accomplished by rotating the head of the sartorius.

Nonoperative Therapy

Nonoperative therapy for arterial infections has been proposed by Kaufman and coworkers[142] for high-risk or debilitated patients. This treatment modality, although effective anecdotally, remains controversial, and further investigation is necessary. Hsu and colleagues[143] reported a series of 22 cases of infected aortic aneurysms treated with antibiotics only and without surgery.[115] The in-hospital mortality was 50%. The event-free survival at 1 year was 32%. The authors noted that these results compared poorly to standard surgical approaches.

Arterial Reconstruction

Restoration of arterial continuity is necessary to control hemorrhage and to provide for perfusion of the distal arterial beds. This can be accomplished with open surgical approaches or by endovascular approaches. Currently, open surgical technique with extraanatomic reconstruction is considered the most conservative approach; however, new reports suggest that this may be changing as familiarity with endovascular technique progresses.

The open surgical management of mycotic aneurysms includes debridement of infected tissues (including the infected artery), along with extraanatomic reconstruction or in situ arterial reconstruction. Reconstruction of the infected arterial tree presents the problem of material interaction with the infectious organisms. Several materials are available for reconstruction: synthetic graft (Dacron), autologous veins, and human cryopreserved arterial allografts.

The material used for reconstruction of the arterial tree in the face of infection represents a significant choice that could influence the outcome of surgery. This is particularly true when the consideration is in situ reconstruction of an infected artery. Reconstruction alternatives include prosthetic grafts, autogenous veins, and cadaveric allografts. Prosthetic grafts are readily available and inexpensive, but present an increased risk of reinfection. Biological grafts are thought to have a better ability to resist infection than do prosthetic grafts. Autologous femoral vein grafts require a time-consuming dissection for graft procurement and may be accompanied by complications related to this dissection. Arterial allograft reconstructions are expensive, are not commonly available, and may be subject to aneurysmal degeneration.

Antibiotic-impregnated grafts. Experimental and clinical evidence suggests that in situ reconstruction with antibiotic-impregnated prosthetic grafts is feasible. Bandyk and colleagues[144] reported 27 patients operated on with rifampin-impregnated grafts as treatment for a variety of arterial infections. At least four recurrent infections were reported, including two that resulted in death. They concluded that in situ replacement using a rifampin-bonded prosthetic graft was most effective for low-grade staphylococcal arterial infection. An added caveat was that in the presence of virulent and antibiotic-resistant bacterial strains, this therapy usually failed. A more recent experience of 27 patients with both graft infections and mycotic aneurysms managed with silver-coated polyester grafts was published by Batt and associates.[145] There were 7 perioperative deaths and 20 long-term survivors. Of the long-term (actuarial period, 24 months) survivors, one developed a recurrent infection. Rifampin may be more readily available than the silver-coated polyester grafts. Rifampin has been shown to have a significant effect in reducing in situ graft reinfection in experimental settings.[146] This approach has been reported from a number of authors who note a low rate of recurrent infections (0% to 8%) involving the reconstruction graft when placed in situ.[147-150]

Vein grafts. Aortoiliac reconstruction with autogenous veins has been performed with both saphenous and femoral veins. An initial experience using femoral veins for aortic and iliac reconstruction was reported by Schulman and associates.[151] The use of superficial femoral and popliteal veins has been advocated by Clagett and associates[152] for a number of infectious indications, including primary aortoiliac arterial infections, has been termed the *NAIS procedure.* In their series of 38 patients with aortofemoral infections who underwent successful reconstruction with autogenous superficial femoral vein, the long-term primary patency was 85% at 5 years.[152]

Human allografts. In situ reconstruction with human allografts for infected aneurysms in the aortoiliac region has been reported with good results: low mortality and good durability. Reinfection rates after prolonged administration of culture-directed antibiotics are generally low. The most common problem associated with allograft reconstruction is the eventual degradation of the allograft, which is subject to aneurysmal degeneration.

Kieffer and associates[153] reported their experience with 43 patients with infected infrarenal aortic prosthetic grafts who underwent in situ replacement using preserved allografts obtained from cadavers. In the early postoperative period, there were five septic complications, including two pseudoaneurysm ruptures; two cases of septic shock; and one instance of peritonitis from colon perforation. In follow-up, one late death may have been related to persistent infection. A report focusing on mycotic aortic aneurysms was published by Leseche and associates.[154] They reported a series of 28 patients operated on for a variety of vascular infections, including five mycotic aneurysms. There were five perioperative deaths, two from sepsis and two from multisystem organ failure. The long-term outcomes were good. There were no recurrent infections and only three instances of aneurysmal degeneration of the allograft. More recent reports of cryopreserved human allograft indicate that the incidence of late aneurysmal degeneration may be further reduced by changes in cryopreservation processing.[155-157]

Extraanatomic Reconstruction

Extraanatomic reconstruction of the arterial tree has become a standard approach to management of graft infection and has been widely advocated for arterial infection in general.[158] In a review of spontaneous abdominal aortic infections, Ewart and associates[159] demonstrated a 23% to 63% reoperation rate for graft infection after immediate in situ reconstruction and a 7% recurrent infection rate when patients were initially treated with arterial debridement and remote reconstruction.

In a review of 51 cases of mycotic aneurysms, Brown and associates[128] noted that the mortality of local graft reconstruction was 32%, whereas extraanatomic reconstruction was associated with a 13% mortality rate. Still, the authors advocated in situ reconstruction in selected cases; they proposed that if no gross purulence was encountered intraoperatively, and if the result was gram-negative, in situ reconstruction using prosthetic material (Dacron) could be performed safely. This approach is predicated on the recommendation that postoperative antibiotics be continued for a minimum of 6 to 8 weeks. Brown and associates[128] demonstrated 63% survival and 19% reinfection rates for aneurysms treated with this approach. In comparison, the rate of infection of extraanatomic bypasses following repair of mycotic aortic aneurysms was as high as 13%.

In situ reconstruction. The benefits of the in situ reconstruction are reduced length of surgery, improved graft patency, and simpler technical management of the case. The risk associated with this reconstruction is that the new arterial prosthesis may become infected.

In situ reconstruction with graft. Experience with in situ reconstruction for primary aortoduodenal fistulas has encouraged some authors to proceed with in situ graft reconstruction of the aorta when there is minimal contamination, no pus, and little extent of the infectious process.[127] Approximately 70% of aneurysms associated with primary aortoduodenal fistulas are not due to arterial infection; the majority of the remaining aneurysms are thought to be infectious in origin.[137] In the case of a primary mycotic aortoduodenal fistula, extensive debridement and extraanatomic bypass graft are recommended for significant infection and obvious involvement of the arterial bed. In situ graft replacement has been performed successfully in cases in which the level of contamination was mild. When the aneurysm is not of infectious origin, in situ reconstruction has been advised by a number of authors.[160,161]

A recent report by Lee and colleagues compares in situ versus extraanatomic reconstructions for infected infrarenal aortic aneurysms.[162] Their series consisted of 28 patients: 15 who underwent extraanatomic bypass and 13 who underwent in situ reconstruction. Early graft infection was noted in one extraanatomic reconstruction and none of the in situ reconstructions. The authors noted that survival was similar in patients who underwent in situ and extraanatomic reconstruction. Late complications were significantly more common in the extraanatomic reconstruction patients. All told, five of the extraanatomic graft patients suffered graft thrombosis, and two of these had graft infections. None of the in situ grafts suffered late infection or other complication. These results are surprising in that in situ reconstructions would be anticipated to have more frequent graft infections. The retrospective nature of the report as well as the limited sample size may partially account for the unexpected findings.

In situ reconstruction with biological grafts. Currently, no large series allograft reconstruction done for mycotic aortic aneurysms exists. All reports are series that combine both primary (mycotic aneurysms) and secondary (aortic graft infection, aortic stent infection, aortic stent-graft) infections.

Brown and associates[156] report the use of arterial allograft in the form of cryopreserved arteries (CPAs) is compared to extraanatomic reconstruction using Dacron grafts or autogenous tissues. This series compared 18 aortic homograft reconstructions and 18 axillofemoral reconstructions done for a variety of aortic infections (both primary 7, and secondary 29 infections). They noted that the in situ cryopreserved aortic homograft group suffered fewer complications (amputation, amputations, death), and no recurrent infections. Although follow-up was limited to a mean of 25 months, no late aneurysmal degeneration was noted in the aortic allograft group. They observed that anastomosis of a cryopreserved allograft to a remnant prosthetic graft in a leg may present a risk of reinfection and graft disruption. They concluded that cryopreserved human aortic allografts represent a viable alternative to reconstruction of the aorta in the presence of an infection. They also caution that this is an early experience and that larger numbers of patients and longer follow-up are required.

Bisdas and associates[157] reported a series of 57 aortic cryograft reconstructions. They report a 30-day mortality of 9%. The actuarial survival at 3 years was 81% and at 5 years was 64%. With a median follow-up of 36 months, they noted one graft occlusion, one graft aneurysmal degeneration, one fistula between a limb of the homograft and duodenum, and one postoperative hemorrhage. The authors note that none of the original infections recurred. They noted that the results from their study suggest aortic cryografts are safe and effective. Cryografts suffer the drawbacks of being costly and at risk of degeneration, and the availability of these grafts is limited.

McCready and associates[163] present a series of 51 aortic reconstructions using cryopreserved arterial homografts. Of these, 15 were primary aortic infections, 28 were aortic graft infections, and 8 were peripheral infections. They report a mean follow-up of 46 months. No aneurysmal degeneration was noted during this period. They did observe 10 graft failures, of which 7 occurred in patients with aortoenteric or bronchial fistulas. They note that the long-term complications of a CPA are uncommon. Finally, they caution that patients with aortoenteric or bronchial fistulas have a high mortality rate.

In situ reconstruction: endovascular repair. The ongoing development of endovascular technique and familiarity with endovascular repair (EVAR) has led to the gradual adoption of endovascular technique to the management of mycotic aneurysms. EVAR offers the advantages of rapid control of hemorrhage, with reduced surgical morbidity and reduced mortality. When coupled with use of antibiotics, EVAR offers an effective means of treating mycotic aneurysms with perioperative and intermediate survival, which is comparable to open repair. A significant concern is that it places a graft in direct proximity to the infection and does not afford the opportunity to debride the infected tissue. This appears to be particularly significant when there may be a source of ongoing contamination such as an aerodigestive aortic fistula, osteomyelitis of the spine, or a psoas abscess. Management of the ongoing infection is critical.

The reports of endovascular treatment indicate that, in combination with prolonged antibiotic administration and the use of drainage, some patients may achieve resolution of the arterial infection, with no infection of the endoprosthesis.[164,165] In 2002, Berchtold and colleagues[164] reported a case of *Salmonella*-associated mycotic infrarenal aortic aneurysm managed with an endovascular graft and prolonged antibiotics. After a 4-year follow-up period, repeated CT scans demonstrated resolution of the aneurysm and no sign of residual infection. More recently, Koeppel and associates[165] reported successful EVAR of a mycotic aneurysm of the infrarenal aorta associated with a retroperitoneal abscess. The aneurysm was treated with an endoprosthesis, and the abscess was drained percutaneously. Antibiotics were continued for 6 months. A CT scan done 1 year after implantation revealed no sign of retroperitoneal inflammation. These investigators noted that EVAR was particularly attractive in critically ill patients who might not be able to tolerate an open surgical repair.

These observations are highlighted by Kan and colleagues in two reviews.[166,167] In 2007, they reviewed the use of EVAR in thoracic and abdominal infected aneurysms. They reported 48 cases that accrued an 89% 30-day survival and an 82% 2-year survival.[166] They noted that fever, age over 65 years, and rupture of the aneurysm were predictors of persistent infection. They concluded that EVAR should be considered a temporary measure in patients who present with fever and rupture. They also noted that the preoperative use of antibiotics for 1 week was a protective measure that appeared to reduce persistence of infection.

In 2010, Kan and associates[167] reviewed the efficacy of EVAR in infected abdominal aortic aneurysms. They reported a series of 41 patients who underwent EVAR or conventional surgery. They noted that early postoperative mortality was similar in both groups. Late mortality, however, was greater in the conventional surgery group (10% vs. 25%). An actuarial analysis indicated that the aneurysm-related event-free survival was the same in both the open and EVAR-treated groups. Factors that predisposed toward poor outcomes included age, *Salmonella* infection, AEF, and shock.

In a similar note, Forbes and Harding[168] noted that *Salmonella*-infected aneurysms might be at risk for late recurrence of the infection. They detailed two cases of *Salmonella* aortic infections that were managed with endovascular aneurysm repair. Recurrence sepsis was noted at 5 months and at 3 years following EVAR.[168] The authors conclude that EVAR should be used with caution in patients with *Salmonella* infections. They suggest that EVAR may be used as an intermediary in these circumstances to stop hemorrhage and allow later definitive reconstruction in a more stable patient.

Lew and associates[169] identified the presence of an aerodigestive fistula in association with a mycotic aneurysm as a significant risk factor for ongoing sepsis and death. They presented a series of nine patients with mycotic aneurysms treated with endovascular stent-grafts. Of these, seven were associated with aerodigestive fistulas. They noted a mortality of 67% within the period of hospitalization. Furthermore, they noted that reoperation for infection of the endograft was required in one of the three long-term survivors. They conclude that EVAR serves to temporize patients with aerodigestive fistulas, but given the ongoing source of infection, other more lasting reconstruction should be attempted.

In the absence of aerodigestive fistula or virulent organisms, EVAR may be definitive. Vallejo and associates[170] recently presented a series of 19 patients with primary mycotic aneurysms of the thoracic and abdominal aorta. The focus of their report is to detail changes on management of these aneurysms resulting from the endovascular approach. All mycotic aneurysms were managed with thoracic endovascular aortic repair (TEVAR), EVAR, and hybrid reconstruction (for aneurysms involving the visceral aorta). They reported three perioperative deaths (17%) from sepsis, cardiac arrest, and bowel ischemia. The median follow-up was 30 months. Three late deaths were noted to result from myeloma, bowel ischemia, and gastrointestinal hemorrhage. They concluded that EVAR is effective, but reconstruction of the visceral aortic segment still requires an open surgical hybrid approach.[170]

Management of Mycotic Aneurysms According to Location

Thoracic Aneurysms

Although not common, thoracic aortic infections may appear with hemoptysis because of a fistula between the mycotic aneurysm and the bronchial tree. In these instances, uncontrolled hemorrhage can lead to asphyxia or secondary pneumonia. Management consists of controlling the hemorrhage and repair of the aneurysm. EVAR offers the most rapid means of controlling the hemorrhage in most instances. Because of the ongoing contamination from the fistula, infection of the aortic endograft is likely. A secondary procedure must be planned to close the fistula, resect the endoprosthesis, and reconstruct the aorta. Given the frequent comorbidities of these patients, these secondary operations are accompanied by considerable morbidity and may present a considerable risk for the patients.[147,162,169,170]

Suprarenal Aneurysms

Because of their unique anatomic characteristics, arterial infections of the paravisceral and suprarenal aorta almost always require immediate in situ arterial reconstruction. It is nearly impossible to bypass the visceral vessels without traversing the bed of the infected paravisceral aorta. Experience gained from the repair of suprarenal mycotic aneurysms has given credence to the concept of in situ repair with adjunctive lifelong antibiotic therapy.

When combined with debridement of grossly infected tissue and appropriate use of antibiotics, most series reporting this type of reconstruction have demonstrated acceptable morbidity and mortality rates. Chan and associates[139] reported a series of 22 patients with mycotic aneurysms of the thoracic and abdominal aorta. Of these, 13 had involvement of the paravisceral aorta, all of which required in situ reconstruction. Twelve of the 13 patients survived surgery and were given lifelong suppressive antibiotics. None had clinical recurrence of the infection. In the overall series, three patients died; two of the deaths were attributed to multisystem organ failure and one to aspiration pneumonia. The authors concluded that in situ reconstruction, along with surgical debridement and lifelong antibiotics, offers the best chance of survival in these patients who are difficult to treat. It should be noted that although this form of therapy (in situ reconstruction) is inescapable in the reconstruction of infected paravisceral aneurysms, its application to arterial infections at other sites (e.g., infrarenal aorta or femoral artery) is less well established and should be approached with caution.

Infected Femoral Pseudoaneurysms

Infections of the vessels of the femoral region are the most common type of arterial infection. In the review by Brown and colleagues,[128] these lesions accounted for 38% of all arterial infections. The most common manifestation is an inflamed, tender, pulsatile inguinal mass. The more common complications include erosion through the skin with hemorrhage, embolization, compression of adjacent structures (femoral vein and nerve), and thrombosis. Of these, erosion and hemorrhage are the most feared complications.

The debate regarding reconstruction is of particular interest in the subset of patients with infected pseudoaneurysms of the femoral bifurcation that are the result of IV drug abuse. Because of the tendency to reuse femoral sites for drug administration, the arterial reconstruction may be in jeopardy of recurrent infection. If the reconstruction required prosthetic material, the resultant reinfection would be all the more complicated and dangerous. Finally, the incidence of graft infection after immediate reconstruction is sufficient by itself to warrant hesitation in such reconstructions. Because of these concerns, some authors have advocated simple arterial ligation and resection of the infected tissues. The problem is that simple ligation of the femoral arteries at the level of the arterial bifurcation can result in a subsequent amputation rate approaching 33%.[134,171]

An alternative approach is to proceed with biological graft reconstruction. The reconstruction should be performed with autogenous tissue if possible. In the course of these reconstructions, the infected arteries and adjacent tissues should be debrided and the reconstruction should be coursed through uninfected tissues.[172]

A third option is to resect, debride, and observe. The artery is ligated, but no reconstructions are performed in the initial setting. The limb is observed for signs of severe ischemia. If the limb appears viable with collateral perfusion alone, no effort is made to reconstruct. If the limb appears severely ischemic, revascularization is attempted. Femoral artery reconstruction should be performed either with in situ saphenous vein interposition grafting or through an extraanatomic approach, such as a transobturator bypass.

Infection and pseudoaneurysm of the common femoral (above the bifurcation), superficial femoral, and deep femoral arteries do not appear to suffer a similar fate. These vessels stand a far better chance of tolerating simple ligation without requiring reconstruction. Wright and Shepard[173] reported a low incidence of amputation following ligation and resection in this circumstance. In a series of 39 patients with such infections, they noted an amputation rate of 5%; these amputations occurred in two patients who had impaired collateral circulation from prior (contralateral) common femoral artery ligation. In the absence of these two cases, the amputation rate in this group of patients was 0%.

Mesenteric Artery Infections

Mesenteric artery infections tend to appear as pseudoaneurysms within the mesentery of the intestine. These lesions may be asymptomatic, but the more common presentation is abdominal pain. These lesions may develop as a consequence of IV drug abuse. Pathophysiologically, they are considered to be the result of mycotic embolization. Because of this, it is necessary to consider the source of the emboli as well as the possibility of other embolic targets. In practical terms, this means that these patients should be screened for both cardiac vegetations and other arterial lesions. Preoperative angiography is recommended if possible. Postoperative angiography should be considered if a preoperative study was not obtained.

Mesenteric artery infections tend to develop rapid expansion and intramesenteric hemorrhage. Alternatively, these aneurysms may result in thrombosis and infarction of the intestine. Management of these vessels is related to the location of the lesion, the available collateral circulation, and the presence and extent of intestinal infarction. Lesions of the proximal mesenteric arteries frequently require reconstruction with autogenous tissues. More distally located pseudoaneurysms can often be managed by simple excision. If a small area of intestinal ischemia develops, a limited bowel resection may also be necessary. In instances of extensive intestinal ischemia, a second-look celiotomy may be advisable after restoration of intestinal perfusion.

Arterial Infections of the Upper Extremity

Infections of the arteries of the upper extremities are fairly rare. Collectively, they represented approximately 10% of arterial infections in the review by Brown and colleagues.[128] Frequently, these lesions are associated with trauma. Like other infections of peripheral vessels, these lesions develop in a number of ways, with the most common presentation being an inflamed, tender, pulsatile mass. In the upper extremities, careful inspection should detect evidence of digital embolization, splinter hemorrhages, and ischemic lesions.

Because of the extensive collateral blood supply to the upper extremities, arterial infections there can often be treated with simple ligation and excision. This is particularly true when the involved segment is between the thyrocervical trunk and the subscapular artery or distal to the deep brachial artery. Reconstruction, when required, should be accomplished with a saphenous vein graft or similar autogenous tissues. As with all mycotic aneurysms, preoperative and postoperative antibiotics should be given for a prolonged period.

Conclusions

Primary arterial infections are relatively rare, but they are frequently lethal. They often follow a rapidly progressive course toward expansion and rupture. Astute diagnosis and correct management can improve a patient's chance of survival. The diagnosis is established by a high index of suspicion, along with identification of risk factors and appropriate testing. Once an arterial infection is identified, management must be tailored to the organism involved and the site and severity of the infection, as well as the condition of the patient. Surgical excision is almost always necessary in the course of management. Long-term (6 weeks) IV antibiotics are almost always required, and the use of lifelong oral antibiotic suppression is strongly recommended for these patients. Optimal care can reduce the mortality of these lesions from nearly 100% to less than 10% to 15%.

Chronic Suppression Therapy

Infection of an arterial graft can be associated with high morbidity and mortality. Excision of the graft has generally been the mainstay of treatment in such patients. However, it has been increasingly recognized that graft explant is not a simple procedure. Often it needs to be combined with extensive alternative vascular reconstructions that can actually be associated with additional morbidity and mortality in some patients and can subject patients to additional stress. Several of these patients may have co-existing advanced medical conditions such as cardiopulmonary disease, advanced malignancy, or their anatomy maybe prohibitively hostile.[174]

An earlier report of the concept of suppressive antibiotic therapy comes from the study published by Chan and colleagues in 1989.[139] As described earlier in the chapter, this study included 22 patents with mycotic aortic aneurysms who were managed with IV antibiotics perioperatively followed by in situ Dacron graft replacement. Postoperatively, antibiotics were continued orally for the rest of the patients' lives. One patient had a recurrent *Proteus* sp. infection involving the intervertebral disc space, which did not appear sensitive to antibiotics. Interestingly, two other patients in this series were noncompliant with antibiotic therapy and had the following postoperative courses. One patient discharged himself against medical advice after the surgical intervention, refused to take antibiotics, and was readmitted with fever and chills. The second patient discontinued antibiotic therapy after discharge and was readmitted with streptococcal aortic infection and aortoduodenal fistula. With in situ prosthetic reconstructions done for arterial infections, lifelong suppressive antibiotics are recommended by several authorities. This chapter dealt primarily with aortic infections, but extrapolation of this concept to infections at other sites should be done cautiously and judiciously.

Chronic suppression of infection with antibiotics has been selectively advocated in some patients. Quite possibly, the greatest benefit of this more conservative approach is derived in patients in whom infection of the graft is suspected but never actually proven. Greatest effort should be made to tailor the long-term antibiotic therapy toward the suspected organism. Antibiotics like rifampicin or clindamycin have high concentration in the leukocytes. Leukocytes may help increase local antibiotic concentrations in the infected graft.[174] Other agents such as TMP-SMX, tetracyclines and quinolones may also be considered because of high oral bioavailability.[175] Partial graft preservation with chronic suppressive antibiotic therapy is also an option.[176]

An important caveat with these patients is to be mindful of the need for close clinical follow-up. There is a possibility of relapse in patients being treated with this approach. In one study of infected aortic grafts treated with graft retention and antibiotics, 59% of the patients had a relapse.[177] Rates of relapse are lower in other reports.[178] Patients with relapse may experience septicemia requiring graft explant or hospitalization with systemic antibiotics. Additionally, some reports have described variable success of this approach with certain types of organisms, for example *Pseudomonas*.[176,179]

The use of chronic suppressive antibiotic therapy has also been described in the literature with aortic endografts. In one small series, there was no statistically significant difference in mortality between patients with aortic endograft infection treated surgically or conservatively.[180] Similar results have been reported by other authors.[181] Most authors have emphasized careful patient selection when attempting conservative management with chronic suppressive antibiotic therapy and endograft preservation.

The risk of *Clostridium difficile* infection, as well as drug reactions and side effects, has to be weighed against the benefit gained from graft preservation.[178]

SUMMATION

The appropriate use of antibiotics in vascular surgery is of critical importance toward a successful outcome. Understanding the causes of infection, the pathogenesis of the organisms, and the strength of the host are all elements that must be taken into consideration in antibiotic selection and use. Ideally, the use of antibiotics should be tailored to the clinical situation and individuated based on local infectious patterns as well as the presence of risk factors.

REVIEW QUESTIONS

1. True or false: Arterial trauma is involved in the pathogenesis of most primary arterial infections.
2. When should prosthetic grafts be used to replace excised mycotic aneurysms?
   a. If the surgical field is laved with antibiotics
   b. In the upper extremities
   c. Only in carefully selected instances
   d. In fungal arterial infections
   e. Never
3. Since 1965, what organism is most commonly associated with microbial aortitis?
   a. *Salmonella* species
   b. Fungi
   c. Mycobacteria
   d. *Pseudomonas* species
   e. *Staphylococcus aureus*
4. In the management of a mycotic mesenteric aneurysm located in the distal arterial arcade (adjacent to the intestine), what is the recommended management?
   a. Reconstruction with a Dacron graft
   b. Reconstruction with a PTFE graft
   c. Reconstruction with an umbilical vein graft
   d. Reconstruction with a vein graft
   e. Ligation and excision without reconstruction
5. True or false: The recommended management of an infrarenal mycotic aneurysm involves the use of antibiotics, debridement of infected tissues, and reconstruction through a remote (extraanatomic) uninfected field.
6. What is the average reported incidence of prosthetic graft infection?
   a. 1% to 6%
   b. 6% to 10%
   c. 10% to 15%
   d. Greater than 15%
   e. 0% to 1%
7. True or false: The study by Pitt and colleagues revealed that intravenous antibiotics were much more effective than antibiotic irrigation.
8. Risk factors for prosthetic graft infection include which of the following?
   a. Multiple reoperations
   b. Inguinal incisions
   c. Open, infected wounds on the extremities
   d. Prior graft infections
   e. Positive arterial wall cultures
   f. All of the above

9. Avenues of infection include which of the following?
   a. Skin
   b. Arterial wall
   c. Open wounds on the distal limb
   d. Intestinal transudate accumulated during aortic bypass
   e. Foley catheter
   f. All of the above

10. What are the most common organisms found in prosthetic graft infections?
    a. *Proteus* species
    b. *Escherichia coli*
    c. *Staphylococcus aureus*
    d. *Streptococcus viridans*
    e. *Staphylococcus epidermidis*

References available online at ExpertConsult.com.

12 CHAPTER

Patterns of Diabetic Vascular Disease

Jayer Chung, Joseph L. Mills

INTRODUCTION

The term *chronic critical limb ischemia* (CLI) was first coined in 1982 and was intended to describe limb-threatening arterial insufficiency in the absence of diabetes mellitus (DM).[1] Since the initial description of CLI, the incidence and prevalence of DM has markedly increased with a current worldwide prevalence of 422 million, which is a fourfold increase from 1980 figures.[2] Since ischemia accompanies DM in approximately half the cases,[3,4] the concept of CLI has undergone a frameshift to recognize the changing pattern of lower extremity limb-threatening ischemia, with an increased contribution of DM to the disease phenotype.[5] An improved understanding of the changing patterns of diabetic vascular disease with respect to pathophysiology, arteriographic patterns, wounds, and infection has enhanced the recognition, management, and outcomes of diabetic vascular disease. This chapter reviews diabetic vascular disease with respect to patterns of disease, distributions of pedal wounds, and infection as well as the common presentation, management strategies, and costs.

EPIDEMIOLOGY OF DIABETES MELLITUS AND VASCULAR DISEASE

Diabetes now affects 9% to 10% of the US adult population, with type 2 DM responsible for over 90% of cases (Fig. 12.1).[6] There is also a rising childhood prevalence of type 2 DM, which now comprises approximately half of all childhood DM cases.[6] The increase in type 2 DM parallels the childhood obesity epidemic and especially affects American ethnic minorities.[6] Type 2 diabetes comprises 90% to 95% of all cases of DM.[6] Worldwide figures mirror those in the United States, with a worldwide prevalence of 9%, and DM is more common in males than in females.[2] Most countries have experienced a dramatic increase in the rates of type 2 DM, with no country having experienced a statistically significant decrease in the prevalence of DM since 1980. Five countries contain approximately half of the world's diabetics: China, India, the United States, Brazil, and Indonesia.[2] Peripheral artery disease (PAD) has also increased in worldwide prevalence, with an estimated 202 million people living with PAD globally as of 2010.[7] With respect to the CLI subpopulation, recent estimates of CLI have also increased, to a current prevalence of 0.2% to 0.4% cited within the US Medicare database.[8,9] The increases in both PAD and CLI, while modest relative to the increased prevalence of DM, remain important due to the synergistic effect of ischemia and DM on major amputation rates.

The prevalence of PAD among adult Americans with diabetes is twofold higher compared with a cohort of similarly aged Americans without diabetes.[10] The 4-year estimate of amputation-free survival (AFS) is approximately 45% among those presenting with diabetic foot ulceration and PAD.[11] This rate is significantly lower than that found in comparable populations of patients with only PAD.[11] Patients with PAD and DM have a 1.5- to 5-fold higher risk of major amputation than comparable patients with either PAD or DM alone.[12,13] These risks amplify the baseline risk, which is already elevated in patients with DM alone and is 10 to 30 times greater than that in similarly aged nondiabetics. These risks are apparent in the United States, with DM having accounted for approximately 60% of nontraumatic lower-limb amputations in patients aged 20 years or older. DM was responsible for approximately 73,000 lower limb amputations in the United States in 2010.[14] Although the age adjusted rate of major amputation in diabetics is decreasing, the explosion in the number of diabetics is such that the overall rate of amputations as a percentage of the population is unchanged.[14] Worldwide there are approximately 1 million lower extremity diabetic amputations each year. Extrapolating from this statistic, a diabetic lower extremity amputation occurs approximately every 20 seconds worldwide.[15] Survival at 4 years is also worse for patients with diabetic foot ulcerations only compared with those with diabetic foot ulcerations and PAD. Although caregivers often focus on limb salvage, these data suggest that practitioners must also focus on efforts to improve mortality in this particularly high-risk cohort.[11]

PATHOPHYSIOLOGY OF VASCULAR DISEASE AND DIABETES MELLITUS

Glucose reacts nonenzymatically with the amino groups of proteins to form Schiff bases, followed by Amadori rearrangement. Nonenzymatic glycosylation is more likely when patients are hyperglycemic, resulting in early glycation products. These become irreversible reactions with dehydration, condensation, and cross-linking, resulting ultimately in advanced glycation end products (AGEs).[16,17] AGEs dissipate only with protein turnover; hence they accumulate in proteins with long half-lives, such as collagen and elastin. AGEs then bind to the receptor for advanced glycation end products (RAGEs), which mediates a variety of processes

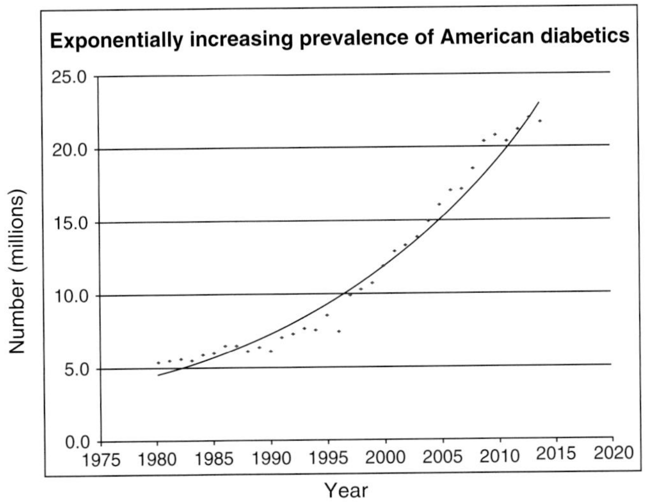

FIG 12.1 Increasing prevalence of type 1 and type 2 diabetes mellitus in the United States from 1980–2014.

to accelerate atherosclerosis. RAGE activation results in increased extracellular matrix production and type IV collagen deposition, increased monocyte migration, and increased expression of cell adhesion molecules, namely vascular cell adhesion molecule-1 (VCAM-1). RAGE's also bind to S-100 proteins, which are highly expressed in atherosclerotic plaque in the context of DM. They likewise increase expression of nuclear transcription factor κB (NFκB), resulting in an increase in a variety of inflammatory cytokines such as tumor necrosis factor α (TNFα), interleukin-1β (IL-1β), and transforming growth factor-β (TGFβ).[16,17] The confluence of these changes is an increase in the development of atherosclerotic plaques in diabetics.

One of the prototypical final manifestations of diabetic vascular disease is calcification of the media in medium-sized arteries. AGEs have been associated with the development of medial calcification by several in vitro studies.[18,19] AGEs bind RAGEs in vascular smooth muscle cells (VSMCs), inducing a change into an osteogenic phenotype. Ultimately it appears that the altered osteogenic VSMCs are responsible for hydroxyapatite deposition within the media of a diabetic's arteries. Although the precise pathway of this phenotypic change is unclear, the VSMC exposure to AGEs mediated by RAGEs appears critical to the development of medial calcification.[19] Medial calcification is more frequently associated with DM, with intimal calcification found mostly in nondiabetic-associated atherosclerosis.

ARTERIOGRAPHIC PATTERNS OF VASCULAR DISEASE IN DIABETES MELLITUS

DM alters the angiographic pattern of atherosclerotic obstructive disease, compared with that which occurs in nondiabetics. There is an increased predilection for disease in the infrapopliteal vessels, especially among elderly males.[20,21] This tendency to the infrapopliteal location may significantly increase major amputation rates among diabetics, especially those whose occlusions are primarily located in the popliteal or infrapopliteal vessels.[21] Graziani et al.[22] retrospectively reviewed 417 patients with diabetes and CLI to characterize the angiographic patterns of disease among diabetics; 2893 lesions were discovered, and 74% were located in the infrapopliteal vessels. Moreover, most of the occlusions were more extensive (>10 cm) and were more prevalent in the infrapopliteal vessels than in the vessels above the knee. The anterior tibial and posterior tibial arteries were most frequently affected, with relative sparing of the peroneal artery. This pattern of disease had been previously observed, but the reasons for this pattern remain unexplained.

The most frequent pattern of disease includes an occlusion of the femoropopliteal artery and concomitant occlusion of one or more of the tibial vessels. The next most frequent pattern involves occlusion of one of the tibial vessels with diffuse disease in the remaining vessels, and occlusion of all crural vessels was found in 28% of patients. The pedal vasculature is frequently spared, however, with 88% of patients having at least one patent pedal vessel.[22] The significance of the arteriographic pattern of atherosclerotic disease in patients with DM is that revascularization of the tibial and pedal vasculature is becoming increasingly relevant.

The microvasculature has been traditionally thought to be occluded in diabetic vascular disease and was viewed as a major contributor to major limb amputation in patients with DM, although this concept is incorrect. Prior researchers extrapolated data from patients with diabetic retinopathy having higher major amputation rates.[23] It was widely assumed that the microvasculature of the foot would behave similarly to that of other microvascular beds in patients with DM. However, the association between diabetic retinopathy and nephropathy may simply be a reflection of poorer long-term glycemic control, with the outcomes reflective of the complications of prolonged hyperglycemia rather than obliterative occlusions of the foot microvasculature. Indeed, subjects with DM do not have extensive occlusions of the microvasculature, as has been traditionally taught.[24] Moreover, the endothelial layer does not appear to have increased proliferative lesions that could obstruct flow at the level of the arterioles.[24]

Arteriolar patency does not signify that the microvasculature is entirely normal in diabetic vascular disease. The microvasculature appears to have increased permeability.[24] This increased permeability may result in a greater deposition of plasma proteins and fluid in the extracellular space, and this process can theoretically decrease oxygen and nutrient diffusion to the tissues, thereby decreasing clearance of infectious or necrotic debris in the soft tissue of the foot. Endothelial function also appears to be abnormal, with reduced availability of nitric oxide, due to increased destruction via free radical overproduction.[24] These changes may decrease the ability of diabetics to augment capillary blood flow to areas of relative ischemia; further study is required to quantify the microvascular dysfunction in diabetic feet and understand the significance of microvascular dysfunction in DM.

DISTRIBUTION OF FOOT WOUNDS IN DIABETIC VASCULAR DISEASE

Changes in the biomechanical pressure profiles on diabetic feet are important to our understanding of the origin of diabetic foot ulceration (DFU) as well as the efficacy of operative reconstructions and adjunctive off-loading strategies to aid ulcer healing. The biomechanical patterns of stress on diabetic feet vary due to alterations in gait as well as changes associated with the loss of sensory feedback and motor weakness of the foot musculature.[25,26] Motor neuropathy results in atrophy of the metatarsophalangeal plantar flexors of the foot and contributes to the development of common diabetic foot deformities, such as hammer toes, claw toes, prominent metatarsal heads, and pes cavus.[25] This can result in sites of abnormally high pressure and ulceration, especially when there is a loss of normal protective sensation (LOPS) coupled with repetitive trauma associated with standing or ambulation.

The role of neuropathy helps to explain the pattern of ulceration at the metatarsal heads (mal perforans ulcers) and hallux. Ledoux et al.[27] examined the interrelationship of neuropathy, DM, and peak plantar pressures with DFU location. The elevated peak pressures were especially pronounced with ulceration on the plantar surface of the foot at the metatarsal heads, especially the fifth and first metatarsal heads. Elevated pressures were also found among patients with a longer duration of DM as well as an increased prevalence of neuropathy.[27] However, the relationship between peak pressure and ulcer location is not perfect. Ledoux et al. also found that ulcerations located on the heel or the hallux had lower peak pressures compared with nonulcerated tissue. This observation suggests that other mechanisms, such ischemia and shear stress, may play a significant role in the ulceration that occurs at nonmetatarsal head portions of the foot.[27]

The multifactorial etiology of DFU is important when looking at the most frequent sites of DFU. Madanchi et al. found that the toe is the most prevalent location of DFU, present in as many as 45% of patients.[28] The next most frequent sites of DFU include the dorsum of the foot, followed by the metatarsal head and other plantar locations. The heel is affected in less than 5% of cases, with the remaining DFUs located in the ankle or other portions of the foot (Fig. 12.2). Neuropathy and foot deformity are significant in patients with DFU and alter the typical pattern of pedal necrosis seen in modern CLI patients without diabetes. The contribution of neuropathy also underscores the importance of appropriate offloading in DFU. Techniques such as total contact casting and orthotics, and foot procedures such as tendon-lengthening have now become increasingly important for modern vascular surgeons to perform to maximize outcomes.

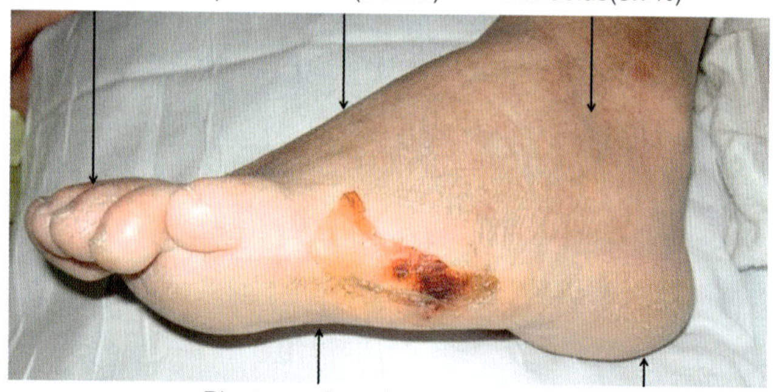

FIG 12.2 Most common sites for diabetic foot ulcerations (DFUs). The toes and areas in between the toes are the most common sites, although 11.3% of patients have multiple sites of ulcerations. This particular patient had an ulcer on the lateral aspect of the foot, a relatively rare site of ulceration (<2%). (Modified from Madanchi N, Tabatabaei-Malazy O, Pajouhi M, et al: Who are diabetic foot patients? A descriptive study on 873 patients. *J Diabetes Metab Disord* 12:36, 2013.)

PATTERNS OF FOOT INFECTIONS IN DIABETIC VASCULAR DISEASE

Microbiology of Diabetic Foot Ulceration

Clinicians should always consider the possibility of a deeper foot infection for any wound in a diabetic patient. Drainage and appropriate antibiotic therapy are critical adjuncts for the management of diabetic foot infections (DFIs).[29] Hence understanding the most common presentations and causal microorganisms is important to guiding therapy, since DM may impair the immune response to infection. DFIs do not always present with classic signs and symptoms of inflammation, such as redness, warmth, swelling, tenderness, pain, purulent secretions, foul odor, or necrotic tissue. Instead, the presentation may be more subtle, including wounds that have been present for more than 30 days, a positive probe-to-bone test, recurrent foot ulcers, a history of minor antecedent trauma, or prior lower extremity amputation. PAD, renal insufficiency, or neuropathy may mask occult infection and should raise the clinician's suspicion of an underlying DFI.[29]

Prospective randomized controlled trial data show that the most frequent pathogen isolated from DFUs is *Staphylococcus aureus*, present in approximately 36% of isolates.[30] The next most frequently isolated organisms include *Enterococcus faecalis* (25%), *Streptococcus agalactiae* (15%), *Pseudomonas aeruginosa* (7%), *Staphylococcus epidermidis* (6%), and other *Enterococcus* species (5%).[30] These data mirror pooled data from other series, with *S. aureus* being the most frequent organism isolated. Methicillin-resistance appears in approximately one-third of *S. aureus* isolates.[31] *P. aeruginosa* may be more prevalent than randomized data would suggest, as it has been found in up to 15% of DFUs from retrospective case series.[2] Typically, ulcers that are deeper and have been present for longer durations have greater microbial diversity as well as a higher prevalence of anaerobic and gram-negative bacteria. Superficial ulcers tend to have more skin flora, such as *Staphylococcus* and *Streptococcus* species.[32]

Identifying the causal microorganisms can be difficult. Ideally, the wound should be debrided prior to obtaining a deep tissue biopsy, or an aspirate of purulent secretions should be obtained. Clinically uninfected lesions should not be swab-cultured, as the culture is likely to be nonspecific, thus misguiding therapy. Wound swabs or samples of wound drainage, especially from wounds that have not been debrided, are often contaminated with normal skin flora. The predictive ability of swab techniques is little better than a coin toss, with a sensitivity of 49%, and a specificity of 62%.[33] Current culture methods also selectively favor the growth of aerobic and gram-negative bacteria and

TABLE 12.1 Distribution of Pathogens Cultured From Diabetic Foot Infections[25,26]

Pathogen	Percentage Range[a]
Staphylococcus aureus	19.1–36.2
Other gram-negative (not *Pseudomonas*) species	16.4–34.8
Enterococcus	8.6–17.7
Streptococcus agalactiae	6.5–15.0
Pseudomonas aeruginosa	6.9–14.9
Staphylococcus epidermidis	5.6–10.0

[a]The range reflects the heterogeneity in sampling techniques, culturing techniques, and the ulcerations themselves.

underrepresent the true prevalence of fastidious organisms and anaerobes in DFUs. Other methods, such as 16S ribosomal ribonucleic acid sequencing, may increase sensitivity and specificity, although the clinical relevance of this enhanced detection is unknown (Table 12.1).[32]

Difficulty remains in distinguishing between benign colonization versus a bioburden that is inhibiting wound healing of the DFU. The distinction between bioburden and more severe overt foot infections or osteomyelitis is also difficult, as there is a significant overlap in the presentation of all of these infectious complications.[29-33] Minimal data exist regarding the prognosis of untreated microbiomes and the associated risk of developing overt diabetic foot infections or osteomyelitis. Although there is growing evidence that the microbiome alters appropriate wound healing in DFUs, it is unclear whether topical or systemic antibiotic therapy directed at the microbiome enhances wound healing.[32] Rather, immunomodulatory therapies that correct the chronic inflammatory state of the nonhealing wound may ultimately prove to be more important. Further study is required to determine the significance of the microbiome with regard to the mechanism of aberrant wound healing as well as the development of more severe infectious complications.

Osteomyelitis Complicating Diabetic Foot Infection

Diabetic osteomyelitis complicates between 20% and 66% of diabetic foot wounds, depending upon the severity of the foot infection.[29,34] Lack of clear consensus definitions of osteomyelitis prevents a more accurate diagnoses and epidemiologic data. Osteomyelitis prevents wound healing and acts as a nidus to sequester microorganisms and increase reinfections. Hence, on a population level, osteomyelitis acts as a risk factor for prolonged hospitalization and amputation by 55-fold and 150-fold respectively.[35] The gold standard of diagnosis remains bone biopsy.[29] Ulcers with exposed bone, or more than 3 mm in depth, or greater than 2 cm^2 with a C-reactive protein (CRP) more than 3.2 mg/dL or an erythrocyte sedimentation rate (ESR) greater than 60 mm/h are also more likely to harbor occult osteomyelitis.[29] Risk factors for the development of diabetic foot osteomyelitis include wounds extending to the bone and/or joint or a history of recurrent/multiple wounds.[34] Suspicion of diabetic osteomyelitis is increased if a well-perfused wound fails to heal after 6 weeks of wound therapy.[36]

Microorganisms most frequently complicating diabetic osteomyelitis are similar to those isolated from DFUs. They are most commonly *S. aureus* and *S. epidermidis*. With respect to gram-negative organisms, *Escherichia coli, Klebsiella pneumoniae, Proteus,* and *Pseudomonas* species are isolated in descending order of frequency. Anaerobic organisms and multidrug-resistant organisms are infrequently cultured.[29] The significance of culture results is that they help to guide antibiotic therapy, with some authors having shown that successful clearance of osteomyelitis is twice as effective with culture-directed antibiotic therapy. However, other studies report success rates of approximately 75% with empiric therapy alone. The specific antibiotics and their duration in diabetic osteomyelitis will continue to be a contentious issue until improved definitions of osteomyelitis and outcomes data from future prospective evaluations can clarify the matter.[29]

PATTERNS OF HEALTH-RELATED QUALITY OF LIFE AND DIABETIC VASCULAR DISEASE

Quality-of-life (QoL) measures are consistently lower for subjects with DFUs.[37,38] Patients requiring a major amputation ultimately had the lowest quality of life compared with all patients with DFUs.[38] Some authors report that up to 25% of patients with DFUs were unable to have their QoL measured owing to cognitive impairment, mental health issues, or illiteracy.[37] This implies that there is a segment of the DFU population whose QoL remains unmeasured. Assuming the worst possible outcome, however, the QoL may in fact be worst in this cohort, suggesting that investigators are systematically underestimating the impact of DFUs on QoL.

Low QoL appears to be predictive of major amputation and death within one year after DFU presentation. Ironically, the converse is not true, as high baseline QoL is not predictive of wound healing.[38] Over time, patients who had chronically nonhealing wounds or major amputations had the lowest QoL as measured by SF-36 scores. This was particularly true for the domains measuring physical functioning and social functioning among those who healed.[37] The implication is that wound healing, regardless of its ultimate impact on amputation-free survival, is a valid patient-centric outcome. Interventions focused on wound healing in this population may have a significant impact upon the patients' QoL and merit further patient-centric research.

COMMON PRESENTATIONS OF DIABETIC VASCULAR DISEASE

The variability of DFI at presentation has been overwhelming due to the heterogeneous contributions of wound severity, ischemia, and foot infection; hence the Society for Vascular Surgery (SVS) developed the Wound Ischemia foot Infection (WIfI) score to quantify the severity of limb threatening ischemia (LTI).[5] This has since been utilized to categorize the presentations of LTI in an effort to improve comparability of outcomes between practitioners and clinical trials. When taken in total, approximately 6.5% of patients presented with WIfI stage I disease. Most patients present with stage 4 disease (37.3%), with the next most frequent presentation being stage 3 patients (28.6%).

Summary of the distribution of wIfI presentations

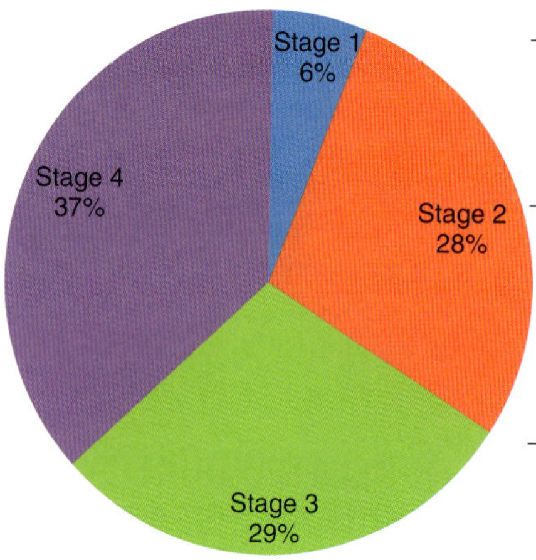

WIfI stage	WIfI spectrum score
Stage 1	W0 I0 fI0,1 W0 I1 fI0 W1 I0 fI0,1 W1 I1 fI0
Stage 2	W0 I0 fI2 W0 I1 fI1 W0 I2 fI0,1 W0 I3 fI0 W1 I0 fI2 W1 I1 fI1 W1 I2 fI0
Stage 3	W0 I0 fI3 W0 I2 fI1,2 W0 I3 fI1,2 W1 I0 fI3 W1 I1 fI2 W1 I3 fI0,1 W2 I0 fI2 W2 I1 fI0.1 S2 I2 fI0 W3 I0 fI0,1
Stage 4	W0 I1,2,3 fI3 W1 I1 fI3 W1 I2,3 fI2,3 W2 I0 fI3 W2 I1 fI2,3 W2 I2 fI1,2,3 W2 I3 fI0,1,2,3 W3 I0 fI2,3 W3 I1,2,3 fI0.1,2,3

FIG 12.3 Summary of published Wound Ischemia foot Infection (*WIfIs*) stages presenting to various tertiary referral institutions as compiled from recent retrospective series.[36-41]

Stage 2 comprised the remainder of the presentations (Fig. 12.3).[39-46] These summary statistics will likely vary significantly among institutions, since they were derived from patient cohorts in tertiary referral practices and therefore subject to significant referral bias. Hence the percentages may overrepresent those at the most severe end of the spectrum of disease. Finally, these are most frequently the patients who were selected for revascularization, with selection bias also skewing the results to the more severe end of the spectrum. The distribution of these stages is remarkably consistent with populations that do not have diabetes[42] as well as in safety net hospitals,[43] further validating the utility of the WIfI classification system for patients with DFUs.

The Eurodiale consortium, a collective database of DFUs at 14 separate European clinics, examined a slightly different patient population. This database included all patients with DFUs, not simply those who had undergone revascularization. Most were male with long-standing DM (>10 years). Over 40% of these patients presented with a deep ulcer, with most ulcers being 1 to 5 cm^2 in diameter. Approximately half of the ulcers were located on the plantar surface and ischemia and infection were prevalent, having been found in approximately 48% and 57%, respectively, of subjects at baseline.[47] Patients with concomitant ischemia were the most severely affected in the overall DFU population, and they were more likely to present with a deep ulcer and have an ulcer present in a nonplantar location. These subjects were also least likely to ambulate independently at baseline and were more likely to present with infection.[47]

Abnormal ankle-brachial indices (ABIs) are frequently found as a consequence of medial calcinosis, with normal ankle pressures and Doppler waveforms present in only 14% of diabetics. Patients may have either stiff arteries with falsely elevated ABIs or reduced ABIs, indicating reduced pressures and perfusion. Almost half (48%) have evidence of occlusive disease, indicative of the relationship between diabetes and atherosclerosis. Evidence of medial calcinosis or mixed disease (atherosclerosis with medial calcinosis) is found in the remainder (38%).[48] Because of the high prevalence of medial calcinosis in DM, adjunctive studies such as toe pressures, Doppler arterial waveforms, pulse volume recordings, or $TcPO_2$ are essential to diagnose concomitant PAD with DM. Due to the extensive burden of disease in the tibial vasculature, some practitioners are nihilistic regarding revascularization outcomes in diabetic patients. However, aggressive revascularization has been shown to be as efficacious as revascularizations performed for traditional atherosclerotic patterns of disease.[49]

PREDICTING PATTERNS OF WOUND HEALING AND AMPUTATION IN DIABETIC VASCULAR DISEASE

In the past, physicians relied on measurements of foot arterial pressures to estimate perfusion and predict wound healing in diabetic vascular disease. Those with absolute ankle pressures 90 mm Hg or more or a toe pressure 55 mm Hg or more were felt to be likely to heal without revascularization.[47] Subjects with a toe pressure equal to or greater than 30 mm Hg, skin perfusion pressure equal to or greater than 40 mm Hg, or a $TcPO_2$ equal to or greater than 25 mm Hg were unlikely to heal.[5] Those with intermediate perfusion values were difficult to predict. Moreover, relying upon pressures and the degree of ischemia alone has failed to account for the effect of infection and the severity of foot wounds.

Recent publications have highlighted the utility of the SVS WIfI classification scheme to predict wound healing and amputation-free survival in diabetic vascular disease. Zhan et al.[39] showed that WIfI stage was predictive of wound healing, with a mean wound healing time of 95 days in WIfI stage 1 limbs compared with 263 days for stage 4 limbs. Revascularization markedly improved outcomes, particularly for WIfI stage 3 limbs, where the mean wound healing time decreased to 94 days with revascularization compared with 238 days without revascularization. Approximately 90% of major amputations occurred in stage 4 limbs, with 10% occurring in stage 3 limbs.[39]

Similarly, Cull et al.[40] found that WIfI was associated with 1-year major amputation rates as well as wound healing. The wound healing, limb salvage, and amputation-free survival rates were 93%, 97%, and 96%, respectively, for WIfI stage 1 limbs. Among stage 4 patients, these rates dropped to 38%, 63%, and 38%, respectively. Causey et al.[41] found that WIfI was predictive of mostly limb outcomes. Other risk scores, such as the PREVENT-III risk score, have helped to predict patient-level outcomes, such as mortality, better than WIfI. Ultimately, to predict all outcomes, a combination of WIfI with other scoring systems may be necessary, as WIfI was designed to predict limb outcome only.

A recent series of over 900 patients undergoing revascularization by Darling et al.[46] suggests not only that the originally proposed WIfI clinical stages correlate with amputation risk and wound healing time but also that WIfI mean and composite scores predict additional important clinical end points. Thus, although the WIfI scoring system may evolve, it seems to contain the key element needed to predict limb outcome and amputation risk.

PATTERNS OF CARE FOR DIABETIC VASCULAR DISEASE

The current standard of care for DFUs is often fragmented, resulting in disjointed evaluations and recommendations with irregular communication between multiple providers. This care model results in heterogeneous, sometimes conflicting therapy, variable surveillance of the wounds, and poor patient adherence to treatment recommendations. Moreover, standard wound care regimens frequently rely on nurses, general practitioners, or the patients themselves, without a wound specialist evaluating and managing the care of the wound and associated medical conditions. Finally, the etiology of DFUs is diverse, with each patient and ulcer requiring the expertise of many specialties and caregivers to optimize care.[50]

In contrast, multidisciplinary care teams provide centralized care pathways with improved access to multiple care providers and communication among different specialists. Many publications have touted the benefits of multidisciplinary care for amputation-free survival, limb salvage, and wound healing in the setting of diabetic vascular disease.[51-54] The specialties required to optimize care on a multidisciplinary team are currently unclear; it will require long-term outcomes and cost-analyses to quantify the incremental benefit of each member of the multidisciplinary team. It appears that a vascular surgeon and podiatrist form the most critical components of a multidisciplinary team, as advocated by the "Toe and Flow" model.[51,55] However, each team will need to recruit the talents of many practitioners so that the optimal limb salvage team can be developed at each institution.

TRENDS IN COST OF CARE OF DIABETIC FOOT ULCERATIONS

Cost of care of DFUs has increased significantly over the last decade. Overall, the United States annually spends approximately $245 billion for diabetic care, most of which relates to the care of the diabetic foot.[56] Estimates of the cost of DFU care vary depending on the registry utilized. In the US Medicare registry, $9 to $13 billion of incremental costs are added for the care of patients with DFUs as compared with the cost of caring for patients with uncomplicated diabetes.[57]

Hicks et al.[58] analyzed the National Inpatient Sample and found that there has been a 10-fold increase in the costs associated with the care of DFUs from 2005 to 2010, reaching more than $790 million in 2010. Statistically significant increases in the median cost per patient for endovascular and open revascularizations, antibiotic use, angiography, x-ray, and minor and major amputation were seen over the study period. After risk adjustment, however, statistically significant factors associated with increasing costs over time were an increase in patient comorbidities and open and endovascular revascularization.[58] Cost-effectiveness research is sparse in the literature regarding diabetic care, so the marginal benefit added by the increased cost of care is unclear. Moreover, the indirect costs associated with the diabetic foot have not been well evaluated. Reduced productivity due to time lost from work by the patients and/or their caregivers appears to account for nearly $70 billion in excess costs associated with DFU care.[56] The cost of wound care is escalating, although the specific contribution of DFU to the total cost is unclear.

CONCLUSIONS

The diabetes epidemic has profoundly changed the phenotype and patterns of presentation of limb-threatening ischemia over the past 35 years, with detrimental population-level effects upon major amputation and mortality rates. DM accelerates atherosclerosis as well as causing calcification of the medium-sized vessels, mostly in the infrapopliteal vasculature. Sensory neuropathy aggravates pressure ulceration, and shear forces on the foot result in characteristic ulcerations. Antibiotics are an essential adjunct to the care of diabetic vascular disease, especially in the setting of DFI and osteomyelitis. The precise role of antimicrobial therapy is unclear, as the distinction between normal flora, colonization, microbiomes, infection, and osteomyelitis remains too imprecise to guide therapy. Health-related quality of life is poor in diabetic vascular disease, and DFU can predict those who have poor outcomes after attempts at limb preservation. The most comprehensive and well-validated classification scheme for limb threat associated with diabetic vascular disease is the SVS WIfI classification system, with most patients presenting as WIfI class 2 or 3 wounds. The WIfI classification system has improved the ability to predict wound healing, as it accounts for the effects of infection as well as pedal wounds. Although it appears that outcomes improve with multidisciplinary care teams centered on vascular surgery and podiatry, further outcomes research will be required to determine the optimal specialties in a multidisciplinary team designed to care for these complex patients.

References available online at ExpertConsult.com.

13 CHAPTER

Medical Management of Vascular Disease—Including Pharmacology of Drugs Used in Vascular Disease Management

John T. Baber, Jr., Jessica Beth O'Connell

INTRODUCTION

Arterial disease is the leading cause of death and significant morbidity in the United States and throughout the world. The American Heart Association estimates that 85.6 million (26.4%) Americans have cardiovascular disease, leading to 787,000 deaths annually. Patients with peripheral arterial disease (PAD) make up a significant proportion of this group, including 795,000 Americans who will have strokes each year. Stroke itself is the third leading cause of death in the Unites States, with an estimated 129,000 patients dying each year. Those who do survive often have significant neurologic deficits, which can become major social and economic burdens to the patients and their families.

PAD is a significant public health issue due to the need for extensive long-term care for patients with these serious disabilities, but also given that much of atherosclerosis and therefore PAD is preventable or diminishable by avoiding tobacco, fatty foods, and taking medications regularly to control hypertension, diabetes, and hyperlipidemia. It is estimated that for 2015, the total direct and indirect cost of cardiovascular diseases and stroke in the United States was $320.1 billion.[1]

In this chapter we will discuss the risk factors for development of atherosclerosis, discuss the clinical relevance of the disease, discuss preventative modalities and evolving medical treatments, and review the pharmacologic agents used in vascular disease management.

ATHEROSCLEROSIS—BASIC PRINCIPLES AND MEDICAL MANAGEMENT

Risk Factors for Atherosclerotic Disease and Modification Strategies

Cardiovascular disease is increasingly recognized as the largest growing burden of disease for health care systems.[2] Although current treatment regimens and surgical outcomes for atherosclerotic disease have improved morbidity and mortality, the current emphasis has been focused on effective clinical guidelines for prevention and modification at an earlier stage in the disease process. Box 13.1 lists the most common risk factors for atherosclerotic cardiovascular disease.

Smoking

Smoking is the greatest contributor to atherosclerotic cardiovascular disease and the number one cause of preventable deaths in the United States per annum.[3] Smoke-related deaths continue to rise, particularly in the developing world.

A dose-related phenomenon has been described for cigarette-smoking that correlates with increased rates of coronary events, ischemic strokes, and peripheral vascular disorders.[4] Despite this dose effect, complete smoking cessation has been demonstrated to be the only significantly effective approach to reducing health risks associated with smoking. As much as a third of cardiovascular mortality can be prevented by abstinence from smoking, an effect that has not yet been realized by pharmaceutical risk-factor management.[5]

Effective holistic treatment plans exist for patients who are motivated to cease smoking, such as nicotine replacement by transdermal patch or chewable gum, behavioral modification, and antidepressant or medical therapy.[6]

Diabetes Mellitus

Diabetes mellitus (DM) rivals smoking in contribution to cardiovascular mortality, as evidenced by the fact that coronary artery disease (CAD) is the principal cause of death in diabetic patients.[7] The rate of coronary and PAD approximately doubles in patients who carry a diagnosis of diabetes.[8] The length of time and severity of diabetic control are strong predictors of atherosclerotic events and have been correlated with the degree of PAD experienced by patients. The microvascular complications of diabetes are beyond the scope of this chapter, but diabetic nephropathy, heralded by microalbuminuria, exacerbates large vessel changes imposed by insulin resistance and hyperglycemia.[9] Atherosclerosis can be shown experimentally to be induced by insulin resistance preceding the development of a clinical diagnosis of diabetes, and has been diagnosed in adolescents and teenagers as part of the metabolic syndrome.

Significant improvements in the glycemic profile and reduction in diabetic complications with prolongation of life expectancy can be achieved through behavioral modification of diabetes. Level 1 data from large randomized national trials of monitored lifestyle modification demonstrate up to 30% reduction in frank

BOX 13.1 Risk Factors for Atherosclerotic Cardiovascular Disease

Well-established	Smoking Diabetes mellitus Hypertension Dyslipidemia Physical inactivity Advanced age Family history of early cardiovascular disease
Emerging	High-sensitivity C-reactive peptide Lipoprotein (a) Fibrinogen and fibrin-degradation products Homocysteine

BOX 13.2 Current Target Guidelines for Diabetic Patients

Fasting blood glucose <110 mg/dL
Hemoglobin A1c <7%
Blood pressure <130/80 (combination HCTZ/ACEI as first-line therapy)
LDL <100 mg/dL (<70 mg/dL considered if established coronary artery disease)
Triglyceride level <150 mg/dL

ACEI, Angiotensin-converting enzyme inhibitor; *HCTZ*, hydrochlorothiazide; *LDL*, low-density lipoprotein.

diabetes with associated reduction in cardiovascular events. The addition of effective glycemic agents such as metformin, sulfonylureas, and thiazolidinediones further contributes to cardiovascular risk reduction. Current glucose targets for diabetic patients are listed in Box 13.2. A causal relationship has been described for long-term blood glucose control, as assessed by the hemoglobin AIc (HbA1c) in the national United Kingdom Prospective Diabetes Study (UKPDS), with an increase in the risk of adverse cardiovascular events for each percentage point above an HbA1c level of 6.2%. The UKPDS recommendations for metabolic control of diabetic patients also focus on other parameters that are known to interact deleteriously with diabetes to increase cardiovascular risk such as hypertension and hyperlipidemia.[10] Physicians now recognize the need for aggressive management of patients with the constellation of diabetes, hypertriglyceridemia, hypertension, and obesity, some of which will fit the definition of the metabolic syndrome.

Hypertension

The prevalence of hypertension in the United States is estimated at one in three individuals. Part of the difficulty in managing hypertension is the racial disparity in prevalence, response to antihypertensive medications, and associated exacerbating factors such as renal disease and diabetes. High-risk groups include African Americans, those older than 60 years of age, and women.[11] A dose phenomenon has been described for hypertension. In general an elevation in blood pressure of 20 mm Hg systolic from a theorized normal of 120 mm Hg systolic confers a cardiovascular risk double that of the normotensive population. A working definition of hypertension is a systolic blood pressure (SBP) greater than 140 mm Hg or a diastolic pressure greater than 90 mm Hg. Prehypertension can be defined further as blood pressure ranging between 120 and 139 mm Hg systolic and 80 to 89 mm Hg diastolic.[12] Almost two-thirds of patients with hypertension have at least one other risk factor for cardiovascular disease, and thus treatment of hypertension should be ideally managed by using therapies that are multivariate in effect—for example, dietary modification or pharmacological agents with benefits for both triglyceride and blood pressure profile.

The 2014 Joint National Committee on Prevention, Detection, Evaluation, and Treatment of High Blood Pressure (JNC-8) panel published guidelines that summarize management goals for the treatment of hypertension.[12] Those recommendations include initiating antihypertensive therapy in patients younger than 60 years of age with SBP greater than 140 mm Hg or diastolic blood pressure (DBP) greater than 90 mm Hg. In patients older than 60, antihypertensive treatment should be initiated for an SBP greater than 150 mm Hg or a DBP greater than 90 mm Hg. All adult patients with DM or chronic kidney disease should have antihypertensive therapy initiated for SBP greater than 140 mm Hg or DBP greater than 90 mm Hg. For the general population, initial therapy should include a thiazide diuretic, calcium channel blocker (CCB), angiotensin-converting enzyme inhibitor (ACEI), or angiotensin receptor blocker (ARB). Initial therapy for black patients without chronic kidney disease (CKD) should be limited to thiazide diuretics or CCBs, while all patients with CKD should use an ACEI or ARB as an initial therapy for hypertension. With regard to lifestyle modifications for the management of hypertension, the JNC-8 does not make specific recommendations, but supports the recommendations of the 2013 Lifestyle Work Group. These recommendations include following the DASH eating plan (Dietary Approaches to Stop Hypertension), consisting of a diet rich in fruits, vegetables, and low-fat dairy products, and limiting intake of sodium, saturated fat, and trans-fat. In addition, they recommend and regular aerobic activity for at least 40 minutes most days of the week.[13]

Dyslipidemia

Low-density lipoprotein (LDL) is firmly established in cardiovascular risk profiling as the major contributor to atherosclerotic disease and is found in abundance in atherosclerotic plaque. Higher serum levels of LDL correlate with a higher risk of cardiovascular disease; data borne out of clinical studies indicate LDL as the main risk factor for coronary disease.[14] The Post-Coronary Artery Bypass Graft (Post-CABG) trial examined this relationship further and attempted to define a threshold target level for LDL.[15] From this work, guidelines were drawn up supporting intensive LDL treatment to a level lower than 100 mg/dL to influence a favorable change in atherosclerotic plaque morphology (see Box 13.2).

Although LDL has been identified as a target for cardiovascular risk reduction, other lipid and lipoprotein abnormalities have been recognized in contributing to the overall risk of atherosclerotic disease. Elevated levels of very-low-density lipoprotein (VLDL), apolipoprotein B, and decreased high-density lipoprotein (HDL) are adverse markers for cardiovascular risk.[16] Clinical evidence for the involvement of these lipoproteins is found in the acceleration of atherosclerotic buildup, seen in patients suffering from inherited forms of dyslipidemia such as familial hypercholesterolemia.

First-line therapies for reducing cholesterol, LDL, VLDL, and increasing HDL involve behavioral modification in the form of dietary changes.[17] Simply reducing body weight toward goal body mass index will produce significant reductions in LDL levels and reduce the overall cardiovascular risk profile.

The main pharmacological modality employed to impair cholesterol metabolism is the hydroxymethylglutarate coenzyme A reductase inhibitors (HMG-CoA reductase inhibitors or "statin" medications). The mechanism of statin action occurs at the hepatocellular level to inhibit cholesterol synthesis in the liver. Statins are powerfully effective in reducing total body LDL levels (from 30% to 60%, depending on dosage). Not surprisingly, these medications have become first-line drug therapy for patients with elevated lipid profiles in the absence of drug contraindications. Myopathy, heralded by a rise in creatine kinase, and transient elevation of hepatic aminotransferases are the most commonly quoted side effects of statin use. These derangements usually resolve with discontinuation of the medication.[17]

Statins, along with four other medications used in the treatment of dyslipidemias (ezetimibe, niacin, fibric acid derivatives, and bile acid sequestrants), will be discussed as follows.

Metabolic Syndrome

Over the past half-century a constellation of metabolic derangements have been seen more frequently occurring in association. Hypertension, DM, obesity, and dyslipidemia are the four entities most commonly described as part of the metabolic syndrome or colloquially known as syndrome X.[18] According to the definition drawn up by the 2001 Adult Treatment Panel III of the National Cholesterol Education Program (NCEP), metabolic syndrome is diagnosed when three of the following criteria are present[17]:

1. Central obesity—waist circumference >102 cm (M), >88 cm (F)
2. Fasting plasma glucose >6.1 mmol/L
3. Hypertension ≥135/85 mm Hg, or the presence of antihypertensive medications
4. Dyslipidemia, including triglycerides ≥1.7 mmol/L, HDL cholesterol <1.0 mmol/L (M), <1.3 mmol/L (F)

For many of the reasons highlighted earlier in the chapter, the metabolic syndrome is strongly associated with the development of cardiovascular disease, portending an approximately 2.5 times risk of fatal cardiovascular events in the population. The single most effective treatment for the metabolic syndrome is the loss of body weight either by nonsurgical or surgical means, which in almost all cases of dramatic weight loss leads to amelioration of all individual components.[19]

Emerging Novel Risk Factors

Although the previously provided well-established risk factors have been strongly linked to the development of cardiovascular disease, there remains a significant proportion of the atherosclerotic population that does not possess these described risk factors. Searches for other contributing factors have focused on molecular biomarkers as diverse as homocysteine levels, high-sensitivity C-reactive protein (hs-CRP), fibrin-degradation products (FDP), and microalbuminuria.

Elevated plasma homocysteine levels have been cited as a defined risk factor for the development of atherosclerotic coronary arterial disease in epidemiological as well as clinical research studies.[20] On a molecular basis, high levels of homocysteine have been demonstrated to occur with disruption of normal methionine metabolism. Homocysteine and related metabolites can be detected in abnormally high levels in the blood and have been linked to an increased risk of stroke, due to carotid plaque buildup, as well as cardiovascular disease.[21] Therapeutic options for individuals diagnosed with homocysteinemia have centered on the replacement of vitamin B12 and folic acid as a primary treatment, with additional restriction of dietary intake of methionine in vitamin B12-insensitive patients. However, studies have not, as of yet, shown that lowering homocysteine levels decreases the risk of cardiovascular disease in these patients.[22]

The elevation of inflammatory markers such as hs-CRP and FDP is considered to be associated with cardiovascular disease.[23] Although originally thought to play a role as potential serum biomarkers of cardiovascular disease, hs-CRP and FDP have only been weakly associated with risk stratification and burden of atherosclerotic disease.

hs-CRP has recently been the subject of much attention with the results of the JUPITER trial—a large multinational, double-blind placebo-controlled trial of more than 17,000 people.[24] The trial was designed to observe the effect that treatment with a statin (rosuvastatin) had on individuals with normal lipid profiles but elevated hs-CRP levels. The study arose from the observation that statins have an antiinflammatory property and decrease hs-CRP levels in an effect that is independent from their cholesterol-lowering ability. The JUPITER trial demonstrated a reduction in both LDL and hs-CRP levels to around half of pretreatment and was terminated prematurely on the basis of this beneficial result. However, the benefit of a normal hs-CRP has not yet been firmly established as a treatment goal in cardiovascular risk profiling and is additionally confounded by the possible benefit of statin therapy in the face of normal lipid profile in certain populations. These findings have, however, motivated further investigation into the association between inflammation and cardiovascular disease in the form of two large placebo-controlled trials: the Canakinumab Anti-Inflammatory Thrombosis Outcomes Study (CANTOS) and the Cardiovascular Inflammation Reduction Trial (CIRT).[25]

Microalbuminuria is a sensitive predictor of mortality and highly associated with cardiovascular adverse events in specific. Diabetic and hypertensive nephropathy can be diagnosed reliably by evidence of proteinuria, which is also associated with an increase in cardiovascular risk profile. Microalbuminuria is similarly associated with an elevated risk of coronary disease, independent of proteinuria, and thus may have clinical utility in patients who do not carry a diagnosis of hypertension or diabetes as a screening tool for atherosclerotic disease.[26] Treatment strategies based on the detection of microalbuminuria are therefore likely to take the form of existing risk-reduction strategies for well-established cardiovascular risk factors.

Surveillance and Secondary Prevention

Given the focus on prevention of atherosclerotic disease, increased surveillance for the development of signs of atherosclerotic disease in those with established risk factors should be included in the routine health care maintenance and follow-up of patients. Regular carotid duplex evaluation for older patients with one or more risk factors for atherosclerosis in addition to at least annual physical examinations is a relatively inexpensive and highly effective screening tool for carotid disease. Similarly, screening aortic ultrasonography, physical examination, and ankle-brachial pressure indices should be considered for at-risk patients in the primary care setting.

For those patients who progress to severe or acute cardiovascular disease, secondary prevention guidelines are well documented and rigorously studied. Many cardiovascular centers have established protocols for treating patients with established disease. One such example is the University of California, Los Angeles CHAMP (Cardiac Hospitalization Atherosclerosis Management Program), which focuses on employing secondary prevention measures while patients are in the hospital in order to improve clinical outcomes.[27] The CHAMP guidelines are summarized as follows:

1. Aspirin 81 to 162 mg daily should be initiated. In the presence of contraindications to aspirin, other platelet agents should be considered—for example, clopidogrel. Combination therapy can be recommended in the setting of acute coronary syndromes (ACS) or post-revascularization therapy.
2. Statin therapy should be initiated in all patients in the absence of contraindications and in all diabetic patients regardless of their lipid profile. Target levels of LDL should be less than 70 mg/dL, HDL greater than 40 mg/dL, and triglycerides less than 150 mg/dL.
3. ACEI or ARB should be commenced in the absence of contraindication, irrespective of the blood pressure or cardiac ejection fraction.
4. Beta blockade should be prescribed for all patients in the absence of contraindication.
5. Fish oil or omega-3 fatty acids should be commenced with dietary instruction for all patients.
6. Aerobic exercise programs that involve 30 to 60 minutes of moderately intense exercise at least five times a week should be prescribed.
7. Smoking cessation should be pursued including access to formal smoking cessation programs.
8. Before hospital discharge and at 6 weeks follow-up, cardiovascular lipid profile and liver enzymes should be checked and routinely thereafter at future follow-up appointments.

PHARMACOLOGY OF DRUGS USED IN THE MANAGEMENT OF VASCULAR DISEASE (Table 13.1)

Anticoagulants

Heparin

Structure and mechanism of action. Heparin is an anticoagulant composed of a heterogeneous group of straight-chain glycosaminoglycans with molecular weights ranging from 5 to 30 kD (mean, 15 kD).[28] It is strongly acidic secondary to its high content of sulfate and carboxyl groups. Heparin is a naturally occurring substance excreted by mast cells and basophils in the process of clot formation. Standard, unfractionated heparin is derived commercially from porcine gut mucosa or bovine lung tissue. Heparin acts at multiple points within the coagulation system. Its major anticoagulant effect is via interaction with antithrombin III, leading to the inactivation of factor Xa and subsequent inhibition of the conversion of prothrombin to thrombin.[29,30] Heparin further inhibits coagulation by inactivating thrombin, preventing the conversion of fibrinogen to fibrin.[31] Heparin also prevents stable fibrin clot formation through the inhibition of fibrin stabilization factor. Heparin has no fibrinolytic activity and therefore does not lyse existing clots.

Heparin's onset of action is immediate with intravenous injection. It can also be administered subcutaneously. The response to heparin is monitored by measuring the activated partial thromboplastin time (aPTT) and activated clotting time (ACT). An aPTT 1.5 to 2.5 times normal has been shown to prevent recurrent thromboembolism.[32] Weight-adjusted nomograms have been shown to be useful in dosing.[33]

The anticoagulant activity of heparin varies greatly among patients. The heterogeneous clinical response is primarily due to the nonspecific binding of heparin to variable concentrations of plasma and cellular proteins, limiting heparin's bioavailability. This leads to marked variability of the anticoagulant response.[29] There also appear to be natural inhibitors of heparin that can be released by sites of active thrombus.[34] Further, the biophysical limitations of the large heparin–antithrombin III complex can block receptors on thrombin to heparin cofactor 2, limiting heparin's effectiveness.[34]

Clinical use. Heparin is indicated for intraoperative anticoagulation in vascular and cardiac surgery, for the prophylaxis and treatment of deep venous thrombosis, for the prevention of pulmonary embolism in surgical patients, and in patients with atrial fibrillation and embolization.[29]

Adverse reactions. Heparin therapy is associated with increased risk of bleeding. It also can cause skin lesions, including papules, plaques, and necrosis.[35] Heparin therapy can lead to hypoaldosteronism,[36] priapism,[37] and osteoporosis.[38] Thrombocytopenia is a known complication of heparin administration. Heparin-induced thrombocytopenia (HIT) can lead to thromboembolic complications, including skin necrosis, extremity gangrene, myocardial infarction, pulmonary embolism, and stroke.[29]

Heparin-induced thrombocytopenia. Two major forms of HIT are recognized. Type I HIT is an early-onset, benign, reversible thrombocytopenia with no associated platelet antibodies. It is non-immune mediated and is usually self-limited without complications.[39] Type II HIT is a more serious immune-modulated thrombocytopenia.[40] It is caused by platelet IgG antibodies that target platelet factor 4, a heparin binding protein, leading to platelet activation.[41,42] The activation of platelets and endothelium and neutralization of heparin all contribute to a highly thrombogenic state.[29] Patients with type II HIT have a high risk of developing thrombotic complications.[29] Fortunately, most patients

TABLE 13.1 Vascular Pharmacology

Medication	Examples/Brand Names	Mechanism of Action	Metabolism	Half-Life	Side Effects	Dosage
Anticoagulants						
Unfractionated heparin	Heparin	• Interacts with antithrombin III which inactivates factor Xa and subsequent conversion of prothrombin to thrombin • Inactivates thrombin preventing conversion of fibrinogen to fibrin • Inhibits fibrin stabilization factor • Varied response due to binding of plasma and cellular proteins	Liver	1.5 h	Bleeding Thrombocytopenia (Type I and II HIT) Skin lesions Hypoaldosteronism Priapism Osteoporosis	VTE prophylaxis 5000 units SQ q 8–12 h VTE treatment: Bolus 80 units/kg IV once, then 18 units/kg per hour and adjust dose to aPTT based on nomogram
Low-molecular-weight heparin	Enoxaparin (Lovenox)	• Inactivate factor Xa by binding to antithrombin III • Reduced ability to inactivate thrombin due to molecular size compared with unfractionated heparin • Decreased nonspecific protein binding • Decreased platelet binding (reduces risk of HIT)	Liver	4.5–7 h	Bleeding Ecchymosis Thrombocytopenia Decreased risk of HIT compared with standard heparin	VTE prophylaxis: 30–40 mg SC q 12 h VTE/PE treatment: 1 mg/kg SC q 12 h Adjust dose for renal impairment
Warfarin	Coumadin	• Inhibits vitamin K dependent clotting factors (II, VII, IX, X) and the anticoagulant protein C and protein S • Response is variable based on genetic factors, drug interactions, various disease states, and diet	Liver	20–60 h	Bleeding Skin necrosis or gangrene Purple toe syndrome	Start 2–5 mg PO daily × 2–4 days, adjust dose based on INR Overlap treatment 4–5 days when transitioning from heparin
Direct thrombin inhibitors	Lepirudin (Refludan)	• Inhibits thrombin directly to prevent conversion of fibrinogen to fibrin	Renal	1.3 h	Hemorrhage Epidural/spinal hematoma Anemia	0.15 mg/kg per hour IV, monitor aPTT
	Desirudin (Iprivask)		Renal	3 h		15 mg SQ q 12 h
	Bivalirudin (Angiomax)		Plasma	25 min		0.2–0.3 mg/kg per hour IV, monitor ACT
	Argatroban		Liver	39–51 min		2 mcg/kg per minute IV, monitor aPTT
	Dabigatran (Pradaxa)		Liver	12–17 h		150 mg PO BID, no routine monitoring Adjust dose for renal impairment
Factor Xa inhibitors	Fondaparinux (Arixtra)	• Bind to antithrombin III, resulting in inactivation of factor Xa, but does not mediate the inactivation of thrombin by antithrombin III	Renal	17–21 h	Hemorrhage Anemia Thrombocytopenia	VTE Prophylaxis: 2.5 mg SC QD DVT/PE Tx: 7.5 mg SC QD
	Rivaroxaban (Xarelto)		Liver	7–11 h		VTE Prophylaxis: 10 mg PO QD
	Apixaban (Eliquis)		Liver	17–21 h		Thromboembolism/stroke prophylaxis: 5 mg PO BID DVT prophylaxis: 2.5 mg PO BID Treatment of DVT: 5 mg PO BID
	Edoxaban (Savaysa)		Renal	10–14 h		Thromboembolism/stroke prophylaxis: 60 mg PO QD Treatment of DVT/PE: 30 mg/60 mg PO qday
Antiplatelet Agents						
Aspirin	Bayer Aspirin, Ecotrin	• Blocks prostaglandin metabolism and synthesis of thromboxane A2, a potent platelet aggregator • The effect on the platelet is permanent, with the platelet life span approximately 10 days	Gut and plasma (ASA), liver (Salicylate)	20 min	Bleeding GI irritation Angioedema Bronchospasm Pancytopenia	75–325 mg PO QD 75–150 mg of aspirin appears to be as effective as higher doses with fewer side effects

Thienopyridines	Clopidogrel (Plavix)	• Inhibit P2Y receptor, an adenosine diphosphate receptor, which results in platelet aggregation	Liver	8 h	Bleeding Diarrhea Skin rash	75 mg PO QD
	Ticlopidine (Ticlid)		Liver	7.9–12.6 h	Neutropenia	250 PO BID
	Prasugrel (Effient)	• Prasugrel is a prodrug that must undergo hydrolysis to be converted to active metabolite	Liver	7 h	Clopidogrel has fewer side effects than ticlopidine	5–10 mg PO QD
Glycoprotein IIb/IIIa inhibitors	Abciximab (Reopro)	• Binds to IIb/IIIa receptors, inhibiting aggregation of platelets	Unknown	10–30 min	Thrombocytopenia Bleeding	0.125–10 μg/kg per minute IV
	Eptifibatide (Integrilin)			2.5 h		1–2 μg/kg per minute IV
	Tirofiban (Aggrastat)			2.0 h		0.1 μg/kg per minute IV
ADP analogs	Ticagrelor (Brillanta)	• Reversibly binds to platelet P2Y12 ADP receptors, reducing platelet activation and aggregation	Liver	9 h	Bleeding Atrial fibrillation Hypersensitivity reaction Hypotension Elevated creatinine	Acute coronary syndrome (ACS): 90 mg PO BID Cardiovascular event prevention: 60 mg PO BID
PAR-1 inhibitors	Vorapaxar (Zontivity)	• Antagonizes platelet protease activated receptor-1 (PAR-1), inhibiting platelet aggregation	Liver	8 days	Bleeding	Thrombotic event prevention: 2.08 mg PO QD for CAD or PAD patients given with ASA and/or clopidogrel
Medical Treatment of Claudication						
Pentoxifylline	Trental	• Lowers blood viscosity, decreasing platelet adhesiveness, and improves erythrocyte flexibility, which increases flow in the microcirculation	Liver	0.4–16 h	Arrhythmias Dyspepsia N/V	Conflicting data regarding benefits and is not currently recommended. 400 mg PO TID Cr Cl 10–50, dose QD to BID Cr Cl <10, give once daily
Cilostazol	Pletal	• Type III phosphodiesterase inhibitor that inhibits platelet aggregation and promotes vasodilation	Liver	11–13 h	Contraindicated with CHF Bleeding Anemia Thrombocytopenia Agranulocytosis	100 mg BID PO 50 mg BID if on CYP3A4 inhibitors
Reversal of Anticoagulation						
Heparin reversal	Protamine Sulfate	• Ionically binds and inactivates heparin molecules	• Liver	• Unknown	• Anaphylaxis • Bradycardia • Circulatory collapse • Pulmonary hypertension	• 1–1.5 mg IV per 100 units of circulating heparin
• Dabigatran reversal	• Idarucizumab (Praxbind)	• Monoclonal antibody fragment which binds the active site of dabigatran	Renal	10.3 h	Headache Hypersensitivity	5 g IV
Thrombolytics						
Tissue plasminogen activators	Alteplase	• Bind to fibrin and converts tissue plasminogen to plasmin, promoting fibrinolysis	Renal	72 min	Bleeding Intracranial hemorrhage Anaphylaxis	STEMI: 15 mg IV ×1, then 50 mg over 30 min, then 35 mg over 60 min Thrombotic stroke: 0.9 mg/kg IV over 60 min PE: 100 mg IV over 2 h
	Reteplase (Retavase)		Renal	13–16 min		STEMI: 10 units IV ×2 separated by 30 min
	Tenecteplase (TNKase)		Liver	90–130 min		STEMI: weight-based dosing. 30–50 mg IV ×1

BID, Twice daily; *CHF*, congestive heart failure; *PO*, per os (by mouth); *QD*, once daily; *SC*, subcutaneous; *STEMI*, ST-elevation myocardial infarction.

who develop HIT antibodies do not develop thrombocytopenia or thrombosis. Furthermore, almost all patients who develop mild to moderate thrombocytopenia during the first 4 days of heparin treatment do not have antibodies. Type II HIT should be considered a clinicopathologic syndrome with a combination of thrombocytopenia and associated clinical events, including thrombosis and confirmation of platelet antibodies.[29] The management of HIT is aimed at preventing thromboembolic complications. All heparin should be discontinued and an alternative anticoagulant initiated.

Protamine

Structure and mechanism of action. Protamine is made up of a heterogeneous group of low-molecular-weight proteins. These proteins are rich in arginine and are strongly basic. They occur naturally in the sperm of salmon and certain other fish species. The mechanism of action for heparin reversal is through electrostatic bonding. Heparin is highly acidic and forms a strong bond with the highly basic protamine molecules, forming an inactive complex.[43]

Clinical use. Protamine is used clinically as a heparin antidote. When administered alone, protamine has an anticoagulant effect similar to that of heparin. However, in the presence of heparin, it forms a stable salt, and the anticoagulant activity of both is lost. Protamine has a rapid onset of action; within 5 minutes of administration, it begins to neutralize heparin.

Adverse reactions. Too rapid administration can have serious side effects, including hypotension and anaphylaxis.[44] Decreased blood pressure, pulmonary hypertension, shortness of breath, flushing, and urticaria have all been associated with rapid administration.[45] Protamine should be administered slowly over 10 minutes, with a goal of 1 mg of protamine to neutralize every 90 units of heparin. Further dosing should be guided by coagulation studies.[43] Severe allergies have been well documented, causing transient systemic hypotension, anaphylaxis, and severe pulmonary vasoconstriction. Patients with risk factors for a protamine reaction include those with fish allergies, vasectomy, and prior protamine exposure, including protamine insulin-dependent diabetics.[46,47]

Low-Molecular-Weight Heparins

Structure and mechanism of action. Low-molecular-weight heparins (LMWHs) are collections of heparin molecules that have significantly lower molecular weights than standard, unfractionated heparin.[48] LMWHs are derived from unfractionated heparin via chemical or enzymatic depolymerization. This produces fragments one-third the size of heparin, with mean molecular weights of 4 to 5 kD (range, 1 to 10 kD). Similar to unfractionated heparin, LMWHs are heterogeneous in terms of both molecular size and anticoagulant activity.[49] The LMWHs have distinct differences from standard heparin. LMWHs have reduced ability to catalyze the inactivation of thrombin, because the smaller fragments cannot bind to thrombin. However, LMWHs retain the ability to inactivate factor Xa. There is a reduction in nonspecific protein binding and subsequent improved predictability in dose-response relationships.[49] LMWHs have an increased half-life compared with standard heparin. This is thought to be secondary to reduced macrophage binding. Similarly, there is reduced binding to platelets and a decrease in the incidence of HIT.[49] LMWHs also have been associated with a reduction in bone loss compared with standard heparin.

Clinical use. The LMWHs have been examined extensively in the prevention of deep venous thrombosis in patients undergoing major abdominal surgery or knee and hip replacement surgery, and in patients with restricted mobility.[48] LMWHs have also been investigated for the treatment of acute deep venous thrombosis and pulmonary embolism.[48] LMWHs are used in patients with ACS and unstable angina.[50] The advantages of LMWHs over standard heparin are longer plasma half-life and a more predictable anticoagulant response, allowing for simple dosing and decreasing the need for laboratory monitoring.[22] LMWHs are also commonly used to bridge patients to oral warfarin therapy.

Adverse reactions. Adverse reactions to LMWHs are similar to those associated with standard heparin. Bleeding, ecchymosis, and thrombocytopenia can all occur with LMWH administration. The incidence of HIT is decreased compared with standard heparin, but LMWHs can cause HIT, and patients should be monitored for this complication.[51]

Warfarin

Structure and mechanism of action. Warfarin is a coumarin derivative that produces an anticoagulant effect through the inhibition of vitamin K–dependent coagulation factors (II, VII, IX, X) and the anticoagulant proteins C and S. Warfarin interferes with the conversion of vitamin K into a 2,3-epoxide.[52] Vitamin K is an essential cofactor for post-ribosomal synthesis of clotting factors, acting through the carboxylation of glutamine residues in the protein.[53] Carboxylation promotes binding of vitamin K–dependent coagulation factors to phospholipid surfaces.[52] Coumarins specifically block vitamin K epoxide reductase, preventing the carboxylation of the factors rendering them inactive.[54] The vitamin K antagonists (VKAs) also inhibit carboxylation of the regulatory anticoagulant proteins C and S.[54]

Warfarin is a racemic mixture of two optically active isomers.[52] Absorption from the gastrointestinal tract is rapid, reaching maximal plasma levels within 90 minutes. Warfarin has a half-life of 36 to 42 hours. Response is variable owing to certain genetic factors, drug interactions, various disease states, and diet. The anticoagulant effect can be overcome by low doses of vitamin K_1, as vitamin K_1 bypasses vitamin K epoxide reductase.[52] Warfarin anticoagulation is monitored via measurement of the prothrombin time (PT). The PT reflects the depression of the vitamin K–dependent factors. PT measurement is laboratory dependent, and therefore the international normalized ratio (INR), a calibration model for reagent thromboplastins used in measuring the PT, was first proposed by Kirkwood in 1983, and soon thereafter was adopted by the World Health Organization as the international PT standardization scheme.[55] It has subsequently become the standard for monitoring the effect of anticoagulant therapy with warfarin.[56]

Clinical use. Warfarin is indicated for the prophylaxis or treatment of venous thrombosis and thromboembolism. It is also indicated for the prophylaxis or treatment of the thromboembolic complications associated with atrial fibrillation and cardiac valve replacement. Warfarin has been shown to reduce the risk of death, recurrent myocardial infarction, and thromboembolic events such as stroke or systemic embolization after myocardial infarction.[52]

Warfarin has been studied in terms of its usefulness in promoting the patency of infrainguinal bypass grafts.[57–60] Although some studies suggest improved patency of infrainguinal bypass grafts with warfarin or a combination of warfarin and aspirin, the American College of Chest Physicians 8th Edition Guidelines for Antithrombotic Therapy for Peripheral Artery Occlusive Disease recommends against long-term anticoagulation in general for extremity reconstructions. The guidelines recommend VKAs not to be routinely used for infrainguinal vein bypass, except in those patients at high risk of bypass occlusion and limb loss where VKAs plus aspirin is recommended. For infrainguinal prosthetic bypass, VKAs are not recommended to be used routinely.[61] These conclusions are based on small improvements in patency in the face of relatively high rates of bleeding complications.

Adverse reactions. Warfarin therapy is associated with an increased risk of hemorrhagic complications. It also can cause necrosis and gangrene of skin or other tissues. It should be used with caution in patients with HIT because it can lead to increased thrombotic complications early in the treatment of HIT.[61]

Direct Thrombin Inhibitors

The direct thrombin inhibitors are small molecules that act directly at the active site of thrombin, without the use of an intermediate such as antithrombin III with heparin. There are five direct thrombin inhibitors currently available for clinical use: lepirudin, desirudin, bivalirudin, argatroban, and dabigatran.

Thrombin is the central enzyme in hemostasis. It is a serine protease that catalyzes the conversion of fibrinogen to fibrin. In addition, thrombin serves many other roles, including the activation of various coagulation factors, platelets, smooth muscle cells, fibroblasts, and endothelium.[62] Thrombin is chemotactic, stimulates secretion of vasoactive proteins from platelets and inflammatory cells, and plays a role in angiogenesis and restenosis.[62]

Antithrombin III, the major regulator of thrombin, forms an irreversible complex with thrombin to block its active site.[49] For years, this has been the main target for thrombin inhibition and anticoagulation via heparin. However, the use of heparin is limited by several major factors: (1) the development of HIT; (2) heparin's inability to penetrate clot, leading to the release of active thrombin from clots; and (3) the variable anticoagulant response, owing to heparin's propensity to bind to plasma proteins.[63] The rationale for the development of direct thrombin inhibitors was to create a small molecule with site-specific thrombin inhibition.[63] With an increased understanding of the detailed molecular structure of thrombin, site-specific agents have been developed with a high specificity for thrombin.[64]

Clinical use. Direct thrombin inhibitors have been studied in the treatment of HIT with thrombosis; the treatment of acute coronary events; and the prevention and treatment of deep venous thrombosis, pulmonary embolism, and stroke.[62,64]

Hirudin. Hirudin, the first direct thrombin inhibitor, was originally isolated from the salivary gland of the medicinal leech (Hirudo medicinalis) after it was noted that leech saliva had anticoagulant properties.[64] It is now produced via recombinant technology as lepirudin and desirudin. It is a 65– to 66–amino acid polypeptide. The amino terminus forms a tight bond with thrombin's active site, and the carboxy terminus binds to the thrombin exosite-1 (fibrinogen binding site).[65] Peak plasma levels are reached after parenteral administration in 20 to 30 minutes. Hirudin is rapidly cleared by the kidneys, having a half-life of 1 to 3 hours. Some hepatic excretion also occurs but is not clinically significant. Hirudin should not be used in patients with renal failure, as no specific antidote exists, should overdosage occur.

Bivalirudin. Bivalirudin is a recombinant protein based on hirudin. It is a 20–amino acid peptide that interacts with the active site of thrombin.[62] It has a short half-life of 25 minutes. In contrast to hirudin, renal excretion is not the major route of excretion.[64]

Argatroban. Argatroban is a synthetic, small-molecule arginine derivative that interacts only with the active site of thrombin.[62,64] It is metabolized by the liver, with a half-life of 45 minutes. Dose reduction may be necessary in patients with liver dysfunction. The anticoagulant effect can be monitored with the aPTT or ACT.

Melagatran/Ximelagatran. Melagatran and Ximelagatran (its prodrug) were the first oral direct thrombin inhibitors. Although initial studies were promising for the use of Ximelagatran, it has since been removed from clinical investigation due to significant hepatotoxicity.

Novel Oral Anticoagulants

The term novel oral anticoagulant (NOAC) has been used to describe a series of medications that have come to market within the last decade that achieve their anticoagulant effect by working at points in the coagulation cascade, other than those targeted by traditional anticoagulants such as warfarin and heparin.[66] The primary benefits of these medications over traditional anticoagulants are their ability to be administered orally and the ability to achieve a consistent degree of anticoagulation with standardized dosing rather than with monitored titration. In addition, the metabolism of these medications is not influenced by dietary intake, such as in the case of warfarin.[66]

These medications also have characteristics that could be considered drawbacks when compared with more traditional anticoagulants. They have relatively short half-lives, and their effect can therefore be interrupted with missed doses.[66] In addition, there are no antidotes to reverse their effects in the case of bleeding or need for emergent surgery or invasive procedure, although prothrombin complex concentrates (PCCs) have been used for this purpose with mixed results.[67,68] The one exception to this rule is dabigatran, which can be counteracted by the recently released idarucizumab.[69] The cost of NOACs is also significantly higher than traditional anticoagulants that are available as generic formulations. As such, these medications are not seen as replacements for traditional anticoagulant medications, but rather alternatives to be considered and used under appropriate circumstances.

Dabigatran

Structure and mechanism of action. Dabigatran etexilate is a synthetic, nonpeptide, direct thrombin inhibitor that inhibits both circulating and clot-bound thrombin and lowers thrombin-stimulated platelet aggregation.[70] It is rapidly absorbed from the gut. Peak concentrations occur approximately 1 hour after oral administration, although when taken with a high-fat meal, they are slowed to approximately 3 hours. The drug is mainly renally excreted and has a half-life of 12 to 17 hours. Renal impairment can increase serum concentrations of dabigatran.[71] The anticoagulation effect is quite stable[72] and monitoring is not required, which makes this drug an appealing alternative to warfarin.

Idarucizumab is a recently approved reversal agent reversal agent for dabigatran to be used in circumstances such as life-threatening bleeding and emergency surgery.[69] Alternatively, PCC can also be administered to reduce dabigatran's efficacy, or the medication can be removed from the bloodstream via hemodialysis.[73] Co-administration of dabigatran with other P-glycoprotein transporter substrates such as Rifampin decreases serum concentrations of dabigatran and may lower its effectiveness. P-glycoprotein inhibitors such as ketoconazole may increase serum concentrations.[39]

Clinical use. Dabigatran has been initially Food and Drug Administration (FDA) approved in the United States for prevention of thromboembolic stroke in patients with nonvalvular atrial fibrillation. The Randomized Evaluation of Long-Term Anticoagulation Therapy (RE-LY) trial studied 18,113 patients with atrial fibrillation considered high risk for stroke and over a median of 2 years of follow-up found a decrease in the rate per year of stroke or systemic embolism with dabigatran compared to warfarin (1.54% vs. 1.71%, $P < .05$).[72] In 2014 dabigatran was approved for treatment of venous thromboembolism (VTE) in patients who have been treated with a parenteral anticoagulant for 5 to 10 days, and to reduce the risk of recurrent VTE in patients who have been previously treated. This approval was based on the results of four global clinical trials: RE-COVER, RE-COVER II, RE-MEDYSM, and RE-SONATE.[74-76] In 2015 dabigatran received FDA approval for prophylaxis against VTE in patients who have undergone hip replacement surgery based on the results of the RE-NOVATE and RE-NOVATE II clinical trials.[77,78]

Adverse reactions. Dyspepsia and gastritis were more common with dabigatran compared with warfarin. In the RE-LY trial, overall major bleeding rates were similar to warfarin, although major gastrointestinal (GI) bleeding was higher with dabigatran.[72] In RE-COVER and RE-COVER II, as well as RE-MEDSYM, use of dabigatran was associated with a lower overall incidence of bleeding events, but an increased incidence of GI bleeding when compared with warfarin.[74-76]

Factor X Inhibitors

Fondaparinux

Fondaparinux is a pentasaccharide that activates antithrombin III in a manner similar to heparin, leading to inactivation of factor X.[79] It differs in one major respect from heparin, in that the pentasaccharide is unable to mediate the inactivation of thrombin by antithrombin III.[79] It is administered subcutaneously and does not require laboratory monitoring. It is renally excreted and is contraindicated in patients with renal failure. Fondaparinux has been evaluated in multiple trials for preventing deep venous thrombosis in patients undergoing major hip fracture and knee replacement surgery.[80-83] It also has been evaluated in the treatment of deep venous thrombosis[84] and ACS.[85]

Rivaroxaban

Structure and mechanism of action. Rivaroxaban is an oral oxazolidinone derivative that binds directly to factor Xa. Rivaroxaban has a high bioavailability of 80% to 100%. Peak serum concentration occurs in 2 to 4 hours, and it has a half-life of 7 to 11 hours. One-third of the active metabolite is renally excreted, and two-thirds is hepatically metabolized by the cytochrome P450 pathway. Strong inhibitors or inducers of the cytochrome P450 pathway can therefore alter serum concentrations. Rivaroxaban can be orally administrated, once or twice daily, without any monitoring or need for dose adjustment. It is contraindication in severe liver insufficiency and not recommended in patients with severe renal impairment.

Clinical use. Rivaroxaban received FDA approval in 2011 for prevention of VTE in hip and knee arthroplasty. A series of phase III trials of rivaroxaban evaluated almost 10,000 patients undergoing elective knee or hip arthroplasty (RECORD 1, 2, and 3 trials).[86-88] In all three trials, rivaroxaban and enoxaparin had comparable safety profiles and low rates of major bleeding. A pooled analysis from RECORD 1, 2, and 3 showed that compared with enoxaparin, rivaroxaban decreases the composite of symptomatic VTE and all-cause mortality after elective total hip or knee arthroplasty, with a small increase in bleeding, no evidence of hepatotoxicity and fewer serious adverse events.[89] Furthermore, rivaroxaban has been shown to have a significantly lower rate of recurrent deep vein thrombosis (DVT) than warfarin-treated patients in the EINSTEIN DVT study.[90] And rivaroxaban has been found to be as effective as warfarin for preventing stroke in patients with atrial fibrillation in the ROCKET-AF study.[91] Throughout all these studies, rivaroxaban has maintained a slightly better safety profile.

Adverse reactions. Adverse reactions with rivaroxaban are related to bleeding, though they may in fact be lower than with other anticoagulants. Epidural and spinal hematomas are associated with the use of rivaroxaban during neuraxial anesthesia or spinal puncture. Hepatotoxicity has not been noted. As with other oral anticoagulants, premature discontinuation of the drug increases the risk of VTE, and therefore bridging therapy with another anticoagulant is recommended unless contraindicated.

Apixaban

Apixaban is an oral Xa inhibitor. It received FDA approval in 2012 for VTE prophylaxis in the setting of nonvalvular atrial fibrillation,[92] followed by approval for prophylaxis against VTE in patients undergoing knee[93,94] and hip[95] arthroplasty and treatment for VTE (AMPLIFY Trial) in 2014.[96] These studies showed apixaban to be equivalent or superior to enoxaparin in prophylaxis against, or treatment of, thromboembolism with a similar safety profile. It is administered as a twice-daily dose of 2.5 mg for prophylaxis against, or 5 mg for treatment of, venous thromboembolism, and 5 mg twice daily for thromboembolic prophylaxis in patients with nonvalvular atrial fibrillation.

Adverse reactions. Apixaban has been associated with an increased risk of bleeding. It has also been known to cause elevation in serum liver enzymes (aspartate aminotransferase [AST], alanine aminotransferase [ALT]), syncope, skin rash, and other hypersensitivity reactions, including anaphylactic reactions such as allergic edema.

Edoxaban

Edoxaban is an oral Xa inhibitor. It received FDA approval for use as prophylaxis against embolic events in patients with nonvalvular atrial fibrillation in 2015.[97] It has been approved for VTE prophylaxis in knee[98] and hip[99] arthroplasty patients in Japan, but has not yet received FDA approval for this indication. It is administered in a once-daily dose of 30 to 60 mg based on body weight.

Adverse reactions. As with other agents with this mechanism of action, edoxaban has been associated with an increased risk of bleeding. It has also been known to cause elevation in serum liver enzymes (AST, ALT) and rash.

Factor XA Inhibitor Reversal Agents

Idarucizumab

Structure and mechanism of action. Idarucizumab is a humanized monoclonal antibody fragment that selectively binds to the active site of dabigatran and its acylglucuronide metabolites, thereby inhibiting their activity. It has an affinity for the active site of dabigatran 350 times greater than that of thrombin, making it a powerful competitive inhibitor of the drug. Once bound, it remains attached to dabigatran, blocking its activity until the drug can be metabolized.

Idarucizumab received expedited FDA approval in October 2015 for use in patients who are taking dabigatran and have an emergent need to reverse the drug's effects, such as in the situations of uncontrolled bleeding or need for emergency surgery. This approval was based on a study of the drug's safety performed in 283 healthy volunteers who were administered dabigatran followed by a single 5 g dose of idarucizumab. Administration of idarucizumab resulted in complete reversal of the effects of dabigatran in 89% of subjects.[100]

This was followed by a cohort case series trial (RE-VERSE AD), which included 123 patients who were taking dabigatran and experienced dabigatran-related life-threatening or uncontrolled bleeding or who required emergency surgery or other procedures. In both groups, the median maximum reversal of the effects of dabigatran was 100%, with 89% of patients achieving complete reversal.[101]

Adverse reactions. Reversal of the effects of dabigatran exposes patients to the thromboembolic risk of their underlying medical condition. Hypersensitivity reactions, including pyrexia, bronchospasm, hyperventilation, rash, and pruritus, have also been reported. As idarucizumab is a protein, the possibility of immunogenicity exists. The recommended dose of idarucizumab contains 4 g of sorbitol; therefore individuals with hereditary fructose intolerance are at risk of adverse events, including death, after administration of idarucizumab.[102]

Andexanet Alfa

Andexanet alfa (PRT064445) is a drug currently under investigation as a potential antidote for factor Xa inhibitors. It is a recombinant derivative of factor Xa, which has been designed to have a higher affinity for factor Xa inhibitors than naturally occurring factor Xa. Phase 2 clinical trials of the drug were completed in 2015 and demonstrated that intravenous administration of andexanet resulted in dose-dependent, rapid, and reproducible reversal of anticoagulant effects of apixaban, rivaroxaban, edoxaban, and enoxaparin in healthy volunteers without evidence of adverse effects. In 2015, the first randomized, double-blind, placebo controlled trials of andexanet were performed in healthy volunteers between 50 and 75 years old (ANNEXA-A and ANNEXA-R).[103] These demonstrated that after a bolus dose of andexanet, the antifactor Xa activity of apixaban and rivaroxaban were reduced by greater than 90% within 2 to 5 minutes. This effect persisted for 1 to 2 hours, and it was prolonged with the administration of a continuous infusion of andexanet after administration of the initial bolus. No serious or severe adverse effects of administration of andexanet were reported.

Antiplatelet Agents

Aspirin

Structure and mechanism of action. Aspirin inhibits platelet aggregation by irreversibly acetylating prostaglandin synthase, inhibiting its cyclooxygenase activity. This blocks prostaglandin metabolism and, most importantly, the synthesis of thromboxane A_2, a potent stimulator of platelet aggregation.[104,105] There are two isoforms of the cyclooxygenase enzyme: COX-1 and COX-2.[106] COX-1 is constitutively expressed in many cell types, including platelets, whereas COX-2 is present only in inflammatory cells. Aspirin is 50- to 100-fold more potent in inhibiting COX-1 than COX-2; thus lower doses are required to obtain antiplatelet compared with anti-inflammatory effects.[106] Several other mechanisms for platelet inhibition have been proposed, including inhibiting neutrophil activation of platelets[107] and interfering with prostacyclin synthesis by endothelium.[108] There are also data suggesting an antioxidant role for aspirin[109,110] and the improvement of endothelial cell function by aspirin.[111] It is primarily the antiplatelet and antithrombotic effects of aspirin that result in cardiovascular benefits. Aspirin is rapidly absorbed by the upper gastrointestinal tract, with measurable platelet effects within 1 hour.[106] Enteric coating significantly impairs its absorption, taking up to 4 hours to reach peak plasma levels. Although the plasma half-life is only 20 minutes, the effect on COX-1 and the platelet is permanent, as the anucleate platelet cannot synthesize new enzyme. The life span of a platelet is approximately 10 days. After a single dose of aspirin and with normal platelet turnover of approximately 10% per days, it may take 10 days for renewal of the platelet population. However, data suggest that as little as 20% of platelets with normal COX enzyme activity are required for normal hemostasis.[106,112]

Clinical use. The benefit of aspirin therapy is determined largely by the patient's absolute risk of vascular events. Those at high risk and those with unstable angina or prior myocardial infarction or stroke derive the most benefit.[113]

Primary prevention. Aspirin for primary disease prevention has been carefully evaluated in multiple clinical trials.[114-119] The combined data demonstrated a significant reduction in myocardial infarction with aspirin but did not demonstrate a decrease in overall mortality. There was a slightly increased risk of bleeding complications with aspirin, so the benefits and risks must be balanced. Generally, the greater the thrombotic risk, the greater the benefits of aspirin for primary prevention.[113]

Secondary prevention. The benefits of aspirin in preventing cardiovascular disease complications have been clearly demonstrated in several large clinical trials.[120] The Antiplatelet Trialists Committee published a meta-analysis that included 287 trials with more than 300,000 patients.[116,121] In high-risk patients—those with a history of myocardial infarction, angina, or stroke—long-term therapy with aspirin significantly decreased the risk of nonfatal myocardial infarction, nonfatal ischemic stroke, and vascular death.[116,117]

Aspirin is also recommended in patients undergoing prosthetic inguinal bypass grafting or carotid endarterectomy and those with asymptomatic and recurrent carotid stenosis.[60] Aspirin has been demonstrated to improve long-term vessel patency in patients undergoing lower extremity angioplasty with or without stenting.[60]

Adverse reactions. The most significant adverse reactions associated with aspirin therapy include bleeding and gastrointestinal irritation. These side effects appear to be dose related. Aspirin dosing varied widely in the Antiplatelet Trialists Committee overview, and there was no significant benefit associated with higher doses.[121] Daily dosing of 75 to 150 mg of aspirin appears to be as effective as higher doses for long-term treatment.[116] Because of the increased side effects with higher doses and the lack of any conclusive data favoring higher doses, the concept of lower dosing is supported.[122]

Thienopyridines (Clopidogrel, Ticlopidine, and Prasugrel)

Structure and mechanism of action. Adenosine diphosphate (ADP) plays a central role in platelet aggregation and activation. ADP released from activated platelets induces further platelet activation and adhesion through binding to the ADP receptor on the platelet surface. The ADP receptor is a membrane-bound, G-protein–coupled receptor.[123,124] There are two main types of ADP receptors, $P2Y_1$ and $P2Y_{12}$.[123] The overall effect of platelet ADP receptor binding is increased platelet activation and aggregation.[123]

Ticlopidine and clopidogrel are selective antiplatelet agents that inhibit the $P2Y_{12}$ receptor. Their chemical structures are similar, with clopidogrel having an extra carboxymethyl side group. Both parent compounds are quickly metabolized in the liver to active metabolites that covalently bind to the ADP receptor. Clopidogrel is six times more potent than ticlopidine. The effect is permanent over the life span of the platelet, and overall platelet function generally recovers within 7 to 10 days after stopping the drug.[123] Prasugrel is a thienopyridine prodrug that must undergo hydrolysis by intestinal esterases and oxidation by CYP3A4 and CYP2B6 to be converted to its active metabolite. The active metabolite then binds to the P2Y12 ADP receptor causing irreversible inhibition of platelet activity.[125]

Clinical use. Ticlopidine has been evaluated in several clinical trials in patients with PAD and has been associated with a reduction in the risk of myocardial infarction, stroke, and vascular death.[126,127] However, ticlopidine's clinical usefulness is limited by the potential for severe hematologic side effects, particularly neutropenia.[128-130]

Clopidogrel, which has fewer side effects than ticlopidine, has been approved for use in patients with recent myocardial infarction, stroke, or established peripheral vascular disease for the reduction of thrombotic events. The FDA has also approved it for use in patients with non-ST elevation ACS and percutaneous coronary interventions. A landmark study of clopidogrel was the Clopidogrel Versus Aspirin in Patients at Risk of Ischemic Events (CAPRIE) trial.[131] This randomized, prospective, double-blinded trial compared the efficacy of aspirin and clopidogrel in reducing the risk of ischemic stroke, myocardial infarction, or vascular death. The study of nearly 20,000 patients with atherosclerotic disease (those with recent stroke, myocardial infarction, or established PAD) found that clopidogrel resulted in an 8.7% relative risk reduction in vascular death, ischemic stroke, or myocardial infarction compared with aspirin. Remarkably, this was not a placebo comparison but a comparison with a known effective antiplatelet agent already proved to confer a 25% risk reduction.[116,132] Subset analyses of CAPRIE showed an even greater benefit in high-risk patients, diabetics, and those with previous vascular interventions.[133]

The newest thienopyridines prasugrel has been compared with clopidogrel in the TRITON-TIMI 38 study, where 13,608 patients with acute coronary syndrome undergoing percutaneous coronary intervention (after coronary anatomy was defined) were randomized to prasugrel or clopidogrel, in addition to aspirin, for up to 15 months. The primary endpoint (cardiovascular death, nonfatal myocardial infarction [MI], or nonfatal stroke) was noted in 9.9% of patients on prasugrel compared with 12.1% with clopidogrel ($P < .001$). This lower incidence was mainly due to a reduction in MI, with no difference stroke rate or cardiovascular death. Coronary stent thrombosis was seen in 2.4% of patients treated on clopidogrel and 1.1% of those on prasugrel.[134-136]

Thienopyridines have been used in vascular surgery practice as antithrombotic therapy for carotid artery and lower extremity balloon angioplasty and stenting, although this has not yet been well examined in randomized clinical trials.[60] Ticlopidine (Ticlid) has been demonstrated to improve the patency of infrainguinal bypass grafts, but its clinical use has been superseded by clopidogrel's significantly fewer adverse effects.[60,137] Currently there are no controlled trials looking specifically at clopidogrel or prasugrel and infrainguinal graft patency, so it cannot be recommended at this time.

Adverse reactions. Side effects of clopidogrel include gastrointestinal complaints and skin rash. Bleeding complications are similar to those associated with aspirin. Neutropenia is a rare complication with clopidogrel but is much more frequent with ticlopidine.[130,138] Neutropenia can be severe and has resulted in fatalities. It generally occurs within 3 months after instituting therapy, and strict hematologic monitoring is recommended.[123] Diarrhea and skin rashes are also common with ticlopidine.[133] Thrombotic thrombocytopenic purpura is a recognized complication of thienopyridine treatment, with an incidence between 1:1600 and 1:5000 patients.[139] With the widespread use of clopidogrel, there has been a subgroup of patients noted to be poor responders to the drug due to genetic polymorphisms of the cytochrome P450 enzyme CYP2C19.[140] At least one of the associated genetic polymorphisms has been found to occur in 15% of Caucasians, 17% of African Americans, and 30% of Asians.[141] At this time there are no clear recommendations for genetic testing for these variants prior to induction of clopidogril therapy;[142] however, if clinical concern exists, genetic testing is available or patients who are taking clopidogrel could have functional platelet aggregation assays to evaluate whether the drug is being activated. Another alternative is to switch to prasugrel, though these same polymorphisms may also affect conversion of prasugrel to its active form by CYP2B6.[143] Another nuance in clopidogrel therapy is the finding that proton pump inhibitors (PPI) may interfere with clopidogrel activation and decrease the antiplatelet effect, increasing the risk of cardiovascular events. A review of four randomized trials has noted that a metabolic drug–drug interaction does appear to exist between clopidogrel and omeprazole but not between clopidogrel and pantoprazole.[144]

It is important to note that prasugrel appears to have a significantly higher risk of bleeding as compared with clopidogrel. In TRITON-TIMI 38, more patients on prasugrel had major bleeding than with clopidogrel (2.4% vs. 1.8%; $P = .03$), life-threatening bleeding, and a small but significant increase in fatal bleeding (0.4% vs. 0.1%; $P = .002$). Among the 4% of patients with ST-elevation MI who required coronary artery bypass graft surgery, major bleeding occurred in 18.8% of prasugrel-treated patients compared with 2.7% of clopidogrel-treated patients ($P = .003$).[136]

Ticagrelor

Structure and mechanism of action. Ticagrelor is a nucleoside analog with an overall structural similarity to adenosine. Like thienopyridines, ticagrelor acts by acting on the ADP receptor subtype P2Y12 found on platelets; however, it binds to an area of the receptor distinct from the binding site of ADP. As a result, ticagrelor functions as an allosteric antagonist to platelet activation, and its action is reversible, which distinguishes it from the thienopyridines.

Clinical use. Ticagrelor received FDA approval in 2011 to be used for the prevention of thrombotic events in patients suffering from acute coronary syndrome with or without ST-segment elevation. This approval was based on the PLATO study, a multicenter double-blinded randomized trial comparing ticagrelor plus aspirin with clopidogrel plus aspirin. This trial demonstrated that patients who experienced these events and were treated with ticagrelor, as compared with clopidogrel, were significantly less likely to die from vascular causes, myocardial infarction, or stroke, without an increased overall rate of bleeding events, but with an increased risk of non-procedure-related bleeding events.[137]

The PEGASUS-TIMI 54 study compared ticagrelor plus aspirin versus placebo plus aspirin in patients greater than 50 years of age with a history of prior MI (1 to 3 years), and at least one risk factor for thrombotic cardiovascular events (CV death, MI, or stroke). The study demonstrated that patients treated with ticagrelor plus aspirin had a significantly lower rate of thrombotic cardiovascular events than those treated with aspirin alone.[138]

Adverse reactions. Side effects of ticagrelor include dyspnea, which occurs in approximately 14% of patients, and is typically self-limiting. As with all inhibitors of platelet function, bleeding is associated with the use of ticagrelor, with a rate of major bleeding of 3.9%. Discontinuation of ticagrelor increases the risk of myocardial infarction, stroke, and death.[139] As ticagrelor is metabolized by CYP3A, its use in patients with severe hepatic impairment is contraindicated, and other drugs that inhibit or induce CYP3A activity can alter serum levels of the drug. Metabolism of digoxin is affected by ticagrelor, and therefore digoxin levels should be monitored upon initiation of ticagrelor therapy or dose adjustment. Maintenance doses of aspirin above 100 mg reduce the effectiveness of ticagrelor, and should be avoided.

Vorapaxar

Structure and mechanism of action. Vorapaxar is a member of a novel group of antiplatelet agents that function by inhibiting protease-activated receptor 1 (PAR-1) expressed on platelets, thereby inhibiting thrombin-induced platelet aggregation. As a result of this novel mechanism, vorapaxar does not inhibit ADP-mediated platelet aggregation, coagulation parameters, or bleeding time.[140] The drug's interaction with the PAR-1 receptor is reversible, but the exceedingly long half-life (3 to 4 days) makes it essentially irreversible.

Clinical use. Vorapaxar is indicated for the reduction of thrombotic cardiovascular events in patients with a history of myocardial infarction or with PAD. This indication was granted by the FDA based on the results of a double-blinded placebo-controlled study in which 26,449 patients who had a history of MI, ischemic stroke, or PAD were randomized to receive standard antiplatelet therapy plus vorapaxar or placebo. Two years after initiation of the study, the use of vorapaxar in patients with a history of stroke was discontinued due to an increased risk of intracranial hemorrhage (1.0% vs. 0.5%). After 3 years, the patients treated with vorapaxar had a significantly lower incidence of myocardial infarction or recurrent ischemia requiring revascularization than those patients who received placebo.[141] A prior study evaluating the use of vorapaxar in patients with acute coronary syndrome demonstrated no benefit in comparison with placebo.[142]

Adverse reactions. Bleeding is the most commonly reported adverse reaction associated with the use of vorapaxar. As described previously, vorapaxar should not be used by patients with a history of stroke, TIA, or intracranial hemorrhage due to an increased risk of intracranial hemorrhage.[143] Use of vorapaxar has also been associated with anemia, depression, and rash, although these reactions are uncommon.[143] As vorapaxar is metabolized by CYP3A4, use of substances that induce or inhibit this enzyme's activity may affect the metabolism of vorapaxar, leading to increased risk of bleeding or thrombotic events.[144]

Glycoprotein IIb/IIIa Receptor Inhibitors

Structure and mechanism of action. The glycoprotein (GP) receptor is an integrin found in high concentrations on the platelet membrane. The GP receptor (GP IIb/IIIa) represents a final common pathway to platelet aggregation and subsequent thrombus formation.[153] Once activated, the receptor undergoes a conformational change that permits the binding of fibrinogen. This allows cross-linking of platelets and aggregation, with the formation of the hemostatic platelet plug.[154] Selective inhibition of the GP IIb/IIIa receptor is a logical target for more specific antiplatelet therapy. There are three main inhibitors approved for clinical use: abciximab (ReoPro), eptifibatide (Integrilin), and tirofiban (Aggrastat).

Abciximab. Abciximab was the first GP IIb/IIIa receptor inhibitor developed. It is a macromolecule composed of the Fab fragment of the chimeric human murine monoclonal antibody c7E3.[155] It has a high binding affinity for the GP IIb/IIIa receptor, which accounts for its prolonged antiplatelet effect after cessation of infusion, with up to 10 days of low-level receptor blockade.[155] Platelet aggregation is almost completely inhibited by 2 hours after infusion, with recovery evident 48 hours after discontinuing the drug. However, a platelet-bound drug can still be detected for up to 10 days.[156]

Tirofiban. Tirofiban is a small, nonpeptide antagonist of the GP IIb/IIIa receptor.[156] It is a tyrosine derivative with a molecular weight of 495 kD. At standard doses, platelet function is inhibited as early as 5 minutes after infusion, with bleeding time and platelet aggregation normalizing within 3 to 8 hours after discontinuation.[156]

Eptifibatide. Eptifibatide is a nonimmunogenic, cyclic heptapeptide that inhibits the GP IIb/IIIa receptor. It is derived from the structure of barbourin, from the venom of a species of rattlesnake.[157] It has a short plasma half-life of 15 minutes, with peak platelet effects within 15 minutes of infusion; platelet function returns to 50% of baseline by 4 hours after terminating the infusion.[158]

Clinical use. The GP IIb/IIIa receptor antagonists have been shown to reduce cardiac event rates in patients with ACS treated by medicine alone or in combination with percutaneous coronary intervention.[159] Evidence supporting their use in percutaneous coronary interventions is good. It confers significant long-term mortality benefits and decreases ischemic events.[153,154,160-162] There are currently no large, randomized clinical trials of GP IIb/IIIa inhibitors specifically in vascular surgery patients.

Adverse reactions. Bleeding is the principal adverse effect of all the GP inhibitors. Nearly all trials demonstrate an increase in serious bleeding rates. Fatal bleeding is rare, less than 0.1%, which is similar to the rate with combined heparin and aspirin therapy.[156] Thrombocytopenia is also associated with GP inhibition. Abciximab causes severe thrombocytopenia (<20,000/μL) in 0.7% of patients, and eptifibatide and tirofiban in 0.2% of patients.[156]

The optimal patients to receive GP inhibitors are those with acute coronary syndrome who undergo percutaneous coronary intervention and are at high risk for early failure. The value of GP inhibition in other vascular interventions is not yet established.[156]

Prothrombin Complex Concentrates

PCCs are lyophilized concentrates of pooled human plasma containing clotting factors. These contain either four (II, VII, IX, X), as in the case of Kcentra, Beriplex, and Octaplex, or three (II, IX, X) coagulation factors, as in the case of Profilnene or Uman complex DI.[163] Prothrombin complex concentrates' concentration of vitamin K–dependent clotting factors is approximately 25 times that of human plasma, and administration of a single dose is equivalent to the administration of approximately 2000 cc of fresh frozen plasma (FFP).[163] These medications have historically been used for the treatment of hemophilia, but have gained recent attention for use in patients suffering from acute bleeding or at high risk of bleeding due to coagulopathy in the place of FFP,[164] particularly with the increased use of the NOACs, as there are very few FDA-approved reversal agents for these new drugs.

The hypothesized benefit of these agents over FFP is due to their lyophilized composition, which allows for dry storage as a powder at room temperature and reconstitution in a highly concentrated solution.[165] This potentially allows for a more rapid and effective reversal of coagulopathy when compared with FFP.[166,167]

Thrombolytics

Structure and mechanism of action. Thrombolytics are a group of medications that are functional analogs of tissue plasminogen activator (tPA). Tissue plasminogen activator is a serine protease found in endothelial cells. It functions by catalyzing the conversion of plasminogen to plasmin, the primary enzyme involved in clot lysis. Plasmin subsequently cleaves cross-linked fibrin proteins, the main structural component of clots, into fibrin degradation products.[168]

Clinical use. Thrombolytics have multiple clinical indications that mostly relate to severe thromboembolic events. There are two subtypes of thrombolytic medications currently in use: recombinant enzymes and naturally occurring enzymes.

Alteplase

Alteplase is a recombinant human tPA. It has been approved for treatment of acute ischemic stroke (AIS), acute myocardial infarction (AMI), and acute massive pulmonary embolism based on multiple randomized control trials.[169-171] It has also been approved for the lysis of clot from dysfunctional central venous catheters.[172,173] Although it has not received FDA approval for this indication, it is commonly employed as a method of peripheral vessel thrombolysis in the setting of acute limb ischemia (ALI) or DVT, when administered via an indwelling catheter.[174,175] Multiple infusion regimens have been evaluated in the literature, and there is currently no consensus on the optimal dose or infusion method; however, an advisory panel convened in 1999 published suggested dosing regimens: (1) a weight-adjusted dose of 0.001 to 0.02 mg/kg/h and (2) a non–weight-adjusted dose of 0.12 to 2.0 mg/h. No formal recommendation was made on the use of weight-adjusted versus non–weight-adjusted dosing. The recommended maximum dosing was no greater than 40 mg for catheter-directed therapy.[176] A minimum effective dose for treatment of ALI has yet to be determined.

Reteplase

Reteplase is a recombinantly derived mutein of tPA consisting of 355 out of the 527 amino acids that form endogenous tPA. It has less affinity for fibrin-bound plasminogen than alteplase, which allows each molecule to bind to plasminogen and activate the plasminogen-to-plasmin conversion, then detach and bind to a new plasminogen molecule, thereby enhancing its fibrinolytic potential over that of alteplase.[177,178] It is currently FDA approved for treatment of AMI, but its use for thrombolysis in ALI and DVT has been evaluated in several small studies.[179-181] An expert consensus meeting held in 2000 suggested that the minimum dose should not be less than 0.25 U/h, with a dose range of 0.25 to 1.0 U/h. Maximum dose amount and infusion time suggested were 20 U and 24 hours, respectively. In a study that examined several doses of reteplase for lower-extremity arterial occlusions, doses of 0.5 U/h, 0.25 U/h, and 0.125 U/h were found to be equally effective, with an increased rate of bleeding events at the highest dose.[182,183]

Tenecteplase

Tenecteplase is a third-generation recombinant plasminogen activator. It is currently FDA approved for treatment of AMI with an improved safety profile in comparison to alteplase, as it has a longer half-life, increased selectivity for fibrin-bound plasminogen, and improved resistance to plasminogen activator inhibitor compared with alteplase.[184] Its use for treatment of ALI and DVT has been evaluated in several small studies, but further evaluation is needed.[184-186] Based on the results of these small studies, the initial bolus dose of tenecteplase should be limited to 1.5 mg, with subsequent continuous infusions of 0.25 and 0.125 mg/h demonstrating similar rates of success and complication.[186]

Streptokinase

Streptokinase is an enzyme that is naturally produced by several species of β-hemolytic streptococci, for which it functions as a virulence factor. Its mechanism of action is analogous to tPA. As streptokinase has been widely available for several decades, it has been used for a variety of applications, from treatment of AMI, pulmonary embolism (PE), DVT, and ALI, to clot lysis from vascular catheters and treatment of loculated pleural effusions.[187-191] As it is a bacterial protein, it is immunogenic and has the potential to precipitate allergic or anaphylactic reactions with repeated exposures. Due to this risk, streptokinase is no longer used in the United States.

Urokinase

Urokinase, also known as urinary plasminogen activator, is a naturally occurring thrombolytic that is produced in the kidney, and was initially isolated from human urine in the 1940s.[192] In contrast to tPA and its derivative medications, urokinase acts on both circulating and fibrin-bound plasminogen. Similar to streptokinase, it has been employed for a wide range of thrombolytic indications, including AMI, ALI, and PE.[193-195] This medication is no longer available in the United States, due to manufacturing issues resulting in a discontinuation of production.

Adverse reactions. Given their common mechanism of action, all thrombolytics share the potential risk of bleeding complications related to systemic fibrinogenolysis and the lysis of normal hemostatic plugs. Bleeding is often noted at a catheterization site, although gastrointestinal and cerebral hemorrhages may occur. Therefore patients who have experienced trauma injury, have recently undergone surgery, or who have a history of cerebral hemorrhagic stroke are not usually administered thrombolytics. Rethrombosis can occur following thrombolysis, and therefore anticoagulants such as heparin are usually coadministered and continued after thrombolytic therapy for a period of time.

Medical Treatment of Claudication

Pentoxifylline

Structure and mechanism of action. Pentoxifylline is an antithrombotic agent whose exact mechanism of action is unknown. It is thought to improve blood flow by increasing red cell deformity, decreasing platelet adhesiveness, and decreasing blood viscosity, leading to increased flow in the microcirculation.[196-198]

Clinical use. Multiple clinical trials of pentoxifylline have demonstrated conflicting results in the treatment of claudication. Some suggested improved walking distance with pentoxifylline,[199-204] while others showed little benefit compared with placebo.[205-208] Based on such conflicting data, it is currently not recommended for use in claudication.

Cilostazol

Structure and mechanism of action. Cilostazol is a type III phosphodiesterase inhibitor that increases cellular cyclic adenosine monophosphate and acts to inhibit platelet aggregation and thrombus formation. It is also a direct vasodilator.[60] Cilostazol has been shown to improve claudication symptoms, but the exact mechanism is unknown. It is absorbed after oral administration and extensively metabolized by hepatic cytochrome P-450 enzymes, with two main active metabolites being produced.[38] Excretion is predominantly urinary.

Clinical use. Cilostazol was approved in 1999 by the FDA for the treatment of intermittent claudication, based on randomized clinical trials that demonstrated increased walking distance and quality of life.[209-211] Compared with those given placebo, patients taking cilostazol experienced significant increases in walking distance. The effect was apparent as early as 2 to 4 weeks after initiating therapy. Cilostazol is more effective than pentoxifylline in improving claudication.[38] Current recommendations are that cilostazol should be used only by those with moderate to severely disabling claudication who are not revascularization candidates.[60] Cilostazol has weak antiplatelet effects, but there are no clinical data to support its use as an antiplatelet agent.[60]

Adverse reactions. Because cilostazol is a phosphodiesterase inhibitor, it should not be used in patients with congestive heart failure. The only adverse effect in study patients leading to discontinuation of the drug was headache, likely secondary to its vasodilatory effects. Other more common side effects include palpitations and diarrhea.

Agents to Prevent Contrast-Induced Nephropathy

Contrast nephropathy (CN) is the third leading cause of acute renal failure in hospitalized patients.[212,213] Most cases of CN are reversible and nonoliguric; however, up to 25% to 30% of patients who develop CN have a permanent decline in renal function.[214] In addition, patients who develop acute renal failure have increased morbidity and mortality.[215] The main risk factors for developing CN are underlying renal insufficiency and diabetes.[216] The exact mechanism behind the development of CN remains unknown but is likely a combination of direct renal tubule epithelial cell toxicity and renal medullary ischemia.[216,217] The use of low volumes of low-osmolar and iso-osmolar contrast agents appears to reduce the risk of CN when compared with the use of high-osmolar contrast agents.[218-220] Multiple trials have demonstrated that saline hydration is also beneficial in preventing CN.[221,222]

Sodium Bicarbonate

Intravenous infusion of isotonic sodium bicarbonate has been demonstrated to be somewhat superior to isotonic sodium chloride (saline) in preventing CN in high-risk patients.[223] This protocol used an infusion of 3 mL/kg per hour for 1 hour before and 1 mL/kg per hour for 6 hours after the procedure. A meta-analysis of seven published clinical trials comparing the use of sodium bicarbonate solution versus saline in patients undergoing contrast-requiring procedures demonstrated a reduced incidence of contrast-induced nephropathy (CIN) in patients who received sodium bicarbonate solution compared with saline (odds ratio [OR] 0.33; $P = .003$); however, significant heterogeneity and bias were identified within the included studies.[224] Based on the available data, no strong recommendations can be made; however, given its low risk for adverse reactions, sodium bicarbonate therapy may be considered in the high-risk patient.

N-Acetylcysteine

Structure and mechanism of action. N-Acetylcysteine (NAC) is the acetylated form of the amino acid L-cysteine. NAC has been in clinical use for more than 40 years, mostly as a mucolytic.[225] NAC is an antioxidant and a free radical scavenger. It can stimulate glutathione synthesis and has vasodilatory properties through its effects on nitric oxide.[226]

Clinical use. Clinical data on the value of NAC in preventing CN are mixed. NAC initially demonstrated a significant reduction in CN in patients with preexisting renal insufficiency.[227] The frequency of CN in patients receiving hydration plus NAC was 2%, compared with 22% in those receiving hydration alone. This was followed by other studies demonstrating similar protective effects of NAC.[228,229] However, subsequent trials have not demonstrated a clear benefit in the prevention of CN.[230,231] Proponents of NAC argue that its ease of administration, relatively low cost, and limited side effects make this an appealing agent in high-risk patients.

Other Agents

A variety of other agents have been used in an attempt to decrease contrast induced nephropathy—theophylline,[238-241] fenoldopam,[232-237] prostaglandin E_1,[216,242] endothelin-1,[212,243,244] CCBs,[245-250] dopamine,[212,251-254] and diuretics such a furosemide and mannitol[221,255]—but none have proven useful to date.

Statins. Statin therapy has been demonstrated to reduce cardiovascular morbidity and mortality in multiple patient populations.[229,256-260] Although the primary mechanism of action is to reduce cholesterol levels, the benefits of statin therapy appear to extend beyond that effect.[261]

Structure and mechanism of action. Statins decrease cholesterol levels through inhibition of the HMG-CoA reductase enzyme, the rate-limiting step through which cells synthesize cholesterol. Inhibition of cholesterol synthesis leads to increased hepatocyte expression of LDL receptors, with increased cellular uptake of LDL and a reduction in plasma LDL and cholesterol levels.[261] Statins also reduce the rate at which apolipoprotein B particles are secreted by the liver.[261]

Clinical use. There are considerable data to support the use of statins in patients with cardiovascular disease. The Scandinavian Simvastatin Survival Study (4S) clearly established that lipid-lowering therapy was safe, and it reduced morbidity and mortality in patients with ischemic heart disease who had elevated cholesterol levels.[257] Statin treatment reduced major coronary events, coronary mortality, and overall mortality. Multiple subsequent studies of patients with elevated cholesterol demonstrated a significant reduction in cardiovascular events and overall mortality with statin therapy.[258,262,263] Statins are also beneficial in patients with cardiovascular disease who have normal lipid levels.[256,260,263,264] In addition, statin therapy is associated with a reduction in the risk of stroke in patients with cardiovascular disease.[265,266]

Besides lowering cholesterol, statins are thought to have significant so-called pleiotropic effects.[261] Statins can improve endothelial cell function[267,268] and reduce inflammation and thrombosis, leading to plaque stabilization.[261,264,269,270]

The majority of studies support the aggressive use of statins in patients at high risk for coronary or cerebrovascular events, particularly in those with established disease, irrespective of their baseline cholesterol levels.

Specific studies focusing on vascular surgery patients are few. Subgroup analysis of patients with peripheral vascular disease in the major statin trials demonstrated a significant decrease in myocardial infarction and cardiovascular events.[271] The 4S trial found that the incidence of new-onset or worsening intermittent claudication was reduced 38% with statin therapy.[257] Statin treatment in patients undergoing noncardiac vascular surgery has been shown to reduce cardiac morbidity and mortality.[272-274] Statins also improve vein graft patency.[275]

Adverse reactions. High-dose statin therapy leads to hepatic necrosis in animal models.[276] In clinical trials, statins have not been demonstrated to cause significant liver enzyme elevations compared with controls.[277] Current recommendations are to monitor hepatic enzymes for 4 to 6 weeks after initiating treatment. In high-risk patients or those taking certain medications, closer monitoring may be warranted. The most serious risks associated with statin therapy are myositis and rhabdomyolysis.[276,278] Cerivastatin was withdrawn from the market, owing to deaths from such complications.[279] Risks for rhabdomyolysis are increased with small body size, advanced age, renal or hepatic dysfunction, diabetes, and hypothyroidism.[279] Patients on statins should be monitored closely for symptoms of myopathy.

New-onset DM in association with statin therapy has been reported in several clinical trials and meta-analyses evaluating the long-term effects of statin therapy.[280-283] Although some of the data are conflicting, the FDA decided there was sufficient evidence to support the addition of a warning label about DM risk to statin packaging in March 2012.[284,285] Multiple mechanisms for this effect have been proposed, including extrahepatic effects of certain subtypes of statin medications,[286] interference with calcium-mediated signaling in pancreatic islet β-cells,[286,287] disruption of glucose transporter 4 (GLUT4) activation by insulin,[288-291] disturbance of intracellular insulin signal transduction,[290,292] interference in adipocyte maturation,[293,294] inhibition of the products of cholesterol biosynthesis,[290,295-298] and alteration of adiponectin and leptin synthesis.[299,300] Uncoupling protein 3 (UCP3) downregulation[301] and microRNA induction[301] are additional proposed mechanisms that require further study.

As the evidence supporting an association between statins and new-onset DM came to light, the resulting question was whether this adverse effect only took place in populations with certain risk factors for developing DM, or in statin-users as a whole. To answer this question, Waters and colleagues pooled data from multiple large randomized trials investigating atorvastatin, and found that baseline fasting glucose higher than 5.6 mmol/L and features of metabolic syndrome (hypertriglyceridemia, body mass index [BMI] >30 kg/m^2, and hypertension) were predictive of new-onset DM.[302] A subsequent re-analysis of the JUPITER trial attempted to determine the relative risks and benefits of statin therapy by grouping participants based on presence of risk factors for DM such as metabolic syndrome, impaired fasting glucose, BMI greater than 30 kg/m^2, and hemoglobin A_1C greater than 6% at enrollment. When none of these risk factors were present, rosuvastatin resulted in a 52% reduction in primary endpoints (MI, stroke, unstable angina, arterial revascularization, or cardiovascular death), with no increased risk of DM. Those subjects with one or more risk factors for DM experienced a 28% increase in DM occurrence with a 39% reduction in primary endpoints, demonstrating that the benefits of statin therapy outweighed the risks, even in high-risk patients.[303] As a result of these findings, no change in clinical practice is currently recommended.

Fish oil. Long-chain, highly unsaturated omega-3 fatty acids, found in cold-water fish and now widely commercially available in capsules, can decrease fasting triglyceride concentrations 20% to 50% by reducing hepatic triglyceride production and increasing triglyceride clearance.[304] With long-term intake, they have been shown to increase HDLs, enhance the antiplatelet activity of aspirin and clopidogrel, improve heart failure, and improve vascular function in diabetes.[304] A large, randomized 5-year trial in more than 18,000 hypercholesterolemic patients already treated with statins showed a significant reduction in major coronary events when eicosapentaenoic acid (EPA) was added.[305] Subanalysis of the JELIS trial demonstrated that specifically in patients with PAD, the incidence of CAD was higher than in controls, and that EPA markedly reduced the occurrence of CAD in those patients.[306] Fish oil benefits the vascular surgical patient through stabilization of the overall cardiovascular system.

Other Lipid-Lowering Agents

Ezetimibe

Ezetimibe is a cholesterol transport inhibitor that acts primarily on the small intestine to reduce cholesterol absorption. Ezetimibe is most effective when combined with statin medications and has been shown to have a synergistic effect on lipid reduction in this setting.[307,308]

Niacin (Nicotinic Acid)

Niacin has been demonstrated to be beneficial in both reducing VLDL and LDL, in addition to increasing levels of HDL. Flushing, diarrhea, and a mild diabetogenic effect are all recognized side effects of niacin use and form the majority of reasons for discontinuation of the medication.[309,310]

Fibric Acid Derivatives

Fibric acid derivatives such as gemfibrozil and fenofibrate have limited applicability in the primary risk-reduction strategy for dyslipidemia, as their effect on LDL levels are marginal but are of marked benefit in patients with pancreatitis associated with hypertriglyceridemia due to their selective reduction in triglycerides.[311,312]

Bile Acid Sequestrants

Bile acid sequestrants are weak cholesterol and LDL lowering medications and act by interrupting the enterohepatic recirculation of bile acids via the inhibition of small intestinal bile acid reabsorption.[313]

CONCLUSIONS

Cardiovascular disease continues to be the most significant cause of mortality in the United States and similarly developed countries. The detection of modifiable risk factors for atherosclerosis continues to remain one of the most promising areas of research in the field of cardiovascular medicine. As the population ages and becomes more obese, there will be a rise in the number of patients with cardiovascular disease. Aggressive risk-factor modification can only occur if there is vigilance and attention to the detection and subsequent treatment of conditions such as diabetes, obesity, dyslipidemia, smoking, and renal disease. Although there are many effective strategies for risk reduction, including an array of pharmacologic agents, once these conditions have been diagnosed, there is a growing body of epidemiological evidence that points toward greater health outcomes when the predisposing factors for these diseases are addressed early, prior to full-blown disease diagnosis.

Preventing individuals from becoming smokers rather than focusing on smoking cessation, educating individuals about diet and exercise strategies to prevent obesity, and modulation of cholesterol intake to reduce hyperlipidemia are all paradigms for reducing the exposure of the population to cardiovascular risk factors. Unfortunately, patients have not embraced these preventative strategies, and public health measures have not been successful in a cost-effective and widespread manner at the present time.

Despite advances in pharmacological treatment of identified risk factors, however, behavioral modification strategies that are effective are limited. Attitude toward health and cultivation of risk-factor avoidance has been difficult to implement; however, it is these very attributes that are most likely to reduce the burden of cardiovascular disease most significantly. These core health traits must be adopted by individuals themselves and supported by education and demonstration of identifiable health benefits before the prevention of cardiovascular disease can be entertained at a population level.

REVIEW QUESTIONS

1. Which of the following risk factors has NOT been reproducibly demonstrated to confer a reduction in cardiovascular risk when modified?
   a. Smoking
   b. Homocysteine levels
   c. HDL, LDL, and triglyceride levels
   d. HbA1c level
   e. Diastolic blood pressure
2. Which of the following targets is NOT part of the guidelines for the management of diabetic patients?
   a. Triglyceride level less than 150 mg/dL
   b. HbA1c level less than 7%
   c. Fasting blood glucose less than 110 mg/dL
   d. Blood pressure less than 140/90 mm Hg
   e. LDL less than 100 mg/dL
3. Which of the following is a well-established side effect of use of HMG-CoA reductase inhibitors ("statins")?
   a. Thrombocytopenia
   b. Stroke
   c. Myositis
   d. Hepatitis
   e. Deep vein thrombosis
4. Which of the following provides the most durable reduction in cardiovascular risk in patients with the metabolic syndrome?
   a. Weight loss
   b. Tight glucose control
   c. Blood pressure less than 130/80
   d. Tight lipid control
   e. Euthyroidism
5. Which of the following is NOT part of the Cardiac Hospitalization Atherosclerosis Management Program (CHAMP) guidelines?
   a. Antiplatelet agents
   b. Beta-blockade
   c. ACE inhibition
   d. HMG-CoA reductase inhibitors
   e. Calcium-channel blockade
6. Which of these therapies has clearly been shown to prevent contrast-induced nephropathy?
   a. High-osmolar contrast agents
   b. Intravenous hydration
   c. Fenoldopam
   d. Theophylline
   e. Lasix
7. True or false: Argatroban, being renally excreted, needs to be dosed carefully in patients with renal failure.
8. Which antigen is thought to be associated with the development of heparin-induced thrombocytopenia?
   a. Platelet factor 4
   b. Von Willebrand factor
   c. Factor X
   d. Platelet ADP receptor
9. Patients with a history of fish allergy may have an increased risk of reaction to which of the following?
   a. Protamine
   b. Heparin
   c. Argatroban
   d. Tirofiban
   e. Clopidogrel
10. Which of the following has clear indications for use in the treatment of intermittent claudication?
    a. Ticlopidine
    b. Clopidogrel
    c. Cilostazol
    d. Pentoxifylline
    e. Tirofiban

References available online at ExpertConsult.com.

CHAPTER 14

Noninvasive Vascular Diagnostic Laboratory

Ankur Chandra, J. Dennis Baker

INTRODUCTION

In the early days of vascular surgery, patient assessment was based on a careful history and physical examination. Although a few clinicians used the Collins oscillometer to estimate the pulse pressure in an extremity, there was little help available in terms of quantitative assessment of arterial or venous disease. Angiography provided the only objective determination of pathologic changes. Early experience with arteriography and venography highlighted some of the limitations of these techniques, especially the problem of underestimating the severity of stenotic lesions on single-plane studies. In addition, the cost, patient discomfort, and risk of complications associated with contrast studies precluded their routine use for screening evaluations and follow-up.

The growing interest in more accurate differential diagnosis, localization of disease, determination of its severity, and documentation of progression stimulated the development of objective measurement techniques. In the 1960s, investigators started working with different plethysmographic techniques to quantify arterial occlusive disease in the leg. Modification of ultrasound equipment to measure blood flow by the Doppler shift principle represented an important step forward in instrumentation and led to the rapid development of noninvasive studies. Additional techniques were designed to evaluate carotid artery disease, as well as deep venous occlusion and insufficiency. This chapter describes the main diagnostic techniques used in the noninvasive laboratory and discusses their clinical application for patients with vascular disease. With an understanding of the merits and limitations of each method, clinicians can make the best use of these tests.

ULTRASOUND PHYSICS AND INSTRUMENTATION

Doppler Effect/Velocity Measurement

High-frequency sound waves (1 to 12 MHz) penetrate soft tissues and are reflected by the different interfaces encountered. Reflection from a moving interface results in the reflected frequency being increased if the motion is toward the point of observation and decreased if the motion is away from it. The magnitude of the shift is determined by the following Doppler equation:

$$f_s = \frac{2Vf_0 \cos\varphi}{C}, \qquad (14.1)$$

where f_s is the frequency shift, V the velocity, f_0 is the transmitted frequency, φ is the angle between the ultrasound beam and the velocity vector, and C is the speed of sound in tissue (1540 m/s). For a given velocity, a greater frequency shift is obtained with a higher transmitting frequency. In contrast, tissue penetration varies **inversely** with probe frequency, so the selection of a frequency for a given application is a balance between depth and velocity requirements.

In some applications, it is more useful to have a measure of velocity rather than the raw frequency data. If the probe angle relative to the direction of flow can be measured, the velocity is estimated using the Doppler equation. The accuracy of the estimate depends greatly on the accuracy of the angle measurement. Errors are greatest when the probe is at a right angle to flow and least when it is at a low angle. Whenever possible, velocities should be measured with an angle equal to or less than 60 degrees.

Continuous Wave Versus Pulsed Wave Doppler

Continuous-wave detectors are the simplest systems. The probe has two separate crystals—one transmitting and one receiving continuously. This system detects all velocities within the intersecting paths of the sound beams. If this zone includes more than one vessel (e.g., an artery and a vein), the resulting signal represents a combination of both velocities. The commonly used bedside Doppler pencil is an example of a continuous wave device. Pulsed wave Doppler systems use a single crystal that repeatedly transmits a short burst of sound followed by a waiting period, during which the crystal functions in a receiving mode. By selecting the time and duration of the listening phase, one can define a sample volume, or the portion of the vessel from which velocity is to be measured. Modern duplex scanners use complex scan probes made up of many elements in an array, but the principle of focal sampling is the same.

Spectral Analysis

The shifted frequency obtained from a vessel is within the audible range, so the data can be presented to the examiner as an audio signal. Although qualitative interpretation is helpful in some patient examinations, quantitative measurements provide objective testing. Spectral analyzers are used to determine the main frequency components obtained from a given vessel. This information is usually displayed on a sonogram, which shows the frequency content in time (Fig. 14.1).

The computational algorithm used to perform the conversion of the amplitude of received frequencies to a frequency over time display is called a fast Fourier transform. This process involves the grouping of frequencies based on quantity for each time unit. This is then converted to a frequency (or proportional velocity) versus time plot where the intensity of the curve (Doppler waveform) corresponds to the amplitude or amount of any given frequency. This has implications in the interpretation of spectral broadening, which implies more turbulent flow with a variety of different frequencies/velocities compared with a more discreet waveform that represents laminar flow with a uniform frequency/velocity for the sampled area.

Duplex Ultrasound

During the 1960s, B-mode ultrasound imaging (B = bright mode, a static image of the tissue) was used for visualization of soft tissue structures. Although early devices had only crude resolution, equipment has improved to the point that clear, detailed images of vessels can be produced in real time (Fig. 14.2). In general, experience shows that when high-quality imaging is obtained, the diagnostic accuracy is very high; however, in patients with advanced atherosclerosis, it is difficult to obtain optimal studies, and diagnostic accuracy is lower. A common problem is incomplete imaging of the vessel wall as a result of calcification, which is present in varying degrees in up to half of patients studied. The extent of interference may be limited, but in some vessels there is no visualization of substantial portions of the artery. Although calcified plaques stand out sharply in the ultrasound image, some atheromas are visualized poorly or not at all. A major source of error is that recent thrombus may have the same echo density as flowing blood, so that an occluded vessel may look normal on the ultrasound image.

To overcome the limitations of ultrasound imaging, the research team at the University of Washington developed the duplex scanner (also called duplex ultrasound), combining a real-time B-mode ultrasound image system with a pulsed wave Doppler detector.[1] The ultrasound image shows not only the vessel under study but also the location of the sample volume of the Doppler beam, so that the examiner can position it to study velocity patterns at specific locations in the vessel. The device can study calcified vessels by analyzing the Doppler velocity signal distal to the areas of calcification. The evaluation of the Doppler signal from the common carotid artery (CCA) and its branches is performed using spectral analysis (Fig. 14.3). Based

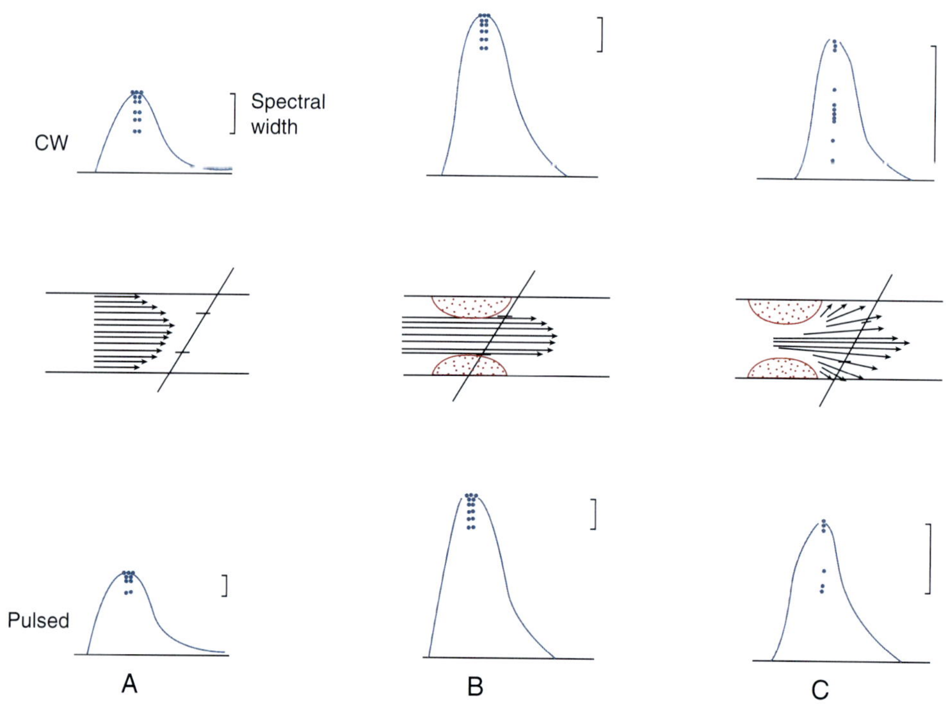

FIG 14.1 Comparison of sonograms from continuous-wave *(CW)* and pulsed Doppler systems. Sonograms display the different frequency contents detected at each point in time. The CW system detects all velocities across the vessel, whereas the pulsed system detects only those velocity vectors within the sample volume, indicated by the marks on the ultrasound beam. (A) Normal arterial signals. CW has more low-frequency content because it detects flow near the walls as well as in the center stream. (B) Within a stenosis, there is increased peak frequency, and the frequency distributions of both types of Doppler systems are similar, because the sample volume encompasses the entire flow stream. (C) Beyond a stenosis, peak frequency is elevated, with increased frequency distribution resulting from turbulent flow. Spectral width is greater with CW systems.

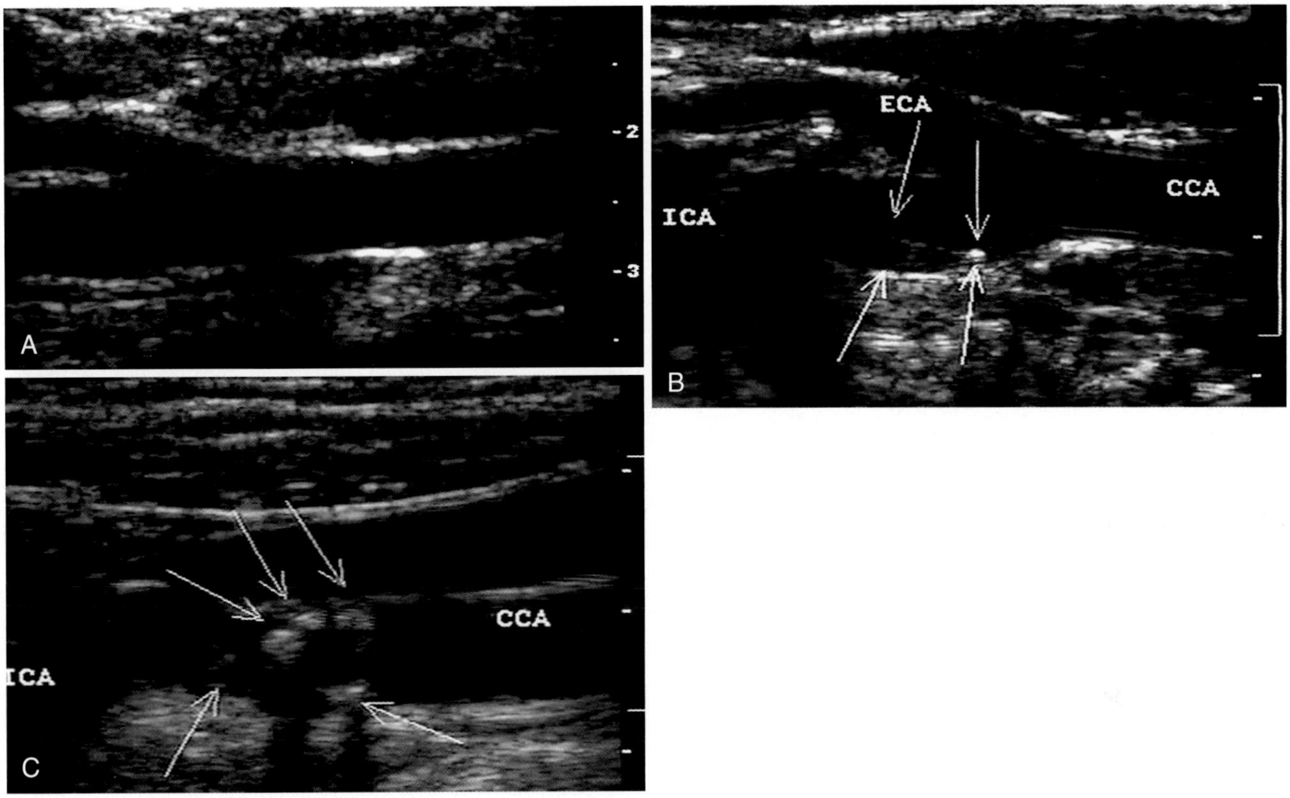

FIG 14.2 B-mode images from carotid duplex scan. (A) Normal bifurcation. (B) Moderate heterogeneous plaque with varying echogenicity. (C) Calcified lesion with high echogenicity and shadowing below the plaque. *CCA,* Common carotid artery; *ECA,* external carotid artery; *ICA,* internal carotid artery.

on the peak systolic velocity (PSV), end-diastolic velocity, velocity ratios, and degree of spectral broadening, a category of stenosis is assigned to the vessel segment.

In the past 20 years, there has been extensive improvement in duplex scanners in terms of both image resolution and Doppler signal processing. The early devices were limited to the study of superficial vessels; however, the availability of low-frequency probes (1 to 5 MHz) permits the evaluation of abdominal vessels, including the aorta, vena cava, and main visceral branches. Study of intracranial artery branches is also possible.

Color Flow Imaging

An important later development was the color-coded Doppler system. A linear array transducer composed of many separate elements is used to produce a grid of sample volumes encompassing the area covered by the B-mode image (Fig. 14.4). A portion of the grid is selected for color-coding of velocity information. Each of the sample volumes within the area is examined. If the returning ultrasound signal has no change in phase or frequency, the amplitude information is used to create the grayscale image at that point in the matrix. If there is a change in phase or frequency, the information is analyzed in terms of velocity. A color is assigned to represent an approximate mean velocity occurring at that point in the field. Red and blue represent flow toward and away from the transducer. The magnitude of the velocity is represented by the hue of the color: a dark shade indicates slow flow, and a lighter shade or white indicates high flow. The aggregate of the color representation from the sample volumes detecting motion produces a real-time representation of the flow patterns within the vessels superimposed on the grayscale image of the stationary tissue. Fig. 14.5 illustrates examples of the advantages of color duplex scans. An additional tool is color-coding of the Doppler power (as opposed to velocity) detected. Power is proportional to the square of the velocity; therefore, this measurement provides more sensitive detection of very slow flow or flow in small vessels. A good example of the benefit of power imaging is the detection of an internal carotid string sign. Squaring the velocity eliminates the positive or negative value, so that power values have no directional representation. Power is represented in a single color, usually orange.

ARTERIAL STUDIES

Carotid Artery Studies

The internal carotid artery (ICA) poses a unique challenge to physical examination, because it is impossible to palpate a distal pulse. It is not uncommon to find a patient whose carotid pulse in the neck is normal to palpation but who has occlusion of the ICA. This limitation stimulated the development of physiologic tests to assess the status of the ICA. Most of the early tests provided indirect measurement by detecting distal changes in blood

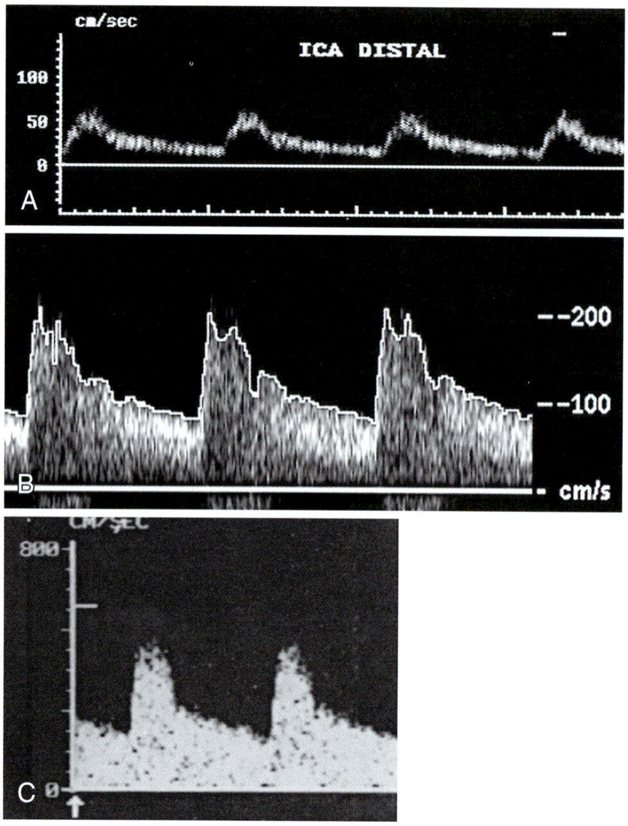

FIG 14.3 Doppler Sonograms From Carotid Duplex Scans. (A) Normal study with normal spectral width. (B) Moderate stenosis with spectral broadening but no increase in peak frequency. (Note that frequency scales are different in the three records.) (C) Severe stenosis with high peak velocity and extensive spectral broadening.

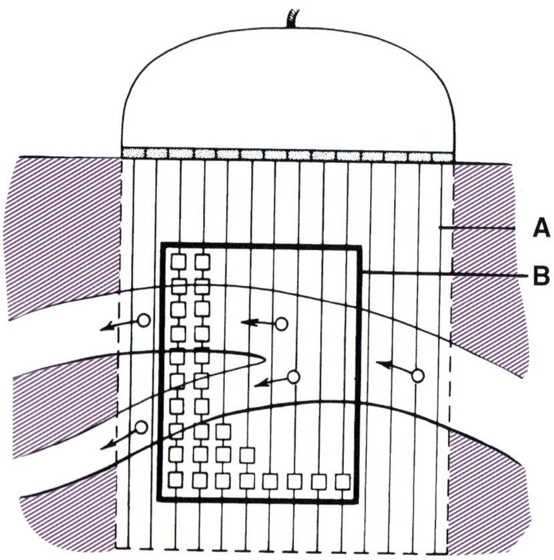

FIG 14.4 Duplex ultrasound system. A linear array transducer is used to create a matrix of sample volumes. A grayscale image is created within area *A*. Most examinations are performed with color-coding of velocities limited to a portion of the image (area *B*). Within this portion of the matrix, ultrasound pulses from sample volumes with a change in frequency are interpreted as velocity data. Otherwise, the data are coded as part of the grayscale image.

flow characteristics produced by advanced stenosis. Common features of the indirect methods are that they detect only lesions that are sufficiently advanced to reduce mean blood flow, and they cannot separate a tight stenosis from an occlusion because the physiologic changes in the distal bed may be indistinguishable. These methods achieved a variable degree of clinical use in the 1970s and 1980s, but were ultimately replaced by duplex scanning.

Duplex Scan (Duplex Ultrasound)

The routine examination covers as much of the CCA and its branches as can be visualized with the configuration of the transducer used. In some patients, the origins of the CCAs can be visualized. Figs. 14.2A and 14.5A show normal carotid bifurcations. The color image demonstrates the reverse velocity detected in the carotid bulb, as a result of the pattern of flow separation at the bifurcation. Many older patients have tortuosity that precludes the CCA, the bulb, and the branches from being visualized in a single plane; in such cases, careful scanning is required to obtain satisfactory imaging. Fig. 14.5B shows an example of tortuosity in an elderly patient. Although such arteries can be studied with a conventional scanner, the application of color flow and power Doppler simplifies the examination. The scan usually identifies the pathologic regions, but with advanced atherosclerosis, it is often difficult to get an adequate image to accurately estimate the degree of stenosis. Much of the classification of stenosis is based on interpretation of the Doppler signal. The two branches are distinguished by the image and the Doppler waveforms. The ICA has a low peripheral resistance at all times, resulting in forward flow throughout diastole, whereas the high resistance in the external carotid artery results in a diastolic flow of zero. Stenoses produce an increased velocity at the site of the lesion and turbulence beyond it (see Fig. 14.1). The turbulence is identified as spectral broadening on the sonogram (see Fig. 14.3). Mild stenoses may not produce a significant increase in PSV but are identified by a moderate degree of spectral broadening.

Stenosis Classification

Based on the PSV and the degree of spectral broadening, the ICA is placed into one of six diagnostic categories. There are two sets of criteria that have been used for many years, and although some laboratories have made modifications or adjustments, the basic principles continue to be applied. The criteria developed at the University of Washington use primarily ICA velocity parameters (Table 14.1).[2] Further improvements in accuracy can be obtained using ratios of ICA velocities to CCA velocities in normal portions of the artery (Table 14.2).[3] The diagnosis of ICA occlusion must be based on image and Doppler information, because the low flow found with some "string signs" is below the velocity detection threshold of many scanners. Contemporary scanners have improved our ability to find small residual flow channels, especially using power Doppler imaging. Both the stippled appearance of chronic thrombus and a small diameter of the ICA indicate occlusion. Overall, low-grade plaques are best assessed with the image, whereas advanced lesions are best evaluated with the Doppler information.

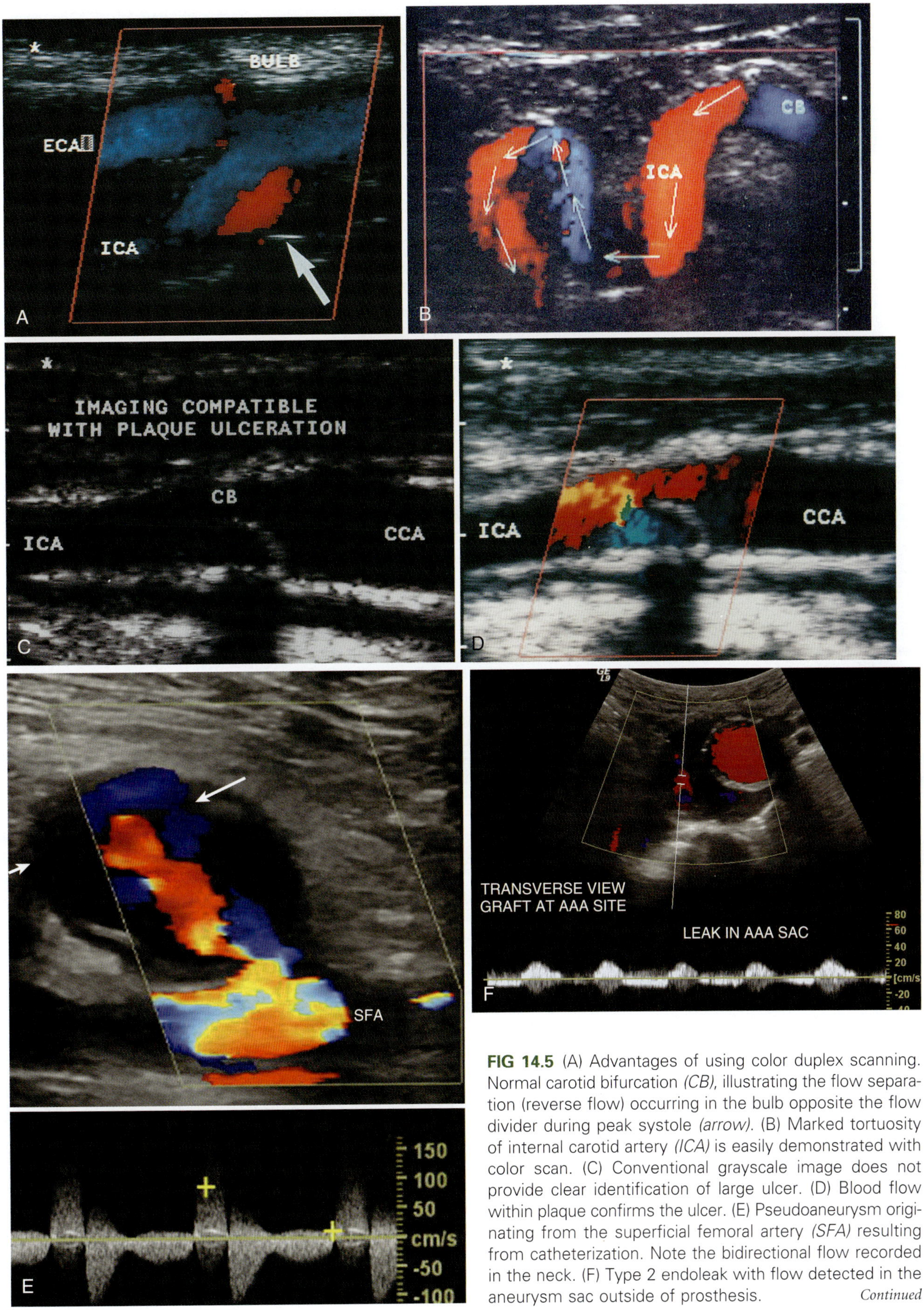

FIG 14.5 (A) Advantages of using color duplex scanning. Normal carotid bifurcation *(CB)*, illustrating the flow separation (reverse flow) occurring in the bulb opposite the flow divider during peak systole *(arrow)*. (B) Marked tortuosity of internal carotid artery *(ICA)* is easily demonstrated with color scan. (C) Conventional grayscale image does not provide clear identification of large ulcer. (D) Blood flow within plaque confirms the ulcer. (E) Pseudoaneurysm originating from the superficial femoral artery *(SFA)* resulting from catheterization. Note the bidirectional flow recorded in the neck. (F) Type 2 endoleak with flow detected in the aneurysm sac outside of prosthesis. *Continued*

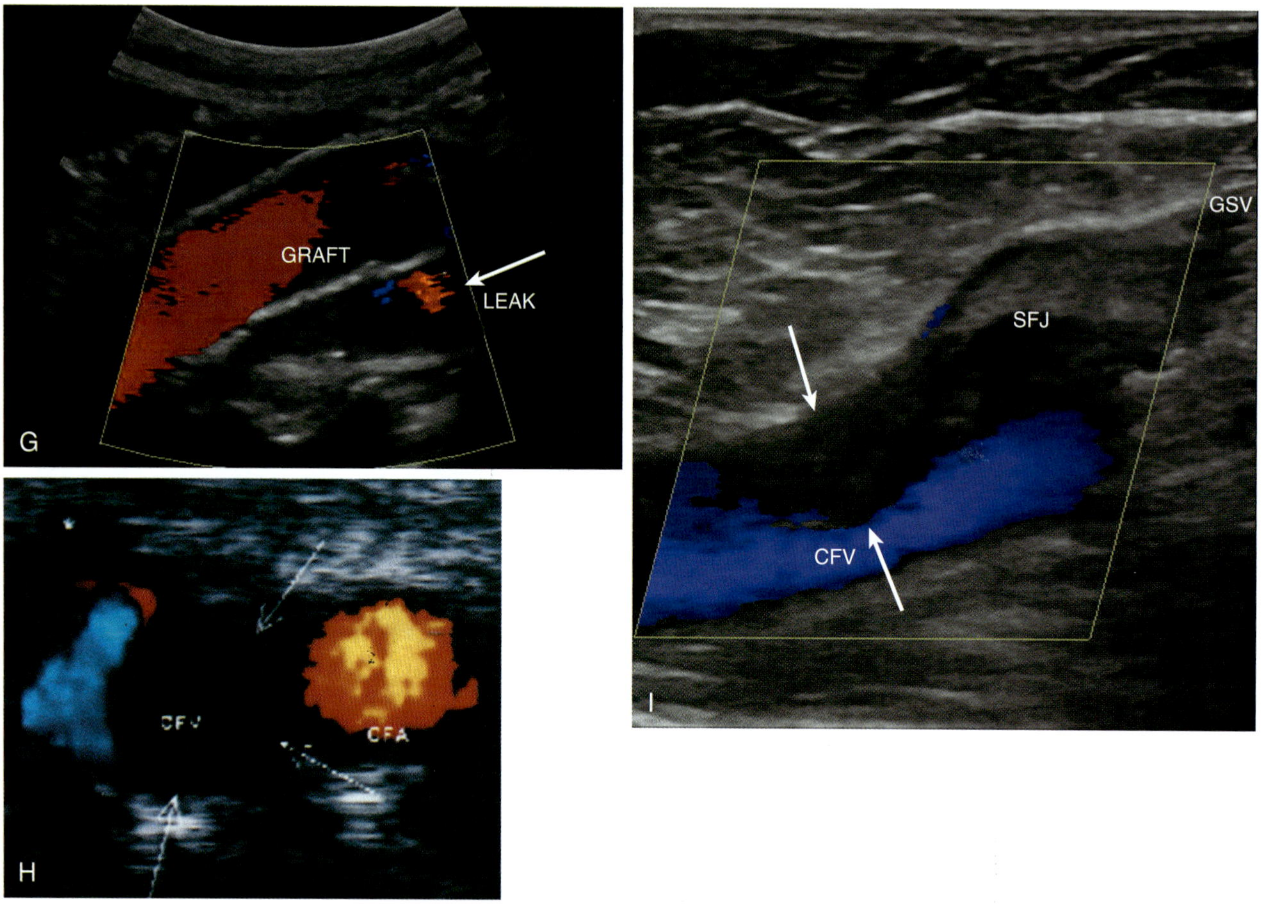

FIG 14.5, cont'd (G) Longitudinal view of same aorta showing leak is posterior to graft. (H) Blood flow around partial occluding thrombus. (I) Thrombus extending into common femoral vein *(CFV)* consistent with a level 4 endothermal heat induced thrombus, seen 2 days after endovascular ablation of great saphenous vein *(GSV)*. *CCA*, Common carotid artery; *CFA*, common femoral artery; *ECA*, external carotid artery; *SFJ*, saphenofemoral junction.

TABLE 14.1 Categories of Internal Carotid Artery Stenosis: University of Washington Criteria

ICA Stenosis	ICA Velocity	Spectrum
Normal vessel	Peak systolic velocity <125 cm/s	No broadening
1%–15%	Peak systolic velocity <125 cm/s	Limited broadening in late systole
16%–49%	Peak systolic velocity <125 cm/s	Broadening throughout systole
50%–79%	Peak systolic velocity >140 cm/s; end-diastolic velocity <140 cm/s	Broadening throughout systole
80%–99%	End-diastolic velocity >140 cm/s (severe stenosis may have very low velocity)	Broadening throughout systole
Occlusion	No ICA Doppler signal; flow to zero in common carotid artery	

ICA, Internal carotid artery.

TABLE 14.2 Categories of Internal Carotid Artery Stenosis: Bluth Criteria

ICA Stenosis	Peak Systolic Velocity (cm/s)	Diastolic Velocity (cm/s)	ICA/CCA Velocity
Normal vessel	<110	<40	<1.8
1%–39%	<115	<40	<1.8
40%–59%	<130	>40	<1.8
60%–79%	>130	>40	>1.8
80%–99%	>250 (severe stenosis may have very low velocity)	>100	>3.7
Occlusion	No ICA Doppler signal	No ICA Doppler signal	No ICA Doppler signal

CCA, Common carotid artery; *ICA*, internal carotid artery.

Duplex scanning has been adopted as the standard for carotid disease diagnosis and screening. Several studies have demonstrated that the technique can be highly accurate. These studies have shown rates of 92% to 96% accuracy in the identification of severe stenosis.[4-6] When these studies are analyzed in terms of correct category of stenosis, exact agreement is found in 77% to 87%, with poor agreement in only 1% to 2%. Of particular importance is the fact that experienced laboratories make few errors in separating severe stenosis from occlusion. Mansour and coauthors[7] reported a 98% positive predictive value and 99% negative predictive value in the correct determination of ICA occlusion.

Although the majority of attention has been focused on the carotid circulation, laboratories routinely investigate the status of the vertebral arteries as well. The examination seeks two types of problems: stenosis in the vertebral artery itself and the abnormal flow produced by subclavian steal, which has both an occlusion of the proximal subclavian artery and reversal of flow in the vertebral artery. In the majority of cases of significant vertebral stenosis, the lesion is located at the origin of the vessel. In some cases of severe occlusive disease, there is sufficient asymmetry in the waveforms of the two vertebral arteries to point to the problem side. However, a more complete assessment is obtained by examining the origins. Because of its deeper location, the left vertebral artery is more difficult to study than the right. Ackerstaff and associates[8] found that the status of the ostium could be studied satisfactorily in about 80% of patients. When adequate evaluation of the prevertebral portion was possible, a sensitivity of 80% and a specificity of 97% were achieved in the detection of reductions greater than 50% in diameter. Most clinical cases of subclavian steal are demonstrated by a reverse flow in the vertebral artery on the affected side. Von Reutern and Pourcelot[9] demonstrated that in some cases of subclavian stenosis there is distortion of the waveform rather than complete reversal of flow. The abnormal waveforms may have attenuation of the systolic component or an alternating pattern with reverse flow in systole and forward flow in diastole (Fig. 14.6). Such cases can be assessed more fully by recording the Doppler signal after arm exercise or the induction of reactive hyperemia. In the presence of advanced subclavian stenosis, this stress test produces full reversal of flow.

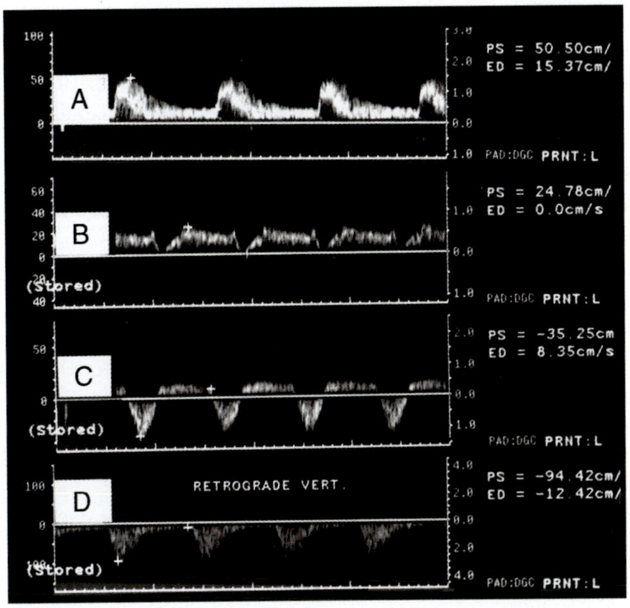

FIG 14.6 Vertebral artery Doppler waveforms. A is normal. B to D are signals recorded on the side of severe subclavian stenosis. (B) Attenuated systolic flow. (C) Reversed flow in systole, with forward flow in diastole. (D) Complete flow reversal.

Plaque Characteristics

In addition to estimating the severity of a stenosis, ultrasound can be used to study the plaque itself. Most investigators merely distinguish between homogeneous- and heterogeneous-appearing plaques and describe the surface as either smooth or irregular. More elaborate approaches to the description of morphology are being evaluated, but no single approach has been widely adopted.

Applications

Symptomatic carotid stenosis. A large number of transient ischemic attacks and strokes are caused by thromboembolization from plaques in the carotid bifurcation. In most situations, a duplex scan is the initial workup, identifying the location and severity of lesions in the carotid system. Many centers use the ultrasound study as the definitive test on which to base the decision to treat. Having an experienced vascular laboratory with a validated record of high accuracy in carotid scanning is the critical element in using duplex scanning as the definitive test. In other settings, additional confirmation is obtained with magnetic resonance or computed tomography angiography (CTA).

Asymptomatic carotid stenosis. Many asymptomatic patients are being referred to vascular laboratories for the evaluation of cervical bruits. Although some of these patients have bruits radiating from the heart or the great vessels, in a considerable number the sound originates from the carotid bifurcation. Duplex scanning can provide accurate separation according to category of stenosis (see Tables 14.1 and 14.2). Patients with severe stenosis are considered at increased risk of stroke and are evaluated for optimal medical and/or surgical treatment for stroke risk reduction. Lesions that fall in the moderate category (>50% stenosis) should have follow-up testing to detect those that progress into the high-risk group. Most people with normal vessels or early disease (<50% stenosis) do not require routine follow-up imaging.

Another indication is the screening of patients with advanced atherosclerotic disease in the coronary or peripheral vessels. Owing to the diffuse nature of atherosclerosis, some of these patients have occult carotid bifurcation lesions, with a resulting increased risk of stroke. Screening is performed most often in patients who are being considered for cardiac or major peripheral arterial operations to detect carotid lesions that may substantially increase the risk of perioperative stroke. Although screening may be appropriate for patients with multiple risk factors or severe occlusive disease in other arteries, routine testing of large populations results in a low yield of stenoses in the 80% to 99% category and is not cost-effective.

Intraoperative assessment. Over the years, there has been increasing use of completion studies to evaluate the status of the operated carotid artery before closing the neck. Contrast angiography is the most common technique used, usually with a single injection into the CCA below the level of the endarterectomy. Another approach is to examine the repair using a simple continuous-wave Doppler unit with subjective evaluation of the signals. This method detects severe residual stenoses but is not sensitive to other problems. Completion duplex scanning is being used to detect residual defects requiring correction, and studies have shown satisfactory results.[10-12] Bandyk and colleagues[13] used a PSV greater than 180 cm/s or a velocity ratio greater than 2.4 as the criterion to perform a confirmatory angiogram or to proceed directly to reopening the artery.[13]

Postoperative follow-up. Recurrent stenosis after carotid endarterectomy remains a clinical problem. Early studies reported as much as 5% symptomatic restenosis and 8% asymptomatic restenosis (as identified by noninvasive testing).[14,15] More recent studies applying life-table analysis have found restenosis rates of 20% to 32% with greater than 50% diameter reduction.[16,17] It has been shown that a substantial proportion of restenoses occur early in the postoperative period. A common practice is to obtain an early postoperative study that can be used as a baseline. Follow-up evaluations are done 6 and 12 months after surgery. If the study remains normal, noninvasive studies are repeated yearly. More recent studies show that in the presence of a normal completion angiogram or duplex scan, follow-up need not be performed until 1 year after operation.[18,19]

Lal and colleagues studied the application of carotid duplex for surveillance for restenosis after carotid artery stenting.[20] They examined 310 studies comparing poststenting duplex with either contrast angiogram or CTA. A PSV greater than 220 cm/s and an ICA/CCA ratio greater than 2.7 corresponded to greater than 50% restenosis. A PSV greater than 340 cm/s and an ICA/CCA ratio greater than 4.15 corresponded to greater than 80% restenosis. In general, the PSV and ICA/CCA ratio cut points were higher than those applied to native atherosclerotic stenosis.

Lower Extremity Arterial Studies and Physiologic Testing

Ankle-Brachial Index

Indirect measurement of extremity pressures has been performed since the beginning of the 20th century using a sphygmomanometer and auscultation of the Korotkoff sounds with a stethoscope. Although this technique is universally used to measure pressures in the brachial artery, its application in the lower extremity is less practical because of the difficulty of listening for Korotkoff sounds in the popliteal space. The technique is certainly not applicable in the distal portions of the extremity because of the small size of the vessels involved. Investigators overcame this limitation by using a variety of plethysmographic devices. In 1959, Winsor[21] first described the clinical measurement of arterial gradients using a plethysmograph. Systolic pressures in the lower extremity are normally higher than those in the upper extremity, due to the greater pulse pressure in the lower extremities. He described the blood pressure index (blood pressure of arm/blood pressure of leg), which in normal persons

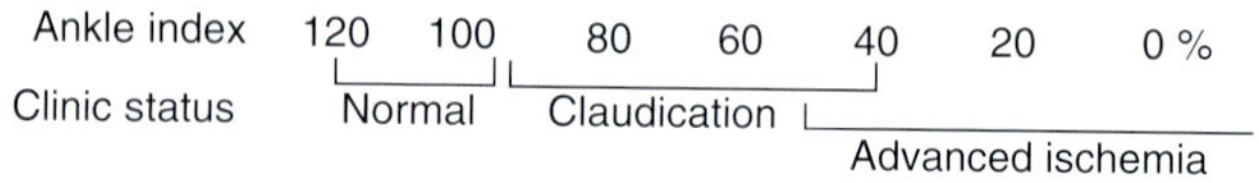

FIG 14.7 Relation of ankle-brachial index to patient symptoms.

is less than 1.0. A value greater than 1.0 indicates clinically significant occlusive disease proximal to the point of measurement. (Note that the ratio Winsor described is the inverse of the currently used ankle-brachial index.) The main limitation of this method is that it detects only occlusive lesions that are sufficiently advanced to reduce the systolic pressure, so that it is not possible to detect early disease. Introduction of continuous wave Doppler greatly simplified the indirect measurement of extremity pressures. For this application, the Doppler device is used merely to detect the presence or absence of the movement of blood in the artery. Measurements made by this method are reproducible, but do not provide diastolic pressure.

In clinical practice, simple screening can be performed by measuring the pressure in the brachial arteries and at the dorsal pedal and/or posterior tibial arteries on each side. The ankle-brachial index (ABI) is determined by dividing the higher ankle pressure on each side by the higher of the two brachial pressures. The resulting value reflects the severity of the occlusive disease for the entire extremity. Normally the ABI should be greater than 1.0, and values less than 0.9 are considered abnormal. Fig. 14.7 summarizes the general relation between ABI values and clinical status. It must be emphasized that this is only a rough correlation and that patients with similar values may have substantial differences in exercise tolerance. Likewise, the index at which rest pain appears varies considerably from patient to patient, ranging from 0.30 to 0.50.

Toe Pressures

An important limitation of the indirect measurement of extremity pressure is seen in patients with abnormal stiffening of the vessel wall, most often due to heavy calcification. Such conditions occur with diabetes mellitus but can also be found with other disorders. In these cases, the systolic pressure measured reflects the cuff pressure required to collapse the vessel wall, in addition to the pressure required to overcome the intraluminal pressure. In a few patients, it is not possible to stop the flow of blood at all. Error due to wall stiffness should be suspected whenever the ABI is greater than 1.3 or its value is out of proportion to the patient's clinical status. In general, a leg with a normal ABI should have an easily palpable ankle pulse. In some patients with stiff arteries, it may be possible to obtain an accurate evaluation by measuring the toe pressure. In a healthy person, there is a normal gradient of 20 to 30 mm Hg between the ankle and the toe; therefore a correction must be made when toe pressures are being used. A toe pressure of less than 30 mm Hg is considered significant, and below this level, wound healing is compromised.

Segmental Pressure Measurements

Localization of occlusive disease can be obtained by measuring the pressures at different levels of the leg. Segmental pressure measurements are usually performed by applying cuffs at the thigh, the upper calf, and immediately above the ankle. A standard adult-sized cuff (12 cm wide) is satisfactory for calf and ankle determinations, but a thigh cuff (18 cm) should be used above the knee. (Using a narrower cuff above the knee results in artificially high pressure measurements as a result of the size discrepancy between the cuff and the diameter of the thigh. Thigh measurements with an arm cuff usually result in determinations that are 20 to 30 mm Hg higher than those obtained with the wider cuff.) A thigh pressure lower than the brachial pressure indicates obstruction proximal to the location of the thigh cuff. Gradients of more than 20 mm Hg between measuring sites are diagnostic of occlusive disease in the intervening segment, and higher gradients are usually associated with more severe lesions.

An important limitation of the use of the wide cuff for thigh measurement is that it is possible to make only a single thigh measurement. As a result, it is not possible to distinguish occlusive disease above the inguinal ligament from that in the proximal portion of the superficial femoral artery, because both conditions can result in the same thigh pressure measurement. To overcome this problem, some investigators have recommended using 12-cm-wide cuffs to obtain two separate thigh measurements. When this is done, it is necessary to take into account the 20- to 30-mm Hg artifact in the results. In a study comparing the wide cuff with the two narrow-cuff techniques in the same group of patients, Heintz and coworkers[22] reported an increased accuracy in the localization of disease using the two-cuff technique. Both methods of thigh pressure measurement are still being used, so it is important to know which method is being reported when reviewing the results of patient studies. Although segmental pressures have been used extensively to detect proximal disease, diagnostic errors may occur in 25% of patients. Other techniques should be used when an accurate determination of the segmental localization is needed.

Stress Testing

Most patients with advanced arterial insufficiency are adequately evaluated by measurements at rest; however, less severe lesions may not produce a sufficient reduction of resting flow rates to be detected by the usual methods. An example of this problem is a patient with typical symptoms of claudication who has normal or borderline leg pressures. A more complete evaluation can be obtained by increasing the flow to accentuate the hemodynamic effect of the stenosis. The simplest and best way to increase blood flow is to have the patient walk. Exercise produces a decrease in vascular resistance in the leg, with a resulting increase in flow to the leg. With moderate levels of exercise, there is no change in distal pressures in a normal extremity, but increasing the flow through a moderate stenosis causes an increased resistance at the lesion. The resulting energy loss can be detected by noninvasive tests such as a pressure gradient or the attenuation of the pulse waveform.

The stress test is performed by having the patient walk on a treadmill for 5 minutes or until symptoms force the patient to stop. Most protocols use a low level of exercise (2 mph with a 10% to 12% grade). This level of stress is sufficient to yield an abnormal result in most claudication patients, without undue cardiac stress. Baseline arm and ankle pressures are measured with the Doppler detector. As soon as walking is completed, the patient lies down on the examining table for repeated pressure measurements, made at 30-second intervals during the first 2 minutes and at 60-second intervals for the remainder of the examination, usually 5 to 10 minutes. The examiner always asks the patient why he or she stopped walking, because in some cases the limiting factor is angina, shortness of breath, or degenerative hip pain rather than true claudication. Identification of these limitations is an important benefit of the stress test because it may uncover or emphasize the significance of these other conditions.

One objective measurement of the severity of occlusive disease is exercise tolerance (i.e., the time the patient walks at the standardized rate). Further assessment is based on the changes in extremity pressures. Fig. 14.8 shows the time-pressure relations seen in control subjects and in different categories of occlusive disease. Healthy people have no significant change or augmentation in ankle pressures, with the modest level of exercise used for the stress test. In contrast, patients with flow-limiting proximal stenoses have a drop in distal pressures as a result of vasodilatation in the muscles. The magnitude of the drop in both ABI and recovery time are increased with more severe occlusive disease. Multiple lesions produce more marked depression of the recovery curve than single lesions.

There are some situations in which treadmill exercise is not practical or does not offer the best evaluation. In such cases, reactive hyperemia can be used to increase blood flow in the extremities. A thigh cuff inflated above systolic pressure produces local circulatory arrest, resulting in hypoxia and local vasodilatation. When the cuff is released, there is a transient increase in flow, the duration of which is related to the period of ischemia and to the total blood flow to the leg. The magnitude of the pressure drop is comparable with that seen after walking, but the recovery is always more rapid with reactive hyperemia. In

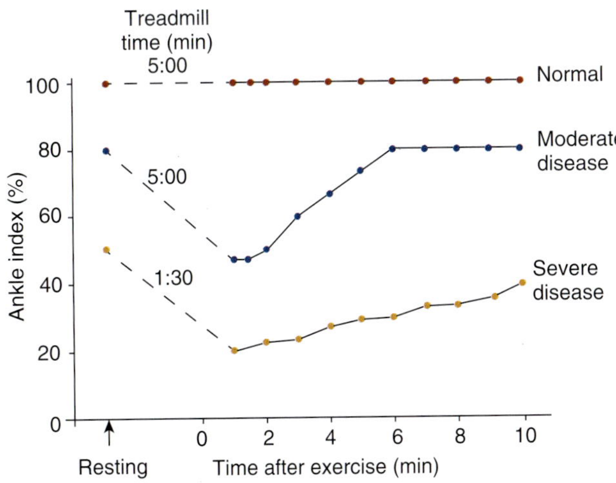

FIG 14.8 Changes in ankle-brachial index with exercise. The severity of the arterial stenosis is related to the exercise tolerance and the magnitude of the drop in ankle pressure and recovery time.

contrast to exercise, reactive hyperemia does produce a transient pressure drop (with a rapid recovery) in normal subjects. Criteria for a normal result are when the lowest ABI is greater than 0.80 and return of the index to 90% of the baseline value occurs within 1 minute.[23] The technique provides a useful test for patients who cannot walk on the treadmill because of disabilities or those who are unwilling to perform adequately on the treadmill, and for the full evaluation of the less-involved limb in patients with marked asymmetry of their occlusive disease.

In general, stress testing is not routinely needed in patients seen in the vascular laboratory. Those with significant abnormalities at rest always have abnormal responses to exercise. An exercise ABI can be reserved for patients with typical symptoms of arterial insufficiency but normal or near-normal resting studies, and those with confusing symptoms in whom one wants to exclude arterial insufficiency as a cause. The stress examination is also useful for research studies in which more sensitivity for the detection of improvement or deterioration is needed.

Doppler Waveform Evaluation

Most commercial Doppler detectors provide an analog signal that is proportional to the velocity of the blood in the vessel studied. This signal can be displayed on a screen or recorded. The overall shape of the waveform reflects the status of the vessel proximal to the point studied (Fig. 14.9). In the lower extremity, the normal velocity wave is triphasic, with reverse flow in early diastole. Proximal stenosis first eliminates the reverse flow; with more severe lesions, there is blunting of the systolic upstroke and increasing flow during diastole. The simplest analysis of Doppler waveforms is a qualitative interpretation of the curves, allowing the identification of broad categories of disease. One specific application has been the assessment of the aortoiliac segment. However, the method suffers from a high false-positive rate, resulting from the fact that an attenuated wave can be caused by proximal disease, distal disease, or a combination of the two.

A variety of techniques for quantitative analysis of the Doppler waveform have been described. These investigations have largely focused on separating significant inflow occlusive disease from that below the inguinal ligament. Although each method evaluated offers some additional diagnostic benefit, none has achieved widespread application. Burnham and colleagues[24] proposed the measurement of common femoral artery acceleration time (onset of systole to peak systole) to identify significant aortoiliac disease. An acceleration time greater than 133 ms is found with proximal stenosis.

Segmental Plethysmography and Pulse Volume Recording

During systole, the blood entering a limb normally causes an increase in the total volume of the extremity, with a return to resting volume during diastole. This phenomenon is responsible for the pulse pressure oscillations seen with the sphygmomanometer while taking blood pressure. The total volume change is small and can be detected only with the aid of sensitive devices. A variety of plethysmographic recorders have been devised using a mercury strain gauge, water displacement, capacitance, and impedance systems, but the majority of these systems have proved to be impractical for routine clinical application. In the early 1970s, the pulse-volume recorder was designed specifically for peripheral arterial diagnosis. The system uses a calibrated recording air plethysmograph, with standard blood pressure cuffs applied at the thigh, calf, and ankle levels. The cuffs are inflated to 65 mm Hg to ensure optimal contact of the cuff around the extremity. A sensitive transducer detects the small increase in pressure within the cuff resulting from the volume increase of the extremity during systole. The recorder provides a hard-copy tracing of the pulse wave, which has been demonstrated to be similar to arterial pressure waves measured directly. The primary diagnosis is based on a qualitative evaluation of the pulse-volume waveform.[25] The tracing from each level is categorized as normal, mildly abnormal, moderately abnormal, or severely abnormal. The normal tracing has a brisk, sharp rise to the systolic peak and usually displays a prominent dicrotic notch (Fig. 14.10). Early disease is characterized by the absence of a dicrotic notch and a more gradual, prolonged downslope. Moderate disease is characterized by a rounded systolic peak. Severe occlusive disease produces a flattened wave with a slow upstroke and downstroke. The absolute amplitude measurements are of limited value from patient to patient, because substantial changes result from variations in cardiac output and vasomotor tone. Comparison of amplitudes from each side in the same patient can be of value in assessing unilateral disease. In the presence of bilateral disease, it can be helpful to standardize the amplitude measurements in the lower extremities by comparing them with arm tracings, because most patients do not have major upper extremity occlusive disease. Serial pulse-volume measurements have been shown to be reproducible in patients with stable disease, so that amplitude changes indicate the progression of disease.

The pulse-volume recorder has received extensive application. In most situations, the plethysmographic studies are used in combination with segmental Doppler pressure measurements. Vascular laboratories report that it is a useful adjunct to routine pressure measurements. One particular advantage is the ability

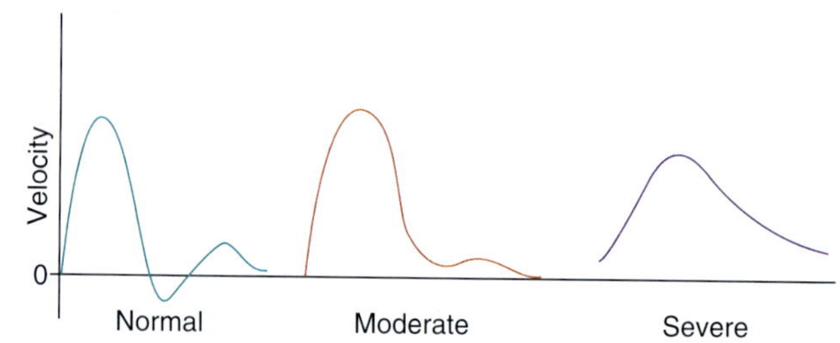

FIG 14.9 Doppler velocity tracings in the leg. Increasing stenosis results in elimination of reverse flow, decrease in systolic peak, and increase in flow during diastole.

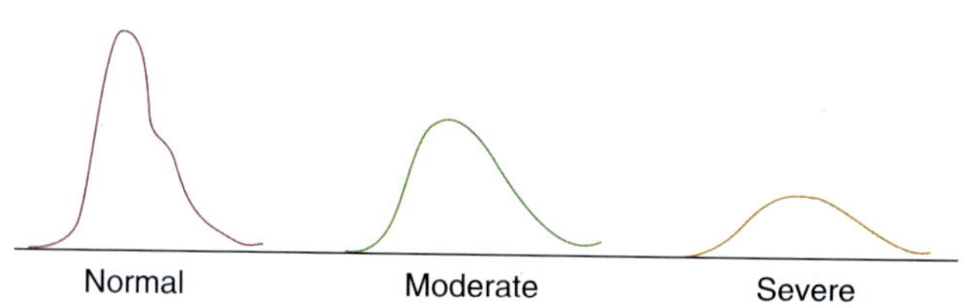

FIG 14.10 Pulse-volume recorder tracings in the leg. Increasing stenosis results in loss of the dicrotic notch and flattening of the curve.

to accurately assess the presence or absence of occlusive disease in patients with rigid arteries. In addition, the pulse-volume recorder has improved the detection of aortoiliac stenosis. Kempczinski[26] reported the correct identification of advanced inflow disease in 95% of extremities.

Arterial Duplex Scan

The duplex scan is now frequently used to evaluate peripheral arteries. With appropriate scan heads, Doppler signals can be obtained from the aorta down to the tibial branches. Screening for occlusive disease can be done by comparing signals from the distal aorta and more distal sites. A more complete assessment is obtained by examining the full length of the segment in question, looking for the increased velocity and spectral broadening produced by a stenosis. The color-coded Doppler scan makes tracking of the vessels and localizing of significant stenoses considerably easier than with conventional scanners. The most common practice is to use the ratio of the PSV recorded at the tightest part of the stenosis to the PSV recorded in a normal portion of the same artery. A ratio greater than 2 defines a greater than 50% diameter reduction of the lumen.[27,28] Some groups have established additional criteria to distinguish stenosis greater than 75%. Cossman and colleagues[29] consider the stenosis to be greater than 75% if the velocity ratio is greater than 4 or the peak velocity in the lesion is greater than 400 cm/s.[29] Gonsalves and Bandyk[30] identify a severe lesion by a velocity ratio greater than 4, a peak velocity greater than 300 cm/s, or an end-diastolic velocity greater than 100 cm/s.

Mesenteric/Renal Testing

Scanning is also used for visceral vessels, including the arteries of normal and transplanted kidneys. The anterior approach to visceral branches can be difficult owing to the presence of bowel gas. Flank approaches and examination of a fasting patient increase the rate of successful studies. Most renal artery stenoses occur at the origins, so it is necessary to obtain recordings from the proximal part of the vessel. As with peripheral lesions, the focus has been on identifying hemodynamically significant stenoses. A PSV greater than 180 cm/s identifies an abnormal vessel, and a ratio of the peak velocity in the stenosis to the peak velocity in the aorta at the level of the renal arteries greater than 3.5 predicts a stenosis with a greater than 60% lumen diameter reduction.[31-33] Another approach has been to use the waveform recorded in the renal hilum.[34] Although recording hilar signals is usually easier than examining the main renal arteries, this approach does not seem to be as accurate in the diagnosis of significant stenoses.[33] An important limitation of the duplex scan in the evaluation of renal disease is that accessory branches are often missed.

Duplex scanning has also been used to study the mesenteric branches. The celiac trunk and the proximal superior mesenteric artery can be located easily. In contrast, the inferior mesenteric artery is often not found unless it provides significant collateral flow because of occlusions in other branches. Unlike the situation with the kidneys, the perfusion to the gut is highly variable, depending on physiologic responses to feeding. Therefore it is important to obtain baseline studies of patients in a fasting state. Severe stenosis is identified by a significant focal increase in velocity, combined with poststenotic turbulence and reduced velocity beyond the stenosis. Moneta and colleagues[35] found that peak systolic velocities greater than 200 cm/s in the celiac artery and 275 cm/s in the superior mesenteric artery indicate stenosis greater than 70%.[35] Zwolak and colleagues found that end-diastolic velocities greater than 55 cm/s in the celiac artery and 45 cm/s in the superior mesenteric artery indicate stenosis greater than 50%.[36]

Applications

Severity and Location of Arterial Lesions

The primary use of noninvasive tests in patients with lower extremity problems is to obtain objective determinations to supplement the physical examination. Such measurements permit reproducibility between different examiners, as well as from one time to another. In addition, the tests are valuable in measuring the progression of arterial disease and assessing arterial reconstructions. Extremity pressures and pulse plethysmographic recordings are valuable to assess disease severity; however, duplex scanning must be used for an accurate determination of the level and extent of lesions. Kohler and associates[27] found a sensitivity of 89% and a specificity of 90% in the identification of iliac stenosis greater than 50%. Legemate and coworkers[37] used a velocity increase of 150% and found a sensitivity of 92% and specificity of 98%. It is possible to estimate common femoral artery blood flow with duplex scan measurements, but the high variability in repeat measurements in individual patients limits the clinical usefulness of this approach.[38] Although further refinement of quantitative criteria is required, it is clear that duplex scanning can play an increasing role in the evaluation of peripheral arterial insufficiency.

Operative Planning

Following the lead of those performing carotid endarterectomy without preoperative angiography, investigators have reported the feasibility of planning arterial peripheral interventions and open operations with only the ultrasound scan.[29,39-42] Wain and coauthors[42] reported that duplex mapping is accurate down to the popliteal level, but in their experience, the technique is not as good at defining an appropriate target vessel at the crural level.[42] More recent studies have shown improved results with mapping of the entire lower leg in order to plan the appropriate bypass operation, including selection of the site of distal anastomosis.[43,44] Adequate visualization of the peroneal artery in the lower calf remains one of the challenges for the examiner.

Procedural Complications

With the increasing frequency of percutaneous revascularization procedures, a need has developed for the evaluation of extremity complications. The duplex scan provides a simple tool to assess the appearance of a mass adjacent to an arterial puncture site. The primary question is whether the mass is simply a hematoma or whether there is an early pseudoaneurysm, possibly complicated by an arteriovenous fistula. Fig. 14.5E shows a pseudoaneurysm originating from the superficial femoral artery. There is a small diameter neck off the artery with flow into the adjacent space. The Doppler waveform from the neck shows a bidirectional pattern typical of a pseudoaneurysm. In the case of a hematoma, there is a homogeneous mass (with no blood flow) adjacent to the vessels, which would appear normal on scan.

Intraoperative Assessment

As with carotid surgery, duplex scanning provides an excellent tool for completion assessment after certain other arterial operations. In many operating rooms, scanning can be done more quickly and provide a more complete examination than can a conventional contrast angiogram. Often, short focal defects such as a retained valve are easily seen on a scan but may not be well demonstrated angiographically, especially with a single film study. Bandyk and associates[45] reported on scanning after infrainguinal bypass grafts. The examination involves scanning the full length of the graft, including both anastomoses. A PSV greater than 180 cm/s or a velocity ratio greater than 2.4 indicates a problem for which revision must be considered. Bandyk and associates[45] reported intraoperative revision rates of 14% to 16%. Fifty-two percent of the legs with significant duplex findings that were not repaired at the time of the original operation underwent subsequent revision.

Intraoperative duplex scanning has also been advocated for renal artery repairs to reduce the risk of early occlusion and possible loss of the kidney. Studies from both Wake Forest and the Mayo Clinic reported an 11% incidence of the detection of defects requiring repair at the time of the original procedure.[46,47] A focal high-velocity jet with a PSV greater than 200 cm/s combined with distal turbulence identifies a tight stenosis, whereas lack of flow in the vessel indicates acute thrombosis.[46] Both these findings mandate immediate revision.

Graft Surveillance

Because of the poor secondary patency of vein grafts that thrombose, close follow-up is recommended after vein graft bypass. As early as 1972, some surgeons advocated postoperative noninvasive testing to identify hemodynamic changes. For many years, graft status was monitored with pressure measurements; however, this technique has limited value in patients with stiff arteries or with small-caliber distal bypasses. In 1985 Bandyk and associates[48] reported good results with graft surveillance using the duplex scanner to measure the PSV. In this study, a peak velocity of less than 40 cm/s was associated with early graft thrombosis. In later years, the surveillance protocol was expanded to include a sampling of the graft velocity and a scan of the entire graft.[49,50] Such mapping permits the identification of the specific site of stenosis. A PSV of 180 to 200 cm/s indicates a problem. Bandyk and Johnson[50] recommended intervention for any lesion with a PSV greater than 300 cm/s or a velocity ratio greater than 3.5. A large proportion of stenoses are found within the first postoperative year; therefore, a program of close surveillance is advocated by many authors.[51-53] The fact that significant problems can appear later is a reason to continue surveillance beyond the first year, albeit at a reduced frequency.

Aortic/Mesenteric Endovascular Stent Surveillance

Over the past 2 decades, there has been an explosion in the use of endograft placement for treating aortic aneurysms. Unlike open repair, the endovascular procedure was found to have a substantial incidence of postprocedure complications, primarily endoleaks (see Chapter 41). From the early days of the procedure, surgeons used CTA to evaluate postoperative results. The common practice was to obtain studies at 6 months, 1 year, and then annually. Increasing concern over the radiation exposure and the repeated administration of nephrotoxic contrast agents to visualize graft patency and endoleaks has led some investigators to evaluate the use of ultrasound for endograft surveillance.[54] Arko and associates compared findings on postoperative CTA and duplex scan.[55] There was a close correlation of aneurysm diameters, and duplex scan had a 90% negative predictive value. Most of the endoleaks missed were type 2 and caused by small lumbar arteries. Improved scanning techniques and equipment have resulted in the increasing use of ultrasound surveillance of endografts. Many surgeons obtain an initial postoperative CTA, and if it is normal, they use duplex ultrasound for routine follow-up.[56] Fig. 14.5F and G shows a typical type 2 endoleak.

AbuRahma and colleagues studied duplex criteria for surveillance after celiac and superior mesenteric artery stenting.[57] They examined patients who underwent concurrent postoperative duplex imaging and angiography and found that the PSV values for significant post-stent restenosis were higher than those for the native vessels. A PSV greater than 363 cm/s for a celiac artery stent corresponded to greater than 70% stenosis with a sensitivity of 88%, specificity of 92%, and accuracy of 90%. A PSV greater than 412 cm/s for the SMA corresponded to greater than 70% stent stenosis with a sensitivity of 100%, specificity of 95%, and accuracy of 97%.

VENOUS DISEASE

The correct diagnosis of venous abnormalities can be challenging. In contrast to arterial occlusive disease, venous disease may be difficult to distinguish from other problems on the basis of physical examination alone. In the past, venous disease diagnoses depended on venography, which, in addition to being painful, can precipitate thrombosis in a normal venous system. In the 1960s Strandness and coworkers[58] and Sigel and colleagues[59] used the simple continuous-wave Doppler to identify normal and abnormal flow patterns in the veins of the leg. With the subsequent development of noninvasive techniques for the arterial system, there was a parallel growth in the methods of venous diagnosis. The 1970s and 1980s saw extensive use of physiologic methods such as impedance phlebography, but these tests have been completely replaced by duplex scanning.

Doppler Venous Examination

The flow in the extremity veins can be evaluated qualitatively with a continuous-wave Doppler detector. The patient is examined in the supine position with the head slightly elevated. The deep veins are found adjacent to the accompanying arteries. A normal vein has spontaneous flow with a phasic variation with respiration. Breath-holding or a Valsalva maneuver decreases or abolishes flow; with release, there is a transient augmentation of the signal. A quick compression of the extremity distal to the probe produces flow augmentation, often followed by a transient decrease on release. Proximal abdominal or leg compression decreases or abolishes the flow signal, with augmentation occurring on release. Examination of a thrombosed segment of vein shows no flow, and adjacent collateral veins have a high-pitched signal. The patent portion of the vein distal to an obstruction has a continuous flow with no respiratory variation, and the Valsalva maneuver produces no change. Limb compression can produce limited augmentation, but clearly less than that in the normal vein. The vein segment proximal to an occlusion may have phasic flow, similar to a normal leg, but distal compression produces little change. The Doppler examination is sensitive to alterations in venous flow patterns, and different forms of extrinsic compression can produce similar changes. Abnormal studies can result from diseases in the vein, as well as extrinsic compression due to large hematomas, massive edema, or ruptured popliteal cysts. A false-positive test can also occur with advanced pregnancy, ascites, morbid obesity, or abdominal masses compressing the inferior vena cava.

The Doppler venous examination can also detect venous valvular insufficiency. Normally there should be no flow produced by compression proximal to the probe, because the valves prevent flow toward the probe. With incompetent valves, proximal compression (or a Valsalva maneuver) produces augmentation, as a result of the retrograde flow. Demonstration of significant reverse flow of greater than 500 ms duration is clear evidence of venous insufficiency and valvular incompetence. The venous examination with a continuous wave device was once an important test for acute deep venous thrombosis (DVT) in the leg, but it has been supplanted by quantitative imaging techniques with pulsed wave Doppler.

Duplex Scan

The high resolution available with duplex scanners makes it possible to visualize venous thrombosis. In this application, the emphasis is on imaging. Thrombus is seen within the vein lumen with varying degrees of echogenicity (Fig. 14.11). On occasion, fresh thrombus may look no different from flowing blood; in these instances, additional assessment is obtained by compressing the vein with the probe. Normally gentle pressure flattens the vein completely (Fig. 14.12). A partially or totally occluding thrombus prevents collapse in response to external pressure. Compression is performed in the transverse mode to ensure accurate evaluation with the maneuver. When examining in the longitudinal orientation, it is possible to move the ultrasound beam off the center of the vein so that the vein appears to collapse when it actually does not. Occluded segments can also be identified by the lack of flow on Doppler examination, and determination of flow characteristics should be part of every study. Abnormalities in Doppler velocity signals either at rest or in response to augmentation maneuvers indicate lesions that might not be evident with imaging. Color-coded Doppler is especially helpful in detecting partial occluding thrombi (see Fig. 14.5H). The color scanner has also improved the examination of the calf veins, which are paired alongside of the arteries, and therefore more difficulty to see without color flow.

Most centers perform a detailed examination from the inguinal ligament to the calf veins. In addition to the deep system, superficial veins can be imaged. The greatest difficulty in many

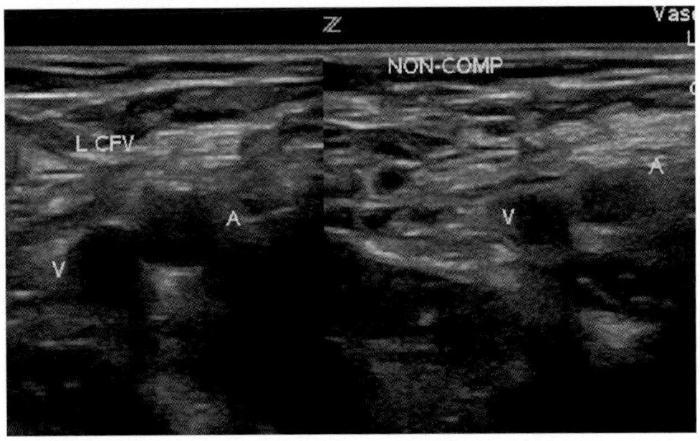

FIG 14.11 B-mode scan of venous thrombus. Note the noncompressibility *(NON-COMP)* of the vein lumen diagnostic for venous thrombosis. *A*, Artery; *V*, vein; *L CFV*, left common femoral vein.

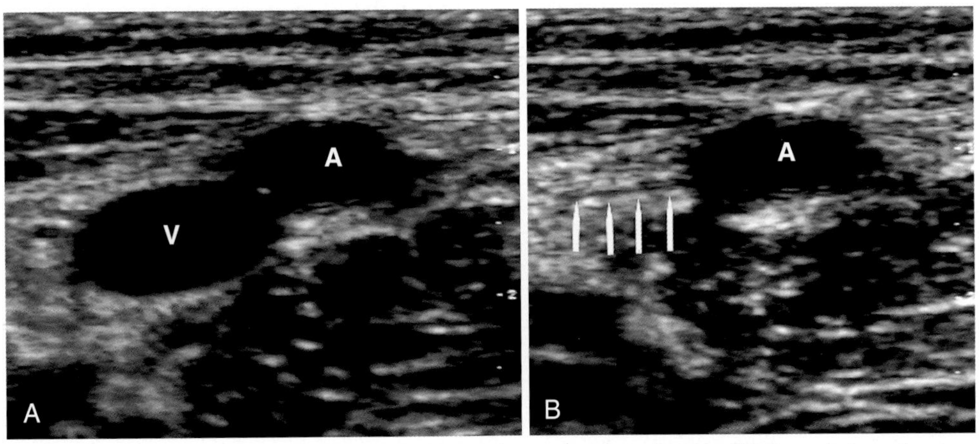

FIG 14.12 Transverse duplex scans. (A) Normal appearance of vein. (B) Complete collapse of vein in response to external compression with the probe. *A*, Artery; *V*, vein.

examinations is following the vein through the adductor canal. The common femoral and femoral veins are examined in the supine position with moderate leg dependency. (The deep femoral vein is usually not followed beyond its origin.) The popliteal vein is best imaged with the patient in the lateral or prone position. Infrapopliteal branches can be difficult to evaluate fully; however, special attention should be given to these whenever the patient has focal calf symptoms. The other problem area is detecting thrombus in the common or external iliac veins. It is difficult to image these veins; therefore one must often rely on indirect evidence, provided by the flow signal from the common femoral vein. Proximal occlusion causes a loss of phasic variation with respiration and limited or no change with the Valsalva maneuver. Vogel and coworkers described using the change in common femoral vein diameter during the Valsalva maneuver—an increase of less than 10% indicates suspicion for iliofemoral thrombosis.[60]

Duplex scanning of the deep leg veins for thrombus is technically difficult and requires considerable experience for an accurate diagnosis. Experienced investigators have reported sensitivities and specificities of approximately 95% for the diagnosis of thrombus.[60-63] Although most studies have focused on acute thrombosis, Rollins and associates demonstrated the same high accuracy in the identification of chronic disease.[62] In addition, they reported 89% accuracy in the evaluation of calf veins, compared with 93% for the proximal veins. When thrombus is identified, the clinician usually wants to know the duration of the process. Currently there is no specific method for determining this age, but generally an acute thrombus has a hypoechoic, homogeneous appearance on grayscale imaging, the vein lumen is distended, and a "floating tail" may be found at the upper end of the thrombus. In the chronic phase, the lesion is more echoic and typically has a heterogeneous appearance. The vein diameter becomes smaller than normal, and venous collaterals may be found.

Ultrasound is also used to evaluate reflux in specific venous segments. Many laboratories perform this evaluation in a casual fashion, examining patients in the recumbent position. Van Bemmelen and associates[64] emphasized the need to examine the patient in the standing position to recreate the maximum stimulus for reflux.[64] In addition, they pointed out the importance of adequate compression. A reverse velocity of 30 cm/s is necessary for consistent valvular closure.[65] Inadequate compression may result in incomplete closure. In such a case, slow reverse flow can occur through a normal valve, leading to the interpretation of an abnormal segment.

Applications

Acute Deep Venous Thrombosis

Clinicians are aware of the fallibility of physical findings in the diagnosis of acute DVT of the leg; therefore most of the effort toward the noninvasive diagnosis of venous disease has focused on acute occlusion. Duplex scanning is the primary modality used to diagnose acute DVT. Many institutions perform alternative imaging studies only in patients with nondiagnostic scans or when the scan cannot be obtained. This practice has been justified by the high accuracy achieved by different investigators.[60-63]

A major advantage of scanning is the ability to identify the specific location of disease, especially when there are thrombi at multiple levels. Another important advantage is the detection of partially occluding thrombi, a key limitation of the physiologic techniques used in the past. In addition to confirming the initial diagnosis, scanning can be used to document changes and resolution during therapy.

Recurrent/Chronic Deep Venous Thrombosis

The diagnosis of recurrent DVT in patients with postthrombotic syndrome presents a great challenge to clinicians. Exacerbation of symptoms can mimic the symptoms of the original thrombosis, and in many cases patients are given anticoagulants without objective evidence of recurrence. Noninvasive testing can be used to obtain an objective diagnosis, and comparison of a new study with an old study can determine if new thrombus has formed. Duplex scanning can also identify residual chronic thrombus by its high echogenicity. Other characteristics include thickened vein walls, fibrosed segments of occluded veins, and valvular insufficiency with reverse flow on Doppler examination. These features allow the examiner to use a duplex scan to distinguish recent from chronic clot; this contrasts with the venogram, which shows all lesions as filling defects.

Venous Insufficiency

The complications of chronic venous stasis are usually obvious, but it may be difficult to assess the relative contributions of outflow obstruction and reflux. Although the initial conservative management is similar, further surgical treatment is directed to the specific cause. Doppler examination can determine the presence of venous reflux. Measurement of reverse blood flow greater than 500 ms in duration provides a quantitative assessment that is not available with the simpler tests.[64,66] Duplex ultrasound of the superficial, perforator, and deep veins can determine the most likely site and cause of the venous insufficiency, and this information can help in the selection of specific interventions.

Preoperative Vein Mapping

For the use of the great saphenous vein as a surgical conduit, knowledge of the patient's specific anatomy is important. Using contrast venograms, Shah and associates[67] demonstrated that only 65% of thighs and 45% of calves had a single saphenous trunk. The rest had variants of double systems and cross-connections. Because of the risks of contrast venography, duplex scanning has become the standard method of mapping the superficial veins in both the arms and the legs.[68,69] High resolution of the images permits a determination of size, course, double segments, and varicosities. These findings correlate closely with superficial venous anatomy found during surgery.

Follow-Up of Endovenous Ablation

Endovenous closure has become the leading treatment for major reflux of the great saphenous vein. Early experience with closure techniques showed a high incidence of vein closure; however, there was concern about possible extension of the thrombosis into the deep system and a chance of subsequent pulmonary embolization (see Chapter 53). Most practitioners obtain a duplex scan in the first week following the procedure, looking for proximal extension. Fig. 14.5I (see color panel) shows thrombus extending from the saphenofemoral junction, adherent to the anterior wall of the common femoral vein without occlusion of this vein. Lawrence and colleagues[70] have established a classification for levels of thrombosis following ablation procedures.

CONCLUSIONS

Development of noninvasive vascular laboratory devices and techniques has increased the amount of objective arterial and venous data that can be obtained noninvasively on a patient. As is the case with other diagnostic modalities, it is critical to remember that these tests should always supplement, and not replace, the information gained from a careful history and physical examination. It is increasingly common to find young physicians relying on vascular laboratory test results before completing a complete history and exam, which allows for a correlation of the vascular lab findings with presenting symptoms and physical findings. In addition, the practice of sending patients to the noninvasive laboratory for "diagnosis of a vascular condition" without an examination results in many inappropriate tests with corresponding unnecessary treatments and costs.

Optimal use of noninvasive test results requires an understanding of both the value and limitations of specific examinations. The choice of noninvasive tests must be based on the clinical questions to be answered; some questions cannot be answered by noninvasive techniques; for example, they cannot currently detect small ulcers in the carotid arteries. In addition, errors, both false-positives and false-negatives, occur with all diagnostic studies; therefore it is important to be aware of the accuracy of the tests being used. Published studies often represent the best that can be obtained, and newly established laboratories often do not achieve optimal results. Therefore, to apply noninvasive results appropriately, it is important to know the accuracy in the laboratory performing the test.

REVIEW QUESTIONS

1. Measuring thigh pressures with a regular arm blood pressure cuff affects the determination in what way?
   a. It is higher than the actual pressure.
   b. It is equal to the actual pressure.
   c. It is lower than the actual pressure.
2. The right ankle index is calculated by dividing the higher ankle pressure by which of the following?
   a. Right brachial pressure
   b. Left brachial pressure
   c. Higher brachial pressure
   d. Lower brachial pressure
3. An ankle-brachial index of 1.60 indicates which of the following?
   a. Normal arterial system
   b. Significant arterial insufficiency
   c. Pathologic vessel wall stiffness
   d. Arteriovenous fistula in the extremity
   e. None of the above
4. When evaluating a patient with an exercise stress test, the severity of occlusive disease is evaluated by what means?
   a. Walking time
   b. Magnitude of drop in ankle-brachial index
   c. Recovery time
   d. All of the above
   e. None of the above
5. Noninvasive cerebrovascular techniques are accurate for all of the following except:
   a. Detecting advanced stenosis of the internal carotid artery
   b. Detecting internal carotid occlusion
   c. Detecting arterial ulceration
   d. Detecting abnormal turbulence in the internal carotid artery
6. For a given arterial velocity, the magnitude of the Doppler frequency shift is related to which of the following?
   a. Distance from the probe
   b. Frequency of the probe
   c. Type of system (pulse or continuous wave)
   d. All of the above
   e. None of the above
7. Which of the following statements is true about spectral broadening of a Doppler signal?
   a. It is greatest proximal to a stenosis.
   b. It is greatest in the stenosis.
   c. It is greatest just beyond a stenosis.
   d. It is the same at all the above sites.
8. When using duplex scanning, very low velocities are best detected by which modality?
   a. Power Doppler imaging
   b. Color Doppler imaging
   c. Sonogram of pulsed Doppler signal
9. Which of these findings is not associated with an acute deep vein thrombosis?
   a. Presence of venous collateral
   b. Enlarge venous diameter
   c. Echolucent mass in vein
   d. "Floating tail" of the thrombus
10. Suitability of a superficial femoral artery for treatment with balloon dilatation can be determined by which of the following?
    a. Segmental pressures
    b. Volume plethysmography
    c. Duplex scan
    d. All of the above
    e. None of the above

BIBLIOGRAPHY

AbuRhama A, Bergan J, eds. *Noninvasive Vascular Diagnosis*. ed 2. New York: Springer-Verlag; 2007.

Mansour MA, Labropoulus N, eds. *Vascular Diagnosis*. Philadelphia: Elsevier; 2005.

Polak J. *Peripheral Vascular Sonography, A Practical Guide*. ed 2. Philadelphia: Lippincott, Williams & Wilkins; 2004.

Zierler RE, ed. *Strandness's Duplex Scanning in Vascular Disorders*. ed 4. Philadelphia: Lippincott, Williams & Wilkins; 2010.

Zwiebel WJ, Pellerito JS, eds. *Introduction to Vascular Ultrasonography*. ed 5. Philadelphia: Elsevier; 2005.

References available online at ExpertConsult.com.

CHAPTER 15

Principles of Imaging in Vascular Disease

Antoinette S. Gomes

Currently there are several imaging techniques used to image the vascular system. These techniques include catheter-based conventional digital subtraction angiography, Doppler ultrasound, magnetic resonance angiography (MRA), and computed tomography angiography (CTA).

Conventional digital subtraction angiography (DSA) has long been the gold standard for arteriography because of its high resolution and rapid image acquisition. In digital radiography, the x-ray signal is electronically detected, digitized, and processed before display. Using subtraction techniques, DSA allows rapid visualization of both the arterial and venous phases and enhancement of the parenchymal phase. Small vessels are well seen. Because image acquisition is rapid, and repeated injections can be made, DSA is invaluable in the performance and assessment of the results of endovascular interventional techniques that are performed at the same time as the diagnostic arteriogram.

Limitations of conventional angiography are its invasive nature, with the requirement for catheter placement; the need for conscious sedation; the length of the study; and radiation exposure. The need for patient monitoring both before and after the procedure and the need for patient recovery time add significantly to the cost of the procedure.

Another limitation is that images are usually acquired in only one plane per contrast injection. Newer developments have helped to overcome this limitation. Newer equipment allows rotational angiography that permits acquisition of an image volume as the image intensifier and x-ray tube rotate around patient. The image volume acquired can be reconstructed to obtain three-dimensional volume-rendered images. This technique is helpful in analyzing complex vasculature and defining vessel branch origins and patterns such as that in aneurysms. The technique is particularly useful in the cerebral circulation. Positioning and timing are more complex in the abdomen. Research in this area is exploring use of this technology for measurement of blood velocity and flow profiles.

Two newer imaging techniques now used for performing angiography are MRA and multislice CTA. These techniques, although representing distinctly different technologies, provide images of the vascular system that are competitive with those obtained from conventional catheter-based angiography. Although the image resolution of these two techniques is less than that of conventional angiography, the image quality is such that these methods have the potential to supplant, and in many instances already do supplant, conventional diagnostic angiography.

MAGNETIC RESONANCE ANGIOGRAPHY

Magnetic resonance imaging (MRI) uses radiofrequency waves and magnetic field gradients to generate images. It is characterized by high contrast between soft tissue and flowing blood. The different pulse sequences used during MRI permit the enhancement or reduction of signal from different tissues based on their hydrogen density and their response to varying magnetic field gradients. MRI can be used to obtain static images of the body and images of the vascular system.

MRA affords visualization of flowing blood in vessels with the option of removing background soft tissues. A variety of pulse sequences have been used to perform MRA. These sequences include two- and three-dimensional time-of-flight (TOF), phase-contrast, and, more optimally, three-dimensional TOF gadolinium-enhanced MRA and time-resolved MRA. With MRA, conventional MRI images are usually acquired before and after any contrast administration as part of a complete magnetic resonance (MR) examination.

Time-of-Flight Angiography

TOF angiography is performed using a flow-compensated gradient refocused sequence. Data are typically acquired as a stack of two-dimensional slices or as a single three-dimensional volume. In this technique, stationary tissues in the slice or volume of interest are saturated from repeated radiofrequency pulses and have low signal intensity.[1-3] Blood flowing into the imaging has not been subjected to these radiofrequency pulses and is therefore fully magnetized (unsaturated). When it flows into the volume, it is bright compared with the stationary background tissues. This two-dimensional inflow technique works well in vessel segments running perpendicular to the imaging plane such as relatively normal arteries and veins, including the carotid arteries, the cerebral vasculature, the inferior vena cava, and iliac veins. Selective saturation pulses can be applied, allowing selective saturation of blood entering the imaging volume, such that either the arterial or the venous signal can be suppressed. With this technique, separate images of the arterial and venous system can be acquired.

A limitation of this technique is in-plane saturation, which results in signal dropout when the long axis of the vessel coincides with the scan plane or in the presence of slowly flowing blood in tortuous arteries. Another limitation is turbulence-induced signal loss in and distal to a stenosis.[4,5] In addition, the relatively long echo times required for gradient moment nulling make TOF imaging sensitive to susceptibility artifacts from bowel gas, implanted metallic objects (e.g., clips), or other air-tissue interfaces. These artifacts are a primary reason for the inaccuracy of TOF MRA. In addition, imaging times are lengthy because vessels need to be imaged perpendicular to the long axis of the vessel and a stack of slices must be acquired. Long acquisition times can lead to artifacts caused by slice misregistration or patient motion. Three-dimensional TOF MRA is used when a small area is being imaged and vessels run in different orientations such as the carotid bifurcation or Circle of Willis. Nearly isotropic volumes may be obtained allowing vessel reformation in any direction. If offers higher spatial resolution and higher signal to noise. Disadvantages include insensitivity to slow flow and saturation effects that limit slab thickness. Imaging times are longer than two-dimensional–TOF techniques and unlike two-dimensional–TOF techniques where motion artifact affect single slices, in three-dimensional–TOF, motion artifact affects all slices.

Phase-Contrast Angiography

Phase-contrast angiography uses velocity-induced phase shifts, which occur as blood flows through a magnetic field in the presence of flow-encoding gradients.[1,6,7] Two images created with opposite bipolar flow-encoding gradients are subtracted from each other; in the phase difference image, the residual phase is proportional to velocity. Stationary tissues do not undergo a velocity-induced phase shift in either image; they are suppressed and therefore subtract completely. The flow-encoding gradients can be in any direction or in multiple directions, depending on the selected flow sensitivity. Phase-contrast angiography can be performed as a two- or three-dimensional gradient refocused sequence and is improved after contrast administration.[8] It has been used in the evaluation of the renal arteries, carotid arteries, and portal veins. It is also used to measure flow velocity. When used with cardiac gating, a time-resolved velocity profile can be generated, providing quantitative measurement of the flow rate.

There are limitations to the technique. The amplitude of the preselected bipolar gradient determines the degree of velocity encoding (VENC). Phase-contrast sequences encode only a specified range of velocities.[9] In occlusive disease, turbulence causes a wide spectrum of rapidly changing velocities, which produce intravoxel phase dispersion and signal loss. Artifactual signal loss at sites of vessel stenosis is common. The sequence is also susceptible to measurement degradation from cardiac, respiratory, and translational motion. Background subtraction can be problematic. Currently, because faster MR angiographic techniques are available, phase contrast techniques are used primarily for the measurement of flow velocity.

Three-Dimensional Contrast-Enhanced Magnetic Resonance Angiography

Three-dimensional TOF gadolinium-enhanced MRA is the most widely used and useful of the MRA techniques. It does not rely on motion of blood to create flow signal. A contrast agent, typically gadolinium chelate, is given to shorten the T1 (spin-lattice) relaxation time of blood so that it is significantly shorter than that of surrounding tissues. Blood is imaged directly using a T1-weighted sequence. Blood is bright relative to background tissues during the arterial phase of three-dimensional contrast-enhanced MRA, because contrast transiently reduces the arterial blood T1 to less than that of the brightest background tissue (fat). This technique reduces the sensitivity to turbulence, and in-plane saturation effects are eliminated.[4,5] With this technique, a number of slices are oriented in the plane of the target vessels, permitting rapid imaging of a large field of view covering a large region of the vascular system. Contrast-enhanced MRA is fast and affords high-quality breath-hold and non–breath-hold angiograms. Dynamic contrast-enhanced MRA exploits the transient shortening in blood T1 after the intravenous (IV) administration of a contrast agent using a fast, three-dimensional spoiled gradient echo sequence. This is a first-pass technique, because the contrast agents currently used are extracellular agents and the gadolinium chelate rapidly leaks into the extravascular space. However, repeated slice volumes over the region of interest can be acquired during passage of the contrast allowing images in both the arterial and venous phases. Typical repetition times for contrast-enhanced MRA are less than 5 ms, with echo times of 1 to 2 ms and total scan times of 10 to 30 seconds. The sequences that use T1-weighted gradient echo, T1 fast field echo, or fast low-angle shot have high spatial resolution and a high signal-to-noise ratio. The images can be acquired in a breath-hold fashion and reformatted in any plane.[10-14] Because intravascular signal is dependent on T1 relaxation rather than inflow or phase accumulation, in-plane saturation and signal loss owing to turbulence are not significant.[4]

During the first-pass arterial phase, imaging is done before vascular contrast equilibration. Using a first-pass technique, steady-state background signal is nearly eliminated. Once the contrast is injected and dynamic imaging is done, however, a second bolus injection of contrast material must be given to repeat the process over, for example, a second region of interest. When the second dose is given, residual soft tissue enhancement can obscure vascular detail.[15] Subtraction techniques, using a precontrast mask, are typically used to remove background tissues. When the second or third dose of contrast is used, subtraction is mandatory. Timing is important in contrast-enhanced MRA. Unlike computed tomography (CT), MRA does not map spatial data linearly over time.[16] With three-dimensional MRI, all the three-dimensional Fourier or K-space data (the information from which the image is constructed) are collected before individual slices are reconstructed. K-space maps spatial frequencies rather than spatial data. Consequently, K-space data do not correspond to image space directly. Different portions of K-space determine the features of the image. The center of K-space, which records low spatial frequencies, affects contrast, whereas the periphery of K-space records high spatial frequencies, which contribute to the fine details, such as edges.[16,17]

Intravascular T1 signal intensity is determined by the gadolinium concentration at the time the center of K-space is collected.[17] The timing is synchronized so that the midportion of the bolus arrives at the desired site as the center of K-space is being collected. Perfect timing produces maximal arterial signal with minimal venous signal. If central K-space data are acquired too early, while arterial gadolinium is increasing rapidly, ringing or banding artifacts may be generated. Acquiring central K-space data too late leads to reduced arterial signal intensity and enhancement of venous structures. Several methods have been used to obtain proper bolus timing, including simple estimates of the travel time of the bolus from the site of injection to the region of interest. For example, in a healthy patient, the travel time from the antecubital vein to the aorta is approximately 15 seconds; in a patient with cardiac disease or an aneurysm, it is 25 to 35 seconds. To estimate contrast travel time more precisely, a test bolus can be used. In this technique, 1 to 2 mL of contrast followed by a 10- to 15-mL saline flush is injected at the same rate as the planned injection. Multiple single-slice fast gradient echo images of the appropriate vascular regions are then obtained as rapidly as possible—typically, every 1 to 2 seconds for a given period—and the time to peak enhancement (contrast travel time) is determined in the region of interest. A limitation of this technique is the setup time; also, the redistribution of the test bolus to the interstitial space may add to the background signal. Other timing techniques used include MR fluoroscopy.[18] In this technique, two two-dimensional sagittal gradient refocused images are obtained rapidly (<1 second per image) throughout the region of interest. Images are generated in near real time and updated at a rate greater than one image every second. The bolus time is watched, and when it arrives, the operator switches over to the three-dimensional MRA sequence. This technique may be helpful in cases of asymmetrical flow because of asymmetrical stenoses.

Another technique is a temporally resolved method in which multiple three-dimensional data sets are rapidly acquired (over 2 to 8 seconds) without any predetermined timing; injection and scanning are begun simultaneously.[19-23] The operator then selects the desired image set. Other techniques used to facilitate MRA involve simply scanning faster using parallel imaging techniques and using alternative K-space acquisition techniques.

Respiratory motion causes image blurring, ghosting, and signal loss. In three-dimensional imaging, blurring occurs in the direction of motion, whereas ghosting is more pronounced in the phase-encoding direction.[24] Before the availability of fast imaging systems, MRA techniques were too long to permit breath holding. Breath holding results in improved images in abdominal and thoracic MRA and facilitates the visualization of small vessels, such as the renal arteries.[25] It does not appear to be as critical in the evaluation of the carotids. Most ambulatory patients can hold their breath 20 to 30 seconds, and imaging is usually done on inspiration.

Another MRA technique that is now widely used is a time-resolved three-dimensional MRA technique with very high subsecond temporal resolution and submillimeter spatial resolution, which allows capture of multiple arterial, mixed, and venous phase images during the passage of contrast agent through the vascular anatomy (e.g., TWIST sequence). No test bolus or bolus timing is required with this technique. Imaging is so fast that venous contamination is eliminated. The technique is helpful for monitoring flow through vascular beds. It is helpful in determining flow patterns through cerebral and peripheral malformations and in delineation of shunt characteristics.

There is also renewed interest in non–contrast-enhanced MRA techniques using inflow inversion recovery techniques, and these sequences are an area of research interest, particularly for assessment of the renal arteries.

Patient Preparation

Patient cooperation is required for optimal contrast-enhanced MRA, because motion and improper breath holding can render the MRA study nondiagnostic. Valuable scanner time is often squandered during attempts to image an uncooperative patient. Patients should be relaxed, and the procedure should be explained to them beforehand. For patients who are particularly anxious, premedication with a sedative such as diazepam or fentanyl may be helpful. The IV catheter should be placed before the imaging is started and before the patient is in the magnet. A 22-gauge IV catheter or larger is placed in the antecubital fossa or below if the arms are to be extended above the head.

Gadolinium-Based Contrast Agents

Currently, almost all contrast-enhanced MRA studies are performed using gadolinium-based contrast agents. Gadolinium is a paramagnetic metal ion. Paramagnetic atoms or molecules possess unpaired electrons that, when placed in a magnetic field, undergo magnetization (attain magnetic susceptibility). The electrons set up circulating currents in response to the externally applied field. These currents induce an internal magnetization that augments or opposes the external field. When the direction of internal magnetization is the same as that of the external field, the effective field within the object is enhanced. This magnetic field enhancement is known as *paramagnetism*.

Gadolinium decreases both spin-lattice (T1) and spin-spin (T2) relaxation times. Because gadolinium is toxic in its natural form, it is chelated with ligands, such as gadopentetate dimeglumine, gadoteridol, or gadodiamide, to form MR contrast agents.[26] These agents are extracellular and pass from the intravascular compartment into the interstitial space in a matter of minutes.[4,5] Measurements of T1 shortening at different cardiac outputs have shown that injection rates greater than approximately 2 mL/s do not increase T1 shortening. Signal intensity increases asymptotically as the injection rate increases, with negligible increases seen beyond a rate of 4 to 5 mL/s.[27,28]

Most contrast-enhanced MR studies are performed with 0.1 mmol/kg of gadolinium or a double dose of 0.2 mmol/kg, or with a set volume of 15 or 30 mL with an injection rate of 1.5 to 2.5 mL/s. Contrast can be injected manually or, preferably, with a power injector. Either technique is followed rapidly by a 15- to 20-mL saline flush.

With contrast-enhanced MRA, once arterial data are collected, the sequence is repeated to capture the venous and equilibrium phases. With longer scanning times, the patient may take a short breath before repeating the sequences.

From their introduction, these agents were found to have a high safety margin and a low rate of adverse effects. It has been estimated that approximately 6 million doses of gadolinium-containing contrast agents are administered annually.[29,30] However, in the late 1990s a new disease was described, and in 2006 was shown to be associated with the use of gadolinium-containing contrast agents.[31] This disease, nephrogenic systemic fibrosis, has a low incidence; there are only several hundred cases reported in the literature.[32,33] It is characterized by fibrosis of the skin, connective tissue, and internal organs, eye changes, and flexion and extension contractures. There is currently no consistently successful treatment, and it is potentially fatal. The majority of cases have occurred in patients with end-stage renal disease, chronic kidney disease, acute kidney injury, and acute renal insufficiency of any severity because of hepatorenal syndrome, and in patients requiring dialysis or those in the perioperative liver transplantation period. These patients and patients with glomerular filtration rate (GFR) of 30 mL/min per 1.73 m^2 or less are at high risk. It is recommended that gadolinium-based contrast agents be avoided in these high-risk patients and alternative imaging methods be used unless the information cannot be obtained with noncontrast MRI or other methods. It is also recommended that all patients undergo screening for renal insufficiency before receiving gadolinium-based contrast agents and package insert doses not be exceeded.[34] The risk in patients with normal renal function is unknown, and to date there have been no reported cases in patients with normal renal function.

Postprocessing Techniques

Three-dimensional contrast-enhanced MRA produces a contiguous volume of data. In most body MRA studies, the volume is asymmetrical (e.g., 400 × 300 × 64). The slice is typically viewed interactively using a computer workstation. Thin multiplanar reformatting (MPR) can be performed,[1,28] and 1- to 2-mm slices can be viewed in multiple planes (axial, sagittal, and oblique).[35,36]

Because the thin sections do not display the entire vessel, the maximum-intensity projection (MIP) processing technique is often used.[37,38] With this algorithm, the user first selects the volume or portion of the volume to be evaluated. The algorithm then generates rays perpendicular to the viewing plane, records the maximum intensity of any voxel encountered along that ray, and assigns that maximum value to the corresponding pixel in the output image. This process results in images similar in appearance to conventional angiograms.

The MIP algorithm has some limitations. A major problem occurs when stationary tissue or structures within stationary tissue have a higher signal intensity than the vessels of interest. This can occur in the presence of crossing vessels, hemorrhage, fat, metallic susceptibility artifacts, or motion artifacts. This results in mapping of these extra signals into the projection image, producing a discontinuity in vessel signal that mimics vessel stenosis.[1] Reducing the thickness of the MIP subvolume to exclude as much extraneous tissue as possible can mitigate this limitation. Underestimation of vessel diameter is another limitation of the technique.

Subtraction techniques are also used to improve vessel visibility. These techniques are performed by a complex subtraction of precontrast and postcontrast raw data sets[39,40] and are routinely used in contrast-enhanced MRA of the extremities. Subtraction is relatively fast and there is good bone removal from the subtracted images. It is important to note that vessel calcifications are not well seen with standard MRI/MRA techniques and calcifications typically appear as dark regions of signal void. Metallic objects such as metallic stents produce artifacts seen as a signal void, limiting assessment of stent patency.

Three-dimensional volume rendering is another postprocessing technique that allows separation of overlapping structures. In many instances, this rendering may provide additional information over standard MIP images.

Clinical Applications

Extracranial Carotid Arteries

The carotid arteries can be well seen with contrast-enhanced MRA (Fig. 15.1). The short circulation time of the carotid circulation (4 to 6 seconds) makes timing critical; otherwise, venous overlap of the images results. Both long and short imaging times have been used to overcome this problem.

High-resolution imaging with short echo time is recommended. A major problem that impedes accurate stenosis assessment is the occurrence of high-speed turbulent jets at the site of stenosis. Specialized coils are recommended. The origins of the vessels from the aorta should be included in the imaging plane. Numerous studies have shown a high degree of correlation between stenosis measurement with contrast-enhanced MRA and DSA.[41-45] MRI has also been used to evaluate atherosclerotic plaque in the carotid arteries.[46,47]

Thoracic Aorta

Contrast-enhanced MRA is used routinely to evaluate the thoracic aorta. It is the standard of practice for following the status of dissections and monitoring aneurysm enlargement (Fig. 15.2).

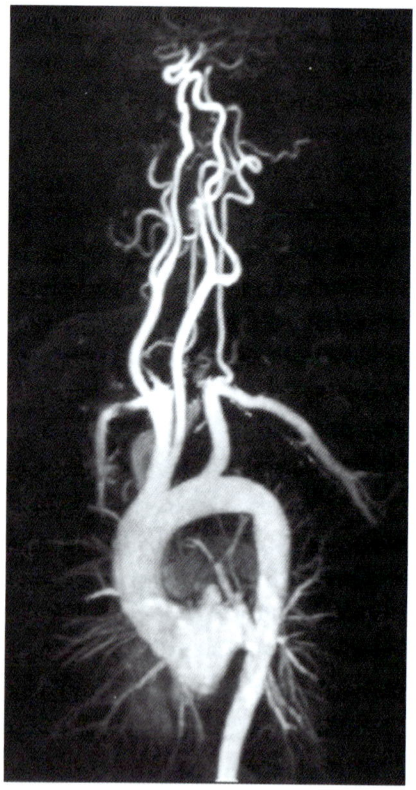

FIG 15.1 Contrast-enhanced magnetic resonance angiography of normal carotid arteries. Sagittal oblique maximum-intensity projection of the thoracic aorta shows normal carotid arteries.

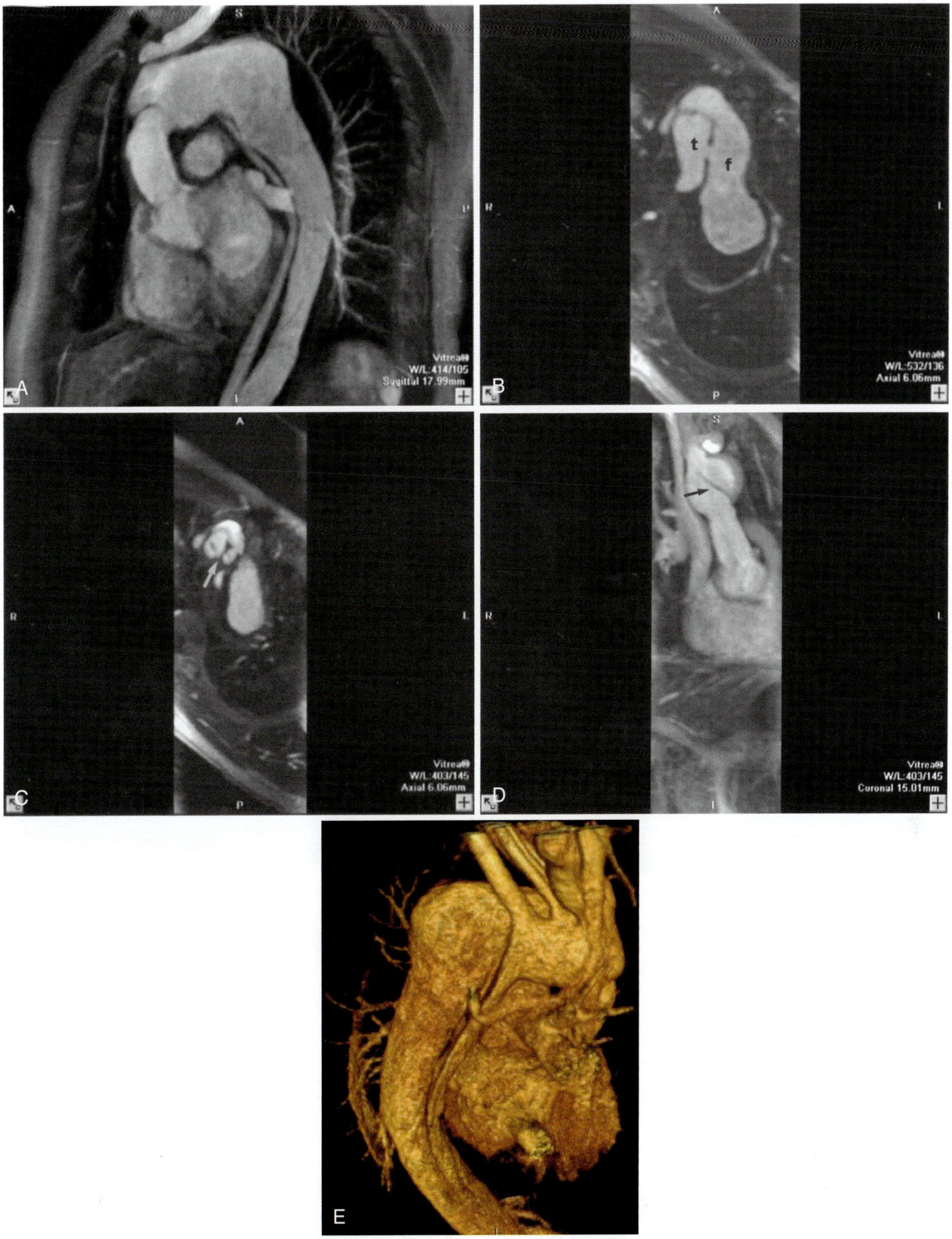

FIG 15.2 Contrast-enhanced magnetic resonance angiography (MRA) of aortic dissection. (A) Sagittal multiplanar reformatting (MPR) in a patient after repair of a type A aortic dissection with valved homograft in the ascending aorta. There is dilatation of the transverse arch. The residual intimal flap is seen as a dark stripe in the descending thoracic aorta. (B) Axial MPR at the level of the transverse aorta shows the intimal flap with a communication between the large false lumen *(f)* and the true lumen *(t)*. (C) Axial MPR at a higher level shows the intimal flap involving the innominate and left common carotid arteries *(arrow)*. (D) Coronal MPR shows that the intimal flap starts just above the homograft *(arrow)*. (E) Three-dimensional volume-rendered MRA of the thoracic aorta shows the compressed true lumen and the dilated false lumen.

Imaging is usually performed in the oblique sagittal plane or coronal plane. In aortic dissection, the origins of the brachiocephalic vessels should be included. A phased array body coil is recommended when the aneurysm is confined to the thoracic aorta. The ascending, descending, and abdominal aortas are evaluated.[48] A full evaluation of the aorta should include multiplanar cardiac-gated black blood imaging of the aortic wall to detect intramural hematoma.

Abdominal Aorta and Pelvic Vessels

Contrast-enhanced MRA is most often performed in this region to evaluate for aortic dissection or abdominal aortic aneurysm or as part of an evaluation for peripheral artery disease (PAD). The images are acquired in the coronal plane using a phased array body coil. A localizer image is obtained first in the sagittal plane, preferably with breath holding, to determine that the entire volume of the aneurysm will be in the field of view (see Fig. 15.2A).

Renal Arteries

Renal contrast-enhanced MRA is performed similarly to an abdominal aortic study, although a thinner coronal slab can be used, allowing decreased slice thickness or acquisition time. High-resolution imaging is preferred. A true slice thickness of less than 2.4 mm is recommended, and breath holding is critical. Otherwise, distal renal artery branches and accessory renal arteries may be difficult to visualize. Typically, renal arteries can be seen out to the interlobar branches. Review of the raw data is critical for full assessment (Fig. 15.3).

Small intrarenal branches are not seen well with current techniques. If resolution is not adequate or if motion occurs, fibromuscular dysplasia might not be detected. Examination of the

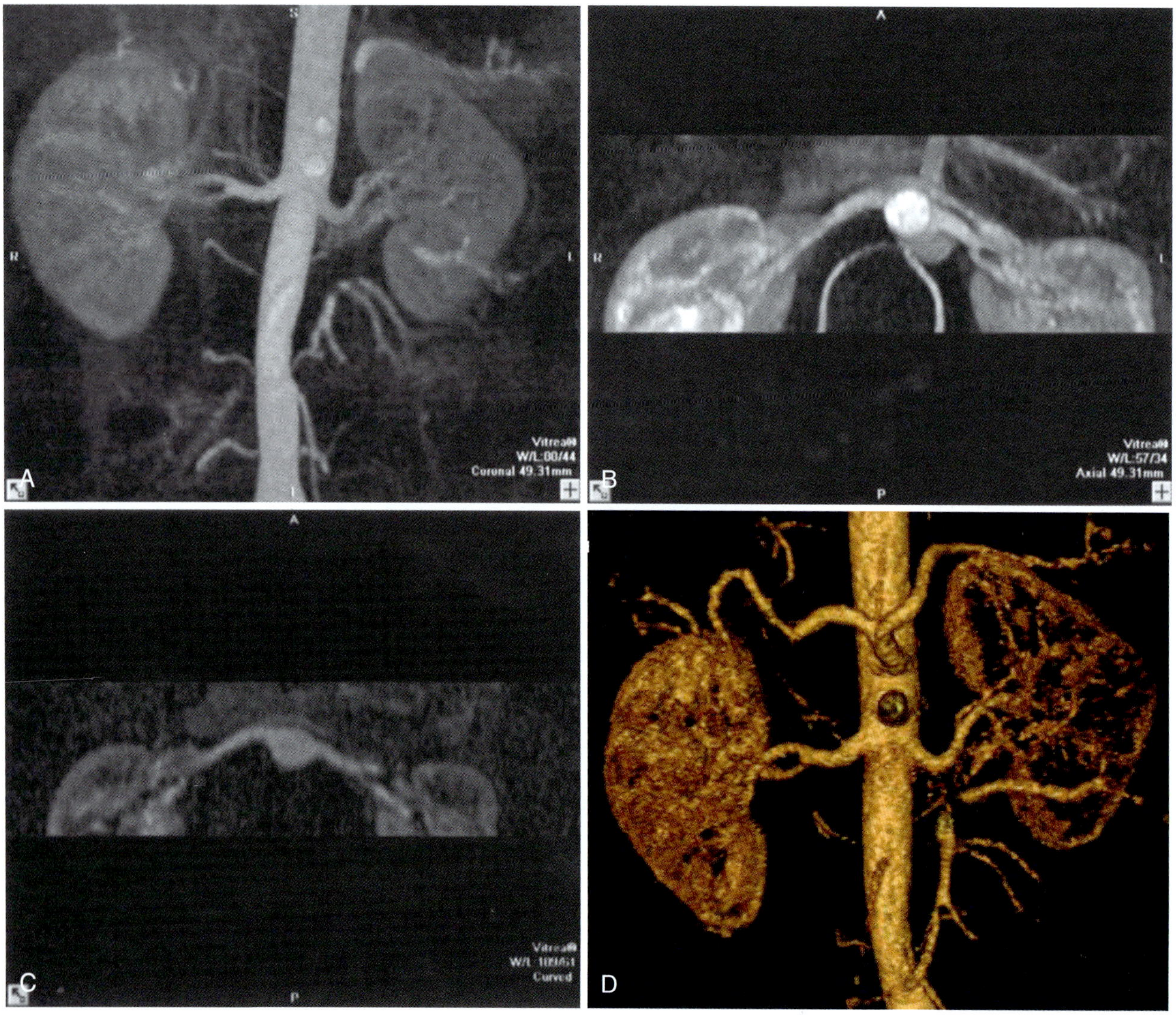

FIG 15.3 Contrast-enhanced magnetic resonance angiography of normal renal arteries. (A) Maximum-intensity projection (MIP) of renal arteries shows normal right and left renal arteries. A plaque is seen in the descending aorta. (B) Thick-slab MIP in the axial plane shows the origins of the right and left renal arteries. (C) Curved multiplanar reformatting allows visualization of the interlobar arteries. (D) Three-dimensional volume-rendered image affords visualization of the right and left renal arteries and the proximal interlobar branches.

source images can provide information regarding renal size and cortical thickness. A transit time can be calculated for each kidney. Newer techniques that shorten acquisition time and reduce motion artifacts should result in improved visualization of the renal arteries. Although there are multiple studies describing the value of renal artery MRA, it is used largely as a screening tool in patients with acceptable GFR. In hypertensive patients undergoing evaluation, conventional arteriography is usually deferred if the renal arteries are normal. If an abnormality is detected, conventional arteriography is usually performed, at which time angioplasty or stent placement can be done (Fig. 15.4). Using conventional angiography as a reference standard, the reported sensitivity and specificity of contrast-enhanced MRA for diagnosing renal artery stenosis are 88% to 100% and 70% to 100%, respectively.[49] Renal transplant arteries can also be evaluated with contrast-enhanced MRA, however if the GFR is reduced, alternate imaging techniques or imaging agents should be considered.

Mesenteric Vessels

The proximal portions of the mesenteric arteries are usually well seen on renal or abdominal MRA. Contrast-enhanced MRA is often used to evaluate for mesenteric ischemia caused by proximal vessel stenosis or occlusion. Evaluation of the source images

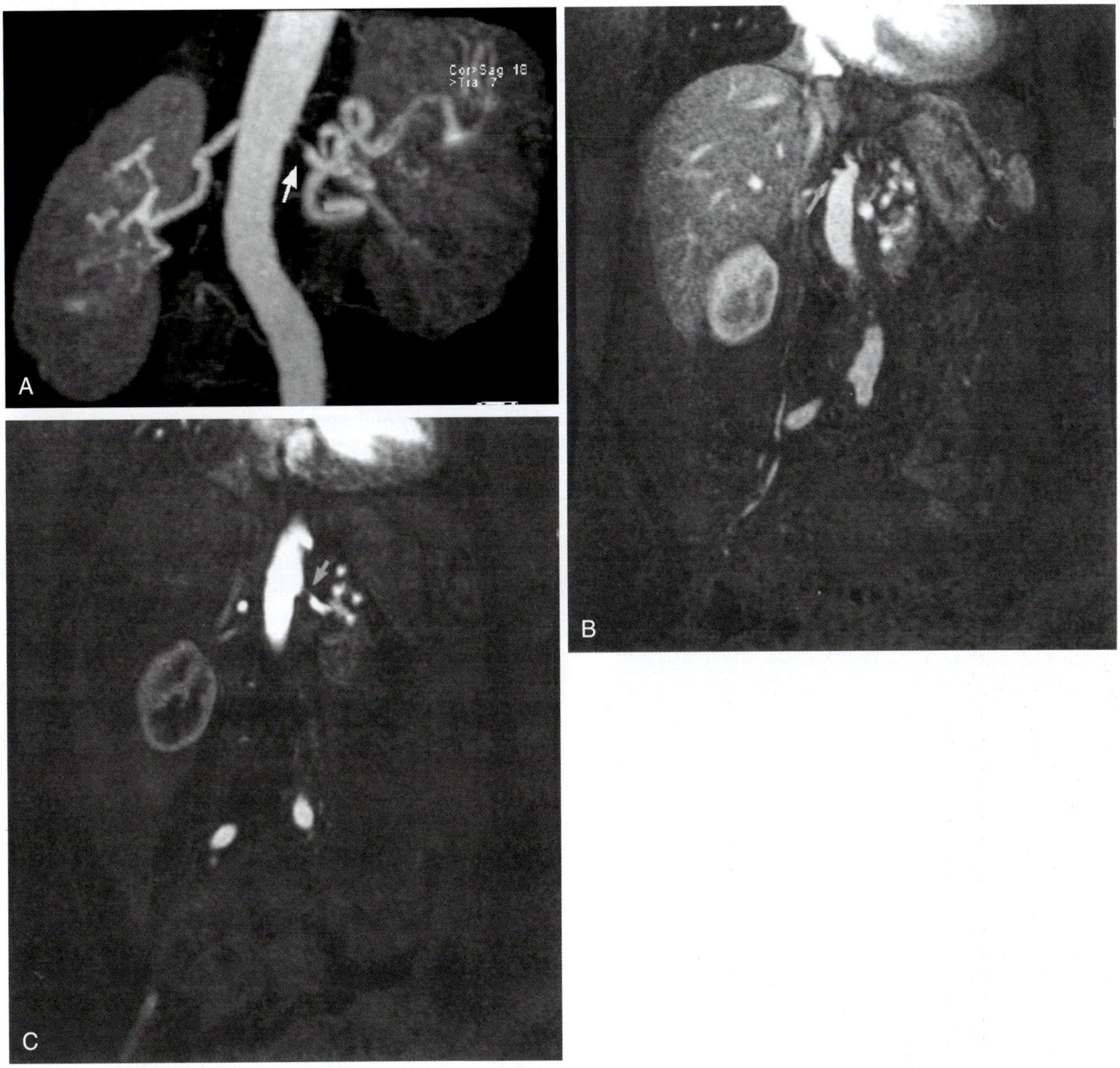

FIG 15.4 Contrast-enhanced magnetic resonance angiography of renal artery stenosis. (A) Anteroposterior view of maximum-intensity projection shows mild irregularity in the right renal artery with high-grade stenosis at the origin of the left renal artery *(arrow)*. (B) Review of raw data shows the origin of the right renal artery. (C) Adjacent slice of raw data shows high-grade stenosis at the origin of the left renal artery *(arrow)*. Inspection of raw data slices from the slab volume is often necessary for accurate diagnosis.

and MPR are useful,[50-53] as is visualization of the images in the sagittal plane. Distal small vessels are usually not visualized well enough to exclude distal small vessel disease. Thin slices are recommended.

Portal Venous System

Contrast-enhanced MRA provides high-quality images of the portal system and hepatic veins. Following arterial phase images, delayed acquisitions are obtained that routinely show the portal and hepatic veins.[53,54] Portal vein thrombosis and collaterals are also seen (Fig. 15.5). Again, a review of the source data thin MIP subvolume and often three-dimensional volume rendering are necessary.

Peripheral Vessels

Initially, contrast-enhanced MRA of the runoff vessels of the lower extremities was limited by the restricted field of view of MR scanners.[55] The field of view of most scanners, typically 400 to 500 mm, required repeated injections to cover the entire lower extremity. This imaging was typically performed by first imaging the smaller vessels of the calf, followed by repeated injections while imaging over the knee and thigh. A complete abdominal aorta and peripheral runoff study could not be performed in one sitting because of soft tissue enhancement from extracellular gadolinium contrast agent. Newer scanners are equipped with a moving table, which allows image acquisition similar to that of conventional arteriography, whereby a single bolus of contrast can be followed and imaged multiple times as it travels from the aorta to the feet (Figs. 15.6 to 15.8). Newer scanners also permit whole-body MRA (Fig. 15.9).

It is important to note that optimal visualization of peripheral vessels requires that they be imaged before venous enhancement occurs and obscures arterial vessels. In addition, because they are smaller than pelvic vessels, calf vessels must be imaged with parameters that afford higher resolution. Typically, with bolus-chase techniques, MRI is performed faster and with lower resolution in the pelvis and thigh, and the infusion rate is low to ensure a long bolus. Injection rates of 0.3 to 2.0 mL/s for 30 to 45 seconds can be used. Subtraction improves image quality. The issue of venous enhancement is related not only to imaging delay and contrast injection but to the underlying disease process. In general, patients with claudication usually do not exhibit venous enhancement until very late, whereas patients with inflammatory processes, such as cellulitis or venous ulcers, tend to have early venous enhancement. The examination must therefore be tailored to the patient. This need has prompted many imagers to perform two injections; the first injection targets the lower station, and the second injection evaluates the upper and middle stations. This technique has proved to be advantageous.[56] In patients with PAD, MRA allows development of an appropriate treatment plan.[57,58]

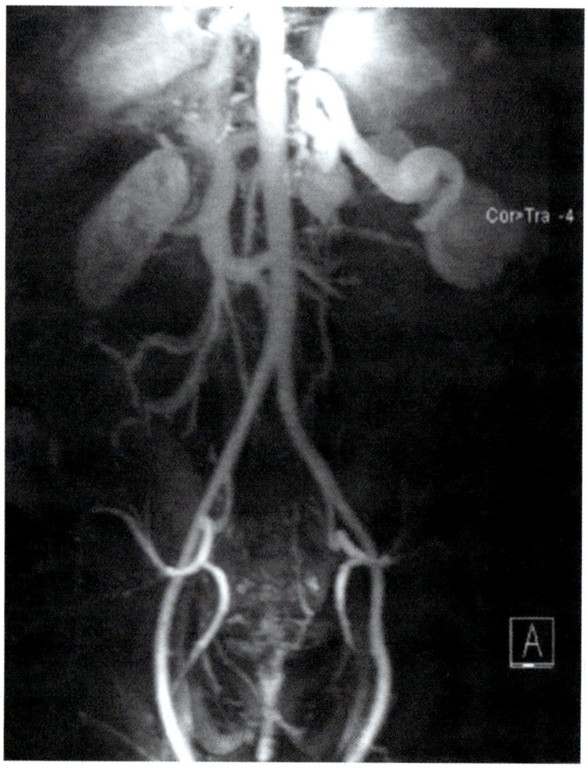

FIG 15.5 Venous phase of abdominal contrast-enhanced magnetic resonance angiography. The superior mesenteric vein and portal vein are seen. Large dilated varices are seen in the splenic bed draining into the left renal vein, producing a spontaneous splenorenal shunt.

Magnetic Resonance Venography

MR venography of the pelvis and extremities can also be obtained during the late phase of a contrast-enhanced MR angiogram. Axial two-dimensional TOF imaging has been used to evaluate venous structures in the upper extremities and venous thrombus in the lower extremities. However, with these studies, vessels parallel to the imaging plane undergo "in-plane saturation," resulting in signal dropout; this can be problematic when evaluating the great veins of the chest because the subclavian and axillary veins are in-plane during an axial acquisition performed to evaluate the superior vena cava. Two-dimensional TOF imaging can also be degraded by patient motion, magnetic field inhomogeneity, and susceptibility artifacts. Despite these limitations, in some circumstances it may be useful to evaluate the pelvic veins and inferior vena cava.[59,60]

Contrast-enhanced MRA overcomes many of the limitations of two-dimensional TOF imaging and is preferred for evaluating the veins of the upper extremity, superior vena cava, jugular veins, inferior vena cava, and renal veins. These structures can be imaged by obtaining delayed acquisition images on a standard contrast-enhanced MRA study (Figs. 15.10 and 15.11). The initial acquisition is timed for the first pass through the arterial system, and multiple acquisitions are obtained following the arterial phase. These late images usually have both arterial and venous enhancement. A selective venous study can be obtained by subtracting the arterial phase study from a mixed venous-arterial phase study.[61,62] Direct venography of upper extremity veins can also be performed by direct injection of a diluted or full-strength gadolinium contrast agent.[63,64]

Text continued on p. 247

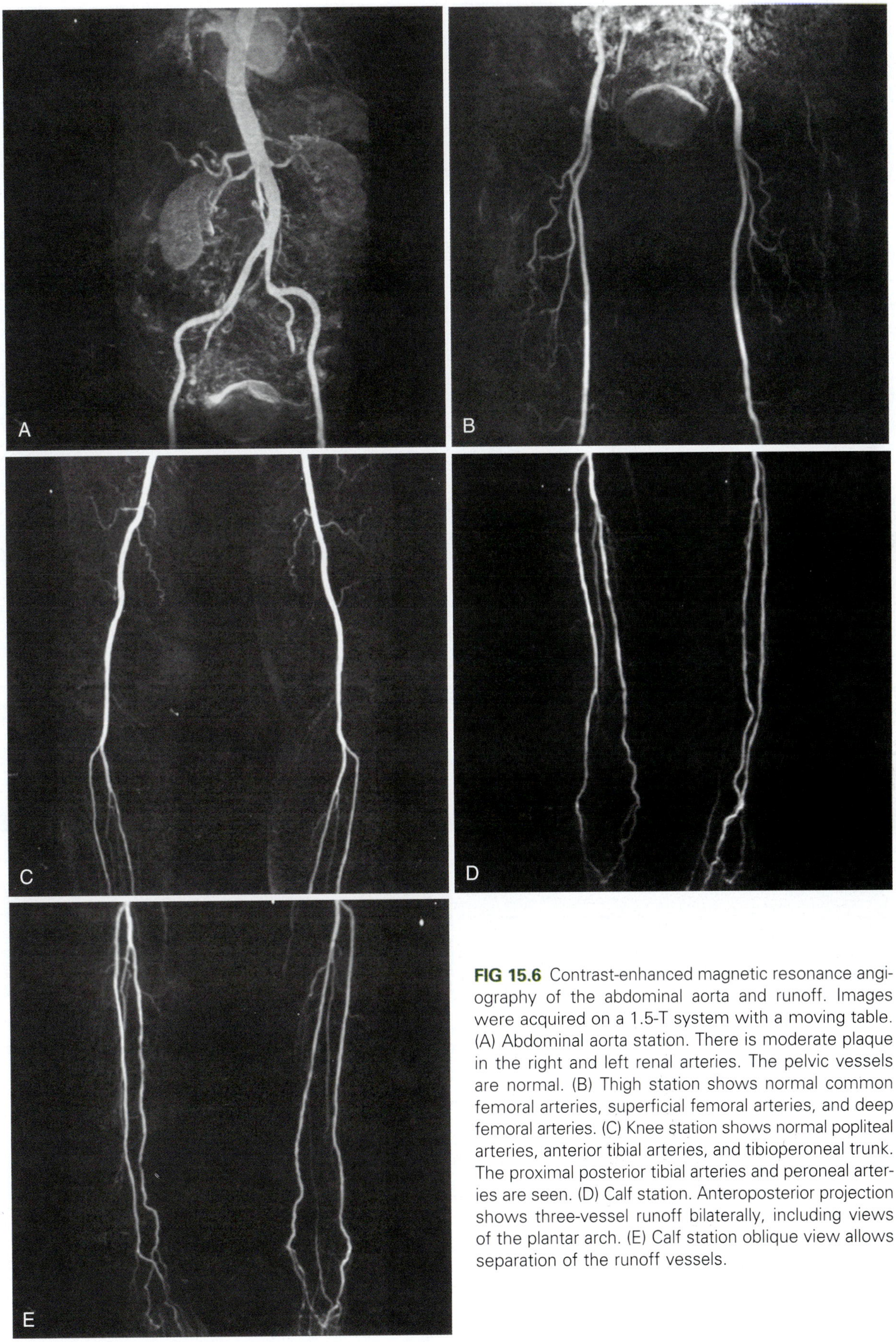

FIG 15.6 Contrast-enhanced magnetic resonance angiography of the abdominal aorta and runoff. Images were acquired on a 1.5-T system with a moving table. (A) Abdominal aorta station. There is moderate plaque in the right and left renal arteries. The pelvic vessels are normal. (B) Thigh station shows normal common femoral arteries, superficial femoral arteries, and deep femoral arteries. (C) Knee station shows normal popliteal arteries, anterior tibial arteries, and tibioperoneal trunk. The proximal posterior tibial arteries and peroneal arteries are seen. (D) Calf station. Anteroposterior projection shows three-vessel runoff bilaterally, including views of the plantar arch. (E) Calf station oblique view allows separation of the runoff vessels.

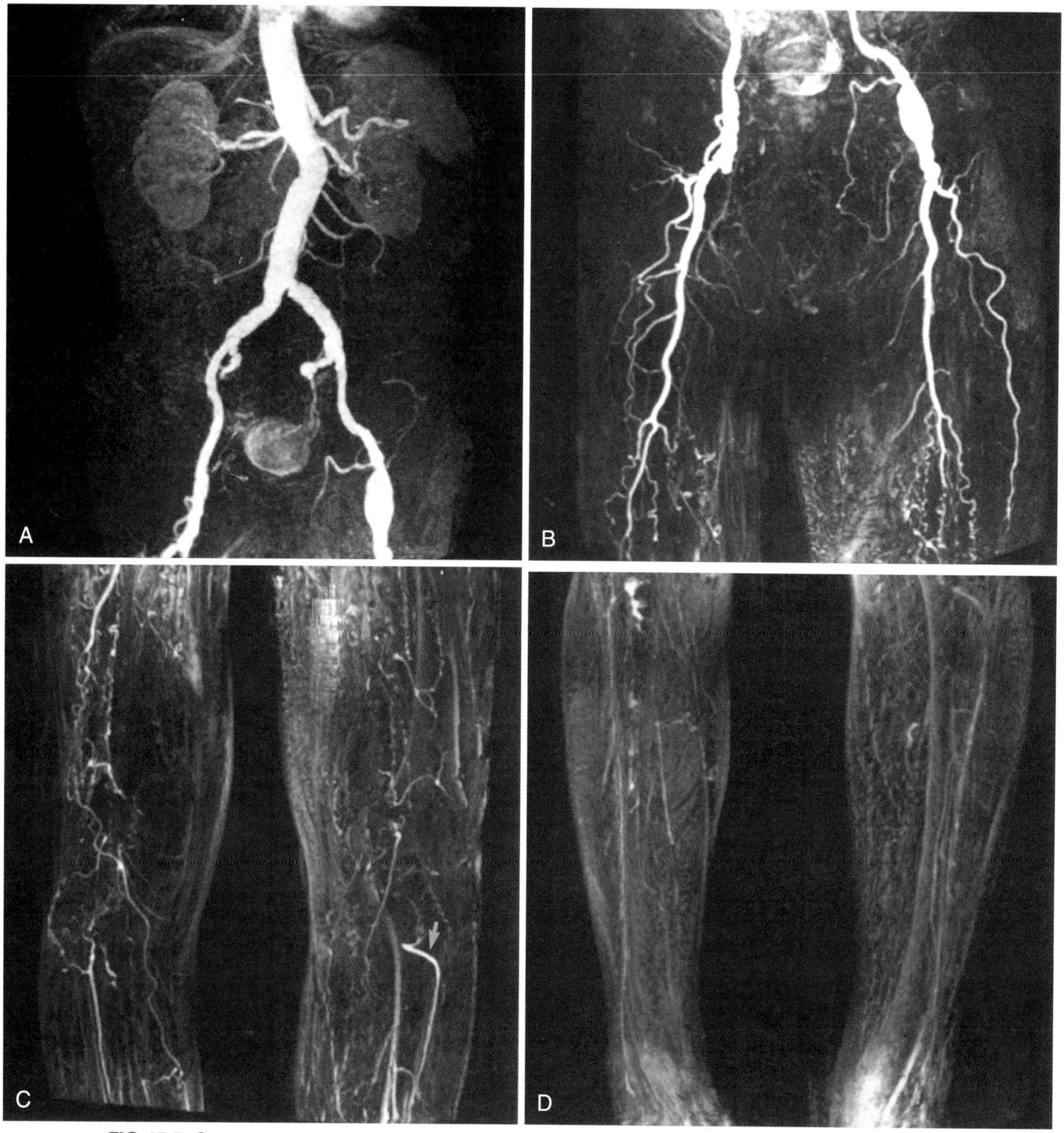

FIG 15.7 Contrast-enhanced magnetic resonance angiography abdominal aortogram and runoff in a patient with severe peripheral vascular disease. (A) Abdominal station shows atherosclerotic changes in the common iliac vessels. An aneurysm is seen in the left common iliac artery. (B) Thigh station shows occlusion of the right and left superficial femoral arteries, with bilateral enlarged deep femoral collaterals. (C) Knee station shows severe occlusive disease. There is no filling of either popliteal artery. On the right, collaterals reconstitute a segment of the anterior tibial artery *(arrow)* and a segment of the posterior tibial artery. On the left, a segment of the proximal anterior tibial artery is reconstituted by collaterals. (D) Calf station. On the right, a diffusely diseased anterior tibial artery is faintly seen. An isolated segment of the posterior tibial artery is identified. On the left, a portion of the anterior tibial artery is faintly seen, and a small portion of the peroneal artery is identified.

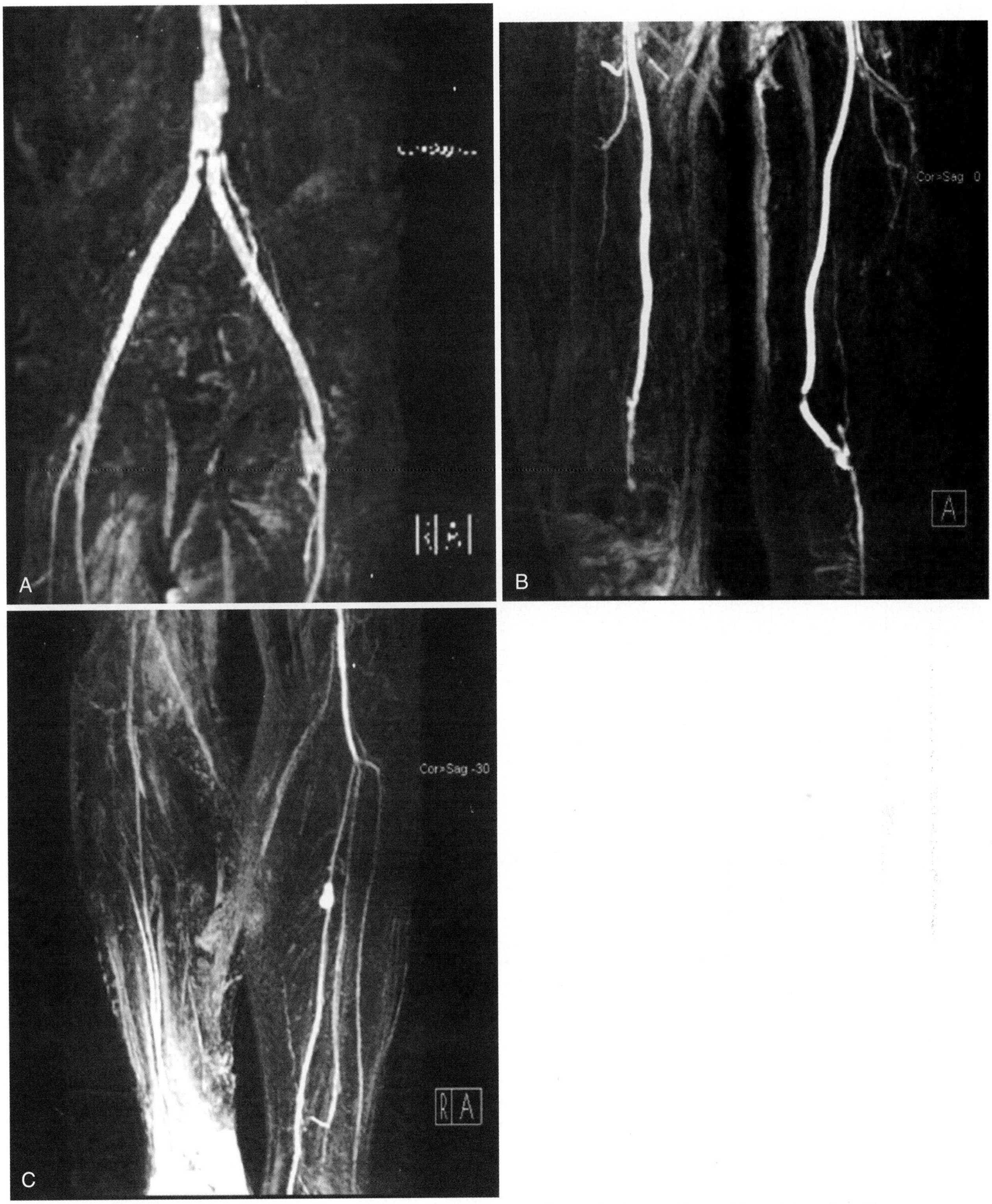

FIG 15.8 Contrast-enhanced magnetic resonance angiography in a patient with peripheral grafts. (A) Aortogram station shows irregularity of the distal abdominal aorta and a patent aortobifemoral graft. A filling defect is seen at the origin of the right limb of the graft. (B) Thigh station shows bilateral superficial femoral artery grafts. The left graft has a tight stenosis proximal to the distal anastomosis. The right graft is occluded distally. (C) Calf station on the right shows poor filling of a portion of the anterior tibial artery. On the left, the popliteal artery is patent, with three-vessel runoff. A small aneurysm is seen in the posterior tibial artery.

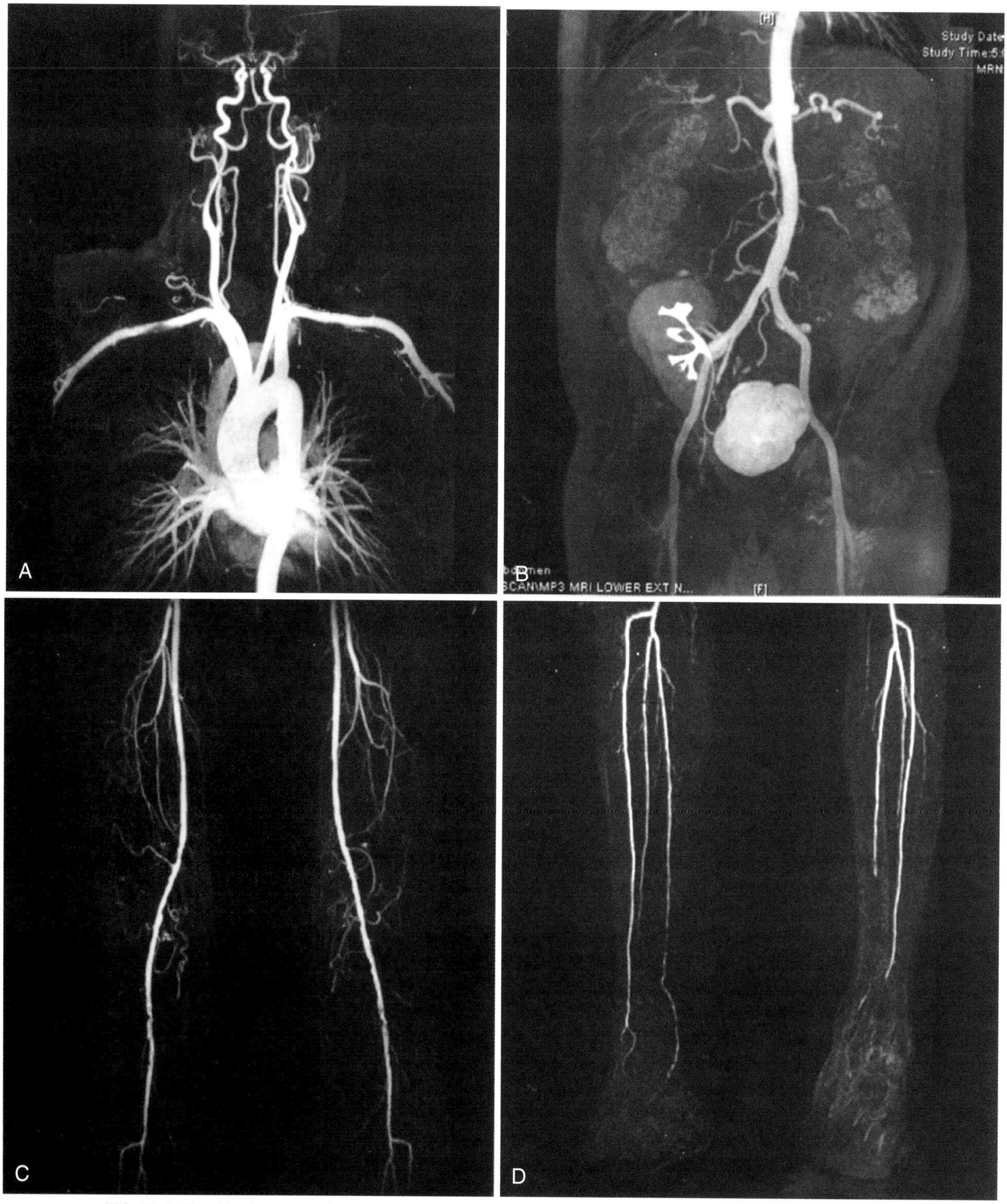

FIG 15.9 Total-body magnetic resonance angiography. (A) The thoracic aorta is normal. (B) Abdominal aorta and pelvis station show right renal transplant. (C) Thigh and knee station show mild atherosclerotic plaque in the superficial femoral arteries. (D) Calf station. Timing is too early on the left, with poor filling of the left calf vessels.

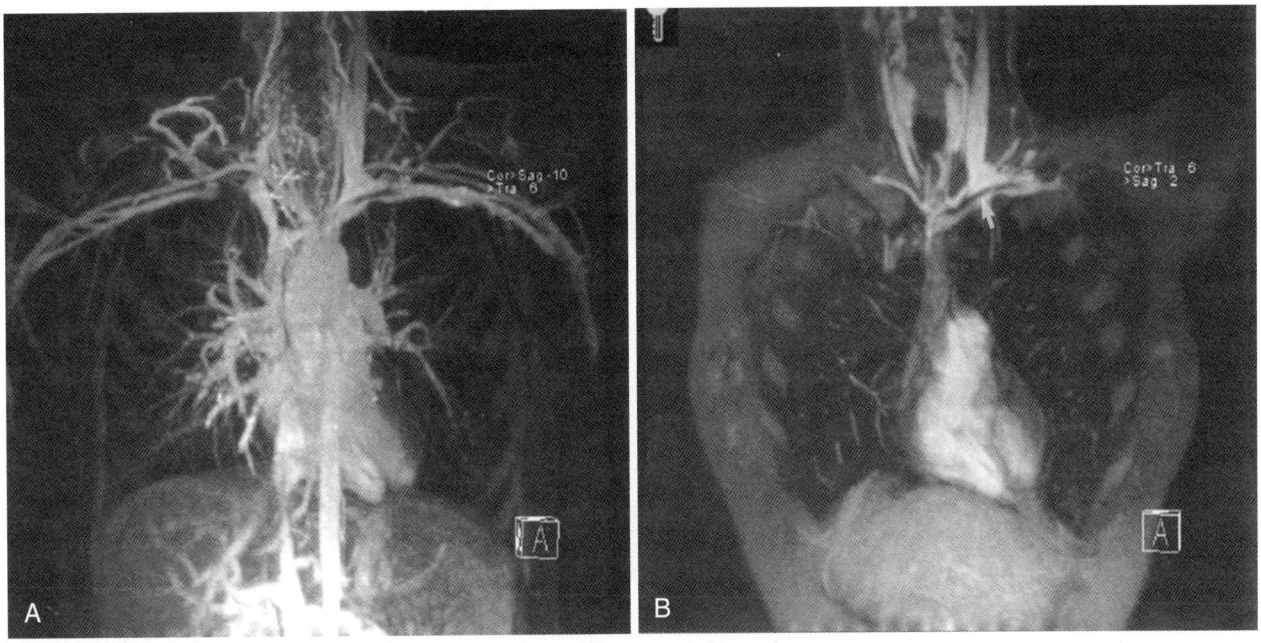

FIG 15.10 Contrast-enhanced magnetic resonance angiography venogram of the upper extremities. (A) Venous phase maximal-intensity projection (MIP) shows occlusion of the right internal jugular vein with multiple collaterals. There is localized occlusion of the right subclavian vein. A dark linear structure is seen in the left subclavian vein and superior vena cava; this represents a catheter. (B) Thin MIP shows the catheter to better advantage *(arrow)*.

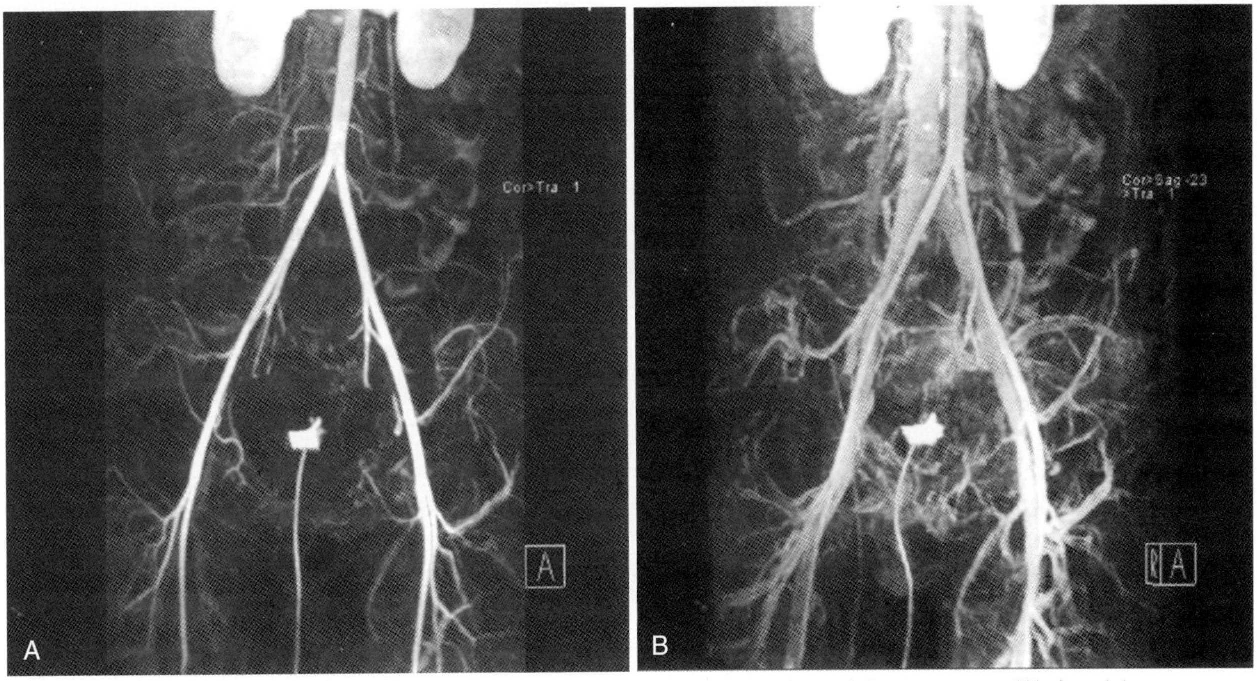

FIG 15.11 Contrast-enhanced magnetic resonance angiography pelvic venogram. (A) Arterial phase shows normal arterial vessels. (B) Delayed phase shows good filling of pelvic veins and inferior vena cava.

Newer techniques, such as true fast imaging with steady-state precession (FISP), a steady-state gradient echo sequence, have also been used with some success to evaluate the arterial and venous systems. A rapidly acquired stack of true FISP images provides thin-section viewing of arteries and veins, which are seen as bright blood.

Source data and postprocessing techniques are important in the assessment of venous thrombus, because low–signal-intensity thrombus might not be seen with MIP. The differentiation of acute and chronic thrombus can be difficult with two-dimensional TOF images. With acute thrombus, contrast-enhanced images may show dense periadventitial enhancement.[65] This enhancement is usually not seen with chronic clots and vessel size reductions. Venous mapping using contrast-enhanced MRA is routine at some centers, and it is also useful for quantifying clot burden and determining the presence and size of collaterals. This information is helpful in assessing alternative access sites in patients with venous obstruction from long-term central venous catheters. Contrast-enhanced MRA can also differentiate bland thrombus from tumor thrombus in patients with neoplasms that extend into the venous system. Tumor thrombus enhancement distinguishes it from bland thrombus that does not enhance. MR venography is routinely used to evaluate the patency of upper extremity veins, jugular veins, and the superior vena cava.

Future Directions: New Contrast Agents

New gadolinium chelate agents formulated at 1.0 M (e.g., gadobutrol), rather than the current 0.5 M, and agents with higher relaxivity due to weak protein interactions (e.g., gadobenate dimeglumine) demonstrate greater intravascular signal than do conventional agents.[66-68] These agents provide better visualization of both large and small vessels. Intravascular blood pool agents are under development, and two main types are currently being evaluated. One type (e.g., MS-325) has a strong affinity for serum albumin,[69-71] and the other type (e.g., gadomer-17) is a macromolecular agent whose size precludes rapid extravasation.[72] Full exploitation of these intravascular agents will necessitate sophisticated subtraction techniques to separate the arteries from the veins. Neither is currently available for use in the United States. Another agent under evaluation is ferumoxytol (Feraheme). Ferumoxytol is a US Food and Drug Administration approved parenteral therapy for treatment of iron deficiency anemia. It consists of an ultrasmall superparamagnetic iron oxide (USPIO) core, which causes T1, T2, and T2* shortening effects, and a carbohydrate shell, which results in a prolonged intravascular half-life.[73]

MULTIDETECTOR ROW COMPUTED TOMOGRAPHY ANGIOGRAPHY

The use of CT for imaging the vascular system has been made possible by the development of multidetector row helical computed tomography (MDCT) scanners. In helical CT, there is continuous CT gantry rotation coupled with continuous table movement through the scanner.[74] This technique permits the rapid acquisition of data and increased data collection with each rotation. Initial spiral scanners were single-row scanners, but the development of multidetector row arrays, faster gantry rotation times, stronger x-ray tubes, and improved reconstruction algorithms has resulted in shorter image acquisition times and improved volume coverage. The three fundamental improvements—speed, volume coverage, and section thickness—are important for CTA. The rapid acquisition speed is such that the contrast bolus can be imaged as it traverses the arterial system. The evolution of 4-, 8-, 16-, 32-, and 64-slice MDCT scanners has resulted in incremental increases in volume coverage and spatial and temporal resolution and reductions in scan time. MDCT scanners with 320 detector rows are now available. With a four-row scanner, the entire thoracoabdominal aorta and iliac arteries can be imaged in 15 to 30 seconds using a 2.5-mm section thickness throughout the entire scan volume. With a 16-row CT scanner, the same anatomic territory can be imaged in 8 to 10 seconds using a 1.25-mm section thickness. CTA is used to image large vessels, such as the thoracic and abdominal aortas, and the major visceral branches of the abdominal aorta, the carotids, and the pulmonary and coronary arteries. With faster scans, MDCT permits the entire abdominal aorta and lower extremity runoff to be imaged in a single, high-spatial-resolution scan. Using a 1.25-mm collimation and a table speed of 27.5 seconds (1.6-mm effective section thickness), a distance of 1300 mm can be covered in less than 30 seconds. Sixteen-slice MDCT permits 100 cm to be covered in 21.4 seconds; with the 64-slice scanner, 153 cm can be covered in approximately 15.6 seconds. Although vascular imaging can be performed on four-row scanners, it is generally accepted that 16-row scanners result in more scans being diagnostic, particularly when large anatomic coverage or small vessel detail is required. Sixty-four–row scanners are currently the most widely used.

The speed of multislice CT shortens breath-hold examination times and reduces the amount of contrast medium needed to achieve consistent high-quality vascular enhancement.[75-77] The speed of MDCT allows large-volume coverage in a short time. This image acquisition speed can also be used to increase spatial resolution with the acquisition of thinner slices to increase the flexibility of a data set. High-resolution imaging requires that thin-slice collimation data be reconstructed to produce a near-isotropic data set of thin, overlapping, transverse images. The 16-row scanner permits the acquisition of 0.625- to 0.75-mm nominal slice thicknesses with nearly isotropic voxels with almost equal in-plane and through-plane resolution. With the 64-slice MDCT, pitch-independent visualization of 0.4-mm isotropic voxels is possible. Although slice thickness of this degree is not necessary for all CT studies, it enhances visualization of small vessels in the central nervous system, coronary and mesenteric vessels, and vessels of the calf.

Acquisition of extensive volumes with submillimeter resolution generates nearly isotropic data that can be arranged in arbitrary imaging planes with the same high spatial resolution as the original axial section. The acquisition of high-resolution data enhances the image quality of two-dimensional displays and three-dimensional volume rendering.[78-83]

The rapid acquisition time of MDCT scans allows image acquisition during a breath hold. Image noise is an important consideration, particularly when images are to be reviewed with three-dimensional volume rendering. The visibility of a structure in the body is dependent on the ratio of that structure and its immediate background to the noise (contrast-to-noise ratio). During CTA, this ratio is affected by the amount of arterial opacification and the noise in the scan. As section thickness is halved, image noise increases by approximately 40%. The goal of decreasing section thickness to visualize small blood vessels and to obtain better detail in large vessels must be balanced with the goal of reducing image noise. Fortunately, image noise is influenced by other factors that do not affect spatial resolution. These include x-ray current and potential and the reconstruction algorithm or kernel used. Depending on the scanner, the pitch can influence scan noise indirectly. According to International Electrotechnical Commission specifications, pitch *(p)* equals the table feed per rotation divided by the total width of the collimated beam. It shows whether data acquisition occurs with gaps ($p > 1$) or with overlap in the transverse direction ($p < 1$). Greater tube current is required to compensate for reconstruction strategies that avoid an increase in the effective section thickness as the pitch is increased. For many acquisitions, an increase in pitch will not affect noise. If the maximum tube current is selected for a scan with a given pitch value, and the pitch value is increased, no more current can be supplied to compensate, and the noise will increase.

With MDCT, slice thickness is a reconstruction parameter rather than an acquisition parameter. The narrowest section thickness that can be reconstructed is dependent on the width of the detector groups. Images can be reconstructed at thicker intervals. When images are acquired with thin sections, as long as the raw data are saved, thicker sections can be reconstructed, and the data set that provides the best diagnostic information can be used.

Contrast Medium Administration

Iodinated contrast material is used for CTA. This is the same contrast material used for conventional arteriography and therefore presents the same risks of idiosyncratic allergic reaction and nephrotoxicity. Optimized vessel opacification is an important aspect of CTA because with each new scanner generation, acquisition time decreases and correct synchronization of CT acquisition relative to arterial enhancement becomes more critical.[84] Care must be taken to match the table speed and helical pitch with the first circulation of contrast material through the anatomic region of interest so that data are acquired during peak enhancement and not before or after the contrast bolus has arrived. Image acquisition techniques are modified depending on the number of detector rows in the scanner. With 16-slice MDCT, the entire chest, abdomen, and pelvis can be imaged in less than 15 seconds. With the 16-slice scanner or higher-row scanners, care must be taken not to outrun the contrast bolus when imaging the peripheral vessels. With MDCT, the scanning delay following an injection of contrast needs to be timed relative to the patient's contrast transit time (from IV injection site to the arterial region of interest). This transit time can be obtained with the injection of a small test bolus. Many scanners have this bolus tracking capability built into the system. When contrast is injected, a series of low-dose scans is acquired while the attenuation in the region of interest is monitored. The transit time equals the time when a predetermined enhancement threshold is reached (e.g., 100 Hounsfield units). The minimum trigger delay to start the CT acquisition after the threshold is reached depends on the scanner (range, 2 to 8 seconds) and on the longitudinal distance between the monitoring series and the starting position of the CT series.[85] Automatic triggering is used, coupled with a dual-head contrast injector that permits a saline flush. The saline flush reduces the total contrast used by eliminating contrast left in the tubing; it also reduces perivenous streak artifacts by removing dense contrast material from the brachiocephalic veins and superior vena cava in thoracic and cardiac CT scans. In routine clinical practice, the injection duration should match the acquisition time. Faster acquisitions require less contrast material volume. Long acquisition times benefit from biphasic injections, with an initially high injection rate followed by a lower one, because they lead to a more uniform enhancement plateau. To ensure adequate vessel opacification with fast MDCT acquisitions, the iodine administration needs to be increased. This is done by increasing the injection flow rate or using contrast material with a higher iodine concentration (e.g., 370 mg/mL of iodine).

Radiation Dose

A variety of measurements have been used to measure or describe CTA dose. Studies using four-slice CTA have shown increased effective collective doses compared with multislice CT. With 16- and 64-row scanners, radiation dose is reduced using dose modulation techniques. In dose-optimized protocols using tube current modulation, the dose is delivered according to the attenuation of the tissues scanned, and the dose is reduced over thinner areas. Depending on scan volume, the dose may be reduced by 10% to 30%.[86] At least two studies have shown an average reduction in dose using the 16-row scanner compared with four-row multislice CT.[86] Nonetheless, the radiation dose from CTA is lower than that of conventional angiography.

Image Reconstruction

The large data sets obtained with multislice CT require three-dimensional workstation viewing. The large number of images prohibits "film" viewing. Typically, comprehensive image analysis is performed, consisting of rapidly scrolling all axial images on a dedicated workstation and performing three-dimensional reconstructions using a variety of algorithms. Postprocessing techniques consist of MPR, MIP, volume rendering, and shaded surface displays. In vascular imaging, heavy calcifications and intravascular stents can impede luminal visualization, but review of the axial transverse images and longitudinal or curved MPR usually permits the evaluation of the vessel lumen.

Dual Energy Computed Tomography

A newer technique is dual-energy CT, in which two x-ray tubes operating at different kilovoltage (kV) acquire data 90 degrees apart; it is based on the energy-dependent tissue attenuation differences. The technique is under evaluation for discrimination of calcified and noncalcified plaque in atherosclerotic vessels.[87]

Applications

MDCT angiography (CTA) is used for imaging most major vessels and even some smaller vessels in the body.

Carotid Arteries

CTA provides high-quality images of the carotid arteries and permits visualization of carotid plaque. CTA with MPR provides views of the plaque and vessel lumen, making it a useful technique for assessing carotid artery stenosis.[88-91]

Quantification of plaque is feasible. The combined use of noncontrast cranial CT with CT perfusion imaging and CTA of the cerebral vessels is safe and feasible,[92] and such a protocol can facilitate the triage of patients with suspected carotid disease.

Coronary Arteries

Coronary artery CTA differs from CTA in other parts of the body in that electrocardiograph (ECG) gating is needed to freeze cardiac motion. Scanners of 64 rows or greater are preferred. Gating may be retrospective or prospective. With retrospective gating, image reconstruction uses only the data acquired during a short segment of the cardiac cycle. The data are then postprocessed to correlate with the ECG and assign cardiac phase to each segment of the reconstructed data. Prospective ECG gating has been implemented in an effort to lower the radiation dose compared with retrospective gating. With prospective gating, information from prior heartbeats is used to estimate the correct time to turn the x-rays off and on during the R-R intervals. The x-rays are turned off completely except during the acquisition phases in diastole when there is less heart motion. The scanner acquires one slab during one heartbeat, repositions the patient during the next heartbeat, and acquires another slab in the next heartbeat. This process requires several heartbeats with 64-row detectors[93] or can be accomplished in a single heartbeat with wider area 320–detector row CT scanners.[94] With CTA, artifacts such as calcium blooming and beam hardening can be problematic in interpreting stenoses in heavily calcified coronary arteries. Dual-energy CT is under evaluation for use in coronary CTA.

Pulmonary Arteries

CTA is used routinely as the first-line imaging technique to assess for pulmonary artery embolism. It has largely replaced conventional invasive arteriography for diagnosis. A main advantage of CTA is that in addition to having a high positive and negative predictive value, it reliably demonstrates alternative or additional disease causing the patient's symptoms. In the past, the major limitation of CTA was inadequate visualization of the peripheral lung bed.[95] Newer MDCT scanners, such as the 16-row scanner, cover the entire thorax with submillimeter slices in one short breath hold (10 seconds), with near-isotropic voxels allowing visualization of the proximal and distal vessels.[86,96] Scans can be acquired with high resolution (thin 0.5- and 1-mm collimation) or in severely dyspneic patients; a faster protocol with wider collimation (2.5 and 1.5 mm) can be acquired. The optimal protocol depends on the equipment used.[86,97-99] MDCT CTA has been used for the combined study of the pulmonary arteries and the deep veins of the legs using the same injected bolus of contrast.[100] Because of the high positive and negative predictive value of CTA of the pulmonary arteries and the added radiation dose required to study the legs, the current recommendation is that if pulmonary embolism is present, the deep venous system should be evaluated with ultrasonography, except in carefully selected patients such as those with suspected involvement of the inferior vena cava.[101,102]

CTA is useful for assessing the presence of other vascular anomalies of the pulmonary arteries, such as pulmonary artery arteriovenous malformations. It is also used for mapping and evaluating abnormalities of the pulmonary veins.

Thoracic Aorta

CT has long been used to evaluate the thoracic aorta. With current scanners, the entire thoracic and abdominal aorta can be imaged with near-isotropic resolution (Fig. 15.12). The traditional helical CT indications for imaging the thoracic aorta have been reemphasized and strengthened with the introduction of MDCT.[103] The availability, speed, and ease of modern MDCT make it the imaging technique of choice for the diagnosis of acute aortic pathology such as aortic trauma, dissection, intramural hematoma, and aneurysm (Fig. 15.13).[104]

MDCTA is faster, more readily available, and less operator dependent than echocardiography, and it provides more complete organ visualization. MDCT CTA is faster than both MRA and conventional arteriography. It is more suitable than MRA for patients in unstable condition, and it is less invasive than conventional arteriography. The ability to perform MPR and the ability to see both the lumen of the aorta and the wall are distinct advantages over conventional arteriography. Imaging of the thoracic aorta typically is done with noncontrast images of the thorax to identify regions of hyperdensity within the aortic wall suggesting intramural hematoma. This imaging can be performed with wider collimation and slice thicknesses of 2.5 to 5 mm. Narrow-slice collimation is necessary for CTA and requires thin slices of 1 to 2.5 mm to provide adequate spatial resolution and image quality for postprocessing.[86] In cases of aortic root pathology, ECG synchronization of the scan acquisition using prospective or, more commonly, retrospective ECG gating removes cardiac motion artifact, allowing evaluation of this region.

Abdominal Aorta and Iliac Arteries

The volume coverage capabilities of MDCT have had a major effect on imaging of the abdominal aorta. With current MDCT scanners, the entire abdominal aorta and iliac vessels can be covered with near-isotropic resolution (Fig. 15.14). The high scan speed allows the use of less contrast material.[105]

In the abdomen, traditional indications for CTA include diagnosis and surveillance of aneurysms, preoperative evaluation of endograft placement and postplacement monitoring, and tumor diagnosis and staging (Fig. 15.15). Other routine uses include evaluation of abnormalities of the mesenteric vessels,[106-108] renal artery stenosis, and portal venous system abnormalities. MDCT CTA is routinely used in the evaluation of potential renal donors[109] and liver donors (Fig. 15.16).[110-112] It is also used in the assessment of patients undergoing liver lesion embolization. The use of thin collimation reduces volume averaging that impedes small vessel visualization; the improved *z*-axis resolution allows clear assessment of small mesenteric vessels and the degree of renal artery stenosis. Using a 0.5-second MDCT scanner, Willmann and colleagues[106] obtained high-quality CT angiograms with 92% sensitivity and 99% specificity for the detection of aortoiliac and renal artery stenosis (Fig. 15.17). The decision to use MRA or CTA to evaluate the abdominal aorta is determined largely by the patient's ability to cooperate, the status of the patient's renal function, and the degree of resolution required for diagnosis.

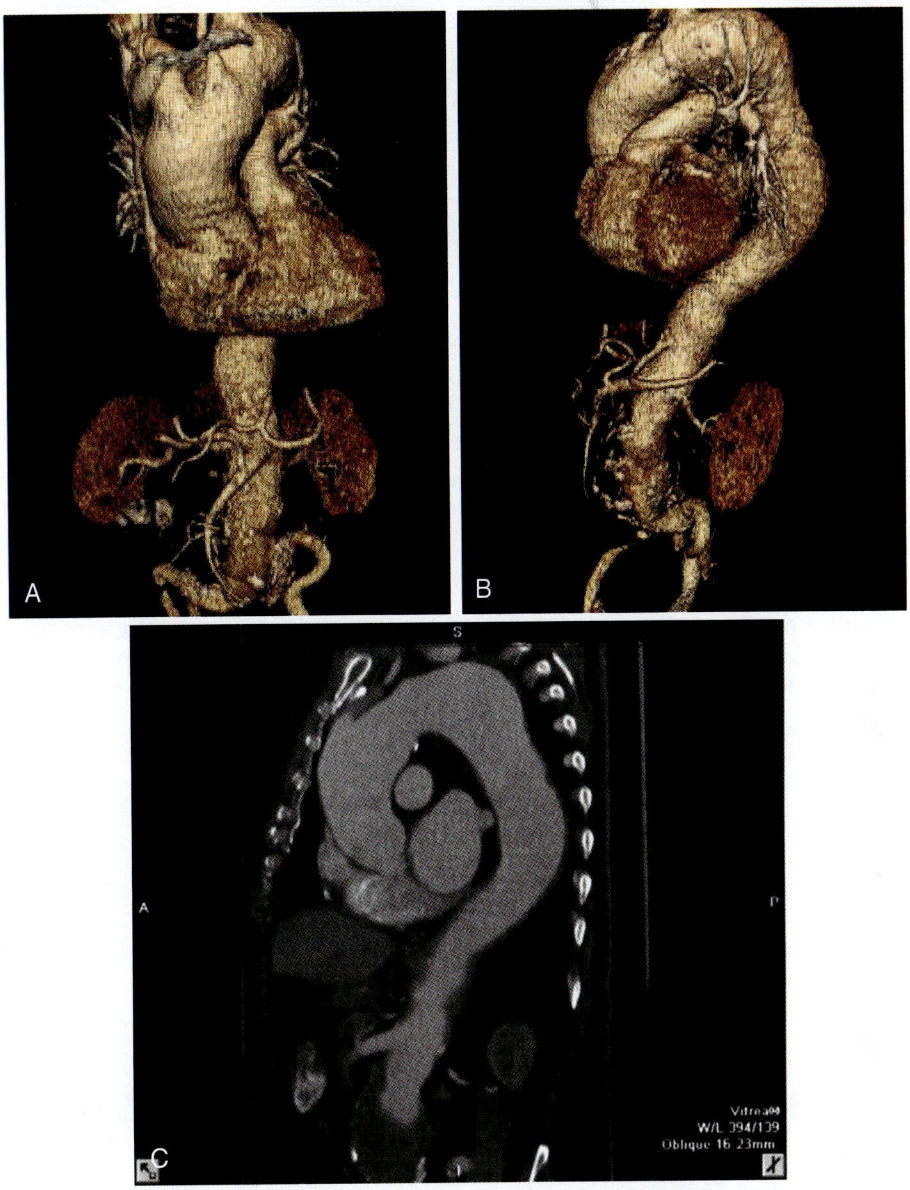

FIG 15.12 Multidetector row helical computed tomography angiography of thoracoabdominal aortic aneurysm. (A) Frontal view shows ascending aorta and abdominal aorta with visceral vessel origins. Calcifications in the aneurysm are seen. (B) Oblique view. (C) Curved multiplanar reformatting.

Peripheral Arteries

Imaging of the peripheral arteries is one of the new and exciting applications of CTA. With multislice CTA, noninvasive imaging of the entire abdominal aorta and runoff vessels can be accomplished with high resolution, providing angiogram-like images of the runoff vessels (Fig. 15.18). Using even four-slice MDCT, a high correlation has been found between MDCT results and DSA in the evaluation of lower extremity atherosclerotic vascular disease.[113-115] The ability to see the relationship of vessel calcifications and the ability to perform MPR are advantages that are not available with conventional arteriography. Although disadvantages such as the use of ionizing radiation, the need for iodinated contrast material, and the demanding postprocessing requirements need to be considered, there are circumstances when MDCT CTA is preferred. Calcifications can be seen and provide useful pretreatment information about whether to use angioplasty alone or stents. Patients who have had prior stent placement are better evaluated with CTA, which allows the vessel lumen to be visualized. In some situations, such as preoperative endograft planning, CTA is sufficient and angiography is unnecessary. Careful bolus timing is required. With four-row scanners, imaging delay can result in venous opacification, obscuring the arteries of the feet. With 16- and 64-row scanners, care must be taken not to outstrip the bolus and acquire images too early, before vessels are filled. Newer dual-energy CT techniques may permit better assessment of vessel stenoses using automatic bone and plaque removal (Fig. 15.19).[116]

Text continued on p. 257

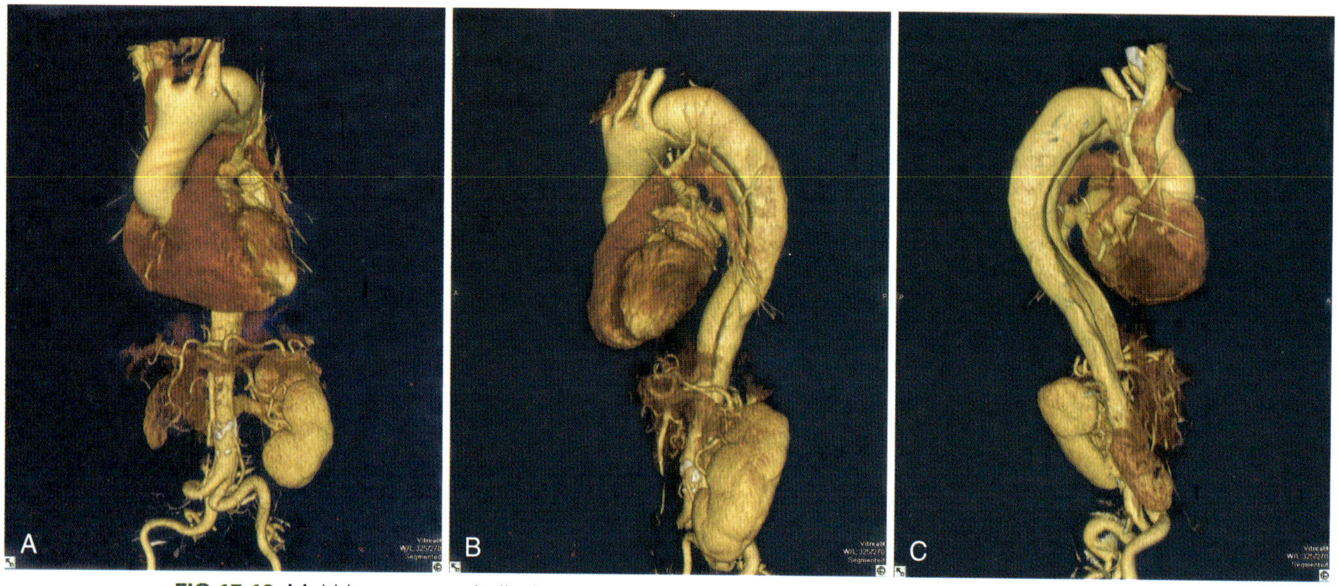

FIG 15.13 Multidetector row helical computed tomography angiography of acute aortic dissection on 16-row multislice computed tomography CT scanner. Three-dimensional volume-rendered images of type B aortic dissection showing the intimal flap and the true and false lumens. Note the clear delineation of the origins of the major branch vessels. (A) Coronal view shows ascending aorta and a black lucency representing the intimal flap arising just distal to the left subclavian artery. (B) Right sagittal oblique view shows a thin black line representing the intimal flap extending down the thoracoabdominal aorta. The false lumen is larger and the true lumen smaller. (C) Left oblique view shows spiraling of the intimal flap, deformity of the compressed true lumen, and involvement of the renal arteries.

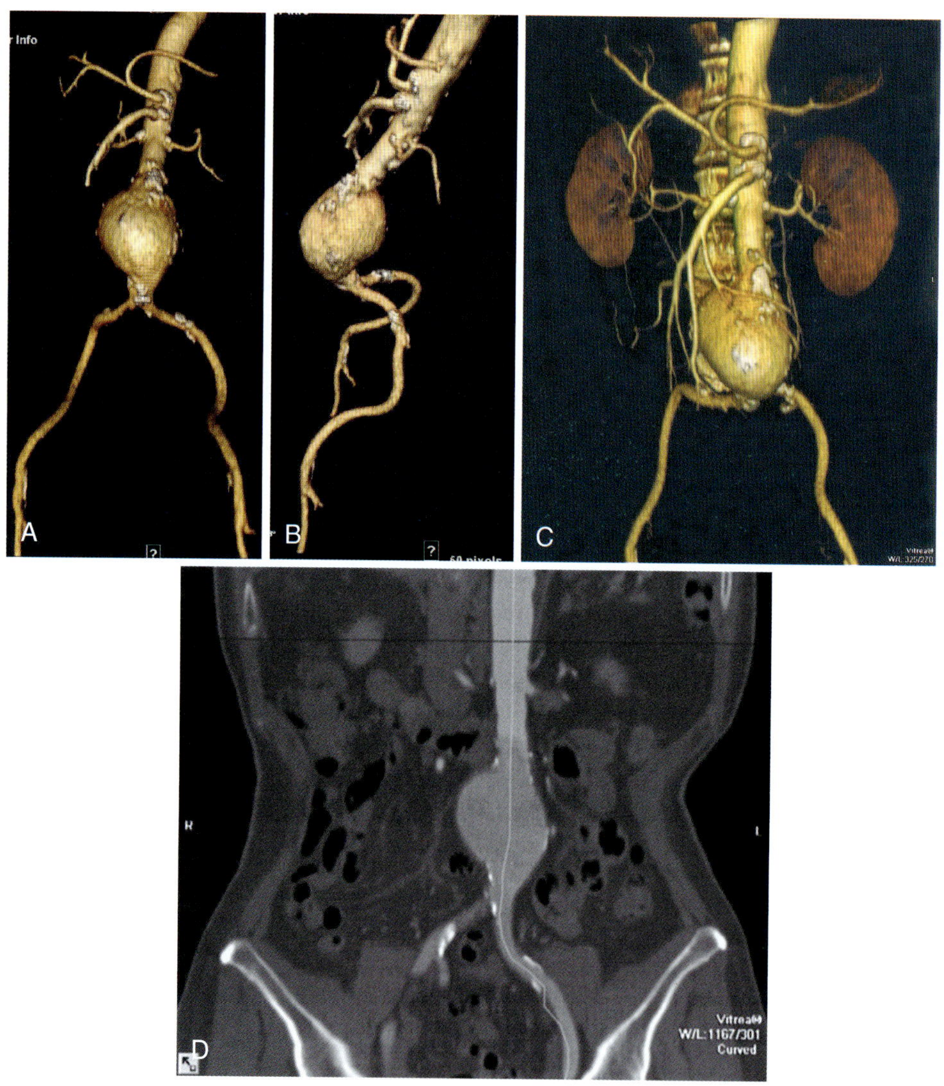

FIG 15.14 Multidetector row helical computed tomography angiography of infrarenal abdominal aortic aneurysm. (A) Three-dimensional volume-rendered image of the abdominal aorta and branch vessels. The celiac artery and superior mesenteric arteries are seen. The infrarenal saccular aneurysm extends to just above the aortic bifurcation. (B) Oblique view of the aorta. (C) Partial removal of bone shows the renal arteries and superior mesenteric artery branches. See color plate. (D) Curved multiplanar reformatting allows measurement of vessel diameter.

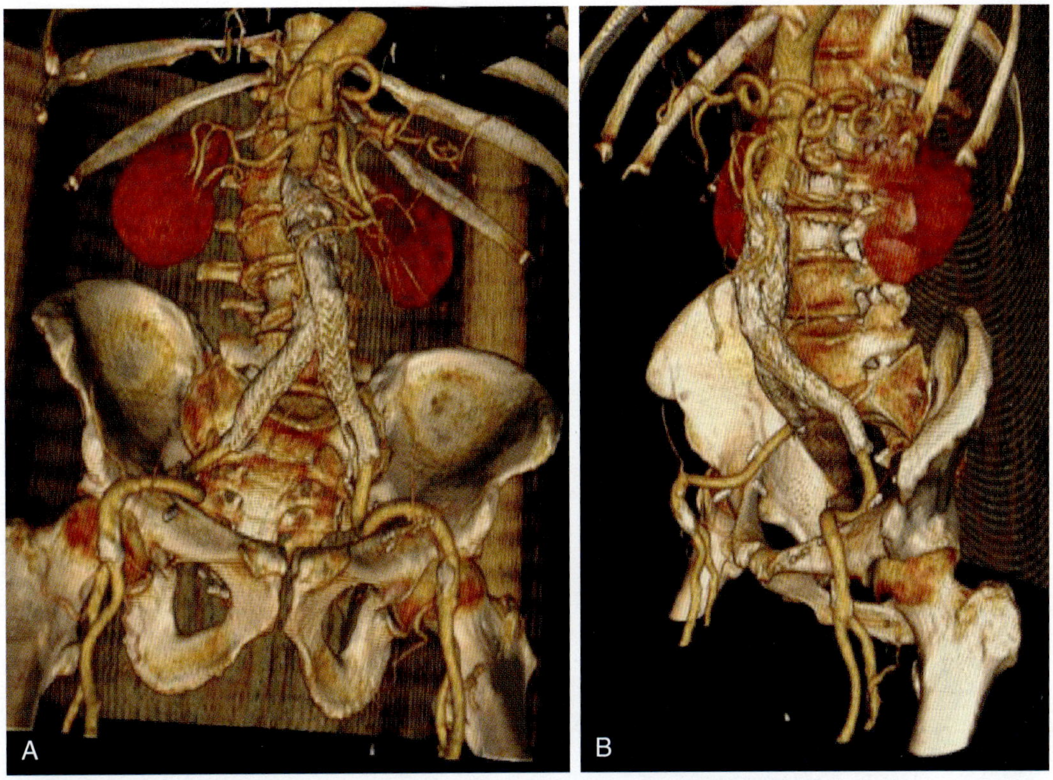

FIG 15.15 Multidetector row helical computed tomography angiography of aortic endograft. (A) Abdominal study shows a bifurcated endograft in the aorta. (B) Oblique view shows that the limbs of the endograft are crossed; no obstruction is seen.

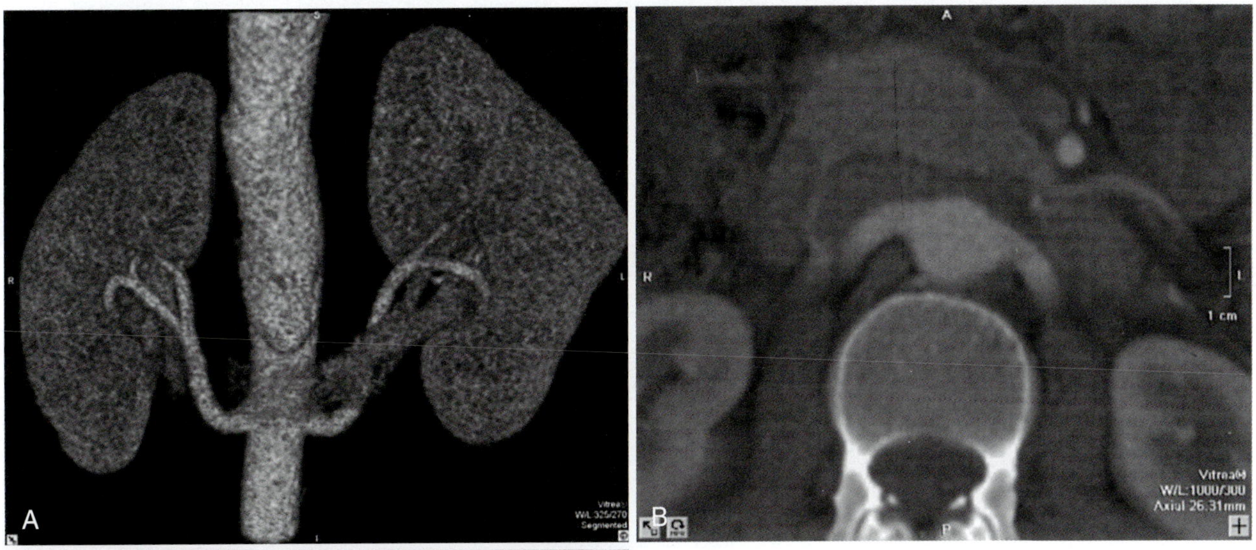

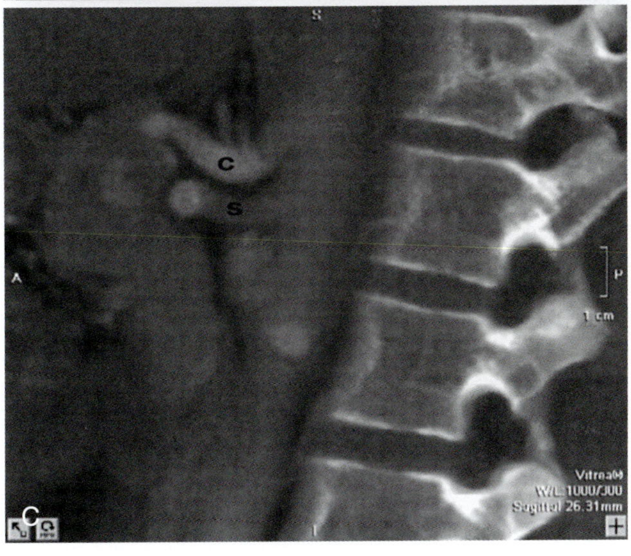

FIG 15.16 Multidetector row helical computed tomography angiography of renal donor. (A) Three-dimensional volume-rendered images of the renal arteries. (B) Multiplanar reformatting (MPR) of the origin of the renal arteries. (C) Note that the origins of the celiac *(c)* and superior mesenteric *(s)* arteries are well seen on sagittal MPR.

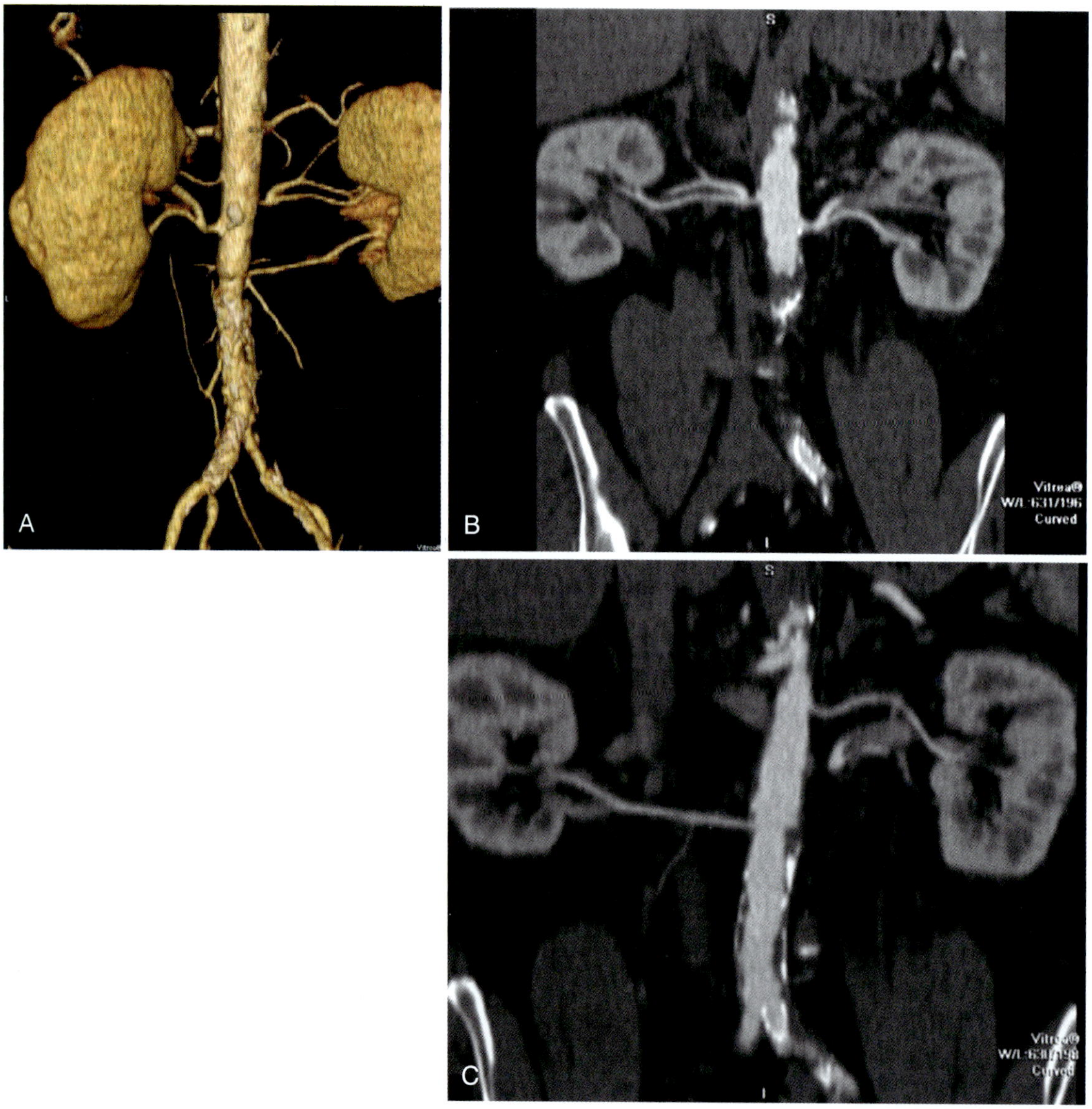

FIG 15.17 Multidetector row helical computed tomography angiography of renal artery stenosis. (A) Three-dimensional volume-rendered image shows high-grade stenosis at the origin of the right renal artery. The left renal artery is normal. An inferior accessory artery is seen on the right, and a superior accessory artery is seen on the left. Note the calcifications in the infrarenal aorta. (B) Curved multiplanar reformatting (MPR) shows the origins of the right and left renal arteries. (C) Curved MPR clearly shows the origins and course of the accessory renal arteries.

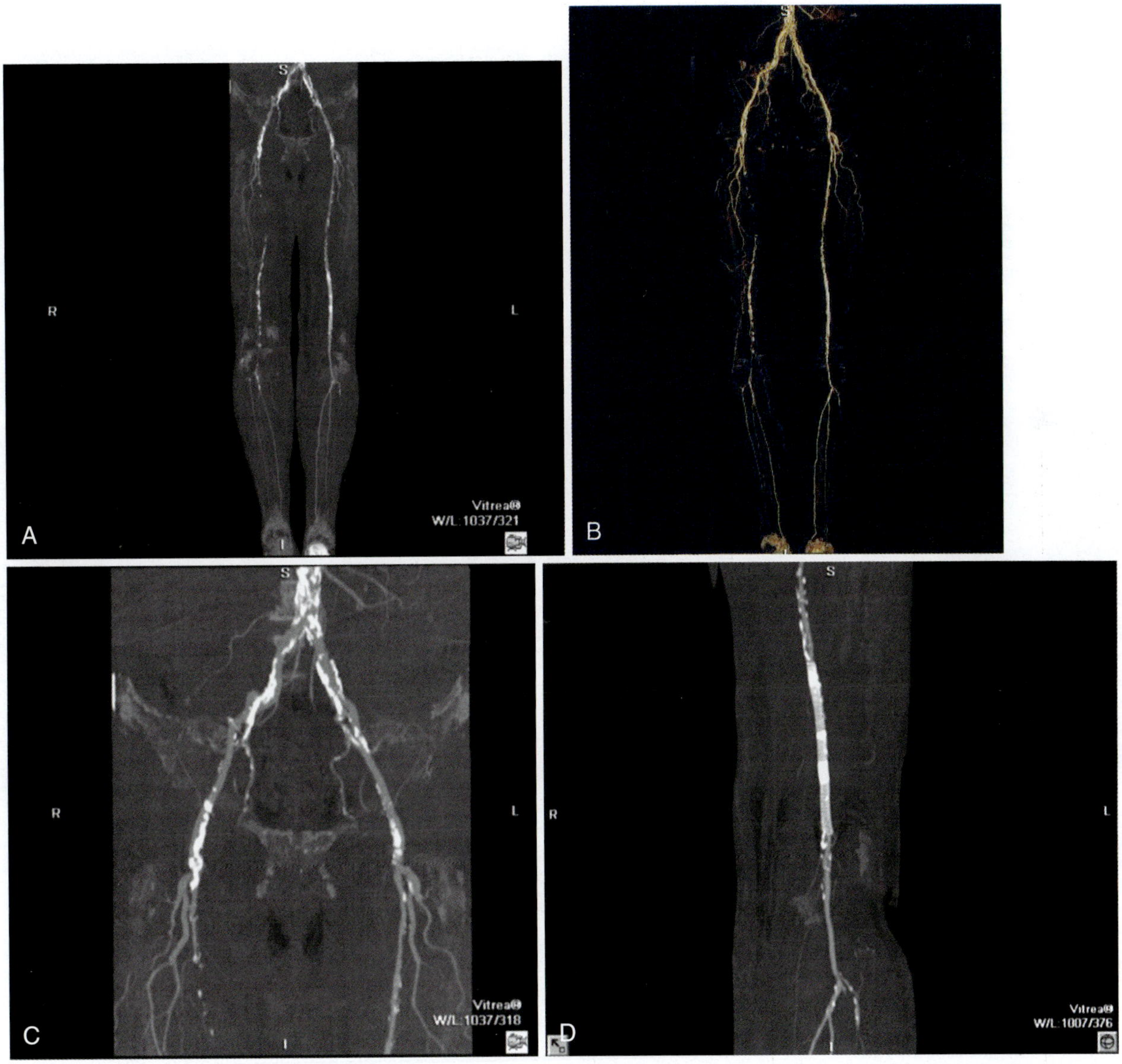

FIG 15.18 Multidetector row helical computed tomography angiography of peripheral runoff. (A) Maximum-intensity projection (MIP) of peripheral runoff study done on a 16-row scanner. Note full coverage of extremities. (B) Three-dimensional volume rendering may also be performed. See color plate. (C) Zoomed images of pelvis station show the dense calcifications in the aorta and pelvic vessels. Occlusion of the right superficial femoral artery (SFA) is seen. (D) Zoomed MIP images of the left distal SFA show the vascular stents.

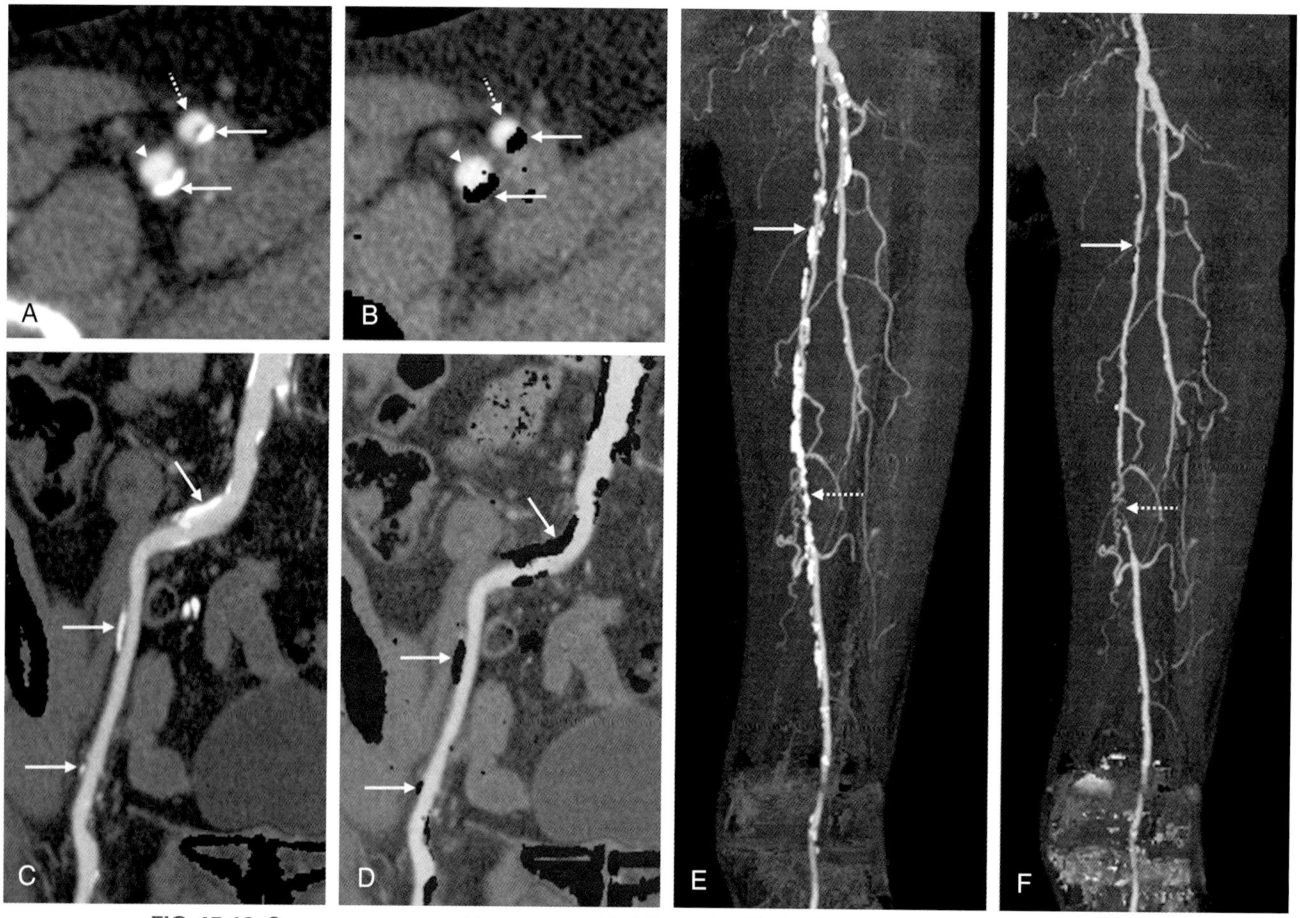

FIG 15.19 Seventy-one-year-old woman with bilateral calf claudication. (A and B) Transversal multiplanar reformatting (MPR) of the superficial *(arrowhead)* and profound femoral artery *(dotted arrow)* without (A) and with dual energy-based plaque subtraction. (C and D) Coronal curved MPR of the pelvic arteries without (C) and with dual energy-based plaque subtraction. (E and F) Maximum-intensity projection of the left thigh (E) after dual energy-based bone subtraction and (F) after additional plaque subtraction. As reflected by the stenosis correlation data, the degree of stenoses in pelvic and thigh arteries is well reflected by the plaque-subtracted images compared to the corresponding native plaques (*arrows* in A to D). The high-grade stenosis of the proximal superficial femoral artery (*arrow* in E and F) and the short occlusion (*dotted arrow* in E and F) is more clearly demonstrated in the plaque-subtracted images. (From Meyer BC, Wernicke T, Hopfenmuller W, et al: Dual energy CT of peripheral arteries: effect of automatic bone and plaque removal on image quality and grading of stenosis. *Eur J Radiol* 68:414–422, 2008.)

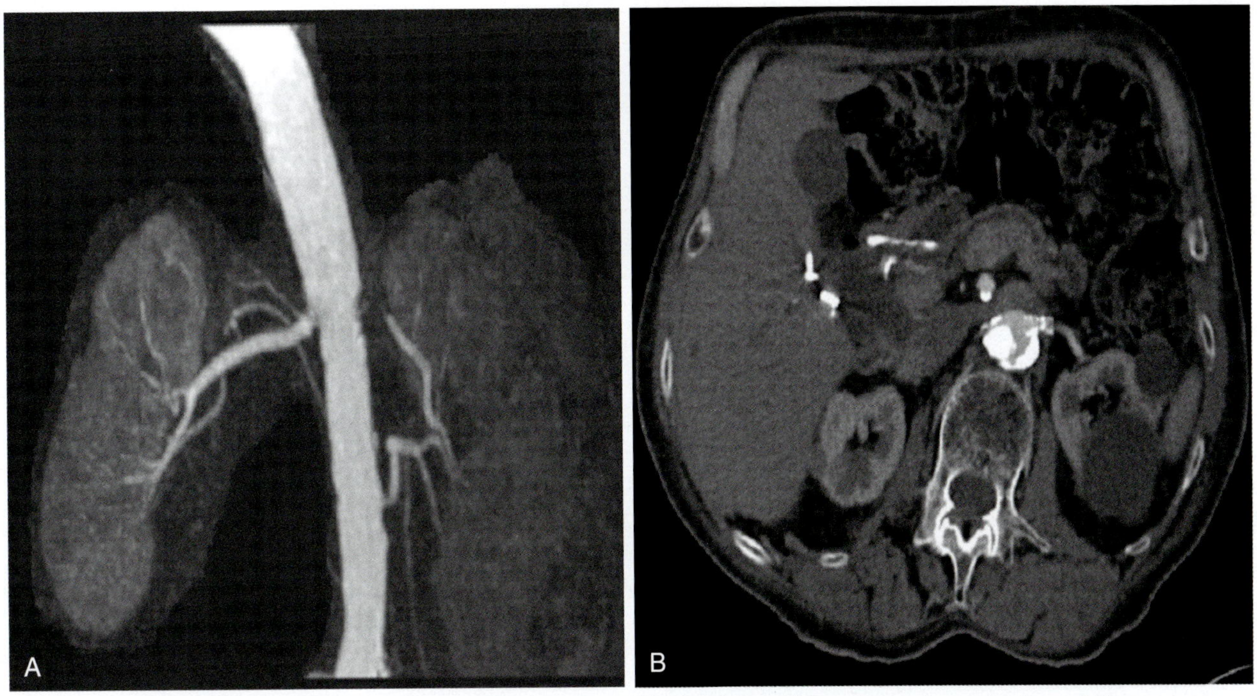

FIG 15.20 Patient with left renal artery stent. (A) Coronal maximum-intensity projection of the aorta shows metal artifact with signal drop-out at the site of a left renal artery stent interfering with assessment of renal artery patency. (B) Computed tomography angiography in the axial plane shows patent stent and left renal artery. Extensive calcifications are seen in the aorta.

MAGNETIC RESONANCE ANGIOGRAPHY VERSUS COMPUTED TOMOGRAPHY ANGIOGRAPHY

The determination to use CTA versus MRA depends on the nature of the vascular bed to be studied, the information to be obtained, and the status of the patient.[117] MDCT CTA is faster, requires less patient cooperation, and affords higher resolution than MRA, but it involves exposure to ionizing radiation and the use of potentially nephrotoxic iodinated contrast material. MRA has lower resolution, takes longer, and requires more patient cooperation, but it does not involve the use of ionizing radiation. Patients with metallic stents and implants are better evaluated with MDCT CTA because of artifacts that occur with MRA (Fig. 15.20). Patients with pacemakers are not routinely studied with MRA unless the information needed cannot be obtained by other means, in which case special precautions are required. If the patient has a newer MRI-conditional device, such as a pacemaker or implantable cardioverter-defibrillator (ICD), standardized protocols are again recommended for MRI imaging.

Both MRA and CTA permit the acquisition of volume data, which can be manipulated with postprocessing techniques. Both techniques provide large data sets that require workstation viewing. Subtraction techniques currently available with MRA make post-processing faster than with CTA, which requires time-consuming background and bone removal (Fig. 15.21). Both these techniques, however, are noninvasive and are likely to supplant conventional angiography in the diagnosis of vascular disease. As technology improves, other applications of CTA and MRA are anticipated, and improved small vessel visualization is expected.

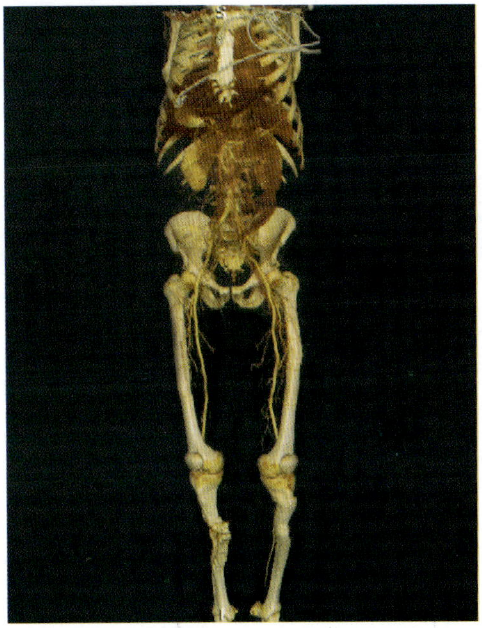

FIG 15.21 Total-body magnetic resonance angiogram. Imaging of the entire body is also possible using 16- or 64-row multi-detector row helical computed tomography scanners. Extensive postprocessing is required to remove bone and soft tissue.

REVIEW QUESTIONS

1. True or false: MRA and CTA provide similar images because they are based on the same technology and use ionizing radiation.
2. Which of the following statements regarding MRA is correct?
   - a. Two-dimensional TOF techniques are best for visualizing tortuous vessels with slow flow.
   - b. Contrast-enhanced MRA techniques use conventional iodinated contrast material.
   - c. Gadolinium-containing contrast material is recommended in patients with GFR ≤30 mL/min per 1.73 m^2.
   - d. Subtraction techniques are used to remove background tissue in both digital subtraction angiography and MRA.
3. Which of the following techniques have been used for MRA?
   - a. Two-dimensional time of flight
   - b. Three-dimensional TOF contrast-enhanced MRA
   - c. Phase-contrast techniques
   - d. All of the above
4. Contrast-enhanced MRA is useful for evaluating which of the following vascular beds?
   - a. Arch vessels
   - b. Abdominal aorta
   - c. Runoff vessels
   - d. Deep veins of the upper and lower extremities
   - e. Tertiary branches of the mesenteric artery
5. Which of the following statements regarding MDCT CTA is true?
   - a. It has lower resolution than contrast-enhanced MRA.
   - b. Image acquisition time is shorter than for contrast-enhanced MRA.
   - c. Postprocessing of images to remove bone and soft tissue is easier with MDCT CTA.
6. Which of the following statements regarding MDCT CTA are true?
   - a. It is frequently used for the diagnosis of acute aortic dissection.
   - b. It is preferred over contrast-enhanced MRA for follow-up studies in patients with chronic aortic dissection.
   - c. It is better than contrast-enhanced MRA in patients with limited ability to cooperate.
7. True or false: Accuracy of stenosis assessment is equal with MDCT CTA and contrast-enhanced MRA.
8. True or false: Peripheral runoff studies can be performed with both MDCT CTA and contrast-enhanced MRA.
9. Which of the following statements regarding MDCT CTA is correct?
   - a. Scanners with four detector rows have larger volume coverage than scanners with 16 detector rows.
   - b. Slice thickness is a reconstruction parameter with MDCT.
   - c. MDCT has higher accuracy than contrast-enhanced MRA for evaluating accessory renal arteries in renal donors.
   - d. All of the above
10. Postprocessing techniques used for MDCT CTA and contrast-enhanced MRA include which of the following?
    - a. MIP
    - b. Three-dimensional volume rendering
    - c. MPR
    - d. All of the above

BIBLIOGRAPHY

Binkert C, Baker P, Petersen B, et al. Peripheral vascular disease: blinded study of dedicated calf MR angiography versus standard bolus-chase MR angiography and film hard-copy angiography. *Radiology*. 2004;232:860–866.

Fleischmann D. High concentration contrast media in MDCT angiography: principles and rationale. *Eur Radiol*. 2003; 13(suppl 3):N39–N43.

Foley WD, Karcaaltincaba M. Computed tomography angiography: principles and clinical applications. *J Comput Assist Tomogr*. 2003;27(suppl 1):S23–S30.

Hartmann IJC, Wittenberg R. Schaefer-Prokop imaging of acute pulmonary embolism using multidetector CT angiography: an update on imaging technique and interpretation. *Eur J Radiol*. 2010;74:40–49.

Holloway BJ, Rosewarne D, Jones RG. Imaging of thoracic aortic disease. *Br J Radiol*. 2011;84:S338–S354.

Idee JM, Port M, Dencausse A, et al. Involvement of gadolnium chelates in the mechanism of nephrogenic systemic fibrosis: an update. *Radiol Clin North Am*. 2009;47:855–869.

Napoli V, Fleischmann D, Chan FP, et al. Computed tomography angiography: state-of-the-art imaging using multidetector-row technology. *J Comput Assist Tomogr*. 2004;28(suppl 1):S32–S45.

Prince M. Body MR angiography with gadolinium contrast agents. *Magn Reson Imaging Clin N Am*. 1996;4:11–24.

Prokop M, Shin HO, Schanz A, et al. Use of maximum intensity projection in CT angiography: a basic review. *Radiographics*. 1997;17:433–451.

Shoepf UJ, Becker CR, Hofmann LK, et al. Multislice CT angiography. *Eur Radiol*. 2003;13:629–636.

References available online at ExpertConsult.com.

CHAPTER 16

Vascular Grafts: Characteristics and Rational Selection

Jeffrey J. Siracuse, Alik Farber

Despite advances in endovascular interventions, the use of surgical bypass is still both relevant and fundamental to the treatment of a wide variety of vascular surgery conditions. The technical details of the bypass procedure and its subsequent outcomes are dependent on the conduit used. The ideal bypass conduit should be as similar as possible to the native vessel it is replacing. It also needs to be readily available, durable, and easy to handle; it needs to hold a low likelihood of infection and thrombosis and be inexpensive. Although such conduit does not exist, autologous blood vessels are closest to the ideal (Box 16.1).

Vein grafts, specifically the great saphenous vein (GSV), are the most commonly used autologous conduit.[1,2] Autologous arterial grafts have been used in selective cases, including coronary revascularization.[3-5] However, because autologous conduits are not always available or appropriate, artificial grafts such as expanded polytetrafluoroethylene (ePTFE, W.L. Gore, Newark, Delaware) and polyethylene terephthalate (Dacron, DuPont, Wilmington, Delaware) have been used in clinical practice. In general, such grafts are harder to handle, best not used in infected fields, and, compared with autologous conduits, are at increased risk for structural deterioration, occlusion, and infection.[2,6] Biological conduits, such as cryopreserved vein, have been used for reconstruction when autologous vein is not available and use of prosthetic graft is judged to be suboptimal.[7] Clinical research involving the use of tissue engineered grafts as conduits is ongoing and holds promise (Table 16.1).[8-10]

AUTOLOGOUS VEIN

Autologous vein has traditionally been the preferred conduit for vascular bypass in multiple anatomic locations and for a variety of indications, the most common of which remain infrainguinal bypass and creation of arteriovenous access.[1] Autologous vein grafts can also be used for vascular reconstructions in other locations, including other peripheral arteries and more central vessels. For example, the carotid artery can be reconstructed using interposition bypass with GSV in the setting of occlusive disease, aneurysmal disease, and traumatic injury.[11-13] Alternatively, autologous vein can be used in the setting of an arm bypass as part of a distal revascularization and interval ligation (DRIL) procedure to treat ischemic steal syndrome after hemodialysis access creation.[14]

Histologically, vein is composed of three layers. The tunica intima consists of the endothelium, plays an important role in vasomotor regulation, and is a barrier and interface for the vein from circulating mediators. The tunica media is composed of smooth muscle cells and elastic fibers, whereas the tunica adventitia is composed of connective tissue which provides structural support for the vessel.[15] Veins have a thinner and less well-defined medial layer compared with arteries, as the venous system is a lower pressure system.[15] The adventitia in the vein comprises the majority of the vessel wall volume, whereas it is only a small part of an arterial wall. Arterial endothelial cells are generally long and narrow, whereas vein endothelial cells are short and wide.[16]

Similar to arteries, arterialized veins can develop intimal hyperplasia, which can lead to graft stenosis and ultimately failure.[17]

Multiple pieces of autologous vein, including saphenous and arm vein, can be anastomosed together to form what are called composite venous grafts. Such grafts are often used in infrainguinal lower extremity bypass. Patency of such grafts is lower than single segment autologous grafts; however, they remain a viable option when the former is not available.[18]

Saphenous Vein

In clinical practice the most commonly used autologous vein conduit is GSV because it is easily accessible, long lengths are available for harvest, and removal is inconsequential.[1] The GSV can be harvested using traditional open techniques, using either continuous or skip incisions. Wound infection rates are similar between continuous and skip incisions.[19] Alternatively, GSV can be harvested endoscopically.[20-23] Comparison of these techniques reveals that, although results are heterogeneous, the overall trend is that endoscopic vein harvest has fewer wound complications but is associated with lower patency rates.[20-23]

GSV conduits have been used in many revascularization scenarios including peripheral artery reconstruction in the lower

BOX 16.1 **Conduit Characteristics**

Ideal Conduit
Readily available
Durable
Easy to handle
Low chance of infection
Low chance of thrombosis
Inexpensive

TABLE 16.1 **Conduit Types**

Conduit Type	Advantages	Disadvantages
Autologous superficial vein	Easily accessible Removal inconsequential Useful for many sites Low risk of infection	Limited availability Potential for size mismatch Limited by length
Autologous deep vein	Reconstruction of larger vessels Useful for many sites Low risk of infection	Limited availability Associated morbidity with removal Limited by length
Autologous arteries	Most similar to arteries being reconstructed Useful for many sites Low risk of infection	Associated morbidity with removal Limited by length Limited donor sites
Prosthetic grafts	"Off-the-shelf" accessible Not limited by length Useful for many sites Available in different diameters and lengths	Lower patency rates Susceptible to infection Harder to handle
Cryopreserved allografts and xenografts	"Off-the-shelf" accessible Available in different diameters and lengths Low risk of infection Useful for many sites	Lower patency rates Expensive At increased risk of aneurysmal degeneration

and upper extremities as well as renal and visceral revascularization. GSV is often used for infrainguinal bypass, using a variety of conduit configurations such as in situ, reversed, and nonreversed reconstruction. Infrainguinal bypass has been applied in both occlusive and aneurysmal disease. The largest series of saphenous vein bypasses analyzed include 2058 in situ bypasses, the majority of which were for critical limb ischemia (CLI).[24] Primary patency rates of 85%, 72%, and 55% were reported at 1, 5, and 10 years, respectively.[24] Taylor reported a series of 516 reversed vein bypass grafts, showing comparable 5-year primary and secondary patency rates of 75% and 81%.[25]

When used for infrainguinal bypass, GSV conduits have been shown to have superior patency to other conduits.[26,27] Subgroup analysis of the Bypass versus Angioplasty in Severe Ischaemia of the Leg (BASIL) trial, the only published randomized trial comparing bypass to endovascular interventions in CLI, showed that vein bypass, of which 90% was performed using GSV, was associated with improved amputation free survival compared with prosthetic conduit.[26,27]

Data from the Project of Ex-vivo Vein Graft Engineering via Transfection (PREVENT) III trial, a large prospective cohort of infrainguinal bypass performed for CLI, revealed that single segment GSV and vein diameter were associated with improved outcomes.[28] Of 1404 total bypass procedures, 604 were performed using single segment GSV greater than 3.5 mm, and 1-year primary patency, primary-assisted patency, secondary patency, and limb salvage rates were 71.5%, 84.4%, 86.9%, and 90.6%, respectively. Conduit characteristics were the main determinant of both early and late graft failure.[28]

The small saphenous vein (SSV) is also an additional source of conduit. It can be used as a single conduit or be spliced with other veins.[29] SSV use can be limited by available length and often requires the patient to be positioned prone for successful harvest.

GSV can be used for vascular reconstructions in other locations. This includes other peripheral arteries and more central vessels. For example, the carotid artery can be reconstructed with GSV in the setting of occlusive disease, aneurysmal disease, or traumatic injury.[11,12] Reconstruction can be either an interposition bypass or an external to internal carotid bypass.[13] GSV can also be used for upper extremity reconstruction for subclavian or axillary occlusive disease or traumatic injury.[30,31] GSV is also often commonly used for DRIL procedures in the setting of steal syndrome after hemodialysis access creation.[14] Finally, GSV can also be used as conduit for renal and visceral bypass for both occlusive and aneurysmal disease.[32-34]

Arm Vein

Arm vein has been used as an alternative to GSV.[35-37] Superficial arm veins include cephalic and basilic veins and are generally thinner than GSV. In the setting of infrainguinal bypass, arm vein has been demonstrated to have adequate long-term patency; however, it often requires creation of a composite conduit.[36,37] Previous peripheral intravenous line placement or blood draws in the arm veins can cause syncitiae or stenoses in a portion of the vein and to that end, intraoperative angioscopy is valuable in identifying such luminal defects and has been shown improve patency outcomes.[37]

One retrospective analysis of arm vein for infrainguinal bypass showed that the distribution of arm vein used was cephalic vein alone in 50.4%, cephalic and basilic vein in 35.6%, and basilic vein alone in 14% of cases. Primary patency at 1 and 3 years was 70.6% and 51.9%, respectively. Vein configuration and composite grafting did not affect patency rates. These authors concluded that arm vein ought to be used as the next option when ipsilateral GSV is not available.[36] A long-term analysis of 520 arm vein bypasses revealed a respective 5-year primary patency, secondary patency, and limb salvage rate of 54.5%, 57.5%, and 71.5%.[37] Single segment or composite reconstruction had similar outcomes.[37] Retrospective comparison of arm vein to prosthetic graft has shown that arm vein has better midterm primary and secondary patency, as well as limb salvage.[38] Subgroup analysis of arm vein bypass shows that patency is best with single segment cephalic vein.[39]

Aside from infrainguinal bypass, arm vein is also essential for creation of arteriovenous access. Either the cephalic, basilic, or even brachial vein can be used to create an autologous arteriovenous fistula (AVF). The basilic or brachial veins often need to be superficialized or transposed for access.[40] Native AVF ultimately require maturation for successful use, and as such, arm vein greater than 3 mm has been associated with increased maturation success.[41] Outflow stenosis develops, not infrequently, in these veins, and treatment is often performed with balloon angioplasty with or without stenting.[42]

Femoral Vein

Femoral vein can be used when a larger-caliber autologous conduit is needed. This vein can be harvested by making an incision approximately 5 cm below the inguinal crease down to the level of the knee. The dissection is performed medial to the sartorius muscle proximally and lateral to it distally. Care must be taken to carefully ligate all venous branches. Bypass using one or both femoral veins has been used to reconstruct the aorta in the setting of aortic graft infection as an alternative to prosthetic material.[43] This procedure may be staged with exposure of bilateral femoral veins performed on the day prior to graft resection and reconstruction. Creation of a neoaortoiliac system (NAIS) involves the harvest of bilateral femoral veins. Successful reconstructions are associated with good patency, yet still carry potential morbidity including venous hypertension and lower extremity thrombosis.[44,45] Femoral veins can also be used for nonaneurysmal abdominal vascular disease, including mesenteric reconstruction.[46]

Femoral vein can also be used in the setting of dialysis access, as a free central venous bypass, and for creation of an AVF via local transposition.[47-49] Brachioaxillary bypass using autologous femoral vein is often performed in patients with a patent central venous system who have failed upper extremity prosthetics access. Preoperative upper extremity venography and arteriography are performed. In one series, primary patency rates of more than 90% at 6 months and secondary patency rates at 18 months have been reported.[47] A 3% 30-day mortality rate and a 57% overall complication rate were noted. Hand ischemia, thigh complications, and arm complications were observed in 43%, 23%, and 17%, respectively. Creation of a lower extremity AVF by directly transposing the femoral vein to the superficial femoral artery has also been shown to have excellent success in patients who have failed upper extremity access.[48] Although the procedure requires a significant incision and dissection, it is associated with less significant risk of infection than a prosthetic groin AVF.[48] Preoperatively, it is recommended that ankle-brachial indices are performed because concomitant peripheral arterial disease is associated with increased risk of ischemic steal. Likewise, intraoperatively, the vein is usually banded to diminish flow and limit the risk of steal. Femoral AVFs have been shown to be associated with excellent 91% and 45%, 1- and 9-year patency rates, respectively.[49]

AUTOLOGOUS ARTERY

Autologous arterial conduits are theoretically ideal to use because they have similar features as the vessel they are replacing. Internal mammary, radial, and gastroepiploic arteries have been used with success for coronary revascularization,[3-5] whereas the internal iliac and radial arteries have been used in the visceral and renal revascularization.[50-52] Finally, the superficial temporal artery has also been used for extracranial-intracranial bypass.[53] Unfortunately, short conduit length and consequences of harvest have limited the use of autologous arterial grafts to a relatively small number of clinical scenarios.

PROSTHETIC GRAFTS

Although autologous vascular grafts are associated with excellent results, there are multiple clinical situations in which such conduits are not adequate, available, or appropriate. The need for conduit in such circumstances has led to the development of artificial, prosthetic grafts. Although multiple materials have been tried, ePTFE and polyethylene terephthalate (Dacron, DuPont, Wilmington, Delaware) are used most commonly.

ePTFE (W.L. Gore) is a paste-extruded fiber in which the PTFE is processed by extrusion and thermal stretch processes. This extrusion process delivers better tensile stretch and less shrinkage compared with nonexpanded PTFE. ePTFE is available in different configurations depending on indication. Grafts are fabricated with or without external ring support. Heparin-bonded ePTFE has emerged and in most cases is the default graft used (Propaten, W.L. Gore, Newark, Delaware). Heparin-bonded ePTFE has been shown to have better long-term patency compared with non-heparin-bonded grafts in femoropopliteal bypass but not in dialysis access.[54-56] Some PTFE grafts are constructed with a premade distal cuff.

Dacron is a collagen-coated polyester graft and is produced in woven and knitted patterns. The woven grafts have less porosity and bleeding but have reduced compliance. Dacron can also be heparin bonded—the Fusion Bioline is a ringed heparin-bonded Dacron graft (Maquet Holding B.V. & Co., Rastatt, Germany).[57]

Prosthetic grafts are currently used in a variety of clinical scenarios. Their use in infrainguinal bypass has had mixed results.[58-60] An early randomized trial by Veith of ePTFE and autologous saphenous vein showed that ePTFE had lower patency rates compared with vein (54% ± 11% vs. 76% ± 9% at 4 years, $P < .05$). Differences for above knee bypass did not reach statistical significance (38% ± 13% vs. 61% ± 12%). Primary patency rates at 4 years for infrapopliteal bypasses showed ePTFE to have a significantly worse performance than vein bypass (12% ± 7% vs. 49% ± 10% vs., $P < .001$).[58] These results fail to support the routine preferential use of ePTFE grafts for either femoropopliteal or more distal bypass. However, this graft may have utility in selected poor-risk patients in need of an infrainguinal bypass, particularly when the target is above the knee joint.

Heparin-bonded grafts have been developed in an attempt to increase graft patency. No systemic effects have been identified from the heparin bonding.[61] There has been one case of heparin-induced thrombocytopenia attributed to heparin boned grafts, although it is unclear whether other exposures to heparin were definitively ruled out.[62,63] A randomized trial comparing heparin-bonded ePTFE (Propaten graft) to standard ePTFE revealed that the heparin-bonded ePFTE had improved patency.[64] Overall, primary patency after 1 year was 86.4% for heparin-bonded and 79.9% for standard ePTFE grafts (odds ratio [OR] 0.627, 95% confidence interval [CI] 0.398; 0.989, $P = .043$). Secondary patency was 88% for heparin-bonded and 81% in standard ePTFE grafts (OR 0.569 [95% CI, 0.353; 0.917, $P = .020$]). A more recent trial looking at long-term data showed a patency benefit at 2 years, with heparin-bonded grafts that disappeared at 5-year follow-up, although patients with CLI had improved patency at 5 years (66.7% vs. 50% $P = .049$).[65] A randomized trial comparing the Fusion Bioline graft with standard ePTFE showed that the primary patency rates at 6 months were 86.4% for the Fusion Bioline heparin-coated vascular graft group compared with 70.0% for the standard ePTFE group, $P = .006$), and the respective rates at 12 months were 76.5% and 67.0% (95% CI, −4.8% to 23.0%; $P = .05$). The mean time to hemostasis of bleeding at the suture hole was 3.5 minutes in the Fusion Bioline group and 11.0 minutes in the standard ePTFE group ($P < .0001$).[57]

Although autologous vein should be used for infrapopliteal bypasses, an ePTFE distal bypass is a potential option when facing a primary amputation. A single-center retrospective analysis of prosthetic bypasses to tibial vessels showed that primary patency rates at 30 days and 1 and 5 years were 87%, 87%, and 60%, respectively. Limb salvage rates at 30 days and 1 and 5 years were 91%, 68%, and 63%, respectively. Survival at 3 and 5 years was, respectively, 53% and 42%. There were no significant differences between diabetics and nondiabetics except for a trend toward decreased patient survival at 3 and 5 years in those with diabetes.[66] These outcomes are worse than those reported by Veith et al., who noted 4-year primary patency rates of infrapoliteal bypass for infrapopliteal PTFE bypass to be substantially lower than similar bypass using vein (12% ± 7% vs. 49% ± 10% vs., $P < .001$).[58]

Prosthetic grafts have also been used with success for replacement and bypass of large- and medium-sized arteries. This includes aortic reconstruction for aneurysmal, occlusive, or trauma indications; inline reconstruction of subclavian, femoral, or carotid arteries; or extraanatomic bypass.

Dacron is used either as a tube graft for aneurysmal disease or a bifurcated graft for aneurysmal or occlusive disease.[67] Aortobifemoral (ABF) bypass, either end to end or end to side, depending on the amount of aortic disease and need for preservation of hypogastric perfusion, is the main bypass treatment for bilateral aortoiliac occlusive disease. Direct inline open repair has been the historical "gold standard," with greater than 80% 10-year patency and relatively low perioperative morbidity and mortality.[68] In cases in which there is a severely diseased infrarenal aorta, a thoracofemoral bypass can also be performed to establish inline flow.

ABF bypass has been shown to have excellent durability and hemodynamic results.[69] A meta-analysis noted that the overall 5-year patency rate is 86.3%, with a 4.1% operative mortality and 16% morbidity. Extraanatomical bypasses for aortoiliac occlusive disease can be performed when inline revascularization is not possible due to prior intraabdominal operations or bypass, current intraabdominal infection, or severe patient comorbidities. Extraanatomical bypasses, including axillary-bifemoral and femoral to femoral artery bypass, are often performed with ePTFE and generally have a higher risk of failure than inline, anatomic bypasses.[70-73]

Prosthetic bypass grafts can also be used in medium-sized arteries. This includes for aneurysmal and occlusive disease of carotid and subclavian arteries.[74] Carotid to subclavian artery bypass have become more frequent with the increased use of debranching as an adjunct for thoracic endovascular aortic aneurysm repair.[75,76] Prosthetic grafts have also been used extensively for dialysis access because many patients may not have adequate autologous vein available for native AVF creation.[77] The most common graft used is ePTFE. Arteriovenous grafts (AVGs) have been shown to have lower patency rates, higher rates of reinterventions to restore patency, and increased risk of infection.[78-80] Tapered AVG have been developed to reduce the risk for steal, but although these grafts have better hemodynamic results, they have not been shown to translate to better clinical outcomes.[81-84] Newer hybrid grafts with self-expanding nitinol-reinforced sections which can avoid a second anastomosis have been developed to aid in areas of difficult anatomy.[85] These grafts have also been used for complex visceral and renal reconstruction.[86,87]

BIOLOGICAL GRAFTS

Limitations of autologous and prosthetic grafts have fueled exploration for other potential conduits, and this investigative effort has led to the evaluation of biological grafts for bypass. These include both allografts (same species graft) and xenografts (different species graft). Biological grafts offer "off-the-shelf" availability, a wide variety of sizes, and excellent handling characteristics. Allografts include cryopreserved GSV, femoral vein, and aorta, whereas xenografts include bovine carotid artery and mesenteric vein grafts. Their use has been hampered by low patency rates, possibly due to immune rejection.

Long-term patency of cryopreserved GSV for infrainguinal reconstruction is low, with rates of approximately 30% at 1 year reported.[88-90] However, limb salvage rates range from 57% to 80% at 1 year.[88,90] Such veins may be used in clinical scenarios when short-term patency is required to heal a wound. It is unclear whether anticoagulation improves patency because there have been contradictory studies.[88,90]

Cryopreserved femoral vein has also been used in multiple sites, including vascular reconstruction in oncologic surgical procedures. Reconstruction of portal vein and superior mesenteric vein has been performed with good results.[91-93] Cryopreserved femoral vein can also be used for dialysis access in cases in which autologous vein is not available and prosthetic is contraindicated.[93] Reported patency rates are equivalent to prosthetic grafts; however, the allografts are susceptible to aneurysm formation.[93] Bovine carotid artery has also been successfully used for hemodialysis access with good patency rates.[94] One prospective randomized study showed superior primary and primary assisted patency with bovine carotid artery compared with ePTFE.[95]

TISSUE-ENGINEERED GRAFTS

The next frontiers in graft development are bioengineered grafts. Such grafts have been created using human vascular smooth muscle cells seeded on polymer scaffolds.[8-10] They consist of human 6-mm acellular vessels with lengths ranging from 35 to 42 cm and were created by using human vascular smooth muscle cells isolated from deceased donors. These cells were expanded and seeded onto polyglycolic acid polymer scaffolds (Biomedical Structures; Warwick, Rhode Island). These were contained within flexible, single-use bioreactors (Charter Medical; Winston-Salem, North Carolina). Developing vessels were subjected to pulsatile cyclic distension for 8 weeks, and then the cells were removed to eliminate immunogenic cellular antigens while preserving the comparatively nonimmunogenic extracellular matrix constituents, specifically collagens type I and III, fibronectin, and vitronectin.[8]

Recently performed phase II human trials show these grafts to be safe and have primary, primary assisted, and secondary patency rates at 6 months of 63%, 73%, and 97% and at 1 year of 28%, 38%, and 89%, respectively. Loss of primary patency is often due to in situ thrombosis.[8]

There is a wide diversity of bypass grafts. Autologous vessels are ideal when available and appropriate. Prosthetic grafts come in a large variety of configurations and can be used but often have lower patency and are prone to infections. Stent-grafts can be used for endovascular repair when a covered stent is required. Biological grafts, including allografts and xenografts, can be used in situations in which autologous and prosthetics are not possible; however, these are hampered by lower patency. Bioengineered grafts have been shown to have good short-term results but require further investigation.

ENDOVASCULAR STENT-GRAFTS

Stent-grafts are increasingly being used for treatment of aneurysms, occlusive disease, and traumatic vascular injury.[96-100] Self-expanding covered stents, such as Viabahn (W.L. Gore, Newark, Delaware), are composed of a heparin-bonded ePTFE liner attached to an external nitinol stent. Stent-grafts have been shown to have improved patency compared with bare metal stents for long segment occlusive femoropopliteal lesions.[99] They have also been increasingly used for repair of popliteal artery aneurysms.[96] Self-expanding stents can also be used for trauma, particularly in areas difficult to access using open surgical techniques.[97,98] Finally, they are also commonly used for recalcitrant stenoses in the venous outflow of AV access.[100]

Balloon-expandable stent-grafts, such as the iCast stent (Atrium, Hudson, New Hampshire), also have been commonly used to treat vascular disease. This stent-graft is composed of stainless steel covered by a thin layer of PTFE. The balloon-expandable stent allows for precision placement; however, it can be susceptible to external compression, and care must be used when advancing the stent through a stenosis to avoid dislodgment. Such stents have been used in fenestrated endovascular aortic repair and have a crucial role in sealing branches of fenestrations.[101] A popular use of balloon-expandable stent-grafts is in the severely diseased, calcified common iliac artery because they protect against rupture. A recent randomized trial demonstrated these stent-grafts to have improved patency over bare metal stents.[102] As such, long-term results of stent-grafting show good patency even in TransAtlantic Inter-Society Consensus C and D iliac lesions.[103]

REVIEW QUESTIONS

1. Which of the following is true about autologous vein grafts:
   - **a.** Greater saphenous vein has historically equivalent patency to arm vein
   - **b.** Endoscopic vein harvesting has been shown to have better patency
   - **c.** There is a potential for mismatched sizing for use of superficial veins for intraabdominal reconstruction
   - **d.** Small saphenous vein is easily accessible
2. Cryopreserved veins
   - **a.** Have poor long-term patency
   - **b.** Have limited section of lengths and diameters
   - **c.** Are inexpensive
   - **d.** Are at low risk of aneurysmal degeneration
3. All the following are true about the femoral vein except:
   - **a.** It is the conduit for neoaortoiliac system (NIAS) reconstruction
   - **b.** It is an option for upper extremity dialysis access
   - **c.** There is low perioperative risk of complications from harvest
   - **d.** Femoral vein-based arteriovenous fistulas have good durability
4. **True or False:** Heparin-bonded PTFE has been shown to have improved patency compared to non-heparin–bonded PTFE.
5. **True or False:** The cryopreserved femoral vein has poor durability for portal vein reconstruction.
6. **True or False:** Tissue-engineered grafts have been shown to have equivalent patency to autologous vein bypass
7. Which of the following is true about stent grafts?
   - **a.** There is no role for them in trauma
   - **b.** They have improved patency for common iliac lesions compared to uncovered stents
   - **c.** The iCAST stent is difficult to precisely deploy
   - **d.** There is no risk of stent-graft infection

References available online at ExpertConsult.com.

17 CHAPTER

Introduction to Endovascular Surgery: Arterial Access, Guidewires, Catheters, Sheaths, Angioplasty Catheters, and Stents

Alan B. Lumsden

The core elements of all endovascular procedures include gaining arterial access safely, placing a sheath with hemostasis valve, and navigating to a selected target using shaped diagnostic catheters and guidewires. In most cases, the intervention itself involves use of an angioplasty balloon and deployment of a stent.[1] We will cover this in the current chapter; other, more sophisticated devices will be described elsewhere in this textbook. Some of the more confusing characteristics of endovascular devices are the sizing measurements and device size compatibilities (an overview is presented in Tables 17.1 to 17.3).

GAINING ARTERIAL ACCESS

The femoral route is selected in the overwhelming majority of cases and the Seldinger technique remains largely unchanged from its original description.[2] This approach is convenient for the operator, safe, and associated with the least likelihood of neurologic impairment. Moreover, the access site can be compressed against the underlying femoral head. We use ultrasound-guided access for all arterial and venous procedures that require vascular access. In our experience, this has been associated with a very low rate of groin complications.

The procedure begins by using fluoroscopy to identify the femoral head. Next, ultrasound is used to identify the common femoral artery and its bifurcation. The anterior rim of the femoral head can also be identified in thin patients. The latter is the only situation in which confirmation using fluoroscopy is not required. We use a micropuncture needle (21-G, 7 cm long) introduced under ultrasound guidance to perform a single wall puncture of the midportion of the common femoral artery. Blood return is observed, but this is not as brisk or as pulsatile as it would be through an 18-G access needle. The micropuncture wire is typically 0.018 in in diameter and 40 cm long. The wire must pass easily and freely in its progression up the iliac artery, and this should be observed fluoroscopically. Any resistance to passage of the wire should result in immediate fluoroscopy to ascertain the wire's location. Once the wire has passed into the common iliac artery, the inner dilator and wire are removed. There should now be brisk arterial bleeding. In our practice, a 0.035-inch Bentson wire is introduced and advanced up into the descending thoracic aorta. Once there is adequate wire support inside the arterial system, the remaining micropuncture sheath is removed and, in most cases, a 5-French access sheath is inserted, its dilator removed, and the side port flushed with heparinized saline.

One exception to the use of a micropuncture kit is in the heavily scarred groin. In this situation, a more robust 18-G needle is used for access to permit immediate placement of a 0.035-inch wire. This wire provides the necessary support to drive a sheath through the scarred groin.

ESSENTIAL TOOLS

Vessel Dilators

Vessel dilators may be necessary when the groin is scarred, when large-bore sheaths are being placed, or when a combination of these circumstances exists. Although they are rarely necessary, their availability can mean the difference between completing and not completing the procedure.

These devices dilate the fascia and tissue to allow easy insertion of an introducer or catheter. Vessel dilators are measured in French sizes and are usually 10 cm long. They come packaged in a range of sizes. Some physicians do not use the introducer sheath during diagnostic studies but may use vessel dilators to prevent arterial damage when a diagnostic catheter is advanced into the artery. It is important not to overdilate to a diameter larger than that of the catheter to be used. However, since the sheaths' outer diameters are larger than their inner diameters, it may be useful to dilate one size larger than the sheath. For example, a 6-French sheath may need a 7-French dilator to allow easy passage. In our practice, we use hemostatic sheaths on every case.

Introducer Sheaths With Hemostasis Valves

Sheaths allow easy passage of guidewires, catheters, and interventional devices into the artery without vessel damage or excessive blood loss. An introducer sheath with a hemostasis valve should be used during all interventional procedures to protect the vessel and allow ease of passage for devices (balloons, stents, and atherectomy catheters) (Fig. 17.1). Sheaths should also be used for diagnostic studies that require multiple catheter exchanges.

Different manufacturers' valves possess different characteristics, such as a self-centering feature for wires to reduce backbleed. Many devices require insertion tools to help cross the valve. Some sheaths may be wire-braided to reduce kinks or include

TABLE 17.1 Calculating French Size

The French size is three times the diameter in millimeters. A round catheter of 1 French has an external diameter of 1/3 mm; therefore the diameter of a round catheter in millimeters can be determined by dividing the French size by 3:

D (mm) = French/3 or French = *D* (mm) *3

For example, if the French size is 9, the diameter is 3 mm.

TABLE 17.2 Units for Sizing Endovascular Devices

Needles	Gauge: thousandths of an inch
Wires	Diameter: thousandths of an inch Length: centimeters
Dilators	Outer diameter: French (divide by Pi to convert to mm)
Sheaths	Inner diameter: French Length: centimeters
Catheters	Outer diameter: French Length: centimeters Lumen: thousandths of an inch
Balloons	Maximal inflated diameter: millimeters Length: centimeters Shaft diameter: French Corresponding wire system: thousandths of an inch
Stents	Expanded size: millimeters Unexpanded size: French Length: centimeters

TABLE 17.3 Guide to the Sizing of Endoluminal Devices

Device	Diameter	Length
Needles	gauge	in/cm
Introducer sheath	French (inner diameter)	cm
Catheter (diagnostic)	French (outer diameter)	cm
Catheter (guide)	French (outer diameter)	cm
Balloons	French (shaft diameter)	cm

a radiopaque tip for visualization. Sizes may range from 4 French to 12 French or larger. Some of the new endoluminal devices will require introducers up to 24 French. The larger sizes may require a cutdown to repair the artery postprocedure. Be aware that the French size relates to the inner diameter of the sheath. The outer diameter is usually 1 to 2 French sizes larger if the introducer has wire-braided reinforcement.

Sheaths also come in a variety of lengths and shapes. For example, in placing a stent in the supra-aortic trunks, a 70- or 90-cm sheath may be necessary. This protects the stent during introduction and allows contrast to be injected directly at the site being treated, thereby providing excellent visualization. It also provides a level of protection should the balloon rupture or the stent be displaced.

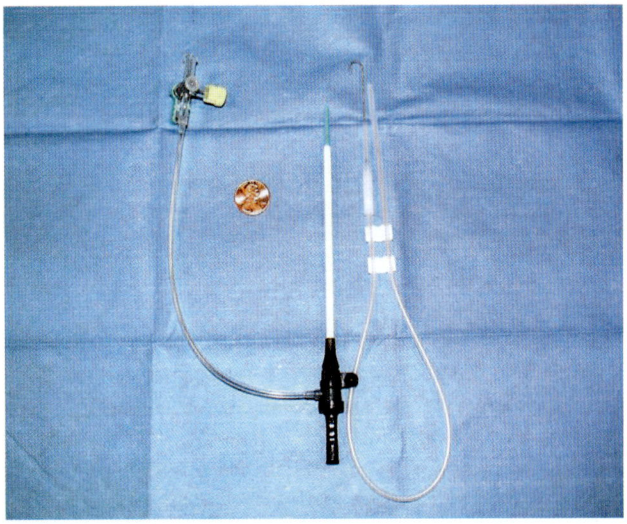

FIG 17.1 Development of a sheath that can provide access to the vascular system without continuous blood loss was a major advance, and it has been widely used during endovascular procedures. The side port allows flushing with heparinized saline to prevent clotting of the sheath. The sheath also protects endovascular devices as they are introduced and recovered from the vascular system.

Guidewires

Two general styles of guidewires are used for vascular access: stainless steel and hydrophilic coated guidewires. Both types are used to gain access, guide catheters into the ostia of vessels, and cross lesions.[3] They have a variety of common characteristics:

- They are available in lengths ranging from 40 to 300 cm.
  - Most common working wires are in the 180-cm range.
  - Shorter wires are used for Monorail balloons.
  - Long wires are used for over-the-wire balloons, thrombectomy catheters, and contralateral tibial interventions.
- "Docking" wires allow an extension to be added to the back end of a wire, thereby "lengthening" the wire.
- Diameter, length, tip configuration, coating, stiffness, and handling properties should be selected for the task at hand.
- They may be used in conjunction with diagnostic catheters to facilitate selective vessel catheterization.
- There are also nonhydrophilic routine access and "working" wires.

In working with any wire, caution is key. If it does not go easily, it should not be forced. When you encounter resistance on removing a wrapped wire, avoid pulling it, as it might unravel. It is better to advance it with catheter support.

Stainless Steel Guidewires

Stainless steel wires may be manufactured as solid steel wires or as wrapped thin steel wires. The wires have a rigid, solid steel core called a *mandrel* and a flexible tip to help prevent vessel injury. Each guidewire has distinct characteristics that allow passage into the target vessel. Guidewires usually have a floppy tip with a stiff body. The distal tip configuration of the stainless steel guidewires is generally straight, angled, or J-shaped.

Diameters are measured in thousandths of an inch, ranging from 0.009 to 0.038. Lengths are measured in centimeters and can range from 80 to 260 cm; however, specialty wires may come in longer lengths. Wires can be broken, but a safety wire built into the construct prevents the components from separating completely.

Hydrophilic Guidewires

- Use hydrophilic wires for passing through tortuosities, crossing tight stenoses, and recanalization.

Similar to stainless steel wires, hydrophilic guidewires also have mandrels but are coated with a special material rendering them very slippery. They are constructed with a central core of superelastic metal alloy that tapers to a soft flexible tip. The kink-resistant core is coated with polyurethane. This polyurethane jacket is bonded with a hydrophilic polymer that becomes slippery when wet. It is essentially a plastic guidewire. Some other hydrophilic guidewires have stainless steel cores with shapeable tips.

There are many manufacturers; choice is dependent on physician preference. These are some general characteristics of hydrophilic guidewires:

- They have Nitinol cores with a hydrophilic polymer coating.
- The tip may be straight, curved, or formed by the operator.
- The coating may shear off if the guidewire is withdrawn through a needle.
- They are particularly valuable in tortuous vessels and in crossing tight stenoses.
- They are used for the recanalization of occlusions—especially with subintimal passage.
- They can be used to cross the aortic bifurcation for contralateral angiography.
- They must be kept wet prior to and during use.
- BUT they are more difficult to handle; they are not adapted for routine access or as working wires, since it is easy to "lose" the wire.

Catheters

Diagnostic and Guide Catheters

Catheters have two purposes: (1) to deliver contrast for arteriography, and (2) to assist in device placement to target lesions for intervention. Diagnostic catheters are usually supplied in small French sizes, 4 or 5 French, whereas guiding catheters are larger, 7 or 8 French, to allow passage of the interventional device. The French size of diagnostic catheters relates to their outside diameters and is usually 4 or 5 French (see Table 17.3). Guiding catheters are also measured by outside diameter; however, the inside diameter is very important so that endovascular devices may pass freely without restriction. Guide catheters are, in many respects, more like sheaths than diagnostic catheters. However, they differ from sheaths in two important respects: they do not have a dilator integrated into the system and they usually do not have a hemostasis valve, so a removable valve must be available. Countless shapes, sizes, and lengths are available from many manufacturers (Fig. 17.2). Selective or diagnostic catheters tips are shaped and have a single end hole for intubating branch vessels.

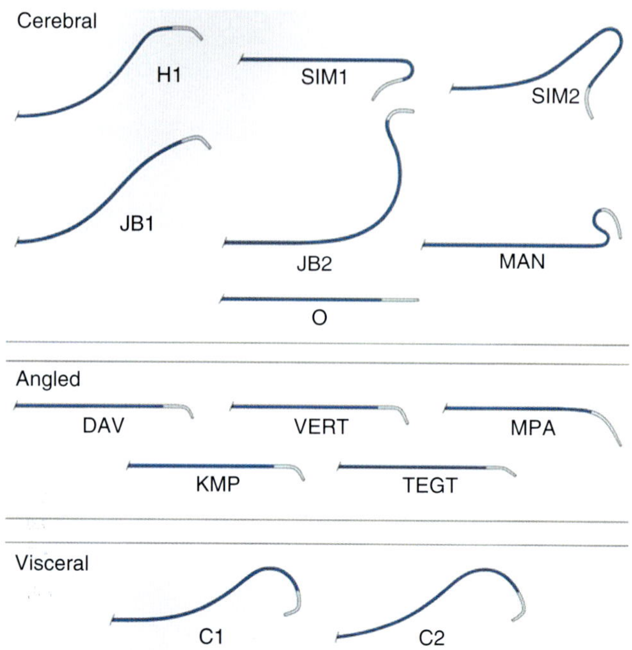

FIG 17.2 Angiographic catheters come in a wide variety of shapes.

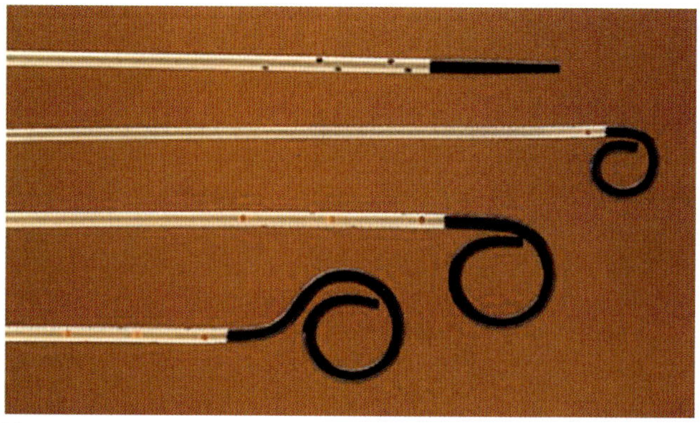

FIG 17.3 Flush catheters have numerous holes on the shaft and end of the catheter to spray contrast across the entire flow field, providing uniform opacification of large blood vessels.

They are best considered as two different devices, even though both are referred to as catheters. Diagnostic catheters are the workhorse catheters, used on every case. They are broadly considered as end-hole and flush catheters (Fig. 17.3). End-hole catheters have a single exit hole at the end of the catheter. This limits the amount of contrast that can be injected, so they are generally not used in very high-flow vessels such as the aorta or inferior vena cava (IVC). On the other hand, flush catheters have numerous holes that spray contrast across a high-flow field; they are used for opacification of the aorta, IVC, and any other high-flow situations. All catheters have their length, guidewire compatibilities, and burst pressures clearly marked on the packaging.

Simple and Complex Curve Catheters

Primary catheterization (first-order branches) is relatively easy but becomes exponentially more difficult as the need to access successively branching vessels increases. The simplest selective catheters have straight and angled curves that do not have to be re-formed inside the vessel. As anatomy becomes more tortuous, more complex curves are required.

The Berenstein catheter is an example of catheter with a simple curve, with the primary curve located near the tip of the catheter.

Complex curves, as in the SIM 2 catheter, are designed for work in tortuous anatomy. Most complex curves must be re-formed or "pulled" into position and are therefore also known as "pull" catheters. Such a catheter may have a primary curve near the tip followed by secondary and tertiary curves. For example, a SIM 2 must be re-formed either in the aorta, using the left subclavian artery, or over the bifurcation. The SIM 2 is designed to abut against the opposite wall of the aorta, so that the tip hunts on the outer curve for the target vessel. A Cobra 2 (C2) catheter's curve is shaped like a Cobra head. It does not have to be re-formed and is especially useful for cannulation of a downward-sloping renal artery or the superior mesenteric artery.

Angioplasty

Balloon Catheter Characteristics

There are two types of angioplasty balloon catheters: compliant and low-compliance, also referred to as noncompliant. Compliance is a measure of how much the balloon surface stretches when force is applied to the catheter. Compliant balloons can be stretched more than low-compliance balloons. Because low-compliance balloons have a limited ability to stretch, they offer significant advantages over compliant balloons. A compliant balloon, because it can stretch more, tends to "hourglass" or "dog bone" around the stenosis. In contrast, because its ability to stretch is limited, a low-compliance balloon retains its shape as it generates force against a stricture. Thus, at the same pressure, a low-compliance balloon will exert greater dilating force at the stricture than a compliant balloon. Because a compliant balloon tends to "hourglass" around the stricture, dilating force is diverted away from the stenosis to areas of less resistance. This decreases the amount of dilating force at the stricture. In contrast, a low-compliance balloon concentrates the dilating forces at the stenosis, thereby generating the greatest force at the stricture.

The balloon must provide strength matched to the type of lesion. The balloon should generate sufficient force over the entire lesion to achieve the desired vessel dilation. The pressure a balloon can withstand without the danger of rupture determines the force a balloon can generate against a lesion.

A dilatation balloon is constructed so that it can withstand the hydrostatic pressure (i.e., the pressure from the fluid used to inflate the balloon) applied during inflation. A balloon's resistance to pressure is considered its burst strength. The "rated burst pressure" indicates the maximum level of pressure, expressed in atm, that the balloon will safely withstand. The manufacturer determines this value, which is always printed on the front of the catheter packaging.

Finally, balloon profile is the quality of shape and diameter. A low profile allows for atraumatic catheter insertion and withdrawal. It also facilitates crossing tight lesions and tracking through small arteries.

Advances in Balloon Construction

The earliest balloons were constructed of latex. However, due to its high compliance, this material, even with refinement, was soon recognized as unacceptable for balloon dilation procedures. In 1974, the Gruentzig polyvinyl chloride (PVC) balloon was developed. However, this early material was again found to be too compliant for successful dilatation. In 1979, the first balloons made of polyethylene (PE) were constructed. This marked a true advance in the level of balloon material noncompliance. Standard balloons today are still constructed of PE. Maximum inflation pressure for these balloons ranges from 3 to 10 atm, depending on balloon diameter.

In 1984, polyester was used to develop the first high-strength, noncompliant balloon. This balloon accepts higher pressure and therefore can be used to deliver additional force to the lesion. Withstanding pressures up to 17 atm, polyester balloons are especially useful for calcified, hard, or fibrotic lesions and tight stenoses where maximum dilating force is required.

In 1987, polyethylene terephthalate (PET) was used to formulate an ultrathin material for balloon construction that combined noncompliance and high strength. This material also offered the lowest deflated balloon profile available, a property that greatly enhanced the interventionalist's ability to reduce trauma during insertion and withdrawal, to cross tight lesions, and to track through small arteries. This combination of noncompliance, strength, and low profile provided interventionalists with their first total-performance balloon.

In 1992, a manufacturer released another advance in balloon material, Poly-5. This exclusive material withstands pressures up to 17 atm and offers a lower profile than conventional high-pressure balloons. Furthermore, it is highly scratch resistant, a critically important quality when tight, calcified lesions need to be crossed, as is commonly the case during high-pressure angioplasty procedures.

Ideal Balloon Catheter

The ideal balloon dilatation catheter should combine the properties desired in the catheter shaft and the dilatation balloon. The catheter shaft should be constructed to provide the high column strength needed for optimal pushability. The shaft should resist buckling even when negotiating tortuous vessels or crossing tight stenoses. The surface of the catheter should be smooth to permit easy movement over the guidewire to the site.

Moreover, the shaft should be downsized to ease advancement through the lumen of the vessel. Concurrently, the inner diameter of the shaft must accommodate a large enough channel for the injection and withdrawal of fluid and permit rapid balloon inflation and deflation. In addition, the shaft must incorporate the channel used for tracking the catheter over the guidewire and the injection of contrast. To combine a small outer diameter with the largest possible double-lumen inner diameter means that the shaft must be made of material that allows thin-walled construction without compromising strength.

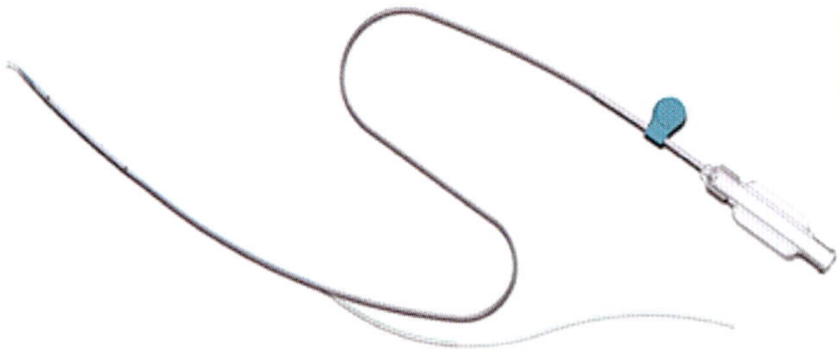

FIG 17.4 Monorail or rapid-exchange systems that have a shorter exposed wire length and may provide faster and greater stability during exchange.

The dilatation balloon must be made of a material that is noncompliant. A highly noncompliant balloon exerts greater radial force on the lesion, producing effective dilatation even on resistant lesions.

Thin-walled balloon construction is another critical characteristic of the ideal balloon dilatation catheter. Such construction allows the balloon to wrap tightly around the catheter shaft, providing the lowest possible profile for ease of advancement and withdrawal.

The ideal balloon dilatation catheter should also be able to safely withstand high pressures. High-pressure balloons are required for resistant lesions.

The ideal balloon catheter should demonstrate excellent refoldability, which will promote easier withdrawal and reduce the potential for hematomas and surrounding complications. This refoldability must be possible whether it is after one inflation or multiple inflations.

Finally, the ideal balloon dilatation catheter should be available in a wide variety of sizes. Safe and successful angioplasty requires that the balloon be sized precisely for the vessel being treated.[4]

New balloon modifications include the following:

- Drug-coated balloons
- Scoring balloons
- Cutting balloons
- Longer balloons
- Lower-profile balloons
- Monorail or rapid-exchange systems that have a shorter exposed wire lengths may provide faster and greater stability during exchanges (Fig. 17.4)

Stents

Next to angioplasty balloons, stents are among the most commonly used endoluminal therapeutic devices. There are two broad categories available: (1) balloon-expandable and (2) self-expanding stents. These can then be subcategorized into covered and uncovered stents. Covered stents used in the peripheral circulation are predominantly covered with polytetrafluoroethylene. Each type of stent has unique deployment characteristics.

Balloon-Expandable Stents

Balloon-expandable stents—which are predominantly made of stainless steel—are mounted on the outside of the balloon (Fig. 17.5). They are typically used when extreme accuracy and

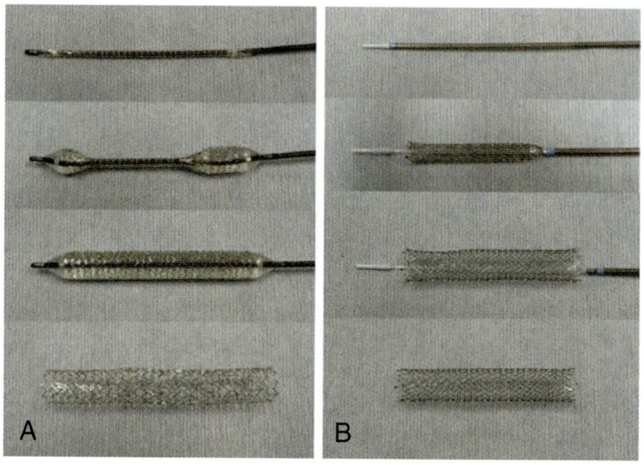

FIG 17.5 (A) Deployment of a balloon-expandable stent; (B) deployment of a self-expanding stent.

high radial force is required, as in a renal artery orifice, a subclavian artery stenosis, or an iliac artery stenosis. Covered balloon-expandable stents are used in combination with fenestrated aortic grafts in restenotic or embolizing lesions. In general, balloon-expandable stents have a higher radial force than self-expanding stents.

Care must be taken during insertion of the stent through the hemostasis valve; the stent is typically delivered to the target site through a long sheath in order to protect it from displacement. Once in place across the lesion, the sheath is retracted, the stent is exposed and positioned, and the balloon is expanded with the stent; throughout this process, it is important to visualize the balloon to ensure that it remains centrally positioned between the two balloon radiopaque markers. If the stent has been displaced, it should be carefully retrieved. As the stent is deployed, carefully visualize the expansion of the angioplasty balloon. Noting that the balloon shoulders expand first ensures that the stent will not be ejected from the balloon during its inflation.

Once the stent has been deployed—usually confirmed by expanding the balloon to its nominal pressure or by visualizing the balloon walls coming up to full expansion—the balloon is deflated. Use a magnification view to observe that the stent remains firmly in place as the balloon is removed from the lumen of the stent. If there is any stent motion, then the sheath is advanced into the stent to collapse and disengage it from the stent struts. Consequently the use of long hemostasis sheaths is highly recommended in using balloon-expandable stents.

Self-Expanding Stents

Self-expanding stents (Fig. 17.6) are made of the nickel-titanium alloy Nitinol. (The Wallstent endoprosthesis is an exception; it is made of braided cobalt-chromium-nickel alloy.) The stent has thermal memory with a predetermined diameter and length, to which it will return when it is unsheathed at body temperature. The stent is constrained on the delivery catheter by a motor-retractable membrane, which, when retracted by the operator, deploys the stent. The stent then attempts to return to

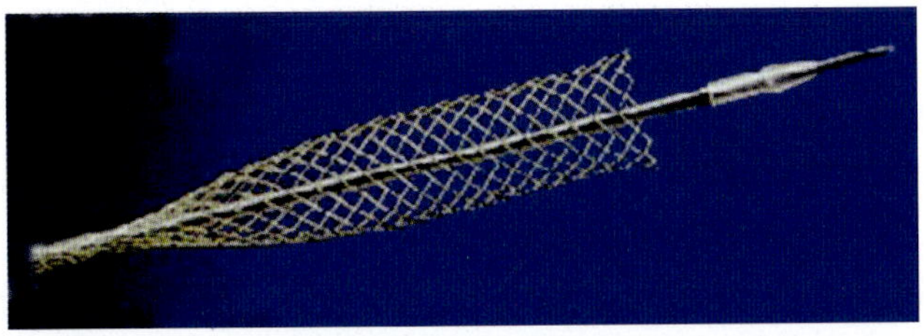

FIG 17.6 Self-expanding stents are constrained within an outer plastic retractable sheath. Exposure to blood at body temperature causes the stent to return to a predetermined diameter.

its predetermined diameter. Postdilation of the stents is generally required to restore an adequate flow lumen, since the hoop strength of the stent alone is inadequate.

Stent Considerations

Stents have now been modified by a variety of manufacturers to permit the delivery of antiproliferative agents from the stent into the wall of an artery. Stent design is also variable among manufacturers. There has been much debate over the relative merits of open-cell versus closed-cell designs, although neither of these technologies has been proven to be more efficacious than the other or to reduce embolization. Here are some of the considerations in selecting a stent:

- High radial force
- Resistance to recoil
- Minimal or no stimulation of intimal hyperplasia
- Longitudinal flexibility
- High radiopacity for visualization
- Ability to conform to the vessel
- Low profile
- Minimal or no foreshortening
- Easy deployment system
- Maintenance of side branches
- Compatibility with magnetic resonance imaging
- Durability

CONCLUSION

The variety of supplies available for endovascular procedures is quite extensive. However, the basics remain the same for most procedures: You will need needles, guidewires, sheaths, balloons, and diagnostic/guiding catheters.[5] That being said, products within those categories can differ greatly or be very similar. Learning to recognize the advantages and disadvantages of each will help you identify the correct tool for the job at hand.

Thus it is important to consider each product's key characteristics and to evaluate their performance. Was a guidewire too stiff? Not stiff enough? Did the wire have torquability? Did catheters slide easily over the wire or were they "sticky"? Are the diagnostic catheters radiopaque? Are they too rigid or not rigid enough? When angioplasty balloons were used, what kind of trackability did they have? What kind of pushability? How fast or slow was inflation/deflation? Did the balloon have a high profile? What was the balloon's appearance when inflated?

Think about the individual suitability of each product used. How did it perform? Was it adequate to perform the procedure or was it a struggle? Know the advantages and disadvantages of each product's characteristics.

There is a bewildering array of catheters, wires, sheaths, balloons, and stents. However, in practice, many are very similar. Learn to use a limited number of workhorse devices and use others only when necessary.

REVIEW QUESTIONS

1. Which of the following artery is not recommended for vascular access?
   a. Brachial artery
   b. Axillary artery
   c. Common femoral artery
   d. None of the above
2. Ultrasound guided access is recommended because:
   a. Of direct visualization of the vessel to be accessed
   b. Of decreased risk of vascular access complications such as arteriovenous fistula
   c. It is useful for access of pulseless arteries
   d. All of the above
3. Compared to the self-expanded stents, the balloon-expanded stents:
   a. Have more radial strength
   b. Are less flexible
   c. Have more hoop strength
   d. All of the above
4. The diameters of the commonly used guidewires are:
   a. 0.014 inch
   b. 0.018 inch
   c. 0.035 inch
   d. All of the above
5. Which of the following is not a mechanism of balloon angioplasty?
   a. Desquamation of endothelial cells
   b. Plaque compression allows for restoration of luminal diameter.
   c. Stretching of the media and adventitia
   d. Longitudinal fracture of the atherosclerotic plaque
6. Which of the following regarding arterial access is false?
   a. Antegrade femoral access allows for intervention of distal lesions in the infrapopliteal arterial system.
   b. Right brachial artery is preferred over left brachial artery.
   c. Retrograde femoral access allows for proximal aortogram and distal intervention of the contralateral lower extremity.
   d. Brachial access is commonly used in patients with aortoiliac disease.

7. Stents with thermal memory:
   - **a.** Are made of nitinol
   - **b.** Are able to expand to a predetermined shape when warmed
   - **c.** Are a subgroup of self-expanded stents
   - **d.** All of the above
8. Which of the following regarding catheters is not true?
   - **a.** Selective catheters have a single hole at the tip.
   - **b.** Flush catheters have multiple side and end holes.
   - **c.** Catheters do not cause intimal injury or dissection.
   - **d.** Flow rate through a catheter varies with its internal radius.
9. Complications at the vascular access site include all of the following except:
   - **a.** Pseudoaneurysms
   - **b.** Arteriovenous fistulas
   - **c.** Intimal hyperplasia
   - **d.** Hematoma
10. The ideal balloon angioplasty catheter has which of the following characteristics?
    - **a.** Pushability and trackability
    - **b.** Easy to rupture to prevent perforation of the artery
    - **c.** High profile when collapsed
    - **d.** Small filling lumen for inflation and deflation of the balloon

References available online at ExpertConsult.com.

CHAPTER 18

Atherectomy and Arterial Closure Devices: Selection, Technique, and Results

Johnathon Rollo, Donald T. Baril

ATHERECTOMY DEVICES

Introduction

Since the early 1990s, percutaneous peripheral atherectomy has provided an ancillary approach to the treatment of atherosclerotic occlusive disease beyond angioplasty and stenting.[1] A variety of technologies have been developed to debulk atherosclerotic lesions, including directional excisional, excimer laser, orbital ablation, and rotational atherectomy. These technologies are designed to treat a variety of lesions from heavily calcified stenoses to soft thrombus-containing occlusions. By removing atherosclerotic plaque, atherectomy provides luminal gain to diseased vessels rather than simply dilating the existing lumen and leaving disease in situ. This can be achieved with a technique that leaves no intraluminal foreign body and facilitates reinterventions if necessary. Furthermore, atherectomy may be used to treat lesions involving joint spaces that are under continuous dynamic stress forces, where stents may be at increased risk of fracture and subsequent failure. The theoretical advantages of atherectomy are apparent, but the data to support its use have been mixed and of poor quality to date. There are a number of commercially available atherectomy devices approved by the US Food and Drug Administration (FDA). Atherectomy devices vary in their mechanism of action and include laser, orbital, rotational, and directional means of removing atherosclerotic plaque. This chapter describes an overview of the clinical data for atherectomy and the indications, ideal lesions, outcomes, and complications are presented.

History

Percutaneous atherectomy as an endovascular modality was initially applied in the coronary bed. However, despite the theoretical advantages, several studies showed unfavorable long-term results compared to angioplasty.[2,3] This same technology was subsequently applied to the first generation of peripheral atherectomy devices, including the Simpson AeroCath (Guidant, Santa Clara, California) and the Auth Rotablator (Boston Scientific, Quincy, Massachusetts). Despite high initial technical success rates of 90%, the first-generation atherectomy devices were associated with poor intermediate and long-term patency rates.[4,5] Subsequent advances have led to the current generation of atherectomy devices, which are now being applied to treat lesions in both the femoropopliteal and infrapopliteal segments.

Overview of Atherectomy Data

The data supporting atherectomy as an adjunct to angioplasty and stenting have been mixed. A 2014 Cochrane Review of atherectomy compared to angioplasty alone was only able to incorporate four studies, including one study performed in 1995 with a first-generation extraction catheter[6] and another performed in 1996 with a cohort of 36 patients.[7] Also included was a more recent study of 58 patients undergoing directional atherectomy versus angioplasty alone that concluded no difference at one year, but fewer bailout stents placed in the atherectomy group, at the cost of higher rates of macroembolization.[8] Orbital atherectomy, by the same author, faired only slightly better in calcified lesions.[9] They concluded that there was no benefit to atherectomy over angioplasty alone. There are a number of retrospective studies that show significant benefit in patients treated with atherectomy, with 1-year primary patency ranging from 60% to 83%, limb salvage of 79% to 95% at 2 years in critical limb ischemia (CLI), complications requiring intervention in 0% to 7% of cases, and target lesion revascularization in up to 28% at 2 years.[10,11,12,13] Data for infrapopliteal intervention using atherectomy are also mixed. One retrospective study comparing 333 percutaneous tibial angioplasty (PTA) to 79 atherectomy interventions (33 laser, 13 directional, and 33 orbital) showed no benefit to PTA with atherectomy compared to PTA alone, but with no difference in complication rates.[14] Another prospective multicenter trial of directional atherectomy demonstrated 90% primary patency of infrapopliteal interventions in claudicants, and 78% in CLI, limb salvage of 95%, and a 3.8% rate of distal embolization. This core-lab adjudicated data compare favorably to primary stent trials.[12] Peripheral interventions in claudicants and nondiabetic patients compare favorably to those who have CLI and diabetes, and the same is true for atherectomy.[15]

DEVICES (Table 18.1)

Directional Atherectomy

SilverHawk, TurboHawk, HawkOne Plaque Excision System (Medtronic, Minneapolis, Minnesota)

The Hawk family of atherectomy catheters was initially approved for peripheral arterial use in 2003 by the FDA (Fig. 18.1). The SilverHawk catheter debulks lesions without the use of a balloon and instead relies on self-apposition against plaque through a

TABLE 18.1 Atherectomy Devices

	TurboHawk Plaque Excision System	CVX-300 Excimer Laser	Diamondback 360 Orbital Atherectomy System	Jetstream Atherectomy System
Manufacturer	Medtronic (Minneapolis, Minnesota)	Spectranetics (Colorado Springs, Colorado)	Cardiovascular Systems Inc. (St. Paul, Minnesota)	Boston Scientific (Marlborough, Massachusetts)
FDA approved	Yes	Yes	Yes	Yes
Mechanism	Directional blade plaque excision	Ultraviolet light plaque dissolution	Centrifugal force plaque sanding	Rotational blade plaque excision and suction
Catheter tip size	1.9–2.7 mm	0.9–2.5 mm	1.25–2.25 mm	1.6–2.4 mm
Sheath size	5–8 French	4–8 French	4–6 French	7 French
Guidewire	0.014 inch	0.014, 0.018, and 0.035 inch	0.014 inch	0.014 inch
Lumen treatment range	3–7 mm	1.4 to >3.8 mm	2 to >5 mm	2.5 to >5 mm

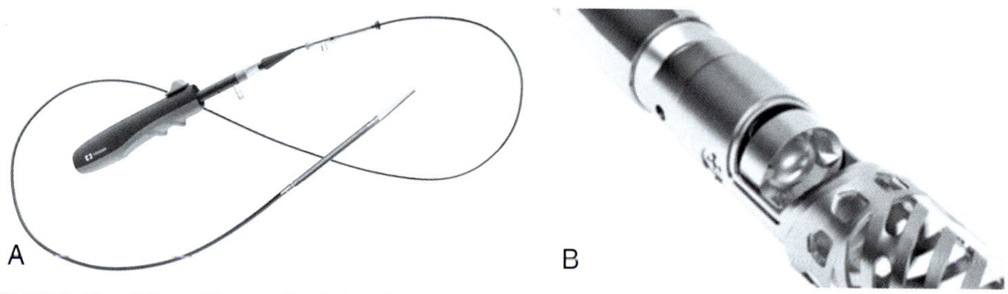

FIG 18.1 HawkOne Plaque Excision System (Medtronic, Minneapolis, Minnesota). (A) Battery-powered motor and catheter. (B) Cutting blade. (Courtesy Medtronic.)

hinged system at the distal end of the catheter. The device consists of a detachable, battery-powered motor that attaches to a 0.014-inch monorail atherectomy catheter. The tip of the catheter contains a rotating blade and a plaque collection chamber. The carbide cutting blade rotates at 8000 rpm when activated. This blade has a concave design that shaves the plaque and then packs it into the nosecone storage compartment. The operator places the tip of the catheter just proximal to the target lesion, activates the blade, and then slowly advances the tip of the catheter through the entire length of the lesion, periodically emptying the nosecone (Fig. 18.2). This process is repeated until an adequate flow channel is achieved. The tip of the catheter may be rotated 360 degrees and thus, plaque excision may be carried out in all four quadrants of the lumen. There is a single (SilverHawk) and double (HawkOne, TurboHawk) jog in the catheter design, which aids in arterial wall apposition. Once the nosecone collection unit is full, the entire catheter must be removed prior to reinsertion and additional passages.

There are several different catheter sizes available to treat target vessel sizes ranging from 2 to 7 mm. All of these require a sheath ranging in size from 5 to 8 French, are introduced over a 0.014-inch guidewire, and have a crossing profile of 1.9 to 2.7 mm. Access may be achieved via a contralateral common femoral arterial puncture or an antegrade approach. The use of a filter to protect against distal embolization is recommended in calcified lesions. The catheter may be used in the flow channel or in a subintimal plane (Fig. 18.3). The TurboHawk device improves on the SilverHawk with a more efficient cutter, more robust driveshaft, and dual jog catheter for wall apposition. The HawkOne device improves the crossing profile, simplifies cleaning, and is more effective in calcium. It is approved for vessels 3.5 to 7.0 mm and is 7 French sheath compatible.

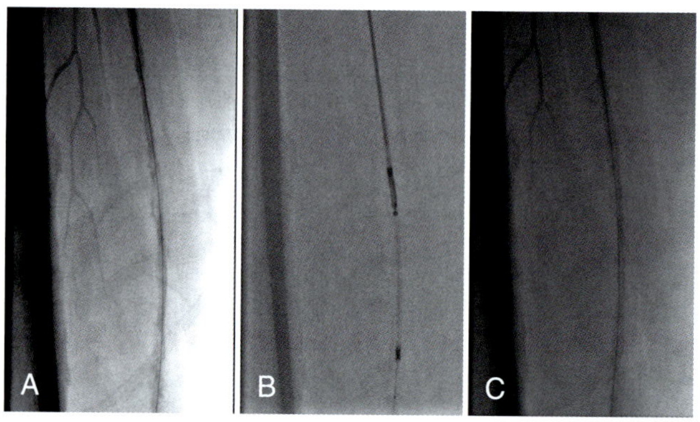

FIG 18.2 Angiogram demonstrating use of TurboHawk system in heavily calcified lesions. (A) Preintervention image demonstrating heavily calcified lesion. (B) Cutting blade as it is engaged in debulking the lesion. (C) Completion angiogram.

Results. There has been one small randomized trial of SilverHawk atherectomy versus angioplasty alone.[16] A two-center prospective randomized trial enrolled 29 patients for atherectomy and adjunctive PTA versus 29 patients with PTA alone. The study found no significant differences in freedom from target lesion

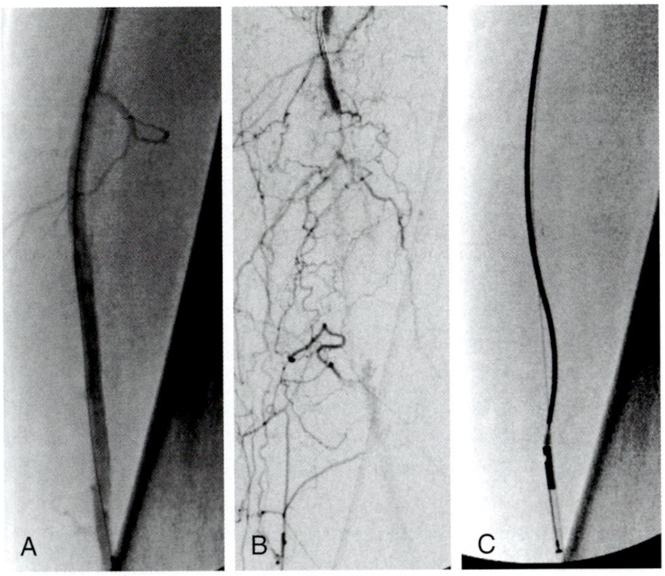

FIG 18.3 Chronic total occlusion of the superficial femoral artery. (A) Preintervention image demonstrating long mixed plaque lesion. (B) Cutting blade as it is engaged in debulking the lesion. (C) Completion angiogram.

revascularization (TLR) between the two groups (89% vs. 83%). There was one clinically significant embolization in the atherectomy arm, requiring intervention at the time of the procedure with no sequelae. Of note, bailout stent rates in the plain old balloon angioplasty (POBA) were 62.1% per patient versus 27.6% in the atherectomy arm. Importantly, this small study excluded lesions greater than 10 cm or heavily calcified lesions, which POBA has traditionally failed.

There have been several reports demonstrating the effectiveness of directional atherectomy for the treatment of atherosclerotic lesions in the femoropopliteal and the infrapopliteal segments. The recent DEFINITIVE LE is a multicenter prospective industry-sponsored database that enrolled 800 patients looking at primary endpoints of 12-month patency and freedom from amputation.[12] The primary patency, defined as peak systolic velocity ratio (PSVR) less than 2.4 by core lab adjudication, was 78% in claudicants and 71% in CLI patients, with 95% rate of limb salvage. The rate of clinically significant embolization was 1.2% to 3.0%, dissection 1.3% to 2.0%, and perforation 1.5% to 5.0%. The bailout stent rate was 3%. Zeller et al.[17] reported 71 lesions treated in 52 patients, with an average lesion length of 48 ± 64 mm. Forty-two percent of these were primary stenoses, 38% were native vessel restenosis, and 20% were in-stent restenosis. The latter was performed outside of the manufacturer's instructions for use. Adjunctive angioplasty was used in 58% of these procedures, whereas stenting was used in 6%. Primary patency rates at 6 months were 80% for primary lesions, 63% for post-angioplasty lesions, and 71% for in-stent restenoses. Zeller et al.[18] subsequently reported longer-term data of 131 lesions in 84 patients with 12-month primary patency rates (defined as < 50% restenoses on ultrasound) of 84% for de novo lesions, 54% for native vessel restenoses, and 54% for in-stent restenoses. At 18 months, these fell to 73%, 42%, and 49%, respectively; however, secondary patency rates were 89%, 67%, and 79%.

The largest outcome data of the SilverHawk atherectomy catheter is the nonrandomized, manufacturer-sponsored TALON registry (Treating Peripherals With SilverHawk: Outcomes Collection), which involved 19 centers in the United States and collected data on 1258 lesions treated in 601 patients.[19] Mean lesion length was 62.5 ± 68.5 mm above the knee and 33.4 ± 42.7 mm below the knee. Procedural success was 97.6% with less than 50% residual stenosis achieved in 94.7% of lesions. Adjunctive angioplasty was used in 21.7% of cases and stenting in 6.3% of cases. Six-month and 12-month freedoms from target lesion revascularization were 90% and 80%, respectively. Predictors of target lesion revascularization included a history of myocardial infarction or coronary revascularization and increasing Rutherford classification.

Recent data from a prospectively maintained database of 559 lesions treated in 255 patients included 228 in the superficial femoral artery (SFA; 106 occlusions), 176 in the popliteal artery (84 occlusions), and 229 in the infrapopliteal arteries (130 occlusions).[8] Eighteen-month primary and secondary patency rates for all lesions were 45.9% ± 3.4 and 80.3% ± 2.5, respectively, with reported 18-month primary and secondary patency rates for claudicants of 59.2% ± 4.9 and 88.1% ± 3.3 and for patients with CLI of 34.3% ± 4.5 and 73.6% ± 3.6. Overall limb salvage was 93.1%.

The use of the SilverHawk atherectomy catheter specifically for the treatment of CLI has also been reported. Kandzari et al.[9] reported the results of 160 lesions in 74 limbs ranging from the external iliac to the dorsalis pedis in patients with Rutherford class 5 and 6 disease. Mean above-knee lesion length was 74 ± 88 mm. Technical success was achieved in 99% of patients, with 17% requiring adjunctive angioplasty and/or stenting. The primary endpoint evaluated was a composite of major adverse events, including death, myocardial infarction, unplanned amputation, or repeat target vessel revascularization. At 6 months, 23% of patients met this endpoint. Amputations that were less extensive than initially planned or avoided completely occurred in 93% of patients at 30 days and 82% at 6 months. Keeling et al.[10] also reported on the use of the SilverHawk atherectomy catheter for the treatment of both claudicants and patients with CLI. The technical success was 87.1% with a 1-year primary patency rate of 61.7%. Restenosis was higher in patients with TASC C or D lesions compared to those with TASC A or B lesions.

Zeller et al.[11] reported additional data on the use of the SilverHawk atherectomy catheter for infrapopliteal lesions alone on 52 lesions in 33 patients. Atherectomy was used alone in 71%. Restenosis (>70% on ultrasound) was observed in 14% of lesions at 3 months and 22% at 6 months, however the cumulative patency rate was 94.1% at 6 months.

Complications. The primary complications associated with this device include perforation and distal embolization. Using the first-generation device, Suri et al.[12] reported a 100% rate of embolic debris in 13 lesions treated with the SilverHawk atherectomy catheter with the concomitant use of a FilterWire (Boston Scientific, Natick, Massachusetts). This embolic debris ranged in size from 0.5 to 10 mm, and, in one patient, led to vessel occlusion that resolved with removal of the filter. Lam et al.[13] also detected emboli during use of the SilverHawk atherectomy catheter using simultaneous Doppler monitoring. Of note, in this study, emboli were detected during the period between passes of the catheter, indicating that debris may shower from the disrupted intimal surface. However, no patient developed any clinically significant sequelae from these emboli.

In more recent studies, the clinically significant embolization rates were significantly lower, particularly in conjunction with an embolic protection device.

Indications and ideal lesions. The Hawk family of atherectomy catheters is indicated for peripheral arterial atherectomy. It is not intended for coronary, carotid, or aortoiliac use. Each catheter has indicated vessel diameters (L 3.5-7, S 2.0-4.0) and cutter blades designed for calcium or soft lesions. In addition, there are nosecones and packing devices designed to more effectively capture debris and shorten treatment time. For example, a long calcified SFA lesion would call for a large device and a cutting blade with a long packer (LX-C). A tibial artery with a soft lesion would be better suited to a small device with a standard tip (SS+). This provides flexibility in treating a variety of lower extremity lesions. The Hawk devices are best suited to long segment, moderately calcified lesions, and are most safely used in conjunction with distal embolic protection devices. These devices can effectively treat dissection, soft or calcified lesions, and in-stent restenosis. It is not indicated in thrombus. They can be used in chronic total occlusion (CTO) lesions and subintimal planes, due to their directional cutting capability.

Orbital Atherectomy

Diamondback (CSI, St. Paul, Minnesota)

The Diamondback 360 Orbital Atherectomy System uses orbiting action to remove plaque and increases lumen diameter by increasing the orbital speed (80,000 to 200,000 rpm). An eccentrically mounted diamond-coated crown rotates at high speed at the end of the catheter to sand away plaque as the crown is slowly advanced through the target lesion. As crown rotation increases, centrifugal force presses the crown against the lesion to effect plaque removal, while the less diseased, more elastic arterial wall flexes away from the crown, minimizing the risk of vessel trauma (Fig. 18.4).[20] It is thought that the "sanding" of lesions creates particles that are too small to cause clinically significant embolization and can be reabsorbed through the reticuloendothelial system[21] and thus the use of embolization protection filters is not needed. This technique emphasizes "plaque modification," that is, emphasizing more effective balloon angioplasty by disrupting the calcium bed over luminal gain. The crown is positioned at the proximal portion of the target lesion and slowly advanced. This crown is manufactured in sizes of 1.25, 1.50, and 2.00 mm in solid micro, classic and solid configurations, to allow for final lumen diameters ranging from 1.25 to 3.50 mm based on the rotational speed. Micro crowns are used in the tibial vessels, and solid or classic crown is used in SFA/popliteal disease.

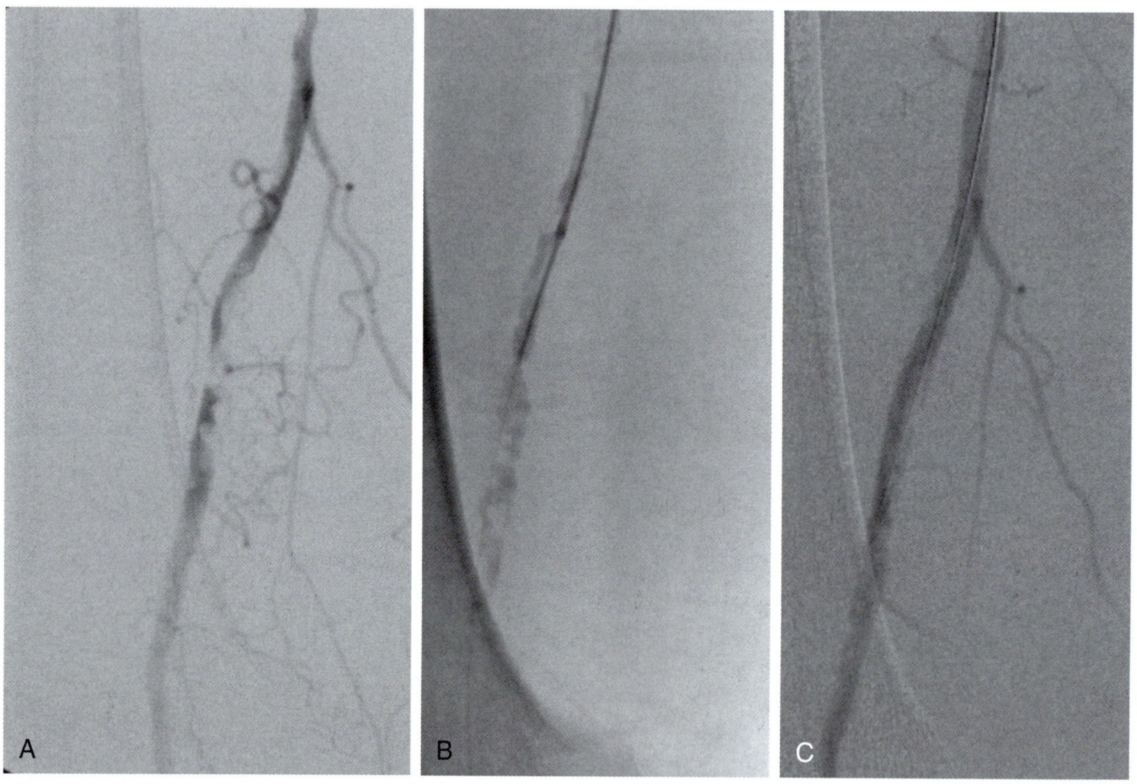

FIG 18.4 Diamondback 360 Peripheral Orbital Atherectomy System (CSI, St. Paul, Minnesota). (A) Preintervention image demonstrating short, heavily calcified lesion. (B) Crown orbital spinning device as it is engaged in sanding the lesion. (C) Completion angiogram.

This device is placed over a 0.014-inch guidewire and requires a 6 or 7 French sheath for access depending on the device size. It is used in conjunction with a lubricant ViperSlide, an emulsion composed of soybean oil, egg yolk phospholipids, glycerin, and water. Allergy to egg is a contraindication for use.

Results. The data regarding orbital atherectomy in the peripheral system are scant and of poor quality. A number of recent trials have evaluated the Diamondback orbital atherectomy system. A small randomized multicenter study evaluated 1-year outcomes in 50 patients with calcified lesions and CLI comparing Diamondback orbital atherectomy with angioplasty to POBA.[9] Bailout stenting occurred in 6% of atherectomy and 14% of POBA patients (not significant). Freedom from TLR in the atherectomy group was 93% versus 80% in POBA (not significant) at 1 year. In the industry sponsored OASIS (Orbital Atherectomy System Investigational Study) trial, a prospective, multicenter database enrolled 124 patients with 201 lesions.[22] Fifty-one percent of these lesions were reported to be noncalcified and 85% were infrapopliteal. This study demonstrated an acute debulking rate, as measured angiographically, of 62%. Device success, as defined by less than 30% residual stenosis on angiography following orbital atherectomy alone, was 78%. The use of adjunctive angioplasty and/or stenting for 84 lesions (42%) increased this to 93%. Ankle-brachial indices were 0.68 at baseline, 0.90 at 30 days, and 0.82 at 6 months. Additionally, the 6-month target lesion revascularization rate was 0.9%. Of note, the mean lesion length in this study was 3.0 cm ± 2.9 cm. The large industry sponsored CONFIRM registry collected data on 3135 interventions with 81% moderate/severe calcium, 36% below the knee (BTK) with mean lesion length 7.2 cm.[21] It revealed high rates of procedural success (defined by target lesion stenosis <30%) but does not report long-term clinical outcomes.

Complications. In the OASIS trial, there was a serious adverse event rate of 8%, although only 3.2% of these were directly device related. These device-related complications consisted of thrombus formation at the site of the treated lesion, perforations (at the site of the target lesion and distal to the lesion), and embolization. In the CONFIRM registry, flow limiting dissection occurred in 1.6% of cases, embolism in 1.8%, and vessel rupture in 0.5%. Interestingly, "slow flow" was listed as a complication in 2.9% of cases, perhaps representing microembolization of small particles causing diffuse small vessel outflow occlusions. In addition, vessel closure and spasm occurred in 1.5% and 4.2% respectively. Hemolysis is a unique complication of orbital atherectomy that occurs in 33% of patients. The clinical significance of hemolysis is unclear, but appears to be minimal including hemoglobinuria (9%) and hypertensive crisis (3%).[23]

Indications and ideal lesions. Instructions for use of the Diamondback 360 device include iliac and infrainguinal calcified atherosclerotic peripheral arterial disease (PAD). Vessel diameter from 2.0 to 10 mm can be treated. The system is designed to modify the plaque, allowing for more effective angioplasty and deemphasizes luminal gain. It is contraindicated in the presence of dissections because the spinning crown can catch and wrap on dissection flaps. It is ineffective in soft lesions or thrombus, and it will cause increased distal embolization. The device is best suited to short heavily calcified lesions with robust tibial runoff. It can also be effective in treating calcified tibial lesions where alternative interventions are limited. Safety can be increased by using short run times and small crown selection.

Rotational Atherectomy

Jetstream (Boston Scientific, Marlborough, Massachusetts)

The Jetstream atherectomy device works by plaque extraction through a rotational cutting blade loaded on a delivery shaft along with active aspiration (Fig. 18.5). The aspiration port is designed to remove debris to minimize the risk of embolization. This is a modification of the Pathway device, which was plagued by high rates of distal embolization. The latest iteration moved the location and increased the suction capacity of the aspiration port. The device is not directed, and thus must be used in true-luminal wire position. It cannot be used in CTO if crossing in subintimal planes. Multiple cutter blade options are available depending on luminal diameter of the treated vessel. There are two cutter designs with the Jetstream device. The Jetstream XC (or eXpandable Cutter Catheters) comes with 2.1- or 2.4-mm tips and is suitable for vessels 3 to 5 mm or larger. The Jetstream SC (or Single Cutter Catheters) comes with 1.6- or 1.85-mm tips (145-cm in length) and are best suited for vessel size 2 to 3 mm. The single cutters have only a front end cutter with no "blades up" feature and are typically used for tibial vessels.[24] It is recommended by some authors to use a saline flush bag with nitroglycerin to prevent vessel spasm around the catheter tip.

Results and complications. Data regarding the Jetstream device are limited and of poor quality. In a large single-center retrospective study of 172 patients treated with a mean lesion length of 2.8 cm, CTO was 29%, and 46% of patients were diabetic.[25] Technical success was achieved in 99% of lesions. Freedom from TLR was 70% to 80% at 12 months. Major adverse events (death, index limb amputation, myocardial infarction, TLR, and target vessel revascularization) occurred in 25% to 31% of patients at 12 months. The same group reported a cohort of 172 patients treated with the Jetstream that demonstrated 82% freedom from TLR at 1 year, with improvement in clinical outcomes and ankle-brachial index (ABI).[26] Rates of embolization were 9.9%, dissection 8%, and there were two scheduled amputations. Specific lesion characteristics were not reported. Jetstream has been

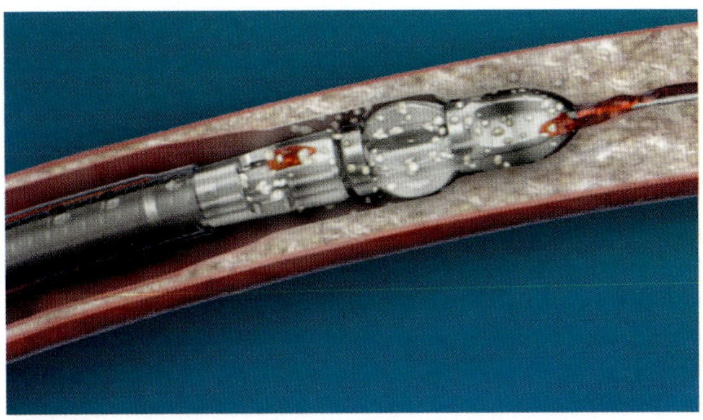

FIG 18.5 Jetstream rotational atherectomy catheter (Boston Scientific, Marlborough, Massachusetts). (Courtesy Boston Scientific.)

specifically studied in in-stent restenosis (ISR). A cohort of 29 patients with a femoropopliteal ISR mean lesion length of 17.4 cm was treated with a 91% angiographic success rate. An embolic filter was used in 50% of cases and macro-emboli were noted in two out of 16 filters. Distal embolization required intervention in 9.4% of limbs. Primary patency by duplex PSVR of less than 2.4 was 72% at 6 months. Freedom from TLR was 59% at 12 months.[27]

Indications and ideal lesions. Given the limited data presently in the literature, the Jetstream device seems suited for short-segment lesions where true-lumen wire crossing can be obtained. It is a relatively easy-to-use device and has comparable rates of embolization compared to other devices. It appears effective for ISR without the risk of creating new stent fractures. The use of an embolic protection device is recommended because macroembolization rates are significant.

Laser Atherectomy

CVX-300 Excimer Laser (Spectranetics, Colorado Springs, Colorado)

The CVX-300 Excimer Laser is used in conjunction with the TURBO-Booster or the TURBO-Elite catheter. The laser removes plaque through photoablation, using light to vaporize and ablate tissue (Fig. 18.6). The CVX-300 uses exact energy control with shallow tissue penetration to decrease the thermal injury to the native artery. The energy is released in short pulses rather than in continuous fashion, as in previous devices. These short pulses reduce tissue that is within 50 µm of the laser tip to molecular particles by breaking molecular bonds, by molecular vibration with resultant heat production, and by expanding and collapsing vapor bubbles at the laser tip. Plaque is broken down into particles smaller than 10 µm.

The CVX-300 Excimer Laser in combination with the TURBO-Booster or the TURBO-Elite catheter can be used for stenoses or complete occlusions. The laser can be used to cross chronic total occlusions by using the "step-by-step" technique whereby the catheter tip is placed in direct contact with the proximal portion of the lesion. The laser is then activated for 5 to 10 seconds and is advanced through the plaque with or without the support of a guidewire. For stenoses, the guidewire is passed beyond the lesion and the catheter is slowly advanced through the lesion at a rate of 0.5 to 1 mm/s. This is typically not a standalone device because the lumen size obtained is generally 1.5 times the size of the probe, and therefore adjunctive balloon angioplasty is almost always required.

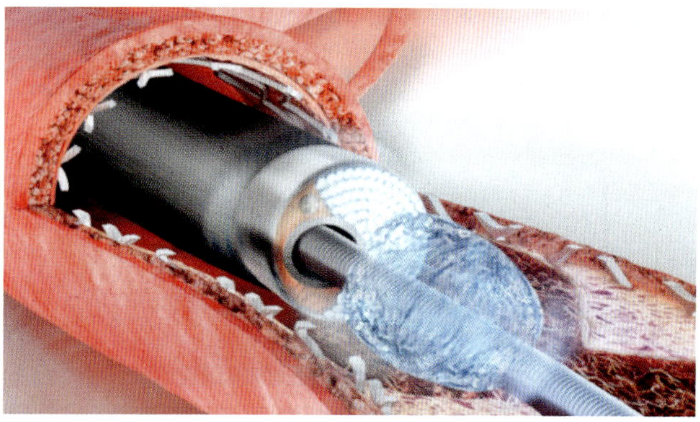

FIG 18.6 Turbo Excimer Laser (Spectranetics) atherectomy catheter debulking an in-stent restenosis. (Courtesy Spectranetics.)

The TURBO-Booster and the TURBO-Elite catheters range in working length from 110 to 150 cm with diameters from 0.9 to 2.5 mm. These are introduced over 0.014- or 0.018-inch guidewires through 4 to 8 French sheaths depending on the catheter size. The TURBO-Booster allows for directional atherectomy, therefore resulting in a large flow channel in the femoropopliteal segment. This modality may therefore prove to be the preferred method for the treatment of in-stent restenosis.

Results. There have been a number of reports demonstrating the safety and efficacy of the Excimer laser for the treatment of infrainguinal occlusive disease. The Peripheral Excimer Laser Angioplasty (PELA) study was a multicenter, prospective, randomized trial comparing laser atherectomy with angioplasty versus angioplasty alone for long SFA occlusions.[28] Procedural success was 85% in the laser group and 91% in the angioplasty-alone group. Complication rates were similar and 12-month primary patency rates were the same for both groups (49%). However, the laser group required less stent implantation compared to the angioplasty group (42% vs. 59%).

Scheinert et al.[29] reported 411 lesions in 318 patients treated with laser-assisted recanalization of chronic SFA occlusions with a 90.5% technical success rate. Stent usage was required in 7.3% of cases. At 1 year, primary patency, assisted primary patency, and secondary patency rates were 20.1%, 64.6%, and 75.1% respectively.

The LACI (Laser Angioplasty for Critical Limb Ischemia) multicenter trial enrolled 145 patients who were deemed poor surgical candidates.[30] A total of 423 lesions were treated in 155 limbs. Adjunctive angioplasty was used in 96% of cases and stenting in 45%. ABIs improved from 0.54 ± 0.21 to 0.84 ± 0.20. Six-month limb salvage was 92.5%.

Stoner et al.[31] reported midterm results of 40 patients treated by laser atherectomy with an average follow-up of 461 ± 49 days. Forty-seven lesions were treated and adjunctive angioplasty was used in 75% of cases. The overall technical success rate (<50% residual stenosis) was 88%. The overall 12-month primary patency was 44% and the 12-month limb salvage rate in 26 patients with CLI was 55%. Chronic renal failure, diabetes mellitus, and poor tibial runoff were all associated with worse outcomes.

Laser atherectomy for ISR has been studied. A dual-center study of 135 patients with symptomatic ISR were treated with excimer laser (ELA) plus angioplasty versus angioplasty alone.[32] There was a significantly lower rate of TLR (14% vs. 44%, P =.05) in patients treated with laser atherectomy at 2 years. A multicenter randomized controlled clinical trial of laser atherectomy in ISR enrolled 250 patients and was stopped early due to efficacy at interim analysis. A total of 169 ELA plus PTA patients compared to 81 PTA alone. Excimer laser and PTA exhibited greater procedural success with fewer complications and 73.5% versus 51% freedom from TLR (52% reduction in TLR).

Complications. As with the other atherectomy devices, laser atherectomy has a risk of perforation, dissection, thrombosis at the atherectomy site, and distal embolization. Scheniert et al. reported a perforation rate of 2.2% and a distal embolization and thrombosis rate of 3.9% in their series. The overall procedural complication rate reported from the LACI trial was 12% and included major dissection (4%), thrombosis (3%), distal embolization (3%), and perforation (2%).

Indications and ideal lesions. Laser atherectomy has been extensively studied in patients with ISR, and is indicated for that use with improved outcomes over POBA alone. Laser atherectomy is ideal for very soft lesions and may be used in soft thrombus. It is less useful in CTO and heavily calcified lesions. Excimer laser technology is not going to deliver significant luminal gain, and will require adjuvant PTA and/or stenting.

Follow-Up After Atherectomy

Residual and recurrent stenoses are common after percutaneous interventions, particularly after atherectomy and a "leave nothing behind" approach whereby stenting is selectively utilized. With improved devices and technique, rates of restenosis can be reduced, but surveillance of these lesions should be robust. To date, no randomized trials have evaluated the utility of duplex ultrasound (DUS) after atherectomy. However, using DUS can identify specific lesions that can be followed over time, and specific predictive cut-off values of peak systolic velocity (PSV) greater than 275 and velocity ratio (Vr) greater than 3.5 have been identified to determine more than 80% restenosis after SFA stenting by Baril et al.[33] In accordance with Society for Vascular Surgery (SVS) guidelines, clinical follow-up is essential. The data regarding timing and clinical utility of DUS after intervention are mixed. A number of studies have shown that serial DUS after interventions did not improve outcomes;[34,35] however, these studies were performed in patients with POBA and stent only. Others have concluded that evidence of restenosis leads to worse outcomes in CLI.[36] We recommend a tailored approach to follow-up DUS and clinical assessment: In patients with CLI, 1-month follow-up with baseline DUS and ABI after atherectomy, with repeat follow-up at 3 months, 6 months, then yearly if no new symptoms develop and wounds are healing. The return of rest pain or nonhealing ulcers should prompt early assessment and reintervention for recurrent stenosis. In patients with claudication, a less rigorous follow-up regimen may be employed, with reintervention reserved for recurrent life-limiting claudication and with reemphasis of lifestyle modifications and exercise regimen. There is no evidence supporting the utility of prophylactic reintervention for asymptomatic restenosis.[37]

Atherectomy as an Adjunct for Challenging Lesions

The data supporting atherectomy in the treatment of PAD are decidedly mixed and of poor quality. There are significant numbers of patients in large company-sponsored registries that provide data in support of a given device. The data should be viewed with caution given the inherent bias and incentives of industry-supported studies. Much of the peer-reviewed data is single center, often single operator, leading to selection bias and expert bias. Further complicating matters, atherectomy is often performed as an adjunct to other interventions, which introduces confounding factors that are difficult to evaluate. In addition, devices change frequently over time, often improving on older models and introducing new potential benefits and complications.

We recommend a lesion-guided approach to atherectomy as an adjunct intervention in the treatment of PAD. Potential advantages of atherectomy include the ability to treat CTO without stenting, leaving no metal behind, and avoiding the risk of stent fracture and occlusion, making reintervention more challenging. Atherectomy also allows for the treatment of ISR and occlusion, and provides an adjunct to POBA in tibial disease. Disadvantages of atherectomy include the risk of distal embolization, the need for embolic protection filters, vessel perforation, and cost. With proper device selection and technical use, these complications can be significantly reduced.

Lesion characteristics should guide device selection. In patients with soft lesions or thrombus burden, excimer laser atherectomy is ideal. Although it will not deliver significant luminal gain, it can be an adjunct to PTA and stenting. Soft lesions are also amenable to the rotational atherectomy devices (Jetstream) because the wire will be likely to remain in the true lumen, but one should avoid orbital atherectomy (Diamondback) in soft lesions and dissections. In ISR lesions, there is level 1 evidence supporting laser atherectomy with PTA over PTA alone. In addition, directional atherectomy (Hawk) can be used, although it should be understood that this is an off-label use of the devices. In moderately calcified non-CTO lesions, the options are numerous, and many devices will provide some benefit to create luminal gain and decrease the bailout stent rate, albeit with relatively decreased rates of freedom from TLR. Long-term, stent occlusion can be a challenging problem and the ability to leave nothing behind allows for much easier reintervention. In short, in heavily calcified lesions, orbital atherectomy performs well, but caution must be taken to avoid long spin times and limit treatment to short-segment lesions. Directional atherectomy performs well in soft, moderate and severely calcified lesions both short and long, albeit with increased risk of embolization in more calcified lesions. When using a calcium cutter, distal embolic protection device use is mandatory. Future studies will evaluate the promising use of the paclitaxel drug-coated balloon (DCB) in conjunction with atherectomy to provide luminal gain with reduced rates of restenosis.[38]

ARTERIAL CLOSURE DEVICES

Introduction

Traditionally, hemostasis following arterial access was achieved using manual compression. However, this method may be complicated by arterial thrombosis or ongoing hemorrhage from the access site leading to hematoma or pseudoaneurysm development. Also, particularly with use of anticoagulation and antiplatelet agents, manual compression may be required for extended periods of time leading to patient discomfort along with discomfort of the operator providing the compression. Following manual compression, bedrest is typically necessary for 4 to 6 hours depending on the sheath size used and the anticoagulation that was given during the procedure. As an alternative to conventional manual compression, arterial closure devices were introduced in the mid-1990s to allow for decreased time to achieve hemostasis, decreased access site complications, and to allow for earlier patient ambulation and discharge in select settings. Since their initial introduction, several different arterial closure devices have been developed that employ a variety of techniques to obtain hemostasis. Additionally, their applications have been broadened to allow for closure of larger access sites, specifically to facilitate percutaneous endovascular abdominal and thoracic aortic repair.

These devices can broadly be categorized into suture closure devices, mechanical nonsuture closure devices, intravascular sealant devices, extravascular sealant devices, and manual compression assistance devices. To date, no study has definitively demonstrated superiority of one device compared to another or to manual compression.[39–41] Additionally, no difference in vascular complications has been demonstrated with the use of closure devices or manual compression alone.[42–46] However, the use closure devices has repeatedly been shown to decrease the time to hemostasis, ambulation, and discharge compared to manual compression.[39–45]

All these devices have been designed and approved for closure of common femoral access sites. Importantly, initial access will help determine the optimal device to use and the ability of these devices to function properly. Specifically, in addition to external anatomic landmarks, ultrasound and fluoroscopic guidance should be used at the time of access to avoid puncture above the inguinal ligament or distal access of the superficial femoral or profunda femoris arteries rather than the common femoral artery. Furthermore, the quality of the artery can be assessed using ultrasound to avoid access of densely calcified portions of the artery, which may impact the efficacy of the closure device. At the time of initial access or at completion of the procedure, angiography of the access artery should be performed with appropriate obliquity of the image intensifier to identify the precise location of the puncture and the intraluminal nature and size of the artery at that site.

Devices

Suture closure

Perclose A-T and Perclose ProGlide. The Perclose A-T (Abbott Vascular, Santa Clara, California) uses a braided suture to provide closure. The device delivers a preformed knot, which allows for closure over the guidewire. This is indicated for closure of up to 8 French access sites. The Perclose ProGlide (Abbott Vascular) uses a monofilament suture to provide closure in a manner similar to the Perclose A-T (Fig. 18.7). This is indicated for closure of up to 8 French access sites but more than one device may be used to close access sites up to 21 French.

Prostar Xl. The Prostar XL (Abbott Vascular) device uses two braided sutures, which are delivered untied to allow for closure over a guidewire (Fig. 18.8). This device is indicated for closure of 8.5 to 10 French access sites but is commonly used off-label to mediate closure of up to 24 French access sites.

Mechanical nonsuture closure

StarClose SE. The StarClose SE (Abbott Vascular) uses an extravascular nitinol clip that grips the adventitial surface of the artery to obtain hemostasis in a circular fashion (Fig. 18.9). This is indicated for closure of up to 6 French access sites.

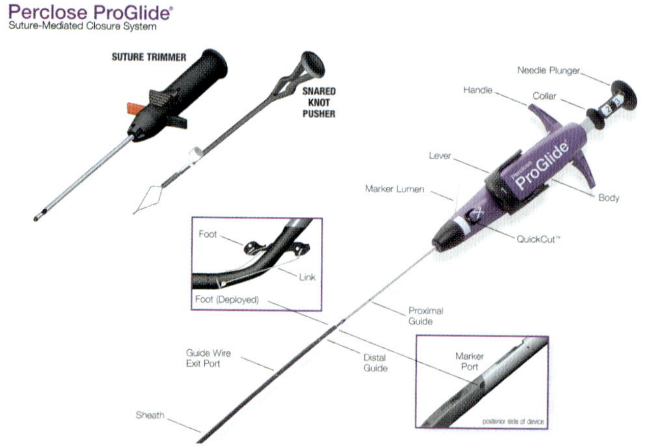

Illustrations are artist renditions. Not drawn to scale.
Courtesy of Abbott Vascular.

FIG 18.7 Perclose ProGlide (Abbott Vascular, Santa Clara, California). (Courtesy Abbott Vascular.)

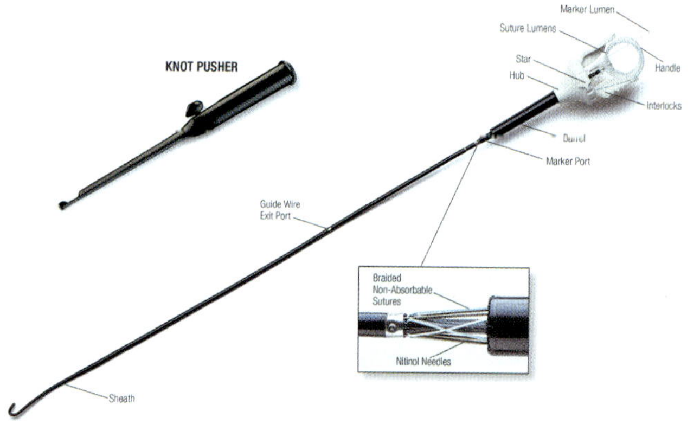

Illustrations are artist renditions. Not drawn to sale.
Courtesy of Abbott Vascular.

FIG 18.8 Prostar (Abbott Vascular, Santa Clara, California). (Courtesy Abbott Vascular.)

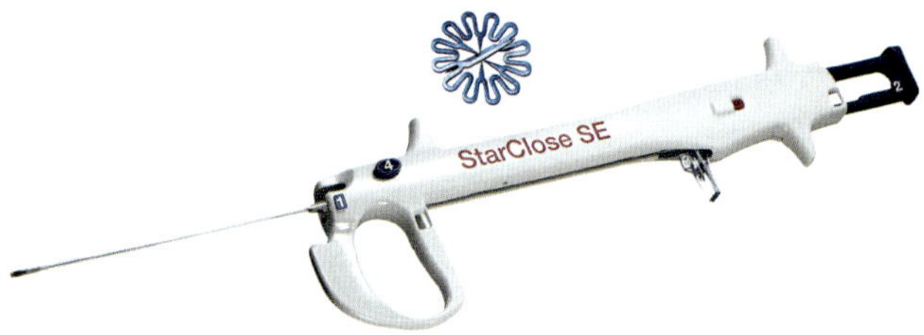

Illustrations are artist renditions. Not drawn to scale.
Courtesy of Abbott Vascular.

FIG 18.9 StarClose SE (Abbott Vascular, Santa Clara, California). (Courtesy Abbott Vascular.)

Extravascular sealant

Cordis Mynxgrip and Mynx Ace. The Mynxgrip (CardinalHealth/Cordis, Santa Clara, California) is delivered through the indwelling sheath and provides closure by delivering an extravascular sealant that adheres to and seals the arteriotomy after a balloon has been deployed via the sheath and pulled on gentle traction to achieve initial hemostasis

(Fig. 18.10). The sealant is composed of polyethylene glycol and dissolves within 30 days. The device is indicated for arterial and venous closure of 5 to 7 French femoral access sites. The Mynx Ace (CardinalHealth/Cordis) is the latest iteration of this device and uses the same sealant via a different deployment system (Fig. 18.11).

Cordis Exoseal. The Exoseal deploys a polyglycolic acid plug outside the arteriotomy via a precise positioning mechanism to prevent intravascular deployment (Fig. 18.12). The plug is resorbed fully within 60 to 90 days. The device is indicated for closure of 5 to 7 French access sites.

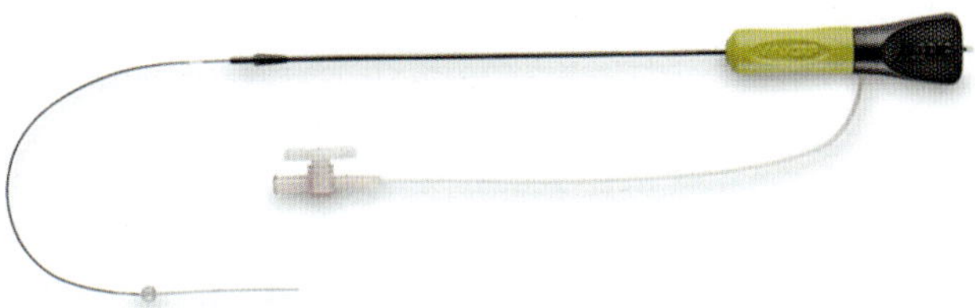

FIG 18.10 Mynxgrip (CardinalHealth/Cordis, Santa Clara, California). (Courtesy CardinalHealth/Cordis.)

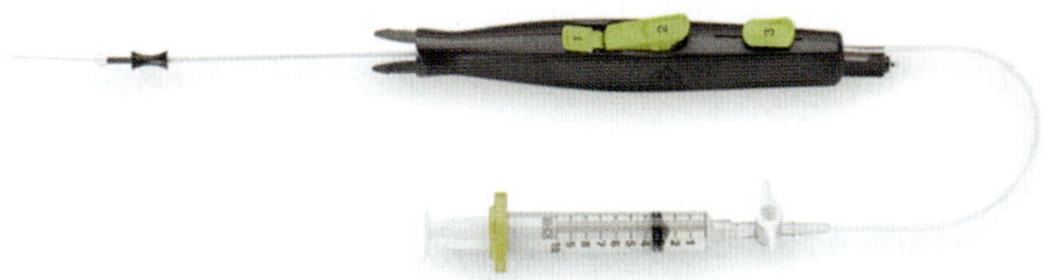

FIG 18.11 Mynxgrip Ace (CardinalHealth/Cordis, Santa Clara, California). (Courtesy CardinalHealth/Cordis.)

Cardiva Vascade. The Vascade Vascular Closure System (Cardiva Medical, Inc., Santa Clara, California) deploys a collagen plug in combination with a tamponade at the access site via a collapsible nitinol disk. The device is indicated for closure of 5 to 7 French access sites.

Intravascular sealant

St. Jude Angio-Seal. The Angio-Seal Evolution, STS Plus, and VIP (St. Jude Medical, St. Paul, Minnesota) use a bioabsorbable anchor combined with a collagen plug to sandwich the arteriotomy. The components reabsorb within 90 days (Fig. 18.13). These devices are available in 6 and 8 French sizes. There is FDA labeling for immediate reaccess of the artery along with 20-minute ambulation and 60-minute discharge for diagnostic cases.

Morris FISH CombiClose and ControlClose. The femoral introducer sheath and hemostasis (FISH) CombiClose and ControlClose devices (Morris Innovative, Bloomington, Indiana) are active closure devices that use a bioabsorbable matrix made from porcine small intestinal submucosa premounted on an access sheath (Fig. 18.14). This patch is deployed via a wire release mechanism and secured via a compression suture at completion of the procedure. The devices range in size from 5 to 8 French.

Manual compression assistance

Cardiva Catalyst II and III. The Catalyst II (Cardiva Medical, Inc., Santa Clara, California) is intended to achieve hemostasis as an adjunct to manual compression. The device is inserted through the indwelling sheath and once it is intraluminal, a nitinol disk is deployed. The sheath is then removed and the disk is pulled up against the arterial wall and then held in place with a tension clip. This also allows for recoil of the puncture site. The Catalyst III uses similar technology with the addition of a protamine sulfate coating to help locally neutralize the effects of heparin in the tissue tract of the puncture. The device is indicated for closure of 5 to 7 French access sites.

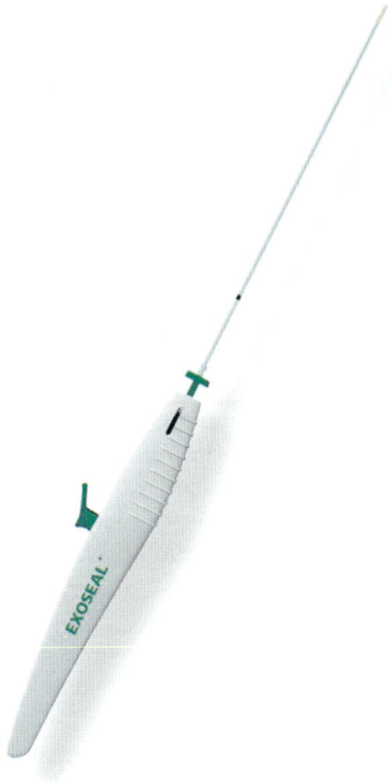

FIG 18.12 Exoseal (CardinalHealth/Cordis, Santa Clara, California). (Courtesy CardinalHealth/Cordis.)

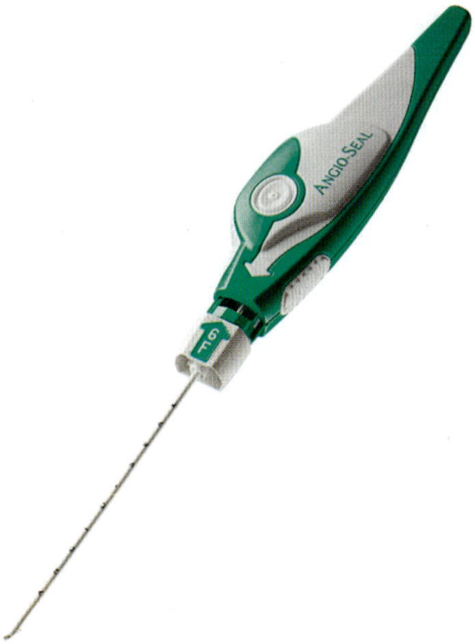

FIG 18.13 Angio-Seal STS Evolution (St. Jude Medical, St. Paul, Minnesota). (Courtesy St. Jude Medical.)

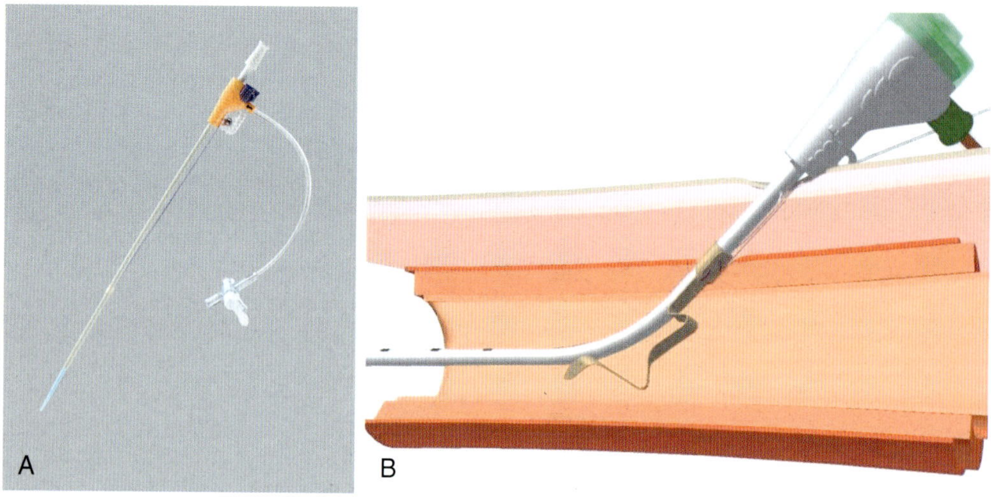

FIG 18.14 (A) FISH CombiClose device (Morris Innovative, Bloomington, Indiana). (B) Deployment of the bioabsorbable matrix. (Courtesy Morris Innovative.)

Self-sealing access

Arstasis Axera Access. The Axera Access (Arstasis, Fremont, California) uses the artery wall at the time of initial access to facilitate closure. The device creates a long, shallow-angle arteriotomy to allow for arterial tissue overlap, at which point a second preprocedure arteriotomy is created. Following removal of the sheath, this overlap of tissue, along with the arterial pressure and abbreviated manual compression, allow for closure without implantation of any foreign material.

Complications

Hemorrhagic

The most frequently encountered complication with arterial closure devices is failure or maldeployment leading to inadequate hemostasis from the access site. Densely calcified arteries may impact the efficacy of suture-mediated closure devices because delivery of the needles may be affected by the calcifications. Select devices, specifically the Perclose and Prostar maintain wire access during the closure process, which allows for the ability to replace a sheath to obtain hemostasis and/or to deploy an additional device or an alternative device. Alternatively, with a sheath in place, anticoagulants may be allowed to become inactive with time or reversal agents can be administered following which the sheath can then be removed and manual compression applied. If a sheath cannot be replaced at the time of closure device failure or maldeployment, manual pressure is applied and anticoagulation can be reversed to decrease the time necessary to achieve hemostasis. Furthermore, despite apparent initial hemostasis, there may be unrecognized incomplete arterial closure leading to delayed hematoma or pseudoaneurysm development, and patients presented with delayed groin swelling and pain following percutaneous access and closure should be appropriately evaluated with duplex ultrasound.

Ischemic

Maldeployment or malfunction of arterial closure devices may lead to lower limb ischemia due to occlusion at the access site or distal embolization. The incidence of ischemic complications has been reported to be less than 0.5% in studies of different devices.[39,47-51] Particularly when treating patients with known PAD, specific attention should be made preprocedure to the pulse examination on the side of access. The exam should be repeated immediately following the completion of the procedure for comparison. Patients with ischemic complications may manifest immediately with new-onset symptoms of claudication or rest pain. Additionally, patients may develop symptoms days to weeks later prompting evaluation of their access site.

The mechanism by which ischemic complications occur tend to be device specific. The suture-mediated devices and the intravascular sealant devices may lead to disruption of the posterior wall intima, particularly in the setting of atherosclerotic plaque leading to arterial dissection and thrombosis. This emphasizes the need for angiography evaluation of the access artery prior to closure to assure that the lumen size and quality are appropriate for the use of certain devices. Small diseased arteries may be more safely closed with the use of extravascular sealant devices. Alternatively, for both the intravascular and extravascular sealant devices, maldeployment of the hemostatic component of the device within the arterial lumen may lead to thrombosis or distal embolization. Following diagnosis of such complications, the most common approach is femoral exploration with thromboendarterectomy with primary closure or patch angioplasty as needed or in certain scenarios, surgical bypass. Additionally, endovascular techniques may be used including thrombolysis, angioplasty, and even atherectomy to remove the intraluminal component of the closure device.

Infectious

Infectious complications of arterial closure devices are unusual and typically occur several days to weeks later. Delayed symptoms of groin pain, swelling, erythema, and fever should prompt immediately evaluation. Definitive treatment involves surgical exploration and excision of all infected tissues and may require arterial reconstruction with autogenous tissue.[47] Strict sterile technique should be adhered to at the time of the procedure to avoid such complications. Additionally, regloving and reprepping the skin and the sheath itself at the time of closure may be beneficial, particularly in the setting of high-risk groins (previous surgery, multiple prior percutaneous accesses, obese, diabetic patients).[52]

Conclusions

Innovations in endovascular therapeutics have continued to advance over the past decade and will likely continue to do so for the foreseeable future. Presently, there are a number of different atherectomy and arterial closure devices that work via different mechanisms with their own advantages and disadvantages. With regard to the atherectomy devices, surgeons should understand the mechanism of action of these and have them in their armamentarium for the management of lower extremity arterial occlusive disease, although their use should be limited to specific anatomic scenarios based on the currently available data. Additionally, surgeons should be aware of the variety of arterial closure devices and their mechanisms and gain comfort with a few of these to allow for safe closure, earlier patient ambulation, and discharge.

REVIEW QUESTIONS

1. All of the following are atherectomy modalities except:
   - **a.** Orbital
   - **b.** Excisional
   - **c.** Rotational
   - **d.** Ultrasonic
   - **e.** Laser
2. The multi-institutional DEFINITE LE study of directional atherectomy found which of the following results?
   - **a.** Primary patency of 90% at 1 year in claudicants
   - **b.** Primary patency of 85% at 1 year in CLI patients
   - **c.** Overall 1-year limb salvage of 95%
   - **d.** Clinically significant embolization in 5% of patients
   - **e.** Arterial perforation in 8% of patients
3. Which of the following lesions would be most amenable to directional atherectomy?
   - **a.** 2-cm calcified popliteal stenosis
   - **b.** 10-cm posterior tibial occlusion
   - **c.** 15-cm in-stent superficial femoral artery restenosis
   - **d.** Intimal hyperplastic stenosis at distal anastomosis of prosthetic femoral-popliteal graft
   - **e.** 20-cm superficial femoral artery occlusion with single vessel (peroneal) runoff
4. The use of arterial closure devices compared to manual compression for hemostasis following percutaneous femoral access has been shown to do which of the following?
   - **a.** Decrease access site pseudoaneurysm or hematoma development
   - **b.** Increase access site infections
   - **c.** Decrease time until ambulation
   - **d.** Decrease time until discharge
   - **e.** Both c and d
5. One week following closure of a femoral access site using a collagen-based device, a patient presents with fever, erythema, and swelling in the groin. Ultrasound reveals a 3-cm fluid collection adjacent to the artery. Which of the following is the most definitive therapy?
   - **a.** Administration of intravenous antibiotics
   - **b.** Device removal and arterial reconstruction with autologous tissue
   - **c.** Ultrasound-guided thrombin injection
   - **d.** Percutaneous drainage
   - **e.** Contralateral access and placement of a covered stent

BIBLIOGRAPHY

Bechara CF, Annambhotla S, Lin PH. Access site management with vascular closure devices for percutaneous transarterial procedures. *J Vasc Surg*. 2010;52(6):1682–1696.

Kalapatapu VR, Ali AT, Masroor F, et al. Techniques for managing complications of arterial closure devices. *Vasc Endovascular Surg*. 2006;40(5):399–408.

Robertson L1, Andras A, Colgan F, et al. Vascular closure devices for femoral arterial puncture site haemostasis. *Cochrane Database Syst Rev*. 2016;(3):CD009541.

References available online at ExpertConsult.com.

19 CHAPTER

Extracranial Cerebrovascular Disease: The Carotid Artery

Wesley S. Moore

HISTORICAL REVIEW

The development of surgery on the extracranial cerebrovascular circulation was dependent on three principal factors: (1) recognition of the pathologic relationship between extracranial cerebrovascular disease and subsequent cerebral infarction, (2) the introduction of cerebral angiography to identify lesions before the patient's death, and (3) the development of vascular surgical techniques that could be applied to the extracranial vessels once the anatomic patterns of disease were understood and described.

The earliest report linking cervical carotid artery disease to stroke is credited to Savory,[1] who in 1856 described a young woman with left monocular symptoms in combination with a right hemiplegia and dysesthesia. Postmortem examination demonstrated an occlusion of the cervical portion of the left internal carotid artery, along with bilateral subclavian artery occlusions. In 1875, Gowers reported a similar case,[2] and subsequent reports of individual cases were made by Chiari in 1905,[3] Guthrie and Mayou in 1908,[4] and Cadwater in 1912.[5] By 1914, in an important publication Hunt[6] emphasized the relationship between extracranial carotid artery disease and stroke. He also described the phenomenon of intermittent cerebral symptoms associated with partial occlusion and used the term *cerebral intermittent claudication* as a characterizing analogy. Hunt also pointed out that the clinicopathologic observations in patients with stroke were hampered by the fact that routine autopsies did not include examination of the cervical carotid arteries (as is often the case today because of the desire to maintain access to the external carotid artery for the mortician). He emphasized that no examination of cerebral infarction can be considered complete without examination of the neck vessels.[6]

The next major step in the evolution of the management of extracranial cerebrovascular disease came with the development of carotid angiography by Moniz in 1927.[7] By 1937, Moniz and colleagues had described four cases of internal carotid occlusion diagnosed by angiography.[8] In 1938, Chao and colleagues added two more cases,[9] and by 1951, Johnson and Walker had collected from the world literature a total of 101 cases of occlusion of the cervical carotid artery diagnosed by angiography.[10] Despite these early observations, the medical world was still slow to appreciate the relationship between extracranial cerebrovascular disease and cerebral symptoms, as emphasized by the fact that when cerebral angiography came into common use for neurologic diagnosis in the 1950s and 1960s, only the intracranial vessels were included on radiographs films. The area of the carotid bifurcation was seldom examined. By the late 1950s, patients with hemiplegia were still commonly receiving diagnoses of a middle cerebral artery thrombosis, without consideration of carotid bifurcation as a source of the problem.

The next major steps in the evolution of understanding came from reports by Fisher in 1951 and 1954.[11,12] Fisher reemphasized the relationship between extracranial arterial occlusive disease and cerebral symptoms. He also pointed out that the lesion could be either total occlusion or stenosis. His most important observation, however, was that the disease was often localized to a short segment of the carotid artery, and he predicted that surgical correction might be possible if patients could be identified in the early stages of the clinical syndrome. Fisher stated, "It is even conceivable that some day vascular surgery will find a way to bypass the occluded portion of the artery during the period of ominous fleeting symptoms. Anastomosis of the external carotid artery or one of its branches with the internal carotid artery above the area of narrowing should be feasible."

The surgical phase of understanding and managing extracranial cerebrovascular disease probably began in 1951, but it was not reported in the literature until 1955. This early report by Carrea and colleagues[13] from Buenos Aires described their experience with the management of a patient with carotid artery stenosis. They resected the diseased internal carotid artery and performed an anastomosis between the external carotid artery and the distal internal carotid, as predicted earlier by Fisher.[11] In 1953, Strully and coworkers[14] attempted a thromboendarterectomy of a totally thrombosed internal carotid artery. This attempt was unsuccessful, but the authors suggested that thromboendarterectomy should be technically feasible before thrombosis occurred, as long as the internal carotid artery is patent distally. The first carotid endarterectomy (CEA) was probably performed by DeBakey and colleagues in an operation done on August 7, 1953, but it was not actually written up until 1959 and then reviewed in 1975.[15,16] The report that was most important in calling the world's attention to the feasibility of carotid artery reconstruction came from Eastcott and associates.[17] Their operation was performed on May 19, 1954, on a patient who was having hemispheric transient ischemic attacks (TIAs) with demonstrable disease at the carotid bifurcation; they used direct, end-to-end anastomosis between the common carotid artery and the internal carotid artery distal to the atherosclerotic lesion.

Although operations on the carotid artery were in the early phase of development, surgical attack was also considered feasible on occlusive lesions of the major arch vessels. In 1956, Davis and colleagues[18] reported their experience with endarterectomy of the innominate artery performed on a patient on March 20, 1954. In 1957, Warren and Triedman reported the second case.[19]

By this time, the stage was set for the explosive development of an aggressive surgical approach to managing extracranial cerebrovascular disease as a means of preventing or treating cerebral infarction.

Thompson,[20] in his 1996 Willis lecture, related in great detail the history of surgery to prevent stroke. Those interested in the definitive history will be rewarded by reading this excellent paper.

NATURAL HISTORY OF EXTRACRANIAL ARTERIAL OCCLUSIVE DISEASE

Therapy aimed at the prevention of cerebral infarction must be compared with the natural history of the disease process. The prognosis for a patient with extracranial arterial occlusive disease differs, depending on the presence or absence of symptoms. When a permanent neurologic deficit is present, the outlook worsens, thus underscoring the importance of prevention. A thorough understanding of the natural history of the disease is essential to formulating a rational and effective therapeutic program. The physician needs to be familiar with the expected results of each available option. This implies that no single alternative is applicable to all situations and that individualization is the key to effective prevention.

In the United States, approximately 600,000 people suffer a first stroke each year. In 200,000 of these cases, death follows, but at any one time approximately 1 million stroke victims are alive and disabled. In 1976, the annual direct and indirect cost of stroke was estimated at $7,363,784,000.[21] Nearly 40 years later, with inflation and the accelerating cost of medical care, this cost has probably quadrupled. The incalculable morbidity of the affected individual adds further to the magnitude of this problem. Prevention remains the most plausible alternative.

The initial mortality of an ischemic stroke ranges from 15% to 33%.[22-24] Survivors remain at an inordinately high risk of subsequent stroke, estimated between 4.8% and 20% per year.[25,26] This implies that half of patients will experience a second event within 5 years.[23,27,28] The average recurrent stroke rate reported in the literature is between 6% and 12% each year. The most common cause of death in patients with extracranial arterial occlusive disease is myocardial infarction (MI). However, in an analysis of 535 stroke victims, the leading cause of death was recurrent stroke, as opposed to the expected myocardial mortality.[26]

Since 1973, public health statistics have documented an accelerating decline in stroke mortality.[29] Stroke used to be considered the third leading cause of death in the United States. The American Heart and Stroke Association recently reported that stroke has now dropped to the fourth leading cause of death. The reasons for this are multifactorial but include successful efforts at primary prevention, including surgical intervention and treatment of carotid bifurcation lesions, improved medical management, and better care for the patient with acute stroke, often in specialized centers. This reduction in stroke mortality has led to the erroneous assumption that a decline has also occurred in stroke incidence, which may not be the case.

In 1989, Wolf and colleagues[30] reported the epidemiologic data from the Framingham Study to the 14th International Joint Conference on Stroke and Cerebral Circulation. They reviewed the experience from three successive decades, beginning in 1953. A decline in stroke fatality in both men and women was observed. However, the 10-year prevalence of stroke actually rose, and the incidence of stroke in men rose from 5.7% to 7.6% to 7.9%, without any apparent change in women. The authors postulated that falling case fatality rates might have resulted from changes in diagnostic criteria, a lessening in stroke severity, or improved care of stroke patients.

Harmsen and colleagues[31] reviewed the stroke incidence and fatality in Gothenburg, Sweden, between 1971 and 1987. They noted that the stroke incidence remained the same during that interval, but the stroke fatality rate declined in both sexes. This was more marked for intracerebral hemorrhage and subarachnoid hemorrhage than for infarction. They concluded that the decline in stroke fatality rates might have been related to a decrease in smoking or better management of blood pressure. They could not explain why no corresponding decline in stroke incidence occurred.

Moden and Wagener[32] examined the epidemiologic aspects of stroke based on death certificate information available from the National Center for Health Statistics' compressed mortality file for all 50 states and the District of Columbia for the period 1968 to 1988. They noted a decline in stroke mortality that continued through the 1970s and 1980s, whereas morbidity remained constant and possibly even increased. They noted similar morbidity and mortality rates in both sexes. They concluded that the observed decrease in stroke mortality rates resulted from improved survival rather than a decline in incidence.[32]

Krishnamurthi and colleagues reviewed the MEDLINE database to determine the incidence of new ischemic and hemorrhagic strokes between various regions over time. They included 119 studies (58 from high-income countries and 61 from low- and middle-income countries) and found that worldwide the incidence of stroke increased significantly between 1990 and 2010. However, the incidence of ischemic stroke in high-income countries reduced significantly by 13% and mortality by 37%.[33] A variety of reasons for the decline in stroke mortality have been postulated, including the more aggressive treatment of hypertension and the use of specialized stroke intensive care units (Fig. 19.1).

Two clinical syndromes deserve special emphasis because of their dismal natural history. Stroke in evolution is also known as *progressing stroke* or *incomplete stroke*; it is an acute neurologic deficit of modest degree that within hours or days progresses to a major cerebral infarct. This can happen in a sequential series of acute exacerbations or in a pattern of waxing and waning signs and symptoms over hours or days, with incomplete recovery eventually leading to a major fixed neurologic deficit. Crescendo TIAs is the pattern that allows complete recovery between ischemic events, suggesting repeated frequent embolization from a point arterial source in the affected territory.

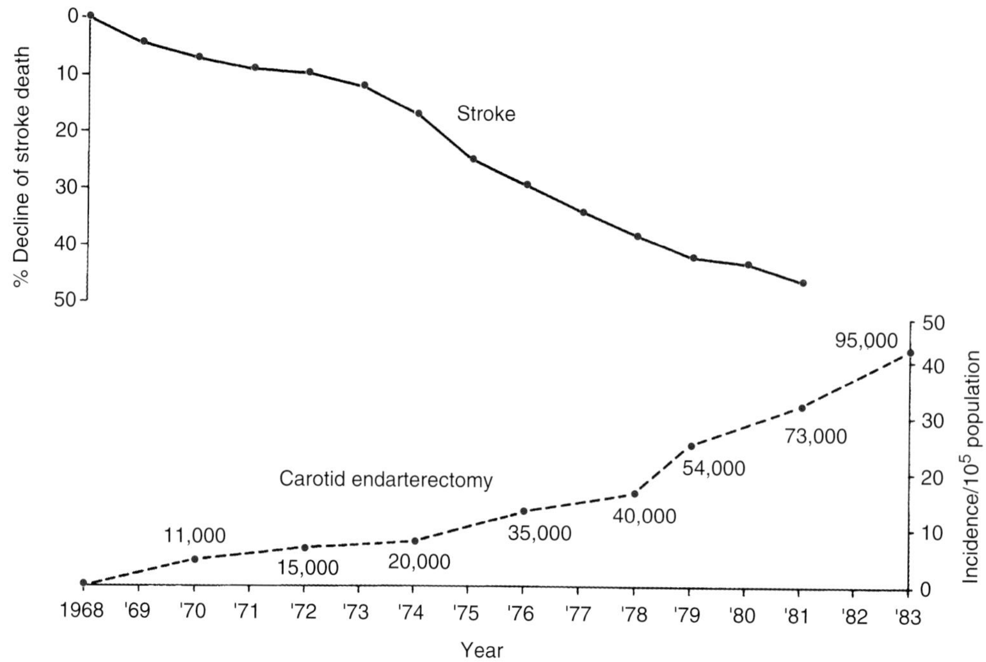

FIG 19.1 The declining incidence of stroke-related death from 1968 to 1981 is compared with the accelerated frequency with which carotid endarterectomy was performed during the same period.

In a review of the literature, Mentzer and colleagues[34] identified 263 reported cases of stroke in evolution managed conservatively. Twenty-three percent had complete resolution or mild neurologic deficit on follow-up. Sixty-two percent had a moderate to severe deficit in the early recovery phase. The overall mortality was 14.5%. In their own series, 26 patients with stroke in evolution were treated conservatively. Mortality was 15%, but more importantly, 66% suffered moderate to severe permanent neurologic deficits, with only five patients recovering completely or experiencing only mild neurologic dysfunction. These results are compared with a series of 17 patients operated on emergently for stroke in evolution. None of these patients had worsening of the preoperative neurologic deficit, four (24%) remained unchanged, and 12 (70%) had complete recovery.[34]

In 1972, Millikan reviewed the natural history of patients with progressing stroke.[35] Of 204 patients, 12% were normal at 14 days, 7% had developed moderate to severe neurologic deficits, and 14% had died. Thus stroke in evolution treated conservatively carries a poor prognosis. More than half of patients develop a severe permanent neurologic deficit within a few days of the onset, and approximately 15% die as a result. Only 10% to 20% recover full or partial neurologic function.[35]

Patients who experience TIAs are also at a higher risk of developing a stroke. In the Mayo Clinic population study,[36] 118 patients with TIAs were monitored as a control group without therapy. The stroke rates at 1, 3, and 5 years were 23%, 37%, and 45%, respectively. Most permanent deficits occurred during the first year. This represents a 16-fold increased risk of stroke compared with an age- and sex-adjusted population. The Oxfordshire project reported an actuarial risk of stroke during the first year after the onset of TIAs to be 11% to 16%.[37] For each subsequent year, the rate was 5% to 9% per year. Some series have reported lower figures,[38,39] but the average reported in the literature is on the order of 30% to 35% at 5 years, or 10% the first year and 6% each year thereafter.

Finally, Toole[40] noted that cerebral infarction in TIA patients goes unrecognized by either patient or physician surprisingly often. These lesions are now identified by better neuroimaging techniques, and there is now evidence to suggest that TIAs are actually small strokes.[40] If TIAs are actually small strokes, the implied benignity of TIAs must be reexamined, and it may be equally important to prevent TIAs. This consideration is further strengthened by the observations of Grigg and colleagues,[41] who correlated cerebral infarction and atrophy as a function of TIAs and percentage of stenosis. They graded carotid stenosis in symptomatic patients from A (no stenosis) to E (occlusion). In patients with amaurosis fugax, the incidence of cerebral infarction rose from 2% in patients with stenosis grades A, B, and C to 40% in grade D and 58% in grade E. The incidence of atrophy increased in parallel, from 10% in grade A to 30% in grade E.

The natural history of asymptomatic patients with significant extracranial or arterial occlusive disease is difficult to predict accurately. Most studies that have addressed this problem used the presence of a cervical bruit as the sole criterion for inclusion. This inevitably includes patients without significant occlusive disease and omits others without cervical bruit but with high-risk lesions in the extracranial circulation.

As noninvasive studies developed, the detection of hemodynamically significant lesions in the carotid system improved. Kartchner and McRae monitored 1130 patients who either were asymptomatic or had nonhemispheric symptoms.[42] The mean interval was 24 months. Of 303 patients with hemodynamically significant lesions, 11.9% had strokes at 2 years. The group with negative noninvasive studies had a much lower stroke rate, on the order of 3% over the same follow-up period. Busuttil and colleagues[43] noted an unfavorable trend toward higher stroke rates in asymptomatic patients with hemodynamically significant lesions in the carotid bifurcation.

In a report by Roederer and colleagues,[44] 167 asymptomatic patients with cervical bruits were monitored with serial duplex scanning, regardless of the degree of stenosis at the time of presentation. During follow-up, 10 patients became symptomatic. The development of symptoms was accompanied by disease progression in 80% of patients. By life-table analysis, the annual rate of symptom occurrence was 4%; however, the presence of progression graded at 80% stenosis was highly correlated with the development of either total occlusion of the internal carotid artery or new symptoms. Thus 89% of the symptoms were preceded by progression of the lesion to greater than 80% stenosis. Progression of a lesion to more than 80% stenosis was an important warning sign, because it carried a 35% risk of ischemic symptoms or internal carotid occlusion within 6 months and a 46% risk at 12 months. Conversely, only 1.5% of the lesions that remained at less than 80% stenosis developed such a complication. These data suggest that careful follow-up with repeated noninvasive evaluation is of great assistance in determining the appropriate management of asymptomatic carotid lesions.[44]

In an analysis of 294 asymptomatic and nonhemispheric patients submitted to cerebrovascular testing, Moore and colleagues[45] found a 15% stroke incidence during the first 2 years in patients with greater than 50% stenosis. In contrast, there was a 3% stroke incidence at 2 years in patients with 1% to 49% stenosis. The difference was found to be statistically significant ($P < .05$). The 5-year cumulative stroke incidence was 21% with greater than 50% stenosis, 14% with 1% to 49% stenosis, and 9% in patients with no noninvasive evidence of carotid artery disease.

Chambers and Norris[46] monitored a group of 500 asymptomatic patients with noninvasive studies and clinical evaluation. They identified two high-risk groups: those with stenosis greater than 75%, and those who showed disease progression between studies. For patients with greater than 75% stenosis, the 1-year neurologic event rate (TIA and stroke) was 22%. The 1-year stroke rate alone was 5%. In a later publication,[47] the authors continued to note that neurologic events correlated with an increasing percentage of stenosis as well as disease progression between test intervals. In the study viewed over 5 years, the annual average neurologic event rate was 10% to 15%, with the highest event rate occurring within the first year of diagnosis. Finally, the incidence of silent cerebral infarction as documented by computed tomography (CT) was studied in the same patient population. The authors noted a 10% incidence of cerebral infarction among patients with mild (35% to 50%) stenosis, 17% with moderate (50% to 75%) stenosis, and 30% in patients with severe (>75%) stenosis. The authors concluded that silent cerebral infarction might be an indication for CEA in asymptomatic patients.[48]

Although the natural history of asymptomatic carotid stenosis remains controversial, studies using serial noninvasive cerebrovascular testing have concluded that an increased risk of stroke exists ipsilateral to a 50% or greater carotid artery stenosis. These lesions appear to carry a risk of subsequent stroke on the order of 4% per year. In addition, progression of the disease carries an even higher risk of stroke, with lesions causing greater than 80% stenosis carrying a 35% risk of subsequent symptoms or carotid occlusion at 2 years.

Other studies have suggested that the composition of the plaque influences the stroke risk of carotid artery lesions. In one analysis, 297 patients with carotid stenosis greater than 75% at the time of initial study were at higher risk than peers without significant narrowing or development of symptoms ipsilateral to the lesion.[49] Even those patients with less than 75% stenosis were at greater risk if the associated plaque was less organized (i.e., soft). This was determined by B-mode ultrasonography, which was used to classify plaques as dense, calcified, or soft. A definite trend toward higher risk was seen in plaques of lower density. Only 10% of those patients with calcified plaque in significantly stenotic vessels developed symptoms, whereas 92% of patients with soft plaques and tight stenosis developed symptoms within the first 3 years of follow-up.[49] The morphology of the atherosclerotic plaque, as documented by B-mode ultrasonography, is emerging as one of the more important factors associated with embolic potential and stroke risk. Two studies have concluded that a heterogeneous plaque carries an increased risk of stroke and is a variable independent from carotid stenosis alone.[50,51]

More recently, attempts have been made to better characterize the asymptomatic patient who is at higher risk for a cerebral ischemic event in order to identify subgroups of patients who would benefit from CEA compared with patients with carotid stenosis, who are at low risk for an ischemic event. In addition to percent stenosis and plaque composition, two factors have been identified as being associated with increased stroke risk in the asymptomatic patient. These factors include the presence of silent brain infarction, as seen on a screening CT scan, and silent brain embolic signals, as documented using transcranial Doppler. Kakkos and colleagues[52] studied 821 patients with CT scans. In patients with 60% to 99% stenosis and without silent brain infarction on CT, the annual rate of TIA and stroke was 1.3%. In patients with silent brain infarction, the annual event rate was 4.4%, suggesting that this subgroup of patients might benefit from CEA, leaving the low-risk group free from an unnecessary intervention.[52] Markus and colleagues[53] evaluated 467 asymptomatic patients with high-grade carotid stenosis in a multicenter study. Transcranial Doppler identified 77 patients with embolic signals. The annual risk of TIA and stroke was 7.13% in patients with embolic signals, compared with 3.04% in patients without embolic signals. For ipsilateral stroke alone, the hazard ratio was 6.37. These findings suggest that screening for silent brain emboli is another method for identifying a high-risk group that is more likely to benefit from intervention.[53]

The embolic potential of ulcerated carotid lesions has been well documented.[54-56] Patients who experience symptoms from these lesions probably have the same prognosis as patients with occlusive lesions. Whether the former patient group responds more favorably to platelet antiaggregants remains to be determined.

Moore and coworkers[57] first pointed out that asymptomatic patients with significant ulceration in a carotid plaque in the absence of stenosis appear to be at higher risk of stroke.[57] In a subsequent report, they expanded their series to 153 patients with asymptomatic, nonstenotic ulcerative lesions in the carotid bifurcation. Patients with deep (grade B) or complex (grade C) ulcerations received follow-up and were found to have a stroke rate of 4.5% and 7.5% each year, respectively.[58] Other reports have suggested a similar stroke risk for complex ulcerations in the carotid bulb. However, a much lower stroke risk was reported for deep (grade B) ulcerations, with no significant added risk of stroke observed in these patients. Controversy still exists about deep ulcerations without complex morphology. However, agreement exists that complex ulcerations in the carotid bulb increase the risk of stroke in asymptomatic patients.[59]

The presence of an asymptomatic hemodynamically significant stenosis may increase the risk of stroke during major surgery. Kartchner and McRae reported their experience with 234 patients, 41 of whom had evidence of significant carotid artery stenosis by oculoplethysmography.[60] Seven postoperative strokes developed in the group with positive criteria (17%), whereas postoperative cerebral infarction developed in 2 of 192 patients (1%) with negative noninvasive studies. The mechanisms of stroke and the territory involved were not specifically reported. This high incidence of permanent neurologic deficits led the authors to conclude that prophylactic CEA should be considered in patients with hemodynamically significant carotid stenosis who are undergoing a major cardiovascular procedure.[61]

Other series have reported results to the contrary.[61-64] Using noninvasive vascular evaluation and, in one series, angiography, patients with 50% or greater stenosis in the carotid bifurcation were compared with patients who had lesser degrees of stenosis undergoing cardiovascular surgery. No increased incidence of perioperative strokes was found in patients with positive criteria. Most of these investigators, however, excluded preocclusive stenosis in their considerations. Lesions causing 90% or greater stenosis were excluded from these series and were subjected to prophylactic endarterectomy before cardiovascular operation.

Cardiac surgeons have long been concerned about the presence of carotid stenosis in patients who will be undergoing cardiopulmonary bypass. Their concern is that during bypass there will be a decrease in pump perfusion pressure and a corresponding and unacceptable drop in cerebral blood flow. In fact, the opposite occurs. Von Reutern and colleagues[65] used transcranial Doppler ultrasonography to study middle cerebral artery blood flow before and during cardiopulmonary bypass in patients with and without carotid artery disease. Surprisingly, middle cerebral artery blood flow actually increased during cardiopulmonary bypass. Although the increase was not as great in patients with carotid artery disease, it was clearly an increase over baseline. This observation should dispel concern about the potential drop in cerebral blood flow in patients with carotid stenosis while using the pump.

Patients with a combination of severe carotid stenosis and symptomatic coronary artery disease represent a cohort that is at high risk of death, MI, and stroke. Brener and colleagues[66] performed an extensive literature review that examined complications associated with different treatment strategies. Patients who underwent staging with CEA first had a high cardiac morbidity and mortality. Patients who had coronary bypass first had higher stroke morbidity. The data suggested that combined or simultaneous coronary artery bypass grafting and CEA might reduce overall morbidity and mortality. However, evidence from retrospective reviews was not sufficiently compelling to make a definitive recommendation.[66] Consensus exists that this is an appropriate topic for a prospective, randomized trial.

The natural history of extracranial arterial occlusive disease cannot be complete without a consideration of the natural history of frequently associated conditions such as coronary artery disease, hypertension, and diabetes. MI remains the most frequent cause of death in these patients. Including these variables in the equation when one is formulating a treatment plan for a particular patient is therefore important. The goal of therapy should be the prevention of a permanent neurologic deficit. When deciding on the most effective way to achieve this, one must consider the life expectancy of the patient and the inherent risk of each particular form of therapy.

PATHOLOGY OF EXTRACRANIAL ARTERIAL OCCLUSIVE DISEASE

The pathology of cerebrovascular disease of extracranial origin can be divided into flow-restrictive lesions and lesions with embolic potential. Each of these can be further subdivided into occlusive and aneurysmal lesions. All entities that have been described as etiologic in extracranial disease fall within these categories.

Atherosclerosis

By far the most common lesion found in patients with extracranial cerebrovascular disease is an atherosclerotic plaque in the carotid bifurcation. This can produce symptoms by reducing blood flow to the hemisphere supplied or, more commonly, by releasing embolic material. Emboli can be composed of clot, platelet aggregates, or cholesterol debris.

The carotid bifurcation appears to be susceptible to the development of atherosclerotic plaques.[67] Frequently, severe changes at the carotid bifurcation occur with minimal or no changes present in the common or internal carotid artery.[68] Several investigators have proposed conflicting theories based on hemodynamic observations in various models. High and low shear stress and fluctuations in shear stress,[69] disordered or turbulent flow, flow separation, and high and low flow velocity have all been implicated.[70-73] It is unknown which of these mechanisms is responsible for plaque formation. Zarins and colleagues[74] used a model of the human carotid bifurcation under steady flow and compared its hemodynamics with those of cadaver specimens. They concluded that carotid lesions localize in regions of low flow velocity and flow separation, rather than in regions of high velocity and increased shear stress. They used their model to explain the propensity of the outer wall of the carotid sinus opposite the flow divider to develop atherosclerotic plaques (Fig. 19.2). This may have further clinical implications, in that an enlarged carotid bulb after endarterectomy may create a region

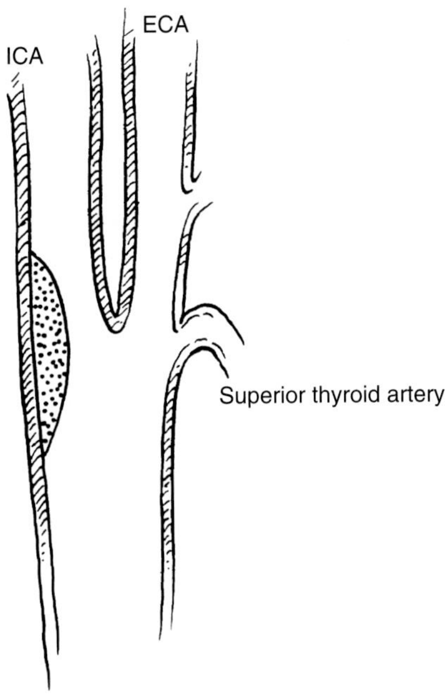

FIG 19.2 The common carotid artery bifurcation, the most common site for atherosclerotic plaque deposition, is located on the wall opposite the divider. *ECA,* External carotid artery; *ICA,* internal carotid artery.

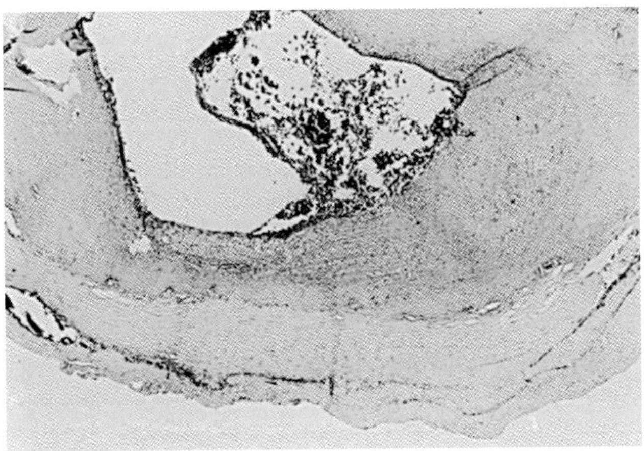

FIG 19.3 Microscopic section of an atherosclerotic plaque removed from the carotid bifurcation. Notice the fibro-intimal proliferation with cholesterol cleft formation. Thrombotic material is adherent to the luminal surface of the plaque.

of reduced flow velocity and increased boundary layer separation, which may favor recurrent plaque deposition.

Once the initial intimal injury is produced by these forces, platelet deposition, smooth muscle cell proliferation, and the slow accumulation of lipoproteins are involved in the reparative process (Fig. 19.3). These eventually lead to plaque formation, which further alters the hemodynamics of the system and favors further injury.

The contribution of platelets to atheroma development can take several forms.[75] Platelets may adhere to one another, to the diseased vessel, or both; this can lead to thrombus formation. This process may narrow the vessel lumen, or the thrombus may dislodge, resulting in distal embolization. Vasoactive substances stored in granules within the platelet may be released, causing vasospasm and also contributing to compromise of the arterial lumen. The platelets' interaction with collagen exposed in an injured intima may include elaboration of a smooth muscle growth factor that can lead to intimal thickening. The activation of enzymes in platelets, by their contact with collagen, initiates the production of highly active prostaglandins. The production of thromboxane A_2 represents the final common pathway of platelet response to diverse stimuli.[76] This substance is a potent stimulant of platelet aggregation and a powerful vasoconstrictor, and is believed to be important in the pathophysiology of plaque formation or the development of symptoms from an already established atheroma.

Hemorrhage into a plaque may also play a significant role in the development of symptoms from an atherosclerotic lesion. Imbalances in wall tension secondary to asymmetrical deposition of plaque can lead to sudden plaque fracture and intraplaque hemorrhage.[77] These can lead to the sudden expansion of the atheroma, with acute restriction of flow or breakdown of the intimal surface and concomitant embolization. An alternative mechanism for sudden intraplaque hemorrhage may be related to an increase in neovascularity within the plaque substance. Hypertension may be responsible for precipitating the rupture of neovascular vessels, leading to intraplaque hemorrhage and expansion.[78] This process may be responsible for a large number of symptomatic lesions. In a prospective evaluation of 79 atheromatous plaques removed from 69 patients undergoing CEA, 49 of 53 (92.5%) symptomatic patients had evidence of intramural hemorrhage.[79] In contrast, only 7 of 26 (27%) asymptomatic patients showed recent or acute intraplaque hemorrhage. Rupture of an atherosclerotic plaque with intraluminal release of atheromatous debris has also been correlated with acute stroke and internal carotid occlusion in an autopsy study.[80]

Fibromuscular Dysplasia

Fibromuscular dysplasia is a nonatherosclerotic process that affects medium-size arteries. It was first described in the carotid artery in 1964,[81] and since then it has been recognized as a cause of cerebrovascular symptoms.[82] It may also affect the intracranial arteries, and approximately 30% of patients with cervical involvement have associated intracranial aneurysms.[83] Up to 65% of patients have bilateral disease,[83] and 25% have associated atherosclerotic changes.[84]

Four histologic types of fibromuscular dysplasia have been described[85]:

1. Intimal fibroplasia accounts for about 5% of cases and affects both sexes equally. It usually appears as long tubular stenoses in young patients and as focal stenoses in older patients. It results from an accumulation of irregularly arranged subendothelial mesenchymal cells with a loose matrix of connective tissue. Medial and adventitial structures are always normal.
2. Medial hyperplasia is a rare form of the disease that produces focal stenoses. The intima and adventitia remain normal, whereas the media shows excess smooth muscle.
3. Medial fibroplasia is the most common pattern of fibromuscular dysplasia, accounting for most, if not all, internal carotid

artery involvement. It may appear as a focal stenosis or multiple lesions with intervening aneurysmal outpouchings. Histologically, the disease is limited to the media, with replacement of smooth muscle by compact fibrous connective tissue. The inner media may show an accumulation of collagen and ground substance separating disorganized smooth muscle cells. Gradation of these changes correlates with the severity of the lesion. Mural dilatations and microaneurysms are common.
4. Perimedial dysplasia is characterized by the accumulation of elastic tissue between the media and adventitia. It affects renal arteries and is associated with macro-aneurysms.

Fibromuscular dysplasia preferentially affects long arteries with few primary branches. Hormonal effects on medial tissue, mechanical stresses on the vessel wall, and unusual distribution of the vasa vasorum in these arteries seem to play a causative role.[85] Some experimental evidence[86] and the fact that women are most commonly affected (92% of cases)[84] support a possible role of hormones in this process. In the appropriate hormonal environment, the normal paucity of vasa vasorum in long, nonbranching arterial segments such as the extracranial carotid artery and the renal artery may predispose to mural ischemia and initiation of the fibroplastic process. Experimental evidence supports this concept.[87]

The exact cause of symptoms is controversial. Thromboembolism from clot, platelets, or both; decreased flow owing to a critical stenosis or a series of noncritical narrowing; intracranial involvement, with or without aneurysm formation; and hypertension have been implicated.[84]

Coils and Kinks

Coils and kinks of the extracranial system on occasion have been associated with fibromuscular dysplasia.[84] More commonly, these are due to embryologic events and changes that occur in the aging process. Most coils are asymptomatic, although neurologic manifestations from these anomalies have been reported in children[88] and in adults.[89-91] Embryologically, the internal carotid artery is derived from the third aortic arch and the dorsal aortic root. In the early stages of development, a normally occurring kink is straightened as the heart and great vessels descend in the mediastinum. Failure of this process may account for the occurrence of coils and loops in children and for its bilaterality in approximately 50% of cases.[91]

In adults, kinking of the extracranial vessels is almost always associated with atherosclerosis. In the aging process, loss of elasticity of the vessel wall occurs, which, in combination with lateral stresses, causes elongation between fixed points—the skull and the thoracic inlet. This produces bowing, with the eventual formation of coils and kinks. Between 5% and 16% of patients submitted for angiographic evaluation have coiling or kinking of one of the extracranial vessels.[89,91] Kinking of the artery is more likely to produce symptoms because of either flow reduction or concomitant plaque formation with distal embolization. Kinking is considered to be an angle of less than 90 degrees between arterial segments (Fig. 19.4). Flow restriction is unlikely to exist in the absence of this configuration. This acute angulation is more likely to occur when the head is turned to the ipsilateral side.[88] In other cases, contralateral rotation, neck flexion, and extension may exaggerate the abnormality, leading to markedly reduced flow. A history of TIAs associated with head motion should lead the clinician to suspect the presence of a kink. Abnormal pulsations in the neck, sometimes suggesting an aneurysmal dilatation, may be present on physical examination. Secondary arteriosclerotic changes can occur because of abnormal flow patterns that predispose to plaque formation and ulceration, accounting for the development of neurologic symptoms. Rarely is the vertebral circulation affected by a kink.[89]

Aneurysms

Aneurysms of the carotid artery can cause neurologic symptoms by several mechanisms. Thrombosis and rupture are rare, but embolization is a frequent event.[92] Pressure on cranial nerves can be seen when expansion is rapid, but more frequently this is associated with acute dissection.

Most extracranial aneurysms are secondary to atherosclerosis. Internal elastic lamina disruption and medial thinning are frequent histologic findings.[93] Two types of aneurysms are recognized: fusiform and saccular. Fusiform aneurysms are more common; they are frequently bilateral and are associated with other arterial aneurysms. Saccular aneurysms are often unilateral and tend to involve the common or internal carotid arteries more often. They may also have a congenital, degenerative, or traumatic origin.[94] Atherosclerotic aneurysms of the extracranial circulation are almost always associated with hypertension.[93]

Trauma is a frequent cause of carotid aneurysms. These are usually saccular and most commonly result from blunt rather than penetrating injury. Hyperextension and rotation of the neck cause compression of the internal carotid artery on the transverse process of the atlas.[95] An intimal injury is produced that frequently leads to thrombosis, but it can also produce aneurysmal dilatation.[93]

Mycotic aneurysms are rare. Syphilis and peritonsillar abscess were once common causes of these aneurysms.[96] *Staphylococcus aureus* is currently the predominant responsible organism.

False aneurysms of the carotid artery may form after penetrating injury, but the most frequent cause is previous carotid surgery. These aneurysms are more common after patch closure of the artery than after primary closure.[92] Disruption of the suture line by infection, suture failure, and technical error are believed to be responsible for their formation. False aneurysms can expand, thrombose, rupture, or lead to distal embolization. The diagnosis of false aneurysm is an indication for surgical or endovascular repair, depending on the location, the presence of intraluminal thrombus, and the experience of the surgeon.

Acute dissection of the carotid artery with or without aneurysm formation is another cause of neurologic events resulting from abnormalities in the extracranial circulation. It can occur secondary to atherosclerosis, fibromuscular dysplasia, or cystic medial necrosis.[97] A history of trauma may or may not be present. On gross inspection, a sharply demarcated transition between the normal color and size of the carotid artery and the dark blue, cylindrical dilatation in the dissected segment is noted.[98] More commonly, the internal carotid artery is affected, and frequently the end of the dissection is not surgically accessible. A double lumen is usually present, with the dissection occurring

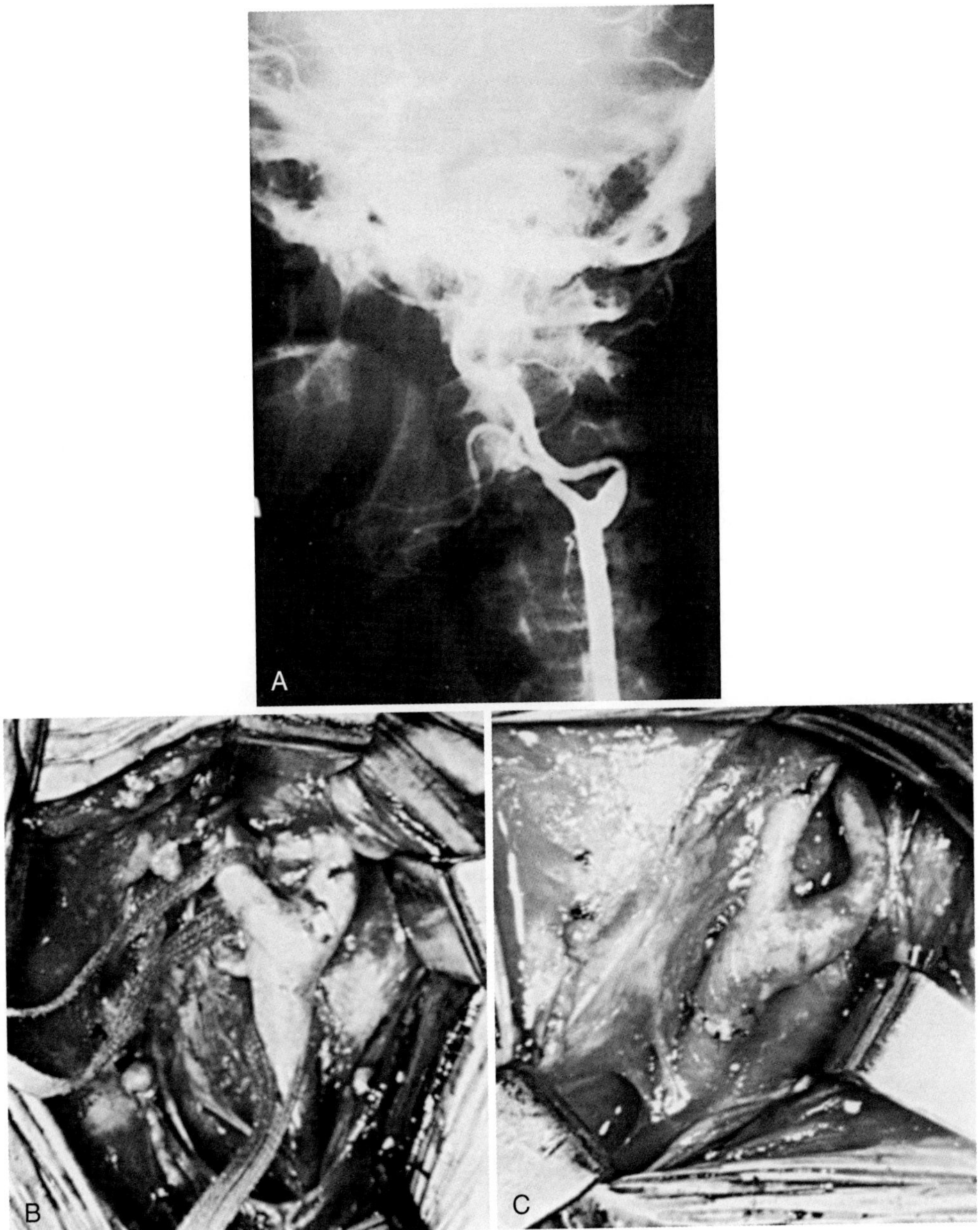

FIG 19.4 (A) Selective left carotid arteriogram demonstrating a kink of the internal carotid artery. Note the angulation of less than 90 degrees and the paucity of contrast material beyond the kink. (B) Operative appearance of the internal carotid artery kink. (C) Operative appearance of the internal carotid artery after connection of the kink by mobilization and segmental resection of the common carotid artery. The carotid bifurcation is pulled down, and an end-to-end anastomosis is constructed.

in the outer layers of the media. Smooth muscle cells are widely separated, and degeneration and fragmentation of the internal elastic membrane occur.[98] The most frequent presentation is a sudden onset of temporal headache or cervical pain associated with a neurologic or visual deficit or Horner syndrome. Acute expansion may cause compression of cranial nerves IX, X, XI, or XII, with concomitant dysfunction.[97] Horner syndrome is thought to be secondary to the disruption of periadventitial sympathetic fibers. The carotid artery is far more frequently affected than the vertebral artery is. Only a few cases of the latter have been reported, with involvement of the segment between C1 and C2 noted consistently.[97]

Takayasu Arteritis

In 1908, Takayasu described ocular changes in a 21-year-old woman with nonspecific arteritis.[99] These changes consisted of a peculiar capillary flush, with rustlike arteriovenous anastomoses around the papilla and blindness owing to cataracts. Similar cases were later described with the absence of pulses in the arm. Since then, Takayasu arteritis has been recognized as a cause of neurologic symptoms secondary to a nonspecific inflammatory process of unknown cause, segmentally affecting the aorta and its main branches. The end result of this process is constriction or occlusion of, and occasional aneurysm formation in, the affected vessels secondary to marked fibrosis and thickening of the arterial wall.[100] Originally thought to be rare in the Western hemisphere, many cases of atypical coarctations of the aorta and other unusual lesions of its main branches are now well recognized as Takayasu arteritis. This explains the many eponyms given to this syndrome.[101]

Four varieties of the disease are recognized.[102] In type 1, involvement is localized to the aortic arch and its branches. Type 2 does not have arch involvement; the lesions are confined to the descending and abdominal aorta. Type 3 has features of both, and type 4 describes any of the first three types, plus involvement of the pulmonary artery. In a retrospective study of 107 patients, 84% were female, and 80% were aged 11 to 30 years.[102]

Two phases of the disease are recognized. In the acute or prepulseless stage, systemic symptoms of a nonspecific nature are present. Skin rash, fever, myalgia, arthralgia, pleuritis, generalized weakness, and other nonspecific symptoms develop, making the diagnosis difficult. These symptoms may resolve and go unrecognized by the patient or physician until months or years later, when the second, or occlusive, stage evolves. Next, symptoms of obstruction of the main aortic branches develop. These lesions are not easily managed by endarterectomy, which makes bypass surgery the treatment of choice.

Other forms of arteritis, specifically giant cell arteritis, can cause neurologic symptoms because of extracranial or intracranial involvement. These patients are older than those with Takayasu arteritis, and both sexes appear to be equally affected.[101] Systemic symptoms are usually present. Tenderness over the carotid artery or other affected areas may occur.[103] The histologic picture is characteristic, with changes confined to the media, where a large number of giant cells interspersed with lymphocytes are seen. Early diagnosis is important, because corticosteroid therapy may abort the latter stages of the process.[103]

Radiation Therapy Injury

External cervical radiation therapy is recognized as a cause of accelerated atherosclerotic changes in the extracranial circulation. Experimentally, atherosclerotic lesions similar to the naturally occurring ones can be produced in the abdominal aorta in dogs by x-ray and electron beam radiation.[104] Injury to the endothelial cell, ground substance, elastic lamina, and smooth muscle appears to alter the vessel wall, increasing its permeability to circulating lipids and impairing its ability to repair elastic tissue, leading to the formation of a plaque characterized by fibrosis, fatty infiltration, and intimal destruction.[105] These changes can occur months to years after the completion of therapy. Lesions occur in locations unusual for atherosclerosis (Fig. 19.5). Blowout of the affected carotid artery may occur, but this is more frequent when surgery is combined with radiation in treating cervical malignancies. Hyperlipidemia and

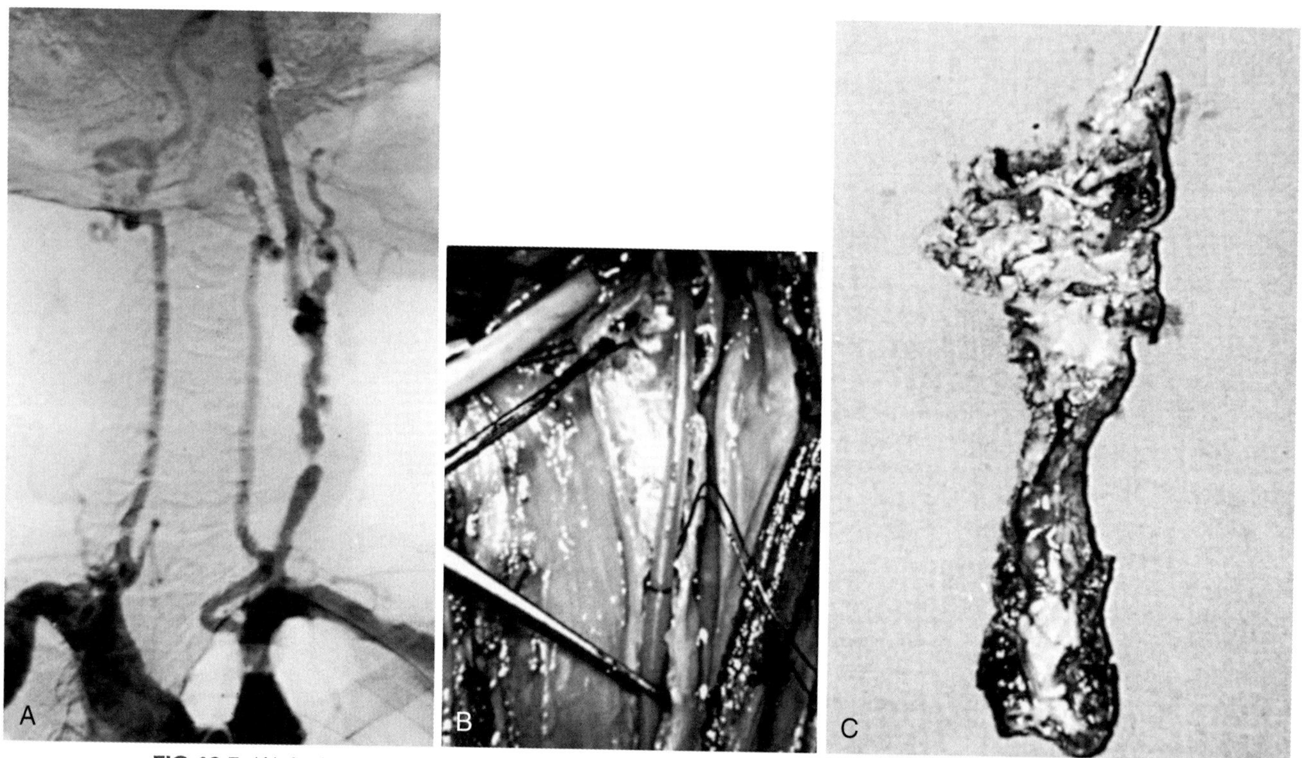

FIG 19.5 (A) Arch angiogram demonstrating carotid artery disease secondary to external cervical radiation. Note complete occlusion of the right common carotid artery. Multiple stenoses are in the left common carotid artery, an unusual site for primary atherosclerosis. (B) Operative appearance of the lesion secondary to external radiation. (C) Intimectomy specimen of the lesion produced by external cervical radiation.

hypercholesterolemia appear to predispose patients receiving radiation therapy to the development of these accelerated changes.[106] Endarterectomy of the affected segments is difficult but can be performed safely.[105,107]

Moritz and colleagues[108] reported their experience with 53 patients who had undergone radiation therapy to the neck an average of 28 months earlier and compared them with a control group of 38 patients who had not had radiation.[108] Thirty percent of the radiated group had moderate to severe lesions of the carotid bifurcation, as detected by duplex scanning, in contrast to only 6% of the control group. Five patients in the radiated group were symptomatic. The authors concluded that patients who receive carotid radiation should undergo periodic follow-up duplex scanning of the carotid arteries.

Recurrent Carotid Stenosis

Recurrent carotid stenosis has been reported to occur in 1% to 21% of cases[109-114] and may yield an incidence of hemodynamically significant stenosis as high as 32% after 7 years.[109] This can lead to neurologic symptoms by producing emboli or restricting flow. The most common lesion developing within the first 2 years after surgery is myointimal hyperplasia. Histologically, a concentric lesion occurs, with no calcium or lipid deposits. A dense accumulation of collagen and mucopolysaccharides surrounds cellular elements. These substances are produced by the myointimal cell in the normal healing process. Their accelerated production seems to be responsible for the development of the fibroplastic lesion leading to luminal stenosis. An endarterectomy plane is almost impossible to develop.

The morphologic characteristics of the early (<2 years) restenosis suggest a lower risk of stroke compared with arteriosclerotic lesions of a similar degree.[115] In addition, regression of stenosis documented by noninvasive tests has been reported. Thus controversy exists over the management of early recurrent stenosis after CEA.[116] In the asymptomatic stage, a restenosis documented by successive noninvasive testing should lead the surgeon to consider surgical intervention if progression to greater than 80% of the diameter occurs. Recurrent symptoms are certainly an indication for reoperation unless a different cause is suspected. Interestingly, Bernstein and colleagues[117] showed an inverse correlation between greater than 50% recurrent stenosis and late stroke and death. Their data suggested that patients with early recurrent stenosis had a better long-term prognosis than those who did not develop recurrent stenosis.

When a stenotic lesion develops more than 2 years after CEA, atherosclerosis is usually the cause. Injury to the vessel by vascular clamps may play a role. Elevated serum cholesterol has a statistically significant association with recurrent carotid stenosis.[110]

These lesions probably carry the same stroke risk as primary arteriosclerotic lesions in the carotid bifurcation. Recommendation for reoperation is thus based on the known risk factors of similar primary arteriosclerotic lesions.

Some investigators have shown that patch closure at the time of the initial CEA may prevent recurrent stenosis. Several prospective, randomized studies, either completed or in progress, suggest a lower incidence of restenosis with the use of patch angioplasty.[111,118-121] The most compelling argument in favor of patch closure comes from a prospective study by AbuRahma and colleagues.[122] The authors identified 74 patients with bilateral carotid stenoses in need of bilateral operation. One side was closed primarily, and the opposite side was closed with patch angioplasty. In this manner, demographic and patient characteristics were controlled. The incidence of ipsilateral stroke for primary closure was 4%, versus 0% for patch closure. In the primary closure group, there was a 22% incidence of recurrent stenosis, versus 1% in the patch group ($P < .003$). There was an 8% incidence of internal carotid artery occlusion with primary closure, versus 0% with patch closure. Restenosis requiring reoperation occurred in 14% of the primary closure group and in 1% of the patch group. In a life-table analysis, the 24-month freedom from recurrence was 75% in the primary closure group, versus 98% in the patch group.[122] A significant benefit of patch angioplasty appears to be a reduction in technical end point problems. Thus patching may be equally important in preventing occurrence and recurrence. The same objective can be achieved by preventing or correcting technical errors at the time of operation when they are identified by completion angiography. Data obtained from experimental hemodynamic studies suggest that an enlarged bulb following patch closure of an endarterectomy site may predispose to areas of low shear stress and therefore recurrent disease. For this reason, it is important not to over-enlarge the bulb when using a patch. Over-enlargement may be responsible for a higher incidence of recurrence after vein patch angioplasty (9%) versus prosthetic patch angioplasty (2%). However, both were superior to primary closure (34%) in a randomized study.[123]

The benefit of patch closure was also seen in a retrospective analysis of other data from the Asymptomatic Carotid Atherosclerosis Study (ACAS). The study examined the incidence of recurrence for three time intervals: within 3 months of operation (residual disease), 3 to 18 months (myointimal hyperplasia), and 18 to 60 months (recurrent atherosclerosis). The use of patch angioplasty reduced the overall risk of restenosis from 21.2% to 7.1%.[124] Factors associated with early recurrence include an incomplete intimectomy, the use of distal tacking sutures, female sex, continued cigarette smoking, and primary closure of an anatomically small internal carotid artery.[125-127] A similar retrospective analysis was carried out using the CREST trial data base. CEA with patch was done in 755 patients and was compared with 328 patients with primary closure. There was a statistically significant reduction in periprocedural stroke, reoperation, the 4-year risk of stroke, and the 2-year risk of restenosis in favor of the patch closure group.[128] Many clinicians routinely prescribe aspirin preoperatively as well as postoperatively, in the hope that embolic events from platelet aggregates can be reduced or eliminated. The rationale is that aspirin will reduce the incidence of myointimal hyperplasia by reducing platelet adhesion or aggregation and interfering with the platelet release reaction. Unfortunately, the carotid artery, like other areas subjected to arterial reconstruction, has not been shown to benefit. A prospective, randomized, placebo-controlled trial failed to show any benefit of aspirin in preventing early carotid restenosis.[129]

PATHOGENETIC MECHANISMS OF TRANSIENT ISCHEMIC ATTACKS AND CEREBRAL INFARCTION

In reviewing the mechanisms for TIA and cerebral infarction, emphasis is placed on those events related to disease in the extracranial vessels. Hemorrhagic stroke is excluded. Cerebral ischemic events related to hypertension and cardiac emboli are briefly reviewed because of their importance in the differential diagnosis and workup of symptomatic patients. Finally, from a pathogenetic standpoint, the difference between TIA and fixed deficit is a matter of degree, duration, and extent of actual infarction. The mechanisms of occurrence are essentially the same. Therefore, for purposes of discussion, we use the general inclusive term *ischemic event*.

Arterial Thrombosis

When an atherosclerotic plaque expands to produce a critical reduction in blood flow, the vessel ultimately undergoes thrombosis. In the case of the internal carotid artery, if this column of thrombus stops at the ophthalmic artery and remains stable, and if collateral circulation is sufficient via the circle of Willis, the thrombotic event may be entirely asymptomatic (Fig. 19.6). If the thrombus propagates beyond the ophthalmic artery to occlude the middle cerebral artery (Fig. 19.7), or if small thrombi rather than a thrombotic column form and are subsequently carried to the intracranial vessels by continuous blood flow (Fig. 19.8), the patient experiences cerebral symptoms that can vary from transient ocular or hemispheric events to a profound hemiplegia, depending on the extent of propagated thrombus or embolus. In addition, if the collateral circulation to the circle of Willis is poor, the sudden loss of flow through a diseased internal carotid artery may incite a precipitous drop in flow to the hemisphere, resulting in ischemic infarction as a consequence of inadequate proximal blood flow.

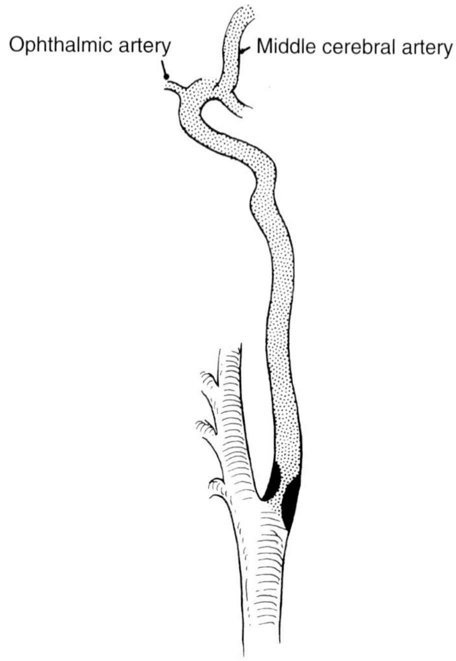

FIG 19.7 Thrombus secondary to an occlusive atherosclerotic lesion of the internal carotid artery progresses beyond the ophthalmic artery to involve the middle cerebral artery.

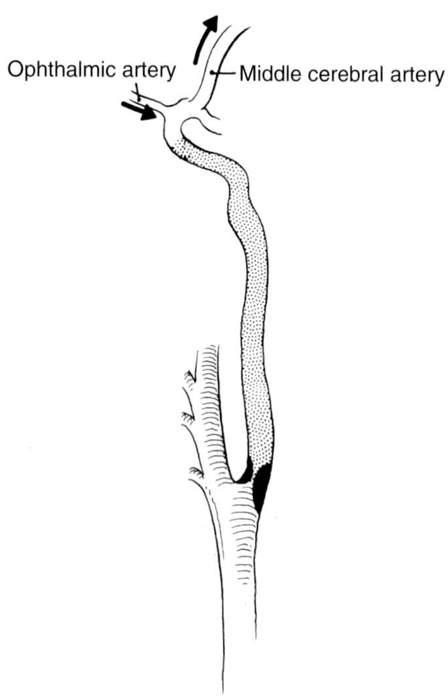

FIG 19.6 Occurring distal to an occlusive lesion of the internal carotid artery. Note that the column of thrombus stops short of the ophthalmic artery, and patency of the middle cerebral artery is maintained.

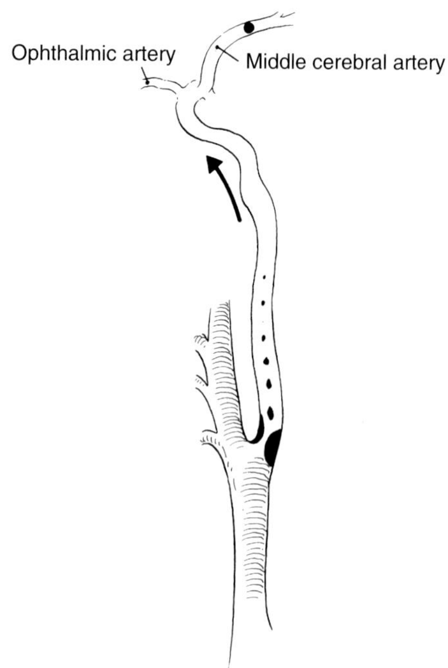

FIG 19.8 Emboli released from a plaque strategically placed at the origin of the internal carotid artery can pass into the middle cerebral artery and lodge in the terminal branch. This results in either a temporary or a permanent neurologic deficit in the distribution appropriate to the arterial occlusion.

Flow-Related Ischemic Events

Although flow-related ischemia used to be considered the most common cause of transient ischemic events, it is actually a rather rare occurrence. Transient drops in hemispheric blood flow or the development of a chronic low-flow state can be responsible for nonspecific symptoms of lightheadedness, presyncope, or intellectual deterioration.[1,130] It must also be recognized that other, nonvascular causes of these symptoms exist and are probably more frequent.

The collateral blood flow to the brain, via the circle of Willis, is an extremely efficient system. Multiple patients have been described who had bilateral internal carotid artery occlusion, perhaps combined with occlusion of the vertebral artery, but were totally asymptomatic from a central neurologic point of view. Experience obtained performing CEA under local anesthesia has shown that approximately 10% of patients experience neurologic symptoms when the carotid artery is clamped.[56] This 10% may have symptoms on the basis of compromised blood flow when the stenosis progresses or goes on to complete occlusion. Another circumstance that can produce symptoms of global ischemia is simultaneous stenosis or occlusion in more than one extracranial vessel—for example, a carotid occlusion on one side combined with a high-grade stenosis in the contralateral carotid artery. Under these circumstances, transient drops in blood pressure, perhaps posturally related, can produce either global or focal ischemic symptoms. Rarely, patients with unilateral carotid occlusion may have a downstream vascular bed that is marginally perfused. Postural changes under these circumstances can also produce focal ischemia and result in a flow-related TIA. Under these conditions, a patient would be a good candidate for extracranial-to-intracranial bypass grafting.

Flow-restricting lesions in the vertebral arteries or in major vessels proximal to the vertebral origin, such as the innominate or subclavian artery, can produce symptoms related to hypoperfusion in the posterior circulation. One of the most dramatic anatomic observations is the so-called subclavian steal syndrome. If a stenosis or occlusion of the subclavian artery is present proximal to the vertebral artery takeoff, the pressure drop distal to the obstruction causes its branches to serve as sources of collateral blood flow by reversing the normal flow direction. The branches now contribute to the flow of the main trunk, rather than receiving flow from the proximally affected artery. The vessels that contribute to collateral blood flow of the distal subclavian artery by reversing flow include the vertebral artery. Under these circumstances, the vertebral artery not only is deprived of the usual antegrade flow but also actually siphons off blood flow from the basilar artery circulation because of flow reversal. This siphoning of blood may be entirely without symptoms if abundant sources of inflow from the other vertebral artery or from the anterior circulation exist. Conversely, if the opposite vertebral artery is small or occluded, a deficiency in basilar artery flow may be present that results in symptoms of basilar artery insufficiency. These symptoms may first appear or become exaggerated if the demand for flow in the affected subclavian artery increases, such as results from active exercise of the arm (Fig. 19.9).

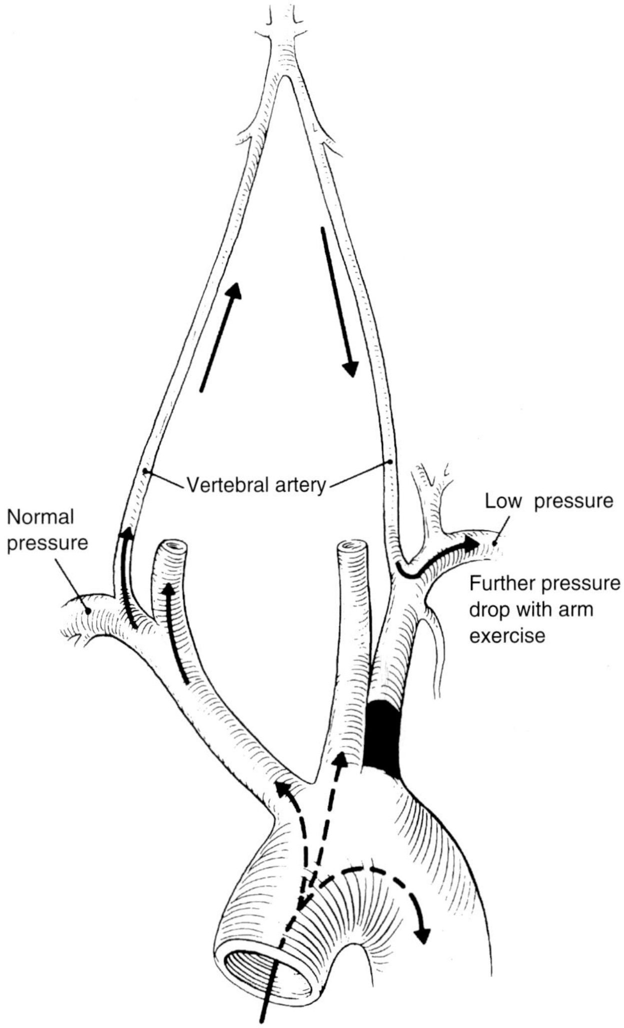

FIG 19.9 Mechanism of the Subclavian Steal Syndrome. Note the occlusion in the origin of the left subclavian artery. This produces a pressure gradient with reversal of blood flow in the left vertebral artery, producing a siphoning or steal from the basilar artery.

Cerebral Emboli

The most common causes of cerebral ischemic events are embolic phenomena, primarily arterial in origin and secondarily from cardiac sources. The emboli of arterial origin occur as a consequence of morphologic change present on the luminal surface of a critical artery.[55,56,131,132] These changes most often are associated with atheromatous plaques but can also occur with other lesions such as fibromuscular dysplasia. When an irregular surface produces turbulence, a stimulus for platelet aggregation is present. If the platelet aggregates become large enough and embolize to an important vessel in the brain, symptoms occur. If the platelet aggregates break up quickly from mechanical forces or from the effect of arterial prostacyclin, the symptoms are transient. If the embolic fragment persists, however, it can lead to focal infarction (Fig. 19.10).

An atherosclerotic plaque may undergo central degeneration or softening. When this occurs, bleeding into the plaque substance

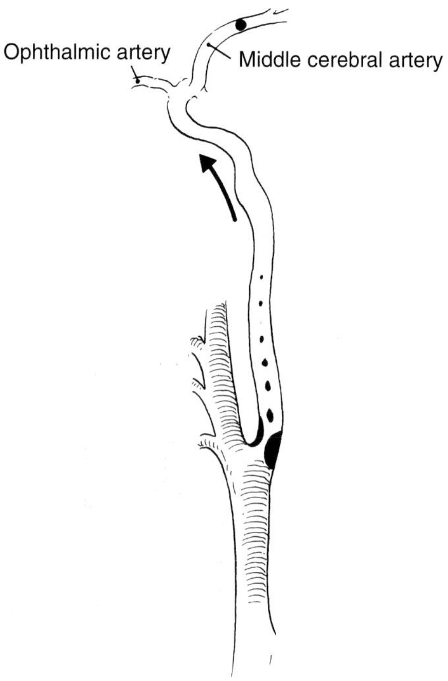

FIG 19.10 Embolic Fragment in the Middle Cerebral Artery. If this persists, it will lead to focal infarction. If the fragment breaks up and distributes itself through the microcirculation, the ischemic event will be transient.

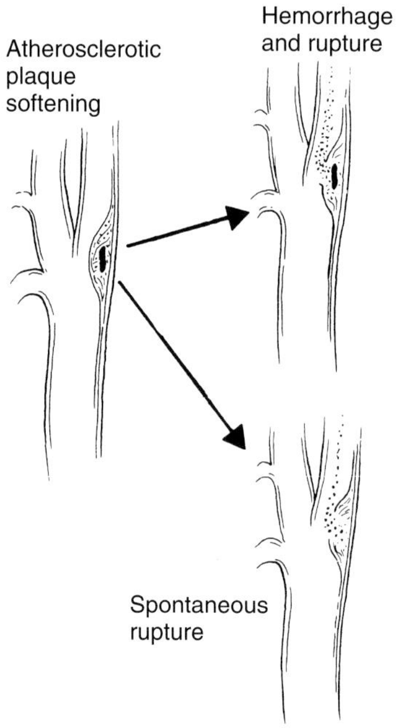

FIG 19.11 Atherosclerotic Plaque Undergoing Central Softening. Spontaneous hemorrhage may occur into the center of the plaque, producing rupture and discharge of embolic fragments, or the plaque may spontaneously rupture as a result of hydrostatic forces, releasing necrotic embolic debris.

can also occur, leading to sudden plaque expansion with intraluminal rupture,[50,78,113,133] or the plaque may spontaneously rupture into the lumen, discharging its contents into the arterial stream. The plaque contents consist of degenerative atheromatous debris, including various mixtures of cholesterol crystals, calcific material, or thrombotic remnants. If the atherosclerotic plaque is located at a critical point, such as the origin of the internal carotid artery, considerable likelihood exists that embolic atheromatous fragments will be carried to important vascular beds of the brain, producing either transient or permanent neurologic events (Fig. 19.11). These events are considered primary embolic events of atherosclerotic plaque origin.

After the plaque has ruptured, a defect is left behind that is called an *ulcer* (Fig. 19.12). Further primary emboli can continue to escape from the raw ulcerated surface, or the ulcer itself may serve as a focal point for thrombus or platelet aggregate material to form. These platelet or thrombotic aggregates may secondarily dislodge, owing to blood flow turbulence, and embolize to the brain (Fig. 19.13). Thus the embolic material from an atherosclerotic plaque can consist of atheromatous debris, platelet aggregates, or blood clot. The emboli of arterial origin can be primary, occurring with plaque rupture or on thrombogenic arterial plaque surfaces,[132,134] or secondary, having developed within ulcerative lesions from previous plaque rupture.[135]

Embolic events may produce dramatic focal neurologic events that are immediately appreciated by the patient, or the embolic fragments may travel to more silent areas of the brain, in which case the results are more subtle and appreciated on a chronic basis, such as cerebral atrophy or multiple-infarct dementia.[136,137] The use of transcranial Doppler ultrasonography has provided

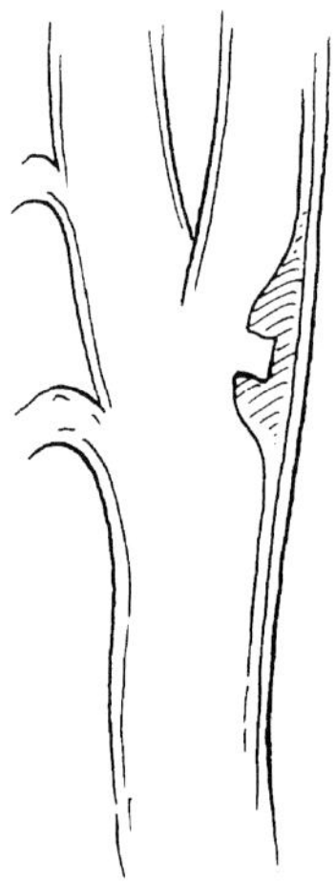

FIG 19.12 Following evacuation of an atherosclerotic plaque, a defect or ulcer is left behind.

more objective evidence of emboli from carotid plaques by discerning discrete noise as an embolic particle passes a point of Doppler insonation.[138] Finally, the occurrence of TIAs in a hemisphere distal to a carotid occlusion raises the question of the importance of decreased flow to arterial border zones. Experimental data have demonstrated that emboli originating from a contralateral carotid artery can cross through the circle of Willis and produce focal infarcts in the hemisphere distal to a carotid occlusion.[139] Thus the contralateral patent carotid artery should always be considered a possible source of emboli when a patient

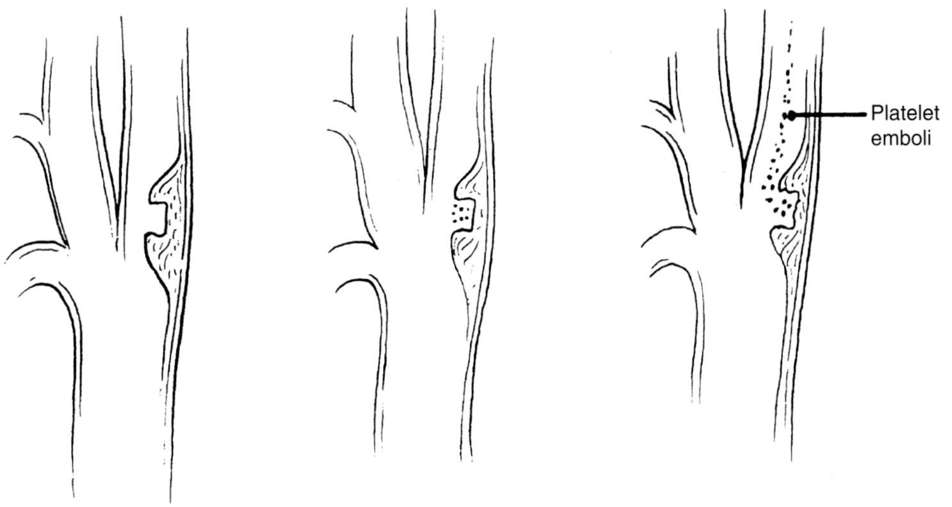

FIG 19.13 The ulcerated lesion within an atheromatous plaque can serve as a nidus for platelet aggregation or thrombotic material. These aggregates can secondarily embolize from the ulcer crypt.

with a carotid occlusion begins to experience symptoms in the hemisphere distal to the occlusion. The stump of an occluded internal carotid artery can also be a source of emboli. Flow to the external carotid artery can sweep platelet aggregate or clot residing in the stump of an occluded into carotid artery into a collateral branch such as the temporal or internal maxillary artery, which may be serving as a collateral to the carotid siphon via reversed flow through the ophthalmic artery.

Emboli can also occur from cardiac sources, which include aortic valvular disease, mitral valve prolapse, cardiac arrhythmias, and mural thrombus after MI. Venous thromboembolism passing through a patent foramen ovale, so-called paradoxical embolism, can also go to the brain. More recently, atherosclerotic plaques of the aortic arch, as seen with transesophageal echocardiography, have been identified as another source of cerebral embolization.[140-142]

Lacunar Infarction

Focal areas of cerebral necrosis occurring in the basal ganglia, internal capsule, or pons have been described as a consequence of end-vessel occlusive disease involving the lenticulostriate or thalamoperforating arteries. The underlying cause is related to uncontrolled hypertension, and the resulting neurologic deficit is often clinically identified as a pure motor or pure sensory stroke.[143] Although descriptions of this phenomenon date back to the early 1900s, current understanding is based on the efforts and writings of Fisher.[144]

The clinical picture may often be confused with arterial-arterial emboli, in that antecedent TIAs may have occurred. The differential diagnosis is best made by the very focal neurologic deficit seen clinically and the typical anatomic location seen on the CT scan of the brain. Evidence shows that the so-called lacunae may also be the consequence of emboli of arterial origin.[145-148] Thus symptoms and imaging of a deep white matter infarct do not rule out atheromatous plaque from the carotid bifurcation as a cause of the event.

CLINICAL SYNDROMES OF EXTRACRANIAL ARTERIAL OCCLUSIVE DISEASE

Extracranial arterial occlusive disease can result in varying symptoms or be completely asymptomatic. A thorough history must be obtained, because this alone can provide clues to the specific nature of the event. Often one discovers the existence of symptoms that the patient has been ignoring. A complete review of symptoms is mandatory, because this may alter the therapeutic alternatives available. Risk factors for atherosclerosis should be specifically recorded.

Patients can be classified into three categories: asymptomatic patients, patients with TIAs, and patients with cerebral infarction. In asymptomatic patients, a hemodynamically significant lesion or a nonocclusive ulcerated arteriosclerotic plaque in the extracranial circulation may be discovered in the absence of transient or permanent neurologic symptoms. The presence or absence of a bruit in the cervical area should not be a criterion for inclusion in this category. It should be recorded as a general marker of a patient at high risk for atherosclerosis.[149]

In an analysis of 1287 patients with cervical bruits, less than one-third of the carotid lesions with bruits proved to be hemodynamically significant by noninvasive criteria.[42] The fact that significant lesions can occur in the absence of a bruit and vice versa is important. The available data on the natural history of asymptomatic bruits cannot be applied to patients with these lesions. This group of patients is usually discovered by angiography while studying other conditions or by noninvasive studies carried out because of the presence of a bruit or for screening before major surgical procedures. Because of what is known about the natural history of these lesions, as discussed later, therapeutic intervention in the asymptomatic stage may be beneficial. The two categories of symptomatic patients with extracranial arterial occlusive disease are discussed separately.

Transient Ischemic Attacks

General Considerations

TIAs are defined as temporary focal neurologic deficits lasting no more than 24 hours, with complete recovery. The event is caused by ischemia in the territory of the brain supplied by a particular artery or branch. Because of its territorial nature, symptoms tend to be stereotyped. Clinically symptoms are of sudden onset and without aura, and resolution is often quick. Disappearance of symptoms ordinarily takes only a few minutes.[150] When symptoms last longer than 6 hours, a permanent abnormality is more likely, although it may not be clinically detectable.[151] The frequency of attacks is variable. The patient may experience only one episode or multiple attacks, with variable symptom-free intervals. The most common cause of these transient territorial deficits is extracranial arterial occlusive lesions. The pathology of these lesions has already been discussed. Other important causes in the differential diagnosis include heart disease; hematologic disorders such as systemic lupus erythematosus, hyperglobulinemia, polycythemia, and sickle cell disease; disseminated intravascular coagulation; subacute bacterial endocarditis; paroxysmal embolism; and several rare connective tissue disorders such as pseudoxanthoma elasticum and Ehlers-Danlos syndrome.[151] Migraine, especially when associated with transient neurologic deficit, can be confused with a TIA. A history of migraine in the family, the throbbing quality of the headache, and its occurrence on recovery from the neurologic deficit can be helpful in the differential diagnosis.

An important concept when evaluating patients with symptoms suggestive of TIA is that the symptoms secondary to emboli from a point source such as the extracranial circulation are often the same with every attack. In contrast, patients whose emboli are from the heart tend to have variable symptoms.

Because only about 9% of patients with TIAs are seen by a physician during an attack,[152] the history remains the main factor in establishing the diagnosis. In this regard, family members may be extremely helpful.

Two important syndromes deserve mention. Occasionally, a patient experiences frequent repeated attacks of a specific neurologic deficit with no interval allowing time for complete recovery. If the deficit is the same with each attack and no deterioration in function is seen, this is known as a *crescendo TIA*. If progressive deterioration is seen with each successive attack, a stroke in evolution may be present. In any case, evaluation must proceed on an emergency basis. If a surgically correctable lesion is present and the neurologic deficit is not dense (no loss of consciousness or dense hemiparesis), serious consideration should be given to proceeding with emergency operation.

Carotid Artery Transient Ischemic Attacks

Manifestations of a transient ischemic episode in the territory of the carotid artery include deficits in areas supplied by the anterior and middle cerebral arteries. In older individuals, both anterior and posterior cerebral arteries may be supplied by one carotid artery.[151]

Ischemia in a cerebral hemisphere often produces contralateral symptoms. Motor dysfunction can include weakness, paralysis, or clumsiness of one or both limbs contralateral to the affected hemisphere. Sensory alterations include numbness, loss of sensation, or paresthesia in the opposite side of the face or in one or both limbs. When a patient is examined during an attack, this sensory loss might not be objectively demonstrable.[152]

Ninety-five percent of patients have a dominant left hemisphere. Both receptive aphasia and motor aphasia can occur. When the former is present, the patient or family may interpret it as confusion. Dysarthria can occur as a function of TIA in the nondominant hemisphere, but when it is the sole symptom, vertebrobasilar TIA is more likely. Other functional deficits of the nondominant side include inattention to the patient's own person and environment on the contralateral side.[151] Loss of function of these areas may also be interpreted as confusion.

Transient visual loss (amaurosis fugax) or blurring of vision in the ipsilateral eye is one of the most reliable symptoms of carotid artery TIAs.[153] This may be described as a curtain coming down (altitudinal) or as quadrant field defects. Conjugate eye deviation, as occurs in seizures or completed strokes, is not seen. Homonymous hemianopsia in combination with any of the above-mentioned symptoms suggests carotid TIAs. This is the result of ischemia in the area of the optic radiation emanating from the optic chiasm, which produces loss of vision in the ipsilateral temporal visual field and the contralateral nasal visual field. When TIAs occur secondary to carotid artery disease, these visual field defects are usually limited to a quadrant corresponding to the distribution of the optic radiation. When hemianopsia is complete, it cannot be distinguished from a vertebrobasilar TIA.[151]

Ischemic optic neuropathy is characterized by blindness and is associated with giant cell arteritis in about 10% of cases. In the other 90% of cases, it has been labeled idiopathic. Berguer[154] found a significant correlation between extracranial occlusive disease and idiopathic optic neuropathy. In fact, of 20 symptomatic eyes examined, significant extracranial arterial occlusive disease was found in 12 (60%). An embolic mechanism was suggested as the cause of the optic nerve infarct. A more severe form is seen in patients with very severe extracranial disease—usually occlusion on one side and a high degree of stenosis on the other. These patients develop an ischemic ophthalmopathy characterized by neovascularization of the iris. The term *rubeosis* has been used to characterize this entity. This suggests that patients with idiopathic optic neuropathy that is not secondary to giant cell arteritis should undergo extracranial vascular evaluation.[154]

Convulsions can occur but are more suggestive of a completed or hemorrhagic stroke. When sensory or motor symptoms are present, they all appear at once, without a march suggestive of focal seizure activity.[151] A combination of symptoms may have more diagnostic reliability than a single symptom alone. In right carotid artery TIA, the combination of ipsilateral visual loss and any contralateral arm symptoms has an increased relationship. In left carotid TIA, diagnostic reliability is increased when language disturbance is combined with right face or extremity weakness or sensory loss.[153]

Altered consciousness or syncope can occur, but it is rarely the only symptom and is more often associated with other disorders, such as cardiac arrhythmias.[151] Other symptoms that make the initial evaluation difficult are dizziness, amnesia, or confusion and impaired vision with alteration in consciousness. These symptoms, without other more specific symptoms, cannot be considered manifestations of TIAs, because they occur most often with other illnesses.

Vertebrobasilar System Transient Ischemic Attacks

Transient ischemia of the area of the brain supplied by the vertebrobasilar system can occur due to flow restriction or emboli from lesions in the vertebral or basilar arteries. Emboli from other sources may also affect this system.

An occlusive lesion at the origin of the subclavian artery can cause vertebrobasilar symptoms as the affected arm is exercised and reversal of flow occurs in the vertebral circulation. This subclavian steal is often accompanied by exertional pain in the arm of the affected side.[151]

Alternating hemiparesis, hemisensory symptoms in repetitive attacks, and bilateral circumoral sensory symptoms associated with unilateral arm or leg weakness or ataxia are highly suggestive of vertebrobasilar TIAs. Symptoms may change from one side to the other with different attacks and may involve all four limbs at one time. Drop attacks, or falling precipitously to the ground without premonitory symptoms, occur in less than 4% of patients.[153] In this syndrome, loss of consciousness is absent or so brief that the patient remembers striking the ground, a feature not present in syncope or seizure.[151]

Equilibratory gait or postural disturbance not associated with vertigo can occur. Complete or partial loss of vision in both homonymous fields or homonymous hemianopsia alone is highly suggestive. Vertigo alone, when not associated with other specific symptoms, should not be considered indicative of TIA. When it occurs in clear relationship to focal weakness of the face, arm, or leg, or to ataxia or persistent diplopia, the existence of TIA is likely. Tinnitus is not a feature of vertebrobasilar TIA and is suggestive of labyrinthine vertigo. Single occurrences of bilateral visual blurring, dysarthria, hoarseness, diplopia, dysphasia, confusion, hiccups, vomiting, loss of consciousness, and vital sign alteration may be manifestations of vertebrobasilar TIAs. These symptoms have so many other causes, however, that the diagnosis is uncertain unless they occur in combination or with additional signs of focal brainstem or posterior hemisphere dysfunction.

Cerebral Infarction

A completed cerebral infarction with or without a clinically apparent neurologic deficit can be another manifestation of extracranial arterial occlusive disease. The specific deficits that are clinically detectable are the same as those discussed earlier as manifestations of TIAs.

Accurately estimating the percentage of strokes that are secondary to lesions in the extracranial circulation is difficult. Available studies differ in terms of population, criteria for diagnosis, and therapeutic approach; thus the estimates range from 15% to 52%.[155,156] Extracranial vascular lesions play a major role in the occurrence of cerebral infarction. Approximately 50% of these events are preceded by TIAs, thus providing a clue to diagnosis.[157]

Lacunar infarcts, emboli from a cardiac source, intracerebral or intracranial bleeding, and some hematologic disorders should be included in the differential diagnosis of the cause of stroke. Cerebrospinal fluid examination, electroencephalography (EEG), echocardiography, Holter monitoring, and brain CT are helpful adjuncts. Angiography should be considered, because noninvasive studies do not exclude ulcerative lesions in the extracranial circulation that may be responsible for the embolic infarction. Identification of a cause of the stroke is essential, because these patients remain at high risk of developing a subsequent cerebral infarction.

ROLE OF THE VASCULAR LABORATORY

The role of the vascular laboratory in the evaluation of patients with suspected cerebrovascular disease has been disputed by some and perhaps misused by others. However, it has an increasingly important role, and this section reviews its current application. The vascular laboratory is covered in detail in Chapter 14.

Asymptomatic Patients

Patients without symptoms may come to our attention as possible candidates for extracranial cerebrovascular disease because of the presence of one or more associated risk factors (advanced age, cigarette smoking, hypertension, diabetes mellitus, coronary artery disease, hyperlipidemia, and peripheral vascular disease), or by the presence of a bruit heard over the carotid artery bifurcation. In the past, the occurrence of a preocclusive carotid stenosis could be ascertained only by carotid angiography, but the incidence of finding a significant lesion by angiographic screening was only 20% to 30%. This means that 70% of the suspect population was subjected to costly and needless hospitalization, plus the risk and discomfort of angiography. Currently the presence or absence of a hemodynamically significant lesion can be ascertained by carotid duplex scanning. This is an inexpensive, noninvasive test with an accuracy of greater than 95% in qualified vascular laboratories.

Symptomatic Patients

Patients may show territorial neurologic events typical of carotid artery or vertebrobasilar disease, or they may have symptoms that are entirely nonspecific or atypical. In the case of a patient with nonspecific symptoms, such as "dizzy spells," these symptoms may be related to global ischemic events as a consequence of decreased blood flow associated with multiple extracranial occlusive lesions, or they may be due to a myriad of disorders unrelated to cerebrovascular disease. The vascular laboratory serves as an effective screen for these patients, avoiding many negative and hence useless angiograms.

Angiography used to be considered mandatory for the workup of symptomatic patients. This is no longer true. Duplex scanning in a qualified laboratory can provide definitive information necessary for both medical and surgical management. For this reason, a carefully performed duplex scan has become a critical part of the evaluation of symptomatic patients. Contrast angiography is now reserved for patients whose symptoms are not explained by findings on duplex scans or other noninvasive imaging tests such as magnetic resonance angiography (MRA) and CT angiography.

In addition, the preoperative baseline data from the vascular laboratory are extremely helpful for monitoring patients immediately after the operation as well as in the late follow-up period. A conversion from a positive to a negative test after operation is expected. If this does not occur, a technical problem is suggested that may require investigation and management. Also, an abnormal study 6 months or a year after surgery in a patient who had a normal study after operation alerts the surgeon to the possibility of recurrent stenosis, often before the onset of symptoms. Finally, the importance of obtaining baseline data on the opposite, asymptomatic carotid artery should not be overlooked. Late strokes that occur in patients who have undergone successful CEA are most often related to the side not operated on. Early identification of progression on the contralateral side permits earlier intervention to prevent contralateral stroke.

BRAIN SCANS AND ANGIOGRAPHY

The advent of CT and magnetic resonance imaging (MRI) has been a benefit in the evaluation of patients with cerebrovascular disease and has virtually eliminated the use of radionuclide scanning. Intracranial space-occupying lesions such as neoplasms, vascular malformations, or subdural hematomas enter into the differential diagnosis of patients with even the most convincing symptoms of transient cerebral ischemia. CT and MRI are quick, noninvasive means of ruling out other abnormalities during the patient workup.

A patient with a TIA may have actually suffered a small cerebral infarction. CT or MRI can identify an unsuspected cerebral infarction and establish a baseline status before operation. The advance knowledge that a small infarction exists is helpful with respect to intraoperative and postoperative management.

Although head scanning may not be a routine part of the preoperative workup, it should become a standard part of the evaluation of symptomatic patients. MRI is replacing CT in some centers. It does not require ionizing radiation or contrast material. It can identify acute cerebral infarction sooner than CT and can image smaller infarcts than CT. Finally, new acquisition programs have enabled the use of magnetic resonance techniques to reconstruct cervical and intracranial arterial anatomy—so-called MRA.

Patients with a clinically overt cerebral infarction should have CT or MRI to document the infarct size and to differentiate between ischemic and hemorrhagic infarction. A hemorrhagic infarction is promptly visible on the CT scan, whereas an ischemic infarction may take several days of evolution before its low-density character is visualized. CT scan data are necessary to determine the proper timing of operation after acute stroke in patients who have had a good neurologic recovery. In fact, of 245 patients with persistent neurologic deficits seen by Dosick and colleagues,[158] 171 were found to have negative CT scan results. Appropriate carotid lesions were found in 110 (64%) of this group. All 110 patients underwent CEA within 14 days of the initial onset of their neurologic deficits. The perioperative morbidity was 0.9%. These investigators concluded that angiography and CEA can be safely performed when indicated in patients with negative CT scan results within the first 2 weeks after a prolonged neurologic deficit.

EEG has generally not been considered helpful in the workup of patients with cerebrovascular disease, with the exception of ruling out seizure disorder in the differential diagnosis. However, a new application of cerebral electrical activity, so-called computerized brain mapping, is of value. This modality uses 32 electrodes (rather than the 16 used with EEG) arranged over both hemispheres. The data are digitized and color-coded. The information is analyzed by computer, and hard-copy integrated data are generated. In a report comparing brain mapping, CT, and MRI, brain mapping was more sensitive in identifying small areas of cortical dysfunction.[159]

Aortocranial angiography was once the cornerstone of diagnosis in the workup of patients with suspected cerebrovascular disease. Today, however, the angiogram is no longer a mandatory preoperative study. Current noninvasive studies are sophisticated enough for diagnosis.

Although aortocranial angiography used to be the gold standard for identifying both extracranial and intracranial cerebrovascular disease, most institutions around the world have elected to forgo angiography, provided that noninvasive preoperative testing is of diagnostic quality and correlates with the patient's clinical presentation. Noninvasive testing, primarily carotid duplex scanning (perhaps supplemented with information from MRA or CT angiography), can clearly identify patients with carotid bifurcation disease. MRA or CT may be more accurate in defining the percentage of stenosis than data from contrast angiography; the contrast angiogram almost inevitably underestimates the percentage of stenosis. Noninvasive testing cannot accurately define carotid ulceration independent of carotid stenosis, but even with angiography, the definition of carotid ulceration is limited. The correlation between the preoperative angiogram and inspection of the plaque at the time of operation was analyzed in the first 540 patients entered into the North American Symptomatic Carotid Endarterectomy Trial (NASCET).[160] The sensitivity and specificity for detecting ulcerated plaques was 45.9% and 74.1%, respectively. The positive predictive value for identifying an ulcer was 71.8%. Thus, even the gold standard of angiography is imperfect in diagnosing ulceration. One possible explanation is that the ulceration may be filled with thrombus when the angiogram is obtained.

The benefit of performing CEA without angiography is that angiography carries a significant risk in patients with extracranial arterial occlusive disease. In the ACAS,[161,162] the neurologic morbidity and mortality was 1.2% for angiography alone. This is almost equal to the risk of operation. Although some express the opinion that this complication rate was abnormally high, all patients had been prescreened with ultrasonography and had documented hemodynamically significant lesions. Therefore this represents a select, high-risk group of patients for angiography. With improved techniques of imaging the carotid bifurcation, there has been increasing acceptance of noninvasive imaging as a substitute for preoperative angiography in patients scheduled for CEA. This change in opinion began with the use of improved-quality duplex scanning, and it continues with the use of MRA and CT angiography. Finally, recognizing the limitations of both of these techniques, some suggest combining duplex scanning and MRA for preoperative assessment. When there is clear agreement between the two techniques, this appears to be a safe substitute for contrast angiography; however, when conflicting information is obtained, when the noninvasive study is unsatisfactory, or when the clinical picture is unexplained by noninvasive imaging, the selective use of contrast angiography is clearly indicated.[163-174]

SURGICAL CONSIDERATIONS AND TECHNIQUE

Anesthesia and Hemodynamic Monitoring

Patients about to undergo cerebrovascular surgery are probably best managed with general anesthesia. Although some surgeons still prefer to perform CEA using local or cervical block anesthesia,[175] a recent Cochrane analysis of randomized trials failed to show any benefit of regional over general anesthesia.[176] General anesthesia has the advantage of reducing the cerebral metabolic demand of the brain and increasing cerebral blood flow. General anesthesia also provides good airway control, reduced patient anxiety, and a quiet surgical field.

Intraoperative blood pressure control and oxygenation are particularly critical during periods of arterial clamping. These parameters are best monitored with an arterial line, usually placed in the radial artery. The judicious use of nitroprusside or vasopressors by the anesthesiologist to maintain blood pressure in the patient's optimal physiologic range is of paramount importance.

Two primary options are available to monitor cerebral perfusion, which might be required during trial clamping of the carotid artery before a decision to use an internal shunt. These options are the measurement of internal carotid artery backpressure[177,178] and the intraoperative use of EEG.[175] Although controversy exists as to which is more effective, excellent results have been reported with both techniques. EEG with CT brain mapping is a sensitive and accurate means of identifying patients who require shunting.[159,179] Another technique, that of somatosensory evoked potentials, has been investigated and does not appear to be as sensitive as EEG.[180] Finally, proponents of no monitoring exist; some advocate the routine use of an intraluminal shunt,[181] and others advocate routine operation without a shunt but done in an expeditious manner.[182,183] The literature currently supports either selective shunting based on clinical and monitoring criteria or routine shunting. The consensus is that either of these techniques provides a safe operation with the best outcome.[184,185]

The argument in favor of selective shunting is as follows: Because only 10% to 15% of patients actually require an intraluminal shunt, as judged by observations during operations carried out under local anesthesia, why expose the other 85% to 90% of patients to the risks of an internal shunt, which include (1) possible air or atheroma embolism, (2) scuffing or dissection of distal intima, (3) difficulty with end-point visualization, and (4) risk of leaving an intimal flap that may lead to thromboembolic complications? The arguments in favor of the routine use of an intraluminal shunt are that, with routine use, operator facility with the technique is increased and there is less likelihood of complications, and the intraluminal shunt acts as a stent, which can aid in the closure of the internal carotid portion of the arteriotomy.

The criteria for mandatory shunting based on backpressure measurement, as originally described by Moore and colleagues,[176,177] include a prior cerebral infarction on the side of operation (regardless of backpressure value) or no prior cerebral infarction but a backpressure of 25 mm Hg or less in a patient who is otherwise neurologically intact. The EEG criteria for shunt use include a loss of amplitude or slowing of rhythm during trial clamping of the carotid artery.

Carotid Bifurcation Endarterectomy

Indications

The indications for CEA have undergone considerable review and analysis. Data based on retrospective reviews, results of prospective, randomized trials, and committee discussions based on expert opinion have been brought together to define the current indications for CEA.[186-188]

In the 1990s, the Stroke Council of the American Heart Association convened a consensus conference on the indications for CEA. Those two reports would constitute the most up-to-date agreement concerning indications.[189,190] The ad hoc committee recognized four categories:

1. Proven—the strongest indication, usually supported by results of prospective, randomized trials
2. Acceptable but not proven—a good indication for operation supported by promising but not scientifically certain data
3. Uncertain—data insufficient to define the risk-benefit ratio
4. Proven inappropriate—current data adequate to show that the risk of surgery outweighs any benefit

The recommendations are further stratified by the symptomatic or asymptomatic status of the patient. Finally, the risk of operation based on the comorbid condition of the patient and the individual surgeon's track record is taken into account. Based on this classification, the general indications for CEA can be classified as follows, for symptomatic good-risk patients with a surgeon whose surgical morbidity and mortality rate is less than 6%:

A. Proven indications
   1. One or more TIAs in the last 6 months and carotid stenosis greater than or equal to 70%
   2. Mild stroke with carotid stenosis greater than or equal to 70%

B. Acceptable but not proven indications
   1. TIAs in the past 6 months and stenosis of 50% to 69%
   2. Progressive stroke and stenosis greater than or equal to 70%
   3. Mild or moderate stroke in the past 6 months and stenosis of 50% to 69%
   4. CEA ipsilateral to TIAs and stenosis greater than or equal to 70%, combined with required coronary bypass grafting

C. Uncertain indications
   1. TIAs with stenosis less than or equal to 50%
   2. Mild stroke with stenosis less than or equal to 50%
   3. Symptomatic acute carotid thrombosis

D. Proven inappropriate indications
  1. Moderate stroke with stenosis less than or equal to 50%, not receiving aspirin
  2. Single TIA, stenosis less than or equal to 50%, not receiving aspirin
  3. High-risk patient with multiple TIAs, stenosis less than or equal to 50%, not receiving aspirin
  4. High-risk patient, mild or moderate stroke, stenosis less than or equal to 50%, not receiving aspirin
  5. Global ischemic symptoms with stenosis less than or equal to 50%
  6. Acute internal carotid dissection, asymptomatic, receiving heparin

For asymptomatic, good-risk patients treated by a surgeon whose surgical morbidity-mortality rate is less than 3%, the indications for CEA are as follows:

A. Proven indications—stenosis greater than or equal to 60% (following ACAS publication)
B. Acceptable but not proven indications—none defined
C. Uncertain indications—high-risk patient or surgeon with a morbidity-mortality rate greater than 3%, combined carotid-coronary operations, or nonstenotic ulcerative lesions
D. Proven inappropriate indications—operations with a combined stroke morbidity-mortality rate greater than or equal to 5%

The Stroke Council of the American Heart Association subsequently updated the report and reaffirmed the indications.[191] Finally, and most recently, multiple specialty societies have contributed their own updated guidelines.[192-194]

Technique

After the induction of satisfactory anesthesia and the placement of appropriate access and monitoring lines, the patient is positioned supine on the operating table with the head turned away from the side of operation. The neck is moderately extended on the shoulders. The head of the table is flexed approximately 10 degrees to reduce venous pressure, which minimizes bleeding.

This author prefers a longitudinal incision placed along the anterior border of the sternocleidomastoid muscle and centered over the carotid bifurcation. This incision can be extended proximally to the sternal notch for more proximal exposure of the common carotid artery and distally to the mastoid process for extensive exposure of the internal carotid artery, when needed. At the present time, we are using on-table, duplex ultrasound to precisely identify the location of the carotid bifurcation. This permits accurate placement of the incision and minimizes the incision length. The dissection plane is maintained along the anterior border of the sternocleidomastoid muscle. If it becomes necessary to extend the incision distally, this will permit anterior mobilization of the tail of the parotid gland rather than dividing its substance, with risk of a salivary fistula. The sternocleidomastoid muscle is mobilized off the carotid sheath, and self-retaining retractors are placed. The jugular vein is visualized through the carotid sheath, and the sheath is opened along the anterior border of the vein. The vein is mobilized until the common facial vein is identified. The common facial vein, when present, is a relatively constant landmark for the carotid bifurcation. The common facial vein is divided between ligatures. In the case of a high carotid bifurcation, particular care must be taken to make sure that the hypoglossal nerve is not lurking behind the common facial vein, because this may lead to its inadvertent injury. Once the common facial vein is divided, the jugular vein can be mobilized laterally off the carotid bifurcation, providing excellent exposure. The vagus nerve usually lies in the posterior portion of the carotid sheath, but on occasion it may spiral anteriorly. Particular care must be taken to watch for this anomalous course to avoid nerve injury. Another anomaly is the occasional presence of a nonrecurrent laryngeal nerve that comes directly off the vagus on the way to innervate the vocal cord. This nerve can cross anterior to the carotid artery and may be mistaken for part of the ansa hypoglossi, resulting in mistaken division and cord paralysis. This anomaly most often occurs on the right side of the neck, but it has also been seen on the left side.

The common carotid artery is mobilized for a sufficient length to get proximal to the atheromatous lesion, as well as to provide sufficient length in case an internal shunt is required. When the dissection approaches the area of the carotid bifurcation, it may be necessary to inject a local anesthetic in the area to block the nerve to the carotid body to prevent or reverse reflex bradycardia. The external and internal carotid arteries are then mobilized for a sufficient length to get completely beyond the atheromatous plaque to a point where the vessels are completely normal circumferentially. When mobilizing the internal carotid artery, particular care must be taken to avoid injury to the hypoglossal nerve (Fig. 19.14).

In the case of a high bifurcation or an extensive lesion, mobilizing the internal carotid artery for its maximum extracranial length may be necessary. Several maneuvers are available to gain additional length. The first and most important maneuver is to divide the nerve to the carotid sinus, along with any adjacent tissue between the internal and external carotid artery. This maneuver allows the carotid bifurcation to drop down, since the nerve acts like a suspensory ligament. Once the bifurcation drops down, additional length of the internal carotid artery can be mobilized. The next maneuver is to extend the skin incision all the way up to the mastoid process, with complete mobilization of the sternocleidomastoid muscle toward its tendinous insertion on the mastoid process. Care must be taken to avoid injury to the spinal accessory nerve (cranial nerve XI), which enters the substance of the sternocleidomastoid muscle at that level. The posterior belly of the digastric muscle comes into view. This muscle can be mobilized anteriorly or, if necessary, divided with impunity, giving additional exposure of the internal carotid artery. If further exposure is needed, the limiting structures are the styloid process and the ramus of the mandible. The styloid process, after suitable preparation, can be divided with bone rongeurs, and the mandible can be displaced anteriorly. Techniques have also been described for dividing the ramus of the mandible to gain additional exposure, but I have not found this maneuver necessary. Once the carotid artery has been sufficiently mobilized, 5000 units of heparin are administered systemically. If the patient is on dual antiplatelet drugs, procedure-related bleeding can be reduced by reducing the usual heparin dose.

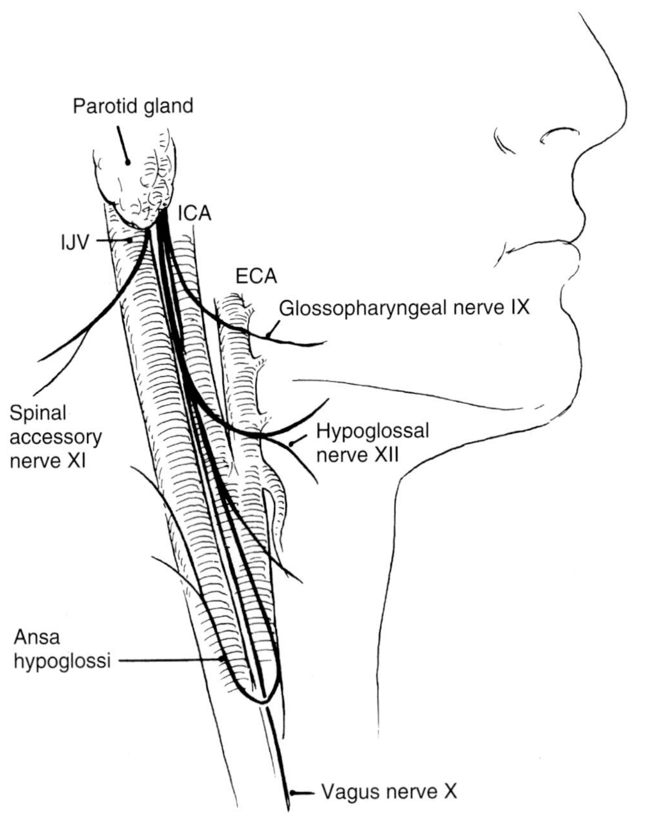

FIG 19.14 Anatomic relationship between the carotid bifurcation and the cranial nerves in the neck. Note the intimate relationship between the hypoglossal nerve and the upper portion of the internal carotid artery *(ICA)*. *ECA,* External carotid artery; *IJV,* internal jugular vein.

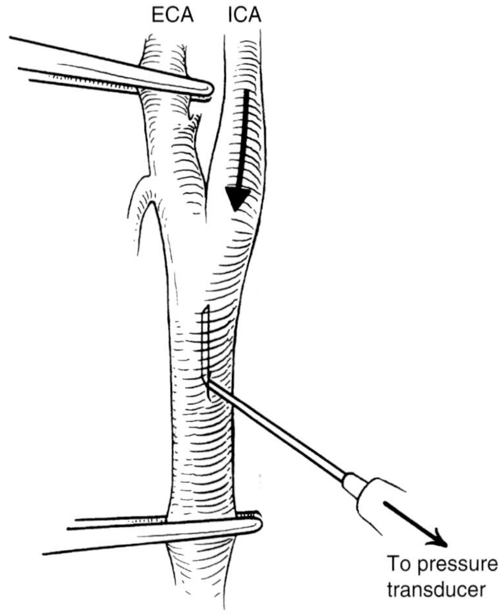

FIG 19.15 Technique of measuring the internal carotid artery *(ICA)* backpressure. Note the needle placement and needle angulation to maintain the tip of the needle in an axial plane with the common carotid artery. A disease-free portion of the common carotid artery is chosen for arterial puncture. *ECA,* External carotid artery.

The decision whether to shunt the patient can be made using EEG or backpressure criteria. If backpressure is selected, a 22-gauge needle is connected to rigid pressure tubing and hooked up to an arterial pressure transducer. The tubing is flushed with saline, and a 0 pressure level is obtained adjacent to the carotid bifurcation. The needle is carefully bent at a 45-degree angle and inserted into the common carotid artery so that the axis of the distal needle is parallel to the axis of the artery and lies freely within the lumen. The free carotid artery pressure is measured and compared with the radial artery pressure to ensure an accurate reading. When the patient's blood pressure is stable and at the optimal level, the common carotid artery is clamped proximal to the needle, and the external carotid artery is also clamped, thus permitting the reading of the internal carotid artery backpressure (Fig. 19.15). If the backpressure is greater than 25 mm Hg, the internal carotid artery is clamped and the needle is withdrawn. If the pressure is less than 25 mm Hg, the clamps on the common and external carotid arteries are temporarily removed, the needle is withdrawn, and preparations are made for the use of an internal shunt.

With the common, external, and internal carotid arteries clamped, an arteriotomy is made on the lateral portion of the common carotid artery with a No. 11 blade and is extended toward the plaque and up the internal carotid artery with Potts scissors. The arteriotomy is extended as far as necessary up the internal carotid artery to get beyond the plaque and to expose a relatively normal artery. An intimectomy plane is then established between the diseased intima and the internal elastic lamina, attempting to leave the circular medial fibers attached to the arterial adventitia. This facilitates getting a clean distal end point. The proximal end point is obtained by sharply dividing the intima. The intimectomy surface is copiously irrigated with heparinized saline solution to allow the visualization of all bits of debris and facilitate their removal.

The arteriotomy can be closed primarily, but overwhelming evidence indicates better results with patch angioplasty closure. Evidence suggests that female patients, patients with small internal carotid arteries, and patients who continue to smoke are at increased risk of recurrent carotid stenosis.[125,126] The use of patch angioplasty in these patients may reduce the risk of recurrent stenosis. Trial results indicate that routine use of a prosthetic patch results in the lowest rates of peripheral complications and recurrent stenosis.[122-124,128] Patch angioplasty should be used routinely when the indication for operation is recurrent stenosis.

Flow is established first to the external and then to the internal carotid artery. I recommend the use of routine completion angiography. There is a 5% to 8% incidence of unsuspected technical errors associated with CEA, and these are best documented with completion angiography.[195,196] Completion angiography is used primarily to identify technical errors involving the internal carotid artery; however, intimal flaps in the external carotid artery occur more commonly and are erroneously considered to be of no consequence. We reported three cases of postoperative stroke secondary to intimal flaps in the external carotid artery: clot formed in the proximal external carotid artery, propagated in a retrograde direction, and then embolized up the internal carotid artery.[197] For this reason, the correction of intimal flaps of the external as well as the internal carotid artery is recommended.

An alternative to completion angiography is the use of intraoperative duplex scanning. Lipski and colleagues[198] reported that the incidence of residual disease and perioperative neurologic complications was statistically significantly reduced in patients who had completion duplex scanning compared with a control group who did not undergo completion imaging.[198] Furthermore, the use of completion duplex scanning identified technical problems and led to their prompt correction in 9 of 39 patients.

Internal Carotid Artery Dilatation

Indications

Internal carotid artery dilatation is uniquely applicable to fibromuscular dysplasia of the carotid artery. It is a major technical advance in simplifying the surgical correction of this lesion.

Technique

The carotid bifurcation is exposed in the usual manner. The internal carotid artery is exposed for its maximal length so that dilatation can be performed under visual and palpable control. Heparin is administered systemically, and the artery is clamped. A transverse arteriotomy, approximately 1/2 the circumference of the carotid bulb, is made adjacent to the internal carotid artery. Coronary artery dilators are introduced and gently passed toward the base of the skull. I usually start with a 2-mm dilator and progress at 0.5-mm increments to a 4-mm dilator. The surgeon has a sensation of intraluminal septal "popping" as the dilator is passed to the base of the skull. Backbleeding is allowed to occur after each passage to allow tissue fragments to be washed out and prevent embolization (Fig. 19.16). On completion, the arteriotomy is closed, blood flow is restored, and a completion angiogram is obtained to ensure adequate dilatation.

Alternatively, intraoperative balloon angioplasty of the affected segment of the internal carotid artery can be performed. This technique is probably safer because traction injury to the intima is avoided. The intraoperative use of balloon angioplasty, through an open arteriotomy, avoids the possibility of forward embolization from the angioplasty site. After the balloon angioplasty is completed, vigorous backbleeding of the vessel is allowed, to retrieve any debris loosened by the dilatation. As with progressive dilatation of the vessel, completion angiography is highly recommended to ensure an adequate technical result.

On occasion, the surgeon might not be sure that the dilator has been advanced fully to the base of the skull. Under these circumstances, the procedure can be monitored with fluoroscopy.

Correction of Kinking of the Internal Carotid Artery

Indications

This procedure is indicated for symptomatic kinking of the internal carotid artery and excessive redundancy of the internal carotid artery after mobilization of that vessel for endarterectomy.

Technique

Redundancy of the internal carotid artery can be corrected in a variety of ways, including (1) resection of the redundant internal carotid artery with an end-to-end anastomosis, (2) division of the internal carotid artery with reimplantation onto the proximal common carotid artery, and (3) resection of a segment of the common carotid artery, thus permitting the redundant internal carotid artery to straighten when the carotid bifurcation is brought down for an end-to-end anastomosis (Fig. 19.17).

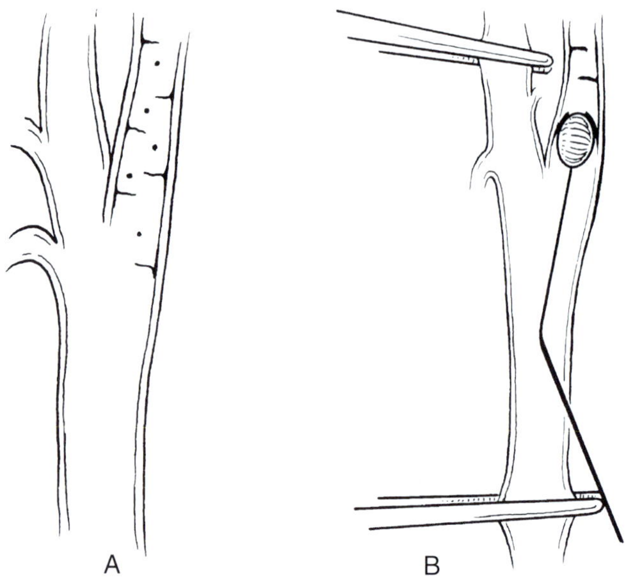

FIG 19.16 (A) Septated lesion of fibromuscular dysplasia. This kind of irregularity leads to symptoms from platelet aggregation and embolization. (B) A coronary dilator is introduced through a small arteriotomy and advanced up the internal carotid artery. The olive tip of the dilator disrupts the small septa of the fibromuscular dysplastic segment. With an open arteriotomy, backbleeding flushes any residual intimal segments or platelet aggregates.

In my experience, the easiest repair is resection of a segment of the common carotid artery, because the anastomosis is the easiest to perform. This requires mobilization of the external carotid artery and division of the nerve to the carotid sinus in order to move the entire bifurcation proximally.

External Carotid Endarterectomy

Indications

External CEA is indicated in the case of TIAs from embolization or flow reduction and for the correction of significant stenosis or ulceration before extracranial-to-intracranial bypass grafting. In addition, if the internal carotid artery is chronically occluded, there is often a proximal stump left behind that can serve as a nidus for clot or platelet aggregate to reside. The potential exists for this material to embolize via the external carotid artery through collaterals to the brain. Removal of the stump as a part of external CEA will correct this problem.

Technique

The carotid bifurcation is dissected out in the usual manner. The internal carotid artery distal to the obstructed plaque is carefully examined because, on occasion, the vessel may still be patent, thus permitting a standard endarterectomy to be performed, with restoration of blood flow to the internal carotid

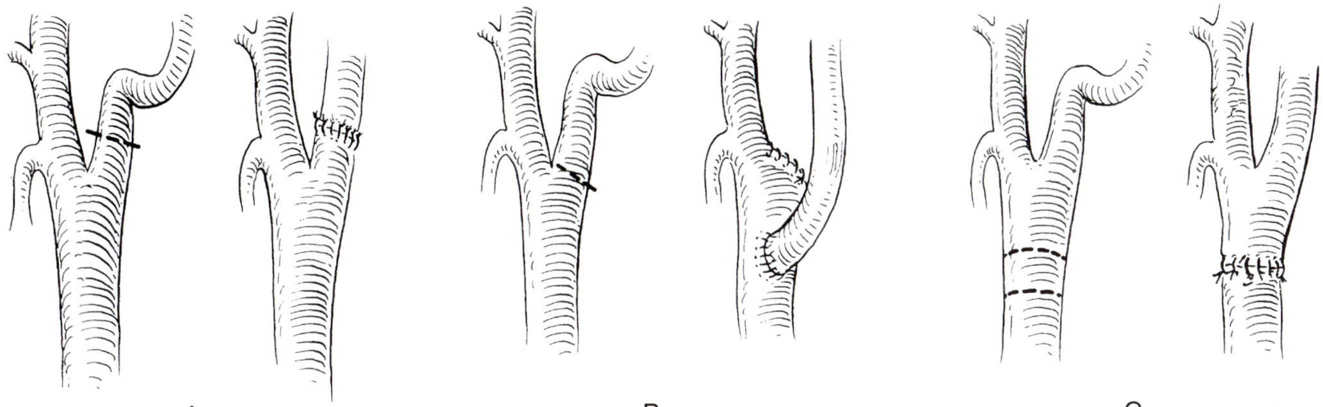

A B C

FIG 19.17 (A) A kink of the internal carotid artery can be repaired by segmental resection of the redundant portion of the artery and direct end-to-end anastomosis. (B) The redundant internal carotid artery can be straightened by dividing it at its origin and moving it proximally to the common carotid artery for end-to-side anastomosis. (C) The kinked internal carotid artery can be straightened by mobilization of the carotid bifurcation, resection of a segment of the common carotid artery, and direct end-to-end anastomosis, resulting in straightening of the kinked vessel.

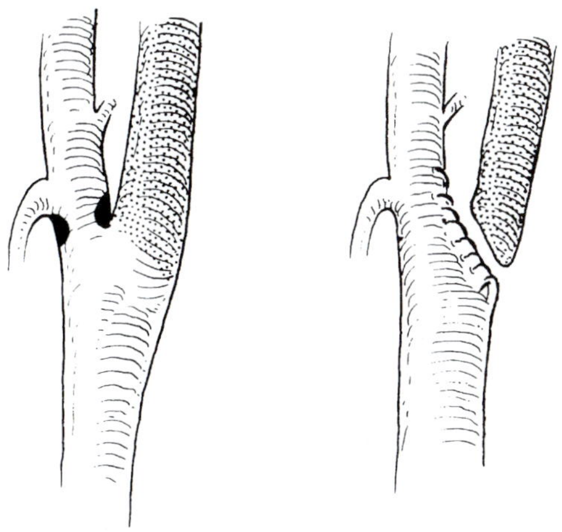

FIG 19.18 External carotid endarterectomy can be performed by removing the occluded internal carotid artery and continuing the arteriotomy past the stenotic lesion. This permits endarterectomy under direct vision and primary closure, leaving a smooth taper between the common and external carotid arteries.

artery. If the internal carotid artery is confirmed to be occluded, it is divided flush with the carotid bifurcation. An arteriotomy is positioned on the posterolateral aspect of the common carotid artery so that its distal extension passes through the divided orifice of the internal carotid artery and onto the external carotid artery, beyond the atherosclerotic plaque in that vessel. An endarterectomy is then performed. The arteriotomy can be closed primarily, leaving a smooth, tapered transition from the common carotid to the external carotid artery (Fig. 19.18). However, the use of a patch is probably preferable. The patch may be of prosthetic material, a vein, or a segment of the occluded internal carotid artery that has been resected and opened. This serves nicely as an autogenous arterial patch.

POSTOPERATIVE CARE

The first 12 hours are the most critical in managing a patient after cerebrovascular reconstruction. In addition to the usual care required for a patient recovering from general anesthesia, the most important factors are observation of the patient's neurologic status, blood pressure control (either hypotension or hypertension must be appropriately treated), and close wound observation. An expanding hematoma should be identified early, and the patient should be returned promptly to the operating room for identification of the bleeding source and evacuation of the hematoma.

Although intensive care monitoring used to be routine, now only a small percentage of patients actually require an intensive care unit. The majority of patients can be sent to a regular room if they are neurologically intact and hemodynamically stable in the recovery room. Most patients can be discharged safely the next morning. This method of case management has reduced hospital costs.[199-201]

Common practice is to resume antiplatelet drugs. One adult or baby aspirin per day is recommended. If this is not tolerated, Aggrenox or clopidogrel (Plavix) can be used. The rationale for the continued use of antiplatelet drugs is to prevent platelet aggregation and embolization from the new intimectomy site, as well as to serve as prophylaxis in the case of residual, unoperated atherosclerotic plaques in other critical cerebral vessels.

COMPLICATIONS AFTER CAROTID ENDARTERECTOMY

Few vascular operations are as well tolerated as a properly performed CEA. The operative trauma, blood loss, and recovery period are minimal after a successful reconstruction. Unfortunately, the benefits of the procedure, especially in asymptomatic patients, can be negated by a high complication rate.

The justification for surgical repair requires that the morbidity of the procedure be kept to a minimum. Possible intraoperative and postoperative complications, their prevention, and their management are discussed.

Intraoperative Complications

One of the most important steps in the prevention of intraoperative problems is adequate preoperative preparation of the patient. Hypertensive patients should have their blood pressure well controlled before the procedure. Patients must be well hydrated, especially if an angiographic procedure has been done within 24 to 48 hours or if they have been receiving continued diuretic therapy. Their myocardial status must be ascertained by careful history, electrocardiography, and other studies such as stress testing as indicated. The use of nitrates during the procedure should be considered in patients with coronary artery disease.

Intraoperative monitoring includes electrocardiographic and continuous blood pressure readings. An intraarterial line can be used to obtain continuous readouts and promptly recognize fluctuations in the patient's blood pressure. The use of Swan-Ganz catheters may be considered in selected patients.

Hypertension and Hypotension

Hypertension and hypotension are frequent during and immediately after CEA. Bove and colleagues[202] found significant hypertension in 19% and hypotension in 28% of 100 consecutive patients undergoing CEA, and reported a 9% incidence of neurologic deficits in this group, as opposed to no neurologic morbidity in normotensive patients. This fact, plus the deleterious effects on myocardial function, underscores the importance of early recognition and immediate treatment of extremes of blood pressure. Taking into account the minimal trauma and blood loss that occur during CEA, other factors must have a role in the development of this fluctuation. Some investigators have found a significant increase in the incidence of this problem in chronically hypertensive patients not well controlled preoperatively.[203] The interference with the baroreceptor mechanisms at the carotid sinus may contribute to postoperative blood pressure fluctuations. The postendarterectomy bulb, which is now distensible, might also have a role.[204] Increased cerebral renin production during carotid cross-clamping has been implicated in the development of postendarterectomy hypertension.[205] In a retrospective study of 100 patients, we found a correlation between the use of halogenated fluorocarbon general anesthesia and the development of postendarterectomy hypertension.[206] In a subsequent study, we demonstrated a correlation between cranial norepinephrine levels in jugular venous blood, but not renin, and the development of postoperative hypertension.[207]

Bradycardia during carotid manipulation usually responds to the local injection of 0.5% lidocaine (Xylocaine) in the soft tissues around the nerve to the carotid sinus. Failure of this maneuver to restore a normal heart rate and blood pressure should be followed by the immediate investigation and correction of other possible causes. Ranson and colleagues[208] suggested that an uncorrected preoperative deficit in intravascular volume is a critical factor in the development of hypotension and bradycardia. Blocking the reflex arc by the administration of atropine sulfate or glycopyrrolate while volume deficits are corrected frequently returns the blood pressure to within normal limits. If no response is seen after this, the use of vasoconstrictor agents should be considered, and they should be routinely available for immediate administration. Use of these drugs can be deleterious to myocardial function in the presence of hypovolemia.[151,209] The use of dopamine hydrochloride titrated by an infusion pump is preferred by this author.

Hypertension during or after endarterectomy also should be treated promptly. It is preferable to use a short-acting β-blocker or nitroglycerine. Sodium nitroprusside by infusion pump is rarely needed but can be used if the hypertension recurs. It is usually started when the systolic blood pressure is greater than 160 mm Hg in normotensive patients and greater than 180 mm Hg in chronically hypertensive patients. It is titrated to keep the systolic levels between 140 and 160 mm Hg. In any case, diastolic pressure is kept at less than 100 mm Hg. The need for intravenous antihypertensive therapy usually lasts less than 24 hours, and patients must be monitored in an intensive care unit during that time. In patients with essential hypertension, oral medications are restarted within that period.

Technical Complications

Technical problems during the procedure can be avoided by careful dissection and adherence to a proven established routine. The occurrence of intimal flaps at the distal end point of the endarterectomized segment usually results from incomplete removal of the plaque or too deep a plane of dissection in the media. Several steps must be taken to ensure that no distal intimal flap develops. Following mobilization of the carotid bifurcation, gentle palpation of the internal carotid artery reveals the distal end of the plaque. The arteriotomy should be carried beyond the visualization of the distal end point. If a shunt is to be inserted, this becomes critical.[210] Only in this manner can the lesion be completely removed under direct vision. As the endarterectomy is carried distally in the internal carotid artery, the most superficial plane in the media that allows complete removal of the plaque should be chosen. In this manner, a tapered end point is almost always encountered. Tacking sutures should virtually never be required. The use of intraoperative completion angiograms is encouraged so that distal end-point defects can be recognized and corrected before completion of the procedure.

Emboli during or after CEA are probably the most frequent cause of neurologic deficits after the procedure. Intraoperatively, these can occur during artery mobilization or shunt insertion or after arteriotomy closure. Care should be taken during the distal insertion of the shunt so that it is done beyond the end of the lesion, as previously mentioned. Failure to do this results in fragmentation of the plaque, with embolization or elevation and wrinkling of the intima. Allowing the shunt to backbleed freely ensures adequate position and removal of all air. Some clinicians prefer proximal insertion with the shunt fully clamped so that slow, careful release allows immediate reclamping if any air or debris are seen flowing through the shunt.

After the endarterectomy is completed, the area should be free of any loose fragments. Careful irrigation with heparinized saline ensures this. Before completion of the arteriotomy closure, the internal, external, and common carotid arteries should be allowed to bleed freely. Flow should be established to the external carotid artery first to ensure that any debris present goes to this system.

Emboli in the immediate postoperative interval, in the absence of an intimal flap or other technical error, are likely to be from fibrin or platelet aggregates formed in the endarterectomized segment. The use of preoperative antiplatelet agents may prevent such occurrences.

Occasionally, once the procedure is completed, a kink is present in the endarterectomized portion of the internal carotid artery. If the angle between the segments is less than 90 degrees, flow restriction can occur, and disturbances that promote recurrent stenosis are likely. Many times this can be anticipated when an elongated or coiled artery is present before the endarterectomy. When this situation develops in severe cases, it is preferable to correct the problem by an angioplasty procedure, usually with resection of a segment of the common carotid artery with pull-down and primary anastomosis (see Fig. 19.17C). Ligation and division of the external carotid artery are rarely required, because dissection of the trunk and main branches allows sufficient mobility to correct the kink. Ligation and division of the nerve of Hering and surrounding bifurcation tissues are always necessary.

A carotid–cavernous sinus fistula is a feared complication when treating acute carotid thrombosis with balloon catheters placed in the internal carotid artery. On the rare occasion when it is necessary, several maneuvers should be attempted before the use of balloon catheters. The clot should be carefully separated from the intima and gently pulled down. The internal carotid backpressure is sometimes helpful in this process, and shunting the external circulation can make a difference, allowing the extraction of the clot. If the use of balloon catheters is necessary, they should never be inserted beyond the proximal intracranial portion of the artery, and the use of traction force is condemned. Although perforating the carotid artery intracranially with the balloon catheter is possible, the most common mechanism of injury that creates a carotid–cavernous sinus fistula is that of traction with the balloon catheter. This shearing force creates a transverse tear in the portion of the intracranial carotid that is intimately adherent to the cavernous sinus and fixed to the petrous portion of the skull. Therefore traction on the inflated balloon catheter should be gentle. Fluoroscopic guidance may be helpful. Failure of these maneuvers makes abandonment of the procedure mandatory and requires the consideration of an extracranial-to-intracranial bypass.

Cranial Nerve Injury

Peripheral cranial nerve injury is another source of morbidity after CEA. In a prospective analysis, Hertzer and colleagues[211] found a 16% incidence of cranial nerve dysfunction after this procedure. Only 60% of injuries were symptomatic. The rest would have gone unnoticed by the patient or physician, had further detailed examination been omitted. A similar overall incidence was found by Evans and colleagues[212] on clinical grounds, but when speech pathologists were added as part of the evaluation team, the incidence increased to 39%, mostly related to superior laryngeal and recurrent laryngeal nerve dysfunction. The majority of these deficits were temporary, and when evaluation was repeated in 6 weeks, the incidence was between 1% and 4%. These injuries can be avoided with careful dissection, the principle being to stay in the periadventitial plane of the artery and to be familiar with the anatomy of the area, including well-recognized anomalies (Fig. 19.19).

The hypoglossal nerve is frequently visualized during CEA. It can be seen descending along the course of the internal carotid, and then crossing the external carotid in a more superficial plane. Mobilization of this nerve may be necessary when a high bifurcation is present or when the lesion extends high in the internal carotid artery. This is accomplished by careful division of small veins that tent the nerve downward. A branch of the external carotid to the sternocleidomastoid muscle is frequently present and requires division. The ansa hypoglossi can frequently be retracted medially, but on occasion it requires division as it comes

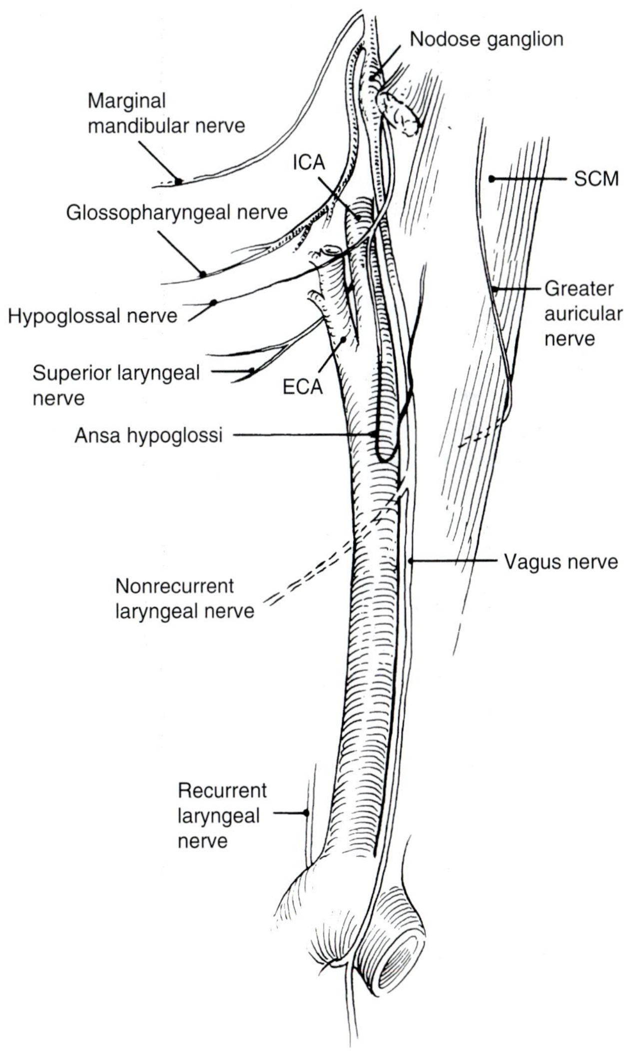

FIG 19.19 Surgical anatomy and relationship of structures encountered during exposure of the carotid bifurcation. *ECA,* External carotid artery; *ICA,* internal carotid artery; *SCM,* sternocleidomastoid muscle.

off the hypoglossal nerve. Traction or retractor injury to the hypoglossal nerve should be avoided. Clinically the deficit is manifested by deviation of the tongue to the ipsilateral side. Speech, deglutition, and mastication problems have been reported.[211]

The spinal accessory nerve is rarely seen during this dissection, but on high dissections it may be seen entering the sternocleidomastoid muscle superiorly. It can be left attached and retracted with the muscle, but care should be taken not to compress it with the retractor.

The vagus nerve is always seen, usually posterolateral to the carotid artery, between the latter and the jugular vein. On occasion, it lies anteromedial to the artery. Keeping the dissection close to the artery prevents injury to this nerve. The recurrent laryngeal nerve usually lies within the trunk of the vagus at this level, but a nonrecurrent laryngeal nerve on occasion traverses the common carotid artery. Injury to these structures can be asymptomatic or manifested by hoarseness, but hoarseness in the postoperative period is due to vocal cord paresis in approximately half of patients.[211] This underscores the importance of laryngoscopic examination in reaching a specific diagnosis. The asymptomatic injury gains significance when bilateral staged reconstructions are planned, in which case routine laryngoscopic visualization of the vocal cords is highly recommended. Detection of a paralyzed vocal cord mandates delaying the procedure until recovery is complete. If vocal cord paralysis is permanent, appropriate precautions should be taken to avoid bilateral injury, and perioperative airway management should be given special consideration.

The superior laryngeal nerve leaves the inferior ganglion of the vagus (nodose ganglion) and courses behind the internal carotid artery, bifurcating into an internal and an external branch. The internal branch is sensitive to the larynx, and the external innervates the inferior constrictor and cricothyroid muscles. The latter is responsible for the quality of voice, specifically the higher pitches. Injury to the external laryngeal nerve can be avoided by keeping the dissection close to the arterial wall, specifically when controlling the superior thyroid artery.

The glossopharyngeal nerve is usually not seen in the dissection but can be injured when dissections are carried high, especially those requiring division of the digastric muscles.[213,214] This nerve courses posterior to the high portion of the internal carotid artery and can be injured with the application of a vascular clamp that includes tissues other than the artery itself. Again, dissection close to the arterial wall is the key to prevention. Clinically the dysfunction is evident when tasks requiring oral pharyngeal muscle activity, mostly deglutition, are examined. Horner syndrome may be produced by injury to the ascending sympathetic fibers in the area of the glossopharyngeal nerve.

The cervical branch of the facial nerve lies beneath the platysma, inferior to the angle of the jaw. In some patients, this nerve sends branches to the mandibular branch, and its injury produces sagging of the ipsilateral corner of the lower lip. The marginal mandibular branch can itself be injured when the incision is carried too close to the jaw. Both of these injuries can be prevented by curving the upper portion of the incision toward the mastoid process.[210] Self-retaining retractors should be carefully placed in this area.

The greater auricular nerve courses deep to the platysma over the sternocleidomastoid muscle at an angle toward the ear in the upper portion of the dissection. Its division should be avoided, but it is frequently necessary in high dissections. Numbness of the earlobe is the usual consequence, although surprisingly some patients have no complaints after its deliberate division.

The parotid gland lies in the superior portion of the incision anterior to the sternocleidomastoid muscle. Again, curving the incision toward the mastoid process prevents injury in high dissections. Troublesome bleeding and the risk of a parotid fistula can be prevented by this maneuver.

Postoperative Complications

On completion of an operation performed with general anesthesia, the patient is awakened in the operating room. A gross neurologic examination is performed. If no deficit is found, the patient is transferred to the recovery room, where a more detailed examination is performed.

Stroke is the most feared complication of CEA. In experienced hands, it occurs in between 1% and 3% of patients, depending on the indication for the procedure.[215] Most of the low rates of stroke have been reported from specialized centers. Early results from pooled data community surveys showed rates of combined stroke morbidity and mortality ranging from 6.5% to 21%.[216-218] Because CEA is a prophylactic operation used to prevent stroke, these higher complication rates erase most benefits and are clearly unacceptable. A committee of the Stroke Council of the American Heart Association reviewed this problem and set standards for upper acceptable limits of stroke and death as a function of indication for operation. Thus, for patients undergoing CEA for asymptomatic carotid stenosis, the combined operative stroke morbidity and mortality should not exceed 3%; for TIA as an indication, 5%; for prior stroke as an indication, 7%; and for recurrent carotid stenosis, 10%.[219] A mechanism for individual surgeon audit was described and recommended. Fortunately, more recent results from individual series, prospective randomized trials, and national databases have shown a marked reduction in stroke morbidity and mortality following CEA. These reports will be discussed in the Results section.

TIAs in the first postoperative week have been reported with a frequency as high as 8%. When a neurologic deficit is found on awakening the patient, the main question to be resolved is the patency of the internal carotid artery. If a completion angiogram was performed and no abnormalities were seen, the event is likely to be embolic, and immediate reoperation would likely be of no benefit. If no completion imaging was performed, immediate patency of the vessel should be assessed. This can be done by noninvasive means,[220] but the most expeditious approach is to return the patient to the operating room for exploration. Immediate reoperation and correction of defect, including thrombectomy, may reverse the deficit.[221] If the vessel appears patent by noninvasive tests, the surgeon needs to determine whether the emboli occurred during the operation or whether a source is present in the operated segment. This is also the case in a patient who is neurologically intact and develops an event in the ipsilateral hemisphere hours or days after surgery. Once

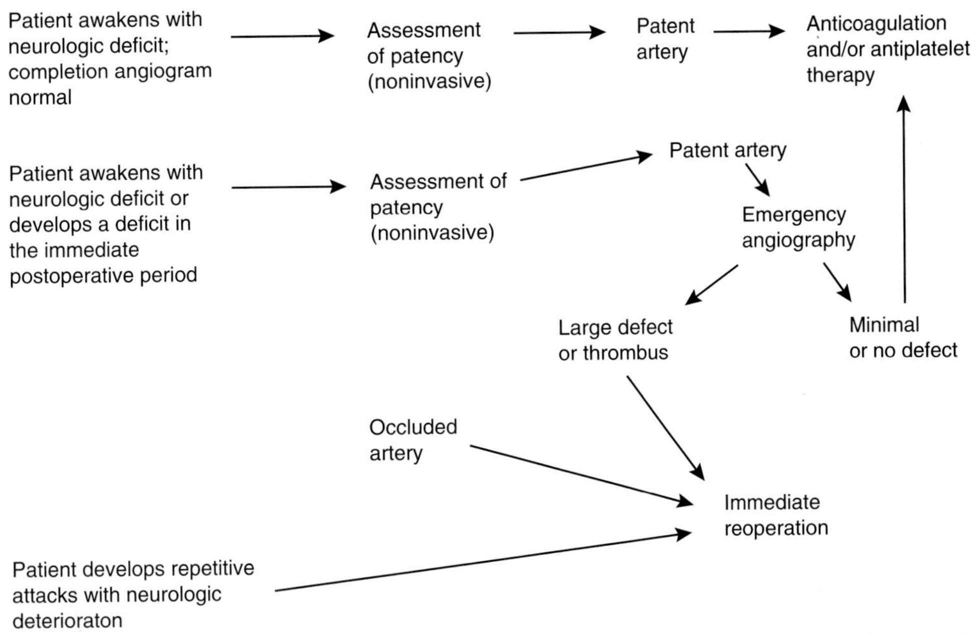

FIG 19.20 Algorithm that can be applied to the management of a patient who awakens with a postoperative neurologic deficit after carotid endarterectomy.

patency is evidenced by exploration or noninvasive means, immediate angiography is indicated. Reoperation is necessary if a significant defect or any clot is present. Otherwise, conservative therapy with anticoagulation, antiplatelet agents, or both is warranted. Other factors inevitably influence the decision to reoperate or observe the patient. The difficulty of the initial reconstruction, the patient's general status, and the availability and reliability of ancillary facilities affect this difficult decision (Fig. 19.20).

Mortality after CEA has declined significantly as the incidence of postoperative stroke has diminished. Pulmonary insufficiency, renal insufficiency, and sepsis are extremely unusual complications owing to the nature of this procedure. MI remains the most frequent cause of death in the early postoperative period, more so in patients with suspected coronary artery disease.[222] Because of this, preoperative assessment is of paramount importance. Postoperatively, electrocardiographic monitoring for the first 24 hours and a 12-lead electrocardiographic tracing should be obtained. Any suspicion of a myocardial event should be investigated and treated aggressively.

Wound infections after CEA are extremely rare. Routine use of prophylactic antibiotics for 24 hours during the perioperative interval is recommended.

Taking into account that the procedure is performed with full heparinization and that many patients have received platelet antiaggregants preoperatively, the incidence of wound bleeding is low. In Thompson's personal series,[215] reoperation for this problem was required in 7/1022 (0.7%) patients.

Large cervical hematomas may form, and reoperation and drainage should be strongly considered in an otherwise stable patient. The routine use of a Silastic drain has not been shown to reduce the incidence of this complication. Bleeding occurs from the suture line rarely. More often, a diffuse ooze is present, requiring the reversal of anticoagulation. In any case, drainage of the hematoma and correction of its cause prevent chronic draining wounds, infection, and the rare occurrence of pseudoaneurysm formation. The last is more frequent when closure is performed with a patch.[215]

Headache after CEA is not unusual. It may be associated with a neurologic deficit, in which case a CT scan should be performed. In the majority of cases, however, it runs a self-limited course and is probably related to altered autoregulatory dysfunction of the cerebral circulation. The use of a β-blocker has been effective in treating troublesome headache. Poorly controlled hypertension can result in encephalopathy. The mildest form is headache, which can progress to seizure, and the most severe form is intracerebral hemorrhage, which is often fatal. The risk of this complication mandates careful preoperative and perioperative management of hypertension.

Complications after CEA can be prevented by careful patient preparation, meticulous technique, and adherence to a rational, well-established routine. An uneventful operation is the best way to effectively change the natural history of extracranial arterial occlusive disease.

RESULTS OF SURGICAL TREATMENT FOR EXTRACRANIAL ARTERIAL OCCLUSIVE DISEASE

The most frequently performed operation for extracranial arterial occlusive disease is endarterectomy of the carotid bifurcation. As experience is gained with this procedure, results have improved, and in experienced hands it can be done with morbidity and mortality rates well below the Stroke Council guidelines. When recommending this procedure, the results of the particular surgeon or institution should be considered, because a higher morbidity and mortality may negate any beneficial effects of surgery.

The first multi-institutional study that compared surgical and medical treatment in a prospectively randomized fashion came from the joint study on extracranial arterial occlusion,[223] in which 1225 symptomatic patients with extracranial arterial occlusive disease were randomly allocated to receive either medical or surgical therapy. The 42-month survival was better in surgically treated patients with unilateral carotid stenosis who were experiencing TIAs or cerebral infarction with minimal residual deficit. The neurologic morbidity in 316 patients who were identified as having hemispheric TIAs as an indication for inclusion in the study was evaluated. The incidence of cerebral infarction at 42 months was reduced in the surgical group. Recurrent TIAs or cerebral infarction usually affected the side not operated on in the surgical patients, in contrast to the medically treated group, where neurologic events occurred chiefly in the distribution of the symptomatic artery at the time of randomization. The differences were statistically significant. The combined postoperative morbidity and mortality in the surgically treated group was approximately 8%, which is considered extremely high by today's standards. This may have affected the results of this study in favor of medical therapy.

The preoperative neurologic status of the patient affects the immediate postoperative results. Asymptomatic patients fare better than patients with TIAs, and the latter have lower morbidity than patients with completed strokes. Rothwell and colleagues[224] reviewed 25 studies and performed a meta-analysis. The combined perioperative risk of death and stroke was 3% to 3.5% in asymptomatic patients, compared with 5.18% for symptomatic patients. These differences were consistent across all studies and indicate that operation on asymptomatic patients is safest. In fact, late results may be similarly affected. Bernstein and colleagues[225] reported a series of 456 carotid endarterectomies monitored for 1 to 11 years, with an average follow-up of 45.3 months.[225] Asymptomatic patients who were operated on had a 1.6% incidence of TIAs and a 3.2% incidence of stroke on late follow-up. Those operated on because of TIAs had a 19.5% and 5.2% incidence of recurrent TIAs and stroke, respectively. Patients with a permanent neurologic deficit preoperatively had a 7.9% incidence of TIAs, and 11% developed a stroke on late follow-up.

Similar results were reported by Hertzer and Arison[226] in 329 patients monitored for a minimum of 10 years after CEA. The cumulative incidence of stroke by the life-table method was 24% at 10 years after operation. Only 10% of patients sustained strokes that clearly involved the ipsilateral cerebral hemisphere. Hypertension, preoperative stroke as an indication, and patients with recognized contralateral carotid stenosis had a much higher incidence of stroke on long-term follow-up. Contralateral hemispheric strokes occurred in 36% of patients with uncorrected contralateral lesions, compared with 8% of those who had elective bilateral reconstruction. This difference was statistically significant. Patients undergoing elective myocardial revascularization had a significant increase in long-term survival when compared with patients with uncorrected coronary artery disease. These results suggest that the annual incidence of late stroke, specifically involving the cerebral hemisphere ipsilateral to the previous carotid repair, is 1.1%, a figure within the expected range for the normal population. Stroke in the subset of patients with bilateral carotid arterial disease was fivefold more common in the contralateral than in the ipsilateral cerebral hemisphere. Therefore staged contralateral endarterectomy should be seriously considered in patients with documented but otherwise asymptomatic advanced contralateral carotid stenosis.[226]

Analysis of the available surgical series with long-term follow-up reveals that a successfully performed CEA places the patient at a significantly lower risk of stroke. The results of the various surgical series are summarized in Table 19.1, according to the indications for operation.[227-236] Asymptomatic patients have a 1.2% per year stroke risk, including perioperative morbidity and mortality. Patients with TIA as an indication for endarterectomy have an initial perioperative morbidity and mortality of approximately 3%, with a long-term risk of stroke of 2% per year. Patients whose indication for operation is cerebral infarction have a higher perioperative morbidity, averaging approximately 5%. Long-term results suggest that these patients have an annual stroke rate of approximately 4% per year. The average recurrence of TIAs is on the order of 8% to 10% at 5 years for all indications. These results represent a clear improvement over the natural history of the disease, including the use of antiplatelet drugs; however, they underscore the importance of maintaining the operative stroke rate at acceptable levels for the various indications. A higher figure negates the early and late beneficial results of surgical therapy.

The results of CEA for nonhemispheric symptoms are less predictable. In a series of 107 patients subjected to CEA, the initial perioperative morbidity and mortality were similar to those in patients with specific indications for operation. CEA was successful in ameliorating symptoms in patients with nonhemispheric symptoms who had greater than 60% diameter reduction of the carotid artery and classic symptoms of vertebrobasilar insufficiency.[237] The same series of 61 patients was updated by Ricotta and colleagues.[238] They compared the results of their cohort of patients with nonhemispheric symptoms to the remainder of their series. Follow-up lasted a mean of 42.3 months. The perioperative stroke rate was 4.9%. Survival was 85.3% at 3 years and 64.9% at 5 years. Stroke-free survival was 77.1% at 3 years and 63.4% at 5 years. During follow-up, 11 patients (18%) developed recurrent nonhemispheric symptoms. These results were not different from the cohort of 553 patients. The authors concluded that CEA provided long-term benefit in this group of patients.

The use of cerebral angiography can also be helpful in selecting patients. The presence of a posterior communicating artery suggests that the anterior circulation may be a major contributor to the vertebrobasilar system. Its presence suggests that removal of a hemodynamically significant lesion in the carotid territory would be beneficial in alleviating posterior circulation systems.

In the absence of significant extracranial carotid artery disease, direct vertebral artery reconstruction is the procedure of choice for patients with vertebrobasilar system lesions secondary to extracranial occlusive disease. The results of direct vertebral artery reconstruction have been good, although the experience is not

TABLE 19.1 Results of Carotid Endarterectomy According to the Indication for Operation

Indication	Author	No. of Patients	Follow-Up	Operative Morbidity (%)	Operative Mortality (%)	Recurrent TIAs, Ipsilateral (%)	STROKE Ipsilateral (%)	STROKE Contralateral (%)
Asymptomatic	Thompson et al.[181]	132	55.1 months	0	1.2	0.75	4.7[a]	NS
	Sergeant et al.[227]	43	6.48 months	2.3	2.3	0	0	0
	Moore et al.[228]	72	6–180 months	0	0	2.7	5.6[b]	2.7
	Bernstein et al.[229]	87[c]	43 months	NS[d]	0	NS	6.3[e]	NS
	Hertzer and Arison[226]	126	10–14 years	NS	NS	NS	9[f]	7[f]
	Lord[230]	226	30–144 months	2.6	1.1	NS	0.4	1.1
TIA	Bernstein et al.[229]	370[g]	12–132 months	NS	0	19.5[h]	5.2	NS
	DeWeese et al.[231]	103	60-months minimum	6.0	0.97	18.4[i]	7.7[j]	10.6
	Thompson et al.[232]	293	Up to 156 months	2.7	1.4	16.3	4.7	0.6
	Takolander et al.[233]	142	5-year actuarial	4.9	1.8	14.7	6.5	4.0
	Hertzer and Arison[226]	123	10–14 years	NS	NS	NS	6[f]	9[f]
Stroke	Thompson et al.[232]	217	Up to 156 months	5.0	7.4	8.2	NS	
	Eriksson et al.[234]	55	21-month average	3.7	3.7	3.8	NS	
	Bardin et al.[235]	127	56-month average	3.9	3.1	20	NS	
	Takolander et al.[233]	60	5-year actuarial	4.9	5.9	11.6[e]	10	NS
	McCullough et al.[236]	50	41-month average	3.4	1.7	3.3	NS	
	Hertzer and Arison[226]	80	10–14 years	NS	NS	NS	6[f]	13

[a]Side of stroke not specified; three strokes were fatal.
[b]Two patients suffered transient postoperative deficits with complete recovery.
[c]Number of procedures; exact number of patients not specified.
[d]Perioperative stroke rate of 3% in the entire series of 370 patients.
[e]Side of neurologic event not specified; risk of stroke at 5 years by life-table analysis.
[f]Does not include perioperative strokes.
[g]Total number of patients in series, including TIA patients.
[h]Territory affected not specified.
[i]Includes patients with nonterritorial symptoms.
[j]Includes operative morbidity.
NS, Not specified; *TIA,* transient ischemic attack.

as extensive as that with carotid artery surgery. In a series of 109 vertebral artery operations, Imparato[239] reported an operative mortality of 3%. Other complications included temporary hemidiaphragm paralysis and Horner syndrome. Two thromboses of the reconstruction occurred; there were no perioperative strokes. Long-term follow-up revealed a stroke incidence of 1.5% per year of follow-up. No controlled series on the natural history of these patients is available for comparison.

The experience with external carotid revascularization is limited; therefore long-term results are not available. In a series of 42 external carotid artery reconstructions, O'Hara and colleagues[240] reported no early morbidity or mortality when the operation was limited to external CEA and patch angioplasty. When the procedure was combined with bypass to the external carotid artery or with an extracranial-to-intracranial bypass, a 33% incidence of stroke was observed. No neurologic symptoms occurred in 25 patients (60%) during follow-up ranging from 1 to 72 months (mean, 27 months). These authors concluded that external CEA can be performed with acceptable risks and long-term effectiveness. When the reconstruction involves bypass to the external carotid artery or extracranial-to-intracranial bypass, a higher operative risk can be expected. A similar note of caution was expressed by Halstuk and colleagues,[241] describing 49 external carotid revascularization procedures performed in 36 patients. Indications included ipsilateral TIAs, amaurosis fugax, and a preparatory procedure in anticipation of extracranial-to-intracranial bypass. Twenty patients had preoperative strokes. Twenty-nine patients underwent unilateral external CEA, with the remaining patients undergoing other procedures in addition to the external revascularization. The incidence of postoperative stroke within 8 days of external carotid revascularization was 13.8%. One operative death occurred, for a mortality rate of 2.7%. Long-term follow-up ranging from 1 to 75 months (mean, 29 months) revealed a 14.2% incidence of late neurologic ischemic events. Three of these were TIAs, one was a reversible ischemic neurologic deficit, and one patient had a stroke 50 months after his initial operation. These results suggest caution in recommending external carotid artery surgery, especially when the revascularization will involve more than just endarterectomy with patch closure.

The perioperative use of aspirin in patients undergoing CEA reduces the risk of stroke and death up to 6 months. Lindblad and associates[242] performed a prospective, randomized trial comparing CEA in patients with and without aspirin. The results

TABLE 19.2 Effect of Perioperative Use of Aspirin

Time After Operation	Complication	CEA With ASA, No. of Patients (%)	CEA Without ASA, No. of Patients (%)
1 week	Stroke	0	7 (6)
30 days	Stroke	2 (1.7)	11 (9.6)
6 months	Stroke	2 (1.7)	11 (9.6)
30 days	Mortality	0.8	4.3
6 months	Mortality	3–4	6

ASA, Acetylsalicylic acid; *CEA*, carotid endarterectomy.

are summarized in Table 19.2. Although the results of individual series are of interest, level 1 data regarding risk and benefit come from prospective randomized trials or population-based analyses.

PROSPECTIVE, RANDOMIZED TRIALS

Despite retrospective data analysis clearly demonstrating the superiority of CEA over medical management in regard to stroke prevention, a number of well-meaning critics point out that retrospective data analysis can be misleading. Retrospective studies compare surgical results with available natural history data. The natural history of a particular disease process can change, often for the better, making the basis of comparison invalid. Likewise, retrospective reviews are often performed in centers of excellence, where surgical complication rates may be lower than the actual risk of operation in the community. For this reason, several prospective, randomized trials were initiated in North America and Europe. The objective of these trials was to scientifically evaluate the efficacy (or lack thereof) of CEA in preventing stroke for a variety of indications when compared with a true, contemporary control group. The trials can generally be categorized into two major classifications: asymptomatic and symptomatic carotid artery disease.

Three asymptomatic trials have completed their data acquisition and reported results: the Veterans Administration (VA) Asymptomatic Carotid Stenosis Study, ACAS, and the European Asymptomatic Carotid Surgery Trial. Three symptomatic trials have been completed: NASCET, the Medical Research Council European Carotid Surgery Trial (ECST), and the VA Symptomatic Trial.

Asymptomatic Trials

Veterans Administration Asymptomatic Carotid Stenosis Study

Ten VA medical centers entered into a prospective, randomized trial designed to test the hypothesis that CEA plus best medical management (aspirin and risk factor control) would result in fewer TIAs than treatment with the best medical management alone. The design of the study was published in 1986.[243] Angiography was performed in 713 patients, 3 of whom (0.4%) sustained a neurologic deficit.[244]

A total of 444 patients were randomized over a 54-month interval. In the surgical group, 211 carotid endarterectomies were performed; these patients also received aspirin therapy. In the medical group, 233 patients were treated with aspirin alone. The study spanned a total of 8 years. The 30-day mortality rate for the surgery group was 1.9%, and the incidence of stroke was 2.4%. The combined stroke and mortality rate was 4.3%.[245]

The data analysis demonstrated that all neurologic events (stroke, TIA, amaurosis fugax) in any distribution (including the study artery), combined with deaths, totaled 30 in the CEA group, which represented 14.2% of that population. For the patients treated medically, a total of 55 events occurred, for an event rate of 23.6%. This difference was statistically significant ($P < .006$). When the data were analyzed for deaths plus ipsilateral events only, a total of 21 events occurred in the CEA group, for an incidence of 10%; in contrast, there were 46 events in the medically treated group, for an incidence of 19.7%. Once again, this difference was statistically significant ($P < .002$). Although the study was not designed to look at stroke alone, this was done retrospectively. A total of 10 strokes occurred in the CEA group ipsilateral to the study artery, for an incidence of 4.7%. A total of 20 strokes occurred in the study artery distribution in the medically treated group, for an incidence of 8.6%. This difference fell just short of statistical significance ($P = .056$), probably because of the small sample size. There was no difference in survival rate between the surgically and medically treated groups. This is not surprising, because the major cause of death in this patient group is MI, and prevention of stroke is unlikely to have a beneficial effect on reducing fatal MI. This lack of difference in survival between the surgically and medically treated groups should not be considered a negative factor when interpreting data results, because the objective of operation is to keep the patient stroke-free during his or her remaining lifetime.[246]

Asymptomatic Carotid Atherosclerosis Study

The ACAS, sponsored by the National Institutes of Health (NIH), was the largest multicenter (34 centers), North American, prospective, randomized trial of surgery for asymptomatic carotid stenosis. It tested the hypothesis that CEA plus aspirin and risk factor control would result in fewer TIAs, strokes, and deaths than would aspirin and risk factor control alone.

The design of the study was published in 1989.[247] Initially 1500 patients were to be randomized, with TIA included as an end point. After criticism of the VA study, the protocol was amended to have stroke and death as the end points. The Data Safety and Monitoring Committee of the NIH gave permission to increase the sample size from 1500 to 1800 patients.

In December 1994, the committee called a halt to the study and informed the investigators, and subsequently the public, that an end point had been reached in favor of CEA,[248] and a full report was published.[161] A total of 1662 patients with diameter-reducing lesions of 60% or greater (as measured by angiography using the North American method; see later) were randomly allocated to receive CEA plus best medical management, including aspirin; the control group received best medical management alone. After a mean follow-up of 2.7 years (4657 patient-years of observation), the aggregate risk over 5 years for ipsilateral stroke, any perioperative stroke, and death was 5.1% for surgical patients and 11% for patients treated medically. The results of surgery, including perioperative morbidity and mortality, reduced the risk of death and stroke by 5.9% absolutely and yielded a 53% risk reduction. This difference was highly significant.

The beneficial effect of surgery in asymptomatic patients was due in large part to the low 30-day perioperative stroke morbidity and mortality. Before the study began, the surgical management committee for ACAS established criteria to audit surgeons who wished to participate in the study.[249] Validation of the audit method was possible on conclusion of the study. Among 825 patients randomized to surgery, the stroke morbidity and mortality rate within 30 days of randomization was 2.3%. However, this included a stroke morbidity and mortality of 1.2% for preoperative angiography. Because of the intent-to-treat design, the angiographic complications were charged to surgery. Of the 724 patients who actually had CEA, mortality was 0.14% and the stroke rate was 1.38%. Thus the true 30-day stroke morbidity and mortality rate was 1.52%.[162]

Asymptomatic Carotid Surgery Trial

A group of European investigators, headed by a team from the United Kingdom, embarked on yet another trial. However, included in their trial were methods designed to try to identify a higher-risk group of patients.[250] The investigators reported their results in 2004.[251] A total of 3128 asymptomatic patients with carotid artery stenoses of 70% or greater, as measured by ultrasonography, were entered into the trial from 1993 to 2003. The patients were equally randomized between immediate CEA and indefinite deferral of operation.

The 30-day risk of stroke or death in the surgical group was 3.1%. When analyzing the 5-year results of the two groups, the stroke risk, excluding perioperative events, was 3.8% in the surgical group, versus 11% in the nonsurgical group ($P < .0001$). Half the stroke events were disabling or fatal. If perioperative events were included, the 5-year stroke rate in the two groups was 6.4% versus 11.8% ($P < .0001$). Comparing fatal or disabling strokes, the event rate was 3.5% in the surgical group versus 6.1% in the nonsurgical group. The investigators found that the results were significant for both men and women when analyzed separately. The authors concluded that in asymptomatic patients 75 years of age or younger with a diameter-reducing stenosis of 70% or greater as measured by ultrasonography, immediate CEA reduced the net stroke risk by half, from about 12% in the control group to 6% (including a 3% perioperative hazard) in the surgical group. Furthermore, half of the 5-year benefit involved the prevention of disabling or fatal strokes.[251]

Symptomatic Trials

North American Symptomatic Carotid Endarterectomy Trial

The NASCET was a large prospective trial designed to test the hypothesis that symptomatic patients (those with TIA or prior mild stroke) with ipsilateral carotid stenosis (30% to 99%) have fewer fatal and nonfatal strokes after CEA than patients treated with medical management alone, including aspirin. Investigators anticipated that approximately 3000 patients would be randomly allocated to receive either medical or surgical management and monitored for a minimum of 5 years. The NASCET was also stratified to study two subsets of patients as a function of the degree of carotid occlusive disease: those with 70% to 99% stenosis and those with more moderate lesions ranging from 30% to 69% stenosis.[252] Included in the design of the trial and required by the granting institution (the NIH) was the establishment of an oversight committee that was responsible for reviewing the results of the data from time to time and calling a halt to the study if a clear difference was observed between the two groups.

On February 25, 1991, a clinical alert was issued by the oversight committee, which reported that a clear difference had developed between the two groups, indicating that CEA was superior to medical management in the high-grade stenosis category (70% to 99%). No clear difference had yet occurred in the moderate stenosis group (30% to 69%), and the latter continued to enter patients for randomization.

In the high-grade stenosis category, 295 patients received medical management and 300 patients received surgical management. Sixteen of the medically treated patients (5.4%) actually crossed over to surgery, but because of the "intent-to-treat" design, these patients continued to be analyzed as if they were managed medically, despite their operations. Crossovers become important if the group that patients are leaving is in fact a disadvantaged group, as is the case in this study.

The 30-day operative morbidity and stroke mortality rate for patients managed surgically was 5%. At the end of 18 months, an interim analysis demonstrated a positive result in favor of surgery. Therefore, this arm of the study was closed. In the surgical group, a 7% incidence of fatal and nonfatal strokes occurred (including perioperative morbidity and mortality). In the medical group, a 24% incidence of fatal and nonfatal strokes occurred. The difference was highly statistically significant ($P < .001$). This represents an absolute risk reduction of 17% in favor of surgical management and a relative risk reduction of 71% with surgical management versus medical management at the end of 18 months.

A surprising finding occurred when the mortality rates were analyzed. To date, no study had shown that CEA patients enjoy greater longevity than those treated medically. However, at the end of 18 months, the mortality rate among the medically treated group was 12%, in contrast to 5% for the surgically treated group. Once again, this difference was statistically significant ($P < .01$). This indicates a relative mortality risk reduction of 58% in favor of CEA. Further analysis demonstrated that for every 10% increase in stenosis between 70% and 99%, a progressive increase occurred in morbidity and mortality in the control group.[237,253]

The NASCET investigators reported their results in the moderate stenosis group (30% to 69%) in 1998.[254] They demonstrated a beneficial effect of surgery in the 50% to 69% stenosis group but not in those patients with less than 50% stenosis. The 30-day mortality and disabling stroke rate was 2.7%, and the nondisabling stroke rate was 4%, for a total of 6.7%. The 5-year rate for ipsilateral stroke in the surgical group was 15.7%, compared with 22% for patients treated medically. Thus 15 patients would need to undergo CEA to prevent one stroke over a 5-year interval.

Medical Research Council European Carotid Surgery Trial

The ECST was a large multicenter trial of symptomatic patients with carotid artery disease that was carried out over a 10-year period and reported at approximately the same time as the NASCET. It confirmed the NASCET results reported to date. A total of 2518 patients were randomized over 10 years, providing a mean follow-up of 3 years. This trial stratified the data into three groups: mild stenosis (10% to 29%), moderate stenosis (30% to 69%), and severe stenosis (70% to 99%). In the mild stenosis category, no apparent benefit was evident for CEA compared with the risk of operation. However, in the severe stenosis category, a highly significant benefit in favor of operation was evident. CEA, despite a 7.5% risk of death and stroke in the perioperative interval, resulted in a sixfold reduction in subsequent strokes over a 3-year interval. This difference was highly statistically significant ($P < .0001$).[255]

One interesting and important difference has come to light between NASCET and ECST: they have different methods of measuring carotid stenosis. In the European method,

$$\% \text{ Stenosis} = (1 - R/B) \div 100,$$

where R is minimal residual lumen diameter through the stenosis, and B is the projected diameter of the carotid bulb. This cannot actually be visualized because it is occupied by plaque; therefore an imaginary line is drawn to outline what is believed to be the bulb.

NASCET uses a method common in North America and was previously described in the VA asymptomatic trial. In this method,

$$\% \text{ Stenosis} = (1 - R/D) \div 100,$$

where D is the diameter of the normal internal carotid artery where the walls become parallel.

The result of this difference is most apparent for moderate stenosis, for which the European method appears to greatly overestimate the percentage of stenosis. Eliasziw and colleagues[256] compared the same angiograms using the European and North American methods. Their findings are partly summarized in Table 19.3.

The ECST found significant benefit of CEA in patients with stenosis of 60% to 90%, which corroborated the results in the NASCET moderate stenosis group. The ECST reported no benefit of surgery in the 30% to 69% group, as measured by the European method. This is not surprising, because a 69% ECST stenosis is only a 40% stenosis, as measured by the North American method.[257]

TABLE 19.3 Comparison of Carotid Stenosis Estimated by European and North American Methods

Percent Stenosis, European	Percent Stenosis, North American
60	18
70	40
80	61
90	80

Data from Eliasziw M, Smith RF, Singh N, et al: Further comments on the measurements of carotid stenosis from angiograms. *Stroke* 25:2445–2449, 1994.

Veterans Administration Symptomatic Trial

The VA symptomatic trial was a prospective, randomized trial designed to test the hypothesis that patients with greater than 50% ipsilateral internal carotid artery stenosis who were experiencing symptoms (including transient cerebral ischemia and mild stroke) would have fewer neurologic events (including cerebral infarction and crescendo TIAs) in the vascular distribution of the study artery after CEA plus best medical management than those receiving best medical management alone. This study was just getting under way when the results of the ECST and NASCET were reported, which led to its being halted earlier than anticipated. Nonetheless, 189 patients with symptomatic carotid stenoses were randomly allocated to receive either medical or surgical management. When the results were analyzed with a mean follow-up of 11.9 months, 7.7% of the patients randomized to surgical care had experienced stroke or crescendo TIAs during the perioperative or follow-up interval. In contrast, those patients randomized to medical management alone experienced a 19.4% incidence of stroke or crescendo TIAs. This difference was statistically significant ($P = .01$). The benefit of operation became apparent within 2 months of randomization.[258]

ALTERNATIVES TO SURGICAL THERAPY

The pathophysiology involved in the development of a stroke from an extracranial lesion has been discussed. The rationale for current medical therapy evolved from an attempt to alter the factors responsible for the development of symptoms secondary to extracranial arterial occlusion. In the past, two forms of therapy were considered mainstays in the medical management of this disease: antiplatelet agents and anticoagulation. At the present time, intensive medical therapy (IMT), as best defined in the SAMMPRIS trial, includes antiplatelet drugs; a statin with dose sufficient to keep the LDL <70 mg/dL; intensive risk factor control, including cessation of tobacco use and tight diabetes control with the HbA1c levels <7%; keeping systolic blood pressure less than 140 mm Hg; and lifestyle changes, including an exercise program.[259-262]

Anticoagulation, mainly with warfarin sodium (Coumadin), has been evaluated in several reports in an attempt to determine whether its use significantly alters the natural history of extracranial arterial lesions. Baker and associates reported a randomized, prospective study in patients with TIAs who were treated with Coumadin.[263] On follow-up, those treated with anticoagulation had a significant reduction in the number of TIAs when compared with control patients. A favorable trend for fewer strokes was noted in the treated group, although the difference in the incidence of cerebral infarction between treated and control patients was not statistically significant.

Two reports from Sweden showed a reduction in the development of TIAs and strokes in patients treated with anticoagulants.

The first study showed a higher incidence of stroke when anticoagulants were discontinued; thus long-term therapy was recommended.[264] In the second study, patients treated with anticoagulants showed an increased mortality rate, and serious bleeding complications were seen in this group.[265] Finally, a meta-analysis of 16 randomized studies of anticoagulation failed to show any benefit in patients suffering from TIA or ischemic stroke compared with untreated control groups. However, evidence suggests that patients with thrombosis in evolution may benefit from anticoagulation.[266]

The available evidence indicates that although the incidence of stroke and recurrent TIAs is reduced in patients treated with anticoagulants, it remains high compared with other available therapies. The need for long-term administration, with the concomitant increased risk of complications, makes anticoagulant therapy less desirable.

Antiplatelet agents, mainly aspirin, have been advocated for use in patients with extracranial arterial occlusive disease. The rationale for this therapy is based on evidence that platelets play a major role in the pathophysiology of this disease. Seven double-blind, randomized, prospective studies have compared the use of platelet antiaggregants with placebo in treating patients with cerebral ischemia secondary to extracranial atherosclerosis. In the Canadian Cooperative Study Group,[267] 585 patients who evidenced cerebral ischemia of extracranial origin were prospectively randomized into four treatment regimens. Each regimen was taken 4 times daily and consisted of a 200-mg capsule of sulfinpyrazone plus placebo, a placebo tablet plus 325 mg of aspirin, both active drugs, or both placebos. Follow-up from 12 to 57 months revealed no statistically significant reduction in TIAs, stroke, or death among patients on sulfinpyrazone. Aspirin reduced the risk for continuing ischemic episodes, stroke, or death by 19%. When analysis was restricted to stroke or death alone, the risk reduction increased to 31%, and when male patients were analyzed separately, the reduction was even higher. No statistically significant differences in stroke or death rate were found among female patients taking any of the four regimens. Based on this observation, the probability of stroke in men taking aspirin was in excess of 5% each year, and in women it was higher than 8% each year.[268] Platelet antiaggregants reduce the incidence of stroke in patients with extracranial lesions. The question still remained whether this reduction equals that achieved by other therapies.

In 1972, a double-blind, randomized, prospective trial of aspirin versus placebo was started in several American centers and continued for 37 months.[269] Sixty percent of these patients had operable lesions in the extracranial territory. The treatment group received 625 mg of aspirin twice daily. At 6 months' follow-up, a statistically significant difference in favor of aspirin was seen when death, cerebral or retinal infarction, and TIAs were grouped together. When each group was considered separately, the difference did not achieve statistical significance. Patients for whom a decision was made to proceed with endarterectomy were also assigned to a randomized, double-blind trial of aspirin during the postoperative period. The results of this trial constitute a separate report.[270] Life-table analyses of these end points at 24 months did not reveal a statistically significant difference in favor of aspirin. When non–stroke-related deaths were eliminated, a significant difference in favor of aspirin emerged. A favorable trend was also noted when the occurrence of TIAs within the first 6 months of follow-up was taken into consideration. In the placebo group, eight brain infarcts occurred among eight patients, reaching an end point in the first 24 months. Eight patients also reached an end point in the aspirin group; however, only two of these suffered a neurologic event.

These two studies showed a favorable trend toward a reduction in the stroke rate among patients receiving aspirin as treatment for symptomatic lesions in the extracranial circulation. In the first, aspirin was used as the principal form of therapy, whereas in the second, aspirin was an adjunct to surgical therapy. The absolute level of cases with an unfavorable outcome in the surgically treated group was about one-fifth the percentage of unfavorable outcomes among those treated medically (2% in the surgically treated group vs. 11.3% in the medically treated group). This difference may reflect the independent favorable effect of surgery.

Two other studies have evaluated the use of aspirin in a randomized, controlled, prospective fashion. In a study from France,[271] 604 patients with arteriothrombotic cerebral ischemic events referable to the carotid or vertebrobasilar circulation were entered in a double-blind, randomized clinical trial comparing aspirin 1 g/day, aspirin 1 g/day plus dipyridamole 225 mg/day, and placebo. A comparison of the placebo and aspirin groups showed a significant reduction ($P < .05$) of cerebral infarction in the aspirin group. Overall, 66 patients in the entire group suffered cerebral infarction during the trial; this corresponds to a cumulative stroke rate for the placebo group of 18% and a rate of 10.5% for each of the aspirin groups. No significant difference in the aspirin plus dipyridamole group was found. Thus the incidence of stroke per year was on the order of 6% for placebo versus 3% for the treatment groups. This represents, again, a 50% reduction in stroke risk. In the dipyridamole-aspirin trial in cerebral ischemia, the American-Canadian Cooperative Study Group found no difference in the stroke risk in patients receiving aspirin or aspirin plus dipyridamole for the prevention of stroke during long-term follow-up.[272] Interestingly, the stroke rate in patients treated with either aspirin or aspirin plus dipyridamole was approximately 20% at 5 years. This yields a 4% per year stroke risk, which is not dissimilar to the lower rates reported in natural history studies.

In 1983, a Danish cooperative study comparing the outcomes of patients with extracranial occlusive disease treated with aspirin or placebo was reported.[273] No favorable influence of aspirin in the prevention of ischemic attacks could be determined. Unfortunately, only 203 patients were monitored, which is probably an insufficient number to achieve any statistically valid data. This study has been criticized and probably suffers from type II statistical error.[274]

The objective of any treatment regimen for carotid artery disease should be the reduction of stroke risk. Although each of the prospective, randomized trials of antiplatelet agents showed a trend toward stroke risk reduction, none achieved statistical significance in regard to that parameter. Only when the end points of TIA, stroke, and nonfatal and fatal MI were lumped together did a statistically significant benefit in favor of aspirin emerge. Individual studies lacked sufficient numbers of patients to show a reduction of stroke risk in favor of aspirin; however, in a meta-analysis combining the patients from the various series, the best that could be shown was a 15% stroke risk reduction in favor of aspirin, and this still failed to achieve statistical significance.[275]

The antiplatelet drug ticlopidine hydrochloride was compared with aspirin in a multicenter, prospective, randomized trial of 3069 patients with recent transient or mild persistent focal cerebral or retinal ischemia.[276] The 3-year event rate for nonfatal stroke or death from any cause was 17% for ticlopidine and 19% for aspirin. The rates of fatal and nonfatal stroke at 3 years were 10% for ticlopidine and 13% for aspirin. The authors concluded that ticlopidine was somewhat more effective than aspirin in preventing stroke in their study population, but that the risks of side effects were greater. One of the disadvantages of ticlopidine is a small but finite incidence of thrombotic thrombocytopenic purpura (TTP). This necessitates frequent blood testing while the patient is taking the drug. Clopidagril (Plavix) has emerged as a safer substitute. Although there have been no specific studies comparing aspirin and Plavix for cerebrovascular disease, Plavix has been shown to be efficacious in reducing morbid events in patients with peripheral vascular disease and coronary disease with a much lower incidence of TTP. Earlier studies using the combination of aspirin and dipyridamole failed to show any benefit over aspirin alone. However, newer studies using the combination in a sustained release form (Aggrenox) have shown a benefit over aspirin alone.[277]

Failures of antiplatelet therapy in the treatment of symptomatic carotid artery disease have been reported.[278] Caution should be used in patients who receive platelet antiaggregants as primary therapy for this disease. Partial disappearance of their symptoms should be considered a failure, and alternative forms of treatment should be considered. Patients who experience complete relief of symptoms should be monitored carefully with annual noninvasive studies. Progression of the lesion may be obscured because of suppression of symptoms by the therapy. In a review of 27 aspirin failures requiring urgent operation,[278] 12 of the surgical specimens showed fresh hemorrhage in the atherosclerotic plaque. Whether this was induced or aggravated by aspirin could not be concluded. This incidence of fresh hemorrhage in an endarterectomy specimen appears to be high compared with the findings in elective cases. Finally, good evidence suggests that aspirin is of no benefit to asymptomatic patients with respect to subsequent neurologic events. Cote and colleagues[279] performed a prospective, randomized trial in asymptomatic patients with carotid stenosis of at least 50%.[279] One hundred patients received aspirin, and 184 patients received placebo. The median follow-up was 2.3 years. The annual rates for vascular events were 11% in the placebo group and 10.7% in the aspirin group.

A 1995 report described the use of lovastatin in an attempt to modify carotid plaques.[280] In patients who were in the 60th to 90th percentiles of low-density lipoprotein cholesterol levels, lovastatin appeared to slow the rate of plaque progression. No evidence of plaque regression existed. More recently, clinical trials have shown a clear benefit in reducing stroke risk with the use of statins.[281,282] The most convincing evidence in support of the use of statins to reduce stroke risk came from the Stroke Prevention by Aggressive Reduction in Cholesterol Levels (SPARCL) trial.[283,284] A total of 4731 who previously had a TIA or stroke within 6 months prior to the study were randomly assigned to 80 mg of Atorvastatin or placebo. During a median follow-up of 4.9 years, there was a 2.2% absolute risk reduction in fatal and nonfatal strokes in the Atorvastatin group. In addition, there was also a 5-year absolute risk reduction of all major cardiovascular events of 3.5%. These and other studies have led to a new concept in the medical management of patients with cerebrovascular disease. It is best called *intensive medical therapy* (IMT). As previously mentioned, it was first described in the SAMMPRIS trial. This prospective trial randomly allocated patients with intracranial atherosclerosis to stenting plus IMT versus IMT alone. The results demonstrated that patients treated with IMT alone did better than those treated with a combination of stenting plus IMT. IMT uses a combination of antiplatelet drugs, a statin dose sufficient to keep the LDL level under 70 mg/dL, strict diabetic control to keep the HbA1c level <7%, blood pressure medication to keep the systolic blood pressure (BP) under 140 mm Hg, absolute tobacco cessation, and lifestyle management, including an exercise program.[259]

The success of IMT in SAMMPRIS has now called into question the contemporary validity of treating asymptomatic carotid stenosis with invasive treatment such as CEA. It has been alleged that the risk of stroke in patients with asymptomatic carotid stenosis has been steadily declining and the results of the previous randomized trials such as ACAS are no longer relevant.[285,286] However, and coincident with improving results with medical management, there has been a steady decline in risk of operation in asymptomatic patients with carotid stenosis. In the CREST trial, the 30-day stroke morbidity/mortality was 1.4%.[287] These excellent results have also been reproduced in the community, as documented in a report by Munster and colleagues.[288] Therefore a new trial in the management of asymptomatic patients with critical carotid stenosis has been initiated and sponsored by the National Institutes of Health (NIH). It is called the Carotid Revascularization and Medical Management for Asymptomatic Carotid Stenosis Trial (CREST2).[289] A detailed outline of the trial can be found online by going to the web site ClinicalTrials.gov. Basically this study has two separate but parallel arms. For patients who are considered candidates for CEA, they are randomly allocated to CEA plus IMT versus IMT alone. For patients who are considered candidates for CAS, they are randomly allocated to CAS plus IMT versus IMT alone. The study is in its early stages and is actively recruiting patients.

In conclusion, the previously available forms of medical management produce a reduction in the stroke rate in patients with significant atherosclerotic lesions of the extracranial circulation. This reduction does not appear to be as significant as that achieved by successful CEA. This is particularly true for symptomatic patients. However, this is no longer clear for asymptomatic patients and is currently the subject of a new trial.

CONTROVERSIAL TOPICS IN CEREBROVASCULAR DISEASE MANAGEMENT

Carotid Endarterectomy for Acute Stroke

Emergent operation after acute stroke was used early in the history of endarterectomy. Because of several reports indicating a risk of converting an ischemic cerebral infarction into a hemorrhagic one, this procedure was abandoned. In reviewing these reports, it is possible to identify several types of patients who experienced such complications, including those with massive cerebral infarctions and in obtunded states, those in whom an attempt was made to open an occluded internal carotid artery several days to weeks after thrombosis, and those with severe, inadequately controlled hypertension.[290]

Later evidence has suggested improved results if carotid artery surgery is delayed for at least 5 weeks after the acute event. Of 49 carotid endarterectomies performed for acute cerebral infarction, 27 were performed within 5 weeks, and 22 were done between 5 and 20 weeks after the acute neurologic event. The latter group showed no morbidity or mortality, whereas patients undergoing early operation had an 18.5% incidence of new postoperative neurologic deficits. The authors concluded that an unstable situation during the early phase of stroke contraindicated endarterectomy. No details about the degree of preoperative neurologic deficit or later recovery were available.[291] Following these guidelines, Dosick and colleagues[158] noted a 21% incidence of recurrent stroke during the 4- to 6-week observation interval. This finding led the authors to select their patients on the basis of CT scans, proceeding with surgery if the scan results were negative. In their series, 110 patients underwent early endarterectomy after a persistent neurologic deficit with negative CT scan results. No patient suffered a neurologic deficit in the territory of the operated artery, and no patient died. Whittemore and colleagues[292] reported a similar experience in 28 patients with small, fixed neurologic deficits undergoing endarterectomy an average of 11 days after the onset of symptoms. There was one postoperative death in this small group of patients and no new perioperative neurologic deficits. The authors recommended proceeding with endarterectomy early in this select group of patients with small cerebral infarcts.

In general, surgical intervention during the acute phase of a stroke is contraindicated. If the patient has a dense neurologic deficit, loss of consciousness, or cardiovascular instability, clearly surgery is not indicated. However, if the patient has a mild to moderate deficit and is fully conscious and otherwise stable, CEA of the responsible lesion can be undertaken soon after the patient has reached a plateau in recovery. This may be days or weeks after the onset of the event. In the small group of patients in whom a clinically unstable lesion exists, manifested by crescendo TIAs or stroke in evolution, emergent endarterectomy should be strongly considered.

Crescendo Transient Ischemic Attacks and Stroke in Evolution

Crescendo TIAs and stroke in evolution used to be considered contraindications to operation. Goldstone and Moore[293] reported experience with a select group of patients with stroke in evolution or crescendo TIAs who were acutely studied with angiography. If an unstable condition such as a free-floating thrombus or a propagating thrombus in the presence of a distally patent internal carotid artery was identified, the patient was taken promptly to the operating room. The net result in a series of approximately 25 patients was no deaths and a return to essentially normal neurologic status, in contrast to the natural history of stroke in evolution, which has an approximately 80% expected mortality.[293]

A similar experience was reported by Mentzer and colleagues,[34] with 17 patients operated on emergently for stroke in evolution.[34] None had worsening of the preoperative neurologic deficit, 4 (24%) remained unchanged, and 12 (70%) had complete recovery. One death occurred, for a 6% operative mortality. This compared favorably with a parallel nonrandomized group of 26 patients with stroke in evolution treated conservatively. The medical group had 15% mortality, but more important, 17 patients (66%) suffered moderate to severe permanent neurologic deficits. This report also presented the collated operative results from 90 cases in the literature. After successful endarterectomy, 55% were improved, 25% had no change, and 10% were worse. A 10% mortality for the collated experience was reported. Thus surgical intervention in the presence of stroke in evolution carries a significantly increased risk of both perioperative stroke and death. However, the results of surgical therapy are considerably better than the natural history of the untreated condition. A specific goal for surgical intervention must be identified by preoperative angiography. Indications for emergent endarterectomy include the presence of an unstable condition such as a free-floating thrombus or propagating thrombus in the presence of a distally patent internal carotid artery. It is highly recommended that CT be used to exclude other associated conditions that could appear to be stroke in evolution. More recently, a derivative report from the VA symptomatic trial identified crescendo TIAs as a surgical imperative.[294]

Carotid Balloon Angioplasty and Stenting

Carotid balloon angioplasty with stenting is being used with increasing frequency in many centers worldwide. Initially, anecdotal reports provided conflicting data for safety and efficacy.[282] The first large series was reported by Dietrich and colleagues.[295] Between April 1993 and September 1995, 110 nonconsecutive patients underwent treatment using balloon angioplasty and stenting in accordance with an approved protocol in a single institution. It is important to note that 72% of the patients in this series were asymptomatic and therefore represented the lowest risk group. There were seven periprocedural (in-hospital) strokes, for an incidence of 6.4%, and there were two in-hospital deaths, for an incidence of 1.8%; thus the combined in-hospital stroke morbidity and mortality was 8.2%. Two patients undergoing stented angioplasty went on to occlusion within 30 days. The same year, Roubin and colleagues[296] reported their experience with 74 patients undergoing placement of 210 stents in 152 vessels. They had one death and nine in-hospital strokes, for a periprocedural stroke morbidity and mortality of 14%.

These and several other anecdotal reports prompted a multidisciplinary group of physicians to write an editorial expressing concern about the proliferation of this procedure without proof of its safety or efficacy. They recommended that a prospective trial comparing stented balloon angioplasty with CEA be performed.[297] Several retrospective comparative studies of CEA and carotid angioplasty with stenting (CAS) have also been reported. Jordan and colleagues[298] compared percutaneous transluminal angioplasty (PTA) with stenting in 107 patients in their institution with 166 carotid endarterectomies done concurrently.[298] The 30-day combined stroke morbidity and mortality for PTA and stenting was 9.3%, versus 3.6% for CEA. In evaluating the late results (>30 days), including such items as amaurosis, recurrent stenosis, TIA, minor stroke, major stroke, and death, the combined adverse event rate for PTA with stenting was 18.7%, versus 6.6% for CEA. These same authors also did a cost comparison and found that the total cost for CEA was $21,670 per patient, whereas CAS cost was $30,140.

Several prospective, randomized trials have also reported their results. The earliest trial, largely from centers in the United Kingdom, noted that the 30-day results were a combined stroke and death rate of 9.9% for CAS and 9.8% for CEA.[299] Because this trial was early in the experience, it has largely been discounted because of the unacceptably high complication rates for both CEA and CAS. Nehler and colleagues attempted to do a single-institution prospective, randomized trial,[300] but the trial was stopped after only 17 patients were entered into the study. Ten carotid endarterectomies were performed without death or stroke; however, five strokes occurred during the course of seven angioplasties.

There were also several industry-sponsored trials. The first of these was the Schneider Wallstent trial, whose results were presented at the 26th International Stroke Conference in February 2001.[301] The 2-day periprocedural stroke and death rate was 7.5% in the stent group and 1.8% in the CEA group; the 30-day stroke and death rate was 12.1% in the stent group and 4.5% in the CEA group; and the primary adverse event rate at the end of 1 year was 12.1% in the stent group and 3.6% in the CEA group. The authors concluded that carotid angioplasty and stenting are not equivalent to CEA.

The trials up to this point had been done without cerebral antiembolism devices. Several devices have since been introduced, and most contemporary trials are now being done in conjunction with their use. The most influential industry-sponsored trial to date has been the SAPPHIRE study, sponsored by Johnson and Johnson and Cordis.[302] Both 30-day and 1-year data have been reported, and based on these reports, the US Food and Drug Administration has given conditional approval for the Johnson and Johnson stent and antiembolism device for use in high-risk patients. The trial randomized 159 patients to stent–balloon angioplasty with cerebral protection versus 151 carotid endarterectomies. All these procedures were performed in what was defined as a high-risk patient group. The authors compared a number of parameters, including death and stroke in the post-procedure interval. They also added nonfatal MI, which included both Q-wave and non–Q-wave MI. Interestingly, there was no difference in the death and stroke rate with angioplasty and stenting versus CEA. However, there was a major, statistically significant difference in the incidence of MI in the two groups. The MI rate in the CEA group was 7.9%, whereas in the angioplasty and stenting group, it was 2.5%. When comparing all patients, both symptomatic and asymptomatic, the combined death, stroke, and MI rate was 5.8% in the stent group and 12.6% in the CEA group. This difference reached statistical significance in favor of angioplasty and stenting for high-risk patients. The difference held at the end of 1 year, when the major adverse event rate was 11.9% in the stent group and 19.9% in the CEA group ($P = .048$). However, after a follow-up interval of 3 years, there was no longer a difference between CEA and carotid angioplasty in this high-risk group.[303] Since this report, several prospective, randomized trials in average risk patients have reported their results. The first report was from France in a trial called EVA-3S. This was a multicenter prospective randomized trial of average risk symptomatic patients. The trial was stopped early by the safety committee because there was a statistically significant difference in favor of CEA over CAS. The 30-day incidence of any stroke and death after CEA was 3.9% versus 9.6% after CAS. These patients have been followed long term, and the 4-year data have now been reported. At 4 years the cumulative death and stroke rate for CEA was 6.2% versus 11.1% for CAS ($P = .03$).[304] The next European trial to report was performed in Germany, Austria, and Switzerland (i.e., the SPACE trial). It was also a multicenter, prospective, randomized trial of average risk, symptomatic patients with severe carotid stenosis. The hypothesis that was being tested was that CAS was not inferior to CEA. After 1200 patients were randomized, the trial was stopped because a futility analysis revealed that the primary hypothesis could not be proved. At the time the trial was stopped, the combined death and stroke rate for CAS was 7.7% versus 6.5% for CEA. Of particular interest was the fact that the incidence of high-grade recurrent stenosis was 10.7% for CAS versus 4.6% for CEA.[305] In 2010, the international carotid stenting study investigators reported their interim results from a multicenter, international trial that involved academic medical centers around the world in a study of symptomatic patients with severe carotid stenosis. A total of 1713 patients were enrolled, making it the largest prospective randomized trial of symptomatic patients to date. The incidence of death, stroke, and periprocedural MI was 8.5% in the CAS group compared with 5.2% in the CEA group ($P = .006$).[306] This trial is of particular interest in that they also studied a subset of 231 patients with preprocedure and postprocedure MRIs looking for new areas of cerebral infarction. In the CAS patients, 50% had at least one new area of infarction, compared with 17% of patients undergoing CEA ($P < .0001$).[307]

The Carotid Revascularization Endarterectomy versus Stent (CREST) trial is a prospective, randomized trial of both symptomatic and asymptomatic patients. It includes 108 centers in the United States and Canada. It is the only trial to date that has included an asymptomatic arm; with those additional patients, the combined study group of 2502 patients is the largest trial to date. The trial has several unique features. One of the most important is a lead-in phase to qualify those wishing to participate as interventionists performing stent/angioplasty. To be eligible, a potential participant first had to submit their prior experience and results for review by the angioplasty management committee. If their data were satisfactory, they then underwent training in the use of the Acunet/Aculink system and had to submit up to 20 lead-in cases done prospectively. If the results of this second or lead-in phase were satisfactory, they were then allowed to join the study and participate in the randomized trial. A total of 427 interventionists applied, but only 227 (52%) were approved, making this a highly selected group of interventionists and ensuring the highest level of competence. The primary end points of the trial were death, stroke in any distribution, MI within 30 days of the procedure, and stroke within the distribution of the study artery afterward. The preliminary results were reported after the last patient entered was followed for 1 year. Because the recruitment spanned 10 years, there was also the opportunity to evaluate cumulative follow-up data, with a mean follow-up of 2.5 years. During the lead-in phase of the trial, the data associated with carotid angioplasty and stenting among the participating centers were reported.[308] Among symptomatic patients, the 30-day morbidity and mortality rate was 5.5%; for asymptomatic patients, it was 2.8%. These results compared well with the surgical series in the NASCET and ACAS. However, it should be recognized that NASCET and ACAS data are 15 to 20 years old, and there is current evidence to indicate that the results of CEA have improved over time. When CREST was unblinded, it was found that the 30-day cumulative results of death, stroke, and MI were 4.5% for CEA and 5.2% for CAS. These differences were not statistically significant. However, when the event rates of death and stroke were analyzed, the combined results for CEA were 2.3% versus 4.4% for CAS ($P = .005$). The longer-term analysis also demonstrated that patients older than 70 years did better with CEA than CAS. Finally, a quality-of-life analysis compared patients with and without an adverse end point. One year following an adverse event, major stroke followed by minor stroke were identified by patients as having the worst effect on their quality of life. MI, after 1 year, did not affect quality of life compared with patients who did not experience the complication. Finally, since it is known that an MI has an adverse effect on long-term survival, it was a surprise to find that despite there being more MIs in the CEA group, long-term survival was the same as CAS. The reason for this was the fact that stroke, even "minor stroke," also resulted in a shortened life expectancy. Therefore it can be concluded that within the CREST trial, CEA continues to hold an edge over CAS regarding lower rate of stroke and death. When meta-analyses are performed using all level 1 trial data, CEA continues to fare better than CAS.[287]

Asymptomatic Carotid Ulceration

Not uncommonly, a large, non-stenotic, ulcerative lesion in a contralateral carotid artery is discovered incidentally when the ipsilateral symptomatic carotid artery is being studied by angiography. Whether to operate on this ulcerative lesion is a common question. My colleagues and I carried out two retrospective reviews of patients with identified non-stenotic ulcerative lesions that were monitored without treatment. We observed that medium and large ulcerative lesions carried a significant stroke risk, usually not preceded by warning TIAs.[57] In the most recent study, the risk of stroke in patients with large ulcerative lesions being monitored expectantly was approximately 7.5% each year of follow-up after initial identification.[58] While there are good data to suggest that medium grade B and large grade C ulcers, when identified, should undergo prophylactic repair, unfortunately, contrast angiography is seldom used at present, and there are no valid studies to suggest that less invasive imaging is accurate in identifying ulceration.

Tandem Lesions

Occasionally there is a stenosis of the origin of the internal carotid artery in conjunction with a significant lesion of the carotid siphon. The question often raised is whether operating on the extracranial carotid artery alone is justified if the siphon lesion is larger than the proximal lesion. Several reports indicate that although tandem lesions exist, the embolic potential of the atherosclerotic plaque at the carotid bifurcation greatly outweighs the thrombotic or embolic risk of the lesion in the carotid siphon.[309] This author's practice is to operate on the carotid bifurcation lesion in symptomatic patients in spite of the presence of a siphon lesion.[310] A retrospective review compared the perioperative morbidity, mortality, and late results in patients undergoing CEA with and without angiographically documented intracranial arterial occlusive disease. There was no difference between the two groups. The perioperative stroke rate was 1.9% versus 1.8%; mortality was 0.5% versus 0.7%; and the 3-, 5-, and 10-year stroke rates were 93% versus 92%, 87% versus 90%, and 79% versus 85%, respectively.[311]

Combined Carotid and Coronary Occlusive Disease

The carotid-coronary area is particularly controversial, and treatment depends on whether symptoms exist in either vascular bed. In patients with symptomatic coronary artery disease in whom an asymptomatic carotid stenosis is found, it is difficult to know whether the carotid artery should be fixed first, followed by coronary artery bypass; whether both lesions should be fixed simultaneously; or whether surgery for the carotid artery lesion should be put off until after coronary artery bypass. The literature is controversial on this subject, and I continue to individualize treatment, depending on which lesion appears to be more critical. For example, if a patient has triple coronary artery disease with unstable angina and an asymptomatic carotid stenosis, I usually recommend that the coronary artery surgery be performed first and that the carotid lesion be evaluated after recovery. Conversely, if a patient has relatively stable angina and symptomatic carotid artery disease or a preocclusive (<90%) stenosis, operating on the carotid artery first and then managing the coronary artery lesions a few days later may be wise. Finally, if a patient has both symptomatic carotid artery disease and unstable angina, a simultaneous, combined approach would be justified. The alternative approach would be the use of carotid angioplasty before coronary bypass. The problem with this approach is that CAS must be done in the presence of dual antiplatelet therapy (aspirin and Plavix). Dual antiplatelet therapy would preclude the use of coronary bypass because of perioperative bleeding problems. Another approach might be to perform CAS, and then go immediately to the operating room for coronary bypass. Currently there are no scientific data to support these alternatives.

Intellectual Testing and Improvement With Carotid Endarterectomy

After CEA, patients and their families often report that the patient appears intellectually brighter and is able to carry out tasks that have been alien for quite some time. Numerous attempts have been made to quantitate this intellectual improvement, usually without success. We must be careful not to regard intellectually impaired patients as routine candidates for CEA, because the majority of these patients are suffering from organic brain disease rather than compromised blood flow. Note that multiple embolization to presume silent areas of the brain has been shown to compromise intellectual function—so-called multiple-infarct dementia.

REVIEW QUESTIONS

1. What is the most common cause of perioperative neurologic deficit after carotid endarterectomy?
   a. Thrombosis of the repair
   b. Lack of cerebral perfusion
   c. Tandem lesions in the carotid system
   d. Low cardiac output
   e. None of the above
2. Carotid endarterectomy for asymptomatic disease (1) is a proven indication for stenosis of 60% or greater, as documented by angiography; (2) carries the lowest perioperative morbidity and mortality; (3) should be considered when progression to 80% stenosis is documented; (4) may prevent stroke, which is the most common initial manifestation of asymptomatic carotid disease. Which of the preceding statements are true?
   a. 1, 2, 3
   b. 1, 3
   c. 2, 4
   d. 4
   e. 1, 2, 3, 4
3. Which of the following statements about tandem lesions in the intracranial carotid system is true?
   a. They carry a similar stroke risk compared with a carotid bifurcation lesion.
   b. They carry a lower stroke risk than a similar extracranial bulb lesion.
   c. They carry a higher stroke risk than a similar extracranial bulb lesion.
   d. They should deter the surgeon from recommending bifurcation endarterectomy.
   e. They are more frequently the source of symptoms when combined intracranial and extracranial disease is present.
4. In regard to fibromuscular dysplasia: (1) it is best described as an atherosclerotic process affecting medium-size arteries; (2) 30% of patients with cervical involvement may have intracranial aneurysms; (3) medial hyperplasia is the most common type affecting the carotid system; (4) it most commonly affects women, suggesting a hormonal factor. Which of the preceding statements are true?
   a. 1, 2, 3
   b. 1, 3
   c. 2, 4
   d. 4
   e. None
5. Which of the following statements about kinks of the carotid artery is true?
   a. They are frequently the cause of cerebrovascular symptoms.
   b. They may be congenital.
   c. They never cause symptoms.
   d. They frequently require excision and grafting for repair.
   e. They are rarely associated with atherosclerosis.
6. Transient ischemic attacks (1) carry a 40% risk of stroke over 5 years when secondary to extracranial arterial occlusive disease; (2) are always secondary to platelet emboli; (3) may be a manifestation of lacunar infarction; (4) as a manifestation of cardiac emboli are usually stereotyped, with similar symptoms with each occurrence. Which of the preceding statements are true?
   a. 1, 2, 3
   b. 1, 3
   c. 2, 4
   d. 4
   e. 1, 2, 3, 4
7. Which of the following statements about the use of an internal shunt during carotid endarterectomy is true?
   a. It is necessary in approximately 50% of patients.
   b. It can be predicted based on angiographic findings.
   c. It carries no added risk.
   d. All of the above.
   e. None of the above.
8. Which of the following statements about external carotid endarterectomy is true?
   a. It carries significant risks when combined with extracranial-intracranial bypass.
   b. It rarely requires patch closure.
   c. It frequently relieves amaurosis but rarely relieves hemispheric transient ischemic attacks.
   d. All of the above.
   e. None of the above.
9. Stroke in evolution (1) may be a manifestation of lacunar infarction; (2) suggests an unstable process requiring urgent evaluation and therapy; (3) has a 10% mortality with surgical therapy; (4) should be treated with prompt medical therapy in view of the increased risk of surgery. Which of the preceding statements are true?
   a. 1, 2, 3
   b. 1, 3
   c. 2, 4
   d. 4
   e. None

10. In regard to carotid endarterectomy for acute stroke, (1) the risks of surgical intervention during the acute phase of a stroke are high, so surgery is never indicated; (2) if a CT scan done within 12 hours of the event is negative, endarterectomy can be safely performed; (3) level of consciousness, hypertension, and severity of the deficit should not influence the timing of surgical intervention; (4) if the patient shows continual recovery without deterioration, endarterectomy can be safely performed once a plateau has been reached. Which of the preceding statements is (are) true?
    a. 1, 2, 3
    b. 1, 3
    c. 2, 4
    d. 4
    e. None

BIBLIOGRAPHY

AbuRahma AF, Robinson PA, Saiedy S, et al. Prospective randomized trial of bilateral carotid endarterectomies: primary closure versus patching. *Stroke*. 1999;30:1185–1189.

Chervu A, Moore WS. Carotid endarterectomy without angiography: personal series and review of the literature. *Ann Vasc Surg*. 1994;8: 296–302.

Dixon S, Pais SO, Raviola C, et al. Natural history of nonstenotic, asymptomatic ulcerative lesions of the carotid artery: a further analysis. *Arch Surg*. 1982;117:1493.

Eastcott HHG, Pickering GW, Rob C. Reconstruction of internal carotid artery in a patient with intermittent attacks of hemiplegia. *Lancet*. 1954;2:994–996.

Executive Committee for the Asymptomatic Carotid Atherosclerosis Study. Endarterectomy for asymptomatic carotid artery stenosis. *JAMA*. 1995;273:1421–1428.

Halliday A, Mansfield A, Marro J, et al. Prevention of disabling and fatal strokes by successful carotid endarterectomy in patients without recent neurological symptoms: randomized control trial. *Lancet*. 2004;363:1491–1502.

Malas M, Glebova NO, Hughes SE, et al. Effect of Patching on Reducing Restenosis in the Carotid Revascularization Endarterectomy Versus Stenting Trial. *Stroke*. 2015;46:757–761.

Moore WS, Barnett HJ, Beebe ME, et al. Guidelines for carotid endarterectomy: a multidisciplinary consensus statement from the ad hoc committee, American Heart Association. *Stroke*. 1995; 26:188–201.

Moore WS, Hall AD. Importance of emboli from carotid bifurcation in pathogenesis in cerebral ischemia attacks. *Arch Surg*. 1970; 101:708.

Moore WS, Kempczinski RF, Nelson JJ, et al. Recurrent carotid stenosis: results of this asymptomatic carotid atherosclerosis study. *Stroke*. 1998;29:2018–2025.

North American Symptomatic Carotid Endarterectomy Trial Collaborators. Beneficial effect of carotid endarterectomy in symptomatic patients with high-grade carotid stenosis. *N Engl J Med*. 1991;325:445–453.

Ricotta JJ, AbuRahma A, Ascher E, et al. Updated Society for Vascular Surgery guidelines for management of extracranial carotid disease: executive summary. *J Vasc Surg*. 2011;54: 832–836.

Thompson JE. The evolution of surgery for the treatment and prevention of stroke: the Willis lecture. *Stroke*. 1996;27: 1427–1434.

References available online at ExpertConsult.com.

20 CHAPTER

Surgical Reconstruction of the Supra-Aortic Trunks and Vertebral Arteries

Enrique Criado

The supra-aortic trunks (SATs) branch from the aortic arch and ascend through the mediastinum to terminate at the carotid bifurcations and the origins of the vertebral arteries. These trunks carry the entire blood supply to the head and upper extremities. The vertebrobasilar system is composed of the two vertebral arteries, the basilar artery, and their branches to the spinal cord, medulla, pons, cerebellum, and cerebral lobes supplied by the posterior cerebral arteries.

The three most common variants in the anatomy of the SATs have implications when considering their reconstruction. These variants include a shared ostium (16%) or a common origin (8%) for the innominate and left common carotid arteries, a left vertebral artery originating from the aortic arch (6%), and a right retroesophageal subclavian artery (~0.5%) arising as the most distal branch of the aortic arch. When the left vertebral artery originates directly from the aortic arch, its entry into the transverse foramina of the cervical vertebra occurs at a higher level, typically at the C4 or C5 transverse foramen. A retroesophageal right subclavian artery is associated with a thoracic duct that empties on the right jugulo-subclavian confluent, a nonrecurrent right inferior laryngeal nerve, a common carotid trunk giving origin to both common carotid arteries in approximately half these patients, and in some instances, an anomalous origin of the right vertebral artery from the right common carotid, in which case the recurrent laryngeal nerve will loop around it.

Through the mechanisms of low flow or atheroembolization, occlusive disease of the SATs can cause symptoms in any of the territories they supply, including the hemispheric (carotid) territory, the posterior cerebral (vertebrobasilar) territory, and, in the case of proximal subclavian disease, the upper extremities. Vertebral artery occlusive disease may restrict inflow into the basilar artery, resulting in vertebrobasilar ischemia. This is more likely if compensatory flow from the carotid system is reduced because of an internal carotid occlusion or diminutive or congenitally absent posterior communicating arteries.

The SATs are afflicted by atherosclerosis mostly in the fifth or sixth decade of life. This results in the development of plaques that can obstruct flow or embolize (atheroembolism). Aneurysmal atherosclerotic disease of the SATs is rare. In some regions of the world, the SATs are a common site for Takayasu arteritis, usually in younger individuals, while giant cell arteritis affects mainly older females. Traumatic and mycotic aneurysms of the SATs are uncommon but potentially life-threatening conditions.

The incidence of atherosclerotic disease is lower in the SATs than in the internal carotid and vertebral arteries. Nevertheless, one-third of patients undergoing arch arteriography have a severe lesion involving one or more of the SATs.[1] The morphology of atherosclerotic lesions of the SATs is not defined as well as that of the internal carotid artery, partly because in earlier decades the SATs were not routinely visualized during arteriography of the cerebral vessels. In addition, while ultrasonography provides valuable morphologic information of the cervical segments of the carotid arteries, the proximal SATs cannot be imaged with ultrasonography. Because there is limited knowledge of the natural history of SAT lesions, surgical indications for their treatment are based partly on inferences. In addition, lesions of the SATs are often found in individuals who have concomitant disease of the carotid or vertebral arteries; a situation that confuses the identification of the lesion responsible for the symptoms. Stenotic lesions of the SATs usually appear at their origin from the aortic arch and often involve more than one artery. Plaques located at the ostia of the SATs often present in continuity with atheroma that extends across the dome of the aortic arch.

The high incidence of concomitant carotid and vertebral artery lesions makes it mandatory to outline the extracranial and intracranial cerebrovascular supply when evaluating a patient for cerebrovascular symptoms. Currently, computed tomography angiography has become the most reliable imaging study for the evaluation of the SATs and the vertebral arteries. However, digital subtraction arteriography is still required in complex cases that may require a dynamic evaluation of the cerebral circulation, as is often necessary in patients with vertebrobasilar ischemia.

Vertebrobasilar ischemia can be caused by poor inflow through the carotid and vertebral arteries, reversal of blood flow in a vertebral artery caused by a proximal subclavian artery occlusion (subclavian steal), reversal of right carotid and vertebral artery flow from an innominate artery occlusion, and embolization from the proximal subclavian, the vertebral arteries, and the basilar artery.

SYMPTOMS OF OCCLUSIVE DISEASE OF THE SUPRA-AORTIC TRUNKS

Patients with occlusive disease of the SATs may show symptoms of carotid, vertebrobasilar, and upper extremity ischemia. Although there is no pathologic evidence to support this view, it has traditionally been taught that in patients with disease of the SATs, cerebral symptoms are due to low flow rather than atheroembolization. This concept runs contrary to clinical evidence, suggesting that the mechanisms of cerebral ischemia from disease of the SATs are similar to those from atheroma of the carotid bifurcation. In addition, patients with subclavian artery stenosis who have a coronary bypass from the internal mammary artery may present with myocardial ischemia because of a coronary steal phenomenon, as flow may reverse in the mammary artery away from the myocardial bed and towards the arm.

Obliteration of the SATs is suggested by absent pulses in the neck (subclavian, carotid) or arm (axillary, brachial) on one or both sides and by the recording of unequal or abnormally low pressures in the upper extremities. Waveforms recorded by Doppler tracings are dampened in arteries which origins are stenotic or occluded, and if so, bruits may be present. In patients with subclavian steal, a pulse lag may be felt between the radial arteries of the two arms or, more precisely, a pulse wave delay of greater than 30 ms can be measured by simultaneously recording both brachial artery waveforms.[2] Claudication of the arm and digital artery embolization may be present in subclavian artery disease. A computed tomographic scan or MRI of the brain with disease of the SATs may reveal clinically silent cerebral infarctions.[3]

In symptomatic vertebral (or basilar) artery occlusive disease, the patient may have any combination of the following symptoms: dizziness, vertigo, diplopia, perioral numbness, blurred vision, tinnitus, ataxia, bilateral sensory deficits, and drop attacks. The mechanism that triggers the symptom (e.g., standing up, rotating or extending the neck) must be sought when evaluating these patients. Patients with orthostatic hypotension have vertebrobasilar symptoms when they stand abruptly after sitting or lying down. Blood pressure measurements taken immediately after they stand up when experiencing symptoms shows a drop in systolic pressure greater than 20 mm Hg. This mechanism is particularly common in diabetic patients with sympathetic paralysis leading to loss of venomotor tone because a substantial amount of blood is pooled in their legs on standing.

The presence of vertebrobasilar ischemia related to neck rotation or extension suggests compression on the vertebral arteries by the bone and/or muscles that surround them, often by vertebral osteophytes. Patients who develop symptoms by extrinsic compression of the vertebral arteries usually require a few seconds with the neck rotated maximally in a particular direction to develop symptoms, while in patients with vestibular disorders, symptoms appear with brief, head-shaking motions. In addition to orthostatism and osteophytic compression, other conditions are capable of causing vertebrobasilar ischemia and must be ruled out. Dissection of a vertebral artery is accompanied by neck pain. In these patients, the symptoms of brain ischemia may be due to critical compromise of the true lumen of the vertebral artery by an intramural dissecting hematoma or embolization of thrombus formed in the true or false lumens, the latter entering through a distal reentry point of the dissection. A number of medical conditions may also present with symptoms of vertebrobasilar ischemia; among the most common are inappropriate antihypertensive medication, cardiac arrhythmia, anemia, brain tumors, and subclavian steal.

INDICATIONS FOR SURGERY

No morphologic database exists for atherosclerotic lesions of the SATs comparable to that available for internal carotid artery disease. It is known from arteriograms and postmortem studies that the SATs are less frequently involved by atherosclerotic disease than is the carotid bifurcation. In general, clinicians do not have the ability to use ultrasonography to study the composition of SAT plaques, and the specimens obtained at operation are few because the interventions to reconstruct the SATs are bypasses rather than endarterectomies. The few specimens available for pathologic study show degenerative features similar to those seen in carotid plaques: surface thrombus, ulceration, and intraplaque hemorrhage. One may reasonably infer that the same pathologic mechanisms operate in both carotid artery plaques and SAT lesions. Until more precise information becomes available, it seems sensible to use criteria similar to those applicable to carotid disease to determine treatment. These criteria, however, must be tempered by the fact that the risk of surgical reconstruction of the SATs is higher than that of carotid endarterectomy, when an endovascular intervention is not applicable.

Currently, perhaps the most common indication for reconstruction of the arch trunks is in combination with proximal thoracic aortic endograft placement. Contemporary vascular surgeons should master the techniques described in this chapter to become comfortable in performing hybrid procedures involving the aortic arch.

The standard indications for surgical repair of SAT lesions include lesions with more than 70% of SAT diameter reduction or plaques with ulceration or surface irregularities in patients with appropriate symptoms (ipsilateral carotid or vertebrobasilar); the same lesions plus ipsilateral internal carotid disease for which an endarterectomy is indicated (the operation should correct both); the same lesions plus a nonacute ipsilateral hemispheric infarction (overt or silent); or preocclusive lesions (>90% cross-sectional area loss) in asymptomatic patients who are good surgical risks. The latter indication often occurs in combination with the need for a carotid endarterectomy and can be done using a retrograde transluminal approach. Proximal subclavian artery stenosis or occlusion causing subclavian steal syndrome with symptoms of posterior cerebral ischemia is an indication for left subclavian revascularization. In patients with stenosis of the subclavian artery and a previous coronary artery bypass using the internal mammary artery, flow may reverse in the mammary artery towards the ischemic arm "stealing" blood from the coronary circulation. These cases should also be treated with immediate left subclavian artery revascularization using the most durable reconstruction, which presently is a carotid-to-subclavian bypass. Asymptomatic subclavian artery stenosis should also be treated when a myocardial revascularization using the left internal mammary artery is necessary.

The primary indication for reconstructing a vertebral artery is to treat vertebrobasilar ischemia. Severe occlusive disease of the vertebral artery found in individuals who have no symptoms of vertebrobasilar ischemia does not require any treatment, surgical or otherwise. Conversely, many systemic causes of vertebrobasilar ischemia are not related to vertebral artery disease.

Therefore, the decision to reconstruct a vertebral artery must be based on a strong anatomic and clinical presumption that the symptom (vertebrobasilar ischemia) is secondary to the anatomic lesion (occlusive disease or extrinsic compression of the vertebral arteries).

Vertebrobasilar ischemia may be due to stenosis or occlusion of the vertebral or basilar arteries, restricting flow in the territory supplied by these arteries. This is the so-called low-flow (or hemodynamic) mechanism. These patients often have repetitive transient ischemic attacks triggered by positional or postural mechanisms. Although their risk for stroke is lower than that in patients with carotid disease, they may suffer serious traumatic injuries because of loss of balance (such as syncopal attack while driving). In patients with low-flow symptoms of ischemia in the vertebrobasilar territory, the surgical indication rests on the assumption that the basilar artery is not receiving adequate inflow from the vertebral arteries. Ischemia of the vertebrobasilar territory may also be due to microembolization (atheroemboli). Approximately one-third of vertebrobasilar ischemic episodes are caused by atheroembolization from plaques or mural lesions of the vertebral arteries. Patients with embolic symptoms are at high risk for infarctions of the brainstem, cerebellum, and posterior cerebral artery territory. The mechanism here is microembolization from the irregular surface or from the core of a plaque in the proximal subclavian or vertebral arteries or from a lesion in the wall of the vertebral artery secondary to repetitive trauma from an osteophyte or from intramural dissection.

In patients with low-flow symptoms, and because two vertebral arteries usually supply the basilar artery, the presence of a normal vertebral artery contraindicates an operation on the opposite artery, regardless of its anatomic condition. A vertebral artery of normal caliber emptying into a basilar artery is enough to adequately supply the basilar territory. This means that for a lesion in the vertebral arteries to be considered significant, it must be severe (>75% stenosis) and the opposite vertebral artery must be equally diseased, hypoplastic, or absent.

The best approach to a patient with low-flow vertebrobasilar ischemia is first to determine whether any other clinical condition (e.g., orthostatism, arrhythmia) capable of producing these symptoms is present. If so, it should be corrected. If symptoms persist after treatment, an arteriogram is indicated. If the arteriogram shows a lesion that fulfills the anatomic criteria listed previously and the operation appears to be technically feasible, a reconstruction of the vertebral artery is indicated.

In patients with vertebrobasilar ischemic symptoms secondary to embolization, typically suggested by the presence of ischemic infarcts in the vertebrobasilar territory, the indication for surgery rests on demonstration of the emboligenic lesion, regardless of the condition of the opposite vertebral artery. The criteria of bilateralism and degree of severity that apply to low-flow lesions are irrelevant when considering treatment for atheroembolic disease.

RECONSTRUCTION OF THE SUPRA-AORTIC TRUNKS

Currently, many focal lesions of the proximal SATs can be treated with transluminal angioplasty and or stenting. When a transluminal intervention on the SATs is indicated and technically feasible, most of these procedures are best done using a retrograde approach via the brachial or axillary artery when treating subclavian lesions, or via the common carotid arteries when treating proximal common carotid or innominate artery lesions. The retrograde approach is in general preferable to the transfemoral route because it avoids instrumentation of the arch and proximal SATs without brain protection. Retrograde trans-carotid transluminal interventions are done through a small cervical incision to expose the common carotid artery proximal to the bifurcation. When retrograde access is established in the common carotid, the artery is clamped proximal to the bifurcation to prevent embolization during lesion crossing and stent placement, and to allow external to internal carotid perfusion. Additionally, this hybrid approach permits external flushing of the common carotid before re-establishing flow into the carotid artery, and ideally, the proximal internal carotid is clamped for a few seconds when cephalad flow is resumed, thereby channeling embolic material generated during the intervention into the external carotid territory. These simple technical principles make retrograde stenting of the SATs a safer approach than the transfemoral route. When indicated, trans-carotid retrograde interventions can be done in combination with a carotid endarterectomy. In these cases, after exposure of the carotid vessels, the proximal carotid or innominate stenting is done first, followed by a standard carotid endarterectomy.

In some patients with extensive or heavily calcified lesions of the proximal SATs a transluminal intervention may not be advisable because of the predictable risk of complications or failure. In those cases, the initial decision should be to decide whether to do a trans-cervical or a transthoracic SAT repair. Cervical repairs are typically done by means of a bypass from a suitable donor vessel to the diseased one. Most of these bypasses run transversely either between vessels on the same side of the neck (carotid to subclavian or subclavian to carotid) or across the neck (carotid to carotid and subclavian to contralateral carotid). Cervical reconstructions include bypass procedures between the ipsilateral carotid and subclavian arteries and transposition procedures that provide the advantage of a single arterial anastomosis without the need for a saphenous vein graft or a prosthetic graft. Transthoracic repairs require a partial or total sternotomy for a direct approach to these vessels. The lesions are corrected with a bypass from the ascending aorta to the innominate, common carotids or right subclavian artery.

Transthoracic repairs are preferred in younger patients who have innominate artery lesions or multiple severe lesions not amenable to endovascular repair (usually innominate and left common carotid). They are also a good choice for patients in whom a simultaneous coronary bypass operation is indicated.

Cervical repairs are preferred in older patients, in those who are at high risk of thoracotomy, in those who have had previous trans-sternal procedures, and in those with calcified plaque in the ascending aorta that makes partial aortic clamping contraindicated. A cervical repair is the choice for all single arterial lesions (other than those of the innominate artery).

Currently, one of the most common indications for reconstruction of the SATs is in conjunction with placement of endografts in the proximal thoracic aorta. These operations are also known as arch "debranching" procedures. The intent of this surgery is to revascularize the supra-aortic trunks whose origins will be covered by a thoracic aortic endograft requiring a proximal landing zone in the arch. Contemporary vascular surgeons should be very familiar with these principles and surgical techniques. When the left subclavian artery origin requires coverage, a left common carotid to left subclavian artery bypass or a subclavian to carotid transposition is indicated. If there is a left vertebral artery arising from the arch, the vertebral artery should be transposed to the left common carotid artery, a critical intervention in patients who have an occluded or hypoplastic right vertebral artery that may prevent a devastating stroke involving the posterior brain. When the left common carotid origin also requires coverage, a retropharyngeal right common carotid to left common carotid is added to the "debranching." Finally, when the innominate artery requires coverage, a transthoracic bypass from the ascending aorta to the innominate, and to the left common carotid is done in addition to a left common carotid to left subclavian bypass done transcervically.

Cervical Repairs

The bypass between the carotid and the subclavian artery is constructed between the proximal cervical segment of the common carotid artery and the retro-scalene segment of the subclavian artery. In some cases, the carotid artery is the donor vessel, to bypass a stenosis of the most proximal portion of the subclavian artery. In others, the subclavian artery is the donor vessel to bypass a proximal common carotid artery lesion. In subclavian-carotid bypasses, an end-to-end anastomosis to the common carotid artery is recommended because with an end-to-side anastomosis there is a possibility of embolization (from the diseased proximal common carotid artery) or of extension of the proximal thrombus across the end-to-side anastomosis.

Carotid-subclavian bypass is the standard operation for the correction of subclavian steal syndrome affecting the vertebrobasilar or coronary territories. However, proximal subclavian artery stenting has become a very acceptable alternative when performed in favorable lesions. In rare cases, when a transluminal intervention or a carotid-to-subclavian bypass are not possible, correction of subclavian steal can be achieved with bypasses between both subclavian arteries or both axillary arteries, albeit with predictably lower patency rates. These remote bypasses are constructed with the graft crossing the neck in front of the sternum, giving a poor cosmetic result, and are subject to external compression. In addition, bypasses coursing the anterior, low-neck may interfere with an eventual tracheostomy or midsternotomy if so required later.

Cervical bypasses are preferably done with prosthetic conduit. Either polytetrafluoroethylene (PTFE) or Dacron grafts provide a good-caliber match, and their patency rates are higher than those of transluminal interventions,[5] probably as a result of the high flow rates usually measured in these arteries.

Anatomic Indications

Innominate artery occlusion or stenosis. A variety of cervical techniques are available to correct flow deficits caused by innominate artery stenosis or occlusion. Subclavian-subclavian and axilloaxillary bypasses can supply the right carotid artery through retrograde flow into the proximal right subclavian or axillary arteries. Carotid-carotid bypasses are technically feasible, but for the correction of severe innominate artery disease they represent an unnecessary risk because both carotid systems will likely be severely hypotensive during the proximal anastomosis of the bypass to the donor left common carotid artery, unless shunted.

If the innominate artery lesion is suspected to be embolizing—or if it exhibits a grossly irregular surface or large ulcerations—the distal innominate artery should be ligated (excluded) at the completion of the remote bypass procedure. This may not be possible using a supraclavicular approach. A complex solution is an end-to-end anastomosis between the proximal subclavian artery and the proximal right common carotid artery, with ligation of the proximal carotid stump, and then revascularization of the middle or distal third of the right subclavian through a remote bypass from the other side of the neck.

Common carotid artery occlusion or stenosis. The common carotid artery can be revascularized by means of a subclavian-carotid bypass from the ipsilateral subclavian artery, with the distal anastomosis being performed end to end to avoid embolization from the diseased proximal common carotid artery. In some cases, the entire common carotid is occluded, with a patent carotid bifurcation maintaining retrograde flow from the external carotid into the internal carotid artery antegradely. Most of these patients necessitate a carotid endarterectomy in conjunction with a subclavian to carotid bypass. This reconstruction can be done placing the distal anastomosis for a graft at the level of the carotid bifurcation in an end-to-side junction (an onlay patch), with or without a concomitant endarterectomy of the carotid bulb (Fig. 20.1). A preferable technique for the distal anastomosis (Fig. 20.2) is to transect the distal common carotid artery at the carotid bulb, doing then a type 2 eversion endarterectomy. The ample cross section of the endarterectomized carotid bifurcation allows a simple end-to-end anastomosis to the bypass arising from the subclavian artery.

If the stenosing lesion of the common carotid artery is located at its origin and its distal two-thirds are free of disease, transposing the midportion of the common carotid artery to the subclavian artery is a better solution than a subclavian-carotid bypass. It requires only one anastomosis and no prosthesis. At times, a thrombosed common carotid artery with a patent bifurcation can be thrombectomized after dividing it low in the neck and doing an eversion endarterectomy up to the bifurcation. The distal portion of the endarterectomy is terminated under direct vision through the standard arteriotomy used for a conventional carotid endarterectomy. After endarterectomy, the common carotid artery is reimplanted into the second portion of the subclavian artery. Subclavian-carotid bypass and transposition of the carotid into the subclavian are easier on the right side, where the subclavian artery is more accessible.

In cases in which the ipsilateral subclavian artery is not a suitable donor vessel, a common carotid artery lesion can be corrected by means of a carotid-carotid bypass. This operation is traditionally done by placing a bypass between both carotids in front of the airway, or preferably using the shorter retropharyngeal route (see later in this chapter).[6]

Subclavian artery occlusion. Reconstruction of the proximal subclavian artery is done (1) to correct symptomatic subclavian steal from the vertebral or the coronary territories, (2) to correct an emboligenic lesion of the proximal subclavian, (3) to revascularize the subclavian before an internal mammary transposition to the coronary arteries, or (4) to revascularize the left subclavian from the left common carotid artery before implanting a thoracic aorta stent-graft across its origin. When not occluded, the subclavian artery must be ligated proximal to the origin of the vertebral artery at the time of the bypass. A direct transposition of the subclavian artery (prevertebral portion) to the common carotid artery is a more complex procedure than the bypass, but it involves only one anastomosis, excludes the diseased proximal subclavian artery when necessary, and does not require a prosthetic graft.

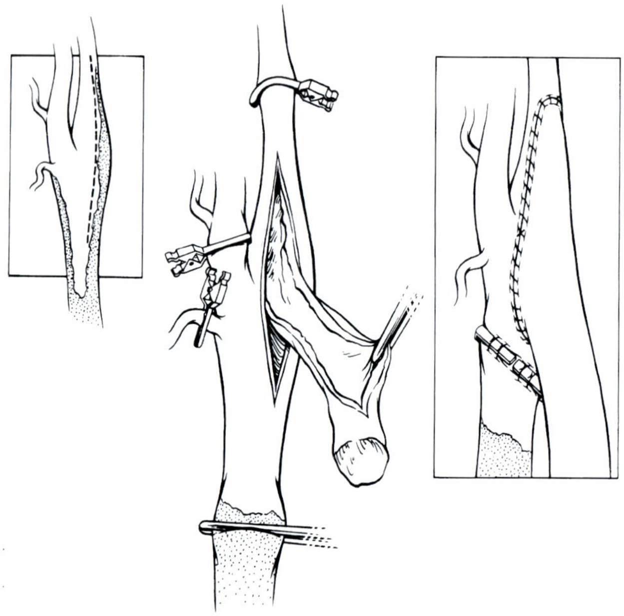

FIG 20.1 Traditional method of anastomosing the distal limb of a graft to the carotid bifurcation following endarterectomy of the latter. Occlusion of the common carotid artery immediately below the anastomosis transforms it into a functional end-to-end junction *(inset, right).*

Techniques

Carotid-subclavian or subclavian-carotid bypass and carotid (or subclavian) transposition. The approach is through a supraclavicular incision, just lateral to the sternocleidomastoid muscle (SCM). The clavicular head of the SCM is divided to improve medial exposure in most cases. The dissection is conducted lateral to the jugular vein, which is retracted medially. The scalene fat pad is mobilized cephalad, and the anterior scalene muscle is exposed. The subclavian artery can be isolated posterior to the anterior scalene (second portion) or lateral to it (third portion) if a bypass is planned. In the first case, the phrenic nerve is dissected from the surface of the anterior scalene, and the anterior scalene is divided to expose the artery. Alternatively, the subclavian artery can be exposed in the third segment, distal to the anterior scalene muscle, with partial division of the latter if necessary.

The dissection is then moved medial to the jugular vein, and the common carotid artery is exposed posterior to the vein. A suitable site is selected for the anastomosis of the graft to the carotid artery. In the case of a carotid-subclavian bypass for subclavian steal, the prosthetic graft is anastomosed to the side

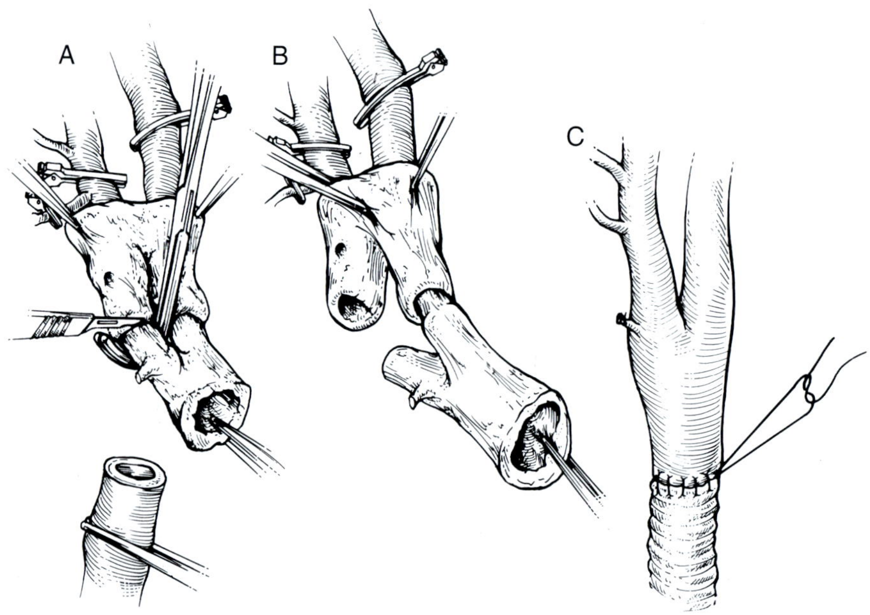

FIG 20.2 My preference for anastomosing the graft to the carotid bifurcation is an eversion endarterectomy followed by an end-to-end anastomosis. (A) Eversion of the external carotid after exposing the flow divider in the plaque. (B) Eversion of the internal carotid component of the plaque. (C) Anastomosis of the graft to everted bifurcation.

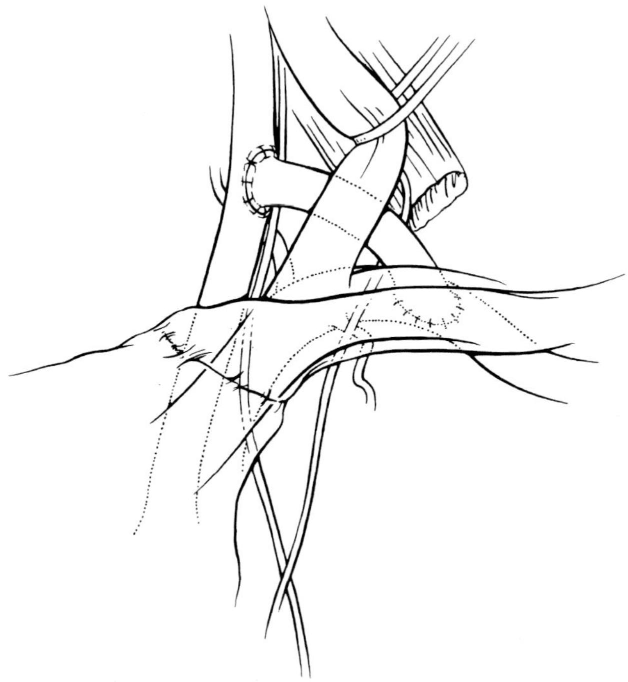

FIG 20.3 Carotid-subclavian bypass graft tunneled under the jugular vein.

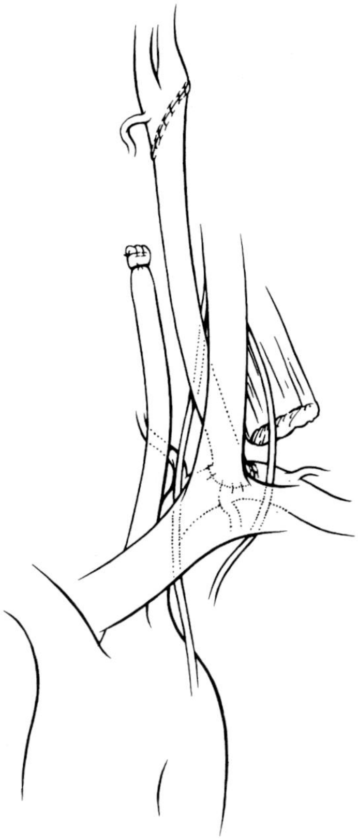

FIG 20.4 Bypass from the left subclavian artery to the left carotid bifurcation.

wall of the carotid artery and then passed under the jugular vein into proximity with the subclavian artery (Fig. 20.3). It is easier to do the subclavian anastomosis first. Both anastomoses are end to side. The graft is then tunneled under the jugular vein and anastomosed end to end to the common carotid artery or to its bifurcation (Fig. 20.4), ligating the proximal carotid stump. Another less hemodynamically sound alternative is to do an end-to-side anastomosis to the common carotid artery and ligate the common carotid artery immediately proximal to the anastomosis, which makes it functionally an end-to-end junction. The proximal exclusion is necessary to avoid embolization from the proximal common carotid artery or extension of the thrombus into the distal common carotid artery.

The bypass technique between the carotid and subclavian arteries is used, in cases of proximal subclavian artery occlusion and in patients with a left internal mammary artery–coronary anastomosis. Transposing one of these arteries into the other is a more elegant surgical solution (Fig. 20.5), in that only one artery-to-artery anastomosis is required. The long-term patency rates for carotid-subclavian transposition are superb. The drawbacks are the greater technical difficulty and the possibility of mediastinal bleeding from improper handling of the stump of the left subclavian artery, which can be quite challenging in some cases. The transposition operation is particularly easy when the common carotid artery is the one being transposed; once freed, the common carotid, which has no branches, moves about the neck with ease. Translocation of the subclavian artery into the common carotid artery may be difficult on the left side, where the subclavian artery may have a deep location or the vertebral artery may have a low origin. When this low origin interferes with good proximal control of the much shorter first portion

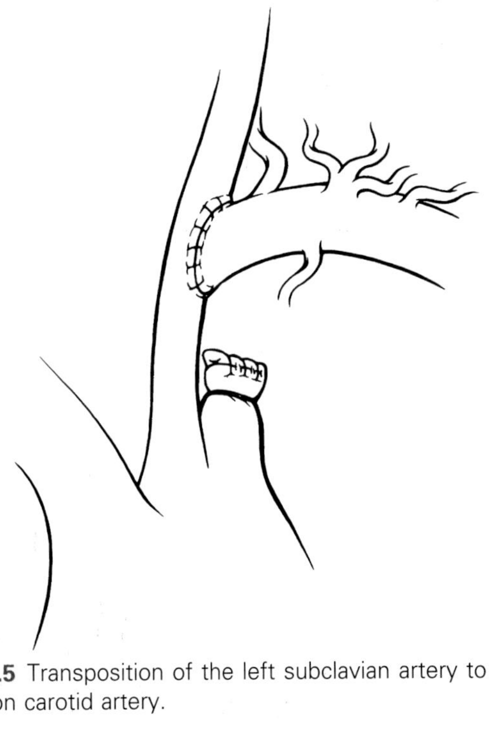

FIG 20.5 Transposition of the left subclavian artery to the left common carotid artery.

of the subclavian, the vertebral artery is divided at its origin and the subclavian artery low in the neck, but distal to the stump of the vertebral artery. The subclavian artery is transposed to the common carotid artery and, separately, the vertebral artery is transposed into either of the two vessels.

When transposing the subclavian artery to the common carotid artery, care must be taken to ensure proper position of the vertebral artery when the subclavian is brought into apposition to the common carotid before the anastomosis. Excessive length of the vertebral artery, once the subclavian artery is freed and moved upward, may cause kinking of this vessel and thrombosis. The division of the left internal mammary artery to facilitate the subclavian transposition is undesirable, as it negates the possibility of a later myocardial revascularization using the left internal mammary artery.

Subclavian-subclavian bypass. There is hardly any indication for subclavian-subclavian bypass. The incision is supraclavicular on both sides, and the second or third portions of the subclavian are approached in the manner described earlier. The tunnel connecting the two subclavian arteries is made behind the sternocleidomastoid muscle, staying as low as possible to protect the graft behind the upper edge of the manubrium. Care is taken to avoid any axial rotation of the graft when tunneling across the neck.

Axilloaxillary bypass. Axilloaxillary bypass is rarely, if ever, indicated. The axillary arteries are exposed through infraclavicular incisions, and the graft is tunneled under the sternal part of the pectoralis major and through presternal subcutaneous tissue into the opposite axillary artery. Both anastomoses are end to side.

Carotid-carotid bypass. Carotid-carotid bypass is used to revascularize a common carotid artery whose origin in the mediastinum is involved by disease. One carotid acts as the donor vessel to the other. Because exposure of the common carotid arteries is a simple procedure, carotid-carotid bypass is a good technique to revascularize one common carotid trunk when the other one is healthy and the ipsilateral subclavian artery is not a suitable donor vessel. The bypass between both common carotid arteries lies low in the midline, partially hidden by the upper edge of the manubrium. Although these grafts make a rather lengthy loop and take off from the donor site at an oblique angle, their patency rate is excellent, provided the donor vessel is free of disease. These bypasses are sometimes cosmetically poor and, as mentioned previously, the grafts run a lengthy trajectory to link two vessels that, anatomically, are only four fingerbreadths apart. It is preferable to tunnel the bypass across the neck through the retropharyngeal space (Fig. 20.6), which is a shorter and straighter path. The tunnel for the bypass is behind the pharynx and in front of the prevertebral fascia. This space is loose and easily admits an 8-mm prosthesis without significant pharyngeal compression.[6]

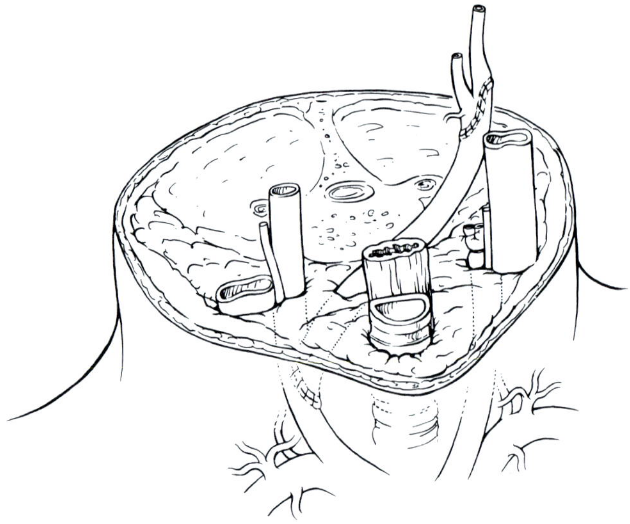

FIG 20.6 Cross section of the neck showing the trajectory of a carotid-carotid bypass through the retropharyngeal space.

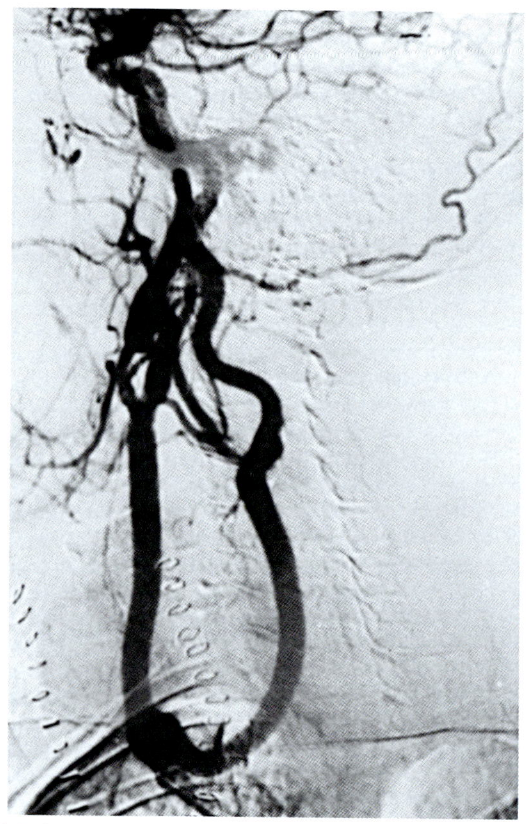

FIG 20.7 Direct transposition of the left carotid artery to the right common carotid artery using the retropharyngeal route. (From Berguer R: The short retropharyngeal route for arterial bypasses across the neck. *Ann Vasc Surg* 1:127–129, 1986.)

The distance between both carotids in the retropharyngeal space (approximately 5 cm) is so short that, in some instances, it permits the direct reimplantation of one carotid into the other without a graft (Fig. 20.7). This procedure has the disadvantage of requiring clamping of both common carotid arteries simultaneously; because of this, it is one of the few instances in which the protection of a shunt may be required to perfuse a clamped (donor) common carotid artery.

Transthoracic Repairs

Endarterectomy was the first technique reported for reconstruction of the innominate artery.[7,8] However, this technique is no longer used because of safety concerns. Its main drawback is the difficulty of clamping the origin of the innominate artery without occluding the left common carotid artery or damaging the plaque that may be present about the ostium of either. A clamp placed to exclude the origin of the innominate artery may result in bilateral hemispheric ischemia when the left common carotid originates from the innominate. With innominate endarterectomy, it is also difficult to achieve a satisfactory proximal end of the endarterectomy in the aortic arch wall, where tacking sutures are often required. Finally, approximately half the patients with symptomatic innominate artery stenosis have severe lesions of either the left common carotid or left subclavian artery, lesions not suited for endarterectomy using the trans-sternal approach.

Rather than endarterectomy, a bypass from the ascending aorta is preferred to correct innominate artery and other proximal trunk lesions that may be present. The technique of bypass from the ascending aorta was introduced by DeBakey and associates.[9]

Technique

Midsternotomy. The anterior mediastinal arteries (innominate and right common carotid) are approached through a midsternotomy (Fig. 20.8). The sternotomy is prolonged through a short incision that follows the right anterior edge of the sternocleidomastoid muscle to expose and obtain control of the proximal right common carotid and right subclavian arteries. After dividing the sternum, the innominate vein is dissected, and the thymic veins are ligated. The thymus is separated through its midline and preserved, to be interposed between the graft and the sternum at the time of closure. The ascending aorta is approached below the innominate vein after opening the pericardial sac. The dissection continues over the origin of the innominate artery and onto its bifurcation. During dissection of the innominate bifurcation, care is taken not to injure the recurrent nerve looping around the origin of the right subclavian artery.

Partial midsternotomy. Approaching the ascending aorta and the anterior trunks can be also done through a partial sternotomy, splitting only the upper three or four sternal segments (Fig. 20.9). The manubrium is sewn down to the third or fourth

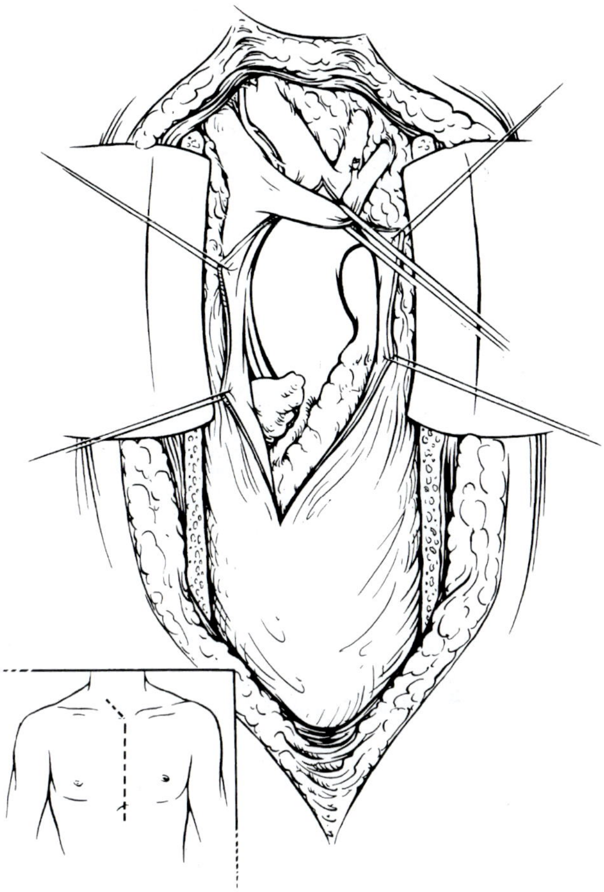

FIG 20.8 Exposure of the ascending aorta and anterior supra-aortic trunks through the traditional full sternotomy (*inset* shows the skin incision).

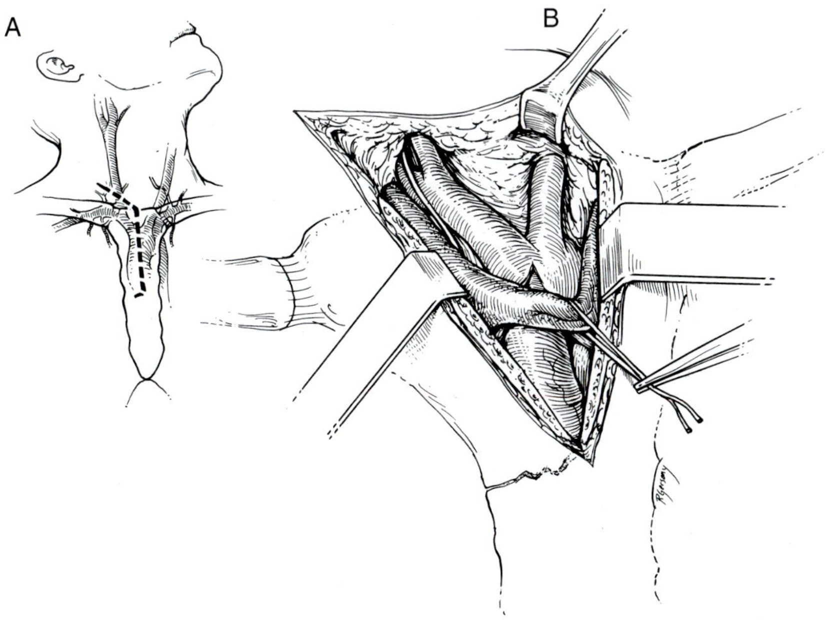

FIG 20.9 Skin incision (A) and exposure (B) obtained through a partial sternotomy.

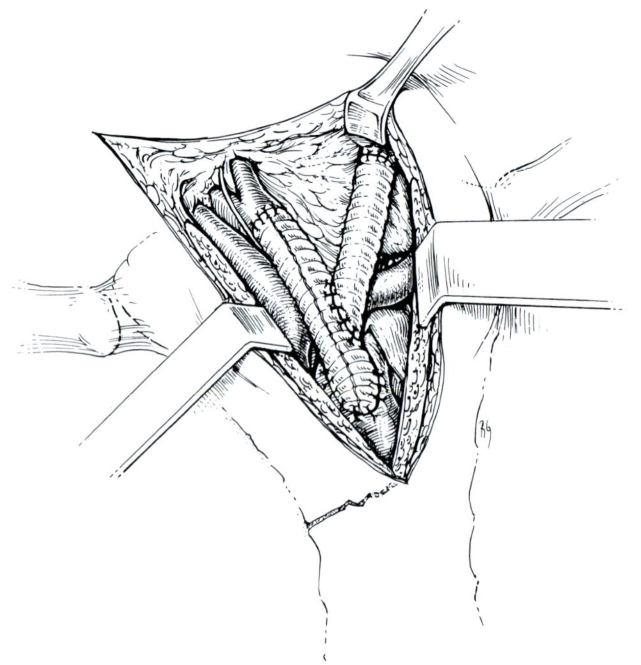

FIG 20.10 Ascending aorta-to-innominate and left common carotid artery bypass completed through a partial sternotomy.

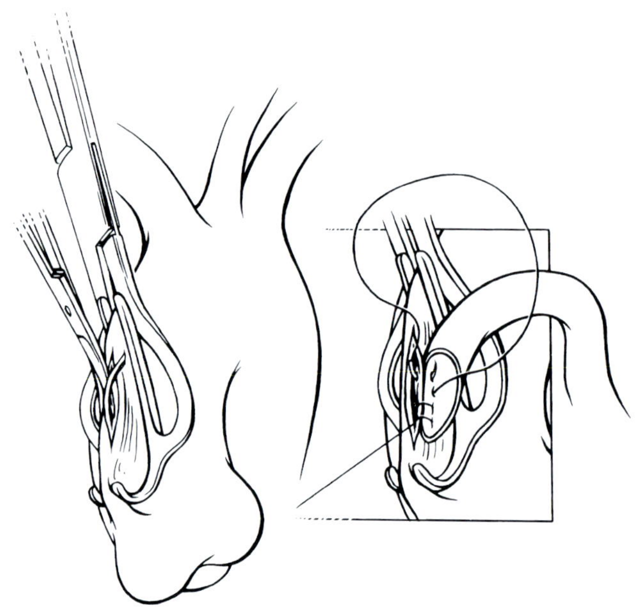

FIG 20.11 Exclusion clamping of the ascending aorta and anastomosis of the main prosthesis to the aortotomy.

intercostal space, where a small notch is made laterally with the oscillating saw. Dissection of the brachiocephalic vein and thymus and exposure of the ascending aorta follow the same steps described for the full sternotomy. The advantages of this partial sternotomy are that the chest cage remains intact and stable in its lower half, postoperative pain is noticeably reduced, and the chance of sternal instability is minimal.

Bypass from the ascending aorta. If the intent is to replace the innominate artery with a bypass (Fig. 20.10), the proximal right subclavian and right common carotid arteries are exposed. More often, however, one and sometimes both carotid bifurcations need to be exposed to be revascularized. The carotid bifurcation in this case is exposed through the standard neck incision used for carotid endarterectomy. After isolating the proximal right subclavian and common carotid arteries, an appropriate prosthetic tube is selected for the bypass. An 8- to 10-mm Dacron graft matches the caliber of the innominate artery, requires only a moderate amount of aortic wall to be clamped, and does not occupy much space in the anterior mediastinum.

The proximal end of the prosthesis is beveled. Partial clamping of the ascending aorta requires the reduction of the systolic pressure to around 100 mm Hg, which is done without heparin administration. The partial occlusion clamp is placed on the proximal aorta (Fig. 20.11). With the clamp secured, the aorta is opened, and the beveled end of the graft is anastomosed to the ascending, longitudinal aortotomy with continuous 4-0 polypropylene sutures. An external cuff of Teflon felt incorporated in the anastomosis is advisable to minimize bleeding and aortic wall tearing. Before unclamping and to avoid air embolization, the patient is transiently placed in Trendelenburg position, the graft is filled with heparinized saline solution, and the proximal anastomosis is then vented and tested. If it is found to be satisfactory, a soft-jaw clamp is placed on the graft immediately above the anastomosis, and the table is returned to the horizontal position.

The patient is then systemically heparinized. Occluding clamps are placed first in the proximal right carotid and subclavian arteries and in the proximal portion of the innominate artery. The innominate artery is divided proximal to its bifurcation through a healthy segment and prepared for anastomosis. The proximal stump of the innominate artery is then closed with a continuous double-running suture, reinforced with Teflon pledgets if necessary. The bypass graft, which is placed over the brachiocephalic vein, is cut to appropriate length and anastomosed to the innominate artery with continuous 5-0 polypropylene sutures. The graft and the distal vessels are back-bled before completing the anastomosis, and flow is reestablished first into the right subclavian artery and last into the right common carotid artery.

In cases in which additional arteries need to be revascularized (usually the left common carotid), an additional 8-mm Dacron side branch is anastomosed at an appropriate angle to the 10-mm main prosthesis after the proximal suture line is completed (Fig. 20.12). Any anticipated side branches are added before the distal anastomosis is done to avoid having to reclamp the innominate portion of the bypass after establishing flow through it. With the side branch anastomosed and excluded, one can perfuse the right carotid and vertebral arteries while constructing the left carotid anastomosis. In multiple branch replacements of the SATs (Fig. 20.13), the main bypass is the one supplying the right-sided trunk (innominate, right carotid, right subclavian). From this trunk emerge the branches supplying the left carotid or left subclavian artery or both.

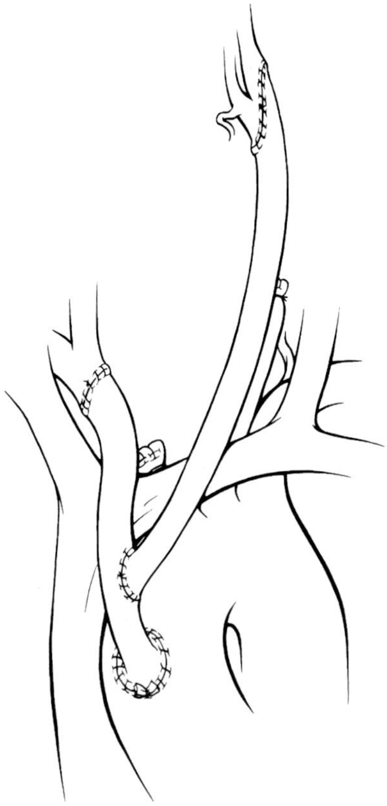

FIG 20.12 Common pattern for revascularization of the anterior supra-aortic trunk: the main prosthesis (10 mm) replaces the innominate artery, and an 8-mm side branch supplies the left carotid system.

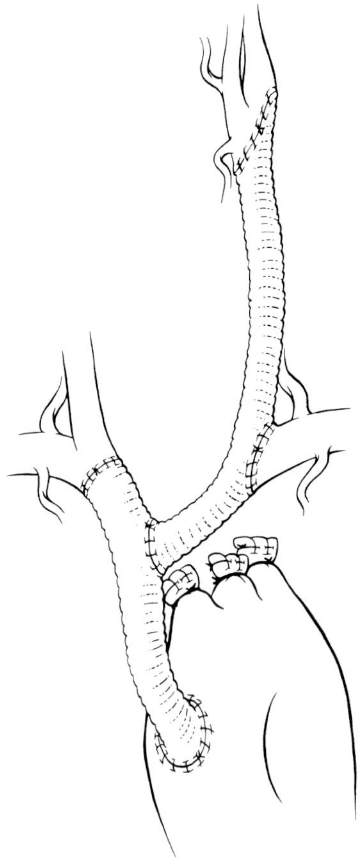

FIG 20.13 Revascularization of all three supra-aortic trunks completed by transposing the left subclavian artery to the prosthesis that replaces the left carotid system.

Results and Complications of Reconstruction of the Supra-Aortic Trunks

Transthoracic reconstructions are generally done in younger patients with multiple-vessel involvement. Cervical repairs are done in older patients who are less likely to tolerate a thoracotomy and in patients with single-vessel disease of the common carotid or proximal subclavian arteries.

Any comparison of the results of the thoracic and cervical approaches must be done considering the differences between the two groups of patients. In addition to age and anatomic extent of disease, other factors affect the choice of the approach, such as pulmonary function, previous coronary artery bypass surgery, and life expectancy.

Reported operative mortality for transthoracic repair ranges from 3% to 19%,[10,11] with most authors reporting series of 20 to 40 patients; some smaller series reported no mortality. Increasing experience, refinement in anesthesia and perioperative care, and better patient selection have reduced the mortality of transthoracic repair from 10% to under 5%.[11–13] Cumulative primary patency rates at 10 years approach 90% for thoracic repairs.

Cervical repairs can be done with both operative mortality and stroke rates under 1% and with graft patency rates exceeding 90 at 5 years.[14] These are outstanding achievements, since patients undergoing these repairs are some of the highest-risk patients among those with cerebrovascular disease, with many of them having previous myocardial revascularization procedures and/or pulmonary disease.

The most frequent and serious complication reported after either cervical or transthoracic repair of the SATs is myocardial infarction.[15,16] The second most frequent complication is stroke, which can develop during the operation or 3 to 4 days afterward. A delayed stroke may be hemorrhagic and is likely related to hyperperfusion and regional hypertension. Perioperative strokes are more common in patients with multiple intracranial and extracranial involvement. Some postoperative strokes may be due to technical flaws resulting in distal embolization or to prolonged clamp ischemia times. The latter can be managed with the usual cerebral protection methods, including administration of steroids prior to clamping, use of heparin at therapeutic levels measuring the activated clotting time, and—in patients with extensive and multiple disease—mild superficial hypothermia. Shunts for SAT repair are not recommended, with the rare exception noted under the description of carotid-carotid bypass.

Technical problems may cause perioperative or postoperative bleeding, which can be severe and life threatening. Suture line bleeding, aortic wall tears from clamp or suture injury, and bleeding from an innominate or carotid artery stump can result in serious perioperative bleeding and severe tension hemothorax. Postoperative graft thrombosis and infections are rare.

The long-term outcome of these patients is largely determined by the progress of their coronary atherosclerotic disease. For patients undergoing cervical and transthoracic repairs, the 10-year survival is 50%.[16–18] Myocardial infarction is the most common cause of death (80%).

Saphenous veins grafts fare worse than synthetics when used for SAT reconstruction; axial rotation, caliber mismatches, kinking, and intimal hyperplasia probably account for this.

In conclusion, cervical reconstruction is indicated in patients with proximal single lesions of the common carotid or subclavian arteries. In this last group, when technically feasible, it is preferable to use transposition techniques between the carotid and the subclavian and, when the midline needs to be crossed, a retropharyngeal bypass. Reconstructive techniques using short (retropharyngeal) bypasses or no bypasses at all (transpositions) have outstanding patency rates, in contrast to the poor patency rates reported for conventional extra-anatomic bypasses that cross the midline. The transthoracic approach is favored for patients with multiple-vessel disease who are of acceptable surgical risk. SAT reconstruction may be done in conjunction with coronary artery bypass grafts.

RECONSTRUCTION OF THE VERTEBROBASILAR SYSTEM

The indications for vertebral artery reconstruction were discussed earlier. The vertebral artery is generally reconstructed at two levels: in its proximal segment for stenotic or embolic disease at its ostium, and in its distal segment (V3 segment) for compression, stenosis, or when a source of embolization is present in the intraspinal (V3) segment of this artery.

Reconstruction of the Proximal Vertebral Artery

Proximal vertebral artery lesions are dealt with by transposition of the artery into the neighboring common carotid artery (Fig. 20.14).[24–26] The appeal of this operation is that it consists of one artery-to-artery anastomosis and does not require a vein graft.

The operation is done through a supraclavicular incision, between the heads of the sternocleidomastoid muscle. The vertebral artery is isolated below the vertebral vein, after dividing the thoracic duct between ligatures. Then, the vertebral artery is dissected cephalad from its origin up to the point where it disappears under the longus colli muscle. This dissection is done with extreme care to avoid transection of the overlying sympathetic ganglion and crossing sympathetic fibers. After choosing the transposition site in the posterolateral wall of the common carotid artery, the patient is heparinized and the vertebral artery is divided above the stenotic area, suture-ligating its proximal stump close to the subclavian artery. The distal segment of the artery is pulled out from the entrapping sympathetic rami and swung on to the common carotid artery (Fig. 20.15). Using an aortic punch, a small arteriostomy is made in the common carotid wall to which the vertebral artery is anastomosed in end-to-side

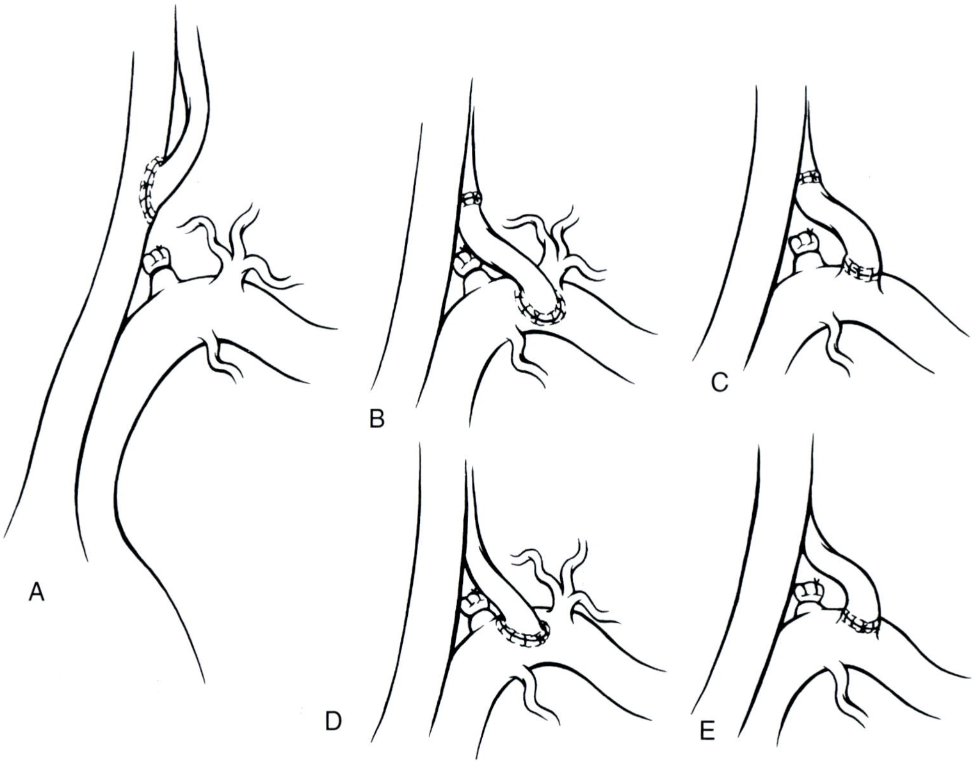

FIG 20.14 Common techniques for reconstruction of the proximal vertebral artery. (A) Transposition of the proximal vertebral artery to the common carotid artery. (B) Bypass from the subclavian to the proximal vertebral artery. (C) Subclavian-vertebral bypass originating in the amputated stump of the thyrocervical trunk. (D) Transposition of the vertebral artery to another subclavian site. (E) Transposition of the vertebral artery to the stump of the thyrocervical trunk.

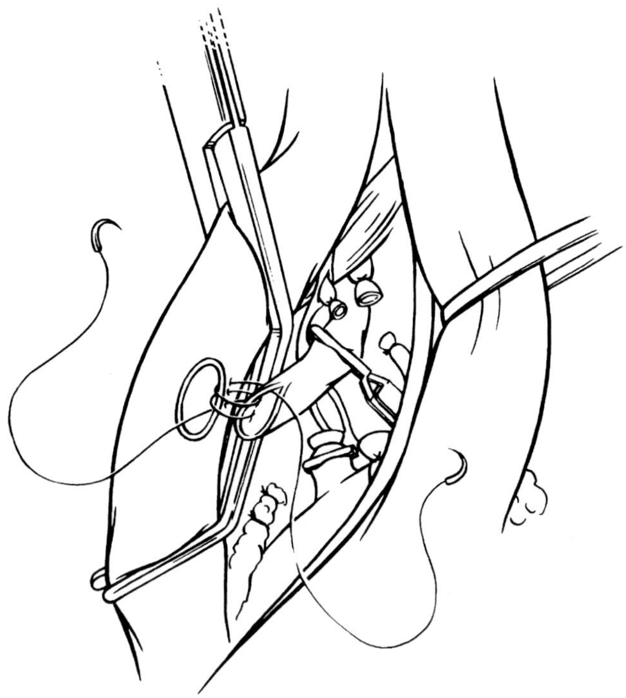

FIG 20.15 Technique for transposition of the left vertebral artery to the left common carotid artery. The thoracic duct has been double ligated. The proximal vertebral artery stump has been clipped and suture-ligated. The sympathetic chain, left intact, is now seen behind the vertebral artery as the latter is brought close to the common carotid artery for anastomosis.

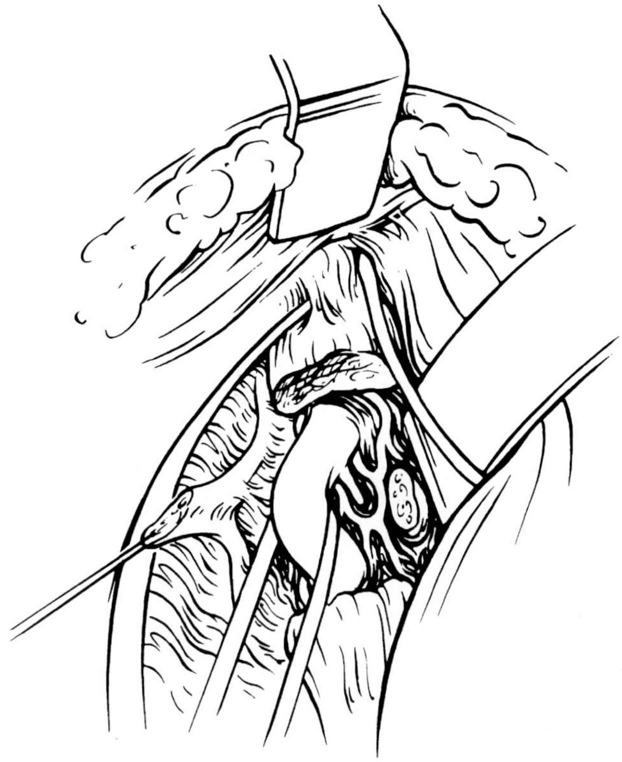

FIG 20.16 Exposure of the vertebral artery between the transverse processes of C1 and C2. The anterior ramus of the C2 nerve has been divided, and its anterior end is retracted with a stay suture. The artery has been dissected away from the surrounding vertebral plexus, which is now seen behind it.

fashion using 7-0 polypropylene sutures, best done using a parachuting open-type anastomosis.

In a few cases, this technique is not possible. The most frequent reason is a contralateral common or internal carotid artery occlusion or an abnormally short first segment of the vertebral artery entering the cervical spine through the transverse process of C7 rather than C6. If the opposite common or internal carotid artery is occluded, clamping the remaining ipsilateral common carotid artery to transpose the vertebral artery to it carries severe risk of brain ischemia. In this situation, a subclavian-to-vertebral artery bypass is preferred. If the vertebral artery is too short to be brought easily to the common carotid artery wall, it can also be bypassed from the subclavian artery using a saphenous vein graft.[22,23] The bypass originates from the subclavian artery lateral to the thyrocervical trunk and is anastomosed end to end to the vertebral artery proximal to the longus colli muscle. This procedure does not require any type of shunting. The most frequent complications from proximal vertebral artery dissection and transposition are partial Horner syndrome from manipulation (or injury) of the intermediate sympathetic ganglion overlying the vertebral artery and an occasional lymphocele from injury to, or failed ligature of, the main or accessory thoracic ducts.

Reconstruction of the Distal Vertebral Artery

Regardless of the level between C6 and C2 where the external compression or occlusive process occurs, the distal vertebral artery is reconstructed at the space between the C1 and C2 transverse processes (Fig. 20.16). This is the widest gap between transverse processes in the neck and is also the segment where the vertebral artery often remains patent by collaterals from the ascending cervical artery when the proximal segment of the artery is occluded.[24–26]

The operation is done through an incision similar to that used for carotid endarterectomy. Exposure of the vertebral artery at this level is done posterior to the jugular vein and identifying the spinal accessory nerve and the levator scapulae muscle. The levator muscle is cut off from its insertion on the transverse process of C1, exposing the anterior ramus of the C2 nerve. The vertebral artery lies under the ramus and is perpendicular to it. The ramus is cut, and the artery is exposed. Dissection of the vertebral artery may be made difficult by the plexus of veins that surrounds it.

Once the artery is isolated, it can be reconstructed in several ways. The most common reconstruction is a bypass from the common carotid artery to the distal vertebral artery immediately below the transverse process of C1 using autogenous vein (Fig. 20.17). This requires dissection of the common carotid below the bifurcation and the availability of a saphenous vein with a caliber approximating that of the vertebral artery. Once the end-to-side anastomosis of the vein graft to the vertebral artery is completed, the latter is ligated immediately below the anastomosis to avoid embolization or flow steal from its proximal segment.

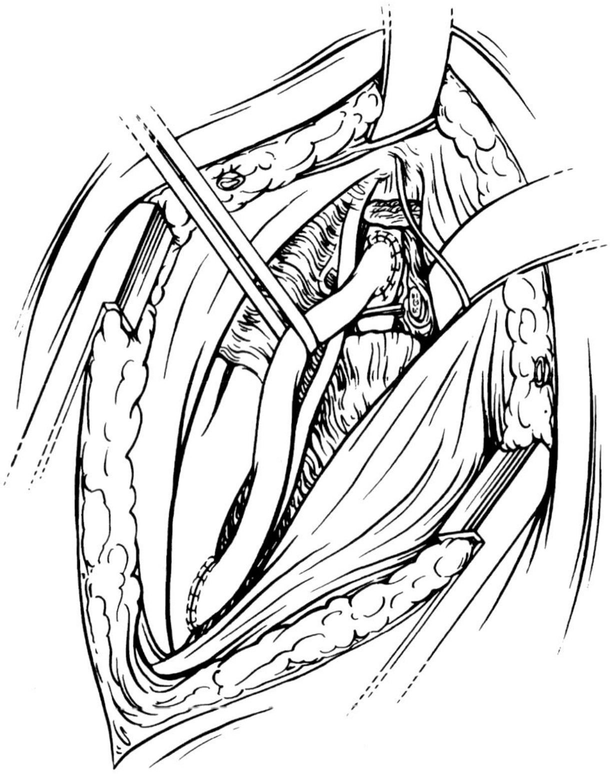

FIG 20.17 Completed common carotid-to-distal vertebral artery bypass graft. A metal clip occludes the distal vertebral artery immediately below the anastomosis, making it function as an end-to-end junction.

Another alternative is to use the external carotid artery (or, in rare cases, the occipital artery) to revascularize the distal vertebral artery (Fig. 20.18). The external carotid is skeletonized and transposed below the jugular vein, anastomosing it end to end to the distal vertebral artery. The appeal of this procedure is that it does not require clamping of the internal carotid supply and that the caliber match between the distal external carotid artery and the vertebral artery is usually good. This choice obviously requires that the external carotid artery and the carotid bifurcation be free of atherosclerotic disease. This type of operation is most suitable for individuals who have external compression or occlusion of the vertebral artery by osteophytes during neck rotation. These patients are generally younger and free of disease of the carotid bifurcation.

A third solution is transposing the distal segment of the vertebral artery to the neighboring internal carotid artery by means of an end-to-side anastomosis. This, again, has the appeal of a limited dissection and no need for a vein graft. The shortcoming is the need to clamp the internal carotid artery for the end-to-side anastomosis. This technique should not be used in patients in whom the opposite internal carotid artery is severely diseased or occluded.

A few patients have extrinsic compression or disease of the vertebral artery above the level of C1. In these patients, the reconstruction is done in the distalmost segment of the extracranial vertebral artery before it penetrates the dura mater as it courses over the lamina of the atlas (the pars atlantica). The approach is posterior through an inverted L-shaped incision

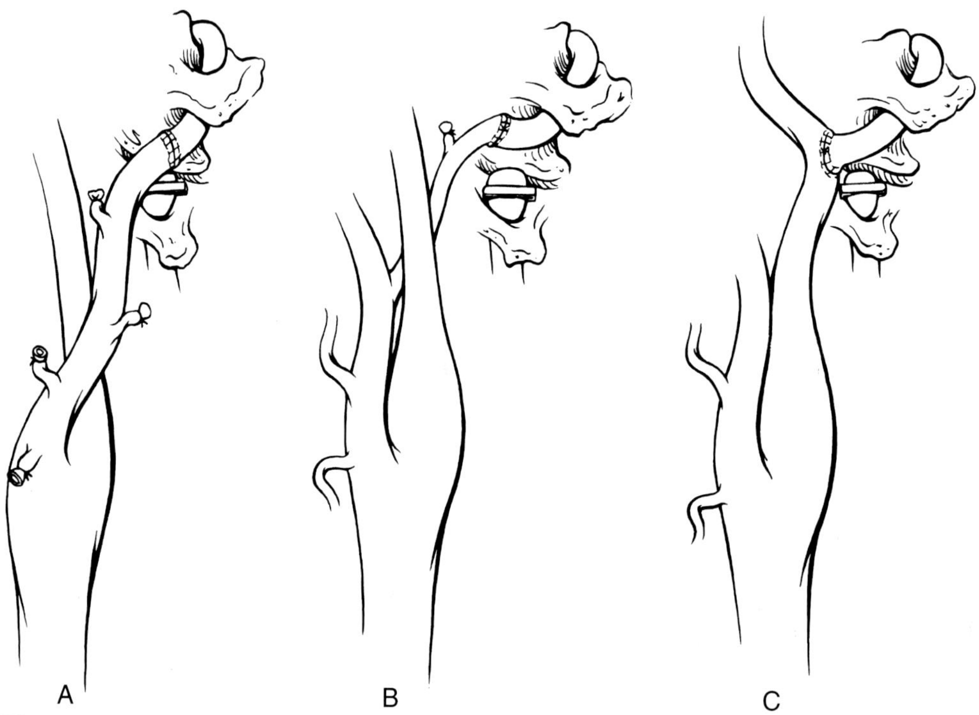

FIG 20.18 Alternative methods for reconstruction of the distal vertebral artery. (A) External carotid transposition to the distal vertebral artery. (B) Occipital artery transposition to the distal vertebral artery. (C) Transposition of the distal vertebral artery to the distal internal carotid artery.

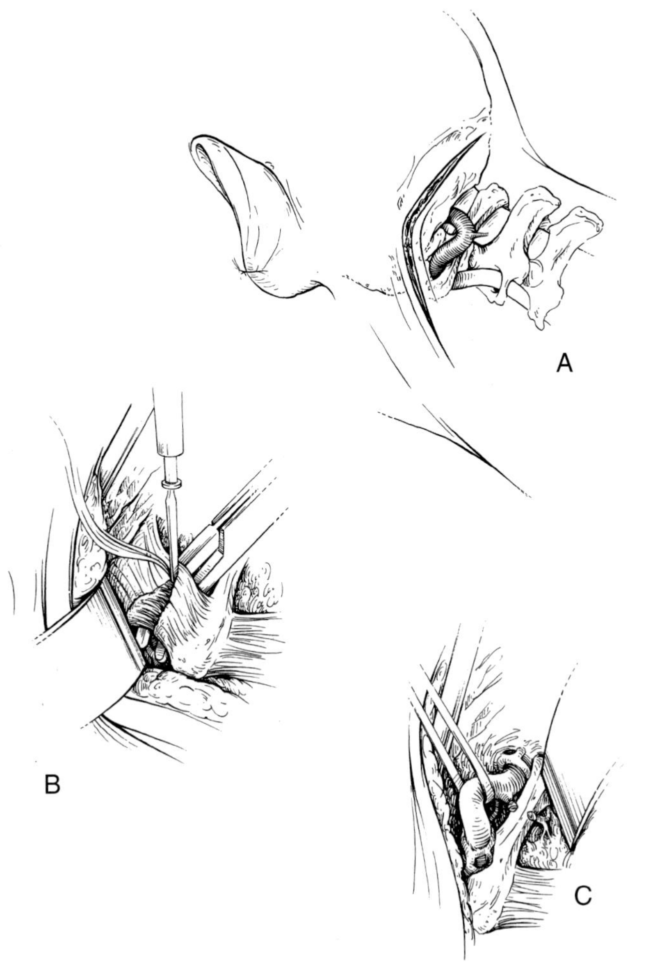

FIG 20.19 (A) Incision to approach the suboccipital segment of the vertebral artery. (B) Division of the obliquus capitis superior. (C) The looped vertebral artery is lifted from the underlying lamina of C1. A descending muscular branch has been ligated and divided. (From Berguer R: Revascularization of the vertebral arteries. In Nyhus LM, Baker RJ, Fischer JE, editors: *Mastery of surgery*, Boston, 1996, Little Brown.)

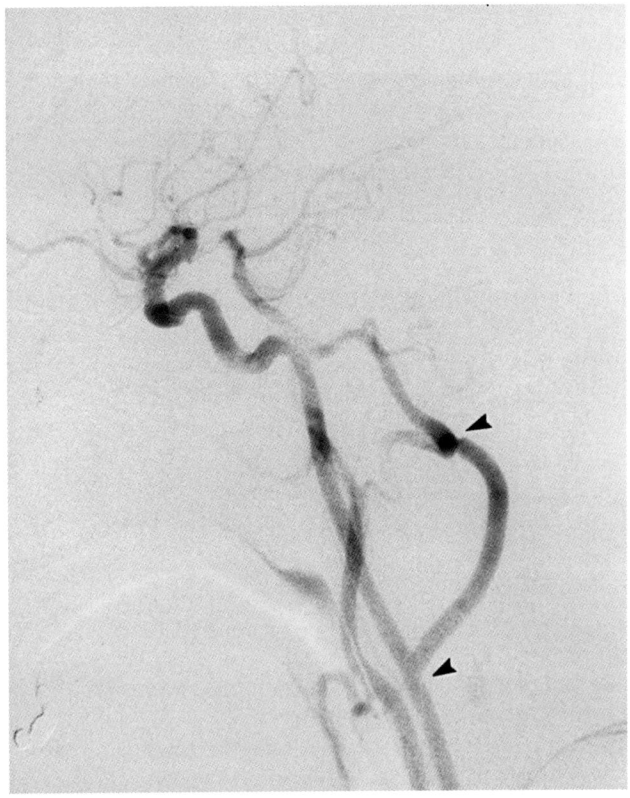

FIG 20.20 Postoperative arteriogram showing a bypass from the cervical internal carotid artery to the suboccipital vertebral artery *(arrowheads)* before its entry into the foramen magnum.

(Fig. 20.19) with the patient in the park-bench position. The semispinalis, splenius, and longus capitis muscles are cut, and the sternomastoid is de-inserted from the mastoid process. The transverse process of C1 is identified, and the obliquus capitis superior muscle is cut. The artery rests on the posterior lamina of the atlas, covered by a dense plexus of veins and tethered by one or two muscular branches, which are divided. The vein bypass is anastomosed end to side to the vertebral artery. The distal cervical internal carotid artery is isolated after dissecting the vagus and hypoglossal nerve trunks, which, in this posterior approach, overlie the internal carotid artery. The proximal end of the vein graft is anastomosed end to side to the distal cervical internal carotid artery (Fig. 20.20). In some patients, the vertebral artery is extrinsically compressed by bony structures between the occipital ridge and the posterior lamina of C1. In this situation, once the vertebral artery is dissected (using the suboccipital approach described here), a laminectomy of C1 eliminates the lower element of compression. Unless there is demonstrable damage to the wall of the vertebral artery by the bony impingement, a bypass is not needed.

The risks and patency rates of vertebral artery operations are different for proximal and distal repairs. Proximal reconstructions are technically easier. Distal reconstructions are more demanding and lengthier procedures. A series of 252 proximal vertebral artery reconstructions[26] reported a combined mortality and morbidity rate of 0.9%. No stroke or death occurred in 159 patients undergoing only a proximal vertebral artery reconstruction. The reported morbidity and mortality occurred in patients undergoing simultaneous carotid and vertebral artery reconstruction. The cumulative secondary patency rate for proximal reconstructions was 92% at 10 years in this series. Symptom resolution of vertebrobasilar ischemia occurred in 83% of patients, and the 5-year stroke-free survival was 97%.

Earlier experience with distal vertebral reconstructions carried combined mortality and morbidity rates between 2.4% and 3.4%, fourfold greater than that for proximal repairs.[27] The more recent experience has reduced the combined morbidity and mortality rates for proximal reconstruction to negligible levels, and to under 2% for distal vertebral reconstructions.

Postoperative thrombosis of a proximal reconstruction is rare. It may occur in cases where a short vertebral artery (entering at C7) may not be repaired by a standard vertebral-to-carotid transposition, and a subclavian-vertebral or carotid-vertebral bypass is performed. Tension at the anastomotic line, or kinking of an interposition vein graft, may result in postoperative graft thrombosis. Other complications of proximal reconstruction are an occasional lymphocele and a partial Horner syndrome from manipulation of or injury to the lower cervical sympathetic chain. During distal vertebral artery exposure, spinal accessory nerve injury may occur from undue traction on the nerve. Technical defects of the vein-to-vertebral anastomosis are more likely during reconstructions at the V3 segment, as exposure is more difficult in this segment. In addition, the vertebral artery can be rather small at this level where it is always a very friable vessel requiring extremely delicate handling.

REVIEW QUESTIONS

1. In a patient with a retroesophageal right subclavian artery, which of the following associated anomalies are expected or likely to occur: (1) nonrecurrent right inferior laryngeal nerve; (2) thoracic duct emptying on the right side; (3) common trunk as the origin of both common carotid arteries; (4) right vertebral artery arising from the right common carotid artery; or (5) left vertebral artery arising from the left common carotid artery?
   a. 1, 3, 4, 5
   b. 2, 3, 4, 5
   c. 1, 2, 3, 4
   d. 1, 2, 3, 4, 5
2. What is the most efficient operation to correct a severe stenosis of the origin of a vertebral artery?
   a. Subclavian-to-vertebral artery autogenous vein bypass
   b. Transposition of the vertebral artery to the common carotid artery
   c. Endarterectomy and patch of the origin of the vertebral artery
   d. Balloon angioplasty of the stenotic origin
3. Vertebrobasilar ischemia may be the result of which of the following: (1) a hemodynamically significant lesion of the vertebral artery; (2) a hemodynamically significant lesion of the basilar artery; (3) microembolization from a vertebral artery lesion; (4) microembolization from a subclavian artery plaque; or (5) microembolization from a dissected vertebral artery?
   a. 1, 3, 4, 5
   b. 1, 3, 5
   c. 1, 2, 5
   d. 1, 2, 3, 4, 5

BIBLIOGRAPHY

AbuRahma AF, Bates MC, Stone PA, et al. Angioplasty and stenting versus carotid to subclavian bypass for the treatment of isolated subclavian artery disease. *J Endovasc Ther*. 2007;14:698–704.

Owens LV, Tinsley EA, Criado E, Burham SJ, Keagy BA. Extrathoracic reconstruction of arterial occlusive disease involving the supraaortic trunks. *J Vasc Surg*. 1995;22:217–222.

Sfyroeras GS, Karathanos C, Antoniou GA, et al. A meta-analysis of combined endarterectomy and proximal balloon angioplasty for tandem disease of the arch vessels and carotid bifurcation. *J Vasc Surg*. 2011;54:534–540.

References available online at ExpertConsult.com.

CHAPTER 21

Endovascular Repair of Extracranial Cerebrovascular Lesions

Danielle E. Cafasso, Peter A. Schneider

Each year in the United States, nearly 800,000 individuals experience a new or recurrent stroke, accounting for direct and indirect costs of more than $40 billion and untold damage to patients and their families. Stroke is responsible for 1 out of every 20 deaths in the United States, making it the fifth leading cause of death. By 2030, it is projected that an additional 3.4 million adults will have had a stroke, a 20.5% increase in prevalence since 2012.[1] Carotid bifurcation stenosis and resultant ischemia producing emboli is a major cause of preventable stroke. Efforts to address this major health issue have focused on risk factor management, including medical therapy, and surgical or endovascular intervention.

Treatment of carotid disease has evolved considerably over the past 60 years with the introduction of the carotid endarterectomy (CEA) in the 1950s and carotid angioplasty in the late 1970s. During the 1990s, several landmark, randomized controlled trials (RCTs) in North America and Europe were published, which demonstrated the superiority of CEA plus medical management over medical management alone, affirming CEA as the gold standard for patients with carotid bifurcation stenosis.[2-9] Carotid stenting was introduced in the mid-1990s and has evolved with advances in technique, equipment, operator experience, and the routine use of cerebral protection devices. Carotid stenting has also been studied in multiple RCTs with long-term results.[10–12] Carotid angioplasty and stenting (CAS) is a viable minimally invasive alternative to CEA for select patient populations, and is continuing to develop as an option for treating carotid bifurcation stenosis. The purpose of this chapter is to describe the techniques available for CAS, provide an overview of current results, and offer perspective as to the value of this treatment in the management of extracranial cerebrovascular disease.

TECHNIQUE

Patient Selection for Carotid Angioplasty and Stenting

Appropriate patient selection for CAS is paramount to a successful procedure, and in minimizing perioperative complications and stroke risk. Part of the motivation in the development of CAS was to address the needs of patients at high risk for CEA in an attempt to improve results of carotid revascularization. In the United States, the Centers for Medicare and Medicaid Services (CMS) has established criteria for patient eligibility for endovascular carotid interventions on the basis of being high risk for CEA, identifying both physiologic and anatomic factors making the patient a high-risk candidate for an open surgical procedure (Box 21.1). Under the current national coverage determination (NCD) policy, CMS coverage for CAS is provided in symptomatic patients with carotid artery stenosis ≥70% or for high-risk patients with symptomatic stenosis ≥50% and asymptomatic stenosis ≥80% who are enrolled in Category B Investigations Device Exemption (IDE) trials or postapproval registries. The NCD requires the use of US Food and Drug Administration (FDA)-approved CAS systems and embolic protection devices, as well as CMS-approved institutions.[13,14] The use of CAS for patients at high risk for CEA is now an established practice; however, CMS coverage has a substantial impact on patient selection and may not have equipoise with evolving techniques and approaches to CAS.[13]

There are also factors that make patients high risk for CAS, which are primarily anatomic. Examples of poor anatomy for CAS include severe tortuosity of the aortic arch, great vessels, or carotid bifurcation, heavy calcification of these vessels, or unsuitable access. Marked angulation, kinks, and coils of the internal carotid artery (ICA) might not allow adequate room for appropriate deployment of cerebral protection devices (CPDs) with adequate wall apposition.[15] If these areas are straightened by stents, the angulation is usually displaced distally and may be more exaggerated. Difficult arch anatomy or severe calcification of the aortic arch and proximal branch vessels may preclude a safe transfemoral carotid intervention. Carotid bifurcation lesions that are recently symptomatic or are composed of soft plaque should also be avoided, if possible. These lesions also can be treated using proximal protection, so that the cerebral circulation is protected from emboli before crossing the lesion. Carotid bifurcation lesions that are too long to treat with a single stent also tend to add risk to the CAS procedure. Poor early results of CAS in older patients have prompted a high level of caution in octogenarians. A recent retrospective review of 135 octogenarians undergoing CAS reported a peri-interventional complication rate of 8.9%, with a low rate of neurological events over 33 months of follow-up. However, a high total death rate was reported, which may be due to the specific patient cohort and comorbidities and not necessarily procedurally related.[16] Extra evaluation for high-risk anatomy, preexisting brain lesions, evidence of cognitive problems, or other factors that may make repair more risky or limit its long-term value should be performed. In the early phases of CAS, these high-risk factors for performing CAS were not yet established. It is now recognized that CAS in its current form and with existing technology is not a direct replacement product for CEA. Nevertheless, the results of CAS have improved steadily over the past 15 years. One of the reasons for this is improved patient selection based on a better understanding of which patients are at high risk for CAS (Table 21.1).

CPDs have also evolved over the last decade from distal occlusion balloons to distal filters and, subsequently, the addition of proximal balloon occlusion or clamp occlusion and flow reversal techniques. Distal filters have replaced distal occlusion balloons that were cumbersome to deploy and compromised visualization of the ICA by occluding flow, and risks of ICA dissection.[17] Distal filter protection requires arch manipulation and crossing the lesion prior to filter placement. Furthermore, unprotected balloon dilation may be required to cross the lesion and place the filter. Thus cerebral embolization may occur before cerebral protection is established. Distal filters may not provide complete protection due to pore size, or lack of wall apposition, and they may become filled with debris, increasing the risk of embolization during retrieval.[17–20] Distal protection systems should not be used in distal ICA tortuosity, which may lead to inadequate vessel wall apposition and retrieval difficulty, or if there is an inadequate landing zone for the device. Proximal protection devices are useful for complex lesions, tortuous anatomy, or a symptomatic or ulcerated plaque that is at higher risk for distal embolization. Proximal occlusion devices stop or reverse flow in the ICA and eliminate crossing the lesion prior to embolic protection. The Medtronic MoMa proximal protection device uses balloon occlusion of the common carotid artery (CCA) and external carotid artery (ECA) to stop flow. The bifurcation is aspirated after stent placement. However, this system requires initial catheterization of the arch and great vessel origins as well as ECA occlusion prior to the establishment of protection, which both pose embolic risks. The direct trancervical approach using the ENROUTE transcarotid neuroprotection system (NPS) is another approach to CAS, which is designed to avoid the risk of embolization during unprotected catheterization of the aortic arch and supra-aortic vessels from a transfemoral approach. In

BOX 21.1 Centers for Medicare and Medicaid Services Criteria: Patients at High Risk for Carotid Endarterectomy

- Age >80 years
- Myocardial infarction
- Left ventricle ejection fraction <30%
- Contralateral carotid occlusion
- New York Heart Association class III or IV
- Unstable angina: Canadian Cardiovascular Society class III or IV
- Renal failure: end stage renal disease on dialysis
- Common carotid artery lesions below clavicle
- Severe pulmonary disease
- Clinically significant cardiac disease (congestive heart failure, abnormal stress test, or need for open-heart surgery)
- Previous neck radiation
- High cervical internal carotid artery lesion
- Restenosis of prior carotid endarterectomy
- Tracheostomy
- Contralateral laryngeal nerve palsy

TABLE 21.1 Summary of Published Results of Observational Studies of Carotid Angioplasty and Stenting

Study	Year of Publication	No. of Lesions	Cerebral Protection (%)	30-DAY OUTCOME Death (%)	30-DAY OUTCOME Stroke (%)
Wholey et al.[57]	1997	114	0	1.8	3.5
Yadav et al.[58]	1997	126	0	0.8	7.1
Henry et al.[59]	1998	174	18	0	2.9
Mathias et al.[60]	1999	799	NG	—	2.1
Shawl et al.[61]	2000	192	0	0	2.6
Wholey et al.[62]	2000	5,210	Very low	1.9	3.9
d'Audiffret et al.[63]	2001	83	18	—	4.4
Reimers et al.[64]	2001	88	100	—	1.1
Roubin et al.[65]	2001	604	0	1.6	5.8
Al Mubarak et al.[66]	2002	164	100	1.2	1.2
Criado et al.[67]	2002	135	0	0	2.2
Guimaraens et al.[68]	2002	194	100	1.9	1.0
Henry et al.[69]	2002	184	100	0.5	2.2
Koch et al.[70]	2002	167	0	—	7.5
Macdonald et al.[71]	2002	150	50	1.3	6.0
Whitlow et al.[72]	2002	75	100	0	0
Cremonesi et al.[73]	2003	442	100	—	2.0
Hobson et al.[74]	2003	114	0	1.8	0.9

this approach, the CCA is exposed through a short supraclavicular incision and cannulated directly. This requires adequate CCA length (a minimum of 6 cm from clavicle to bifurcation) and minimal atherosclerotic disease in the CCA to permit safe sheath placement and arterial clamping. A reversed-flow circuit is established between the CCA sheath and a femoral vein cannula. The minimal supraclavicular incision required for this approach remains a viable option in patients who are poor candidates for standard CEA due to poor arch anatomy, hostile neck anatomy, or medical unsuitability.[21]

The patient must be neurologically intact and able to follow commands to permit safe carotid stenting. Patients who cannot lie flat on the fluoroscopy table because of shortness of breath from cardiac or pulmonary problems will not tolerate intervention. Morbid obesity makes femoral access more challenging, as well as control of the access site after the procedure. Patients who cannot be treated safely with antiplatelet agents before and after the procedure, or who are at high risk for hemorrhagic complications, should not undergo endovascular carotid interventions.

Preprocedure Evaluation

Thorough evaluation and preparation of the patient before the procedure is essential for safe carotid intervention. The brachiocephalic anatomy is studied before the procedure to assess candidacy for the percutaneous approach. A thorough understanding of the arch, carotid, and cerebral arterial anatomy can be obtained with catheter-based arteriogram, computed tomographic angiogram (CTA), or magnetic resonance angiography (MRA). CTA is advantageous for multiple reasons. It is fast, depicts the arch anatomy well with good vessel wall and lumen definition, identifies calcifications, and can be used to measure the distance from the clavicle to the carotid bifurcation, which is important for the transcervical approach. MRA offers anatomical detail without radiation exposure, but it is slow and may be uncomfortable for some patients. Both CTA and MRA provide information on plaque morphology. Several anatomic factors can be considered relative contraindications to CAS, as mentioned previously, and these are well identified using preoperative imaging.

A National Institutes of Health (NIH) stroke scale or other objective evaluation is completed before to CAS. A CT or magnetic resonance image (MRI) of the brain is obtained in symptomatic patients and in those 80 years of age or older to evaluate for preprocedure cerebral pathology. Octogenarians have a higher risk of stroke with CAS; therefore, it should be performed with caution.[22] Antiplatelet therapy is administered: aspirin daily, and clopidogrel (Plavix) 75 mg/day for 5 days before the procedure. In all cases, patients should have received clopidogrel (total dose of 300 mg) before the intervention. Antihypertensive medication is held or decreased on the day of the procedure. If an antihypertensive is required during the procedure, it is best to use a short-acting agent. Postoperative hypotension or bradycardia can occur after CAS as a result of baroreceptor stimulation. Patients with aortic stenosis may have cardiovascular collapse in this setting, and external pacing pads or a temporary internal pacemaker should be placed. In patients with absent femoral pulses owing to aortoiliac occlusion or hostile groin anatomy, a transbrachial or transcervical approach may be considered.

The CAS procedure is performed using local anesthesia with minimal or no sedation to facilitate patient cooperation and continuous neurologic monitoring. Continuous arterial pressure monitoring is required. Techniques, such as squeezing a rubber toy, aid in simple and effective neurologic monitoring during the procedure.

Approved carotid stenting systems are limited to use in patients with symptomatic ≥50% stenosis, or asymptomatic ≥80% stenosis (Table 21.2). CAS in standard risk patients and those at high risk for CEA but who are asymptomatic are not currently approved for reimbursement under Medicare guidelines, unless it is performed as part of an approved clinical research protocol. Reconsideration of the extent of coverage of CAS by the CMS is likely to take place as a result of recent data accumulated through recent RCTs.

Access for Transfemoral Approach

Femoral artery access is the usual approach when planning to use a distal filter or proximal balloon occlusion for cerebral protection. The majority of CAS cases have been performed through

TABLE 21.2 High-Risk Prospective Registry Data

Name	Company	No. of Patients	Stent	Embolic Device	MAE (%)	Stroke (%)	Year Presented
ARCHER 1	Guidant	158	Acculink	None	7.6	4.4	2003
ARCHER 2	Guidant	278	Acculink	Accunet	8.6	6.8	2003
ARCHER 3	Guidant	145	Acculink	Accunet	8.3	7.6	2003
BEACH	BSC	480	Wallstent	Filterwire	5.8	4.4	2005
CABERNET	BSC	454	Nexstent	Filterwire	3.9	3.4	2005
CREATE	EV3	160	Acculink	SPIDERX	5.6	4.4	2005
SECuRITY	Abbott	305	Xactstent	Emboshield	7.5	6.2	2003
MAVErIC	Medtronic	399	Exponent	PercuSurge	5	3	2004

ARCHER, The Acculink for Revascularization of Carotids in High-Risk Patients; *BEACH,* Boston Scientific EPI: a carotid stenting trial for high-risk surgical patients; *CABERNET,* Carotid Artery Revascularization Using the Boston Scientific Filterwire EX system and the EndoTex NextStent Carotid Stent; *CREATE,* Carotid Revascularization with the EV3 Arterial Technology Evolution; *SECuRITY,* Registry Study to Evaluate the Neuroshield Bare Wire Cerebral protection System and X-act Stent in Patients at High Risk for Carotid Endarterectomy; *MAE,* major adverse event; *MAVErIC,* Evaluation of the Medtronic Self-Expanding Carotid Stent with Distal Protection of Carotid Artery Stenosis.

femoral artery access. The right common femoral approach is the most convenient for catheter manipulations by the right-handed surgeon, but the left is acceptable as well if the right side is hostile. A micropuncture set (21-gauge needle) can be used for the initial femoral access; this has significantly reduced the number of femoral access complications. The use of ultrasound during puncture has become routine, and it has enhanced the ability to use closure devices at the conclusion of the procedure. Following guidewire access, an introducer sheath is placed in the common femoral artery, which is the same size as that intended for the carotid stent placement (typically 6 or 7 French) or CPD (8 or 9 French for the MoMa device). If a brachial approach is planned, access to the CCA is usually best obtained from the contralateral brachial artery. Transcervical access will also be discussed later in this chapter.

Arch Evaluation

Arch manipulation carries a risk of neurologic events. In several studies of CAS, up to 1% of patients sustained a stroke in the contralateral hemisphere, suggesting that carotid access is a contributor to morbidity.[23,24] Systemic heparin should be administered before aortic arch manipulation. An activated clotting time (ACT) of 250 seconds or greater is desired.

Following systemic anticoagulation, an arch aortogram is performed using a multi-sidehole flush catheter (e.g., pigtail catheter) with the image intensifier in a left anterior oblique (LAO) position. The goal is to obtain an en face view of the aortic arch as it traverses posterior and laterally toward the patient's left. An angle of 30 to 45 degrees LAO usually provides an optimal view of the origins of the arch vessels. The pigtail catheter is subsequently withdrawn over a 260-cm angled Glidewire. The guidewire and pigtail catheter should be pulled back together into the descending aorta where the pigtail can then be removed and the guidewire can be advanced into the ascending aorta. As few manipulations as possible are performed in the aortic arch and great vessels to lower the risk of an iatrogenic embolic event.

Hypertension and advanced age are associated with increased tortuosity of the access pathway to the carotid bifurcation. This makes no difference in the performance of CEA, but directly influences the challenges posed for transfemoral CAS. Negotiating the tortuous arch requires more manipulation for catheterization, a more embedded position of the exchange guidewire, and more maneuvers to achieve sheath placement. The tortuosity of the arch can be assessed rapidly by drawing a horizontal line across the apex of the inner curvature of the arch.[25] Vessels that originate below the horizontal line at the apex of the aortic arch (e.g., branches that arise from the ascending aorta) are more difficult to selectively cannulate (Fig. 21.1). The authors caution against transfemoral carotid stenting in the setting of a "difficult arch" until the operator has become expert with selective cannulation of the common carotid arteries in this situation. Even then, the

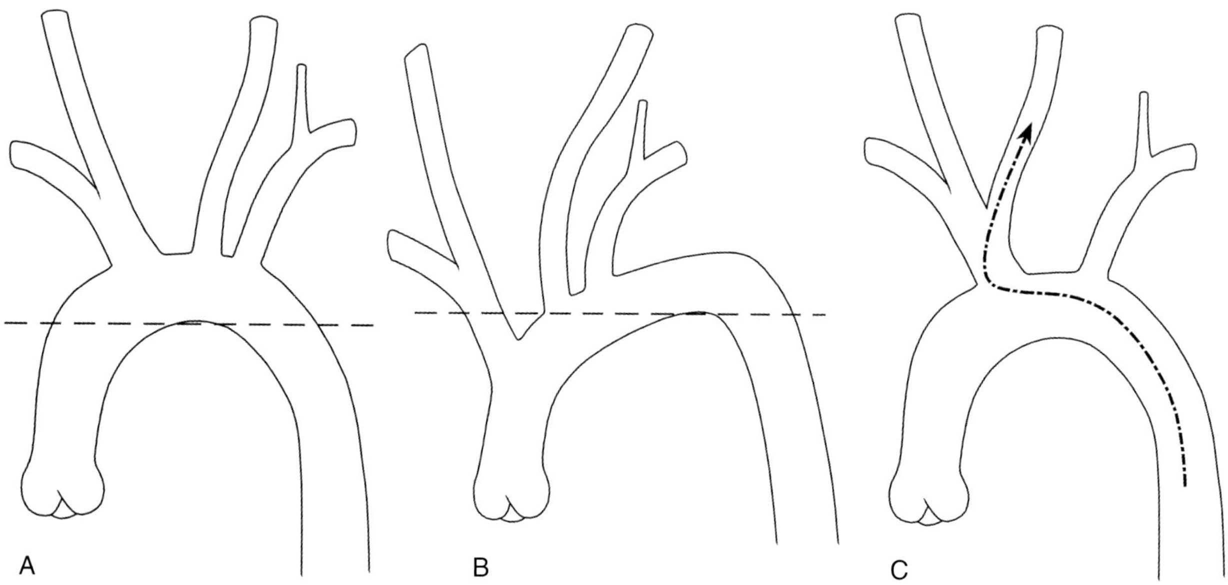

FIG 21.1 Evaluation of the Aortic Arch. The arch of the aorta can be assessed rapidly for anticipated challenge in selective catheterization of the arch branches. Draw a horizontal line across the upper, inner crest of the aortic arch. (A) When arch branches originate from the top of the arch, they are usually straightforward to selectively catheterize. (B) When arch branches originate from the upslope of the ascending aorta, the upper, inner aspect or crest of the arch serves as a fulcrum over which the cerebral catheter must work to achieve selective access. This is the situation in which a reversed curve catheter is particularly helpful. This can be assessed easily by drawing a horizontal line across the upper inner aspect of the arch of the aorta. (C) The bovine arch configuration can be a challenge when treating the left carotid artery. The origin of the artery is displaced toward the patient's right and the vessel path courses to the patient's left, creating a sharp turn from the arch into the left common carotid artery (see *dotted line*).

tortuous arch likely poses a slight increase in the overall risk of CAS. Training and credentialing documents suggest varying numbers of carotid arteriograms as a prerequisite to initiating CAS training.[26,27]

SELECTIVE COMMON CAROTID CANNULATION

Selective cannulation can be accomplished using one of two preshaped catheters; a simple curve catheter such as a vertebral catheter or a complex curve catheter such as the reversed-angle Vitek catheter (VTK). The image intensifier is maintained in its fixed position (i.e., LAO) and landmarks or roadmapping can be used to guide vessel cannulation. The first-choice catheter in most cases is a simple curve catheter. The simple curve catheter is passed into the ascending aorta. The guidewire is retracted into the shaft of the catheter to permit the catheter tip to function on its own, without the added stiffness of the wire. The catheter is withdrawn slowly into the arch, and its tip is rotated superiorly. When the catheter tip engages the arch branch, the catheter is rocked gently side to side to allow it to "seed" itself into the CCA. These are very slight movements while visualizing the catheter tip to see that it is taking a shape consistent with position in the arch branch. The guidewire is advanced, slowly at first to ensure that it does not catch on the wall and kick the catheter tip out of the artery. Once the guidewire has accessed the CCA, the simple curve catheter is advanced over the guidewire into the mid-CCA for selective angiograms of the carotid artery and its bifurcation. Be careful to avoid inadvertently passing the guidewire into the carotid artery bifurcation. As the cerebral catheter rounds the turn from the arch into the CCA, it tends to straighten the wire out and may prompt the catheter and wire to jump forward. Meticulous adherence to the fundamentals of wire and catheter handling is essential to avoid unintentional movement of devices in the carotid artery or to introduce air bubbles.

Complex curve or reversed-angle catheters such as the VTK are usually required when the aortic arch is tortuous, the common carotid arteries are retroflexed toward the patient's left, or there is a bovine arch configuration (Fig. 21.2). Complex curve catheters are best reformed in the proximal descending aorta and then pushed proximally into the arch. The catheter is advanced into the arch with the tip angled anteriorly and then the tip is angled superiorly as the branch of choice for catheterization is approached. After the tip is engaged into the CCA of choice, the catheter is adjusted slightly, usually with a gentle pull, to allow the elbow of the catheter (located at the second curve of a reversed curve or complex curve catheter) to reach its optimal intended configuration and seed itself in the artery origin. Arteriography can be performed from this position, and the catheter is unlikely to slip out. However, reversed-angle catheters cannot be as easily advanced into the branch vessels after cannulation of the origin. They are used mainly to access the origin of the branch vessels for a selective angiogram of the carotid arteries. Advancing the reverse curve catheter into the ECA requires that as much wire as possible be placed beyond the catheter tip. Because of the reverse angle, a forward push on the catheter shaft when it does not have a reasonably robust rail of wire to pass along will advance the catheter shaft further proximally into the aortic arch and actually drag the tip out of the CCA.

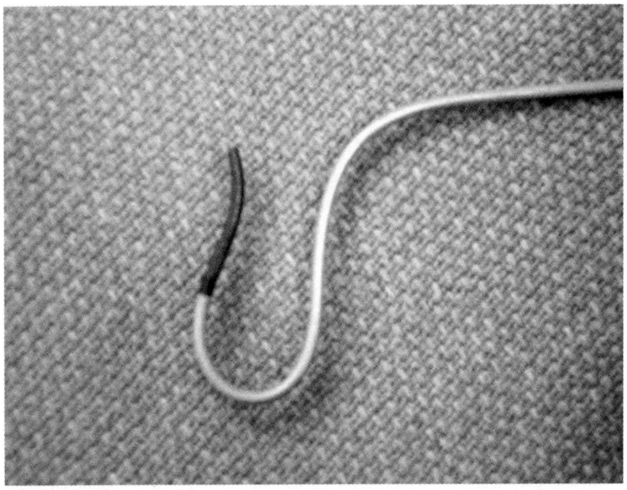

FIG 21.2 Complex-curve or reversed-curve cerebral catheters, such as the Vitek, can be used to catheterize branches arising from a tortuous arch. A severely retroflexed common carotid artery or a bovine arch configuration may also be approached with the Vitek catheter. There is a first bend near the tip of the catheter and a second, more acute bend to approximately 180 degrees (an elbow shape), which allows the tip of the catheter to point in a direction opposite from the direction of the catheter shaft.

After selective cannulation of the CCA, angiograms are usually performed with half-strength contrast. The carotid bifurcation usually is best visualized in the ipsilateral oblique or lateral position. Multiple views may be required to best unfold the carotid bifurcation. This is necessary since the next step usually involves selective cannulation of the ECA. If an arteriogram or CT angiogram was performed before the CAS procedure, optimal angles for viewing the open carotid bifurcation can usually be derived from these studies. If a lateral view of the carotid bifurcation is required to open the carotid bifurcation and cannulate the ECA, after the exchange guidewire is anchored in place, the sheath is best advanced using an LAO view. This permits the operator to best visualize the pathway of the sheath as it crosses from the arch to the CCA. This is the location where the sheath is most likely to encounter an obstacle.

Lateral and craniocaudal anteroposterior intracranial images are obtained if cerebral artery imaging has not already been done before CAS to identify any intracranial pathology and to document the intracranial circulation before CAS. Contrast is administered at 3 to 5 mL/s for 2 seconds with a rate of rise of 0.5 seconds.

CAROTID SHEATH ACCESS THROUGH TRANSFEMORAL APPROACH

Carotid sheath access requires placement of an adequate length of exchange guidewire into the CCA. When the arch is straightforward and there is no tortuosity and the CCA is of

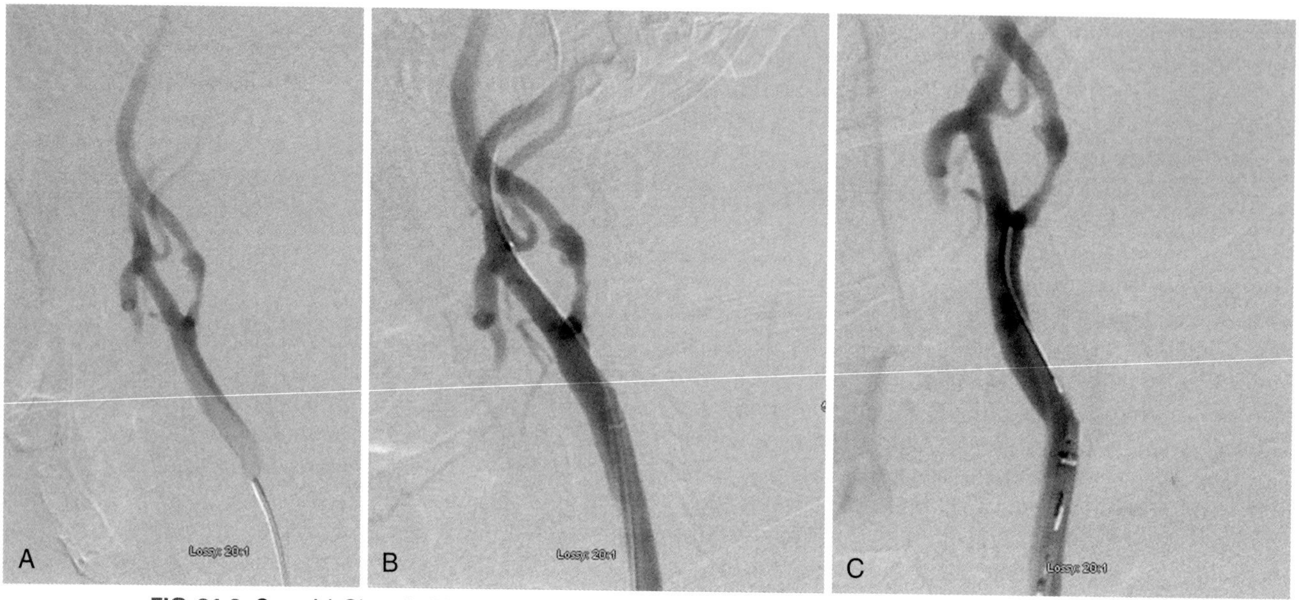

FIG 21.3 Carotid Sheath Placement. (A) A landmark is selected from the carotid angiogram performed before sheath placement, and this is used to help decide where to place the tip of the sheath and to stop sheath advancement. (B) The external carotid artery is usually catheterized and a stiff exchange guidewire is placed. The cerebral catheter is withdrawn and the exchange guidewire is used as a rail over which to place a 6- or 7-French 90-cm-long carotid access sheath. (C) During sheath advancement, the image intensifier is placed in the left anterior oblique position, and the tip of the exchange guidewire is observed. The progress of the sheath tip is monitored as it makes the turn from the aortic arch into the common carotid artery. If the tip of the guidewire begins to back up, sheath advancement should be stopped because this is a sign that the rail is not adequate for sheath passage.

adequate length, this can be accomplished by placing the tip of the exchange guidewire in the distal CCA. However, more often, it is necessary to place a greater length of exchange guidewire than what can be provided by advancing the exchange wire to the distal CCA. This can be accomplished by placing the exchange guidewire into the ECA and using it to anchor the stiff guidewire to create an adequate rail for sheath advancement (Fig. 21.3). Selective external carotid cannulation can be accomplished with a 260-cm angled guidewire and the vertebral catheter. An attempt should be made to reach as distal as possible in the ECA. This allows adequate guidewire length for the subsequent placement of the carotid sheath. The Glidewire is then withdrawn from the vertebral catheter, and a 260-cm Amplatz Super Stiff or other exchange guidewire is passed into the ECA. Passage of the stiff exchange guidewire into the small ECA branches must be done with caution to avoid injury or perforation to these branches. Caution should also be used during wire exchanges. Removing the wire too quickly can create a vacuum, resulting in introduction of air bubbles along the luminal surface of the catheter. It is sometimes helpful to administer contrast into the catheter to confirm external carotid placement. Contrast injections into the carotid system should not be done unless free backflow of blood is present at the hub of the diagnostic catheter. Otherwise there is a risk of pushing microbubbles into the system. In the ECA, back bleeding can at times be diminished by the tight fit of the catheter in the small ECA branches. In this event, the cerebral catheter is slowly withdrawn until adequate backflow is noted.

The vertebral catheter is withdrawn, leaving the Amplatz guidewire in the ECA. The groin access sheath is removed. A 90-cm-long sheath (Destination by Terumo [Somerset, NJ] or Shuttle Sheath by Cook [Bloomington, IN]) is advanced over the Amplatz guidewire into the CCA. Image the tip of the Amplatz guidewire in the ECA and the last turn from the arch into the CCA during sheath passage. If the tip of the advancing sheath hangs at the turn into the CCA or the tip of the guidewire moves back, it indicates that the sheath is not advancing appropriately over the guidewire. Reassess the curvature in the system and ensure that an adequate length of stiff exchange guidewire is present. The dilator tip for the 90-cm carotid sheath is long and not well visualized during fluoroscopy. Identify the optimal length for the dilator to protrude from the sheath and lock the Y-adaptor on the back end of the dilator in this position. After the dilator and sheath are advanced fully into the CCA, and if a position closer to the bifurcation is needed, the dilator is held steady while the sheath is advanced over it. The stiff exchange guidewire and the dilator are withdrawn, and the carotid angiogram is repeated through the carotid sheath with a road map of the carotid bifurcation stenosis in preparation for filter placement.

CEREBRAL PROTECTION USING DISTAL FILTERS

There are no large, randomized trials comparing CAS with and without cerebral protection devices, although their use has become

BOX 21.2 Commercially Available Cerebral Protection Devices by Category

Distal Filter
- Angioguard XP
- Emboshield
- FilterWire EX, EZ
- AccuNet
- SPIDER
- Fibernet

Distal Occlusion
- PercuSurge Guardwire

Proximal Occlusion
- MoMa

BOX 21.3 Advantages and Disadvantages of Distal Filter

Advantages
- Preservation of antegrade flow
- Less spasm than distal occlusion devices
- Angiographic evaluation of lesion during procedure

Disadvantages
- Larger crossing profile
- Potential thrombosis or occlusion of filter
- Unprotected during passage of filter
- Must pass retrieval catheter through stent

the standard practice after early data suggested a decrease in embolic complications.[15] The CMS also mandates CPD use for endovascular carotid interventions. There are numerous commercially available CPDs (Box 21.2) that are categorized as follows: distal filter, distal occlusion balloon, and proximal occlusion balloon.

Distal filter placement has been the most commonly used CPD. The filter is placed distal to the lesion before stent placement, on a 0.014-inch guidewire system. These devices vary in shape and deployment, but once in place, they permit continuous antegrade flow into the intracranial ICA while serving as a barrier to embolic debris. Distal filters generally capture particles greater than 100 μm in size. Filters may be fixed to the wire or separate from the initial guidewire. The fixed-guidewire systems are simpler and require fewer steps. However, in the fixed-guidewire system, any guidewire movement after the filter is deployed results in movement of the filter itself. In addition, the attachment of the filter to the guidewire limits the handling of the guidewire during lesion traversal. The free-guidewire systems permit a choice of guidewires. When there is substantial tortuosity, a complex lesion, or other challenges, the free-guidewire systems have an advantage. The advantage of filters is that they allow continued cerebral perfusion, particularly in patients who have inadequate collateral circulation to permit temporary carotid occlusion (Box 21.3).

Proximal balloon occlusion devices do not require crossing the lesion before establishing embolic protection (Box 21.4). Such devices provide protection by occluding the common and external carotid arteries, after which collateral flow through the circle of Willis creates a back-pressure that prevents antegrade flow into the ICA.

BOX 21.4 Advantages and Disadvantages of Proximal Occlusion

Advantages
- Complete protection prior to lesion manipulation
- Not limited by tight or tortuous lesions
- No guidewire restrictions
- Angiographic evaluation of lesion during procedure

Disadvantages
- Larger sheath introducer size
- Interruption of flow during procedure
- Potential dissection/spasm in common carotid artery or external carotid artery

TECHNIQUE FOR USE OF DISTAL FILTERS

The distal filter should be placed only after the sheath is in a stable position in the CCA. Any movement of the sheath after filter placement could also move the filter. If the sheath should flip back into the arch during the procedure while the filter is deployed, the filter may be withdrawn into the lesion or tangle with the stent. The supporting guidewire for the filter is not sturdy enough to support a repeated advancement of the sheath, so the sheath must be placed in its optimal position during initial approach. After placement of the CCA sheath, the appropriate guidewire for the selected filter is used to cross the target lesion. The tip of the leading guidewire is hand-shaped with a curve, usually a hockey-stick shape, to provide directionality for crossing the lesion. Most lesions that are isolated to the proximal ICA are posterior wall plaques. In passing the guidewire tip to cross the lesion, the best pathway is usually anterior in the proximal ICA, just behind the flow divider. Bifurcation lesions that involve the distal CCA are often more complex and contain a less predictable pathway for the wire. The key is to lead with the guidewire tip; do not make a loop, and be gentle in probing the lesion. Each encounter with the lesion is an opportunity to produce a neurologic event. Once the lesion is crossed with the guidewire tip, the filter device is advanced across the target lesion into a straight, normal segment of the distal extracranial ICA distal to the lesion by a few centimeters, and deployed. When using a fixed-wire filter system, there is an abrupt transition in device size and stiffness from the floppy wire tip to the filter fixed to the wire. In a tortuous or critically stenotic lesion, the filter may not cross the lesion, even though the leading wire tip is safely across. In this case, it is advisable to go slowly with gentle forward pressure, and it is sometimes helpful to slightly rock the catheter back and forth, and carefully observe the system under a magnification view to ensure that the system is tracking and not buckling. Placing the filter into a landing zone that is tortuous may be difficult and could impede filter function. The landing zone for the filter is assessed in advance; it must be reachable with the proposed filter and be long enough and straight enough to accommodate the filter. An ACT of 250 seconds or higher is required before placing filter devices.

The crossing profile of the constrained filter may be larger than the residual lumen in a tight stenosis. Occasionally it may be difficult to cross extremely stenotic, tortuous, or calcified lesions. A "buddy wire" may be helpful in providing extra support during filter placement. A slightly larger sheath is needed to accommodate a buddy wire, such as a 7-French sheath. If tortuosity is the issue, sometimes it can be improved by placing a stiff but low-profile guidewire into the ECA. Tortuosity may also be improved by having the patient change the neck position, capitalizing on the natural mobility of the carotid artery. When a tight lesion cannot be crossed with a filter, occasionally a balloon predilation with a 2.0- or 2.5-mm-diameter angioplasty balloon is required. When critically stenotic carotid lesions or highly tortuous carotid bifurcations are involved, the use of a "free-wire" filter system (e.g., Emboshield [AbbottVascular, Santa Clara, CA], Spider [Medtronic, Minneapolis, MN]) has advantages over a fixed-wire system (e.g., Accunet [AbbottVascular, Santa Clara, CA], Filterwire [Boston Scientific, Natick, MA]).

The image intensifier is positioned so that the tip of the sheath is visible on the inferior aspect of the monitor screen and the filter is visible on the superior aspect. In this manner, the stability of the system can be observed during treatment of the lesion. If the filter becomes filled with debris, it must be aspirated. When removing a full filter following the completion of an angiogram, it is important not to recapture it completely, because debris may be extruded from it and embolize distally. If there is evidence of a filling defect within the filter, or some indication that it may contain debris, catheter aspiration is performed prior to retrieval. The usual tendency during the procedure is for any tension on the guidewire to result in partial withdrawal of the filter; this can induce spasm or spill any debris that the filter holds. Another potential problem is for the filter to tangle with the stent (Box 21.5).

The Mo.Ma Ultra cerebral protection device is a proximal occlusion device that prevents antegrade flow in the ICA. The system is compatible with an 8- or 9-French sheath. Femoral access is obtained, the CCA is cannulated and an exchange guidewire is placed into the ECA. The Mo.Ma catheter is placed into the CCA. The Mo.Ma Ultra system is advanced over the wire under fluoroscopy until the distal marker is positioned in the ECA. The distal marker is on the ECA balloon, which should be positioned far enough into the ECA so it does not slip back into the CCA upon inflation but less than 1.5 cm from the bifurcation so the CCA balloon does not interfere with stent deployment. Remove the mandrel and gently inflate the ECA balloon. Confirm ECA occlusion with a contrast injection. The 0.035-inch guidewire can then be removed and CCA balloon inflated. Inflation of the CCA balloon is performed gradually and the shape of the balloon is observed. If it is overinflated, the balloon may prolapse over the tip of the sheath. Flow cessation can be confirmed by first aspirating 10 mL of blood and then slowly injecting contrast medium through the working channel. The contrast medium will stagnate in the occluded segment, verifying that cerebral protection is achieved, and the remaining portion of the carotid artery stent procedure can be performed. A 0.014-inch guidewire of the operator's choice is then passed across the carotid lesion after proximal protection has been established. At the completion of the procedure, debris removal by aspiration is performed while the occlusion balloons remain fully inflated. Debris removal should aspirate 60 mL of blood and continue aspiration until no additional debris is visible. Once debris removal is completed, restoration of antegrade flow is established by deflating the ECA and then the CCA balloons under fluoroscopy.[28]

DIRECT CERVICAL ACCESS TO THE COMMON CAROTID ARTERY

Proximal protection can also be achieved using direct open cervical access to the CCA. Transcarotid stenting with dynamic flow reversal is a novel technique that may decrease the risk of cerebral embolization. The technique requires a transcervical CCA exposure through a supraclavicular incision and percutaneous femoral vein access. A flow reversal circuit is created by placing an 8-French sheath in the CCA and another one in the common femoral vein. The CCA is exposed using a short supraclavicular incision; this is usually performed in a transverse fashion (Fig. 21.4). The sternal head of the sternocleidomastoid muscle is divided. At this level, the jugular vein is usually anterior to the CCA. The jugular vein is mobilized laterally to expose the CCA for a few

BOX 21.5 Advantages and Disadvantages of Distal Occlusion

Advantages
- Complete protection of distal ICA
- Low crossing profile
- High flexibility
- No sizing issues

Disadvantages
- Interruption of blood flow during protection
- Potential dissection/spasm in distal ICA
- Potential embolization via external carotid artery
- No angiographic evaluation of lesion during procedure
- Prolonged procedure time
- Unprotected during passage of balloon

ICA, internal carotid artery.

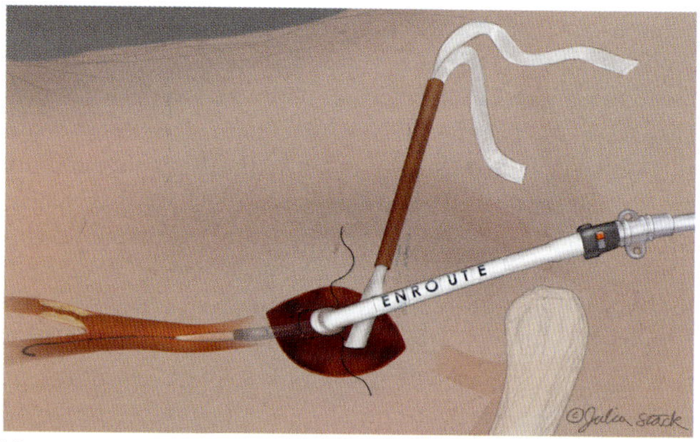

FIG 21.4 Transcervical Exposure. A short transverse supraclavicular incision is performed. The proximal common carotid artery is exposed and looped in preparation for direct access.

cm. A 5-0 pursestring suture is place in the anterior wall of the CCA. A micropuncture needle is placed through a pursestring suture for later closure. During preoperative evaluation with CTA or duplex, the distance from the clavicle to the bifurcation is measured and must be a minimum of 6 cm for this technique to be applicable. When the initial wires are introduced, care must be taken to avoid passage of the wire inadvertently into the bifurcation. The CCA sheath has a stopper on the tip that allows its insertion only 3 cm into the artery to avoid encroaching upon the bifurcation. After placement of the sheath in the CCA and the sheath in the femoral vein, the sheaths are connected by a large-bore regulated flow line to create an arteriovenous shunt (Fig. 21.5). There is a filter in the circuit to capture any debris that may be liberated from the treatment site. The flow in the circuit can be modified for high or low flow or for temporary cessation of flow for angiography. The CCA is proximally occluded with a vascular clamp or Rummel tourniquet. The circuit creates a low-pressure gradient creating flow reversal in the ICA. After proximal protection with reversed flow is established, a guidewire of the operator's choice is advanced across the lesion. The CAS procedure is completed through the CCA sheath during flow reversal. After stent placement and completion angiography, the reversal of flow may be continued for a few minutes, if desired, to help ensure that all the removable debris have exited the site. The CCA is then unclamped and the sheath removed, using the previously placed pursestring suture to close the puncture site. The neck incision is closed in standard fashion. The femoral vein sheath is also removed and direct pressure held for hemostasis.

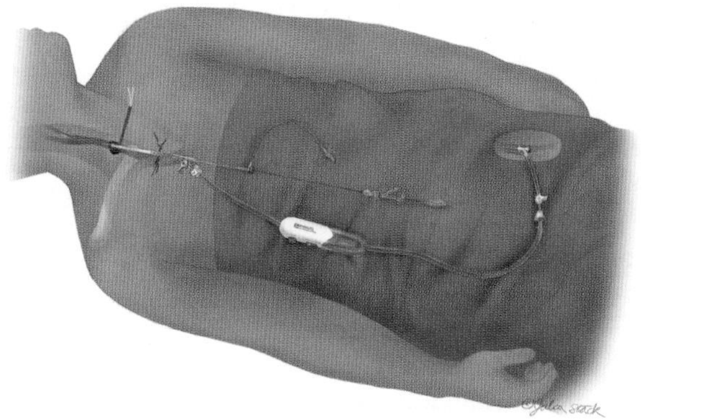

FIG 21.5 Establishment of a Reversed-Flow Circuit. The common carotid artery (CCA) sheath is connected to the common femoral vein sheath using tubing with an in-line filter and the capability of regulated flow. Prior to crossing the carotid lesion, the CCA is clamped.

STENT PLACEMENT

Predilation is performed selectively before stent placement with a 3-mm rapid exchange balloon, usually 4 cm in length to avoid "watermelon seeding" of the balloon upon inflation (Fig. 21.6). Some operators routinely administer small doses of atropine or glycopyrrolate before balloon dilation, except in patients with a recurrent stenosis, because the carotid bulb is already denervated in these patients. The pressure used for predilatation is nominal for the balloon used. Use higher pressure (14 to 16 atm) in heavily calcified stenoses. The duration of the predilation depends on the appearance and behavior of the balloon. If the balloon immediately attains its full shape, which it usually does, the predilation time is shorter. Observe the monitor for bradycardia if a prolonged inflation is required. If there is significant bradycardia with predilation, there is a high likelihood that bradycardia will occur after stent placement and dilation.

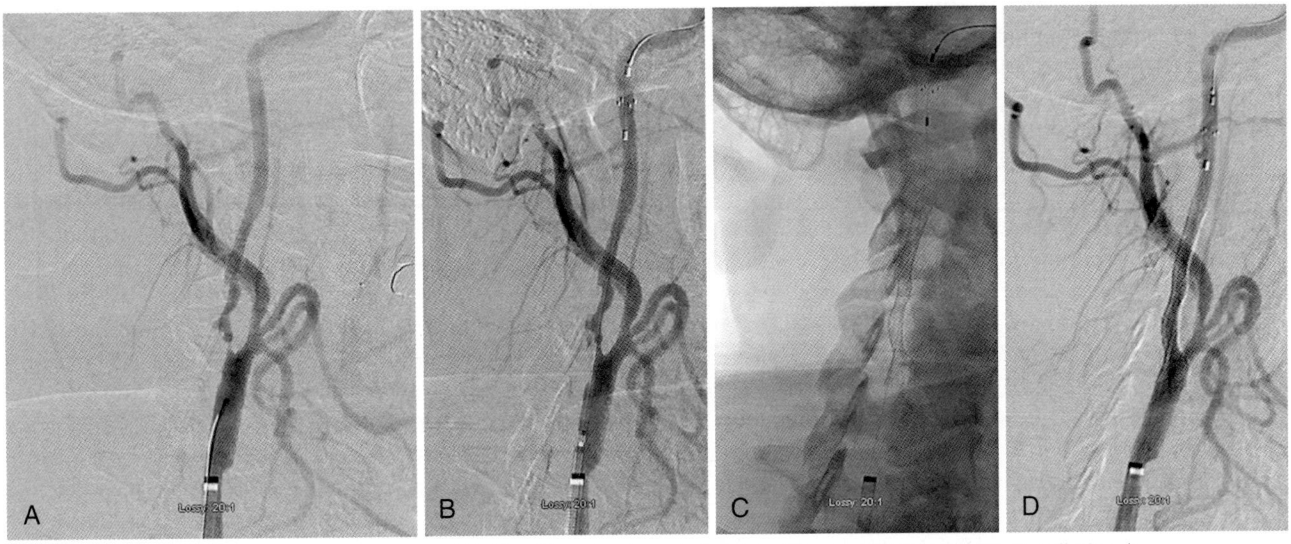

FIG 21.6 Stent Placement. (A) The filter is placed distal to the carotid lesion. (B) Predilation is performed. (C) The carotid stent is placed across the lesion, from nondiseased internal carotid artery (ICA) distal to the lesion to the common carotid artery. (D) After poststent dilation, there is excellent prograde flow across the ICA and a widely patent stent.

A variety of self-expanding stents are available for use and are approved by the FDA. Self-expanding stents are classified as open cell or closed cell. The open-cell stents have larger cells, in general, and there is suggestion that this may invite more late-stage emboli through the tines of the stent. However, post-CAS neurologic events are multifactorial, and specific variables are difficult to isolate. The open-cell stents are also more easily contoured than the closed-cell stents and can handle tortuosity better. Closed-cell stents have smaller cells, more outward radial force in general, and are less flexible. Closed-cell stents are also easier to cross with the filter retrieval catheter. Mesh-covered stents are designed to prevent plaque protrusion and embolization after stent implantation while also providing the flexibility of an open-cell stent. None of the mesh-covered stents are approved for use in the United States, but several are currently being evaluated. The self-expanding stent is deployed using a bifurcation roadmap. The stent is placed from normal artery distal to the lesion to normal artery proximal to the lesion. The stent length is usually 30 or 40 mm. The stent should be selected and placed so that the proximal end of the stent has at least several millimeters of adherence and apposition to the CCA wall. In most cases, the stent is placed across the bifurcation; therefore, the stent diameter is sized for the CCA diameter. For example, an 8- or 9-mm diameter CCA may prompt the selection of a 10-mm diameter stent, since the self-expanding stent must be oversized to adhere properly to the wall of the healthy artery juxtaposed to the lesion. The self-expanding stent is usually postdilated with a 5-mm balloon; rarely is a 6-mm balloon required after stent deployment. Each step of the stent procedure is associated with the potential for transcranial doppler (TCD) hits, but postdilation seems to produce more TCD hits than other steps. Following stent deployment, shorter (2-cm) balloons are used to dilate the narrow portion of the stent where the residual stenosis is visible using fluoroscopy. If the stent has assumed a reasonable profile after placement, postdilation may not be required. Avoid overdilation, even though this is how lesions in multiple other vascular beds are treated. The difference in the carotid is that the stent is used as scaffolding; it provides continuous expansile energy after the procedure, and there is a desire to avoid disrupting the lesion more than necessary. The patient may again be pretreated with a small dose of vagalytic to blunt the carotid sinus response to stretching. A mild to moderate residual stenosis may be accepted. The balloon used for postdilation after stenting is always maintained within the stent to avoid dissection. Nominal pressure is used to fully expand the balloon and the stent. In the majority of the cases, the stent is placed across the bifurcation into the CCA, crossing the origin of the ECA. Deployment of the stent across the ECA has not resulted in adverse events; follow-up arteriograms and duplex studies have demonstrated that the ECA remains patent in most patients.

Kinks and bends in the ICA may pose a problem with stent implants. Deploy stents across significant bends only if they are isolated. Avoid placing the distal end of the stent into kinks and tortuous segments of the ICA, especially if more than a single bend is noted. Quite commonly, there is a significant bend in the artery just distal to the lesion. As the carotid lesion becomes harder it also lengthens a bit. The efferent turn back toward the normal trajectory of the carotid artery occurs at the location where the artery reaches its first softer segment. When placing a stent in this situation, the distal end must go beyond the location of this efferent turn. Tortuosity cannot be eliminated; it is usually displaced distally, and can become more exaggerated when a stent is placed, and it results in stiffening of a segment of artery. A highly tortuous ICA should be considered a relative contraindication for CAS. In addition, there may be difficulty in advancing the stent delivery catheter into place in this situation. Be aware that placement of the access sheath into the CCA can also exacerbate tortuosity by stiffening the artery proximally and temporarily making the tortuosity at the bifurcation or distal carotid appear worse.

AFTER STENT PLACEMENT: COMPLETION ANGIOGRAM, ACCESS SITE MANAGEMENT, POSTOPERATIVE CARE

The filter is maintained in place until the carotid reconstruction is evaluated and continued flow through the filter is documented. Following stent placement, completion angiograms are acquired in the projection that had demonstrated the maximum stenosis. Attention is paid to the ICA immediately distal to the stent. Spasm in this segment may be encountered, especially where the filter is located (Fig. 21.7). If significant spasm is encountered, a small dose of intraarterial nitroglycerine (50 to 100 μg) is administered directly into the ICA. Distal dissections are rare and when present can be remedied with an additional stent that is sized for the distal ICA. Reasonable prograde flow through the stented segment and the filter should be present. If there is slow flow or a filling defect within the filter, an aspiration catheter is used before filter removal. The filter retrieval catheter is passed carefully through the stent to capture the filter. Open-cell stent designs have excellent contour ability, but also have diamond-shaped points that protrude into the lumen that can snag the retrieval catheter. If the retrieval catheter catches on the stent, do not push the catheter forward, because this will tend to withdraw the filter down toward the stent. Have the patient rotate or extend the neck to permit a straight shot of the retrieval catheter along the wire through the stented portion. After filter retrieval, intracranial angiograms are obtained after CAS by most operators as a routine, and these may be compared with preoperative studies. The neurologic status of the patient is monitored during the procedure and is assessed at its conclusion.

In suitable patients, access site hemostasis is achieved at the end of the procedure using one of several approved closure devices. A femoral arteriogram is performed in the oblique projection. If a closure device cannot be used, the long sheath is exchanged for a short sheath of the same caliber that is removed when the ACT is less than 180 seconds, and manual pressure is held for the appropriate time period.

Patients are monitored in the hospital overnight. It is not uncommon for patients to respond to carotid sinus distension with bradycardia and hypotension. Occasionally, 24 to 48 hours of inotropic support is required before the carotid sinus adapts to the radial force of the self-expanding stent. Avoidance of

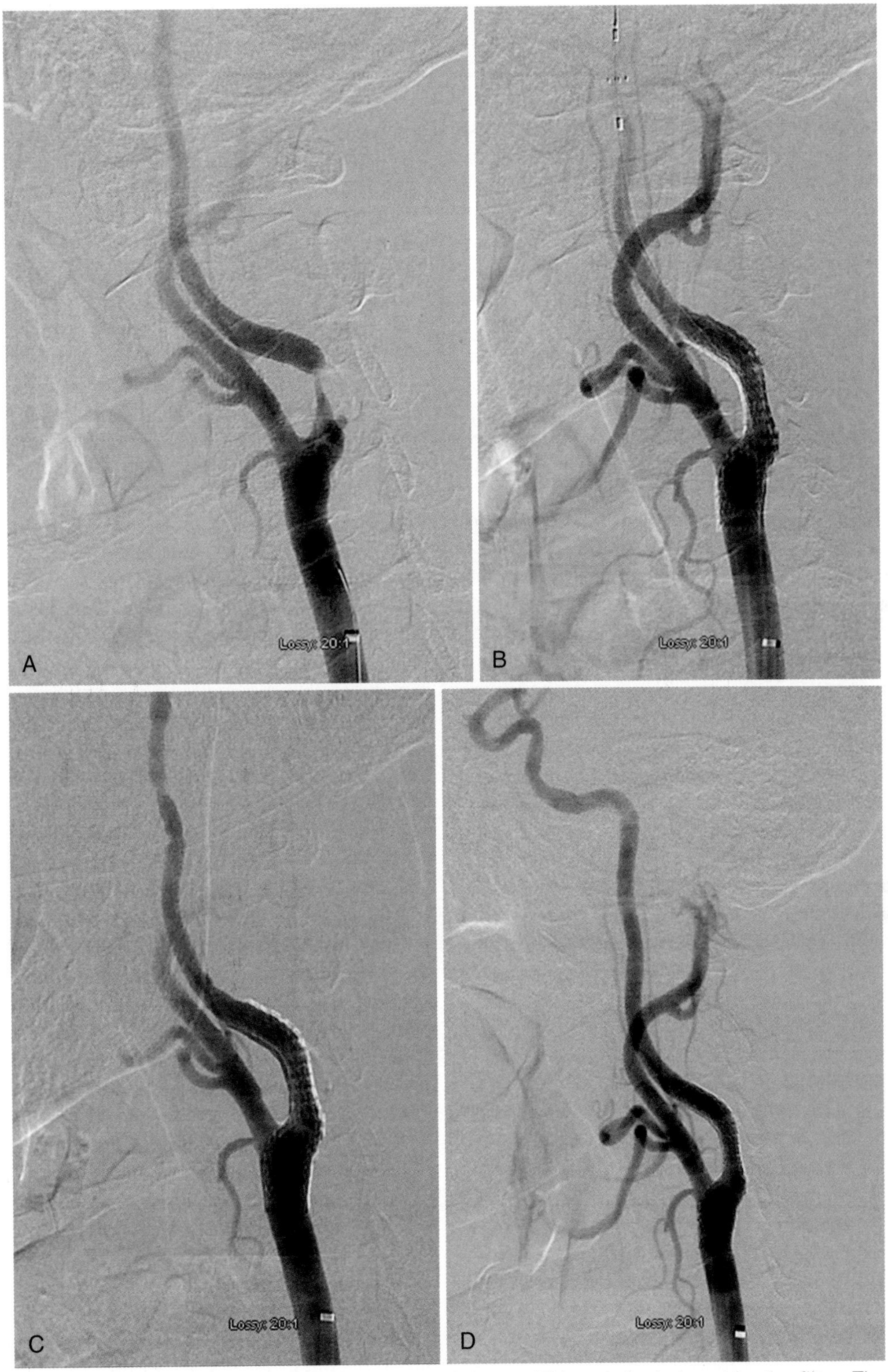

FIG 21.7 Spasm of the Distal Internal Carotid Artery. This may be induced by the filter. The key is to finish the case and retrieve the filter in an expedited manner. However, if spasm occurs in the middle of the procedure, it may be helpful to administer small doses of nitroglycerine while completing the stent procedure. (A) ICA pre-treatment. (B) ICA post-stent placement with distal filter in place. (C) ICA after filter retrieval with distal arterial spasm. (D) Completion angiogram after nitroglycerin administration.

extreme oversizing of the stents likely helps to decrease the incidence of bradycardia and hypotension following CAS. The presence of significant hypotension in the absence of bradycardia is unusual in the immediate postprocedure period, and other causes (e.g., retroperitoneal bleed related to access site problems) should also be considered. Other potential perioperative complications include stroke, myocardial infarction (MI), and access site complications. A predischarge evaluation and an NIH stroke scale are completed. Medications include aspirin (325 mg/day indefinitely) and clopidogrel (75 mg/day for 3 months). Follow-up includes 1-month, 6-month, and yearly clinical evaluations and duplex examinations.

UNIQUE COMPLICATIONS OF CAROTID ANGIOPLASTY AND STENTING

Perioperative cerebral embolization remains a feared complication of CAS. Studies of transfemoral, distal-filter mediated stents are reviewed in the next section. These have generally shown that periprocedural stroke is more frequent, especially with respect to minor stroke; is more likely to occur after stenting of a symptomatic lesion; and may occur in a delayed fashion (24 hours to 30 days). Aside from the obvious concern for clinically apparent neurological complications, silent brain lesions, as demonstrated by diffusion-weighted MRI (DW-MRI), may also be related to long-term deterioration in cognitive function. It appears that most DW-MRI brain lesions are temporary, but the presence of ischemic lesions on DW-MRI may be used as a surrogate endpoint for neurological risk. Arch and bifurcation manipulation, the lesion composition, cerebral protection devices, and stent types all play a role in the risk of stroke or silent brain infarction, but it can be challenging to separate these variables.

A recent meta-analysis on the occurrence of postprocedural new diffusion-weighted imaging (DWI) lesions after CAS versus CEA reported 40.3% versus 12.2%, respectively.[37] These data are consistent with previously reported trends,[38] and includes studies done prior to routine cerebral protection. The International Carotid Stenting Study (ICSS) demonstrated a higher incidence of stroke within 30 days of stenting compared to endarterectomy, and approximately 3 times more ischemic lesions on DWI posttreatment scans. Of 231 patients in the brain MRI cohort, 50% of the stenting group versus 17% of the endarterectomy group had at least one new DWI lesion detected on posttreatment scans. Among those stenting group patients with new DWI lesions, 71% had more than one lesion. Also, 45% of patients in the stenting group had lesions in the contralateral carotid or vertebrobasilar circulation, suggesting an embolic pathogenesis potentially during arch manipulation. The use of distal embolic protection with a filter was actually associated with a higher incidence of ischemic lesions identified, although this could also have been patient selection.[39] Manipulation of the carotid bifurcation prior to cerebral protection leads to an increased risk of cerebral embolization and silent brain lesion on DW-MRI. The PROFI study compared proximal balloon occlusion with the Mo.Ma device to distal filter protection, and showed a higher incidence of ischemic lesions on DW-MRI in the filter group (87.1%) versus the balloon occlusion group (45.2%).[40] A meta-analysis comparing the two neuroprotection systems in preventing embolization during CAS mirrored these results showing significantly lower lesions on DW-MRI in the proximal balloon occlusion group as compared to the distal filter group.[41]

Aortic arch instrumentation during diagnostic procedures has been shown to produce silent ischemic brain infarcts as high as 26% in either hemisphere.[42] For example, Carotid Revascularization Endarterectomy versus Stent Trial (CREST) reports rates of all stroke at 4.1% for CAS versus 2.3% for CEA, while ipsilateral stroke is 2% for CAS versus 2.3% for CEA.[43] These numbers signify the increased risk of stroke with arch manipulation as seen in CAS. Transcervical CAS with proximal protection carotid flow reversal permits avoidance of the arch. This approach was evaluated in the ROADSTER 1 Trial, which included 141 patients in the pivotal arm and reported no major strokes and two minor strokes for an overall stroke rate of 1.4%.[21] The PROOF study evaluated 44 patients undergoing transcervical CAS with flow reversal, and reported 5 patients (16%) with evidence of silent ischemic brain lesions on DW-MRI.[44] Leal and colleagues[45] reported the results of 31 patients undergoing CAS with this approach and had no clinically apparent strokes, and only 4 patients (12.5%) with postprocedural DW-MRI ischemic infarcts were identified. These infarcts were all ipsilateral to the treated hemisphere, which signifies a significant improvement in cerebral embolization risk associated with arch manipulation. Finally, Leal and colleagues[46] then compared transcervical CAS to transfemoral CAS in a small study and found a much higher incidence of new DW-MRI ischemic infarcts in the transfemoral (33.3%) versus the transcervical (12.9%) group.

The stent type may influence neurologic events as well. Open-cell stents have been associated with plaque prolapse more often than with closed-cell stents. Multiple reports have evaluated open versus closed-cell stents and the rates of new DW-MRI lesions. Park and colleagues[47] evaluated almost 100 patients undergoing transfemoral CAS and found new lesions on DW-MRI significantly more frequently in the open-cell stent group (51.5%) versus the closed-cell stent group (27.3%). Schnaudigel and colleagues[38] reported similar findings in a meta-analysis of CAS versus CEA where stent design, filter protection, and shunting were also examined. The authors reported a significant increase in the incidence of new ipsilateral DW-MRI lesions in the open-cell stent design versus the closed-cell stent design. In a 2007 report, Bosiers examined the Belgian-Italian registry of more than 3000 patients who underwent CAS to determine if carotid stent design had an impact on neurologic events. The overall combined rates of adverse events were 4.2% in the open-cell group and 2.3% in the closed-cell group. Postprocedural complications rates were highest for the open-cell stent types compared to the closed-cell stent types (3.4% vs. 1.3%) and rates increased with larger free-cell area. However, the difference between the open-cell and closed-cell stents was mainly seen in symptomatic patients.[48]

Hypotension and bradycardia can occur after CAS due to the stretching of the carotid sinus baroreceptors by the balloon and stent. This can be worrisome in the high-risk patients that are typically referred for CAS, who may be more vulnerable to cardiac or cerebrovascular hemodynamic changes and may require drug intervention. The rates of hypotension and bradycardia after CAS vary from 10% to 42% and 27% to 37%, respectively.[49–51] Vasopressor treatment or atropine treatment may be required in 18% of patients, with 7% of patients requiring both medications.[49] Persistent hemodynamic depression is associated with increased risks of periprocedural major adverse events.[49] Independent predictors of hypotension and bradycardia after CAS include asymptomatic stenosis, less than 10 mm from stenosis to bifurcation, stenosis severity, and aggressiveness of balloon dilation.[50] Calcified plaque has also been suggested as a high-risk feature.[49] A history of CEA is associated with lower risk.[49,50] Freedom from hypotension or bradycardia episodes increases with time; 80% and 73%, respectively, in the first 3 hours, and 97% and 91% at 6 to 12 hours, respectively.[50]

RESULTS OF CAROTID STENTING RANDOMIZED CONTROLLED TRIALS

Landmark RCTs comparing CEA plus best medical therapy versus best medical therapy alone were published in the early 1990s and provided level I evidence for the use of CEA as the standard for treatment of carotid occlusive disease.[2-9] In the more recent era, multiple RCTs comparing CAS to CEA have been conducted, which inform our current practice (Table 21.3).

The Stenting and Angioplasty with Protection in Patients at High Risk for Endarterectomy (SAPPHIRE) trial demonstrated promise for CAS and was the first randomized trial to evaluate patients who were at high risk for CEA.[23] SAPPHIRE was also the first randomized trial of CAS to use mandatory distal embolic protection. The majority of patients (more than 70%) were asymptomatic. The 30-day combined periprocedural adverse event rate was 4.8% for CAS patients and 9.8% for CEA patients ($P = .09$). At 1 year, the combined major adverse event rate was 12.2% for CAS patients and 20.1% for CEA patients ($P = .004$ for noninferiority analysis; $P = .05$ for intention-to-treat analysis).[23] These data showed noninferiority of CAS for patients at high risk for CEA. A significant difference in event rates between CAS and CEA was due to the greater association of CEA with non-Q-wave MI. Excluding MI, there was no significant difference found between CAS (5.5%) and CEA (8.4%) patients. The long-term follow-up data at 3 years revealed a substantial cumulative incidence in death from cardiac and nonneurologic causes (18.6% CAS vs. 21.0% CEA).[29] Nevertheless, SAPPHIRE was viewed as the trial that proved the noninferiority of CAS in high-risk patients. CAS continues to be a mainstay in treatment in most US centers for patients with compelling indications for carotid repair, but who are at high risk for conventional repair with CEA.

Two European RCTs, Stent-Protected Angioplasty versus Carotid Endarterectomy (SPACE) and Endarterectomy Versus Stenting in Patients with Symptomatic Severe Carotid Stenosis (EVA-3S), sought to establish noninferiority in standard-risk, symptomatic patients.[30,31] In the SPACE trial, the primary endpoint was ipsilateral stroke or death, or both, at 30 days. A variety of different stents were used, and embolic protection was not mandated. The initial aim of the study was to enroll 950 patients per group to achieve a power of 80%. The interim analysis in the SPACE trial comprised 1183 patients and reported a primary event rate of 6.84% in the CAS group versus 6.34% in

TABLE 21.3 Randomized Controlled Trials

Trial	Year	No. of Patients	CPD (%)	Asymptomatic (%)	F/U (Months)	Completed
CAS vs. CEA	1998	23	0	0	1	No (harm)
Wallstent	2001	219	0	0	12	No (futility)
Brooks	2001	104	0	0	48	Yes
CAVATAS	2001	504	0	3	36	Yes
Brooks	2004	85	0	100	48	Yes
SAPPHIRE	2004	334	96	71	36	No (slow enrollment)
EVA-3S	2004	527	92	0	6	No (futility/harm)
SPACE	2006	1,200	—	0	1	No (funding)
TESCAS-C	2006	166	100	—	6	Yes
BACASS	2006	20	—	0	45	Yes
Steinbauer	2008	87	0	0	64–66	Yes
CREST	2010	2,502	96	47	30	Yes
ICSS	2010	1,703	72	0	3	Yes

BACASS, Carotid artery stenting versus carotid endarterectomy. A prospective, randomised trial with long-term follow-up; *CAS,* carotid angioplasty and stenting; *CAVATAS,* Carotid and Vertebral Artery Transluminal Angioplasty Study; *CEA,* carotid endarterectomy; *CPD,* Cerebral protection device; *CREST,* Carotid Revascularization Endarterectomy versus Stent Trial; *EVA-3S,* Endarterectomy Versus Stenting in Patients with Symptomatic Severe Carotid Stenosis; *F/U,* follow-up; *ICSS,* International Carotid Stenting Study; *SAPPHIRE,* Stenting and Angioplasty with Protection in Patients at High Risk for Endarterectomy; *SPACE,* Stent-Protected Angioplasty versus Carotid Endarterectomy; *TESCAS-C,* trial of endarterectomy versus stenting for the treatment of carotid artery atherosclerosis in China.

Modified from Brott TG, Hobson RW, 2nd, Howard G, et al; CREST investigators: stenting versus endarterectomy for treatment of carotid-artery stenosis. *N Engl J Med* 363:11–23, 2010.

the CEA group (P = .09 for noninferiority analysis).[30] Although SPACE CAS patients were treated variably with embolic protection, there was no significant difference in results between those who were treated with and without CPD. Furthermore, in most endpoints there was a favorable trend toward the surgical arm, although none was statistically significant. After this interim analysis, the steering committee decided to terminate the study on the basis of both futility and financial constraints because it was revealed that 2500 patients would be needed to adequately power the study to achieve trial endpoints. Thus, the SPACE trial failed to prove noninferiority of CAS compared with CEA, despite the similar perioperative stroke and death rates for the two procedures. The authors concluded that CEA should remain the preferred treatment for patients with symptomatic stenosis, because evidence was lacking to support equivalent endovascular treatment. Subsequent subgroup analysis from the SPACE trial revealed that there was an excess risk in stenting in men than in women (P = .03) and in patients older than 70 years (P = .08).[32]

Similarly, the EVA-3S trial failed to demonstrate noninferiority of CAS in symptomatic patients. The primary endpoint was defined as a composite of any stroke or death occurring within 30 days after treatment. The goal was to enroll 872 patients per group to achieve a power of 80%. A variety of different stents was used at different centers, and cerebral protection was initially not required until the safety committee instituted a protocol change as a result of a 25% 30-day rate of stroke or death in patients treated without embolic protection devices (EPDs).[33] The study randomized 527 patients and was subsequently ended prematurely for safety reasons after an interim analysis revealed a significantly higher 30-day event rate in the CAS group (9.6%) compared with the CEA group (3.9%; P = .01). These results persisted at 6 months, with an event rate of 11.7% in the CAS arm versus 6.1% in the CEA group (P = .02).[31] The EVA-3S results have been criticized for the significantly higher 30-day stroke rate observed in the CAS arm of the study compared with other published results. Also, the trial did not compare groups of physicians with equal experience. Whereas the surgeons performing CEA had performed at least 25 endarterectomies within 1 year before trial entry, interventionists were certified after performing less than half that number of CAS and were allowed to enroll study participants while completing their training and certification, a factor that could also increase stroke risk in the CAS arm. However, despite these claims, subgroup analysis failed to show any statistically significant difference between operators based on level of experience.[31] The conclusion from the EVA-3S authors supported the notion that CEA remains an excellent option for symptomatic carotid stenosis with low complication rates that were not matched by CAS.

The ICSS enrolled 1713 symptomatic patients with at least 50% ICA stenosis to compare efficacy of CEA and CAS.[12,34] Surgeons were required to have performed at least 50 CEA operations, and interventionists were required to have performed at least 50 stenting procedures with at least 10 in the ICA. Evaluated endpoints were stroke, MI, and death. Interim analysis of data at 120 days demonstrated that the incidence of stroke, MI, or death in the CAS group was significantly higher than in the CEA group (8.5 vs. 5.2, respectively; P = .006).[34] A subgroup of the ICSS patient cohort underwent DW-MRI brain imaging after treatment, and patients who underwent stent placement had a significantly higher incidence of asymptomatic lesions on cerebral imaging. The ICSS study had been criticized for bias toward the surgical arm because of the poor experience level of those performing CAS. Long-term data up to 10 years after randomization showed similar long-term functional outcome and risk of fatal or disabling stroke between stenting (cumulative 5-year risk 6.4%) and endarterectomy (cumulative 5-year risk 6.5%) for symptomatic carotid artery stenosis. The CAS group had a significantly higher number of strokes overall, but there was no significant difference in the number of fatal or disabling strokes between the CEA and CAS groups. There was also no significant difference between the groups in long-term rates of severe carotid restenosis (>70%) or occlusion.[12]

The Carotid Angioplasty and Stenting Versus Endarterectomy in Asymptomatic Subjects who are at Standard Risk for Carotid Endarterectomy with Significant Extracranial Carotid Stenotic Disease Study (ACT I) was a prospective, randomized, multicenter trial comparing CEA and CAS in asymptomatic patients with severe stenosis at a standard risk for CEA.[10] The trial was a noninferiority study and was halted early, after randomization of 1453 patients, due to slow enrollment. The ACT I carotid stent platform included the Xact, Abbott Vascular closed-cell stent in conjunction with distal embolic protection (Emboshield, Emboshield Pro, or Emboshield NAV6, Abbott Vascular). The primary composite endpoint included death, stroke, or MI within 30 days, or ipsilateral stroke with 1 year. ACT I investigators reported noninferiority of CAS to CEA in the primary composite endpoint (3.8% vs. 3.4%; P = .01). Also, there was no significant difference in the composite endpoint in an analysis of up to 5-year follow-up.[10]

The CREST is an NIH-sponsored, prospective, randomized, multicenter trial comparing the efficacy of CEA and CAS in both symptomatic and asymptomatic patients.[11,35] The primary endpoint includes a 30-day periprocedural composite of stroke, MI, and death, or any ipsilateral stroke during the 4 years following randomization.[35] The long-term extension study arm evaluated outcomes every 6 months for up to 10 years.[11] A total of 2502 symptomatic and asymptomatic patients from 117 centers in Canada and the United States were enrolled. To address concerns from previous trials, CREST required rigorous credentialing for surgeons and interventionists. Surgeons had to document that they had performed at least 12 CEAs in the previous year with rates of complications and deaths less than 3% and 5% for asymptomatic and symptomatic patients, respectively. Interventionists were certified after satisfactory evaluation of their endovascular experience, CAS results, participation in hands-on training, and participation in a lead-in phase of up to 20 cases.[22,36]

CREST investigators reported no significant difference between the CAS and CEA arms in regard to the combined endpoints of stroke, MI, and death (Table 21.4).[36] Analysis of each endpoint individually showed a higher rate of stroke after CAS at 30 days (4.1% vs. 2.3%; P = .01) and a higher rate of MI after CEA (2.3% vs. 1.1%; P = .03). The estimated 4-year rates of combined primary

TABLE 21.4 **CREST Trial Results: Endpoints According to Treatment With Carotid Angioplasty and Stenting or Carotid Endarterectomy**

Endpoint	CAS (n = 1262)	CEA (n = 1240)	P value
Any periprocedure stroke or postprocedure ipsilateral stroke (%)	4.1 ± 0.6	2.3 ± 0.4	**.01**
Major stroke (%)	0.9 ± 0.3	0.6 ± 0.2	.52
Minor stroke (%)	3.2 ± 0.5	1.7 ± 0.4	.01
Myocardial infarction (%)	1.1 ± 0.3	2.3 ± 0.4	.01
Death (%)	0.7 ± 0.2	0.3 ± 0.2	.18
Primary study endpoint[a] perioperative (%)	5.2 ± 0.6	4.5 ± 0.6	.38
Primary endpoint[a] to 4 years (%)	7.2 ± 0.8	6.8 ± 0.8	.51
Cranial nerve palsy	0	5%	—

[a]Primary study endpoint was any periprocedural stroke or myocardial infarction or death or postprocedural ipsilateral stroke.
CAS, Carotid angioplasty and stenting; *CEA,* carotid endarterectomy; *CREST,* Carotid Revascularization Endarterectomy versus Stent Trial.
From Berkefeld J, Chaturvedi S: The International Carotid Stenting Study and the North American Carotid Revascularization Endarterectomy Versus Stenting Trial: fueling the debate about carotid artery stenting. *Stroke* 41:2714–2715, 2010.

TABLE 21.5 **CREST Results: Asymptomatic and Symptomatic Patients**

Endpoint	CAS	CEA	P value
Any Periprocedural Stroke or Postprocedural Ipsilateral Stroke (%)			
Asymptomatic	2.5 ± 0.6	1.4 ± 0.5	.07
Symptomatic	5.5 ± 0.9	3.2 ± 0.7	.25
Primary Study Endpoint[a] (%)			
Asymptomatic	3.5 ± 0.8	3.6 ± 0.8	.56
Symptomatic	6.7 ± 1.0	5.4 ± 0.9	.69

[a]Primary study endpoint was any periprocedural stroke or myocardial infarction or death or postprocedural ipsilateral stroke.
CAS, Carotid angioplasty and stenting; *CEA,* carotid endarterectomy; *CREST,* Carotid Revascularization Endarterectomy versus Stent Trial.
From Berkefeld J, Chaturvedi S: The International Carotid Stenting Study and the North American Carotid Revascularization Endarterectomy Versus Stenting Trial: fueling the debate about carotid artery stenting. *Stroke* 41:2714–2715, 2010.

endpoints was 7.2% versus 6.8% for CAS and CEA, respectively (P = .51). Cranial nerve injury occurred in 5% of CEA patients and none after CAS. Both CEA and CAS outcomes were within the American Heart Association (AHA) guidelines for periprocedural stroke and death for carotid repair (≤3% for asymptomatic patients and ≤6% for symptomatic patients; Table 21.5). Long-term results show no significant difference in the rate of postprocedural ipsilateral stroke over 10-year follow-up in the CAS group (6.9%) and the CEA group (5.6%), and no significant difference between groups in restenosis rates. Also, the rate of postprocedural ipsilateral stroke did not differ between symptomatic or asymptomatic groups or between genders.[11]

The carotid stenting systems used during the CREST, the Accunet filter and Acculink stent, were established at the initiation of the trial and used for the course of the study. Over the ensuing decade, other carotid stenting systems became available and other methods of cerebral protection were developed but were not included in the trial. During the CREST enrollment period (2000 to 2008), concurrent registry studies demonstrated a steady decrease in the risk of adverse outcomes with CAS. This may reflect better patient selection based on an improved understanding of which patients are at high risk for CAS (e.g., tortuous or heavily calcified arch, great vessels or carotid bifurcation). Because the equipment used in CREST was held static for the study, any improvement in results over time may be due to better technique, more experience, and especially improved patient selection for CAS.

CREST was a huge, lengthy, and largely successful undertaking—the results of which will significantly influence carotid practice going forward. CREST showed excellent results for both CAS and CEA. This was also the first major randomized trial to use rigorous credentialing standards for study operators and to provide long-term follow-up with published 10-year data. Some potential disadvantages of the study design: the CAS systems used were rigidly established so that other options for cerebral protection and stenting were not included, and there is concern about the potential lack of generalizability to the community. Additional arguments that have been prompted by the CREST Trial include the value of a composite endpoint that contains MI, since the effects of stroke and MI on the patient are probably not interchangeable.[35] CREST included symptomatic and asymptomatic patients while ICSS, SPACE, and EVA-3S included symptomatic patients, and ACT 1 studied asymptomatic patients. During the study design of this standard risk trial, there were significant data and clinical experience to determine which patients were at high risk for CEA, but there was a paucity of data on which patients were at high risk for CAS.

Among currently completed RCTs, study arms compared CEA and CAS without an additional arm for best medical therapy, especially as an alternative for treatment of asymptomatic carotid stenosis. The ongoing Carotid Revascularization and Medical Management for Asymptomatic Carotid Stenosis Trial (CREST-2; Clinical Trials.gov number, NCT02089217) is a multicenter, RCT of carotid revascularization. It has a unique study design containing two related trials of medical management alone versus medical management plus carotid bifurcation repair in patients with asymptomatic high-grade carotid artery stenosis. One trial will randomize patients to CEA plus medical management versus no medical management alone, and the other trial will randomize patients to CAS plus medical management versus medical management alone. The European Carotid Surgery Trial 2 (ECST-2; Current Controlled Trials number, ISRCTN97744893) will include asymptomatic patients as well as symptomatic patients who have been deemed at low risk for stroke and will compare medical management plus repair versus medical management alone. The results of these ongoing trials will undoubtedly influence the future of carotid artery disease management and revascularization.

RESULTS OF PROXIMAL BALLOON OCCLUSION AND FLOW REVERSAL

Proximal balloon protection gained widespread use in CAS as it eliminates traversal of the lesion without cerebral protection, and thus, theoretically decreases the risk of cerebral embolization. The proximAl pRotection with the MO.Ma device dUring caRotid stenting trial (ARMOUR) is a prospective, multicenter trial that evaluated the safety and effectiveness of the MO.Ma Proximal Cerebral Protection Device (Medtronic) in patients undergoing CAS. To be included in the trial, patients were deemed at high risk for CEA. The primary endpoints included MI, stroke, or death through 30 days. The registry enrolled 262 patients, of which 15.1% were symptomatic and 28.9% were octogenarians. The trial demonstrated that the device is safe and effective, with a 98.2% device success rate and 93.2% procedural success rate. The primary endpoint rate was 2.7% and the 30-day risk of major stroke was 0.9%. Of note, no symptomatic patient suffered a stroke during the trial.[28] In an earlier European trial evaluating the feasibility of the Mo.Ma device, 7.6% of patients had transient intolerance to flow cessation.[52] Proximal occlusion with distal protection can be used as an adjunct in this circumstance, or in patients for whom ECA branches cannot be occluded due to stenosis or tortuosity.

The Prevention of Cerebral Embolization by Proximal Balloon Occlusion Compared to Filter Protection During Carotid Artery Stenting (PROFI) Study is a prospective, randomized trial comparing proximal balloon occlusion (MO.Ma, Invatec) to distal filter protection (Emboshield, Abbott Vascular) in patients undergoing CAS. A total of 62 patients were randomized with 31 in each group. The primary endpoint was the incidence of new cerebral ischemic lesions assessed by DW-MRI. The secondary endpoint was major adverse cardiovascular and cerebral events (MACCE). There was a significant reduction in the incidence of new cerebral ischemic lesions in the proximal balloon occlusion group (45.2% vs. 87.1%; $P = .001$). Contralateral cerebral lesions were significantly higher in the distal filter group than the proximal balloon group (29% vs. 6.5%, $P = .047$). However, the difference in MACCE was insignificant.[53] A more recent meta-analysis of eight studies including 357 patients also compares proximal balloon occlusion and distal filter protection during CAS. The incidence of new ischemic lesions detected by DW-MRI is significantly lower in the proximal balloon occlusion group.[41]

Transcarotid stenting with dynamic flow reversal has the unique advantage of avoiding the arch and theoretically significantly decreasing the periprocedural CAS stroke risk. The Safety and Efficacy Study for Reverse Flow Used During Carotid Artery Stenting Procedure trial (ROADSTER) is a prospective, single-arm multicenter clinical trial performed to evaluate the safety and efficacy of the ENROUTE Transcarotid NPS (Silk Road Medical Inc.) during CAS procedures. The primary endpoint was the composite of MI, stroke, or death at 30 days postprocedure. In the pivotal cohort 141 patients were enrolled, 26% were symptomatic and 75% were asymptomatic. Device and technical success was 99%. The composite endpoint was 3.5%, the all-stroke rate 1.4%, and the stroke and death rate 2.8%. The overall stroke rate of 1.4% is the lowest reported for any prospective, multicenter clinical trial of CAS.[21] The ROADSTER 2 Trial is currently enrolling in the United States with plans to treat more than 600 patients at high risk for CEA using the transcervical approach.

HYBRID CAROTID STENTS

Long-term stroke prevention and restenosis after the first 30 days are similar between CEA and CAS.[11,35] Stroke prevention in the first 30 days is paramount to the success of CAS. Currently available stents are either open cell or closed cell. The struts of the stent are the only protection against postprocedural neurologic events. The ideal carotid stent must comprise sufficient radial force, vessel conformability, and adequate scaffolding. Open-cell stents provide flexibility and conformability but inadequate scaffolding and subsequently, higher rates of neurologic events in the first 30 days.[48] Plaque prolapse between stent struts has been shown on optical coherence tomography, more frequently in open-cell stents (61.5%) than closed-cell stents (17.6%).[54,55] Closed-cell stents provide better scaffolding and wall coverage, but are limited in flexibility and conformability and have been associated with stent malapposition.[54] The evolution of hybrid carotid stents combines the quality of the open-cell frame with an outer mesh layer. There are three mesh-covered stents in development that have reached the phase of clinical evaluation.

The Carotid Embolic Protection Using Micronet Trial (CARENET) is a prospective, multicenter study of 30 patients undergoing CAS in which the CGuard Carotid Embolic Protective Stent system was placed.[56] This stent is wrapped with a MicroNet mesh. The primary endpoint was procedural success combined with the number and volume of new lesions on the ipsilateral side as assessed by DW-MRI. Procedural success was 100% with zero complications. The 30-day MACCE rate was 0%. New ipsilateral MRI lesions occurred in 37% of patients and all but one lesion completely resolved by 30 days.[56]

The Roadsaver (Terumo) CAS is a nitinol dual layer micromesh stent that is repositionable and is part of The Carotid Trial Investigating the Efficacy of Endovascular Treatment of Carotid Arterial Disease with the multilayer Roadsaver stent trial (CLEAR-ROAD; Clinical Trials.gov number, NCT02529345).

The GORE Carotid Stent Clinical Study for the Treatment of Carotid Artery Stenosis in patients at Increased Risk For Adverse Events from Carotid Endarterectomy Study (SCAFFOLD) is a prospective study evaluating a heparin bonded PTFE mesh-covered open-cell nitinol stent.

CONCLUSION

CEA has a long track record of success in carotid revascularization, and CAS now has multiple RCTs showing equipoise in appropriately selected patients. CAS is established therapy for patients at high risk for CEA, especially those with a hostile neck. According to the National Center for Health Statistics, CAS is a routinely performed procedure in both academic and community settings. Whether CAS will be expanded to standard-risk populations awaits further evaluation and analysis of ongoing clinical trial data. As these and long-term data reflecting the durability of CAS continue to accumulate, greater operator experience is acquired, and new stenting technology develops, the application of CAS will continue to mature and likely expand.

REVIEW QUESTIONS

1. Carotid stenting is approved for use in the United States for patients with characteristics that make the patient at high risk for carotid endarterectomy. These factors include which of the following?
   a. Patient chooses to have carotid stent
   b. Patient has an extensive history of gastrointestinal (GI) bleeding
   c. Patient is a nonresponder to clopidogrel
   d. Patient has a tracheal stoma
   e. Patient has an asymptomatic moderate stenosis
2. Anatomic factors that increase the periprocedural risk of carotid stenting include all of these, except:
   a. tortuous arch
   b. highly calcified arch
   c. recently symptomatic critical carotid stenosis
   d. restenosis after previous carotid endarterectomy
   e. fresh thrombus at the site of the bifurcation lesion
3. Periprocedural medications for use in the carotid stent procedure includes all of these, except:
   a. aspirin
   b. papaverine
   c. clopidogrel
   d. nitroglycerine
   e. atropine
4. A common method of establishing carotid sheath access is:
   a. Place a stiff exchange guidewire in the ECA and advance the carotid sheath over the exchange guidewire.
   b. Advance the carotid sheath over the soft guidewire used for selective catheterization of the CCA.
   c. Place the stiff guidewire into the ICA beyond the lesion and advance the carotid sheath over the exchange guidewire.
   d. Advance the sheath into the arch and then cannulate the CCA using a stiff exchange guidewire.
5. Which of the following is true about the use of cerebral protection devices?
   a. Only one filter is approved for use with CAS
   b. CMS mandates the use of cerebral protection devices during CAS
   c. Filters have been shown in large randomized trials to provide a lower risk of periprocedural stroke than when no filter is used.
   d. The dwell time for a filter has no correlation with periprocedural risk of stroke.
   e. Filters are just as simple to place when the artery distal to the bifurcation is extremely tortuous.
6. In the first few hours after carotid stent placement, an average patient's vital signs are more likely to trend toward:
   a. bradycardia and hypotension
   b. hypertension and tachycardia
   c. hypertension and bradycardia
   d. no significant change from prior to stent placement
7. Randomized, controlled trials of carotid stenting and carotid endarterectomy include all of these, except:
   a. NASCET
   b. CREST
   c. SAPPHIRE
   d. ICSS
   e. SPACE
8. The primary endpoint for the CREST Trial was:
   a. stroke and death at 30 days
   b. stroke, death, MI, and cranial nerve injury at 30 days
   c. stroke, death, and MI at 4 years
   d. stroke, death, and MI at 30 days and postprocedural ipsilateral stroke at long-term follow-up
   e. stroke, death, and MI, cranial nerve injury and positive diffusion-weighted MRI at 30 days
9. The CREST results showed that:
   a. the risk of periprocedural MI was higher with stenting than with endarterectomy
   b. the risk of minor stroke was higher with endarterectomy than with stenting
   c. the risk of persistent cranial nerve injury beyond 6 months after carotid endarterectomy was 0%.
   d. there was no significant difference in the risk of major stroke or death between carotid stenting and carotid endarterectomy
10. Name some of the advantages of the use of embolic protection during carotid stenting.
    a. Distal filters permit preservation of prograde flow to the brain during the CAS procedure.
    b. Proximal occlusion can be performed with a smaller caliber carotid sheath than other types of protection.
    c. When using proximal protection, it is simple to avoid patients who are at high risk for intolerance of reversed flow by evaluating cerebral collaterals based on preprocedure MRI scanning.
    d. Distal filters permit the use of any guidewire the operator would like to use for passage of the balloon and stent into the carotid artery.

SELECTED REFERENCES

10. Rosenfield K, Matsumura JS, Chaturvedi S, et al. Randomized trial of stent versus surgery for asymptomatic carotid stenosis. *N Engl J Med*. 2016;374(11):1011–1020.
11. Brott TG, Howard G, Roubin GS, et al. Long-term results of stenting versus endarterectomy for carotid-artery stenosis. *N Engl J Med*. 2016;374(11):1021–1031.
12. Bonati LH, Dobson J, Featherstone RL, et al. Long-term outcomes after stenting versus endarterectomy for treatment of symptomatic carotid stenosis: the international carotid stenting study (ICSS) randomised trial. *Lancet*. 2015;385(9967):529–538.
21. Kwolek CJ, Jaff MR, Leal JI, et al. Results of the ROADSTER multicenter trial of transcarotid stenting with dynamic flow reversal. *J Vasc Surg*. 2015;62(5):1227–1234.
29. Gurm HS, Yadav JS, Fayad P, et al. Long-term results of carotid stenting versus endarterectomy in high-risk patients. *N Engl J Med*. 2008;358(15):1572–1579.
30. SPACE Collaborative Group, Ringleb PA, Allenberg J, et al. 30 day results from the SPACE trial of stent-protected angioplasty versus carotid endarterectomy in symptomatic patients: a randomised non-inferiority trial. *Lancet*. 2006;368(9543): 1239–1247.
31. Mas JL, Chatellier G, Beyssen B, et al. Endarterectomy versus stenting in patients with symptomatic severe carotid stenosis. *N Engl J Med*. 2006;355(16):1660–1671.
34. International Carotid Stenting Study investigators, Ederle J, Dobson J, et al. Carotid artery stenting compared with endarterectomy in patients with symptomatic carotid stenosis (international carotid stenting study): an interim analysis of a randomised controlled trial. *Lancet*. 2010;375(9719):985–997.
35. Brott TG, Hobson RW 2nd, Howard G, et al. Stenting versus endarterectomy for treatment of carotid-artery stenosis. *N Engl J Med*. 2010;363(1):11–23.

References available online at expertconsult.com.

CHAPTER 22

Carotid Body Tumors: Diagnosis and Surgical Management

Peter F. Lawrence, Rameen S. Moridzadeh

INTRODUCTION

Carotid body tumors (CBTs) are rare and usually benign neuroendocrine neoplasms that have a predictable but slow growth rate and a low potential for malignancy. They arise from the carotid body, which functions as the body's sensor, primarily to O_2 partial pressure. Through afferent fibers of the glossopharyngeal nerve, the carotid body transmits information to the central nervous system. The carotid body is made up of a small cluster of chemoreceptor cells, located near the bifurcation of the carotid artery, which detect not only changes in pO_2 but also CO_2, pH, and temperature in the arterial blood flowing past it. It is composed of two types of glomus cells, type I (chief) cells and type II (sustentacular cells); chief cells are derived from neural crest and release neurotransmitters, including acetylcholine, adenosine triphosphate, and dopamine, while type II cells function as a supporting structure.[1] Due to its function, the carotid body contains some of the most vascular tissue in the body.

PATHOLOGY

A paraganglioma is a neuroendocrine neoplasm arising from chemoreceptor cells. While the term "paraganglioma" is the most widely accepted to describe these tumors, they were previously called chemodectomas.[1] Over 85% of paragangliomas develop in the abdomen, while 13% develop in the chest, and only 3% develop in the head and neck region; 95% are benign.[2,3]

CBTs are the most common of the head and neck paragangliomas and are located exclusively in the carotid bifurcation. Other sites in the neck where the paragangliomas may occur include the parasympathetic and sympathetic nerves. When neoplasms arise in these locations, they are often called glomus tumors, and although they behave in a similar clinical pattern to CBTs, they are not CBTs.

INHERITANCE/GENETICS

Approximately 75% of paragangliomas are sporadic, while 25% are hereditary (Table 22.1).[2,4] They more commonly occur in patients living at a high altitude. Succinate dehydrogenase gene mutations have been found among families with a high incidence of head and neck paragangliomas and CBTs. Power and colleagues recently demonstrated that mutations in the succinate dehydrogenase gene are highly correlated with a family history of CBTs as well as bilateral CBTs. Specific mutations of the succinate dehydrogenase genes have been associated with increased risk of malignant paragangliomas. Patients with succinyl dehydrogenase (SDH)-positive tumors more often have bilateral, functional, malignant, systemic, recurrent, and metachronous tumors.

DIAGNOSIS

Most patients diagnosed with a CBT initially have minimal symptoms, so the most common finding in the early stages is a painless neck mass.[5] It is often discovered by the patient or after a thorough physical exam. As the neck mass enlarges, it becomes more painful, and with gradual enlargement specific nerve compression may lead to neck or jaw pain, facial droop, or voice hoarseness.

Imaging is the best method of diagnosis, starting with duplex ultrasound, which identifies the typical finding of a mass in the carotid bifurcation with "splaying of the carotid arteries." Duplex ultrasound can also determine the location of the mass with respect to other structures, such as the thyroid, and whether the mass shows the high degree of vascularity present in CBTs. Because of its vascularity, a needle biopsy should never be performed on a CBT. Many surgeons will proceed with treatment based solely on the duplex ultrasound results, although large CBTs—those encasing the internal carotid artery (ICA) and those close to the base of the skull—may need additional imaging.

For most patients, the next diagnostic study is a computed tomography (CT) scan, which is often performed with contrast, and which provides significant additional information (Fig. 22.1). The tumor's vascularity, size, relationship to the carotid arteries and base of the skull, and its intracerebral cross circulation can all be assessed with a CT angiogram. In addition, balloon occlusion can be performed to determine the impact of clamping and/or ligating the carotid artery. Preoperative embolization can be used before surgery to reduce bleeding during resection. As an alternative, a magnetic resonance imaging or magnetic resonance angiography can substitute for the CT scan, particularly if other pathology is suspected. An angiogram is rarely needed in CBT patients, unless embolization or carotid balloon occlusion is being performed. The imaging tests performed should be done in a systematic fashion with an algorithm approach used to limit the number and types of imaging studies.

TABLE 22.1 Patient and Tumor Characteristics (n = 356)

Patient Characteristics	Mean ± SD (Range) or No. (%)
Age	51.2 ± 14.5 (range, 20–84)
Female	257 (72.2%)
Ethnicity	
White/Caucasian	138 (38.8%)
Black/African American	9 (2.53%)
Asian/Pacific Islander	16 (4.49%)
Hispanic/Latino	149 (41.9%)
Unknown	44 (12.4%)
Family history of CBT	23 (6.46%)

CBT, Carotid body tumor.
Modified from Kim GY, Lawrence PF, Moridzadeh RS, et al: New predictors of complications in carotid body tumor resection. *J Vasc Surg* 65(6):1673–1679, 2017.

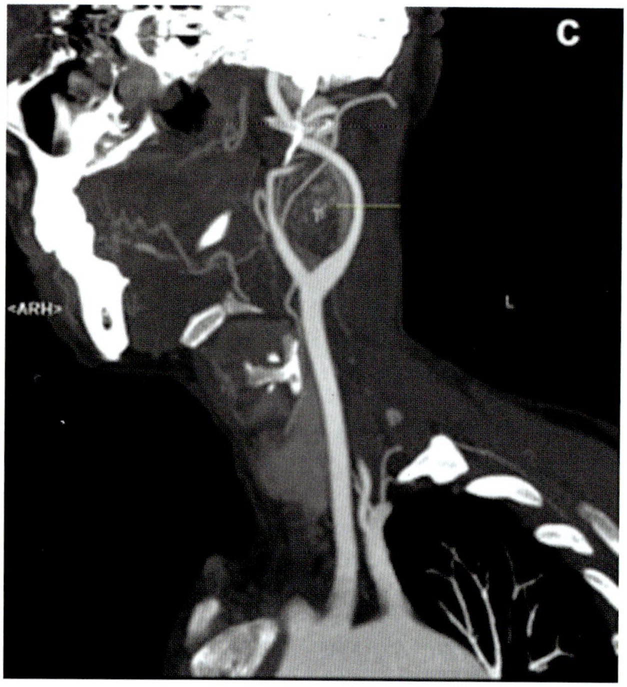

FIG 22.1 Carotid body tumor on computed tomography (CT) scan. This representative sagittal cross section on CT imaging demonstrates the relationship between the carotid body tumor and the carotid arteries. The tumor arises from the carotid body, which is located at the posterior-medial aspect of the carotid bifurcation. As the tumor enlarges, it causes splaying of the internal and external carotid arteries. If the tumor continues to grow without resection, it can eventually encase the carotid arteries as well as adjacent nerves. (Originally published in Jin ZQ, He W, Wu DF, Lin MY, Jiang HT: Color Doppler ultrasound in diagnosis and assessment of carotid body tumors: comparison with computed tomography angiography. *Ultrasound Med Biol* 42:2106–2113, 2016.)

TABLE 22.2 Shamblin Classification at Presentation (n = 356)

Shamblin Grade (n = 349)	No. (%)
I	113 (31.7%)
II	154 (43.3%)
III	82 (23.0%)

Modified from Kim GY, Lawrence PF, Moridzadeh RS, et al: New predictors of complications in carotid body tumor resection. *J Vasc Surg* 65(6):1673–1679, 2017.

LABORATORY TESTS

The most important lab study, in addition to routine preoperative studies, is the SDH deficit blood study. This test shows whether the CBT is associated with a genetic defect, which may lead to development of another paraganglioma or the likelihood that other family members will develop a CBT. Certain mutations of the SDH gene, specifically SDHB mutation, have been shown to be associated with an increased risk of malignancy.

CAROTID BODY TUMOR CLASSIFICATION

The Shamblin classification system has been used over the past 50 years to classify CBT, based on their relationship to the ICA. The system is quite simple, with only three classes (Fig. 22.2), based on the degree of encasement of the ICA: Shamblin 1, with no carotid artery encasement; Shamblin 2, with partial encasement; and Shamblin 3, with complete encasement of the ICA (Table 22.2).[1] The Shamblin classification system has been correlated with many factors, including the estimation of the volume of blood loss, the need for embolization of the branches to the CBT to reduce blood loss, the risk of stroke, the need for carotid artery reconstruction, and the likelihood of cranial nerve injury (Fig. 22.3). Many studies have also demonstrated that higher Shamblin grades are associated with a higher incidence of complications.[3-9] Many investigators have suggested the need to improve on this classification system. One proposed modification uses the Shamblin system but adds to it the size (volume) of the tumor, as well as the distance from the base of the skull, and is based on the theory that large tumors high in the neck are more difficult to resect, even when they do not encase the ICA.[5] Measuring the tumor size, volume, and relationship to the base of the skull can additionally help quantify the risks of bleeding and cranial nerve injury. For every 1 cm the CBT is located closer to the base of skull, there is 1.8 times the increase in risk of greater than average intraoperative blood loss, 1.4 times increased risk of transfusion, 1.5 times increased risk of cranial nerve injury, and 2.7 times increased risk of multiple cranial nerve injuries. Knowing the risks of complications preoperatively can greatly assist in patient education, and may lead to different surgical strategies.

PREOPERATIVE PREPARATION

Counseling is an important aspect of a patient's preparation, since nerve injuries are the most common complication, and

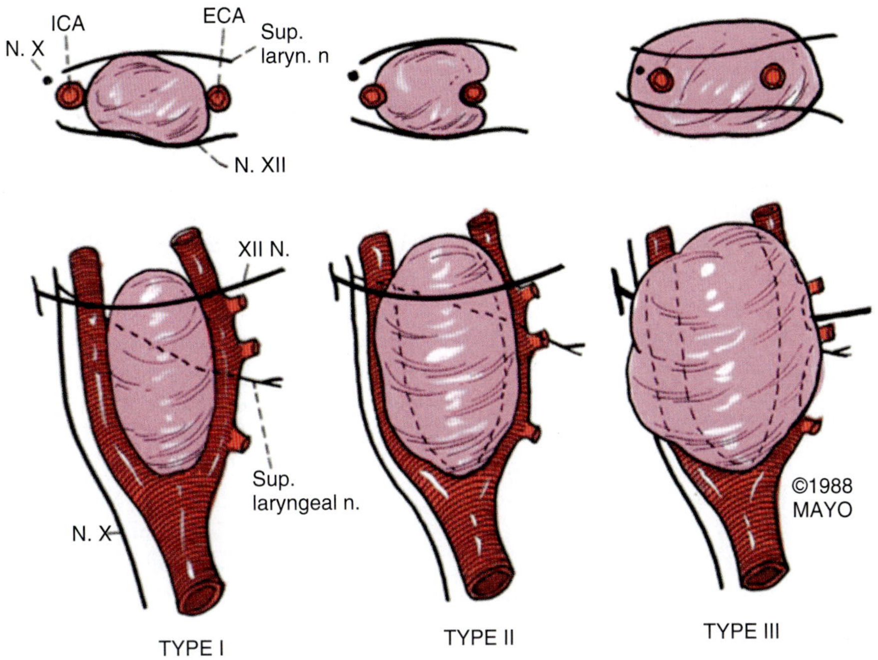

FIG 22.2 Shamblin classification of carotid body tumors. The Shamblin classification describes the relationship between the carotid body tumor and the surrounding structures. Shamblin I tumors are small and confined the carotid bifurcation. Shamblin II tumors are larger, but they do not entirely encase the carotid vessels. Shamblin III tumors are the largest and often encase the internal and external carotid arteries (*ICA* and *ECA*) as well as adjacent nerves. (Originally published in Power AH, Bower TC, Kasperbauer J, et al: Impact of preoperative embolization on outcomes of carotid body tumor resections. *J Vasc Surg* 56:979–989, 2012.)

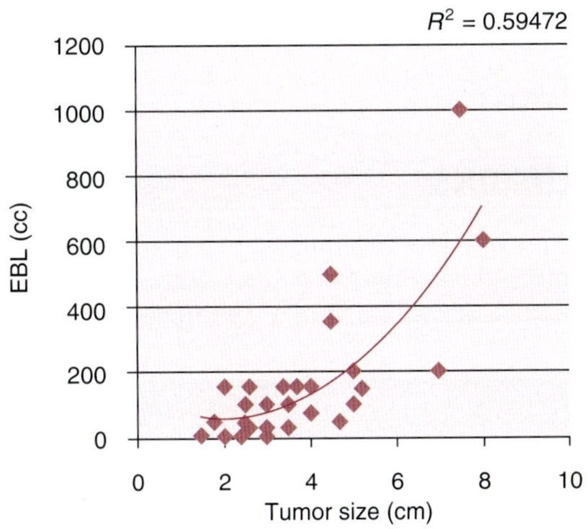

FIG 22.3 Carotid body tumor size and estimated blood loss (*EBL*). In this single-center study from the University of California Los Angeles, tumor size is plotted against EBL from 43 carotid body tumor resections in 37 patients. EBL increases with a given increase in carotid body tumor size. In addition, tumors greater than 5 cm in size were found to be significantly associated with an increased risk of cranial nerve injury. For this reason, some surgeons endorse the use of preoperative embolization and the use of bipolar cautery to reduce blood loss in large tumors.

some can be debilitating and permanent. Surgical planning is also critical, since blood loss and intraoperative bleeding often occur during CBT resection. Inadequate control of bleeding can also lead to adjacent nerve and carotid artery injury, as well as stroke.

EMBOLIZATION

Preoperative embolization is often utilized to improve the success of surgical resection for CBTs. It has been reported to reduce blood loss and is thought to be helpful for also decreasing cranial nerve injuries. However, there are no guidelines for which CBT patients should receive embolization prior to resection. Some surgeons do not embolize, while others embolize all CBTs. Many of the tumors that have preoperative embolization are located close to the base of skull.

TREATMENT

Surgical resection is the primary treatment of CBT before they become painful and involve cranial nerves; studies have found little utility in primary radiotherapy, chemotherapy, or embolization for definitive therapy. Although surgical resection is the recommended treatment modality, it is associated with significant risk, with up to 30% to 40% morbidity and mortality.[3-9]

Tumor resection of CBT requires significant preoperative and operative planning. If carotid clamping is anticipated, then electroencephalogram (EEG) monitoring is often used to monitor cerebral function and is set up prior to anesthesia induction. If a tumor is close to the base of the skull, there are several options to provide the best exposure, including nasotracheal intubation and subluxation of the mandible. Once anesthetized, the incision used is surgeon dependent, but often along the anterior border of the sternocleidomastoid muscle, although several other incisions may also be used. After entering the carotid sheath, most surgeons agree that initial proximal control of the common carotid artery is important, as well as distal ICA control. The external carotid artery is also important to clamp early in the dissection, since the external carotid artery is the source of the blood supply to the CBT. It can also be ligated to facilitate both the control of bleeding and the dissection. When dissecting the carotid artery off of the surrounding tissues, bipolar cautery is often helpful. If the tumor cannot be dissected from the ICA, carotid reconstruction may be necessary. This is required in ~5% of CBT cases in most series, and the artery can be replaced with either a polytetrafluoroethylene graft or saphenous vein. Although stroke is rare in CBT resection patients, even when carotid reconstruction is necessary, EEG monitoring is helpful to determine when a carotid shunt is needed.

COMPLICATIONS

Mortality is rare in virtually every large study of CBT resection (Table 22.3). Trends in morbidity associated with CBT resection have improved with advances in technique; however, there have been no improvements in cranial nerve injuries. Many studies report that patients often experience changes in their voice, difficulty with tongue movement and speech articulation, and difficulty swallowing; these deficits are associated with injuries to the superior laryngeal, hypoglossal, and vagus nerves, respectively. Intraoperative bleeding is another important complication associated with CBT resection, since inadequate control of bleeding can have serious consequences, including adjacent nerve injury and carotid artery injury, as well as stroke. Although previous studies have documented some of these complications, there is a lack of preoperative information that can help quantify an individual's risk for cranial nerve injury and bleeding. However, overall complications occur in ~25% of patients.

TABLE 22.3 Outcomes of Carotid Body Tumor Resection

Outcomes	
Cranial nerve injury	87 (24.4%)
Stroke	5 (1.40%)
Death	1 (0.281%)

Adapted from Kim GY, Lawrence PF, Moridzadeh RS, et al: New predictors of complications in carotid body tumor resection. *J Vasc Surg* 65(6):1673–1679, 2017.

Meticulous sharp dissection is the best method of reducing nerve injury, although it is not always possible to prevent nerve injury with large CBTs. When nerve involvement is anticipated, a nerve stimulator can both prevent injury by identifying nerves before dissections and by identifying injured or cut nerves after nerve injury occurs.

LONG-TERM RESULTS

Recurrence is rare when CBT resection is complete and tumor is not intentionally left behind. In rare cases of malignancy, lymph node resection is indicated for the diagnosis of metastasis, although recurrence is much more likely. Most nerve injuries are temporary, but a few are permanent (Table 22.4).[5] The most disabling symptoms occur with glossopharyngeal nerve injury, since difficulty swallowing and aspiration are disabling. Voice changes with vagus and superior laryngeal nerve injury are often temporary, but can be managed with procedures that improve voice, when needed.

CONCLUSIONS

CBTs are infrequently encountered in a head and neck or vascular surgery practice, but when they occur, it is important to follow vascular principles with a comprehensive preoperative

TABLE 22.4 Cranial Nerve Injuries After Carotid Body Tumor Resection

Injured Cranial Nerves (n = 85)	No. (%)	Temporary No. (%)	Permanent No. (%)
CN VII (facial n.)	10 (2.80%)	10 (100%)	0 (0%)
CN IX (glossopharyngeal n.)	12 (3.37%)	10 (83.3%)	2 (16.7%)
CN X (vagus n.)	39 (11.0%)	17 (43.6%)	21 (53.8%)
Superior laryngeal n.	19 (5.34%)	11 (5.26%)	8 (42.1%)
Recurrent laryngeal n.	3 (0.842%)	1 (33.3%)	2 (66.7%)
CN XI (accessory n.)	4 (1.12%)	4 (100%)	0 (0%)
CN XII (hypoglossal n.)	35 (9.83%)	24 (68.6%)	11 (31.4%)
Sympathetic ganglion	10 (2.80%)	6 (60.0%)	3 (30.0%)
Any CN injury (at least 1 injury)	87 (24.4%)	—	—
Multiple CN injuries (>1 injury)	35 (9.83%)	—	—

CN, Cranial nerve.
Adapted from Kim GY, Lawrence PF, Moridzadeh RS, et al: New predictors of complications in carotid body tumor resection. *J Vasc Surg* 65(6):1673–1679, 2017.

evaluation. Appropriate patient counseling includes discussion of the risks of stroke, bleeding, and nerve injury. With appropriate preoperative planning, several options exist to reduce bleeding risk, including embolization of the tumor and carotid balloon occlusion, although it is unclear if either of these maneuvers actually reduce bleeding and stroke risk, since they are commonly used in the largest and highest CBT. In the operating room, meticulous technique and sharp tissue dissection, early control and/or clamping of the external carotid artery, and distal ICA control usually facilitate resection without extensive bleeding or nerve injury. Carotid repair or resection is rarely needed but should be anticipated in all Shamblin 2 and 3 tumors, where it partially or fully encases the ICA. When resection is required, the interposition graft can be either prosthetic or autogenous tissue, since both have excellent long-term results. Postoperative complications are rare, except for temporary cranial nerve injury, which occurs in less than 10% of patients. Succinate dehydrogenase mutation testing has been recommended for young patients with CBT to help predict the likelihood of bilateral tumors and familial CBT in first-degree relatives.

REVIEW QUESTIONS

1. The gene mutation most commonly associated with carotid body tumors is:
   - **a.** Succinate dehydrogenase
   - **b.** Pyruvate kinase
   - **c.** Lactate dehydrogenase
   - **d.** Aldolase
   - **e.** Hexokinase
2. All of the following statements regarding the carotid body are true except:
   - **a.** It transmits information to the central nervous system via afferent fibers of the glossopharyngeal nerve
   - **b.** It is located at the carotid bifurcation
   - **c.** It detects changes in pH, pO_2, and CO_2
   - **d.** It is a largely avascular structure
   - **e.** It releases acetylcholine and dopamine
3. Carotid body tumors are more frequent in patients who reside in which of the following areas?
   - **a.** Sea level
   - **b.** Rural regions
   - **c.** High altitude
   - **d.** Metropolitan cities
   - **e.** Cold climates
4. What is the most common presentation of carotid body tumors?
   - **a.** Stroke
   - **b.** Facial nerve palsy
   - **c.** Dysphagia
   - **d.** Painless neck mass
   - **e.** Pulsatile neck mass
5. Which is the most common complication following carotid body tumor resection?
   - **a.** Stroke
   - **b.** Mortality
   - **c.** Hemorrhage requiring blood transfusion
   - **d.** Cranial nerve injury
   - **e.** Tumor metastasis
6. Which of the following statements regarding carotid body tumors is true?
   - **a.** Most are malignant
   - **b.** They are associated with squamous cell carcinoma
   - **c.** Most are sporadic and not familial
   - **d.** The majority are bilateral
   - **e.** Most are functional tumors secreting catecholamine
7. The preferred initial diagnostic modality for CBT is which of the following:
   - **a.** MRI
   - **b.** MR angiography
   - **c.** CT angiography
   - **d.** Duplex ultrasound
   - **e.** Catheter based angiography
8. Which of the follow statements best describes the Shamblin classification?
   - **a.** It describes the relationship between the CBT and the common carotid artery
   - **b.** It dictates the need for vascular reconstruction
   - **c.** It describes the relationship between the CBT and the vagus nerve
   - **d.** It describes the relationship between the CBT and the external carotid artery
   - **e.** It describes the relationship between the CBT and the carotid arteries
9. Definitive treatment of carotid body tumors requires which of the following?
   - **a.** Surgical resection with or without arterial reconstruction
   - **b.** Chemotherapy
   - **c.** Embolization
   - **d.** Radiation
   - **e.** No treatment given; most tumors are benign
10. Which of the following is the predominant blood supply to the carotid body tumor?
   - **a.** Common carotid artery
   - **b.** Superior thyroid artery
   - **c.** Internal carotid artery
   - **d.** Branches of the thyrocervical trunk
   - **e.** External carotid artery

References available online at ExpertConsult.com.

23 CHAPTER

Surgical Management of Aortoiliac Occlusive Disease

Dean J. Arnaoutakis, Michael Belkin

In the Western world, atherosclerotic occlusive disease of the abdominal aorta and iliac arteries is a common cause of lower extremity ischemia in middle-aged and elderly patients. Although not as common as occlusive disease of the femoropopliteal arterial system, with which it may be combined, aortoiliac occlusive disease may be more disabling because of the greater number of muscle groups subjected to diminished perfusion. The initial manifestation of occlusive disease of the distal aorta or iliac arteries is intermittent claudication of the buttock, hip, thigh, and/or calf. Because the calf muscles are usually the only muscle groups affected by intermittent claudication caused by superficial femoral artery occlusion, the involvement of more proximal muscles in the symptom complex may help to distinguish aortoiliac occlusive disease from femoropopliteal occlusive disease. However, relatively few patients with aortoiliac disease complain of only calf claudication; male patients with aortoiliac occlusive disease often complain of impotence because of pelvic ischemia with inadequate perfusion of the internal pudendal arteries. In addition to impotence, these men may develop buttock claudication, atrophy of the leg muscles, lower extremity pallor, and absent femoral pulses, a constellation of symptoms first described by Rene Leriche in the 1940s.[1]

Patients with aortoiliac occlusive disease can develop ischemic rest pain or tissue loss; however, this presentation is uncommon, because patients develop a rich collateral circulation reconstituting the infrainguinal system, thereby providing adequate tissue perfusion at rest. Collaterals often form between the hypogastric and lumbar arteries to the circumflex iliac, femoral, and profunda vessels as well as between the mesenteric arteries and hemorrhoidal vessels. Arteriosclerotic plaque in the aorta and iliac arteries can also embolize, causing the so-called blue toe syndrome (i.e., microembolization of arteriosclerotic debris to the terminal vessels in the foot).[2-5] Such symptoms can occur in a patient who otherwise appears to have adequate distal perfusion, including palpable pedal pulses. Under these circumstances, a workup should ensue with a computed tomography (CT) angiogram, looking for a proximal source of microembolization. When there is concomitant femoropopliteal occlusive disease in the setting of aortoiliac disease—a combination more prevalent in elderly patients with diabetes and hypertension—rest pain or tissue loss may ensue.[6] As in any arterial system, tandem lesions in the periphery are more significant than single lesions.

Aortoiliac occlusive disease usually afflicts older patients who have a history of tobacco use, hypertension, and hyperlipidemia.[7-18] In our experience, patients reporting symptoms of claudication caused by aortoiliac occlusive disease are on average nearly a decade younger than those complaining of claudication from superficial femoral artery occlusion. However, patients with rest pain from concomitant multisegmental occlusive disease are usually older (i.e., in the seventh decade of life) than those who present with rest pain from isolated femoropopliteal disease.

The initial lesions of aortoiliac occlusive disease usually begin at the terminal aorta and the proximal portions of the common iliac arteries or at the bifurcations of the common iliac arteries (Fig. 23.1). The lesions then progress proximally and distally. Approximately 33% of patients treated for symptomatic aortoiliac disease have disease at the origin of the deep femoral arteries, and more than 40% have superficial femoral artery occlusions. The natural history of aortoiliac occlusive disease is one of slow progression.[19,20] The ultimate anatomic result of aortoiliac atherosclerosis is variable, as occlusion of the distal abdominal aorta can occur with progression of the thrombus up to the level of the renal arteries (Fig. 23.2). Although occlusion of the terminal aorta may remain stable for years, it does not always have a benign course.[21] Starrett and Stoney observed that more than one-third of patients with aortic occlusion went on to develop thrombosis of the renal arteries over a period of 5 to 10 years (Fig. 23.3). However, many years later, authors from the same institution[22] found no evidence of renal thrombosis in 21 patients who were followed with arteriography after a mean of 27.7 months.

Variants in the pattern of aortoiliac occlusive disease can occur, including relatively circumscribed occlusive lesions of the midabdominal aorta described in early to middle-aged female smokers (Fig. 23.4). Although the upper abdominal aorta is ordinarily spared in patients with aortoiliac occlusive disease, a minority of these patients have marked involvement of this aortic segment, with occlusive disease at the origins of the major visceral vessels and renal arteries (Fig. 23.5).

DIAGNOSIS

The diagnosis of aortoiliac occlusive disease should be made after a thorough history and physical exam. Complaints of thigh claudication, with or without accompanying sexual dysfunction in males, suggest this disease process. Claudication symptoms, however, must be differentiated from symptoms of nerve root irritation caused by spinal stenosis or intervertebral

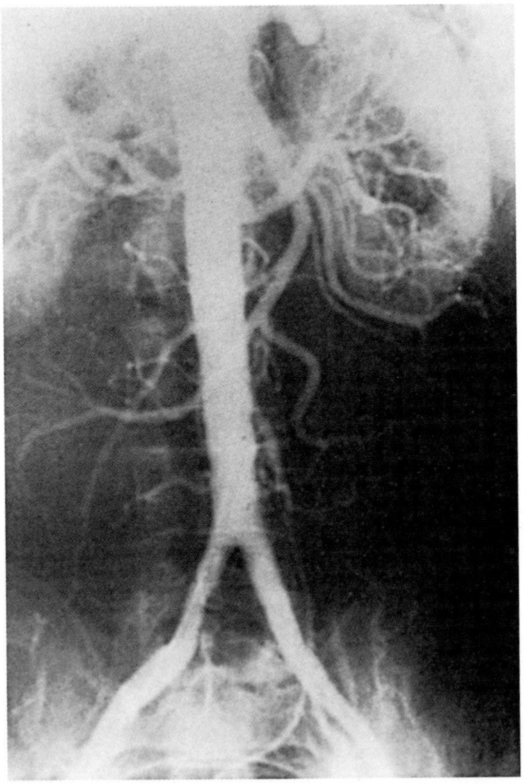

FIG 23.1 The earliest manifestations of aortoiliac occlusive disease are evident in the terminal aorta and proximal common iliac vessels.

disk herniation, which may be associated with activity and relieved by rest.[23] Patients with spinal disease can ordinarily be distinguished from patients with vasculogenic claudication because of the typical sciatic distribution of their pain, which is equally reproducible with standing and walking. An even more sensitive finding in patients with lumbar spinal stenosis is that prolonged standing in an erect posture will exacerbate symptoms.

Over time, a patient with intermittent claudication may develop atrophy of the lower extremity muscles from chronic disuse; however, the soft tissue of the extremities will usually appear healthy and well perfused at rest. Diminished or absent femoral pulses is a critical physical exam finding that can indicate the level of the occlusive disease. Bruits heard in the groin can also call attention to proximal occlusive lesions. However, stenotic lesions at the origins of the superficial or deep femoral arteries can also cause femoral bruits. Palpable pedal pulses at rest may be found in patients with severe claudication from aortoiliac occlusive disease even when the femoral pulses are barely discernible. This reflects a rich collateral circulation that can develop over time.

Segmental Doppler pressures at all levels in the lower extremity are lower than the brachial pressure; in the absence of concomitant superficial femoral occlusive disease, no significant gradient between the upper thigh pressure and the ankle pressure will be present. However, disabling symptoms can occur in patients with aortoiliac disease who have near-normal resting ankle pressures

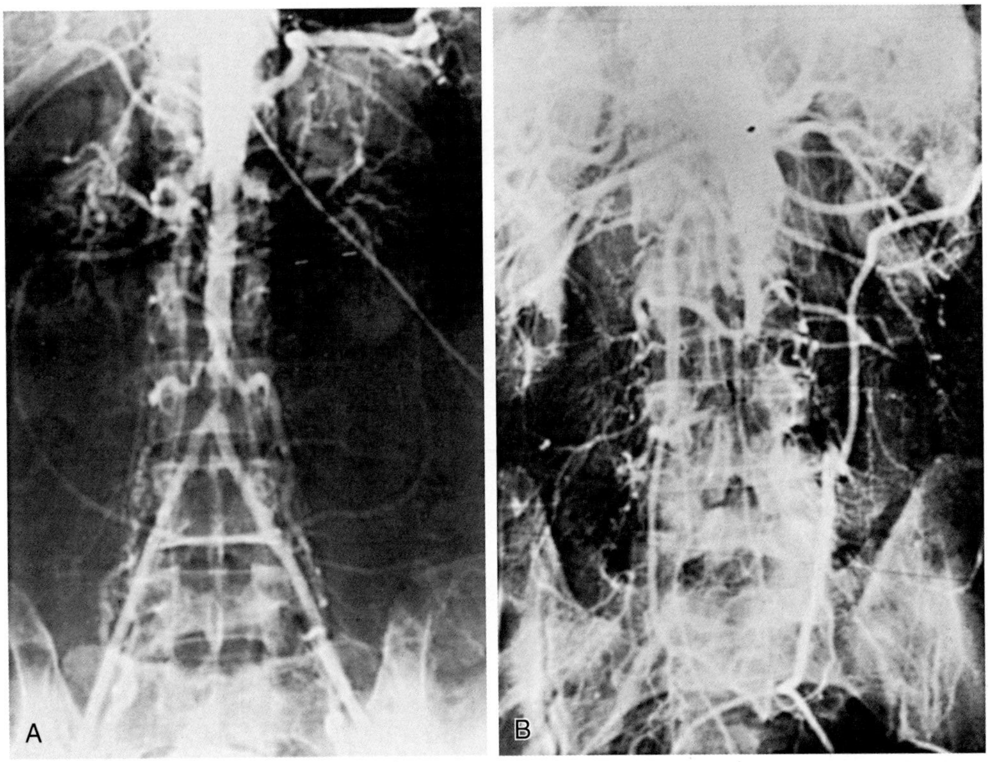

FIG 23.2 Aortoiliac occlusive disease results in a variable degree of collateralization, shown as a discrete channel from a lumbar artery to the deep iliac circumflex artery (A) and as a multiplicity of small vessels that supply the hemorrhoidal and gluteal arteries that reconstitute the femoral vessels via iliac and femoral circumflex arteries (B).

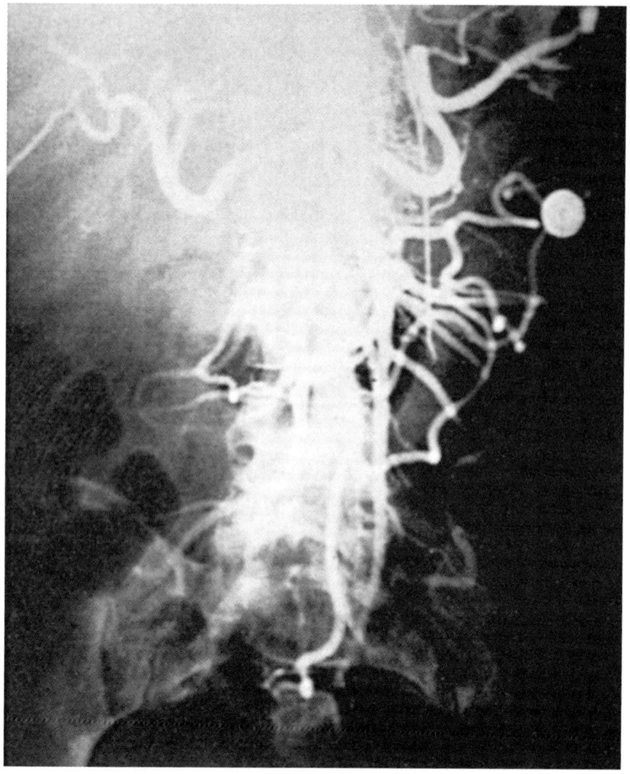

FIG 23.3 The end result of aortoiliac occlusive disease consists of total aortic thrombosis, which may include the origins of the renal arteries.

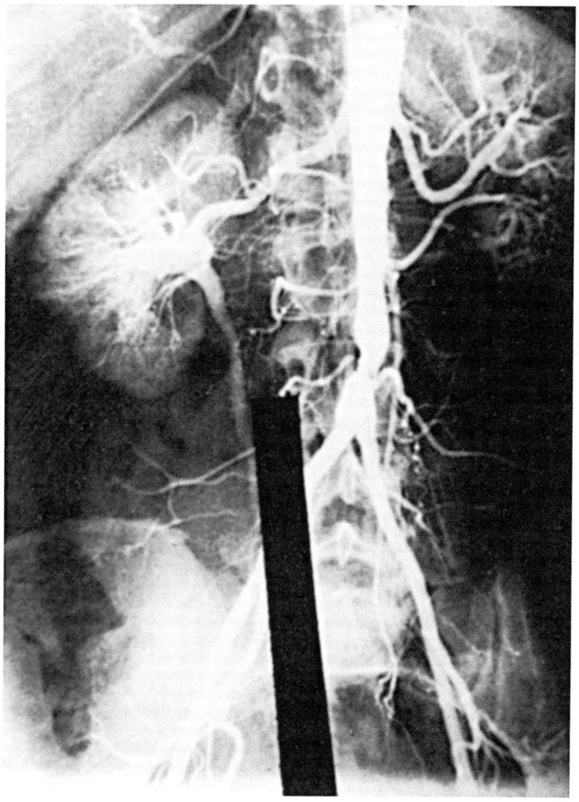

FIG 23.4 Aortoiliac occlusive disease may consist of a short-segment circumferential lesion, especially common in younger women. Such a lesion may be amenable to localized endarterectomy.

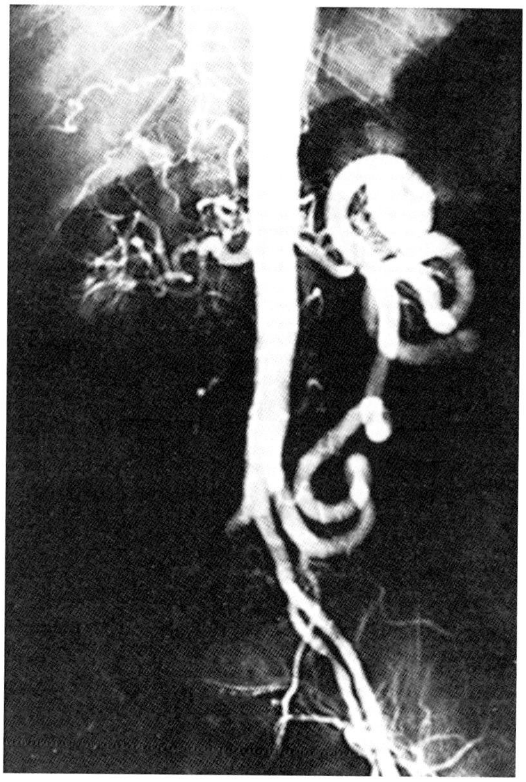

FIG 23.5 A large meandering mesenteric artery associated with total superior mesenteric artery celiac occlusion, renal artery stenosis, complete occlusion of the right common iliac artery, and distal left external iliac stenoses with a single patent hypogastric artery. End-to-side proximal anastomosis may best preserve both the mesenteric and pelvic circulation.

and a normal ankle-brachial pressure index at rest. Therefore it can be helpful to repeat pressure measurements after a period of graded exercise, because a marked decrease will occur in patients with significant aortoiliac disease.[24] More sophisticated Doppler waveform analysis or the use of a pulse-volume recorder may reveal patterns suggestive of proximal occlusive lesions.[25-27] We have found, however, that resting and postexercise Doppler pressure measurements are satisfactory for the evaluation of most patients.

Indications for intervention include disabling claudication despite optimal medical therapy, ischemic rest pain, or tissue loss. For those with lifestyle-limiting claudication, emphasis should initially be placed on optimal medical therapy of hypertension, elevated cholesterol, and glucose control as well as risk factor modification with smoking cessation and weight loss. In addition, exercise therapy may relieve symptoms adequately to allow a lifestyle acceptable to the patient; intervention is then not needed or recommended, particularly in elderly patients or those with cardiac, pulmonary, neurologic, or other comorbidities. In contrast, patients with critical limb ischemia should be more aggressively and expeditiously treated by open or endovascular means as long as their medical risk and life expectancy warrant such intervention.

PREOPERATIVE EVALUATION

The preoperative evaluation of a patient with aortoiliac occlusive disease includes a careful evaluation of any accompanying cardiopulmonary disease. In the authors' experience, approximately 40% of patients with symptomatic aortoiliac occlusive disease have clear clinical and electrocardiographic evidence of coronary artery disease. Symptomatic unstable coronary artery disease in such individuals demands investigation, including stress testing and cardiac catheterization in many cases. If coronary revascularization is indicated, this procedure should take precedence; the aortoiliac occlusive disease can be repaired later. Patients with mild or stable coronary artery disease can ordinarily undergo aortoiliac reconstruction without great risk. Older patients with severe cardiopulmonary disease who are not candidates for coronary artery intervention are probably best managed with an extraanatomic bypass as opposed to direct reconstruction. Patients with severe restrictive pulmonary disease may require a period of preoperative preparation that includes bronchodilators, broad-spectrum antibiotics, and abstinence from cigarette smoking.

Angiography, most often performed through a retrograde femoral approach, has historically been deemed the "gold standard" in the preoperative evaluation of patients with symptomatic aortoiliac disease.[28] However, axial imaging with CT angiography (CTA) or magnetic resonance angiography (MRA) is now the most common diagnostic imaging study. CTA and MRA are well suited for evaluating the aorta and the mesenteric, renal, and iliac arteries, affording careful operative planning. Faster acquisition techniques and high-quality three-dimensional postprocessing capabilities make MRA an attractive, noninvasive modality. However, the question of which is the most cost-effective imaging modality remains controversial. Regardless of the imaging technique, the goal of the radiographic examination is to provide views of the entire abdominal aorta in two planes and to look for unexpected lesions of the celiac axis or superior mesenteric artery origins, to provide anteroposterior and oblique views of the pelvis to define any iliac artery lesions in more than one plane, and to demonstrate possible lesions at the origins of the deep femoral arteries. It is critical to preoperatively identify and ultimately preserve a large inferior mesenteric artery in the setting of severe superior mesenteric artery disease in order to prevent bowel ischemia (see Fig. 23.5). Views of the distal runoff vessels should also be obtained to demonstrate associated femoropopliteal occlusive disease. If catheter angiography is used, at the time of angiography, obtaining pull-back pressures across iliac artery lesions of unclear significance can help to elucidate the clinical significance of such lesions. Measurements should be taken at rest and after papaverine injection or during a period of reactive hyperemia after tourniquet ischemia to mimic the hemodynamic situation that occurs with exercise.[29]

Open surgical reconstruction and percutaneous balloon angioplasty with or without stenting are the main treatment options for aortoiliac occlusive disease. The choice of treatment approach should be based on the durability of the intervention for the occlusive lesion or lesions as well as the patient's ability to safely tolerate a particular intervention. The TransAtlantic Intersociety Consensus (TASC) II guidelines delineated which anatomic lesions are best served by percutaneous versus open surgical therapy.[32] In general, TASC A and B lesions (focal, short-segment lesions [≤3 to 10 cm], unilateral or bilateral) are best treated with endovascular options. Conversely, TASC D lesions (long-segment occlusions and diffuse, severe long-segment disease, particularly bilateral) are best treated with open surgery. Intermediate TASC C lesions can be treated appropriately with either technique; however, these lesions and even some TASC D lesions are increasingly being treated by percutaneous stenting.

AORTOFEMORAL BYPASS GRAFT

The aortofemoral bypass graft, given its long-term durability, remains the gold standard for the treatment of severe symptomatic aortoiliac occlusive disease. This procedure's 30-day operative mortality rate of 5% to 8% in the early 1970s has been reduced to less than 2% over the past two decades, a level similar to that observed in patients undergoing elective abdominal aortic aneurysm repair.[33-39] Much of the reduction in operative mortality is due to the prevention of early cardiac deaths in patients with heart disease through improvements in perioperative care. These advances include selective utilization of preemptive cardiac surgery, sophisticated pharmacologic management of the damaged myocardium, continuation of certain antiplatelet agents, and more precise perioperative fluid management tailored to the myocardial reserve.[39]

Surgical Technique

After the administration of appropriate antibiotics, the femoral vessels are often exposed first through bilateral groin incisions to reduce the time of an open abdomen and the insensible fluid loss and hypothermia that occur with an exposed abdomen. The proximal extent of the dissection should be carried to the inguinal ligament. Often, partial division of the inguinal ligament is necessary to identify a soft segment of vessel that will be suitable for clamping. Control of the epigastric and circumflex iliac vessels with Silastic tapes is often necessary, as these vessels are often enlarged from years of receiving collateral flow. Distally, the superficial femoral and deep femoral arteries are also controlled. The extent of their exposure depends on the extent of concomitant femoropopliteal disease. Once the femoral dissection is complete, the inferior aspect of a retroperitoneal tunnel in each groin is bluntly created, ensuring that this tunnel remains directly anterior to the external iliac artery.

Next, the aorta is exposed through a midline transperitoneal incision, although some prefer a transverse incision. Others expose the infrarenal aorta through a left retroperitoneal exposure, which is an attractive alternative for patients with multiple prior intraabdominal procedures. Once the duodenum and small bowel have been mobilized and retracted to the right, a self-retaining retractor is placed and the infrarenal aorta is exposed from the left renal vein down to the inferior mesenteric artery and until soft areas for clamping are identified. The softest part of the aorta is often located right below the renal arteries. Dissection of the distal aorta and iliac arteries should be minimized to prevent injury to the iliac veins and hypogastric plexus. Injury to the nerve plexus can cause men to have difficulty achieving an erection and ejaculating. Once all vessels are exposed, tunnels are created bluntly from the peritoneal cavity toward each groin incision using the anterior surface of the common and external iliacs arteries as a guide. By doing so, the tunnels will be behind the ureters, and they will not be mistakenly incorporated into the tunnel passage. Note that the tunnel on the left side is created deep to the sigmoid mesentery and lateral to the nerve plexus overlying the terminal aorta. Systemic heparin sodium is administered prior to the application of atraumatic vascular clamps. It may be necessary to apply the clamp in an anteroposterior configuration in the event of severe posterior calcification in order to prevent traumatic clamp injury.

A bifurcated, knitted Dacron prosthetic graft, usually impregnated with collagen or gelatin, is used by most surgeons, although polytetrafluoroethylene (PTFE) grafts are used by some. There is some evidence that a knitted graft may provide a more stable pseudointima than a woven prosthesis.[43,44] The graft size—typically 18 by 9 mm, 16 by 8 mm, or 14 by 7 mm—is selected to best match the native aorta and femoral arteries. The graft is trimmed accordingly and then the proximal anastomosis is constructed either end to end or end to side, using a running 3-0 polypropylene or PTFE suture, just inferior to the renal arteries. After completion of the proximal anastomosis, the limbs are flushed with heparinized saline, clamped, and then passed through the retroperitoneal tunnels to the groin. In the groin, end-to-side anastomoses are fashioned onto the distal common femoral artery with a running 5-0 polypropylene suture. Often, the anastomoses are carried down onto the deep femoral arteries for a short distance. Prior to completing the anastomoses, graft flushing maneuvers are used; then the clamps are removed, one side at a time, while monitoring the blood pressure as reperfusion can result in hypotension.

An important factor contributing to improved outcomes has undoubtedly been recognizing the role of the deep femoral artery in providing sustained patency of the aortofemoral graft limb.[33,36,45,46] The current practice of extending the distal anastomosis onto the origin of the deep femoral artery to ensure an adequate outflow tract is critical in patients with tandem superficial femoral occlusions or stenosis of deep femoral origin. If a profundaplasty or endarterectomy is necessary, the vessel should be closed with a patch of saphenous vein, bovine pericardium, or endarterectomized superficial femoral artery as opposed to creating a long deep femoral patch with the distal end of the aortofemoral prosthesis.[45]

The incidence of graft infection has been minimized with perioperative antibiotic administration.[33,47-49] Aortoenteric fistulas can be minimized by closing the retroperitoneal tissue and posterior parietal peritoneum over the graft and proximal suture line, thereby preventing erosion of the graft into the duodenum.[33,50,51] In thin patients, it may be difficult to primarily close the retroperitoneum over the graft; an omental flap can be utilized in such scenarios.

Controversy remains over the proper configuration of the proximal anastomosis as it has several ramifications.[33,52,53] Most favor an end-to-end configuration, during which the aorta is transected between clamps approximately 1 to 2 inches below the renal arteries and the distal stump is oversewn or stapled (Fig. 23.6). This technique permits a comprehensive endarterectomy or thrombectomy of the proximal native aorta under direct vision before constructing the anastomosis. Excluding flow from a heavily diseased distal aorta, which may have had plaque or thrombus dislodge during clamp application, may prevent intraoperative emboli to the lower extremities. Additionally, this configuration theoretically creates a better inflow pattern with less turbulence.

Furthermore, the end-to-end technique does not project anteriorly, thereby affording easier closure of the retroperitoneum, which arguably results in lower rates of aortoduodenal fistulas. However, this configuration relies on patent external iliac arteries in order for the pelvis to receive retrograde perfusion. In comparison, an end-to-side configuration (Fig. 23.7) is best suited for those with heavily diseased external iliac arteries, such that preservation of antegrade aortic flow is necessary to supply the hypogastric or inferior mesenteric artery.[52] In addition, an end-to-side anastomosis should be constructed in those with a critically large inferior mesenteric artery (IMA) or accessory renal arteries to preserve flow in these crucial vessels. With this technique, a longitudinal aortotomy is made on a nondiseased segment of aorta just below the renal arteries. Great care is taken to remove all loose debris and mural thrombus from the segment of clamped aorta. At completion of an end-to-side anastomosis, adequate backflushing of all loosened debris and clot from the distal aorta is essential before forward flow is reestablished. Unfortunately controlled studies have not been conducted to substantiate that the results of one technique is superior to the other. Arteriographic studies in patients with indications for an end-to-side anastomosis are shown in Figs. 23.5 and 23.8.

Despite significant advances in laparoscopic and robotic surgery, applications of these techniques to vascular surgery have been limited. Nonetheless, several authors have applied laparoscopic techniques to aortofemoral reconstruction. Whether performed completely via the laparoscopic approach or through limited incisions with laparoscopy-assisted dissection, the procedure has proved to be time-consuming and technically challenging.[55,56] As the technology evolves and intracorporeal anastomotic techniques are refined, the future role of laparoscopic or robotic aortofemoral bypass will become defined.

In patients with focal aortoiliac lesions, aortoiliac endarterectomy is a suitable albeit uncommon treatment option. This tedious operation, even in the hands of enthusiasts, is confined to patients whose aortic disease ends distally near the bifurcation of the common iliac arteries (Fig. 23.9; see also Fig. 23.4).[33] This group of patients characteristically consists of middle-aged women with small aortas and occlusive disease of the midabdominal aorta that ends at the aortic bifurcation or in the proximal portions of the common iliac arteries. Aortoiliac endarterectomy is typically avoided in males because such a technique will interfere with the autonomic nerve plexus at the terminal aorta. There is little evidence to suggest that endarterectomy is superior to a properly performed aortofemoral bypass graft in terms of early or late results. Furthermore, in the current endovascular era, most patients will focal lesions are treated with percutaneous balloon angioplasty with or without stenting.

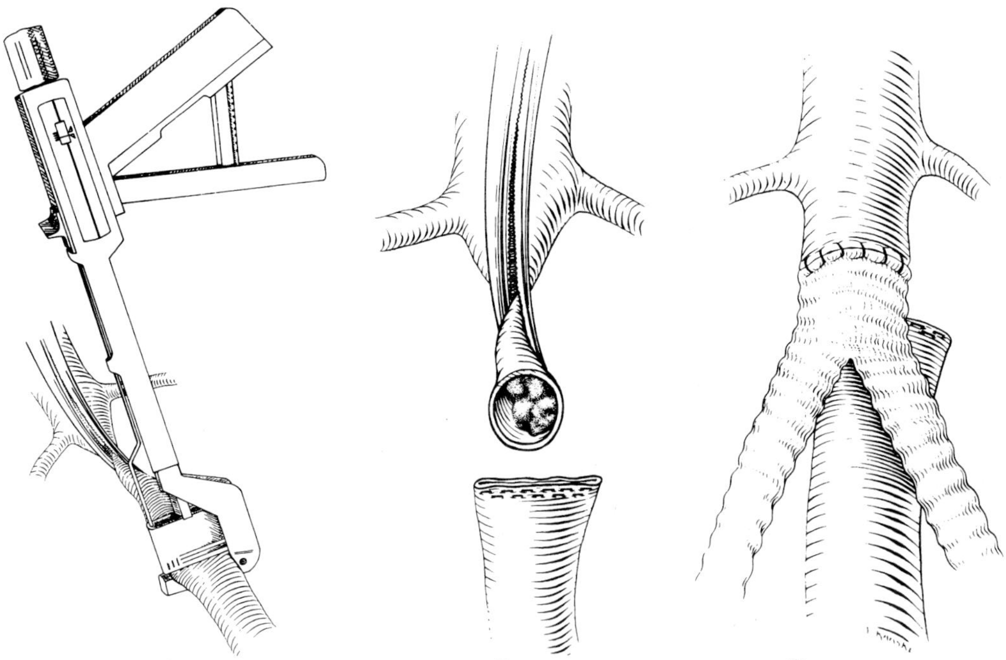

FIG 23.6 End-to-end proximal anastomosis for aortofemoral reconstruction can be initiated with the infrarenal aortic cross-clamp placed in an anteroposterior direction, with minimal dissection as close to the origin of the renal arteries as possible. The aorta is then stapled or occluded with a second clamp just proximal to the origin of the inferior mesenteric artery (A). After transection of the infrarenal aorta and complete thromboendarterectomy of the proximal infrarenal aortic cuff (B), end-to-end anastomosis is completed with continuous 3-0 polypropylene sutures (C).

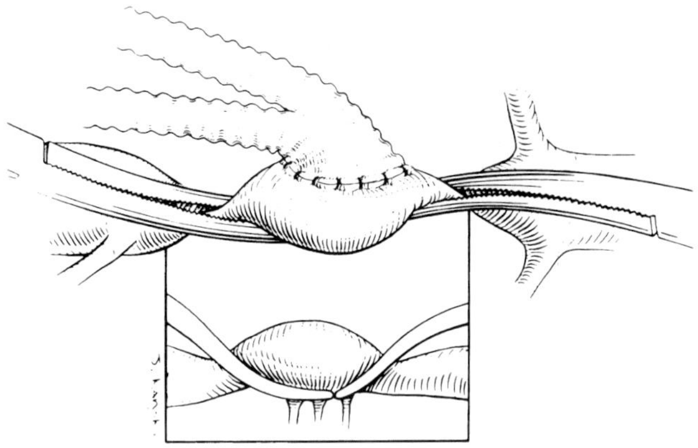

FIG 23.7 End-to-side proximal anastomosis for aortofemoral reconstruction is required to preserve antegrade pelvic perfusion when retrograde perfusion from distal femoral anastomoses is doubtful. The infrarenal aorta is occluded proximal to the origin of the inferior mesenteric artery and just distal to the origin of the renal arteries. After longitudinal arteriotomy and thorough thromboendarterectomy, if required, the anastomosis is constructed using continuous polypropylene sutures.

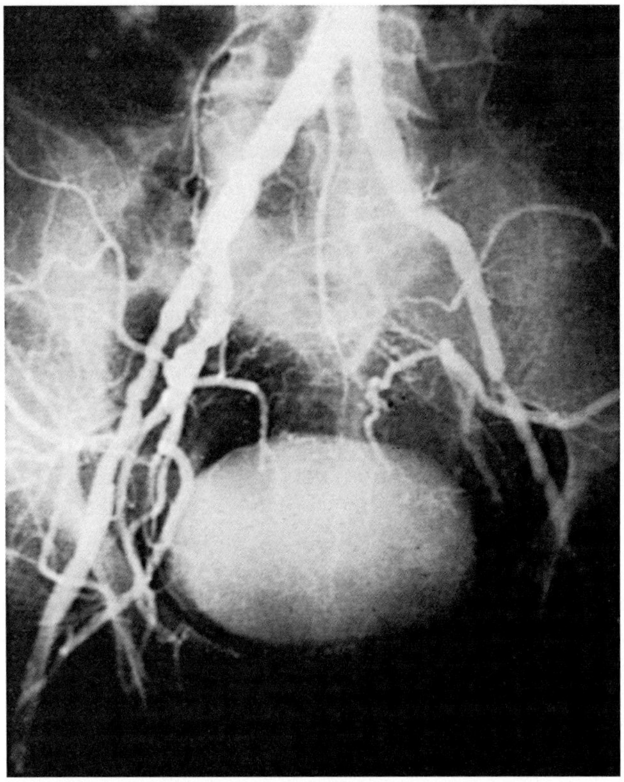

FIG 23.8 Diffuse aortoiliac disease with left hypogastric occlusion and minimal left pelvic collateralization may warrant end-to-side proximal anastomosis to preserve the right hypogastric system.

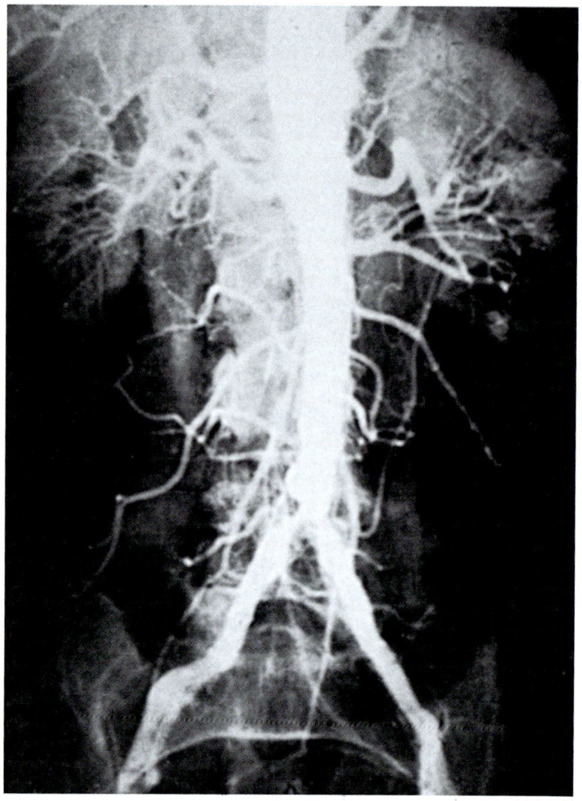

FIG 23.9 Aortoiliac occlusive disease with significant lesion confined to the origin of the right common iliac artery, amenable to either local endarterectomy or percutaneous transluminal angioplasty.

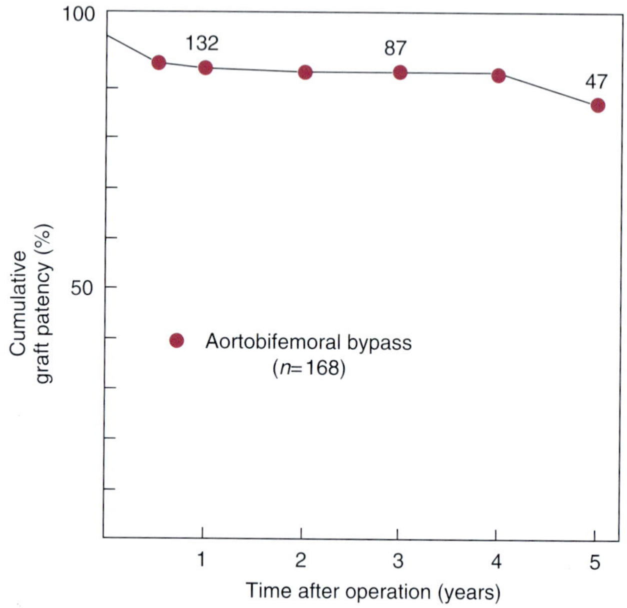

FIG 23.10 For 168 aortobifemoral graft limbs inserted in 84 consecutive patients, the 5-year cumulative patency was 86%.

Complications

In contemporary series evaluating aortobifemoral bypass grafting, the perioperative mortality rate is exceptionally low (1%); the morbidity ranges from 17% to 35%.[33,34,36,57,58] Wound complications—including surgical site infections, hematomas, and lymphoceles—are the most common postoperative events, being reported in up to 15% of patients. Cardiopulmonary events occur with less frequency, but their occurrence is certainly associated with mortality. Renal failure is unlikely to develop if the clamp position is infrarenal; however, injury or kinking of the ureters during tunneling can cause postobstructive renal failure. Ischemia to the spinal cord, bowel, or lower extremities can happen, although rarely, from atheroemboli released after clamp removal. Several late, uncommon complications include aortoenteric fistula, anastomotic false aneurysm, and graft thrombosis. Graft thrombosis typically occurs in a unilateral fashion as a result of neointimal hyperplasia at the distal anastomosis or from progressive native femoral disease.

Results

Outcomes after aortobifemoral graft bypass are excellent— early patency rates approach 100% and the 5-year patency is greater than 80%.[33,34,36,57,58] Durability is sustained, with 10-year patency rates approaching 75%.[33] These findings remain true regardless of indication, approach, or anastomotic configuration. A number of operative refinements have aided in decreasing graft limb thrombosis. The more prevalent use of the aortobifemoral graft, as opposed to aortoiliac bypass or extended aortoiliac endarterectomy, has negated the effect of unsuspected or progressive atherosclerosis in the external iliac vessels. Avoiding graft limb redundancy and selecting a graft diameter that is most compatible with the native vessel have also helped to maintain long-term patency.

Our results with aortofemoral bypass grafting are illustrated in Fig. 23.10. The 5-year cumulative patency of 86% is comparable with that reported in a number of other studies.[33,34,36,57] Thirty-day operative mortality was slightly less than 1%, which reflects careful patient selection as well as improved perioperative management and anesthetic technique. However, because aortoiliac occlusive disease is rarely life threatening (although it may be limb threatening), it is preferable to treat high-risk patients with procedures of lesser magnitude. With regard to survival, 80% of patients are alive at 5 years, whereas only 50% reach 10 years. The 5-year cumulative survival for a patient undergoing aortofemoral bypass grafting is approximately 14% lower than the expected survival for a normal age-corrected person.[53]

There is a subset of patients, however, who do not enjoy such excellent results. Younger patients and those with small aortas are vulnerable to late graft failure. A study of aortofemoral reconstructions in 73 patients younger than 50 years documented a 5-year primary patency rate of only 50%.[53] The authors also found that patients with aortas less than 1.8 cm in diameter had significantly lower patency rates (6-year patency of 20%) than did those with aortic diameters greater than 1.8 cm (6-year patency of 60%). Similarly, we have documented lower patency rates in young patients: 5-year patency was only 66% in patients younger than 50 years, compared with 87% for 50- to 60-year-olds and 96% for those older than 60 years.[59] Younger patients also had significantly smaller aortas, corroborating the influence of aortic size on long-term outcomes. Neither gender nor indication (limb salvage versus claudication) was found to significantly affect long-term patency rates.

Although graft patency does not directly correlate with functional outcome, approximately 95% of patients are initially improved or asymptomatic following surgery; after 5 years, about 80% remain in this category.[36,57] A study from the United Kingdom indicated that among patients fully employed before aortobifemoral bypass, 85% returned to full employment at an average of 4 months after surgery, and more than 50% of those not previously employed returned to work after bypass.[60] Other studies have documented a more sobering functional outcome after successful aortofemoral arterial reconstruction. One study, employing the SF-20 questionnaire, found that patients after aortobifemoral bypass had decrements in physical function and general health perception similar to patients with congestive heart failure or recent myocardial infarction.[61] Clearly more functional outcome analysis is necessary after the treatment of aortoiliac occlusive disease.

Concomitant Distal Reconstruction

When patients have threatened limb loss from a combination of aortoiliac and femoropopliteal occlusive disease, restoring suprainguinal inflow is necessary to salvage the extremity. However, performing a concomitant distal reconstruction, such as femoropopliteal bypass, at the time of the initial operation is debated. Results suggest that repairing the aortoiliac disease alone, thereby restoring perfusion into the deep femoral system, will achieve limb salvage in the vast majority of patients with ischemic rest pain.[46,62] However, patients with significant tissue loss of the foot, particularly individuals with diabetes, will typically require pulsatile flow to the foot in order to heal the ulcer. Under these circumstances a concomitant distal reconstructive procedure is necessary at the time of the aortobifemoral bypass. The additional distal bypass procedure adds operative time and therefore risk to the patient, but utilizing a two-team operative approach in conjunction with modern anesthetic management can mitigate the risks.

ALTERNATIVES FOR HIGH-RISK PATIENTS

Although aortobifemoral bypass grafting can be performed successfully with low morbidity and mortality, less extensive procedures may be preferable in patients who are high risks for major vascular surgery under general anesthesia. In such patients, distal aortic and proximal iliac occlusions can be treated by an axillofemoral bypass.[63-67] If the occlusive disease is limited to one common or external iliac artery, then the contralateral, patent iliac system can be used as the origin for a bypass graft. Such a technique permits a shorter graft segment and arguably affords better long-term patency compared with an axillofemoral bypass. The femorofemoral bypass is an example of such a procedure.[68] An anatomically similar procedure, the iliofemoral graft, has received little attention in the literature.

Ilioiliac and Iliofemoral Bypass Grafts

Patients with multiple medical issues who have occlusive disease involving mostly the external iliac artery but sparing the aorta and the proximal common iliac artery are candidates for reconstruction using a patent common or external iliac artery for the proximal anastomosis (see Fig. 23.5). The distal anastomosis can be taken to the contralateral external iliac artery or the ipsilateral femoral artery, depending on the location of occlusive disease. Constructing an ilioilial bypass is advantageous in that it avoids a groin incision with its inherent complications, preserves the native femoral artery for future use, minimizes postoperative ileus, and avoids potential injury to the presacral nerves.

The operation begins with a curvilinear incision parallel to and above the inguinal ligament, identical to the approach for renal transplantation. The retroperitoneal exposure of the iliac vessels is technically simple, even in obese patients. A limited iliac endarterectomy may be necessary. For an ilioiliac bypass, symmetrical incisions are made to expose the iliac vessels and the graft is positioned in the retroperitoneum (Fig. 23.11A). If an ileofemoral bypass is necessary, a separate vertical groin incision is made to expose the common femoral artery. The graft is tunneled under the inguinal ligament (see Fig. 23.11B and C). For patients undergoing bilateral iliofemoral reconstruction, the crossover limb is placed from the iliofemoral graft retroperitoneally in the iliac fossa or, in a few cases, subcutaneously to the contralateral femoral artery (see Fig. 23.11C).

Our institution reviewed a series of 94 patients undergoing ilioiliac or iliofemoral bypass grafting from 1982 to 1992. The patients were on average 60 years of age and suffered from the typical cardiovascular comorbidities. Of the cohort, 58% had claudication and 42% had critical limb ischemia. The majority underwent an iliounifemoral bypass and the remainder had iliobifemoral or ilioilial grafts. No patients died within 30 days. The 4-year cumulative patency for the ilioiliac grafts (23 limbs) and iliofemoral grafts (91 limbs) was 96% and 72%, respectively (Fig. 23.12). The 4-year patency for iliobifemoral grafts (72%) was nearly identical to that of the iliounifemoral grafts (71%). If both the superficial and deep femoral arteries were patent, the 4-year cumulative patency rate for iliofemoral grafts was higher (85%) than if only the deep femoral artery was patent (62%). Aortofemoral grafts enjoy slightly superior 4- and 5-year patency rates compared with iliofemoral grafts, although this is not statistically significant. An iliofemoral bypass is a durable alternative for elderly, poor-risk individuals in the rare circumstance where occlusive disease is confined mostly to the external iliac arteries or to one iliac system.

Femorofemoral Bypass Graft

A femorofemoral bypass can be used in patients whose occlusive disease is confined to one iliac artery but the aorta and contralateral iliac system are free of hemodynamically significant lesions. One of the most common indications for femorofemoral bypass is for patients undergoing endovascular aortounifemoral repair of aortic aneurysms, necessitating contralateral revascularization, or in patients having a previous endoprosthesis relined and converted to an aortouni-iliac device. Multiple authors[66,68,69,70] have demonstrated that this operation yields satisfactory long-term results (60% to 80% 5-year patency). It is uncommon for these grafts to fail because of progressive proximal atherosclerosis. Disease progression may be stunted by increased flow through

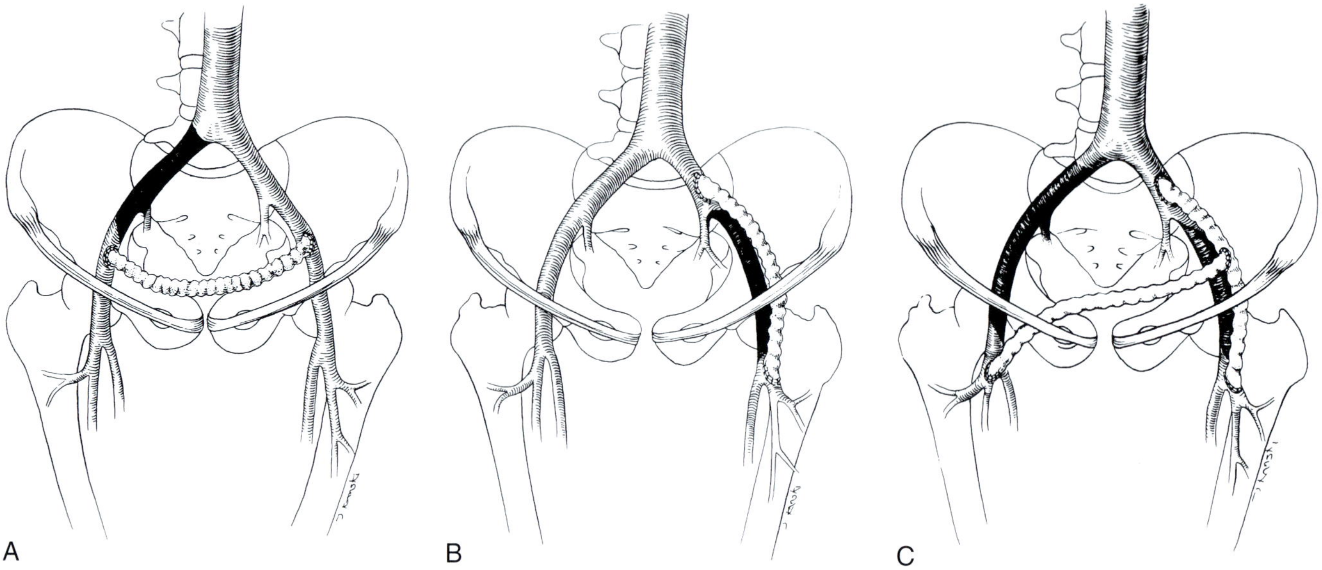

FIG 23.11 A patent common or external iliac artery may be used as a donor vessel for ilioiliac (A), iliofemoral (B), or iliobifemoral (C) bypasses in appropriate patients who would otherwise require axillofemoral reconstruction.

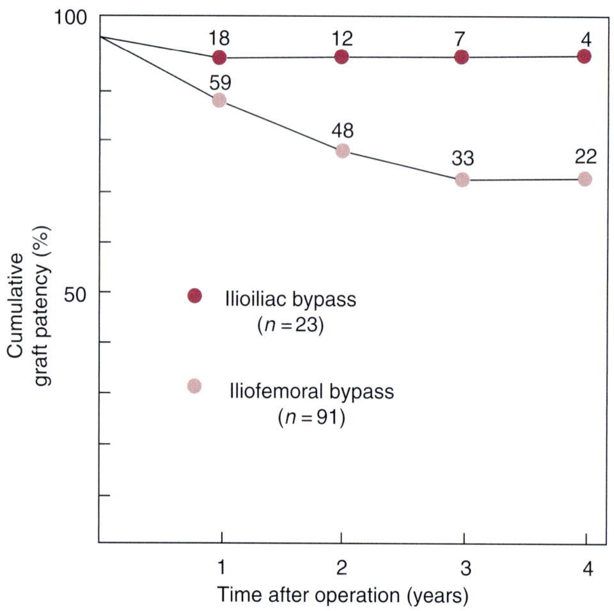

FIG 23.12 Using a patent iliac vessel as the donor artery, the 4-year cumulative graft patency for 23 ilioiliac grafts was 96%, whereas the patency for 91 iliofemoral graft limbs was 72%.

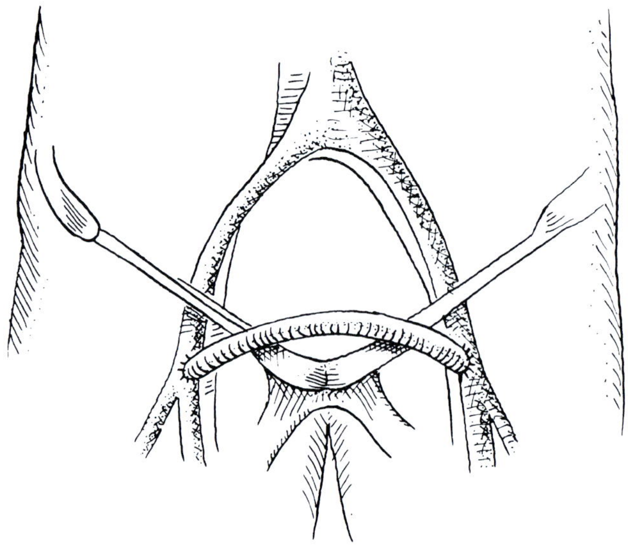

FIG 23.13 The femorofemoral bypass graft is illustrated, with the preferred C configuration of the subcutaneous tunnel constructed well above the pubis.

the donor iliac system, which is required to supply blood to both of the lower extremities. Berguer and coworkers[71] reported experimental support for this hypothesis by demonstrating in animals that intimal hyperplasia correlates inversely with blood flow and shear stress. However, experimental results yielding the opposite conclusion have also been reported.[72]

The femorofemoral graft is particularly applicable to high-risk patients because it can be performed easily under epidural, spinal, or even local anesthesia. The common femoral arteries are exposed through short groin incisions. A subcutaneous suprapubic tunnel is bluntly created anterior to deep fascia in order to connect the two incisions. It is preferable to have the graft form a C configuration, with the anastomoses placed in the distal common femoral arteries and the graft traveling proximally up through the suprapubic tunnel and down to the opposite common femoral artery (Fig. 23.13). In our experience with femorofemoral bypass, the majority of patients were elderly and suffered from coronary artery disease, diabetes, and/or hypertension and presented with critical limb ischemia. The 5-year cumulative graft patency was 80%, which is lower, although not statistically significant, than that for aortofemoral bypass grafting (Fig. 23.14). In selected patients with focal common iliac artery stenosis, donor limb

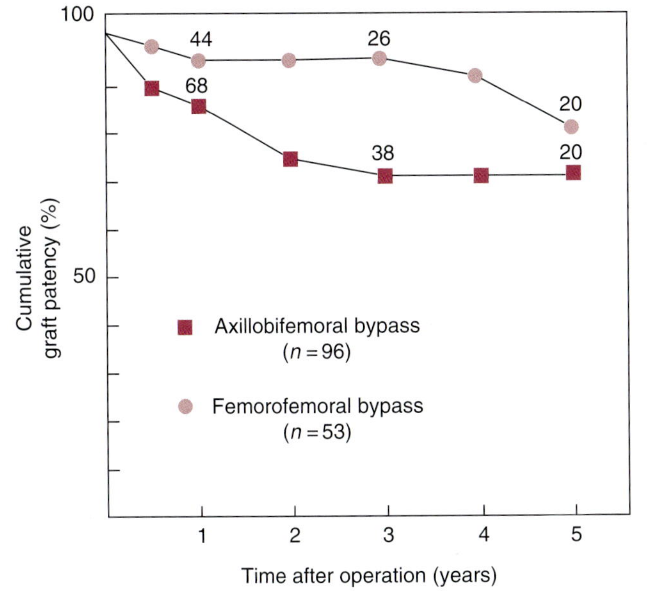

FIG 23.14 The 4-year cumulative graft patency for 53 femorofemoral grafts was 80%, and the patency for 48 axillobifemoral grafts (96 limbs) was 70%.

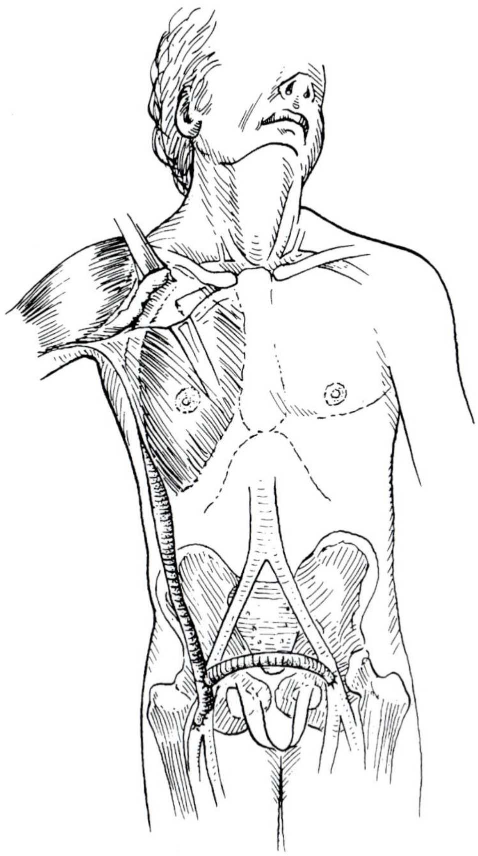

FIG 23.15 Subcutaneous axillobifemoral bypass graft completed with proximal anastomosis to the right axillary artery, right distal anastomosis to the common and deep femoral arteries, and extension of the prosthesis with a side limb to the left common femoral artery.

angioplasty and stenting followed by a femorofemoral bypass is safe and efficacious.[73] This hybrid approach expands the patient population eligible for femorofemoral bypass. The reasonably good long-term results, ease of performance, and low morbidity associated with femorofemoral bypass suggest that it can be used in good- and poor-risk patients who have proximal occlusive disease confined to one iliac arterial segment. Although it is difficult to argue against this point of view, the fact that the groins have been operated on and the common femoral arteries dissected during the performance of a femorofemoral graft makes an aortobifemoral reconstruction in such individuals technically more difficult if progression of proximal disease causes a return of symptoms or late failure of the femorofemoral bypass. Therefore, in good-risk patients with evidence of arteriosclerotic disease in the aorta or in the patent iliac system, the recommendation is for aortobifemoral bypass at the outset in an attempt to avoid possible future reoperation.

Axillofemoral Bypass Graft

Extraanatomic reconstruction with an axillofemoral bypass graft is an important part of the vascular surgeon's armamentarium, since it is one of the only treatment options for ill, elderly patients with aortoiliac occlusive disease who have critical limb ischemia. Additionally, axillofemoral bypass can prove useful in patients with multiple prior abdominal procedures, previous pelvic irradiation, infected prosthetic arterial grafts, or aortoenteric fistulas. Because this operation is relatively noninvasive, patients typically recover quickly as their ability to breathe, cough, or take oral feedings is not impaired. On the first postoperative day, most patients are ambulatory and on a regular diet.

An axillobifemoral bypass is the most common configuration, as opposed to an axillounifemoral graft, because several reports[65] showed that the axillobifemoral graft has a better 5-year cumulative patency.[67] The likely explanation for this discrepancy is that the axillobifemoral graft has approximately twice the flow rate in its axillary limb as compared with the axillounifemoral graft. However, other investigators found no significant difference in patency between bilateral and unilateral reconstructions, probably reflecting patient selection and status of distal outflow.

In constructing an axillobifemoral graft, the proximal axillary artery is exposed through an infraclavicular incision located over the insertion of the pectoralis minor (Fig. 23.15). A muscle-splitting technique should be used to dissect through the pectoralis major. Often, the pectoralis minor is divided to provide both exposure of the axillary artery and additional space for the graft as it emerges from the axilla into the subcutaneous plane. The common femoral arteries are exposed through bilateral short groin incisions. A tunnel is then created from the axilla to the groin, coursing posterior to the pectoralis major and then in a subcutaneous plane along the abdominal wall in the midaxillary line. It is important to direct the tunnel anterior to iliac crest and then in front of the inguinal ligament into the ipsilateral groin incision. An externally supported Dacron or PTFE prosthesis, usually 8 mm in diameter, is used, and the proximal anastomosis is carried out in an end-to-side manner as medially onto the axillary artery as possible. Some redundancy in the graft is needed to minimize anastomotic tension when the arm is abducted. The distal anastomosis with the femoral artery is created in an end-to-side fashion and the femorofemoral graft is then attached to the distal anastomotic hood of the axillofemoral graft. The contralateral groin anastomosis is then completed after the graft has been passed through a subcutaneous suprapubic tunnel.

Patency rates associated with axillofemoral reconstruction range from 30% to 85%.[74-76] This variability in patency can be explained in large part by patient selection, indication, and status of the outflow vessels. Extraanatomic reconstruction for nonocclusive disease, as in patients with intraabdominal sepsis or an infected aneurysm, yields better patency than does reconstruction for occlusive disease. Patients with claudication fare better than those requiring limb salvage because of inherent outflow restriction in the latter group. In a similar fashion, patients who undergo simultaneous distal femoropopliteal reconstruction do better than those whose infrainguinal disease is not addressed.

From 1982 to 1992, we performed elective axillobifemoral grafts in 48 poor-risk patients for symptomatic aortoiliac occlusive disease that resulted in critical limb ischemia. The 5-year cumulative graft patency was 70% (see Fig. 23.14). Although this patency rate is acceptable, it is inferior to that achieved with aortobifemoral bypass grafting during the same period.

Some of the most favorable results were reported by Harris and colleagues in 1990.[75] They achieved an 85% patency rate after 4 years in a group of 76 patients, 26% of whom had nonocclusive disease and 20% had simultaneous outflow reconstruction. Of note, this series was performed in a single institution using a technique that had been standardized over many years. Similar excellent 5-year patency and limb salvage rates of 74% and 89%, respectively, were reported by Passman and colleagues, leading these authors to conclude that a more liberal application of the axillobifemoral bypass is warranted.[77] In contrast, a less favorable patency rate (29%) was reported by Donaldson and colleagues[74] for 72 patients managed in several institutions by a group of 30 surgeons operating on patients with predominantly occlusive disease. Finally, many series report reasonable secondary patency rates. When axillofemoral grafts fail, thrombectomy can be successful if the patient presents promptly after the onset of symptoms. Approximately 25% of grafts thrombectomized in this fashion go on to long-term patency.[65] Thus the functional results achieved with axillobifemoral grafting may be somewhat better than the 70% graft patency figure indicates. In general, axillofemoral grafts should be reserved for poor-risk individuals in danger of limb loss and should be avoided in those with claudication alone.

Thoracofemoral Artery Bypass

The descending thoracic aorta can be used as an inflow source to bypass to the femoral artery.[78,79] Although seldom indicated as a primary procedure, this bypass offers a durable alternative after aortic failure, aortic graft infection, or other problems that necessitate avoidance of the abdominal aorta. The thoracic aorta is usually exposed through an incision along sixth- or seventh-rib interspace. A 10-mm synthetic graft is tunneled through the diaphragm at the posterior pleural reflection and then into the retroperitoneal space, terminating in the left groin. A small lateral flank incision can facilitate safe tunneling through the retroperitoneum. The descending thoracic aorta is generally of good quality and is usually clampable with a partially occluding clamp. The procedure is then completed with a femorofemoral bypass. Although there are only a few reports in the literature focusing on this procedure, they report excellent outcomes. McCarthy and colleagues[78] achieved a 100% 4-year patency rate with 21 thoracofemoral artery bypasses, while Criado and Keagy[79] reported an 83% 6- to 8-year secondary graft patency rate.

REVIEW QUESTIONS

1. Symptoms of the Leriche syndrome include all of the following except
   a. Claudication of the thigh and buttock
   b. Rest pain of the feet
   c. Impotence
   d. Diminished femoral pulses
2. Blue toe syndrome is usually characterized by which of the following?
   a. Severe claudication symptoms
   b. Absence of distal palpable pulses
   c. Palpable pedal pulses
   d. Severe tibial artery occlusive disease
3. Which of the following statements is true of patients with isolated aortoiliac occlusive disease?
   a. They generally do not suffer from ischemic rest pain.
   b. They often have relatively normal ankle-brachial indices at rest.
   c. They frequently have palpable pedal pulses.
   d. All of the above.
   e. None of the above.
4. Advantages of the end-to-end technique for proximal anastomosis of an aortobifemoral bypass graft include all of the following except
   a. Decreased incidence of aortoduodenal fistula
   b. More complete endarterectomy of the proximal aortic stump
   c. More complete preservation of pelvic blood flow
   d. Decreased incidence of distal atheroemboli
5. The end-to-side technique for aortobifemoral bypass grafts is preferred in patients with which of the following?
   a. Extremely calcified infrarenal aortas
   b. Occluded inferior mesenteric arteries
   c. Common iliac artery occlusions
   d. External iliac artery occlusions
6. Reported results of aortobifemoral bypass surgery suggest which of the following?
   a. Five-year cumulative patency rates greater than 80%
   b. Poor patency rates for patients with small (<1.8 cm) aortas
   c. Significant decrements in physical and social role function despite successful bypass
   d. All of the above

7. Reported results of aortobifemoral bypass surgery suggest which of the following?
   a. Younger patients enjoy superior long-term results.
   b. Aorta size is not a major predictor of long-term outcome.
   c. Results are relatively equal between the genders.
   d. Superficial femoral artery outflow is an important predictor of long-term patency.
8. Success rates for percutaneous transluminal angioplasty of the iliac arteries are better for which of the following?
   a. Common iliac rather than external iliac lesions
   b. Patients with claudication rather than rest pain
   c. Stenotic rather than occlusive lesions
   d. All of the above
9. Which of the following statements is false regarding extraanatomic reconstruction for aortoiliac disease?
   a. The postoperative recovery following an axillobifemoral bypass is usually quicker than direct reconstruction.
   b. Long-term patency rates following axillobifemoral bypass grafting are wide-ranging, likely a reflection of patient selection and indication.
   c. The suprapubic tunnel for a femorofemoral bypass is typically created below the fascia.
   d. A hybrid approach utilizing a femorofemoral bypass in conjunction with transluminal angioplasty and stenting of the donor iliac artery is an effective treatment option for patients with iliac disease.
10. Concomitant inflow and infrainguinal revascularization is indicated in which of the following situations?
    a. In all patients with complete superficial femoral artery occlusion
    b. For patients with severe rest pain
    c. For patients with extensive tissue necrosis
    d. For patients with diabetes

References available online at ExpertConsult.com.

24 CHAPTER

Angioplasty and Stenting for Aortoiliac Disease: Technique and Results

Ruth L. Bush, William D. Jordan, Jr.

HISTORY OF ENDOLUMINAL TREATMENT

The concept of endovascular therapy of atherosclerotic occlusive disease was introduced in the 1960s when Dotter performed the first transluminal angioplasty in a patient with ischemic extremities.[1] His novel technique, however, could not reliably maintain luminal patency and did not receive wide acceptance as a treatment of vascular occlusive lesions. Subsequent device modifications led to the development of an angioplasty balloon composed of latex material. The clinical success of this new construct was limited, in part because of its improved compliance, and could not fully dilate a calcified lesion. The introduction of an angioplasty balloon made of polyvinyl chloride in 1976 by Gruntzig and Hopff,[2] followed by rigid balloons composed of polyethylene and polyethylene terephthalate, marked a significant advance in endovascular therapy. The latter angioplasty balloons displayed a low compliance and high radial force in a fully inflated condition. As the technology and techniques of endovascular therapy continued to improve and become more widely accepted as outcomes data became available, transluminal balloon angioplasty evolved to an important modality in the treatment of peripheral vascular disease.

Despite numerous studies demonstrating the short-term clinical success of transluminal angioplasty, it has several limitations, in part because of the architectural variation of atherosclerotic lesions. Early restenosis or occlusion following angioplasty can occur because of elastic recoil of the arterial wall or intimal dissection.[3,4] Vessels that are heavily calcified, completely occluded, or that contain ulcerated plaques might not be amenable to balloon angioplasty. Moreover, residual luminal irregularities following angioplasty occasionally trigger mural thrombus formation, leading to thrombotic occlusion.[5,6] Late restenosis following angioplasty can occur as a result of intimal hyperplasia or atherosclerotic progression.[7–9]

In an effort to improve the results of transluminal angioplasty, researchers proposed the concept of intravascular stents as a means of maintaining vessel patency against the restenotic process and improving the clinical outcome of balloon angioplasty. Since Dotter first reported his successful deployment of intravascular stents in canine femoral and popliteal arteries in 1969,[10] a variety of stent devices composed of various materials have been introduced.[11–14] Intravascular stenting is recognized as a potentially effective modality in overcoming elastic recoil of the arterial wall, stabilizing intimal dissection at the site of angioplasty, and maintaining the luminal patency of arteries with calcified and eccentric atherosclerotic plaques.

CLASSIFICATION OF AORTOILIAC OCCLUSIVE DISEASE

The 2000 Trans-Atlantic Inter-Society Consensus (TASC) guidelines were developed to assist physicians in the management of peripheral arterial disease.[15] The classification of inflow of aortoiliac lesions was updated in 2007 as TASC II to reflect the advances in endovascular technology. General guidelines included in the TASC II document state that lesions classified as TASC A (Table 24.1) should be treated preferentially with endovascular techniques, whereas lesions classified as TASC D should be treated preferentially with open surgery. The recommendations for lesions classified as TASC B or C are not as clear. Good surgical judgment including surgical experience, available technology, and patient overall health needs to be considered when deciding on the appropriate initial treatment plan.

GENERAL PRINCIPLES OF ENDOLUMINAL STENTS

The desired characteristics of an intravascular stent depend on the anatomic placement and lesion characteristic for which it will be used. In general, the optimal stent needs to be encased in a low-profile device to cross high-grade lesions, and the stent should be deployed easily and accurately. Flexibility and durability are important characteristics that need to be combined with a low thrombogenic nature and high radial force. Moreover, the stent should have noticeable radiographic opacity to facilitate visualization. Finally, the ideal stent would be biocompatible, to promote endothelialization without causing intimal hyperplasia.

Intravascular stents can be separated into three distinct types: self-expanding stents, balloon-expandable stents, and covered stents (Table 24.2). Within each of these categories, there are numerous stents with different structural materials, deployment devices, and biocompatible characteristics.[11,12,16–19] In addition, there are many stents undergoing clinical trials. Table 24.3 lists the commercially available stents that can be used to treat aortoiliac occlusive disease with the US Food and Drug Administration (FDA) indication status. Some stents are tested and marketed in noniliac positions but have found use in the clinical world for arterial occlusive disease. Additionally, medicated stents and

TABLE 24.1 Trans-Atlantic Inter-Society Consensus II: Morphologic Stratification of Iliac Lesions

Type	Definition	Treatment Choice
A	Unilateral or bilateral stenoses of CIA Unilateral or bilateral single short (<3 cm) stenosis of EIA	Endovascular
B	Short (≤3 cm) stenosis of infrarenal aorta Unilateral CIA occlusion Single or multiple stenoses totaling 3–10 cm involving the EIA not extending into the CFA Unilateral EIA occlusion not involving the origins of the internal iliac or CFA	Endovascular preferred
C	Bilateral CIA occlusions Bilateral EIA stenoses 3–10 cm long, not extending into the CFA for good-risk patients Unilateral EIA stenosis extending into the CFA Unilateral EIA occlusion that involves the origins of the internal iliac and/or CFA Heavily calcified unilateral EIA occlusion with or without involvement of origins if internal iliac and/or CFA	Open surgery preferred
D	Infrarenal aortoiliac occlusion Diffuse disease involving the aorta and both iliac arteries requiring treatment Diffuse multiple stenoses involving the unilateral CIA, EIA, and CFA Unilateral occlusions of both CIA and EIA Bilateral occlusions of EIA Iliac stenosis in patients with AAA requiring treatment and not amendable to endograft placement or other lesions requiring open aorta or iliac surgery	Open surgery

AAA, Abdominal aortic aneurysm; *CFA*, common femoral artery; *CIA*, common iliac artery; *EIA*, external iliac artery.

TABLE 24.2 Characteristics of Stents

Self-Expanding	Balloon-Expandable	Covered Stent
Flexible	Rigid	Flexible
Low radial force	High radial force	Low radial force
Longer lengths	More effective at short lengths	Longest lengths available
Covering sheath in delivery system	Premounted on a balloon	Sheath or balloon premounted
Shortening is variable	Some shortening	Minimal shortening
Nitinol frame	Steel frame	Nitinol or steel frame
Radiopacity is low	Radiopacity is moderate	Radiopacity is moderate
Less accurate placement	Accurate placement	Variable accuracy

TABLE 24.3 Available Stents for Aortoiliac Disease

Device Name	Manufacturer	Stent Type	FDA Approved for:
Omnilink	Abbott	Balloon Expandable	Iliac
Herculink	Abbott	Balloon Expandable	Renal
Express LD	Boston Scientific	Balloon Expandable	Iliac
Express SD	Boston Scientific	Balloon Expandable	Renal, biliary
Formula	Cook Medical	Balloon Expandable	Renal, biliary
Palmaz	Cordis/Cardinal	Balloon Expandable	Iliac
iCast	Atrium/Maquet	Covered, Balloon Expandable	Tracheobronchial
Assurant Cobalt	Medtronic	Balloon Expandable	Iliac
Visipro	Medtronic	Balloon Expandable	Iliac
Absolute Pro	Abbott	Self-Expanding	Iliac
Supera	Abbott	Self-Expanding	SFA/popliteal
Luminexx	Bard	Self-Expanding	Iliac
LifeStent	Bard	Self-Expanding	Iliac/SFA
Epic	Boston Scientific	Self-Expanding	Iliac
Innova	Boston Scientific	Self-Expanding	SFA
Wallstent	Boston Scientific	Self-Expanding	Iliac
Zilver	Cook Medical	Self-Expanding	Iliac
Smart	Cordis/Cardinal	Self-Expanding	Iliac
Complete SE	Medtronic	Self-Expanding	Iliac, SFA. popliteal
Everflex	Medtronic	Self-Expanding	Iliac, SFA, popliteal
Protégé	Medtronic	Self-Expanding	Iliac
Misago RX	Terumo	Self-Expanding	SFA, popliteal
Fluency	Bard	Covered, Self-Expanding	AV grafts
Viabahn	W.L. Gore	Covered, Self-Expanding	SFA, popliteal
Zilver PTX	Cook Medical	Drug Eluting, Self-Expanding	SFA

AV, Arteriovenous; *SFA*, superficial femoral artery.

drug-coated balloons have been approved for arterial occlusive disease but are currently FDA approved only for iliac lesions. The Bard Lutonix balloon catheter (Bard Peripheral Vascular, Tempe, Arizona) and the Impact Admiral balloon catheter (Medtronic Vascular, Santa Rosa, California) have also been approved to treat superficial femoral artery (SFA) lesions, but they have also been reported for use in the iliac arteries.

Self-Expanding Stents

Self-expanding stents are generally manufactured so that the stents are constrained within a delivery sheath. The prosthesis is placed intravascularly through an introducer sheath that is advanced over a guidewire for deployment. Deployment is achieved by withdrawing the constraining sheath while keeping

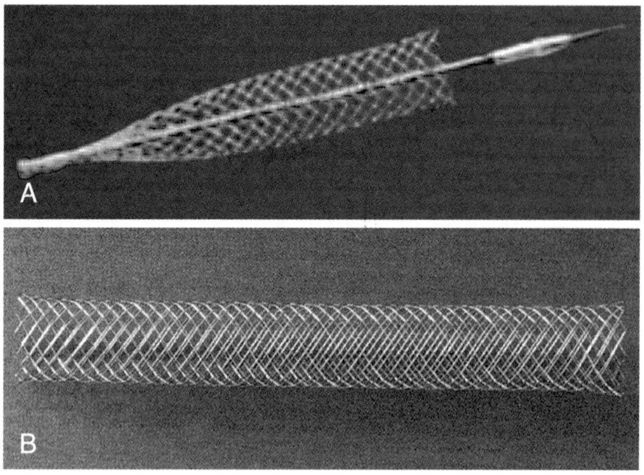

FIG 24.1 (A) Deployment of the Wallstent is achieved by withdrawing the constraining sheath. (B) The fully deployed Wallstent.

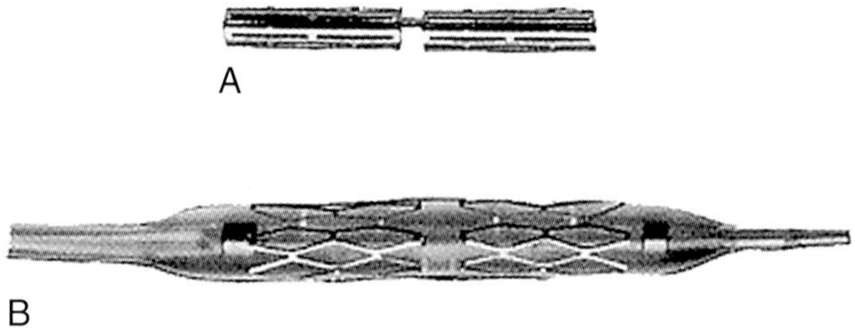

FIG 24.2 (A) The Palmaz stent is crushed to a small caliber and mounted on an angioplasty balloon. Sizes most commonly used for iliac interventions are already premounted by the manufacturer. (B) The Palmaz stent is deployed by inflating the angioplasty balloon.

the stent in position, thus permitting the stent to self-expand and anchor to the vessel lumen (Fig. 24.1). Stents in this category are generally noted for their ease of deployment and high degree of flexibility for meandering around the curves typically found in an iliac artery. These characteristics are advantageous because self-expanding stents can be used across arteries of varying diameters, specifically from the common to the external iliac. Compared with balloon-expandable stents, however, they may have lower radial force, or resistance to radial compression. These stents require oversizing by 2 to 3 mm to maintain outward radial force after deployment. Most self-expanding stent delivery systems have a smaller diameter compared with those of balloon-expandable stents. In addition, the Wallstent and the Gianturco-Z stent (Cook, Bloomington, Indiana) are available.

Another type of self-expanding stent is the nitinol stent, which was first introduced by Dotter and colleagues in 1983.[20] Nitinol is a nickel-titanium alloy that has a unique temperature-associated memory property. The nitinol wires can be shaped into a coil spring configuration to serve as a stent when heated to 500°C. As it cools down to 0°C, the nitinol coil straightens into a linear alignment that can be constrained into a delivery catheter for stent deployment. The exposure to warm body temperature after deployment causes the nitinol stent to resume its original coil spring shape. Several clinical studies have evaluated the application of these stents in vascular occlusive lesions.[20–23]

Balloon-Expandable Stents

The balloon-expandable stent is first mounted and compressed onto an angioplasty balloon. The original stents were all operator mounted; newer stents are premounted by the manufacturer. Once the stent is positioned intraluminally, it is deployed by inflating the balloon to expand the stent (Fig. 24.2). Unlike a self-expanding stent, the balloon-expandable stent can be expanded beyond its nominal diameter by using a larger angioplasty balloon catheter. Most balloon-expandable stents are characterized by excellent radial strength because of intrinsic stent rigidity once deployed, which can be advantageous in treating stenotic vessels containing calcified plaques. The rigid property of such a stent, however, can create a technical dilemma when treating lesions in tortuous vessels. Moreover, it makes a contralateral approach for iliac artery stenting a challenge, although newer stents are more trackable and flexible.

Covered Stents

The first covered stent approved by the FDA for use in the iliac system was the Gore Viabahn stent (Gore, Flagstaff, Arizona). It is a flexible Nitinol stent lined with expanded polytetrafluoroethylene. The flexibility of nitinol, as in self-expanding stents, allows it to closely conform to the vessel shape. In addition, it has a heparin-bioactive surface that is thromboresistant. It is important to conduct predeployment percutaneous transluminal angioplasty (PTA) of the affected area with subsequent coverage of the entire PTA-treated area with the covered stent. This stent is deployed by untwisting the screw-connector at the base of the deployment knob and slowly pulling the knob away from the adapter. In the Gore Viabahn Endoprosthesis Feasibility Study, 45 limbs in 42 subjects were treated for iliac artery occlusive disease.[24] There was a 12-month primary patency of 86% and a procedural success rate of 93%. This was the first-generation endoprosthesis without the heparin bioactive surface. The Gore VBX stent-graft is a balloon-expandable covered stent with more flexible design. The stent has been recently approved for iliac artery indication.

The main argument for the use of a covered stent rather than an uncovered stent is that the layer material will provide a direct barrier to tissue ingrowth from neointimal hyperplasia.[25] However, restenosis can develop at edges that are not covered by graft material where intima injury may have occurred.[26,27] Covered stents are also sometimes used when there is concern about the integrity of the arterial wall, such as cases involving perforation.

Interim results from the Covered versus Balloon Expandable Stent Trial (COBEST) conducted in Australia have provided excellent results for challenging aortoiliac occlusive disease.[28] Patients with a classification of TASC B, C, or D in the iliac level were randomized to the Advanta V12 group versus a bare metal stent group. They were followed with duplex ultrasound at various intervals and freedom from stent occlusion was assessed. The covered stent group had a significantly lower restenosis rate and greater freedom from stent occlusion than the bare metal stent group. The covered stent also showed superiority when treating TASC C and D lesions.

BOX 24.1 Indications for Intravascular Stent Placement

- Residual stenosis of 30% or greater
- Unstable intimal flaps
- Dissection
- Transstenotic pressure gradient of 10 mm Hg or greater
- Early restenosis following percutaneous transluminal angioplasty
- Nearly or totally occluded iliac arteries
- Ulcerative plaques
- When combined with an infrainguinal bypass operation

BOX 24.2 Contraindications to Intravascular Stent Placement

- Arterial disruption not related to dissection (covered stent may treat this complication)
- Severely calcified vessels
- Coexistent aneurysmal disease requiring surgical intervention
- Successful balloon angioplasty
- Presence of hypercoagulable disorder (relative contraindication)
- Target vessels that may serve as the proximal or distal site of an open surgical procedure

INDICATIONS FOR STENT PLACEMENT

Indications approved by the FDA for iliac stent placement include stenotic or occlusive atherosclerotic lesions or failed or inadequate balloon angioplasty in the iliac artery (Box 24.1). The latter condition can be assessed by angiography, intravascular ultrasound (IVUS), or hemodynamic means. Angiographic or IVUS detection of residual stenosis of 30% or greater, unstable intimal flaps, and dissection along the subintimal or medial layers are all considered inadequate angioplasty results that warrant intraluminal stent placement. Furthermore, a transstenotic pressure gradient of 10 mm Hg or greater following angioplasty is considered an indication for iliac stent placement. Provocative testing using pharmacologic agents that stimulate vasodilation may be necessary to identify a hemodynamically significant lesion. Up to 75% of patients without a translesion pressure gradient will have a significant gradient following injection of a vasodilator. Either 100 to 200 µg/mL of nitroglycerin or 30 to 60 mg of papaverine can be injected directly into the vessel in question. Immediate arterial dilatation is induced, thus mimicking exercise. A pressure drop of 10 mm Hg or more is considered indicative of a hemodynamically significant stenosis.

In addition to the FDA-approved indications for iliac artery stenting, certain other arterial conditions may be considered for stent placement. In the case of early restenosis following balloon angioplasty, stent placement is appropriate rather than repeated angioplasty alone. The 2-year patency rate of the iliac artery following angioplasty is between 65% and 81% and is affected by numerous factors, such as the degree of stenosis, the length of the lesion, and the distal vessel patency.[3,29,30] Restenosis of the iliac artery frequently occurs at the original angioplasty site,[7,9,11,31] which can be caused by neointimal hyperplasia or rapid atherosclerotic progression. Iliac artery stenting in such a condition can delay the restenotic process.

Primary stent placement, as opposed to stenting following inadequate angioplasty, has been used more frequently in the treatment of difficult iliac lesions. Nearly or totally occluded iliac arteries may be appropriate for primary stenting because angioplasty alone in these situations generally yields poor long-term patency rates.[14,32–36] Stenotic iliac vessels with ulcerative plaques can cause distal embolization when treated with balloon angioplasty.[6,37] It is appropriate to perform primary stent placement in such a condition to prevent plaque dislodgment. Moreover, primary stenting can be used as an adjunct procedure to improve iliac inflow when combined with a planned infrainguinal bypass operation.[38–40] A randomized controlled trial comparing primary stent placement versus primary angioplasty followed by selective stent placement found similar cumulative patency at 2 years (71% vs. 70%, respectively; $P = .6$).[41] The authors concluded that because angioplasty followed by selective stent placement is less expensive than primary stent placement, the former seems to be the treatment of choice for intermittent claudication as a result of iliac artery occlusive disease.

CONTRAINDICATIONS TO STENT PLACEMENT

Box 24.2 summarizes the contraindications for intravascular stent placement. Arterial perforation as a result of balloon angioplasty, as evidenced by contrast extravasation, is considered a contraindication unless a stent can stabilize the dissection. In these challenging situations, placement of a covered stent may be more appropriate.[42,43] Stent placement should also be avoided in aneurysmal arteries, because persistent blood flow around the stent can lead to further aneurysm expansion unless a covered stent is used. Because balloon-expandable stents, such as the Palmaz stent, are relatively rigid, they are less than ideal in tortuous vessels. Self-expanding stents, such as the Wallstent, have greater flexibility and are more appropriate in vessels with marked tortuosity. Severely calcified arteries are often not amenable to balloon angioplasty; similarly, stent placement should not be expected to restore the normal vessel lumen, because stent deployment requires the same basic techniques as balloon angioplasty. Finally, stent deployment should be avoided in arteries that might serve as either the proximal or distal site of a bypass grafting procedure. In a stented artery, application of vascular clamps might cause significant damage to the arterial wall, and might also crush the stent so that reexpansion is impossible. If vascular control is needed in a stented artery, an intraluminal occlusion balloon catheter should be considered rather than vascular clamps.

AORTOILIAC OCCLUSIVE DISEASE

In the infrarenal aorta, short segment stenoses can occur that are unrelated to the bifurcation. Atherosclerotic occlusive disease is the cause in the vast majority of cases. Primary stent implantation for the endovascular treatment of such focal atherosclerotic stenoses has been demonstrated in small studies to be technically

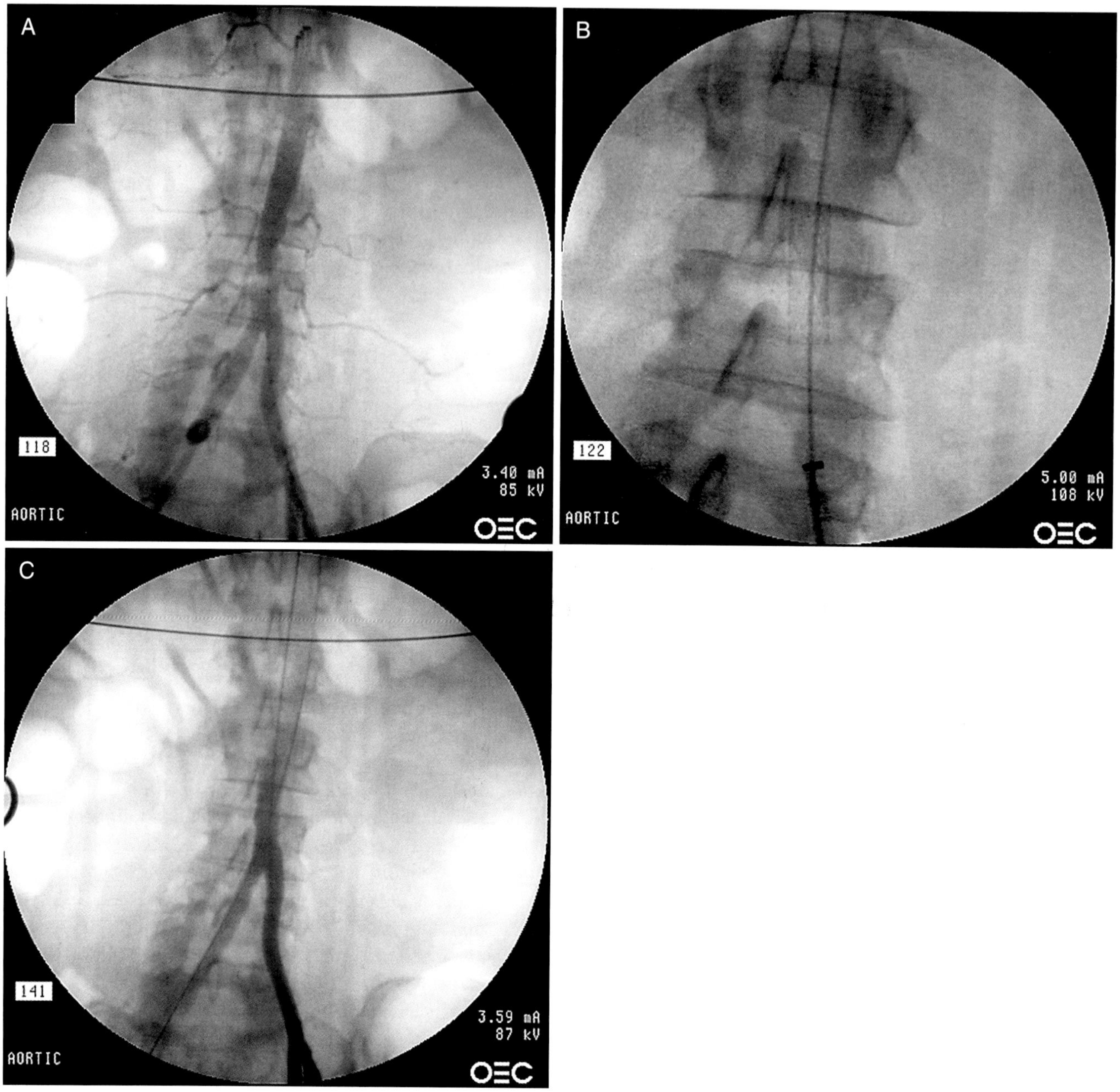

FIG 24.3 (A) Focal atherosclerotic "apple core" lesion of the distal aorta in a woman with relatively small vessels and disabling claudication. A pressure gradient of 50 mm Hg existed across the lesion. (B) Unilateral femoral access was gained, and a balloon-expandable stent was placed across the lesion. (C) Follow-up imaging demonstrates no residual stenosis, with no further pressure gradient measures.

feasible, relatively easy to perform, and with satisfactory midterm results (Fig. 24.3).[44-46] These patients usually exhibit disabling claudication and are between 30 and 70 years of age. The disease may be a focal infrarenal stenosis or, more commonly, involve the origins of the common iliac arteries.

The spectrum of symptoms is commonly referred to as the *Leriche syndrome,* a combination of diminished or absent femoral pulses, thigh and buttock claudication, and erectile dysfunction in men. Women may exhibit these types of lesions because of the intrinsically small caliber of their vessels. Female patients tend to be younger, be heavy smokers, and have elevated lipid levels. Alternatively, distal embolization presenting as blue toe syndrome may be the first manifestation of disease.

In patients deemed appropriate for intervention, noninvasive studies to determine the physiologic nature of the obstruction and angiography (conventional, MRA, or computed tomographic angiography) are valuable in analyzing the extent of the lesion and planning appropriate treatment. The type of lesion, patient characteristics, concomitant comorbidities, and acuteness of symptoms are all factors to consider in choosing percutaneous therapy versus surgical modalities. Percutaneous techniques are a viable alternative to major surgical reconstruction, with lower costs, morbidity, and mortality. Evaluation of aortic lesions with IVUS and subsequent evaluation after stent deployment has improved long-term clinical outcomes of balloon angioplasty and stented aortic lesions.[47]

AORTIC STENOSIS

Techniques used for angioplasty, with or without stenting, of the aorta and iliac segments are similar. Although PTA has demonstrated excellent results in focal stenoses of the abdominal aorta and iliacs, primary stenting may reduce the degree of restenosis with PTA alone and decrease distal embolization, especially if there is significant irregularity on the vessel surface and a substantial amount of plaque.[32,35,43,46,48–50] Focal aortic stenoses are treated by mounting a balloon-expandable stent on a larger-caliber angioplasty balloon or using a large self-expanding stent. When using a balloon-expandable stent, the operator should consider passing a sheath and dilator through the lesion to avoid dislodgement of the stent off the balloon by the lesion. Often the stent is initially mounted on a smaller balloon and then serially dilated until the angiographic result or hemodynamic gradient is improved. In addition, a heavily calcified lesion has a high risk of rupture if it is aggressively dilated, and a self-expanding stent or covered stent may be the safer option. Self-expanding stents have a large diameter relative to the size of the sheath; therefore a larger self-expanding stent than a balloon-expandable stent will fit through the same sheath. As a result, the length of the lesion to be covered needs to be carefully measured, and the operator must be familiar with the behavior of these stents. The role of covered stents, such as cuffs made for endoluminal abdominal aortic aneurysm repair, has gained some recent attention. Maldonado and colleagues reported a multicenter review of 91 patients with TASC II D lesions (long segment occlusions) treated with endografts and found 88% of patients had assisted patency at 2 years. However, there was a 22% early complication rate and 10% reintervention rate to maintain this success.[51]

The aortic diameter should be sized with a calibrated catheter, with IVUS, or by preintervention computed tomographic scanning to avoid undersizing. Balloon size usually ranges between 12 and 18 mm. A single stent is generally required in most cases, with no special technical requirements. Large Palmaz-type stents (Palmaz XXL) and endograft aortic cuffs have been used successfully and can be dilated up to an appropriate diameter. Concentric aortic stenosis may encroach on the inferior mesenteric artery; coverage of this vessel may be unavoidable. Furthermore, only midabdominal aortic lesions should be treated in this fashion. Different techniques (described later) are used when the lesion involves the aortic bifurcation. For focal aortic stenoses, technical success, safety, and adequate patency rates have been reported with primary stent placement.[35,45,46,52,53] Durability appears satisfactory in properly selected patients.

ILIAC STENOSIS OR OCCLUSION

Patients with iliac lesions exhibit a wide spectrum of symptoms, depending on the amount of involvement of the iliac arteries, whether the lesions are focal or multisegmental, and the degree of infrainguinal disease. Indications for intervention are severe disabling claudication, rest pain, tissue loss, or blue toe syndrome. Individual risk factors and possible adverse outcomes associated with each procedure must also be taken into consideration when deciding on the best treatment option. Initially, iliac artery angioplasty with subsequent stent placement was used only for focal lesions; however, with technologic advances, more complex multisegmental lesions are now approached endoluminally with varied results.

RESULTS OF ILIAC ANGIOPLASTY AND STENTING

Multiple studies have documented excellent results following both focal and complex iliac artery stenting procedures, with most reporting superior results over angioplasty alone (Figs. 24.4 and 24.5).[a] In a large, representative systematic review by Bosch and Hunink,[62] technical success with angioplasty alone was 91%; with stent placement, it was 96%. This report of more than 2100 patients compared the PTA cohort (n = 1300) with the stent cohort (n = 816) and demonstrated similar complication rates between the two groups; however, the patients with stents had improved long-term patency rates. When performed for claudication, 4-year primary patency rates were 65% for stenosis and 54% for occlusion after angioplasty, versus 77% for stenosis and 61% for occlusion after stenting. The rate differential was similar, although the overall percentages were lower, when procedures were performed for critical limb ischemia. Statistical analysis showed a 39% reduction in long-term failure after stent placement compared with PTA.

As seen in Table 24.2, there is currently no consensus about the best treatment for moderately severe iliac artery lesions (TASC type B and C lesions). In a review of their experience with percutaneous and surgical treatment of these complex iliac lesions, Timaran and colleagues[29] evaluated the primary outcome of patency and also analyzed potential variables that may preclude successful revascularization.[29] At all time points (1, 3, and 5 years), patients with surgical reconstruction (n = 52) had higher patency rates than patients with stents (n = 136). Poor runoff was the only independent predictor of primary failure in either cohort. Furthermore, in patients with poor runoff, iliac stenting was associated with inferior outcomes compared with surgical reconstruction. This finding has been supported by other studies of surgical or endovascular interventions.[56,64,65] In a review of the treatment of TASC type D lesions, the most severe type, Ballard and colleagues[65] found that ipsilateral SFA obstruction was also an independent predictor of both stent and bypass graft failure.

The endovascular management of complex iliac artery occlusions targeting TASC C and D lesions was evaluated by Leville and colleagues.[63] They reported on 89 patients with symptomatic iliac occlusions classified as TASC B, C, or D. Twenty-four percent of the patients in the TASC C and D groups required hybrid procedures with femoral artery endarterectomy and patch

[a]References 13, 14, 22, 29, 32, 39, and 54–63.

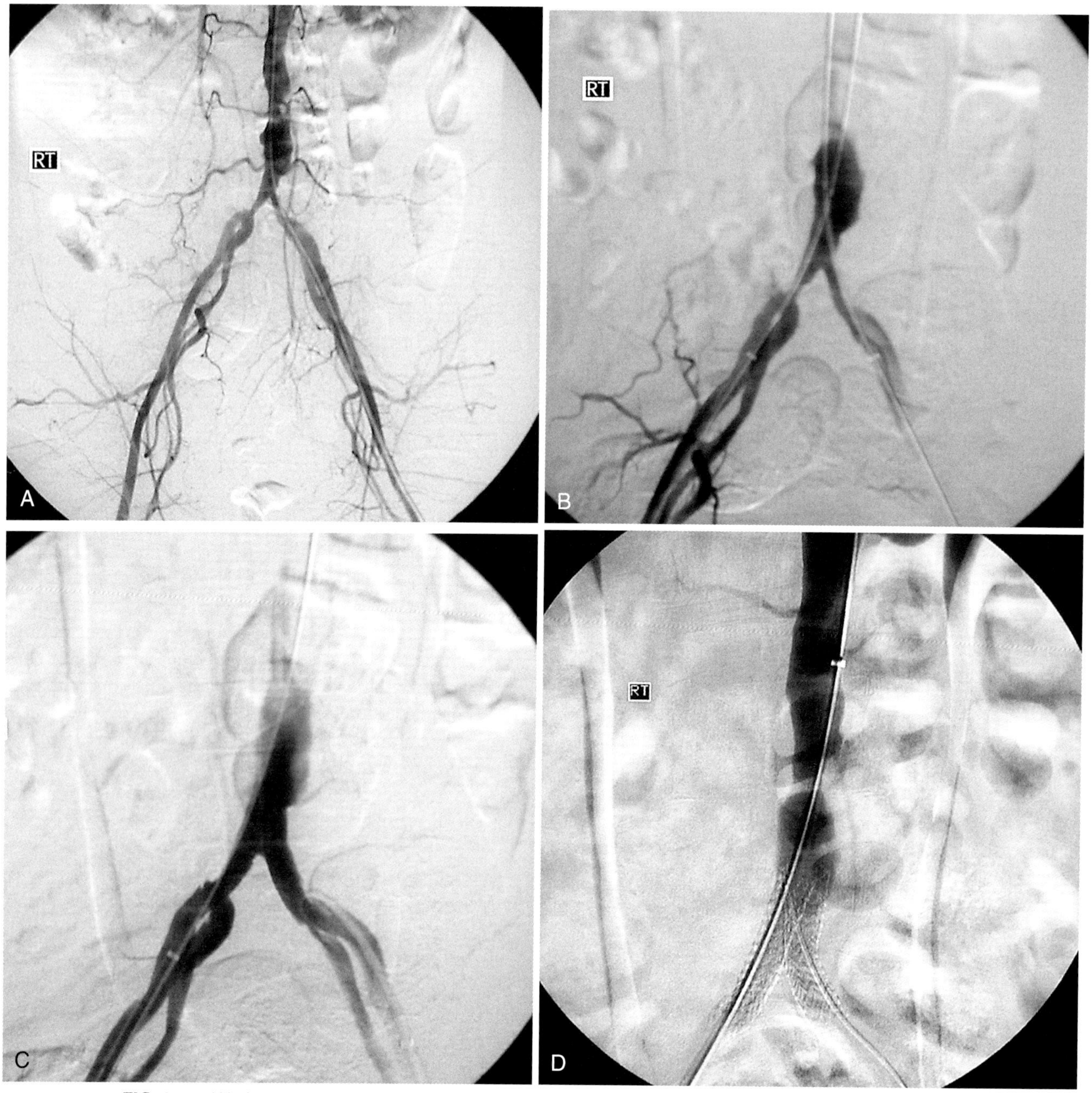

FIG 24.4 (A) Angiogram in a man with Leriche syndrome demonstrates focal atherosclerotic disease at the distal aorta and proximal common iliac arteries. (B) Bilateral percutaneous femoral access was obtained with placement of 6-French sheaths. (C) Initial improved result after angioplasty of the common iliac arteries. (D) Completion angiogram after deployment of bilateral "kissing" balloon-expandable stents.

angioplasty and half required multiple access sites. However, the 3-year primary patency was 76%, and secondary patency was 90% with a 97% limb salvage rate. The authors concluded that complex iliac occlusions can be treated safely with endovascular means with results comparable to open reconstruction.

In most gender-based comparisons, women have inferior results following iliac stent placement compared with their male counterparts.[65-67] Conversely, in a retrospective study of 44 women having iliac angioplasty compared with men matched for comorbidities, female gender was not a negative predictor of outcome. Although women in this series had smaller vessels and a higher incidence of pretreatment total occlusion, no statistically significant difference existed in 2-year primary patency, percutaneous primary-assisted patency, or limb salvage rates. However, stent placement was not performed in these patients. Perhaps the use of stents in smaller vessels in women should be limited. Full critical evaluation awaits future randomized prospective trials or larger retrospective series or registries.

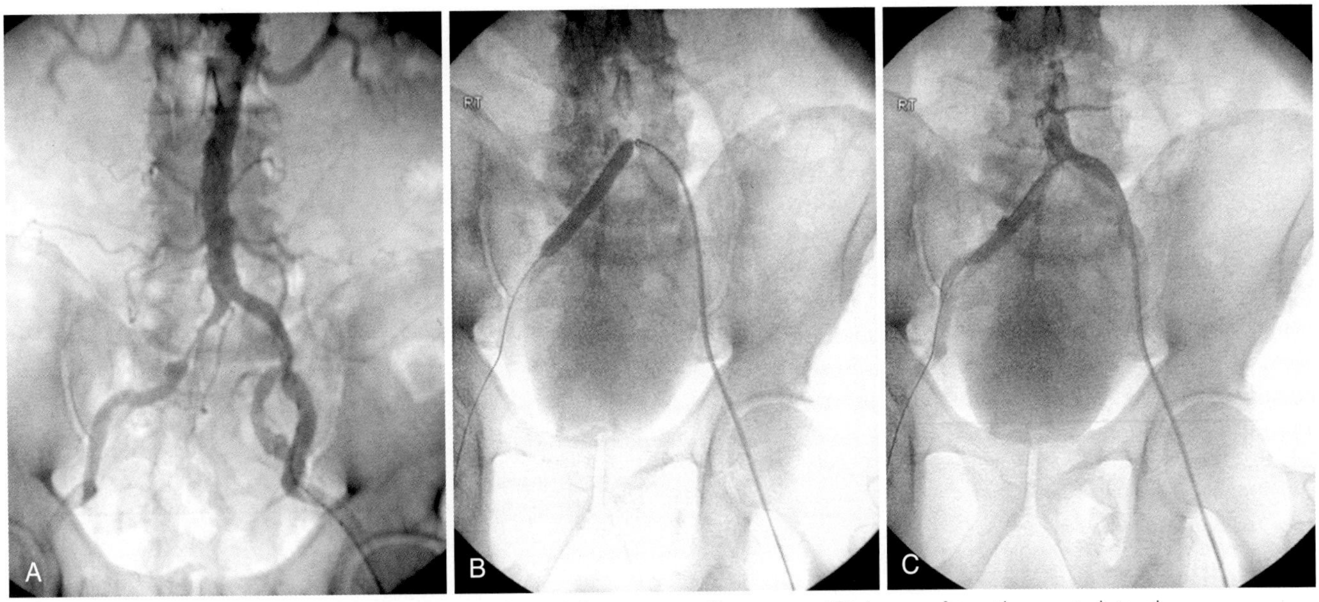

FIG 24.5 (A) High-grade lesion of the right common iliac artery. (B) Access from the contralateral femoral artery was used for initial angioplasty. (C) Results after balloon angioplasty, with no apparent residual stenosis. The patient went on to have a self-expanding stent placed across the lesion (not shown).

CHRONIC TOTAL OCCLUSION OF THE ILIAC ARTERY

The use of endovascular techniques to treat stenotic common and external iliac arteries is well established.[b] However, endovascular techniques for chronic total occlusions of these arteries continue to be described. Recanalization of the common and external iliac arteries has many challenges, but likely the most important is crossing the lesion safely, particularly in the area of the aortic bifurcation. This is often achieved through subintimal recanalization. In recent years, this specific technique has been shown to be achieved with the new so-called reentry devices such as the Pioneer catheter (Medtronics, Minneapolis, Minnesota) or the Outback catheter (Cordis, Miami, Florida).

APPROACHES TO COMMON AND EXTERNAL ILIAC ARTERY OCCLUSIONS

Approaches for complete occlusions of the iliac artery include using the contralateral or ipsilateral iliac artery in a retrograde manner or the transbrachial artery technique. When using the contralateral retrograde crossover approach, a curved catheter can be used to approach the occlusion by engaging the stump of the common iliac artery. At this point, a stiff hydrophilic 0.035-inch wire can be used to cross the occlusion followed by percutaneous balloon angioplasty and stenting. This approach has the disadvantage that there is minimal support from the catheter; therefore there might not be enough support to successfully cross the lesion. In addition, this approach may not adequately align the balloon and stent with the aortic bifurcation leaving suboptimal results. Finally, it may also impede the use of any reentry devices because of the angulation.

The transbrachial approach, usually from the left brachial artery, has several advantages including improved support, pushability, and a straight approach to the involved iliac artery. Disadvantages include the need to use longer sheaths (at least 90 cm) to reach the aortic bifurcation, the risk of cerebral embolization, and limited sheath size (maximum recommended size of 6 French). However, as technology continues to improve, more devices, catheters, balloons, and stents become available at lower profiles.

The ipsilateral retrograde iliac artery approach may be a difficult access site because it is distal to the occlusion in a pulseless femoral artery. Ultrasound and fluoroscopy combined with roadmapping may be necessary to cannulate the pulseless femoral artery. In addition, subintimal recanalization may be taken into the aorta and can create a retrograde dissection that limits the success of the procedure. Therefore this approach may be the least desirable to recanalize the occluded iliac artery. Of course, confirmation or entry back into the true arterial lumen should be performed with contrast visualization or IVUS. The subintimal plane can also be traversed with the aid of reentry devices or techniques.

REENTRY DEVICES

Reentry devices such as the Pioneer catheter (Medtronics, Minneapolis, Minnesota) or the Outback catheter (Cordis, Miami, Florida) may occasionally be needed if there is not a successful reentry into a nondiseased artery. These devices help by saving time and avoiding complications if other maneuvers have been unsuccessful. More importantly, if the subintimal space

[b]References 13, 14, 22, 29, 32, 39, and 54–63.

is excessively dissected, then the reentry device will not work as well or at all. Therefore the subintimal space must remain relatively small for the successful use of a reentry device.

The Outback catheter has an external marker to help orient the needle into the lumen using fluoroscopy. The Pioneer catheter uses IVUS technology to guide the reentry needle toward the true lumen. Once the needle is in the true lumen, a 0.014-inch wire may be advanced, and the reentry catheter is removed and angioplasty and stenting can be conducted as planned.

Multiple small series report success and rapid reentry times (routinely <3 minutes) with both catheters.[68,69] In addition, they report no patients requiring conversion to open surgery. Most authors believe that this technology has opened the endovascular world to TASC C and D lesions, which would otherwise require management with open surgical approaches.

BOX 24.3 Complications Associated With Intravascular Stent Placement

- Local complications
- Hematoma
- Pseudoaneurysm
- Arteriovenous fistula
- Plaque distal embolization
- Stent dislodgment in delivery system
- Stent migration and embolization
- Stent misplacement
- Contrast allergic reaction
- Vessel perforation
- Side branch occlusion
- Accelerated intimal hyperplasia
- Extrinsic compression of stent
- Stent infection

COMPLICATIONS OF INTRALUMINAL STENT PLACEMENT

The complication profile is similar for aortic or iliac interventions (Box 24.3), and premature dislodgment of the stent from the balloon and catheter delivery system may occur. Although this problem can usually be managed with endovascular techniques, the self-expanding stents do not have this problem. Similar complications occur that are nonspecific for percutaneous procedures, including those related to puncture sites, arterial dissection, and vessel rupture. Unlike with self-expanding stents, which constantly exert an outward radial force, external compression on balloon-expandable stents because of vascular clamping injury can result in stent deformity that may create an occlusive lesion if not redilated. Although short-term failure is mainly due to thrombosis in the stented vessel, long-term patency can be adversely affected by restenosis induced by intimal hyperplasia. Factors associated with stented artery thrombosis are baseline iliac artery occlusion, multiple stent deployment, and hypercoagulable disorders. Stent placement in an occluded iliac artery is particularly prone to restenosis, in part because of the lack of an endothelial lining in the occluded vessel. Stent deployment may further denude the intimal lining, thereby reducing the protective antithrombotic function of endothelium. In addition, the incidence of distal embolization following the stent placement is 2.4% to 7.8%.[37] As with all radiographic interventions, transient contrast-induced nephropathy can occur after an interventional procedure.

CONCLUSIONS

Intravascular stent placement has proved to be an invaluable tool in both the primary treatment of aortoiliac occlusive disease and the management of complications of balloon angioplasty. Clinical application of iliac stents has also extended to the treatment of patients with total iliac occlusion and restenosis. Although balloon angioplasty alone has met with limited success in treating totally occluded iliac arteries, the use of intravascular stents has improved the success rate to approximately 80% at 3 years, with a late occlusion rate similar to that of stenotic lesions. The benefit of primary stenting of the iliac artery has been demonstrated in several series, with a favorable 5-year patency rate of greater than 90%, which is comparable to conventional surgical reconstruction. The primary weakness of intravascular stenting is related to the biologic response of neointimal hyperplasia, which may be exacerbated by a metal stent placed into the arterial circulation. There are many focus areas for future research in attempting to solve this dilemma, including covered stent technology. Promising techniques, including the use of drug-eluting stents, drug-coated balloons, cutting balloons, and aggressive antiplatelet regimens, are being tested to improve clinical outcomes.[70–76]

REVIEW QUESTIONS

1. All of the following are indications for stent placement, except:
   - **a.** Intimal dissection
   - **b.** Residual stenosis greater than 15%
   - **c.** Recurrent stenosis following angioplasty alone
   - **d.** Symptomatic atherosclerotic iliac lesions
2. Which of the following statements about pharmacologic agents in angiography are true?
   - **a.** They may induce peripheral vasodilatation that unmasks significant stenosis.
   - **b.** Either papaverine or nitroglycerin may be used.
   - **c.** They are injected directly into the intraarterial catheter or sheath in the vessel under investigation.
   - **d.** They cause significant vasospasm.
3. Covered stents may be used in the iliac arteries in all of the following conditions except:
   - **a.** Arteriovenous fistulas
   - **b.** Vessel ruptures
   - **c.** Aneurysms
   - **d.** Mycotic aneurysms
   - **e.** Atherosclerotic occlusive lesions

4. Complications of iliac stent placement include which of the following?
   a. Distal embolization
   b. Thrombosis
   c. Stent malposition
   d. Vessel rupture
   e. All of the above
5. The classic definition of Leriche syndrome consists of all of the following except:
   a. Decreased femoral pulses
   b. Blue toe syndrome
   c. Buttock claudication
   d. Impotence
6. Iliac stenting has been recommended as the primary treatment for which of the following lesions?
   a. TASC type A
   b. TASC type B
   c. TASC type C
   d. TASC type D
7. The outcome after stenting of which vessel most closely approximates surgical results?
   a. Common iliac artery
   b. External iliac artery
   c. Common femoral artery
8. Long-term patency of intravascular stents is limited by which of the following?
   a. Vessel size
   b. Neointimal hyperplasia
   c. Progression of atherosclerosis
   d. Stent durability
9. Complications common to percutaneous procedures include which of the following?
   a. Contrast-induced nephropathy
   b. Puncture site hematoma
   c. Vascular injury
   d. Nerve damage
10. All of the following are (relative) contraindications for intravascular stent placement except:
   a. Target area across from an area of flexion, such as the knee joint
   b. Arterial perforation with contrast extravasation
   c. Residual stenosis of 40% following balloon angioplasty
   d. Multisegmental iliac disease

BIBLIOGRAPHY

Ballard JL, Bergan JJ, Singh P, et al. Aortoiliac stent deployment versus surgical reconstruction: analysis of outcome and cost. *J Vasc Surg*. 1998;28:94–101.

Brewster DC. Current controversies in the management of aortoiliac occlusive disease. *J Vasc Surg*. 1997;25:365–379.

Dotter CT, Judkins MP. Transluminal treatment of arteriosclerotic obstruction: description of a new technique and a preliminary report of its application. *Circulation*. 1964;30:654–670.

Greiner A, Dessl A, Klein-Weigel P, et al. Kissing stents for treatment of complex aortoiliac disease. *Eur J Vasc Endovasc Surg*. 2003;26:161–165.

Harnek J, Zoucas E, Stenram U, et al. Insertion of self-expandable nitinol stents without previous balloon angioplasty reduces restenosis compared with PTA prior to stenting. *Cardiovasc Intervent Radiol*. 2002;25:430–436.

Martin D, Katz SG. Axillofemoral bypass for aortoiliac occlusive disease. *Am J Surg*. 2000;180:100–103.

Mohamed F, Sarkar B, Timmons G, et al. Outcome of "kissing stents" for aortoiliac atherosclerotic disease, including the effect on the non-diseased contralateral iliac limb. *Cardiovasc Intervent Radiol*. 2002;25:472–475.

Murphy TP, Ariaratnam NS, Carney WI Jr, et al. Aortoiliac insufficiency: long-term experience with stent placement for treatment. *Radiology*. 2004;231:243–249.

Norgren L, Hiatt WR, Dormandy JA, et al. Inter-society consensus for the management of peripheral arterial disease (TASCII). *J Vasc Surg*. 2007;45(suppl S):S5–S67.

Schneider JR, Besso SR, Walsh DB, et al. Femorofemoral versus aortobifemoral bypass: outcome and hemodynamic results. *J Vasc Surg*. 1994;19:43–55.

Stoeckelhuber BM, Meissner O, Stoeckelhuber M, et al. Primary endovascular stent placement for focal infrarenal aortic stenosis: initial and midterm results. *J Vasc Interv Radiol*. 2003;14:1443–1447.

Tetteroo E, van der Graaf Y, Bosch JL, et al. Randomised comparison of primary stent placement versus primary angioplasty followed by selective stent placement in patients with iliac-artery occlusive disease. Dutch Iliac Stent Trial Study Group. *Lancet*. 1998;351:1153–1159.

Timaran CH, Prault TL, Stevens SL, et al. Iliac artery stenting versus surgical reconstruction for TASC (TransAtlantic Inter-Society Consensus) type B and type C iliac lesions. *J Vasc Surg*. 2003;38:272–278.

Timaran CH, Stevens SL, Freeman MB, et al. Infrainguinal arterial reconstructions in patients with aortoiliac occlusive disease: the influence of iliac stenting. *J Vasc Surg*. 2001;34:971–978.

Treiman GS, Schneider PA, Lawrence PF, et al. Does stent placement improve the results of ineffective or complicated iliac artery angioplasty? *J Vasc Surg*. 1998;28:104–112.

Waksman R. Vascular brachytherapy vs drug-eluting stents for the treatment of in-stent restenosis: the jury's still out. *Catheter Cardiovasc Interv*. 2004;62:290–291.

References available online at ExpertConsult.com.

25 CHAPTER

Diagnosis and Surgical Management of the Visceral Ischemic Syndromes

Aamir S. Shah, Lewis B. Schwartz, James F. McKinsey, Bruce L. Gewertz

Although the causal relationship between mesenteric vascular occlusion and intestinal gangrene was suspected in the 15th century, the first successful case of intestinal resection for infarction was not reported until 1895.[1] Recognition of the chronic form soon followed, with the term angina abdominis applied by Goodman to illustrate the similarities to the newly described angina pectoris.[2] Indisputable evidence was provided in 1936 by Dunphy,[3] a surgical resident at the Peter Bent Brigham Hospital in Boston, who described the clinical course of a 47-year-old man with weight loss and periumbilical pain out of proportion to the findings on physical examination. The patient died suddenly in the hospital, and postmortem examination revealed chronic mesenteric disease with fresh thrombus completely occluding the celiac trunk. Dunphy reviewed twelve other deaths from mesenteric vascular occlusion and found an antecedent history of chronic recurrent abdominal pain in seven.

The first successful reports of mesenteric revascularization for chronic mesenteric ischemia appeared in 1958.[4] In that year, Shaw and Maynard[4] from the Massachusetts General Hospital reported two cases of superior mesenteric artery (SMA) thrombosis superimposed on atherosclerotic occlusive disease. Both patients were treated with SMA thromboendarterectomy and survived. The surgeons made the astute observation that although the responsible atherosclerotic lesions involved all three mesenteric arteries, they were confined to the proximal segments, such that vascular reconstruction was technically feasible.

Since that time, intestinal ischemic disorders have been recognized as uncommon but clinically important causes of abdominal pain. Although their incidence is estimated at only a few cases per 100,000 population, their lethal nature requires vigilance and a high index of clinical suspicion to avoid catastrophe. This chapter reviews the pathophysiology, clinical presentation, diagnostic evaluation, and treatment of both acute and chronic intestinal ischemic disorders. The surgical and endovascular techniques of treatment and outcomes are discussed in detail.

VASCULAR ANATOMY

The mesenteric circulation consists primarily of three branches of the abdominal aorta (Fig. 25.1): the celiac axis, the SMA, and the inferior mesenteric artery (IMA). The mesenteric vascular bed is "privileged"—that is, it exhibits very low resistance to both mean and oscillatory blood flow and has the potential for extensive collateralization when its main trunks are compromised. Their multiple branch points and interconnections form such a rich anastomotic network that compromises two of the three major arteries that are usually required for the development of chronic ischemic symptoms. Knowledge of the normal and variant anatomy is essential for surgical diagnosis and revascularization.

Celiac Axis

The celiac axis supplies the foregut including the stomach, liver, spleen, portions of the pancreas, and the proximal duodenum. It originates from the ventral portion of the abdominal aorta, near the level of T12 to L1, between the diaphragmatic crura. Its origin is encased in the median arcuate ligament, a dense, fibrous portion of the central posterior diaphragm draped across the aortic hiatus. In most patients, the celiac axis branches soon after its origin into the common hepatic, splenic, and left gastric arteries. In 1% of cases, the SMA arises from the celiac axis as well, forming a common celiomesenteric trunk.

The hepatic artery is usually the first branch of the celiac axis. It may also arise from the SMA (the so-called replaced right hepatic artery) in approximately 12% of cases. Additional variants include the replaced common hepatic artery (approximately 2.5%) and direct origin of the common hepatic artery from the aorta (approximately 2%). The common hepatic artery gives rise to the right gastric artery and the gastroduodenal artery, which further divides into the right gastroepiploic and superior pancreaticoduodenal arteries. The remaining proper hepatic artery gives rise to the cystic, right hepatic, and left hepatic arteries, which serve the gallbladder, the right and caudate hepatic lobes, and the middle and left hepatic lobes, respectively.

The second branch of the celiac axis is the splenic artery. Its first named branch is the dorsal pancreatic artery, supplying the posterior body and tail of the pancreas. Just before entering the splenic hilum, the splenic artery gives rise to the left gastroepiploic artery and multiple short gastric arteries, providing blood flow to the gastric fundus.

The final branch of the celiac axis is the left gastric artery. It courses cephalad and to the left to supply the gastric cardia and fundus along the lesser curvature of the stomach, joining centrally with the right gastric artery from the hepatic artery. In approximately 12% of the population, the left hepatic artery originates from the left gastric artery.

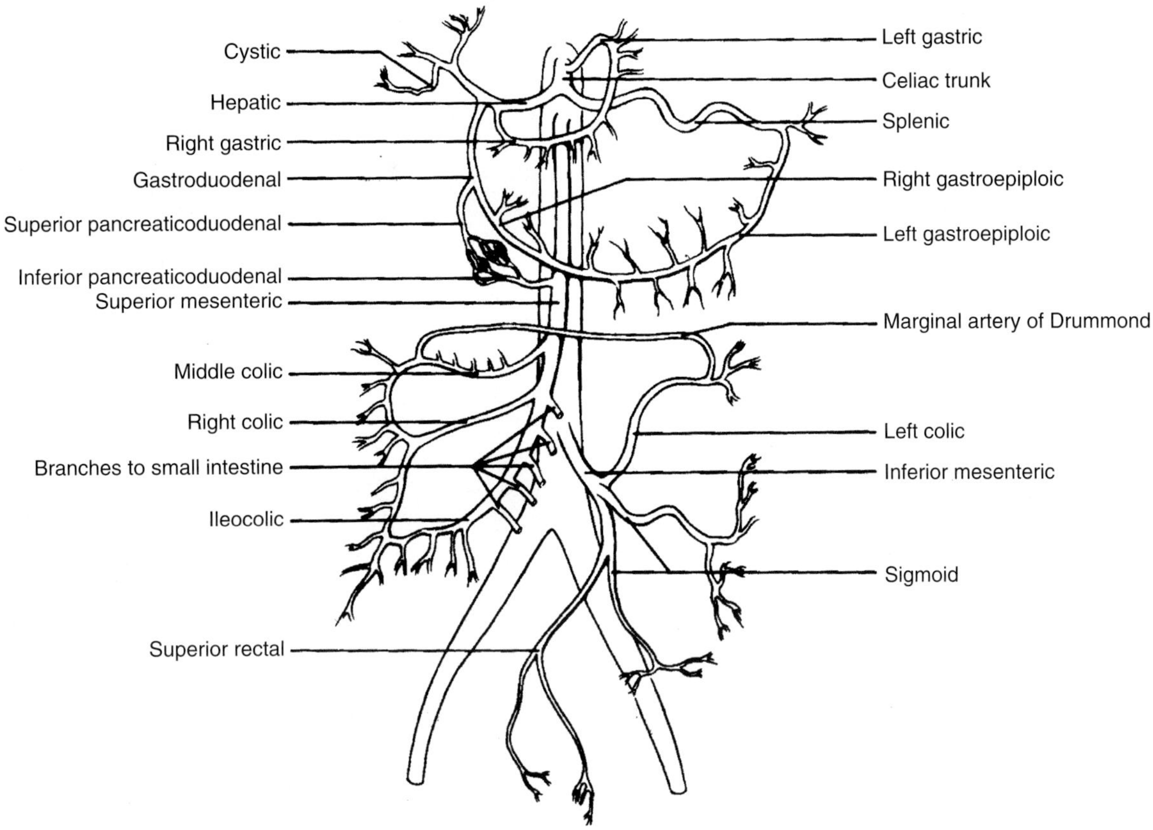

FIG 25.1 The mesenteric circulation. (From Schwartz LB, Davis RD Jr, Heinle JS, et al: The vascular system. In Lyerly HK, Gaynor JW Jr, editors: *The Handbook of Surgical Intensive Care*, ed 3, St Louis, 1992, Mosby Year Book, p 287.)

Superior Mesenteric Artery

The SMA arises from the aorta just distal to the celiac axis at the level of L1 to L2. It passes behind the neck of the pancreas, in front of the uncinate process, and over the third portion of the duodenum. Its first branch, the inferior pancreaticoduodenal artery, courses superiorly to join the superior pancreaticoduodenal artery (from the gastroduodenal artery) and forms the most proximal collateral pathway with the celiac axis. The central branches of the SMA supply the midgut from the ligament of Treitz to the midtransverse colon. These include the middle colic (serving the proximal two-thirds of the transverse colon), right colic (mid-ascending and distal ascending colon), and ileocolic (distal ileum, cecum, appendix, and proximal ascending colon).

Inferior Mesenteric Artery

The IMA arises from the left side of the aorta 8 to 10 cm distal to the SMA at the level of L3. It travels caudad and to the left before dividing into the left colic and sigmoid arteries. The IMA supplies the distal third of the transverse colon, the descending and sigmoid colons, and the proximal rectum. It has anastomotic communications with the left branch of the middle colic from the SMA and with portions of the middle and inferior rectal arteries from the internal iliac.

Collateral Circulation

The mesenteric circulation has a redundant collateral network that serves to maintain perfusion, even with compromise of the proximal main channels. The celiac axis and SMA communicate primarily via the superior and inferior pancreaticoduodenal arteries (via the gastroduodenal artery). The SMA and IMA communicate via the centrally located arch of Riolan (often referred to as the *meandering mesenteric artery*), and by the multiple communications at the periphery of the colon called the *marginal arteries of Drummond*. In addition to these collateral pathways, muscular branches of the aorta may contribute to intestinal perfusion, including the lumbar arteries, internal mammary arteries (via the deep epigastric arteries), middle sacral artery, and internal iliac arteries (via collaterals between the inferior and superior rectal arteries). Because of this plentiful collateral network, it is understandable that in most instances of gradual occlusion, at least two of the three major mesenteric artery orifices must be blocked to produce the clinical syndromes of chronic intestinal ischemia. In contrast, sudden occlusion of one widely patent vessel can cause acute ischemia because collaterals may be underdeveloped.

ACUTE ISCHEMIA

Pathophysiology

Acute mesenteric ischemia (AMI) is caused by an abrupt reduction in or cessation of the delivery of oxygen to the intestine. This can result from an occlusion of the mesenteric arterial supply or venous drainage as well as hypoperfusion during shock states. The most common pathophysiologic mechanisms include acute embolization to the SMA (approximately 50% of all cases), in situ SMA thrombosis of a preexisting atherosclerotic lesion at the origin of the vessel (20%), nonocclusive mesenteric ischemia (20%), most often associated with low-flow states such as shock and/or mesenteric vasospasm, and mesenteric venous thrombosis (10%).[5,6] In earlier series, the phenomenon of nonocclusive mesenteric ischemia was not well appreciated and was frequently misdiagnosed as acute venous occlusion. For example, Cokkinis[7] reported in 1935 that acute mesenteric venous thrombosis accounted for the majority of cases of AMI.

Other unusual arteriopathies, such as Takayasu arteritis, fibromuscular dysplasia, and polyarteritis nodosa, may first present with intestinal ischemia. Isolated dissections of the SMA also have been reported,[8] although the more common mechanism is extension of dissections of the descending thoracic aorta into the SMA and celiac axis.[9,10]

If untreated, acute intestinal ischemia commonly leads to intestinal infarction. Tissue loss may result from both hypoxia during flow interruption and reperfusion injury once intestinal arterial blood flow is restored. Reperfusion injury is principally mediated by activation of the enzyme xanthine oxidase and the recruitment and activation of circulating polymorphonuclear neutrophils (PMNs).[11,12] In the presence of oxygen and hypoxanthine (a by-product of adenosine triphosphate metabolism), xanthine oxidase produces oxygen-derived free radicals that cause severe local tissue injury through lipid peroxidation, membrane disruption, and increased microvascular permeability.[13] PMNs are attracted to reperfused tissue by the local secretion of cytokines (tumor necrosis factor-α, interleukin-1, platelet-derived growth factor) by ischemic endothelium.[14-16] Subsequent rolling, adherence, and activation of the PMNs in the microcirculation result in the secretion of myeloperoxidase, collagenases, and elastases that can further injure the already ischemic and vulnerable tissue.[17-19] Activation of the inflammatory cascade may also have systemic effects, with cardiac, pulmonary, and other organ system dysfunction.[20]

Acute Mesenteric Arterial Embolism

Most mesenteric arterial emboli originate from left atrial or ventricular mural thrombi or cardiac valvular lesions. These thrombi are usually associated with cardiac dysrhythmias such as atrial fibrillation or hypokinetic regions from previous myocardial infarctions. The majority of mesenteric emboli lodge in the SMA because of its high baseline flow rate and nearly parallel course to the abdominal aorta. Only 15% of SMA emboli remain impacted at the origin of the vessel. The majority of emboli progress distally 3 to 10 cm to the tapered segment of the SMA just past the origin of the middle colic artery (Fig. 25.2). The middle colic and ileocolic branches may remain patent and the resulting pattern of bowel ischemia may be less extensive, with the proximal jejunum and transverse colon being spared, than after in situ thrombosis, where the ascending colon and more of the small bowel are involved. A substantial fraction (10% to 15%) of mesenteric emboli are associated with concurrent emboli to another arterial bed.[21] Intestinal ischemia due to embolic arterial occlusion can be compounded by reactive mesenteric vasoconstriction, which further reduces collateral flow and aggravates the ischemic insult.

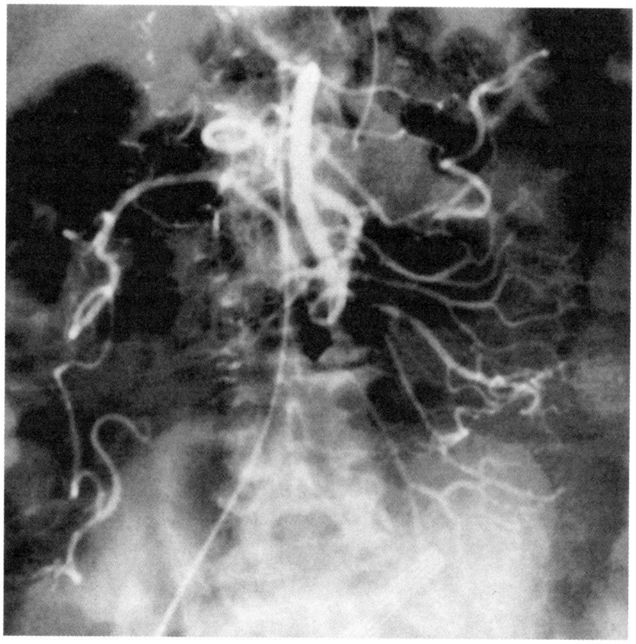

FIG 25.2 Anteroposterior view of the aorta revealing embolic occlusion of the proximal superior mesenteric artery (SMA). Note the normal-appearing proximal jejunal arterial branches and then an abrupt cutoff of the SMA. (From McKinsey JF, Gewertz BL: Acute mesenteric ischemia. *Surg Clin North Am* 77:307–318, 1997.)

Acute Mesenteric Arterial Thrombosis

Thrombosis of the SMA or the celiac axis is usually associated with preexisting arterial lesions. When carefully questioned, many of these patients have histories consistent with chronic mesenteric ischemia (CMI), including postprandial pain, weight loss, "food fear," bloating, and early satiety. By far, the most common underlying lesion is an atherosclerotic plaque that slowly progresses to a critical stenosis over years, until the residual lumen suddenly thromboses during a period of low flow. Unlike embolic occlusions, thrombosis of the SMA generally occurs flush with the aortic origin of the vessel.

As noted previously, visceral malperfusion resulting from acute aortic dissection or visceral artery dissection can also result in acute mesenteric ischemia. The intimal flap of the dissection can exclude, compress, or extend into the visceral vessels, resulting in acute thrombosis. Dynamic obstruction of the visceral artery ostia resulting from compression of the aortic true lumen by the pressurized false lumen of the aortic dissection or by prolapse of the dissection flap into the visceral artery ostium can be treated by endovascular stenting of the true lumen of the aortic dissection or fenestration of the intimal flap. This may result in decompression of the false lumen and reexpansion of the aortic true lumen with resulting increased perfusion of the aortic side branches and resolution of visceral malperfusion. A static visceral artery obstruction can be caused by propagation of the dissection flap into the mesenteric vessels resulting in either decreased distal perfusion or thrombosis of the visceral vessel. This will not likely resolve by increasing perfusion of the aortic true lumen alone with an aortic stent graft, and very likely will require open surgical revascularization distal to the point of obstruction or endovascular stenting of the visceral vessel.

The symptoms of bowel ischemia may be masked by the pain associated with the aortic dissection, leading to a delay in diagnosis and treatment. Acute mesenteric ischemia following coronary artery bypass grafts is rare but highly lethal, with mortality rates as high as 70%. Ischemia occurs in severely stenotic mesenteric vessels that occlude during the nonpulsatile perfusion of extracorporeal bypass.[22,23]

Nonocclusive Mesenteric Ischemia

Mesenteric ischemia unassociated with anatomic arterial or venous obstruction can occur during periods of low cardiac output. Such low-flow states can result from cardiac failure, sepsis, or administration of α-adrenergic agents or digitalis compounds. Although less common, mesenteric vasospasm can also follow elective revascularization procedures for chronic SMA occlusion, in which case vasoconstriction of small and medium-size vessels is precipitated by early enteral feeding.[24] The older mean age of the population has produced a group of people with severe medical problems at risk for this type of mesenteric ischemia. The diagnosis is made at the time of angiography. Radiographic criteria suggesting the diagnosis include (1) narrowing of the origins of multiple branches of the SMA; (2) alternate dilatation and narrowing of the intestinal branches (the "string-of-sausages" sign); (3) spasm of the mesenteric arcades; and (4) impaired filling of the intramural vessels.[25] The mortality of this specific subset of patients is relatively high regardless of treatment, owing to the serious underlying medical conditions and the frequent delay in diagnosis.[26]

Mesenteric Venous Thrombosis

Mesenteric venous thrombosis (MVT) is thrombosis of the veins draining the intestine (inferior mesenteric, superior mesenteric, splenic, and portal veins). Acute mesenteric venous thrombosis (AMVT) was once thought to be an uncommon cause of acute intestinal ischemia. However, with newer imaging modalities, it is now estimated that approximately 10% to 15% of AMI results from AMVT. The obstruction in venous return leads to edema, distension, and eventual infarction of affected segments. In advanced cases, there may be associated spasm of the SMA that further compromises bowel viability.

Primary MVT is idiopathic, although given the improved understanding of predisposing conditions, the number of patients in this category is diminishing. Patients in whom a causative factor is identified are said to have secondary MVT. These factors include myriad clinical syndromes, including trauma, surgery, cancer, cirrhosis, pancreatitis, dehydration, and increasingly recognized hypercoagulable syndromes such as polycythemia vera, thrombocytosis, protein C and S deficiency, antithrombin III deficiency, antiphospholipid antibody syndrome, and factor V Leiden mutation (activated protein C resistance).[27] Cirrhotic patients who are awaiting liver transplantation have a 15% incidence of mesenteric and portal venous thrombosis.[28]

Patients with MVT have a somewhat different presentation from those who have ischemia caused by arterial obstruction; the onset of symptoms with MVT may be insidious and the findings more subtle. Pain out of proportion to the physical examination is still an essential feature. The test of choice to confirm the diagnosis is contrast-enhanced computed tomography (CT), although duplex scanning and magnetic resonance imaging (MRI) with and without contrast are gaining popularity. Thrombus is located in the superior mesenteric vein in 70% of patients, with portal and inferior mesenteric vein thrombus found in about 30%.[29] Symptomatic acute MVT is a lethal disease, with a previously reported 30-day mortality of about 25% and a 3-year survival of 35%.[29] Patients with evidence of chronic thrombosis fare somewhat better, because collateral venous channels form to augment intestinal venous drainage.

The widespread availability of diagnostic imaging technologies has enabled earlier diagnosis and modest improvement in outcomes. Morasch and colleagues reported a series of 31 patients diagnosed with MVT from 1985 to 1999.[30] The 30-day mortality rate was 23%; 72% of patients were initially treated with heparin and one patient received thrombolytic therapy. Thirty-two percent of patients underwent bowel resection, and the overall mortality rate for surgery was 27%. Acosta and colleagues reported a series of 51 patients identified with MVT between 2000 and 2006 with a 30-day mortality of 20% and an overall survival rate of 67%.[31]

Outcomes data on the use of thrombolytic therapy are limited and not yet sufficient to guide the clinical management of patients with AMVT. Hollingstead and associates reported a large retrospective series with 20 patients diagnosed with acute or subacute portal vein or mesenteric vein thrombosis (MVT) from 1990 to 2001 treated with transcatheter thrombolytic therapy.[32] Resolution of symptoms was observed in 85% of patients. Complete lysis of thrombus was noted in 15%; partial lysis in 60%, and 25% had no lysis of thrombus. Major bleeding complications were noted in 60% of patients with one death occurring due to gastrointestinal hemorrhage. The authors concluded that thrombolytic therapy should be reserved for patients with advanced disease due to the high complication rate.

Clinical Presentation and Diagnosis

AMI can appear precipitously with decompensation over hours or insidiously with progression over days. Classic symptoms of AMI include sudden abdominal pain out of proportion to the physical examination, with gut emptying at the onset of pain. The subacute pattern of mesenteric ischemia is characterized by a more gradual development of vague abdominal signs and symptoms. These include less intense and nonspecific abdominal pain with nausea, vomiting, and changes in bowel habits. The abdomen may become distended but still have active bowel sounds.

Predictably, physical signs intensify as the syndrome progresses. In the early phases, signs of peritoneal irritation such as abdominal guarding and rebound are absent. As the bowel becomes more ischemic, necrosis progresses from the mucosal layers to the seromuscular layers. After full-thickness bowel infarction, the abdomen is often grossly distended, with absent bowel sounds and exquisite tenderness to palpation. Bowel infarction can impart a feculent odor to the breath.

Ancillary laboratory evaluations often reveal an increase in hemoglobin and hematocrit, consistent with hemoconcentration.

There is a marked leukocytosis with a predominance of immature white blood cells (left shift). Although no specific laboratory findings are diagnostic, serum levels of amylase, lactic dehydrogenase, creatine phosphokinase, and alkaline phosphatase are often elevated, along with a metabolic acidosis with a persistent base deficit.[33] Unfortunately, most of these abnormalities do not develop until after bowel necrosis has occurred. Electrocardiography may be helpful if it reveals an atrial dysrhythmia.

Plain abdominal radiographs are used to exclude other potential causes of abdominal pain, rather than confirm the diagnosis of AMI. In fact, completely normal plain abdominal films are seen in more than 25% of patients with mesenteric ischemia.[34] Subtle signs of AMI on plain abdominal films include a dynamic ileus and distended air-filled loops of bowel. Bowel wall thickening from submucosal edema or hemorrhage can be prominent, especially in cases of acute MVT. In advanced stages, pneumatosis of the bowel wall and portal vein gas portend an extremely poor prognosis.

Barium contrast evaluations of the upper and lower gastrointestinal tracts are contraindicated because residual intraluminal contrast material can limit visualization of the mesenteric vasculature during diagnostic angiography. On the rare occasion when barium studies are performed in a patient with the gradual development of abdominal pain, the submucosal edema and hemorrhage of intestinal ischemia are manifest by thickening of the bowel wall, strictures, or ulcerations.

Duplex ultrasonography may be of some benefit in visualizing flow in the SMA and celiac axis. These tests can document proximal stenoses in the SMA or celiac axis or complete occlusion of these vessels.[35] In newer series, color Doppler ultrasonography has been shown to be a valuable screening tool for AMI; it is far more specific than clinical evaluation alone.[36,37] Unfortunately, a significant percentage of patients at risk for mesenteric ischemia have dilated air-filled loops of bowel that make ultrasonography difficult, if not impossible.

Multidetector CT angiography (MDCTA) has become the definitive diagnostic study for the detection of occlusive AMI due to its widespread availability and the rapidity with which it can be performed. With high resolution, vital diagnostic information regarding the central visceral arterial and venous circulation can be obtained. Other potential causes of abdominal pain can also be excluded and bowel perfusion can also be evaluated. CT of the abdomen and pelvis can delineate subtle changes consistent with subacute bowel ischemia such as focal or segmental bowel wall thickening.[38] Thrombus within the mesenteric veins or the lack of opacification of the veins after intravenous contrast administration (Fig. 25.3) is often seen in MVT.[39] Nonenhancement of the arterial vasculature with timed intravenous contrast injections is seen in acute mesenteric arterial thrombosis or embolization. CT scans can also vividly demonstrate pneumatosis or portal vein gas in advanced stages. Kirkpatrick and colleagues have reported MDCTA to have a sensitivity of 96% and specificity of 94% for the diagnosis of AMI.[40]

Advances in contrast-enhanced and cine phase magnetic resonance angiography have allowed better visualization of the visceral vasculature and have an important role in the diagnosis of AMI.[41] Specifically, when MRI is coupled with magnetic resonance oximetry, both anatomic and physiologic information regarding the mesenteric circulation can be obtained.[42]

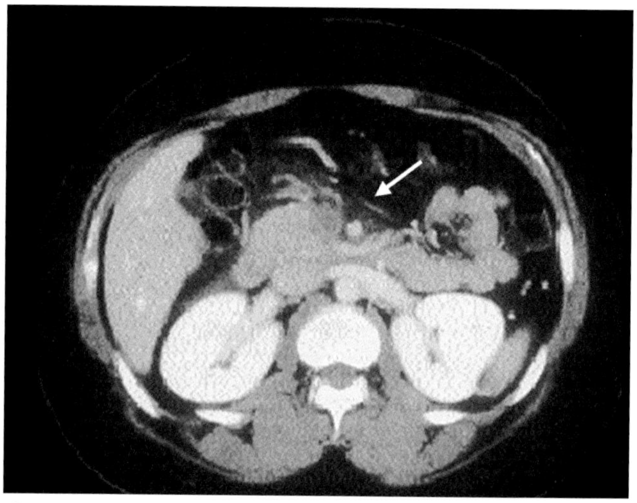

FIG 25.3 Contrast-enhanced computed tomography scan demonstrating acute mesenteric venous thrombosis of the superior mesenteric vein, which is thrombus filled and has an enhancing rim *(arrow)*.

Despite these aforementioned developments, the definitive diagnostic study remains mesenteric angiography via CT angiography or catheter-based studies if the former is not available. Image manipulation (three-dimensional reconstruction) or multiple views are often needed for adequate assessment of the vessels at risk. The origins of the celiac axis and the SMA can be visualized only by lateral views, whereas the more distal celiac axis and SMA distributions are best viewed through anteroposterior projections. On occasion, selective cannulation of the origins of the celiac axis and SMA is often required to completely define the anatomy and pathophysiology. Thorough aortography is also needed to evaluate potential inflow and outflow sites for bypass grafts, and to clarify the extent and location of other atherosclerotic lesions in the iliac artery and the IMA.

In patients with nonocclusive ischemia, angiography usually reveals multiple areas of narrowing and irregularity in major branches. The small- and medium-size arterial branches may be decreased or absent, and the vasculature is diffusely pruned, with an absent submucosal "blush." In MVT, selective angiograms may demonstrate reflux of contrast material back into the aorta because of extremely slow flow and heightened outflow resistance. A prolonged arterial phase with accumulation of contrast and thickened bowel walls is also characteristic. In extreme cases, angiographic contrast may extravasate into the bowel lumen, which is indicative of active bleeding. The definitive diagnosis of MVT is made during the venous phase; a filling defect is noted within the portal vein or, in more severe cases, the entire venous phase is absent.

In patients presenting with suspected advanced stages of AMI with clinical evidence of peritonitis requiring emergent laparotomy, diagnostic arteriography performed in a hybrid operating suite may establish the diagnosis and provide valuable information on the location and nature of arterial lesions, thereby enabling endovascular therapy (ET) if technically feasible or immediate surgical exploration and revascularization. Selective injections can generally differentiate among arterial embolism, in situ thrombosis, and mesenteric vasospasm.

Diagnostic arteriography may also offer endovascular therapeutic options including pharmacologic vasodilatation, visceral artery angioplasty and stenting, or intervention with mechanical thrombectomy and catheter directed thrombolysis. Mechanical thrombectomy can be initially performed to achieve restoration of visceral perfusion, followed by adjunctive thrombolysis if there are significant residual arterial thrombotic occlusions.[43] The majority of patients undergoing ET for AMI still require laparotomy for bowel wall assessment, underscoring the complementary nature of endotherapy and open surgery for the treatment of AMI as well as the need to perform these procedures in a hybrid surgical operating suite.[43,44] Retrograde open mesenteric stenting, which is discussed in the next section, can also be performed to restore perfusion of a thrombotic occlusion of the SMA during laparotomy.[45,46]

Treatment Options

Initial treatment of AMI includes volume resuscitation, correction of acidosis, and administration of appropriate antibiotics. Systemic anticoagulation should be started immediately to prevent further propagation of thrombus. A urinary catheter, as well as a peripheral arterial catheter, should be placed for monitoring intravascular volumes and hemodynamic status. A nasogastric tube should be placed to decrease the chance of aspiration. Patients who have profound acidosis, hemodynamic instability, or clinical evidence of peritonitis should be taken immediately to the operating suite for abdominal exploration. In these advanced cases, correction of acidosis may not be possible until the ischemic bowel has been removed or revascularized. Perioperative morbidity and mortality in these patients is significant, with the reported mortality ranging from 20% to 50%.[43,44,47]

Contrast-enhanced imaging studies, such as CT angiography, should be performed immediately, if the patient's clinical condition allows. In selected patients with an early diagnosis of SMA embolus unassociated with bowel necrosis, a trial of thrombolytic therapy and angioplasty may be appropriate.[48,49] Such treatments are usually limited to patients with abdominal pain for less than 8 hours' duration without signs of peritoneal irritation. If lysis is not accomplished within 4 hours of commencing thrombolytic therapy or if peritoneal signs develop, the infusion should be discontinued and immediate surgical exploration should be performed.

An increasing number of case reports and series have detailed the use of percutaneous angioplasty to dilate significant atherosclerotic plaques of the SMA that are unmasked by thrombolytic therapy.[50–52] Due to the variable angle of the origin of the SMA from the aorta, placement and removal of the angioplasty catheter and stent placement may be more difficult than for lower extremity angioplasties.[10] Restenosis rates range from 25% to 50% in earlier series,[50,51] but recent reviews report more promising results.

In a 9-year series of 70 consecutive patients with AMI from 1999 to 2008, the Cleveland Clinic achieved an 87% success rate in endovascular treatment of AMI (65% thrombotic occlusions and 35% embolic occlusions).[43] ET was the preferred treatment in the majority of patients, with 81% undergoing ET and 19% undergoing open surgical repair (OSR), with the treatment modality determined by surgeon preference. Patients in the endovascular group were slightly older (65 ± 12 vs. 60 ± 13 years), were weighted with more thrombotic occlusion cases (72% vs. 64%), and had longer duration of symptoms (median, 62 vs. 26 hours). The primary mode of endovascular treatment was thrombolysis in 48%, mechanical thrombectomy in conjunction with thrombolysis (12%); additional therapy included vasodilator (papaverine or nitroglycerin) therapy (51%), and percutaneous transluminal angioplasty (PTA) plus stent (33%). Successful endovascular therapy, defined as successful return of bowel perfusion, resulted in fewer laparotomies (69% vs. 100% in traditional therapy), lower rates of acute renal failure (27% vs. 50%) and pulmonary failure (27% vs. 64%), and lower mortality rates (36% vs. 50%). Those who failed endovascular treatment had the same elevated 50% mortality rate as the open surgical group.

Ryer and colleagues at the Mayo Clinic recently reported a series of 93 patients who underwent emergency arterial revascularization for acute mesenteric ischemia from 1990 to 2010.[44] The majority of patients were treated with OSR. The etiology of AMI included in situ thrombosis in 54% and embolism in 31% of patients. ET alone or as a hybrid procedure was performed in 11 patients. There was no significant difference in outcomes between open and endovascular revascularization. Thrombolysis or mechanical thrombectomy was performed in five patients and visceral PTA in seven patients. There was no significant difference in outcomes among patients treated in the 1990s ($n = 45$ patients) and the 2000s ($n = 48$ patients) with the overall 30-day mortality being 22%. Major adverse events were observed in 47% of patients. Of the 88% of patients who underwent OSR, mesenteric thromboembolectomy was performed in 45%, prosthetic bypass grafting in 40%, endarterectomy in 7%, and autologous saphenous vein bypass grafting in 7%. If the use of a prosthetic graft was required in the presence of necrotic bowel, grafts were soaked in rifampin and excluded with omentum prior to performing an enterectomy.

Still, while ET is increasingly used for AMI at major centers, open surgical revascularization remains the predominant treatment across the United States.[53] Outcomes comparing open and endovascular treatment of AMI utilizing the National Inpatient Sample database from 2005 to 2009 were reported by Banlieu and associates.[54] A total of 4665 patients were identified who underwent interventional treatment, with a mean age of 70.5 years. Seventy-six percent underwent open surgery and 24% underwent endovascular treatment. The severity of comorbidities did not differ significantly between the groups. Mortality (39% OSR vs. 25% ET), need for bowel resection (33% OSR vs. 14% ET), and length of stay (17.1 days OSR vs. 12.9 days ET) were significantly greater following open revascularization, compared with endovascular treatment.

Wyers and colleagues described a series of six patients with AMI with acute atherosclerotic thrombosis of the SMA treated with retrograde open mesenteric stenting (ROMS).[45] The hospital mortality rate was 17%. An advantage of this approach is that the increased "pushability" allowed by sheath access in close proximity to the obstruction can facilitate treatment of some occlusive lesions that cannot be successfully treated via antegrade access. Blauw and colleagues recently reported a series of 15 patients undergoing ROMS for AMI from 2007 to 2011.[46] The 30-day and 12-month mortality were 20%; the 12-month primary stent patency was 83%, and secondary patency was 100%. This method is a viable alternative to open bypass and may also be considered as a bridge to more durable open revascularization following recovery.

When an aortic dissection involves the origin of one or more of the visceral vessels, endovascular repairs have been attempted through stent placement[55,56] and balloon fenestration of the dissection septum.[57] Although these less invasive treatments are attractive, they are currently limited by the rapid onset of ischemic symptoms, inability to gain access to the dissection channel, or the need for surgical repair of an associated aortic aneurysm.

Regardless of the cause, most patients with acute arterial occlusion require early surgical exploration and reestablishment of mesenteric flow to prevent or minimize bowel infarction. A generous midline incision should be made, and the extent of mesenteric ischemia and necrosis should be assessed. If the entire small bowel is gangrenous, enterectomy with lifelong hyperalimentation is the only option. If the process is more segmental, portions of frankly ischemic and nonviable intestine should be resected and controlled while further exploration is continued. After locating all infarcted segments, the cause of the intestinal ischemia should be sought.

To achieve adequate exposure, the transverse colon is retracted superiorly, and the fourth portion of the duodenum is mobilized to the ligament of Treitz. The SMA is identified by palpation of the root of the mesentery. If the cause of mesenteric ischemia is an embolus, a more proximal SMA pulse is often noted. The SMA is encircled at or just distal to the level of obstruction (Fig. 25.4), and a transverse arteriotomy is made. Balloon-tipped embolectomy catheters are inserted retrograde, and the embolus is extracted. Embolectomy catheters should also be passed distally to ensure that no fragmentation of the clot or discontinuous thrombosis has occurred. Transverse arteriotomies are closed primarily with interrupted fine monofilament sutures to ensure that the vessel is not stenosed. If a longitudinal arteriotomy is required, closure is best accomplished with a vein patch. Appropriately selected longitudinal arteriotomies can also be used for distal anastomoses of bypass grafts if thrombectomies are unsuccessful in obtaining arterial inflow.

When flow is restored, the bowel is reinspected for persistent regions of ischemia. Segments that previously demonstrated equivocal viability may improve with revascularization, and resection may be avoided; lengths of bowel that are obviously nonviable must be removed. Bowel continuity can be restored primarily, or stomas may be exteriorized if the patient is unstable. In most instances, a second-look operation should be performed at 24 to 36 hours to assess the cumulative effects of reperfusion. Planning for this reexploration allows the surgeon to minimize the amount of bowel resected primarily and to ensure that the final bowel anastomoses are performed with viable bowel.

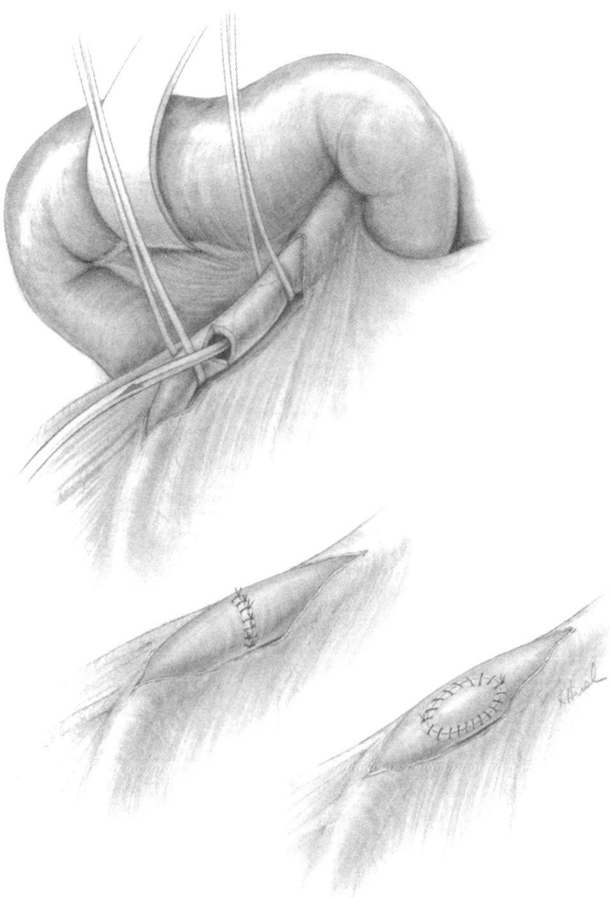

FIG 25.4 Exposure of the superior mesenteric artery (SMA) at the root of the small bowel mesentery with the SMA encircled with silastic tapes. Balloon-tipped catheter extraction of a mesenteric embolus is performed through a transverse arteriotomy. Primary closure of the arteriotomy is then completed transversely or with a vein patch to prevent stricture. (From Zarins CK, Gewertz BL. *Atlas of Vascular Surgery*, 2nd ed, Philadelphia, 2005, Elsevier Churchill Livingstone, pp 176–177.)

The management of SMA thrombosis caused by underlying atherosclerotic lesions is more challenging, because simple surgical thrombectomy is unlikely to be durable.[58] The length of the SMA should be palpated and interrogated with continuous wave Doppler imaging to identify a patent distal artery that is acceptable as an outflow source. The proximal SMA should be opened through a longitudinal arteriotomy. If thrombectomy is temporarily successful, an intraarterial shunt is placed while the exposures needed for definitive revascularization are performed. The longitudinal arteriotomy in the SMA can serve as the distal anastomotic site for both antegrade bypasses originating in the supraceliac aorta and retrograde bypasses from the infrarenal aorta or iliac vessels. If there is a high likelihood of bowel resection, an autologous conduit should be used for the bypass. If bowel necrosis is present and a suitable autogenous vein is not available for conduit, then a prosthetic graft may be soaked in rifampin antibiotic solution prior to use.[44]

If there is thrombosis of the SMA with a high-grade proximal occlusive lesion, then a hybrid procedure for acute atherosclerotic thrombosis of the SMA with ROMS can be performed during the laparotomy procedure.[45,46,59] Utilizing an identical exposure approach as described above, open thromboendarterectomy of the SMA is performed. Subsequent retrograde cannulation of the SMA toward the aorta is then carried out. After wire access into the abdominal aorta beyond the proximal SMA occlusive lesion is achieved, angioplasty of the orificial occlusive lesion is performed with a balloon-expandable stent. Finally, after adequate inflow is restored, primary closure or patch angioplasty of the SMA arteriotomy is performed. This technique has also been successfully applied by the authors in a patient with visceral malperfusion and static obstruction of the proximal SMA caused by acute type B aortic dissection in whom flow could not be restored to the SMA utilizing antegrade access.

In syndromes of nonocclusive ischemia, the primary therapy is selective arterial administration of vasodilating agents such as papaverine. Such treatment must be coupled with the cessation of α agonists or other vasoconstrictors. Heparin should also be administered to prevent thrombosis in the cannulated vessel, but the drug must be infused through a peripheral intravenous catheter to avoid precipitation when mixed with papaverine. If a patient demonstrates signs of continued bowel ischemia or necrosis, as evidenced by peritonitis or guarding, surgical exploration is required. All necrotic bowel should be resected while arterial infusions of vasodilators continue. The room temperature should be elevated, and the bowel should be kept in moist laparotomy pads to minimize vasoconstriction during exploration. Most patients should undergo a second-look operation in 24 to 48 hours to reassess bowel viability.

The surgical treatment of MVT is restricted to fluid resuscitation, correction of any underlying coagulopathy, and resection of nonviable bowel. Unfortunately, venous thrombectomy is of limited durability and has not proved effective in most instances. The extent of bowel resection should be generous, and repeated exploratory laparotomy is often required to ensure that adequate bowel resection has been performed. Because many patients succumb despite these measures, a more aggressive stance toward early surgical thrombectomy or fibrinolysis has been advocated by some.[32,60,61] The risks of these maneuvers are considerable, however, and intervention should be reserved for patients who do not improve with conventional therapy.

Although the detection of frankly necrotic bowel is not difficult, the determination of viability in marginally perfused bowel is more challenging. Simple indicators of viability include visible peristalsis as well as a pink and normal color of the serosa. Along with palpation of the distribution of the SMA for arterial pulsations, Doppler ultrasonography can be used to further evaluate arterial signals within the vascular arcades. If any question remains, the bowel should be reassessed at a minimum of 30 minutes after revascularization. Administration of intravenous fluorescein followed by illumination with a Wood ultraviolet light will confirm perfusion of the bowel. The primary limitation of fluorescein is that it is eventually absorbed in fat; therefore it can be administered only once before it diffuses throughout all tissue and loses its specificity. Unfortunately, no combination of tactics is sufficiently sensitive or specific for error-free evaluation of bowel viability.[62]

Long-term patient outcomes after acute intestinal ischemia are strongly dependent on the timeliness of diagnosis, the underlying lesion, and the associated cardiovascular status. In a comprehensive report by Klempnauer and colleagues of 90 patients suffering from intestinal ischemia, 31 patients survived and were discharged from the hospital.[63] Cumulative 5-year survival was approximately 50% (16 of 31). Mortality was greatest during the first year after the incident. The worst survival (20% at 5 years) was seen in patients who suffered mesenteric arterial thrombosis, and the best survival was seen in patients with emboli or nonocclusive ischemia (about 70%). Only one patient who survived the first episode of arterial thrombosis died because of recurrent bowel ischemia. Remarkably, 8 of the 15 surviving patients returned to work.

CHRONIC MESENTERIC ISCHEMIA

In contrast to the varied causes of AMI, CMI is a result of end-stage atherosclerosis in more than 90% of cases. The lesions usually represent extensions of aortic atheroma rather than intrinsic disease of the mesenteric arteries. Risk factors parallel those of atherosclerosis in general, including a positive family history, smoking, hypertension, and hypercholesterolemia. Interestingly, in most series, there is a slight female preponderance, and nearly 50% of patients have a history of prior cardiovascular surgery.[64] Nonatherosclerotic causes of CMI include thrombosis associated with thoracoabdominal aneurysm, aortic coarctation, aortic dissection, mesenteric arteritis, fibromuscular dysplasia, neurofibromatosis, middle aortic syndrome, Buerger disease, and extrinsic celiac artery compression by the median arcuate ligament.

Clinical Presentation

The sine qua non of CMI is postprandial abdominal pain. The pain is characteristically dull and crampy, occurring primarily in the epigastrium or midabdomen. The discomfort results from activation of visceral afferent nerves that respond to distension and ischemia but that poorly localize pain. The pain occurs 15 to 45 minutes after eating, with increasing severity according to the size and nature of the meal. The temporal relationship between pain and food ingestion often leads to "food fear" (sitophobia), a classic but variable complaint.

Weight loss is the second classic symptom of CMI. Although malabsorption can contribute to malnutrition in severe cases, most weight loss is simply due to the patient's fear of eating. Many patients become so emaciated that they undergo extensive evaluations for occult neoplasms.

Other less common symptoms of CMI include diarrhea, nausea and vomiting, and constipation. The variability in signs and symptoms is due in part to the region of the gut affected. Foregut ischemia (celiac axis distribution) is usually accompanied by nausea, vomiting, and bloating, whereas midgut ischemia (SMA) causes classic postprandial abdominal pain and weight loss. The infrequent findings of constipation, occult blood in the stool, and ischemic colitis on colonoscopic biopsy may signify hindgut (IMA) involvement. The lack of specificity of the signs and symptoms of this syndrome often leads to a delay in diagnosis, and it is common for affected patients to have undergone myriad interventions, including antacid or antireflux therapy, cholecystectomy, hysterectomy, and adhesiolysis.

The findings on physical examination are also nonspecific, but the astute clinician can recognize several clues indirectly suggesting the diagnosis. Unexplained weight loss and emaciation alone should arouse suspicion of the syndrome. Manifestations of atherosclerosis in other vascular beds are common, including a cervical or peripheral bruit, decreased peripheral pulses, and signs of chronic lower extremity ischemia. An abdominal bruit can be heard in up to 70% of affected patients.

Diagnosis

Routine laboratory evaluation is rarely helpful, although malnutrition may be accompanied by hemoconcentration, immunoincompetence, hypoalbuminemia, hypoproteinemia, or hypocholesterolemia. Tests for malabsorption, such as stool fat content, D-xylose tolerance, or vitamin B_{12} absorption, may be positive but are nonspecific. Plain abdominal films may reveal aortic or arterial calcification, suggesting mesenteric atherosclerosis. Additional imaging studies, such as endoscopy, gastrointestinal contrast examination, and CT, rarely establish the diagnosis but are useful in excluding more common clinical syndromes.

Ultrasonography has added a new dimension to the diagnostic evaluation of patients with suspected CMI. The ability to screen patients with chronic abdominal pain without incurring the risk of contrast arteriography has been a significant advance in the identification of affected patients. Predictive values in excess of 80% have been documented using peak systolic velocity criteria of greater than 275 cm/s for the SMA and greater than 200 cm/s for the celiac axis.[65,66] End diastolic velocity (EDV) has also been found to be an important indicator of significant stenosis. Zwolak and associates reported that for the SMA, EDV greater than 45 cm/s had sensitivity, specificity, and positive and negative predictive values of greater than 90% for detecting angiographic stenosis of greater than 50%.[67] For the celiac artery, retrograde flow demonstrated in the common hepatic artery was found to be 100% predictive of severe stenosis or occlusion. The high sensitivity and negative predictive values of duplex ultrasound suggest that it may be an appropriate modality for excluding the diagnosis of CMI and may avoid the need for unnecessary arteriography.

With regard to duplex surveillance following prior ET, there are no well-established criteria for determination of significant in-stent restenosis. Baker and colleagues reported the peak systolic velocity (PSV) in successfully stented SMAs to be higher than the PSV criteria of greater than 275 cm/s used for the diagnosis of significant SMA stenosis in nonstented vessels.[68] It is recommended to obtain a baseline surveillance duplex study early after ET to compare to future surveillance studies. The authors suggested an increase above this baseline or an in-stent PSV greater than 500 cm/s to be suggestive of significant in-stent restenosis.

For positive or equivocal ultrasound examinations, diagnostic arteriography is required for more exact lesion localization and for planning revascularization. A complete examination consists of anteroposterior and lateral aortic views, as well as selective injections of the celiac axis, SMA, and IMA (Fig. 25.5). Occlusion of two or three of the main trunks is generally required for development of the CMI syndrome (Fig. 25.6). Significant mesenteric occlusive disease combined with the development of large collateral vessels is essentially pathognomonic (Fig. 25.7). Celiac axis occlusion by the median arcuate ligament may also be readily demonstrated by contrast arteriography during provocative maneuvers including expiration, and may be responsible for CMI in younger patients (Fig. 25.8).[69]

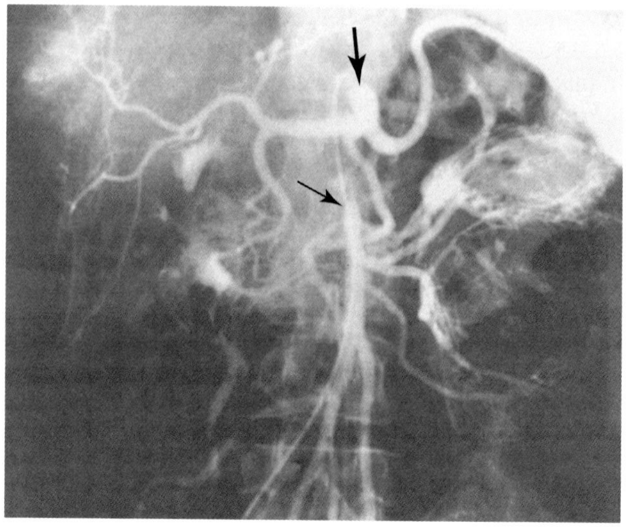

FIG 25.5 Chronic mesenteric ischemia in a 67-year-old woman who underwent antrectomy, vagotomy, and cholecystectomy, and presented with nausea, vomiting, and a 40-pound weight loss. Anteroposterior arteriogram with direct celiac injection shows critical stenosis of the celiac axis *(thick arrow)* and distal reconstitution of an occluded superior mesenteric artery *(thin arrow)*. (From Schwartz LB, Gewertz BL: Chronic mesenteric arterial occlusive disease: clinical presentation and diagnostic evaluation. In Perler BA, Becker GL, editors: *Vascular Intervention: A Clinical Approach,* New York, 1998, Thieme Medical, p 522.)

More recent developments in CT and image processing have allowed such detailed reconstructions of the visceral aortic branches that catheter-based arteriography may become unnecessary in many cases. As demonstrated in Figs. 25.9 and 25.10, identification of a highly calcified plaque at the SMA origin prompted contrast-enhanced CT reconstruction. Significant orificial lesions with poststenotic dilatation of both the celiac axis and the SMA were demonstrated in this patient with symptoms of CMI and a large abdominal aortic aneurysm.

Treatment Options

Because there is no effective medical therapy for CMI, its treatment is focused on the mechanical relief of occlusive lesions and restoration of blood flow. Open mesenteric bypass has been the gold standard of treatment in the past; however, endovascular therapy, consisting of percutaneous transluminal angioplasty and stenting (PTA/stent), has emerged recently as the most favored

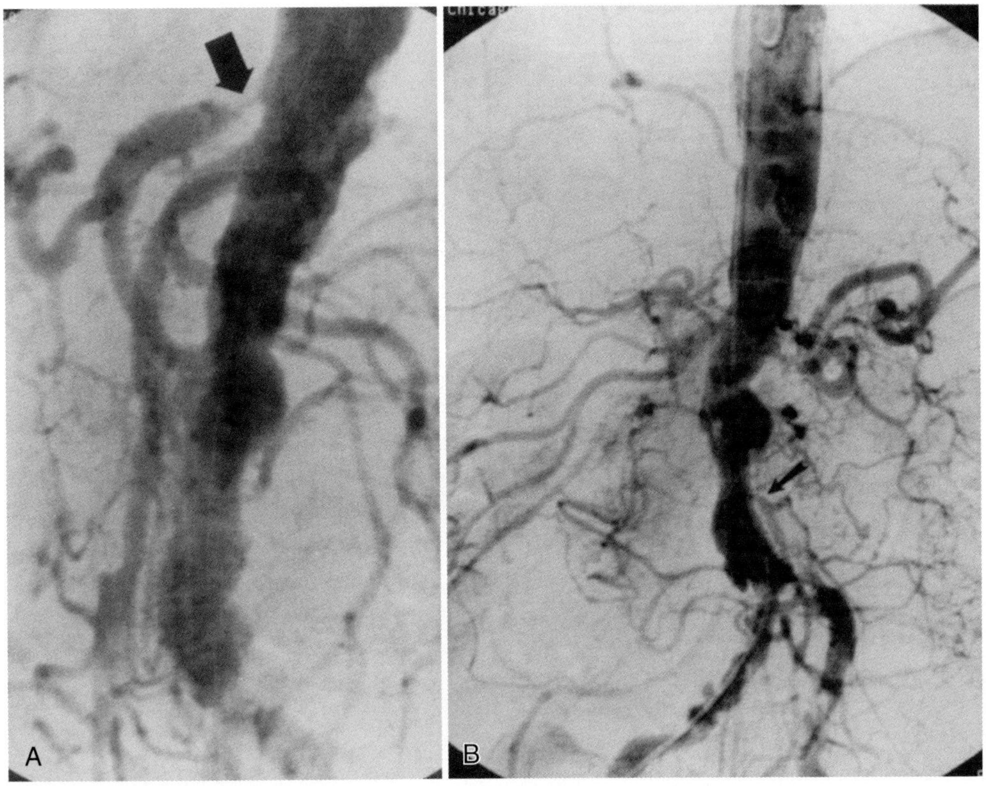

FIG 25.6 Chronic mesenteric ischemia in a 78-year-old woman who underwent a coronary artery bypass and carotid endarterectomy, and presented with claudication, a 30-pound weight loss, and postprandial pain. (A) Lateral aortogram shows critical celiac axis stenosis *(arrow)*. (B) Anteroposterior aortogram shows severe infrarenal aortic disease and critical inferior mesenteric artery stenosis *(arrow)*. (From Schwartz LB, Gewertz BL: Intestinal ischemic disorders. In Yao JST, Pearce WH, editors: *Modern Trends in Vascular Surgery,* Stamford, CT, 1999, Appleton and Lange, pp 347–367.)

treatment modality for CMI (Fig. 25.11).[70] The utilization of ET has been progressively increasing, with data from the Nationwide Inpatient Sample (NIS) database from 1988 to 2006 indicating that the annual number of ETs performed for chronic mesenteric ischemia surpassed OSR in 2002 and more than doubled it by 2005.[53] The NIS data demonstrated that although there were 6342 cases of endovascular intervention and 16,071 OSRs for all causes of mesenteric ischemia (both acute and chronic), patients with CMI were more frequently treated endovascularly than with open bypass (62% vs. 38%). The mortality rate for all procedures captured by the NIS database was lower for ET than after OSR (3.7% vs. 13%, $P < .01$). Compared to OSR, patients undergoing ET were older, more likely male, and had higher comorbidities.

Turba and associates reported a retrospective series of 166 consecutive patients undergoing ET for CMI.[71] The technical success rate was 97% and was higher for stenting than PTA (99.4% vs. 86%; $P = .0001$). Multiple mesenteric arteries were treated in 46 patients. The 30-day mortality was 3%, and the 5-year survival was 76%. Immediate clinical improvement was observed in 88% of patients. During follow-up, 28 of 166 patients had recurrence of symptoms with imaging evidence of restenosis. The 5-year cumulative primary patency rates for the celiac artery, SMA, and IMA were 68%, 67%, and 84% respectively, whereas the primary assisted patency rates for the celiac artery, SMA, and IMA were nearly 100%. Of particular interest, the outcome of SMA treatment was better with PTA alone than with PTA with stenting ($P = .014$).

Major academic centers have demonstrated comparable outcomes for both open and endovascular repairs.[72-74] In 2009, the Mayo Clinic group published their analysis of risk-stratified outcomes in their retrospective review of 229 CMI patients who underwent open or endovascular treatment. Patients who underwent percutaneous intervention were significantly older and of higher risk. Interestingly, the mortality rate was not statistically different, although open surgical patients had higher cardiac and pulmonary complication rates (36% vs. 18%) and longer hospital stays.[74]

Despite the documented advantages of percutaneous therapy, OSR has been shown to have superior durability; therefore the choice of therapy should be tailored to the patient's comorbidities and disease process. In general, ET is associated with fewer complications, but it does demonstrate lower primary patency rates and a greater need for earlier reintervention.[72-74] One of the largest series with intermediate-term (3 years) follow-up describes 49 patients treated endovascularly for symptomatic

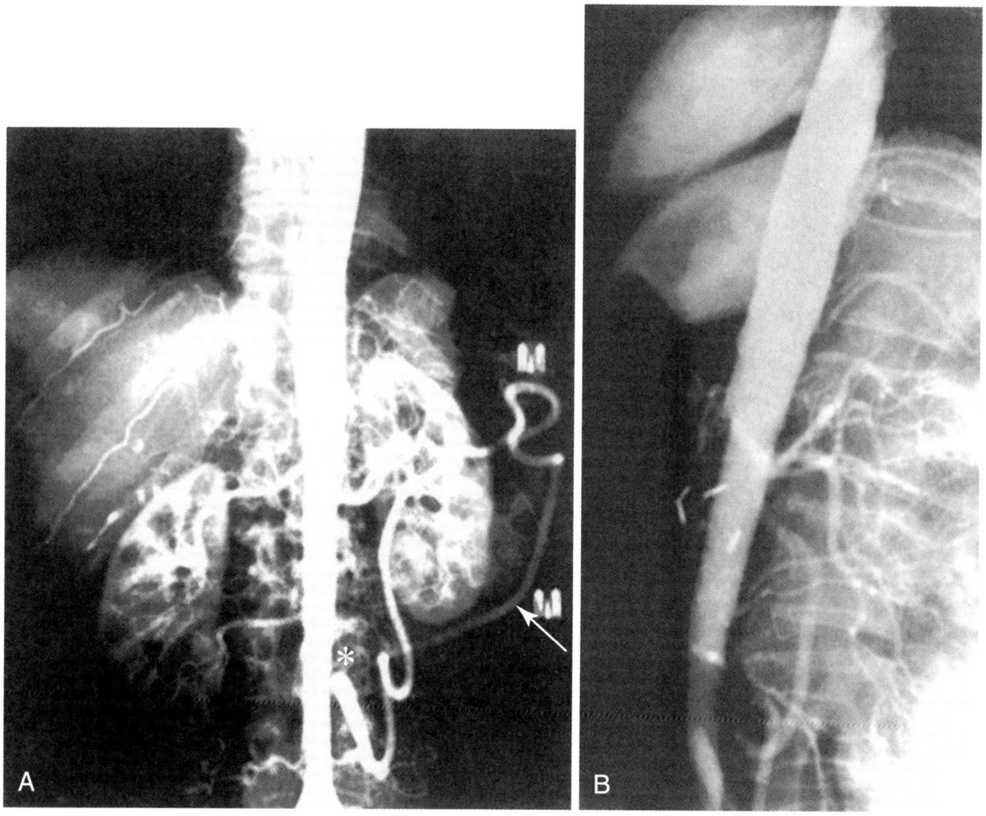

FIG 25.7 Chronic mesenteric ischemia in a 67-year-old woman with postprandial abdominal pain and a 30-pound weight loss. (A) Anteroposterior aortogram (early phase) shows occlusion of the celiac axis and superior mesenteric artery, along with critical stenosis of the inferior mesenteric artery origin *(asterisk)*. Note the presence of a meandering mesenteric artery *(arrow)*. (B) Lateral aortogram demonstrating occlusion of both the celiac and superior mesenteric arteries at the origin. (From Schwartz LB, Gewertz BL: Chronic mesenteric arterial occlusive disease: clinical presentation and diagnostic evaluation. In Perler BA, Becker GL, editors: *Vascular Intervention: A Clinical Approach,* New York, 1998, Thieme Medical, p 521.)

CMI. Primary patency was 64% and approximately 30% of patients required reintervention.[75] The extensive plaque burden from aortic atherosclerosis has been proposed as the principle mechanism for the high restenosis rate.

Surgical revascularization remains the most durable treatment for CMI. Early reports emphasized single-vessel reconstruction using autologous vein and a retrograde approach with bypass grafts originating from the infrarenal aorta.[76,77] Although this procedure avoids supraceliac aortic dissection and clamping, the geometry of a retrograde bypass is theoretically unfavorable, with the potential for compression by the overlying abdominal viscera. In the modern era, antegrade bypass using grafts originating in the supraceliac aorta has become the preferred surgical technique.[78]

Regardless of the method of revascularization, proper patient selection is critical to optimize results. Other common gastrointestinal disorders should be excluded, and the diagnosis of CMI should be ascertained. Concurrent extracranial carotid and coronary artery disease should be evaluated and treated appropriately. Medical or percutaneous treatment for myocardial ischemia is preferred, because patients with CMI are at increased risk for intestinal infarction during and after coronary artery revascularization.

Although hypoproteinemia with serum albumin of less than 3 mg/dL frequently accompanies CMI, postponement of operative therapy to nourish the patient is rarely helpful. The risk of intestinal infarction during the preoperative period is significant and is often associated with catastrophic results. In patients with life-threatening malnutrition, consideration should be given to ET as a temporizing measure before surgical reconstruction.

Antegrade Bypass

Aortic-celiac-mesenteric bypass is best performed through a transperitoneal approach. After a thorough exploration of the abdomen, attention is directed toward exposure of the distal thoracic aortic inflow source. This portion of the aorta is usually spared from atherosclerosis. The triangular ligament of the left lobe of the liver is divided, and moist laparotomy packs are inserted to protect the liver parenchyma. Although exposure is greatly facilitated by the use of self-retaining retractor systems, care should be taken to avoid excessive force. The lesser sac is entered by division of the gastrohepatic ligament. The esophagus

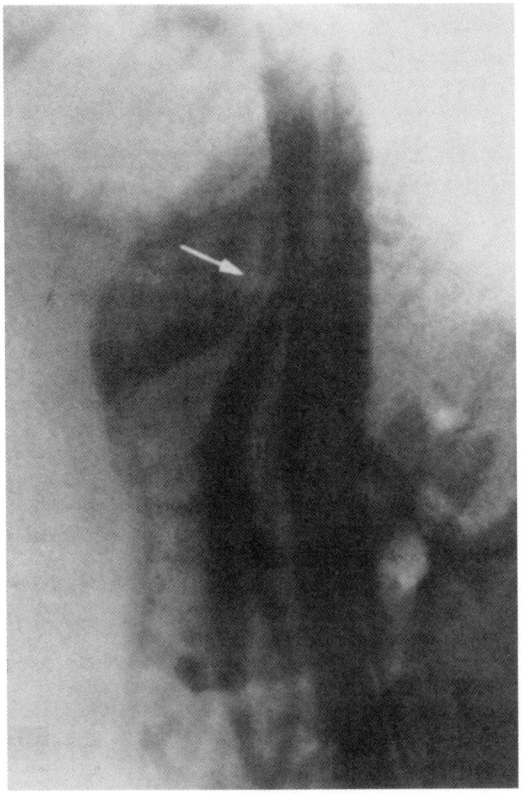

FIG 25.8 Median arcuate compression syndrome. Lateral aortogram in a 27-year-old woman with postprandial abdominal cramping, bloating, and occasional nausea and vomiting. Note the compression of the celiac axis and superior mesenteric artery *(arrow)*. Her twin sister had similar complaints and arteriographic findings. (From Bech F, Loesberg A, Rosenblum J, et al: Median arcuate ligament compression syndrome in monozygotic twins. *J Vasc Surg* 19:935, 1994.)

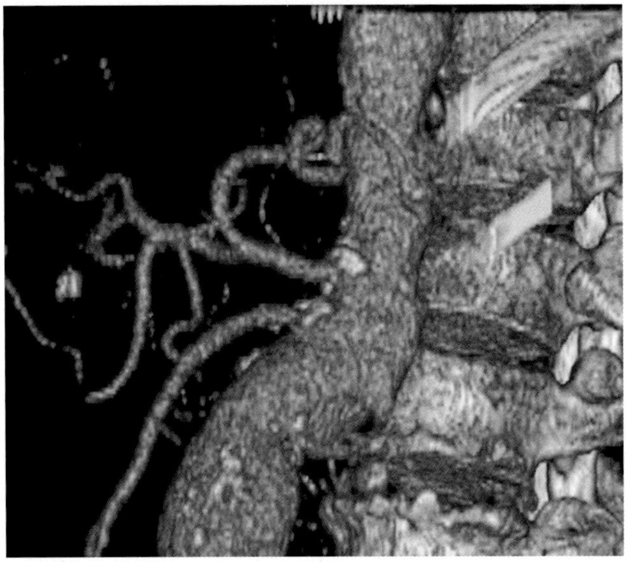

FIG 25.10 Contrast-enhanced reconstruction of computed tomography scan confirms the hemodynamic significance of orificial lesions of the celiac axis and superior mesenteric artery. Note the detail of the distal vessels on the image, allowing operative planning.

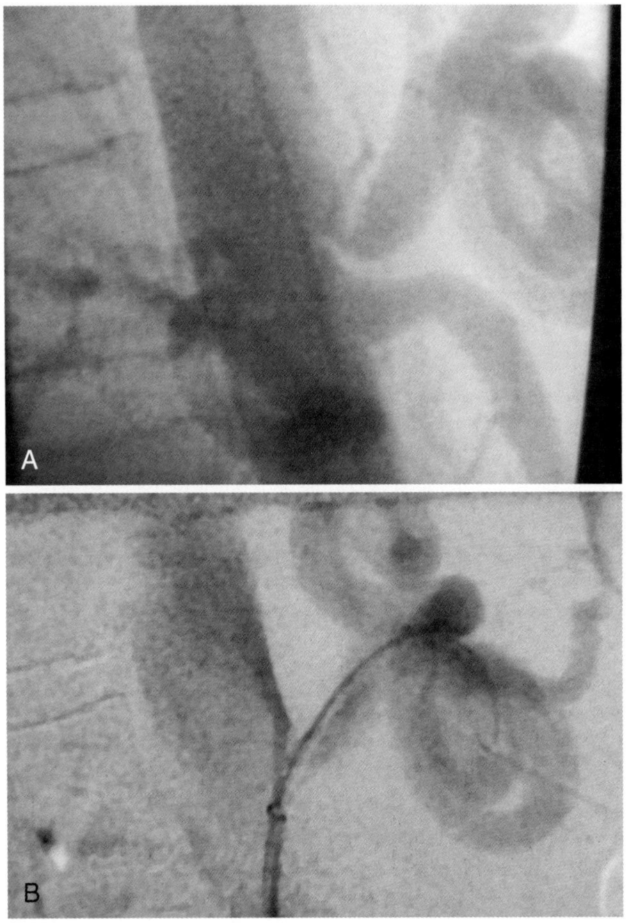

FIG 25.11 (A) Severe stenosis of the celiac axis in a patient with foregut ischemic symptoms. (B) Successful angioplasty with stent placement despite angulation of the artery origin.

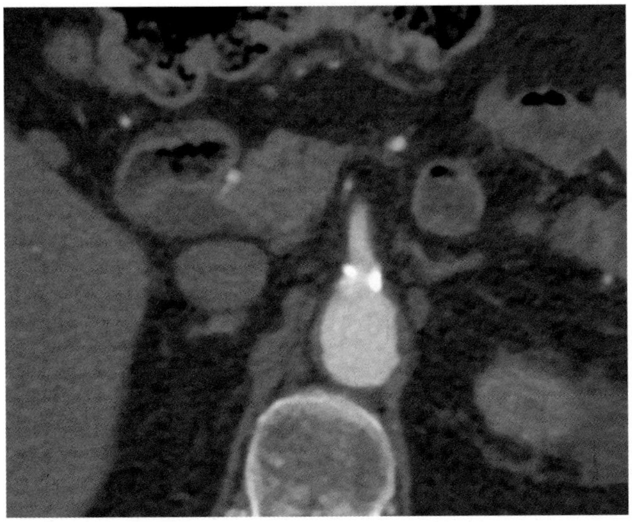

FIG 25.9 Calcified plaque is noted at the origin of the superior mesenteric artery.

is retracted to the left, and final aortic exposure is achieved by division of the diaphragmatic crura and median arcuate ligament. This allows isolation of 8 to 10 cm of the distal thoracic aorta without division of the diaphragm.

The mesenteric arterial branches are identified next. The origin of the celiac axis is already substantially exposed during the aortic dissection. Dissection along its length is continued until a soft patent distal target is appreciated (usually within the distal celiac axis before its branching). Following this, the operative field is temporarily shifted to the midabdomen by lifting and superiorly displacing the transverse colon. The small bowel and the fourth portion of the duodenum are retracted to the right. The SMA is palpated in the small bowel mesentery as the vessel courses from the retroperitoneum at the inferior margin of the pancreas. The peritoneal membrane is incised, and a suitable segment is isolated. Blunt dissection is used to develop a tunnel behind the pancreas on the left side of the aorta.

Intravenous heparin (100 units/kg) and mannitol (25 g) are administered. A longitudinal incision is made in the aorta, and additional arterial wall is removed as needed. A bifurcated Dacron or polytetrafluoroethylene graft (typically 14 × 7 mm) is delivered to the field. Proximal aortic followed by distal celiac axis anastomosis is performed, and the viscera are reperfused. SMA anastomosis is performed last, after the second limb of the graft is tunneled beneath the pancreas (Fig. 25.12). An alternative but equally effective technique involves sequential bypass using a single 7-mm Dacron graft (Fig. 25.13).[78-80]

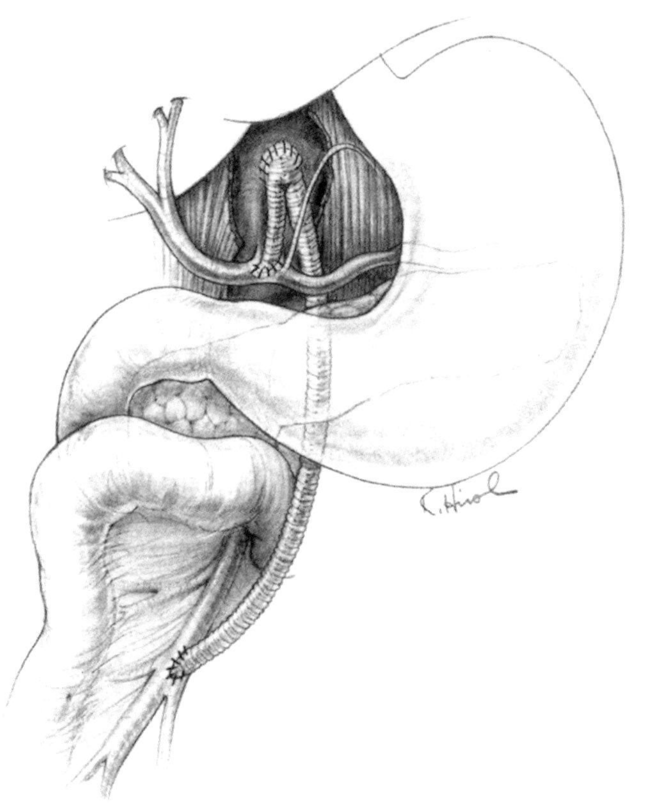

FIG 25.12 Aorta–celiac artery–superior mesenteric artery bypass using a bifurcated Dacron graft. (From Zarins CK, Gewertz BL: *Atlas of Vascular Surgery*, New York, 1989, Churchill Livingstone, p 109.)

Retrograde Bypass

Mesenteric bypass grafts originating from the infrarenal aorta or iliac arteries (retrograde bypass) were the first techniques used in surgical correction of mesenteric arterial lesions.[6] This approach offers the advantages of limited dissection and avoidance of supraceliac aortic occlusion. Despite these features, retrograde bypass has been used less frequently in recent years. Results from a number of clinical series suggest (but do not prove) that retrograde bypass is less durable than its antegrade counterpart.[81,82] This is presumed to be due to the tendency for SMA grafts to kink or twist when the viscera are returned to their normal anatomic positions. Although the use of stiffer prosthetic conduits and meticulous technique can improve the orientation of these reconstructions, retrograde bypass should be considered a third option to be used only if antegrade bypass and aortomesenteric endarterectomy are not feasible. Specific indications for retrograde bypass currently include (1) emergency revascularization in patients undergoing laparotomy for AMI, (2) inaccessible supraceliac aorta due to previous surgery or subphrenic inflammation, (3) severe cardiac disease with contraindications to supraceliac aortic occlusion, and (4) the need for simultaneous infrarenal aortic and mesenteric revascularization.

Retrograde mesenteric bypass begins with exposure of the most proximal suitable segment of the SMA as it exits from beneath the pancreas. The more proximal the anastomosis in the SMA, the less likely it is that kinking will occur, because the graft will lie geometrically parallel to the aorta. The mesentery is then returned to its normal position as the graft is pulled taut to lie adjacent to the aorta. A soft portion of the aorta or iliac

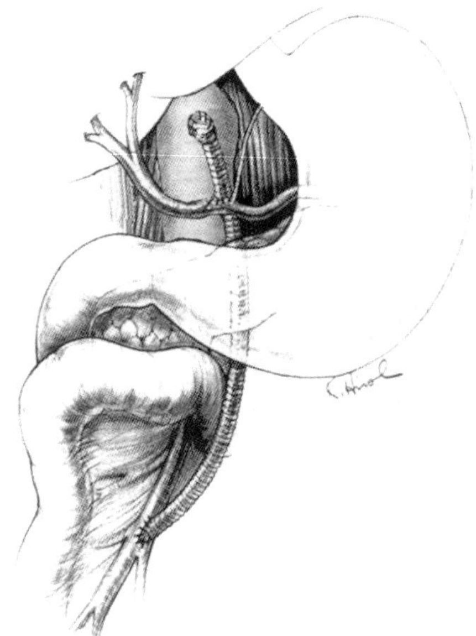

FIG 25.13 Sequential aorta–celiac axis–superior mesenteric artery bypass using an 8-mm Dacron graft configured in sequential fashion. (Modified from Zarins CK, Gewertz BL: *Atlas of Vascular Surgery*, New York, 1989, Churchill Livingstone, p 109.)

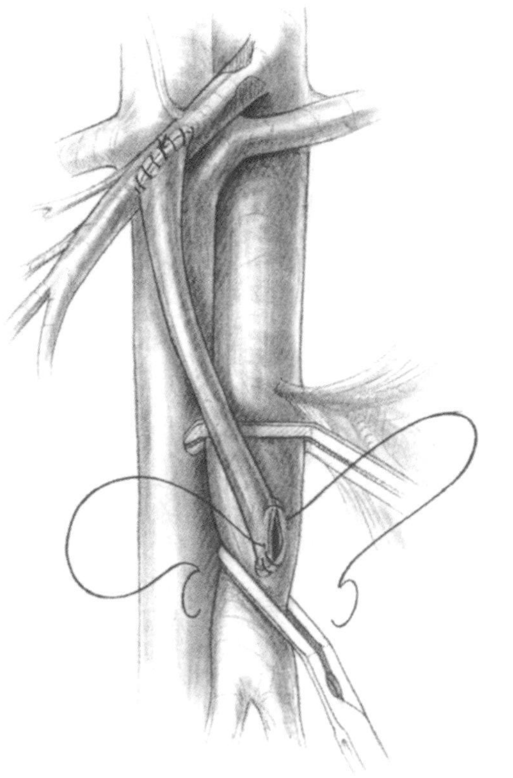

FIG 25.14 Retrograde infrarenal aorta–superior mesenteric artery bypass using autologous vein. (From Zarins CK, Gewertz BL: *Atlas of Vascular Surgery*, New York, 1989, Churchill Livingstone, p 107.)

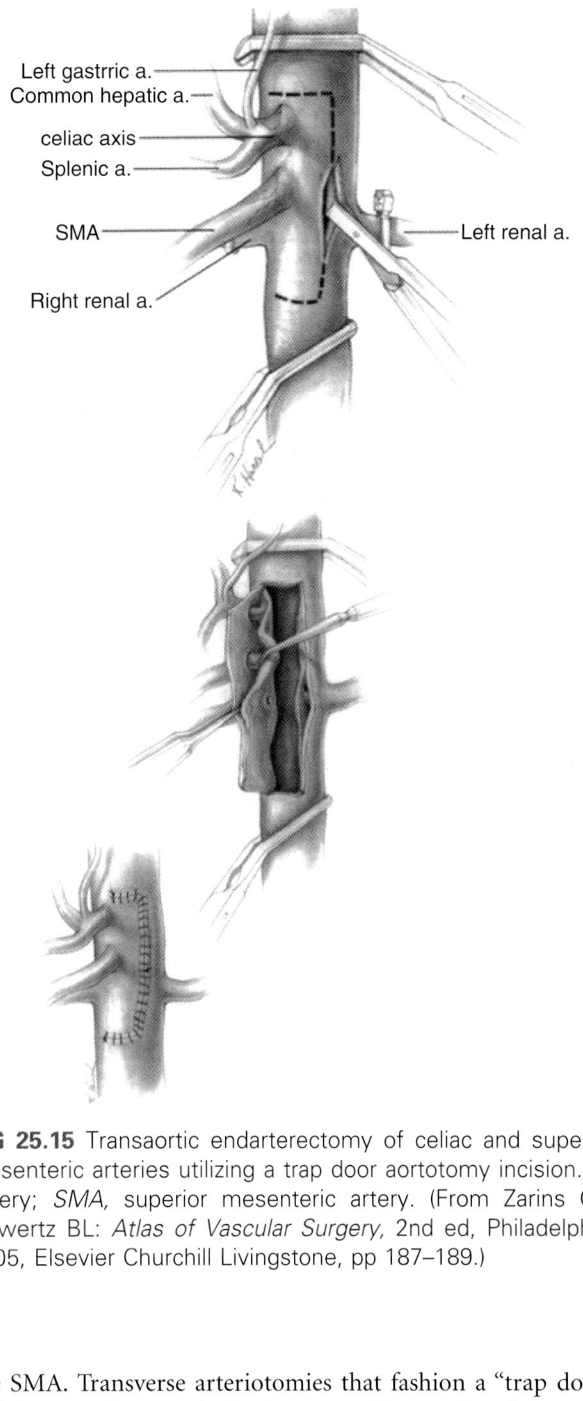

FIG 25.15 Transaortic endarterectomy of celiac and superior mesenteric arteries utilizing a trap door aortotomy incision. *a.*, Artery; *SMA*, superior mesenteric artery. (From Zarins CK, Gewertz BL: *Atlas of Vascular Surgery*, 2nd ed, Philadelphia, 2005, Elsevier Churchill Livingstone, pp 187–189.)

artery is located, and the proximal anastomosis is performed; a fair amount of tension must be maintained on the graft to avoid laxity and kinking when the abdomen is closed (Fig. 25.14).

Access to the celiac axis is problematic with this approach; therefore celiac revascularization is usually performed via anastomosis to the common hepatic artery or, less commonly, the splenic artery. The common hepatic anastomosis (distal anastomosis) is performed in an end-to-side fashion. After the Kocher maneuver, the graft can be tunneled behind the duodenum and head of the pancreas, en route to the infrarenal aorta. In this position, torsion and kinking are minimized. When the less robust splenic artery is used, grafts are tunneled behind the tail of the pancreas and anterior to the left renal vein.

Aortic Endarterectomy

Orificial occlusive lesions involving both the celiac and SMA are usually best endarterectomized through a transaortic approach (Fig. 25.15).[83] This technique has the advantage of removing atheroma from the aorta and visceral branch orifices during the same procedure. The perivisceral aorta can be exposed through a transperitoneal or retroperitoneal approach. After medial visceral rotation is performed, continuous exposure of the aorta, celiac axis, SMA, IMA, and both renal arteries is obtained. After both renal arteries are controlled, a longitudinal arteriotomy is made in the aorta anterior to the left renal artery. The incision is continued cephalad above the celiac axis, and caudad below the SMA. Transverse arteriotomies that fashion a "trap door" incision are then made in the aorta. The aortic atheroma is removed, and eversion endarterectomies of the plaque extensions into the orifices of the celiac artery and SMA are performed. If satisfactory distal endpoints are not obtained on all vessels, the distal endpoint must be exposed and intimal tacking sutures placed to avoid dissection and postoperative thrombosis. An alternative is to place a stent from the open aorta to tack the distal endpoint. The aortotomy is closed with a continuous 3-0 or 4-0 monofilament suture.

Endovascular Therapy

ET to the visceral vessels can be performed via femoral or brachial arterial access. The brachial approach may be advantageous because the acute and caudally directed angle between the aorta and visceral vessels may limit the "pushability" required to advance a guidewire across a stenosis from a femoral approach. Disadvantages of the brachial approach include the need for longer catheters and devices due to increased distance from the target vessels, limited maximal sheath size of 7 French without surgical exposure of the brachial artery, and the risk of embolic stroke from wire manipulation in the aortic arch. One recent study has shown that the type of guidewire or device platform, brachial versus femoral access, and the presentation (stenosis versus total occlusion) had no impact on mortality or primary patency.[71]

Like open revascularization, endovascular treatment of both the celiac trunk and SMA is preferred. Orificial lesions may be refractory to treatment by PTA alone and may require treatment with balloon-expandable stents, with increased radial force and more controlled deployment, rather than self-expandable stents. For midsegment lesions, PTA with selective stenting may be employed. Covered stents have been used to reduce restenosis, although there are no controlled studies that compare restenosis between covered and uncovered stents. Potential disadvantages of ET include access site complications, contrast nephropathy, and mesenteric vessel perforation. Similar to open surgical revascularization, reperfusion hemorrhage has also been described following mesenteric PTA.[84]

Outcomes of Surgical Treatment

A review of collected series of the surgical treatment of CMI during the 1980s and 1990s reveals an overall operative mortality rate of 6%, with 20% of patients sustaining major complications.[85] Most clinicians agree that recurrence is less likely if more than one vessel is revascularized. This concept was first championed by Robin and colleagues,[61] who noted differential recurrence rates corresponding to the number of vessels treated. Subsequent reports confirmed this finding,[86,87] making complete revascularization the standard.

Although many clinicians report excellent symptomatic relief after surgical revascularization for CMI, only a few have rigorously examined graft patency.[78,88,89] McMillan and coworkers used duplex scans and arteriography to document graft patency in 25 patients undergoing mesenteric bypass.[88] Their series included 16 patients treated for CMI and 9 treated for AMI, in whom the perioperative morbidity was predictably higher. Considering the 22 patients who survived for more than 1 month, graft patency after a mean of 35 months was approximately 90%. The success rates of retrograde and antegrade grafts were indistinguishable, as were the outcomes of prosthetic and autogenous vein reconstructions. It was noted that two of the three patients experiencing occluded grafts were asymptomatic, emphasizing that patency cannot be inferred from clinical criteria alone.

Expected results in the modern era are typified by the University of Chicago experience with 24 consecutive patients undergoing mesenteric revascularization over a 10-year period.[78] All patients had significant SMA involvement, and 21 also had lesions of the celiac axis. Seventeen antegrade and seven retrograde bypasses were performed. Calculated 5-year primary patency was 78%, documented by duplex scans, arteriography, or both; 5-year patient survival by life-table analysis was 71% (Fig. 25.16).

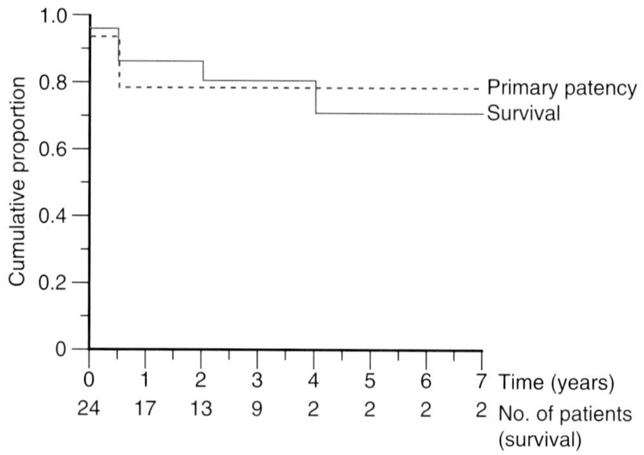

FIG 25.16 Symptom-free survival (n = 24) and primary patency (n = 19) in patients undergoing surgical revascularization for chronic mesenteric ischemia. Calculation was done using the life-table method. Number of patients per interval is shown at the bottom. (Modified from Moawad J, McKinsey JF, Wyble CW, et al: Current results of surgical therapy for chronic mesenteric ischemia. *Arch Surg* 132:616, 1997.)

More recent operative series have also documented excellent surgical outcomes. Park and colleagues reported a series of 98 patients who underwent open revascularization for CMI from 1989 to 1998.[90] In this series, 81% underwent two or three mesenteric vessel revascularizations, 19% underwent single-vessel revascularization of the SMA alone, and 79% underwent antegrade configuration bypasses. The in-hospital mortality was 5% with cardiac complications the cause in 60% of deaths. Symptom-free survival was achieved in 95% at 1 year and 92% at 5 years. Kruger and associates reported a series of 39 patients undergoing open revascularization for CMI from 1992 to 2006.[91] Multivessel revascularization was performed in all patients when anatomically feasible, with 61% undergoing multivessel reconstruction. Perioperative mortality was 2.5%, and primary graft patency was 92% at 5 years.

Outcomes following aortic and mesenteric endarterectomy for CMI were reported by Mell and colleagues in a series of 80 patients, with 37 patients undergoing endarterectomy alone (34 transaortic endarterectomy, 3 local mesenteric endarterectomy), 29 patients undergoing mesenteric bypass, and 14 undergoing a combined procedure.[92] Concurrent aortic reconstruction was required in 16%. The hospital mortality was 3.8%, 1-year survival was 92%, and 5-year survival was 65%. The 5-year symptom-free survival was 82%. On multivariate analysis, freedom from symptomatic recurrence correlated with performance of endarterectomy as the method of revascularization, indicating in this study that endarterectomy provided the most durable symptomatic relief in patients with CMI.

Endovascular Versus Surgical Revascularization

Tallarita and colleagues at the Mayo Clinic recently reported a large series of 343 patients between 1991 and 2010 and compared OSR (n = 187) and ET (n = 156).[93] From 2002 onward the annual number of patients treated with ET exceeded those treated with

OSR. There were more low-risk patients (67% vs. 38%) in the OSR group and more high-risk patients (26% vs. 5%) in the ET group. The overall 5-year survival was greater in the OSR group than the ET group (69% vs. 44%; $P < .001$). Multivariate analysis revealed age greater than 80 years, diabetes, chronic kidney disease (stage IV or V), and home oxygen therapy as independent predictors of death. A propensity score–matching analysis revealed no difference in 5-year survival between the two groups (OSR 60%, ET 57%; $P = .7$). The reintervention rate for symptomatic recurrence or high-grade stenosis (OSR 14%, ET 21%; $P = .6$) and late mesenteric-related deaths (OSR 5.8%, ET 4.1%) were no different among the treatment groups. The authors concluded that late patient survival is not influenced by the type of reconstruction, and that the treatment modality should be based on the likely durability of the procedure.

Atkins and colleagues at the Massachusetts General Hospital reported a series of 80 consecutive patients with symptomatic CMI undergoing elective revascularization with OSR performed in 49 patients and ET in 31 patients.[73] The ET group had fewer vessels revascularized (1.5 vs. 1.8 vessels, $P = .001$) and had shorter length of stay (5.6 vs. 16.7 days, $P = .001$). There was no difference noted in major morbidity or mortality between the groups. There was no difference in symptomatic recurrence between the groups (ET 23%, OSR 22%) and actuarial survival was similar at 2 years (ET 88%, OSR 74%, $P = .28$). Primary patency and primary assisted patency were lower at 1 year in the ET group (primary patency 58% vs. 90%, $P = .001$; primary assisted patency 65% vs. 96%, $P < .001$).

A systematic literature review of the last 25 years including all studies evaluating 10 or more patients undergoing OSR, ET, or both modalities for CMI was recently reported by Pecoraro, Veith, and associates.[94] A total of 1795 patients were included in the analysis, with 786 undergoing ET and 1009 OSR. Perioperative morbidity and mortality were both significantly greater for the OSR group versus the ET group (mortality 7% vs. 3.5%; morbidity 33% vs. 13%), though this was not a risk-adjusted analysis. Survival data at 1 and 5 years showed no difference between the groups, with 5-year survival with OSR of 65% and ET of 69%. Primary and secondary patency rates at 5 years were significantly greater for OSR versus ET. At 5-year follow-up, primary patency was 81% in the OSR group and 49% in the ET group with secondary patency of 98% and 88% respectively. Symptomatic recurrence of CMI was statistically greater following ET and the authors postulated that this may be because a significantly higher number of mesenteric vessels were revascularized in the OSR group. The authors recommend that the treatment modality for CMI should be based on lesion anatomy, nutritional status, and life expectancy of the patient. They also suggest that ET should be used as a bridge therapy to OSR in malnourished patients if it does not preclude subsequent OSR.

The outcomes of surgical and endovascular reinterventions in patients with previous failing open mesenteric revascularizations was recently reported by Kanamori and associates in a combined series from Cleveland Clinic and the Mayo Clinic.[95] There were 238 patients who underwent OSR for CMI at these two institutions from 1991 to 2013. Forty-seven patients presented with failing open revascularizations and underwent reintervention (38 patients presented with CMI, 9 patients with AMI) with open surgical reintervention performed in 28 patients (CMI in 19 patients, AMI in 9) and ET in 19 patients (all with CMI), with mean follow-up of 50 months. For patients with AMI, 30-day mortality was 22%, and all patients were treated with open reintervention. For patients with CMI, 30-day mortality was 0% for patients undergoing open surgical reintervention or ET. The 5-year survival was 60% in the entire group. There was no significant difference in primary patency at 1 year between the two groups (open surgical reintervention 61%, ET 77%; $P = .41$). When comparing patients undergoing first-time OSR to those undergoing open surgical reintervention, case control matching revealed that primary patency at 1 year was lower in the open surgical reintervention group (66% vs. 94%; $P < .05$), but early morbidity, mortality, and freedom from reintervention were similar.

Summary

Visceral ischemic syndromes are rare but potentially catastrophic disorders. In acute presentations, treatment of AMI includes systemic anticoagulation, thrombolytic therapy, open surgical revascularization, and percutaneous endovascular therapy. Open surgical mesenteric revascularization with thromboembolectomy or bypass remains the mainstay of modern therapy. This is due in part to the need for laparotomy with bowel inspection or resection in the majority of patients. Increasingly, ET has been successfully utilized for patients with AMI, with treatment options including a combination of thrombolytic therapy, mechanical thrombectomy, balloon angioplasty, and ROMS. ET as the primary modality may be associated with lower morbidity and mortality than open surgical revascularization. However, laparotomy for inspection of the intestines is still required in the majority of patients undergoing endovascular therapy.

ET has also now become the preferred treatment option for patients with chronic mesenteric ischemia with the annual number of ETs performed for chronic mesenteric ischemia, with ET significantly exceeding the number of OSRs. Open surgical revascularization has traditionally been associated with outstanding long-term outcomes. Although earlier studies demonstrated lower primary patency and higher reintervention rates associated with endovascular treatment, more recent analyses have demonstrated no difference in midterm reintervention rates or symptomatic recurrence compared with open surgical therapy. As such, ET should be considered the first line of therapy for patients with anatomically suitable lesions or excessive open surgical risk. In patients with life-threatening comorbidities, ET may also be considered as a temporizing measure or bridge to definitive open surgical reconstruction.

ACKNOWLEDGMENT

Thanks to Drs. Tina T. Ng and Brian Funaki for their contributions to previous versions of this chapter.

REVIEW QUESTIONS

1. What is the incidence of a "replaced right hepatic artery" arising from the SMA rather than the celiac axis?
   a. 2%
   b. 5%
   c. 12%
   d. 20%
   e. 40%
2. What is the most common site of origin of a mesenteric embolus?
   a. Midthoracic aorta
   b. Left ventricle
   c. Aortic valve
   d. Supraceliac aorta
   e. Pelvic veins (paradoxical embolus)
3. Nonocclusive mesenteric ischemia is associated with all of the following except:
   a. Digitalis toxicity
   b. Low cardiac output
   c. Administration of α-adrenergic agents
   d. Sepsis
   e. Inotropic administration
4. What is the most common cause of mesenteric venous thrombosis?
   a. Leukemia
   b. Hypercoagulable states
   c. Intraabdominal abscess
   d. Primary portal hypertension
   e. Pancreatic cancer
5. What is the most common location for a clinically significant acute embolic obstruction of the mesenteric circulation?
   a. Origin of the celiac axis
   b. Origin of the SMA
   c. Origin of the IMA
   d. Mid-SMA just distal to the origin of the middle colic artery
   e. None of the above
6. What is the most common location for a clinically significant chronic obstruction of the mesenteric circulation?
   a. Origin of the celiac axis
   b. Origin of the SMA
   c. Origin of the IMA
   d. Mid-SMA just distal to the origin of the middle colic artery
   e. None of the above
7. What is the best clinical indicator of the presence of acute intestinal ischemia?
   a. Severe leukocytosis
   b. Severe abdominal pain without rebound tenderness
   c. Acidosis
   d. Atrial fibrillation
   e. Hyperamylasemia
8. All of the following statements about angioplasty for mesenteric vascular disease are true except:
   a. The immediate failure rate is less than 5%.
   b. The periprocedural mortality is lower than that for operative therapy.
   c. Percutaneous transluminal angioplasty is useful in ischemia related to aortic dissection.
   d. Durability (defined as relief of symptoms) is less than that with operative repair.
   e. Stenting has improved patency.
9. What is the principal advantage of antegrade mesenteric bypass versus retrograde bypass for chronic mesenteric ischemia?
   a. Lower operative mortality
   b. Higher blood flow in grafts
   c. Allows use of autogenous conduits
   d. Avoids potential kinking of grafts
   e. Lower cardiac stress
10. What is the most reliable sign or symptom when making the clinical diagnosis of chronic mesenteric ischemia?
    a. Postprandial pain
    b. Weight loss
    c. Melena
    d. Postprandial vomiting
    e. Hypoalbuminemia

References available online at ExpertConsult.com.

CHAPTER 26

Diagnosis and Management of Renal Vascular Occlusive Disease

Ryan A. Haqq, Benjamin J. Pearce

HISTORICAL BACKGROUND

Renovascular Hypertension

In 1934, Goldblatt[1] demonstrated that constriction of the renal artery (renal artery stenosis [RAS]) produced atrophy of the kidney and hypertension in dogs. As a clinical pathologist, Goldblatt noticed that extensive vascular disease was often present at autopsy in patients with hypertension and was frequently severe in the renal arteries. In his own words: "Contrary, therefore, to what I had been taught, I began to suspect that the vascular disease comes first and, when it involves the kidneys, the resultant impairment of the renal circulation probably, in some way, causes elevation of the blood pressure."[1] Goldblatt's elegant experiments introduced a new era by demonstrating that renal artery stenosis could produce a form of hypertension that may be corrected by nephrectomy.

In 1938, Leadbetter and Burkland[2] described the first successful treatment of this correctable form of hypertension. They cured a 5-year-old child with severe hypertension by removal of an ischemic ectopic kidney. The photomicrographs published from that renal artery specimen were the first documentation of a renovascular origin of hypertension. In subsequent years, numerous patients were treated by nephrectomy, based on the findings of hypertension and a small kidney on intravenous pyelogram. Smith reviewed 575 such cases in 1956 and found that only 26% of patients were cured of hypertension by nephrectomy.[3] This led him to suggest that nephrectomy should be limited to strictly urologic indications.

In 1954, Freeman performed an aortic and bilateral renal artery thromboendarterectomy in a hypertensive patient, which resulted in resolution of the hypertension.[4] This first cure of hypertension by renal revascularization, in combination with the widespread use of aortography, was followed by enthusiastic reports describing blood pressure benefit after renal revascularization.[5–8] Nevertheless, by 1960 it became apparent that renal revascularization in hypertensive patients with renal artery stenosis was associated with a beneficial blood pressure response in fewer than half of individuals. These clinical results fostered general pessimism regarding the value of operative renal artery reconstruction for the treatment of hypertension and have not been altered with the introduction of endovascular correction of renal artery stenosis.

Contemporary operative management of renovascular hypertension (RVH) began with the introduction of tests of functional significance. Split renal function by Howard and Connor,[9] Stamey and associates,[10] Page and Helmes,[11] and others[12–14] identified the role of the renin-angiotensin system in blood pressure control, thus describing the pathophysiology of RVH. After accurate assays for plasma renin activity became available, physicians could accurately predict which renal artery lesion was producing RVH.

Ischemic Nephropathy

Until the current era, the pathophysiology and management of renovascular disease (RVD) focused solely on hypertension; however, contemporary reports have emphasized the relationship between RVD and renal insufficiency.[15–23]

The term *ischemic nephropathy* has been adopted to recognize this relationship. By definition, ischemic nephropathy describes the presence of severe occlusive disease of the extraparenchymal renal artery in combination with excretory renal insufficiency. In 1962, Morris and associates reported on eight azotemic patients with global renal ischemia who experienced improved blood pressure and renal function after renal revascularization.[24] Novick, Libertino, and Dean and their groups found a similar beneficial functional response when bilateral renal lesions were corrected in azotemic patients.[17–21] These early reports and the reports that followed suggested that ischemic nephropathy could mediate renal insufficiency that was *rapidly* progressive, contributing to end-stage renal disease. In this chapter, diagnostic studies and methods of management for RVD, RVH, and ischemic nephropathy are reviewed.

PATHOLOGY

The majority of interventions performed for RVD are due to atherosclerosis and fibromuscular dysplasia; however, renal artery aneurysm (RAA), aortic dissection, and traumatic injury have all been implicated in RVD. Atherosclerosis of the renal artery is not unique. The pathogenesis parallels atherosclerotic lesions elsewhere, with cholesterol-rich lipid deposition and intimal thickening. Later, this atheroma may undergo central degeneration and even calcification. Atheromas typically occur at or near the renal artery ostium (Fig. 26.1). This ostial lesion reflects aortic atheroma that spills over into the renal artery orifice. Most commonly, these lesions are found on the left and account for approximately 70% of patients with RVH. Like atherosclerosis elsewhere, angiographic findings that are pathognomonic for a hemodynamically significant lesion include poststenotic dilatation and the presence of collateral vessels. Often there is simultaneous angiographic involvement of the abdominal aorta and its bifurcation. Most commonly, the renal artery lesion is only one manifestation of generalized atherosclerosis.

Fibromuscular dysplasia of the renal artery encompasses a variety of hyperplastic and fibrosing lesions of the intima, media, or adventitia. They are most frequently seen in young women. This is of no predictive value, however, because fibrodysplastic lesions can be found at any age and in either sex. Medial fibroplasia is the most common lesion, accounting for 85% of dysplastic lesions. The right renal artery is more commonly affected than the left, but bilateral involvement is present in the vast majority of patients. The basic cause of medial fibroplasia remains unknown, but its frequent occurrence in multiple arteries suggests a systemic arteriopathy. It often involves long segments of the renal artery and its branches, producing a characteristic "string-of-beads" appearance angiographically. Embryologic variations, hormonal influences, autoimmune mechanisms, and even recurrent trauma during youth have been suggested as possible causative factors. None of these explanations is adequate, however, and the supporting evidence remains mostly conjectural.

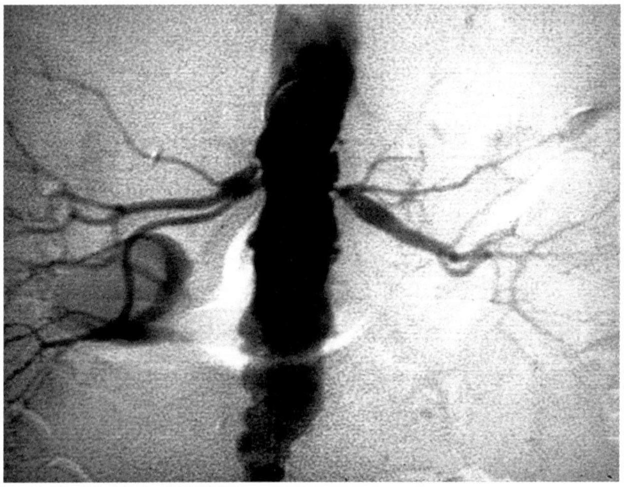

FIG 26.1 Arteriogram showing typical appearance of ostial atherosclerotic renal artery stenosis. Aortic atheroma spills over into the renal artery to create stenosis.

Based on the angiographic appearance of fibromuscular disease, several methods of categorization have been suggested. To establish a uniform terminology, Harrison and McCormack[25] combined their experience and developed a classification of these lesions correlating the histologic and angiographic appearance. Depending on the layer predominantly involved, lesions may be categorized as intimal, medial, or adventitial (Fig. 26.2). Clinically, however, it may be difficult to segregate individual lesions into one of these categories. The most common variety of fibromuscular dysplasia is medial fibroplasia (85%) with mural microaneurysms (Fig. 26.3). Less commonly, the dysplastic lesions may appear as a single mural stenosis (see Fig. 26.2), which is consistent with intimal fibroplasia (5%). Perimedial dysplasia (10%) demonstrates the same gender predilection and arterial septa as medial fibroplasia; however, mural microaneurysms are absent.

With the widespread acceptance of thoracic endografting as appropriate therapy for type B aortic dissection (TBAD), surgeons are more frequently being involved in the care of these patients. Dissection can result in obstruction of the renal ostia via a dynamic or static obstruction. Dynamic obstruction occurs when the aortic flap temporarily occludes the renal ostia due to alterations in lumen pressure during the cardiac cycle. Conversely, a static obstruction can occur when the dissection flap carries out into the main renal vessel proper. Both pathologies can lead to acute renal failure and worsening of hypertensive control.

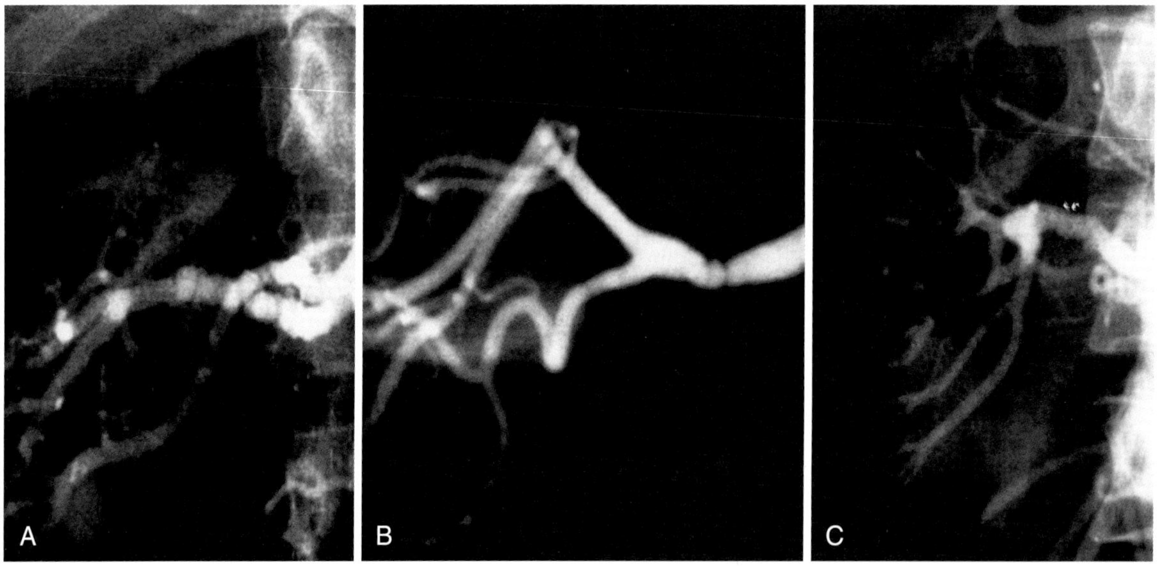

FIG 26.2 Angiographic appearance of fibromuscular dysplasia: alternating septa and mural microaneurysms of medial fibroplasia (A), focal stenosis of intimal fibroplasia (B), and fine septa without microaneurysms characteristic of perimedial dysplasia (C).

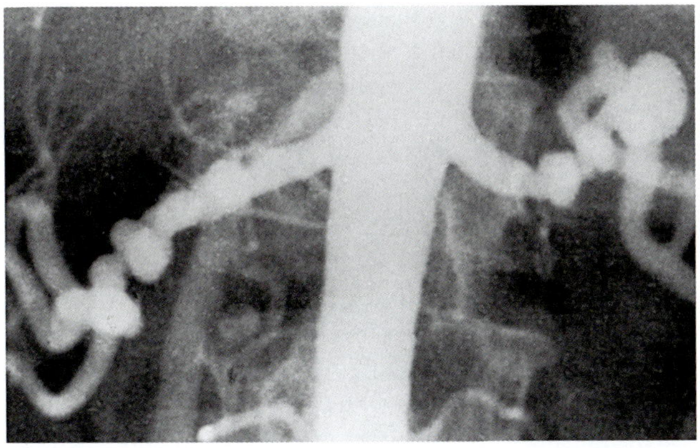

FIG 26.3 Arteriogram demonstrating typical "string-of-beads" appearance of medial fibroplasia with fine septa and microaneurysm.

RAA has been implicated in RVH in the past. In fact, the most common reason for repair of symptomatic RAA in the Society for Vascular Surgery's Low Frequency Disease Consortium's evaluation of RAA[26] was hypertension. No obvious causal effect has been linked between RVH and RAA; however, embolization and artery kinking are posited to play a role.

PATHOPHYSIOLOGY

The kidney, because of its influence on circulating plasma volume and on the modulation of vasomotor tone, is a dominant site of blood pressure regulation. To examine the pathophysiology of RVH, a review of the normal homeostatic activities of the kidney in blood pressure regulation is appropriate.

Renin-Angiotensin-Aldosterone System

The renin-angiotensin-aldosterone system is a complex feedback mechanism that normally acts to maintain a stable blood pressure and blood volume under varying conditions. Richly innervated modified smooth muscle cells located along the afferent arterioles in juxtaposition to the renal glomerulus (juxtaglomerular apparatus) are sensitive monitors of perfusion pressure. Diminished perfusion pressure stimulates these cells to release renin, a proteolytic enzyme. Renin interacts with angiotensinogen, an α-globulin manufactured in the liver, to produce angiotensin I. Angiotensin I, an inactive and labile decapeptide, is converted to the potent vasoconstrictor angiotensin II by angiotensin-converting enzyme, which is abundant in the lungs and other tissues. In addition to its potent vasoconstrictor properties, angiotensin II, through its conversion to angiotensin III, also increases blood pressure by stimulating aldosterone release from the zona glomerulosa of the adrenal cortex. This, in turn, increases plasma volume by increasing sodium and water resorption in the renal tubules. Through these actions of angiotensin II and III, blood pressure, plasma volume, and plasma sodium content are increased. In addition, the adjacent cells of the distal convoluted tubule (macula densa) may play a role by acting as sensors of sodium concentration in the distal tubules and exerting a positive feedback mechanism on renin release. As these mechanisms increase perfusion pressure in the juxtaglomerular cells, further renin production and release are suppressed, and blood pressure is modulated within a narrow range.

Goldblatt Kidneys: One-Clip Two-Kidney and One-Clip One-Kidney Hypertension

Potentially, two forms of hypertension may be produced by hemodynamically significant RVD: renin-dependent hypertension and volume-dependent hypertension. In the original Goldblatt experiments, renovascular insufficiency was induced through two methods. The first mimicked unilateral RAS by creating a stenosis in one kidney and leaving the other kidney normal. Decreased perfusion activates the renin-angiotensin-aldosterone axis and the angiotensin II–mediated increase in peripheral resistance and blood pressure as well as the aldosterone-mediated volume expansion. When the contralateral renal artery and kidney are normal, the feedback mechanisms in the normal kidney produce a natriuresis and compensatory reduction in circulating plasma volume. In this scheme, an angiotensin II–vasoconstrictive source of hypertension is created.

In contrast, when the contralateral renal artery or kidney is also diseased as replicated by removing one kidney and creating a stenosis in the remaining one, this compensatory diuresis is lost and volume expansion occurs, producing an angiotensin-aldosterone–mediated, volume-dependent hypertension. Modification of renal perfusion by renal revascularization can effectively diminish or abolish the underlying mechanism producing either of these varieties of RVH.

It would be simplistic to think that these factors provide a complete description of all the mechanisms activated by the onset of renal hypoperfusion. In the clinical context, however, the pathophysiology of renal hypertension can be characterized by a sustained elevation in peripheral vascular resistance that is mediated by the activation of both the renin-angiotensin and the sympathetic nervous systems and their concomitant contribution to vascular endothelial dysfunction. Although the contribution of increased renin secretion and angiotensin II production is a sustaining stimulus for the hemodynamic and hormonal response, the actions of angiotensin II on the vascular endothelium may play the biggest role in sustained blood pressure elevation. Both the renin-angiotensin and the sympathetic nervous systems appear to act in concert to regulate the integrated hormonal response that operates to regulate sodium and potassium balance and arterial pressure.

It is well accepted that RVH is caused by increased activity of the renin-angiotensin system produced initially by hypersecretion of renin from the juxtaglomerular apparatus of the ischemic kidney. However, as hypertension evolves into a chronic stage, adaptive cardiovascular changes may become an essential mechanism for the maintenance of elevated blood pressure and peripheral vascular resistance. The effect of hypertension on precapillary resistant vessels triggers a myogenic response that is evidenced by the combination of hypertrophy and hyperplasia of the vascular smooth muscle.[27,28] This augments vascular reactivity to pressor agents. There is also evidence that renin may be trapped in structural elements of the vascular wall.[29] Local production of angiotensin II by tissue renin-angiotensin systems may contribute to the remodeling of resistance vessels.[30]

Angiotensin-converting enzyme exists in the plasma membrane of vascular endothelial and smooth muscle cells. Thus the necessary components for the production of angiotensin II may be found in both vascular and cardiac tissue. In the chronic phases of the hypertension process, hypersecretion of renin from the ischemic kidney may be less important than increased production of vascular angiotensin II as the mechanism that sustains the elevation in arterial pressure.

Ischemic Nephropathy

The pathophysiology of renovascular renal insufficiency (i.e., ischemic nephropathy) is incompletely understood.[31] The earliest clinical reports suggested a "glomerular filtration failure" based on hypoperfusion of the kidney,[32] but the molecular basis for ischemic nephropathy is poorly characterized. Like RVH, the renin-angiotensin system likely contributes to ischemic nephropathy through its paracrine effects—intrarenal angiotensin peptides increase efferent arteriolar tone.[33] In the presence of a pressure-reducing renal artery lesion, this paracrine effect increases glomerular capillary pressure to support glomerular filtration. In contrast to these positive effects, angiotensin peptides have also been shown to promote tubulointerstitial injury in the presence of a renal artery lesion.[34] This observation is supported by the induction of transforming growth factor-β and interstitial platelet-derived growth factor-β, which are associated with increased extracellular matrix and interstitial fibrosis.[35–38] Disruption of the tubular cell cytoskeleton and the loss of tubular membrane polarity have also been suggested. Besides these potentially reversible contributors to excretory renal insufficiency, an atherosclerotic renovascular lesion can also be a source of atheroemboli.[39] The inability to distinguish potentially reversible ischemic nephropathy from irreversible renal parenchymal disease has enormous clinical importance. Recovery of renal function after renovascular intervention has proved to be the strongest predictor of dialysis-free survival.[16,19]

PREVALENCE OF RENOVASCULAR HYPERTENSION AND ISCHEMIC NEPHROPATHY

RVH is generally thought to account for 5% to 10% of the hypertensive population. Tucker suggested an even lower prevalence.[40] Likewise, Shapiro and colleagues[41] suggested that the identification and successful operative treatment of RVH in patients older than 50 years are so unlikely that diagnostic investigation for a correctable cause in that group should be undertaken only when hypertension is severe and uncontrollable. Estimates of the prevalence of hypertension in the United States from all causes range from 60 to 80 million people, and hypertension may be present in 25% to 30% of the adult population.

The actual contribution of RVD to hypertension or renal insufficiency has been uncertain because the population-based prevalence of RVD was unknown. Past prevalence estimates of RVD were extrapolated from case series, autopsy examinations, or angiography obtained to evaluate diseases of the aorta or peripheral circulation.[24,42–48]

Recently, the population-based prevalence of RVD has been estimated for participants in the Cardiovascular Health Study (CHS) sponsored by the National Heart, Lung, and Blood Institute. The CHS is a longitudinal, prospective, population-based study of coronary heart disease and stroke in elderly men and women. This study showed that hemodynamically significant RVD was present in 6.8% of this elderly, free-living cohort.[49] Multivariate analysis demonstrated that increasing participant age (P =.028; odds ratio [OR], 1.44; 95% confidence interval [CI], 1.03 to 1.73) and increasing systolic blood pressure at baseline (P = .007; OR, 1.44; 95% CI, 1.10 to 1.87) were significantly and independently associated with the presence of RVD. Moreover, renal insufficiency was associated with RVD, but only when renal artery disease coexisted with significant hypertension. Contrary to historical assumptions, RVD demonstrated no significant relationships with gender or ethnicity.[49]

As in the general population, the incidence of RVH is undoubtedly low when all patients with hypertension are considered. Because RVH tends to produce relatively severe hypertension, its prevalence in the large population of mildly hypertensive patients (diastolic blood pressure <105 mm Hg) is probably negligible. In contrast, however, it is a frequent cause of hypertension in the smaller group of patients with severe hypertension. In the Wake Forest experience, the presence of severe hypertension at the two extremes of life carried the highest probability of its being RVH. Their review of the causes of hypertension in 74 children admitted for diagnostic evaluation over a 5-year period showed that 78% of the children younger than 5 years had a correctable renin-dependent cause.[50] In 1996, the same group screened 629 hypertensive adults older than 50 years for RVD (Table 26.1). Overall, 25% of subjects demonstrated significant renal artery disease. However, 52% of those older than 60 years whose diastolic pressure was greater than 110 mm Hg had significant renal artery stenosis or occlusion. When serum creatinine was elevated in conjunction with this age and blood pressure, 71% of subjects demonstrated hemodynamically significant RVD.

The presence of RAS itself is fairly common in a number of disease states such as peripheral vascular disease, congestive heart failure, and abdominal aortic aneurysm. However, the presence of hemodynamically significant RAS leading to RVD is more dramatic in presentation than essential hypertension and can be predicted by thorough patient history.[51]

TABLE 26.1 Results of Renal Duplex Sonography in 629 New Hypertensive Adults

Renal Vascular Disease	No. Present (%)	Absent (%)	Total (%)
All patients	154 (24)	475 (76)	629 (100)
<60 years + DBP ≥110 mm Hg	98 (52)	91 (48)	189 (30)
DBP ≥110 mm Hg + SCr ≥2.0 mg/dL	53 (71)	22 (29)	75 (12)

DBP, Diastolic blood pressure; *SCr*, serum creatinine.
From Deitch JS, Hansen KJ, Craven TE, et al: Renal artery repair in African-Americans. *J Vasc Surg* 26:465–473, 1997.

CHARACTERISTICS OF RENOVASCULAR HYPERTENSION

Because of the small proportion of RVH among the entire hypertensive population, many reports have focused on the value of demographic factors, physical findings, and screening tests to discriminate between essential hypertension and RVH. Most frequently cited as discriminate factors suggesting the presence of RVH and a need for further study are recent onset of hypertension, young age, lack of family history of hypertension, and presence of an abdominal bruit. The most complete study comparing the clinical characteristics of patients with RVH to those with essential hypertension was the Cooperative Study of Renovascular Hypertension.[52] In that study, the prevalence of certain clinical characteristics in 339 patients with essential hypertension was compared with their prevalence in 175 patients with RVH secondary to atherosclerotic lesions (91 patients) and fibromuscular dysplasia (84 patients). Although the prevalence of several characteristics was significantly different in RVH compared with essential hypertension, none of the characteristics had sufficient discriminant value to be used to exclude patients from further diagnostic investigation for RVH. Certainly, the finding of an epigastric bruit in a young white female with malignant hypertension is strongly suggestive of a renovascular origin of the hypertension. The absence of such criteria, however, does not exclude the presence of RVH, and such criteria should not be used to eliminate patients from further diagnostic study.

Therefore, the decision to undertake diagnostic study should be based on the severity of hypertension. Mild hypertension has a minimal chance of being renovascular in origin. In contrast, the more severe the hypertension, the higher the probability that it is from a correctable cause. With this in mind, we evaluate all adult patients with diastolic blood pressures greater than 105 mm Hg who would be considered for intervention to evaluate for a renovascular lesion as a correctable origin of hypertension. Children are evaluated when their blood pressure exceeds the 95th percentile for height and age.[53] Other hallmarks for RVH include sudden worsening of long-standing hypertension, acute worsening of chronic kidney disease in the absence of other inciting factors, acute pulmonary edema, and acute renal dysfunction when starting angiotensin-moderating medications.[51]

NATURAL HISTORY OF ATHEROSCLEROTIC RENOVASCULAR DISEASE

Historically, RVH was thought to mimic other atherosclerotic processes and progression to occlusion was considered in decision for intervention. However, this has not been borne out in the literature. A prospective study by Pillay and colleagues[54] described the change in blood pressure and serum creatinine among patients with atherosclerotic RVD. Ninety-eight patients in this multicenter, nonrandomized observational study were noted to have greater than 50% renal artery stenosis during aortography to evaluate peripheral vascular disease. On a minimum duration of 2 years of follow-up, 64 patients with unilateral renal stenosis and 21 patients with bilateral disease were managed medically. Twelve patients with bilateral disease underwent percutaneous intervention or open operative repair. The overall 2-year estimated mortality was 32%. Mortality was equivalent for patients treated with renal artery intervention and for those treated medically. There was no change in median blood pressure, number of anti-hypertensives, or change in renal size in follow-up among survivors. A small but statistically significant increase in serum creatinine was observed in patients who underwent renal artery intervention. Patients with bilateral RVD treated medically had stable serum creatinine over 2-year follow-up. This study lacked a specific measure of glomerular filtration; however, it demonstrated stable length and stable serum creatinine with controlled hypertension in medically managed patients who had anatomic disease but no clinical indication for RVH.

A series of consecutive reports described prospective duplex studies performed at the University of Washington.[55–56] These authors first reported on serial duplex examinations performed on 80 patients with hypertension. Renal arteries were classified according to four categories: normal, stenosis less than 60%, stenosis greater than 60%, or renal artery occlusion. The rate of progression to greater than 60% stenosis during 3 years of follow-up was 8% for renal arteries that were initially classified as normal and 43% initially classified as having less than 60% diameter-reducing stenosis. Incidental renal artery occlusions were observed only in arteries previously categorized as having 60% diameter-reducing stenosis. The 3-year risk for occlusion among the entire group was 7%. Lesion progression was associated with increasing patient age, increasing systolic blood pressure, smoking, female sex, and poorly controlled hypertension.

Davis and colleagues[57] reported on 119 participants in the Cardiovascular Health Study with 235 kidneys followed over an 8-year period. None of these subjects demonstrated severe hypertension. Controlling for within-subject correlation, the overall estimated change in RVD among all 235 kidneys was 14% (95% CI, 9.2% to 21.4%) with hemodynamically significant RVD in 4% (95% CI, 1.9% to 8.2%).[57] No hemodynamically significant stenosis at baseline progressed to renal artery occlusion on follow-up. Increased blood pressure and decrease in renal length were not associated with RVD at baseline examination. These findings cast doubt on the value of renal artery intervention in the absence of RVH or renal insufficiency.

The most difficult decision in evaluation of RAS in patients with hypertension is parsing out essential hypertension from true RVH. As demonstrated above, the presence of RAS and hypertension together is of infrequent clinical significance. However, the systemic cardiovascular effects of true RVH, such as congestive heart failure, renal insufficiency, severe hypertension, and cerebrovascular accident, result in a significant increase in the likelihood of early cardiac death in patients with true RVH.[51] Thus, in patients with the spectrum of symptoms that are of concern for RVH, appropriate workup is important.

DIAGNOSTIC EVALUATION

The general evaluation of all hypertensive patients should include a careful medical history, physical examination, serum electrolyte and creatinine determination, and electrocardiography. Electrocardiography is important to gauge the extent of secondary myocardial hypertrophy or associated ischemic heart disease. Serum electrolyte and serial serum potassium determinations can effectively exclude patients with primary aldosteronism if potassium levels are greater than 3.0 mg/dL. One must remember, however, that hypokalemia is often due to salt-depleting diets and previous diuretic therapy. Finally, estimation of renal function is mandatory. Preexisting renal disease may reduce renal function and cause hypertension. Conversely, renal dysfunction may reflect ischemic nephropathy.

Screening Studies

Identification of a noninvasive screening test that accurately identifies all patients with RVD that may warrant interventional management remains an elusive goal. Prior methods such as peripheral plasma renin activity, rapid-sequence intravenous pyelography, and saralasin infusion have been abandoned. Screening studies are basically of two types: functional studies or anatomic studies. Of the functional type, isotope renography continues to be proposed as a valuable screening test, but the methods used are continually modified with the hope of improving its sensitivity and specificity. The newest versions of isotope renography consist of renal scans performed before and after the administration of an inhibitor to angiotensin I–converting enzyme. Of these, only captopril renal scanning has gained widespread use and acceptance as a screening tool. Anatomic screening studies include renal duplex sonography and arteriography.

Captopril Renal Scanning

To understand the basis of captopril renal scanning, one must consider some of the features of renal physiology and the importance of the renin-angiotensin system in the maintenance of homeostasis. Glomerular filtration is governed partially by the relative tone of the afferent and efferent arterioles. During periods of reduced blood pressure recognized by the juxtaglomerular apparatus (e.g., proximal renal artery stenosis), increased renin is released, which ultimately leads to an increase in the level of intrarenal angiotensin II. Angiotensin II acts predominantly to constrict the efferent arteriole to maintain renal glomerular perfusion pressure and filtration. When an angiotensin I–converting enzyme inhibitor such as captopril is given in this circumstance, an acute reduction in the amount of angiotensin II occurs. This leads to a reduction in constriction of the efferent arteriole and a decrease in the glomerular filtration rate (GFR). Captopril renal scanning is composed of a baseline renogram and a repeat renogram obtained after a dose of captopril. A test is considered positive when a normal baseline scan becomes abnormal after captopril administration—that is, when the time to peak activity increases to more than 11 minutes or when a normal glomerular filtration ratio between the two sides increases to greater than 1.5:1 (Fig. 26.4). In experienced hands, this study is reported to be highly reliable.[58] Unfortunately, it is less reliable when significant parenchymal disease is present. For that reason, we do not rely on its results to eliminate RVD in azotemic patients.

Renal Duplex Sonography

Through continued improvements in probe design and duplex sonographic technology, imaging and Doppler shift interrogation of deep abdominal vasculature have been introduced as screening methods to identify and quantify visceral and renal artery occlusive disease. We have evaluated the role of duplex sonography as an initial surface screening test, as an intraoperative study to confirm the technical success of reconstructive procedures, and as a postoperative surveillance method to follow progression of disease and stability of reconstructions.[53,59–62]

Technically successful studies, defined as a complete main renal artery interrogation from aortic origin to renal hilum, can be obtained in almost 95% of cases. These results are ensured by proper patient preparation and method of examination. Details of the conduct of the procedure are covered elsewhere.[59]

The criteria for identifying renal artery stenosis by renal duplex sonography are given in Table 26.2. Assuming that renal artery peak systolic velocity (PSV) varies with the degree of renal artery stenosis and aortic PSV (i.e., inflow), most authors have advocated using the ratio of renal artery PSV to aortic PSV (the renal-to-aortic ratio) of 3.5 to define critical renal artery stenosis.[63–66] Focal renal artery PSV of 1.8 m/s or more in combination with distal poststenotic turbulence correlates highly with the angiographic presence of diameter-reducing renal artery

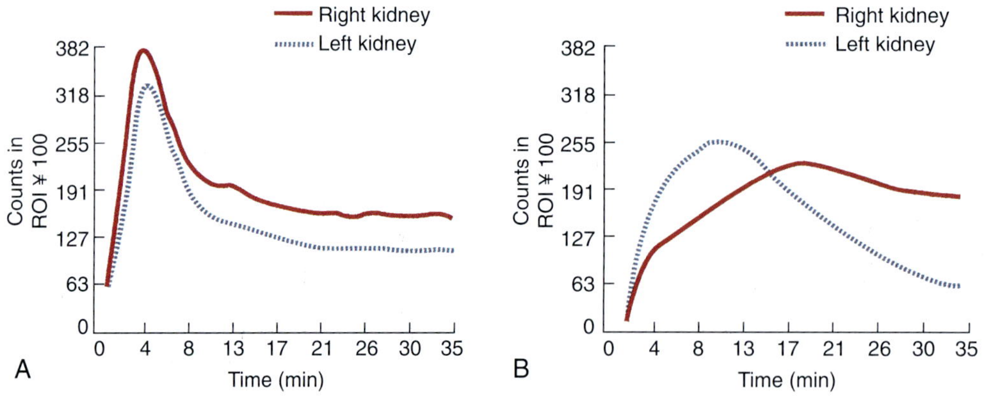

FIG 26.4 Captopril renal scintigraphy before (A) and after (B) captopril administration demonstrates the positive finding of a time delay in reaching peak radioactivity after captopril. *ROI,* Region of interest.

TABLE 26.2 **Doppler Velocity Criteria for Significant Stenosis and Occlusion**

Defect	Criteria
<60% diameter-reducing RA defect	RA-PSV from entire RA <1.8 m/s
≥60% diameter-reducing RA defect	Focal RA-PSV ≥1.8 m/s and distal turbulent velocity waveform
Occlusion	Doppler-shifted signal from RA B-scan image
Inadequate study for interpretation	Failure to obtain Doppler samples interpretation from entire main RA

RA, Renal artery; *RA-PSV,* renal artery peak systolic velocity.
From Hansen KJ, Tribble RW, Reaves SW, et al: Renal duplex sonography: evaluation of clinical utility. *J Vasc Surg* 12:227–236, 1990; and Motew SJ, Cherr GS, Craven TE, et al: Renal duplex sonography: main renal artery versus hilar analysis. *J Vasc Surg* 32:462–471, 2000.

stenosis of 60% or greater.[59] In 122 kidneys with single renal arteries and renal angiography for comparison, renal duplex sonography correctly identified 67 of 68 kidneys with normal arteries or less than 60% renal artery stenosis, and 35 of 39 kidneys with 60% to 99% renal artery stenosis. All 15 renal artery occlusions were correctly identified by failure to obtain a Doppler-shifted signal from an imaged renal artery. Using this method and these criteria for interpretation, renal duplex sonography was 93% sensitive and 98% specific.

Renal Angiography

Angiography continues to be the most sensitive diagnostic method to assess RAS. In patients with an abnormal screening duplex exam, contrast radiography can provide anatomic details and be useful in operative or interventional planning. Although computed tomography (CT) and magnetic resonance (MR) modalities have been validated as appropriate for evaluating RAS in patients with suspected RVH,[67] catheter angiography can more precisely control for total contrast administration.

The fact that angiography in patients with severe renal insufficiency (especially those with concomitant diabetes mellitus) can aggravate renal failure is widely recognized. Nevertheless, we believe that this risk is justified in patients with severe or accelerated hypertension and in those with positive renal duplex sonography results. In these circumstances, the potential benefit derived from the identification and correction of a functionally significant renovascular lesion exceeds the risk of contrast exposure.

Because the mortality and the morbidity of contrast nephropathy leading to dialysis dependence are high, measures to protect renal function during angiography should be taken. Conventional contrast agents have iodine incorporated into their structure to absorb x-ray photons, thereby achieving visualization of the vasculature. The nephrotoxicity of such iodinated contrast agents has been recognized for many years. The principal site of contrast-induced nephrotoxicity is the renal tubule from transient regional renal ischemia, whereas the effect on glomerular function appears to be mild.[68,69] It was believed that the ionization and high osmolarity of early contrast agents may have contributed to their nephrotoxicity. Nonionic contrast agents (e.g., iohexol) are available that provide comparable absorption of x-ray photons, but are significantly less charged than traditional agents. It was hoped that the reduced ionic nature would decrease their nephrotoxicity, but the occurrence of severe adverse renal events did not differ between ionic and nonionic contrast media in a large randomized clinical trial.[70]

Renal nephrotoxicity after exposure to ionic agents occurs most commonly in patients with preexisting renal insufficiency (3.3 relative risk) alone or in combination with diabetes mellitus, especially juvenile-onset diabetes.[70] Other risk factors such as dehydration, volume of contrast used, and simultaneous exposure to other nephrotoxins contribute to the likelihood of acute contrast nephrotoxicity.[71] Other risk factors include multiple myeloma and heavy proteinuria. Overall, the incidence of acute renal dysfunction following contrast angiography varies from 0% to 10%, although these estimates are skewed by several studies that included only juvenile diabetics. In one study, hospital-acquired nephropathy occurred in 12% of patients.[72] In patients with normal renal function, however, the incidence of contrast nephropathy is only 1% to 2%.[73] The effect of diabetes on the risk of acute renal failure following angiography appears to be dependent on the type of diabetes and the magnitude of secondary diabetic nephropathy.

Adjuncts or alternatives to angiography are appropriate in many instances. In addition to the use of digital subtraction techniques, carbon dioxide gas can be used for angiography with minimal renal risk.[74] Because it offers limited detail, carbon dioxide angiography is often used to identify the site of disease, which is then better defined with conventional contrast agents.

Finally, high-dose loop diuretics, angiotensin-converting enzyme inhibitors, and angiotensin II receptor antagonists are held for at least 72 hours before aortic reconstruction or exposure to arterial contrast agents. Selective β-blockers and calcium channel blockers are substituted when necessary.[75]

Both aortography and selective renal angiography using multiple projections may be necessary to adequately examine the entire renal artery. The proximal third of the left renal artery usually courses anteriorly, the middle third transversely, and the distal third posteriorly, whereas the right renal artery arises from the anterior aorta and then pursues a more consistent posterior course. Lesions in the renal artery that are coursing anteriorly or posteriorly are frequently not seen or may appear insignificant in an anteroposterior aortogram. Oblique aortography or oblique selective renal angiography projects these portions of the vessels in profile and reveals the stenosis. Fig. 26.5 illustrates how the delicate septal lesions of fibromuscular dysplasia may be unrecognizable or appear insignificant in the anteroposterior projection, whereas the true severity is demonstrated in the oblique projection.

Functional Studies

Historically, two functional studies—renal vein renin assays and split renal function studies—have proved valuable in confirming the functional significance of renal artery stenosis diagnosed with imaging. Neither has great value, however, when severe bilateral disease or disease in the renal artery supplying a single

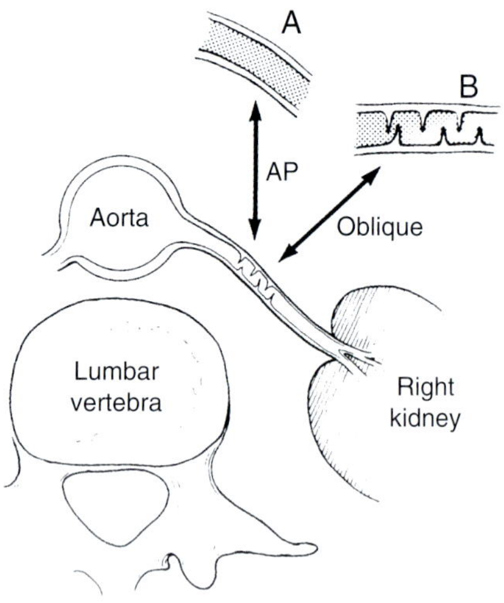

FIG 26.5 Graphic illustration of how the septa of medial fibroplasia can be missed. (A) When the vessel is viewed with an anteroposterior *(AP)* arteriogram, the septa are masked by the overlying dye column. (B) In the oblique projection, the septa are demonstrated because they are parallel to the direction of the x-ray.

kidney is present. In these circumstances, the decision for operation is based on the severity of hypertension and the degree of renal insufficiency. In most centers, the decision to treat RVH is made based upon the clinical scenario and presence of significant stenosis as outlined above.

MANAGEMENT OPTIONS

Appropriate treatment of RVH remains controversial. There are no prospective, randomized trials that compare all available treatment options. In the absence of level I data, advocates of medical management, percutaneous transluminal angioplasty and stenting (PTA+S), or operative intervention cite selective clinical data to support their particular views.

A majority of the medical community evaluates patients for RVH only when medications are not tolerated or hypertension remains severe and poorly controlled. However, many of the single-center studies erroneously report the effects of therapy on patients with essential hypertension versus those with true RVH. However, when this distinction is addressed, the benefit of intervention is demonstrated. Hunt and Strong[76] reported a direct comparison of patients with diagnosed RVH to assess the comparative value of medical therapy and operation. In this nonrandomized study, the results of operative treatment in 100 patients were compared with the results of drug therapy in 114 similar patients. After 7 to 14 years of follow-up, 84% of the operated group was alive, compared with 66% of the drug therapy group. Of the 84 patients alive in the operated group, 93% were cured or significantly improved, compared with only 21% of the surviving patients in the drug therapy group. Death during follow-up was twice as common in the medically treated group as in the operated group, resulting in differences that were statistically significant in patients with either atherosclerosis or fibromuscular dysplasia of the renal artery.

The detrimental changes that can occur during medical therapy alone are often cited as supporting evidence for intervention for all renovascular lesions. It should be emphasized, however, that the only prospective angiographic data were obtained from patients with proven RVH (i.e., high-grade renal artery stenosis with severe hypertension and positive physiologic studies).[77] Accordingly, these data should not be applied to asymptomatic patients. Indications for interventional management include all patients with severe, difficult-to-control hypertension[78,79]; this includes patients with complicating factors such as branch lesions and extrarenal atherosclerotic disease, including those with associated cardiovascular disease that would be improved by blood pressure reduction. Moreover, young patients whose hypertension is moderate, who have no associated end-organ disease, and who have easily correctable atherosclerotic or dysplastic main renal artery lesions are also candidates for operative intervention. The chance of curing moderate hypertension is good in such patients, and it remains to be proved that medical blood pressure control is equivalent to the cure of hypertension.

Similarly, select populations of patients with fibromuscular dysplasia (FMD) can have an excellent response to intervention. The strongest predictors of good outcomes are the age of the patient and duration of hypertension.[80] In general, favorable results can be obtained with treatment of renal FMD in patients younger than 50 years, duration of hypertension less than 8 years, and absence of FMD in other arterial beds.

Likewise, the outcome of surgical and endovascular correction of RAA has been shown to have acceptable morbidity and mortality.[81–84] Further, in the largest pooled series of RAA repair,[26] the authors advocate offering correction of renal artery aneurysm when indication for repair is hypertension.

RESULTS OF INTERVENTION

As with all other vascular beds, endovascular technique has rapidly gained acceptance in treatment of RVH. In fact, for typical ostial stenosis, RPTA+S has essentially replaced the need for surgical bypass. Likewise, renal angioplasty (RPTA) alone with adjunct stenting is now the method of choice for intervention for FMD or arteritis-driven lesions.

Percutaneous Transluminal Angioplasty/Stent

Isolated percutaneous transluminal angioplasty (PTA) for atherosclerotic RAS was the initial endovascular procedure of choice, but this technique had limited durability because of a higher restenosis rate. An early report by Miller and colleagues[85] in 1985 noted that only 45% of ostial and mixed lesions improved after 6 months; Sos and colleagues reported only a 14% benefit rate when bilateral ostial lesions were treated.[86] These results show that PTA alone has little value in the treatment of this type of lesion; one must accept the risks of cholesterol embolization, vessel thrombosis, and loss of renal function for only a minimal chance of prolonged benefit from PTA.

Recognizing the poor immediate success of PTA alone for ostial atherosclerosis, current practice involves the primary placement of endoluminal stents for these lesions.[87] Table 26.3 summarizes single-center reports on renal function and angiographic

TABLE 26.3 **Renal Artery Revascularization With Angioplasty and Stenting**[a]

Reference	Year	Patients	Bilateral Treatment (%)	Preprocedure Renal Dysfunction (%)	Renal Function Response (%): Improved	Renal Function Response (%): Unchanged	Renal Function Response (%): Worsened	Hypertension Response (%): Cured	Hypertension Response (%): Improved	Hypertension Response (%): Failed	Periprocedure Mortality (%)	Periprocedure Morbidity (%)
Burket and colleagues[89]	2000	126	NR	29	43	24	56	8	NR	NR	2	4
Lederman and colleagues[88]	2001	265	41	37	7.5	78	14	NR	70	30	<1	2
Bush and colleagues[90]	2001	73	16	68	23	51	26	6	89	5	1.4	9
Rocha-Singh and colleagues[91]	2002	51	55	100	77	18	5	NR	91	9	0	14
Gill and Fowler[92]	2003	100	26	75	31	38	31	4	79	17	2	18
Zeller and colleagues[93]	2004	456	NR	52	34	39	27	NR	46	54	<1	NR
Nolan and colleagues[94]	2005	82	NR	59	23	53	24	0	81	0	0	7
Kayshap and colleagues[95]	2007	125	36	100	42	23	25	0	0	0	1.6	6
Corriere and colleagues[96]	2008	99	11	75	28	65	7	1	21	78	0	5.5
Mean%[b]			31	55	28	38	31	4	54	29	1	6.6

[a]Series selected based on publication in 2000 or later, use of angioplasty and stenting, and inclusion of more than 50 patients, and categorical reporting of renal function or hypertension responses, or both.
[b]Weighted mean based on number of patients with reported data categorized according to column; references where data was not reported or categorical response categories were combined were not included in calculation.
NR, Not reported.

follow-up after treatment of ostial atherosclerosis by PTA in combination with endoluminal stents in 1377 patients since 2000.[88–95] These studies differ in regard to criteria for ostial lesions, evaluation of the clinical response to intervention, and parameters for significant restenosis. Despite these differences, these cumulative results provide estimates of early hypertension response, change in renal function, and primary patency. The overall hypertension cure rate was 4%, with a range of 0% to 8%; 54% of the patients had improved blood pressure control (less medications needed to control BP), with a range of 0% to 91%.

Concerning improvement of renal function, defined as a 20% or greater decrease in serum creatinine concentration, response rates ranging from 7.5% to 77% were observed (mean, 28%). A number of authorities also make use of the concept of "stabilized" renal function, defined as a less than 20% change in serum creatinine concentration. By this definition,[88–96] renal function was stabilized in the majority of patients included in the studies published between 2000 and 2008 (range, 18% to 78%; mean response rate, 38%; see Table 26.3). Again, these results are similar to those reported in the meta-analysis from 2000 (range, 0% to 64%; mean response rate, 38%).[49,96] A significant percentage of treated patients (range, 0% to 56%; mean, 31%) also experienced post-PTA+S worsening of renal function. The periprocedural morbidity was 6.6% and periprocedural mortality was 1% for these patients.

To date, only one prospective, randomized, controlled study has compared endovascular treatment with surgical revascularization for the treatment of RVH.[97] In this report, 58 patients with RVH were randomly assigned to either surgical revascularization or angioplasty. In both groups, hypertension was cured or improved in approximately 90% of patients. However, more than half of the patients in whom angioplasty failed were switched to the surgical arm for revascularization. On the basis of these results, the authors recommended angioplasty as the treatment of choice for selected renovascular lesions contributing to RVH, with aggressive follow-up and repeat intervention (endovascular and surgical) carried out as needed.

A more contemporary meta-analysis published in 2014 summarized all randomized controlled trials of endovascular treatment versus medical management for management of hypertension and encompassed 2222 patients. The studies were not designed to discriminate between high-risk groups for RAS-driven hypertension as opposed to essential hypertension. As such, the overall difference in hypertensive medication requirement was not significantly different between the two groups. However, these data do demonstrate that intervention can be carried out with a low mortality of less than 1%. Another important finding was the role that statin agents play in reducing restenosis in treated vessels.

Reported experience with PTA of medial fibroplasia shows early results similar to those of open surgical repair. Beneficial blood pressure responses have been reported to be as high as 100% after PTA in properly selected patients, and although vessel perforation, hemorrhage, and branch occlusions have been reported, their incidence is less than 5%.[98] One would anticipate that such complications would be most likely in patients with diffuse fibromuscular dysplasia affecting both the distal main renal artery and its branches. When the procedure is performed by an experienced interventionist, the cure rate of fibromuscular dysplasia after PTA ranges from 37% to 51%.[99] Fibromuscular dysplasia involving the branch level is best managed primarily by an open operative approach, and PTA should be reserved for the subgroup of patients with medial fibroplasia limited to the main renal artery.

Stenotic lesions occurring in children are usually discrete narrowings and therefore appear to be ideal for PTA. However, the stenotic area is commonly a congenital hypoplasia of the entire vessel wall and is composed predominantly of elastic tissue. When such a hypoplastic vessel is subjected to PTA, the original diameter returns after dilatation or, if the vessel has been overdistended, rupture of the vessel wall is likely. Therefore PTA is an inappropriate method of intervention in children with renal artery stenosis, and lifelong success is best achieved by operative correction.

Contemporary Randomized Control Trials

The heterogeneity of the existing data regarding the benefits of RPTA+S versus medical therapy alone in the treatment of RVD led to two contemporary randomized controlled trials intended to elucidate the difference. Because these trials offer the most oft-quoted data in the justification for management of RVD in contemporary practice, special attention is given to them here.

ASTRAL Trial

The Angioplasty and Stenting for Renal Artery Lesions (ASTRAL) trial was a prospective, randomized, unblinded clinical trial that was designed to determine whether revascularization combined with best medical therapy improved renal function when compared to medical therapy alone, in patients with atherosclerotic renal artery stenosis.[100] The benefits of treatment of RVH were a secondary endpoint.

Patients were screened if clinical findings, such as refractory/uncontrolled hypertension or unexplained renal dysfunction, suggested a diagnosis of renal artery atherosclerosis. Patients were eligible to participate if they had substantial atherosclerotic stenosis in at least one renal artery that was considered potentially suitable for endovascular revascularization. Hemodynamically significant lesions (>70%) were defined by angiography, CT angiography, MR angiography, or duplex ultrasound. Patients were excluded if *their physician was uncertain that the patient would definitely have a clinical benefit from revascularization*. Patients were also excluded if they had nonatheromatous cardiovascular disease or had undergone prior renal artery revascularization.

The primary outcome was the change in renal function, which was assessed by measuring the mean slope of the reciprocal of the serum creatinine over time. Secondary outcomes included blood pressure, time to first cardiovascular/renal event, and mortality. Renal events were defined as new onset of acute kidney injury, initiation of dialysis, renal transplantation, nephrectomy, or death from renal failure. Cardiovascular events were defined as myocardial infarction, stroke, hospitalization or death from cardiovascular causes, or coronary-artery revascularization.

Patients were randomized to undergo revascularization and medical therapy versus medical therapy alone. Local practitioners determined the precise revascularization procedure (angioplasty alone or with stenting) and best medical therapy (typically statins, antiplatelet agents, and antihypertensives). Neither the intervention technique nor medical management were standardized. Renal protection devices were not used.

The trial was designed to detect a reduction of 20% in the mean slope of the reciprocal of the serum creatinine level. Target recruitment was initially set at 1000 patients to allow for crossover from the medical therapy group to the revascularization group. However, the number was subsequently reduced to 750 patients due to lower rates of crossover than anticipated. During a 7-year period, 806 patients were enrolled (403 patients in each group) in 57 hospitals. Average patient age was 70 years and participants in both groups were similar in terms of baseline demographics, comorbidities, blood pressure, and renal function. Interestingly, 40% of patients did not have significant baseline renal dysfunction or a hemodynamically significant lesion (<70% stenosis), with the remainder having normal renal function and 50% to 70% stenosis. The median follow-up was 33.6 months. In the revascularization group, the procedure was attempted in 83% (335/403) of patients, with a technical success rate of 95%. The majority of patients received a stent. Twenty-four patients (6%) of the medical-therapy group crossed over to undergo revascularization.

At 1 year, the average number of antihypertensive agents was slightly higher in the medical therapy group, whereas more patients in the revascularization group received renin-angiotensin blockers. During the 5-year study period, both groups demonstrated no difference in the primary endpoint (change in creatinine). Both groups demonstrated a decrease in blood pressure over the 5-year period, which was not significant. There was also no difference in time to first renal event or acute kidney injury between the two groups. The number of cardiovascular events was not significant between the two groups. The overall survival rate was 58% at 5 years and was similar between the two groups. The major complication rate in the revascularization group was 9%, and 20% for less serious complications.[101]

The authors concluded that there was no worthwhile clinical benefit for revascularization in patients with renal artery atherosclerosis. Revascularization carried substantial risk and was not associated with any added benefit because both groups demonstrated similar rates of blood pressure reduction, renal/cardiovascular events, and overall mortality.

The ASTRAL trial has been the subject of intense scrutiny given its design and procedural aspects. Perhaps the greatest critique of this trial is the exclusion of patients based on an uncertainty that the patient would definitely have a clinical benefit from revascularization. Thus, the exact group that this study should have focused on, those who would have the best response to revascularization, were excluded. Furthermore, 40% of patients that underwent treatment did not have baseline renal dysfunction or a hemodynamically significant lesion. Thus, these patients would have less of a benefit from treatment compared to those with significant renal artery atherosclerosis or worse renal function. The best medical therapy and the specific intervention planned was left up to the local practitioner. Although patients were followed for 5 years, the follow-up did not include arterial imaging or patency rates. Long-term success of the stents was based solely on a biochemical marker (reciprocal of serum creatinine).

CORAL Trial

The Cardiovascular Outcomes in Renal Atherosclerotic Lesions (CORAL) trial was a prospective, randomized, unblinded study that attempted to improve on the weaknesses of the ASTRAL trial and clarify the utility of revascularization compared to medical therapy in patients with atherosclerotic renal artery stenosis and elevated blood pressure, chronic kidney disease, or both.[102] Patients were eligible if they had hypertension while receiving two or more antihypertensive medications, or severe renal artery stenosis defined angiographically as stenosis of at least 80% of the diameter of an artery. All angiograms were analyzed by a core laboratory. Patients with renal artery fibromuscular dysplasia, baseline serum creatinine greater than 4.0 mg/dL, affected kidneys less than 7 cm in length, or stenotic lesions not amenable to a single stent, were excluded. Medical therapy consisted of an angiotensin-receptor blocker, with the use of a diuretic or amlodipine for additional blood pressure control. All patients received an antiplatelet, a statin, and diabetes was managed according to local practice guidelines. By the end of the enrollment period, a number of changes were made, including lowering the threshold for defining systolic blood pressure, inclusion of patients without hypertension but with evidence of chronic kidney disease, and by defining severe renal artery stenosis with noninvasive imaging.[102]

The study randomized 947 patients over a 5-year period to medical therapy alone or medical therapy plus stenting. The primary endpoint was the occurrence of a major cardiovascular or renal event (stroke, myocardial infarction, hospitalization for congestive heart failure, progressive renal insufficiency, or the need for permanent renal-replacement therapy). Stents were placed in 94% of the of the stent group (434/459 patients). The most common angiographic complication was arterial dissection (2.4%).

The mean age was 69 years with an even distribution in gender. At a median length of follow-up of 43 months, there was no significant difference in the occurrence of a major cardiovascular or renal event between the stent group and the medical therapy-only group. Additionally, the number of antihypertensive medications did not differ between the two groups. The systolic blood pressure demonstrated a modest yet statistically significant decrease in the stent group.

The authors concluded that when combined with high-quality medical therapy, renal artery stenting offers little benefit with respect to cardiovascular/renal events, mortality, and the need for renal-replacement therapy. The intent of the CORAL trial was to demonstrate a difference in treatment arms. The use of a core lab and a defined protocol for medical management were clear advantages over ASTRAL. However, the change in inclusion criteria due to low enrollment led to the inclusion of patients with chronic kidney disease without significant hypertension. As with the ASTRAL trial, the patient cohort ultimately studied would not be expected to benefit from intervention and that was borne out in the results.

Conclusion

In a time of increasing interventions for atherosclerotic renal artery stenosis, the ASTRAL and CORAL trials attempted to evaluate the utility of renal artery stenting as compared to medical therapy alone. The overall conclusion in these trials was that renal artery stenting offered little clinical benefit when compared to medical therapy, but was associated with significant risk. Although both studies had weaknesses, they highlighted the importance of careful evaluation and avoidance of "drive-by" stenting.

Ultimately, the patients who were most likely to benefit from intervention were not represented in this dataset. These trials demonstrate well that patients with more moderate hypertension and stable chronic kidney disease do not warrant renal intervention just because of the presence of RAS. However, the data say nothing about patients with severe hypertension, recent worsening of hypertension control, precipitous renal decline, or flash pulmonary edema in the setting of severe (>80%) RAS. It is this cohort that will likely benefit from either endovascular or surgical intervention.

OPERATIVE TECHNIQUES

Renal Angioplasty and Stenting (RPTA+S)

As discussed above, the majority of RAS occurs in the setting of aortic atherosclerosis and is localized to the renal artery ostia. As such, they are easily amenable to endovascular correction and this should be the first line of therapy in cases excluding those involving branch vessels, aneurysm, or need for surgical correction of other aortovisceral occlusive lesions. As discussed above, the technique of renal angioplasty without stent is preferred for FMD or arteritis cases. However, the conduct of those cases can easily mimic the steps of RPTA+S without stent placement unless a suboptimal result is obtained.

The basic steps of endovascular access and imaging are discussed in Chapter 17. The renal vessels can be easily accessed from a femoral or brachial approach. However, there is great variability in angulation due to variability in kidney migration during gestation. The Stanford group has demonstrated a significant difference in delivery of stents to renal vessels based on degree of ptosis in the renal artery. In general, an angle of more than 30 degrees has preferred access from the brachial artery, otherwise the femoral approach is more efficient.[103] In addition, when evaluating renal ostia, it is critical to remember to correct the gantry angle for the individual take-off of the renal vessels (Fig. 26.6).

Once the approach and gantry angle are selected, we fully heparinize the patient before any attempts to manipulate the renal ostia. It is worth mentioning here that randomized data has demonstrated that intraoperative platelet inhibition[104] is the most useful adjunct in prevention of intraoperative embolization and decline in renal function. We choose to have patients initiate dual antiplatelet therapy with aspirin and Plavix at least 5 days prior to the surgery date. If this is not feasible, intravenous glycol-protein IIb/IIIa inhibition can be performed.

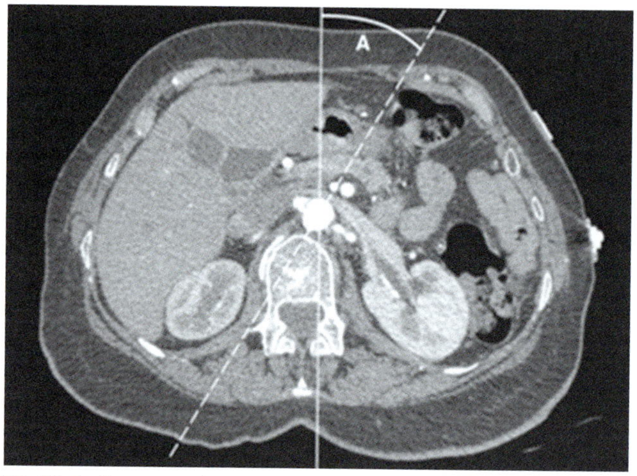

FIG 26.6 Computed tomography imaging demonstrating the proper gantry angle for visualizing renal ostia to ensure orthogonal imaging and not miss critical pathology.

We place a long sheath in the aorta to alleviate the need for sheath exchange once the renal artery is selected. We prefer the use of hydrophilic guide catheters and wires for selection. Once access to the renal artery is obtained, the sheath is advanced past the plaque over a polytetrafluoroethylene (PTFE)-coated support wire. If the dilator and sheath will not track, we then use a low-profile 4 mm × 20 mm angioplasty balloon and advance the sheath by "swallowing" the balloon with the sheath as it is deflated. We do not routinely use distal protection devices for renal intervention; however, if the lesion has concerning factors for embolization, then use of a filter wire is feasible. Often the filter can be deployed through a 0.035-inch catheter placed once the sheath is in the main renal artery. If the balloon-expandable stent (BES) cannot be tracked due to lack of stability, a 0.018-inch stiff buddy wire can be placed next to the filter and a 0.035-inch system BES can be loaded onto both wires simultaneously because the total diameter of the two wires is only 0.032 inch. Once in place, the BES should traverse the entire lesion with at least two stent struts prolapsed back into the aorta. The sheath is pulled back and the BES is deployed to a nominal size chosen as 1:1 of the native renal vessel where it is free of disease. We then postdilate the aortic component of the stent with a short balloon 2 mm larger than the stent diameter to flare it at the renal ostia.

A completion angio is performed through the sheath. It is critical at this juncture to identify any renal dissection (Fig. 26.7). As long as wire access is maintained to the true lumen, most dissections can be managed by extension with a nitinol self-expanding stent (SES) out to the main renal bifurcation. Conversely, if the dissection appears to extend beyond the first major branch, the flap can be tacked with prolonged inflation of an appropriately sized balloon. Because of the continuous flow in the renal artery, the corrected flap will usually stay in place and renal perfusion maintained.

Once adequate perfusion is confirmed, all wires/filters are removed from the renal artery and devices retracted in standard fashion. We maintain DAPT for at least 6 weeks and will often extend Plavix therapy as opposed to aspirin to avoid use of nonsteroidal antiinflammatory drugs (NSAIDs) in patients with renal insufficiency.

Open Surgical Correction

Although the mainstay of therapy is now endovascular, an appreciation and understanding of the open approach to renal revascularization is still pertinent. A variety of operative techniques have been used to correct renal artery stenoses. From a practical standpoint, three basic operations are most frequently used: aortorenal bypass, thromboendarterectomy, and reimplantation. Bypass is most versatile. Endarterectomy has particular application to ostial atherosclerosis, especially when visceral arteries are also involved. When the renal artery is sufficiently redundant, reimplantation is technically easiest and has particular application in children (Fig. 26.8).

Antihypertensive medications are reduced during the preoperative period to the minimum necessary for blood pressure control. Frequently, patients requiring large doses of multiple medications for control have significantly reduced requirements while hospitalized and on bed rest. If continued therapy is required, vasodilators (e.g., nifedipine) in combination with selective β-adrenergic blockers (e.g., atenolol) are the drugs of choice. There is little effect on hemodynamics when these agents are combined with anesthesia. If the patient's diastolic blood pressure exceeds 120 mm Hg, the pressure must be brought under control, and operative treatment must be postponed until this is accomplished. If blood pressure is difficult to control, the patient may be transferred to the intensive care unit, where intravenous nitroprusside therapy with continuous intraarterial monitoring of blood pressure is instituted for 24 hours before operation. Similarly, if the patient has a significant history of heart disease, then pulmonary artery wedge pressure and cardiac performance are monitored to maintain optimal cardiac hemodynamics and recognize and correct adverse changes before they become clinically significant.

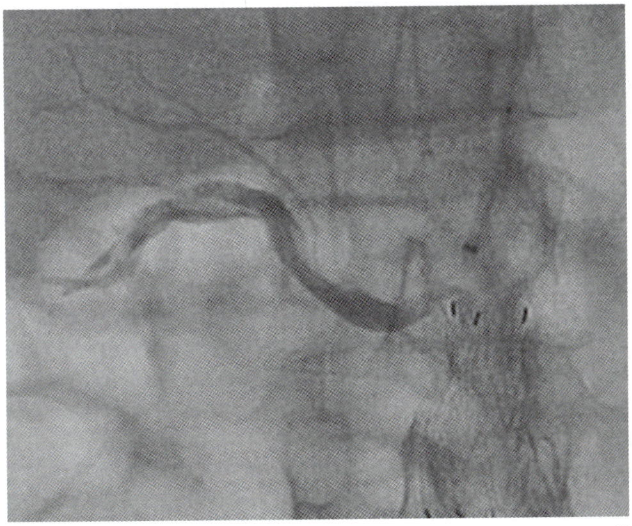

FIG 26.7 Intraoperative image demonstrating renal artery dissection after angioplasty.

Certain measures and maneuvers are applicable to almost all renal artery operations. Mannitol (12.5 g) is administered intravenously early in the operation. Just before renal artery cross-clamping, heparin (100 units/kg) is given intravenously, and systemic anticoagulation is verified by activated clotting time.

Mobilization and Dissection

Through a midline xiphoid-to-pubis incision, the posterior peritoneum overlying the aorta is incised longitudinally, and the duodenum is reflected to the patient's right to expose the left renal artery (Fig. 26.9). By extending the posterior peritoneal incision to the left along the inferior border of the pancreas, an avascular plane behind the pancreas can be entered to expose the entire renal hilum on the left (Fig. 26.10).

This exposure is of special significance when distal lesions must also be managed. The left renal artery lies behind the left renal vein. In some cases, the vein can be retracted cephalad to expose the artery; in other cases, caudal retraction of the vein provides better access. Usually the gonadal and adrenal veins,

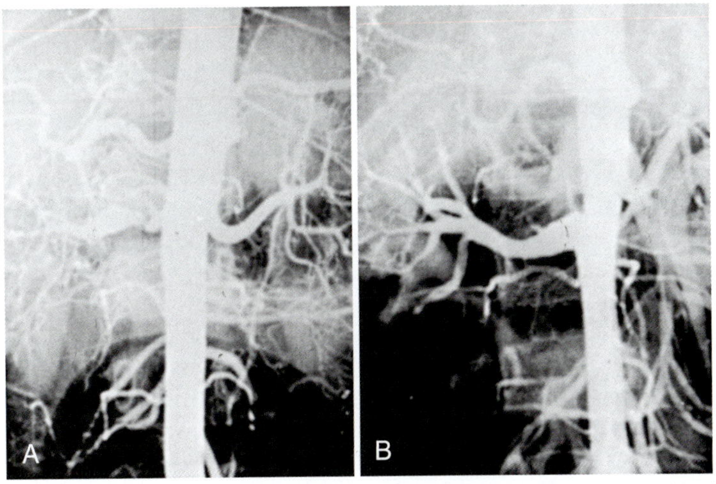

FIG 26.8 Preoperative (A) and postoperative (B) arteriograms in a 5-year-old child who underwent right renal artery reimplantation.

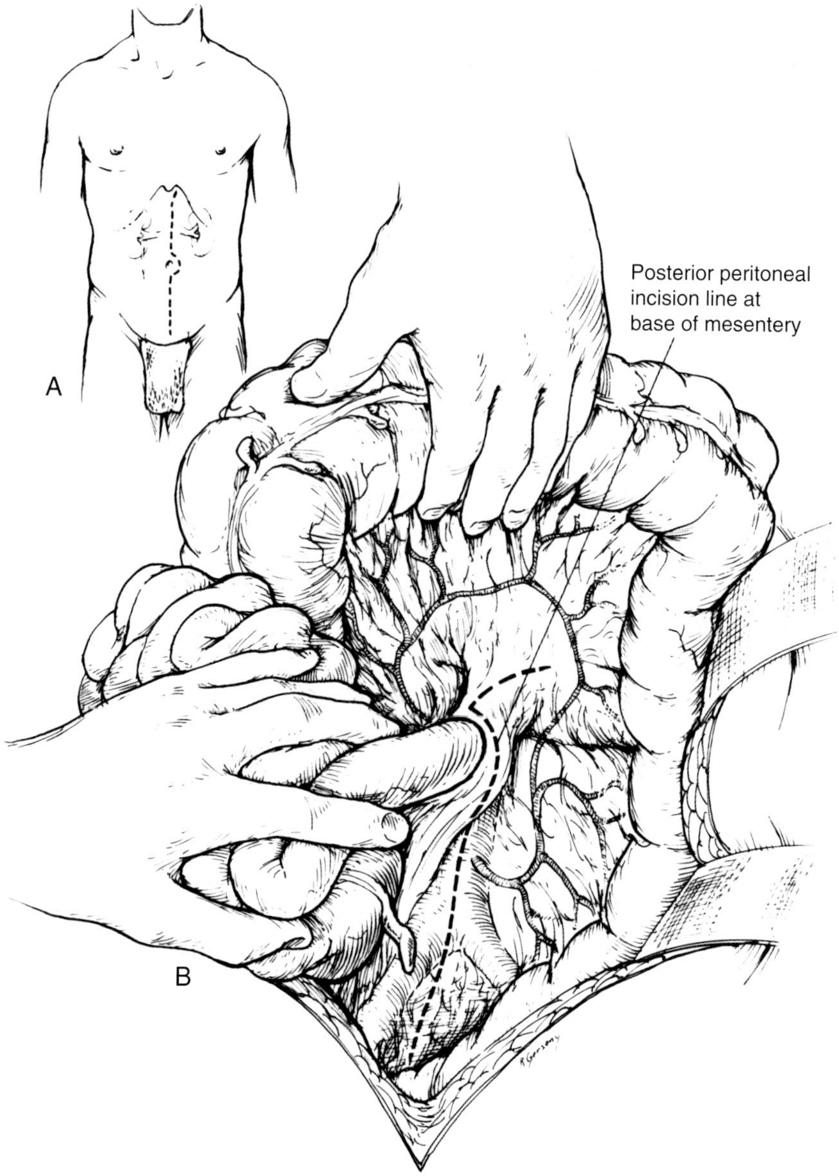

FIG 26.9 (A) Skin incision. (B) Exposure of the aorta and left renal hilum through the base of the mesentery. Extension of the posterior peritoneal incision to the left, along the inferior border of the pancreas, provides entry to an avascular plane behind the pancreas. This allows excellent exposure of the entire left renal hilum and the proximal right renal artery. (From Benjamin ME, Dean RH: Techniques in renal artery reconstruction: part I. *Ann Vasc Surg* 10:306–314, 1996.)

which enter the left renal vein, must be ligated and divided to facilitate exposure of the artery. Frequently, a lumbar vein enters the posterior wall of the left renal vein, and it can be avulsed easily unless special care is taken while mobilizing the renal vein. The proximal portion of the right renal artery can be exposed through the base of the mesentery by ligating two or more pairs of lumbar veins and retracting the left renal vein cephalad and the vena cava to the patient's right. However, the distal portion of the right renal artery is best exposed by mobilizing the duodenum and right colon medially (Fig. 26.11). Next, the right renal vein is mobilized and usually retracted cephalad to expose the artery.

When bilateral renal artery lesions are to be corrected, and when correction of a right renal artery lesion or bilateral lesions is combined with aortic reconstruction, we modify these exposure techniques. First, we extend the base of the mesentery exposure to allow complete evisceration of the entire small bowel and the right and transverse portions of the colon; in this exposure, the posterior peritoneal incision begins with division of the ligament of Treitz and proceeds along the base of the mesentery to the cecum and then up the lateral gutter to the foramen of Winslow (Fig. 26.12). Second, we extend the incision to the left along the inferior border of the pancreas to enter a retropancreatic plane, thereby exposing the aorta to a point above the superior

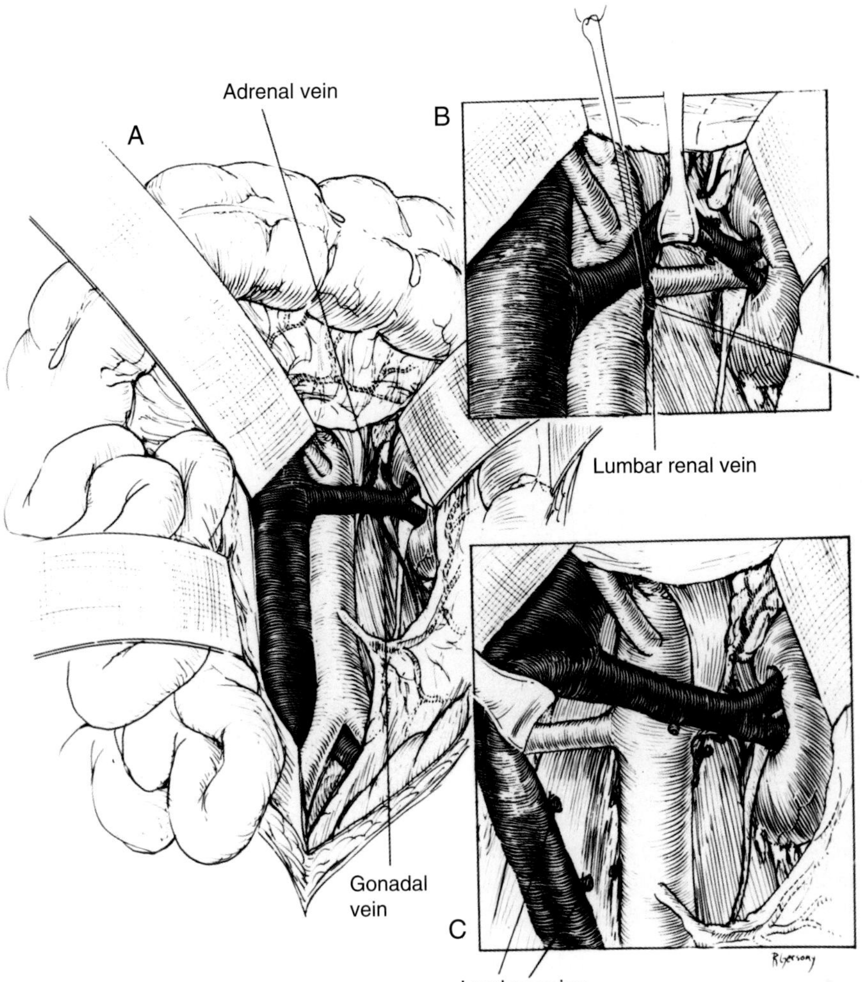

FIG 26.10 (A) Exposure of the proximal renal arteries through the base of the mesentery. (B) Mobilization of the left renal vein by ligation and division of the adrenal, gonadal, and lumbar renal veins allows exposure of the entire left renal artery to the hilum. (C) Two pairs of lumbar vessels have been ligated and divided to allow retraction of the vena cava to the right, providing adequate exposure of proximal renal artery disease. (From Benjamin ME, Dean RH: Techniques in renal artery reconstruction: part I. *Ann Vasc Surg* 10:306–314, 1996.)

mesenteric artery. Through this modified exposure, simultaneous bilateral renal endarterectomies, aortorenal grafting, or renal artery attachment to the aortic graft can be performed with wide visualization of the entire area.

Another technique is to partially divide both diaphragmatic crura as they pass behind the renal arteries to their paravertebral attachment. By partially dividing the crura, the aorta above the superior mesenteric artery is easily visualized and can be mobilized for suprarenal cross-clamping.

Aortorenal Bypass

Three types of graft are usually available for aortorenal bypass: autologous saphenous vein, autologous hypogastric artery, and synthetic prosthesis. The decision of which graft to use depends on a number of factors; the saphenous vein is preferred by some. However, if it is small (<4 mm in diameter) or sclerotic, the hypogastric artery or a synthetic prosthesis may be preferable. A thin-walled, 6-mm PTFE or polyester graft is satisfactory when the distal renal artery is of large caliber.

When an end-to-side renal artery bypass is used, the anastomosis between the renal artery and the graft is done first. Silastic slings can be used to occlude the renal artery distally. This method of vessel occlusion is especially applicable to this procedure. In contrast to vascular clamps, these slings are essentially atraumatic to the delicate renal artery. The absence of clamps in the operative field is also advantageous. Furthermore, when tension is applied to the slings, they lift the vessel out of the retroperitoneal soft tissue for more accurate visualization.

The length of the arteriotomy should be at least three times the diameter of the renal artery to guard against late suture-line stenosis. A 6-0 or 7-0 monofilament polypropylene suture material is employed with loop magnification.

After the renal artery anastomosis is completed, the occluding clamps and slings are removed from the artery, and a small

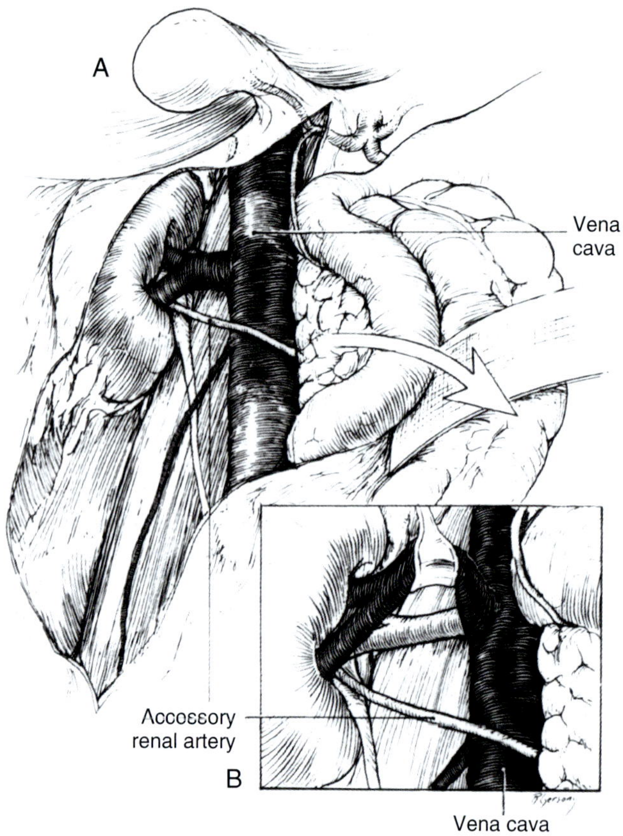

FIG 26.11 (A) Not uncommonly, an accessory right renal artery arises from the anterior aorta and crosses anterior to the vena cava. (B) The right renal vein is typically mobilized superiorly for exposure of the distal right renal artery. (From Benjamin ME, Dean RH: Techniques in renal artery reconstruction: part I. *Ann Vasc Surg* 10:306–314, 1996.)

bulldog clamp is placed across the vein graft adjacent to the anastomosis. The aortic anastomosis is then done. First, an ellipse of the anterolateral aortic wall is removed, and then the anastomosis is performed. If the graft is too long, kinking of the vein and subsequent thrombosis may result. If any element of kinking or twisting of the graft occurs after both anastomoses are completed, the aortic anastomosis should be taken down and redone after appropriate shortening or reorientation of the graft. In most instances, an end-to-end anastomosis between the graft and the renal artery provides a better reconstruction. This is especially true for combined aortorenal reconstruction. In this circumstance, the renal artery graft is attached to the Dacron aortic graft before its insertion. After the aortic graft is attached and flow is restored to the distal extremities, the renal artery can be transected and attached to the end of the saphenous vein graft without interrupting aortic flow.

Thromboendarterectomy

Thromboendarterectomy is used only for atherosclerotic renal artery stenosis. It is not applicable in fibromuscular disease. Transaortic endarterectomy of bilateral main renal artery lesions has been strongly advocated by Wylie and colleagues[105] (Fig. 26.13). In today's practice, this procedure is applicable to the subset of patients with combined visceral and renal occlusive plaque such as the "coral reef" aorta. In this procedure, the proximal aortic clamp must usually be placed above the superior mesenteric artery or celiac artery. If it is placed below this artery, it seriously compromises the exposure of the orifices of the renal arteries. Visualization of the distal end of the renal artery endarterectomy is facilitated by inversion of the renal artery into the aorta yielding specimen as seen in Fig. 26.14. Alternatively, a transrenal endarterectomy uses a transverse aortotomy, carrying the incision across the stenoses and into each renal artery. By this method, the entire endarterectomy can be performed under direct vision with or without patch closure.

Extraanatomic Bypass

Extraanatomic procedures have become increasingly popular as an alternative method of renal revascularization for high-risk patients. We do not believe that these procedures are equivalent to direct reconstructions, but they are useful in a highly select subgroup of high-risk patients.

Hepatorenal Bypass

A right subcostal incision is usually used to perform the hepatorenal bypass. The hepatoduodenal ligament is incised, and the common hepatic artery both proximal and distal to the gastroduodenal artery origin is encircled. Next, the descending duodenum is mobilized with the Kocher maneuver, the inferior vena cava is identified, the right renal vein is identified, and the right renal artery is encircled where it is found, either immediately cephalad or caudad to the renal vein.

A greater saphenous vein graft is usually used to construct the bypass. The hepatic artery anastomosis of the vein graft can be placed at the site of the amputated stump of the gastroduodenal artery or proximal to this branch when it must be saved as a collateral for gut perfusion. After completion of this anastomosis, the renal artery is transected and brought anterior to the vena cava for anastomosis end to end to the graft.

Splenorenal Bypass

Splenorenal bypass can be performed through a midline or a left subcostal incision. The posterior pancreas is mobilized by reflecting the inferior border cephalad. When the retropancreatic plane has been entered, the splenic artery can be mobilized from the left gastroepiploic artery to the level of its branches. The left renal artery is exposed as described earlier. After the splenic artery has been completely mobilized, it is divided distally, spatulated, and anastomosed end to end to the transected renal artery.

Ex Vivo Reconstruction

Ex vivo management is necessary in patients with fibromuscular dysplasia and aneurysms or stenoses involving renal artery branches; patients with fibromuscular dysplasia, renal artery dissection, and branch occlusion; patients with congenital arteriovenous fistulas of renal artery branches requiring partial resection; and patients with degeneration of previously placed grafts to the distal renal artery. Several methods of ex vivo hypothermic perfusion and reconstruction are available. A midline xiphoid-to-pubic incision is used for most renovascular procedures and is

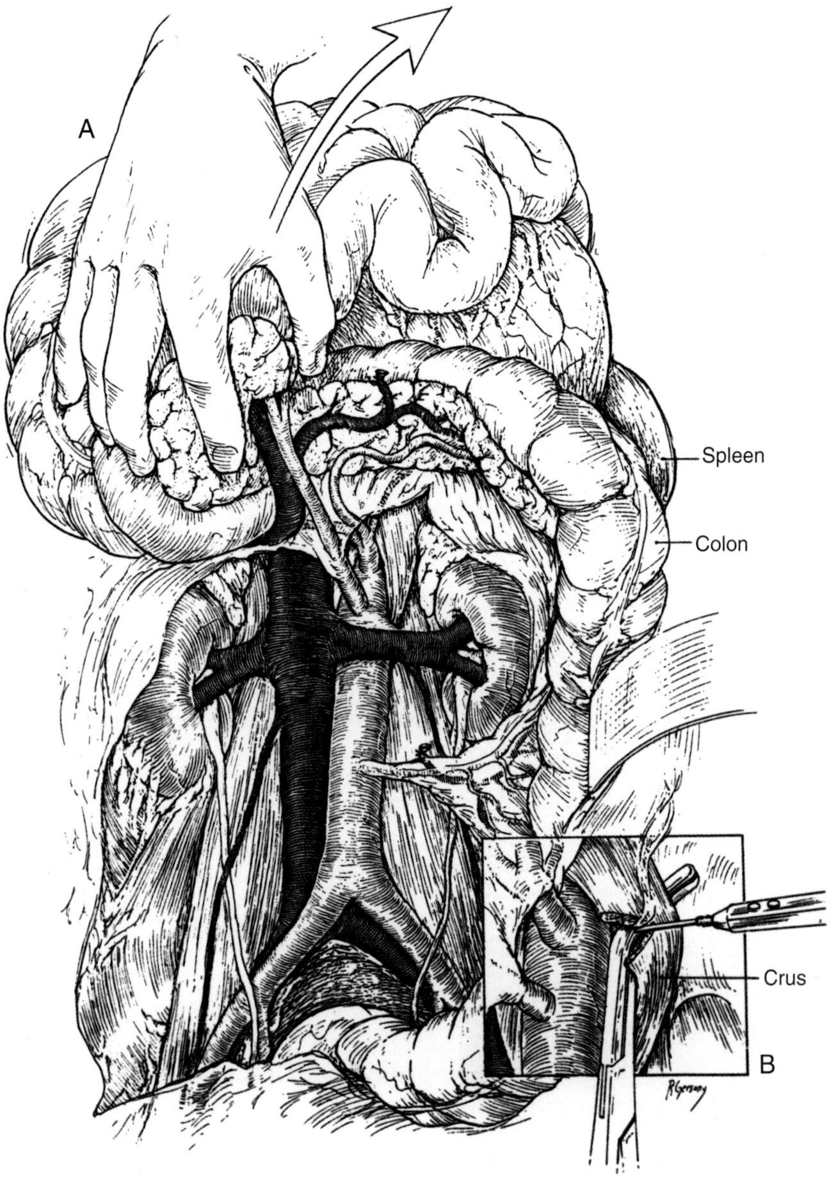

FIG 26.12 (A) For bilateral renal artery reconstruction combined with aortic repair, extended exposure can be obtained with mobilization of the cecum and ascending colon. The entire small bowel and right colon are then mobilized to the right upper quadrant and placed onto the chest wall. (B) Division of the diaphragmatic crura exposures the origin of the mesenteric vessels. (From Benjamin ME, Dean RH: Techniques in renal artery reconstruction: part I. *Ann Vasc Surg* 10:306–314, 1996.)

preferred when autotransplantation of the reconstructed kidney or combined aortic reconstructions are to be performed. An extended flank incision made parallel to the lower rib margin and carried to the posterior axillary line is used for complex branch renal artery repairs and is the preferred approach for ex vivo reconstructions without autotransplantation. The ureter is always mobilized but left intact, and an elastic sling or noncrushing clamp is placed around it to prevent collateral perfusion, inadvertent rewarming, or continued blood loss through the ureteric collaterals.[106]

After the kidney is mobilized and the vessels divided, the kidney is placed on the abdominal wall and perfused with a renal preservative solution. Continuous perfusion during the period of total renal ischemia is possible with complex perfusion pump systems and may be superior for prolonged renal preservation during storage periods. However, simple intermittent flushing with a chilled preservative solution provides equal protection during the shorter periods (2 to 3 hours) required for ex vivo dissection and complex renal artery reconstructions. For intermittent flushing, refrigerate the preservative overnight, add the additional components immediately before use to make up 1 L of solution, and hang the chilled (5°C to 10°C) solution on an intravenous stand to provide gravitational perfusion pressure of at least 2 m. Five hundred milliliters of solution

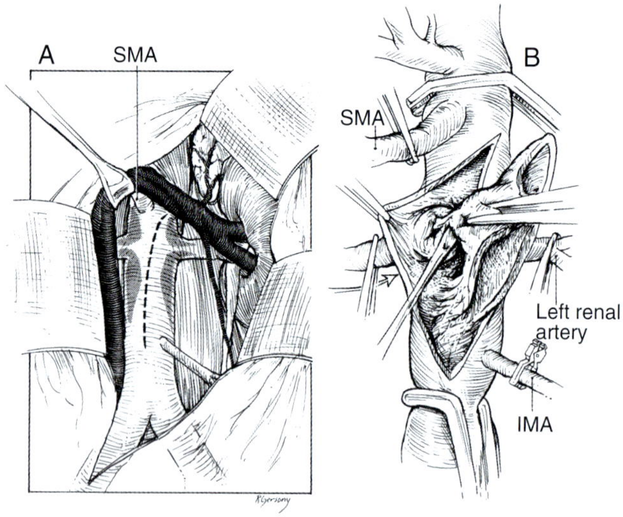

FIG 26.13 Exposure for a longitudinal transaortic endarterectomy is through the standard transperitoneal approach. The duodenum is mobilized from the aorta laterally in standard fashion or, for more complete exposure, the ascending colon and small bowel are mobilized. (A) The dotted line shows the location of the aortotomy. (B) The plaque is transected proximally and distally, and with eversion of the renal arteries, the atherosclerotic plaque is removed from each renal ostium. The aortotomy is typically closed with a running 4-0 or 5-0 polypropylene suture. *IMA,* Inferior mesenteric artery; *SMA,* superior mesenteric artery. (From Benjamin ME, Dean RH: Techniques in renal artery reconstruction: part I. *Ann Vasc Surg* 10:306–314, 1996.)

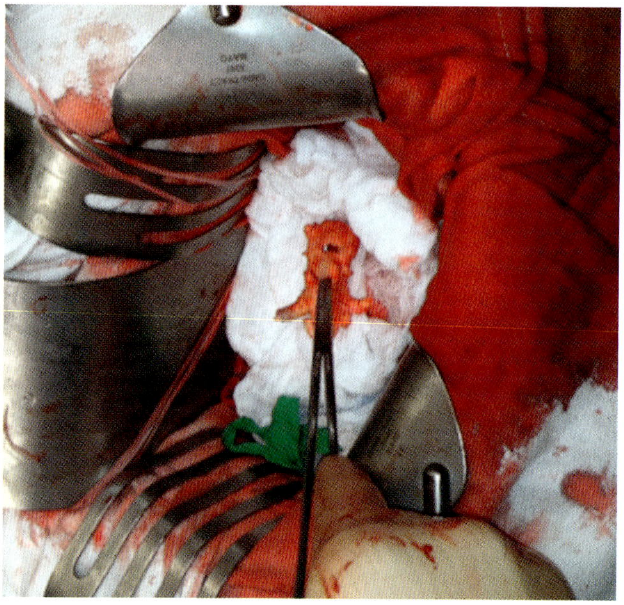

FIG 26.14 Postop specimen demonstrating successful thromboendarterectomy. (Courtesy William D. Jordan Jr., MD.)

is flushed through the kidney immediately after its removal from the renal fossa. If arterial exposure is adequate, the vein may be left intact, controlled with an atraumatic clamp, and a small venotomy made for the egress of perfusate. Regardless of whether the vein is divided or left intact, as each anastomosis is completed, an additional 150 to 200 mL of solution is flushed through the kidney, a procedure that also shows any leaks at the suture line.

Surface hypothermia is used to maintain constant hypothermia during ex vivo renal artery reconstruction. One method of surface hypothermia consists of the following steps.

- Place two 1-L bottles of normal saline solution in ice slush overnight.
- After removing the kidney, place it in a watertight plastic sheet from which excess saline solution can be suctioned away, and place laparotomy pads over the kidney.
- Keep it cool and moist by a constant drip of the chilled saline solution.

With this technique, it is possible to maintain renal core temperatures of 10°C to 15°C throughout the period of ischemia.

When both the renal artery and renal vein have been divided, autotransplantation to the iliac fossa is not necessary for most ex vivo reconstructions, even though it is an accepted method for reattachment of the ex vivo reconstructed renal artery. Autotransplantation of the reconstructed kidney to the iliac fossa was adapted from renal transplant surgeons, with no thought given to the significant difference between the two patient populations. Reduction in the magnitude of the operative exposure, manual palpation of the transplanted kidney, potential use of irradiation for episodes of rejection, and ease of removal when treatment of rejection has failed are all historical and practical reasons for placing the transplanted kidney into the recipient's iliac fossa, but none of these advantages apply to patients requiring ex vivo reconstruction.

For replacement of the kidney in its original site, the Gerota capsule must be opened during mobilization. Before transection of the renal vein begins, a large vascular clamp is placed to partially occlude the vena cava where it is entered by the renal vein. An ellipse of vena cava containing the entrance site of the renal vein is then excised, and the kidney is removed for ex vivo perfusion and reconstruction. When the distal renal artery–graft anastomoses are completed and the kidney is replaced in its bed, the ellipse of vena cava is reattached. This technique protects against stenosis of the renal vein anastomosis as a result of technical error. The renal artery graft is then attached to the aorta in the standard manner.

Nephrectomy

Nephrectomy is a procedure that should be limited to a subgroup of patients with RVH in whom the kidney responsible for the hypertension has nonreconstructable vessels and negligible residual excretory function. In these circumstances, nephrectomy can be of benefit because it controls hypertension without diminishing overall excretory function. In all other circumstances in which significant residual excretory function is present, the price of nephrectomy (loss of functioning renal mass) is greater than the potential benefit. This extreme conservatism regarding nephrectomy is based on the knowledge that more than 35% of patients with atherosclerotic lesions develop severe contralateral lesions during follow-up. Such lesions place the patient at risk for clinically severe renal failure and recurrent hypertension. This risk is even more important in children, because 50% of those who initially show a unilateral lesion subsequently develop contralateral disease.

EFFECT OF OPERATION ON HYPERTENSION

Most of the controversy surrounding the role of open surgical treatment of RVH relates to the morbidity and mortality associated with operation, the frequency of technical failure, and the low rate of a favorable blood pressure response to operation. Certainly, the literature documents the fact that poorly performed operations in poorly selected patients seldom result in a blood pressure benefit. Current results of operative intervention in centers experienced with the management of RVD, however, underscore the high rate of long-term patency and benefit to both blood pressure and renal function. Although our cumulative experience spans more than 40 years and includes the operative management of more than 1500 patients, a review of the results of a recent series of 500 consecutive atherosclerotic patients exemplifies current experience.[16]

Among patients with nonatherosclerotic RVD, 92% had a beneficial hypertension response, but only 43% were considered cured—a lower cure rate than that reported in the earlier surgical series.[23,107] This difference may be explained by the number of older patients, the number of patients with uncorrected contralateral lesions, and the duration of hypertension in many of these patients with nonatherosclerotic RVD. In contrast to the blood pressure results obtained in the entire group, patients younger than 45 years who had all anatomic renal artery lesions corrected and who had been hypertensive for less than 5 years had a cure rate of 68% and an improvement rate of 32%. This response rate is comparable with results from earlier reports.

Although operation was accomplished in the nonatherosclerotic RVD group without death, the operative mortality of 4.7% among 1076 patients with atherosclerotic RVD was high.[16,19,108–111] Blood pressure benefit (i.e., cured and improved) was observed in 88% of patients, of which 49% were cured and 39% improved. Unfortunately, 13% of the patients failed to see a benefit.

EFFECT OF RENAL REVASCULARIZATION ON RENAL FUNCTION

Little information is available regarding the incidence, prevalence, or natural history of ischemic nephropathy. Nevertheless, circumstantial evidence suggests that it may be a more common cause of progressive renal failure in the atherosclerotic age group (55 years or older) than previously recognized. In a 1988 report, 73% of patients with end-stage renal disease were in the atherosclerotic age group.[112] In a report by Mailloux and colleagues,[113] a presumed renovascular cause of end-stage renal disease increased in frequency from 6.7% for the period 1978 to 1981 to 16.5% for the period 1982 to 1985. The median age at onset of end-stage renal disease for that group was the oldest of all groups, falling in the seventh decade of life.

In 1076 patients (Table 26.4), 44% experienced improved renal function with a range of 23% to 58% among the individual studies. In addition, 44% experienced no change in their renal function after open repair. Renal function worsened in 12% of the patients.

To improve understanding of ischemic nephropathy, Dean and colleagues[114] undertook a retrospective review of data collected during a 42-month period from 58 consecutive patients with ischemic nephropathy who were admitted for operative management. They examined the rate of decline in their renal function during the period before intervention and the effect of operation on their outcome. Their ages ranged from 22 to 79 years (mean, 69 years). Based on serum creatinine values, immediate preoperative estimated GFR ranged from 0 to 46 mL/min (mean, 23.85 ± 9.76 mL/min). Patients with at least three sequential measurements for the calculation of estimated GFR changes during the 6 months before operation ($n = 50$) and the first 12 months after operation ($n = 32$) were used to describe the preoperative rate of decline in estimated GFR and the effect of operation on this decrease in the operative survivors. In addition, comparative analyses of data from patients with unilateral versus bilateral lesions and patients classified as having improvement in estimated GFR versus no improvement after operation. Comparison of the immediate preoperative and immediate postoperative estimated GFRs for the entire group showed significant improvement in response to operation. Likewise, the rate of deterioration in estimated GFR for the total group improved after operation. A similar improvement in the rate of deterioration in estimated GFR was seen in the subgroup of patients who had an immediate improvement in response to operation.

From this review, it was found that the site of disease (unilateral or bilateral), the anatomic status of the distal renal artery, and the rate of deterioration in renal function were significant predictors of a beneficial effect on renal function. Conversely, unilateral disease, absence of severe hypertension, and diffuse branch vessel occlusive disease were negative predictors of such benefit.

The data presented in this retrospective review argue that ischemic nephropathy is a rapidly progressive form of renal insufficiency. The effect of renal revascularization on renal function, however, was heterogeneous. Nevertheless, the frequency of both retrieval of renal function and slowing the rate of its deterioration during follow-up was gratifying and encourages continued study of the role of operation in properly selected patients.

EFFECT OF BLOOD PRESSURE RESPONSE ON LONG-TERM SURVIVAL

The rationale for the management of hypertension of any cause is to decrease long-term cardiovascular morbidity and improve event-free survival. The Wake Forest group has the greatest longitudinal follow-up of revascularization in this subset of patients. Dean and colleagues evaluated the outcome of 71 patients who underwent operative management of RVH 15 to 23 years previously.[115] Complete follow-up was available in 66 of the 68 patients who survived operation. Comparison of the initial blood pressure response after operation (1 to 6 months postoperatively) with the blood pressure status at the time of death or current date (up to 23 years later) showed that the effect of operative

TABLE 26.4 **Surgical Renal Artery Revascularization**[a]

Reference	Year	Patients	Bilateral Repair (%)	Preoperative Renal Dysfunction (%)	RENAL FUNCTION RESPONSE (%)			HYPERTENSION RESPONSE (%)			Perioperative Mortality (%)	Perioperative Morbidity (%)
					Improved	Unchanged	Worsened	Cured	Improved	Failed		
Fergany and colleagues[109,b]	1995	175	2.3	92.3	35	47	18	46	54	0	2.9	NR
Geroulakos and colleagues[108,b]	1997	38	NR	47	45	37	18	3	53	44	2.6	23.6
Hansen and colleagues[19]	2000	232	64	100	58	35	7	11	76	13	7.3	30
Cherr and colleagues[16]	2002	500	59	48.8	43	47	10	73	12	15	4.6	16
Marone and colleagues[110]	2004	96	27	100	42	41	16	NR	NR	NR	4.1	NR
Grigoryants and colleagues[111,b]	2007	35	57	46	23	60	17	9	79	12	2.8	NR
Mean %[c]					44	44	12	49	39	13	4.7	20.6

[a]Renal function and hypertension responses expressed percentage of patients surviving operation.
[b]Weighted mean based on number of patients with reported data categorized according to column.
[c]References in which data were not reported or categorical response categories were combined are not included in calculation.
NR, Not reported.

treatment is maintained over long-term follow-up. In patients who required repeated renovascular operation for recurrent RVH during follow-up, the majority of the operations were performed for the management of contralateral lesions that had progressed to functional significance (i.e., produced RVH).

Assessment of the effect of blood pressure response on late survival produced results that are not surprising. Although the subgroup of nonresponders was small, they experienced a significantly more rapid death rate during follow-up than did patients who had a positive blood pressure response to operation. This finding confirms the validity of the premise that inadequate management of RVH leaves the patient at higher risk of early death from cardiovascular events. The presence of angiographically diffuse atherosclerosis at the time of evaluation and operation was predictive of a more rapid rate of death during follow-up.[114]

This difference in subsequent death rate was present even though a comparison between patients with diffuse atherosclerotic disease and those with focal atherosclerotic disease was undertaken only in patients experiencing a significant blood pressure response. In view of the suggestion by some physicians that the presence of diffuse disease precludes a high rate of blood pressure response to operation, it is important to note that no significant difference occurred in the frequency of response between the focal (80%) and diffuse (77%) groups in this study. In addition, although the presence of diffuse disease was associated with a more rapid death rate, it does not preclude the probability of a longer survival in this subgroup compared with a similar group of patients who either did not undergo operation or received no blood pressure benefit from such intervention. Furthermore, if one considers that diffuse disease is only a later stage of focal disease, it is not surprising that the endpoint of clinically significant disease—namely, death from cardiovascular events—arrives sooner when one begins follow-up or removes a risk factor that causes its acceleration later in its natural history.

In contrast, a contemporary group of 500 atherosclerotic patients did not demonstrate improved event-free survival in association with beneficial blood pressure response to operation.[16] As noted earlier, only atherosclerotic patients who are cured (i.e., normotensive without medications) have demonstrated increased survival. Although there are a number of possible explanations for this observed difference, renal function response among contemporary patients demonstrated a significant and independent association with follow-up survival. Global renal disease treated with complete renal artery repair after rapid decline in renal function provided the best opportunity for improved glomerular filtration. Patients whose renal function was unimproved or worse remained at increased risk for eventual dialysis dependence. In the contemporary population, progression to dialysis dependence was the single strongest risk factor for death.

CONCLUSION

The role of intervention for RVH and ischemic nephropathy continues to be muddled due to the lack of appropriate randomized data. Enthusiasm for endovascular intervention has not been met with overwhelmingly favorable results in the general hypertensive population. However, when appropriate patient selection is made, as seen in historical surgical groups, significant patient benefit exists for diagnosis and treatment of RVD.

In young patients, those with precipitous decline in renal function or increase in hypertension, FMD, the pediatric population, and others with hallmark signs of symptomatic RVH, appropriate intervention can be a life-saving measure. It is clear that the cardiovascular side effects of prolonged renin-angiotensin activation can lead to mortality. A modern vascular practice should incorporate renal intervention in this select population.

REVIEW QUESTIONS

1. Unilateral renovascular hypertension (RVH)—two kidney, one clip model—results in:
   a. Renal failure
   b. Aldosterone-mediated volume-dependent hypertension
   c. Angiotensin II–driven vasoconstrictive hypertension
   d. Well compensated heart failure
2. The prevalence of renal artery derived hypertension in the overall hypertensive population is:
   a. 5% to 10%
   b. 25%
   c. 50% to 60%
   d. >80%
3. Which of the following is clinically correlated to possible RVH?
   a. Young age at onset
   b. Recent onset or acute change in blood pressure control
   c. Abdominal bruit
   d. All of the above
4. Which duplex ultrasound findings are consistent with renal artery stenosis?
   a. Renal to aortic ratio of ≥ 3.5
   b. PSV > 200
   c. Reversal of flow on color imaging
   d. Increase in grey scale median
5. The ASTRAL trial of renal artery stenting demonstrated:
   a. Significant improvement in number of medications needed to treat hypertension in treated patients
   b. Renal function preservation and avoidance of dialysis in stented patients
   c. Increased mortality in the observation arm
   d. None of the above

6. The most useful adjunct for prevention of embolization with renal angioplasty and stents:
   a. Double filter technique
   b. Use of self-expanding stents
   c. Intraprocedural platelet inhibition
   d. Use of 0.018-inch balloon platform

7. Proven operative technique for surgical correction of RVH is:
   a. Thromboendarterectomy
   b. Aortorenal bypass
   c. Renal artery reimplantation
   d. All of the above

BIBLIOGRAPHY

ASTRAL Investigators, Wheatley K, Ives N, et al. Revascularization versus medical therapy for renal-artery stenosis. *N Engl J Med.* 2009;361(20):1953–1962.

Barnes RW. Utility of duplex scanning of the renal artery. In: Bergan JJ, Yao JST, eds. *Arterial Surgery: New Diagnostic and Operative Techniques.* Orlando, Fla: Grune & Stratton; 1988:351–366.

Cherr GS, Hansen KJ, Craven TE, et al. Surgical management of atherosclerotic renovascular disease. *J Vasc Surg.* 2002;35:236–245.

Cooper CJ, Haller ST, Colyer W, et al. Embolic protection and platelet inhibition during renal artery stenting. *Circulation.* 2008;117(21):2752–2760.

Cooper CJ, Murphy TP, Cutlip DE, et al, CORAL Investigators. Stenting and medical therapy for atherosclerotic renal-artery stenosis. *N Engl J Med.* 2014;370(1):13–22.

Klausner JQ, Lawrence PF, Harlander-Locke MP, et al. The contemporary management of renal artery aneurysms. *J Vasc Surg.* 2015;61(4):978–984.

Main J. Atherosclerotic renal artery stenosis, ACE inhibitors, and avoiding cardiovascular death. *Heart.* 2005;91(4):548–552.

Pillay W, Kan Y, Crinnion J, et al. Prospective multicentre study of the natural history of atherosclerotic renal artery stenosis in patients with peripheral vascular disease. *Br J Surg.* 2002;89:737–740.

Trinquart L, Mounier-Vehier C, Sapoval M, Gagnon N, Plouin PF. Efficacy of revascularization for renal artery stenosis caused by fibromuscular dysplasia: a systematic review and meta-analysis. *Hypertension.* 2010;56(3):525–532.

References available online at ExpertConsult.com.

CHAPTER 27

Angioplasty and Stenting for Mesenteric and Renal Artery Disease

Gustavo S. Oderich, Giuliano de A. Sandri, Emanuel Junio R. Tenorio

MESENTERIC ARTERIAL DISEASE

Chronic mesenteric ischemia (CMI) is an uncommon disorder, accounting for fewer than 1 per 100,000 hospital admissions in the United States.[1] Since the first successful mesenteric endarterectomy by Shaw and Maynard in 1958, techniques of revascularization have evolved.[2] The first endovascular angioplasties for mesenteric stenoses were performed in 1980.[3] Similar to renal artery stenosis (RAS), endovascular approach has become the first line of treatment, relegating open surgery to patients who are not suitable for this procedure or fail an angioplasty and stenting.[4]

Etiology

The most common cause of CMI is atherosclerotic disease, accounting for over 90% of cases in most series. Atherosclerotic lesions usually affect the origin or the proximal 2 to 3 cm of the mesenteric arteries, frequently with associated plaque in the aorta and renal arteries. Nonatherosclerotic lesions can also affect the mesenteric arteries. The differential diagnosis includes vasculitis, systemic lupus, Buerger disease, spontaneous dissections, fibromuscular dysplasia, neurofibromatosis, radiation arteritis, coarctation, mesenteric venous stenosis or occlusion, and drug-induced arteriopathy from the use of cocaine or ergot.

In the resting state 20% of the cardiac output passes through the mesenteric arteries; but during the digestive process there is a hyperemic postprandial response and the output increases to 150%.[5] Patients with mesenteric ischemia fail to provide the postprandial hyperemic response that is required to supply oxygen for the metabolic processes of digestion.[6] The term "intestinal angina" was coined to describe postprandial pain after a meal, which is a direct analogy to angina pectoris, since the mechanism of pain is an imbalance between supply and demand of oxygen and metabolites. Because the mesenteric circulation has an extensive collateral network, symptoms usually start once obstructive lesions affect at least two or three visceral vessels (Fig. 27.1). However, contrary to what has been described in many medical texts, some patients can suffer from CMI with a single diseased vessel.[7] The clinical significance of ischemia correlates not only with the extent of disease but also with the adequacy of the collateral pathways, acuteness of symptoms, and presence of arterial steal.

Asymptomatic mesenteric stenosis tends to have a benign course, although 15% to 50% of patients with acute mesenteric ischemia from in situ thrombosis of preexisting lesions have no previous signs or symptoms.[8,9] The prevalence of mesenteric stenosis or occlusion in male patients older than 65 years is 18% by duplex ultrasound. Most patients have single-vessel lesions and remain asymptomatic.[10] Severe mesenteric artery disease was identified in 6% of patients submitted to aortography.[11] In a small series of 15 patients with severe three-vessel disease, 4 (27%) developed symptoms, of whom 3 underwent successful revascularization and 1 died from acute ischemia.

ENDOVASCULAR MANAGEMENT

The diagnosis of CMI is discussed in Chapter 34. There is no role for a conservative approach in patients who develop symptoms. An excessive delay in proceeding with definitive revascularization or prolonged use of parenteral nutrition alone has been associated with clinical deterioration, bowel infarction, or risk of sepsis from catheter-related complications.[12,13] Revascularization is indicated in all patients with symptoms of CMI. Treatment goals are to relieve symptoms, restore normal weight, and prevent bowel infarction.

The indication for prophylactic revascularization in patients with asymptomatic lesions remains controversial. This may be considered in patients with severe three-vessel disease, especially if access to medical care is difficult for those who live in remote or underserved areas.[11] Our approach has been to counsel patients regarding symptoms of mesenteric ischemia and to have a low threshold to proceed with revascularization if any gastrointestinal symptoms (e.g., bloating, diarrhea, atypical pain) arise. Revascularization may also be considered in asymptomatic patients with severe three-vessel disease undergoing open surgical aortic reconstructions.

Choice of Open Versus Endovascular Revascularization

Selection of the open versus the endovascular approach is based on careful review of preprocedure CTA and clinical risk. The superior mesenteric artery (SMA) is the primary target for revascularization; therefore the anatomy of the SMA is the most important determinant of choice of therapy. The ideal lesion for angioplasty and stenting is a short, focal stenosis or occlusion with minimal to moderate calcification or thrombus. Celiac axis (CA) angioplasty and stenting carries a higher risk of restenosis[14]

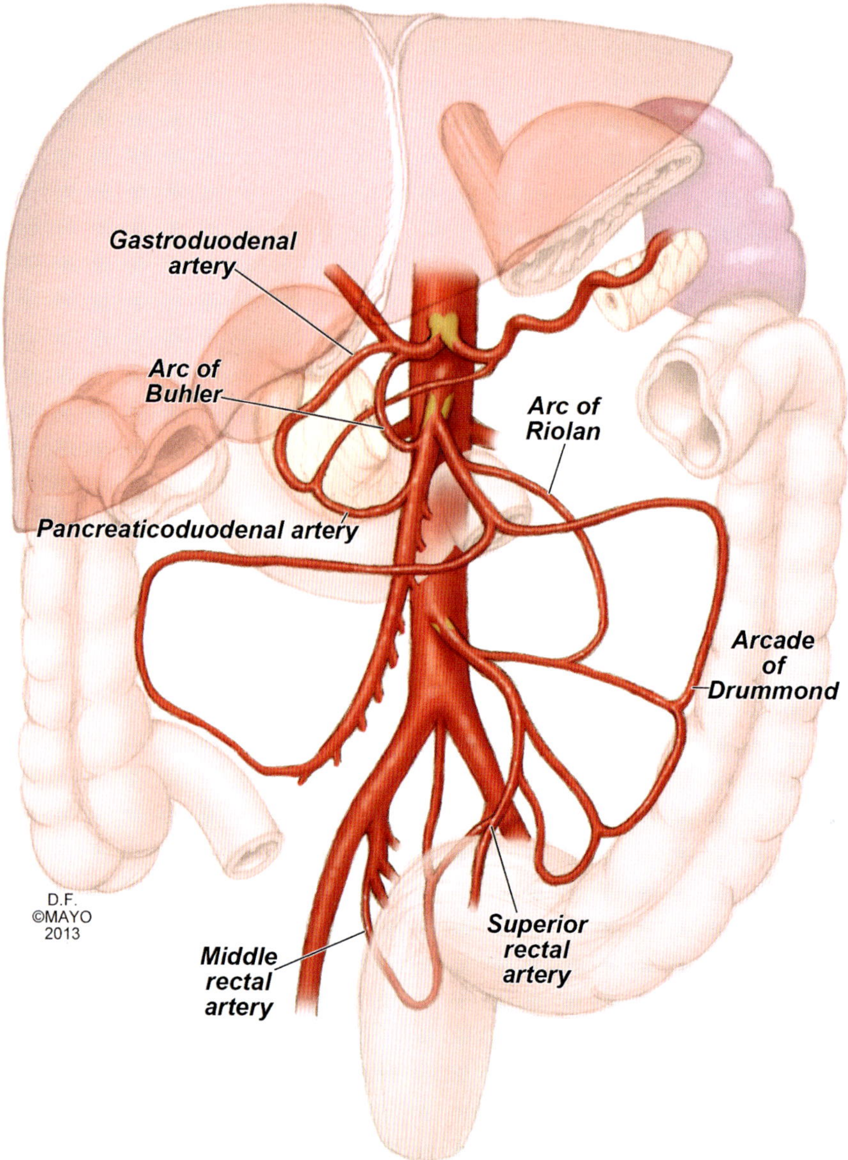

FIG 27.1 Schematic representation of the collateral circulation between the celiac axis, superior mesenteric, inferior mesenteric, and internal iliac arteries.

and should not be performed if there is active compression by the median arcuate ligament unless this has been surgically released.

The technical difficulty of endovascular procedures can be anticipated by the presence of severe eccentric calcification, flush occlusion, and in dealing with patients who have longer lesions, small vessels, and tandem lesions affecting branches. These anatomic features are associated with worse technical results, increased risk of arterial complications (e.g., distal embolization, dissection), and restenosis.[15,16] Our preference in these patients is to offer open revascularization if the anatomy is unfavorable for angioplasty and stenting, particularly if the clinical risk is low. Open reconstruction has also been used in younger patients with nonatherosclerotic lesions and in those who have failed percutaneous intervention or have had multiple recurrent in-stent restenoses.

Preprocedure Evaluation

Preoperative evaluation should focus on a critical review of surgical risk, nutritional status, and anatomic factors that affect the choice of reconstruction. Optimization of clinical and nutritional status should be sought as long as no significant delay is caused. Evaluation and management are tailored to each patient. Optimal medical therapy in these patients ideally should include cessation of cigarette smoking, acetylsalicylic acid, beta-blocker, and lipid-lowering medication.

Revascularization should not be excessively delayed. Patients who present with deterioration of symptoms should be admitted, started on intravenous heparin, and treated urgently within 24 to 48 hours. Patients with iodinated contrast allergy should be premedicated with a steroid preparation. Those with chronic kidney disease who have a serum creatinine level above 1.5 to

2.0 mg/dL (133 to 177 mmol/L) should undergo intravenous hydration with sodium bicarbonate and oral acetylcysteine starting the day prior to intervention. Gentle bowel preparation may be used prior to open reconstruction but should be avoided in those with severe or subacute ischemia.

Technique of Endovascular Revascularization

Arterial access can be obtained using either the femoral or brachial approach, preferentially with ultrasound guidance and a micropuncture set. Choice of access is based on physician preference, the presence of mesenteric occlusion, and angle of origin. Diagnostic angiographies are usually done as part of the intervention and rarely indicated to establish the diagnosis. Brachial access offers more catheter support in patients with very acute origins and occlusions. To minimize risk of access-related complications, the authors' preference is to surgically expose the brachial artery with a small 1- to 2-cm incision under local anesthesia.[17]

Initial arterial access is obtained with a 5 French sheath. Diagnostic angiography is done using a 5 French flush catheter positioned approximately at the level of T12. The patient is anticoagulated with intravenous heparin (80 UI/kg) prior to crossing the lesion for any intervention. Use of a low-osmolar contrast agent (e.g., Visipaque) minimizes the abdominal discomfort that occurs during selective injections. A complete diagnostic study should include an abdominal aortogram with anteroposterior and lateral views to define the location, severity, and extent of visceral artery involvement and to identify concomitant lesions in the aorta or the renal or iliac arteries. The optimal projection to display the proximal CA and SMA is a lateral view; for the origin of the inferior mesenteric artery (IMA), it is usually a 15-degree right-lateral-oblique view. Diagnostic angiography may not be needed if the preprocedure CTA has documented the extent of disease.

Mesenteric interventions are usually done using a 6 or 7 French sheath. If the brachial access is selected, a 90-cm hydrophilic sheath is positioned in the descending thoracic aorta. Choice of catheter shape for selective catheterization is dependent on access site, angle of origin, and individual preference. A multipurpose A (MPA) catheter is ideal for selective catheterization from the brachial approach, whereas a secondary curve catheter (e.g., SOS, VS1, or Simmons) can be used from the femoral approach. The initial selective angiography should demonstrate the area of stenosis and the distal runoff branches for comparison with postintervention views. In patients with questionable lesions, pressure gradients can be measured using pressure wire, "pull-back," or a simultaneous pressure measurement technique.[18] The target lesion is initially crossed using a 0.035-inch soft angled hydrophilic guidewire, which is exchanged for the interventional wire of choice. The tip of the guidewire should be visualized and positioned within the main trunk of the SMA rather than within small secondary branches, which are prone to perforate or dissect (Fig. 27.2). Embolic protection may be useful in selected patients who present with acute or subacute symptoms, particularly those with occlusions, long lesions (>30 mm length), severe calcification, or thrombus. In these cases, the authors' preference is to use a 320-cm working-length 0.014-inch filter wire (Spider RX, Medtronic Covidien, Plymouth, MN). If a 0.035-inch stent is selected, a two-wire technique can be used by combining a 0.014-inch filter wire with a 0.018-inch "buddy wire." Most recently, our practice has changed to covered stents (0.035-inch) in patients with lesions that do not involve side branches. Covered stents offer superior patency rates compared with bare metal stents.[4] If a two-wire technique is used, the stent is introduced via both wires for better support and to facilitate subsequent retrieval of the embolic protection device (Fig. 27.3). Predilatation is recommended only if there is tight stenosis, occlusion, or severe calcification, or to gauge the size of stents. A balloon-expandable stent with diameter from 5 to 8 mm is used in more than 95% of cases, allowing precise deployment and greater radial force. The stent should cover slightly more than the entire length of the lesion and should go 1 to 2 mm into the aortic lumen. Ideally the stent should be flared gently into the aorta to prevent missing the ostia and to facilitate recatheterization if needed. Occasionally a self-expandable stent is used if the treated segment is tortuous or long, extending across proximal jejunal branches.

The primary goal of percutaneous treatment is to restore antegrade flow into at least one of the three mesenteric arteries, preferentially the SMA. In most cases primary stenting is recommended because of elastic recoil and restenosis, which occurs with angioplasty of ostial lesions. Routine use of two-vessel stenting is not recommended, since it adds cost and potential risk of complications without any evidence of better outcomes.[14,19]

Recanalization of chronic occlusions poses a special challenge. The technique requires a stiffer support system to cross the lesion and deliver the stent. A coaxial support system uses a 7 French sheath, 7 French MPA guide catheter, and 5 French MPA catheter (Fig. 27.4). Attempting difficult recanalization from the femoral approach adds time, contrast, and catheter manipulations and is fraught with failure. The tip of the MPA catheter engages the stump of the occluded SMA, whereas the support system allows the lesion to be crossed using a straight-tipped hydrophilic, soft 0.035-in Glidewire. Occasionally, 0.018- or 0.014-in guidewires are needed. It is important to avoid the subintimal plane owing to the risk of dissection or disruption; it is best achieved using straight-tipped guidewires. A Quick-cross catheter (Spectranetics, Colorado Springs, CO), an alternative support catheter, or even a small coronary balloon may be needed to cross a tight lesion. Once the lesion has been crossed, access into the true lumen should be confirmed. Our preference has been to use an embolic protection device with a two-wire technique routinely in cases of total occlusion.

Following deployment and flaring of the stent, the embolic protection device is retrieved with careful attention to avoid entrapment into the stent. The basket is examined for debris. A formal completion angiography should be obtained, including a focal magnified view of the stent with the sheath in the aorta to demonstrate the vessel origin and a panoramic view of the entire SMA and its branches to rule out embolization or perforation. The stiff guidewire should be retracted and nitroglycerin may be administered via the sheath to minimize spasm or kinks caused by the guidewire tip.

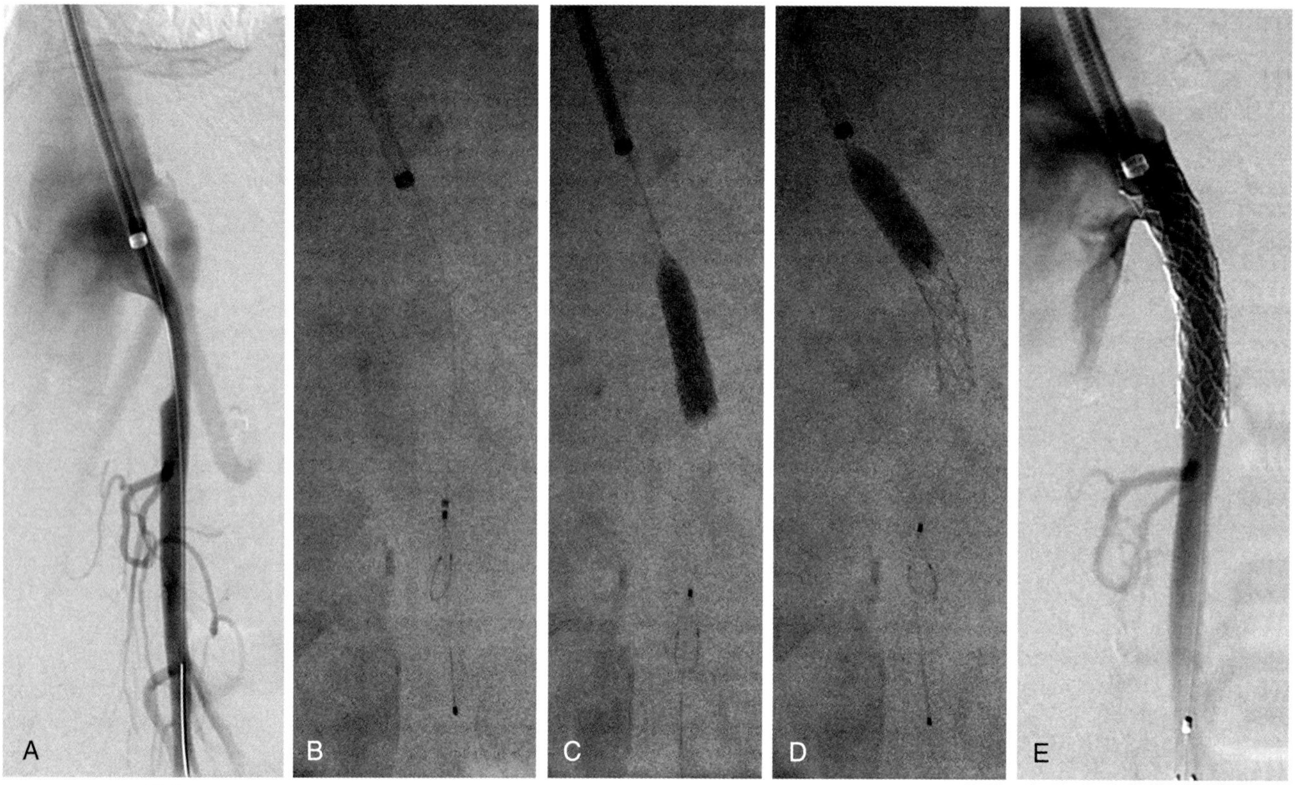

FIG 27.2 Angioplasty using the brachial access of the superior mesenteric artery. A 6 or 7 French main pulmonary artery catheter is positioned in the descending thoracic aorta. (A) Selective catheterization with choice of catheter and initial selective angiography demonstrating the area of stenosis and distal runoff branches. (B) Placement of distal embolization protection device. (C and D) Following deployment and flaring of the covered balloon expandable stent. (E) Control angiography without residual stenosis or distal embolization.

A number of adjunctive techniques can be used to optimize results in complex lesions, but the authors acknowledge that these techniques are anecdotal. The presence of acute and subacute symptoms suggests fresh thrombus or a complicated plaque. In these cases local administration of tissue plasminogen activator (t-PA) into the diseased segment 20 to 30 minutes prior to stent placement may improve technical success. For eccentric, calcified lesions, percutaneous atherectomy has been used in very select cases.[20] It is critical to have an appreciation for the limitations of this technique when it is applied as an off-label use in the mesenteric arteries.

Complications

The most commonly reported complications are access-related problems in 3% to 16%, renal insufficiency in 2% to 8%, acute bowel ischemia in 1% to 7%, gastrointestinal bleeding in 1% to 5%, cardiac events in 1% to 7%, and respiratory complications in 1% to 7% of cases.[19,21-34] Mortality is usually related to cardiac events, gastrointestinal bleeding, and bowel ischemia. The last is typically associated with intraprocedural complications such as distal embolization, thrombosis, or dissection. Distal embolization occurs in 8% of patients treated by SMA stents without embolic protection, with higher rates among patients with subacute symptoms, occlusion, long lesions (>30 mm), and severe calcification.

Postprocedure Management

All patients are admitted for observation overnight. Worsening abdominal pain after the procedure is unusual and warrants evaluation to rule out thrombosis, embolization, or a mesenteric hematoma from jejunal branch perforation (Fig. 27.5). Patients are allowed to resume a regular diet within 6 to 8 hours. Antiplatelet therapy is typically started prior to the intervention with acetylsalicylic acid and continued indefinitely thereafter. Clopidogrel is started the day of the intervention with a loading dose of 300 mg and continued for 6 to 8 weeks as dual antiplatelet therapy or indefinitely if a covered stent is used. A duplex ultrasound scan prior to discharge or within the first few days after the procedure serves as a baseline for future comparison. Follow-up includes clinical examination and duplex ultrasound every 6 months during the first year and annually thereafter.

RESULTS

Endovascular revascularization has been associated with decreased morbidity, length of stay and convalescence time, but similar mortality compared to open repair.[35,36] Morbidity and length of stay averages 11% and 3 days with endovascular intervention compared with 33% and 14 days with open surgery. Mortality

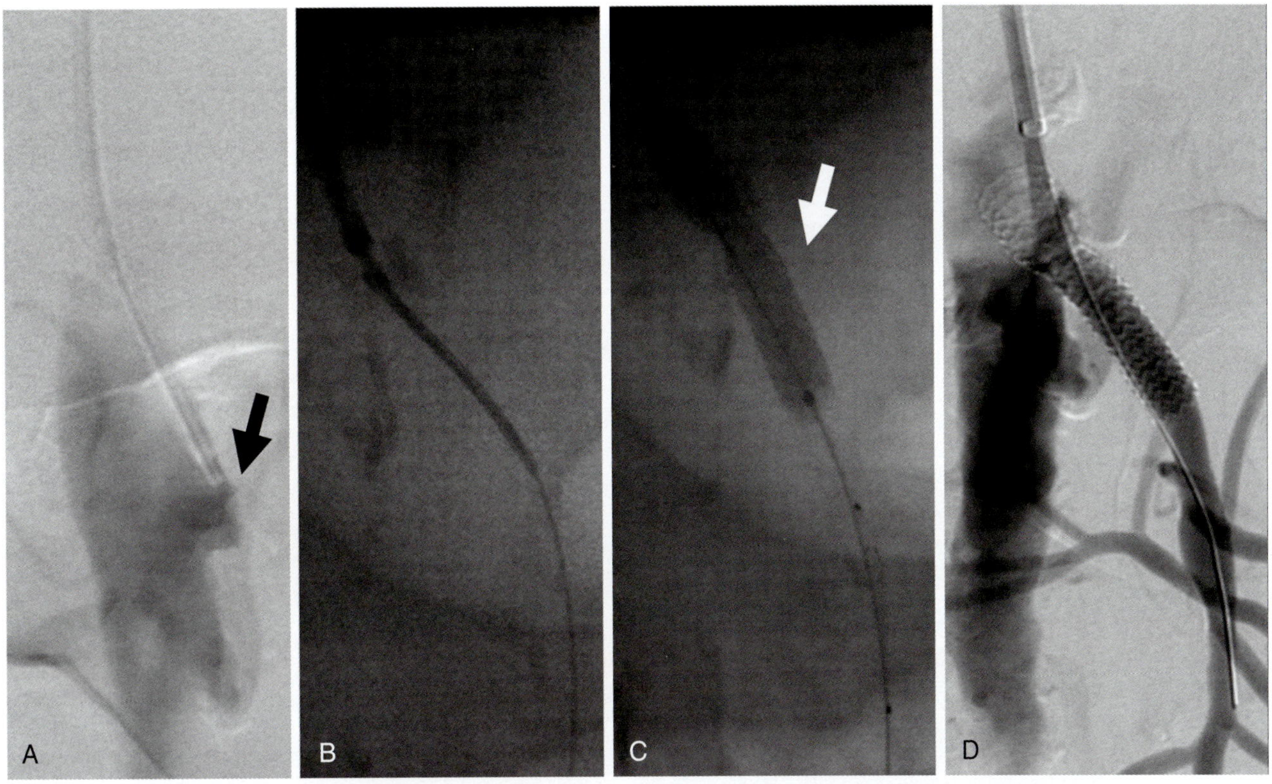

FIG 27.3 Recanalization technique. This technique requires a stiff support system to cross the lesion and to deliver the stent. (A) Coaxial support system using a 7 French sheath, 7-French multipurpose A (MPA) guide catheter, and 5 French MPA catheter. *Black arrow* indicates stump of occluded SMA. (B) Recanalization with placement of distal embolic protection device; (C) Angioplasty and stenting *(white arrow)*. (D) Angiogram after flaring of the covered balloon expandable stent.

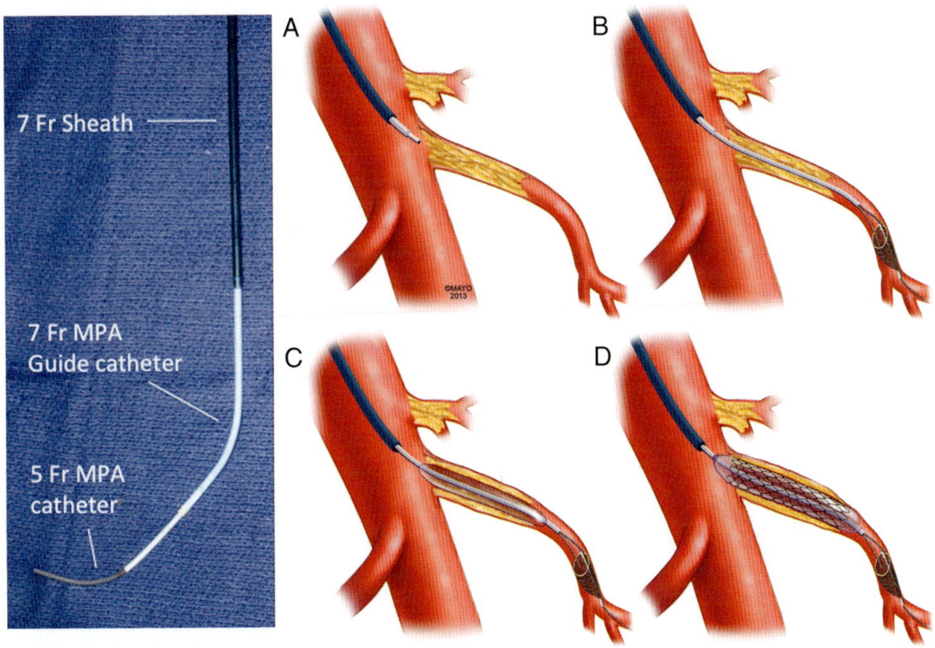

FIG 27.4 Technique of recanalization using a coaxial system with a 7 French sheath, 7 French guide catheter, and 5 French multipurpose A catheter. The occluded superior mesenteric artery stump is engaged with the coaxial system (A). The lesion is crossed using a guidewire and catheter (B), followed by predilatation (C) and stent placement (D).

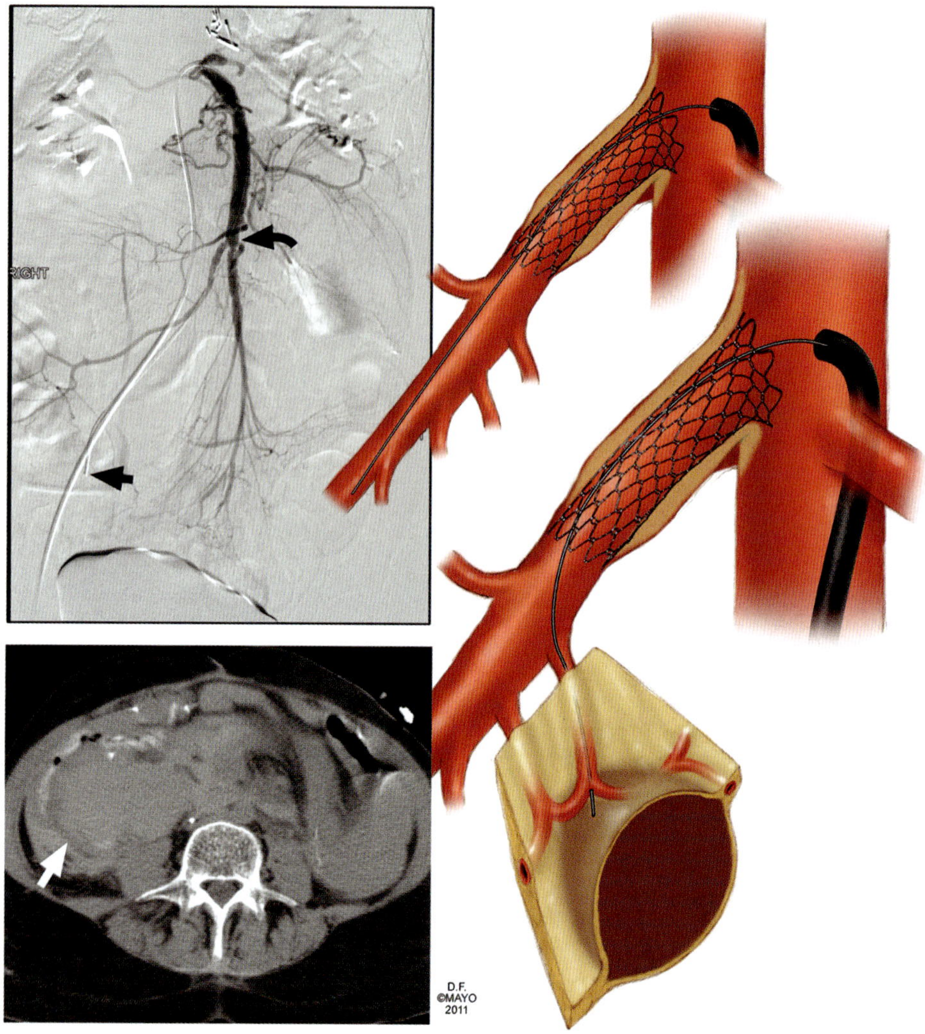

FIG 27.5 Angiography demonstrates patent superior mesenteric artery after stenting, without obvious perforation. Note the guidewire is within a small jejunal branch *(straight arrow)* instead of the main trunk *(curved arrow)*. Computed tomography demonstrating mesenteric hematoma *(white arrow)* after jejunal branch perforation.

rates are similar, averaging 6% (0% to 15%) for open and 5% (0% to 21%) for endovascular revascularization.[36]

In regard to symptom relief, angioplasty alone has been associated with lower rates of technical success (78%) compared with primary stenting (>95%).[37] Symptom improvement is noted immediately after revascularization, but it is not uncommon for patients to complain of modest bloating and worsening diarrhea. Persistent abdominal pain may suggest other diagnoses.

Endovascular treatment has been plagued by higher rates of restenosis affecting as much as 20% to 66% of the patients, not matching the excellent patency rates reported for open reconstructions (Table 27.1).[4,19,21-33,35,38,39] The average 3-year primary patency rate for bare metal stents is 52% (range, 30% to 81%) calculated from pooled literature.[37] Reinterventions can yield secondary patencies as high as 90%.[16,37] Oderich and associates reported a nonrandomized comparison of covered versus bare metal stents in 225 patients treated for CMI.[4] In that study, covered stents had 92% ± 6% primary and 100% secondary patency rates at 3 years, rivaling the results of open bypass. Covered stents outperformed bare metal stents, with less restenosis, symptom recurrences, or reinterventions and with better patency rates. These observations stood both in primary interventions for native artery lesions and in reinterventions for in-stent or native artery restenosis after an endovascular procedure. Independent predictors of restenosis were use of bare metal stents, cigarette smoking, advanced age, and female gender.

The type of revascularization has not been shown to affect survival, but comparative analysis is limited by selection bias favoring open bypass in good-risk cases and endovascular revascularization in higher-risk patients. Poor prognostic indicators for long-term patient survival after mesenteric revascularization include advanced age and the presence of severe cardiac, pulmonary, or renal disease.[35,40] Tallarita and associates reported long-term survival in a cohort of 343 patients treated for CMI, with nearly identical 5-year survival rates using propensity matched scores for patients treated by open (57%) or endovascular (60%) revascularization.[40] Five-year patient survival averaged 71% ± 4% for low-risk, 49% ± 6% for intermediate-risk,

TABLE 27.1 **Results of Contemporary Reports of Angioplasty and Stenting for Treatment of Chronic Mesenteric Ischemia**

Author (Year)	N	Vessels	Stented Vessels (%)	Technical Success (%)	Mortality (%)	Morbidity (%)	Recurrence (%)	Reintervention (%)	Primary Patency (%)	Follow-Up (Months)
Bare Metal Stents										
Kasirajan et al. (2001)[21]	28	32	82	100	11	18	34	—	73 at 3 years	24
van Wanroij et al. (2004)[22]	27	33	94	93	0	11	—	19	81 at 19 months	19
Silva et al. (2006)[19]	59	79	100	96	2	—	17	17	71	38
Biebl et al. (2007)[23]	23	40	96	—	0	4	26	22	—	10
Atkins et al. (2007)[24]	31	42	87	100	3.2	13	23	16	58	15
Sarac et al. (2008)[25]	65	87	100	—	8	31	—	31	65	12
Lee et al. (2008)[26]	31	41	—	98	14	6	44	10	69 at 7 years	32
Oderich et al. (2009)[35]	83	105	72	95	2.4	18	31	31	41 at 5 years	36
Dias et al. (2010)[27]	43	49	100	98	0	23	12	33	—	43
Fioole et al. (2010)[28]	51	60	100	93	0	4	25	22	86	25
Peck et al. (2010)[29]	49	66	89	100	2	16	29	29	64 at 3 years	37
Schoch et al. (2011)[30]	107	116	78	100	0	—	42	42	67	16
Turba et al. (2012)[31]	166	221	74	92	3	10	17	19	67	34
AbuRahma et al. (2013)[32]	83	105	100	97	2	2	35	30	19	31
Grilli et al. (2014)[33a]	47	41	100	87	2	7	17	17	78 at 24 moths	19.1
Barret et al. (2015)[38]	43	—	77	95	0	19	37	37	—	63
Zacharias et al. (2016)[39]	116	143	—	—	5.2	—	23	23	74 at 36 months	37
Covered Stents										
Schoch et al. (2011)[30]	14	14	100	100	0	—	—	0	100	16
Oderich et al. (2013)[4]	42	42	100	98	0	12	10	10	92 at 3 years	19

[a]Considering only occluded superior mesenteric arteries. In one case a covered stent was used, and in others bare metal stents.

and 38% ± 7% for high-risk patients. Freedom from mesenteric-related death was 91% ± 2% after open and 93% ± 4% after endovascular revascularization at 5 years. Independent predictors of any-cause mortality were age greater than 80 years (odds ratio [OR] 3.3, confidence interval [CI] 1.03–1.06, $P = <.001$), chronic kidney disease stage IV or V (OR 5.5, CI 1.4–16.6, $P <.01$), diabetes (OR 1.7, CI 1.2–2.6, $P <.01$) and home oxygen therapy (OR 3.7, CI 1.2–9.1, $P <.001$). Chronic kidney disease stage IV or V (OR 3.4, CI 3.3–345, $P = .003$) and diabetes (OR 4.2, CI 1.7–10.5, $P = .005$) were independently associated with mesenteric-related death. In that study, the most common causes of late death were cardiac events, followed by cancer, respiratory complications, and mesenteric-related complications. The combined rate of early and late mesenteric-related death was 8% for patients treated by the open technique and 6% for those who had endovascular revascularization.

RENAL ARTERY DISEASE

The role of renal revascularization to restore kidney function and improve blood pressure control in patients with RAS has been a topic of controversy in the literature. Open surgical revascularization of renal artery occlusive disease is associated with satisfactory results in patients with renovascular hypertension and ischemic nephropathy but carries higher morbidity and mortality. Endovascular treatment has emerged as a less invasive alternative and is currently the first choice of treatment in most patients when indicated.[41] Improvements in endovascular technology with lower-profile rapid-exchange systems and premounted balloon-expandable stents have increased technical success with these procedures and relegated open surgical repair to patients with unsuitable lesions, multiple recurrences, or complex branch-vessel disease.

The development of endovascular techniques has led to an explosion in renal artery interventions, often with poorly defined indications. In order to address that issue, prospective randomized trials have compared the role of primary stenting with best medical therapy.[42,43] A number of criticisms have been raised with respect to study design and methodology. Nonetheless, it is critical that vascular interventionists understand the rationale for disease management and which endovascular techniques should be applied to revascularize critical renal artery lesions when indicated.

NATURAL HISTORY

Atherosclerosis affecting the renal arteries is a progressive disease that is often an extension of aortic plaque into the renal artery origin.[44] The prevalence of significant atherosclerotic renal artery lesions is estimated at 6.8% in individuals above 65 years of age.[45] Once RAS becomes hemodynamically significant (>60%), progression to renal artery occlusion occurs at an average of 5% per year.[46] Caps and associates[47] showed that 49% of patients with RAS greater than 60% measured by duplex ultrasonography showed disease progression over a 3-year period. Zierler and colleagues[48] also reported progression to occlusion in 5% of patients in the first year and 11% in the second year of follow-up. Renal artery occlusion is associated with kidney atrophy resulting in a mean decrease in kidney length of 1.8 cm in Zierler's report. Renal atrophy can also occur in association with stenotic but nonoccluded renal arteries. Patients with RAS have decreased overall survival, with up to 30% mortality in 2 years, especially if there is concomitant peripheral arterial disease (PAD).[49,50]

DIAGNOSIS

Atherosclerotic RAS affects more often males older than 60 years of age. Patients often have risk factors for atherosclerosis, including diabetes, hyperlipidemia, tobacco use, and hypertension. RAS should be suspected in adults who present with severe or difficult-to-control hypertension despite use of multiple antihypertensive drugs. Progressive deterioration of renal function may result from significant arterial (ischemic) nephropathy. However, the deterioration of renal function without accompanying hypertension makes RAS unlikely. Development of malignant hypertension in a patient with previously well-controlled hypertension is also suggestive of RAS. A less common clinical scenario is flash pulmonary edema from decompensated congestive heart failure in the setting of accelerated hypertension. Physical examination may reveal abdominal bruit and diminished peripheral pulses. Laboratory findings consistent with RAS include refractory hypokalemia and an elevated peripheral renin assay, but these are not sensitive or specific to establish the diagnosis. However, any of these clinical findings, alone or in combination, may raise the index of suspicion and should prompt diagnostic imaging of the renal arteries.

IMAGING STUDIES

Renal duplex ultrasonography is the recommended screening study for RAS. Although it requires significant technical expertise, it is safe and associated with low cost and no radiation exposure. Renal duplex ultrasound provides information on kidney size, cortical thickness, renal artery hemodynamics, and velocity profiles as well as nonvascular anatomic renal abnormalities such as cysts. A peak systolic velocity (PSV) greater than 180 cm/s along with a renal-aortic velocity ratio greater than 3.5 is usually used in most vascular laboratories to determine a greater than 60% stenosis (Fig. 27.6). Sensitivity, specificity, and overall accuracy are 72%, 81%, and 78%, respectively.[51] PSV seems to be the most important factor to be analyzed,[52] and increasing PSV criteria to 220 cm/s may yield better sensitivity and specificity with a negative predictive value of 95%.[53] Ultrasound is limited in patients with a large body habitus and overlying bowel gas obscuring identification of the renal arteries.

The renal resistive index (RRI) may be useful to help predict response to revascularization. In a study by Radermacher and colleagues, a RRI greater than 0.8 indicated poor blood pressure control, progression to dialysis in 46% of patients, and a mortality rate of 29%.[54] A high resistive index could be indicative of intrinsic renal disease not amenable to improvement by revascularization. However, results of the Radermarcher study have not been replicated in other studies.[55]

Cross-sectional imaging is often obtained to confirm RAS or plan treatment using magnetic resonance angiography (MRA) or computed tomography angiography (CTA). MRA with gadolinium has a sensitivity of 90% to 100% and a specificity of 76% to 94% in identifying significant RAS compared with conventional arteriography.[56,57] As a screening modality, MRA is more expensive and less well tolerated by patients compared with duplex scanning or CTA. A concern in patients with advanced renal dysfunction is the risk of nephrogenic systemic fibrosis.[58]

CTA provides accurate reconstructions of abdominal vascular anatomy and pathology with high sensitivity and specificity.[59] This modality is particularly appealing because it combines the accuracy of arteriography with the low risk of intravenous contrast use. The major limitations to widespread use of CTA include the need for iodinated contrast, exposure to ionizing radiation, and significant cost. These factors also limit the use of this modality for serial surveillance of known subcritical stenoses. Nonetheless, CTA is often indicated for planning the procedure when duplex ultrasound shows unusual anatomy, multiple renal artery lesions, or small accessory renal arteries (see Fig. 27.6). It is also useful for demonstrating the severity of calcifications or mural thrombus, which can limit the application of endovascular therapy.

Conventional angiography is currently rarely used to make a diagnosis, but it may be used in conjunction with planned intervention. In the presence of renal insufficiency, carbon dioxide has been used instead of an iodinated contrast agent.[60] Modern endovascular intervention suites and proper planning can also minimize the use of iodinated contrast without sacrificing image quality and procedural safety.[61] Physiologic tests such as peripheral or renal vein renin sampling and nuclear scanning have not been proved sufficiently reliable to be of value in selecting patients for treatment.

ENDOVASCULAR MANAGEMENT

Preprocedure planning and preparation is similar to what has been described for patients with mesenteric artery disease. There are many different combinations of sheaths, guidewires, and other devices that can be used in performing the procedure.

Percutaneous femoral artery access is used in most patients, although a brachial or radial artery approach may be needed in patients with difficult renal artery lesions or if there is caudal angulation or severe aortoiliac occlusive disease. Femoral access is often obtained in the side opposite to the RAS. Following percutaneous arterial access and placement of a 5-French sheath, a flush catheter is placed in the abdominal aorta and positioned at the level of the L1-L2 vertebral interspace for aortography. Contrast can be diluted with saline at 50%. Complete visualization of the renal artery's origins usually requires anteroposterior

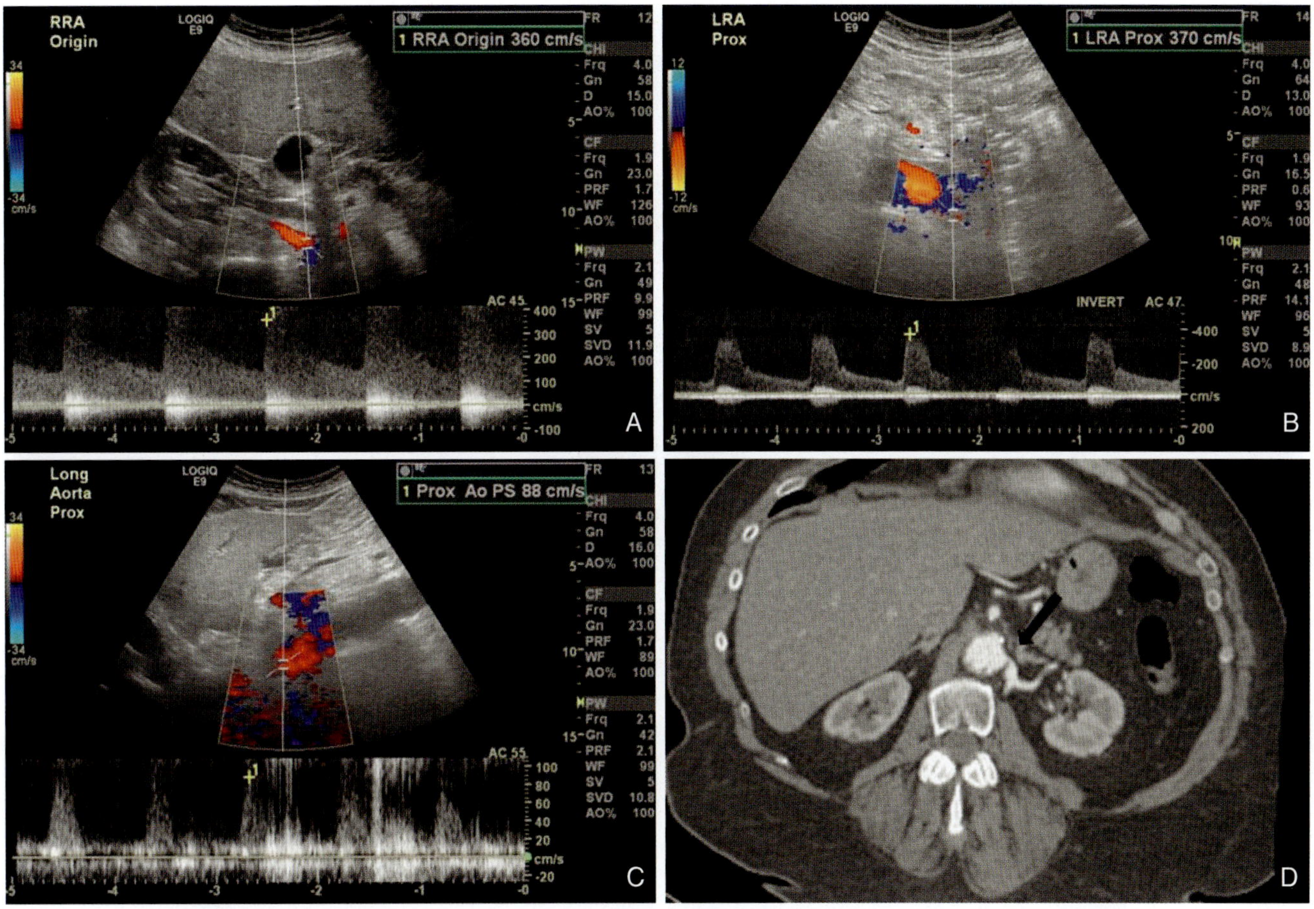

FIG 27.6 Renal duplex ultrasonography and computed tomography angiography (CTA) of a patient with bilateral renal artery stenosis. Right renal artery with peak systolic velocity (PSV) of 360 cm/s and renal-aortic velocity ratio of 4.1 (A). Left renal artery with a PSV of 370 cm/s and renal-aortic velocity ratio of 4.2 (B). Abdominal aorta with PSV of 88 cm/s (C). CTA showing the left renal artery stenosis *(black arrow)* (D).

and oblique views. If a previous high-definition CTA or MRA has been performed, formal aortography may be avoided. In these cases, selective angiography of the targeted vessel is appropriate and can be done using a guide catheter. The angle of gantry projection can be obtained from a review of preoperative imaging studies, thus minimizing contrast use and radiation exposure. The patient should be systemically heparinized prior to selective catheterization or intervention.

The suspected renal artery target is catheterized using a guide catheter of choice with single or two-wire ("no touch") technique (Fig. 27.7). Selective angiography demonstrates the location and severity of the stenosis. Pressure gradient measurements may be obtained across the lesion if there is questionable hemodynamic significance. In most centers, the technique has evolved from use of 0.035-in premounted stents (over a 6 or 7 French sheath) to use of 0.014- to 0.018-in balloon expandable stents via 6- or 7-French guide catheters. The ideal guide catheter is selected based on angle of origin and aortic diameter. In most patients, a left internal mammary artery (LIMA) catheter or renal double curve (RDC) guide catheter is used (Fig. 27.8). The lesion is engaged by the guide tip. The two-wire "no touch"

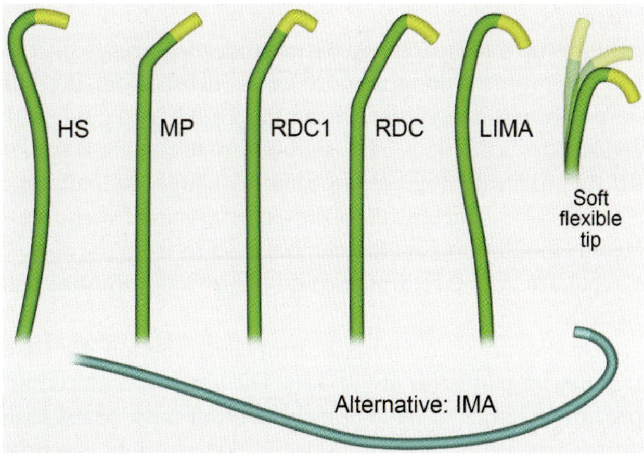

FIG 27.7 Guide catheter shapes for selective catheterization of renal and mesenteric arteries. *HS,* Hockey stick; *IMA,* inferior mesenteric artery; *LIMA,* left internal mammary artery; *MP,* multipurpose; *RDC,* renal double curve; *RDC1,* renal double curve 1.

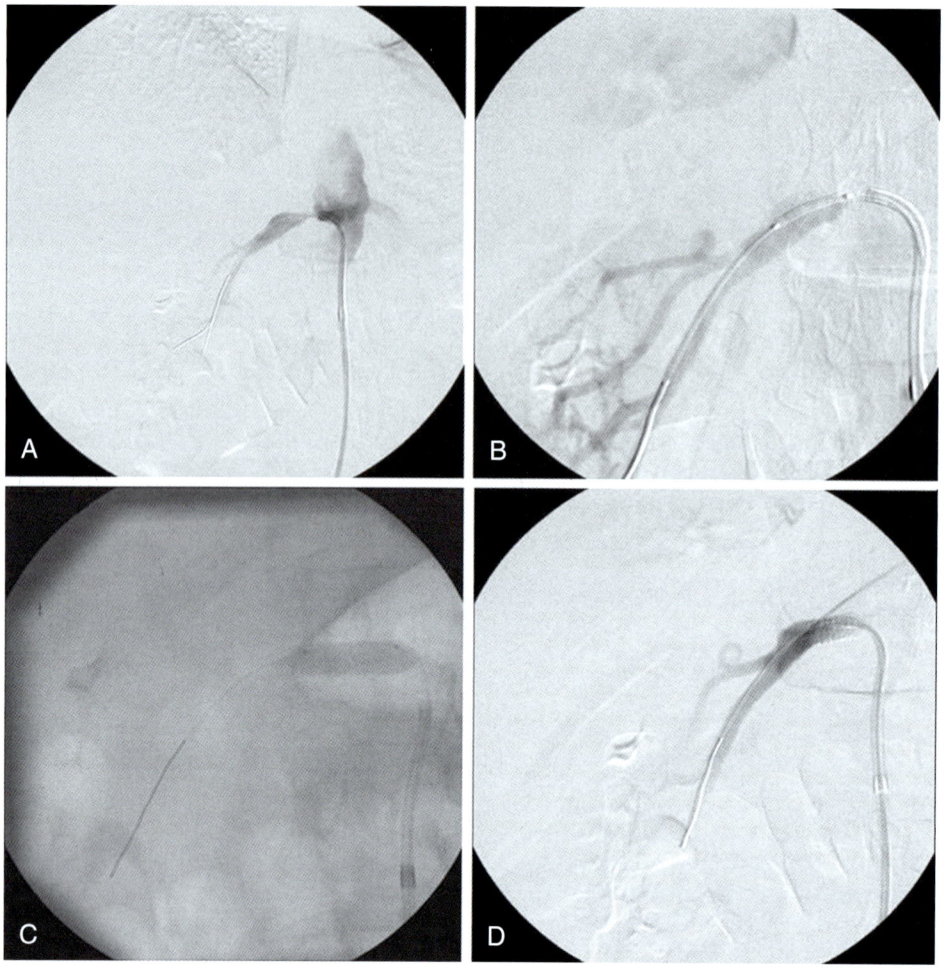

FIG 27.8 Angioplasty using the femoral access of the right renal artery. A 6 or 7 French LIMA guide is positioned in the abdominal aorta. (A) Selective catheterization with choice of catheter and initial selective angiography demonstrating the area of stenosis and distal runoff branches; (B and C) Following deployment and flaring of the bare metal balloon expandable stent. (D) Control angiography without residual stenosis or distal embolization.

technique uses a separate 0.035-in guidewire placed into the aorta to prevent dislodgement of aortic debris from excessive manipulation of the guide catheter tip. The shaped guide catheter provides a stable coaxial support to advance a 0.014- to 0.018-in guidewire, followed by rapid exchange of a balloon or stent. Selective catheterization should be executed with finesse to avoid embolization of atheroembolic debris from the aorta or the renal artery orifice, which could further compromise renal function.

Most systems used for renal artery intervention are based on guidewire platforms of 0.014 in. The wire tip is placed into a proximal segmental renal branch. Caution must be exercised with the passage of any wire to avoid dissection or parenchymal perforation. Atherosclerotic lesions generally require stent placement, whereas fibromuscular dysplasia is usually treated with balloon angioplasty alone. Premounted rapid-exchange balloon-expandable stents are preferred owing to their radial force and precise deployment. These low-profile systems are flexible and usually come in a rapid-exchange configuration. Predilatation is generally not required and may be associated with microembolization of plaque fragments to the renal parenchyma. Stent dimensions range from 12 to 20 mm in length and 4 to 7 mm in diameter. The stent should not be oversized and should be positioned across the lesion, with 1 to 3 mm projecting into the aorta for ostial lesions. Once the stent is deployed, the balloon is deflated and withdrawn. A useful maneuver is to advance the sheath or guide over the balloon as this is being deflated. Wire access across the lesion must be carefully maintained throughout the procedure. A completion angiogram is performed with contrast injected through the side arm of the sheath or guide catheter. The completion study should be critically assessed for technical success (<30% residual stenosis) and for complications such as dissection, thrombosis, emboli, or perforation.

RESULTS

Technical success is most commonly defined as residual stenosis of less than 30%, with no evidence of flow-limiting dissection, perforation, or branch vessel compromise. The most common cause of technical failure is inability to traverse the lesion with a guidewire in 2% to 5% of patients.[62] The use of stents has resulted in increased technical success (>95%) and improved patency rates as compared with balloon angioplasty alone. van de Ven and coworkers[63] performed a randomized, prospective study to compare stent versus plain balloon angioplasty in 84 hypertensive patients. Primary stenting resulted in a higher immediate success rate (88% vs. 57%), primary (75% vs. 29%) and secondary patency (80% vs. 51%) in 6 months as compared with balloon angioplasty, with no difference in complications or long-term clinical results. Currently primary stenting has been established as the treatment of choice in most patients with ostial RAS, when indicated.

A meta-analysis of primary renal artery stenting by Isles and associates[64] documented a technical success rate of 96% to 100%. Restenosis occurred in 9% and 39% at 6 and 12 months. Sivamurthy and colleagues[65] reported primary patency of 82% and primary assisted patency of 100% at 5 years. Complication rates are low in most reports, but there is a risk of inadvertent dissection, perforation, or thrombosis, which can result in loss of a kidney. Martin and associates[66] reviewed complication rates in 2994 patients treated by endovascular revascularization. Periprocedural complication rates ranged from 12% to 36%. The most common complications were groin hematoma and puncture-site trauma, both occurring in approximately 5% of patients. The incidence of symptomatic renal artery embolization varied from 1% to 8%, with renal artery occlusion rates between 0.8% and 2.5%.

Blood Pressure Response

The ASTRAL trial[42] randomized 806 patients with atherosclerotic renovascular disease to receive either endovascular revascularization with medical therapy or medical therapy alone. The primary end point was renal function and the secondary outcomes were blood pressure control, time to renal and major cardiovascular events, and any-cause mortality. The CORAL trial[43] randomized 947 patients with RAS and hypertension with use of at least two medications or chronic kidney disease to receive either stent and medical therapy or medical therapy alone. Neither study showed any clinical difference between groups, although the CORAL trial did show a small but statistically significant decrease in systolic blood pressure over time.

These two trials are considered landmark investigations in the management of renovascular disease. Nonetheless, both suffered major critiques because of several methodologic flaws. The ASTRAL trial enrolled 41% of patients with moderate stenosis (<50%) that otherwise would not have required treatment. Other major critiques of the ASTRAL study included the low level of recruitment per center, with 67% of centers recruiting less than nine patients over a 7-year period.[67] The CORAL trial made many changes in the enrollment criteria in order to achieve the planned number of patients. These included a change in the minimal systolic hypertension threshold of 155 mm Hg to a nonspecific level or even a normal level. In addition, one-third of patients had well-controlled hypertension, one-third had less than 60% RAS, and one-third had diabetes. Last, both studies might have suffered from preselection bias by the investigators, meaning that patients who were seen as potentially benefiting the most were preselected for treatment without randomization.[67,68] Nonetheless, despite these methodologic shortcomings, similar results were found in other randomized trials.[69,70] At least three recently published meta-analyses[71-73] from the most relevant trials have failed to identify any benefit from renal artery stenting over best medical therapy alone.[71] Results of these published reports are summarized in Table 27.2.

TABLE 27.2 Characteristics of Selected Randomized Clinical Trials Published for Renal Artery Angioplasty

Trial (Year)	*N*	PI	MT	Design	Inclusion Criteria	Assessment Point	Technique of Intervention	End Points
DRASTIC (2000)[70]	106	56	50	Prospective, single center, randomized	Resistant HTN with CRI	3 and 12 months	Angioplasty (no stent in 96.4%)	Primary: BP at 3 and 12 months Secondary: Treatment score, SCr, SCr Clearance
ASTRAL (2009)[42]	806	403	403	Prospective, multicenter, randomized	Resistant HTN with CRI	1–3 months, 6–8 months, and 1, 2, 3, 4 and 5 years	Angioplasty (used stent in 93%)	Primary: change in renal function Secondary: BP, time to first renal event, time to first cardiovascular event and mortality
STAR (2009)[69]	140	64	74	Prospective, multicenter, randomized	CRI	3–24 months	Angioplasty (used stent in 98%)	Primary: 20% or greater reduction in creatinine clearance Secondary: BP, cardiovascular morbidity and mortality
CORAL (2013)[43]	947	442	478	Prospective, multicenter, randomized	Resistant HTN with CRI	3, 6, 9 months and 1, 2, 3, 4, 5 years (mean of 43 months)	Renal artery stenting	Primary: composite of death, stroke, myocardial infarction, hospitalization for congestive heart failure, progressive renal insufficiency, or the need for permanent renal replacement therapy Secondary: all-cause mortality, in detail

MT, Medical therapy; *PI*, percutaneous intervention.

Changes in Renal Function

Even before the ASTRAL and CORAL trial "era," results of endovascular intervention for ischemic nephropathy were not compelling. Both the ASTRAL and CORAL studies failed to identify a difference in renal function outcomes compared with medical therapy. A review of pooled data from randomized trials and other reports has also demonstrated lack of a beneficial effect in patients with RAS.[71-73]

Despite the negative findings from the randomized trials, some retrospective studies suggest that selected subgroup of patients may benefit from revascularization. Beutler and colleagues[74] found that stent placement resulted in the stabilization of renal function in 87% of patients with rapidly declining renal function. No effect on renal function was evident when patients with stable renal function were treated. Burket and colleagues[75] reported that 43% of patients with baseline renal insufficiency showed significant improvement in renal function after intervention. Small case series have demonstrated the recovery of dialysis patients after stenting.[76-78]

Surgical revascularization remains an option available for the treatment of ischemic nephropathy in select patients. Large single-center reports have documented that surgical revascularization provides substantial improvement in renal function, particularly if the RAS is bilateral or affects a solitary kidney.[79-81] In addition, the more severe the renal insufficiency, the greater the benefit seen. A randomized series of 50 patients comparing open surgical reconstruction and stenting for RAS showed longer durability and lower morbidity for open reconstructions.[82]

Patient Survival

There is no evidence that renal artery stenting improves survival over medical therapy alone. The CORAL trial was designed specifically with the following primary end points: death from cardiovascular or renal causes, myocardial infarction, stroke, hospitalization for congestive heart failure, progressive renal insufficiency, or the need for renal replacement therapy. It also analyzed noncomposite survival and other complications as secondary end points. With a mean follow up of 43 months, there was no difference in patient survival between the two treatment arms.[43] Whether a difference in survival will appear with further observation between groups remains to be seen.[71-73]

Current Indications for Renal Artery Revascularization

The reported results of the randomized trials have tempered the liberal indications for renal artery stenting. Nephrologists and endovascular interventionists share a common understanding that there are select groups of patients that probably benefit from revascularization. These patients may not have been adequately identified in the randomized studies because of the limitations already discussed. Consequently the decision to intervene is ultimately a clinical judgment and can never be made with absolute certainty of benefit.[83] Table 27.3 shows a list of clinical situations where revascularization is currently recommended.

TABLE 27.3 List of Accepted Indications for Renal Revascularization

Patients With High Likelihood of Benefiting From Renal Intervention

Unilateral Stenosis
- A short duration of blood pressure elevation prior to the diagnosis of renovascular disease, since this is the strongest clinical predictor of a fall in blood pressure after renal revascularization;
- Failure of optimal medical therapy to control the blood pressure;
- Intolerance to optimal medical therapy (e.g., deterioration of renal function during antihypertensive drug therapy);
- Recurrent flash pulmonary edema and/or refractory heart failure.

Bilateral Stenosis (and Unilateral Stenosis in a Single Viable Kidney)
- All the criteria for unilateral stenosis;
- Otherwise unexplained progressive renal insufficiency

CONCLUSIONS

Mesenteric disease and renal artery disease share similar anatomic features and etiology in that both are usually atherosclerotic lesions. For mesenteric disease, endovascular treatment is safe and effective, and it significantly reduces morbidity. Open surgical reconstruction is considered for patients who are not suitable for or have failed the endovascular approach.

The indications for renal angioplasty and stenting have changed since the report of randomized trials, which indicated no benefit in patients with RAS. Despite their methodologic flaws, the most recent randomized trials have at least drawn the line, which separates a group of patients that clearly have no benefit to receive invasive treatment from another group that is very unlikely to ever be analyzed in the light of higher level of evidence because it would simply be unethical to do so. The technical aspects of renal artery angioplasty and stenting are well developed and well refined, being safely executed in the hands of experienced surgeons and interventionists. To adequately identify the individuals with a higher likelihood of benefiting from the intervention is as important as the procedure itself for the achievement of good clinical results.

REVIEW QUESTIONS

1. Which of the following alternatives is correct with respect to the management of patients with mesenteric arterial disease?
   - **a.** The most common etiology is ostial atherosclerotic disease.
   - **b.** Patients with two-vessel asymptomatic mesenteric artery stenosis benefit from prophylactic revascularization.
   - **c.** Long-term parenteral nutrition is an acceptable treatment option.
   - **d.** Computed tomography angiography is the recommended imaging modality for screening.
   - **e.** A and D are correct.
2. Endovascular revascularization for chronic mesenteric ischemia has gained acceptance as the first treatment option in most patients. Based on the reported literature, which alternative is correct with respect to mesenteric angioplasty and stenting?
   - **a.** Primary angioplasty offers a similar rate of symptom relief and restenosis as stenting.
   - **b.** The primary target vessel for revascularization is the superior mesenteric artery whenever possible.
   - **c.** Covered stents are associated with lower patency rates due to a higher rate of intimal hyperplasia as compared with bare metal stents.
   - **d.** Self-expandable stents are used in most patients.
   - **e.** The procedure is contraindicated in the presence of mesenteric occlusion.
3. Which of the following conditions would be most amenable to mesenteric stenting?
   - **a.** Chronic epigastric pain and extrinsic compression of the celiac axis in a 50-year-old female
   - **b.** Three-vessel mesenteric disease and long-segment occlusion of the SMA in a healthy 65-year-old male
   - **c.** Giant cell arteritis affecting the proximal SMA in a 55-year-old female.
   - **d.** Focal stenosis of the SMA and celiac axis in a 75-year-old female with no symptoms
   - **e.** Postprandial pain and high-grade stenosis of the SMA and celiac axis in a 63-year-old female
4. Which alternative is an accepted indication for renal artery angioplasty and stenting?
   - **a.** Bilateral renal artery stenosis with recurrent flash pulmonary edema
   - **b.** Failure of four-drug medical therapy to control blood pressure
   - **c.** Intolerance to multidrug antihypertensive therapy
   - **d.** Difficult-to-control hypertension in a young patient with bilateral renal fibromuscular dysplasia
   - **e.** All of the above

References available online at expertconsult.com.

28 CHAPTER

Surgical Management of Femoral, Popliteal, and Tibial Arterial Occlusive Disease

Frank J. Veith, Neal S. Cayne, Gregg S. Landis, Nicholas J. Gargiulo III, Evan C. Lipsitz, Enrico Ascher

This chapter discusses open surgical options for femoral, popliteal, and tibial arterial occlusive disease. Although some of these procedures may also be performed for disabling intermittent claudication, the vast majority should only be performed for critical lower limb ischemia, which is defined as sufficiently poor arterial blood supply to pose a threat to the viability of the lower extremity. Manifestations of critical ischemia are rest pain, ulceration, and gangrene. These manifestations typically occur due to arteriosclerotic occlusive disease of large, medium-sized, or small arteries, although other etiologies can produce or contribute to these ischemic conditions. For example, many nonvascular causes result in limb pain at rest, infection may cause or contribute to gangrene, and trauma and decreased sensation may produce ulceration. Although thromboembolism and other etiologies can produce acute critical limb ischemia, this chapter will address only chronic lower extremity ischemia owing to obliterative arteriosclerosis. Over the last 3 decades, it has become increasingly apparent that limbs that are threatened by this process almost always have multilevel occlusive disease, which often includes occlusions of arteries in the thigh, leg, and foot.[1]

Surgical options for chronic critical lower limb ischemia include local amputations of toes and other portions of the foot, a variety of debriding procedures including open amputations of portions of the foot to control infection, and a variety of traditional surgical revascularization procedures, primarily vein and prosthetic arterial bypasses above or below the inguinal ligament. Occasionally these procedures may be supplemented with localized endarterectomies with or without patch angioplasties, except for an occasional patient with common femoral artery (CFA) or deep femoral artery (DFA) lesions, these operations are rarely sufficient to save a severely ischemic limb.

TOE AND FOOT AMPUTATIONS, DEBRIDEMENTS, AND CONSERVATIVE TREATMENT

Although a detailed description of these procedures is beyond the scope of this chapter, certain principles should be emphasized. Gangrenous and infected toes can be successfully amputated by closed or open techniques in patients with good circulation, manifested by pedal pulses. Extensive debriding and partial foot amputations will usually heal in patients if all infected and necrotic tissue is excised. Such procedures will result in patients regaining effective walking. Amputation of one or more gangrenous or ulcerated toes or limited debriding may also result in a healed foot in patients without distal pulses and substantial arterial occlusive disease (e.g., an occluded superficial femoral artery [SFA]). Determination of moderately good collateral circulation by ankle-brachial indices or pulse volume recordings may be helpful in predicting healing; however, sometimes in patients with borderline circulation, a trial at local procedures is warranted before proceeding with a major effort at revascularization. If prompt healing does not occur, revascularization is justified and should be performed without delay.

Some patients with critical ischemia, manifested by mild ischemic rest pain or limited gangrene or ulceration, can be treated conservatively with good foot care, antibiotics, analgesics, and limited ambulation.[2] Conservative treatment is indicated in patients who might not tolerate revascularization procedures because of major comorbidities. Long periods of palliation and occasional healing of small ulcerations or gangrenous patches may occur in a few patients with critical ischemia.[2]

HISTORY OF AGGRESSIVE APPROACH TO LIMB SALVAGE

In the 1960s and 1970s, major below-knee or above-knee amputation was regarded as the safest and best treatment for gangrene and ulceration from arteriosclerotic occlusive disease below the inguinal ligament,[3] despite the effectiveness of reconstructive arterial surgery (bypass and endarterectomy) for aortoiliac occlusive disease and despite some occasional positive results from femoropopliteal and even femorotibial bypasses. Because we had access to unusually good arteriography that visualized all the arteries in the leg and foot (Fig. 28.1), we developed and promoted an aggressive approach to salvage threatened limbs, including those with extensive gangrene.[4] More than 96% of patients with threatened limbs were subjected to an effort to save the limb. Only 4%, those with severe dementia or gangrene extending beyond the midfoot, were excluded. Only 6% of all patients with threatened limbs, when examined by arteriography, had no patent artery in the leg or foot that could serve as an outflow site for a bypass.[4] With improvements in technique, this proportion of patients with arteries unsuitable for a bypass fell to 1% to 2%.[1,5-11] Successful foot salvage was achieved in 81% to 95%

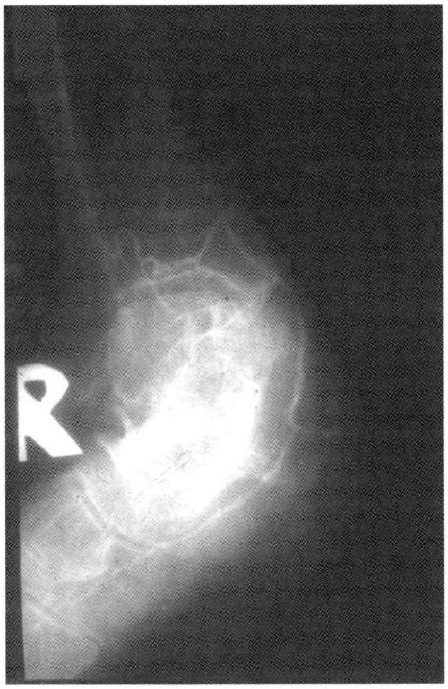

FIG 28.1 This 83-year-old patient with diabetes had a gangrenous great toe. A vein bypass to the posterior tibial artery in 1971 resulted in limb salvage for 10 years after the limb-threatening event. (From Veith FJ, Cayne NS, Gargiulo NJ III, et al: Surgical options for critical limb ischemia. In Bosiers M, Schneider P, editors: *Critical Limb Ischemia*, New York, 2009, Informa Healthcare, pp 195–208.)

of patients in whom bypasses were performed for the period that they lived, up to 5 years.[1,4] However, 52% of these limb salvage patients had medical comorbidities and died, usually from cardiac causes, within the first 5 years after their initial bypass.[4] More than two-thirds of the patients who lived beyond 5 years retained a useable limb and were able to ambulate beyond the 5-year time point.[4] However, to maintain limb salvage, many of these patients required reoperation or reintervention because they developed a failed (thrombosed) or failing (threatened but patent) graft from a lesion in their graft or its inflow or outflow tract.[1,4,5] These limb salvage results were achieved because of a myriad of improvements in the surgical techniques,[1,4-11] developed to facilitate the reoperations these patients required,[12-14] and because of improved anesthetic and intensive care management of limb-salvage patients who often had advanced cardiorespiratory disease, poor kidney function, and diabetes. Collectively, these improvements made it possible to attempt limb salvage in almost every patient with a threatened limb and intact brain function.[1,4,9] Many vascular centers throughout the world adopted these policies and were able to achieve equally good results.

EARLY USE OF ENDOVASCULAR TECHNIQUES WITH BYPASS SURGERY

In the mid-1970s, some centers embraced the use of percutaneous transluminal angioplasty (PTA) to treat elderly patients with critical limb ischemia.[4] Initially, PTA was used to correct hemodynamically significant iliac artery stenosis. In most instances, it was combined with some form of infrainguinal bypass. However, as PTA techniques improved, balloon angioplasty was used to treat short iliac occlusions and some SFA lesions. Approximately 20% of patients with a threatened limb could be treated with PTA alone without an adjunctive bypass, whereas another 14% required some form of open surgical revascularization along with their PTA.[1] These percentages increased and results improved with the introduction of iliac stents. As technical improvements in endovascular technology were developed, it became possible to use popliteal, infrapopliteal, and tibial PTA to treat some of these limb salvage patients less invasively and to avoid some of the systemic and local complications of the lengthy and sometimes difficult distal operations in these high-risk elderly patients.[15-17] These endovascular techniques could also be used to treat patients with failed or failing bypasses, because reoperative procedures are often more difficult than primary bypass operations.[1,4,18,19] Sometimes (in approximately 20% of patients) PTA eliminated the need for a secondary bypass: more often it made the secondary bypass simpler. In addition, we developed a number of unusual approaches to lower extremity arteries to facilitate reoperations by eliminating the need to redissect previously dissected arteries.[12-14,20]

CURRENT AND FUTURE RELATIONSHIP BETWEEN ENDOVASCULAR TREATMENTS AND OPEN BYPASS SURGERY

Recent improvements in catheter, guidewire, stent, and stent-graft technology have transformed the treatment of lower limb ischemia from a primarily open surgical modality, supplemented by catheter-based treatments, to a primarily endovascular modality supplemented by surgery. Most who treat critical ischemia regard endovascular treatments as the first option to treat chronic obstructive arteriosclerosis at all levels, including disease in the leg and foot. Indeed, there are some endovascular enthusiasts who mistakenly believe they have originated the limb salvage concept, and some maintain that if a limb cannot be salvaged by endovascular treatment, the next option should be a major amputation.

Although endovascular treatment should be the first therapeutic option to revascularize a critically ischemic limb in most patients, some patients whose leg and foot cannot be saved by endovascular treatment can undergo an open surgical bypass procedure to salvage a foot.

Although there are still some indications for open surgical bypasses for limb-threatening ischemia, there is wide variation in opinions about the proportion of patients with critical ischemia that require an open bypass at some point in their disease process. We believe that at least 20% to 35% of patients with critical ischemia will require open surgery at some point in the course of their disease, although endovascular techniques continue to improve, so that this proportion may decrease in the future. We also believe that such procedures will usually be indicated after failures of one, or usually more, endovascular treatments, although there are some patients with extensive foot gangrene, long occlusions, limited target outflow arteries, and a good greater saphenous vein in whom a bypass is the best initial treatment option.[21,22]

The initial surgical option depends on many factors, such as the age and health of the patient, the pattern of disease, and the skills of the involved interventionalist and surgeon. One real concern is that, as fewer bypasses are performed, fewer surgeons will be skilled in these demanding bypass techniques, particularly in the difficult circumstances in which they will be needed. Perhaps referral centers for bypasses should be established for the same reasons that such centers have been recommended for patients who require open thoracoabdominal aneurysm repair.

It has been recognized for many years that repetitive or redo procedures are an important component of care for patients with critical ischemia.[1,4,5] Endovascular procedures may be used to salvage limbs after failed or failing open surgical bypasses,[1,18,19] and this tendency will increase as technology improves. Similarly, bypass operations or partially open thrombectomy will be required after early or late failure of endovascular procedures or prior bypasses in patients in whom no further endovascular options are available. Most of the 20% to 35% of critical ischemia patients who require an open surgical bypass or thrombectomy will require it in such a setting.

There are certain principles and precautions that should be followed by those performing endovascular interventions for limb ischemia. These interventions should be performed in a way that preserves at least one good target outflow artery, leaving the option of an open surgical rescue if the intervention fails. In addition, care must be taken not to render initially patent arterial segments unusable, thereby necessitating a more distal bypass than would have been required before the endovascular procedure. Moreover, key collateral vessels should be preserved so that the patient will not be worse than he originally was if the intervention fails.

SPECIFIC OPEN SURGICAL REVASCULARIZATION PROCEDURES

Open surgical revascularization procedures fall under two major headings: bypass procedures with and without thrombectomy and revision of failed (thrombosed) prior bypasses that cannot be rescued by endovascular means. The latter circumstance is usually associated with an organized fibrinous plug that cannot be lysed, dilated, or removed at the proximal or distal anastomosis of a prosthetic bypass.

SUPERFICIAL FEMORAL ARTERY AND ABOVE-KNEE POPLITEAL OCCLUSIVE DISEASE

With the introduction of improved techniques for crossing total occlusions, subintimal or intraluminal PTA can be used to treat most occlusions of the SFA and above-knee popliteal artery. Nitinol self-expanding stents and stent-grafts (Viabahn, W. L. Gore, Flagstaff, AZ) can be used as adjuncts to these procedures.[23-25] When performing these procedures, care must be taken not to violate the principles and precautions outlined previously and to preserve important collateral vessels, such as the DFA. In the unusual instance when these endovascular interventions fail and cannot be restored to patency or when technical difficulty is encountered, a femoropopliteal bypass can be performed to the below-knee popliteal artery or tibioperoneal trunk via standard medial approaches.[26] This bypass is best performed with a reversed great saphenous vein, harvested via skip incisions, although endoscopic vein harvest has been described[27]; however, this technique requires special equipment and technical expertise. In situ vein bypass offers no advantage in the femoropopliteal position. If the groin is heavily scarred or infected, the distal two-thirds of the DFA can be accessed directly in the thigh and used for bypass inflow (or outflow if a bypass ends in the groin).[13] In circumstances in which the medial approach to the popliteal artery is difficult or impossible because of scarring or infection, both the above-knee and the below-knee popliteal arteries can be accessed via lateral approaches and used for bypass outflow.[14] If this is done, the graft can be tunneled laterally in a subcutaneous plane. If patients do not have a saphenous vein or arm vein or if their veins are too small (<3.5 mm in distended diameter) or involved with preexisting disease[28] and they require a femoropopliteal bypass, a 6-mm polytetrafluoroethylene (PTFE) conduit may be used.[29] If a vein conduit is used, postop duplex surveillance is warranted and reintervention is justified for a failing (threatened) graft. However, if the graft has failed (thrombosed), reintervention is indicated only if the failure results in critical ischemia, which occurs in approximately 65% of cases in whom the original bypass was performed for critical ischemia.[12]

TIBIAL AND PERONEAL ARTERY BYPASSES

Tibial and peroneal artery bypasses may be indicated after multiple failures of endovascular treatments. Some also believe that these bypasses are indicated when long segments of all three crural vessels and the below-knee popliteal or tibioperoneal trunk are occluded, especially if extensive foot necrosis is present. However, even in this circumstance, long-segment tibial subintimal PTA is effective.[30] However, no one has been able to duplicate some tibial artery results, despite enthusiasm for subintimal PTA for shorter lesions and in the SFA and popliteal arteries.[31]

For tibial and peroneal bypasses, autologous vein is the graft of choice, if it is disease-free.[28] The source of the superficial vein can be from any limb or site, and the vein can be used in the reversed or in situ configuration. A randomized comparison of reversed and in situ vein grafts to crural arteries demonstrated no significant patency or limb salvage differences, except for veins less than 3 mm in distended diameter.[32] In this circumstance, in situ grafts performed better, but the difference was not statistically significant. To facilitate the use of vein as the conduit, the grafts should be as short as possible. In addition, the SFA, the popliteal artery, and even tibial arteries have proved to be effective sites of origin for these distal bypasses, when there is no significant proximal disease (Figs. 28.2–28.4).[6-8,10] If proximal disease is present, it can often be treated with PTA, enabling a distal short vein graft without compromising patency.[33] Moreover, if there is a patent popliteal blind or isolated segment (without tibial or peroneal outflow) and limited lengths of autologous vein, a composite sequential bypass may be performed, with the distal component being a vein graft from the isolated popliteal to a patent tibial artery and the proximal component being a PTFE graft from a femoral artery to the proximal end of the

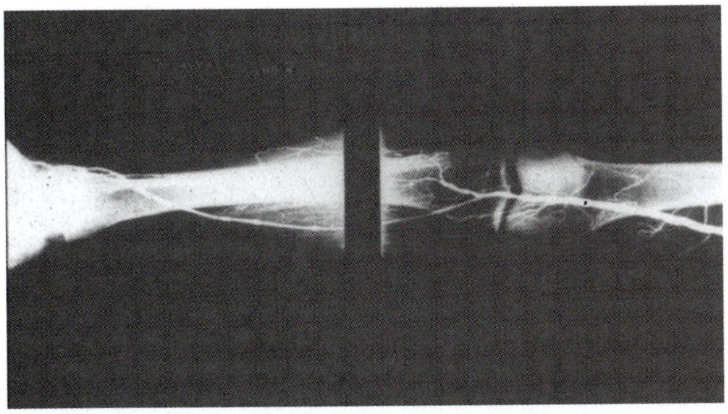

FIG 28.2 This arteriogram was obtained 10 years after a reversed vein bypass from the below-knee popliteal artery to the distal anterior tibial artery. (From Veith FJ, Cayne NS, Garbiulo NJ III, et al: Surgical options for critical limb ischemia. In Bosiers M, Schneider P, editors: *Critical Limb Ischemia*, New York, 2009, Informa Healthcare, pp 195–208.)

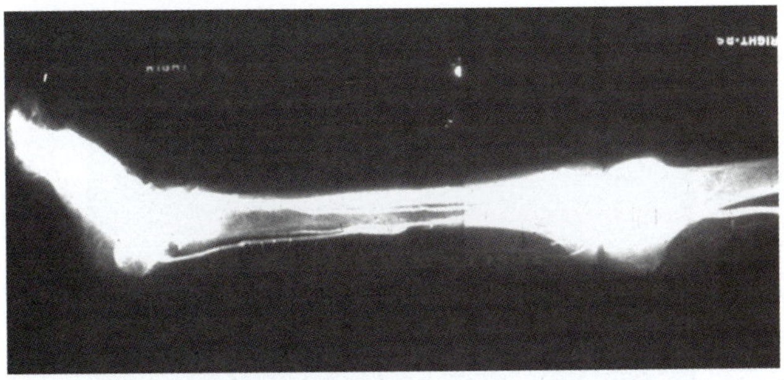

FIG 28.3 This tibiotibial bypass performed with a reversed vein graft was patent after 12 years. (From Veith FJ, Ascer E, Gupta SK, et al: Tibiotibial vein bypass grafts: a new operation for limb salvage. *J Vasc Surg* 2:552–557, 1985.)

vein graft.[34] If a patient with critical ischemia is faced with an imminent amputation and is without satisfactory autologous vein, a PTFE tibial bypass is an acceptable option, and good secondary patency and limb salvage results have been demonstrated (43% 5-year secondary patency and 66% 5-year limb salvage) in this setting (Figs. 28.5 and 28.6).[29,35] Although some advocate the use of a distal vein patch or cuff to improve patency,[36] others are not convinced that any of these adjunctive procedures improve patency results more than a carefully constructed distal PTFE anastomosis. In the authors' recent experience, PTFE bypasses to leg arteries have a role in achieving and maintaining limb salvage when other options are not available.[37] The graft must, however, be implanted into a leg artery that has luminal continuity to its normal terminal branches and preferably richly supplies the foot, and the surgeon must be willing to do a secondary or redo prosthetic tibial bypass if the original graft fails.[37] Many groups have not been able to duplicate these results, although others have.[38,39]

BYPASSES TO FOOT ARTERIES AND THEIR BRANCHES

In the late 1970s and early 1980s, it was realized that many patients who were thought to have patterns of arteriosclerosis

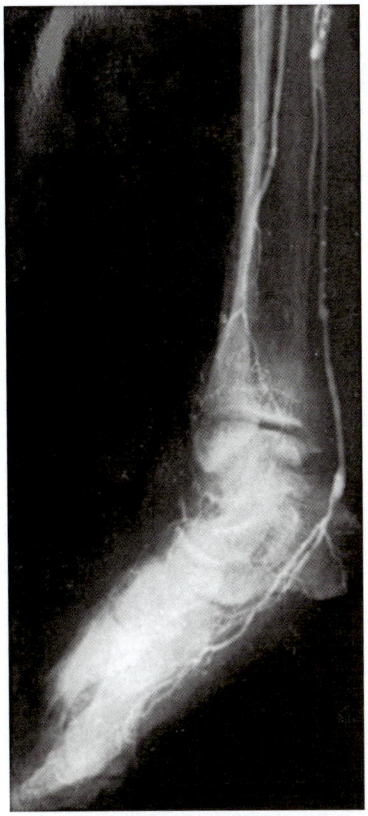

FIG 28.4 A magnified arteriographic view of the foot of the patient shown in Fig. 28.3. Twelve-year limb salvage was achieved despite an incomplete plantar arch. (From Veith FJ, Ascer E, Gupta SK, et al: Tibiotibial vein bypass grafts: a new operation for limb salvage. *J Vasc Surg* 2:552–557, 1985.)

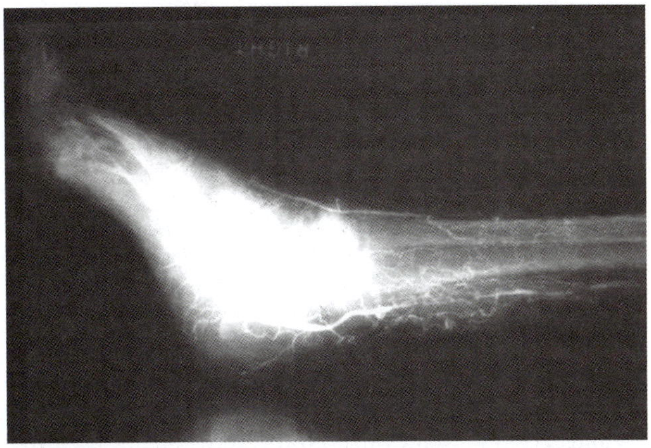

FIG 28.5 This arteriogram is from a patient with great toe gangrene. There is only an isolated posterior tibial artery segment. No other patent arterial segments were available as targets for revascularization, and no autologous vein available for a bypass. (From Veith FJ, Cayne NS, Gargiulo NJ III, et al: Surgical options for critical limb ischemia. In Bosiers M, Schneider P, editors: *Critical Limb Ischemia*, New York, 2009, Informa Healthcare, pp 195–208.)

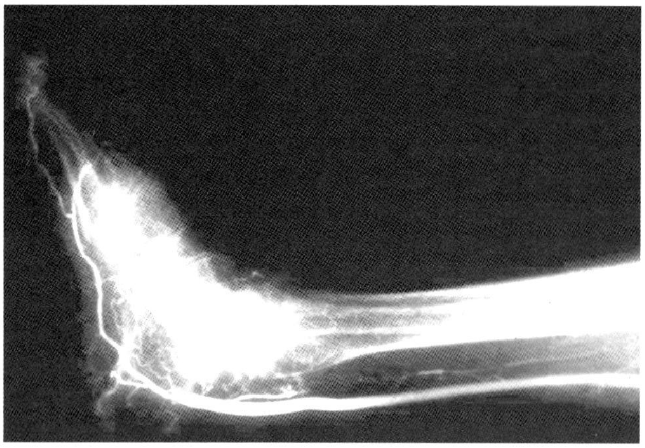

FIG 28.6 A prosthetic bypass with a polytetrafluoroethylene graft was performed to the isolated segment shown in Fig. 28.5. This arteriogram was obtained 4 years after the original operation. Patency was maintained until the patient's death 6 years after the operation. (From Veith FJ, Cayne NS, Gargiulo NJ III, et al: Surgical options for critical limb ischemia. In Bosiers M, Schneider P, editors: *Critical Limb Ischemia*, New York, 2009, Informa Healthcare, pp 195–208.)

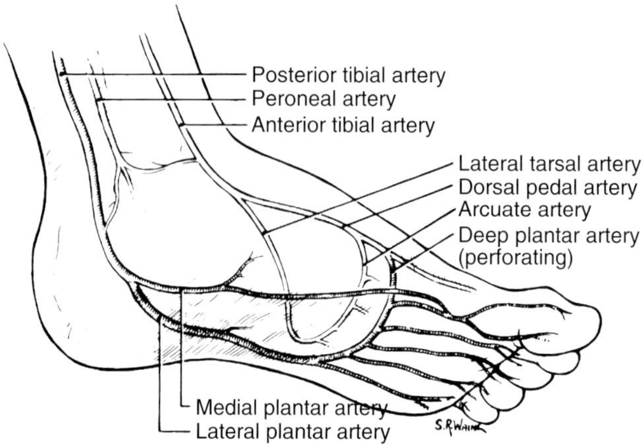

FIG 28.7 Diagram showing important pedal arteries. All these named arteries can be used for limb salvage revascularizations. (From Ascer E, Veith FJ, Gupta SK: Bypasses to plantar arteries and other tibial branches: an extended approach to limb salvage. *J Vasc Surg* 8:434–441, 1988.)

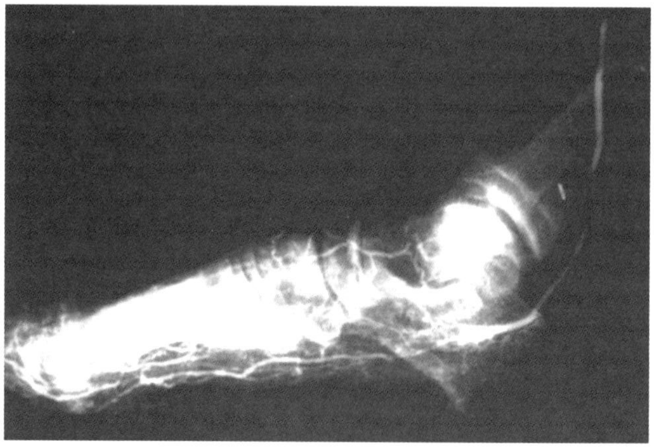

FIG 28.8 This arteriogram was obtained 4 years after a reversed vein graft to the lateral plantar artery. (From Veith FJ, Cayne NS, Gargiulo NJ III, et al: Surgical options for critical limb ischemia. In Bosiers M, Schneider P, editors: *Critical Limb Ischemia*, New York, 2009, Informa Healthcare, pp 195–208.)

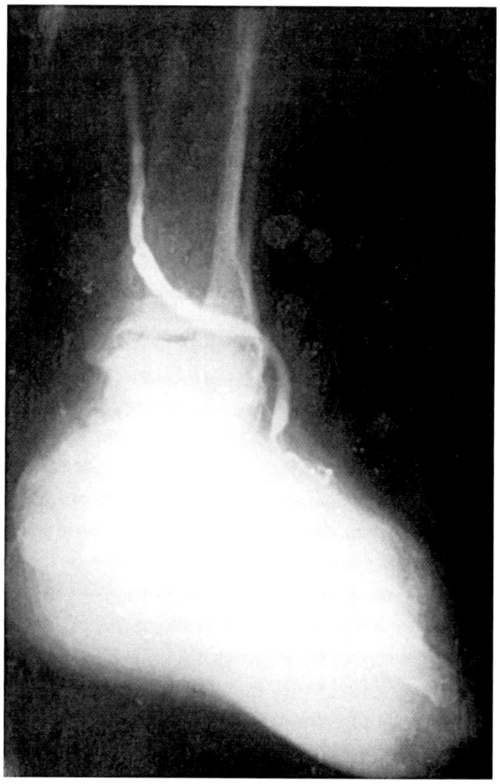

FIG 28.9 This arteriogram was obtained 12 years after a reversed vein bypass to the lateral tarsal artery. Note the forefoot amputation required to obtain healing. Despite this, the patient walked normally. (From Ascer E, Veith FJ, Gupta SK: Bypasses to plantar arteries and other tibial branches: an extended approach to limb salvage. *J Vasc Surg* 8:434–441, 1988.)

totally unsuited for revascularization actually had patent arteries in their foot that could be used as outflow sites for distal bypasses (Fig. 28.7).[1,4,7,10] By performing bypasses to these vessels, it was possible to substantially increase the number of critical ischemia patients whose threatened limb could be saved (Figs. 28.8 and 28.9).[1,7,10] Many other groups subsequently confirmed these initial results.

These distal grafts should only be performed with vein as a conduit; however, many of these grafts may originate from the below-knee popliteal artery or even from patent proximal tibial arteries (see Figs. 28.2–28.4).[1,6,7,10] As with all infrainguinal bypass grafts, and especially those to crural arteries, the procedures must be performed with care and technical perfection. Any technical error in graft preparation, tunneling, or anastomotic construction will result in failure. Good lighting (headlight), a dry field, and patience are essential. Magnification and microsurgical instruments are often required, and care must be taken to treat outflow arteries atraumatically and to preserve all outflow branches, even the small ones that are unnamed. Completion arteriography (cinefluoroscopy) is also essential, as with all infrapopliteal bypasses, to assure good anastomotic configuration and bypass flow rates. If spasm or decreased flow is noted, vasodilators (nitroglycerin, papaverine) may be helpful.[40] Additional technical details and illustrations are provided in a recent textbook chapter that goes beyond the scope of this chapter.[26]

Although these foot artery procedures were developed before endovascular approaches existed to revascularize these very distal arteries, they still have a role. Coronary balloons, 0.14-inch guidewire-based systems, and stents are now being used to revascularize patent arteries in the lower leg and foot. Although these techniques can work well in the short term, long-term results are unclear, and it remains to be determined how these results will compare with bypass operations.

NEWER TECHNIQUES FOR REDO PROCEDURES AFTER FAILED BYPASSES

It is well known that infrainguinal revascularization procedures, both endovascular and open surgical, are associated with progressive failure due to a diminished luminal caliber, followed by thrombosis. This is due to both intimal hyperplasia, which is largely a reaction to vascular injury, and progression of the arteriosclerotic process. When bypasses or PTAs that have been performed for critical ischemia fail after a patency interval of 6 months or longer, the originally threatened limb is only threatened again in approximately 65% of patients. This may be due to healing of the original gangrenous or ulcerated lesion and greater blood flow is required to achieve healing than to maintain it. Alternatively, the maintenance of a healed foot after a revascularization failure may be due to improved collateral blood flow or absence of the trauma or infection that initially contributed to the gangrene or ulceration.

Management strategies for patients with failed revascularization procedures should be influenced by the understanding that critical ischemia might not recur. Only if critical ischemia is present should a secondary intervention be undertaken, because secondary procedures are generally more difficult and have worse results than primary procedures. Thus redo procedures are not indicated to prevent critical ischemia. The one exception is when a primary procedure is determined by physical examination, symptoms, or noninvasive testing to be in a failing mode (i.e., threatened by the development of a new or recurrent lesion that reduces flow but without thrombosis of the revascularization).

A full description of all possible redo procedures that are indicated when a primary bypass (with vein or prosthetic) fails is beyond the scope of this chapter and is available elsewhere.[12] Nevertheless some principles deserve emphasis, in addition to those already mentioned. First, endovascular interventions should always be considered as the first option in patients requiring a redo procedure, even if the original revascularization was a bypass. Improved technology that was previously unavailable may provide sufficient increased blood flow to maintain foot viability.

Second, redissection of previously dissected arteries, particularly in the groin, should be avoided because they are difficult to perform and prone to an increased risk of infection. If a totally new bypass is required, as is usually the case when a failed vein graft cannot be freed of clot, alternate or new approaches to patent arteries should be used.[12-14,20]

Third, complete preprocedure arteriography (magnetic resonance angiography [MRA], computed tomography angiography [CTA], or catheter) should precede any reoperative procedure; planning can be optimized only when the surgeon or interventionist is fully aware of the location and extent of all occlusive and stenotic arterial disease throughout the aortoiliac system and the entire lower extremity.

Fourth, if the failed bypass is a prosthetic conduit, an effort should be made to restore patency percutaneously, using mechanical thrombectomy devices and lytic agents. This is often facilitated if the proximal anastomotic hood of the original graft can be seen angiographically to facilitate guidewire passage. Only if interventional procedures fail should reoperation be undertaken; this is generally required when the proximal or distal organized thrombotic plug cannot be lysed or removed by percutaneous means. In this circumstance the PTFE graft is best approached at its most accessible midportion, usually in a subcutaneous position and remote from any anastomosis. The graft is opened longitudinally, and the liquefied clot is removed gently with balloon catheters. Next, using fluoroscopic guidance, guidewires and catheters are gently used to traverse the anastomosis. Fluoroscopy with contrast injections is used to identify any inflow or anastomotic lesions and similarly any outflow lesions. A double-lumen balloon catheter is then passed over the guidewire across the anastomosis, the balloon is inflated with dilute contrast, and under fluoroscopic control the balloon is withdrawn gently to remove free clot. By observing the distortion of the balloon, hyperplastic and arteriosclerotic lesions can be identified and corrected by PTA with or without stent placement.[41,42] Balloon distortion within the proximal graft indicates the presence of an organized gelatinous or fibrinous plug that usually cannot be removed with a balloon catheter.[42] In that case, and because loose clot has been removed, there may often be some flow in the opened graft, presenting a problem with hemostasis. If so, a 9 French hemostatic sheath is placed into the graft, and bleeding around the sheath is controlled with doubled Silastic loops. The sheath and its dilator are passed over the wire across the anastomosis. The dilator is removed and an adherent clot removal catheter (Edwards Laboratory) is passed within the sheath under fluoroscopic control. The sheath is retracted and the wires of the clot removal catheter are deployed within the graft, under fluoroscopic control to engage the adherent plug and remove it without injuring the adjacent artery.[42] Angiography should be used to demonstrate the absence of residual luminal defects. A similar procedure is then performed distally. If unobstructed distal flow cannot be obtained after PTA and stent placement, the proximal graft (now with unobstructed inflow) is transected and used as the origin for a partially new bypass to another patent distal artery accessed via a virginal approach.[12,14,20] Completion contrast fluoroscopy should be used to confirm an adequate lumen without defects and unimpeded flow through the graft and into the outflow tract.

MULTIPLE REDO PROCEDURES

Some patients are subject to repetitive failure of lower extremity revascularization procedures, including bypasses. Some believe that patients who have failure of two or more bypasses in the same lower extremity should, if they redevelop critical ischemia, undergo a major amputation. Lipsitz and colleagues[43] have recently demonstrated the value of repetitive redo bypasses, performed over several years, in preserving the limb of these patients. They observed that the duration of patency following more than three bypasses was substantial and resulted in more than 3 years of extended limb salvage in more than 50% of the patients who would otherwise have required an amputation.[43] These beneficial results were obtained only when the repetitive bypasses were performed according to the principles already outlined. Moreover, these repetitive bypasses should be performed only when the patient would otherwise require an immediate major amputation.

CONCLUSIONS

All surgical treatment efforts should be used to salvage the threatened foot in elderly, high-risk patients who will not walk well after one major amputation and certainly will not after bilateral amputations. Although the surgical methods to save limbs and maintain limb salvage may be time consuming and technically demanding, and although they require a continuing commitment on the part of the vascular surgeon, they are gratifying to those who perform them. They are particularly rewarding to patients who are able to maintain an ambulatory life style in the presence of advanced atherosclerosis.

REVIEW QUESTIONS

1. True or false: Multiple reinterventions and redo bypasses are often indicated and worthwhile after a failed primary vein bypass.
2. Bypasses to arteries below the popliteal artery should be performed for limb salvage with PTFE grafts in which of the following circumstances?
   a. When no acceptable autologous vein is present in the involved lower extremity
   b. Only when no autologous vein is available in any of the patient's four extremities
   c. In no circumstances
   d. Only to the posterior tibial artery
   e. None of the above
3. True or false: Heavily calcified, incompressible tibial arteries are unsuitable for use in limb salvage arterial bypasses.
4. True or false: Studies have clearly shown that in situ vein bypasses are superior to reversed vein bypasses.
5. True or false: The standard arteriogram for femoropopliteal occlusive disease should visualize all arteries from the renal arteries to the forefoot.
6. True or false: Vein and PTFE bypasses to isolated popliteal artery segments have a poor chance of being successful in treating critical limb ischemia and should be avoided if possible.
7. When is bypass to a tibial artery at the ankle level or in the foot indicated for disabling intermittent claudication?
   a. Always
   b. Almost never
   c. Almost always
   d. Frequently
   e. Never
8. True or false: Toe amputation or foot debridement should never be combined with arterial revascularization.
9. True or false: The presence of pedal pulses is evidence of sufficiently good circulation in the foot that a toe amputation for infection is likely to heal.
10. True or false: In patients with a failed infrainguinal bypass and a threatened limb, there is a poor chance of saving the foot by performing a secondary revascularization.

References available online at ExpertConsult.com.

CHAPTER 29

Endoscopic Harvesting of the Saphenous Vein

Juan Carlos Jimenez, Christian Eisenring

Open vein harvest (OVH) for coronary artery bypass grafting (CABG) and infrainguinal bypass procedures is associated with increased patient morbidity and postoperative wound complications.[1] In the limb salvage population, patients exhibit severe peripheral arterial occlusive disease, marginal distal perfusion, poor nutrition, and infected wounds. These factors make it difficult to heal the lower-extremity skin incisions that are required to harvest long, continuous segments of saphenous vein required for optimal bypass patency. Over the past decade, endoscopic harvest of the saphenous vein and the radial artery has been increasingly used by cardiac surgeons for CABG and has become the standard of care within this specialty.

More recently, these techniques have been used increasingly for minimally invasive harvest of autogenous conduits in conjunction with peripheral vascular surgery. Because longer, continuous segments of conduit are required for infrainguinal revascularization, especially infrapopliteal bypass, certain technical modifications have been required to facilitate use for lower extremity limb salvage procedures.[2]

RESULTS

Endoscopic Vein Harvesting: Coronary Artery Bypass Grafting

Several prospective, randomized trials have compared endoscopic vein harvest (EVH) with traditional open saphenous harvest during CABG and have demonstrated superior outcomes for EVH. Advantages include lower wound complication rates, decreased postoperative pain, increased patient satisfaction, improved cosmesis, and equivalent graft patency rates.[3–8] Griffith and colleagues[9] performed a histologic analysis of veins harvested by open techniques and EVH. There was no difference in endothelial, smooth muscle, and elastic lamina continuity between the two groups, and medial and adventitial connective tissue uniformity was not significantly altered.

In a meta-analysis of 267,525 patients, Sastry and colleagues found that there was no statistical difference in vein graft stenosis or occlusion between open and endoscopically harvested veins when considering evidence only from randomized studies. EVH was associated with less pain and leg wound complications. At a median of 2.6 years, there was no significant difference in mortality, myocardial infarction, repeat revascularization, angina recurrence, or vein graft stenosis and occlusion.[10]

Despite multiple supportive studies validating EVH for CABG, a recent study by Lopes and colleagues[11] questioned the superiority of this technique. They reviewed the outcomes of 1753 patients who underwent EVH for CABG and compared them to 1247 patients in the open harvest group. They demonstrated a higher rate of vein-graft failure at 12 to 18 months in the EVH group compared with the open cohort (46.7% vs. 38%, respectively). At 3 years, EVH was also associated with higher rates of death, myocardial infarction, and repeated revascularization. Critics of this study highlighted the elevated vein-graft failure and death rates in both open and EVH groups compared with similar published series. Additional criticisms included an overall lower use of internal mammary artery conduits, which are associated with superior patency compared with vein grafts, and that 20% of the procedures in this patient cohort were performed off-pump.

A recent study performed by the Northern New England Cardiovascular Disease Study Group demonstrated a decreased risk of leg wound infections with EVH, but an increased adjusted risk of bleeding requiring a return to the operating room.[12] Endoscopic harvest was also associated with a significant reduction in long-term mortality in these patients. The results also demonstrated that between 2001 and 2004, the use of EVH increased from 34% to 75% in patients requiring CABG.

Endoscopic Vein Harvesting: Infrainguinal Revascularization

Several studies have demonstrated similar favorable results for EVH during distal arterial bypass for limb salvage, although no randomized controlled trials have been conducted (Table 29.1).[13,14,16,17] Jordan and colleagues[13] performed 164 saphenous vein EVHs for lower extremity arterial reconstructive procedures over a 6-year period.[13] A review of patency rates using Kaplan-Meier analysis at 1, 3, and 5 years demonstrated vein graft patencies of 85%, 74%, and 68%, respectively. Fourteen patients (8.5%) developed wound infections during the 30-day postoperative period, and two patients developed harvest site hematomas. None of these wound complications led to graft failure or limb loss. The limb salvage rate was 89%.

A review by Erdoes and Milner[16] examined the outcomes following EVH for infrainguinal arterial bypass in 214 limbs over a 6-year period. The indication for bypass was limb salvage in 88.3%, claudication in 9.3%, and trauma and aneurysm in 2.4%. Assisted primary patency at 18 months was 77.2% by

TABLE 29.1 Results of Endoscopic Vein Harvest Used in Conjunction With Peripheral Arterial Bypass

Study	Year	Mean Operative Time (Min)	Primary Patency (%)	Overall Limb Salvage (%)	Overall Wound Complication Rate (%)
Jordan and colleagues[13]	2001	NA	69 (12 mo)	89	0.9
Suggs and colleagues[14]	2001	295	93 (12 mo)	92	4
Illig and colleagues[15]	2003	NA	60 (12 mo)	98	20.4
Erdoes and Milner[16]	2005	248	71.5 (18 mo)	91	7.5
Gazoni and colleagues[17]	2006	241.5	92.8 (21 mo)	96.5	13.8
Pulatt and colleagues[18]	2006	NA	30 (12 mo)	85	6
Jimenez and colleagues[2]	2007	410.4	78.5 (12 mo)	100	14
Hines and colleagues[19]	2010	NA	73.2 (72 mo)	63	37
Juilliard and colleagues[20]	2011	NA	42.2 (36 mo)	81	20.2
Eid and colleagues[21]	2014	392.1	43.2 (36 mo)	97.5	15.4
Santo and colleagues[22]	2014	316	41 (36 mo)	91	37

NA, Not available; *mo,* months.

Kaplan-Meier analysis. Wound complication rates were 7.5%, with 2.5% of patients requiring readmission to the hospital. Only one patient early in the series required conversion to an open harvest.

Gazoni and colleagues[17] reported results for patients who underwent femoral to below-knee arterial bypass grafting over a 27-month period.[17] Fifty-nine patients underwent traditional open saphenectomy, and 29 had EVH. There was a trend toward improved patency rates in the EVH group compared with open harvest, although no statistically significant difference was noted (92.8% vs. 80.6%). No significant differences were found between the two groups in postoperative complications, operative time, length of hospital stay, patency rates, limb salvage, and death. The incidence of wound complications was 3.4% in the EVH group and 15.3% in the open harvest group, although this difference also was not statistically significant. Similarly, Hines and colleagues examined outcomes over a 5-year period for 27 patients who underwent femoral-popliteal bypass with EVH in patients with Trans-Atlantic Inter-Society Consensus (TASC) D disease of the superficial femoral artery.[19] Kaplan-Meier primary and primary assisted patency rates were 73.2% and 80.8% at 1 year, respectively, and these rates were maintained for 70 months. Only one patient developed a superficial wound infection.

Following formal systematic training by vascular surgeons and implementation of technical modifications specific to limb salvage procedures at our institution, we noted 30-day primary and primary-assisted patency rates of 85.7% and 92.9%, respectively.[2] Kaplan-Meier primary assisted patency was 63.6%. No patients required primary amputation at 19 months. One graft occlusion occurred within 30 days as a result of a tunnel hematoma in a patient who sustained a postoperative myocardial infarction and required therapeutic anticoagulation. One late hematoma was noted, and one patient demonstrated skin necrosis at the level of the ankle requiring prolonged hospitalization. Complete wound healing was achieved in 75% of patients with preoperative tissue loss due to critical limb ischemia.

The long-term durability of EVH for lower-extremity bypass has been questioned following a study by Julliard and colleagues.[20] Over a period of 8.5 years, 363 patients underwent infrainguinal bypass; 170 patients underwent EVH and 193 underwent traditional open saphenous vein harvest. No differences in indication for surgery were noted between groups. Primary patency rates were significantly lower in the EVH group compared with the open group at 6, 12, and 36 months. There were no differences in length of stay or wound complication rates. Limb salvage and survival were also identical between groups. The differences were not significant in patients with claudication and in those without diabetes.

Two more recent studies have demonstrated inferior patency rates when using the EVH technique for lower extremity bypass. Eid and colleagues from the University of Pittsburgh noted a graft patency rate of 43.2% in the EVH group and 69.4% in the OVH group at three years ($P = .007$). However, the authors did demonstrate a decreased rate of wound complications with similar limb salvage and secondary patency rates associated with EVH compared to OVH. Santo and colleagues from the University of Oregon also demonstrated impaired primary patency at 1 and 3 years in the EVH group (71% and 52% respectively) when compared to the OVH group (58% and 41% respectively). EVH was also associated with increased need for intervention, longer operative times, shorter hospital stays, and decreased harvest site complications. Limb salvage rates and amputation-free survival was similar in both groups.[21,22]

Thus despite mixed outcomes with regard to vein graft patency following EVH for infrainguinal revascularization, the decision to implement this technique must be weighed against decreased wound complication rates, diminished postoperative pain, and similar limb salvage rates compared with EVH. It is likely that graft patency rates following EVH are influenced by the surgeon's experience and technique and may improve in the future as newer technology emerges.

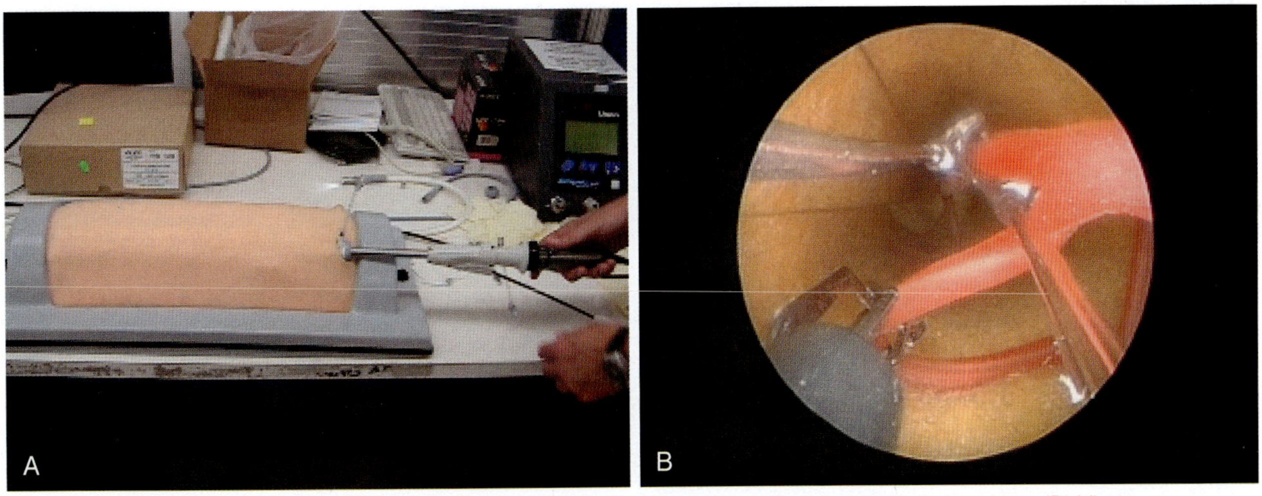

FIG 29.1 (A) Endoscopic vein harvest (EVH) simulator in our Surgical Skills Laboratory. (B) View of the harvest tunnel and the great saphenous vein during EVH simulation.

TECHNIQUES

Endoscopic Harvest of the Greater Saphenous Vein

Currently, there are several systems available for endoscopic vein harvesting including Terumo VirtuoSaph (TERUMO Medical Corporation, NJ) and Venapax (Saphena Medical, MA). Although several endoscopic vein-harvesting systems are currently available, at the University of California, Los Angeles (UCLA), the Vasoview Hemopro II Harvesting system is used (Maquet, Wayne, NJ). Of note, we used vein harvest simulators in the Surgical Skills Lab at our institution to train our vascular residents and fellows in techniques for EVH (Fig. 29.1A and B). Preoperative color duplex mapping is performed to assess vein diameters, caliber, patency, and location of branches. In addition, intraoperative ultrasound is performed to mark the course of the vein under sterile conditions before EVH to maximize incision placement accuracy.

An incision is made three fingerbreadths posterior to the medial femoral or tibial condyles, depending on whether harvest will be performed above or below the knee. A longitudinal 2-cm incision is made and the greater saphenous vein (GSV) is identified. A silastic vessel loop is placed around the GSV for mobilization (Fig. 29.2). At this time, several more centimeters of vein are bluntly dissected and mobilized from the surrounding subcutaneous tissue to ease placement of the blunt tip trocar (BTT) in the direction of intended vein harvest. The BTT is placed into the subcutaneous space overlying the GSV, and the port balloon is sufficiently inflated to ensure a good seal with the adjacent skin. Leakage of CO_2 outside the harvest tunnel can lead to suboptimal visibility and bleeding during vein mobilization. A CO_2 cannula is then attached to a port on the BTT and continued at a flow rate of 3 to 5 L/min up to a maximum pressure of 10 to 15 mm Hg. Carbon dioxide insufflation should not exceed central venous pressure to avoid embolism. Insufflation of the vein harvest tunnel facilitates placement of the 5-mm camera through the main port of the BTT and enhances visualization of the GSV within the subcutaneous space.

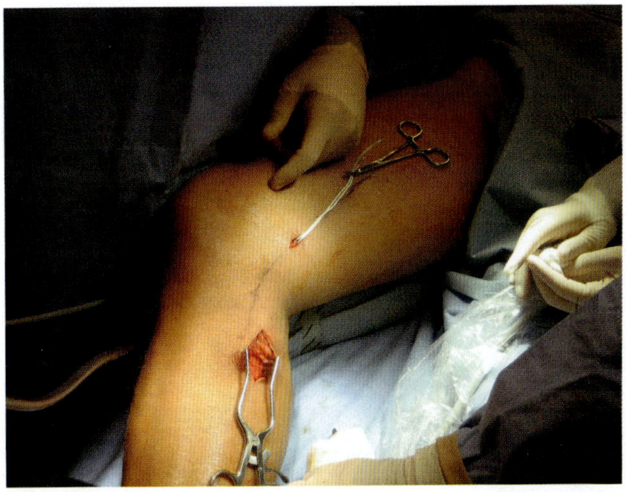

FIG 29.2 A 3-cm longitudinal incision is made above or below the knee for initial mobilization of the greater saphenous vein and placement of the blunt tip trocar.

A conical tip is placed on the tip of the camera, and the vein is dissected bluntly along its anterior and posterior surfaces (Fig. 29.3). Branches are skeletonized from surrounding soft tissue and exposed to maximal length before division with the bipolar dissector. The main goal before division of branches is to suspend the entire length of the vein by its branches in the center of the harvest tunnel and allow maximal CO_2 insufflation for good visibility (Fig. 29.4). Care must be taken at this time to avoid avulsion of large branches. Generally the disruption of minor venous branches is not problematic, because the insufflation tends to control bleeding from these tributaries without the need for additional cauterization.

Following complete blunt dissection, the BTT is replaced with the vein-harvesting cannula, which serves to retract, cauterize, and divide all branches. The Vasoview system provides a retractable C-ring that is used in conjunction with the harmonic scalpel

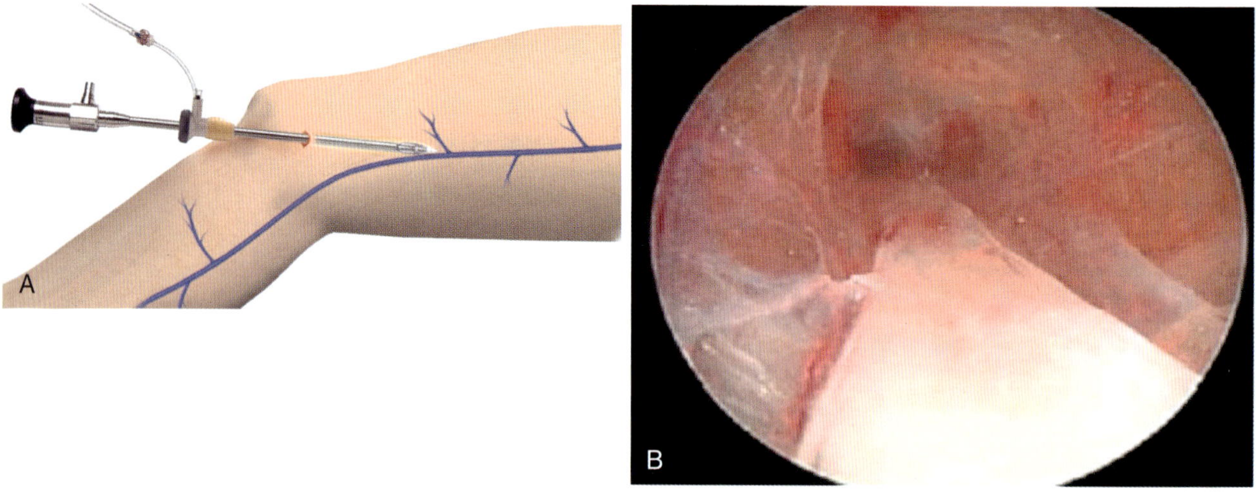

FIG 29.3 (A) Cartoon depiction of blunt dissection and tunnel insufflation during endoscopic vein harvest. (B) Blunt mobilization of the anterior and posterior planes of the greater saphenous vein using the conical tip of the 5-mm camera.

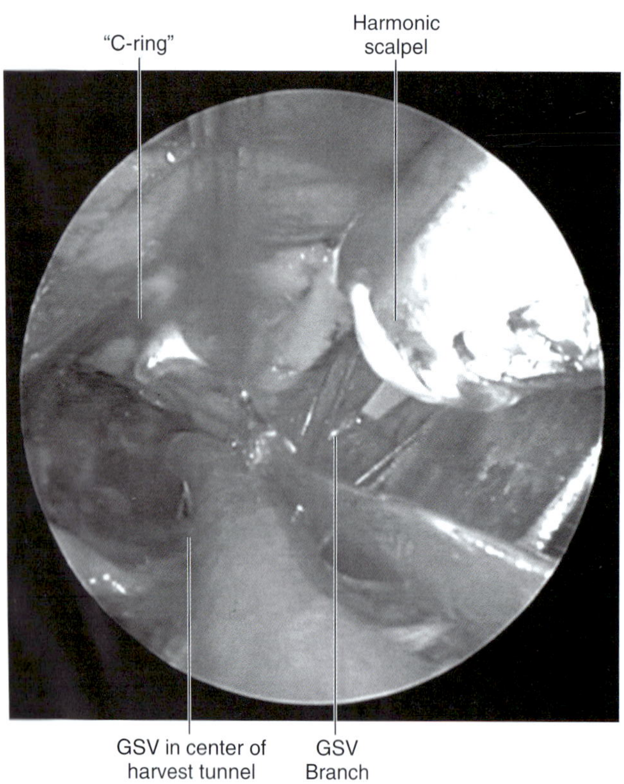

FIG 29.4 Branch ligation in the insufflated endoscopic harvest tunnel following circumferential vein dissection. *GSV*, Greater saphenous vein.

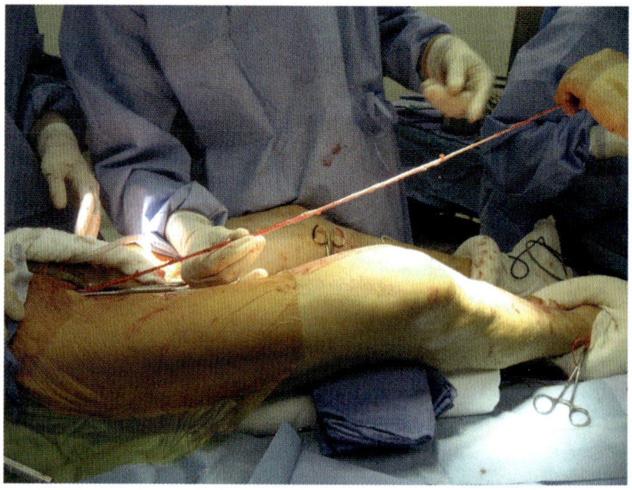

FIG 29.5 Long, continuous saphenous vein segments required for infrainguinal revascularization can be obtained using endoscopic vein harvest.

dissector to mobilize the main vein and provide counter-tension at each individual branch site. A retractable harmonic dissector is then used to cauterize and divide all branches while avoiding direct or collateral thermal injury to the vein wall. Care must be taken to avoid overly aggressive retraction at this time, which can result in branch avulsion and bleeding within the tunnel. Once all branches are cauterized and divided, the vessel cradle (the C-ring) is run along the entire length of harvested vein to ensure that no branches remain. The vein can then be removed through a proximal and distal stab incision made directly at opposite ends of the harvest tunnel (Fig. 29.5). All cauterized side branches should be reinforced before limb salvage bypass with individual silk and Prolene sutures. Injured segments of the vein must be repaired directly with Prolene suture and, if luminal compromise is present, the affected segment of the vein must be excised and venovenostomy is performed. The vein is then prepared and flushed in usual fashion.

Endoscopic Harvest of the Small Saphenous Vein

EVH of the lesser saphenous vein (LSV) is performed in the prone position. Preoperative vein mapping can be useful to determine length, diameter, and caliber of this vessel for use in lower extremity limb salvage procedures. The LSV usually has more large branches than the GSV, and it lies deeper within the subfascial plane. Care must be taken to avoid injury to the sural nerve, which lies adjacent to the LSV in the leg. A 2-cm transverse incision is made in the upper leg below the knee joint distal to where the LSV dives deep and joins the popliteal vein. The vein is harvested and removed in similar fashion. A stab incision can then be made in the distal calf to remove the vein in its entirety (see Fig. 29.5). Minimally invasive popliteal-to-posterior tibial artery bypass can also be performed in this position with placement of the vein through the harvest tunnel in reversed or nonreversed fashion (following treatment with a semiclosed valvulotome.)

Technical Modifications in the Limb Salvage Population

Although the techniques of harvest are similar for cardiac surgeons and those performing limb salvage procedures, certain technical adjustments have been applied to infrainguinal bypass for limb salvage. At UCLA, vascular surgeons and fellows underwent formal training on operative simulators before implementation in the operating room. This training included familiarization with the different components of the device during formal sessions with industry representatives and the review of video and other interactive materials during didactic sessions.

Certain technical modifications have been implemented during EVH by vascular surgeons; these modifications facilitate use during lower-extremity limb salvage procedures. Longitudinal vein harvest incisions are preferred over the traditional transverse incisions performed during cardiac surgery procedures, because they can be extended proximally or distally, or both, and used to simultaneously expose arterial targets for bypass. A medial EVH incision just above the knee at the level of the femoral condyle can be used subsequently to expose the above-knee popliteal artery after the GSV has been removed. A harvest incision just below the knee at the level of the tibial condyles can also be used for exposure of the below knee popliteal artery, the tibioperoneal trunk, and the proximal peroneal and posterior tibial arteries. A longitudinal incision just proximal to the medial malleolus can be extended to expose the distal posterior tibial artery.

When ipsilateral GSV harvest is performed for limb salvage procedures, the harvest tunnel is frequently used for subcutaneous placement of the vein. It can be reversed or left in situ with subsequent valve lysis with the use of a semiclosed valvulotome. Meticulous hemostasis must be ensured within the harvest tunnel because bleeding and hematoma formation can jeopardize graft patency. Compression bandages should be avoided when ipsilateral harvest is performed for limb salvage procedures, whereas this technique is frequently used following EVH for CABG. Patients are instructed to discontinue oral clopidogrel (Plavix) 7 days before the operation to minimize bleeding risk. Immediate postoperative therapeutic heparin drips or subcutaneous low-molecular-weight heparin should be avoided. Platelet antiaggregation therapy with aspirin or clopidogrel can usually be reinstated safely 24 to 48 hours after the operation.

COMPLICATIONS OF ENDOSCOPIC VEIN HARVEST

All wound complications associated with open saphenous vein harvest can occur with minimally invasive techniques. These complications include infection, dehiscence, hematoma, lymphocele, and limb swelling. A metaanalysis of randomized trials conducted by Athanasiou and colleagues[23] compared minimally invasive versus conventional vein harvesting and found that EVH techniques were associated with an overall reduced risk of wound infections. However, infections occurring within the harvest tunnel following EVH usually require drainage of fluid collections contained in a closed space. Allen and colleagues[24] identified three closed-space tunnel infections out of 1259 patients who underwent EVH. These three patients also had early postoperative hematomas and wound cultures that were positive for *Staphylococcus aureus*. Two patients were treated by unroofing the tunnel with an incision over its entire length. One patient was managed successfully using closed-space irrigation with a Blake drain irrigated every 8 hours and gradually withdrawn over a 10-day period.

Carbon dioxide insufflation during EVH can result in hypercarbia,[25] pneumoperitoneum,[26] and CO_2 embolus, especially when the insufflation pressure exceeds central venous pressure.[27] Chiu and colleagues[27] randomly assigned 498 patients to high (15 mm Hg) and low (12 mm Hg) CO_2 insufflation groups for EVH during CABG. Transesophageal echocardiography (TEE) with transgastric inferior vena cava views was used to monitor for the appearance of CO_2 bubbles. The incidence of CO_2 embolus was significantly elevated in the high-pressure insufflations group (13.3% vs. 6.5 %; $P < .05$). Two patients in the high-pressure group required immediate cessation of insufflation. Although no patient exhibited hemodynamic alterations in either group in this study, massive CO_2 embolus with circulatory collapse has been noted in separate reports. All patients with visible CO_2 bubbles on TEE were converted to open harvest and these patients all exhibited subclinical injury to the vein wall.

When EVH is performed on the ipsilateral GSV during minimally invasive distal arterial bypass, care must be taken to avoid postoperative tunnel hematomas because the compressive effects may compromise vein graft patency. Because the vein graft is usually placed within the EVH tunnel, meticulous hemostasis in the subcutaneous tissue and reinforcement of all ligated branches must be ensured. Extension of existing incisions should be used in selected instances when significant bleeding is noted. Immediate postoperative anticoagulation should be avoided, as well as compression wraps when the ipsilateral GSV is used for graft tunneling because of possible compression of the vein within its subcutaneous position.

Although rare, skin necrosis has been reported following EVH, especially in the lower leg at the level of the ankle where minimal subcutaneous fat exists. Conversion to open harvest at this level should be performed if excessive resistance is noted during blunt dissection. At UCLA, one patient exhibited full thickness skin necrosis requiring flap coverage and ultimately leading to late graft failure. Early recognition and flap coverage is crucial, especially when the harvest tunnel is used for graft placement.

REVIEW QUESTIONS

1. A 2011 study by the Northern New England Cardiovascular Disease Study Group demonstrated which of the following results?
   a. A significant reduction in long-term mortality
   b. A decreased risk of leg wound infections
   c. An increased adjusted risk of bleeding
   d. An increase in the use of EVH between 2001 and 2004
   e. All of the above
2. A 2009 study published in the *New England Journal of Medicine* by Lopes and colleagues demonstrated which of the following results?
   a. Equivalent outcomes following both EVH and open harvest
   b. Higher rates of vein graft failure with open harvest
   c. Higher rates of vein graft failure following EVH
   d. Lower rates of death with EVH
   e. Lower rates of myocardial infarction with EVH
3. Complications following EVH include which of the following?
   a. Tunnel hematoma
   b. Skin necrosis
   c. Hypercarbia
   d. Lymphocele
   e. All of the above
4. Specific technical modifications to EVH that facilitate use in limb salvage procedures include which of the following?
   a. Longitudinal harvest incisions
   b. Avoidance of the harvest tunnel for placement of the vein graft
   c. Routine use of compression Ace bandages following bypass
   d. Transverse harvest incisions
   e. Routine therapeutic heparinization following bypass
5. When harvesting the small saphenous vein, which of the following is true?
   a. Branches are encountered less frequently than EVH of the great saphenous vein.
   b. Care must be taken to avoid injury to the sural nerve.
   c. Care must be taken to avoid injury to the epigastric vein.
   d. Dissection is performed deep to the muscular fascia.
   e. The small saphenous vein connects directly with the femoral vein in most patients.
6. Closed space wound infections following EVH should be treated with:
   a. Warm compresses
   b. Warm compresses and aspirin
   c. Warm compresses and ibuprofen
   d. Unroofing of the harvest tunnel and drainage
   e. All of the above
7. Technical details of EVH for limb salvage procedures should include which of the following considerations?
   a. A medial EVH incision can be used for exposure of the above- or below-knee popliteal artery.
   b. A longitudinal EVH incision at the medial ankle can be used for both vein harvest and exposure of the anterior tibial artery.
   c. The GSV should never be harvested through the femoral incision.
   d. Only reversed GSV bypasses can be performed following EVH.
   e. Reinforcement of cauterized vein branches is not usually necessary for hemostasis prior to bypass.
8. Technical differences between EVH for coronary artery bypass surgery and limb salvage procedures include which of the following?
   a. The preferred use of longitudinal incisions in limb salvage procedures
   b. Longer lengths of vein are usually required for limb salvage procedures
   c. Harvest of the great and small saphenous veins can be performed for both
   d. Overall decreased risk of wound infections has been demonstrated for both
   e. All of the above
9. Carbon dioxide insufflation during EVH has been known to cause which of the following?
   a. Hypercarbia
   b. Pneumoperitoneum
   c. CO_2 embolus
   d. Circulatory collapse
   e. All of the above
10. Which of the following statements are true regarding EVH?
    a. Randomized controlled trials have demonstrated superior outcomes for EVH compared with OVH following limb salvage procedures.
    b. No histologic studies have been performed following both types of harvest.
    c. Endoscopically harvested GSV has superior patency compared with the internal mammary artery.
    d. Lower extremity skin incisions in the limb salvage population are difficult to heal due to poor nutrition, infected wounds, and atherosclerotic disease.
    e. All of the above

References available online at ExpertConsult.com.

CHAPTER 30

Infrainguinal Endovascular Reconstruction: Technique and Results

Johnathon Rollo, Brian G. DeRubertis, Peter A. Schneider

Management of infrainguinal arterial occlusive disease continues to move away from open surgery and toward percutaneous procedures, and the number of percutaneous options is growing rapidly. This chapter focuses on standard techniques for arterial access, diagnostic imaging, lesion crossing, and options for treating occlusions and stenoses of the femoropopliteal and tibial circulation.

PATIENT SELECTION AND PREOPERATIVE IMAGING

Infrainguinal occlusive disease can usually be diagnosed by history and physical examination. Confirmatory studies are usually performed—duplex mapping, computed tomography angiography (CTA), or magnetic resonance angiography (MRA)—to plan the therapeutic approach and limit the amount of contrast required for arteriography. Diagnostic arteriography does not currently exist in many practices, because most patients do not undergo arterial access unless there is an intention to treat. Occasionally, what initially appeared to be a lesion appropriate for angioplasty based on duplex scanning, MRA, or CTA turns out to be more complex, and only an arteriogram is obtained.

Infrainguinal occlusive disease can be classified by its morphology, which assists in determining which patients are best managed with endovascular intervention and which ones require surgery. The Trans-Atlantic Inter-Society Consensus (TASC) classification (Box 30.1) and others have defined disease morphology in an effort to clarify the issue of lesion severity.[1] The general concept is that endovascular techniques are preferred in patients with less severe forms of disease and among those with shorter life expectancies or greater periprocedural risk factors. Conversely, open surgical approaches have a better risk-benefit profile in patients with fewer medical comorbidities or more severe forms of disease, such as long-segment occlusions or heavily calcified lesions, in which endovascular procedures are less durable. The TASC document recommends that type A lesions be treated with endovascular intervention, type D lesions be treated with surgery, and types B and C lesions be treated with either, depending on the patient's comorbidities, general medical condition, expected longevity, and availability of conduit for bypass. These recommendations have been challenged by reports of high technical success obtained with endovascular revascularization for complex TASC D lesions.

Over the past decade, many practices have seen a steady movement toward the use of endovascular techniques for infrainguinal arterial occlusive disease, to the point that some approach all patients with an "endovascular first" strategy with open surgical bypass reserved for failures of endovascular therapy. This approach appears reasonable provided that attempts at endovascular therapy do not result in loss of bypass targets, distal embolization, or other complications that limit future surgical options, and there remains a recognition that certain lesions, such as common femoral disease or popliteal occlusions with distal tibial reconstitution, are generally best treated with open surgical techniques.

Approaches

Percutaneous intervention for infrainguinal occlusive disease is usually performed through the contralateral femoral artery using an up-and-over approach or through the ipsilateral femoral artery using an antegrade approach (Table 30.1). Infrainguinal interventions can also be performed through the brachial artery, but this approach is rarely required and may be more challenging because of the longer distances involved and the higher likelihood of access-related complications. More recently, pedal approaches have been used for distal tibial interventions or when antegrade access is not possible. The primary advantages of the up-and-over approach, which is most commonly used, are the following: An aortogram with runoff can be easily converted to endovascular therapy; it permits evaluation of the inflow aortoiliac arteries before treatment of infrainguinal lesions; only a simple retrograde femoral puncture is required; and it facilitates selective catheterization of the superficial femoral artery (SFA) orifice and treatment of proximal SFA lesions, which can be difficult via the ipsilateral antegrade approach. Furthermore, puncture site management is contralateral to the intervention site rather than proximal to it. The antegrade approach may be used for better guidewire and catheter control in infrapopliteal intervention and in patients who have contraindications to the up-and-over approach. The likely approach is determined before the procedure to facilitate room setup and the availability of supplies, but both groins are always prepared in case an alternative approach is required during the procedure.

Platforms

Percutaneous intervention in the infrainguinal circulation can be achieved with 0.035-inch, 0.018-inch, or 0.014-inch platforms,

BOX 30.1 Trans-Atlantic Inter-Society Consensus Classification of Femoropopliteal Lesions

Type A Lesions
- Single stenosis <3 cm

Type B Lesions
- Single stenosis 3–10 cm long, not involving the distal popliteal artery
- Heavily calcified stenosis up to 3 cm
- Multiple lesions, each <3 cm (stenosis or occlusion)
- Single or multiple lesions in the absence of tibial runoff to improve inflow for distal surgical bypass

Type C Lesions
- Single stenosis or occlusion >5 cm long
- Multiple stenoses or occlusions, each 3–5 cm

Type D Lesions
- Occlusion of the common femoral artery, popliteal artery, proximal trifurcation arteries
- Occlusion of the superficial femoral artery >10 cm long

From Schneider PA, Nelken N, Caps MT: Angioplasty and stenting for infrainguinal lesions. In Yao JST, Pearse WH, Matsumura JS, editors: Trends in Vascular Surgery, Chicago, 2003, Parmentier Publishing, p 292.

TABLE 30.1 Comparison of Approaches to Infrainguinal Interventions: Up-and-Over Versus Antegrade

	Up-and-Over Approach	Antegrade Approach
Puncture	Simple retrograde femoral	More challenging, less working room
Catheterization	Challenging with tortuous arteries, narrow or diseased aortic bifurcation; easier to catheterize SFA when going up and over femoral	Entering SFA from antegrade approach requires proximal puncture and selective catheter
Guidewire and catheter control	Fair	Excellent
Catheter inventory	More supplies needed	Minimal, shorter catheters
Specialty items	Up-and-over sheath, long balloon catheters	None
Indications	Proximal SFA disease, CFA disease ipsilateral to infrainguinal lesion, obesity	Infrapopliteal disease, patients with contraindication to up-and-over approach

CFA, Common femoral artery; *SFA,* superior femoral artery.
From Schneider PA: The infrainguinal arteries—advice about balloon angioplasty and stent placement. In Schneider PA, editor: *Endovascular Skills*, ed 2, New York, 2003, Marcel Dekker, p 316.

using sheath sizes ranging from 4 to 7 French. Most diagnostic angiograms and interventions are begun with a standard 0.035-inch platform. This platform has several advantages: the guidewires and catheters are easy to handle, the inventory is usually readily available, the fluoroscopic visualization of these larger-caliber devices is simpler, and the larger guidewires and catheters are often more helpful than the smaller diameter devices when crossing chronic or heavily calcified occlusions. However, there are also some significant disadvantages of 0.035-inch systems: the larger-caliber guidewires and catheters may not easily cross critically diseased segments and may be more prone to cause arterial damage; at longer distances, these catheters lose their "pushability" because of high friction; and in small arteries such as tibial vessels, the standard platform devices may be too big. In addition to their smaller crossing profiles, the smaller 0.018- and 0.014-inch platforms tend to be more trackable in small, tortuous vessels at locations distant from the access site, especially when using monorail (rapid-exchange) systems with longer guiding sheaths or catheters. Most of the coronary devices are on a 0.014-inch or 0.018-inch platform, as are current atherectomy systems; therefore the array of available balloon catheters and stents is much broader with this system. Monorail balloon catheters permit better pushability because the friction of the guidewire on the balloon catheter lumen occurs over a much shorter distance than with coaxial balloon catheters. Monorail systems have the additional advantages of greater ease of use (especially with a single operator), shorter required guidewire lengths, and less guidewire movement during catheter exchanges.

Sheaths

For initial diagnostic angiography, a 5 French sheath is generally used in conjunction with 5 French diagnostic catheters (Omni Flush [AngioDynamics, Queensbury, NY] or VCF [Cook Medical, Bloomington, IN] catheter for aortography with runoff; Kumpe or Angled Glide [Cook Medical] catheter for selective angiograms). Although angioplasty alone can be performed through 4 or 5 French sheaths, especially when using balloons designed for 0.014- or 0.018-inch platforms, most stents and atherectomy devices require larger sheaths. As a result, most interventionists will change to a larger sheath for intervention once diagnostic angiograms have been performed and the operator has decided to proceed with intervention. It is important to note that with the advent of better percutaneous closure devices, sheath size has become a less important consideration because the larger puncture holes can be closed safely and easily in a percutaneous fashion in most patients, without the need for manual compression.

Technique

Up-and-Over Approach

Supplies required for an up-and-over approach are listed in Table 30.2. This approach requires longer guidewires, catheters, and sheaths than the antegrade approach. A standard retrograde common femoral artery puncture is performed contralateral to the symptomatic side. A floppy-tipped guidewire is passed into the aorta. A hook-shaped, multi–side-hole flush catheter, such as a 65-cm Omni Flush (AngioDynamics), is passed into the aorta, and an aortoiliac arteriogram is obtained. If bilateral runoff

TABLE 30.2 Supplies for Up-and-Over Approach to Infrainguinal Intervention

Category	Type	Function	Diameter	Length	Other Features
Guidewires	Bentson	Starting	0.035 inch	145 cm	
	Glidewire	Selective, therapy	0.035, 0.018 inch	150, 260 cm	Steerable
	Rosen	Exchange	0.035 inch	180 cm	Sheath placement
	Amplatz	Exchange	0.035 inch	180 cm	Sheath placement
	Ironman	Therapy	0.014 inch	190, 300 cm	
Catheters	Omni-flush	Flush, selective	4 French	65 cm	
Straight	Flush, exchange	5 French	90 cm	Multi–side hole	
Glidecath	Selective, exchange, 4, 5 French	100 cm	Angled tip		
Sheaths	Destination	Guide sheath	5, 6 French	45 cm	Straight
	Rabbe	Guide sheath	6 French	45, 70 cm	Straight
Balloons	Multiple	PTA infrainguinal	0.035, 0.018, 0.014 inch	75, 90, 110 cm OTW Rapid exchange	Balloon diameters, 2–6 mm Balloon lengths, 2, 4, 5, 10 cm
Stents	SMART	Stent SFA, popliteal Self-expanding	0.035 inch	80, 120 cm OTW	Stent diameters, 7–8 mm Stent lengths, 4, 6, 10 cm
	Precise	Stent SFA, popliteal Self-expanding	0.018 inch	120 cm Rapid exchange	OTW, Stent diameters, 7–8 mm Stent length, 4 cm
	Multiple	Stent tibials Balloon-expandable	0.014 inch	150 cm Rapid exchange	Stent diameters, 2.5–4 mm Stent length, 2 cm

OTW, Over the wire; *PTA*, percutaneous transluminal angioplasty; *SFA*, superficial femoral artery.

is required, it can be performed at that time with the catheter head placed in the infrarenal aorta. When only unilateral runoff on the symptomatic side is indicated, the catheter is passed over the aortic bifurcation, and lower extremity arteriography is performed. After evaluating the infrainguinal lesions, determining that the aortic bifurcation can accommodate an access sheath, and deciding that the up-and-over approach is best, an up-and-over sheath is placed (Fig. 30.1).

The aortic flush catheter is withdrawn to the aortic bifurcation, and its tip is rotated toward the contralateral side to direct the guidewire into the contralateral iliac artery. The advancing guidewire, usually a steerable, angled-tip Glidewire (Terumo Medical, Tokyo, Japan), must be steered into the external iliac artery and then into the infrainguinal arteries. From this approach, the guidewire usually tends to select the contralateral internal iliac artery if there is tortuosity of the iliac system. The guidewire also tends to select the SFA rather than the deep femoral artery. Either of these destinations for the guidewire is satisfactory from the standpoint of sheath placement, as long as the guidewire is well anchored distal to the groin. The catheter is advanced over the bifurcation, and a stiffer exchange-length (260 cm) guidewire (Stiff Angled Glidewire [Terumo Medical], Supra-Core Wire [Abbott Vascular, Abbott Park, IL] or Rosen Wire [Cook Medical]) is placed. The tip of the exchange guidewire should be distal to the groin as far as it will easily travel. If there is a proximal SFA lesion that is planned for treatment, the guidewire is usually directed into the deep profunda femoris artery. If there is excessive iliac tortuosity, an Amplatz Superstiff guidewire (Cook Medical) may be required.

Dilators can be used to enlarge the arteriotomy prior to sheath placement. Because dilators are sized by their outside diameter and sheaths are sized by their inside diameter, if a 6 French sheath is planned for placement, the tract should be dilated using a 7 French dilator. This step is often not necessary for the placement of contemporary sheaths as they generally have a smooth transition between the sheath and inner dilator, though the use of dilators prior to sheath placement can be invaluable for patients with scarred groins from prior surgery or heavily calcified arteries. Upon placing the sheath, it is carefully advanced over a fixed stiff guidewire; when a curved sheath is used, it is oriented such that its curved end is pointing toward the contralateral side and the side arm of the sheath is on the side of the operator. The sheath is advanced over the guidewire using fluoroscopy, alternatively watching the sheath tip and the distal wire tip to prevent injury to the aorta and iliac segments or the infrainguinal vasculature. Passage over a narrow or diseased aortic bifurcation is performed with care and patience. The sheath is advanced to its hub, if possible. It is important to remember that the tip of the dilator extends beyond the radiopaque marker on the end of the sheath tip for a short distance, and injury to the arteries can occur if this dilator advances beyond the end of the guidewire. The tip of the sheath will generally terminate somewhere between the mid-external iliac artery and the very proximal SFA, depending on the height of the patient. Heparin is usually administered (100 U/kg) as the sheath is placed, and an activated clotting time (ACT) is checked (goal ACT >250 seconds).

Fig. 30.2 demonstrates the steps required for infrainguinal intervention using an up-and-over approach. The exchange guidewire is replaced with a steerable 260-cm Glidewire (Terumo Medical). The diseased infrainguinal segment is road-mapped through the side arm of the sheath, and the Glidewire is used to cross the lesion to be treated. Lesion crossing is facilitated by supporting the Glidewire with a hydrophilic catheter, such as a

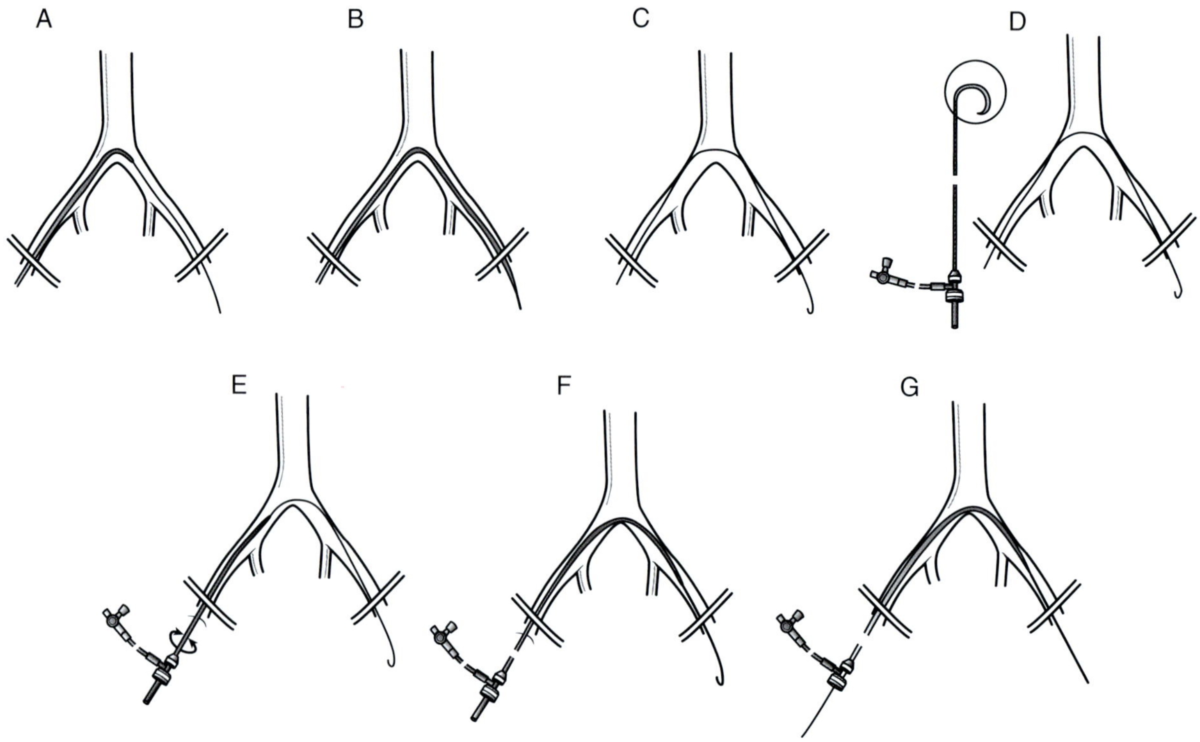

FIG 30.1 Placement of an up-and-over sheath. (A) A guidewire and catheter are passed over the aortic bifurcation. (B) The catheter is advanced to the contralateral femoral artery. (C) An exchange guidewire is placed, and the catheter is removed. (D) The sheath is oriented with its tip pointing toward the contralateral side. (E) The sheath is advanced over the guidewire. This is visualized using fluoroscopy. (F) The sheath is advanced to its hub. There must be enough guidewire ahead of the sheath tip to permit a smooth advance. (G) The dilator is removed, and the sheath is ready to use. (From Schneider PA: The infrainguinal arteries—advice about balloon angioplasty and stent placement. In Schneider PA, editor: *Endovascular Skills*, ed 2, New York, 2003, Marcel Dekker, p 195.)

5 French Angled Glidecath (Cook Medical) or Quick Cross catheter (Spectranetics). If treatment of tibial lesions is planned, a 5 French, 100-cm-long catheter is advanced into the distal popliteal artery, and road mapping is performed through this catheter. A low-profile guidewire, usually a 0.014-inch hydrophilic wire such as a Command wire (Abbott Vascular) is used to cross the tibial lesions, and the 5 French diagnostic catheter is exchanged for a 135-cm-long, 0.014-inch Quick Cross catheter (Spectranetics) to support the wire. Interval arteriography may be performed through the side arm of the sheath or through the selective catheter using a Tuohy-Borst adapter during attempts at lesion crossing. Once the lesion has been crossed, the supporting catheter is advanced down to the level of the reconstituted artery, the wire is removed to assess for blood return from the catheter lumen, and confirmatory angiography is performed to demonstrate the intraluminal position of the catheter.

Antegrade Approach

Supplies required for an antegrade approach are listed in Table 30.3. An antegrade common femoral artery puncture is performed ipsilateral to the symptomatic side. This approach is well suited to patients who have normal aortoiliac inflow, especially if tibial angioplasty is required or if there is a need to limit the use of contrast material. The puncture should be performed as proximally as possible along the common femoral artery to leave some working room between the puncture and the origin of the SFA. A steerable guidewire, such as the Wholey guidewire (Mallinckrodt, Hazelwood, MO), is used; the shaft of this guidewire is more supportive for catheter and sheath passage than a Glidewire. The Wholey guidewire can often be steered anteromedially into the SFA. If not, the guidewire is advanced into the deep femoral artery, and an angled-tip catheter is placed over it (Fig. 30.3). The image intensifier is placed in the ipsilateral anterior oblique position to open the femoral bifurcation, and the catheter is withdrawn enough to perform road mapping by refluxing contrast material into the SFA. The catheter is used to steer the guidewire into the SFA.

If the lesion is in the proximal to mid-SFA, the artery is road mapped using the catheter, and the guidewire is advanced across the lesion (Fig. 30.4). The same guidewire can be used for sheath placement. If the lesion is more distal in the artery, the guidewire is advanced without crossing the lesion, and the sheath is placed. The sheath size required may be 4, 5, or 6 French, depending on the platform used and treatment modality desired. An appropriately sized dilator is used to enlarge the arteriotomy before sheath placement.

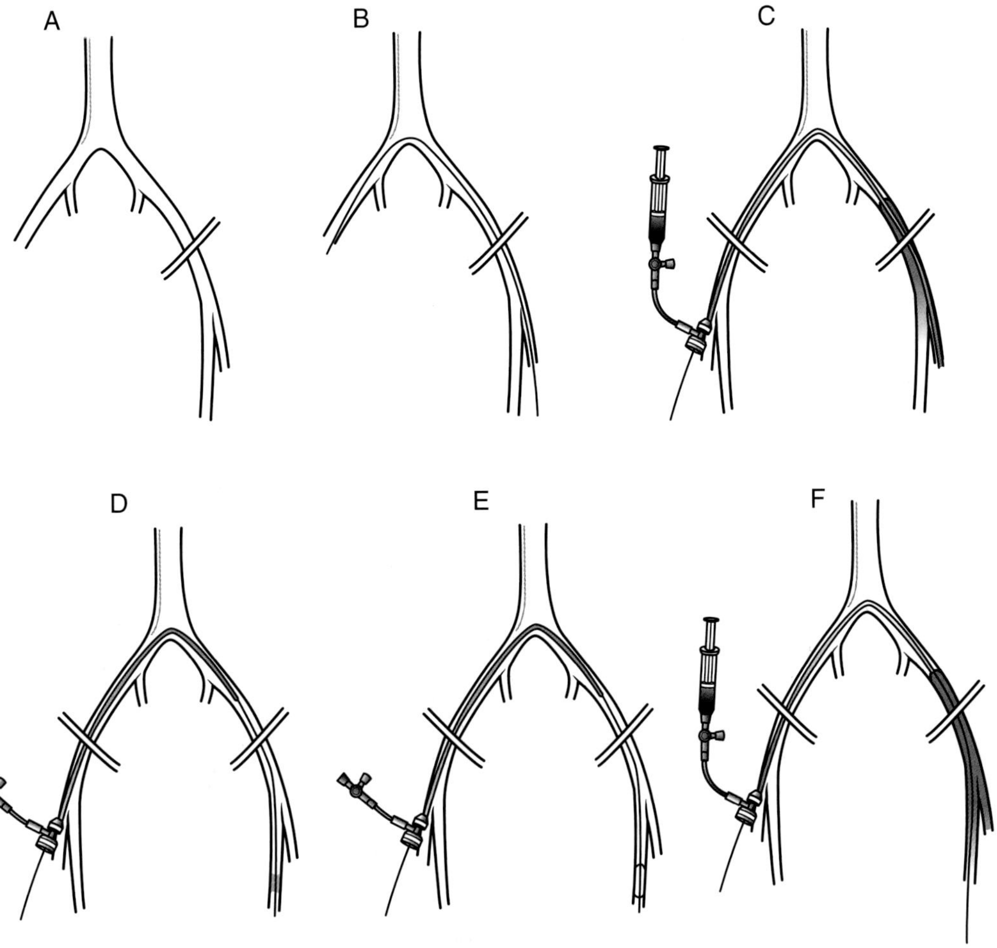

FIG 30.2 Balloon angioplasty of the femoral and popliteal arteries through an up-and-over approach. (A) A superficial femoral artery lesion is identified. (B) A guidewire is introduced through the contralateral femoral artery and passed over the aortic bifurcation. (C) An up-and-over sheath is placed, and arteriography is performed. (D) The guidewire crosses the lesion. (E) Balloon angioplasty is performed. (F) Completion arteriography is performed through the sheath. (From Schneider PA: The infrainguinal arteries—advice about balloon angioplasty and stent placement. In Schneider PA, editor: *Endovascular Skills*, ed 2, New York, 2003, Marcel Dekker, p 323.)

TABLE 30.3 Supplies for Antegrade Approach to Infrainguinal Intervention

Category	Type	Function	Diameter	Length	Other Features
Guidewires	Wholey	Starting, selective	0.035 inch	145 cm	Steerable
	Glidewire	Selective, therapy	0.035 inch	150, 180 cm	Steerable
	Rosen	Exchange	0.035 inch	180 cm	Sheath placement
	Ironman	Therapy	0.014 inch	190 cm	
Catheters	Kumpe	Selective, exchange	5 French	40 cm	Short, angled tip
Glidecath	Selective, exchange	4, 5 French	70 cm	Angled tip	
	Straight	Flush, exchange	5 French	70 cm	Multiside hole
Sheaths	Standard	Access, guide	5, 6 French	12–20 cm	Straight
Balloons	Multiple	PTA infrainguinal	0.035, 0.018, 0.014 inch	75, 90 cm	Balloon diameters, 2–6 mm; balloon lengths, 2, 4, 6 cm
Stents	SMART	Stent SFA, popliteal Self-expanding	0.035 inch	80 cm OTW	Stent diameters, 7–8 mm Stent lengths, 4, 6, 10 cm
	Precise	Stent SFA, popliteal Self-expanding	0.018 inch	80 cm OTW Rapid exchange	Stent diameters, 7–8 mm Stent length, 4 cm
	Multiple	Stent tibials Balloon-expandable	0.014 inch	100 cm Rapid exchange	Stent diameters, 2.5–4 mm Stent length, 2 cm

OTW, Over the wire; *PTA,* percutaneous transluminal angioplasty; *SFA,* superficial femoral artery.

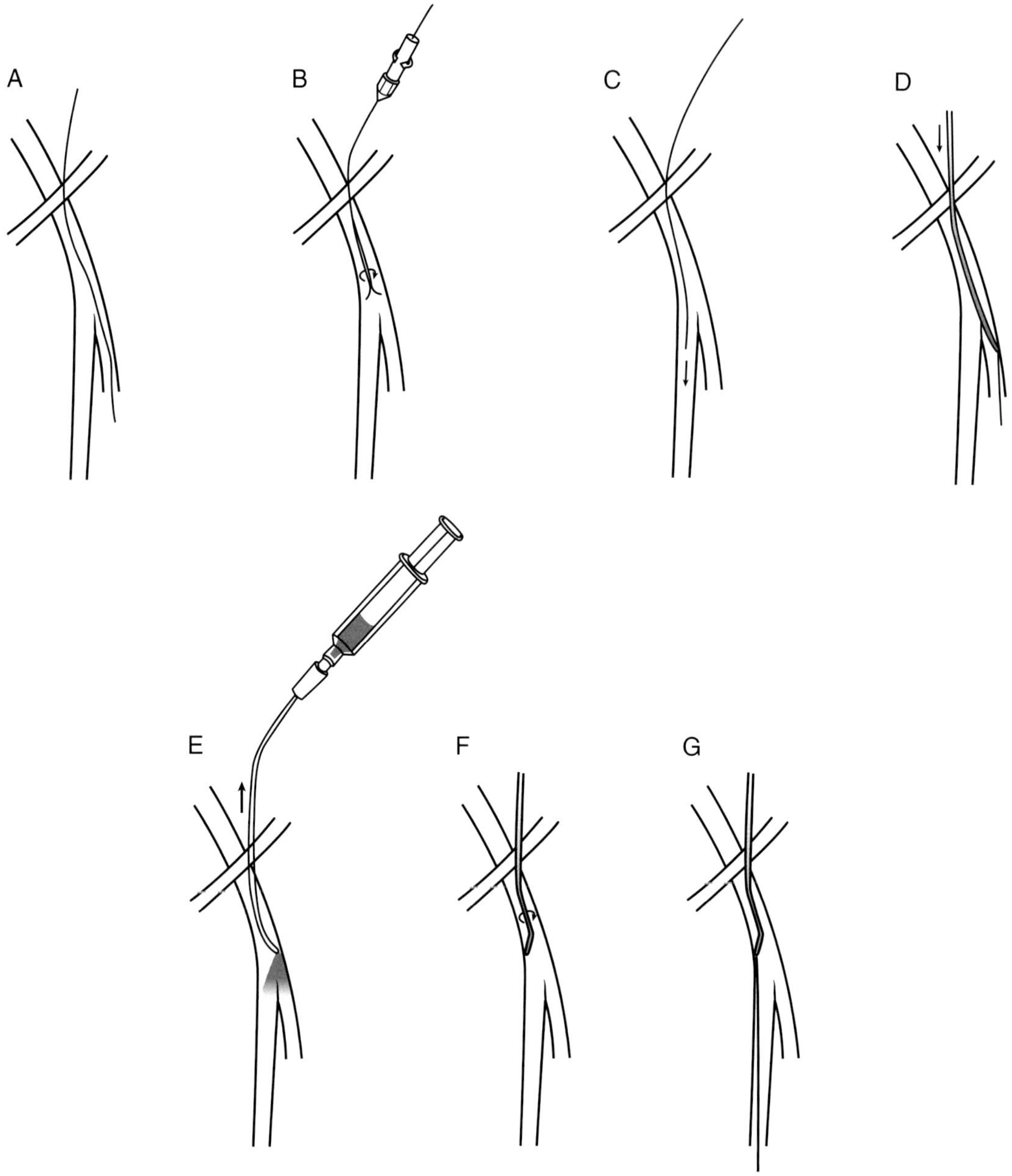

FIG 30.3 Catheterization of the superficial femoral artery (SFA) through an ipsilateral antegrade approach. (A) After antegrade femoral puncture, the guidewire tends to advance into the profunda (deep) femoral artery (PFA). (B) A Wholey guidewire can be used with a torque device to direct the guidewire into the SFA. (C) The guidewire tip is rotated anteriorly and medially to enter the SFA. (D) Another option is to pass an angled-tip catheter into the PFA. (E) The guidewire is removed, and the catheter is slowly withdrawn while puffing contrast material to demonstrate the femoral bifurcation. (F) The catheter tip is rotated toward the SFA. (G) The guidewire is advanced through the catheter into the SFA. (From Schneider PA: The infrainguinal arteries—advice about balloon angioplasty and stent placement. In Schneider PA, editor: *Endovascular Skills*, ed 2, New York, 2003, Marcel Dekker, p 109.)

After the sheath is placed, femoral arteriography is performed through its side arm. Heparin is administered (100 mg/kg) and the ACT is assessed. Standard-length, 180-cm, 0.035-inch guidewires may be used for lesions above the knee. Longer 260-cm, 0.014- or 0.018-inch guidewires are used for infrageniculate intervention, especially in tall patients. As with the contralateral approach, the lesion is then evaluated angiographically, and a steerable guidewire and supportive hydrophilic catheter is used to cross the lesion. Arteriography is repeated after the guidewire is across the lesion to be certain that the guidewire is in the distal artery and not in a perigenicular collateral. The lesion is then treated with the operator's preferred treatment modality, and the completion arteriography is performed through the sheath while maintaining guidewire control until the results are assessed.

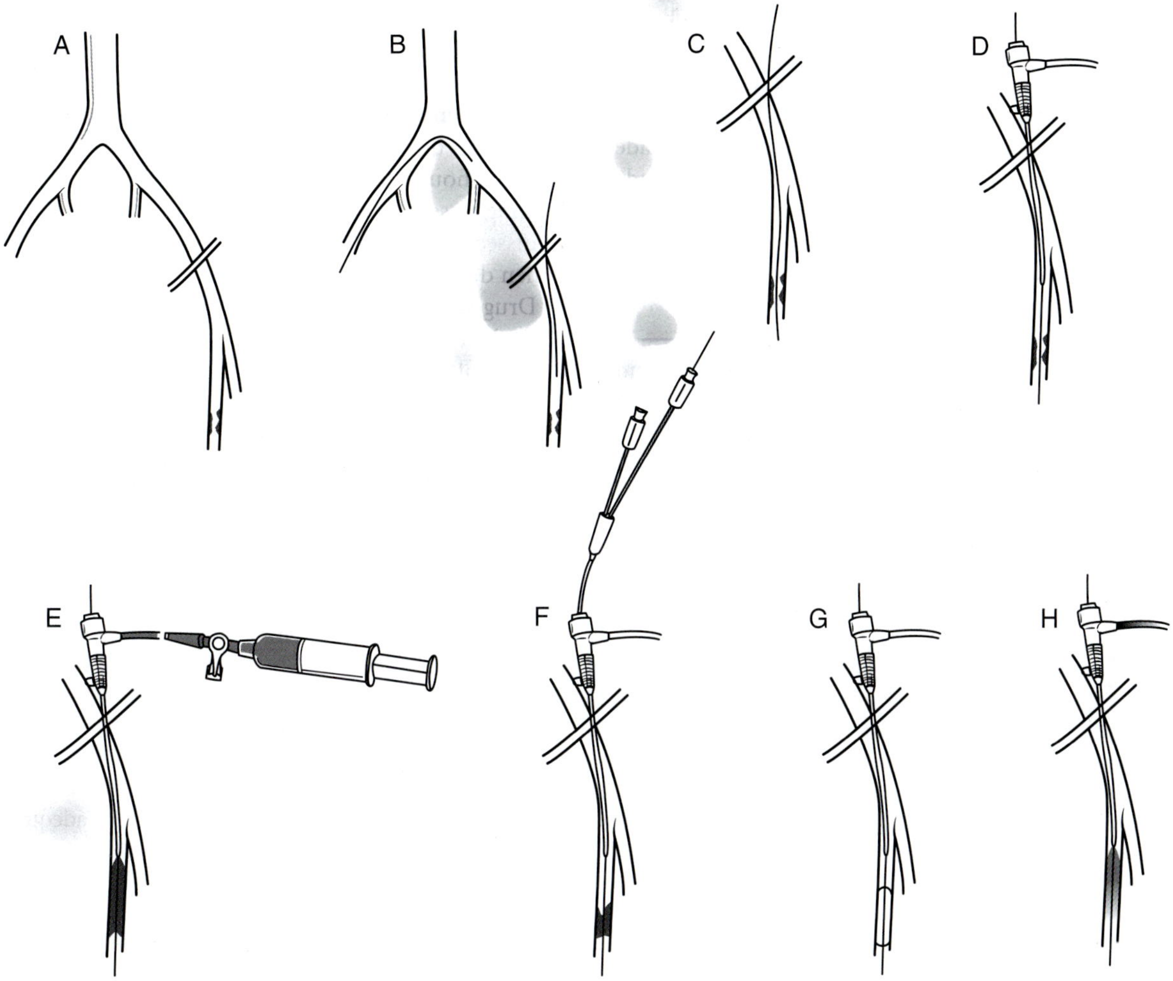

FIG 30.4 Balloon angioplasty of the superficial femoral artery (SFA) and popliteal artery through an antegrade approach. (A) Stenosis of the SFA is suitable for balloon angioplasty. (B) The lesion may be approached from either the contralateral or the ipsilateral femoral artery. (C) The guidewire is placed across the stenosis through an antegrade approach. (D) An access sheath is placed into the proximal SFA. (E) Arteriography is performed through the side arm of the sheath to evaluate the lesion and confirm guidewire position. (F) The balloon angioplasty catheter is passed over the guidewire and advanced into the lesion. (G) Balloon angioplasty is performed. (H) Completion arteriography is performed. Guidewire position is maintained until the results are assessed. (From Schneider PA: The infrainguinal arteries—advice about balloon angioplasty and stent placement. In Schneider PA, editor: *Endovascular Skills*, ed 2, New York, 2003, Marcel Dekker, p 318.)

Retrograde Approach

In cases of particularly challenging lesions where dense calcium is present, or chronic occlusions prevent access from an antegrade approach, the retrograde pedal or tibial access may be employed. Typically reserved for critical limb ischemia (CLI) patients in whom in-line pedal flow is critical to limb salvage, this technique has gained wider acceptance and utilization since first described in 2003.[2] After failure of antegrade recanalization, the antegrade wire and catheter are left in place as a target for retrograde recanalization. Based on angiogram findings, a patent tibial vessel is identified that would provide in-line flow to the foot, ideally with an intact plantar arch. Typically, the dorsalis pedis or posterior tibial is accessed, but peroneal access has also been described.[3] Using a standard 4 French micropuncture kit (Cook, Bloomington, IN) and a combination of duplex ultrasound (DUS) and fluoroscopic guidance, the tibial or pedal vessel is accessed as proximally as possible in a patent portion of the vessel. The 0.018-inch guidewire is advanced and the 4 French micropuncture dilator is inserted over the wire. Using only the dilator minimizes trauma to the vessel before intraluminal cannulization is confirmed with a gentle angiogram. Once the tibial lumen is accessed, the 0.018-inch micropuncture wire is exchanged for a 0.018-inch Connect wire (Abbott Vascular, Santa Clara, CA). For added support, a 0.018-inch CXI catheter (Cook) is advanced in tandem with the V18 wire, and this catheter can either be inserted through the Cook Pedal access sheath, or can be used "bare-back" without a sheath to minimize the arteriotomy size. Using standard subintimal crossing techniques, the wire and catheter are advanced until true lumen access is obtained. At this point, the retrograde crossing wire can be snared from the antegrade approach and one end can be externalized ("flossed") through the femoral sheath. Using the flossed wire, balloon angioplasty can be performed and devices delivered to restore a lumen. Then, a catheter is advanced over the flossed wire to the point of retrograde puncture, the flossed wire is removed, and a new antegrade 0.014-inch or 0.018-inch wire is advanced into the distal tibial vessels. Standard tibial interventions follow, as described below.

TREATMENT MODALITIES

Selection of approach and technique of sheath placement and lesion crossing are performed similarly regardless of the ultimate treatment modality that is chosen. Once the lesion has been crossed and confirmation of true-luminal reentry has been ascertained, the operator can choose from an increasing number of percutaneous treatment modalities. Although much of this decision is based on operator preference and comfort level, certain modalities are better suited for specific disease patterns.

Balloon Angioplasty and Drug-Coated Balloons

Balloon angioplasty has been used since the 1980s and has the advantage of being technically simple and quick to perform, thus minimizing contrast usage and radiation exposure. Most superficial femoral and popliteal artery lesions are treated with balloons ranging from 4 to 6 mm in diameter, and a number of vendors provide balloons in lengths up to 250 mm. Tibial arteries range from 1 to 4 mm in diameter, but most are treated with balloons ranging from 2 to 3.5 mm in diameter and up to 150 mm in length. Increased balloon lengths allow long-segment lesions to be treated faster by minimizing the number of inflations and reducing the number of times a recently treated area is subjected to stagnation of blood flow because of a balloon inflation proximal or distal to it. Most modern angioplasty balloon catheters are relatively noncompliant in nature, thus ensuring that the balloon diameter varies little, even at high-pressure inflations.

Catheter length must be anticipated before selecting the balloon. Most of the standard 0.035-, 0.014-, or 0.018-inch platform balloons are on shafts that are either 75 to 80 cm long or 120 to 150 cm long. A 75-cm balloon catheter shaft passed up and over the bifurcation will reach anywhere from the common femoral artery to the distal SFA, depending on the patient's height. An estimation of the distance to the lesion can be obtained by using a 75-cm-long straight exchange catheter for guidewire exchanges. The up-and-over sheath also provides clues because its length is known.

When performing angioplasty of an infrainguinal lesion, the balloon catheter is passed over the guidewire and into the lesion. The location of the lesion may be marked using road mapping or an external marker. The balloon is then inflated until the waist on the balloon profile is resolved, which generally requires inflations up to 6 to 10 atm. The duration of balloon inflation is anywhere from a few seconds to several minutes. If the waist caused by a lesion fails to resolve even at high inflation pressures, this can sometimes be remedied by exchanging a long balloon for a short (2 cm long) balloon, which is then centered directly at the waist and inflated to the balloon's rated burst pressure. Following treatment, the completion arteriogram is obtained through the side arm of the sheath. Balloon angioplasty of the superficial femoral and popliteal arteries almost always produces some evidence of dissection on completion arteriography. In this setting, deciding which patients require a stent may be challenging, though stents are generally used in patients with flow-limiting dissections, large spiral dissections, or residual stenoses or dissections resulting in greater than 30% reduction in flow lumen diameter.

Drug-coated balloons (DCBs) have recently become available in the United States, and these devices use existing angioplasty balloon platforms that are coated with a combination of an excipient and the antineoplastic drug paclitaxel. Paclitaxel is a highly lipophilic drug that has been shown to inhibit smooth muscle cell proliferation and thereby intimal hyperplasia, and the excipient aids in delivery of the drug from the balloon to the vessel wall.[4] Prior to use of the DCB, vessel preparation with plain old balloon angioplasty (POBA) or atherectomy should be performed to pretreat the lesion and to prevent the lesion from stripping the drug from the balloon while the balloon is in transit through the lesion. Care must be exercised to avoid getting the balloon wet prior to insertion in the sheath, and overmanipulation of the balloon should be avoided to prevent drug loss. Once inserted into the sheath and delivered to the target lesion, the balloon is inflated in standard fashion, but is kept inflated for at 2 to 3 minutes to ensure that adequate transfer of the drug into the vessel wall occurs.

Stent Implantation

Early reports of stent use in the infrainguinal circulation were plagued with poor patency outcomes, mostly because of a high number of stent fractures and subsequent occlusions owing to the use of balloon-expandable stainless steel stents. Most contemporary series of femoropopliteal stent implantation demonstrate improved patency results, likely because of the use of self-expanding laser-cut nitinol stents or stents comprised of woven nitinol wires that have increased flexibility and resistance to stent fractures.

Laser-cut nitinol stents can be oversized between 1 and 3 mm larger than the intended artery segment, allowing for increased versatility of these devices, although there is some evidence that oversizing increases chronic inflammation and may be a trigger for restenosis. Self-expanding nitinol stents are available for 0.035-inch platforms ranging in diameter from 4 to 7 mm and lengths of 20 to 250 mm for the femoropopliteal circulation. These stents generally require a 6 French delivery sheath, although some can be delivered via smaller sheaths. Current laser-cut nitinol stents foreshorten only minimally and have markers on the ends for better visualization. Stent delivery catheters are 80 or 120 cm long, based on stent diameters and intended target vessel. During deployment, the constrained stent is usually passed slightly beyond the lesion and pulled back with a fine-tuning adjustment as its tip end begins to open. Self-expanding stents deploy by unsheathing the stent from the tip end of the catheter, back toward the hub end. Stent delivery systems include pin-and-pull systems, in which the push rod is held steady while the stent delivery catheter hub is pulled back to unsheath the stent,

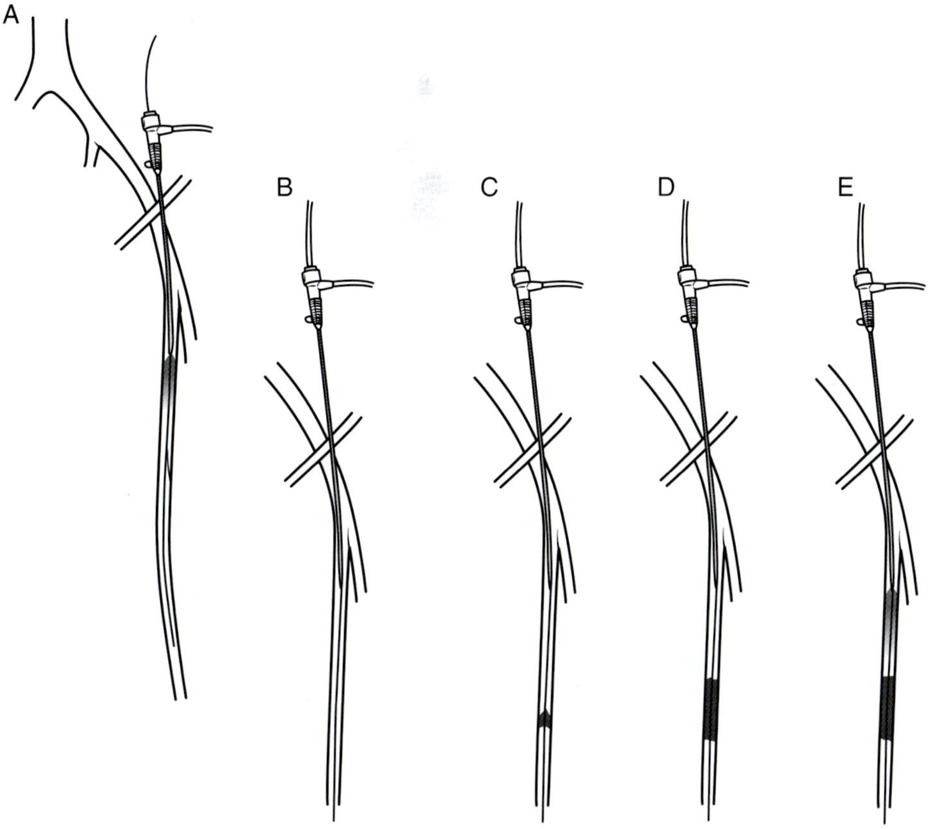

FIG 30.5 Stent placement in the superficial femoral artery. (A) Dissection is present after balloon angioplasty. (B) A self-expanding stent delivery catheter is placed over the guidewire and advanced into the segment of dissection. (C) The stent is deployed from the tip end to the hub end of the catheter. (D) Poststent balloon angioplasty is performed to bring the stent to its appropriate profile. (E) Completion arteriography is performed. (From Schneider PA: The infrainguinal arteries—advice about balloon angioplasty and stent placement. In Schneider PA, editor: *Endovascular Skills*, ed 2, New York, 2003, Marcel Dekker, p 321.)

or click-wheel systems, in which a trigger or wheel is activated to deploy the stent in a controlled fashion (Fig. 30.5). After the stent is deployed, balloon angioplasty is repeated to ensure wall apposition.

Woven nitinol stents (Supera, Abbott Vascular) have the advantage of improved flexibility that appears to resist stent fractures, as well as improved crush resistance without exerting chronic outward radial force on the vessel. These stents come constrained in the delivery catheter at three times their nominally deployed length, and optimal results with these stents require that proper technique is employed so that they are delivered to within 10% of their intended length. This requires adequate vessel preparation to enlarge the lumen of the artery enough to accommodate the stent, generally employing an angioplasty balloon measuring 0.5 to 1.0 mm larger than the outer stent diameter. The stent is delivered by slowly advancing a thumb-slide under direct fluoroscopic visualization while applying gentle forward pressure on the delivery catheter to "pack" the coils of the stent into the proper geometry, thus ensuring proper nominal length.

Stents can be used as a primary modality or selectively following angioplasty as described previously for flow-limiting dissections (with or without contrast trapping in the wall of the artery), spiral dissections, or residual stenosis of the artery lumen greater than 30%. Primary stent placement has been shown in a single randomized trial to result in improved patency rates relative to angioplasty alone, although many continue to use selective stenting preferentially. Primary stent implantation is also used in most cases following recanalization of long-segment occlusions where there is greater likelihood of early rethrombosis.

Atherectomy

Atherectomy, whether performed by excisional, orbital, rotational, or laser atherectomy devices, has the advantage of allowing for plaque debulking with the potential for improved results over angioplasty alone without leaving behind a stent. This advantage has particular importance in specific areas, such as the popliteal circulation, where stents are subject to a number of dynamic forces. In addition, atherectomy systems have the ability to treat vessels without changing the options for subsequent open surgical revascularization. The most commonly used atherectomy systems currently available include the SilverHawk and TurboHawk excisional atherectomy systems (eV3, Plymouth, MN), the Diamondback 360 orbital atherectomy system (Cardiovascular

Systems, St. Paul, MN), and the TurboElite excimer laser catheter (Spectranetics, Colorado Springs, CO).

The SilverHawk excisional atherectomy system received US Food and Drug Administration (FDA) approval in 2003. This single-use, battery-powered atherectomy catheter allows for directional atherectomy in which the plaque is excised by a rotational cutter and packed into the nose cone of the device. It is compatible with 6 to 7 French sheaths and is used with a 0.014-inch platform in a monorail fashion. Although the original SilverHawk catheters offer treatment ranges from 1.5 to 7 mm vessel diameter, the newest iterations of the device (TurboHawk, HawkOne) offer improved cutter efficiency and wider vessel diameter treatment ranges, allowing a single catheter to treat vessel diameters of 2 to 4 mm (TurboHawk SX-C) or 3.5 to 7 mm (TurboHawk LX-C, HawkOne).

The Diamondback 360 atherectomy catheter received FDA approval in 2007 for the treatment of arterial lesions in the peripheral vasculature. This device consists of a diamond-tipped burr or crown that is positioned eccentrically on a flexible drive shaft of the catheter that runs over a 0.018-inch platform. The drive shaft generates an orbital speed of 80,000 to 200,000 rpm, which allows the crown to sand down plaque into debris that is small enough (2 to 6 μm) to pass through the capillary circulation. This mechanism of action makes this device well suited for tough fibrous lesions or heavily calcified lesions; therefore, it has been applied most frequently to infrageniculate lesions.

The TurboElite laser atherectomy system is composed of the catheter and a separate generator that creates a xenon laser in the ultraviolet wavelength that vaporizes plaque. Tissue penetration is 10 μm, thus resulting in minimal temperature change to neighboring tissue. The catheters range in diameter from 0.9 to 2.5 mm, but can be used in conjunction with the TurboBooster catheter, which allows directional orientation of the laser catheter to create a significantly larger lumen than the catheter alone. As a result, lumen diameters can range from 1.5 to 6 mm. The catheters require 0.014- or 0.018-inch platforms and are compatible with 6 to 8 French sheaths, depending on whether the TurboBooster catheter is used.

The steps required for atherectomy in the infrainguinal circulation begin in a similar fashion as for angioplasty and stenting. An appropriately sized up-and-over sheath for the device of choice is placed following diagnostic angiography. Next, the patient is given 100 units/kg of intravenous heparin for systemic anticoagulation, and the lesion must be crossed. Although the stenosis or occlusion can be crossed with any size guidewire, 0.035-inch wires must then be exchanged for a 0.014- or 0.018-inch wire depending on the system chosen. Atherectomy is then performed, generally with slow and deliberate advances of the catheter to avoid distal embolization. Some clinicians prefer to use distal embolic protection devices during atherectomy, but most systems do not require this and rates of clinically relevant embolization are low in most series. After several passes of the atherectomy catheter, generally in different orientations when using directional catheters, the device is removed and angiography is repeated. Areas of residual luminal irregularity because of dissections or residual plaque can be postdilated with low-pressure balloon angioplasty. Rarely, stent implantation may be necessary after plaque debulking if residual flow-limiting lesions exist. In general, all atherectomy systems are more complex and require somewhat longer procedure times relative to balloon angioplasty and stenting. In addition, increased contrast usage is typical because of the multiple passes required and the repeated angiography needed to assess treatment response. However, benefits of atherectomy include minimization of the barotrauma associated with angioplasty and avoidance of stent implantation in most cases.

Covered-Stent-Grafting

The most common mode of failure following percutaneous interventions for the infrainguinal circulation results from restenosis as a result of intimal hyperplasia. To combat this process, some clinicians have adopted the placement of covered stent-grafts in the SFA. This technique prevents ingrowth of intimal hyperplasia and excludes other thrombogenic material on the surface of the treated artery from the arterial lumen. Currently available stents include expanded polytetrafluoroethylene-covered nitinol self-expanding stents (Viabahn [W.L. Gore, Flagstaff, AZ] and Fluency [Bard, Murray Hill, NJ]) and balloon-expandable stainless steel stents (iCast [Atrium Medical Group, Hudson, NH] and Jostent [Abbott Vascular]). Of these, the Viabahn endoprosthesis is used most frequently and is available in a range of diameters and lengths appropriate for the SFA. Increasingly smaller delivery catheters are available, allowing treatment of most patients with sheaths as small as 6 French. The technique for placement of these stents is similar to that of nitinol stents, although there are additional issues that should be considered to ensure that the risk of stent-graft thrombosis and resultant ischemia is minimized. First, as with any surgical bypass, it is important that the patient has adequate inflow and distal tibial runoff. Second, debulking with atherectomy or predilatation with balloon angioplasty, as well as postimplantation angioplasty, is important to allow full expansion of the stent-graft. In addition, oversizing should be avoided to prevent infolding and kinking of the graft. Finally, although all diseased segments of the artery should be covered, care should be taken to avoid unnecessary coverage of significant collaterals if at all possible because the coverage of such collaterals can result in acute limb-threatening ischemia if the graft occludes. Antiplatelet therapy with aspirin and clopidogrel is important in all percutaneous interventions, but it should be considered mandatory in patients undergoing stent-grafting of the SFA.

RESULTS OF PERCUTANEOUS INFRAINGUINAL INTERVENTION

Balloon Angioplasty for Femoropopliteal Lesions

The patency of percutaneous transluminal angioplasty (PTA) of a short femoropopliteal lesion under favorable circumstances is 70% to 80% at 1 year and 50% to 60% at 5 years.[5-15] This type of lesion is ideally suited to PTA. Endovascular intervention is cost effective compared with surgery in this setting and is the treatment of choice.[16] Unfortunately, most situations in which femoropopliteal balloon angioplasty is considered are more complex and factors are not as favorable. The technique of

TABLE 30.4 Meta-analyses of Femoropopliteal Balloon Angioplasty: Effect of Lesion Type and Clinical Stage

				PRIMARY PATENCY (%)		
Reference	**Number of Limbs**	**Lesion Type**	**Clinical Stage**	**1 Year**	**3 Years**	**5 Years**
Hunink and colleagues[7]	4800	Stenosis	Claudication	79	74	68
		Stenosis	Limb threat	62	54	47
		Occlusion	Claudication	52	43	35
		Occlusion	Limb threat	26	18	12
Muradin and colleagues[10]	923	Stenosis	Claudication	61		
		Stenosis	Limb threat	43		
		Occlusion	Claudication	48		
		Occlusion	Limb threat	30		

From Schneider PA, Nelken N, Caps MT: Angioplasty and stenting for infrainguinal lesions. In Yao JST, Pearse WH, Matsumura JS, editors: *Trends in Vascular Surgery*, Chicago, 2003, Parmentier Publishing, p 293.

subintimal angioplasty for long-segment occlusions of the femoropopliteal arteries, which involves the intentional entry into a subintimal dissection plane followed by reentry into the true lumen after the occlusion is crossed, was first described in the late 1980s. Technical success rates with this procedure range from approximately 70% to 90%.[17-21] The major obstacle to technical success is the difficulty in reentering the true lumen distal to the occlusion. Preliminary results using two commercially available systems designed for true lumen reentry are promising and may improve technical success rates.[22,23] In one of the largest studies of long-segment femoropopliteal lesions treated with subintimal recanalization with long-term follow-up, patency rates following technically successful procedures were 71% at 1 year and 58% at 3 years.[20]

Data accumulated over 20 years provide a deeper understanding of femoropopliteal balloon angioplasty across a variety of patient and lesion characteristics. In a summary of studies covering 1241 patients, the pooled results (weighted averages) for femoropopliteal balloon angioplasty were as follows: 90% technical success rate, 4.3% complication rate, 1-year patency of 61%, and 5-year patency of 48%.[1] In a review of several large studies published in the early to mid-1990s, before the broad availability and use of stents, patency rates ranged from 47% to 63% at 1 year and 26% to 48% at 5 years.[5] Multiple factors affect the results of femoropopliteal PTA, including lesion length, clinical stage (claudication vs. limb salvage), runoff, lesion type (stenosis vs. occlusion), proximal location, and lack of residual stenosis after PTA (Tables 30.4 and 30.5).[6-8] Meta-analyses have demonstrated the effect of lesion type and clinical stage (see Table 30.4).[9,10] Lesion length is not addressed in as many studies, and length classifications have not been standardized; however, it appears that length also has a significant effect on results (see Table 30.5).[11-14]

TABLE 30.5 Effect of Lesion Length on Results of Femoropopliteal Balloon Angioplasty

Reference	Lesion Length (cm)	Patency (%)	Follow-Up
Murray and colleagues[11]	<7	81	6 months
	>7	23	6 months
Currie and colleagues[12]	<5	59	6 months
	>5	4	6 months
Jeans and colleagues[13]	<1	76	5 years
	>1	50	5 years
Krepel and colleagues[14]	<2	77	5 years
	>2	54	5 years

From Schneider PA, Nelken N, Caps MT: Angioplasty and stenting for infrainguinal lesions. In Yao JST, Pearse WH, Matsumura JS, editors: *Trends in Vascular Surgery*, Chicago, 2003, Parmentier Publishing, p 293.

Drug-Coated Balloon Angioplasty for Femoropopliteal Lesions

With the advent of paclitaxel-coated balloons, the treatment paradigm of SFA lesions has shifted. There are multiple randomized studies comparing DCB angioplasty POBA and the results favor DCB. In LEVANT II, 476 patients were randomized to the Lutonix DCB (Bard, New Hope, MN) or POBA at a 2:1 randomization ratio to evaluate the clinical efficacy and safety profile of this DCB. Importantly, this study excluded patients who were stented after predilation before randomization and required a blinded clinician in follow-up. Primary patency was found to be significantly higher in the DCB group at 12 months (65.2% in the DCB group and 52.6% in the POBA group; $P = .02$), although there was no difference in target lesion revascularization (TLR).[24] In the INPACT-SFA trial, patients were randomized to treatment with the paclitaxel-coated IN.PACT Admiral DCB (Medtronic, Minneapolis, MN) or POBA, again at a 2:1 randomization ratio. Primary patency was significantly higher in the DCB group compared to the POBA group at 24 months, (78.9% vs. 50.1%, respectively), and clinically driven TLR was significant lower (9.1% and 28.3% respectively). There were no differences in adverse events, and at the end of 24 months, DCB patients had 58% fewer reinterventions.[25] A Cochrane review of DCB versus POBA found 11 trials with 1838 patients, and high-quality evidence showing an advantage for DCB in primary vessel patency (OR 3.51 at 24 months) and rate of TLR (0.44 at 24 months).[26]

There is increasing interest in treating SFA lesions with DCBs prior to stenting with nitinol bare metal stents (BMSs) to reduce restenosis rates and prevent the need for lesion revascularization. In the Drug-Eluting Balloon in Peripheral Intervention (DEBATE-SFA) trial, 110 limbs were randomly assigned to DCB with BMS or POBA with BMS. The primary endpoint was restenosis, and mean lesion length was 94 ± 60 mm. Binary restenosis was defined as greater than 50% luminal narrowing by arteriography or peak systolic velocity (PSV) ratio greater than 2.5 by DUS. At 12 months, restenosis was 17% and 47.3% in the DCB and POBA groups, respectively. Freedom from TLR trended in favor of the DCB-treated group ($P = .07$).[27] In addition, there is retrospective data that suggest the use of DCB in conjunction with directional atherectomy improves primary patency in restonic vessels.[28] Overall, the data suggest that treating femoropopliteal lesions with DCB reduces restenosis rates, leads to fewer reinterventions, and improves primary patency over POBA. Treating SFA lesions with DCB in the setting of stent placement appears to improve BMS stent patency.

Stent Implantation for Femoropopliteal Lesions

Over the past 10 years, stent placement has been integrated into infrainguinal intervention. This evolution has been prompted by the development of a variety of simple, low-profile, user-friendly, self-expanding stents that can be easily placed when needed or when the immediate results of PTA or DCB are not satisfactory. Earlier studies showed no patency benefit to primary stent implantation over selective stenting, but these studies focused on the use of rigid stainless steel balloon-expandable stents, which are not well suited for the femoropopliteal circulation (Table 30.6).[29-32] More recent data suggest that modern self-expanding nitinol stents may significantly improve patency results over balloon-expandable stents because nonrandomized studies have shown 70% to 80% primary patency at 3 years.[33-35] In addition, a randomized trial comparing primary stenting of the SFA with self-expanding nitinol stents to selective stenting for residual stenoses or dissections suggested that primary stenting of all lesions is associated with decreased rates of restenosis and increased ankle-brachial indices compared to selective stenting.[36] In this study of 104 patients with severe claudication or limb-threatening ischemia because of lesions in the SFA, the rate of restenosis on angiography at 6 months was 24% in the stent group and 43% in the angioplasty group ($P = .05$); at 12 months the rates on duplex ultrasonography were 37% and 63%, respectively ($P = .01$).

TABLE 30.6 Results of Randomized Trials Comparing Primary Versus Selective Stent Placement for Femoropopliteal Occlusive Disease

Author	Year	PATENCY AFTER STENT PLACEMENT (%)		Follow-Up (Years)
		Primary	Selective	
Vroegindeweij and colleagues[29]	1997	74	85	1
Cejna and colleagues[30]	2001	65	65	2
Grimm and colleagues[31]	2001	62	68	3
Becquemin and colleagues[32]	2003	44	57	4
Schillinger and colleagues[36]	2006	63	37	1

Modified from Schneider PA, Nelken N, Caps MT: Angioplasty and stenting for infrainguinal lesions. In Yao JST, Pearse WH, Matsumura JS, editors: *Trends in Vascular Surgery*, Chicago, 2003, Parmentier Publishing, p 293.

Although the merits of primary stent placement continue to be debated, it is clear that selective stent placement has an important role in successful percutaneous intervention. The immediate success of intervention is higher with the availability of stents. Approximately 15% of patients undergoing PTA alone require selective stent placement or experience immediate failure.[30-32] The least favorable results of PTA come from the treatment of long lesions, occlusions, residual stenoses, and limb-threatening ischemia. Stents are an essential tool if endovascular intervention is to be an option in treating these complex lesions and unfavorable clinical situations. A meta-analysis of 423 stent implantations for femoropopliteal occlusive disease demonstrated 66% patency at 3 years, which was not dependent on clinical indication or lesion type.[10] Stents have also yielded promising results with long, chronic occlusions.[37]

Just as self-expanding nitinol stents appear to provide additional benefit over stainless steel stents, advances in stent technology continue to offer promise of improved results. Another new stent design is demonstrated in the Supera stent (Abbott Vascular, Santa Clara, CA), which is composed of six pairs of nitinol wires interwoven in a helical fashion with a closed cell geometry that is delivered through a 6 to 7 French sheath over a 0.014- or 0.018-inch platform, with diameters from 4 to 8 mm and lengths up to 150 mm. The interwoven nitinol helix provides the stent with fourfold the radial force and more than threefold the crush resistance of standard self-expanding nitinol stents, and early European data suggest that the stent may perform well in long lesions. Recently presented data on 159 patients who underwent stenting of femoropopliteal arteries and 23 patients who underwent isolated popliteal stenting demonstrated a 74% and 83% 12-month patency rate (by duplex), respectively. Moreover, the average lesion length in the femoropopliteal group was 240 mm, with 40% TASC D classification and 57% total occlusions, suggesting that these patients had long complex lesion anatomy. Finally, subgroup analysis showed no stent fractures at 24 months.[38] In the SUPERB trial, 264 patients with SFA lesions of length 83 ± 33 mm were treated with woven nitinol stents. Primary patency was 86.3% at 12 months.[39]

Drug-Eluting Stent Implantation for Femoropopliteal Lesions

Drug-eluting stents have been used extensively in the coronary circulation and have been shown to result in reduced restenosis after intervention. Currently available balloon-expandable drug-eluting coronary stents include the Taxus stent (Boston Scientific, Natick, MA), which is a paclitaxil-coated stent in diameters of 2.25 to 4 mm and lengths of 8 to 38 mm; and the Cypher stent (Cordis; Johnson and Johnson, Miami Lakes, FL), which is a sirolimus-coated stent in diameters of 2.25 to 3.5 mm and lengths of 8 to 33 mm. The first such stent studied in the periphery was a sirolimus-coated SMART stent (Cordis; Johnson and Johnson), which was implanted for SFA lesions in claudicants and patients with limb-threatening ischemia in the SIROCCO I and SIROCCO II trials.[40,41] These randomized trials did not show a statistically significant benefit for the sirolimus-coated stents relative to BMS at 6 months, and at 24 months the restenosis rates were nearly identical.

More recently, the Zilver PTX trial, which evaluated the paclitaxel-eluting Zilver (Cook Medical) self-expanding nitinol stent in the SFA,[42,43] was a multicenter randomized trial in which 479 patients were treated with primary Zilver PTX stent placement versus angioplasty alone, or by secondary randomization to provisional stenting with the Zilver BMS versus the Zilver PTX stent in those patients who failed to have adequate results with angioplasty alone. Long-term follow-up data demonstrated a 50% reduction in restenosis in patients treated with the drug-eluting stent at 2 years. The primary patency of Zilver PTX compared to standard of care was 84.4% versus 67.4% at 2 years and 66.4% versus 43.4% at 5 years, respectively. In the provisional stent randomization group, 81.2% of the arteries treated with the drug-eluting stents remained patent compared with 62.7% of those treated with BMS alone at 2 years and 72.4% versus 53% at 5 years.[43,44]

Covered Stent-Grafting of the Femoropopliteal Arteries

Several groups have reported outcomes following the use of these covered stent-grafts in the SFA with follow-up periods of up to 4 years.[45-48] The only published data from a randomized trial using covered stent-grafts for the treatment of infrainguinal occlusive disease compared percutaneous placement of the Viabahn stent-graft (W.L. Gore) with surgical femoropopliteal (above-knee) bypass with expanded polytetrafluoroethylene and found favorable results for the use of covered stents in this setting.[48] This study randomized 100 limbs (86 patients) to treatment with either Viabahn stents or bypass and followed the patients postoperatively with ankle brachial index and arterial duplex up to a median of 18 months. The two groups had equivalent primary and secondary patency rates at 12 months (74% and 84%, respectively, for the stent-graft group and 74% and 84%, respectively, for the bypass group). More recently, a dual-center retrospective review of 315 patients with covered stent placement in SFA lesions (50% TASC C/D) showed primary patency rates of 72.2%, 51.8%, and 47.6% at 1, 3, and 5 years respectively.[49] The VIASTAR trial of 141 patients with long lesions (189 ± 63 mm) treated with standard BMS versus the Viabahn self-expanding stent showed a primary patency benefit to the Viabahn group (69.4% vs. 40.0% at 2 years).[50] No freedom from TLR or clinical outcome differences were demonstrated. A continued concern in using covered stent-grafts in the femoropopliteal circulation is the risk of acute limb ischemia following occlusion of these grafts. Although this problem does occur, the rates of acute ischemia remain relatively low in published studies.

Balloon Angioplasty and Stent Placement for Infrapopliteal Lesions

The patency of infrapopliteal balloon angioplasty is not as well established as that for more proximal lesions. Most of these patients have limb-threatening ischemia, multilevel disease, and multiple or diffuse tibial lesions that require treatment. Results have been assessed most often by evaluating limb salvage rather than patency. A meta-analysis of 1282 treated limbs demonstrated a technical success rate of 93% and a 2-year limb salvage rate of 74%.[51] Stent placement is technically feasible using low-profile, balloon-expandable coronary stents on a 0.014-inch platform. More recently, drug-eluting stents have been used for the treatment of infrapopliteal disease, with encouraging results.[52] There have been two randomized trials comparing BMS versus sirolimus-eluting stent (SES) for infrapopliteal disease demonstrating improved patency for SES at 1 year[53] and 3 years.[54] Indeed, novel everolimus-eluting bioresorbable scaffolds have been developed for coronary lesions and are being applied to below-the-knee interventions with promising 12-month outcomes in 33 patients.[55]

Balloon Angioplasty for Infrainguinal Bypass Graft Stenosis

The results of balloon angioplasty for failing infrainguinal bypass grafts have been mixed,[56,57] in part because of the nature of lesions caused by myointimal hyperplasia. These lesions are smooth and fibrous and are often not sufficiently remodeled by standard balloon angioplasty; there is a relatively high probability of elastic recoil. Preliminary studies on the use of cutting balloons for infrainguinal bypass graft stenoses have demonstrated promising results.[58,59] Cutting balloons (Flextome Cutting Balloon; Boston Scientific) are available on a 0.014-inch platform and contain three or four longitudinally placed atherotomes designed to create a controlled series of incisions in the lesion, thereby promoting more effective remodeling. Currently, cutting balloon diameters range from 2 to 4 mm and are available in lengths of 6, 10, and 15 mm. Cutting balloon angioplasty is frequently followed by larger standard balloon angioplasty to improve luminal diameter.

Atherectomy for Femoropopliteal and Tibial Lesions

Like most data concerning percutaneous intervention in the infrainguinal circulation, much of the efficacy data available on atherectomy come from nonrandomized registries or retrospective studies. Among the largest studies of the use of the SilverHawk system in both femoropopliteal and infrageniculate disease is a recent prospective single-center series that evaluated 579 lesions in 275 patients.[60] Sixty-three percent of patients were treated for CLI; lesion distribution included femoropopliteal disease in 53.4%, tibia disease in 37.6%, and multilevel disease in 9.0%. At a mean follow-up of 12.5 months, 18-month primary and secondary patency was 58% and 83%, respectively, for claudicants, and 49% and 70%, respectively, for patients with CLI. Limb salvage at 18 months in patients with CLI was 92.4%

The DEFINITIVE LE study[61] is the first prospective, multicenter trial with independent lab–adjudicated results evaluating directional atherectomy with 12-month follow-up. Of the 800 patients enrolled, 201 had CLI (25%), with a mean lesion length of 8.3 ± 5.7 cm. Of the 1022 lesions treated, occlusions were present in 17.4% and 30% in claudicants and CLI, respectively, and heavy calcium in 37.1%. Procedural success (91.3% vs. 83.0%) and primary patency (78% vs. 71%) were improved in claudicants compared to CLI patients. There was no difference in 12-month primary patency for diabetic patients (77% vs. 78%). Patency for lesion lengths 5 to 9.9 cm was 83% in the SFA, 74% in the popliteal artery, and 88% in the infrapopliteal segment. Limb salvage was 95% at 12 months in the CLI cohort, and the bailout stent rate was very low at 3.2%. Periprocedural events were rare, with embolization occurring in 3.8%, abrupt closure in 2.0%, and dissection in 2.3%. Primary patency, clinical outcomes, and adverse event rates were comparable to second-generation nitinol stent studies despite significantly more advanced and multilevel disease in this cohort of patients.

Among the most widely cited studies regarding outcomes following laser atherectomy with the Spectranetics excimer laser is the Laser Angioplasty for Critical Limb Ischemia trial.[62] This international multicenter trial evaluated the excimer laser in patients who were deemed poor open surgical bypass candidates because of poor bypass targets, lack of available conduit, or presence of severe comorbid illness putting the patient at high risk for surgical complications. One hundred fifty-five limbs were treated in 145 patients with limb-threatening ischemia. Popliteal or infrageniculate vessels were treated in more than 50% of the limbs, and mean treatment length per limb was greater than 150 mm. The 6-month limb salvage rate in this group of patients was 93%, despite their severe degree of disease. In addition to the use of this laser atherectomy device in patients with CLI, some have used the Spectranetics laser in claudicants. In the Peripheral Excimer Laser Angioplasty trial, 251 patients with claudication were randomized to either excimer laser–assisted angioplasty or balloon dilation alone. The 12-month patency rates and functional status were similar in both groups.[63] Laser atherectomy for in-stent restenosis (ISR) has been evaluated in multiple studies and shown to have benefit over POBA.[64] A multicenter randomized controlled clinical trial of excimer laser atherectomy (ELA) with angioplasty versus POBA alone in ISR enrolled 250 patients and was stopped early due to the efficacy of laser atherectomy at interim analysis.[65] In this study, mean lesion length was 19.6 ± 12 cm and 30.5% versus 36.8% exhibited total occlusion in laser versus POBA respectively. Patients treated with ELA had a significantly increased success rate (93.5% vs. 82.7%), freedom from TLR (73.5% versus 51.8%), and decreased major adverse events (5.8% vs. 20.5%) compared to POBA. Overall, ELA with PTA was associated with a 52% reduction in TLR.

CONCLUSIONS

Although the results of endovascular intervention for occlusive disease of the iliac arteries are excellent, whether this success can be extrapolated to the infrainguinal arteries remains controversial. It is clear, however, that the lower periprocedural morbidity and rapid recovery associated with endovascular approaches make them attractive to physicians and patients, and establish them as an important tool in the vascular surgeon's arsenal in combatting lower extremity arterial occlusive disease. A full-service vascular surgery practice must include a broad variety of both endovascular and surgical options for treating infrainguinal arterial occlusive disease. Infrainguinal endovascular intervention and its growing cadre of associated options have a high likelihood of improving the care of patients with vascular disease in the years to come.

REVIEW QUESTIONS

1. Which of the following is an advantage of endovascular intervention over open surgery for infrainguinal arterial occlusive disease?
   a. Less morbidity
   b. Improved patency
   c. Superior durability
   d. All of the above
2. The ipsilateral antegrade femoral approach for infrainguinal intervention is preferred over the contralateral up-and-over approach in which of the following circumstances?
   a. Preprocedural imaging demonstrates absence of iliac inflow disease.
   b. There is chronic renal insufficiency.
   c. Infrapopliteal intervention is planned.
   d. All of the above
3. Which of the following is an advantage of the smaller (0.014- or 0.018-inch) platforms over standard (0.035-inch) systems in infrainguinal endovascular intervention?
   a. Smaller crossing profiles
   b. Better fluoroscopic visualization
   c. Improved ability to cross chronic occlusions
   d. All of the above
4. When using smaller platforms, why are monorail (rapid-exchange) catheters preferred over coaxial catheters?
   a. Less friction and improved trackability
   b. Reduced guidewire movement during catheter exchanges
   c. Shorter required guidewire lengths
   d. All of the above

5. Which of the following statements regarding sheath selection for infrainguinal endovascular intervention is true?
   a. Balloon angioplasty requires a sheath sized 6 French or larger.
   b. Stent placement requires a sheath sized 6 French or smaller.
   c. Sheaths are sized according to their outer diameter.
   d. All of the above
6. Which of the following factors is associated with improved outcomes in patients undergoing femoropopliteal balloon angioplasty?
   a. Long lesions
   b. Absence of residual stenosis after angioplasty
   c. Poor outflow
   d. All of the above
7. Which of the following statements regarding the use of stents for femoropopliteal disease is true?
   a. All stenotic lesions should be stented primarily.
   b. Balloon-expandable stents are more effective than self-expanding stents.
   c. Postangioplasty dissection with contrast trapping should be stented.
   d. All of the above
8. Major obstacles to technical success with infrainguinal subintimal angioplasty include which of the following?
   a. Entering the subintimal plane from the true lumen above the occlusion
   b. Reentering the true lumen below the occlusion
   c. Perforation
   d. All of the above
9. Endovascular intervention for infrainguinal bypass graft stenoses differs from de novo atherosclerotic lesions in which of the following respects?
   a. Increased incidence of elastic recoil
   b. Increased incidence of dissection
   c. Increased need for stents
   d. All of the above
10. Which of the following statements regarding infrapopliteal balloon angioplasty is true?
   a. Patency rates are well established.
   b. Unsuccessful PTA can be salvaged with balloon-expandable coronary stents.
   c. Contralateral up-and-over approach is preferred over ipsilateral antegrade approach.
   d. All of the above

BIBLIOGRAPHY

Becquemin JP, Favre JP, Marzelle J, et al. Systematic versus selective stent placement after superficial femoral artery balloon angioplasty: a multicenter prospective randomized study. *J Vasc Surg*. 2003;37:487–494.

Dake MD, Ansel GM, Jaff MR, et al. Durable Clinical Effectiveness With Paclitaxel-Eluting Stents in the Femoropopliteal Artery: 5-Year Results of the Zilver PTX Randomized Trial. *Circulation*. 2016;133(15):1472–1483.

DeRubertis BG, Faries PL, McKinsey JF, et al. Shifting paradigms in the treatment of lower extremity vascular disease: a report of 1000 percutaneous interventions. *Ann Surg*. 2007;246(3):415–422.

Dippel EJ, Makam P, Kovach R, et al. EXCITE ISR Investigators. Randomized controlled study of excimer laser atherectomy for treatment of femoropopliteal in-stent restenosis: initial results from the EXCITE ISR trial (EXCImer Laser Randomized Controlled Study for Treatment of FemoropopliTEal In-Stent Restenosis). *JACC Cardiovasc Interv*. 2015;8.

Laird JR, Schneider PA, Tepe G, et al. IN.PACT SFA Trial Investigators. Durability of Treatment Effect Using a Drug-Coated Balloon for Femoropopliteal Lesions: 24-Month Results of IN.PACT SFA. *J Am Coll Cardiol*. 2015;66(21):2329–2338.

Lammer J, Zeller T, Hausegger KA, et al. Sustained benefit at 2 years for covered stents versus bare-metal stents in long SFA lesions: the VIASTAR trial. *Cardiovasc Intervent Radiol*. 2015;38(1):25–32.

Liistro F, Grotti S, Porto I, et al. Drug-eluting balloon in peripheral intervention for the superficial femoral artery: the DEBATE-SFA randomized trial (drug eluting balloon in peripheral intervention for the superficial femoral artery). *JACC Cardiovasc Interv*. 2013;6(12):1295–1302.

McKinsey JF, Zeller T, Rocha-Singh KJ, et al. DEFINITIVE LE Investigators. Lower extremity revascularization using directional atherectomy: 12-month prospective results of the DEFINITIVE LE study. *JACC Cardiovasc Interv*. 2014;7(8):923–933.

Rosenfield K, Jaff MR, White CJ, et al. LEVANT 2 Investigators. Trial of a Paclitaxel-Coated Balloon for Femoropopliteal Artery Disease. *N Engl J Med*. 2015;373(2):145–153.

Schillinger M, Sabeti S, Loewe C, et al. Balloon angioplasty versus implantation of nitinol stents in the superficial femoral artery. *N Engl J Med*. 2006;354(18):1879–1888.

References available online at ExpertConsult.com.

31 CHAPTER

Endovascular Repair of Infrapopliteal Arterial Occlusive Disease

Miguel Montero-Baker, Joseph L. Mills

Endovascular therapy (EVT) has increasingly become the initial clinical option for treating both claudication and critical limb ischemia (CLI).[1] Similar to the evolution of open bypass surgery, EVT began above the knee and has been progressively extended to the infrapopliteal segment, now even including the pedal and arch vessels. Enthusiasm for infrapopliteal EVT was tempered by poor initial results,[2] but advances in technique, equipment, and patient selection have led to improved outcomes and more widespread EVT application. This chapter discusses standard techniques for infrapopliteal EVT and reviews the contemporary results of tibial angioplasty, stenting, and atherectomy.

PATIENT SELECTION

The revised Trans-Atlantic Inter-Society Consensus (TASC II) guidelines provide the current consensus recommendations for EVT.[3] TASC II guidelines do not delineate specific anatomic criteria for infrapopliteal disease and do not formally recommend infrapopliteal EVT, whereas previous TASC guidelines included anatomic criteria for infrapopliteal lesions (Table 31.1).[4] TASC II guidelines mention growing evidence to support EVT for infrapopliteal occlusions in patients with comorbidities in whom in-line flow to the foot can be reestablished. In addition, the guidelines also point out that failed angioplasty does not usually preclude subsequent bypass. Graziani and colleagues[5] also proposed a classification system for patients with CLI secondary to multilevel infrainguinal disease (Fig. 31.1).[5] Arterial lesions were graded class 1 to class 7, indicating progressive disease severity with decreasing transcutaneous oxygen tension ($TcPO_2$).

The decision to proceed with infrapopliteal EVT is based on many factors gathered from a complete history, physical examination, laboratory studies, noninvasive imaging, and frequently diagnostic angiography. A surgeon must carefully consider the indication (claudication vs. CLI), disease severity, functional status, age and medical comorbidities, availability and quality of an autologous vein conduit, and prior extremity interventions. EVT is preferred in patients with less severe disease, more comorbidities, shorter life expectancy, and absent suitable autologous vein. Open bypass surgery is more strongly considered for younger, healthier patients, especially when a good autologous vein conduit is available.

TECHNIQUE

Infrapopliteal EVT is best performed through the ipsilateral common femoral artery (CFA) using an antegrade approach. The proximal CFA should be accessed to allow working room between the puncture site and superficial femoral artery (SFA). Accessing the contralateral CFA for an up-and-over approach is also possible, but is probably better reserved for treating lesions above the knee. The antegrade approach has distinct advantages: better wire and catheter control and "pushability" using shorter devices, no routine use of a long sheath, and no requisite crossing of the aortoiliac vessels. Both groins should always be prepared in case an alternative approach is required.

Once the ipsilateral CFA has been accessed, a guidewire is manipulated anteromedially to cannulate the SFA. If this is not possible, the wire can be advanced down the profunda femoris artery, and a short, angled-tip catheter is advanced over the wire. Lateral anterior oblique positioning of the image intensifier helps open the femoral bifurcation. The catheter is withdrawn slowly while puffing contrast until the femoral bifurcation is clearly demonstrated. The catheter tip is steered medially and anteriorly toward the SFA, and the guidewire is advanced into the SFA. The access sheath diameter is typically 5 French, although tibial angioplasty with 0.014- and 0.018-inch platforms can be performed through a 4 French sheath. If an up-and-over approach is used, a long sheath with its tip in the popliteal artery facilitates tibial interventions.

After sheath placement, a diagnostic angiogram is performed through its side port. Lesions above the knee are well delineated in this manner. A short 0.035-inch guidewire is maneuvered into the popliteal artery below the knee, and a 4 or 5 French Glidecath (Medi-Tech, Watertown, MA) is advanced to the end of the wire. Digital subtraction angiography is then used to identify lesions in the trifurcation and distal runoff vessels into the foot. Lateral views of the foot are routinely obtained.

Both transluminal and subintimal approaches can be used for infrapopliteal angioplasty. When choosing a wire for crossing infrapopliteal lesions, several characteristics must be considered, including size (0.035, 0.018, or 0.014 inches), length (180 to 300 cm), coating (bare or hydrophilic), base metal construction (stainless steel, nitinol), stiffness, weight, and tip construction (stiffness, length, coating, shape). Smaller caliber wires (0.014 or 0.018 inches) with a hydrophilic coating and floppy tip are

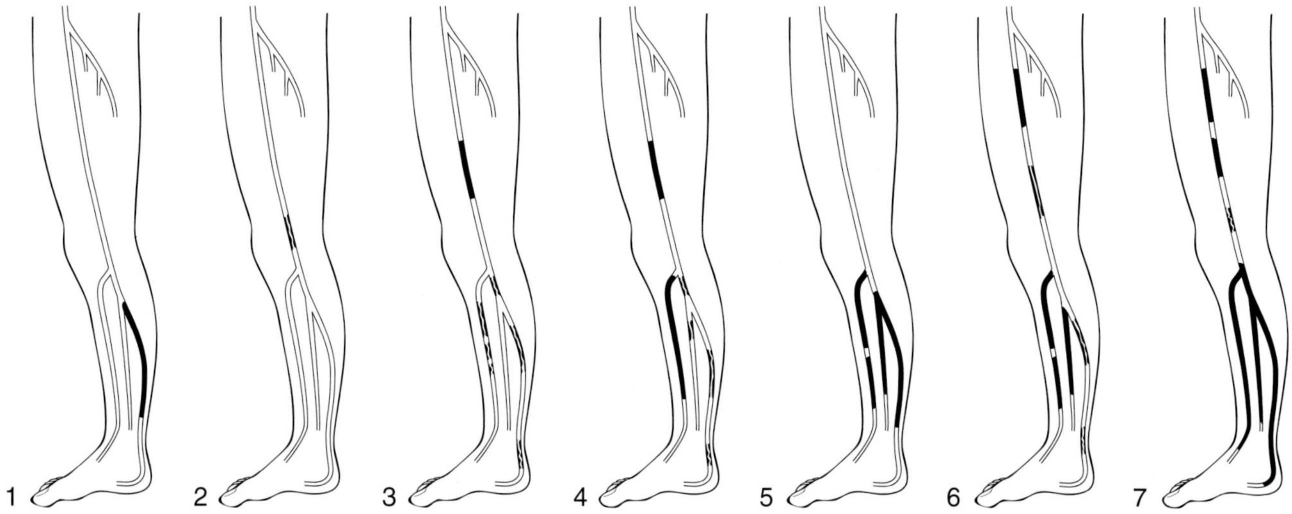

FIG 31.1 Graziani classification scheme for multilevel infrainguinal disease. (From Graziani L, Silvestro A, Bertone V, et al: Vascular involvement in diabetic subjects with ischemic foot ulcer: a new morphologic categorization of disease severity. *Eur J Vasc Endovasc Surg* 33:453–460, 2007.)

TABLE 31.1 Trans-Atlantic Inter-Society Consensus I Classification of Infrapopliteal Lesions

Classification	Lesions Characteristics
TASC A	Single stenosis <1 cm long in tibial or peroneal vessels
TASC B	Multiple focal stenoses of tibial or peroneal vessels <1 cm long One or two stenoses <1 cm long involving the trifurcation Short tibial or peroneal stenosis with femoropopliteal PTA
TASC C	Stenoses 1–4 cm long in tibial or peroneal vessels Occlusions 1–2 cm long in tibial or peroneal vessels Extensive stenosis of the trifurcation
TASC D	Occlusion >2 cm long in tibial or peroneal vessels Diffusely diseased tibial or peroneal vessels

PTA, Percutaneous transluminal angioplasty; *TASC,* Trans-Atlantic Inter-Society Consensus.

often used to cross tibial lesions. The preferred wires are 0.014-inch, nonhydrophilic, medium-weight with short floppy tips for crossing tibial stenoses. Occlusions, particularly when calcified and long, are more difficult to cross. The V18 wire (Boston Scientific, Natick, MA) is particularly useful for crossing tibial occlusions. Contemporary use of the retrograde pedal approach has increased technical success rates when confronting complicated anatomy.

If difficulty arises when attempting to cross stenotic lesions or occlusions with a particular wire, several additional maneuvers are available to facilitate success. Particularly hard or calcified plaque can cause 0.014- and 0.018-inch wires to coil, especially if they have floppy tips. Upsizing to a 0.035-inch wire may give the additional support needed to navigate across the difficult lesion. Another option is the use of a catheter, such as the hydrophilic Glidecath, which can be advanced to the end of the wire and lend additional support. Crossing catheters, such as the Quick-Cross (Spectranetics, Colorado Springs, CO), feature a firmer, tapered tip, which facilitates lesion crossing. These micro-catheters have also been reinforced with a metallic braid, resulting in increased pushability, such as is seen in the CXI family (COOK, Bloomington, IN). Predilation with a small, 2- to 2.5-mm–diameter coronary balloon may fracture a particularly difficult lesion and subsequently allow passage of a wire or low-profile crossing catheter. Guidewires with dilatable tips are also available for this technique. Devices specifically designed for crossing a chronic total occlusion (CTO) are a more recent development. These devices use different strategies to facilitate lesion crossing, including plaque microdissection (Frontrunner XP CTO Catheter; Cordis, Bridgewater, NJ), fast and bidirectional catheter spinning (CrossBoss CTO Catheter; BridgePoint Medical, Plymouth, MN), and catheter tip deflection capability with spiral wedges to facilitate advancement (Wildcat Catheter; Avinger, Redwood City, CA).

Subintimal angioplasty is a useful technique first described by Bolia and coworkers[6] in 1989 for the treatment of long-segment femoropopliteal occlusions.[6] This technique may also be successfully applied to infrapopliteal lesions (Fig. 31.2, see color insert). A wire is used to intentionally create a subintimal dissection plane just proximal to an occlusion. The wire is typically formed into a short J shape and is advanced in the subintimal plane until the occlusion has been passed. If reentry into the true lumen is difficult, it may be facilitated by a special reentry device, such as the Outback LTD (Cordis, Dublin, OH) or the Enteer reentry system (Medtronic, Minneapolis, MN)

Once a stenosis or occlusion has been crossed successfully, balloon angioplasty is possible (Fig. 31.3, see color insert). Balloon angioplasty stretches the arterial wall causing plaque fracture and

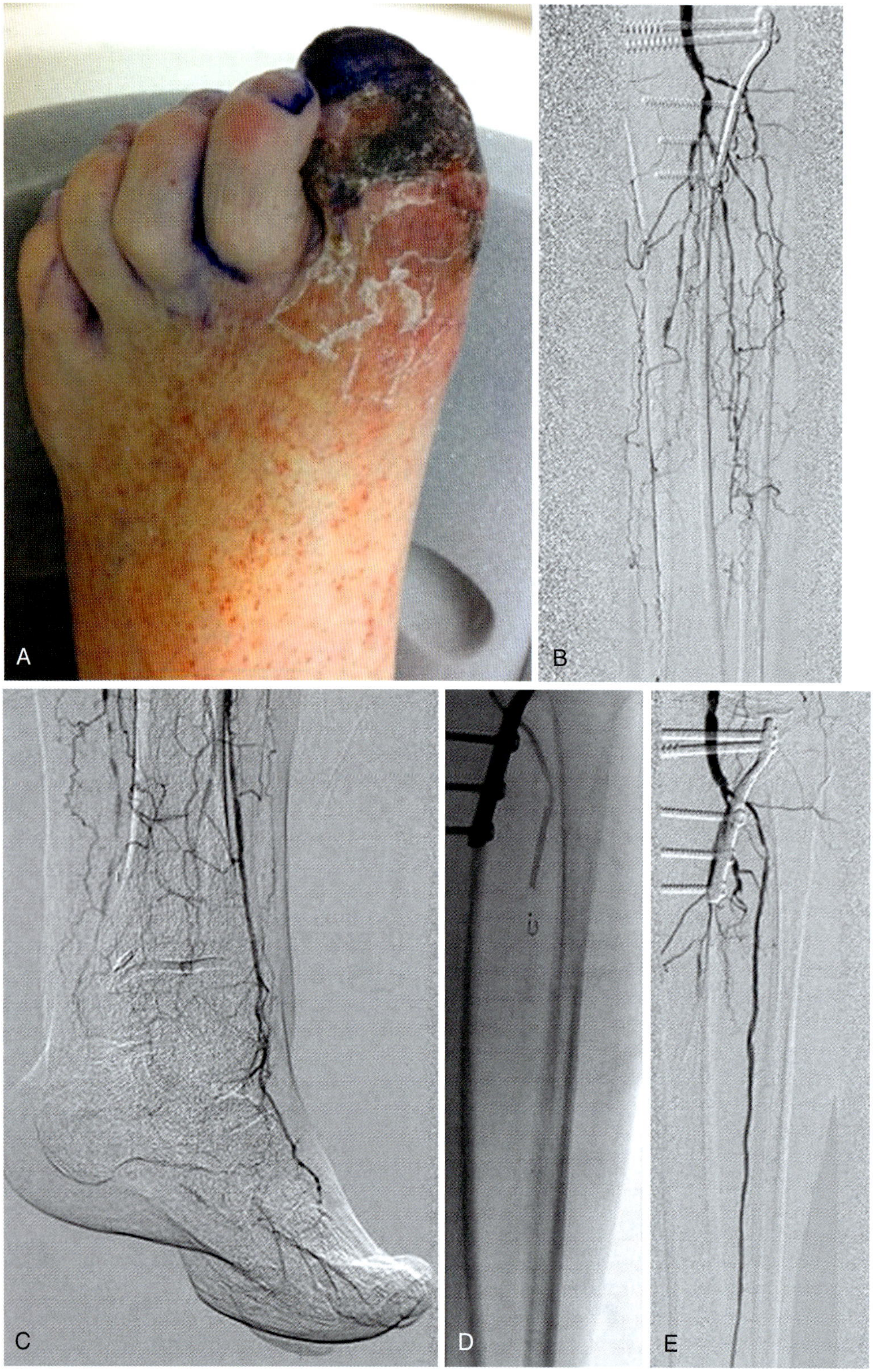

FIG 31.2 A 77-year-old high-risk patient with diabetes and great toe gangrene. (A) Critical limb ischemia with ankle-brachial index (ABI) of 0.39. (B) Three-vessel long-segment (>25 cm) tibial artery occlusions, with (C) distal anterior tibial artery reconstitution. (D) Subintimal angioplasty of long-segment occlusion. (E) Anterior tibial artery after long-segment subintimal angioplasty with ABI improved to 0.81. Toe amputation healed and the vessel remains patent 6 months after intervention.

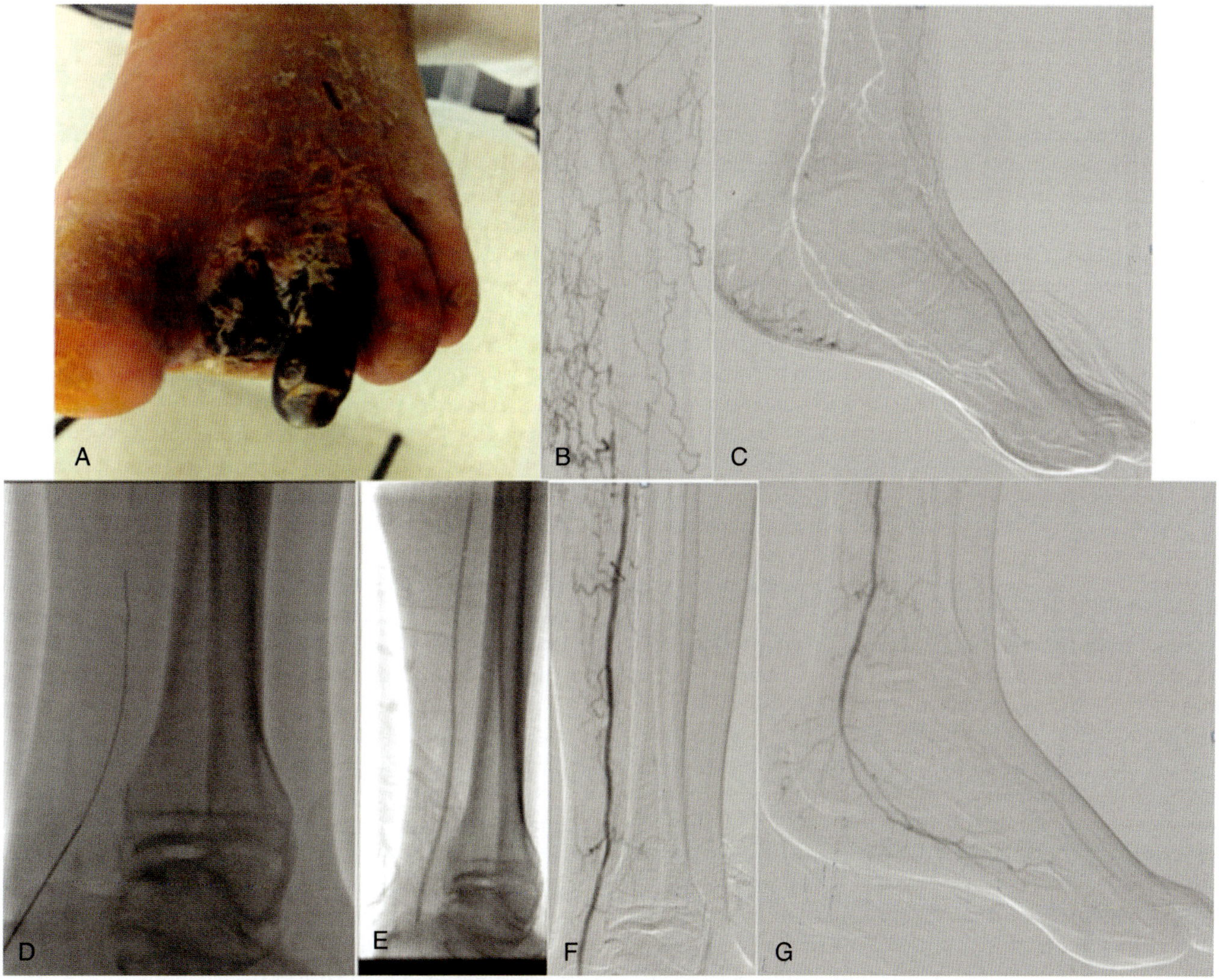

FIG 31.3 (A) A 69-year-old frail patient with diabetes, renal failure, and nonhealing toe amputation site. The patient had nonpalpable pedal pulses and a toe pressure of 12 mm Hg. (B) Diagnostic angiogram showed occluded popliteal and tibioperoneal arteries. (C) Distal reconstitution of the posterior tibial artery by means of collaterals at the ankle level. (D) Retrograde access of the ankle-level posterior tibial artery and further crossing of the long-segment occlusion with a V-18 control wire supported by a 0.018-inch CXI angled microcatheter. (E) Angioplasty with a 3.5 mm × 220 mm low-profile balloon. (F) Technical success and linear flow down to the foot after multilevel intervention. (G) Widely patent and perfused pedal plantar loop after retrograde recanalization and treatment of the posterior tibial artery.

sometimes local dissection, which is usually not flow limiting. Treating long-segment tibial lesions with longer balloons is a useful technique, but some short, focal lesions require a shorter balloon with more directed dilation force. A cutting balloon (Boston Scientific), which features three to four microsurgical blades fixed longitudinally along the outer surface of a noncompliant balloon, is particularly useful for the intimal hyperplasia near graft anastomoses. Creating controlled cuts in the intima theoretically allows less vessel wall disruption, less neutrophil activation, and more controlled balloon dilation.[7] The drug-coated balloon (DCB) is another emerging technology that has been primarily used in markets outside of the United States and has yet to receive US Food and Drug Administration (FDA) approval.[8]

Stenting in the infrapopliteal segment has traditionally been reserved for obviating emergency surgery because of poor angioplasty results, such as a flow-limiting dissection. More recently, drug-eluting stents have been used for the treatment of infrapopliteal disease, with encouraging results.[9] Other infrapopliteal maneuvers, such as atherectomy and cryotherapy, may add more cost than real benefit compared to angioplasty alone.[10]

THE RETROGRADE TECHNIQUE

In 2008, Montero-Baker and colleagues[11] reported that antegrade revascularization failed in up to 62 (17.8%) of 343 limbs with complex total occlusions of the popliteal and/or infrapopliteal vascular territory. Retrograde transpedal access has increased technical success during complex tibioperoneal interventions.

Various authors have published their own series. A total of 881 patients are currently accounted for in peer-reviewed journals.[11–21] In general terms, all of these papers conclude that transpedal access is safe and effective. Transpedal access was initially used as an adjunctive access site when preceded by unsuccessful attempts at antegrade recanalization. It is noteworthy that CTOs were present in more than 90% of patients with average occlusion lengths greater than 220 cm, demonstrating the effectiveness of this technique since the technical success rate remained greater than 90% with relatively low contrast volume, reasonable procedure times, and low rates of procedural complications. Retrograde access is increasingly used primarily rather than serving as a bailout approach, especially when anatomic difficulties are anticipated.

In essence, the technique has evolved and is based on ultrasound-guided retrograde distal access, although some operators still advocate the use of fluoroscopy to guide access. Once the needle is placed in the intraluminal space, access can be secured with or without a sheath. In cases in which a sheath is used, experienced users advise the use of 4 French or smaller sheaths. Most authors agree that this access can usually be done in a sheathless fashion; the objective is to cross the lesion from below, but deliver therapy in an antegrade fashion once the wire has been snared from above.

RESULTS

The outcome of infrapopliteal EVT depends on many factors, including indication for the procedure, lesion characteristics, runoff status, comorbidities, and technical factors such as dissection or persistent stenosis (Table 31.2). Poorer outcomes appear to be predicted by the following factors: CLI versus claudication,[22] longer lesion length,[23–25] poor runoff status,[22,23,26] comorbidities of diabetes[27,28] and renal failure,[22,29] smoking,[28] and untreated intraprocedure flow-limiting dissection and persistent stenosis greater than 30%.

Angioplasty

Giles and associates[23] retrospectively reviewed 163 consecutive patients (176 limbs) who underwent infrapopliteal EVT for CLI; 102 patients (58%) also had concomitant femoropopliteal angioplasty or stenting, or both[23]; and 97 lesions (55%) were TASC C or D. Subintimal angioplasty was performed only for complete occlusions that could not be crossed transluminally. The technical success rate was 93%, and 1- and 2-year primary patency rates were 53% and 51%, respectively. The 3-year limb salvage was 84%. On multivariate analysis, predictors of restenosis were TASC D lesions and lack of a bypass target, whereas multilevel intervention was protective. Sadek and colleagues[30] retrospectively reviewed 85 patients (89 limbs) who underwent either single-level tibial (29 limbs) or multilevel (60 limbs) interventions. Overall, 77% of patients had CLI. The technical success rate was 91%, and 12- and 18-month primary patency rates were 34% and 27%, respectively, in the single-level interventions and 58% and 48%, respectively, in the multilevel interventions. The 12- and 18-month limb salvage rates in the single-level interventions were 75% and 67%, respectively, and in the multilevel interventions they were 84% and 63%, respectively. The difference of primary patency and limb salvage between the two groups did not reach statistical significance. Peregrin and associates[26] retrospectively reviewed 1268 patients (1445 limbs) who underwent infrapopliteal angioplasty for CLI. Almost all lesions were classified as TASC D. The technical success rate was 89%, and the primary and secondary limb salvage rates at 1 year were 76% and 84%, respectively. Interestingly, the number of patent infrapopliteal arteries at the end of angioplasty significantly correlated with 1-year limb salvage rates. As the number of patent crural arteries increased from 0 to 3, the 1-year limb salvage rate increased from 56% to 83%. Conrad and colleagues[22] retrospectively reviewed 144 patients (155 limbs) who underwent infrapopliteal angioplasty; 133 limbs (86%) were treated for CLI, and 116 limbs (75%) had TASC C or D lesions. The technical success rate was 95%, and the 24- and 40-month primary patency rates were 71% and 62%, respectively. Multivariate analysis showed poor runoff, CLI, and dialysis as negative predictors of patency. The 40-month limb salvage rate was 86%; negative predictors of limb salvage included dialysis and failure to improve runoff.

Data are also available regarding angioplasty for long-segment infrapopliteal disease. Schmidt and coworkers[31] studied 58 patients (62 limbs) with CLI who underwent infrapopliteal angioplasty for lesions 8 cm or greater in length.[31] The technical success rate, defined by restoration of flow in at least one infrapopliteal vessel, was 95%. At short-term follow-up of 3 months, angiography demonstrated restenosis of less than 50% in 31% of treated arteries, restenosis greater than 50% in 31%, and occlusion in 38%. Clinical improvement (wound healing or improvement of rest pain) was present in 76% of treated limbs. All arteries with restenosis greater than 50% or occlusion were retreated. At 15 months, 77% of limbs showed further clinical improvement, and the limb salvage rate was 100% without bypass.

Subintimal Angioplasty

Groups have also published specifically regarding subintimal angioplasty. Tartari and colleagues[32] reported on 117 subintimal angioplasty procedures for complete occlusions, 82 (15 TASC C and 67 TASC D) of which were infrapopliteal. Technical success, defined as recanalization of at least one tibial vessel with adequate flow to the foot, was possible in 83% of cases. At a mean follow-up of 13.5 months, 12.5% of this cohort underwent major amputation and 11.3% underwent surgical bypass. Vraux and coworkers[24] reviewed 46 patients (50 limbs) with CLI and tibial occlusions. Technical success was possible in 82% of cases. Primary patency was 46% at 12 months and 42% at 24 months. Limb salvage was 87% at 12 and 24 months. Longer lesion length and the need to extend treatment to the popliteal artery were associated with lower clinical patency rates. Ingle and colleagues[33] retrospectively reviewed 67 consecutive patients (70 limbs) who underwent infrapopliteal angioplasty for occlusive lesions; 61 patients (91%) had CLI. The technical success rate was 86% and the limb salvage rate at 3 years by Kaplan-Meier life-table analysis was 94%.

TABLE 31.2 **Results of Infrapopliteal Angioplasty, Stenting, and Atherectomy**

Author	Year	Number Treated	CLI	Mean Lesion Length	Technical Failures	Primary Patency	Limb Salvage Rate
Angioplasty							
Giles and colleagues[23]	2008	176	100%	NR	7%	53%, 1 year 51%, 2 years	84%, 3 years
Conrad and colleagues[22]	2009	155	86%	NR	5%	71%, 2 years 62%, 3.3 years	86%, 3.3 years
Sadek and colleagues[30] (Single vs. multilevel PTA)	2009	89	77%	NR	9%	34%, 1 year Single level 58%, 1 year Multilevel	67%, 1.5 years Single level 63%, 1.5 years Multilevel
Peregrin and colleagues[26]	2010	1445	100%	NR	11%	NR	76%, 1 year
Schmidt and colleagues[31]	2010	62	100%	18.3 cm	5%	50%, 3 months	100%, 15 months
Subintimal Angioplasty							
Ingle and colleagues[33]	2002	70	91%	NR	14%	NR	94%, 3 years
Vraux and Bertoncello[24]	2006	50	100%	78% >10 cm	18%	46%, 1 year 42%, 2 years	87%, 1 year 87%, 2 years
Tartari and colleagues[32] (SFA only in 27 limbs)	2007	109	100%	59% ≥10 cm	17%	NR	87%, 1 year 85%, 2 years
Cutting-Balloon Angioplasty							
Engelke and colleagues[35]	2002	16	31%	NR	6%	67%, 1 year	93%, 10 months
Ansel and colleagues[36]	2004	73	71%	2.7 cm	0%	NR	89%, 1 year
Vikram and colleagues[34]	2007	11	NR	NR	18%	50%, 1 year	NR
Drug-Coated Balloon[a]							
Tepe and colleagues[8]	2008	48	15%	7.5 cm	2% All cases	80%, 6 months	96%, 6 months
Stenting							
Feiring and colleagues[44]	2004	92	68%	NR	7%	NR	87%, 1 year
Bosiers and colleagues[42]	2006	300	100%	NR	NR	76%, 1 year	99%, 1 year
Donas and colleagues[45]	2009	34	100%	6.5 cm stenosis; 7.5 cm occlusion	3%	91%, 10 months	100%, 10 months
Randon and colleagues[43]	2010	16	100%	38% ≥10 cm	13%	56%, 1 year	92%, 1 year
Drug-Eluting Stent							
Scheinert and colleagues[9]	2006	30	63%	NR	0%	100%, 6 months	100%, 9 months
Feiring and colleagues[48]	2010	130	100%	NR	9%	NR	88%, 3 years
Karnabatidis and colleagues[28]	2011	51	100%	7.7 cm	0%	30%, 3 years	NR
Rastan and colleagues[46]	2011	82	51%	3.0 cm	0%	81%, 1 year	98%, 1 year
Atherectomy							
Zeller and colleagues[25]	2007	36	53%	4.6 cm	2%	67%, 1 year 60%, 2 years	100%, 2 years
Safian and colleagues[49]	2009	124	32%	3.0 cm	2.5%	NR	100%, 6 mo

[a]Femoropopliteal.
CLI, Critical limb ischemia; *NR*, not reported; *PTA*, percutaneous transluminal angioplasty; *SFA*, superficial femoral artery.

Cutting Balloon Angioplasty

Data from cutting balloon angioplasty are also available. Vikram and associates[34] compared conventional and cutting balloon angioplasty in 36 patients with failing infrainguinal vein grafts. Short-term primary patency seemed to be better in the cutting balloon cohort; however, primary patency for angioplasty at 1 year was not significantly different between the two groups. Engelke and colleagues[35] treated 16 anastomotic stenoses after infrainguinal bypass. Cutting balloon angioplasty was successful in 15 lesions (94%), including 6 lesions that were resistant to conventional angioplasty; there were no perforations. The primary lesion patency at 12 months was 76%. Ansel and coworkers[36] reviewed their treatment of 73 patients (93 vessels) with cutting balloon angioplasty, 52 (71%) of whom had CLI. Most vessels treated (71%) were infrapopliteal. Technical success was possible in 81%, with all failures being successfully stented. There were no perforations. At 1-year follow-up, the limb salvage rate was 89%.

Drug-Coated Balloon Angioplasty

At present, there are no FDA-approved DCBs for treatment of below-the-knee vessels in the United States. Randomized trials evaluating the performance of this technology have reported inconsistent results: some trials demonstrated benefit,[21,37] others equivalence,[38,39] and one potential harm.[40]

Cassese and colleagues.[41] pooled all appropriate patients in a meta-analysis. A total of 641 participants (378 randomized to DCB and 263 to control therapy) were studied. They concluded that DCBs have similar clinical efficacy and favorable angiographic outcomes when compared with uncoated balloons or drug-eluding stents (DESs) at 1-year follow-up.

The encouraging results of antirestenotic therapy in the femoropopliteal segment have not been replicated in this territory, likely due to the complexity of the plaque, especially in long-standing diabetic and renal failure patients. The results of ongoing research of plaque-modulating technologies that may improve luminal gain is awaited. One current hypothesis to explain the lack of sustained patency in below-the-knee vessels is related to the use of very small diameter drug-coated balloons, which may have not achieved ideal luminal expansion.

Stenting

Bosiers and colleagues[42] prospectively collected data on 443 patients (681 lesions) who underwent infrapopliteal EVT for CLI. Patients were allocated to percutaneous transluminal angioplasty (PTA) plus stenting (300 patients), PTA alone (79 patients), or excimer laser atherectomy (64 patients) groups. Mean lesion length was not specifically reported, but 21% of treated lesions were occlusive. Laser atherectomy was generally used for single, long lesions. At 1-year follow-up, primary patency rates for PTA, PTA plus stenting, and laser atherectomy were 68.6%, 75.5%, and 75.4%, respectively. Limb salvage rates at 1 year for PTA, PTA plus stenting, and laser atherectomy were 96.7%, 98.6%, and 87.9%, respectively. Randon and colleagues[43] enrolled 35 patients (38 limbs) with CLI for randomization to angioplasty (22 limbs) or primary stenting (16 limbs); 64% of treated lesions were occlusive, with most occlusions greater than 2 cm in length. At 1-year follow-up, there was no difference between angioplasty and stenting in regard to primary patency (66% vs. 56%), limb salvage (90% vs. 92%), or survival (69% vs. 74%). The only significant difference between the cohorts was an increased need for redo angioplasty in the PTA group after 6 months (3 vs. 0 in the stenting group). Feiring and colleagues[44] reviewed their experience treating 82 patients with infrapopliteal lesions; six occlusions could not be crossed, leaving 76 patients (86 limbs) treated with infrapopliteal stents. CLI was the indication for stenting in 68% of patients. A total of 197 stents were deployed in the study including an assortment of balloon expandable and self-expanding coronary stents. At 1-month follow-up, CLI patients had a significantly improved mean ankle-brachial index (ABI; 0.32 to 0.9). Between 6 and 12 months of follow-up, two patients developed in-stent restenosis, which was successfully treated. At 1-year follow-up, the limb salvage rate for CLI patients was 96%; however, expressed on an intention-to-treat basis, the 1-year limb salvage rate was 87%. Donas and coworkers[45] treated 34 CLI patients with infrapopliteal stenting. Indications for stenting were long-segment stenoses or occlusions, or flow-limiting dissection or elastic recoil after PTA. Immediate (12 to 24 hours) improvement in ABI was realized (0.45 to 0.92), which was partially sustained at 6 months (0.77). The 6-month limb salvage rate was 100%, and primary patency was 91% at a mean follow-up of 10.4 months.

Drug-Eluting Stents

Scheinert and colleagues[9] studied 60 consecutive patients with infrapopliteal obstructions treated with a bare-metal stent (BMS) or sirolimus-eluting stent (SES).[9] At 6 months follow-up, the SES cohort had a significantly lower mean degree of in-stent restenosis (1.8% vs. 53.0%). Likewise, Rastan and colleagues[46] conducted a randomized, double-blinded, multicenter study of 161 patients with infrapopliteal disease who received either a BMS (79 points) or SES (82 points). The 1-year primary patency rate was significantly higher in the SES cohort (80.6% vs. 55.6%). In addition, the median change in the Rutherford classification[47] was −2 in the DES cohort compared with −1 in the BMS cohort. Karnabatidis and colleagues[28] prospectively studied 81 patients with CLI and long segment (>4.5 cm) infrapopliteal lesions treated with a BMS (34 points) or everolimus-eluting stent (47 points). At 3-year follow-up, the everolimus-eluting stent cohort had a significantly higher primary patency rate (30% vs. 21%). Regression analysis revealed that smoking and diabetes were significant predictors for increased restenosis and reduced patency. Feiring and colleagues[48] prospectively enrolled 118 patients (130 limbs) with CLI for treatment with at least one infrapopliteal DES. A total of 228 stents were deployed in the study, and 35% of patients received overlapping stents. On an intention-to-treat basis, the 3-year limb salvage rate was 88%.

Atherectomy

Data on infrapopliteal atherectomy are lacking, but Zeller and associates[25] studied infrapopliteal directional atherectomy with the SilverHawk device (FoxHollow Technologies, Redwood City, CA) on 36 patients (49 lesions). CLI was the indication for intervention in 19 (53%) patients. The mean lesion length was 46 mm, and the mean percent diameter stenosis was 89%; there were 11 (22%) occlusions. Predilation was performed in 16 (33%) lesions, and following atherectomy, 19 lesions (38%) were treated with additional balloon angioplasty. After atherectomy, there was an immediate increase in mean ABI (0.48 to 0.81), which was partially sustained at 1-year follow-up (0.72). Primary patency was 67% at 1 year and 60% at 2 years. Lesions with a length of 50 mm or greater had a significantly higher restenosis rate (44% vs. 26%). Safian and colleagues[49] studied 124 patients (201 stenoses) in a nonrandomized, prospective fashion. They used the Diamondback 360° Orbital Atherectomy System (Cardiovascular

Systems, St. Paul, MN) to perform infrapopliteal atherectomy; CLI was the indication to intervene in 40 (32%) patients. The mean lesion length was 30 mm, and the mean percent diameter stenosis was 87%. Following atherectomy, adjunctive angioplasty was performed in 79 (39%) lesions. At 6-month follow-up, there was an increase in mean ABI (0.68 to 0.82), and 78% of patients had improvement in chronic limb ischemia based on the Rutherford-Becker ordinal scale.

POSTPROCEDURAL MANAGEMENT

Following EVT, patients should be maintained on their preprocedure medical regimens for control of hypertension, congestive heart failure (CHF), angina, and arrhythmia. Diligent fluid management is especially important in patients with CHF, who may easily become volume overloaded. Beta blockade should be continued if there are no contraindications; in this same moderate and high-risk population, targeted heart rate control has been shown to reduce cardiac complications and improve mortality after open vascular operations.[50,51] Metformin, a commonly prescribed antihyperglycemic drug, should be withheld around the time of contrast administration because of the possibility of lactic acidosis with worsening renal function.[52] For patients with normal renal function, metformin should be withheld immediately before contrast administration and for 48 hours after the study. For patients with renal dysfunction, metformin should be withheld 48 hours before and 48 hours after contrast administration. In both cases, metformin should only be restarted in the absence of an acute decline in renal function.

ANTIPLATELET THERAPY

Patients with claudication or CLI are usually already taking aspirin (81 or 325 mg daily). Aspirin has well-established cardiac and cerebral protective effects and may improve patency after PTA and stenting.[53–55] Aspirin has a rapid onset of action, within minutes, with a peak action of less than 30 minutes; it produces approximately 20% platelet inhibition, lasts 5 to 7 days, and is the most cost-effective antiplatelet therapy.[56] Clopidogrel is another antiplatelet option,[57] which can be added to aspirin to provide up to 40% platelet inhibition. It takes 5 days to reach peak activity, which can be reduced to hours with a loading dose of 300 mg.[58] Clopidogrel is significantly more expensive than aspirin and may have an increased risk of complications compared with aspirin alone.

CONCLUSIONS

A growing body of evidence supports the use of infrapopliteal EVT for CLI. Advances in technique, technology, and patient selection have fostered short-term results similar to bypass. Infrapopliteal EVT for CLI maximally benefits older, higher-risk patients with shorter life expectancies who do not require the durability of a bypass, but rather the shorter-term augmentation in blood flow to heal a wound or resolve ischemic rest pain. Newer technologies, such as DCBs, DESs, and atherectomy, have shown promise for infrapopliteal application and may further increase the ability to successfully treat CLI in an endovascular fashion.

REVIEW QUESTIONS

1. Which of the following projections of the left common femoral artery usually best delineates the origin of the left deep femoral artery?
   a. Straight anteroposterior (AP)
   b. Left anterior oblique (LAO)
   c. Right anterior oblique (RAO)
   d. 30-degree craniocaudal
   e. True lateral
2. Antegrade femoral access would be of greatest utility when performing endovascular therapy for which of the following lesions?
   a. Proximal common femoral to posterior tibial bypass graft stenosis
   b. SFA origin stenosis
   c. Profunda femoris artery (PFA) stenosis
   d. Aortobifemoral graft limb stenosis
   e. Below-knee popliteal artery stenosis
3. Which of the following best describes a TASC (I) C infrapopliteal artery lesion?
   a. Multiple focal posterior tibial artery stenoses less than 1 cm long
   b. 1.5-cm–long midperoneal artery occlusion
   c. 4-cm–long anterior tibial artery occlusion
   d. Two less than 1 cm long stenoses in the tibioperoneal trunk
   e. Solitary tibial stenosis less than 1 cm in length
4. Poorer outcomes of infrainguinal angioplasty are associated with all of the following *except:*
   a. Poor runoff
   b. Diabetes mellitus
   c. End-stage renal disease
   d. Claudication
   e. Residual stenosis greater than 30%

5. Which of the following statements about tibial angioplasty is most correct?
   a. Initial technical success rates are less than 80% in most series.
   b. One-year patency rates are generally poor (<50%).
   c. Limb salvage rates in patients with critical limb ischemia are less than 75% at 1 year.
   d. Runoff does not have a major impact on patency.
   e. Cutting balloon angioplasty patency rates are better at 1 year compared to angioplasty with standard balloons.
6. All of the following are advantages of the antegrade approach for infrapopliteal angioplasty *except:*
   a. Wire pushability
   b. Avoidance of iliac artery disease and tortuosity
   c. Catheter control
   d. Ease of access in obese patients
   e. Sheath passage
7. Based on most published data, improved results following tibial angioplasty are most strongly suggested for which one of the following therapies or adjuncts?
   a. Cutting balloon angioplasty
   b. Atherectomy
   c. Subintimal angioplasty
   d. Bare-metal stents
   e. Drug-eluting stents

References available online at ExpertConsult.com.

CHAPTER 32

Thoracic and Lumbar Sympathectomy: Indications, Technique, and Results

Peter Gloviczki

Minimally invasive endoscopic technology has rapidly transformed both thoracic and abdominal surgery, and the field of surgical sympathectomies is no exception. For thoracic sympathectomy, the thoracoscopic procedure is used almost exclusively.[1–3] Laparoscopic[4] and retroperitoneoscopic techniques[5,6] have also been developed for ablation of the lumbar sympathetic chain. Because of its relatively less invasive nature, the open technique for lumbar sympathectomy is still performed, but with rapidly decreasing frequency.[7,8] Indications for both thoracic and lumbar sympathectomies have changed over the past decades. Earlier indications such as claudication, uncomplicated primary Raynaud syndrome, or scleroderma are not used.[9] Refractory palmar and plantar hyperhidrosis, chronic pain syndrome, Buerger disease, frostbite, and complicated primary Raynaud syndrome and secondary Raynaud phenomenon with nonhealing digital ulcerations have become the most common indications for endoscopic sympathectomy.[2,8,10]

HISTORICAL BACKGROUND

Although Jabouley suggested sympathetic denervation for vasospastic disorders as early as 1899, periarterial sympathectomy was introduced by Leriche only in 1913 for ischemic lesions caused by vasospasm.[11] The first lumbar sympathectomy was performed by Royle in 1923 to treat a patient with spastic paralysis of the lower limb.[12] The concept of sympathectomy was soon adopted by Adson and Brown,[13] who performed lumbar sympathectomy to relieve vasospasm of the lower extremities. Adson and Brown[14] were the first to perform cervicothoracic sympathectomy in 1929.

Using the single-scope technique, thoracoscopic sympathectomy was popularized by Kux[15] in Austria as early as 1954. With the advent of endoscopic surgery, both thoracoscopic[1–3] and laparoscopic or retroperitoneoscopic procedures[5,6] have been developed for sympathetic denervation.

ANATOMY AND PHYSIOLOGY

The peripheral nervous system includes both somatic and autonomic components. The somatic efferent motor nerves control the voluntary striate muscles and the afferent nerves transmit somatosensory information to the brain. The autonomic nervous system transmits information from the abdominal viscera as well as the smooth and cardiac muscles and the exocrine glands. Autonomic nerves are composed of the sympathetic and parasympathetic nervous systems.

Anatomy

The sympathetic nervous system consists of the central autonomic network—which includes the brain stem, diencephalons, and cortex—and the peripheral sympathetic pathways. The peripheral sympathetic pathway consists of preganglionic and postganglionic neurons. Information from the brain stem and hypothalamus descends through the lateral funiculus of the spinal cord to the preganglionic sympathetic fibers. The preganglionic sympathetic neurons originate in the anteromedial column of the thoracolumbar cord, between T1 and L2. These myelinated white nerve fibers travel in the ventral root of the spinal cord to the paravertebral sympathetic ganglia, where they synapse onto the postganglionic unmyelinated gray fibers. It is likely that each preganglionic axon innervates about 10 postganglionic neurons.[16] The postganglionic axons can leave the parasympathetic ganglia at the level of the synapse or can travel first up or down in the sympathetic chain before exiting the ganglion via gray rami. The regional activity of the sympathetic chain is the product of reflex arcs between somatic afferent fibers and preganglionic efferent fibers. For sympathetic denervation of the upper limbs, interruption of the sympathetic chain from T2 to T4 is required. Although the stellate ganglion has some innervation to the upper limbs, resection of the stellate ganglion results in Horner syndrome (ptosis, myosis, and enophthalmos). Because of this associated morbidity, the stellate ganglion is not removed surgically. The nerves of Kuntz (Fig. 32.1) are important because they provide direct collaterals from the T2 and T3 ganglia to the upper limbs. Resection of T2 and T3 ganglia (sympathectomy) is thought to be essential to achieve good and durable sympathetic denervation of the arms. The preganglionic fibers may bypass the paravertebral ganglia to synapse with more distal intermediate ganglia or may cross over to innervate the contralateral side as well. Therefore, as mentioned previously, a complete sympathectomy includes division of the preganglionic fibers and excision of the relay ganglia T2 and T3 and the intercommunicating fibers (the nerve of Kuntz). Several authors advocate T4 and T5 resection, especially in patients who undergo the operation for axillary hyperhidrosis.[3]

Fig. 32.2 depicts the finer anatomy of the nerves and illustrates the difference between T2 sympathectomy and T1 to T2 sympathotomy at the level of the second rib. Atkinson and colleagues[2]

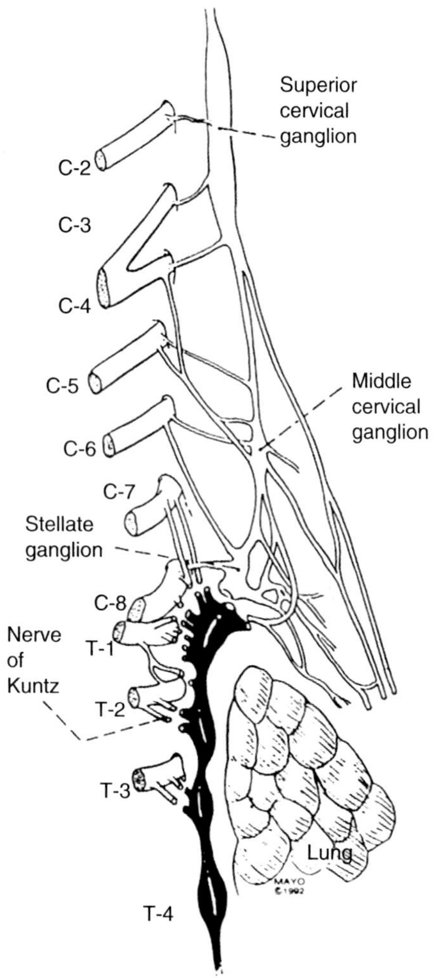

FIG 32.1 Lower cervical and upper thoracic sympathetic chain. The nerve of Kuntz, originating at the level of T2, provides direct communicating fibers to the brachial plexus. (From Lowell RC, Gloviczki P, Cherry KJ, Jr, et al: Cervicothoracic sympathectomy for Raynaud's syndrome. *Int Angiol* 12:168–172, 1993. With permission of Mayo Foundation)

advocate performing sympathotomy by severing all visualized sympathetic branches between the T1 (and C8) ganglion and the T2 ganglion so as to minimize axonal and potential neuronal injury, which may increase side effects, particularly compensatory postsympathectomy hyperhidrosis.[2]

In addition to the paravertebral ganglia, there is another subtype of peripheral sympathetic ganglia: the prevertebral ganglia. These include the celiac, aortorenal, and superior and inferior mesenteric ganglia located in the abdominal cavity, on the top of and around the aorta. These ganglia send postganglionic fibers to the abdominal and pelvic organs.

Physiology

The sympathetic nervous system modifies basal organ functions and mediates the body's response to stress ("fright, flight, and fight response"). The primary function of the peripheral sympathetic nervous system is to prevent heat loss by reducing the blood flow to the skin and subcutaneous tissue of the limbs. The increased activity of the postganglionic sympathetic nerves, mediated by norepinephrine, results in decreased blood flow because of stimulation of the vasoconstrictor fibers innervating the blood vessels. There is increased sweating caused by stimulation of the sudomotor fibers innervating the exocrine glands (an activity mediated by acetylcholine, adenosine, and other neuropeptides) as well as piloerection mediated through the activity of the pilomotor fibers that innervate the erector pili muscles.[16] The sympathetic system antagonizes the vasodilatory effect of the parasympathetic nerves on the arterial resistance vessels, the cutaneous precapillary sphincters, and the capacitance venules.

As a result of sympathetic denervation, the blood flow to the skin increases, there is a loss of sweating and piloerection, and the hands after thoracic sympathectomy/sympathotomy and the feet after lumbar sympathectomy become warm, pink, and dry. Sympathectomy also results in decreased pain in the ischemic limb, likely owing to an enhanced tolerance to pain stimuli. The pain tolerance is better because of decreased tissue concentration of norepinephrine and reduced spinal augmentation of pain transmission to cerebral centers.

The maximal effect of the sympathectomy/sympathotomy is immediate, although vasodilation will be less after 1 week because of compensatory mechanisms. Blood flow changes recorded at 6 months following sympathectomy are minimal because of incomplete denervation, regeneration of fibers, and hypersensitivity of the receptors to circulating catecholamines.

Several authors have investigated the effect of sympathectomy on blood flow of the limbs. Cronenwett and colleagues[17] found no increase of nutrient capillary perfusion as a result of sympathectomy. Using intradermal xenon clearance, Moore and Hall[18] observed increased flow to the cutaneous capillary circulation. Rutherford and Valenta[19] failed to confirm increased muscle flow as a result of sympathectomy. Dalessandri and colleagues,[20] however, described increased collateral circulation in patients who underwent sympathectomy.

It is evident that the effect of sympathectomy on cutaneous blood flow is transient, but this period may be sufficient to heal superficial ulcerations. The more lasting effects of sympathectomy are on sweating, abnormal vasomotor tone, and pain relief.

THORACIC SYMPATHECTOMY

Indications

In an earlier study from the Mayo Clinic, Lowell and colleagues[9] reviewed indications for cervicothoracic sympathectomy in 68 patients. The most frequent indications were atheroembolism followed by Raynaud syndrome, causalgia, hand ischemia, reflex sympathetic dystrophy, and Buerger disease. The most frequently used indications for thoracic sympathectomy are medically refractory palmar-plantar hyperhidrosis and causalgia.[2,3] Additional indications include distal digital occlusion, vasospastic disorders with digital ulcerations not responding to medical treatment, Buerger disease, and frostbite.[1,10,21–23] There is also a beneficial effect of sympathectomy on facial blushing.[10] Uncomplicated Raynaud disease and scleroderma are contraindications to cervical sympathectomy (Table 32.1).

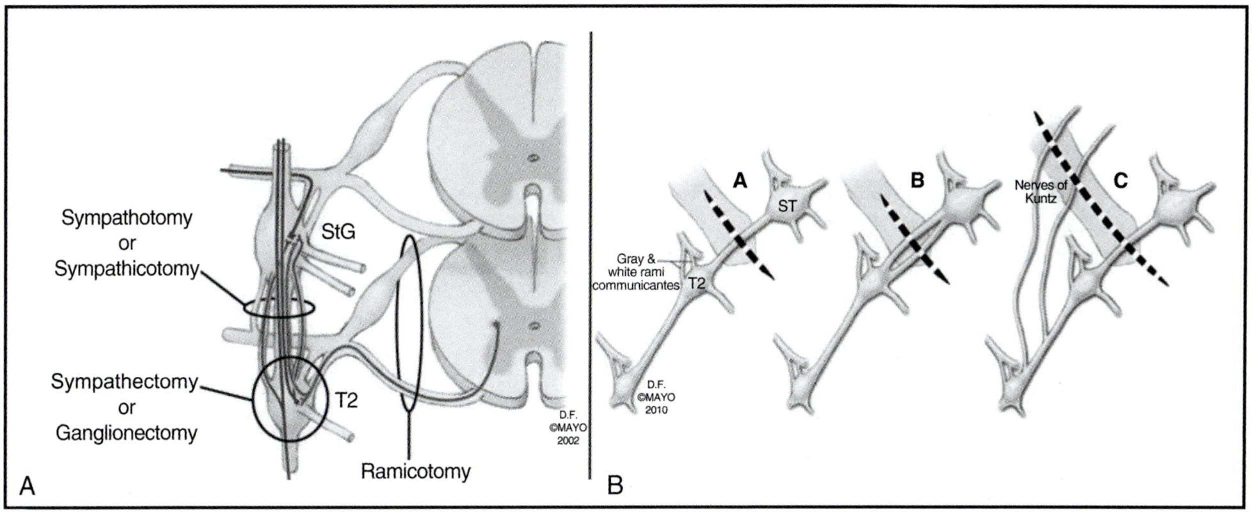

FIG 32.2 (A) Illustration of the two techniques for interrupting the sympathetic chain. (1) T1 to T2 sympathotomy has less chance of causing compensatory hyperhidrosis and axonal injury *(red)* from the neuron in the spinal cord. (2) Sympathectomy has a higher chance of causing axonal injury, which may also lead to neuronal injury, and more chance of causing compensatory hyperhidrosis. (B) During sympathotomy, all nerves are severed, including the nerves of Kuntz that run across the second rib between the stellate ganglion *(StG)* and the T2 ganglion. A, Single sympathetic trunk. B, Multiple trunks. C, Trunk with lateral nerves of Kuntz (16 patients). (With permission from Atkinson JL, Fode-Thomas NC, Fealey RD, et al: Endoscopic transthoracic limited sympathotomy for palmar-plantar hyperhidrosis: outcomes and complications during a 10-year period. *Mayo Clinic Proceed* 86:721–729, 2011.)

TABLE 32.1 Indications for Sympathectomy

Indication	Thoracic Sympathectomy	Lumbar Sympathectomy
Best	Hyperhidrosis Causalgia Frostbite Buerger disease Raynaud phenomenon caused by stable arterial occlusions (e.g., traumatic subintimal fibrosis, distal emboli, digital gangrene) Facial blushing	Hyperhidrosis Causalgia Frostbite Buerger disease Atheroembolism (blue toe syndrome)
Acceptable	Primary Raynaud syndrome with digital ulcerations or distal arterial occlusions	Inoperable Buerger or atherosclerotic arterial occlusions with limited tissue loss Rest pain in nondiabetic patient owing to small arterial occlusions (e.g., distal Buerger atherosclerosis, arterial emboli) with or without Raynaud phenomenon
Contraindications	Uncomplicated Raynaud disease	Claudication Diabetes with neuropathy

Surgical Technique

Thoracic sympathectomy can be performed using open surgical technique, via transaxillary transthoracic approach or cervical approach, or using the thoracoscopic approach. Open techniques are rarely performed, usually only if thoracotomy or cervical incision is needed for another reason, such as vascular reconstruction or cervical or first rib resection.

Open Surgical Techniques

Transaxillary approach. Patients who are treated by the transaxillary approach to the thoracic sympathetic chain are placed into a 90-degree lateral decubitus position with the arm elevated by the surgical assistant or with the help of an arm board. The transverse skin incision is made in the axillary fossa, just distal to the axillary hairline. The dissection is carried down to the third rib, avoiding injury to the long thoracic nerve anteriorly and the subscapular artery and thoracodorsal nerve posteriorly. The pectoralis major muscle is retracted anteriorly, and the latissimus dorsi is retracted posteriorly. A 6-cm-long segment of the third rib is dissected from its periosteum and removed. The pleura is entered, and the lumbar sympathectomy chain is dissected in the paravertebral region posteriorly by incising the posterior pleura (Fig. 32.3). The chain is located

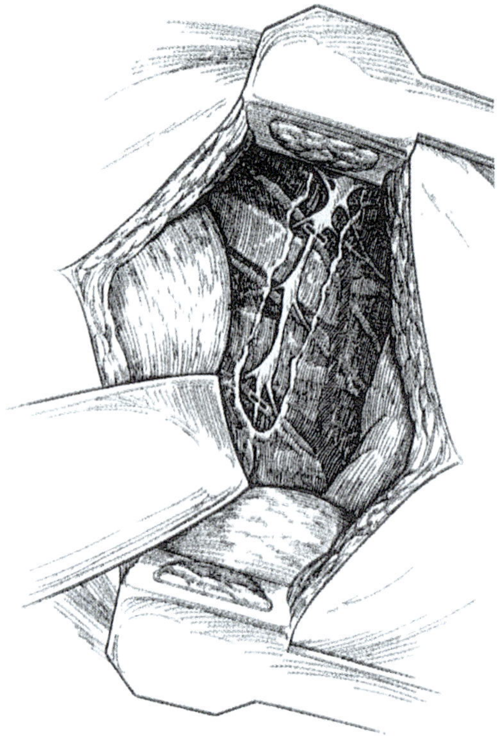

FIG 32.3 Transaxillary minithoracotomy through the third intercostal space performed with resection of a 6-cm-long segment of the third rib. After opening the pleura, the sympathetic chain distal to the stellate ganglion is resected, including the T2 and T3 segments. (With permission from Rutherford RB: *Atlas of Vascular Surgery*, Philadelphia, 1993, WB Saunders.)

2 to 3 cm lateral to the azygos vein. The chain between T1 and T5 is sharply dissected, and the sympathetic chain with the T2 to T3 and usually T4 ganglia is removed. The stellate ganglion should not be removed, and dissection toward the neck should be avoided.

Cervical approach. The cervical approach is through a supraclavicular skin incision. A 6-cm-long transverse incision is made 2 cm proximal to the clavicle, and the posterior belly of the sternocleidomastoid muscle is divided. The external jugular vein is ligated and divided, and the anterior scalene muscle is divided while also carefully retracting the phrenic nerve medially. The subclavian artery is gently retracted caudally, and the stellate ganglion is exposed medial and anterior to the brachial plexus. It usually lies immediately lateral to the vertebral artery (Fig. 32.4). The stellate ganglion is preserved, and dissection is carried down into the thoracic cavity, retracting the pleural dome as much as possible. The T1, T2, and T3 ganglia can usually be removed through this approach. On the left side, the dissection is similar, but attention must be paid to avoid injury to the thoracic duct. If the thoracic duct or one of the larger cervical ducts is injured and leak of chyle is identified, ligation of the duct is warranted to avoid the complications of a chylocutaneous cyst or fistula.

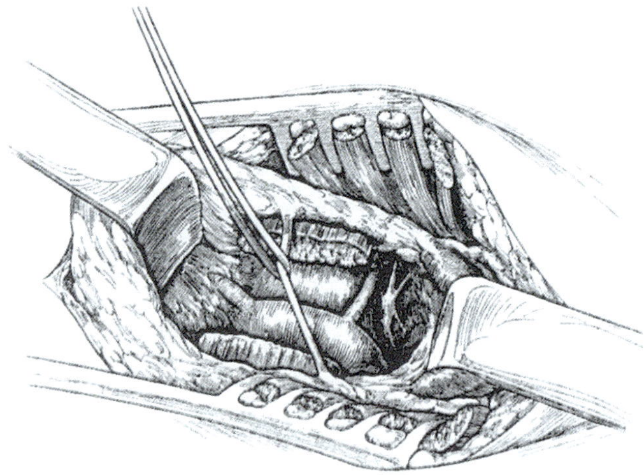

FIG 32.4 Right supraclavicular approach for thoracic sympathectomy. The stellate ganglion is just lateral to the vertebral artery, which is exposed after transection of the anterior scalene muscle. Note the phrenic nerve on a vessel loop. T1 to T3 is resected, thus gaining further exposure with downward retraction. (With permission from Rutherford RB: *Atlas of Vascular Surgery*, Philadelphia, 1993, WB Saunders.)

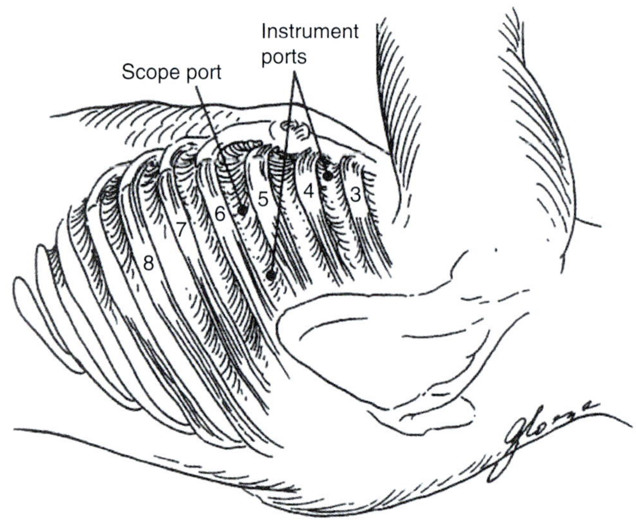

FIG 32.5 Thoracoscopic sympathectomy using three endoscopic ports: two instrument ports in anterior and posterior axillary line and a scope port in midaxillary line. (With permission from Ahn SS, Machleder HI, Concepcion B, Moore WS: Thoracoscopic cervicodorsal sympathectomy: preliminary results. *J Vasc Surg* 20:511–519, 1994.)

Thoracoscopic Sympathectomy

The technique of thoracoscopic sympathectomy was first described in detail by Kux in 1978 using a single-scope technique.[15] Modern endoscopic instrumentation resulted in significant modification of the original technique, using multiple ports, as reported by Ahn and colleagues[1] (Fig. 32.5). There have been many subsequent modifications to this technique, and currently a large number of patients, primarily with hyperhidrosis,

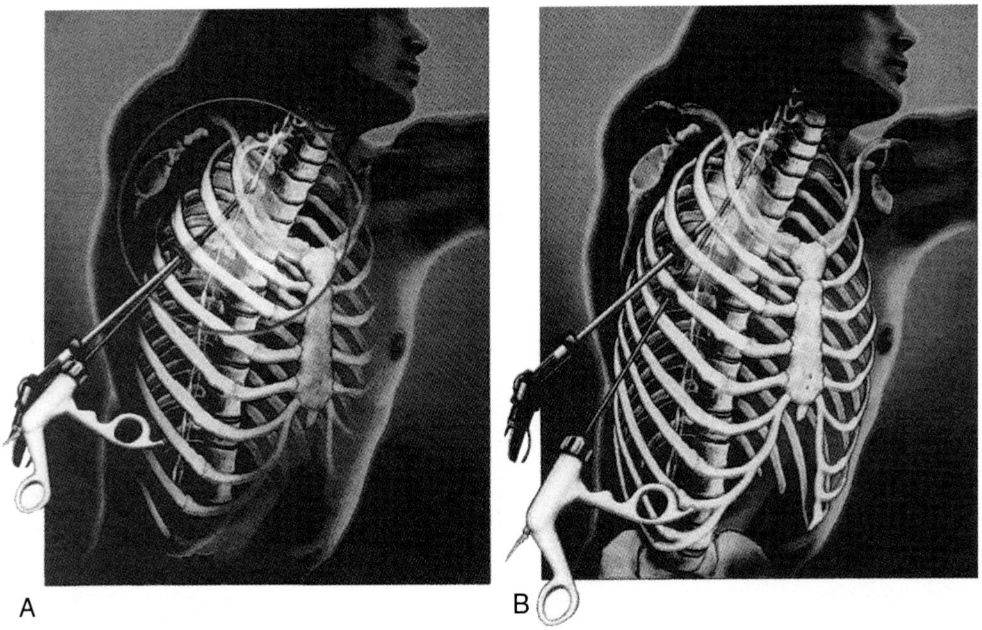

FIG 32.6 (A) Port location and instrument placement for uniportal thoracoscopic sympathectomy. (B) Port locations and instrument placement for biportal thoracoscopic sympathectomy. (With permission from Johnson JP, Patel NP: Uniportal and biportal endoscopic thoracic sympathectomy. *Neurosurgery* 51:78–79, 2002.)

undergo thoracoscopic sympathectomy using one, two, or three endoscopic ports.

An excellent description of uniportal and the biportal sympathectomy has been given by Johnson and Patel[24] (Fig. 32.6A, B). The operation is performed under general anesthesia using a double-lumen endotracheal tube for deflation of the ipsilateral lung during the procedure. For bilateral procedures, the patient is positioned supine with the arms abducted bilaterally. For unilateral procedures, the patient is laid on the side.

Standard thoracoscopic instrumentation is used, with a 5-mm rigid scope (with 30-degree and right-angle camera), electrocautery, and Harmonic scalpel (Ethicon Endo-Surgery, Cincinnati, OH) for dissection and ablation of the sympathetic ganglia and fibers. The port is placed through the third intercostal space for the uniportal procedure; the third and fifth spaces are used for the biportal operation, both placed in the anterior axillary line (see Fig. 32.6A, B). Some surgeons use three thoracoscopic ports to help with retraction of the lung during sympathectomy.[1] The uniportal procedure is performed with the instruments placed through the port beside the endoscope. The sympathetic chain courses over the rib heads just lateral to the vertebral bodies. The sympathetic chain and ganglia are well visualized through the posterior pleura. The sympathectomy procedure by this and many other groups involves incision of the posterior pleura and cauterization of the T2 and T3 ganglia, which provide most of the sympathetic innervation to the arm and hand via the nerve of Kuntz. Most authors suggest ablating the T4 ganglia as well. The azygos vein on the right and the hemiazygos vein on the left side of the ganglia should be avoided. Sometimes intercostal veins cross over the sympathetic chain, and injury or cauterization can result in bleeding from these vessels.

Recommendations of the Society of Thoracic Surgery and the International Society of Sympathetic Surgery include treatment at R (rib) 3-R4 level for palmar and R4-R5 level for axillary hyperhidrosis. Craniofacial hyperhidrosis should be treated at the R2 and R3 levels.[25]

A recently introduced technique at Mayo Clinic by Atkinson and colleagues[2] has been gaining popularity because it is aimed at decreasing the side effects of sympathectomy, such as post-sympathectomy neuralgia and reactive hyperhidrosis. The technique of T1 to T2 sympathotomy differs in some detail from the previously described procedure.

The operation is performed using general anesthesia, followed by placement of a double-lumen endotracheal tube. Both of the patient's arms are abducted to 90 degrees and the back is elevated to 40 degrees. The chest wall is perforated through a small (<1 cm) transaxillary skin incision or, occasionally, it is perforated in the anterior midclavicular area between the second and third ribs in order to place a small endoscope and attached monopolar cautery. There is no gas insufflation with this technique (Fig. 32.7). Sympathotomy is performed above the T2 ganglion and below the T1 ganglion (or the stellate ganglion) by transection of all nerve fibers across the second rib using an electrocautery. Once both sides are done, bilateral pediatric feeding tubes are placed and the wounds are closed. The intrapleural air is aspirated through the bilateral pediatric feeding tubes, which are then removed. Most patients are discharged within 23 hours.

The Mayo group also uses a Doppler palmar blood flow device to confirm the elevation of skin blood flow after sympathotomy. This technique provides immediate feedback to the surgeon about the efficacy and completeness of the operation.[2]

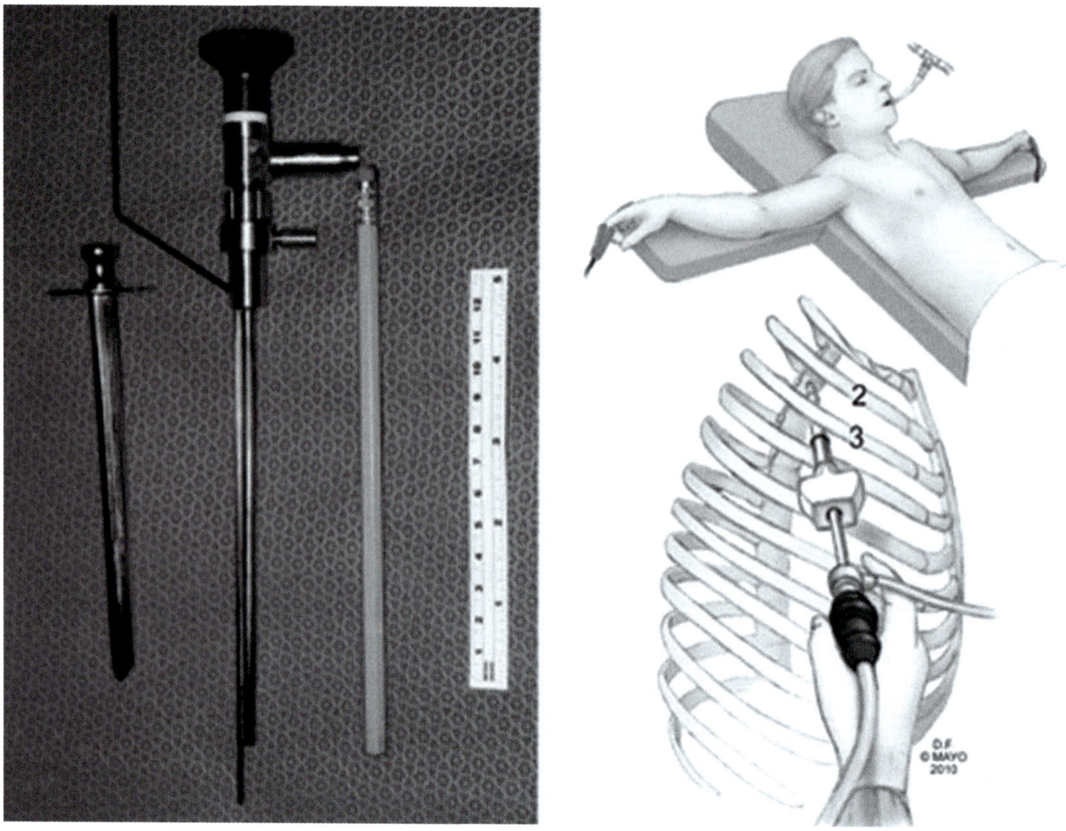

FIG 32.7 *Left,* Instruments used for sympathotomy at Mayo Clinic. Hollow trocar with obturator for perforating the chest wall allows penetration of the chest wall through a small (<1 cm) incision, removal of the inner obturator, and passage of the endoscope with attached monopolar cautery probe (second object). A pencil and tape measure provide perspectives of size. *Right, upper,* Position of patient at surgery. *Lower,* Single small incision and uniportal access with endoscope and cautery combined. (With permission from Atkinson JL, Fode-Thomas NC, Fealey RD, et al: Endoscopic transthoracic limited sympathotomy for palmar-plantar hyperhidrosis: outcomes and complications during a 10-year period. *Mayo Clinic Proceed* 86:721–729, 2011.)

Transumbilical Thoracic Sympathectomy

Natural orifice transluminal endoscopic surgery (NOTES) has become popular in recent years, while for thoracic sympathectomy embryonic natural orifice transumbilical endoscopic surgery (E-NOTES) was introduced. Long-term results using an ultrathin flexible endoscope have recently been reported.[26] The operation is performed under general anesthesia and intubation with a double-lumen endotracheal tube. Access to the abdominal cavity is obtained through the umbilicus and the diaphragm is crossed through the muscular parts of the left and then right diaphragmatic dome using contralateral lung ventilation during the procedure. Hot biopsy forceps are used to grasp and ablate the T3 and T4 sympathetic ganglia.

Results

Hyperhidrosis

Zacherl and colleagues[27] reported on the long-term results of 630 operations performed in 352 patients. Complications included pneumothorax in 1.3%, Horner syndrome in 3.8%, and subcutaneous emphysema in 2.1%. The median follow-up of this study was 16 years; 68% of the patients were fully satisfied and 26% were partially satisfied with the procedure. Permanent cure was obtained in 93% of the patients, although 67% complained of compensatory sweating. Just like other authors, this article also reported a lower success rate in axillary hyperhidrosis.[27]

Drott and colleagues[22] published results of 850 thoracic sympathectomies performed for hyperhidrosis of the palms, axillae, and face.[22] For palmar hyperhidrosis, cure is almost 100% after thoracoscopic sympathectomy, and the success rate was dependent on resection or ablation of the T2 ganglion.

Compensatory hyperhidrosis appears to be frequent, although according to some authors, avoiding resection of T3 and T4 likely decreases the risk of this complication. The overall satisfaction rate following the operation for palmar hyperhidrosis has been reported to be between 87% and 95%. For axillary hyperhidrosis, the satisfaction rate is much lower (60%), and some surgeons avoid sympathectomy completely. Resection of T4 and T5 is frequently required to achieve good results. Panhofer and colleagues found severe compensatory hyperhydrosis at 5 years in 6.7% of 163 patients operated on for primary hyperhidrosis.[28] This was twice as common in patients who were operated on for paloaxillary sweating than in those who had palmar hyperhidrosis only.

A consensus document of The Society of Thoracic Surgeons' General Thoracic Workforce reviewed 1097 published articles on this topic, including 12 randomized controlled trials and 90 comparative studies. The document concluded that primary hyperhidrosis of the extremities, axillae, or face is best treated by endoscopic thoracic sympathectomy. Interruption of the sympathetic chain can be achieved either by electrocautery or by clipping. The literature suggests that the highest success rates occur when interruption is performed at the top of the third rib (R3) or the top of R4 for palmar-only hyperhidrosis. R4 may offer a lower incidence of compensatory hyperhidrosis[29] but moister hands. For palmar and axillary; for palmar, axillary, and pedal; and for axillary-only hyperhidrosis, interruptions at R4 and R5 are recommended. The top of R3 was thought to be best for craniofacial hyperhidrosis.

Wolosker and colleagues[30] prospectively followed 453 patients with hyperhidrosis who underwent endoscopic thoracic sympathectomy to evaluate long-term improvement in quality of life. Quality of life improved immediately after surgery in 91% of the patients, and this improvement was sustained after 5 years.

Atkinson and colleagues[2] performed a retrospective review of 155 patients who underwent thoracoscopic T1 to T2 sympathotomy disconnection surgery for medically refractory palmar-plantar hyperhidrosis. No patient had Horner syndrome, intercostal neuralgia, or pneumothorax. Two patients (1.3%) developed hemothorax. All 155 patients had immediate improvement. At a mean of 40 months after surgery, 97% had successful control of palmar sweating and 69% experienced decreased axillary sweating. Compensatory hyperhidrosis did not occur in 32%; it was mild in 62%, moderate in 5%, and severe in 1%.

Reflex Sympathetic Dystrophy

In patients who have complex regional pain syndrome or reflex sympathetic dystrophy, sympathectomy has been reported to effectively decrease pain. Singh and colleagues[31] analyzed long-term results in 42 patients. Thirty-two underwent thoracoscopic and 10 had open cervicothoracic sympathectomy. Early improvement was reported in all patients. There was no morbidity and no major early complications. The hospital stay was shorter in the thoracic sympathectomy group, and these patients had a better outcome. These authors did not find preoperative stellate ganglion blockade predictive of postoperative clinical outcome. Because of the obvious benefit of thoracoscopic sympathectomy, they recommended it over open surgical sympathectomy as a procedure of choice for patients with complex regional pain syndrome.

Raynaud Syndrome

Lowell and colleagues[9] have reported on results of open surgical treatment of 20 patients who underwent open cervicothoracic sympathectomies for Raynaud syndrome. No mortality was reported, but Horner syndrome was observed in five patients (transient in three and mild in two). Three patients had post-sympathectomy neuralgia, two had phrenic nerve palsy, and one had pneumothorax. Of the 20 patients, 19 had immediate improvement following surgical treatment. This early benefit, however, disappeared in all patients at 6 months, and the authors concluded that cervicothoracic sympathectomy in patients with uncomplicated Raynaud syndrome is not recommended.

In a recent systematic review, Coveliers and colleagues[32] analyzed the evidence for a total of 728 thoracic sympathectomies in the management of digital ischemia caused by both primary Raynaud disease (PRD) and secondary Raynaud phenomenon (SRP). Early improvement was reported in 92% of PRD patients and in 89% of SRP patients, but long-term beneficial effects were found in only 58% of patients with PRD and 89% of those with SRP. Most benefit in PRD patients was limited to the first 6 months, and no improvement was noted thereafter in 42%. Ulcer healing or early improvement was still achieved in 95%, suggesting that thoracic sympathectomy may maximize tissue preservation or prevent amputation; it remains a useful treatment for both PRD and SRP. However, most patients with uncomplicated primary Raynaud syndrome should not undergo thoracic sympathectomy, as emphasized in a recent review by Landry.[33]

Conclusions

The technique of thoracoscopic sympathectomy is currently the operation of choice for patients who need surgical denervation of the thoracic sympathetic chain. Of the open techniques, if needed in the occasional patient, the best is the transaxillary transthoracic sympathectomy. Resection or thoracoscopic ablation of at least the T2 to T3 ganglia is reported to achieve good results. Highly selective T1 to T2 sympathotomy for palmar hyperhidrosis offers a high long-term success rate and low complication rate.

The best indications for cervical sympathectomy include refractory palmar hyperhidrosis and causalgia resulting in chronic pain syndrome. Chronic occlusive arterial disease caused by arteritis (e.g., Buerger disease or Raynaud disease) with nonhealing superficial ulcerations is also a good indication for sympathectomy. Preoperative stellate block does not always predict outcome, and complications of the operation include compensatory sweating, Horner syndrome, and postoperative neuralgia. Compensatory sweating appears to be less frequent with sympathotomy. Compensatory sweating can be such a disabling condition that techniques for reversal of the thoracic sympathectomy have recently been entertained. These include reconstructions using nerve grafts and the application of clips to the nerves during the first operation with the idea of removing them at a later stage should compensatory sweating develop. New surgical techniques using transumbilical thoracic sympathectomy to decrease side effects of transthoracic access, such as chronic pain or paresthesia, are currently being developed.

LUMBAR SYMPATHECTOMY

Indications

Causalgia, plantar hyperhidrosis, frostbite, Buerger disease, pain from atheroembolism (blue toe syndrome), and digital ulcerations are current indications for lumbar sympathectomy. Patients who have critical limb ischemia but an ankle-brachial index greater than 0.3 have also been suggested as candidates for lumbar sympathectomy. Patients who have claudication or diabetes with diabetic neuropathy should not undergo lumbar sympathectomy.

Techniques

Open Surgical Lumbar Sympathectomy

The operation is performed in a semilateral decubitus position (Fig. 32.8). An 8-cm oblique flank incision is made from the tip of the 11th rib either toward the umbilicus or slightly lower halfway toward the umbilicus and the pubis. The dissection is carried down to the abdominal muscles; the muscles are split along their fibers, and the retroperitoneum is entered. On the right side, the peritoneum with the ureter is retracted medially, and the lumbar sympathetic chain is identified between the inferior vena cava and the psoas muscle (see Fig. 32.8C, D). On the left side, the sympathetic chain is located between the aorta and the psoas muscle. The genitofemoral nerve that lies over the psoas muscle is identified and carefully preserved (Fig. 32.9A, B). Attention is paid to avoid any retractor injury to the aorta that may cause embolization into the lower limbs, not infrequently into the right leg. The sympathetic chain is dissected from the rim of the pelvis all the way up to the level of L1. Usually three ganglia (L2 to L4) are removed with the intervening sympathetic chain. Frequently the chain runs under the lumbar vessels, and dissection has to be done carefully to avoid injury to these vessels. To avoid sexual dysfunction in males, L1 must be preserved; bilateral resection of the L1 ganglia should not be performed at all in young males. After excision of the ganglia and the chain, careful hemostasis is performed and the muscles, subcutaneous tissue, and skin are closed in layers.

Endoscopic Lumbar Sympathectomy

This technique was well described by Beglaibter and colleagues[6] and more recently by Rieger and colleagues.[34,35] The procedure is performed with anesthesia and endotracheal intubation, with the patient's flank hyperextended (Fig. 32.10). Balloon dissection of the retroperitoneal space is done by inserting the balloon through a small incision in the flank. Two or three ports are used for retraction and dissection. The chain is ablated with excision and electrocautery. To facilitate localization of the various levels of the lumbar sympathetic trunk, Rieger recommends that projection of the lumbar vertebral bodies onto the anterior abdominal wall be marked fluoroscopically.

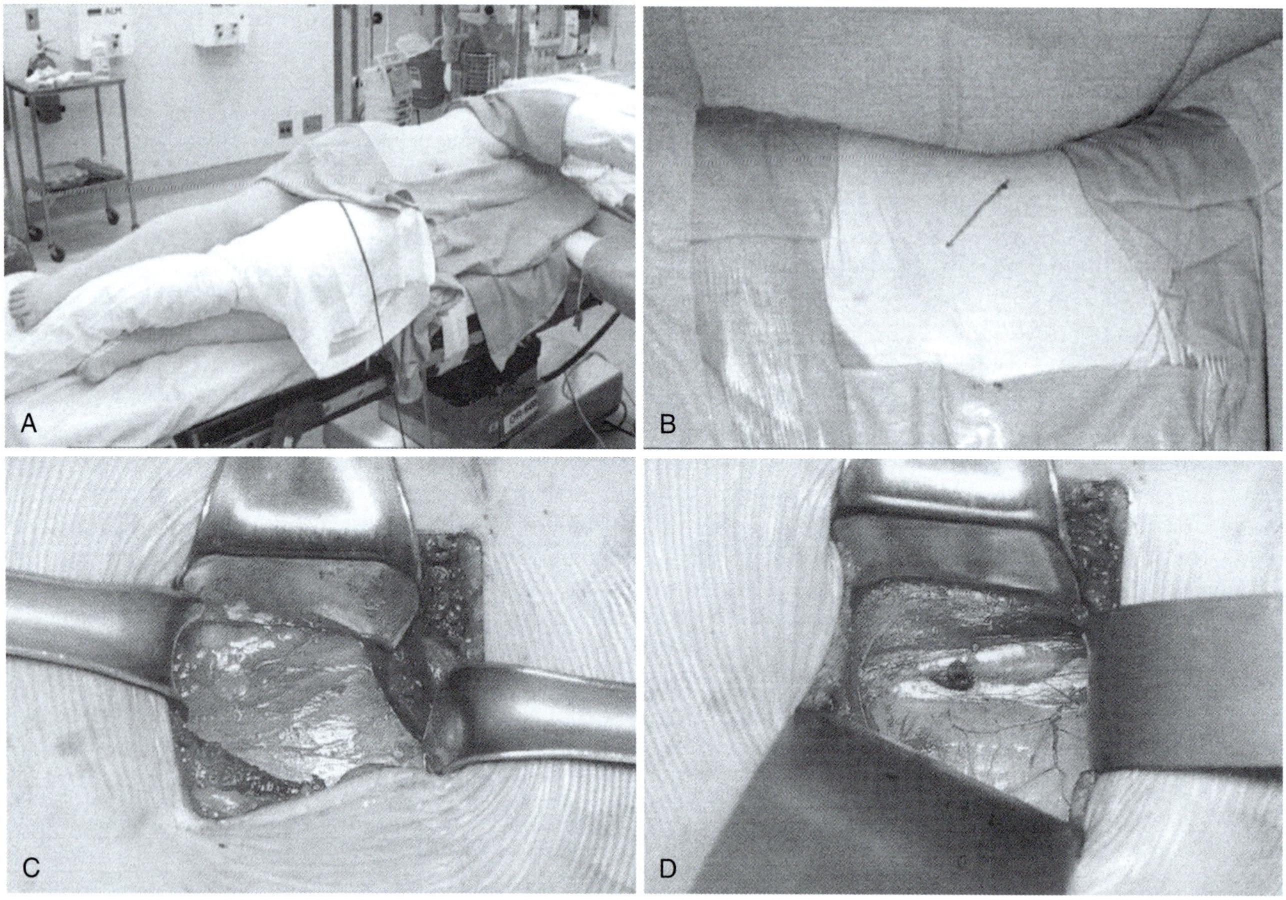

FIG 32.8 (A) Position of the patient on the operating table for right lumbar sympathectomy. (B) An 8-cm skin incision is made from the tip of the 11th rib toward halfway between the umbilicus and the pubis. (C) The abdominal muscles are split along their fibers. (D) Blunt retroperitoneal dissection is made to explore the space between the medial edge of the psoas muscle and the inferior vena cava.

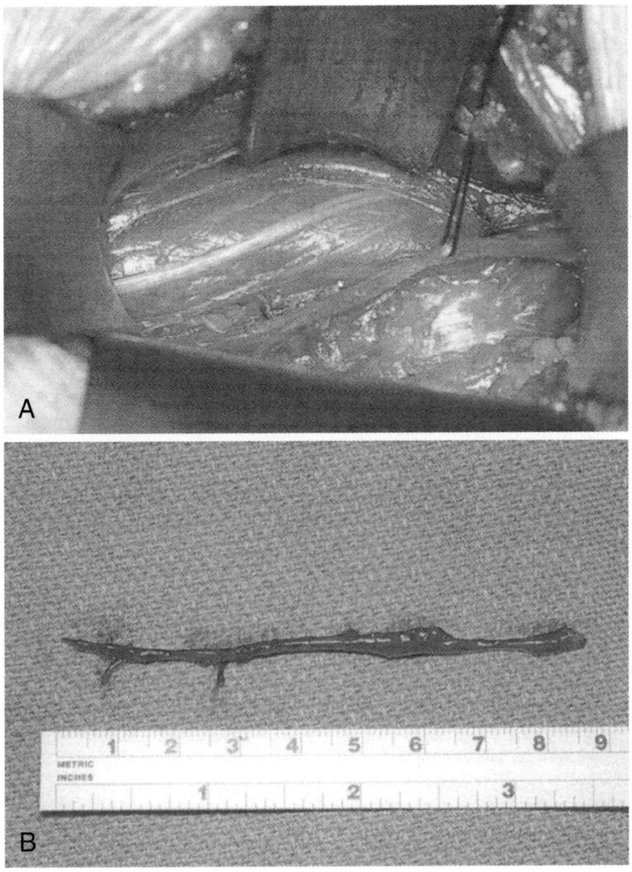

FIG 32.9 (A) The lumbar sympathetic chain is on a black silk. Note the genitofemoral nerve over the psoas muscle. (B) The resected sympathetic chain with T2, T3, and T4 ganglia.

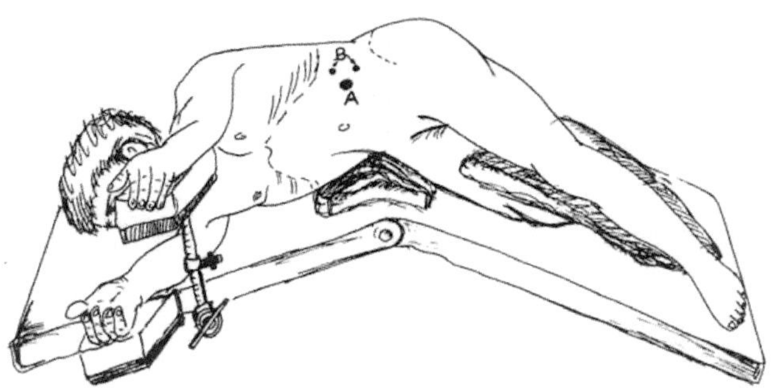

FIG 32.10 Position and port placement for retroperitoneoscopic lumbar sympathectomy. (With permission from Beglaibter N, Berlatzky Y, Zamir O, et al: Retroperitoneoscopic lumbar sympathectomy. *J Vasc Surg* 35:815–817, 2002.)

Results

The most frequent early complication of lumbar sympathectomy is postsympathectomy neuralgia, which has been described in 20% to 50% of the patients.[8] Paradoxic gangrene is usually the result of embolization from the aortoiliac vessels; careful retraction of the tissues during the operation will prevent this complication. As mentioned previously, bilateral resection of the L1 sympathetic ganglia may result in the disturbance of ejaculation or potency.

Persson and colleagues[36] have reported on the results of lumbar sympathectomy for ischemic rest pain and ulcers in 37 patients who had inoperable disease. All patients had an ankle-brachial index greater than 0.3. There was no neuropathy, and patients had limited tissue loss; 78% of these patients had long-term pain relief, and only 11% required amputation. On the contrary, Fulton and Blakeley[37] reported no effect of sympathectomy on amputation in patients with severe distal ischemia. Seventeen unselected patients in this series with advanced arteriosclerosis underwent lumbar sympathectomy; the 70% rate of amputation discredited this operation. This report and others caused significant controversy regarding this operation and decreased the use of lumbar sympathectomy for the indication of critical limb ischemia.

Bandyk and colleagues[8] reported on the results of sympathectomy in 73 patients who underwent surgical treatment for reflex sympathetic dystrophy. Forty-seven of these patients underwent thoracic sympathectomy, and 37 had lumbar sympathectomy. The authors found that a greater than 50% reduction in pain score for more than 2 days after sympathetic block predicted a good response to the operation. No mortality or major morbidity was reported. Transient neuralgia was noted in 20% of the patients after lumbar sympathectomy and 90% of patients reported excellent results at 3 months. At 1 year, 25% still had significant pain relief and 50% had improvement. Overall patient satisfaction was 77%.

Beglaibter and colleagues[6] presented the results of 29 retroperitoneoscopic lumbar sympathectomies performed in 27 patients. Of these, 22 had ischemia of the lower limb, 5 because of Buerger disease; 5 had severe reflex sympathetic dystrophy. Improvement in symptoms was noted in all patients.

Five patients in the series previously underwent computed tomography–guided chemical sympathectomy. It should be noted that reported complications related to attempts at chemical sympathectomy using phenol or alcohol injections resulted in complications related to the injection itself and to the effects of the chemicals that are injected. Ureteral damage—including stricture and necrosis, retroperitoneal abscess formation, and fibrosis—have been reported.[38]

Rieger and colleagues[34] performed 178 endoscopic lumbar sympathectomies at the L3 and L4 levels for plantar hyperhidrosis in 90 patients. Postsympathetic neuralgia occurred in 42% and compensatory sweating in 42%. Postsympathetic neuralgia, however, was only minor and temporary, and only one patient had severe compensatory sweating. One patient had temporary loss of ejaculation. At 24 months, 97% of the patients had been cured of hyperhidrosis. Endoscopic lumbar sympathectomy is effective and safe, and a recent review found that plantar hyperhidrosis can be treated with excellent results in in more than 95% of cases with a low risk of morbidity and side effects.[39]

Conclusion

Lumbar sympathectomy is effective and durable in patients with plantar hyperhidrosis. Lumbar sympathectomy also has good results in patients who have causalgia, Buerger disease, or frostbite. Patients with reflex sympathetic dystrophy with confirmed sympathetically mediated pain syndrome can have long-term benefit from this operation. With the advent of lower limb revascularizations, indications for critical limb ischemia have decreased significantly. Good results have been reported with Buerger disease and in nondiabetic patients with distal atherosclerosis who have rest pain, limited tissue loss, and an ankle-brachial index better than 0.3. The most frequent complication of the operation is postsympathectomy neuralgia, which is usually transient and responds well to pain medications. Open lumbar sympathectomy will soon be completely replaced by retroperitoneoscopic procedures.

QUESTIONS

1. The peripheral nervous system includes all components except
   - **a.** Somatic efferent motor nerves
   - **b.** Somatic afferent motor nerves
   - **c.** Somatic efferent nerves to the exocrine glands
   - **d.** Autonomic nerves to the abdominal viscera
   - **e.** Autonomic sympathetic and parasympathetic nerves
2. Most experts agree that for sympathetic denervation of the upper limb, interruption of the sympathetic chain at the following level is required:
   - **a.** Stellate ganglion
   - **b.** Stellate ganglion and T1
   - **c.** T2 to T4
   - **d.** T4–T5
   - **e.** T5
3. In patients with axillary hyperhidrosis, resection of the following ganglions as extension of a T2–T3 sympathectomy is recommended:
   - **a.** T4
   - **b.** T4–T5
   - **c.** T1
   - **d.** C8
   - **e.** C8–T1
4. Indications for thoracoscopic sympathectomy include all of the following except
   - **a.** Hyperhidrosis
   - **b.** Buerger disease with digital ulcers
   - **c.** Uncomplicated Raynaud syndrome associated with scleroderma
   - **d.** Frostbite
   - **e.** Causalgia
5. The right sympathetic chain with T2 to T5 ganglia is located 2 to 3 cm lateral to the
   - **a.** Phrenic nerve
   - **b.** Azygos vein
   - **c.** Hemiazygos vein
   - **d.** Long thoracic nerve
   - **e.** Right atrium
6. Direct collateral sympathetic fibers to the arm at the T2 to T3 levels are located in the
   - **a.** Nerve of Herring
   - **b.** Intercostobrachial nerve
   - **c.** Nerve of Kuntz
   - **d.** Paravertebral ganglia
   - **e.** Brachial plexus
7. The right lumbar sympathetic chain is located
   - **a.** Lateral to the psoas muscle
   - **b.** Medial to the inferior vena cava
   - **c.** Lateral to the genitofemoral nerve
   - **d.** Between the psoas muscle and the inferior vena cava
   - **e.** Just lateral to the aorta
8. To avoid sexual dysfunction, lumbar sympathetic ganglia at what level must be preserved in males
   - **a.** L1
   - **b.** L2
   - **c.** L3
   - **d.** L4
   - **e.** L5
9. Which of the following is usually a contraindication to lumbar sympathectomy?
   - **a.** Digital gangrene
   - **b.** Causalgia
   - **c.** Frostbite
   - **d.** Diabetic neuropathy
   - **e.** Buerger disease
10. Sympathectomy results in all of the following changes in a limb except:
    - **a.** Decreased sweating
    - **b.** Increased skin circulation
    - **c.** Decreased pain
    - **d.** Increased circulation to the skeletal muscles
    - **e.** Increased parasympathetic tone

BIBLIOGRAPHY

Atkinson JL, Fode-Thomas NC, Fealey RD, et al. Endoscopic transthoracic limited sympathotomy for palmar-plantar hyperhidrosis: outcomes and complications during a 10-year period. *Mayo Clin Proc*. 2011;86(8):721–729.

Bandyk DF, Johnson BL, Kirkpatrick AF, et al. Surgical sympathectomy for reflex sympathetic dystrophy syndromes. *J Vasc Surg*. 2002;35:269–277.

Cerfolio RJ, De Campos JR, Bryant AS, et al. The Society of Thoracic Surgeons expert consensus for the surgical treatment of hyperhidrosis. *Ann Thorac Surg*. 2011;91(5):1642–1648.

Coveliers HM, Hoexum F, Nederhoed JH, et al. Thoracic sympathectomy for digital ischemia: a summary of evidence. *J Vasc Surg*. 2011;54(1):273–277.

Rieger R. Management of Plantar Hyperhidrosis with Endoscopic Lumbar Sympathectomy. *Thorac Surg Clin*. 2016;26:465–469.

Sternbach JM, DeCamp MM. Targeting the sympathetic chain for primary hyperhidrosis: an evidence-based review. *Thorac Surg Clin*. 2016;26:407–420.

References available online at ExpertConsult.com.

CHAPTER 33

Thoracic Outlet Syndrome and Vascular Disease of the Upper Extremity

Hugh A. Gelabert, David A. Rigberg

INTRODUCTION

To many physicians, the diagnosis and management of thoracic outlet syndrome (TOS) is confusing. Part of the confusion arises because TOS is a term applied to three distinct clinical entities, which may share common anatomical elements yet may present with a variety of symptoms. In addition, there has been lack of agreement as to the defining criteria, the indications for intervention, and the anticipated outcomes. This has led to a wide spectrum of opinions as to the identification of TOS and the results of subsequent management. In response to these issues, the Society for Vascular Surgery recently published reporting standards for TOS.[1,2] The goal of this chapter is to provide an overview of TOS and vascular diseases of the upper extremity. Although not comprehensive, it will serve as a sound foundation and provide direction for further study.

BACKGROUND

History

Although symptoms associated with neurovascular compression of the upper extremity have been present throughout the ages, it has only been in relatively recent times that the concept of TOS has taken a unified form. Galen is attributed with the first mention of cervical ribs in the second century AD, but descriptions of cervical rib syndrome in the English literature date to the early 19th century. Sir Astley Cooper is credited with description of cervical rib syndrome (London 1821).[3] Coote reported resection of a cervical rib in 1861, heralding the recognition of skeletal abnormalities in upper extremity pain syndromes.[4] With time, the role of soft tissue compression by the scalene muscles came to the fore after reports by Adson and Coffey at the Mayo Clinic.[5] This was named Scalenus Anticus (Nafziger) Syndrome by Ochsner, Gage, and Debakey in 1935, giving credit to Naffziger for the concept.[6,7]

The recognition of venous thrombosis of the subclavian vein was initially described independently by Sir James Pager (London 1875) and Leopold Von Shcroetter (Vienna 1884). The designation Paget-Schroetter syndrome (PSS) was devised by Hughes (London 1948) when reviewing 320 cases of spontaneous subclavian vein thrombosis.[8] Arterial presentations of TOS (aTOS) were likewise evolving during this period.

The unifying term TOS was used by Peet (1956) and Rob (1958) to describe neurovascular compression at the thoracic outlet.[9,10] Their idea was to consider compression of neurovascular structures at the thoracic outlet as a common etiology that presented different manifestations according to those elements most severely impacted.

This concept of TOS preceded a further shift in therapeutic approach toward these maladies. Instead of identifying bony anomalies (cervical rib syndrome) or muscular compression (scalenus anticus syndrome), the concept of thoracic outlet compression emphasized the interaction of these elements.

The surgical approach to TOS evolved apace with these conceptual developments. The cervical rib syndrome was managed by cervical rib resection. This was first reported by Coote in 1861.[4] Scalenus anticus syndrome was managed with scalenectomy. TOS led to the adoption of first rib resection.

Murphy performed a first rib resection in 1908,[11] but concerns with nerve complications led to its abandonment until it was reintroduced by Clagett in 1962.[12] He applied his experience with thoracoplasty done for treatment of tuberculosis (TB) to a posterior approach to first rib resection. This was a technically difficult operation with considerable morbidity. The description of the transaxillary approach by Roos in 1966 presented a dramatically superior approach. Transaxillary surgery had far less morbidity than the posterior rib resection and was subsequently widely adopted. The principal problem was that it was a technically challenging operation.

The supraclavicular approach to first rib resection experienced a surge of interest because it combined supraclavicular surgical exposure and scalenectomy, which was more familiar to vascular surgeons, with partial removal of the posterior aspect of the first rib. Subsequent evolution of the supraclavicular approach has led to inclusion of a secondary infraclavicular incision to allow further resection of the anterior portion of the first rib.

Anatomy

The skeletal thoracic outlet is that space defined by the first ribs, sternum, and spine circumscribing the top of the thoracic cage. It forms the floor to which are attached the muscular elements of the thoracic outlet. The clavicle forms a superior boundary, riding over the neurovascular structures. The muscular elements include the anterior scalene, middle scalene, and subclavius muscles (Fig. 33.1).[13,14]

Taken together these structures give rise to two areas of potential compression: the *scalene triangle* and the *costoclavicular space*. The scalene triangle is formed by the anterior scalene muscle,

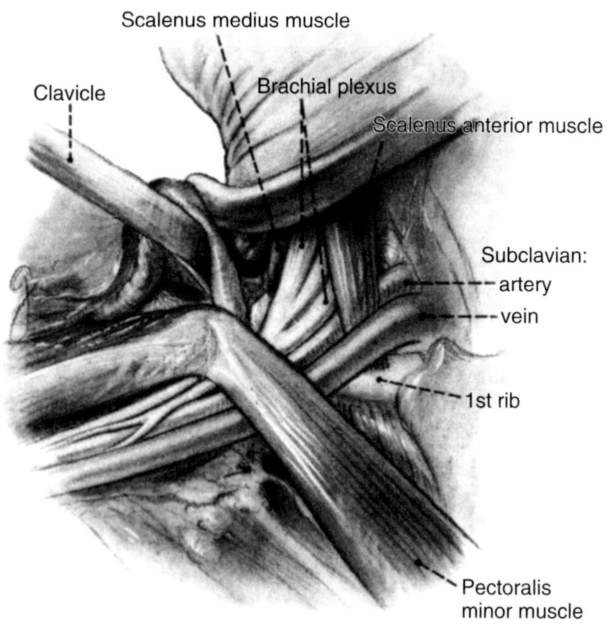

FIG 33.1 Anatomic dissection showing the anatomy at the thoracic outlet. The cadaver's head is turned to the left, and the clavicle is reflected laterally. (From Machleder HI, editor: *Vascular Disorders of the Upper Extremity*, ed 3, Mt. Kisco, NY, 1998, Futura Publishing.)

the middle scalene muscle, and the first rib. Through this triangle pass the brachial plexus and the subclavian artery. The anatomic configuration where the brachial plexus and subclavian artery travel through the scalene triangle accounts for some of the confusion in defining symptoms of TOS. Any compression of the brachial plexus will also result in some compression of the subclavian artery. Consequently, arterial and neurogenic TOS (nTOS) are at times confused. The costoclavicular space is formed by the first rib and the clavicle. These form an open-ended triangle that joins at the hinged junction of these two bones. The subclavian vein crosses through the apex of this triangle and may be subject to compression at this location.

The *anterior scalene* muscle is unique in separating the subclavian artery and vein: the subclavian vein travels outside the scalene triangle in a venous channel bordered anteriorly by the subclavius muscle and posteriorly by the anterior scalene muscle. The anterior scalene muscle forms the anterior border of the scalene triangle. The phrenic nerve courses on the anterior aspect of the anterior scalene muscle. It descends from the superior lateral border of the muscle and crosses toward the inferior medial portion of the scalene and enters the chest behind the subclavian vein.

The *middle scalene* muscle forms the posterior border of the scalene triangle. The anterior scalene muscle is innervated by the C5 and C6 cervical spinal nerves. It originates from the anterior transverse processes of C3 to C6 and inserts onto the first rib on the scalene tubercle. The middle scalene muscle is the largest of the scalene muscles. It is innervated by nerves arising from nerve roots C4 to C6. The middle scalene originates from the transverse processes of the C2 to C7 cervical vertebrae. The muscle occupies a broad insertion on the dorsal aspect of the first rib from the posterior aspect of the rib extending toward the mid portion of the rib. The dorsal scapular, suprascapular, and long thoracic nerves traverse the body of the middle scalene muscle. In this location, they are at risk of injury in the course of middle scalene resection and supraclavicular rib resection.

Both scalene muscles are important elements in the genesis of thoracic outlet compression because spasm and contraction of these muscles will result in elevation of the first rib and muscular compression of the structures traversing the scalene triangle.

The *scalenus minimus* is a small muscle that most often arises from the middle scalene muscle, traverses between the nerve roots, and inserts on the first rib and thickened dome of the pleura (Sibson fascia). As such, it is a muscular sling that envelops the lower trunks of the brachial plexus and may contribute to genesis of symptoms.

The *subclavian vein* travels in a *venous channel* that is bordered anteriorly by the *subclavius muscle tendon* and posteriorly by the *middle scalene muscle*. The subclavius muscle arises from the undersurface of the clavicle and inserts on the first rib in front of the costoclavicular ligament. It is innervated by a nerve to the subclavius arising from nerve roots C5 and C6.

The *brachial plexus* arises from nerve roots C5 to C8, and T1. These roots then form three trunks (upper [C5 and C6], middle [C7] and lower [C8 and T1]). The trunks then intermix to form divisions (three anterior and three posterior), which are intermediaries to the formation of cords. The cords (posterior, medial, and lateral) then lead to the terminal nerves, which supply the arm (median, radial, ulnar, and musculocutaneous).

Several *important nerve branches* arising from the brachial plexus traverse this space: among these are the phrenic nerve, the long thoracic nerve, the dorsal scapular nerve, the suprascapular nerve, and the thoracodorsal nerve.

The *suprascapular nerve* arises from nerve roots C5 and C6 and innervates the supraspinatus and infraspinatus muscles. It courses through the body of the middle scalene muscle. The supraspinatus muscle forms part of the rotator cuff and abducts the arm at the shoulder. The infraspinatus muscle forms part of the rotator cuff of the shoulder and serves to externally rotate the arm and stabilize the shoulder.

The *dorsal scapular nerve* arises from the C5 nerve root. It courses through the body of the middle scalene muscle and innervates the rhomboid and levator scapulae. The rhomboid muscles pull the scapular toward the midline. The levator scapula elevates the scapula and lifts the scapula toward the head.

The *phrenic nerve* arises from nerve roots C3 to C5 and innervates the diaphragm. The nerve arises on the superior lateral border of the anterior scalene muscle, courses across the front of the anterior scalene muscle, and reaches the medial inferior border of the anterior scalene. Loss of function will result in paralysis of the hemidiaphragm. Most patients are quite symptomatic with loss of the hemidiaphragmatic function, making this an easily identified nerve injury. In about 13% of the population the phrenic nerve forms two separate bundles, which course in parallel across the anterior scalene muscle.

The *long thoracic nerve* arises from nerve roots C5 to C7, travels through the body of the middle scalene muscle, and innervates the serratus anterior muscle. Damage to this nerve results in instability of the scapula when the arm is raised or used to push. This defect is noted with the medial border of the scapula pushing backward and is called a winged scapula. Because of the prominence of this defect, it is easy to identify.

The *thoracodorsal nerve* arises from nerve roots C6 to C8, and innervates the latissimus dorsi muscle. The latissimus dorsi muscle is a broad muscle that attaches from spine to humerus and serves to extend, abduct, and stabilize the shoulder. The latissimus dorsi may occasionally give rise to the axillary arch—a slip of the muscle that may cross in front of the axillary vessels resulting in neurovascular compression.

The following are additional structures of importance in upper extremity neurovascular syndromes:

The *pectoralis minor muscle* arises from the chest wall over the anterior aspect of ribs 3 to 5. It inserts on the coracoid process in the undersurface of the scapula. Along its course it crosses over the neurovascular bundle as this exits the thoracic outlet and enters the arm. In this manner it may generate symptoms of nerve or vascular compression in the arm, giving rise to pectoralis minor syndrome.

The *quadrilateral space* is a muscular space bordered by the heads of the teres major and teres minor muscles, as well as the triceps muscle and the neck of the humerus. Coursing through this space is the axillary nerve and the posterior humeral circumflex artery. The posterior humeral circumflex artery is subject to injury at this location resulting in a well-documented thromboembolic syndrome.

Anatomical Variants

Many TOS presentations are associated with acquired or developmental anomalies of the muscular elements within the thoracic outlet. Hypertrophy of the scalene and subclavius muscles is associated with venous TOS (vTOS). Overdevelopment or chronic spams of the anterior and middle scalene muscles may be associated with arterial and nTOS.

The most clinically significant variations in thoracic outlet structure consist of alterations in the size and insertion of the muscles, variations in the number and shape of the bony elements, and presence of tendinous bands. David Roos described nine variants, which he termed bands.[15] These include varying attachments of cervical ribs, scalene muscles, and ligaments onto the pleura and first rib. Machleder recorded anatomical variants in 200 consecutive cases. Variations in scalene muscle development or insertion accounted for 43% of cases. Anomalies of the subclavian muscle and tendon accounted for 19%, and an accessory scalene minimus muscle was noted in 10%.[16] The scalenus minimus muscle is an accessory muscle that separates the brachial plexus and subclavian artery. It most often arises as a fascicle of the middle scalene muscle and traverses the lower roots of the brachial plexus. The net effect is that it may form a muscular tendinous band that essentially encircles the lower brachial plexus roots (Fig. 33.2).

Cervical ribs are a well-recognized anatomical variant associated with TOS. The cervical rib is a supernumerary rib that

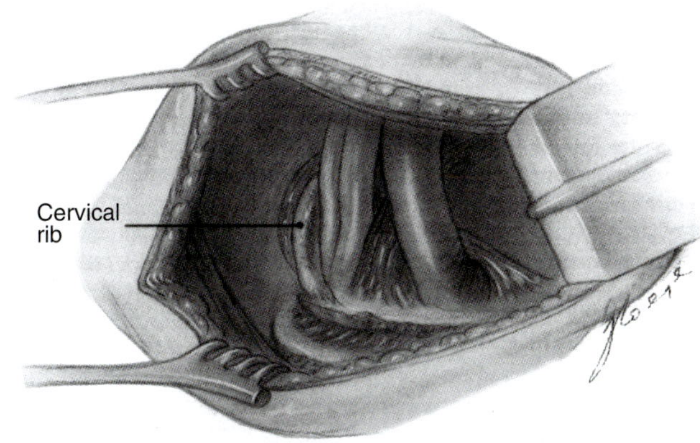

FIG 33.2 Appearance of the scalenus minimus abnormality from the transaxillary surgical approach. (From Makhoul RG, Machleder HI: Developmental anomalies at the thoracic outlet: an analysis of 200 consecutive cases. *J Vasc Surg* 16:534–545, 1992.)

arises from the transverse process of the C7 vertebral body. The presence of cervical ribs is noted in about 0.5% to 1% of the population.[17-19] These are noted to occur in women with twice the frequency as with men and are bilateral in almost half of the cases.[14,20] Cervical ribs arise as a developmental anomaly in early embryogenic development. In the course of body segmentation, early embryogenic cervical ribs C5 to C7 will normally regress as the nerve roots of the brachial plexus form. If this process does not occur, or if it occurs with incomplete regression, then a cervical rib remains. There is a considerable variety in the formation of cervical ribs, from fully ossified ribs joining with the sternal border to shortened partial ribs with fibrous bands completing their course to the first rib, to an elongated transverse process of the C7 vertebral body associated with a fibrous band. The Gruber classification is a simple system that organizes cervical ribs according to size: less than 2.5 cm (class I), greater than 2.5 cm (class II), and junction of a full-sized rib with the first rib: fibrous union (class III; Fig. 33.3) or full articular junction (class IV; Fig. 33.4).[1] Although as many as 45% of people with cervical ribs are asymptomatic, cervical ribs are associated with arterial and nTOS symptoms.[20] The presence of a cervical rib reduces the space within the scalene triangle. Partially formed cervical ribs are often associated with fibrous bands that constrict the lower trunks of the brachial plexus.

A developmental consequence of cervical rib persistence is noted in abnormal first rib growth. In cases with fully formed cervical ribs, the first rib will simulate a normal second rib in its growth: it will reside more laterally and may have a form similar to the normal second rib. Variations of this effect are seen with the various permutations of cervical ribs: smaller cervical ribs or an elongated transverse process may not alter the first rib development. Intermediate-sized cervical ribs will have an intermediate effect.

Abnormal First Rib Development

A number of anatomical variations of first rib growth have been associated with TOS. Most of these result in bony compression

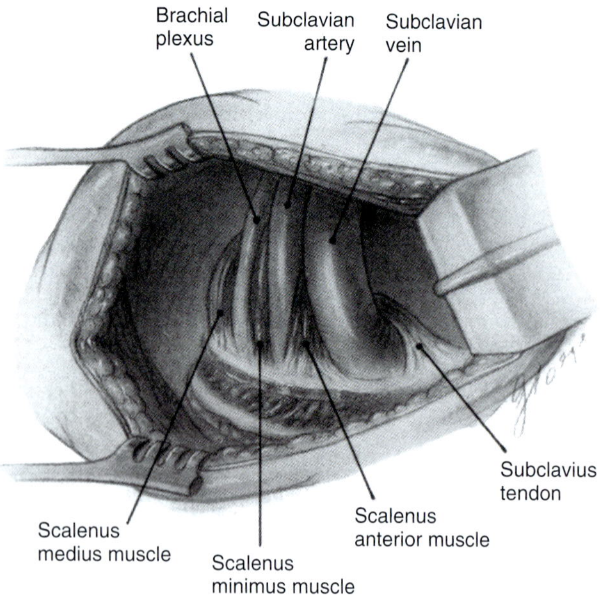

FIG 33.3 View of a fibrocartilaginous band from the tip of the right-sided seventh cervical transverse process from the trans-axillary surgical approach. This abnormality can compress the brachial plexus and subclavian artery, causing symptoms identical to those resulting from a cervical rib. The fibrocartilaginous band commonly occurs with an elongated C7 transverse process and represents partial formation of a cervical rib. (From Makhoul RG, Machleder HI: Developmental anomalies at the thoracic outlet: an analysis of 200 consecutive cases. *J Vasc Surg* 16:534–545, 1992.)

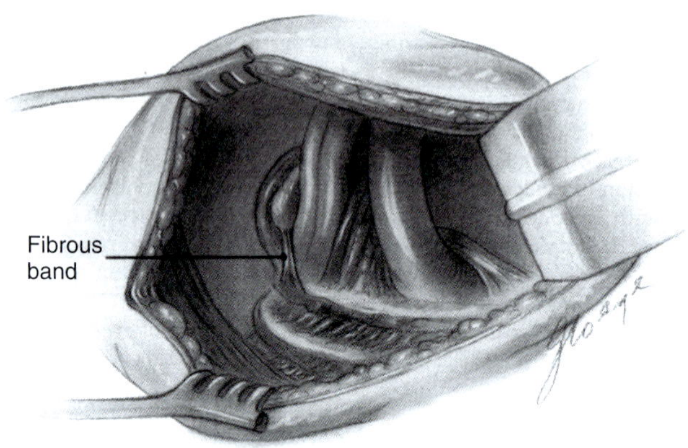

FIG 33.4 View of thoracic outlet structures from the transaxillary surgical approach. The brachial plexus and subclavian artery are compressed and displaced by a right-sided cervical rib. This cervical rib articulates in the center of the first thoracic rib. (From Makhoul RG, Machleder HI: Developmental anomalies at the thoracic outlet: an analysis of 200 consecutive cases. *J Vasc Surg* 16:534–545, 1992.)

of the neurovascular structures. Abnormalities include variations in the length of the rib, its curvature, and presence of exostosis or pseudoarthrosis. In a similar manner, fracture of the first rib or clavicle may result in callous formation with consequent impingement on the thoracic outlet structures.

DEFINITIONS: THORACIC OUTLET SYNDROME

TOS may be best defined as symptoms and findings that result from compression of the neurovascular structures as they traverse the thoracic outlet. Accordingly, the presentations will include neurogenic, arterial, and venous symptoms.[1,2]

Neurogenic Thoracic Outlet Syndrome

nTOS is the symptomatic presentation of compression of elements of the brachial plexus as they cross the thoracic outlet. Cardinal symptoms include pain, paresthesia (numbness, tingling, and alteration of sensation). Weakness and loss of dexterity are also common. When compression at the thoracic outlet affects the sympathetic fibers, color changes, temperature instability (mostly coldness), and mottling are noted. It should be noted that some of these symptoms are strongly associated with arterial insufficiency, but in this instance arise from nerve compression. Atrophy of the muscles of the hand and (less commonly) the forearm are noted in cases where motor denervation results from nerve compression.

Venous Thoracic Outlet Syndrome

vTOS commonly arises from compression of the subclavian vein as it crosses between the clavicle and first rib, bound by the anterior and middle scalene muscles. The most common of these presentations is that of acute subclavian vein thrombosis. In addition to acute thrombosis, some presentations include acute chronic thrombosis, chronic obstructive venous congestion, and nonthrombotic positional intermittent venous occlusion (McLeery syndrome).

Arterial Thoracic Outlet Syndrome

aTOS are a result of chronic compression with damage to the subclavian artery. These presentations include aneurysmal degeneration, acute and chronic embolization to the upper extremity, and arterial thrombosis. Intermittent positional compression, without evidence of arterial thrombosis or embolization (which may occur when a patient raises their arm overhead), is not considered an arterial presentation of TOS.

SYMPTOMATIC PRESENTATIONS

Neurogenic Thoracic Outlet Syndrome

The *typical presentations* of nTOS include numbness, tingling, weakness, and pain in the upper extremity. These are usually along the distribution of the nerve trunks. The symptoms tend to course along the ulnar or radial aspect of the limb with involvement of the hand and fingers.[21-23]

In addition to paresthesia, sensation of coldness and color changes are often noted in the affected hand. Headaches are a frequent accompanying symptom. There seems to be an association of migraine where the development of nTOS will exacerbate migraine.

Atrophy of the musculature of the hand is a relatively unusual but well-recognized presentation of nTOS. When atrophy is associated with presence of a cervical rib and shows evidence of denervation on electromyography (EMG) the presentation is sometimes termed the Gilliatt-Sumner (1970) hand.[24]

Core symptoms of nTOS include pain or paresthesia from the base of the neck to the fingers. In addition to these, many patients will present with *associated symptoms* including migraine, ocular, ear, facial, parascapular, pectoral, and axillary symptoms. A further subdivision of symptoms into upper plexus and lower plexus presentations is based on the predominance of radial or ulnar symptom distribution. This distinction is sometimes used to direct the choice of operations.

Atypical presentations may include incomplete presentations as well as presentation with unusual symptoms. Incomplete presentations might be pain and paresthesia limited to the neck and shoulders but not including the arm and hand. Unusual presentations may include chest pain with repeated emergency room evaluations for angina along with pain or paresthesia in the arm.

Diagnosis of Neurogenic Thoracic Outlet Syndrome

TOS is a clinical syndrome. The diagnosis of TOS is based on the summation of patient symptoms and the findings of physical examination. The diagnosis does not rest on any one pathognomonic symptom or finding. The diagnosis may be supported by appropriate testing. Testing is directed toward evaluating both the diagnosis of TOS and the competing differential diagnosis. There is no test that is considered a gold standard. There is no single finding on exam that is clearly diagnostic. Clinical acumen and appreciation of diagnostic patterns is probably most important in identifying patients who have TOS. Testing for TOS needs to be individualized—not all patients require all tests. In addition to supporting the diagnosis, testing may also provide insight into the likely result of treatment.

Patients presenting with nTOS represent the most complex group to diagnose. This is partially due to the overlap of symptoms and exam findings between nTOS and other neurocompressive syndromes affecting the upper extremity. The first step in diagnosis is to recognize elements of a typical presentation. The typical symptoms of nTOS include pain, numbness, tingling, and weakness in the upper extremity. The pain and paresthesia tend to be centered over the brachial plexus in the base of the neck and will then radiate down the arm. In many instances there may be symptoms in the upper trapezius, parascapular area, chest wall, and the side of the head. In a minority of cases, atrophy of the musculature of the hand is a prominent feature.

Differential Diagnosis

The differential diagnosis of nTOS includes any cervical spine disease that may result in radicular symptoms: spondylolisthesis, disk herniation, foraminal stenosis, and ostephyte formation. In addition, peripheral nerve compression syndromes such as carpal tunnel, cubital tunnel, Guyon tunnel, and radial tunnel compression may result in neuralgia and should be considered in the differential diagnosis. Other disease processes that are characterized by pain including fibromyalgia and myofascial pain syndromes should be considered. Shoulder pathology may cause positional triggering of symptoms but would not be expected to result in pain or paresthesia radiating down the extremity along a neural pathway.

Physical Examination

Physical evaluation requires a complete neurovascular exam of the upper extremity. This should include evaluation of sensory function, motor function, and reflexes. The next step is evaluation of sensitivities over the compressive sites by palpation and percussion. The hands should be assessed for strength and muscular atrophy. Function of the opponens muscles in the thumb and fifth fingers, as well as grip strength and interosseous function are routinely done.

Percussion over the nerves eliciting radiating pain or paresthesia is referred to as Tinel sign and is an indication of irritability of a given nerve. At minimum, Tinel testing is performed over the Erb point (at the anterior base of the neck over the scalene muscle), over the ulnar nerve at the elbow as it courses through the olecranon groove, and over the median nerve at the wrist where it travels through the carpal tunnel. Additional points of evaluation may include the radial tunnel in the forearm or Guyon canal at the wrist, if clinically indicated.

In addition, palpation and percussion should evaluate tenderness over the pectoralis muscle. If pressure over the pectoral muscle results in pain in the muscle along with pain or paresthesia down the arm, then pectoralis minor syndrome should be considered.

Provocative examination includes maneuvers that use different positions of the arm to elicit positional compression of arteries or to place tension on the nerves and elicit positional exacerbation of symptoms. These tests include the Adson maneuver, the abduction external rotation (AER) test, the costoclavicular compression test, the elevated arm stress test (EAST), the upper extremity limb tension test (UELTT), and the Wright hyperextension test.[23]

The *Adson test* consists of abduction of the limb with head turning, deep breath holding, and assessment of radial pulse. Turning the head and taking a deep breath engages the scalene muscles resulting in loss of pulse. In a positive test the pulse is lost and symptoms may be reproduced.[14]

The *AER test* raises the arm laterally to the level of the shoulder or above while assessing the radial pulse and auscultating for subclavian bruit. A positive test includes loss or severe reduction of pulse, development of a bruit, and pallor of the hand.[25]

The *costoclavicular compression test,* or military brace test, places arms at the side while retracting the shoulders and extending the neck. The radial pulse is assessed. Loss of pulse and reproduction of symptoms indicates a positive test.

Positional loss of pulse must be evaluated in the context of presenting symptoms. Almost 50% of the normal population will demonstrate positional loss of radial pulse. The positional loss of pulse is significant only in those patients who have nTOS symptoms. The rationale for these tests is recognition that the brachial plexus and subclavian arteries are in immediate proximity to one another as they course through the scalene triangle. Thus the positional loss of pulse is seen as a proxy for nerve compression.

The *EAST* requires the patient to raise the arms above the head with the arms at shoulder level, then open and close the hands repeatedly. This is continued for 1 to 3 minutes while recording symptoms. A positive test includes reproduction of radiating symptoms in the arms and hands. Pallor of the hands is often noted with hyperemia when the arms are lowered.[26]

The *UELTT* is designed to place gradually increased stretch on the nerves in the upper extremity to try to reproduce symptoms of pain or paresthesia radiating down the arm. This is performed by having the patient extend the arms out to the sides at shoulder level. The next step is to have the patient dorsiflex the hands. The third step is to have the patient lean their head from side to side. A typically positive test will rapidly result in pain or paresthesia down the arm.

The *Wright hyperextension* test is performed by having the patient reach both arms downward behind the torso. This places the pectoralis minor muscle on tension and results in accentuating compression of the neurovascular bundle as it courses down the arm. A positive test will result in pain in the pectoral region and pain or paresthesia down the arm.

In addition to the above noted tests, evaluation of cervical spine disease is done with rotation, extension, and flexion of the neck with evaluation of any resulting symptoms. The *Spurling maneuver* is an additional test done to assess possible nerve root compression. This is done by exerting downward pressure on the patient's head while leaning the head slightly toward each side. A positive result is that of pain or paresthesia down the arm.

Evaluation of these tests may show sensitivity over the thoracic outlet and not in the arm and thus may be helpful in supporting the diagnosis of nTOS. As noted before, there may be considerable overlap of nerve compression syndromes of different source. Once a nerve is irritated at one point, it may be irritated along the entire course, thus making differentiation of a peripheral nerve compression and TOS clinically difficult. Finally, not all presentations are typical. Some patients may have pain in the neck, shoulder, and upper arm without continuation to the hand and fingers.

Testing

Testing as part of evaluation of nTOS serves two purposes: to identify concurrent disease processes that may mimic nTOS presentations and to support the diagnosis of nTOS.

Tests that are done to assess possible concurrent problems include cervical spine magnetic resonance imaging (MRI) and peripheral nerve conduction and EMG testing.

Testing that supports the diagnosis of nTOS includes imaging studies: x-ray evaluation for presence of cervical ribs and abnormal first ribs, and MRI to assess anatomical evidence of nerve and vascular compression. Additional testing that may confirm a diagnosis of nTOS includes electrophysiologic testing and scalene muscle blocks.

Imaging

Cervical x-ray imaging is fundamental to evaluation of TOS patients. Chest x-rays should be reviewed to assess the presence of cervical ribs and abnormal first ribs. If there is uncertainty, a cervical spine series should be done in addition to the chest x-rays. Chest or cervical films taken with a 15-degree apical-lordotic view will offset the cervical rib and make it more readily apparent.

Imaging used for evaluation of nTOS has included MRI, duplex ultrasound, and catheter-based arteriography. *MRI imaging* is popularly considered to be a definitive modality to assess most neurological maladies. In the instance of nTOS, however, its promise remains unfulfilled. In general, TOS MRI studies have not been standardized across the nation. Accordingly, there is a wide variation in how these tests are performed and evaluated. The most complete evaluations will include a magnetic resonance arteriogram (MRA) and a magnetic resonance venogram (MRV) along with MRI of the brachial plexus. Careful examiners will note the course of the brachial plexus structures, the presence of edema within the nerves, and anatomical abnormalities. Compression of the subclavian artery or vein may be documented.[27-29] Further refinement includes measurement of muscle sizes (anterior scalene, middle scalene, subclavius), and measurements of the distances between structures within the thoracic outlet. Because of the variation in how these exams are conducted, these tests may not prove helpful unless performed at a center with a dedicated interest in diagnosis of TOS.

Catheter-based imaging has been used as a proxy to identify neurological compression. Past experience shows this to be an unreliable means of identifying nTOS.[30] Catheter-based imaging does not establish a diagnosis of nTOS. In the absence of evidence suggesting arterial thromboembolic disease or venous thrombosis, it serves no diagnostic role (Fig. 33.5).[1]

Similarly, *arterial duplex ultrasonography* is not a reliable means of establishing the diagnosis of nTOS. Although it may identify positional loss or reduction of arterial signals, this may also be seen in normal asymptomatic subjects and so is not considered sufficiently specific to be diagnostic.

Electrophysiologic testing may provide evidence of nTOS. Indirect evidence of compression at the thoracic outlet may be provided by findings of delayed antidromic f-waves. Although the presence of positive findings among these tests does not exclude TOS, the presence of coexisting problems needs to be taken into account in formulating a treatment plan.[27-29]

Somatosensory evoked potential (SSEP) testing has been shown to have considerable specificity in the diagnosis of nTOS. Unfortunately, the sensitivity of this test may limit the number of patients diagnosed. The test involves using a peripheral stimulating electrode on the hand and recording electrodes placed over the Erb point, the cervical spine, and the contralateral cerebral cortex. The test is done to assess both median and ulnar conduction both with the arm at the side and with the arm in a stress position. Evaluation includes measurement of conduction velocity and amplitude across the thoracic outlet.[28,29] In a review of experience at the University of California–Los Angeles (UCLA), Machleder and Newer reported return of normal amplitude and latency in up to 92% of patients following surgical relief of symptoms.

More recently, assessment of *median antebrachial cutaneous sensory nerve action potentials* (MAC SNP) has generated interest. This test, evaluating a branch of the median nerve, has been used to help establish the diagnosis of TOS.[30] As with all nerve conduction testing, there are significant limitations in sensitivity and specificity. Also, familiarity with the testing methodology is not widespread and so the exam is not generally available.

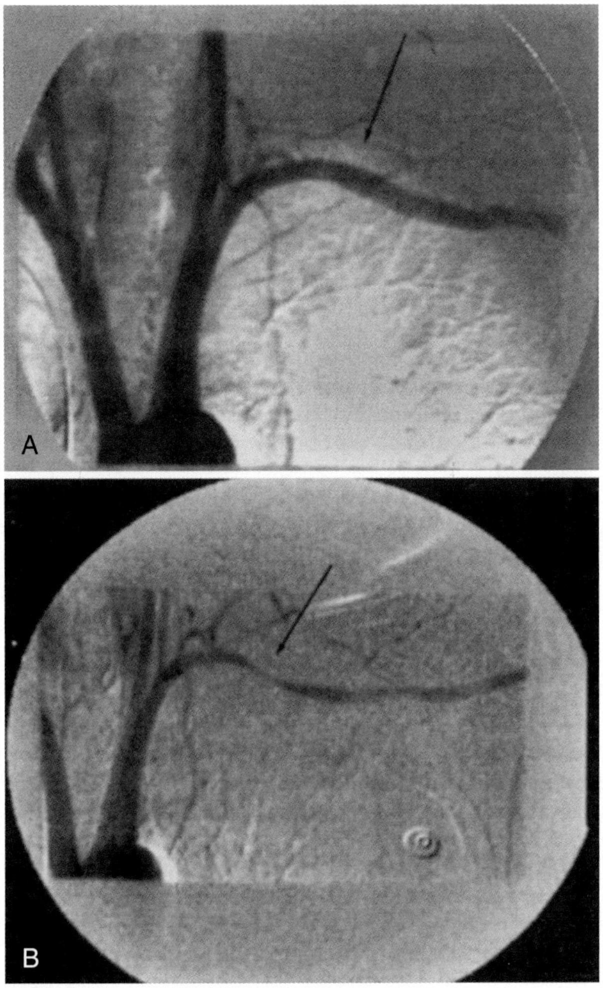

FIG 33.5 Digital intravenous axillosubclavian angiogram obtained in the supine (A) and sitting (B) positions to demonstrate thoracic outlet compressive changes *(arrows)*, which are often seen only in the sitting position.

The *anterior scalene muscle block* is the only test that relates the patient's symptoms to the dynamic anatomy at the thoracic outlet. It is the only test that associates a test intervention with the effect on the patient's symptoms. With this test, a local anesthetic such as lidocaine or Marcaine is injected into the anterior scalene muscle and the patient is asked to report the impact of the injection on upper extremity symptoms. It is important that the test be performed with the assistance of imaging such as ultrasound, fluoroscopy, or computed tomography (CT) to accurately guide needle placement in the body of the scalene muscle. Variations in the test include addition of associated muscles to the target set (middle scalene, subclavius, upper trapezius) and the use of blinded controls (long-duration versus short-duration local anesthetics).

The methods of performing an anterior scalene muscle block have been carefully reported by Jordan and Machleder.[31] Anesthetic blocks of the anterior scalene muscle have been used as a method of confirming TOS and predicting the likely benefit from surgical decompression.[26] When a local anesthetic agent is injected into the anterior scalene muscle and paralyzes it temporarily, the patient's symptoms caused by compression are relieved for a few hours to a few days. However, the technique of using surface landmarks often results in inadvertent somatic and sympathetic block because there is no reliable way to verify needle tip localization.[26] For this reason, a guided technique using electrophysiology, ultrasound, CT, or fluoroscopy is recommended.

Jordan and Machleder[27,31] reported that electrophysiologic guidance facilitates accurate needle tip placement in the performance of anterior scalene muscle blocks. A Teflon-coated, 25-gauge hypodermic needle, bared at the tip, is advanced through the sternocleidomastoid muscle. Electromyographic activity is monitored as the needle is advanced through the tissue layers; the anterior scalene muscle can be activated with lateral neck bending against resistance and with deep inspiration. In most patients, a twitch of the scalene muscles is visible with electrical stimulation. The patient is asked whether pain is produced and whether insertion at this depth produces pain that is similar in quality and location to the usual pain experienced. After an injection of 2 mL of 2% lidocaine into the anterior scalene muscle, the arm is placed into a stress position and exercised for 1 minute; the patient is then asked to rate the pain. Attempts to activate the anterior scalene muscle are performed again with lateral neck movement and with deep inspiration, but only distant motor action potentials can be identified. Electrical stimulation can no longer produce a visible twitch of the scalene muscles. A positive test occurs if the patient has greater than 50% improvement in the elevated arm stress pain score after anesthetic injection of the anterior scalene muscle compared with a baseline examination. The results of these blocks correlate with surgical outcomes; a positive result predicts a good outcome to surgical decompression. Note that the absence of pain relief does not exclude the presence of TOS as long as the patient has symptoms and clinical findings, but the probability of surgical success is significantly reduced.

Treatment

nTOS is usually treated initially with physical modalities and medication. A large number of these patients will require no surgical intervention.

Initial management of nTOS should include evaluation of causative factors. Many repetitive motion injuries at work are related to poor ergonomic conditions. In the office this may be the result of ergonomically improper workstations, computers, and desks. Ergonomic workplace assessment and correction is important for such instances. Workplace restrictions may help alleviate symptoms in some. Avoidance of overhead reaching and lifting may help allow an injured limb to rest and recover.[18,32,33]

Physical modalities are an important part of treating TOS patients. Included in this are physical therapy, acupuncture, massage, and chiropractic care. Physical therapy is believed to be helpful in about 85% of TOS patients. The fundamental goals of PT include balancing of muscle strength, stretching of the scalene muscles, and correction of posture.[34-36]

Postoperative PT is helpful in the majority of patients. The postoperative PT goals include assistance with range of motion, strengthening, and posture correction.

Medication used in managing TOS patients include antiinflammatories, muscle relaxers, pain medication, and medication to reduce nerve sensitivity. In more severe and chronic situations, consultation with pain management is advised. *Therapeutic scalene muscle blocs* may be indicated in patients who are not interested in surgery, or for some reason cannot undergo surgery. These are done with combinations of local anesthetics (Marcaine), steroids, and antiinflammatory agents (platelet-rich plasma [PRP]). The goals are to reduce inflammation, edema, and muscle spasm.

Botox has been used with the intention of limiting the scalene muscle's ability to contract. Success rates of Botox are believed to be about 85% with a duration of about 3 to 4 months. Botox often requires ongoing administration. The number of patients whose nTOS is permanently relieved by Botox administration is not clearly established.[37,38]

Surgical Goals for Neurogenic Thoracic Outlet Syndrome

Surgery for nTOS is reserved for cases that are severe and do not respond to other less invasive modalities. Physical therapy, workplace accommodation, avoidance of triggering activities, use of medication, and injections should generally precede a decision for surgery. Ultimately the decision for surgery is based on an assessment of the severity of symptoms, the degree of disability, and the likely benefit of surgery.

The surgical goals vary for each of the TOS presentations. For those patients presenting with nTOS (pain and paresthesia), the goal is to alleviate symptoms. For those whose presentation includes atrophy and weakness, the goal is to forestall progressive loss of function. The fundamental surgical goal is decompression of the neural elements as they cross the scalene triangle. To accomplish nTOS decompression, the scalene triangle is deconstructed and anomalous muscular and fibrous bands are resected. Removal of either muscle or rib accomplishes this goal. If a cervical rib is present, then the goal includes addressing the cervical rib as well. In instances where a long or complete cervical rib is present (Gruber II, III, or IV), the cervical rib should be removed. For small partial cervical ribs (Gruber I) or elongated transverse processes, the residual fibrous band arising from the rib is the source of compression and is the target of decompression and must be removed. Cases involving anomalous first ribs should be managed with removal of the anomalous first rib.

SURGERY FOR THORACIC OUTLET SYNDROME DECOMPRESSION

Choice of Operations

There are a surprising number of surgical alternatives for TOS decompression. These are essentially combinations of rib resection and scalene muscle resection and vary as to the extent of resection and the approach to the resection. The surgical approaches for TOS decompression include scalenectomy (supraclavicular anterior scalene muscle resection or anterior and middle scalene muscle resection), posterior rib resection (partial first rib resection from a posterior approach), claviculectomy, transaxillary first rib resection (partial scalene muscle resection and complete first rib resection via axillary approach), supraclavicular rib resection (complete anterior and middle scalene muscle and partial first rib resection), paraclavicular first rib resection (complete anterior and middle scalene muscle and complete first rib resection by means of additional infraclavicular incision), and anterior infraclavicular partial first rib resection. Kashyap and colleagues[39,40] reviewed some of the advantages and disadvantages of different surgical approaches.

A surgeon's choice of operation is largely based on familiarity with the procedure. Additional elements may favor one approach over the other: presence of a cervical rib, presence of an anomalous first rib, vTOS presentation, aTOS presentation may require specific interventions.

Some authors have suggested that presentations be grouped as upper plexus (symptoms along radial distribution) and lower plexus (symptoms along ulnar distribution), and that surgery be guided according to these groupings: supraclavicular scalenectomy approach for upper plexus symptoms, and first rib resection for lower plexus symptoms. Finally, an estimation of risk for each operation may favor one approach over another; the supraclavicular approaches have greater risk of injury to the brachial plexus and its branches, and if such injuries would be particularly difficult in a given patient, then perhaps it is better proceed with the transaxillary approach.

Scalene muscle resections include resection of the anterior scalene muscle alone or both anterior and middle scalene muscles. The decision between these two operations is based largely on familiarity of the surgeons and considerations of risk. Scalenectomy is accomplished via a supraclavicular approach. *Resection of the anterior scalene muscle* dates to the era of Adson, Nafziger, and Oschner. This operation is fairly successful in relieving TOS symptoms, but a number of patients may have residual symptoms related to the middle scalene muscle and the first rib. The principal risk of anterior scalene muscle resection is injury to the phrenic nerve. Additional concerns include lymphatic leak from thoracic duct injury and vascular injury to the subclavian artery and vein. The principal limitation is the rate of significant persistent and recurrent symptoms.

Resection of the anterior and middle scalene muscles is a more extensive operation. It requires mobilization of the brachial plexus to reach the middle scalene muscle. As the muscle is resected, there is risk of injury to the long thoracic nerve, suprascapular nerve, and the dorsal scapular nerve. These risks are in addition to those noted with anterior scalene muscle resection alone. The result of resection of both anterior and middle scalene muscles are slightly better that those of anterior scalene resection alone.

Scalenectomy without resection of the first rib is generally attended by a reduced success rate when compared to operations that include resection of the first rib. First rib resections are most commonly accomplished via the supraclavicular or transaxial approach. A posterior approach to first rib resection has been largely abandoned due to its potential morbidity and the superiority of other approaches. An anterior infraclavicular resection is used by some as treatment of vTOS.

Supraclavicular first rib resection requires resection of the anterior and middle scalene muscles to reach the first rib. Supraclavicular rib resection does provide effective decompression of the neural structures across the thoracic outlet. Another advantage is the ability to address cervical ribs from this approach. Because the cervical ribs attach to the transverse process of the C7 vertebral body, the attachment of the cervical rib to the spine can be exposed in the course of a supraclavicular operation. This is particularly helpful in small (Gruber I) cervical ribs, which are not as easily approached by transaxillary means.

The limitations of the supraclavicular approach lies principally in the inability to resect the anterior portion of the first rib. Supraclavicular rib resection normally allows the anterior portion of the first rib to remain in place. Thus, in cases of vTOS, it does not provide adequate decompression. In cases of vTOS, surgeons who prefer the supraclavicular approach will add an anterior infraclavicular incision to remove the anterior portion of the first rib and resect part of the subclavius muscle. This approach has been referred to as a "paraclavicular approach." Another concern with supraclavicular rib resection is the potential risk to the brachial plexus and its cervical branches, especially the phrenic nerve, the long thoracic nerve, and the dorsal scapular nerve.

Transaxillary first rib resection approaches resection of the first rib from beneath the arm, traveling along the chest wall beneath the brachial plexus and its nerve branches. The entire first rib may be resected from the transaxillary approach.[41] Larger cervical ribs (Gruber II, III, and IV may also be resected via the transaxillary approach. The transaxillary approach allows for effective decompression of the subclavian vein in cases of vTOS. Because the approach courses below the neural structures, the incidence of brachial plexus, long thoracic, and phrenic nerve injuries is accordingly lower than that seen with supraclavicular operations.

The principal limitations of transaxillary rib resection arise from the inability to reach the upper portions of the scalene muscles. In the course of transaxillary rib resection, the lower 25% of the scalene muscle is resected. This allows removal of the first rib and allows for resection of that portion of the muscles that overlaps and attaches to the neural and vascular structures. The residual portion of the scalene muscle may eventually require removal in a minority of cases. Similarly, small cervical ribs are not readily removed via the trans-axillary approach. If these are believed to result in persistent symptoms, then a supraclavicular approach is required.

Description of Operations

Transaxillary Rib Resection and Partial Scalenectomy

The transaxillary rib resection and partial scalenectomy was originally described by Roos in 1966 and is arguably the most common approach used for thoracic outlet decompression.[41] First rib resection is recommended mainly for the lower type of TOS with C8 to T1 root symptoms.[27] Supraclavicular scalenectomy is applicable in patients with the upper type of TOS involving C5 to C7 roots[22] or in those with recurrence after first rib resection, thought to be due to scarring of the scalenes.[22] The surgical strategy for nTOS is (1) transaxillary first rib resection and subtotal lower scalenectomy as a primary procedure and (2) completion scalenectomy with a supraclavicular approach for patients with recurrent symptoms who need surgery.

Technique. The patient is placed in the semisupine lateral position (45 to 60 degrees) with a soft axillary roll placed under the dependent axilla. The ipsilateral arm, neck, chest wall, and axilla are prepared. The arm is covered with a sterile cotton stockinette, wrapped with a gauze bandage, and placed in a sterile arm holder for retraction. Retraction of the arm to the contralateral side and upward provides better visualization of the neurovascular structures in the axillary tunnel. However, it is important to avoid overzealous arm retraction with this approach, and occasional intermittent release of traction prevents arm ischemia or brachial plexus injury.

A transverse incision is made just below the hair-bearing area in the axilla between the pectoralis major and latissimus dorsi muscles (Fig. 33.6). The incision is deepened in the subcutaneous tissue until the chest wall is reached. The thoracoepigastric vein should be divided for adequate exposure. The brachiointercostal nerve may also have to be sacrificed to gain adequate exposure. A tissue plane deep to the axillary fascia and on top of the serratus anterior is bluntly dissected superiorly and anteriorly through loose areolar tissue. The highest thoracic artery, a branch from the axillary artery penetrating the first intercostal space, should be identified, ligated, and divided to avoid troublesome bleeding. Using further blunt dissection with a sponge-tipped hemostat, the loose tissue is cleared to identify the first rib. The subclavian vein, anterior scalene muscle, subclavian artery, brachial plexus, and middle scalene muscle are carefully dissected (see Fig. 33.6). The phrenic nerve anterior to the anterior scalene muscle must be identified and carefully protected. It is necessary to lift the arm carefully to facilitate the exposure. To avoid serious injury, the blade of the retractor must not apply traction to the nerve roots or the brachial plexus.

Once the anterior scalene muscle is dissected and the vessels are free, a right-angled clamp placed under the muscle elevates it away from other structures as the muscle is divided with scissors as far from the first rib as possible. The smallest scalene muscle, if it exists, is divided off the Sibson fascia and the C7 transverse process. The middle scalene muscle is dissected and divided with scissors at the highest level feasible, with a right-angled clamp placed to hook the muscle. The long thoracic nerve posterior to the middle scalene muscle must be identified and

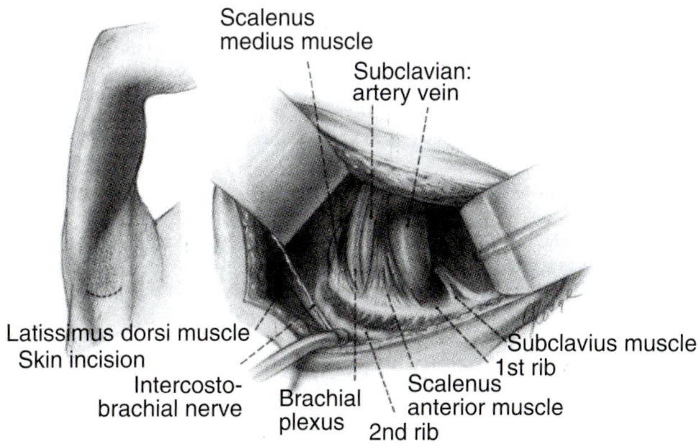

FIG 33.6 View of thoracic outlet structures from the transaxillary approach to first rib resection. (From Machleder HI, editor: *Vascular Disorders of the Upper Extremity*, ed 2, Mt. Kisco, NY, 1989, Futura Publishing.)

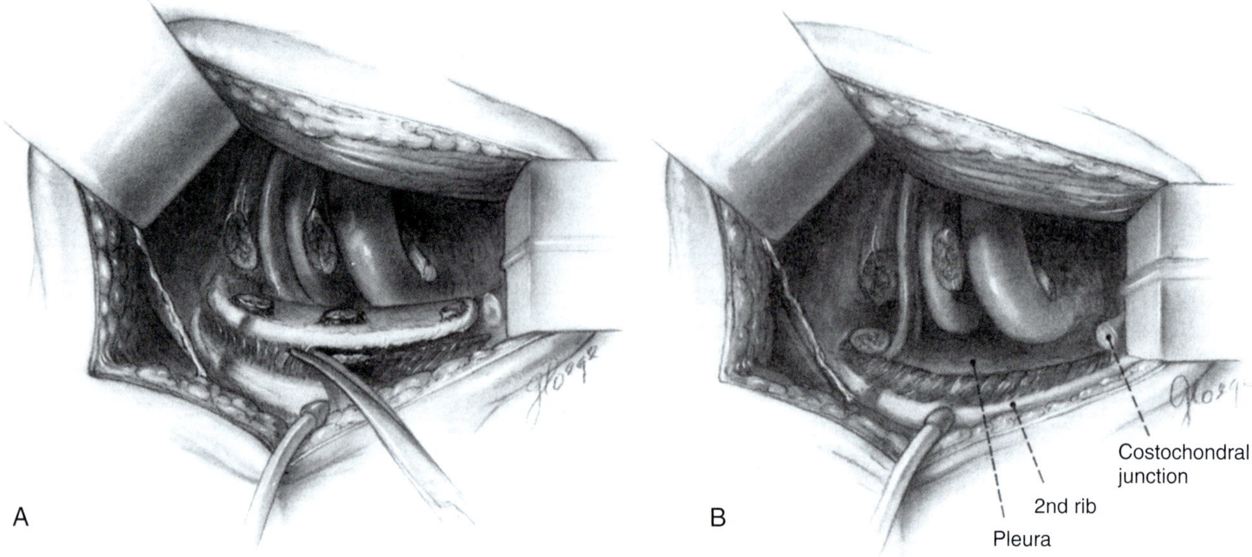

FIG 33.7 Steps in transaxillary first rib resection. (A) Division of subclavius, anterior scalene, and middle scalene tendons, and initial incision of the intercostal muscle. (B) Relationship of structures after removal of the first rib.

carefully protected. The first rib resection is performed in an extraperiosteal fashion, except in areas where the vein or artery may be adherent to the periosteum and prone to tearing, where subperiosteal dissection is required. The intercostal muscle is pushed away by blunt dissection with a periosteal elevator (Fig. 33.7A). The first rib is then freed circumferentially by the periosteal elevator and a blunt-tip right-angled clamp anteriorly and posteriorly. With a Roos nerve protector shielding the C8 and T1 nerve roots, an angled bone-cutting instrument is carefully placed on the posterior neck of the rib and applied to cut the rib posteriorly. The subclavius tendon is divided sharply to the sternal joint space with a scalpel under direct vision, with careful protection of the vein. The rib is then divided anteriorly with a Bethune rib shear. The rib is thus detached and removed from the field (see Fig. 33.7B). A large-angled bone rongeur is used to trim the anterior remaining end of the rib to the sternal joint. The posterior stump of the first rib is further truncated close to the transverse process using a box-shaped bone cutter. Any sharp bony fragments must be identified with visual inspection or palpation and removed. Any additional soft tissue bands crossing the brachial plexus nerve roots are sought and carefully divided. The remaining anterior and middle scalene muscles are trimmed further until the stumps are above the neurovascular bundle.

A drainage tube connected with closed suction is brought out through a separate stab wound below the incision. After closure of the subcutaneous tissue, the skin is closed using monofilament polypropylene suture with plastic surgery technique.

During the performance of this operation, adequate lighting and visualization need to be maintained because of the configuration and depth of the operative field. Cautery must not be used after reaching the first rib to avoid injuring the neurovascular structures.

Advantages and limitations. This approach allows rapid exposure of the first rib without much manipulation of the subclavian vessels or brachial plexus. The incision itself is cosmetically appealing and allows for rapid recovery, and most patients leave the hospital on the first postoperative day. Many groups have used this procedure with short- and long-term success.[22,25,41,42] A cervical rib can also be managed through the axillary approach.

The drawbacks of this approach are directly related to the operative view. Visualization is through a long axillary tunnel that must be adequately lighted to prevent injury, which occurs most commonly to the axillary vein or T1 nerve root.[43] A supplementary light source from a headlight is indispensable, and a fiber-optic lighted retractor is paramount for the safe conduct of this operation. Recent addition of high-definition videoendoscopy to assist visualization indicate a significant advance.[44]

In patients with vasomotor presentations or chronic arterial occlusion, sympathectomy can be added easily. Satisfactory exposure of the subclavian artery or vein with intention of open surgical reconstruction is not advised with this approach.

Supraclavicular Scalenectomy With or Without Rib Resection

Procedures performed through a supraclavicular approach include anterior and middle scalenectomy alone or combined with first rib resection.

Technique. A simple scalenectomy has been advocated by some and requires division of the muscle close to its origin at the cervical transverse processes.[45-47]

The patient is placed in the semi-Fowler position, with the head turned away from the operative side and the ipsilateral arm draped over the chest.

An incision is made in the supraclavicular area approximately 1 to 2 cm above and parallel to the clavicle between the internal

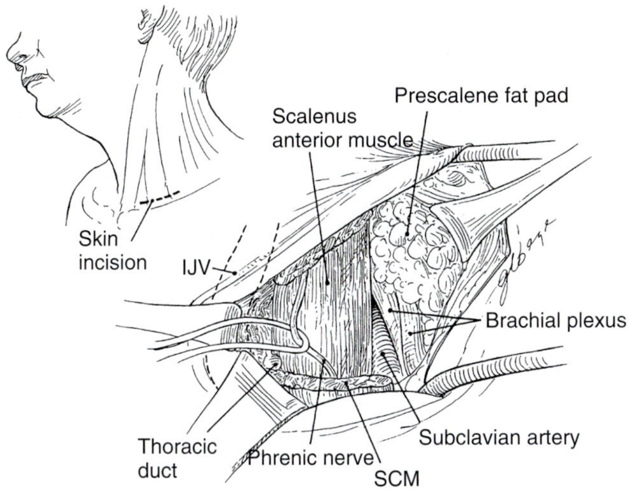

FIG 33.8 Transcervical approach to scalenectomy for relief of thoracic outlet compression syndrome. The relationship of major surrounding anatomic structures is depicted. *IJV,* Internal jugular vein; *SCM,* sternocleidomastoid muscle. (From Machleder HI, Moll FL: Surgery for Thoracic Outlet Syndrome. In Trout HH 3rd, DePalma RG, editors: *Reoperative Vascular Surgery*, New York, 1987, Marcel Dekker.)

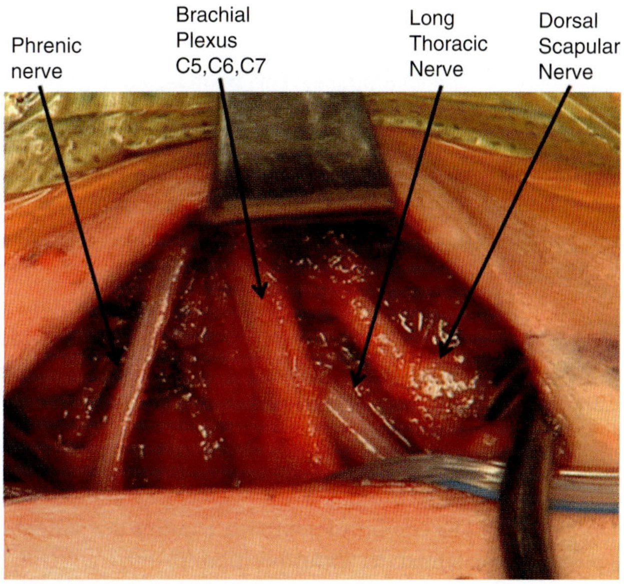

FIG 33.9 Intraoperative photo of left supraclavicular approach, showing nerves exposed after resection of anterior and middle scalene muscles.

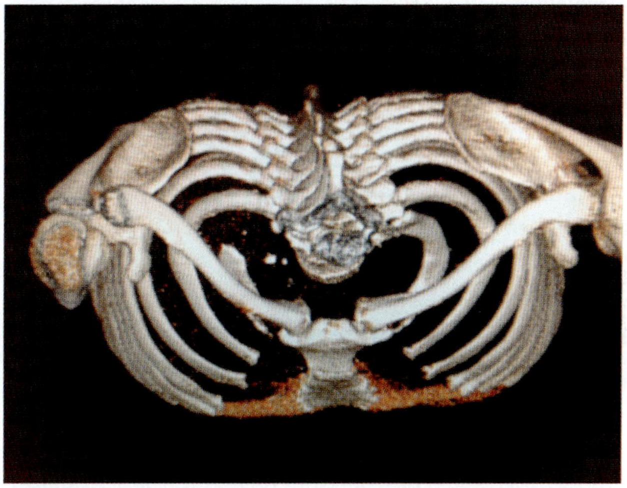

FIG 33.10 Computed tomography scan showing the extent of resection of first rib following a supraclavicular right first rib resection.

and external jugular veins. Subplatysmal flaps are constructed, and the clavicular head of the sternocleidomastoid may be divided if needed. The internal jugular vein is retracted medially. Dissection continues parallel and lateral to the jugular vein. The scalene fat pad is mobilized laterally to expose the anterior aspect of the anterior scalene muscle and the associated phrenic nerve.

The phrenic nerve is carefully identified using a nerve stimulator. It must be dissected away from the anterior scalene muscle by incising the epimysium and connective tissues, which bind these together. The practice of placing a vessel loop around the phrenic nerve to mark its location is controversial because this maneuver may by itself render the nerve more vulnerable.

Next, the muscle is transected at a point near the insertion onto the first rib, with care to avoid injuring the underlying subclavian artery. The scalene muscle is reflected cephalad to its origins and then transected. Any fibrous adhesions between the scalene muscle and brachial plexus should be removed. The wound should then be carefully inspected for lymph leakage or bleeding. Once these are attended, the wound is closed by reapproximating the scalene fat pad. Platysma and skin are sutured closed in separate layers.

Many practitioners advocate a more complete TOS decompression by removing the first rib as well as the anterior and middle scalene muscles. Rib resection requires mobilization of the brachial plexus and division of the middle scalene muscle (Figs. 33.8 and 33.9). The long thoracic nerve, dorsal scapular, and suprascapular nerves may traverse the body of the middle scalene muscle. They need to be carefully identified using nerve stimulation to confirm the nerve function. The middle scalene muscle is resected from around these nerves.

If a cervical rib is present, it will be found within the fibers of the middle scalene muscle.

The first rib is resected by dividing the intercostal muscle attachment. The posterior aspect of the rib is divided with rongeurs near the articulation with the transverse process. Division of the first rib posteriorly is done as close to the transverse process as possible and requires gentle retraction of the brachial plexus anteromedially.

The pleura and subclavian vessels are separated from the rib with blunt dissection. The rib is divided as anteriorly as possible with a rib shear or rongeur. From the supraclavicular approach, only the posterior portion of the first rib cannot be resected (Figs. 33.10).

In instances where anterior decompression is required, an infraclavicular counterincision is made for rib division close to the costochondral junction, which is usually required for vTOS. This is called the "paraclavicular approach."[48]

Advantages and limitations. The main advantages of the supraclavicular approach are an excellent view of the structures in the thoracic outlet, with wide exposure and the ability to perform arterial reconstruction if necessary. Cervical ribs or prolonged transverse processes are easily removed with this approach.[49] Long-term success in correcting compressive symptoms has been documented.[50,51]

This approach requires the dissection and mobilization of the phrenic nerve, brachial plexus, and long thoracic nerve, which leads to its major disadvantage—the risk of nerve damage caused by traction injury or transection of these structures.[43] This approach is also limited for vTOS.

Combined Transaxillary and Supraclavicular Approach

Technique. The combined approach requires the patient to be placed in the lateral decubitus position for the transaxillary approach and then moved to the supine position for the supraclavicular approach. Once the first rib resection is complete, the anterior and middle scalenectomy can be performed easily because most of the distal insertions were already released from the first rib during resection.

Advantages and limitations. The transaxillary approach allows removal of the first rib in a safe and expeditious manner, and the supraclavicular approach allows complete scalenectomy and arterial reconstruction. The combination of both procedures allows complete decompression of the thoracic outlet and correction of the arterial source of embolization in one setting. This approach can be used in selected patients but is not needed for most patients with TOS.[52,53]

Posterior Approach

Technique. The posterior approach requires a posterior periscapular incision, with division of the trapezius muscle and elevation of the scapula. With superior retraction, the thoracic outlet can be reached and the first rib freed from the surrounding structures. In Clagett's original description,[12] the rib is essentially removed subperiosteally, but then as much periosteum is removed as necessary to prevent bony regeneration.

Advantages and limitations. Experience with this approach indicates that it might have a role in a few selected patients needing exposure of the proximal brachial plexus roots, particularly at the intraforaminal level.[54] Patients with prior anterior irradiation and tissue fibrosis who require exposure of the thoracic outlet or those requiring reoperations for TOS may also benefit from this approach.

This approach has not been widely accepted because of the relatively high morbidity compared with other surgical options. The incision and posterior dissection lead to considerable postoperative pain and shoulder disability. Furthermore, visualization of the anterior structures is difficult, and arterial reconstruction is impossible with this approach.

Postoperative Care

An upright chest radiograph is performed in the recovery room to detect pneumothorax or phrenic nerve injury. A large pneumothorax may need transthoracic aspiration, but small air collections usually resolve spontaneously. Pain medication should be prescribed. Most patients leave the hospital on the first postoperative day. The closed suction drain is usually removed in the outpatient clinic once the total amount of lymphatic fluid discharge is less than 30 mL per 24 hours. Showering with sutures in place is allowed once drain sites are closed. Patients are encouraged to use the affected side to perform activities of daily living and to begin a home exercise program (arm exercises at least three to four times per day) starting on day 1. These exercises help to prevent a "frozen" shoulder. Heavy lifting (more than 5 lb) should be avoided until 3 to 4 weeks after surgery. Patients are usually seen for a follow-up visit within 2 weeks after surgery. Many patients return to work in 4 to 6 weeks. Sutures with plastic surgery technique should be removed 3 to 4 weeks postoperatively to prevent hypertrophic scars and keloids. Typically, patients undergoing surgery have had symptoms for a long time, and even after decompression surgery, they often have some residual or intermittent symptoms of dysesthesia, numbness, or other tolerable symptoms that may need ongoing attention.

Surgical Complications

Vascular, nervous, and lymphatic injuries can occur from decompression surgery for TOS.

Pneumothorax

Because first rib resections are technically variants of thoracotomy operations, the violation of the pleura with air entry to the chest is not by itself a complication. It should be considered a complication if a large volume of air enters the chest and is not evacuated prior to closing the incisions. Pleural tear has been reported in up to one-third of cases of transaxillary first rib resection.[55] It may also occur in the course of a supraclavicular resection.

Small residual air collections following rib resection usually resolve spontaneously. Additionally, postoperative radiographs frequently confuse postoperative changes from rib resection with small pneumothorax. Rib resection will result in the pleura settling to a lower position because the support provided by the first rib is lost with removal of the rib. Routine use of closed suction drains often eliminates the need for a chest tube in cases of small pneumothorax. Large residual intrathoracic air collections are best managed by aspiration with a small-caliber (8F to 12F) chest tube. In the absence of a parenchymal injury to the lung, these may be removed once the lung fully reexpands.

Nerve Injuries

Although uncommon, nerve injuries may result in devastating impairment. Fortunately, the majority of nerve injuries are the result of bruising or minor traction and will resolve spontaneously in the course of 3 to 12 months. Injuries that occur as a result of transection or disruption tend to be more profound and even after repair have a higher chance of resulting in permanent impairment.

Brachial plexus injury, either temporary or permanent, represents one of the most serious complications. Most commonly, this is a traction injury and occurs as a result of excessive and prolonged distraction of the brachial plexus. It may occur in the course of transaxillary or supraclavicular approaches. Far less common, inadvertent surgical transection may also occur. In these instances, the lower plexus (C8 and T1) is more likely injured because these nerves are in close proximity to the first rib. These injuries are usually permanent, and result in loss of the lower plexus function to the arm and hand. The motor deficit includes the long flexors of the fingers and the intrinsic muscles of the hand, although the sensory deficit involves only the small finger in the hand and the medial side of the forearm.[55] In large series, the incidence of permanent brachial plexus is less than 1% with each approach.[41,45,56]

The *phrenic nerve*, because of its proximity to the anterior scalene muscle, is prone to injury during scalenectomy. Although phrenic nerve injuries have been reported with transaxillary approaches, they are far more commonly associated with the supraclavicular approach. Although most injuries are temporary, they may take up to a year to resolve. The consequence of a phrenic nerve injury is loss of function in the ipsilateral diaphragm. This loss results in dyspnea with exertion. The incidence of phrenic nerve injury is less than 1% with transaxillary approaches and about 3% to 8% with supraclavicular approaches. In patients with bilateral TOS requiring operation on the contralateral side, it is essential to ensure that phrenic nerve paresis has completely resolved before a second operation. If not, it can result in complete diaphragmatic paralysis and severe ventilatory incapacity.[57]

Long thoracic, dorsal scapular, and suprascapular nerve injury can occur in the course of resection of the middle scalene muscle. The nerves should be identified before excising the muscle. Injury to the long thoracic nerve may result in instability of the scapula, an injury often referred to as a winged scapula. Injury to the dorsal scapular and suprascapular nerves will result in difficulty with lateral abduction of the arm. The incidence of these injuries is uncertain because they have often not been noted in surgical series.

The *intercostobrachial cutaneous* nerve usually originates from the second intercostal nerve. It appears under the second rib in the midaxillary line at the midpoint of the transaxillary incision. Injury to this nerve results in temporary or permanent numbness or paresthesias on the medial aspect of the arm. The incidence of injury to this nerve is thought to be about 50%. The vast majority of these injuries are transient unless the nerve is sacrificed. Some surgeons will routinely deliberately sacrifice this nerve to allow better exposure of the thoracic outlet structures.

Injury to the Subclavian Artery and Vein

Vascular injuries may be difficult to visualize, because the exposure for TOS decompression is limited, and the rib or the muscle may hide the injury. If the field becomes bloody, it is prudent to pack the operative field for a few minutes rather than proceeding. Most venous injuries are initially managed with tamponade and may thrombose. If bleeding persists, balloon occlusion may allow development of the exposure required to repair the vessel. In transaxillary approaches, occasional additional supraclavicular exposure may be needed for visualization or control. To manage bleeding in supraclavicular approaches, extension of the exposure medially may be required for similar reasons.

Lymphatic Leakage

The thoracic duct usually empties into the venous system at the junction of the left subclavian vein and the internal jugular vein. However, the anatomy may be variable; there may be double ducts or significant branches.[58] Injury to the thoracic duct most commonly occurs with left supraclavicular approaches. There are instances of developmental variants with large lymphatic vessels noted in the right supraclavicular fossa. Accordingly, lymphatic leaks are also possible with right supraclavicular approaches. Lymph leakage is rare with the transaxillary approach. If identified, the lymph vessel is best managed with ligation or clipping. In the event of persistent lymph leakage, endolymphatic embolization should be considered as a minimally invasive approach prior to open reexploration.

Results of Surgical Treatment for Neurogenic Thoracic Outlet Syndrome

Decompression surgery for TOS has few standard objective criteria for evaluation, and most postoperative results are reported with a subjective grading of success that relies on the patient's response to treatment. Functional outcome is an important parameter, as is improvement of symptoms. Thus, the patient's ability to return to the same job provides a good index of operative success. Use of standardized assessment instruments such as the Disabilities of the Arm, Shoulder, and Hand (DASH) questionnaire, Short Form-36 (SF 36), and the Cervico-Brachial Symptoms Questionnaire (CBSQ) will allow more reliable reporting of results.[1,2,59,60]

Primary success can be defined as 50% improvement or greater of ipsilateral symptoms or the patient's return to preoperative work status without the need for an additional ipsilateral procedure. Secondary success is similarly defined following an additional ipsilateral procedure. Altobelli and colleagues conducted a review of 9 years of experience with 254 primary first rib resections with partial scalenectomy via a transaxillary approach, followed by 80 secondary operations for recurrent symptoms using the supraclavicular scalenectomy in 185 patients.[61] The initial success rate at 2 months was 86.6% for primary procedures. Life-table analysis revealed that the primary success rates were 46.9% at 18 months, 37.6% at 36 months, and 36.0% at 72 months. The secondary success rates were 71.7% at 18 months, 58.9% at 36 months, and 49.1% at 72 months (Fig. 33.11). In evaluating these results, length of follow-up is a crucial factor, because recurrent TOS usually occurs within 18 months after the initial surgery; 90% and 65% of failures occurred within 18 months of primary and secondary success, respectively. Therefore reports with short-term follow-up could mask the overall success rate of the procedures performed.

Reported results in the literature were similar. Improvement of nTOS symptoms may be noticed shortly after surgery, sometimes immediately.[26] The initially high percentage of improvement generally decreases after a few years. When comparing different approaches, Sanders's review of the surgical results for TOS showed some interesting data.[62] Transaxillary, supraclavicular,

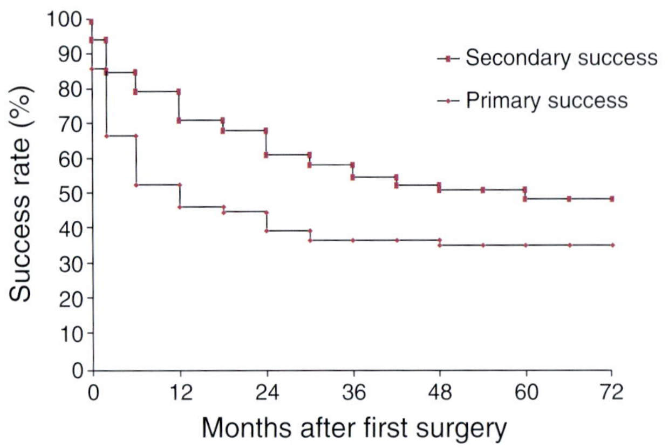

FIG 33.11 Life-table analysis for primary and secondary clinical success rates after transaxillary first rib resection with partial scalenectomy followed by supraclavicular scalenectomy. Note that 90% and 65% of failures occur within 18 months of primary and secondary success, respectively. (From Altobelli GG, Kudo T, Haas BT, et al: Thoracic outlet syndrome: pattern of clinical success following surgical decompression. *J Vasc Surg* 42:111–117, 2005.)

infraclavicular, posterior, and transpleural first rib resection, as well as scalenectomy and combined rib resection, all had similar success rates. In addition, in Sanders and coworkers' own series,[56,63] which included transaxillary first rib resection, anterior and middle scalenectomy, and combined scalenectomy and rib resection, the 3- to 5-year success rate was approximately the same, and the overall improvement was 70% using life-table methods. *Success* in these series was defined as enough symptomatic improvement for the patient to believe that the surgery was worthwhile.

The most important cause of failure of surgical decompression is inadequate decompression. In cases managed with transaxillary decompression, this may relate to inadequate resection of the first rib or reattachment of the scalene muscles.[64] In cases managed with scalenectomy alone, recurrence often reflects the need for first rib resection. In cases where both first rib resection and scalenectomy have been performed, recurrence may be associated with inadequate rib resection or scar formation directly on the brachial plexus. The second most common cause for failure of surgical decompression is the presence of a secondary source of symptoms.

Occupational injuries are associated with poorer outcome following TOS surgery.[31] Other studies have found that preoperative depression and surgeries for some other compression syndrome, such as carpal or cubital tunnel syndrome, were associated with a worse outcome. Psychological testing has indicated that depression is associated with poor outcomes.[65]

On the other hand, a recent study reported that compliance with TOS-specific physical therapy, improvement in quality-of-life scores after physical therapy, young age, and competitive athletics were associated with improved surgical outcomes.[66]

In patients with recurrent TOS, symptoms may develop several weeks or months after the primary surgery. After 2 years, symptoms of recurrence occur less frequently.[67] In Sanders and colleagues' series of 134 operations in 97 patients for recurrent TOS using the transaxillary and transcervical approach over 22 years, the 84% initial success rate dropped to 59% at 1 to 2 years, 50% at 3 to 5 years, and 41% at 10 to 20 years.[40]

Vascular Thoracic Outlet Syndrome

Venous Thoracic Outlet Syndrome (Paget-Schroetter Syndrome)

Spontaneous, or effort-related, thrombosis of the axillosubclavian vein is a disabling disorder of young, otherwise healthy individuals.

VENOUS THORACIC OUTLET SYNDROME

vTOS commonly arises from compression of the subclavian vein as this crosses between the clavicle and the first rib, bound by the anterior and middle scalene muscles. The most common of these presentations is that of acute subclavian vein thrombosis. In addition to acute thrombosis, there are presentations that include acute or chronic thrombosis, chronic obstructive venous congestion, and nonthrombotic positional intermittent venous occlusion (McLeery syndrome).

Incidence

Upper extremity deep venous thrombosis (DVT) accounts for about 10% of all DVT. Of these, vTOS accounts for about 60% of acute upper extremity DVT. The incidence of vTOS ranges from 0.1 to 2 per 100,000. Associated with this are pulmonary emboli, which are believed to occur in about 5% to 15% of cases. Pulmonary embolism from axillosubclavian vein thrombosis has been well documented,[68-70] and deaths from pulmonary embolism from these sources have been recorded in the surgical literature. Furthermore, severe thromboembolic pulmonary hypertension is an infrequent but potentially fatal complication of PSS.[71]

Causes and Pathophysiology

vTOS is more commonly associated with repeated upper extremity exertion. Laborers and athletes form a large portion of this patient group. The fundamental pathological processes include reduction of the dimensions of the venous channel between the subclavius muscle and the anterior scalene muscle. This is the result of hypertrophy of these two muscles. Any hypertrophic expansion of the muscle requires these to expand their attachment to the first rib. As this occurs, the muscles effectively grow closer to each other and reduce the space where the subclavian vein may cross the first rib. In addition, the compression may be accentuated by approximation of the clavicle and first rib. This is the result of hypertrophied muscles pulling these two bones toward one another.

The compression of the subclavian vein then results in a repetitive injury to the intimal and endothelium. This results in a fibrotic response and loss of normal endothelial function. The damaged endothelium is then thought to be a nidus for thrombus formation. The reduced flow in the subclavian artery as a result of the reduced venous diameter sets the stage for thrombus propagation. While these events are slowly developing, patients are often asymptomatic. Symptoms develop when thrombus occludes the subclavian vein. The thrombus may then propagate

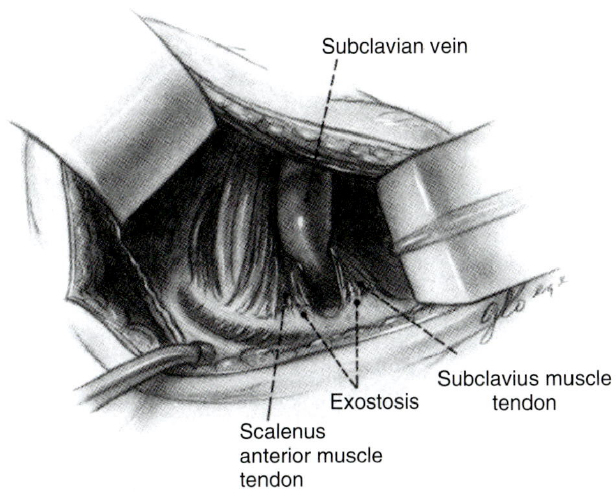

FIG 33.12 Typical Paget-Schroetter abnormality. Hypertrophy of the subclavius tendon and associated exostoses are seen at the subclavius and anterior scalene insertions to the first rib (visualized from the transaxillary surgical approach). The vein is compressed in the most medial area of the thoracic outlet.

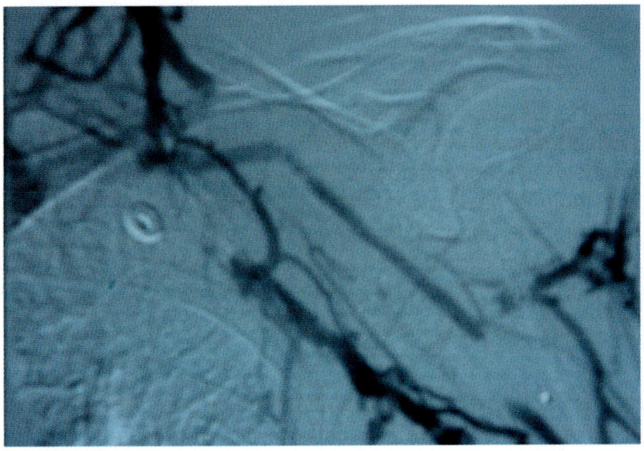

FIG 33.13 Axillosubclavian vein thrombosis characteristic of Paget-Schroetter syndrome or the effort thrombosis variant of thoracic outlet compression syndrome. Note the collateral vessels and intraluminal thrombus.

and obstruct many of the venous collaterals in the arm, resulting in acute venous congestion (Figs. 33.12 and 33.13).

Presentations Venous Thoracic Outlet Syndrome

The most common presentation of vTOS is that of acute spontaneous venous thrombosis involving the subclavian vein: PSS. It is important to recognize that spontaneous venous thrombosis is not always associated with vTOS. It is estimated that up to 33% of PSS is not associated with extrinsic venous compression at the thoracic outlet. These cases are secondary to coagulation abnormalities and tumors. In most cases (66%), the subclavian vein thrombosis is secondary to extrinsic compression of the subclavian vein at the thoracic outlet.

The hallmark of vTOS is venous congestion of the upper extremity with cyanosis, edema, venous distension, and development of venous collateralization across the shoulder and chest. During the acute presentation, the arm may be painful and have dramatic swelling. With the passage of time and development of collateralization, the pain and swelling recede. In later more chronic stages, congestion with exertion or use of the limb becomes the primary symptom.

Diagnosis of Venous Thoracic Outlet Syndrome

Historical elements in the diagnosis of vTOS include a review of patient activities and avocation. vTOS is often associated with heavy labor, muscular development, and athletic avocation. As a prodrome, patients may report intermittent symptoms of venous congestion prior to the acute thrombotic event. Some patients may present prior to thrombosis and their intermittent venous congestion is the primary symptom.

Physical Examination

Physical exam findings for vTOS are consequent to the acute venous occlusion: limb edema, discoloration, engorgement of superficial veins, and presence of collateral veins across the shoulder.[69,70]

These symptoms of congestion—swelling, venous prominence, and discoloration—are often exacerbated by mild effort. In the course of a physical exam—exercise testing such as EAST may lead to display of these symptoms. Additionally, venous congestion despite arm raising may be present. In severe cases, the patient's ability to flex the elbow or wrist, and the ability to close the hand in a grip may be impeded by the edema alone.

Differential Diagnosis

The principal diagnostic dilemma in acute primary subclavian vein thrombosis is differentiating thromboses arising from coagulation disorders from those that are related to extrinsic compression (vTOS). Thrombolysis offers the ability to clear a thrombus from the venous lumen and then allows diagnostic imaging to demonstrate extrinsic compression. In cases that are not afforded thrombolysis and are managed with anticoagulation alone, it is necessary to allow sufficient time to pass for autologous clot lysis while the patient is anticoagulated, which may clear the venous lumen. At that point venography may be diagnostic.

In instances where no evident venous compression is seen after thrombus resolution, coagulation abnormalities and presence of tumors should be evaluated.

Other points of venous compression should be considered in addition to the thoracic outlet. Pectoralis minor impingement may occasionally lead to axillary vein thrombosis. Innominate vein compression may lead to thrombosis of innominate, jugular, and subclavian veins.

Evaluation of Coagulation

A significant number of patients presenting with subclavian vein DVT have been found to have coagulation abnormalities. Cassada and colleagues identified the presence of common coagulation conditions in 67% of their patients.[72] Thrombophilia may be related to the use of exogenous steroids for oral contraception.[73] Abnormalities of endogenous coagulation factors has been identified as a cause of upper extremity DVT in 15% of cases.[74] Because of this, evaluation of the patient coagulation factors is commonly done. The use of anticoagulants is then adjusted according to the results of such information.

Imaging

The diagnosis of venous thrombosis is readily established with ultrasonography or venography (Fig. 33.14). Ultrasonography is limited in evaluation of the intrathoracic venous segments and will occasionally fail to detect subclavian venous obstruction. The widespread availability, noninvasive nature of the exam, and low cost make it a frequent first evaluation for the swollen upper extremity.

Additional diagnostic imaging includes magnetic resonance (MR) and CT venography. These have the advantage of providing a larger field of evaluation. CT pulmonary angiography is done when clinically indicated to assess possible pulmonary embolization.

Venography is generally considered to be more accurate than ultrasonography in diagnosing upper extremity venous thrombosis. Ultrasonography may occasionally miss the presence of stenosis or occlusion of the subclavian vein as it travels behind the clavicular head.

Venography may include catheter-, CT-, and MR-based imaging. Catheter venography has the advantage of allowing administration of thrombolytic agents for treatment of acute thrombus. Thrombolysis for acute venous thrombosis alleviates venous congestion more rapidly and by clearing the venous lumen of thrombus allows visualization of extrinsic compression at the thoracic outlet. By analogy to experience with iliofemoral DVT, thrombolysis is thought to reduce the degree of inflammation and postthrombotic stenosis of the subclavian vein. The success of thrombolysis after 2 to 3 weeks decreases significantly so that many authors advise against thrombolysis at an intermediate or late stage of presentation.[75]

Findings on venography that support the diagnosis of vTOS include irregularity or indentation of the subclavian vein at the point where it crosses the thoracic outlet. Collateralization across the thoracic outlet is noted to varying degrees. The size and extent of collateral vein formation is believed to be an index of

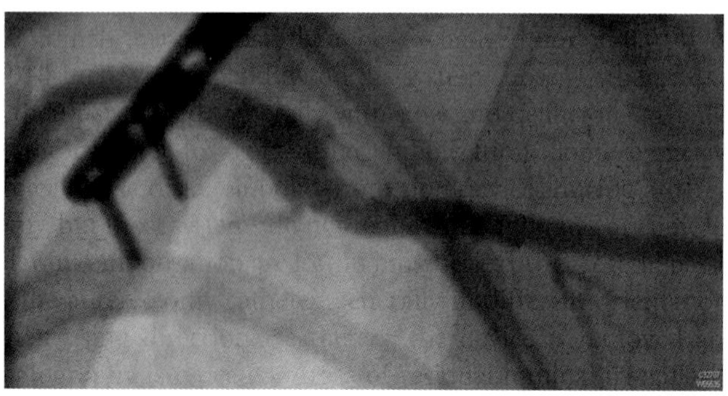

FIG 33.14 Subclavian artery aneurysm associated with arterial compression at the thoracic outlet.

the chronicity of the venous compression. Presence of collateral veins is taken as evidence of hemodynamic impairment to flow in the subclavian vein and therefore confirmation of significant impingement at the thoracic outlet. Absence of such collateral veins would suggest no significant impingement is present and would suggest further evaluation is needed.

Venography in the setting of chronic vTOS presentations is helpful in assessing the presence of venous compression, the development of venous collaterals, and the positional compression of both the subclavian vein and the venous collaterals. In nonthrombotic presentations of vTOS (McLeery syndrome), demonstration of positional changes in venous compression and flow, and correlation of this finding to clinical symptoms is essential in making the diagnosis.

Imaging modalities such as MR venography, CT venography, and intravascular ultrasound (IVUS) can provide cross-sectional assessment of venous diameters and patency. This may be helpful in selected instances where a conventional venogram does not clearly indicate compression at the thoracic outlet. CT imaging is often selectively used for evaluation of pulmonary embolization where clinical suspicion is significant.[76] CT venography is particularly helpful in evaluation of cases of recurrent vTOS following surgical intervention. The ability of CT imaging to resolve the extent and adequacy of rib resection and the relative locations of remnant rib and subclavian vein make this modality particularly helpful in these cases.

Treatment of Venous Thoracic Outlet Syndrome

The initial treatment for vTOS is predicated on the presentation. Acute subclavian vein DVT is treated with *anticoagulation* and *thrombolysis*. A subacute (within 1 to 8 weeks of DVT) presentation should be managed with anticoagulation.[77-79] Thrombolysis after 2 to 3 weeks is unlikely to be beneficial.[75] A chronic presentation (after 3 months) would not require anticoagulation and would not be expected to benefit from thrombolysis.

The duration of anticoagulation following acute subclavian vein thrombosis is dependent on the stage of presentation and the condition of the subclavian vein. Acute subclavian vein thrombosis is managed, like all DVTs, with anticoagulation for at least 3 months.[77-79] A rational argument can be made for subacute presentations to be anticoagulated for 3 months. Duration of anticoagulation may also be affected by the presence of hypercoagulable factors, some requiring lifelong use of anticoagulants.

The duration of anticoagulation use may be affected by anatomical factors. Toward the end of the initial 3 months of anticoagulation for treatment of acute DVT, subclavian veins should be assessed for stenosis and patency prior to completion of anticoagulation. In unoperated patients, the factors leading to thrombosis must be assumed to remain present and unmodified. In such instances where the subclavian vein has autolysed and is patent but remains compressed, cessation of anticoagulants would be expected to result in recurrence of the acute DVT. In these cases, anticoagulation should be continued until the extrinsic compression is resolved. Otherwise a recurrent thrombosis would be highly likely.

If patients have been treated surgically, then a postdecompression venogram should be done with the intention of assessing the subclavian vein for residual stenosis. The process of extrinsic compression over a prolonged period of time results in an injury to the vein wall with resultant fibrosis. Once the extrinsic compression is relieved, the fibrosis may impede the vein's ability to fully expand. The result is a persistent fibrotic stenosis of the vein that could potentially result in recurrent thrombosis. In these instances, balloon angioplasty will resolve the stenosis and restore the vein to normal patency. Anticoagulation is beneficial in preventing recurrent thrombosis prior to angioplasty. Beyond that point, anticoagulation should be continued for a short period of time (usually 2 to 4 weeks) to allow the vein to reendothelialize following angioplasty.

Physical modalities are most helpful following surgery for vTOS. Preoperatively, PT will not serve to effectively relieve the compression of the subclavian vein. The processes that lead to vTOS are longstanding and involve dramatic hypertrophy of muscles and growth of bony exostosis. These processes are not reversible with physical therapy.

Thrombolysis

The role of thrombolysis has been established in acute subclavian vein thrombosis, particularly in those clinical settings where vTOS is suspected. The efficacy of thrombolysis of the subclavian vein in the acute setting is high.[80] With the passage of time, the efficacy and benefit of thrombolysis decreases, so that it is not recommended to proceed with thrombolysis if the acute event is past 2 to 3 weeks. As noted, the benefit of thrombolysis is to help clarify the cause of subclavian vein DVT, to expose the underlying venous compression in vTOS, and to reliably reestablish venous flow in the subclavian vein.[77,78] There is no role for stenting of the subclavian vein in the region of the thoracic outlet before operative decompression, and the persistent mechanical forces in this region likely lead to stent malfunction and failure, thus making the situation worse.

Initial thrombolytic protocols called for lysis to be followed by a period of 3 months anticoagulation to allow regeneration of endothelium and resolution of inflammation.[77,78] More recent studies have validated the success of immediate surgical decompression following thrombolytic therapy.[79,80]

Surgical Goals

Goals for vTOS patients include restoration of subclavian vein patency and improvement of venous drainage of the arm. For this to succeed, compression at the costoclavicular space must be alleviated. Then the venous injury may be repaired. In cases of vTOS, it is imperative that the bony elements impinging on the vein be relieved. This is accomplished by first rib resection or claviculectomy. For cosmetic reasons, most patients prefer first rib resection. The muscular elements, which may by themselves result in venous compression, should be removed. To accomplish this, partial resection of the subclavius and anterior scalene muscles is required.

Following decompression, the next issue is restoration of venous patency. Because vTOS is the result of chronic compression of the subclavian vein, the pathophysiology includes fibrosis of the vein wall at the point of compression. Additionally, the thrombotic events that lead to many vTOS presentations often result in fibrosis of the subclavian vein wall with synechia and occlusion.

Several approaches have been taken to restore venous patency including balloon angioplasty, open venous endoluminal resection of fibrous material and patch angioplasty, and venous graft reconstruction. Subclavian vein graft reconstruction with adjunctive arteriovenous fistula is generally reserved for patients with severe congestion and significant extensive venous occlusion.[81,82] Controversy remains as to which, if any, of these procedures are required. Our approach has been to proceed with postoperative venography at about 2 weeks post decompression. This time point is chosen because it allows for thrombolysis should an interval rethrombosis occur. At the time of venography, if angioplasty is required, then it may proceed. Approximately 60% to 70% of patients will have residual venous stenosis and will benefit from angioplasty. Stenting is avoided as it is usually unnecessary. Occasionally an occluded vein cannot be recanalized at this point. Should that occur, patients are maintained on anticoagulation and reevaluated after 3 months.

ARTERIAL THORACIC OUTLET SYNDROME

Incidence

Arterial TOS is thought to account for 1% to 3% of most TOS series. In general estimation, it is believed to occur in 0.03 to 0.9 per 100,000.

Causes and Pathophysiology

In aTOS, the focus of compression is the subclavian artery. This is frequently mediated by the presence of a cervical rib, however cervical ribs do not inexorably result in development of aTOS. Anomalous first ribs are also associated with aTOS. It has been reported that about 90% of aTOS is associated with a cervical rib or an anomalous first rib.[83-85]

The fundamental pathological process is that of repetitive compressive injury to the subclavian artery. The artery is compressed between the scalene muscle and the first or cervical rib. This compression results in intimal injury. Subsequent events include aggregation of platelets and thrombus. A second mechanism for generation of embolic material involves the development of a subclavian artery aneurysm. In some instances arterial compression will result in poststenotic arterial dilation, resulting in formation of a subclavian artery aneurysm. A thrombus may then form within the aneurysm. If the embolic particles are small, repeated embolization may occur and still remain largely undetected. If the emboli are large, an acute ischemic presentation is noted.

The consequences range from relatively minor microembolic events to major vessel thromboembolic complications resulting in potentially limb-threatening ischemia.[86]

Even when TOS has been recognized, the arterial manifestations may be overlooked because of the belief that nerve compression is causing the patient's symptoms.[85,87] As a result, the appropriate diagnosis might not be made until obvious ischemic changes of the upper extremity occur.

Presentation

Arterial TOS most often presents with acute onset arterial ischemia of the upper extremity, evidenced by pain, pallor, paresthesia, and weakness. This is the result of an acute thrombotic event: thrombosis of a subclavian artery aneurysm or embolization of thrombus from a subclavian artery aneurysm. Occasionally the acute thrombotic episode occurs in the presence of chronic embolization to the upper extremity. In these instances, much of the arterial architecture of the hand and forearm are chronically occluded, and the acute thrombosis is a result of loss of runoff. Unlike nTOS and vTOS presentations, acute arterial ischemia is a vascular emergency requiring urgent revascularization.

Occasionally aTOS is identified as an asymptomatic aneurysm of the subclavian artery. Like aneurysms elsewhere, it is treated according to standards of size and evidence of thrombus formation and embolization.

Diagnosis of Arterial Thoracic Outlet Syndrome

Most aTOS presentations are characterized by abrupt onset of arterial insufficiency. A prodrome of arm pain and accompanying neurogenic symptoms such as paresthesia in the arm or pain in the upper back, chest, or shoulder may be noted.

The principal diagnostic dilemma in evaluating acute upper extremity ischemia is identifying the source cause of the ischemic event. Typically the limb will require urgent revascularization. After that evaluation of potential sources may proceed. Duplex ultrasonography and arteriography are used to help evaluate potential lesions.

Differential Diagnosis

The differential diagnosis of acute upper extremity ischemia includes emboli from sources other than the thoracic outlet. This includes peripheral arterial lesions such as injury to the brachial artery or its major branches. The assessment of these possible sources should be done in the context of the patient's age and associated medical conditions. Arterial TOS is a disease of adults in early to middle age. This is a group that is not characterized by cardiac disease or advanced atherosclerosis. Although possible cardiac arrhythmia and aortic arch stenosis are considerations, these are rare in this age group.

Physical Examination

Arterial TOS presentations may include both acute and chronic findings. The diagnosis of acute limb ischemia is often clinically evident with presentation of pain, pulselessness, pallor, and delayed capillary refill. Neurological examination should focus on the presence of motor and sensory function. An important part of the exam is evaluation of the severity of ischemia and determination of the timeframe toward intervention. Acute limb-threatening ischemia will require urgent revascularization. Indolent, chronic ischemic presentations with evidence of microembolization, Roth spots, splinter hemorrhages, or digital ulceration may not require emergent revascularization and may allow more time for diagnostic evaluation.

Imaging Modalities

Radiography should be done in cases of upper extremity acute arterial occlusion to evaluate the presence of a cervical rib. This is necessary due to the high correlation with cervical ribs and aTOS syndrome. A chest x-ray will readily identify a large cervical rib. To improve visualization of a cervical rib, an anteroposterior (AP) chest x-ray done with 15 degrees of apical lordosis will offset the upper chest and optimize the view of cervical ribs. A cervical spine series of x-rays will also provide an optimal view.

Noninvasive testing with duplex ultrasound is most commonly used to confirm the arterial occlusion and to help establish the extent of arterial thrombosis. In aTOS, duplex ultrasonography is particularly helpful in evaluating aneurismal enlargement of the subclavian artery. The presence of a subclavian artery aneurysm ipsilateral to an acutely ischemic upper extremity suggests the ischemic event is related to the aneurysm.

Catheter-based angiography allows for diagnosis of aneurysm, stenosis, or occlusion. In some instances where an aneurysm lumen is occupied by thrombus, arteriography may fail to detect aneurysmal dilation (Fig. 33.15). Catheter arteriography may allow for interventions such as thrombolysis. In the event of acute upper extremity ischemia, the degree of ischemia and extent of thrombosis need be taken into consideration in electing thrombolysis versus open thrombectomy.

CT angiography is beneficial in establishing the relationship of bony structures to the point of arterial stenosis. CT angiography done with the arm in neutral and stress positions is very effective in identifying extrinsic arterial compression at the thoracic outlet. CT angiographies allow definitive identification of bony abnormalities such as cervical ribs and abnormal rib growth.

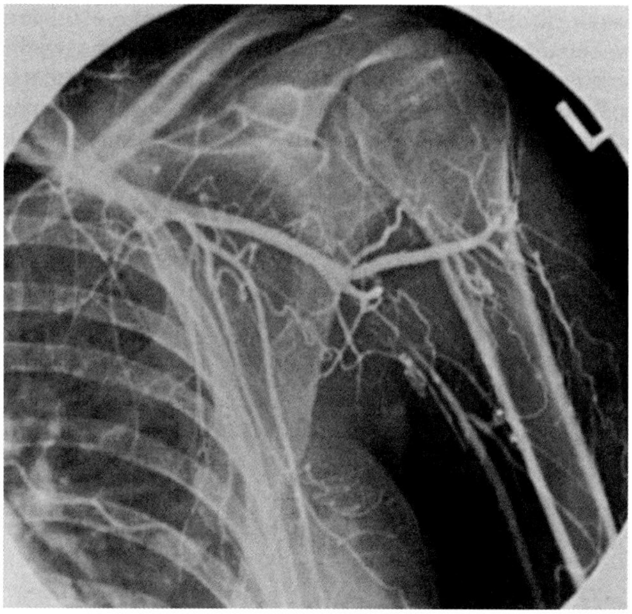

FIG 33.15 Intimal dissection and occlusion of the axillobrachial artery at the level of the brachial plexus cords. This lesion is best repaired by reverse vein grafting, with care being taken to avoid entrapment of brachial plexus elements.

CT angiography may detect aneurysmal enlargement of the subclavian artery, but given the size of the artery, the density of adjacent bone, and the resolution of the scan, small aneurysmal dilation may be missed. MR angiography is not as useful in aTOS, because it does not readily demonstrate bony anomalies and does not visualize aneurysmal enlargement as well as CT angiography or duplex ultrasound.

Treatment of Arterial Thoracic Outlet Syndrome

Acute aTOS presentations are managed with anticoagulation and prompt restoration of arterial perfusion.

Restoration of circulation is done by thrombolysis or thrombectomy. The role of arterial thrombolysis is based on evaluation of the severity of limb ischemia. In patients with profound acute limb ischemia, surgical thrombectomy may be preferable. In patients with moderate ischemic changes, thrombolysis may be attempted. As with lower extremity arterial occlusion, use of angiography is essential to assessing the extent of thrombosis and the result of thrombectomy. In upper extremity cases, it is imperative to assess flow into the hand and digits.

Once arterial perfusion is restored, imaging is required to identify the source of thromboembolism. Diagnostic imaging with CT, MR, or catheter arteriography is central to establishing a diagnosis. Careful evaluation of the entire upper extremity arterial tree should be done with the specific intent to assess the most common sources of arterial embolization: the subclavian artery at thoracic outlet, the axillary artery across the humeral head, and the humeral circumflex arteries at the neck of the humerus. Imaging of the hand and digits is important to assess aneurysmal degeneration of the radial and ulnar arteries. Imaging of digital arterial arcades will often provide evidence of chronic embolization. The typical findings of chronic embolization include loss of one or both digital arteries, abrupt loss of arterial segments, and reconstitution of distal arterial segments.

Arterial imaging will assist in establishing the diagnosis of aTOS. Typical findings include focal arterial deficits caused by impingement at the thoracic outlet. Cervical spine imaging has a high probability of identifying the presence of cervical ribs. Evaluation for aneurysmal degeneration is done with ultrasound or CT scan. Once the evaluation is completed, surgical correction is the next step.

Surgical Goals

For aTOS patients who have suffered embolization, the goal is to prevent further loss of arterial circulation. Surgical goals are complex: the embolic source is identified, and the underlying arterial lesion is repaired in addition to decompression of the thoracic outlet. Decompression often requires resection of the cervical rib and first rib. Repair of the arterial lesions often requires reconstruction of the subclavian artery.

Options for the surgical treatment of vTOS consist of (1) management of ischemia of the extremity, (2) decompression, (3) repair of the arterial lesion, and (4) dorsal sympathectomy. Surgical thrombectomy or catheter-based thrombolysis should be done after diagnostic angiography in the operating room. Usually, decompression surgery, including rib resection and scalenectomy, should be performed later to reduce the risk of hemorrhage. Vessels with aneurysmal changes or poststenotic dilation of more than 2 cm should be resected and reconstructed with autogenous saphenous vein or synthetic prosthesis using the supraclavicular approach with an infraclavicular incision. An arterial lesion less than 2 cm can be left alone, and only rib resection and scalenectomy should be performed using the transaxillary approach. Dorsal sympathectomy can be performed through the axillary incision or under thoracoscopic guidance.[87] Increased cutaneous perfusion and improved pain threshold can be observed. Generally, excellent outcomes can be expected with timely diagnosis and treatment.[83,84]

VASCULAR DISEASE OF THE UPPER EXTREMITY

The upper extremities are subject to a variety of unique intrinsic arterial and venous disorders, as well as the peripheral manifestations of systemic collagen vascular diseases. Patients developing arterial insufficiency of the upper extremities generally demonstrate one of three different clinical patterns: (1) attacks of Raynaud disease symptoms, (2) digital ischemia and gangrene, or (3) crampy pain with exercise, often referred to as *claudication*. The initial examination of the upper extremity should begin with inspection, palpation, and auscultation. Noninvasive vascular testing, such as segmental systolic pressure measurement with Doppler flow detector, digital plethysmography, and duplex scan, can be used to further document the disorder.

Afflictions of the Major Vascular Structures

Approximately 50% of cases of acute arterial insufficiency of the upper extremity are secondary to embolization; of the remainder, 25% are the result of primary arterial thrombosis and 25% are iatrogenic in origin, including arterial blood pressure monitoring, sampling of arterial blood gases, and creation of an arteriovenous fistula for dialysis. Brachial artery catheterization is a well-documented cause of upper extremity ischemia.[88] Trauma to the brachial vessels generally carries a poor prognosis secondary to the commonly associated nerve injury. When signs of ischemia accompany an upper extremity fracture, fracture reduction should be done as a primary maneuver, and reassessment of arterial integrity should be done promptly. Takayasu arteritis should be considered, particularly in a relatively young female patient. The vast majority of embolic arterial occlusions in the upper extremity are of cardiac origin, but brachiocephalic aneurysmal disease occasionally results in embolic episodes.

Other less common causes include quadrilateral space syndrome and humeral head syndrome, where the axillary artery or the posterior humeral circumflex branches are injured and give rise to arterial emboli. Most often associated with throwing athletes, these injuries represent a discrete set of lesions that respond to surgical intervention.[89]

The diagnosis of upper extremity ischemia is straightforward. The triad of symptoms—pain, paresthesias, and pallor—is generally accompanied by a loss of radial and ulnar pulse and diminished segmental pressures on noninvasive testing. Diagnostic and therapeutic measures must be prompt in episodes of acute upper extremity embolization. It has been documented that patients treated within 12 hours of the embolic episode have excellent long-term results.[90,91] Two modes of therapy may produce satisfactory results: the immediate administration of continuous intravenous heparin with careful monitoring of the thromboplastin time, and embolectomy with careful observation for the development of compartment syndrome. High-dose local infusion of thrombolytic agents such as urokinase or tissue plasminogen activator (TPA) by transarterial catheter has been effective in the lysis of intraarterial thrombi.[92] This technique can be used intraoperatively to more effectively remove thrombotic material from the very vasoactive vessels of the upper extremities. If there is any clinical or radiographic evidence of vasospasm, vasodilator agents such as papaverine or nitroglycerin can be infused via the same catheter.[93] Experience has also been accumulating on the use of recombinant tissue-plasminogen activator.[94]

Arterial quadrilateral space syndrome arises as the humeral artery is partially avulsed from the axillary artery. The injured segment may develop to form a pseudoaneurysm or a dissection. Both of these may then become the source of emboli. In addition to thrombolysis or thrombectomy, the surgical management of arterial quadrilateral space syndrome includes careful identification of the injured humeral circumflex artery, then flush ligation and division of the artery. This is done to prevent recurrent embolization.[89]

In humeral head syndrome, the axillary artery is repeatedly stretched over the head of the humerus with hyperabduction of the arm. This results in dissection or aneurysmal degeneration of the axillary artery and these lesions give rise to arterial emboli. The surgical management of these lesions requires appreciation of the complex motions of the arm and artery. Arterial reconstruction with a saphenous vein graft is the solution of choice.[89]

Small Vessel Occlusion in the Upper Extremity

The collagen vascular diseases manifest themselves by deposition of immune complexes in the intimal and subintimal surfaces of small vessels. In addition, obliterative, proliferative processes characterize diseases such as scleroderma and diabetes. Scleroderma is the most common entity manifesting with digital ischemia. The fact that digital ischemia may precede systemic manifestations of these diseases adds to the difficulty of the initial diagnosis and emphasizes the need for a logical approach, which may have to be repeated during the evolution of the patient's disease.[95,96] The response to cigarette smoking, particularly in men suspected of suffering from Buerger disease, is characteristic in this group of patients. The presence of digital gangrene in a young patient without evidence of atherosclerosis or aneurysmal disease, and particularly in the presence of normal upper extremity segmental pressures, should lead one to suspect a generalized collagen vascular disease. The process of gangrene in the fingers is quite different from that of necrosis, which is a wet suppurative process. Fingertip gangrene is more often a process of desiccation and mummification. Serologic tests are the basis of the diagnostic workup in these patients. Plain radiographs of the hands are also indicated. Evidence of skin atrophy and shiny tenseness or calcinosis of the skin are also valuable diagnostic findings. In cases in which skin biopsy is performed, immunofluorescence staining is extremely helpful. Specific arteriographic findings of collagen vascular diseases have been well documented: bilateral lesions; arterial obstruction without calcification; absence of atherosclerotic changes; smooth narrowing of the arterial lumen; total arterial occlusion or a stringlike appearance; multiple lesions, predominantly in the forearm and hand; less collateral circulation, giving a winding, corkscrew appearance; and small, attenuated terminal digital branches having the appearance of a "tree root."[97] Arteriography is also useful in excluding proximal lesions, although it rarely demonstrates specific changes characteristic of certain types of arteritis (Fig. 33.16). Medical management includes avoidance of cold exposure, use of gloves, discontinuation of tobacco use, and medication such as nifedipine, which is useful in relieving arterial spasm and associated digital ischemia.

Raynaud disease is a vasospastic condition. Although associated with the collagen diseases, it can also be idiopathic. The chief symptom is a peculiar blanching and cyanosis of the fingertips owing to profound vasoconstriction of the capillary beds caused primarily by exposure to cold and aggravated by the use of tobacco and caffeine. The diagnosis is confirmed by arteriography. Intraarterial injection of 25 mg tolazoline (Priscoline) during arteriography relieves the spasm momentarily and elucidates the spastic process. Initial treatment is with calcium channel blockers, such as nifedipine (30 to 60 mg daily). Surgical treatment is a dorsal sympathectomy, often performed by a thoracoscopic approach.

Arteriography

Arteriography can be useful in the diagnosis and assessment of vascular disorders of the upper extremity. The transfemoral route is preferred, particularly to enable visualization of the proximal aortic vessels and to avoid the need to traverse a potentially diseased axillosubclavian vessel. Proximal aneurysmal dilation and atherosclerotic occlusive disease, as well as thrombosis and ulcerating plaques, are generally well identified radiographically. Proximal subclavian occlusion with subclavian steal phenomenon and retrograde flow in the vertebral artery is easily demonstrated.

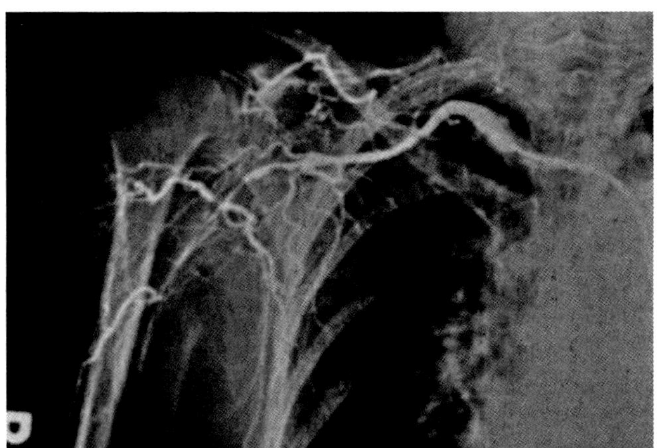

FIG 33.16 Typical pattern of axillosubclavian arterial occlusive disease seen in giant cell arteritis.

This lesion should be suspected whenever there is a pressure discrepancy greater than 20 mm Hg in the contralateral brachial artery pressure.

Magnification views of the hand during arteriography, particularly if augmented by hand cooling or warming, or injection of intraarterial vasodilating drugs such as papaverine or nitroglycerin, can differentiate between Raynaud phenomenon, which is generally associated with segmental occlusions, and Raynaud disease, which is generally identifiable only by vasospastic hypersensitivity. The angiographic characteristics of arterial vasospasm are marked delay in flow, a threadlike appearance, and tapered areas of occlusion relieved by the injection of vasodilating drugs or hand warming.

Iatrogenic Venous Insufficiency of the Upper Extremity

Although thoracic outlet compression can lead to axillosubclavian vein thrombosis, the vast majority of venous occlusive processes result from trauma or iatrogenic injury. Long-term intravenous alimentation, upper-extremity intravenous access for therapy, or procedures such as central venous pressure monitoring and Swan-Ganz monitoring can result in axillosubclavian thrombotic episodes. It is important to recognize that chronic axillosubclavian vein thrombosis may be an indolent and relatively silent process and is seldom associated with symptoms in the upper extremity. Whenever this problem has been examined prospectively, however, the incidence of venous thrombosis in the major upper extremity veins approaches 25%. Heparin therapy rarely leads to lysis, but it might prevent extension of thrombosis with removal of cannulas. Thrombolytic therapy with streptokinase or recombinant tissue plasminogen activator may prove efficacious. Reports of successful surgical therapy by thrombectomy or interposition grafting do not demonstrate any superiority over conservative management, and the failure rate is sufficiently high that enthusiastic recommendation of surgical intervention cannot be supported.

REVIEW QUESTIONS

1. The Allen test is useful in evaluating which of the following?
   a. Thoracic outlet compression
   b. Presence of cervical rib
   c. Integrity of palmar arch
   d. Digital blood flow
   e. Acute effort thrombosis
2. Which of the following structures compose the skeletal frame of the thoracic outlet?
   a. The sternum
   b. First thoracic rib
   c. First thoracic vertebral body
   d. Subclavian artery
   e. Subclavius tendon
3. The scalene triangle is traversed by which of the following structures? (More than one may be correct.)
   a. Subclavian artery
   b. Brachial plexus
   c. Anterior scalene muscle
   d. Pectoralis major tendon
   e. Middle scalene muscle
4. Digital gangrene is not associated with which of the following?
   a. Buerger disease
   b. Vasculitis
   c. Raynaud disease
   d. Arterial thoracic outlet syndrome
   e. Paget-Schroetter disease
5. Digital plethysmographic tracings are most apt to be misinterpreted secondary to which of the following?
   a. Cuff malfunction
   b. Transducer malfunction
   c. Segmental arterial occlusions
   d. Changes in sympathetic activity
   e. Poor light
6. Which of the following is a common cause of prominent right-sided supraclavicular pulsation?
   a. Common carotid aneurysm
   b. Subclavian aneurysm
   c. Subclavian tortuosity or elongation
   d. Innominate artery aneurysm
   e. Mycotic aneurysm
7. Effort thrombosis of the subclavian vein is often associated with which of the following?
   a. Straining at bowel movement
   b. Hypercoagulation syndrome
   c. Thoracic outlet compression syndrome
   d. Calcinosis cutis, Raynaud phenomenon, sclerodactyly, and telangiectasia (CRST syndrome) or scleroderma
   e. Collagen vascular disease in general
8. Regarding the diagnosis of aTOS, which of the following are true?
   a. aTOS commonly presents with acute onset of unilateral upper extremity ischemia.
   b. Cervical ribs associated with development of subclavian artery aneurysms.
   c. Surgical decompression is the first step in management of acute upper extremity ischemia related to aTOS.
   d. Thrombolysis or arterial thrombectomy are the first steps in management of acute upper extremity ischemia related to aTOS.
   e. None of the above

9. Diagnosis of neurogenic thoracic outlet syndrome should include which of the following criteria?

a. Symptoms appropriate to compression of the neurovascular bundle at the thoracic outlet
b. Physical exam findings that indicate neurovascular compression
c. Testing that supports the diagnosis of nTOS
d. History of injury consistent with development of nTOS
e. All of the above

10. When diagnosing neurogenic thoracic outlet syndrome, the single best test to determine whether symptoms are related to the compression of the neurovascular bundle at the thoracic outlet is which of the following?

a. Magnetic resonance angiography
b. Magnetic resonance venography
c. An electrophysiologic test, such as electromyogram or somatosensory evoked potential test
d. EMG-guided scalene muscle stimulation and block test
e. Provocative Adson or abduction and external rotation test

References available online at ExpertConsult.com.

CHAPTER 34

Natural History and Nonoperative Treatment of Chronic Lower Extremity Ischemia

Olamide Alabi, Amir F. Azarbal, Erica L. Mitchell, Gregory J. Landry, Gregory L. Moneta

Despite the focus on operative and endovascular interventions in vascular surgery, most patients with chronic lower extremity ischemia do not require surgical intervention. Nonoperative therapy and risk factor modification remain the primary components of management for the majority of patients. Less than 2% of people below 50 years of age suffer from symptoms of intermittent claudication; this increases to 5% in those aged 50 to 70 years and to 10% in those above age 70.[1-3] Overall, 8 to 12 million people in the United States[4] and 27 million people in North America and Europe[5] have symptomatic peripheral arterial disease (PAD), and this number will certainly increase as the population ages.

STRATIFICATION AND EPIDEMIOLOGY

Chronic lower extremity ischemia represents a clinical spectrum ranging from asymptomatic disease and atypical symptoms to classic intermittent claudication and critical limb ischemia with impending limb loss. Various classification systems for acute and chronic limb ischemia—such as those of Fontaine,[6] and Rutherford,[7] and others—have been developed over the years. Many focused on ischemia whereas others have been used solely for describing chronic wounds. The Wound Ischemia foot Infection (WIfI) classification system,[8] introduced in 2014, was created to include multiple aspects of wound status and arterial occlusive disease by grading wound descriptions, burden of infection, as well as stratifying hemodynamic indices. At present, classification systems are primarily used in clinical research and communication among clinicians and are not intended to dictate therapy.

Intermittent claudication is typically reported as the number of blocks a patient can walk on level ground at a normal speed and without stopping. Patients, however, are often poor judges of objective walking distance; pharmaceutical trials therefore have generally stratified patients based on walking distances (initial or absolute claudication distances) or claudication times using either fixed or graded load treadmill testing. Disease-specific health-related quality-of-life tools such as the Walking Impairment Questionnaire (WIQ)[9] or Vascular Quality of Life questionnaire (VascuQOL)[10] stratify intermittent claudication symptom severity as well as providing a validated, comparable assessment of the psychosocial/emotional well-being and functional status of the PAD patient.[11] Combining the objective measurements of ischemia (ankle-brachial pressure index, toe pressure, pulse-volume recordings) with clinical parameters helps to define the natural history of various patient groups with chronic lower extremity ischemia.

Atherosclerotic cardiovascular disease is a systemic process affecting multiple arterial beds, including the coronary, and cerebrovascular, upper and lower extremities, and visceral arteries with significant disease overlap. PAD is a well-recognized independent risk factor for cardiovascular morbidity and mortality.[12,13] Large, epidemiologic studies have described the incidence and prevalence of PAD, with results dependent on the definition of PAD employed.[14-17]

Asymptomatic Arterial Insufficiency

Asymptomatic PAD is defined as a decreased ankle-brachial index (ABI) without lower extremity symptoms. Most studies use an ABI below 0.9 as the reference standard for PAD.[5] The presence of asymptomatic lower extremity occlusive disease varies, but available data indicate that for every patient with intermittent claudication, there are probably three others with similar disease who do not complain of symptoms or have atypical symptoms.[14] Estimated ratios of symptomatic to asymptomatic patients range from 1 : 1.8 to 1 : 5.3.[1,2,15,16]

The prevalence of asymptomatic PAD was 25.5% among 1537 participants in the Systolic Hypertension in the Elderly Program.[17] Data from a nationwide cross-sectional study, based on more than 350 primary care practices, demonstrated that 13% of 6979 patients older than 50 years had abnormal ABIs, with or without symptoms of intermittent claudication.[12] Only 24% of patients identified with chronic lower extremity ischemia had a previous diagnosis of PAD, and asymptomatic patients accounted for 48% of newly diagnosed PAD.

Incidence of Symptomatic Peripheral Arterial Disease

The majority of epidemiologic studies of PAD have focused on patients with intermittent claudication, defined as leg pain with walking (most often calf pain, but it can involve the thighs and buttocks well). Pain is induced by exercise and relieved by rest. Reported incidences of PAD depend on age and the definition of intermittent claudication and vary from 2.2% in a population aged 33 to 82 years to 17% in a population aged 55 to 70 years.[1,2] In the Framingham Heart Study,[18] the incidence of PAD was based on symptoms of intermittent claudication in subjects 29 to 62 years old. The annual incidence of intermittent claudication per 10,000 subjects at risk rose from 6 in men and 3 in women aged 30 to 44 years to 61 in men and 54 in women aged 65 to 74 years. The average rate of development of intermittent claudication over a 2-year period in subjects older than age 50 was 0.7% in men and 0.4% in women.

In the Edinburgh Artery Study of almost 1600 subjects older than 55 years, the 5-year cumulative incidence of PAD was 9%.[19] In a study of 8400 Israeli men over a 21-year period, the cumulative incidence of PAD was 43.1 per 1000 population.[20] In the Quebec Cardiovascular Study of 4570 men followed over 12 years, an incidence of 41 per 10,000 population per year was noted.[21] In the Physicians' Health Study, 433 incident cases of PAD were reported among 22,071 relatively healthy men.[22]

Prevalence of Symptomatic Peripheral Arterial Disease

Epidemiologic studies have used both questionnaires and noninvasive vascular laboratory screening to estimate the prevalence of PAD in the elderly adult population. Before the development of reliable noninvasive testing, the diagnosis of PAD was based on patient questionnaires. Among questionnaires, the World Health Organization/Rose Questionnaire and the Edinburgh Classification Questionnaire (ECQ) have been the most extensively utilized. The ECQ appears to be more robust, with a sensitivity of 91% and a specificity of 99% for the diagnosis of intermittent claudication.[23] Using the ECQ, the prevalence of lower extremity arterial disease was estimated to be 4.6% in the Edinburgh Artery Study in men and women between the ages of 55 and 74 years.[2] Other studies have found the prevalence of intermittent claudication in adults older than age 45 to be approximately 1% to 5% (Table 34.1).

When the ABI is used as a reference standard, the detected prevalence of lower extremity arterial occlusive disease is greater, likely because of the inclusion of patients who are asymptomatic or have atypical symptoms. The overall age-adjusted prevalence of PAD diagnosed on the basis of the ABI is approximately 12%; for intermittent claudication, it is 1% to 2% up to age 50 and 5% to 7% above the seventh decade.[24] In the Cardiovascular Health Study, the prevalence of a decreased ABI (<0.9) was 12.4% in adults aged 65 years or older in four US communities.[17] Using the same criteria, investigators in the Rotterdam Study reported a PAD prevalence of 19% in subjects older than 55 years.[15] In the Edinburgh Artery Study, the prevalence of lower extremity arterial occlusive disease diagnosed using the ABI was 17% in subjects between the ages of 55 and 74 years.[2] In a Danish study, the prevalence of lower extremity arterial occlusive disease in 60-year-old subjects was 16% for men and 13% for women (Table 34.2).[25] Thus objective standards of measurement identify a greater number of patients with PAD than does reliance on patient description of symptoms.

Several factors might explain the lack of sensitivity of questionnaires and the increased prevalence of PAD with noninvasive testing.[2,26] First, symptoms might not occur until the disease is advanced. This is particularly relevant in older patients, who may rarely walk more than one or two blocks at a time in the performance of their activities of daily living or who may assume

TABLE 34.1 Prevalence of Intermittent Claudication by History or Questionnaire in Large Population Studies

Study	No. of Patients	Age (Years)	Intermittent Claudication Prevalence (%)
Schroll and Munck (1981)[16]	360 men	60	5.8
	306 women	60	1.3
Reunanen et al. (1982)[258]	5738 men	30–59	2.1
	5224 women	30–59	1.8
Fowkes et al. (1991)[2]	1592 men and women	55–74	4.5
Stoffers et al. (1991)[259]	3654 men and women	45–54	0.6
		55–64	2.5
		65–74	8.8
Smith et al. (1990)[116]	18,388 men	40–64	0.8
Skau and Jonsson (1993)[260]	7254 men and women	50–89	4.1
Newman et al. (1993)[17]	5084 men and women	65–85	2.0
Stoffers et al. (1996)[24]	1719 men	55–75	1.5
	1935 women	55–75	2.8
Zheng et al. (1997)[261]	15,106 men and women	45–64	1.0
Meijer et al. (1998)[15]	3052 men	70	2.2
	4663 women	70	1.2

TABLE 34.2 Prevalence of Peripheral Arterial Disease Based on Ankle-Brachial Index Abnormalities in Large Population Studies

Study	No. of Patients	Age (Years)	Intermittent Claudication Prevalence (%)
Schroll and Munck (1981)[16]	360 men	60	16.0
	306 women	60	13.0
Criqui et al. (1985)[1]	613 men and women	38–82	11.7
Hiatt et al. (1990)[262]	950 men and women	44–68	11.9
Newman et al. (1991)[263]	1592 men and women	55–74	24.6
Coni et al.et al. (1992)[26]	265 men and women	>65	9.1
Newman et al. (1993)[17]	2214 men	>65	13.9
	2870 women	>65	11.4
Stoffers et al. (1991)[259]	1719 men	55–75	11.0
	1935 women	55–75	8.6
Meijer et al. (1998)[15]	2589 men	>55	16.9
	3861 women	>55	20.5

that leg pain while walking is a natural part of the aging process. Second, patients with PAD may have other comorbidities, such as arthritis, cardiac disease, or pulmonary disease, affecting their walking ability to a greater degree than PAD.

RISK FACTORS

Smoking

The specific mechanisms by which tobacco exerts its adverse effects on arteries remain poorly understood; however, a direct relationship between tobacco smoking and peripheral arterial disease is well established.[27] All epidemiologic studies of lower extremity arterial disease have confirmed cigarette smoking as a strong risk factor for the development of such disease, with relative risk ratios ranging from 1.7 to 7.5.[1,15,17,28-32] A case-control study revealed a sevenfold higher risk of developing PAD in ex-smokers compared with those who had never smoked, and the risk increased to 16-fold in current smokers compared with those who had never smoked.[33] The diagnosis of lower extremity arterial disease is made up to a decade earlier in smokers compared with nonsmokers. More than 90% of all patients referred to vascular clinics for PAD have a history of smoking.[34]

In addition to the chronic effects of smoking on the development of atherosclerosis, smoking has acute effects on lower extremity function. Smoking two cigarettes within a 10-minute period results in an acute lowering of the ABI in chronic smokers from 0.64 ± 0.14 to 0.55 ± 0.11 ($P = .008$).[35] In addition to having adverse influences on atherosclerosis, tobacco smoke may directly contribute to claudication. Smoking is associated with acute drops in treadmill walking distances, presumably related to the effects of carbon monoxide.[36] An immediate and significant decrease in the time or distance patients can walk on the treadmill before they manifest claudication symptoms has been demonstrated when they breathe air containing carbon monoxide.[36,37] Smokers have an increased risk of peripheral arterial disease progression,[38] myocardial infarction, stroke, and death.[39] Smokers also have an increased risk of major amputation.[40,41]

Diabetes Mellitus

There is a strong association between diabetes mellitus and PAD. Two types of vascular disease are seen in patients with diabetes: microcirculatory dysfunction involving the capillaries and arterioles of the kidneys, retina, and peripheral nerves and a macroangiopathy involving the peripheral and coronary arterial circulations.[42] The Framingham Study was one of the first major epidemiologic studies to demonstrate the association between diabetes and PAD. Diabetes increased the risk of claudication by a factor of 3.5 in men and 8.6 in women.[43] Numerous subsequent studies have associated impaired glucose tolerance with a two- to fourfold increase in the risk of developing intermittent claudication.[44-49] In an elderly white population, 20.9% of patients with diabetes mellitus and 15.1% of those with an abnormal glucose tolerance test had an ABI less than 0.9.[50] In a Swedish study, 21% of patients with diabetes had signs of PAD.[51] The duration and severity of diabetes mellitus correlate strongly with the incidence and severity of PAD.

Patients with diabetes mellitus more often develop symptomatic forms of PAD and have poorer lower extremity function than do those with PAD alone.[52] The prevalence of diabetes in patients undergoing lower extremity revascularization ranges from 25% to 50% compared with a prevalence of 6% in the general population.[53] The rate of lower extremity amputation is 7- to 10-fold higher in diabetic patients than in those without diabetes,[28,54-55] with diabetes being the leading cause of nontraumatic lower extremity amputations. In addition to diabetes, insulin resistance and hyperinsulinemia are also risk factors for PAD.[31,56] There is an increased mortality risk in PAD patients, but compared with PAD patients without diabetes, PAD patients with diabetes still have an almost threefold increased risk of death within 10 years.[57]

Gender

Early epidemiologic studies focused on PAD in men. The popular notion, based on the Framingham Study, was that symptomatic PAD in women lagged behind men by 10 years and that women were generally not affected by PAD until after menopause.[58] Recent epidemiologic studies, however, indicate that the prevalence and incidence of PAD in men and women are similar, with the age-adjusted incidence of intermittent claudication equal in both genders.[25,59] However, the frequency of PAD among diabetic women is markedly higher than that among diabetic men.[25] In patients with a low ABI, coronary artery disease is less prevalent among women. Women also had a lower frequency of cerebrovascular disease.[59] In another study, the prevalence of PAD was essentially identical in men and women, with other cardiovascular disease twice as prevalent in men.[12] Progression of PAD, as measured by changes in ABI, appears to be the same in men and women.[60]

Women with PAD may suffer a faster functional decline and have a somewhat varied distribution of atherosclerotic lesions. A prospective trial of 380 men and women showed that at 4-year follow-up, women were more likely than men to have a decline in walking distance and to develop mobility-related disability. Functional differences may be attributable to a smaller baseline calf muscle area in women,[61] and women may be more susceptible than men to the development of aortoiliac arterial occlusive disease.[62] Autopsy findings indicate, that women, compared with men, have more fatty streaks in the abdominal aorta but not in the coronary arteries.[63]

It is likely that PAD is underdiagnosed in women to a greater degree than in men. Women are less likely than men to have diagnosed PAD on the basis of symptoms, even if clinically significant PAD is present on noninvasive examination.[64,65] In addition, infrainguinal arterial reconstructions in women, compared with men, tend to be performed for more advanced disease, and such women tend to be older.[66,67]

The reasons for the more advanced presentation of PAD in women are unclear. Some speculate that women more frequently assume a caretaker role and therefore are more likely to ignore their own medical care; or perhaps women are more likely to ignore mild to moderate pain, attributing it to a consequences of old age.[68] It is clear that, as more data accumulate on PAD in women, the previous dictum of PAD being primarily a disease of men is proving to be incorrect.

Race

Few studies have assessed differences in PAD prevalence among different ethnic groups. One early study indicated that African American patients with PAD typically had a higher prevalence of infrapopliteal atherosclerosis, which was associated with a greater incidence of limb loss.[69] PAD may be underreported in the African American population. In the Atherosclerosis Risk in Communities Study, more than 4000 African American men and women were screened for PAD. Despite a greater prevalence of hypertension and diabetes, the prevalence of PAD measured by questionnaire was lower among African American men than among white men. However, 3.3% of African Americans had an ABI below 0.9, compared with only 2.3% of whites.[59] In the Cardiovascular Health Study, the nonwhite population had a 3.5-fold increased frequency of an ABI below 0.8.[17]

Hyperlipidemia

Up to 50% of patients with lower extremity arterial disease have hyperlipidemia. In the Framingham Study, a fasting cholesterol level above 270 mg/dL was associated with a doubling of the incidence of intermittent claudication.[58] Population studies have demonstrated that the relative risk of PAD is 2 times greater in patients with hypercholesterolemia,[70] 1.7 times increased in patients with hypertriglyceridemia,[29] and 2.0 times increased in patients with elevated levels of lipoprotein(a).[71] On the other hand, triglyceride level is not an independent risk factor for PAD when corrected for other serum lipid variables.[29,72] In an evaluation of multiple plasma lipid constituents on the risk of developing PAD, the ratio of total cholesterol to HDL cholesterol was the strongest predictor of PAD development, and the addition of screening for other lipid abnormalities did not improve predictive values.[72] The addition of screening for two nonlipid variables—C-reactive protein and fibrinogen—did, however, improve the prediction of PAD risk.[73]

Hyperhomocysteinemia

Prospective and retrospective studies have suggested an association between elevated levels of plasma homocysteine and premature vascular disease in the coronary, cerebrovascular, and peripheral circulation.[74-77] Early studies suggesting this association, however, were based on small numbers of patients. Darius and colleagues[78] evaluated plasma homocysteine level as an independent risk factor for PAD in 6880 primary care patients older than 65 years. Although PAD (defined as an ABI <0.9) was more frequently diagnosed in patients in the highest quintile of homocysteine levels (24.3%) than in those in the lowest quintile (13.0%; crude odds ratio 2.1), the association was less strong after adjusting for other atherosclerotic risk factors (odds ratio 1.4). Thus the association between hyperhomocysteinemia and atherosclerosis is mild.

Serum Markers

Fibrinogen and C-reactive protein have been implicated in the pathogenesis of PAD.[39,79-84] Their role in the pathogenesis of atherosclerosis is unclear; however, they are thought to be potential markers of endothelial dysfunction,[85] and elevated fibrinogen levels have been found to be an independent risk factor for PAD.[15,86] C-reactive protein is an acute-phase reactant that is elevated in acute inflammatory conditions. Persistent elevations are observed in chronic inflammatory disorders, consistent with the modern concept of atherosclerosis as an inflammatory disorder. Other atherogenic risk factors such as age,[87,88] smoking,[89] diabetes,[90] and hyperlipidemia[91] are associated with elevated levels of C-reactive protein in the absence of PAD. Elevated C-reactive protein may be an epiphenomenon associated with, but not causative of, an atherogenic state.

Elevated C-reactive protein and D-dimer, a marker of ongoing fibrin formation and degradation, are associated with poorer physical functioning in PAD patients.[92,93] Measurements of walking distance, walking speed, and balance are significantly worse in patients with elevated C-reactive protein and D-dimer. Other inflammatory biomarkers, such as soluble adhesion molecules and tumor necrosis factor-α (TNF-α), have also been studied with monocyte expression of TNF-α and found to be associated with a decrease in maximal treadmill walking time.[94]

Infection

Although controversial, there is evidence that atherosclerosis may be associated with an inflammatory process caused by chronic infection with *Chlamydia pneumoniae* or other infectious agents.[95-97] A meta-analysis of pooled data from 38 studies calculated an overall odds ratio of 1.6, suggesting only a mild causative role at best.[98] *C. pneumoniae* may therefore be primarily an innocent bystander in the atherosclerotic process rather than a cause. In support of this argument, the association between atherosclerosis and *C. pneumoniae* infection appears to be higher in retrospective cross-sectional and case-control studies than in prospective case-control studies, and the association is inversely proportional to length of follow-up.[98]

Alcohol Consumption

Mild to moderate alcohol consumption is associated with a reduced risk of cardiovascular disease and reduced cardiac mortality,[99-102] with an inverse relationship between alcohol consumption and PAD.[22,103-106] The beneficial effects of alcohol are thought to be due to its influence on hemostasis,[86] lipid profiles,[107] and the decreased generation of oxygen free radicals.[108]

NATURAL HISTORY

Once the diagnosis has been made, many patients and physicians fear both disease progression and limb loss, in addition to the functional limitations imposed by intermittent claudication.[109-112]

Cardiovascular Overlap

Because atherosclerosis is a systemic process, significant overlap exists between PAD and other forms of cardiovascular disease—primarily coronary artery and cerebrovascular disease. Hertzer and colleagues[113] clearly demonstrated a high incidence of coronary artery disease in vascular surgery patients. Their conclusions were based on a series of 1000 patients undergoing major vascular surgery in whom they performed preoperative coronary angiography, regardless of a history of coronary artery disease or

TABLE 34.3 Incidence of Coronary Artery Disease in 1000 Consecutive Patients With Peripheral Vascular Disease Screened by Angiography

	UNSUSPECTED		SUSPECTED	
Extent of Disease	**No. of Patients**	**(%)**	**No. of Patients**	**(%)**
Normal coronary arteries	64	14	21	4
Mild to moderate CAD	218	49	99	18
Advanced compensated CAD	97	22	192	34
Severe correctable CAD	63	14	188	34
Severe incorrectable CAD	4	1	54	10

CAD, Coronary artery disease.
Data from Hertzer NR, Beven EG, Young JR, et al: Coronary artery disease in peripheral vascular patients: a classification of 1000 coronary angiograms and results of surgical management, *Ann Surg* 199:223–233, 1984; table from Taylor LM Jr, Porter JM: Natural history and nonoperative treatment in chronic lower extremity ischemia. In Moore WS, editor: *Vascular Surgery: A Comprehensive Review*, Philadelphia, 1993, WB Saunders.

TABLE 34.4 Concomitant Cerebrovascular and Coronary Artery Disease in Patients With Peripheral Arterial Disease

Study	Cerebrovascular Disease (%)	Coronary Artery Disease (%)
Ogren et al. (1993)[264]	33	51
Szilagyi et al. (1986)[265]	19	47
Mendelson et al. (1998)[266]	35	62
Aronow and Ahn (1994)[13]	34	58
CAPRIE (1996)[128]	19	40
Meijer et al. (1998)[15]		
Men	9	39
Women	8	14

CAPRIE, Clopidogrel versus Aspirin in Patients at Risk of Ischemic Events.

cardiac symptoms. More than 90% of patients had significant coronary artery disease, much of which was asymptomatic. The authors also found an increased frequency of severe coronary artery disease with age, from 22% among patients younger than 50 years to 41% among patients 70 years of age or older (Table 34.3).

The well-recognized overlap between PAD and other types of cardiovascular disease has been confirmed in numerous large epidemiologic studies and clinical trials (Table 34.4). In the Cardiovascular Health Study, 60% of patients with PAD had a history of other symptomatic cardiovascular disease, such as myocardial infarction, angina, or stroke.[19] Forty percent of patients with coronary artery or significant cerebrovascular disease also had PAD. Similar findings were reported in a large epidemiologic study[13] in which 1886 patients aged 62 years or more were screened for cardiovascular disease. Seventy percent of patients with PAD had associated coronary artery or cerebrovascular disease (34% cerebrovascular, 58% coronary artery).

TABLE 34.5 Relative Risk of Mortality in Patients With Peripheral Arterial Disease Compared With Those Without

Study	No. of Patients	Follow-Up (Years)	Relative Risk
Reunanen et al. (1982)[258]	5738 men	5	3.0
McKenna et al. (1991)[118]	744 men and women	5	2.4
Criqui et al. (1992)[115]	565 men and women	10	3.1
Ogren et al. (1993)[264]	477 men	10	2.5
Vogt et al. (1993)[119]	1492 women	4	4.0
Kornitzer et al. (1995)[120]	1592 men	10	3.3
Leng et al. (1996)[19]	1592 men and women	5	1.6

Progression of Symptoms

Knowledge of the natural history of PAD is essential when planning therapeutic strategies. When patients with intermittent claudication are followed for 5 years, approximately 50% to 75% have either no change in symptoms or experience improvement. Approximately 25% experience symptom progression, with 5% to 25% requiring therapeutic intervention and only 2% to 4% needing major amputation.[24,114] Both continued tobacco use[38] and diabetes mellitus[114] are correlated with deterioration in the most consistent predictor of an adverse outcome—that is, the severity of objectively determined arterial occlusive disease at the first patient encounter.[56]

Life Expectancy

In contrast to the relatively benign lower extremity prognosis in most patients with PAD, the prognosis for morbidity and mortality from other manifestations of cardiovascular disease is worse. Life expectancy is reduced in patients with PAD, primarily due to cardiovascular disease (Table 34.5).[a] The relative risk of a patient with intermittent claudication having a fatal or nonfatal myocardial infarction or stroke is two- to threefold that of a nonclaudicant. All-cause mortality is also two- to fourfold higher, with 60% of deaths from myocardial infarction and 15% from stroke.[115,117] The 5-year mortality of the average claudicant is 30%, with the majority of deaths caused by manifestations of cardiovascular disease.[25] An additional 5% to 10% will experience a nonfatal cardiovascular event.[24]

The prevalence of asymptomatic carotid artery disease in patients with chronic lower extremity atherosclerotic disease has also been examined. Screening carotid duplex scans in patients requiring infrainguinal revascularization have demonstrated a 30% incidence of asymptomatic internal carotid artery stenosis greater than 50%.[121,122]

[a]References 1, 2, 17, 19, 25, and 115-120.

Multiple risk factors have been defined as important contributors to the increased long-term cardiovascular mortality of patients with lower extremity arterial occlusive disease. These include advanced age, continued tobacco use,[39] diabetes,[123] and dialysis dependence.[124-126] Of these, end-stage renal disease is the most pronounced, with 2-year survival rates of only 50% to 65%.

Survival is inversely related to the degree of objectively determined chronic lower extremity ischemia at presentation.[127] Patients with an ABI less than 0.3 have a significantly higher mortality than those with an ABI of 0.3 to 0.9 (relative risk 1.8).[127] In a group of patients followed for 10 years, there was progressively decreasing survival with increasing PAD severity.[115] Among patients with a normal ABI, asymptomatic PAD, moderately symptomatic PAD, and severe symptomatic PAD, 10-year survival rates were approximately 85%, 55%, 40%, and 25%, respectively. In another study, patients with multilevel PAD had a relative mortality risk of 7.2 compared with controls,[119] whereas patients with PAD confined to the aortoiliac arterial segment had a relative mortality risk of 2.0 compared with controls. Aggressive risk factor modification reduces near-term cardiac mortality in PAD patients.[128-133]

Critical Limb Ischemia

Critical limb ischemia (CLI) occurs when arterial blood flow is inadequate to accommodate the metabolic needs of resting tissue. Clinically, CLI describes a group of patients with limb-threatening ischemia and includes those with rest pain, ischemic ulcerations, and gangrene. Objective circulatory measurement of CLI populations provides the best stratification of prognosis. The likelihood of near-term limb loss is related to the severity of ischemia at the time of patient presentation, associated infection, and the presence of tissue loss. Data on the incidence and prevalence of CLI are less definitive than data on intermittent claudication. Using multiple different extrapolation methods, it is estimated that between 500,000 and 1 million new cases occur each year.[134,135] This means that 1 new patient per year develops CLI for every 100 patients with intermittent claudication. Few epidemiologic studies of CLI exist as compared with the myriad of studies addressing the epidemiology of intermittent claudication. In a 7-year prospective study from the Lombardy region of northern Italy, CLI was estimated by three methods: conversion of intermittent claudication to CLI in prospectively followed patients, hospital admissions for CLI over a 3-month period, and rates of major limb amputation.[134] Similar results were obtained with each method, with the incidence of CLI ranging from 450 to 650 cases per 1 million population per year. A national survey of the Vascular Surgical Society of Great Britain and Ireland found a similar incidence of 400 patients per 1 million population per year.[135]

Patients with CLI and those with intermittent claudication share similar risk factors, but most patients with CLI do not have a clear history of intermittent claudication. Major risk factors for advanced limb ischemia include age, smoking, and diabetes. The incidence of major amputation rises markedly with age. A Danish national discharge survey reported that the incidence of major lower extremity amputation increased from 0.3 per 100,000 per year for patients younger than 40 years to 226 per 100,000 per year for those older than 80 years. Patients with diabetes who smoke require amputation earlier in life than diabetics who do not smoke.[135]

Not all CLI is truly critical. Clearly patients with progressive gangrenous changes and constant ischemic pain have an unstable clinical situation requiring prompt therapy. However, abundant clinical experience indicates that patients who have CLI manifested by intermittent rest pain may experience noticeable improvement over time, perhaps secondary to improved cardiac hemodynamics. Small ulcerations may heal with protective dressings alone. Several randomized pharmacologic trials have documented ulcer healing in up to 40% of CLI patients randomized to placebo,[136,137] although in most of these trials fewer than half the control patients were alive without a major amputation after 6 months.[138,139]

Chronic Lower Extremity Ischemia in Younger Patients

Lower extremity ischemia in patients younger than 40 years old is infrequent. Peripheral vascular disease in young patients has several unique features that must be considered (Table 34.6).[140-146] Such patients are almost always heavy smokers. In addition, evaluation for hypercoagulable states in younger patients with chronic lower extremity ischemia suggests that up to 90% have laboratory abnormalities of coagulation (deficiencies in natural anticoagulants, defective fibrinolytic activity, or the presence of antiphospholipid antibodies),[143] and there are often also significant abnormalities in LDL cholesterol oxidation in younger patients with CLI PAD compared with older PAD patients.[140]

Despite attempts at revascularization, younger patients who manifest limb-threatening symptoms frequently progress to limb loss. The limited patency of reconstructions and need for more frequent operative revisions characterizes these patients.[140,147] Although survival is reduced in younger patients with peripheral

TABLE 34.6 Chronic Lower Extremity Ischemia in Younger Patients

Study	No. of Patients	Follow-Up (Years)	Stable/Improved (%)	Worse (%)	Dead (%)	Amputated (%)
McCready et al. (1984)[146]	21	4–6	38	52	10	—
Pairolero et al. (1984)[145]	50	13.5	64	36	10	30
Evans et al. (1987)[144]	153	5.5	—	—	17	16
Valentine et al. (1990)[141]	22	2.2	76	24	4.5	0
Levy et al. (1994)[267]	109	2.3	—	—	—	27

vascular disease compared with age-matched controls, on balance, coronary atherosclerosis in younger patients with severe PAD does not appear to be as aggressive as the atherosclerosis affecting their lower extremities.[148,149]

Nonoperative management with aggressive risk factor modification (cessation of tobacco use, lipid control) is the initial therapy of choice in younger patients with claudication. However, the greater functional expectations and frequent limitations on gainful employment experienced by younger patients with claudication complicate their ability to tolerate a prolonged course of nonoperative therapy. Despite this, revascularization attempts should be made judiciously, with an understanding of the diminished longevity of these procedures in this age group and the higher amputation rate after failure.

Amputation

CLI patients who undergo major amputation often have not experienced a steady disease progression from claudication to rest pain to tissue necrosis to amputation. The incidence of major lower extremity amputation appears to have reached a plateau or decreased in the last decade, possibly owing to improved methods of revascularization and limb salvage, reduction in smoking, and improved diabetes control.[150-153] In a review of 713 patients who underwent below-knee amputations for ischemia, more than half had experienced no ischemic symptoms as recently as 6 months before the amputation.[154]

Overall, the ratio of below-knee amputations to above-knee amputations is equal and has not significantly changed in several decades.[148,154-156] However, the introduction of aggressive limb salvage teams has increased the rate of below-knee amputations at selected centers.[157] Primary healing of below-knee amputations ranges from 30% to 90%.[157,158] An attempt at below-knee salvage varies from 4% to 30%,[159-161] and half of all below-knee amputees who fail to achieve primary healing ultimately require an above-knee amputation.[162-164]

More below-knee than above-knee amputees achieve ambulation.[155,165,166] Overall, however, only a small number of major amputees for ischemic disease achieve meaningful independent ambulation, and initial rehabilitation can take 9 months or longer. After 2 years, 30% of amputees who had been walking no longer use their prostheses.[155] Advanced age and female gender bode poorly for ambulation.[167] Fifteen percent of amputees require contralateral amputation, and another 20% to 30% die within 2 years.[155,157,168]

NONOPERATIVE TREATMENT

The nonoperative treatment of chronic lower extremity ischemia includes risk factor modification, exercise, and pharmacologic therapy.

Management of Risk Factors

The first step in the management of PAD patients is treatment of atherosclerotic risk factors. Multiple randomized trials in large populations at high risk for coronary disease indicate that aggressive risk factor modification (lipid reduction, antiplatelet therapy, diabetes management, and blood pressure control) reliably reduces near-term cardiac mortality.[128,130-133] Table 34.7 describes basic guidelines for risk factor modification based on these trials.

TABLE 34.7 Recommendations for Risk Factor Reduction in Patients With Chronic Lower Extremity Ischemia

Parameter	Target Goal	Therapy
Blood pressure	Systolic <130	β-blockers
Diastolic	<85	ACE inhibitors
Antiplatelet therapy	All patients on some form	Aspirin, clopidogrel
Diabetes	HbA_{1c} <7%	Insulin, ↑insulin sensitivity
Tobacco cessation	Complete abstinence	Nicotine replacement, antidepressant

ACE, Angiotensin-converting enzyme; *Hb A_{1c}*, glycosylated hemoglobin.

Smoking Cessation

Smoking cessation is by far the most important treatment for patients with PAD. PAD symptoms are unlikely to progress and may even improve once smoking is stopped completely.[169] In patients with intermittent claudication, improvement in walking distance up to 40% has been reported with smoking cessation.[169,170] Improved patency of arterial repairs in nonsmokers has been demonstrated for both aortofemoral and femoropopliteal reconstructions,[171-174] and the degree of tobacco use (measured by carboxyhemoglobin levels) bears directly on the incidence of graft occlusion.[175]

Patients with PAD are often unaware of the strong association between smoking and lower extremity disease. In one study, only 37% of smokers with PAD recognized smoking as a risk factor.[176] The initial effort, therefore, on the part of all physicians must be to educate patients about the relationship between tobacco use and PAD and to inform patients unequivocally that smoking is the most important factor responsible for their leg condition. Studies have shown that strong and repeated advice by physicians to quit smoking results in abstinence in more than one-third of smokers.[177]

Physicians must be prepared to provide a plan to help patients achieve the goal of smoking cessation. Reassurance is extremely important. Multiple attempts at quitting are common; for most people who eventually quit, 2 to 5 years and an average of six abstinence-relapse cycles are required.[178] Although half of all smokers make an attempt to discontinue tobacco use each year, as few as 3% to 5% remain abstinent at 1 year.[179] A recent randomized controlled trial demonstrated that patients enrolled in an intensive smoking cessation program—consisting of education, counseling, behavioral therapy, and advice regarding pharmacologic adjuncts—were threefold more likely to abstain from smoking at 6 months compared with patients only receiving advice from their physician.[180]

Pharmacologic adjuncts for the treatment of smoking addiction may be helpful in facilitating cessation. Current adjuncts include nicotine replacement therapy, partial nicotine receptor agonists, and antidepressant therapy. Most nicotine replacement agents provide up to 30% of a smoker's regular daily nicotine intake and reduce or prevent withdrawal symptoms. Nicotine gum is the oldest form of nicotine replacement and is currently available without a prescription. Drawbacks include the requirement of specific chewing techniques to maximize nicotine release and drug inactivation with pH changes if beverages are consumed during use. Nicotine transdermal patches (dose ranging from 7 to 21 mg per 24 hours) are easier to use. Reviews of randomized double-blind nicotine replacement trials for smoking cessation therapy in younger patients (30 to 40 years old) document biochemically confirmed 6-month abstinence rates of 20% to 45% in the treatment groups compared with 5% to 25% in the control groups, depending on the setting (with treatment initiation in a smoking cessation clinic superior to that in a primary care office).[181,182] No benefit was derived from treatment longer than 8 weeks or from the tapering of nicotine. Intermediate-dose (14 mg per 24 hours) nicotine patches have been used cautiously in patients with symptomatic coronary artery disease.[183]

Partial nicotine receptor agonists, such as varenicline, have recently gained popularity as adjuncts to smoking cessation. A recent Cochrane database meta-analysis indicated that varenicline appears to be superior to placebo and bupropion for smoking cessation but not significantly better than nicotine replacement therapy.[184] Finally, nicotine and citrate inhalers have been used in several small randomized trials with or without nicotine patches.[185,186] These devices maintain reinforcement of the ritual and sensory phenomena of smoking. Although short-term abstinence with these devices has been achieved in 20% to 30% of cases, long-term results have been disappointing.

Smoking cessation programs now focus on depression as an important component of the smoker profile and as a major factor in withdrawal symptoms.[187] The antidepressant agents bupropion and fluoxetine have been used in randomized trials with 12-week biochemically confirmed cessation rates of 30% to 40%.[188] In addition to diminishing withdrawal symptoms (which share many characteristics with chronic depression), these agents appear to attenuate some of the weight gain observed with smoking cessation. They have also been used in combination with nicotine replacement (patch or inhaler), with improved results compared with either agent alone.[189]

Treatment of Diabetes

Although diabetes is clearly recognized as a risk factor for PAD, it is not clear how optimizing glycemic control affects the progression of PAD. Although glycemic control prevents the microvascular complications of diabetes, its effect on macrovascular complications is less clear.[190] In the Diabetes Control and Complications Trial comprising patients with type 1 diabetes who were randomized to intensive versus conventional insulin therapy, patients receiving intensive insulin treatment had fewer cardiovascular events, with no effect on PAD progression.[191] Similarly, in the United Kingdom Prospective Diabetes Study of patients with type 2 diabetes, intensive treatment resulted in fewer deaths from myocardial infarction but no difference in amputation or death from PAD.[192] Recommendations for optimal glycemic control (hemoglobin A_{1c} <7%) in the PAD patient are therefore based primarily on beneficial cardiac effects rather than peripheral arterial end points.

Treatment of Hyperlipidemia

In general lipid-lowering therapies are associated with stabilization or regression of PAD as measured by angiography and severity of symptoms.[190,193] In the Cholesterol Lowering Atherosclerosis Study, 188 men with PAD and coronary artery disease were randomized to treatment with colestipol and niacin versus placebo. Lipid-lowering therapy was associated with stabilization of femoral artery atherosclerosis.[194] In the Program on the Surgical Control of the Hyperlipidemias study, 838 patients with a history of myocardial infarction and hyperlipidemia were randomized to ileal bypass surgery versus placebo and followed for 10 years. A significant reduction in PAD progression was noted in the surgical group, with a 44% risk reduction in development of an abnormal ABI (i.e., <0.95) and a 30% risk reduction in development of intermittent claudication.[195] Similar results were found in the Scandinavian Simvastatin Survival Study, in which cholesterol reduction was associated with a 38% reduction in the risk of new or worsening symptoms of intermittent claudication.[196] Recommendations regarding lipid-lowering therapy goals, however, continue to evolve. The 2013 American College of Cardiology/American Heart Association (ACC/AHA) Guideline on the Treatment of Blood Cholesterol to Reduce Atherosclerotic Cardiovascular Risk in Adults moved away from targeting specific LDL or non-HDL cholesterol goals.[197] Instead, multiple randomized controlled trials were reviewed, and specific groups of patients who demonstrated significant benefit from 3-hydroxy-3-methylglutaryl-coenzyme A reductase (HMG-CoA) inhibitors (i.e., statins) therapy were recommended to take moderate- or high-intensity statins for primary and secondary prevention of atherosclerotic cardiovascular disease. Niacin can also be an important adjunct in increasing HDL levels and decreasing triglyceride levels.[198] However, it is important to note that there is no evidence available that states that an improvement in one's lipid fractions translates to an advantage in peak walking time or claudication onset time.[199]

Treatment of Hypertension

Although hypertension is a risk factor for PAD, there is little evidence that management of hypertension alters disease progression. As a result, the goal of hypertension management in patients with PAD is to reduce the risk of myocardial infarction and stroke. There has been concern that the use of β-blockers might result in a worsening of PAD symptoms; this was based on early reports of reduced blood flow to the lower extremities with β-blocker therapy.[200] However, there is no evidence that β-blockers adversely affect mild to moderate claudication.[201]

Treatment of Hyperhomocysteinemia

Hyperhomocysteinemia is a recognized risk factor for PAD and other manifestations of cardiovascular disease. Elevated plasma homocysteine levels can be lowered with vitamin B and folate supplements. There is, however, no evidence that treatment of hyperhomocysteinemia alters the course of PAD.

Antiplatelet Therapy

Although there is no clear evidence of improvement in PAD symptoms with antiplatelet therapy, patients with PAD benefit from antiplatelet therapy to reduce the risk of cardiovascular morbidity and mortality. The most frequently used antiplatelet medications include aspirin and the thienopyridines.

Aspirin

The Antiplatelet Trialists' Collaboration reviewed 189 controlled studies involving the prevention of cardiovascular events in more than 100,000 patients with clinical evidence of cardiovascular disease. Overall, there was a 25% relative risk reduction of fatal and nonfatal myocardial infarction, stroke, and cardiovascular death associated with antiplatelet therapy at 3 years of follow-up.[202] However, in a subgroup analysis of 3295 claudicants, the risk reduction in these end points after a mean follow-up of 27 months was not significantly different. The small number of patients in the subgroup analysis may have accounted for this lack of statistical difference. Similar benefit was shown for aspirin doses ranging from 75 to 350 mg per day. However, in the Physicians' Health Study of 22,071 male physicians, aspirin at a dose of 325 mg every other day, compared with placebo, resulted in a 54% risk reduction in the subsequent need for peripheral arterial surgery.[203] Based on these findings, aspirin has been recommended as antiplatelet therapy in patients with PAD by groups such as the American College of Chest Physicians[204] and the TransAtlantic Inter-Society Consensus.[25] The efficacy of aspirin therapy in the primary prevention of cardiovascular events in patients with asymptomatic PAD has yet to be demonstrated. In fact, a recent randomized controlled trial of 3350 patients without evidence of cardiovascular disease and an ABI below 0.95 showed no difference in myocardial infarction, stroke rate, or all-cause mortality between the aspirin-treated group and the control group.[205]

Thienopyridines

Drugs in this class include ticlopidine, prasugrel, and clopidogrel. These agents block the adenosine diphosphate (ADP)-dependent aggregation of platelets through inhibition of the $P2Y_{12}$ receptor. No reversal agents are currently available for these agents in the event of acute bleeding episodes.

Ticlopidine. Ticlopidine has been shown to significantly lower the risk of ischemic cardiovascular events, including stroke and fatal and nonfatal myocardial infarction.[206] Ticlopidine compared with placebo also decreases the need for lower extremity revascularization procedures in patients with PAD.[207] However, ticlopidine is infrequently utilized because of rare but severe hematologic side effects including thrombotic thrombocytopenic purpura, thrombocytopenia, and neutropenia.[208]

Prasugrel. Much of the available evidence for this medication is in the cardiology literature, with many comparisons between prasugrel and clopidogrel. The TRial to assess Improvement in Therapeutic Outcomes by optimizing platelet inhibitioN with Prasugrel-Thrombolysis in Myocardial Infarction (TRITON-TIMI) 38 was a phase 3 trial in patients with acute coronary syndrome. Prasugrel was associated with fewer ischemic events than clopidogrel; however, it also led to higher rates of major bleeding. Overall mortality was the same for both groups.[209] A murine model of hindlimb ischemia treated with prasugrel demonstrated gradual recovery of blood flow and gait abnormalities after femoral artery injury.[210]

Clopidogrel. The most extensively studied medication of this class in reference to PAD is clopidogrel. In the Clopidogrel versus Aspirin in Patients at Risk of Ischemic Events (CAPRIE) trial, 19,185 patients with recent stroke, myocardial infarction, or stable PAD were randomized to receive clopidogrel (75 mg daily) or aspirin (325 mg daily).[128] There was a significant relative risk reduction of 8.7% ($P = .04$) for subsequent cardiovascular events (myocardial infarction, ischemic stroke, or vascular death) in the patients treated with clopidogrel. In the subgroup of more than 6000 patients with PAD, the relative risk reduction was even greater, at 24%.

The safety profiles of aspirin and clopidogrel were comparable in the CAPRIE study. Clopidogrel and ticlodipine have similar antiplatelet effects, but clopidogrel is associated with fewer hematologic side effects. The risk of thrombotic thrombocytopenic purpura in patients taking clopidogrel is estimated at 4 per 1 million population, so routine hematologic monitoring is not considered necessary.[211]

Exercise Therapy

Patients with intermittent claudication typically reduce their walking in response to their exercise-induced leg pain, leaving some severely affected individuals essentially housebound. Patients may believe that the pain manifested as claudication indicates injury and therefore avoid walking to prevent perceived adverse consequences. Contrary to that belief, exercise therapy is the best documented noninvasive therapy in the treatment of claudication and is an essential component of nonoperative management. Regular walking results in a measurable improvement in maximal and pain-free walking distance as well as community-based functional capacity in most patients with intermittent claudication.[212-215] The major limitation of exercise therapy is the presence of associated medical conditions that limit the ability to exercise. Initial evaluation includes functional assessment followed by exercise to determine pain-free and maximal walking distances. Success is defined as improvement in pain-free and maximal walking distances, improvement in scores on quality-of-life questionnaires, or both.

Exercise programs can increase walking distances from 80% to 234%.[212,213] A meta-analysis of supervised exercise programs found a mean increase of 179% in the distance that patients can ambulate prior to claudication and a mean increase of 122% in maximal walking distance.[214] Most studies show that supervised exercise is more effective than unsupervised exercise in improving maximal walking distance and the distance prior to onset of claudication.[215,216] However, home-based and physician-recommended programs are also of benefit. Use of a step-activity monitor in an unsupervised setting can be as effective in increasing peak walking time and claudication onset time as supervised exercise therapy.[217] Further research by this group directly compared 12 weeks of a step-watch home-exercise program, supervised exercise program, and a control group. The home and supervised exercise groups both had significant gains in all ambulation indices; however, only the home-exercise group demonstrated significant improvements in large artery elasticity index and high-sensitivity C-reactive protein (hsCRP) levels. The home-exercise group also had low attrition and an 81% adherence rate.[218]

The optimal frequencies and durations of exercise as therapy for intermittent claudication are unclear, but significant benefits in claudication symptoms are detectable with supervised exercise for 30 to 60 minutes 2 or 3 days a week.[219] Surgical intervention may be more effective than exercise in some patients; however, the economic burden, attendant morbidities, and potential mortality must be considered.[220]

The mechanism by which walking exercise improves symptoms of claudication is not completely understood. Neither ankle blood pressure nor calf muscle blood flow are objectively improved in claudicants with improved walking tolerance after an exercise program.[213,217-221] Elevated levels of proangiogenic vascular endothelial growth factor have been detected in exercised muscle.[222] The current belief is that adaptation of the muscle cells, likely by enzyme induction, to the relatively decreased oxygen delivery in an ischemic limb is largely responsible for the improved muscle performance seen with exercise training.[223] Other possible mechanisms include improved hemorheologic blood cell characteristics, changes in gait with more efficient use of muscle groups, better fatty acid metabolism, and an increased ratio of muscle fibers to capillaries after regular exercise.[222-225]

Pharmacologic Therapy

Intermittent Claudication

Pharmacologic therapy should also be considered and is occasionally useful in improving symptoms. A number of drug classes—including vasodilators, hemorheologic agents, prostaglandins, antiplatelet agents, and anticoagulants—have been studied in recent years for the treatment of claudication symptoms. Two drugs, pentoxifylline and cilostazol, have been approved by the US Food and Drug Administration for the treatment of patients with intermittent claudication.

Pentoxifylline. Patients with chronic lower extremity ischemia have abnormal hemorheology. Blood from patients with claudication demonstrates reduced flow rates through filters with uniform pore size.[225] Multiple studies have demonstrated decreased erythrocyte and leukocyte deformability, increased platelet aggregation, increased leukocyte and platelet adhesion, and increased blood viscosity in patients with chronic lower extremity ischemia.[226,227] Pentoxifylline is a hemorheologic agent that decreases blood viscosity and platelet aggregation and improves red blood cell flexibility. A modest improvement in claudication symptoms can be anticipated in some patients treated with pentoxifylline[227,228]; however, fewer than 10% of patients demonstrate improved walking distances greater than 100%. Patients with ABIs less than 0.80 and symptoms of less than 1 year's duration appear to experience the most benefit. The most common side effects are gastrointestinal complaints and headaches.

Cilostazol. Cilostazol is a phosphodiesterase inhibitor that has many possible mechanisms of action, including vasodilatation, inhibition of platelet aggregation and smooth muscle proliferation, and improvement of lipid profile. Randomized multicenter placebo-controlled trials have demonstrated the superiority of cilostazol over placebo in improving initial and absolute claudication distances in patients with intermittent claudication.[229-232] These trials demonstrated improvements in initial claudication distance of 35% to 59% and absolute claudication distance of 41% to 51% after 12 to 24 weeks of treatment with cilostazol versus placebo. These positive effects disappear after discontinuation of the drug.[233] The usual dose of cilostazol is 100 mg orally twice a day.

One randomized prospective trial comparing pentoxifylline to cilostazol demonstrated significantly greater improvement in walking distance in patients receiving cilostazol versus pentoxifylline or placebo.[234] In 54 centers, 698 patients were randomized to receive pentoxifylline ($n = 232$), cilostazol ($n = 227$), or placebo ($n = 239$). After 24 weeks of treatment, mean maximal walking distance in patients receiving cilostazol increased by 107 m, compared with 64 m in patients receiving pentoxifylline and 65 m in those receiving placebo. Quality-of-life assessments using Medical Outcome Study SF-36 questionnaires also demonstrated the efficacy of cilostazol. Side effects include headache, diarrhea, and dizziness.

Other pharmacologic agents. A number of additional pharmacologic agents have been investigated in the treatment of intermittent claudication. Although each has exhibited some benefit in limited, small trials, none has proved efficacious in large randomized trials.

Naftidrofuryl. Naftidrofuryl is a vasoactive drug frequently used for intermittent claudication in Europe but not available in the United States. Naftidrofuryl is a serotonin antagonist that improves aerobic metabolism in oxygen-depleted tissues (via stimulation of carbohydrate and fat entry into the tricarboxylic acid cycle). It may also reduce both erythrocyte and platelet aggregation.[235] Systematic reviews of randomized controlled trials comparing naftidrofuryl with placebo revealed modest but statistically significant increases in both pain-free walking distance and total walking distance. Treatment with naftidrofuryl does not change ABI.[236]

Carnitine. Intermittent claudication is the result of blood flow abnormalities to the lower extremities and metabolic abnormalities in skeletal muscle. Carnitine metabolism has been shown to be abnormal in patients with intermittent claudication; they have an accumulation of acylcarnitines (intermediates of oxidative metabolism) in skeletal muscle that inhibits the transport of free fatty acids into the mitochondria.[237] Treatment of such patients with carnitine analogs (L-carnitine or propionyl L-carnitine) has resulted in significant improvements in treadmill walking distance and quality of life compared with placebo[238-240]; however, carnitine is not approved for PAD treatment in the United States.The amount of acylcarnitine in muscle corresponds to the degree of walking impairment. This has led to the hypothesis that carnitine supplementation acts by improving muscle performance. Possible biochemical mechanisms of action include promoting pyruvate entry into the citric acid cycle and facilitating the transport of free fatty acids into the mitochondria.

Prostaglandin analogs. Prostaglandin analogs (synthetic prostaglandin E_1 and prostaglandin I_2, or prostacyclin) are potent vasodilators that also inhibit platelet aggregation.[241] Prostaglandins have been evaluated primarily for the treatment of critical limb ischemia with fewer trials performed in patients with claudication. Intravenous prostaglandin E_1 was evaluated in two randomized controlled trials that demonstrated significant improvements in maximal walking distance (371% increase in absolute claudication distance) and quality of life compared with placebo.[242,243] Side effects include frequent vasoactive flushing and headache.

Because intravenous preparations are not practical for widespread use in patients with intermittent claudication, oral prostaglandin analogs have been developed. Beraprost sodium is an oral prostacyclin analog with vasodilatory and antiplatelet effects. A European trial suggested that beraprost increased walking distance in claudicants.[244] However, a large trial in the United States failed to show any statistical benefit.[245]

Vasodilators. Vasodilator drugs were the first class of drugs used to treat intermittent claudication. Examples include α-blockers, calcium channel blockers, and direct-acting vasodilators such as papaverine. Controlled trials, however, indicate that vasodilators have no efficacy in treating intermittent claudication.[246] One explanation is that ischemic muscle beds are already maximally vasodilated during exercise, so vasodilators may not augment arterial flow in muscle beds distal to stenosis and may cause vasodilatation of nonischemic muscle beds, creating a "steal" phenomenon that takes blood away from ischemic tissue.

Anticoagulants. Anticoagulants (heparin, low-molecular-weight heparin, oral anticoagulants) result in no significant improvement in either pain-free or maximal walking distances. An increased risk of bleeding has been noted with these agents. Anticoagulants are not indicated for the treatment of intermittent claudication.[247]

Buflomedil. Buflomedil, a vasoactive hemorheologic agent, has been used for the treatment of intermittent claudication in Europe for many years, despite scant clinical evidence demonstrating efficacy. Blufomedil reduces vasoconstriction through both α_1 and α_2 adrenolysis. Although modest improvements in walking distance have been reported, the data are not strong enough to support recommending this medication for the treatment of intermittent claudication. It is not available in the United States.[248]

L-Arginine. L-Arginine is an amino acid that has been demonstrated to enhance nitric oxide formation and endothelium-dependent vasodilatation in patients with atherosclerosis. Two small trials demonstrated improvements in initial and absolute claudication distances, but larger trials are needed to define the role of L-arginine in the treatment of claudication.[249,250]

Critical Limb Ischemia

The mainstay of treatment for chronic CLI is either surgical or endovascular revascularization; however, this is not always required when the only manifestations are intermittent rest pain or shallow ulcers. The natural history of intermittent rest pain is not necessarily one of inevitable progression to gangrene and limb loss. This was clearly shown in randomized controlled trials of prostaglandin treatment in patients with CLI, in which approximately 50% of patients with rest pain or ulcers improved on placebo.[136,251] Patients who refuse surgery or are not surgical candidates (owing to severe comorbidities or lack of target vessels, small ulcers, or rest pain) can sometimes improve without revascularization.

Novel nonoperative therapies for CLI have focused on three main areas: intermittent pneumatic compression (IPC) devices, stem cell therapy, and gene-directed therapy. Intermittent pneumatic compression devices aim to increase blood flow to ischemic limbs by increasing the arteriovenous pressure gradient of the limb. Hemodynamic improvement of limbs with CLI has been demonstrated with the use of IPC devices.[252] There are randomized controlled trials demonstrating improved ABI, claudication distance, and quality of life in stable claudicants randomized to IPC therapy compared with controls[253]; however, there are no randomized trials of IPC therapy for limb salvage in patients with CLI.

Stem cell therapy arose from the discovery that a subset of bone marrow–derived mononuclear cells are able to differentiate into endothelium and thus to promote new vessel growth. Currently progenitor cells can be obtained from bone marrow aspiration or peripheral blood apheresis. These progenitor cells are then delivered to the ischemic limb via intra-arterial or intramuscular injection. A meta-analysis of more than 701 patients treated with stem cell therapy showed significant benefit in ABI, transcutaneous partial pressure of oxygen (TCO_2), pain-free walking distance, pain scale, ulcer healing, and amputation rates.[254] Intramuscular administration appears to be superior to intra-arterial administration, but the preference of bone marrow– versus peripheral blood–derived stem cells is controversial.

Gene-induced angiogenesis introduces angiogenic genes or gene products into an area of ischemia using gene transfer approaches and viral and plasmid vectors. Trials of the angiogenic potential of stem cells and the utilization of vascular endothelial growth factor (VEGF), fibroblast growth factor (FGF), hepatocyte growth factor, and the *DEL1* gene have been reported.[255,256] A meta-analysis identified one trial of gene therapy (using basic fibroblast growth factor) that reported clinical benefit. All other trials and the pooled data showed no benefit in patients with claudication or CLI when only gene therapy trials were included.[257]

CONCLUSION

An understanding of the natural history of lower extremity PAD is important for patient education and management. Patients with peripheral vascular disease often have concomitant atherosclerotic disease affecting other vascular beds. Appropriate nonoperative management of patients with chronic lower extremity ischemia is complex. Risk factor modification is aimed at preventing both disease progression and adverse cardiovascular events. Intermittent claudication usually confers a low risk of limb loss, and initial treatment is generally nonoperative with a trial of exercise and pharmacologic therapy. The risk of limb loss is greater in patients with CLI, and patients with CLI generally require surgical or endovascular revascularization. Newer treatments including gene and progenitor cell–derived therapies are emerging, but there is limited evidence for their use.

REVIEW QUESTIONS

1. An abnormal ABI is present in approximately what percentage of patients older than 50 years?
   - a. 1%
   - b. 2%
   - c. 15%
   - d. 25%
   - e. 35%
2. What is the increased risk of developing peripheral arterial disease in current smokers versus those who have never smoked?
   - a. Two times
   - b. Four times
   - c. Six times
   - d. Sixteen times
   - e. Thirty-two times
3. What disease process leads to the most nontraumatic amputations in the United States?
   - a. Diabetes
   - b. Buerger disease
   - c. Tobacco abuse
   - d. Obesity
   - e. Connective tissue disorders
4. What is the prevalence of peripheral arterial disease in women versus that in men?
   - a. 10% that in men
   - b. 50% that in men
   - c. 75% that in men
   - d. Equal to that in men
   - e. 150% that in men
5. The relative risk of a patient with intermittent claudication having a myocardial infarction or stroke compared with a nonclaudicant is increased by what factor?
   - a. One to two times
   - b. Two to three times
   - c. Four to five times
   - d. Six to eight times
   - e. Ten times
6. What proportion of patients undergoing amputation for ischemia experienced ischemic symptoms 6 months before the amputation?
   - a. Less than 50%
   - b. 60% to 70%
   - c. 70% to 80%
   - d. 80% to 90%
   - e. 100%
7. The relative risk reduction for myocardial infarction, ischemic stroke, or vascular death in patients with peripheral arterial disease managed with clopidogrel versus aspirin is approximately which of the following?
   - a. 5%
   - b. 10%
   - c. 15%
   - d. 20%
   - e. 25%
8. The most likely mechanism by which exercise therapy improves walking distance in patients with intermittent claudication is which of the following?
   - a. Increase in ankle-brachial index
   - b. Muscle cell adaptation to decreased oxygen delivery
   - c. Increased collateral formation
   - d. Improved cardiac output
   - e. Improved blood hemorheology
9. Which of the following is currently the most effective drug available in the United States for improving walking distance in patients with peripheral arterial disease and intermittent claudication?
   - a. Cilostazol
   - b. Pentoxifylline
   - c. Warfarin
   - d. Aspirin
   - e. Carnitine
10. Which of the following is a contraindication to the use of cilostazol for the treatment of intermittent claudication?
    - a. Congestive heart failure
    - b. Walking distance less than 100 feet
    - c. CYP 3A inhibitors
    - d. Warfarin therapy
    - e. Use of β-blockers

BIBLIOGRAPHY

Beebe HG, Dawson DL, Cutler BS, et al. A new pharmacological treatment for intermittent claudication: results of a randomized, multicenter trial. *Arch Intern Med.* 1999;159:2041–2050.

CAPRIE Steering Committee: A randomised, blinded, trial of clopidogrel versus aspirin in patients at risk of ischaemic events (CAPRIE): CAPRIE Steering Committee. *Lancet.* 1996;348:1329–1339.

Criqui MH, Langer RD, Fronek A, et al. Mortality over a period of 10 years in patients with peripheral arterial disease. *N Engl J Med.* 1992;326:381–386.

De Haro J, Acin F, Lopez-Quintana A, et al. Meta-analysis of randomized, controlled clinical trials in angiogenesis: gene and cell therapy in peripheral arterial disease. *Heart Vessels.* 2009;24: 321–328.

Fowkes G, Price J, Stewart M, et al. Aspirin for prevention of cardiovascular events in a general population screened for a low ankle brachial index. *JAMA.* 2010;303:841–848.

Fowl RJ, Gewirtz RJ, Love MC, et al. Natural history of claudicants with critical hemodynamic indices. *Ann Vasc Surg.* 1992;6:31–33.

Gardner AW, Parker DE, Montgomery MS, et al. Step-monitored home exercise improves ambualtion, vascular function, and inflammation in symptomatic patients with peripheral artery disease: a randomized controlled trial. *J Am Heart Assoc.* 2014;3: 1–11.

Hennrikus D, Joseph A, Lando H, et al. Effectiveness of a smoking cessation program for peripheral artery disease patients. *J Am Coll Cardiol.* 2010;56:2105–2112.

Mills JL Sr, Conte MS, Armstrong DG, et al. The Society for Vascular Surgery Lower Extremity Threatened Limb Classification System: risk stratification based on wound, ischemia, and foot infection (WIfI). *J Vasc Surg.* 2014;59:220–234.

Murabito JM, D'Agostino RB, Silbershatz H, et al. Intermittent claudication: a risk profile from the Framingham Heart Study. *Circulation.* 1997;96:44–49.

Stone NJ, Robinson JG, Lichtenstein AH, et al. 2013 ACC/AHA guidelines on the treatment of blood cholesterol to reduce atherosclerotic cardiovascular risk in adults: a report of the American College of Cardiology/American Heart Association task force on practice guidelines. *J Am Coll Cardiol.* 2014;63: 2889–2934.

References available online at ExpertConsult.com.

35 CHAPTER

Thrombolysis for Arterial and Graft Occlusions: Technique and Results

Gener Augustin, William J. Quiñones-Baldrich, Vikram Kashyap

Thrombolytic therapy is an important modality in the treatment of patients with peripheral arterial and venous thrombosis. Randomized clinical trials have compared thrombolytic therapy with traditional surgical options, thus providing guidelines for patient selection. As a therapeutic intervention, lytic therapy may be the best alternative in certain clinical situations. In many other cases, it is just one aspect of the overall care of patients with thrombotic complications of peripheral vascular disease.

This chapter provides an overview of the fibrinolytic system and the available agents. This information can be translated into guidelines to help clinicians select patients who may benefit from thrombolytic therapy. Methods, dosages, complications, and promising new areas are also discussed.

HISTORY

The fluidity of blood post mortem is an observation that dates to the Hippocratic school in the 4th century BC.[1] Almost 2000 years later, it was rediscovered by the Italian anatomist Malpighi.[2] In 1761 Morgagni noted that blood does not retain its liquid state after death but frequently forms clots.[3] This is followed by partial or complete reliquefaction.

In 1906 Morawitz observed that postmortem blood destroys fibrinogen and fibrin in normal blood.[4] Thus the presence of an active fibrinolysin was postulated. The term *fibrinolysis* had been coined by Dastre in 1893 to describe the disappearance of fibrin in unclottable blood obtained from dogs subjected to repeated hemorrhage.[5] From the latter part of the 19th century until the present, intense investigation has been undertaken to elucidate the complex and vital functions of the fibrinolytic system. Charles Dotter was the first to describe intraarterial drug delivery into thrombus for thrombolysis.[5a] The role of the fibrinolytic system from a homeostatic point of view is fully appreciated. The interplay of components, activators, and inhibitors are becoming more appreciated. The potential to harness the fibrinolytic system for therapeutic means has emerged in the past few decades, and results from prospective clinical trials are now available, providing guidelines to patient selection and therapy. For the vascular specialist, thrombolytic therapy represents one of the most promising therapeutic modalities for arterial and venous thrombosis, but careful dosing and monitoring of thrombolytic therapy are required. In addition, careful attention and observation of the patient, renal dysfunction, systemic effects, and often the limb undergoing treatment are required.

FIBRINOLYTIC SYSTEM

The complex and intricate relationships among all components of the fibrinolytic system are only partially understood. However, much progress has been made, mostly owing to recognition of the importance of the fibrinolytic system as a homeostatic system. This same process has been harnessed for a therapeutic effect in cases of clinical thrombosis. The concept of dynamic equilibrium was proposed by Astrup in 1958.[6] In a delicate balance, fibrinolysis breaks down fibrin, which is continuously being deposited throughout the cardiovascular system. This is the result of limited activation of the coagulation system. This baseline fibrinolytic activity is probably under local and central control mechanisms. The feedback loop that prevents systemic fibrinolysis involves both inhibitors at the activator level and specific inhibitors of the proteolytic enzyme plasmin.

The final common pathway in the fibrinolytic system is the conversion of the proenzyme plasminogen to the active enzyme plasmin. Plasminogen is a glycoprotein produced by the liver. Full-sized plasminogen can be divided into a heavy N-terminal region that consists of five homologous but distinct triple-disulfide–bonded domains (kringles) fused to a lighter catalytic C-terminal domain. At least four forms occur in plasma, based on variations in the N-terminal and the degree of glycosylation. The two main forms are Glu-plasminogen and Lys-plasminogen.[7] Glu-plasminogen contains glutamic acid and exists in high concentrations in plasma. Lys-plasminogen, containing mostly lysin in the N-terminal, results from limited proteolysis of the Glu form; it has a shorter half-life and is found in higher concentrations in thrombus, most likely secondary to its higher affinity for fibrin.[8] A schematic view of the fibrinolytic system is presented in Fig. 35.1.

The kringle portion of plasminogen is a nonprotease, or heavy chain, consisting of five homologous domains. These domains exhibit a high degree of sequence homology with one another and with domains found in prothrombin, tissue plasminogen activator (t-PA), urinary plasminogen activator, and factor XII. Kringle-4 shares homology with apolipoprotein A. The function of these kringles is thought to be of paramount importance in the binding of plasminogen and plasmin to fibrin, α_2-antiplasmin, and other macromolecules.[9,10] In addition, the kringle portion of plasminogen has been implicated in mediating neutrophil adherence to endothelial cells.[11] On binding, conformational changes occur that transform a closed structure into an open

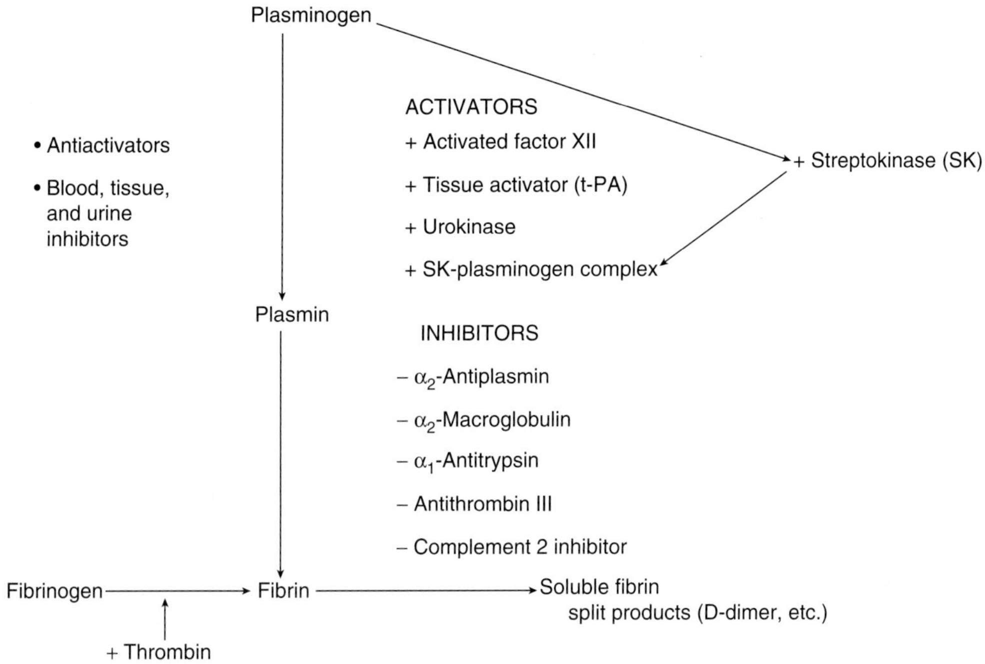

FIG 35.1 Simplified scheme of the fibrinolytic system with endogenous and exogenous activators.

structure. ε-Aminocaproic acid and tranexamic acid induce this change from the closed structure to the open structure. Because of this change, plasminogen is far more readily cleaved to the active enzyme plasmin by plasminogen activators. The open conformation also binds more readily to exposed lysine residues on fibrin's surface. Concentrations of lysine analogs, such as tranexamic acid and aminocaproic acid, that actually promote the more active, open conformation of Glu-plasminogen also prevent its binding to fibrin and therefore exhibit an antifibrinolytic effect.[12]

The primary substrates for the proteolytic activity of plasmin in circulation are fibrinogen and fibrin. Circulating fibrinogen is composed of three polypeptide chains known as the α, β, and γ chains. These chains are bonded together by disulfide bonds, which are also linked to a second identical chain, thus making fibrinogen a dimer of trimers. Thrombin, the common pathway of the coagulation cascade, removes several amino acid peptides from the end terminal of the α chain, the β chain (fibrinopeptide B), to form fibrin. As new sites are exposed, staggered polymerization is initiated.[7] Through catalysis by factor XIIIa, the domains are brought together and chemically cross-linked. Plasmin catalyzes the hydrolysis of these bonds, producing peptides that can be assayed in circulation. Specifically, those produced after the cleavage of fibrinogen consist of truncated polypeptides collectively known as *X fragments*. X fragments can be incorporated into both newly forming and existing thrombi, causing them to be more fragile. This has been proposed as a possible explanation of why fibrin-specific fibrinolytic agents such as t-PA do not result in fewer bleeding complications compared with nonspecific agents. Because t-PA is such a potent fibrinolytic activator, the accumulation of these X fragments could make existing thrombi more susceptible to its fibrinolytic action. Several fragments are specifically produced by the action of plasmin on fibrin, as opposed to fibrinogen. Unique fragments such as D-dimers can be assayed, documenting fibrinolysis as opposed to fibrinogenolysis.[13]

Plasmin is a relatively nonspecific protease and thus can hydrolyze many proteins found in plasma and extracellular spaces. Known targets of plasmin are factors V and VIII and von Willebrand factor.[1] Prothrombotic activity can be shown with the initial administration of fibrinolytic agents (specifically t-PA and streptokinase, which may relate to the release of fibrinopeptide A). Plasminogen can also cause the release of kinin from high-molecular-weight kininogen. In addition, it can directly and indirectly activate prekallikrein, again inducing kinin formation.[14,15] Plasmin can also attack protein components of the basement membrane, as well as other active proteases within the matrix, including fibronectin, collagen, and laminin.[7]

Activation of factor XII by various stimuli results in initiation of the coagulation cascade, conversion of prekallikrein to kallikrein and kinin (inflammatory response), and formation of plasmin from plasminogen. This intrinsic mechanism of activation is complemented by a second intrinsic pathway that is not dependent on factor XII. The main pathway for plasminogen activation is known as the extrinsic system. Two activators are recognized in humans: urokinase-type plasminogen activator (u-PA) and t-PA. Their physiologic activity is controlled by inhibitors, mostly plasminogen activator inhibitor (PAI) type 1 (PAI-1) and type PAI-3. These inhibitors control the activity of the activators in plasma and possibly at the cellular level. PAI-1 is synthesized in the liver and vascular endothelial cells and is normally present in trace amounts in plasma. PAI-1 elevation leading to prothrombotic states is becoming increasingly recognized. When pharmacologic dosages of these agents are administered, the inhibitor activity is suppressed. It is estimated that one-third to one-half of the initial pharmacologic dosage of urokinase, for example, becomes inactivated shortly after administration.[11] Once plasminogen has been converted to plasmin, inhibitors of plasmin come into play. The main physiologic inhibitor of plasmin is α_2-antiplasmin. This protease inhibitor is a single-chain glycoprotein that inhibits plasminogen in two steps: a fast reversible binding step, followed by the formation of a covalent complex involving the active site of plasmin.[7] The half-life of this complex is approximately 12 hours.[16] Other inhibitors of plasmin include α_2-macroglobulin, protease nexin, and aprotinin.

This complex system is capable of maintaining a balanced equilibrium between clotting and lysis, so that blood fluidity is ensured. It is important to recognize that although plasmin is highly selective for fibrin, it also digests fibrinogen and other plasma proteins. Circulating plasmin inhibitors prevent this otherwise disordered lytic action and preclude free circulating plasmin under normal conditions.

A link between lipoprotein metabolism and fibrinolytic function has been suggested by the demonstration of significant homology between the amino acid sequence of apolipoprotein A and the structure of plasminogen. Thus a prothrombotic function by virtue of interference with the numerous physiologic functions of plasminogen has been suggested in patients with increased levels of apolipoprotein A. Apolipoprotein A has also been found to competitively inhibit the binding of plasminogen to fibrinogen and to the plasminogen receptor on endothelial cells.[26]

Plasma levels of both t-PA and PAI-1 exhibit circadian variations. For example, t-PA activity is lowest in the early morning and highest in the afternoon. Plasma PAI activity peaks in the early morning and passes through a trough in the afternoon. Thus overall there is decreased fibrinolytic activity in the morning.[27-30] Differences in patterns have been observed between men and women, suggesting a hormonal influence.[31] Furthermore, PAI activity has been noted to vary secondary to diet, with caffeine-containing beverages possibly enhancing fibrinolytic activity. Conversely, cigarette smoking induces an acute increase in t-PA; this increase in t-PA may deplete normal stores and thus paradoxically decrease fibrinolytic capacity.

From the foregoing discussion, it is evident that the fibrinolytic (plasminogen-plasmin) system plays a vital role in biological homeostasis. In addition, it has a pivotal role in certain disease states, ranging from atherosclerosis to carcinogenesis.

From a therapeutic standpoint, drugs capable of converting plasminogen to plasmin achieve their lytic effect to a great extent by overwhelming circulating plasmin inhibitors and generating an abundance of plasmin (exogenous fibrinolysis). Circulating plasmin not only produces the desired fibrinolysis but also proceeds to digest circulating fibrinogen. A more desirable situation results in the activation of thrombus-bound plasminogen (endogenous fibrinolysis) by these agents. Thrombus-bound plasminogen is, to a certain extent, protected from circulating inhibitors and thus proceeds with fibrin digestion much more effectively. Current investigations are concentrated on producing agents with a high affinity for thrombus-bound plasminogen and little activation of the circulating zymogen. Clinical experience to date has failed to demonstrate this theoretical benefit. With better understanding of the complexity of the fibrinolytic system, it is possible that these benefits can be realized.

THROMBOLYTIC AGENTS

The use of thrombolytic agents has clearly resulted in a significant improvement in the outcome of patients with acute cardiac ischemia, myocardial infarction, and cerebral infarction. It has also resulted in a modification in the treatment algorithm for patients with peripheral arterial occlusion. Thrombolytic therapy is an important treatment option for patients with vascular occlusive disease. Table 35.1 summarizes the characteristics of some of the common thrombolytic agents. Several schemes may be used to classify thrombolytic agents. The agents can be grouped by their mechanism of action—those that directly convert plasminogen to plasmin versus those that are inactive zymogens and require transformation to an active form before they can cleave plasminogen. Agents can be classified by their mode of production. In addition, thrombolytic agents can be classified by their pharmacologic actions—those that are fibrin specific (i.e., bind to fibrin but not to fibrinogen) versus those that are nonspecific, and those that have a great degree of fibrin affinity (i.e., bind

TABLE 35.1 Thrombolytic Agents

Characteristics	Streptokinase	Urokinase	Tissue Plasminogen Activator	Reteplase
Source	β-Hemolytic *Streptococcus*	Fetal renal cell culture	Recombinant DNA technology	Plasminogen activator
Metabolism	Liver	Liver	Liver	Liver
Advantages	Low cost	Direct activator; no allergic reaction	Fibrin-selective direct activator	Plasminogen activator in presence of fibrin
Disadvantages	Allergic reactions; complex mechanism of action	High cost	High cost	High cost
Regional infusion dosage	Low dose: 5000–10,000 units/h High dose: 30,000–60,000 units/h	30,000–50,000 units/h 2000–4000 units/min for 1–2 h, then 1000–2000 units/min	0.05–0.1 units/kg per hour	0.5 units/h IV; no bolus Rate may be adjusted up to 0.75–1.0 units/h or down to 0.25 units/h

IV, Intravenously.

avidly to fibrin) versus those that do not. Another useful classification of thrombolytic agents is groups based on their origin: the streptokinase compounds, the urokinase compounds, the t-PAs, and an additional group consisting of novel agents. In the following sections, we have divided thrombolytic drugs chronologically.

First-Generation Thrombolytic Drugs

First-generation thrombolytic agents—namely, streptokinase and urokinase—are highly effective at thrombolysis, but their potency is limited by the fact that they are not fibrin specific. They also convert circulating plasminogen to plasmin, but because circulating plasminogen and the plasminogen in thrombus are in equilibrium, the plasminogen in thrombus would be depleted, thus limiting the efficacy of the agent. This has been termed *plasminogen steal* and is thought to reduce clot lysis.

Streptokinase

Streptokinase is a single-chain nonenzymatic protein produced by β-hemolytic streptococci. Its discovery by Tillett and Garner[32] in 1933 revived an interest in fibrinolysis that has spanned the past 7 decades. Early clinical experience was complicated by a multitude of pyogenic and allergic reactions. This prompted manufacturers to refine the drug, achieving the currently purified product and a marked reduction in febrile and allergic reactions.

The mechanism of action of streptokinase is complex. It initially forms an equimolar complex with plasminogen to form a plasminogen activator. Thus it requires plasminogen as a cofactor and a substrate. Once the activator complex is formed, it is an excellent activator of all mammalian plasminogen. Besides converting uncomplexed plasminogen to plasmin, plasminogen within the activator complex is converted to plasmin, and during this conversion, streptokinase undergoes rapid progressive degradation.

The kinetics of these reactions have been studied in vitro. In vivo a more complicated series of reactions occurs. Infusion of streptokinase is followed initially by neutralization by circulating antistreptococcal antibodies. The remaining drug then combines with circulating plasminogen to form the activator complex. This then converts uncomplexed plasminogen to plasmin, which combines with any excess free streptokinase, is neutralized by circulating antiplasmins, or binds to preformed fibrin. The last produces the desired effect of thrombolysis. However, when activity is measured, two half-lives are detected—16 minutes and 83 minutes—indicating that these complex interactions have a significant effect on the concentration and activity of the drug.

From the foregoing discussion, it is evident that precise control of thrombolysis is not possible because the dose-response relationship of streptokinase varies from patient to patient. Initially, clinical use was guided by titers of antistreptococcal antibodies and measurement of the various components or products of the system. This proved impractical, and current practice relies on standardized dosages that achieve the desired effect in the great majority of cases. A potential drawback of this approach is that excess amounts of drug could use most of the circulating plasminogen to form activator complex; this might leave inadequate amounts of zymogen to convert to plasmin. This problem of exceeding plasminogen availability may be important during regional, rather than systemic, administration. Some investigators have combined streptokinase with plasmin administration, resulting in improvements in measured parameters such as plasminogen level, fibrinogen level, and potential fibrinolytic capacity.[33] Similar results are obtained by intermittent rather than continuous infusion of the drug. Unfortunately, the results of these noncontrolled trials have raised doubts about the effectiveness of such regimens. Streptokinase has largely fallen out of favor, partly because of the immunogenicity of even the refined form, which can result in fever, allergic reactions, and acquired drug resistance.

Streptokinase is the only thrombolytic agent approved by the US Food and Drug Administration (FDA) for use in peripheral arterial and venous thrombolysis, but it is rare to find it being used for that purpose, for the reasons stated earlier. The newer thrombolytic agents have much better safety profiles and better therapeutic efficacy; therefore off-label use of these alternative thrombolytic agents is the norm.

Urokinase

Urokinase is a serine protease with direct activator activity; it is normally present in urine as a product of renal tubular cells. It was originally isolated by MacFarlane and Pilling in 1947.[34] Urokinase is present in varying molecular weights, with variable activity. Original purification was done from urine, yielding small amounts of the enzyme at a considerable cost. Newer production methods use human fetal kidney cell culture.

Urokinase is nonantigenic, and its mechanism of action is much more direct compared with that of streptokinase. Urokinase cleaves plasminogen (its only known protein substrate), by first-order reaction kinetics, to plasmin. It is pH and temperature stable. The lack of circulating neutralizing antibodies and its direct mechanism of action allow for a predictable dose-response relationship. Although allergic reactions are rare, over the past few years a febrile response to drug administration has become more common. It has been suggested that this may be related to interleukins that are still present in recently manufactured drug batches. In the past, when the use of urokinase was less common, aging of the drug actually allowed the interleukins to become inactive. These febrile reactions respond readily to antipyretics. Interestingly, urokinase does not contain any lysine-binding sites and therefore does not have any fibrin-binding properties.[35] However, high-affinity receptors for urokinase have been demonstrated in several cell types and have been postulated as a mechanism by which cells can invade the intracellular matrix and play a role in other physiologic and pathologic processes.[36-38]

Urokinase is a serine protease and hydrolyzes synthetic esters containing arginine and lysine. Unlike streptokinase, urokinase directly activates plasminogen by cleaving the Arg560-Val561 activation bond. The activation of plasminogen by urokinase occurs by proteolysis. When administered intravenously, urokinase is rapidly removed from the circulation, mainly via hepatic clearance. It has been estimated that the half-life of urokinase in humans is on the order of 14 minutes. Urokinase also reacts with other proteins, including fibrinogen. Urokinase is much more effective in cleaving the susceptible site in plasminogen when it is in the Lys form than in the Glu form. However, the activation reaction of the latter by urokinase may be enhanced by the presence of fibrin.[39] Administration of exogenous plasminogen may also accelerate thrombolysis by urokinase.

Controversy exists regarding the actual thrombolytic effect of urokinase when administered in vivo. Experimental studies have suggested exogenous fibrinolysis as the main pathway, with limited activation of plasminogen within the thrombus (endogenous fibrinolysis).[40] In clinical practice, the results of urokinase therapy have paralleled those achieved with streptokinase, with a decreased incidence of bleeding complications suggested by several investigators.[42-44] Although major bleeding complications are seen in 15% to 20% of patients treated with streptokinase, such complications have been reported in only 5% to 10% of patients treated with urokinase. Thus the benefits observed in laboratory results and the reduced incidence of significant plasminemia with urokinase seem to translate into a decreased incidence of bleeding complications in clinical practice. Although the cost of urokinase remains high compared with that of streptokinase, when complications are considered, the cost of therapy for streptokinase and urokinase is comparable.[45]

Residual thromboplastic activity was detected in the early urokinase preparations,[46] and this may account for the initial hypercoagulable state reported by Kakkar and Scully.[47] At present, this does not appear to be a clinically significant problem.

Despite the drug's record of safety and efficacy accrued over the years, the FDA halted the release and use of urokinase, manufactured by Abbott Laboratories (Chicago, IL), on the grounds of deviations from the FDA's current good manufacturing practices guidelines, developed to prevent the manufacture of unsafe products. The FDA inspection of Abbott's manufacturing facility in North Chicago in 1998 raised concerns about the neonatal kidney cells that were being used as a source of urokinase.[48,49] The cells originated from Cali, Colombia, and were obtained through a separate company. The source population was thought to be at high risk for various diseases, including tropical ones, although there were no documented cases of infectious transmission resulting from urokinase administration. The FDA stated that any connection between the drug and such cases might have gone unrecognized.

In October 2002 the FDA approved the reintroduction of urokinase to the market after Abbott made significant changes in its quality control and manufacturing practices. Urokinase was approved for use in the treatment of pulmonary embolism (PE). Although it has not been approved for use in the peripheral arterial and venous systems, many practitioners have experience with off-label use in the periphery. During the time that urokinase was unavailable, increased experience and familiarity were gained with other agents, such as recombinant tissue plasminogen activator (rt-PA) and reteplase.[50] Now, the use of urokinase in the United States has dwindled as most practitioners are using other agents.

Second-Generation Thrombolytic Drugs

Unlike first-generation thrombolytic drugs, second-generation agents are supposed to be fibrin selective. These agents were developed to avoid systemic depletion of circulating fibrinogen and plasminogen and the consequent systemic thrombolytic state; these agents are represented by t-PA, or alteplase, and single-chain u-PA, or pro-urokinase. There is considerable evidence that the plasminogen activator agents are not appreciably fibrin or thrombus specific and that they activate the complement system and damage the cell membranes of platelets and endothelial cells.

Tissue Plasminogen Activator

t-PA is a naturally occurring enzyme present in all human tissues. Its concentration is variable, with high levels detected in the uterus and moderate amounts in the heart, skeletal muscles, kidneys, ovaries, lungs, thyroid, pituitary, and lymph nodes. Scant amounts of t-PA are found in the liver, spleen, brain, and testes.[51] It is thought to originate from vascular endothelium, and, with the exception of the liver and spleen, tissue concentration correlates with vascularity.

Isolation and purification of t-PA were initially hampered by inadequate sources and procedures. In 1979 Rijken and associates[52] were successful in obtaining 1 mg of t-PA from 5 kg of human uterine tissue. Recognizing the potential of this drug, investigators have concentrated on other sources.

At present, there are two main sources of t-PA. The Bowes melanoma cell line is uniquely efficient in producing large quantities of t-PA,[53] which was subsequently proved to be identical to uterine t-PA.[54] Another source has emerged from the use of recombinant DNA technology, and efforts in the cloning and expression of the t-PA gene from the melanoma cell line have been successful. Since 1987, when rt-PA was approved for the treatment of acute myocardial infarction, it has been used for peripheral thrombolysis as an alternative to urokinase.

In general, plasminogen activators do not cause clot dissolution directly; they must first find and activate molecules of plasminogen in the vasculature at the site of the clot. t-PA is a direct plasminogen activator. Its main advantage is its high affinity for thrombus-bound fibrin. The agent exhibits significant fibrin specificity. t-PA is a poor enzyme in the absence of fibrin. However, the presence of fibrin strikingly enhances the activation rate of plasminogen by t-PA. Two types of t-PA are recognized, with a commercial preparation being a mixture of both types. A single-chain form is cleaved by plasminogen to yield two-chain t-PA. The one- and two-chain forms of t-PA are comparable in activity, with the one-chain form being quickly converted to the two-chain type as lysis proceeds. Most of the circulating t-PA is in the single-chain form. Its selective action promises to produce fewer systemic effects when compared with streptokinase or urokinase.[55] The half-life of t-PA has been estimated to be between 4 and 7 minutes in vivo.[56] With its presumed nonantigenicity and high affinity for fibrin, t-PA theoretically should produce improved clinical results.

When fibrin-selective agents are used for regional infusion, most of the thrombolytic effect is secondary to fibrin-bound plasminogen. However, the importance of a fresh supply of plasminogen to maintain the fibrin-bound plasminogen pool has been emphasized. Experimental studies have suggested that clot lysis induced by the activation of plasminogen is dependent on clot-associated plasminogen, which in turn depends on the concentration of plasminogen in plasma. Depletion of both contributes to less frequent and less rapid recanalization, which is more noticeable with non–fibrin-selective agents than with fibrin-selective ones, likely the result of the depletion of plasminogen induced by the nonselective agents.[57]

Trials comparing rt-PA with streptokinase in patients with acute coronary thrombosis have failed to establish that this more specific drug is a better thrombolytic agent. Systemic bleeding complications have been similar, despite a milder homeostatic defect by laboratory evaluation in the rt-PA groups.[58] Questions still exist regarding proper dosage to achieve effective local lysis with minimal systemic effects.

t-PA may also bind and be activated on platelet surfaces.[59] Owing to this binding to platelet receptors, platelets can direct t-PA action on their surface, leading to rapid cleavage of glycoprotein Ib and the loss of platelet binding to von Willebrand factor. This may explain why concentrations of t-PA achieved early in therapy may inhibit.

In a study in which 17 patients were infused with rt-PA at a rate of 0.1 mg/kg per hour, all patients demonstrated thrombolysis, with 16 showing clinical improvement.[61] More important, there were no systemic complications, with a mean fibrinogen drop of 42% of baseline. The infusion time was 1 to 6 hours, compared with the usual 48 to 72 hours necessary for streptokinase infusion. One patient died from an intracranial hemorrhage during postinfusion heparin therapy. Experience in randomized trials has suggested that a lower dosage is just as effective, with a decreased risk of bleeding. The recommended lower dose is 0.05 mg/kg per hour.[62]

Systemic complications may be more related to dosage and method of administration with t-PA than with urokinase or streptokinase. It appears that t-PA is more potent and faster than the older agents, perhaps because of its high fibrin affinity. In this regard, t-PA may be ideally suited for intraarterial administration, because a 4- to 6-hour trial could be followed by timely surgical intervention. In addition, intraoperative use could be a welcome adjunct to surgical embolectomy.

Pro-Urokinase

Saruplase, also known as recombinant single-chain u-PA, or pro-urokinase, is a prodrug produced from a naturally occurring physiologic protease.[62] Pro-urokinase is a single-chain polypeptide of 411 amino acids that is converted by plasmin into an active, low-molecular-weight form of urokinase with 276 amino acids.[63] Pro-urokinase functions as a potent plasminogen activator of fibrin-bound plasminogen without requiring extensive systemic conversion to two-chain urokinase. Thus the entire thrombolytic process is confined to the fibrin clot itself. Administration of pro-urokinase causes decreases in α_2-antiplasmin and fibrinogen and an increase in fibrinogen degradation products. Pro-urokinase is highly effective in the conversion of Lys-plasminogen to plasmin. In contrast, it has little or no activity in the conversion of Glu-plasminogen to plasmin. Because Lys-plasminogen is present in high concentrations in thrombus, this gives pro-urokinase fibrin-specific properties. In addition, plasminogen that is absorbed in thrombus changes its configuration to a pseudo–Lys-plasminogen, which is also attacked by pro-urokinase, converting it to Lys-plasmin. Circulating pro-urokinase is very stable in plasma because of its resistance to plasma inhibitors and ionized calcium.[64] The fibrin specificities of t-PA and pro-urokinase appear to rely on different mechanisms. Although t-PA is fibrin clot binding, the fibrin-selective properties of pro-urokinase are thought to be secondary to its preference for activation of Lys-plasminogen or Lys-like–plasminogen substrate found in thrombus. This effect prolongs half-life, which has been estimated to be several days. Such a prolonged half-life has theoretical advantages in clinical situations in which prolonged activity is desired. However, in peripheral arterial occlusions, if the regional infusion fails to produce the desired result and the patient must go to the operating room shortly after discontinuation of the infusion, this prolonged effect may be undesirable.

A recombinant form of pro-urokinase is Prolyse (Abbott Laboratories). This urokinase compound has the advantage of not originating in a human cell source. Many of the clinical trials using this drug have been studies of patients with myocardial infarction, where the notable finding was an increased incidence of intracranial hemorrhage (0.9%).[65] The most recent trial was the Prolyse in Acute Cerebral Thromboembolism II (PROACT II) study, which evaluated intraarterial prourokinase for acute ischemic stroke.[66] Early intracranial hemorrhage with neurologic deterioration within 24 hours occurred in 10% of pro-urokinase patients and 2% of control patients. Although pro-urokinase is effective at thrombolysis, the increased bleeding risk has limited its widespread use. A phase II trial evaluating pro-urokinase versus urokinase for thrombolysis of acute peripheral arterial occlusion showed that pro-urokinase had a greater efficacy but an increased risk of bleeding complications at a dose of 8 mg/h; with a dose of 2 mg/h, there was a slightly lower rate of thrombolysis, combined with a lower incidence of bleeding complications and fibrinogenolysis.[67]

Third-Generation Thrombolytic Drugs

The last few years have seen the development of a new generation of thrombolytic drugs, including mutant molecules of single-chain u-PA and t-PA; chimeric plasminogen activators; conjugates of plasminogen activators with monoclonal antibodies against fibrin, platelets, or thrombomodulin; and plasminogen activators of animal and bacterial origin.[50]

Reteplase

Reteplase is a single-chain deletion mutant of alteplase, consisting of just the kringle-2 and protease domains.[68] Reteplase is produced by recombinant genetic technology in *Escherichia coli* cells.[68a] It has a fivefold decrease in fibrin binding and a half-life of 14 to 18 minutes because of the aforementioned structural differences. Reteplase has less binding to endothelium and monocytes compared with t-PA, and this reduced binding results in increased circulating levels in the bloodstream.[69] Reteplase catalyzes the cleavage of endogenous plasminogen to generate plasmin. The activation of plasminogen is stimulated in the presence of fibrin and is mediated by the kringle-2 domain.[10,70] Plasmin then degrades the fibrin matrix of the thrombus, thus exerting its fibrinolytic action.

The fact that plasminogen activators generally activate plasminogen molecules in or near the clot allows efficient lysis in small clot burdens, such as the coronary circulation. The absolute dependence on a sufficient amount of available plasminogen limits the dose-related efficacy when the clot burden is large. Long, retracted (i.e., organized) clots, such as those in the peripheral arterial circulation, are often deficient in plasminogen. Despite this deficiency, plasminogen activators such as reteplase and t-PA are efficacious when delivered through a catheter directly into the thrombus rather than systemically.

Reteplase has increasingly been used in the treatment of peripheral vascular occlusion, given the unavailability of urokinase for a few years. Nevertheless, published studies regarding its use in controlled trials are relatively few in number. There are two pilot studies that evaluated the dosing regimen of reteplase in the treatment of myocardial infarction.[71,72] These studies demonstrated that reteplase produced significantly higher TIMI-3 (Thromboembolism in Myocardial Infarction) flow rates at 60 and 90 minutes than did front-loaded alteplase. However, in two subsequent trials—the International Joint Efficacy Comparison of Thrombolytics (INJECT)[73] and Global Use of Strategies to Open Occulated Coronary Arteries (GUSTO III)[74] trials—despite the higher TIMI-3 flow rates, this did not translate into a lower mortality in the reteplase-treated patients (7.5% for reteplase vs. 7.2% for alteplase).[15] Reteplase penetrates the clots and activates plasminogen inside the clot, whereas t-PA binds tightly to the fibrin matrix and accumulates on the surface of the clot. This difference is possibly due to the lower affinity of reteplase for fibrin compared with t-PA, resulting in faster clot lysis. Pharmacodynamic differences and pharmacokinetic differences between reteplase and t-PA may account for the higher initial clot lysis rates reported with reteplase.[5a]

Thrombolytics may also cause platelet activation, and this may have been responsible for some of the previously noted lack of efficacy. The addition of glycoprotein IIb/IIIa inhibitors appears to increase the efficacy of thrombolytic agents, as well as speed the lysis.

Tenecteplase

Tenecteplase (TNK-t-PA) is a t-PA mutant in which a threonine molecule (^{100}Thr) is replaced by Asn, and the sequence Lys-His-Arg-Arg is changed to Ala-Ala-Ala-Ala. This change confers high fibrin selectivity and prolongs the half-life to 15 to 19 minutes. TNK-t-PA is highly effective in arterial, platelet-rich thrombi and is more resistant to PAI. Although most of the published data regarding TNK-t-PA have been related to acute coronary syndromes, there is increasing experience in peripheral arterial thrombolysis. One group published its experience with continuous tenecteplase infusion in conjunction with glycoprotein IIb/IIIa inhibition with tirofiban for peripheral arterial thrombolysis.[75] The dose of TNK-t-PA infusion was 0.25 to 0.50 mg/h, with a mean infusion time of 7.5 hours. Of 48 patients with iliofemoral arterial thrombosis, complete lysis was achieved in 35 patients (73%). There were no deaths, no intracranial bleeding, and no embolic events. It appears, at least from this study, that lysis time is shorter; however, the longer half-life has implications for surgical intervention, as addressed earlier.

Staphylokinase

Staphylokinase is a plasminogen activator produced by certain strains of *Staphylococcus aureus* and was first described as having fibrinolytic properties in 1948.[76] The gene has been cloned from genomic DNA of a lysogenic strain of *S. aureus*. When exposed to a fibrin clot in human plasma, staphylokinase reacts with plasmin at the clot-plasma interface; this staphylokinase-plasmin complex activates thrombus-bound plasminogen and exerts its fibrinolytic activity. Any plasmin that is liberated from the clot is rapidly inactivated by α_2-antiplasmin. In this manner, plasminogen activation by staphylokinase is confined to the thrombus, and the collateral effects of fibrinogen depletion and serum plasminogen activation are minimized. However, patients treated with staphylokinase do develop neutralizing antibodies, the titers of which can remain elevated for several months.[77]

Immunofibrinolysis

In an attempt to develop fibrin-specific agents, monoclonal antifibrin antibodies have been bonded to urokinase or streptokinase, rendering these agents fibrin selective. These monoclonal antibodies do not appear to cross-react with fibrinogen and thus show a marked increase in in vitro fibrinolysis compared with unmodified activator.[78] The clinical applicability of these agents remains to be determined; they may significantly alter the current approach to the management of thrombotic disease. Nevertheless, repeated therapy would require different monoclonal antibodies to prevent adverse immunologic reactions.

Fibrolase is a direct-acting fibrinolytic enzyme. It is a metalloprotease isolated from the venom of the southern copperhead snake, which dissolves fibrin through rapid hydrolysis. There are some data to suggest that fibrolase dissolves thrombi much quicker than the plasminogen activators. An added advantage of fibrolase is the rapid inactivation by α_2-macroglobulin, which is relatively abundant in the systemic circulation. Alfimeprase (Nuvelo, Inc., San Cerlos, CA), a recombinant variant of fibrolase, underwent evaluation in clinical trials of peripheral arterial occlusion, with inconclusive results. In addition, amediplase (Menarini Group, Florence, Italy) is undergoing evaluation in clinical trials. Amediplase is a chimeric protein that combines part of the t-PA and part of the single-chain urokinase plasminogen activator (sc-UPA). In animal models, amediplase is a more potent and longer-lasting thrombolytic than alteplase.

Summary

Most of the clinical experience to date has been with streptokinase, urokinase, and, most recently, t-PA. The effectiveness and complication rates of each of these agents are discussed later in the specific sections dealing with the various clinical entities. Based on the experience to date, streptokinase seems to be a less desirable agent for use in peripheral vascular thrombosis, probably because of its complex mechanism of action, which translates into dosage difficulties and clinical complications.

Bleeding associated with thrombolytic therapy, regardless of the agent used, is most frequent at sites used for cardiac catheterization, arterial blood gas studies, intravenous infusion, or venipuncture. At any invaded site, the vascular endothelium is disrupted, resulting in an inflammatory reaction. The major components of an inflammatory reaction are fibrin and two different cell types that form the hemostatic plug. The fibrin in the hemostatic plug is identical to the fibrin in a pathologic thrombus in freshly (recently) formed thrombi and is much more susceptible to lysis. Thus, if a fibrin-specific thrombolytic agent is infused into the circulation, it will interact with molecularly identical fibrin in both the hemostatic plug and the pathologic thrombus; this brings about dissolution of the hemostatic plug, thereby inducing bleeding. This may be the reason why, in all recently completed studies comparing first- and second-generation thrombolytic agents, there is as much if not more bleeding with the newer, second-generation agents as with the older ones.

The degradation products of fibrinogen or fibrin are the absolute index of the degree of activation of the fibrinolytic system. When there are high levels of these fibrin degradation products, they are easily detected and signify an intense activation of the plasminogen-plasmin proteolytic system. There is good evidence that all the newer agents, despite assertions to the contrary, do induce the systemic fibrinolytic system, and this probably explains why the rate of distant hemorrhage is no different from that of older generation agents. Regional administration of agents (vs. systemic), dosage, and duration of therapy could have an important role in realizing the clinical benefits of a fibrin-specific agent.

VENOUS THROMBOLYSIS INCLUDING SYSTEMIC THROMBOLYTIC THERAPY

This section briefly discusses systemic thrombolytic therapy for venous thromboembolism and venous occlusions. Treatment of acute coronary thrombosis and stroke are purposely omitted. Although systemic thrombolytic therapy has been used for peripheral arterial occlusions, results have been disappointing, with bleeding complications outweighing any benefit obtained. Local intraarterial administration prevents many of the systemic complications and is used for peripheral arterial and graft occlusion. This route allows directed thrombolytic therapy to the site of occlusion, minimizes the dose and duration of thrombolytic agent, and is highly effective. Even venous thrombolysis is most effective when it is catheter directed. Patient selection is probably the most important factor in obtaining good results with either modality.

Patient Selection

During the course of systemic thrombolytic therapy, a systemic lytic state is achieved in which fibrin is lysed wherever it has been deposited in the body. Thus hemostatic plugs are as vulnerable as the clot or thrombus for which therapy was initiated. Selection of patients for systemic lytic therapy is based on the presence of an appropriate documented indication and careful evaluation for the presence of contraindications.

Contraindications to systemic therapy are listed in Box 35.1. Absolute contraindications are active internal bleeding and recent (within 2 months) cerebrovascular accident or other intracranial condition. Relative major contraindications include recent (within 10 days) major surgery, trauma, obstetric delivery, organ biopsy, or puncture of a noncompressible vessel; recent gastrointestinal bleed; and severe hypertension. Relative minor contraindications carry a higher risk of complications, but the benefits of therapy may still outweigh the hazards. Peripheral embolization from a central source is a potential hazard of systemic lytic therapy. Therefore valvular heart disease, atrial fibrillation, and previous history of emboli are relative contraindications to systemic lytic therapy. The presence of a mural thrombus is a relative contraindication to fibrinolytic therapy because of the potential for peripheral embolization due to fragmentation, which could have devastating consequences. In patients with a thrombus in the left side of the heart demonstrable by echocardiography, alternative forms of treatment should be considered. However, it must be recognized that successful lysis of ventricular thrombi with urokinase has been reported.[79] Severe liver disease affects drug metabolism, making the response unpredictable. During pregnancy, a systemic lytic state may precipitate abruptio placentae or lead to hypofibrinogenemia in the fetus, with an increased risk of bleeding. Streptokinase is specifically contraindicated in patients with known allergy, previous therapy within 6 months, or recent streptococcal infection.

One of the most devastating complications of fibrinolytic therapy is intracranial hemorrhage. The incidence of this complication is approximately 1% of treated patients in trials for acute myocardial infarction. The median time between the start of thrombolytic therapy and the onset of clinical signs of intracranial hemorrhage ranges from 3 to 36 hours, with a mean of 16 hours. Mortality is high for this complication, with an estimated mortality of 66%. Factors predictive of intracranial hemorrhage by multivariate logistic regression analysis include oral anticoagulation before admission, body weight less than 70 kg, and age older than 65 years. An increased incidence of intracerebral hemorrhage has been observed in patients receiving

BOX 35.1 Contraindications to Systemic Lytic Therapy

Absolute
- Active internal bleeding
- Recent (<2 months) cerebrovascular accident
- Intracranial pathologic condition

Relative Major
- Recent (<10 days) major surgery, obstetric delivery, or organ biopsy
- Active peptic ulcer or gastrointestinal disorder
- Recent major trauma
- Uncontrolled hypertension

Relative Minor
- Minor surgery or trauma
- Recent cardiopulmonary resuscitation
- High likelihood of left heart thrombus (e.g., atrial fibrillation with mitral valve disease)
- Bacterial endocarditis
- Hemostatic defects (e.g., renal or liver disease)
- Pregnancy
- Diabetic hemorrhagic retinopathy

higher doses of t-PA. In the Thrombosis in Myocardial Infarction (TIMI) trial,[80] 1.3% of patients receiving 150 mg of t-PA suffered an intracerebral hemorrhage, as opposed to 0.4% of patients receiving 100 mg of the drug. Interestingly, in the TIMI-II trial, patients who received immediate beta-blockade as part of their regimen had no incidence of intracerebral hemorrhage when given 100 mg of t-PA, compared with 0.5% in the group that did not receive beta-blockade. However, this was not true for patients treated with 150 mg of t-PA. The mechanism by which beta-blockers may protect against intracerebral bleeding has not been established.[81]

In the Surgery versus Thrombolysis for Ischemia of the Lower Extremity (STILE) trial, patients were randomized to thrombolytic therapy with t-PA or urokinase versus surgery for the treatment of lower limb ischemia.[82] When evaluated with an intent-to-treat analysis, the incidence of life-threatening hemorrhage was 5.3% to 5.7%. When analyzed on a per-protocol basis, the incidence of this complication was 7.8% in the thrombolysis group. The incidence was similar in patients treated with t-PA and urokinase; these patients also received aspirin and heparin, which may have added to the risk. However, patients with bleeding complications did not receive more heparin or a higher dose of lytic agent; they appeared to respond differently to the therapy. At the end of the infusion, patients with bleeding complications had a significantly lower fibrinogen level than did patients without hemorrhagic complications (188 vs. 310 mg/dL). Measurement of fibrinogen levels, along with the international normalized ratio and partial thromboplastin time (PTT), may be helpful in guiding dose and duration of therapy.

Indications

Pulmonary Embolism

In 1968 a cooperative, controlled, randomized study to evaluate the use of urokinase in PE was initiated.[83] By 1970, 160 patients were entered and assigned to one of two therapeutic arms. Pulmonary angiography was performed on all patients before and after therapy, with lung scans repeated at 3, 6, and 12 months. The minimal eligibility was occlusion of at least one segmental pulmonary artery on angiography. Excluded from the trial were patients who had recent operations and those with contraindications to heparin or thrombolytic therapy. Seventy-eight patients received anticoagulants alone (heparin 75 units/lb loading dose, 10 units/lb per hour for 12 hours), and 82 received urokinase (2000 units/lb per hour for 12 hours). After the 12-hour infusion, all patients received heparin for a minimum of 5 days to maintain a prolonged bleeding time.

The randomization produced a reasonably good balance between the treatment groups. Urokinase therapy resulted in a significantly accelerated resolution of pulmonary emboli at 24 hours, as shown by pulmonary arteriograms, lung scans, and right-sided pressures. No significant differences in mortality or recurrence rates were observed. Patients receiving urokinase tended to respond better if they were younger than 50 years old, the embolus was less than 48 hours old, or the embolus was large, especially if shock was present.

Bleeding complications were significant in both groups (heparin, 27%; urokinase, 45%). This high complication rate is likely the result of demands in the protocol for multiple, frequent invasive procedures, including cutdowns performed for pulmonary angiography. The study group concluded that further study was needed before specific therapeutic recommendations could be made.

In 1974 the second phase of this cooperative study was reported.[84] This study followed the same guidelines as in phase I, comparing 12 hours of urokinase therapy with 24 hours of urokinase therapy and 24 hours of streptokinase therapy. A group treated with heparin alone was not included because the protocol was almost identical to that in the phase I trial, which showed urokinase to be superior to heparin in clot resolution. Fifty-seven patients were given urokinase (2000 units/lb loading dose, 2000 units/lb per hour for 24 hours), and 61 patients received the same regimen for 12 hours. Fifty-eight patients received streptokinase (250,000 units loading dose, 100,000 units/h for 24 hours).

As expected, the drop in plasminogen during therapy was steeper for patients receiving streptokinase; otherwise the lytic effect was similar. Patients receiving 12 hours of urokinase infusion had nearly equivalent results to those in the phase I trial receiving urokinase. No benefit was seen from extending the urokinase infusion to 24 hours. However, in patients with massive embolism, the greatest improvement was seen with 24-hour urokinase infusion, although the differences were not statistically significant. Streptokinase and urokinase yielded similar results, with small differences favoring urokinase. The study group concluded that all three regimens were more effective in accelerating the resolution of pulmonary thromboemboli than heparin alone.

One of the major problems with the use of thrombolytic therapy for PE is that these patients usually have major contraindications to thrombolytic therapy. For example, this is the case with PE in a postoperative patient. In 1992 an experience with 13 patients treated for angiographically proven PE within 14 days of surgery was reported.[85] The protocol used urokinase (2200 units/kg body weight) injected directly into the clot through a catheter positioned in the pulmonary artery. A continuous infusion at the same dosage was then maintained for up to 24 hours, with the simultaneous administration of heparin at 500 units/h. The fibrinogen level was maintained at less than 0.2 g/dL. No deaths or bleeding complications were seen, with complete lysis achieved in all patients. This selective therapy for PE may be appropriate for patients in the early postoperative period who suffer a major life-threatening pulmonary embolus.

The long-term results of patients randomized to the Urokinase Pulmonary Embolism Trial (UPET) suggest the clinical importance of resolution of the obstructive process in the pulmonary circulation. Several patients from this study were reexamined 7 years after the original pulmonary embolus. Those assigned initially to thrombolysis had significantly higher pulmonary capillary blood volumes and preservation of the normal pulmonary vasculature response to exercise at 7 years. In contrast, patients who had been treated with anticoagulants alone demonstrated a lower pulmonary capillary blood volume at 1 year and a markedly abnormal increase in pulmonary artery pressure and pulmonary vascular resistance when undergoing exercise testing during right heart catheterization.[86] These data suggest that initial management with thrombolysis can offer improved quality of life years after the event.

More recently, rt-PA has been evaluated in the treatment of acute massive PE. In a multicenter trial the intravenous administration of rt-PA was compared with intrapulmonary administration in 34 patients with massive pulmonary emboli.[87] All patients were systemically anticoagulated with heparin. The patients received 50 mg of intravenous or intrapulmonary rt-PA over 2 hours, with 22 patients receiving another 50 mg over the subsequent 5 hours. No difference was noted between the intrapulmonary group and the intravenous group, and 7-hour administration was superior to a single infusion of 50 mg over 2 hours. In all groups, up to 38% resolution of the angiographically determined embolism occurred. A decline in the pulmonary arterial pressure was documented in all groups. Fibrinogen levels dropped significantly, and bleeding complications were limited to puncture or operative sites; only four patients required blood transfusions.

In a separate trial, 36 patients with angiographically documented pulmonary emboli received 50 mg of rt-PA over 2 hours, followed by repeated arteriography and, if necessary, an additional 40 mg of rt-PA over 4 hours.[88] Thirty-four of the 36 patients had angiographic evidence of clot lysis, with marked improvement in 24 of the 36. Two bleeding complications occurred, one related to a pelvic tumor and the other 8 days after coronary artery bypass surgery. Again, significant improvement in the clinical condition of these patients was documented.

A randomized controlled trial of rt-PA versus urokinase in the treatment of acute PE was reported in 1988.[89] Forty-five patients were randomized to 100 mg of rt-PA over 2 hours versus urokinase at systemic doses. At 2 hours, 82% of the rt-PA patients had complete lysis, as opposed to 48% of patients receiving urokinase. Eight of 23 urokinase patients required premature termination of the infusion because of bleeding complications. There was no difference in plasma fibrinogen level or improvement in lung scans between the two groups.

In 1980 the National Institutes of Health Consensus Development Conference concluded that thrombolytic therapy results in greater improvement and normalization of the hemodynamic responses to pulmonary emboli than that observed with heparin alone.[90] Lytic therapy may prevent permanent damage to the pulmonary vascular bed by lysing emboli and restoring the pulmonary circulation to normal. The conference report also stated that, although the incidence of bleeding complications was high, contemporary clinical experience suggested an incidence of approximately 5%, which was certainly within the acceptable range.

The thrombolytic agents currently approved by the FDA for use in the treatment of patients with PE are t-PA, given in a 100-mg dose over 2 hours, and since 2002 the newly reintroduced urokinase. As stated earlier, there is no evidence of improved survival or outcomes in patients with PE who are hemodynamically stable. Tebbe and colleagues[91] evaluated the efficacy of reteplase, given as two 10-unit boluses 30 minutes apart, compared with t-PA in the 100-mg dose. There was no difference in clinical outcomes, complications, or mortality. The rates of stroke and intracranial hemorrhage were similar. However, reteplase reduced pulmonary vascular resistance more quickly than t-PA did. However, it should be emphasized that there is no level I evidence that thrombolysis for the improvement of PE offers any survival advantage, except in cases of massive embolism with hemodynamic compromise.

In current clinical practice, thrombolytic therapy should be considered in all patients with an established diagnosis of PE, any evidence (clinical or monitoring) of hemodynamic compromise, and no absolute contraindication to systemic lytic therapy. This excludes small pulmonary emboli in a patient who remains clinically stable after the initial episode. In this situation the benefits of thrombolytic therapy over heparin alone are not clear.

In 2015 a systemic review and meta-analysis of 15 randomized control trials comparing systemic thrombolytic therapy plus anticoagulation versus anticoagulation alone for the treatment of patients with acute PE demonstrated that, compared with heparin alone, the use of thrombolytic therapy was associated with a significant reduction in overall PE-related mortality; however, it is associated with increase in fatal, intracranial, or major hemorrhage, therefore having a narrow and likely insignificant overall benefit.[91a]

It is important that the diagnosis of pulmonary emboli be well documented. Helical or spiral computed tomography (CT) scans are increasingly being used to detect PE. With current technology, image acquisition can be done in 20 seconds, the equivalent of a single breath-hold. The sensitivity and specificity of helical CT in the diagnosis of acute PE range from 69% to 92% and 86% to 96%, respectively.

Under these guidelines a patient who has a large PE and evidence of right ventricular dysfunction should be considered for a trial of lytic therapy. Systemic anticoagulation with heparin is critical as soon as the diagnosis is strongly suspected. Pulmonary embolectomy is then reserved for hemodynamically compromised patients who fail lytic therapy or have an absolute contraindication to thrombolytic therapy. Once again, it should be emphasized that thrombolytic therapy has not been shown to affect mortality after PE; its efficacy is reflected in secondary end points, not in survival.

Deep Venous Thrombosis

The goal of therapy for deep venous thrombosis (DVT) is the prevention of PE and of long-term sequelae characterized by the postphlebitic syndrome. Anticoagulation has been highly effective in achieving the former but ineffective in preventing valvular damage and thus avoiding the latter. The incidence of such long-term complications can be as high as 90%.[92]

Several well-controlled, randomized, prospective studies have compared systemic lytic therapy with conventional heparin therapy in the treatment of DVT.[93-97] All concluded that dissolution of DVT with lytic therapy is faster and more complete than that observed with heparin alone. On average, complete lysis was seen in 35% of patients, compared with 4% of those treated with heparin alone. At 3 to 6 months' follow-up, valve function was preserved in 7% of heparin-treated patients, compared with 50% of patients treated with thrombolytic agents. The incidence of PE was similar for both regimens, with no difference in mortality. Bleeding complications averaged 4% and 17% for heparin and lytic therapy, respectively. In one study, phlebography at a mean of 7 months after treatment suggested an improved outcome for patients treated with fibrinolytic agents. Normal venograms were found in 40% of streptokinase-treated patients, compared with 8% of those who had received heparin. Clinical symptoms were related to therapeutic results and previous thrombosis. Longer follow-up was reported by Arnesen and colleagues,[98] who phlebographically evaluated 35 patients at a mean observation period of 6.5 years after they had randomly received streptokinase or heparin. Only seven patients had phlebographically normal veins, and all were in the streptokinase group. On clinical examination, 76% of patients in the streptokinase group had normal legs, compared with 33% of patients in the heparin group. Contrasting results were reported from a small prospective study in which 24 patients with major proximal DVT treated with heparin were compared with 25 patients similarly afflicted and treated with streptokinase.[99] After 2.5 years of follow-up, no major difference in hemodynamic status, as measured by foot volumetry, was seen between the two groups. The authors questioned the validity of treatment with lytic therapy, given its higher complication rate. In all these studies, thrombi older than 3 to 5 days were less likely to respond.

A randomized trial of rt-PA for the treatment of proximal DVT was performed by Turpie and colleagues.[100] Twenty patients with proximal DVT were randomized to intravenous rt-PA (0.5 mg/kg) or placebo over 4 hours, following initiation of a therapeutic dose of intravenous heparin. Patients were randomized to rt-PA (0.5 mg/kg) or saline over 1 hour if repeated venography within 72 hours did not show complete lysis. Five of 10 patients treated with rt-PA under this protocol showed partial or complete lysis, compared with 1 of 10 patients treated with heparin. A systemic lytic effect was demonstrated by a drop in plasma fibrinogen and α_2-antiplasmin concentration, with positive fibrin degradation split products and elevated euglobulin lysis time. Thus modest effectiveness was demonstrated in this study, similar to that achieved by urokinase or streptokinase. Long-term follow-up data on these patients are not available. Three other randomized trials have yielded similar results.[101-103]

Use of systemic thrombolysis for DVT is hampered by concerns over bleeding risk, but regional thrombolytic therapy for DVT is increasingly popular. The concept of regional thrombolytic therapy for DVT is attractive because it can relieve the obstructive process and aid in the preservation of valvular function. These two features are established predictors of the development of the postthrombotic syndrome (PTS).[104] The early reports of success with thrombolysis for DVT led to the development of a national multicenter registry for the evaluation of catheter-directed thrombolysis for lower extremity DVT.[105] The early results in 473 patients were published in 1999 and demonstrated that the methods used to deliver the lytic agent (in this case, urokinase) affect the anatomic result. Attempts to lyse the thrombus by a pedal infusion were remarkably unsuccessful, with a failure rate of 80%. In contrast, catheter-directed lysis, with the agent laced directly into the clot, achieved substantial lysis in 83% of cases and complete lysis in 33%. This experience provides a strong argument in favor of abandoning systemic infusion for thrombolysis because the rates of lysis are not improved, but the dose of lytic agent administered is higher with systemic infusion. Major bleeding complications occurred in 11% of patients, most at the puncture site, and mortality was less than 1%. Comerota and colleagues[106] published a report evaluating health-related quality-of-life variables in patients with iliofemoral DVT treated with thrombolysis versus those treated with anticoagulation alone. Patients treated with thrombolysis reported better overall physical functioning, less health distress, less stigma, and fewer postthrombotic symptoms ($P < .05$ for each outcome measure).

Whether preservation of valve function is achieved by this more aggressive form of therapy is uncertain. Nevertheless, it is difficult to ignore the significant improvement in the obstructive component of DVT with thrombolysis, considering that the combination of obstruction and valvular incompetence likely results in the most severe form of postphlebitic syndrome. In view of this, should lytic therapy be offered to all patients with DVT? Recently, the ATTRACT (Acute Venous Thrombosis: Thrombus Removal with Adjunctive Catheter-Directed Thrombolysis) trial has been initiated. This study involves randomization of consecutive symptomatic patients with acute proximal DVT to best endovascular therapy plus standard DVT therapy or standard DVT therapy alone. The primary objective is to determine whether catheter-directed thrombolytic therapy reduces the occurrence of PTS compared with anticoagulation alone. This study may answer lingering questions about thrombolytic efficacy in DVT.

Of note, when thrombolytic therapy is started more than 5 days after the onset of symptoms, effectiveness is significantly decreased. The incidence of DVT is highest in postoperative patients, women during pregnancy or after childbirth, trauma victims, and patients suffering cerebrovascular accidents or spinal injuries. Lytic therapy is contraindicated in these instances, as well as in septic thrombophlebitis. Prior episodes of thrombophlebitis are likely to have destroyed delicate vein valves, making the benefits of lytic therapy in recurrent attacks uncertain. If clinical evidence of valve competence is present, an attempt to prevent further damage from a recurrent attack and resolve the obstructive component is a reasonable goal. In addition, lytic therapy seems to offer an advantage in more proximal thrombosis (i.e., popliteal vein or higher); thus, treatment of isolated calf thrombi with lytic therapy is of questionable value.

Phlegmasia cerulea dolens at onset causes massive iliofemoral thrombosis with limb-threatening venous outflow occlusion. Historically, the results of venous thrombectomy have been variable, with a significant incidence of rethrombosis and mortality, although more recent experience has been encouraging.[107,108] A much more compelling argument can be made for the use of thrombolytic therapy in the treatment of phlegmasia cerulea dolens. There is no real consensus on treatment, but the advent of catheter-directed thrombolysis presents an attractive and effective treatment option for this disease, which historically resulted in 20% to 40% mortality and a significant amputation rate in survivors.[109] Patel and colleagues[110] reported on two patients with phlegmasia cerulea dolens who were successfully treated with catheter-directed thrombolytic therapy and stenting, without limb loss. This is one of many case reports that demonstrate the feasibility and efficacy of this approach. Lytic therapy offers an important advantage over surgical thrombectomy, because multiple peripheral thrombi not accessible to the catheter may be dissolved. In addition, a general anesthetic, frequently required for venous thrombectomy, is avoided. Although the experience with thrombolytic therapy in this disease is limited, 13 of 14 reported cases were judged to have achieved excellent results, with no mortality.[93,111-113]

It is important to mention the possible acute renal dysfunction that can occur with the use of pharmacomechanical thrombolysis in patients with more proximal DVT, such as those with femoral vein and iliac vein thrombus. Although this topic has not been born out in any randomized control trials, there have been several papers and case reports discussing the effects of hemolysis, particularly with high-volume injection and aspiration on kidney function.[113a] Intravascular hemolysis can cause acute tubular necrosis secondary to hemoglobunuria. Patients can experience red urine, elevated creatinine, and elevated serum lactate dehydrogenase levels. It is unclear of the exact mechanism that results in acute tubular necrosis; however, it is thought that heme proteins precipitate cast formation and obstruction of renal tubule.[113b] Close monitoring of urine output, creatinine trends, bicarbonate, and lactate levels are critical, and the early involvement of a renal specialist when recovery is slow or obsolete is recommended.

Upper Extremity Venous Thrombosis: Axillary and Subclavian Vein

Upper extremity venous thrombosis involves venous thrombosis of the brachial, axillary, or subclavian vein that can extend into more proximal vessels of the brachiocephalic, superior vena cava, and jugular veins. They can be divided into primary or secondary causes. Primary causes included thoracic outlet syndrome, Paget-Schroetter syndrome, or thrombophilia. Secondary causes include iatrogenic causes such as indwelling catheters, pacemakers, pregnancy, trauma, or cancer-related disease. Secondary causes account for the overwhelming majority of upper extremity deep venous thrombosis (UEDVT).[113c]

Axillary vein thrombosis (effort thrombosis) usually occurs in young individuals, and its sudden clinical manifestations lead the patient to seek early medical attention. As a result, this entity is ideally suited for thrombolytic therapy. Anticoagulation rarely leads to resolution and merely arrests the process, allowing for collateral drainage and amelioration of symptoms. This frequently leads to some degree of disability. Catheter-induced axillary subclavian vein thrombosis usually has a more gradual presentation, with slow, progressive occlusion allowing for collateral venous drainage. The clinical presentation aids in the decision whether to offer lytic therapy to a patient with catheter-induced axillary subclavian vein thrombosis. When symptoms develop rapidly over the course of a few days, there is a good probability that the thrombotic material will be sensitive to lytic agents. A combination of infusion through the catheter and in the ipsilateral peripheral vein is most effective. However, if symptoms develop over weeks or months, they tend to be milder in nature and less responsive to fibrinolytic agents. This is likely a result of organization of the thrombotic material.

Both forms of axillary thrombosis have been successfully managed with lytic therapy (Fig. 35.2).[114-116] Either systemic or local low-dose infusion appear to be effective.[114] Local infusion requires that the catheter be lodged in thrombus; otherwise, venous collaterals will decrease its effectiveness. A systemic lytic state is avoided in the majority of patients treated by local infusion.

After complete resolution of the clot is achieved, repeated venography with the extremity in abduction and external rotation is recommended. If an underlying thoracic outlet compression is identified, surgical correction should be advised. Surgical decompression of the thoracic outlet can be performed at the same admission (i.e., after thrombolysis), because no increase in bleeding complications or rethrombosis rates have been noted. In a study reviewing 12 series of papers looking at patients undergoing treatment for Paget-Schroetter syndrome, UEDVT, or effort thrombosis, more than 40% of patients who underwent endovascular therapy without surgical intervention such as first rib resection eventually required rib resection for recurrent symptoms, suggesting that, despite thrombolytic therapy, permanent symptom relief and long-term patency were strongly dependent on surgical intervention.[67,116a] After thoracic decompression, a repeat venogram is obtained at 2 weeks. If a stenosis of the vein is identified, balloon dilatation may be successful in avoiding rethrombosis.[114]

Superior Vena Cava Thrombosis

Superior vena cava thrombosis is frequently the result of neoplastic, traumatic, or infectious processes in the mediastinum. In these instances, external compression or inflammation precludes successful resolution of the process with lytic agents. Thrombosis secondary to an indwelling catheter is usually a slow process, allowing for organization and fibrotic replacement of the clot. It is unlikely that this thrombosis will respond to lytic therapy, and surgical decompression may be an option in these patients. Conversely, patients who develop rapidly progressive symptoms may respond to lytic therapy by means of dissolution of the most recently formed clot, which is likely to be sensitive to lysis.

Thrombosis is idiopathic in approximately 4% of patients. Successful resolution of idiopathic vena cava thrombosis has been reported with systemic thrombolytic therapy.[117]

Complications

Bleeding is the most frequent and important complication of systemic lytic therapy. However, most lytic treatments for peripheral arterial or venous thrombosis are done by catheter-directed techniques rather than by systemic administration of thrombolytics. The major exceptions are thrombolytics for stroke and myocardial infarction, which are administered via a bolus and short-term infusion rather than prolonged infusion. The reported incidence of major bleeding (requiring transfusion or discontinuation of the drug) varies from 7%[118] to as high as 45%.[83] Major bleeding occurs in an average of 15% of cases and correlates with the number and type of invasive procedures during therapy. Duration of therapy also seems to influence the incidence of bleeding.

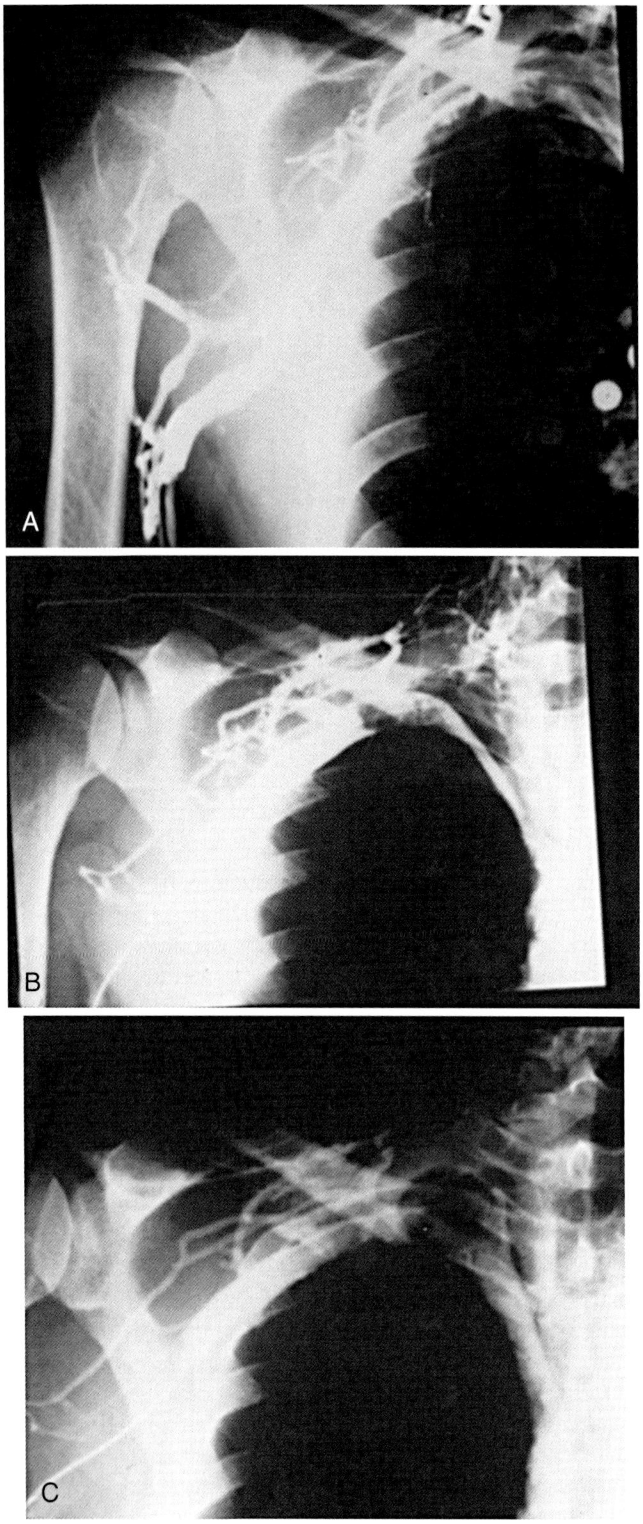

FIG 35.2 Venograms of a 28-year-old man with acute onset of pain and swelling in the right upper extremity. (A) Ascending venogram confirms axillary vein thrombosis. Low-dose streptokinase infusion (10,000 units/h) was initiated. (B) Twenty-four hours later, intraluminal thrombus is seen, with patency of the system. (C) Forty-eight hours later, there is complete resolution of the occlusion.

Two broad categories of bleeding are observed. Superficial bleeding, seen at invasive sites, is frequently controlled with pressure. Avoidance of unnecessary procedures and preservation of an intact vascular system are the best preventive measures. Internal bleeding, usually seen in the gastrointestinal tract or the intracranial space, is frequently the result of poor patient selection. Internal bleeding should be suspected with unexplained drops in hematocrit. As a rule, any change in the neurologic status of a patient receiving fibrinolytic therapy is considered a complication of therapy until proved otherwise. The infusion is discontinued immediately, and appropriate diagnostic and therapeutic measures are instituted.

Superficial bleeding, which is controlled by local measures, can be tolerated in the final stages of therapy. Its occurrence early in the infusion, or any significant bleeding requiring transfusion, should lead to discontinuation of therapy. The hemostatic defect is corrected by the administration of fresh frozen plasma or cryoprecipitate. These two components are rich in fibrinogen and usually result in resolution of the lytic state. ε-Aminocaproic acid administration (plasmin inhibitor) is rarely recommended and carries a significant risk of aggravating the process for which lytic therapy was instituted. Increasing the dose of streptokinase to decrease its proteolytic effect is scientifically correct but unnecessary. It is interesting to note that bleeding tends to occur in the lag period between termination of lytic therapy and anticoagulant administration.[53,119] Thus heparin administration should be delayed until the thrombin time or PTT is less than twice normal, and it should be initiated without a loading dose.

Laboratory parameters correlate poorly with the risk of bleeding. However, extremely low fibrinogen levels (<20% of baseline or <100 mg/dL) in the presence of an otherwise minor bleeding complication do increase the chances of continued bleeding, requiring cessation of therapy. An alternative is to temporarily discontinue the drug, administer fresh frozen plasma or cryoprecipitate, and restart the infusion several hours later.

Allergic reactions are not infrequent with streptokinase, although most are minor febrile episodes of no clinical consequence. Serious allergic reactions are extremely rare with the current preparations, and the few reported cases have responded well to conventional therapy.[90]

PE can occur during treatment for DVT. The incidence appears to be similar to that seen with conventional heparin therapy. In the absence of other complications, continuation of lytic therapy is the treatment of choice. If recurrent emboli are observed, discontinuation of the fibrinolytic agent, heparin administration, and placement of a caval filter may be life-saving.

REGIONAL INTRAARTERIAL THROMBOLYTIC THERAPY

The management of acute arterial and graft occlusions by the intraarterial local administration of fibrinolytic agents has emerged as an alternative and a frequent adjunct to surgical therapy in a selected group of patients. Recently completed prospective, randomized clinical trials have helped to establish the role of lytic therapy in the treatment of patients with peripheral vascular disease. Excellent results with low morbidity and mortality are now possible with modern vascular techniques. It is difficult to estimate the effects of intraarterial lytic therapy based on cases in which surgical management has traditionally been successful.

Emerging from the literature are guidelines that help to define the role of intraarterial lytic therapy. Unquestionably, patient selection is the most important factor in achieving good results with this nonoperative approach. As experience in manipulating the fibrinolytic system increases, improvements in areas where surgical results are poor may follow.

Patient Selection

As a rule, intraarterial fibrinolytic therapy should be considered when the surgical alternative carries a high risk of morbidity or mortality or when the surgical approach has traditionally yielded poor results. In patients with previous multiple vascular reconstructions, lytic therapy may offer an alternative to a difficult and unpredictable surgical intervention. In some cases, it may facilitate such an undertaking, thus serving as a true adjunct to surgical therapy.

In the early experience of intraarterial fibrinolytic therapy, low doses of the agent were administered close to the thrombus to minimize systemic effects. With a low-dose regimen, dissolution of intraarterial thrombi is a slow, gradual process, requiring 12 to 72 hours or longer. If this method is chosen, the viability of the ischemic tissues should be ensured. Otherwise, these patients are better managed surgically because prompt revascularization can be accomplished. Candidates for intraarterial lytic therapy must be able to tolerate ischemia for the duration of the infusion. With the advent of multiple percutaneous mechanical thrombectomy devices, restoration of some blood flow can be accomplished early after initiation of the endovascular procedure.

Cumulative retrospective and prospective analysis has helped to define guidelines for patient selection. In a prospective study of 80 consecutive patients receiving intraarterial urokinase for acute (<14 days) ischemia, successful lysis was accomplished in 71% (57 patients).[120] Most of these patients required additional adjunctive procedures to maintain patency; only 28% of patients avoided the need for additional interventions. Prosthetic graft and native arterial occlusions responded equally well (78% and 72%, respectively), whereas vein graft occlusions were less likely to respond (53%). Diabetics fared significantly worse compared with nondiabetics. Most important, placement of the catheter within the substance of the thrombus and passage of the guidewire through the occlusive process were the best predictors of success. The location of the occlusion influenced the need for adjunctive procedures. Although 88% of aortoiliac and 82% of infrainguinal occlusions required adjunctive procedures, only 17% of upper extremity procedures required additional interventions. The investigators underscored the importance of patient selection, noting that unsuccessful thrombolysis not only delays revascularization but also increases the risk of bleeding complications.[120]

Absolute and relative contraindications to intraarterial fibrinolytic therapy are listed in Box 35.2. Approximately 50% of patients receiving low-dose intraarterial infusion of lytic drugs will develop a systemic lytic state. Thus patients with active internal bleeding, recent cerebrovascular accidents (within 2 months), or intracranial lesions are not candidates for any form of fibrinolytic therapy.

> **BOX 35.2 Contraindications to Intraarterial Fibrinolytic Therapy**
>
> **Absolute**
> - Active internal bleeding
> - Cerebrovascular accident within 3 months
> - Intracranial pathologic condition
>
> **Relative**
> - Recent major surgery or trauma
> - Minor gastrointestinal bleeding
> - Severe hypertension
> - Valvular heart disease
> - Atrial fibrillation
> - Endocarditis
> - Coagulation disorder
> - Pregnancy
> - Minor surgery
> - Severe liver disease
> - Axillofemoral graft or knitted Dacron graft

Relative contraindications represent risk factors associated with a higher incidence of complications. Recent major surgery or trauma significantly increases the risk of bleeding in the presence of a systemic lytic state. Individual judgment is required, but the presence of relative contraindications should not deter the clinician from using regional lytic therapy if significant benefit is anticipated.

Several cases of embolization to the ipsilateral extremity during intraarterial lytic therapy for occluded axillofemoral grafts have been reported.[120] The length of these grafts makes them less suitable for lytic therapy, so that surgical thrombectomy remains the therapy of choice. Dissolution of the fibrin layer that seals Dacron prostheses can occur with systemic absorption of the drug, leading to oozing through these porous prostheses. Discontinuation of therapy usually results in stabilization of the hematoma by the surrounding capsule.

Indications

Thrombosis After Endovascular Therapy

Percutaneous angioplasty is frequently performed for stenotic arterial lesions in the iliac and femoral systems. Thrombosis after balloon angioplasty is relatively infrequent, but when it occurs, local thrombolytic therapy is highly effective in restoring patency. The onset of occlusion is usually within 24 hours of dilatation; thus the thrombotic material is fresh and highly sensitive to fibrinolysis. The underlying stenosis has been relieved by the angioplasty, and when thrombosis occurs immediately, it is a simple matter to change catheters so that proximal infusion is promptly initiated.

More than 80% of cases of post–balloon dilatation thrombosis can be treated successfully with intraarterial lytic therapy.[121-123]

The duration of therapy is short because the infusion is started early and the thrombotic material is fresh; thus thrombectomy of a friable, recently dilated artery can be avoided. If dilatation of an iliac lesion was performed through an ipsilateral puncture, there is a risk of bleeding and pseudoaneurysm formation (Fig. 35.3). If patency was restored by the infusion, repair of the pseudoaneurysm can consist of simple closure of the puncture site without embolectomy.

Native Vessel Occlusion

Acute occlusion of a native artery can be the result of thrombosis secondary to an underlying stenosis or embolization from a central source. In selecting patients for intraarterial lytic therapy, it is important to attempt to delineate the mechanism of occlusion. Lytic therapy appears to be more effective when applied to peripheral embolization.[120] Although 50% to 60% of thrombotic occlusions resolve with thrombolytic therapy, approximately 80% of embolic occlusions can be lysed effectively. Conversely, surgical management of proximal lower extremity emboli by transfemoral embolectomy is highly successful, with low morbidity and mortality. In addition, some investigators have noted that emboli secondary to atrial fibrillation may have well-organized components and thus be resistant to fibrinolysis.[124] For these reasons, surgical embolectomy is preferred for proximal (iliac, femoral) emboli secondary to atrial fibrillation. If the embolus is secondary to a recent myocardial infarction (i.e., the surgical risk is increased and the embolus is usually fresh clot), intraarterial fibrinolytic therapy should be considered. It must be kept in mind that the presence of mural thrombus in the ventricle, usually secondary to a recent myocardial infarction, is a relative contraindication to lytic therapy. Although the absence of such findings on echocardiography does not absolutely exclude the possibility, their presence should raise the level of concern about performing lytic therapy.

The management of multiple distal emboli must be individualized, depending on the viability of the extremity and the surgical risk. Intraarterial lytic therapy is a reasonable option in these patients when the extremity is viable and the anticipated surgical reconstruction is difficult. If the ischemia is not well tolerated, proceed with popliteal exploration, thrombectomy, and, on occasion, intraoperative lytic therapy (discussed later).

The use of local fibrinolytic therapy for thrombotic arterial occlusions should be based on the anticipated difficulty, morbidity, and mortality of the surgical alternative. The success rate of fibrinolytic therapy alone in thrombotic occlusion is variable. Of 25 patients with atherosclerotic occlusion, Risius and associates[125] succeeded in treating 13 (52%); of these 13, only four required no further therapy, three had successful percutaneous transluminal angioplasty, and the remaining six required surgery or distal amputations. Of 40 patients with thrombotic occlusions treated by Katzen and colleagues with intraarterial lytic therapy, 32 (80%) achieved successful outcomes.[122] Successful lysis was achieved by Graor and colleagues[121] in 25 of 45 patients (56%) with thrombotic arterial occlusions. Eighteen of these 25 patients required secondary procedures. Seventy-eight percent of patients whose thrombi were less than 30 days old were successfully lysed, compared with 37% of patients with older occlusions. This trend has been observed by others and confirmed by recently completed randomized, prospective clinical trials (see later).

Careful analysis of the reported series reveals that, although the lytic infusion may reestablish patency, additional procedures are often required. If surgical management becomes necessary, this is often simplified because better preoperative planning is possible. Thus, if the ischemia is well tolerated, the anticipated surgical intervention complex, the occlusion fairly recent (within 2 weeks), and the patient at significantly increased surgical risk, thrombolytic therapy seems justified. Based on the reported experience, long-term results depend mainly on whether a correctable lesion is identified and on the location of the occlusion. Larger vessel occlusions resolved by intraarterial lytic therapy tend to do better, with an expected patency of 60% at 2 years. Similarly treated superficial femoral and popliteal occlusions have a lower long-term patency of approximately 30% at 2 years.[126] If a correctable lesion is identified and appropriately treated, long-term results are significantly improved. Patencies as low as 20% at 2 years have been reported when no causative lesion was identified.[127]

There are specific instances when surgical intervention has traditionally achieved poor results. Emboli or thrombosis of the popliteal artery with distal clot propagation or multiple tibial emboli carry a risk of amputation of 40%, despite prompt surgical embolectomy.[3,128,129] In patients with a viable extremity at presentation in whom no major runoff vessels are seen on angiography, a trial of local fibrinolytic therapy may improve these results. Surgical correction of the underlying lesion (stenosis or aneurysm) can be performed in a timely fashion. When severe ischemia precludes lytic therapy, it is best to proceed with popliteal exploration and embolectomy. Intraoperative intraarterial infusion of lytic agents in an attempt to lyse clots that are inaccessible to the embolectomy catheter may improve the results of embolectomy alone.

Thrombosis or embolization to the renal arteries is a promising area in which thrombolytic therapy may offer significant advantages over surgical intervention (Fig. 35.4). As a complication of myocardial infarction, an embolus to the renal artery carries an inordinate risk with surgical intervention. Capsular collaterals frequently maintain viability of the renal parenchyma to allow sufficient time for success with thrombolytic therapy. The clot material is sensitive to lysis, and the length of the occlusion is short. The reported experience is limited but has been highly successful.[122,130] If a stenosis is uncovered during infusion, percutaneous dilatation or elective surgical repair may be undertaken, as deemed appropriate.

Acute mesenteric artery occlusion has been treated successfully with local intraarterial streptokinase infusion (Fig. 35.5).[131] In contrast to the kidneys, the bowel is exquisitely sensitive to ischemia and reperfusion. It is difficult to clinically assess the tolerance to ischemia on presentation and during therapy. If lytic therapy is elected for acute mesenteric ischemia, any deterioration in the overall clinical status, persistent acidosis, or sepsis mandates emergency exploration. Otherwise, frequent angiographic assessment, as often as every 6 hours, is advisable. Failure to show progress during these intervals should trigger early, rather than delayed, exploration.

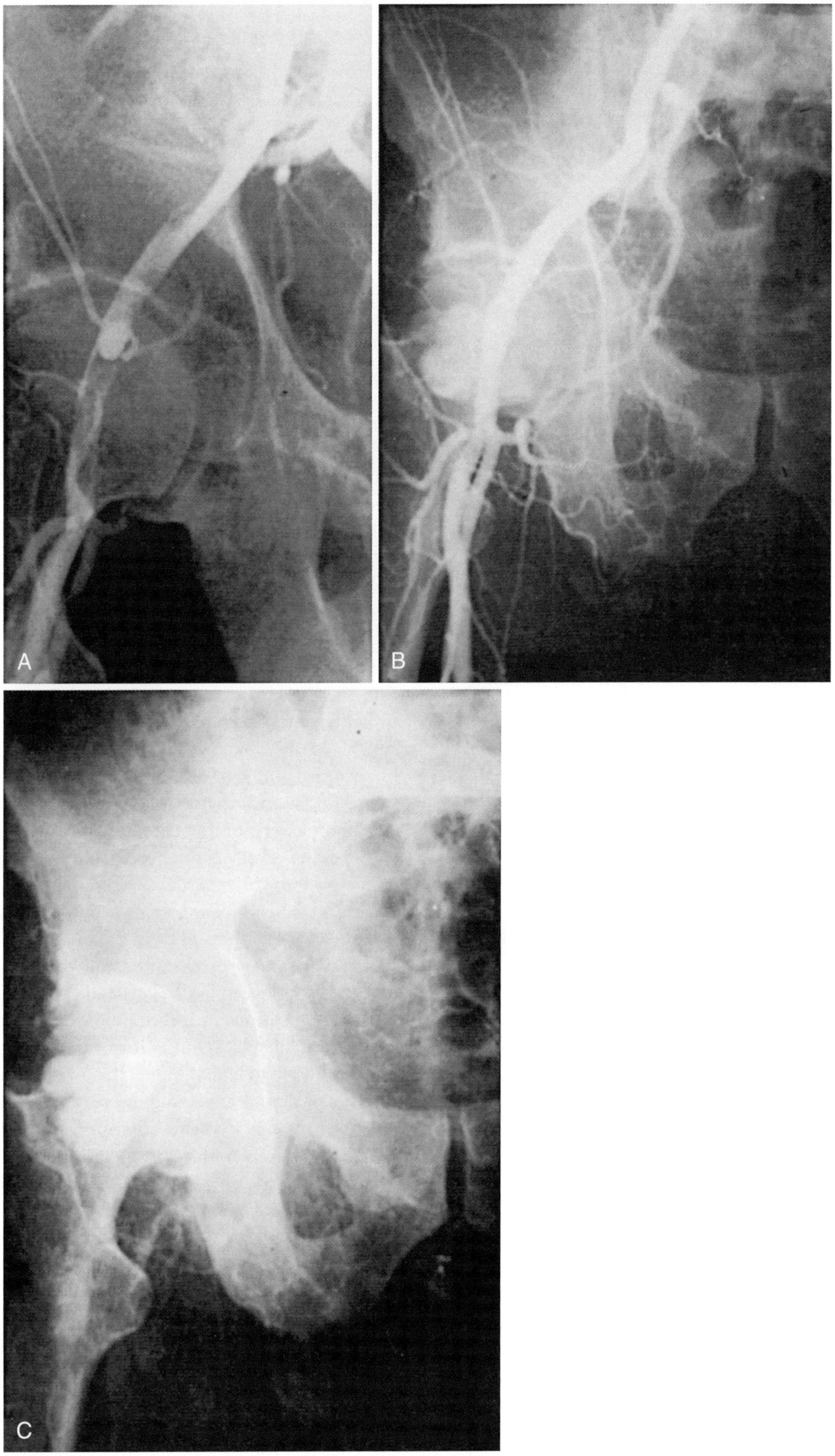

FIG 35.3 This 63-year-old man underwent balloon angioplasty of a right external iliac artery stenosis. (A) Postprocedure angiogram shows thrombosis of the dilated segment. (B) After 12 hours of intraarterial streptokinase, there is complete resolution of the thrombus. (C) A pseudoaneurysm is evident on angiography. Repair was limited to suture closure of the perforation, with no need for thrombectomy.

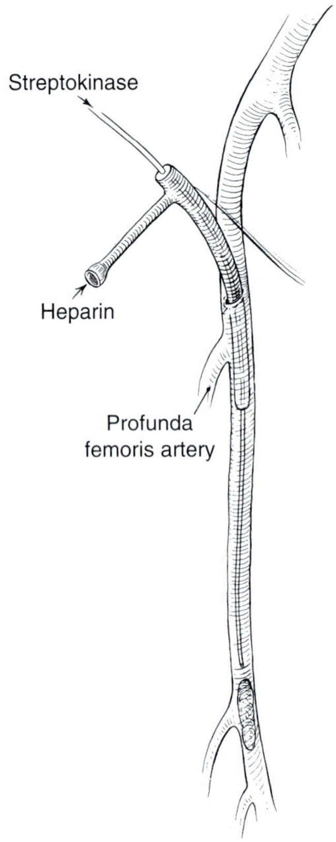

FIG 35.4 Preferred delivery method for intraarterial lytic therapy for distal lower extremity occlusions. Low-dose heparin is infused through the coaxial system to avoid upstream thrombus.

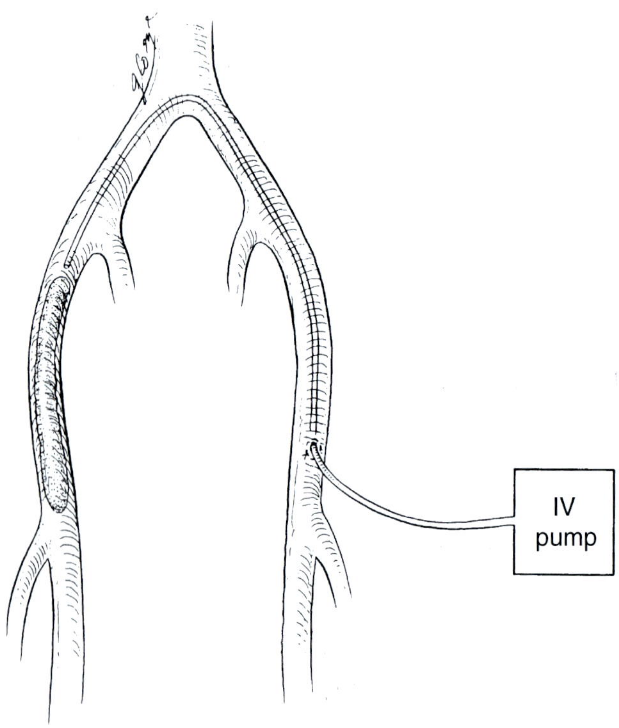

FIG 35.5 Preferred method of intraarterial lytic therapy for proximal (iliac, common femoral) occlusions. If possible, the catheter tip should be within the thrombus. *IV*, Intravenous.

Acute Graft Occlusion

Acute occlusion of an arterial graft frequently leads to recurrent symptoms and, on occasion, limb-threatening ischemia. Thrombectomy, with or without revision, achieves excellent results in prosthetic grafts and variable results in autogenous vein grafts.[132] Autogenous vein grafts frequently require extensive revision and replacement. Intraarterial thrombolytic therapy, in contrast, has been highly unsuccessful in resolving prosthetic graft occlusions. Of 25 patients with prosthetic graft occlusions treated with local lytic therapy by Sussman and coworkers,[120] the treatment was successful in only six patients, five of whom required surgical correction of the offending lesion. In the 19 failures, amputation followed in 12 patients. In the experience reported by Van Breda and colleagues,[129] among 19 patients with 20 prosthetic graft occlusions, only 4 patients were managed nonoperatively, 2 of whom required percutaneous transluminal angioplasty. Despite this, lytic therapy was considered beneficial because it allowed elective surgery in 12 patients and improvement in the surgical risk in an additional 2 patients. An adjunctive role for lytic therapy was proposed. Although achieving successful lysis in 7 of 10 polytetrafluoroethylene (PTFE) grafts with thrombolytic therapy, Graor and associates[121] noted that surgical revision was required in most of these patients.[121] In view of the excellent results obtained with surgical thrombectomy, one must seriously question the value of thrombolytic therapy in the management of prosthetic graft occlusions.

The results obtained with lytic therapy in the management of occluded autogenous grafts have been somewhat more gratifying. In the experience of Perler and colleagues,[133] occluded vein grafts were more susceptible to lytic therapy than were PTFE grafts. This experience is shared by others.[134] However, Graor and coworkers[121] observed a similar response between PTFE and vein grafts, reporting a 75% success rate in vein grafts occluded for less than 14 days. Taking into account the variable results with surgical thrombectomy in the management of occluded autologous grafts, a trial of lytic therapy is an attractive alternative if the event is recent. However, long saphenous vein grafts to tibial vessels in the lower third of the leg or ankle are less responsive to lytic therapy; this may have to do with limited supplies of plasminogen in these very low-flow grafts. Nevertheless, even in unsuccessful attempts, it is not unusual to find liquefied, thickened blood in the graft at operation, thus minimizing the need for mechanical thrombectomy. The operation may actually be limited to removal of the most distal occlusive material and revision of an identified lesion. Retrieving an occluded vein graft in these circumstances is possible with minimal mechanical trauma to the endothelium.

A study of acute limb ischemia (ALI) of the lower extremities delineated outcomes in 129 limbs treated in 119 patients.[159] Technical success was achieved in 82% cases. The 30-day mortality rate was 6.0%, with all 30-day deaths occurring in females. One (0.76%) central nervous system hemorrhage was noted in this cohort. Primary patency for the entire cohort at 12 and 24 months was 50.1% (95% confidence interval [CI], 39.5 to 60.7) and 37.7% (95% CI, 26.2 to 49.1), respectively, whereas secondary patency was 74.0% (95% CI, 64.9 to 83.1) and 65.3% (95%

CI, 54.5 to 76.2), respectively. Multivariable analyses identified patients presenting with femoropopliteal (hazard ratio [HR], 2.63) or tibial thrombosis (HR, 2.80); graft thrombosis (vs. native artery thrombosis; HR, 2.57) and long-term dialysis (HR, 3.66; 95% CI, 2.35 to 5.71; $P < .001$) were associated with poorer primary patency rates. Cumulative limb salvage at 24 months was 68.8% (95% CI, 59.5 to 78.1), with female gender (HR, 3.34; $P = .002$) and thrombolysis for 3 days or greater (HR, 2.35; $P = .019$) associated with an increased risk of limb loss. Overall 36-month survival was 84.5% (95% CI, 77.5 to 91.6). Women had decreased survival rates both in the short and mid term (HR, 6.29; 95% CI, 1.78 to 22.28; $P = .004$). This study highlighted that endovascular therapy with thrombolysis remains an effective treatment option for patients presenting with lower extremity ALI. However, thrombolysis should be limited to shorter than 3 days. Female gender negatively affected the rates of limb salvage and survival.

It is important to consider several factors when deciding whether to use lytic therapy for an occluded graft. Certainly, surgical risk must be assessed. Infrequently, surgery is avoided altogether. If delaying surgical intervention allows an improvement of the overall risk, lytic therapy should be considered. If little improvement is expected, it is preferable to proceed with thrombectomy in a timely fashion. When dealing with a prosthetic graft occlusion, thrombectomy remains the therapy of choice. In patients in whom multiple previous reconstructions make a surgical approach less desirable, a trial of lytic therapy is a reasonable option; however, one must realize that the chances of success without eventual surgical correction are low. The management of an occluded vein graft differs, in that the results of surgical thrombectomy are less predictable. Thus, if the ischemia is well tolerated, a trial of lytic therapy may help to restore patency of the vein graft. Correction of the causative lesion may then be undertaken without the need for thrombectomy of the graft. This can be accomplished percutaneously if the lesion is less than 0.5 cm long; surgery is preferable for longer lesions. Long-term results of this approach tend to correlate with preocclusion history of the bypass. Grafts that fail within the first year after implantation fare worse than those that have been patent for longer periods. Thus an early failure of a vein bypass graft in which a complex lesion is identified may be best treated with a new reconstruction if autogenous tissue is available. Failure of a vein graft beyond 1 year may be best treated with a trial of lytic therapy and correction of the causative lesion.

Results of Randomized Trials

Lower Extremity Ischemia

Despite a multitude of retrospective reviews of the results of thrombolytic therapy in the management of thrombotic complications of peripheral arterial disease, the precise role of this form of therapy could not be clearly established. For this reason, several investigators embarked on prospective, randomized trials comparing surgery to thrombolysis for ischemia of the lower extremities.

The largest trial to date (STILE) randomized 393 patients with native arterial or bypass graft occlusion to either optimal surgical therapy or intraarterial, catheter-directed thrombolysis with rt-PA or urokinase.[82] Outcomes were analyzed on an intention-to-treat basis to maintain statistical validity. The dosage of rt-PA was 0.05 mg/kg per hour for up to 12 hours; for urokinase, a 250,000-unit bolus injection was followed by 4000 units/min for 4 hours, then 2000 units/min for up to 36 hours. End points measured included death, ongoing or recurrent ischemia, major amputation, and major morbidity. Additional end points included reduction in surgical procedure, clinical outcome classification, length of hospitalization, and outcome by duration of ischemia. The randomization produced equivalent groups in terms of risk factors and comorbid conditions. A monitoring committee terminated the study before its anticipated patient recruitment because a significant primary end point occurred in the first interim analysis. Failure or inability to place the catheter in the thrombolytic group occurred in 28% of patients who were randomized, and these were considered treatment failures. A significant benefit of surgical therapy compared with thrombolysis occurred at 30 days, primarily because of a reduction in ongoing or recurrent ischemia. Clinical outcome classification at 30 days was similar. Stratification by duration of ischemia suggested that patients with ischemia of less than 14 days' duration had lower amputation rates with thrombolysis and shorter hospital stays. Patients with ischemia of longer duration (more than 14 days) who were treated surgically had less ongoing or recurrent ischemia and trends toward lower morbidity. At 6 months, there was an improved amputation-free survival in acutely ischemic patients treated with thrombolysis. However, chronically ischemic patients who were treated surgically had lower major amputation rates. Fifty-five percent of patients treated with thrombolysis had a reduction in the magnitude of their surgical procedure. No difference between rt-PA and urokinase was noted, with fibrinogen depletion being a predictor of hemorrhagic complications.

Other investigators concluded that surgical revascularization of patients with ischemic symptoms of less than 6 months' duration was more effective and safer than catheter-directed thrombolysis. Crossover to surgical treatment from the thrombolytic group probably accounted for the clinical outcomes being similar in both groups at 30 days. Patients with fewer than 14 days of ischemia who were treated with thrombolysis had an improved amputation-free survival compared with patients who underwent surgical treatment. Of concern was the 28% of patients in the thrombolytic arm who did not receive thrombolytic therapy because of failure to place the catheter within the thrombus. Subsequent analysis revealed that even if these patients were eliminated from the analysis as failures in the thrombolytic arm, the results and conclusions did not change.

Further analysis of those patients in the STILE study who had native, nonembolic arterial thrombosis has been completed.[135] Two hundred thirty-seven patients with lower extremity ischemia owing to iliofemoral or superficial femoropopliteal native artery occlusion, with symptomatic deterioration within 6 months, were randomized to either thrombolytic therapy or surgical revascularization. Before randomization, the optimal surgical procedure was determined for subsequent comparison with eventual outcome. For patients randomized to lytic therapy, the catheter could be properly positioned and the lytic agent delivered in 78% of patients; thus 22% of patients in that group did not receive lytic therapy owing to an inability to position the catheter. A reduction in the subsequent surgical procedure performed occurred in 58% of patients with femoropopliteal occlusions and in 51% of patients with iliofemoral occlusions. Urokinase and rt-PA were equally effective and safe, but lysis time was shorter with rt-PA than with urokinase (8 vs. 24 hours). At 1 year, the incidence of recurrent ischemia was significantly higher in patients treated with thrombolytic therapy than in those treated with surgery (64% vs. 35%). Major amputation rates were also higher in the thrombolytic therapy group, with 10% of patients eventually requiring a major amputation in the thrombolytic arm of the study versus no patients in the surgical arm. Factors associated with poor lytic outcome included femoropopliteal occlusion, diabetes, and presence of critical ischemia. There was no difference in mortality observed at 1 year between the surgical and lytic therapy groups. The investigators concluded that surgical revascularization for lower extremity native arterial occlusions is more effective and durable than thrombolysis. A reduction in the planned surgical procedure occurred for the majority of patients treated with thrombolysis. However, long-term outcome was inferior, particularly in those patients with femoropopliteal occlusions, diabetes, or critical ischemia.

A prospective, randomized comparison of thrombolytic therapy and operative revascularization in the initial management of acute peripheral arterial ischemia was performed in a single institution and published in 1994.[136] In this study, patients with limb-threatening ischemia of less than 7 days' duration were randomly assigned to intraarterial, catheter-directed urokinase therapy or operative intervention. If an anatomic lesion was unmasked by the thrombolytic infusion, this was treated with either balloon angioplasty or surgery. Primary end points included limb salvage and survival. A total of 114 patients were randomized; 57 received thrombolytic therapy, and an equal number had surgery. Thrombolytic therapy resulted in dissolution of occluding thrombus in 70% of patients in the lytic group. Cumulative limb salvage was similar in the two treatment groups, at 12 months (82%). However, cumulative survival was significantly improved in patients randomized to thrombolysis (84% vs. 58% at 12 months). The higher mortality in the surgical arm was primarily due to an increased frequency of in-hospital cardiopulmonary complications. The benefits of thrombolysis appeared to be accomplished without significant differences in the duration of hospitalization and with a modest increase in hospital costs (median, $15,672 vs. $12,253). Intraarterial thrombolytic therapy was associated with a reduction of in-hospital cardiopulmonary complications and therefore improved patient survival.

Based on these results, and to further elucidate the possible effect of thrombolytic therapy on 1-year survival, a multicenter, randomized, prospective trial comparing thrombolysis and peripheral arterial surgery was carried out.[137] Phase I was designed to be a dose-ranging trial to evaluate the safety and efficacy of three doses of recombinant urokinase in comparison with surgery. Two-hundred thirteen patients who had acute lower extremity ischemia of less than 14 days' duration were prospectively randomized to one of two groups. The first group received one of three dosages of recombinant urokinase (2000, 4000, or 6000 IU/min for 4 hours, then 2000 IU/min for a maximum of 48 hours). The second group underwent surgical revascularization. Successful thrombolytic therapy was followed by either surgical or endovascular intervention when a lesion responsible for the occlusion was recognized. Follow-up on an intent-to-treat basis was performed for 1 year. The most effective dose of recombinant urokinase was found to be 4000 IU/min. This dose accomplished complete thrombolysis in 35 of the 49 patients (71%) who were randomized to this dose in the lytic therapy group. Mean infusion time was 23 hours. Patients who received 2000 IU/min had a 67% success rate, whereas patients who were randomized to the highest dose (6000 IU/min) had a 60% success rate. Hemorrhagic complications were 2%, 13%, and 16% in the 4000-, 2000-, and 6000-IU/min groups, respectively. When comparing the 4000-IU/min group with the surgical group, the 1-year mortality rate was similar (14% vs. 16%), and amputation-free survival was not statistically different (75% vs. 65%). Again, patients treated with lytic therapy had a decrease in the planned surgical procedure that was statistically significant. The investigators concluded that recombinant urokinase is most effective at 4000 IU/min. Thrombolytic therapy and surgical therapy had similar rates of survival and limb salvage.

From the foregoing results, it is evident that in patients with relatively acute ischemia, thrombolytic therapy is an important and effective treatment, with results that compare favorably with those of surgery. Considerable judgment is required in patient selection, which should account for the duration of the ischemia, the complexity of the anticipated surgical intervention, the presence of contraindications to thrombolytic therapy, and the tolerance of the limb to ischemia (Fig. 35.6). Although the number of vein grafts included in these trials was not sufficient to allow specific recommendations, retrospective information suggests that the long-term outcome of thrombolytic therapy in the management of thrombosed vein grafts is best when the vein graft has failed late (more than 1 year) and when a specific lesion can be identified and corrected after completion of the lytic infusion.

Hemodialysis Access

Thrombosed arteriovenous fistulas can be managed successfully with intragraft administration of fibrinolytic agents. Usually the diagnosis is established early, when the patient notices the absence of a thrill; thus the thrombotic material is very sensitive to lysis. Administration is by direct puncture because there are no collaterals to dilute the effect of the agent. It is usually best to lace the intragraft thrombus with the lytic agent and then proceed with high-dose intragraft administration. Graor and colleagues[121] were successful in treating 40 of 46 arteriovenous fistulas (87%); PTFE and vein fistulas were equally responsive.[121] Thrombi older than 4 days were less susceptible to lysis (29%). Unfortunately, most patients required surgical revision of the venous anastomosis, and lytic therapy was only a temporizing intervention. However, in some patients, this allowed better preoperative preparation and elective, rather than urgent, operation.

A new method of opening thrombosed grafts is pulse-spray pharmacomechanical thrombolysis, followed by balloon

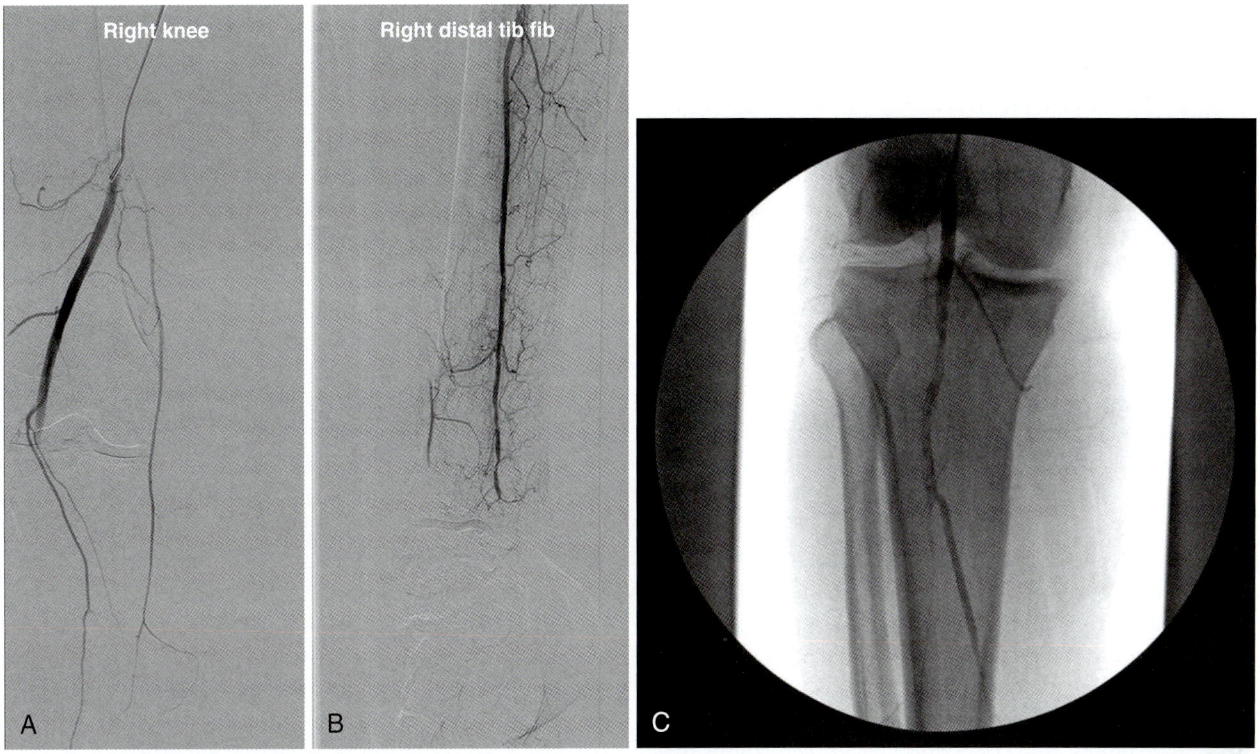

FIG 35.6 (A) Selective angiography of the right leg in a 73-year-old female with acute limb ischemia documents an embolic cutoff in the popliteal artery. (B) Distal imaging reveals pedal emboli as well with absence of runoff vessels to the foot. (C) Catheter-directed thrombolytic therapy is initiated, which partially resolves the proximal embolic material but fails to clear the runoff preventing limb salvage.

maceration. This allows successful lysis of the graft but more quickly than with intragraft administration and with a smaller dose of lytic agent. The pulse-spray can be done with heparinized saline or with a thrombolytic agent. A relatively underappreciated but well-documented phenomenon resulting from pulse-spray thrombolysis of clotted hemodialysis access grafts is the development of PE. A prospective, randomized, double-blinded study was conducted to evaluate the incidence of PE following the use of this technique with urokinase versus heparinized saline. Although PE occurred in both groups, as documented by lung perfusion scan, the incidence was 18.2% with urokinase and 64.3% with heparinized saline ($P = .04$).[138] All the patients, it should be noted, were asymptomatic.

Many studies have attempted to perform cost-benefit analyses of thrombolysis versus surgical thrombectomy. The most common reason for dialysis graft failure is a lesion, usually neointimal hyperplasia, at the venous anastomosis. The interventional techniques allow thrombolysis and identification of the underlying anatomic lesion; this can be treated with balloon angioplasty. Although angioplasty is successful in many cases, surgical revision is usually required at some point in the future.

Acute Stroke

In June 1996 the FDA approved t-PA as a safe and effective treatment for acute stroke if given within 3 hours of the onset of symptoms.[139] Since then, there has been a proliferation of large clinical trials testing the efficacy of antiplatelet and antithrombotic treatment regimens. The approval of the use of intravenous t-PA was based on the results of the National Institute of Neurological Disorders and Stroke (NINDS) Recombinant Tissue Plasminogen Activator Stroke Study, in which 624 patients with ischemic stroke were treated with 0.9 mg/kg of t-PA within 3 hours of the onset of symptoms.[140] Of the t-PA group, 31% to 50% had complete or near-complete recovery at 3 months, compared with 20% to 38% of the placebo group. This benefit prevailed for 1 year. However, there was a 6.4% incidence of symptomatic brain hemorrhage in the t-PA group, versus 0.6% in the placebo group. The mortality rates were similar between the groups. The presence of a mass effect or a greater severity of initial neurologic deficit presented an increased risk of hemorrhage. The beneficial effect of t-PA was not observed in three other large trials (the European Cooperative Acute Stroke Study I and II and the Alteplase Thrombolysis for Acute Noninterventional Therapy in Ischemic Stroke [ATLANTIS] trial).[141-143] However, patients in these three trials were treated much later (only 14% treated within 3 hours) than those in the NINDS rt-PA study (622 of 624 enrolled within 3 hours, and 48% treated within 90 minutes).

There have been two large randomized trials evaluating intra-arterial thrombolytic therapy for stroke. PROACT II evaluated patients with angiographically documented occlusion of the middle cerebral artery or a first-order branch.[66] By 2 hours, there was partial or complete lysis in 67% of patients in the pro-urokinase group, compared with 18% in the heparin-only group

($P < .001$). The primary outcome measure analyzed was the ability to live independently 3 months after the stroke. The percentage of patients able to attain this end point was 40% in the pro-urokinase group and 25% in the heparin group ($P < .05$). Intracerebral hemorrhage with neurologic deterioration occurred in 10% of patients in the pro-urokinase group and in 2% in the heparin group ($P = .06$). This trial was the first to show a clinical benefit from the use of intraarterial thrombolysis of a middle cerebral artery occlusion. To date, there are no randomized controlled trials comparing the efficacy of intravenous versus intraarterial thrombolytics. However, it is clear that thrombolytic therapy for acute ischemic stroke can no longer be considered experimental. It has been shown to have clinical benefit as long as patient selection is strictly in accordance with the criteria set forth in the trials and the NINDS guidelines.

Technique

A plethora of strategies for thrombolysis have been used and are described in a recent consensus document.[160] In this comprehensive review, 33 recommendations were made by a panel of experienced surgeons and interventionists from North America and Europe. The areas covered in this publication cover management of patients with lower limb arterial occlusion from presentation to postoperative monitoring. The critical recommendations that deserve emphasis are that thrombolysis for peripheral arterial occlusion should be via a catheter-directed delivery of agent and that systemic thrombolysis should no longer be used. The likelihood of success with thrombolysis is related to the ability to cross the thrombosed region ("guidewire traversal test"), and placement of an infusion catheter and/or wire embedded into the thrombus. Perhaps, most importantly, identifying and treating the culprit lesion that led to the thrombotic episode is paramount for a long-term successful outcome. Of note, more than 40 dosage schemes were reviewed and described for thrombolytic infusion. These schemes included strategies of continuous versus stepwise infusion, bolusing or lacing the clot, and intraoperative thrombolysis. The most popular strategies included using urokinase 4000 units/min for 4 hours, and then decreasing to 2000 units/min for a maximum of 48 hours, t-PA at a dose of 1 mg/h and lacing the clot to increase thrombolytic efficiency.

The preferred current technique is described later. First, and of particular importance, thrombolysis should not be attempted in any patient whose ischemia has been of sufficient severity or duration to cause severe motor or sensory impairment or in patients whose ischemia cannot tolerate the anticipated duration of the infusion. Because a systemic lytic state can occur with prolonged regional intravascular thrombolytic therapy, absolute contraindications include active internal bleeding, recent surgery or trauma to the area to be perfused, recent cerebrovascular accident, or documented left heart thrombus. Relative contraindications include gastrointestinal bleeding, severe hypertension, mitral valve disease, endocarditis, hemostatic defects, or pregnancy. After a decision to proceed with thrombolysis, expeditious management in an endovascular suite should ensue.

The chosen approach should maximize access to the occlusion and minimize morbidity. Arterial punctures distal to the presumed occlusion are avoided. Sites where bleeding may cause serious morbidity (e.g., axillary, translumbar) are avoided. When the suspected occlusion is below the superficial femoral artery (strong femoral pulse), an antegrade ipsilateral puncture is preferred (Fig. 35.7). When the suspected occlusion is at the femoral level or above, a contralateral puncture with passage of the catheter around the aortic bifurcation is preferred (Fig. 35.8). Multiple puncture attempts can be avoided with the use of Duplex ultrasound in patients with diminished pulses or scarring. Infusions in the upper extremities or aortic branches are carried out through a transfemoral approach. Multi–side-hole catheters are used for infusion, with the infusion length portion of the catheter imbedded in the thrombus. When the infusion is at the popliteal level or below, small (3 French) catheters or infusion wires are used

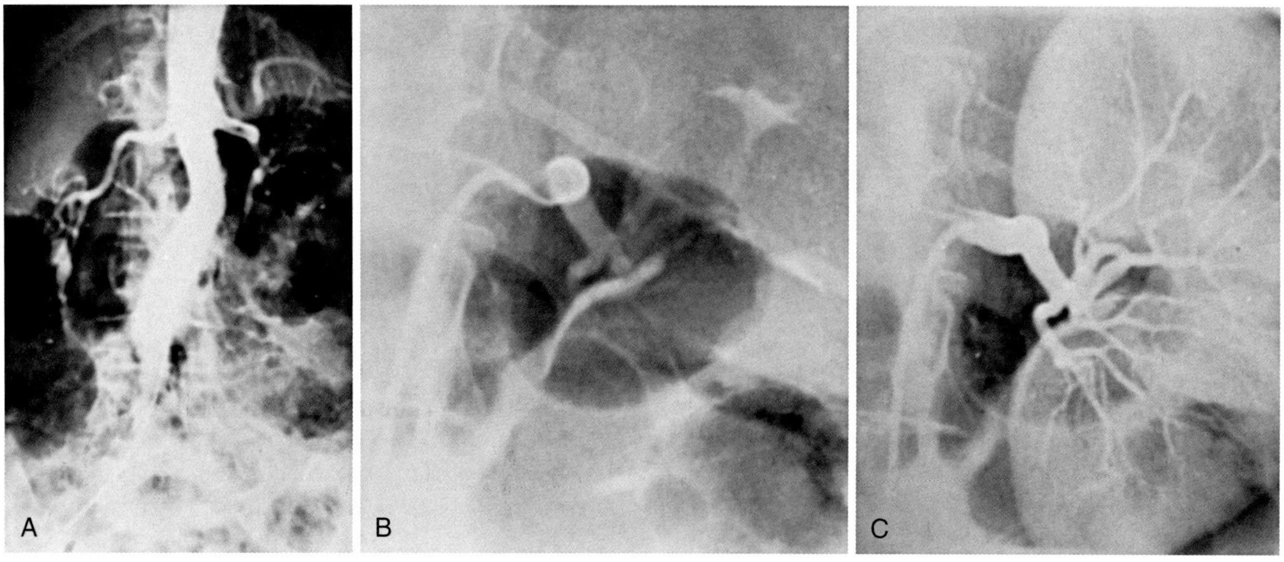

FIG 35.7 (A) Aortogram showing left renal artery embolus. (B) After 1 hour of high-dose intraarterial urokinase, there is partial clearing and improved perfusion to the left kidney. (C) Complete clearance of embolus after 3 hours of high-dose intraarterial urokinase.

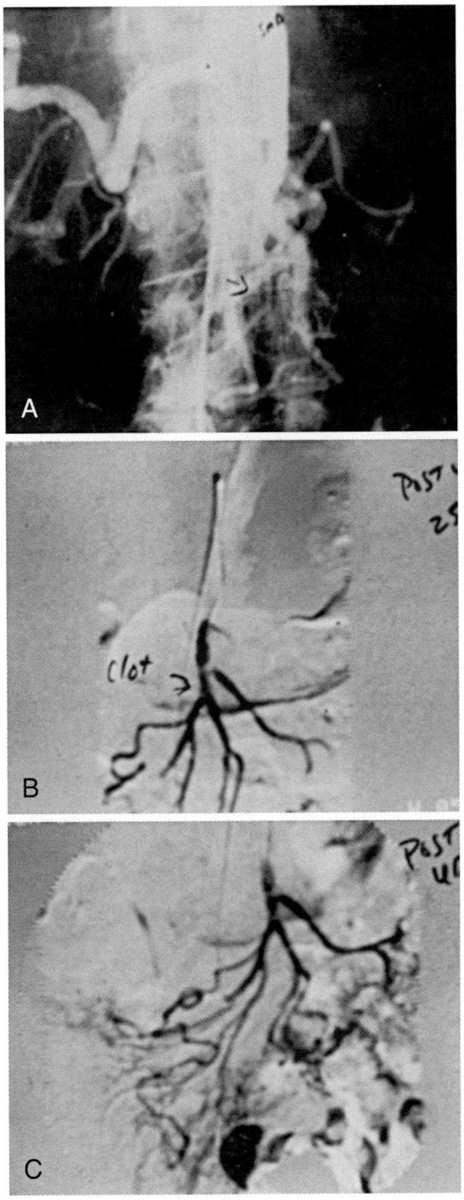

FIG 35.8 (A) Selective superior mesenteric artery angiogram showing occlusion of the distal tree. (B) Partial clearing of embolus after 250,000 units of intraarterial urokinase administered over 1 hour. (C) Complete resolution of superior mesenteric artery occlusion after 2 hours (500,000 units) of intraarterial urokinase therapy.

through a coaxial system to prevent upstream clot formation (Fig. 35.9). A flush heparin infusion is maintained through the coaxial catheter. If the catheter does not properly penetrate the thrombus, lysis is slowed and inefficient because the lytic agent is "washed out" through collaterals.

Creation of a channel into the thrombus with the angiographic guidewire is of prognostic significance and is technically necessary. Failure to pass the guidewire through the occlusion implies either plaque or a well-organized thrombus, which may be resistant to fibrinolysis. Easy passage of the guidewire through the occlusion not only establishes a channel in which the fibrinolytic agent can concentrate but also implies soft thrombi that can be dissolved. After confirmation of distal arterial patency, the next step is usually power-pulse thrombolysis using a percutaneous mechanical thrombectomy system (i.e., the Possis AngioJet system). This step is performed with a minimal amount of thrombolytic agent (2 mg in 50 mL of saline) that is laced throughout the clotted region with short bursts of the catheter. After 20 minutes, mechanical thrombectomy can be performed without any lytic agent to restore a channel and blood flow into the distal vasculature. The next step is thrombolysis with t-PA. Bleeding complications appear to correlate most closely with duration of therapy rather than with the total dosage of the agent. Therefore it believed that higher-dose, short-term infusions are better tolerated than longer-term, low-dose infusions. A higher dose initially (urokinase 4000 units/min, t-PA 1 mg/h) appears to be effective with switching to a lower-dose regimen when there is remnant thrombus on lytic check angiography (urokinase 1000 to 2000 units/min, t-PA 0.2 to 0.5 mg/h). Valved infusion catheters and infusion wires are used singly or in combination to achieve the appropriate infusion length for intrathrombus infusion. After dissolution of the thrombus, treatment of the culprit lesion is critical to durable patency of the thrombolytic procedure.

Duration of the infusion is guided by periodic angiographic and clinical monitoring but should rarely exceed 72 hours.[159] The patient is monitored in an intensive care unit, and angiography is repeated daily or more often, depending on the clinical response. Before initiating therapy, baseline fibrinogen, thrombin time, PTT, and fibrin degradation product measurements are obtained. These are repeated 12 hours after commencing the infusion and then daily. It is expected that the fibrinogen level will drop and fibrin degradation products will become positive. Prolongation of the PTT or thrombin time suggests a systemic lytic state and occurs in approximately 50% of patients. Although specific parameters do not correlate with the risk of bleeding, presence of a systemic lytic state increases the risk. If good progress is being made by the infusion, a low fibrinogen value (<50% of baseline) or evidence of a lytic state in the absence of bleeding complications is tolerated, and therapy is continued. In the absence of a systemic lytic state when little progress is evident, the dosage is increased and the result reassessed. Therapy should be discontinued if there is no improvement in any 24-hour interval, persistent or worsening ischemia, or a major bleeding complication.

The administration of heparin during regional thrombolytic therapy is advocated by most investigators. Clearly, in patients with profound ischemia and very low flow in the extremity, and when pericatheter thrombus formation would be significant (e.g., when 3 to 4 cm of the catheter is in a vessel with low or no flow), concomitant heparin administration should be strongly considered. Heparin administration may also be useful in increasing thrombolysis and minimizing the adverse consequences of a potential episode of distal clot migration or embolization. However, heparin therapy may increase the incidence and severity of pericatheter bleeding during lytic therapy and may increase the risk of distant bleeding. For these reasons, it is common to proceed with heparin administration via a continuous infusion to maintain a prolonged PTT at 1.5- to 2.0-fold the control only

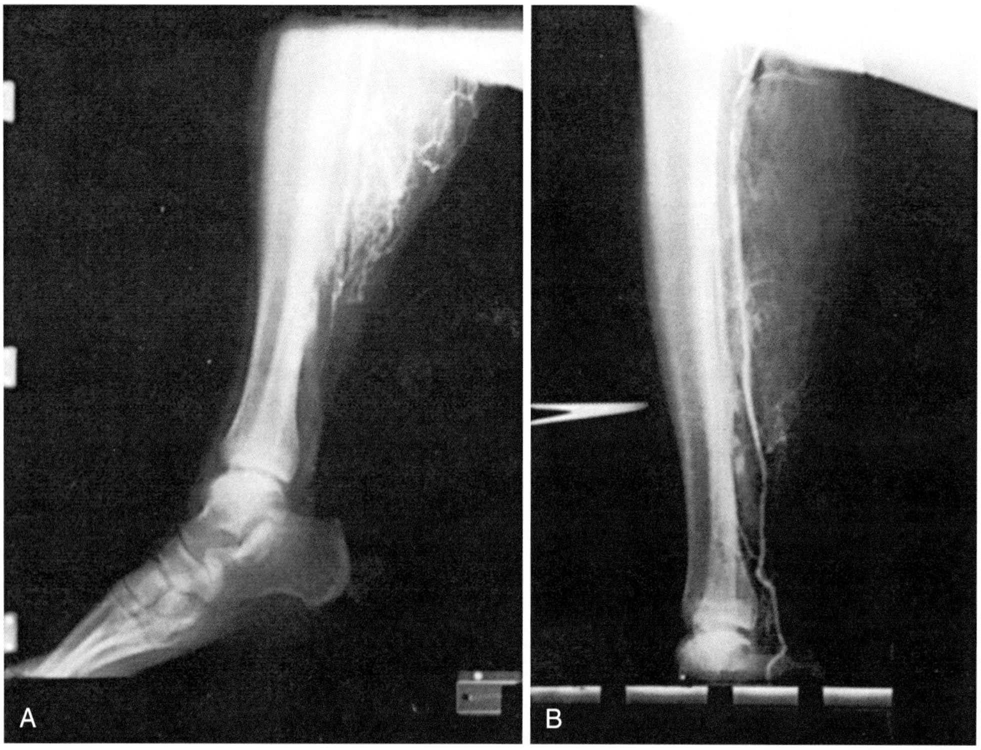

FIG 35.9 (A) Intraoperative completion angiogram after popliteal embolectomy. Note the absence of runoff vessels to the foot. (B) Repeated angiogram after intraoperative infusion of streptokinase 60,000 units and heparin 1000 units over 30 minutes through the same catheter used for angiography. Note the remarkable improvement in runoff.

till thrombolysis is initiated. After lysis begins, a lower dose of heparin is administered, usually 500 units/h through the sheath side arm. It is important that the PTT not exceed 60 seconds at the time of catheter and sheath removal. Heparin can then be restarted without a bolus.

When emergency surgery is required, the lytic agent is discontinued and fresh frozen plasma is administered if the fibrinogen level is less than 100 mg/dL. The half-life of these agents is short and is usually not a problem in this setting.

Complications

As with any form of lytic therapy, bleeding is the most feared and frequent complication of low-dose fibrinolytic therapy. The risk of major bleeding (requiring cessation of therapy or blood transfusion) ranges from 5% to 15% when appropriate precautions are observed.[121,144] Bleeding is usually related to systemic effects of the drug, and management was discussed earlier in this chapter.

Considering that high-risk patients may be treated preferentially by this nonsurgical approach, the incidence of bleeding with intraarterial lytic therapy must be considered. The most recent experience indicates that the risk of bleeding correlates more with duration than with total dosage. It is therefore preferable to use higher-dose protocols, especially when a short occlusion is being treated. Although specific coagulation parameters do not correlate with the risk of bleeding, the presence of a systemic lytic state increases this risk. It is important to document whether systemic effects of the drug are present, because such knowledge helps to determine the most appropriate course of action. Systemic effects are heralded by a 50% drop in fibrinogen from baseline, a prolongation of the thrombin time to twofold greater than normal (or higher), or both. If significant progress is being made, continuation of therapy is warranted, despite systemic fibrinolysis. If no significant improvement is noted within the last interval, reassessment should be made, weighing the risks and benefits of the alternatives.

Treatment of hemorrhagic complications depends on their severity and on the progress made during lytic therapy. A small amount of oozing around the catheter entry site, without hematoma formation during the final stages of the infusion, can be controlled locally, keeping the patient under close observation until therapy is completed. The same situation in the early stages of the infusion, when more than 12 to 24 hours of therapy are anticipated, should lead to discontinuation of the drug. Development of a significant hematoma or bleeding at a remote site warrants cessation of therapy. Fibrinogen should be replaced by the administration of fibrinogen-rich components, such as cryoprecipitate or fresh frozen plasma. This usually suffices because the half-life of both urokinase and streptokinase is short.

Distal embolization occurs more frequently than is clinically appreciated. Continuation of therapy is preferable, with perhaps a temporary increase in the hourly dose. When severe ischemia is seen as the result of distal emboli, discontinuation of lytic therapy with prompt surgical embolectomy is indicated.

Several cases of embolization to the ipsilateral extremity have been reported during intraarterial lytic therapy for occlusion of axillofemoral grafts.[121] The length of these grafts makes them unsuitable for lytic therapy; therefore surgical thrombectomy remains the therapy of choice.

Allergic reactions to streptokinase were discussed earlier. Routine administration of 100 mg of intravenous hydrocortisone may prevent some of these reactions and is recommended.

Pseudoaneurysm formation is rare but may occur secondary to bleeding from an arterial puncture site. Surgical repair is recommended.

Intracranial bleeding is a recognized complication of any form of lytic therapy. Any change in the patient's neurologic status during therapy should be viewed as related to the fibrinolytic agent until proved otherwise. Bleeding from an unrecognized intracranial lesion must be ruled out. Lytic therapy should be discontinued while the evaluation is proceeding.

Fatal pulmonary emboli have been reported during intraarterial fibrinolytic therapy.[123] A possible mechanism for this complication is decreased venous circulation in the ischemic extremity, with clot formation, partial lysis, and eventual pulmonary embolization. This is a rare occurrence. Treatment options include cessation of lytic therapy with heparinization or a switch to systemic intravenous lytic therapy. If the latter is chosen, leaving the intraarterial catheter in place may decrease the risk of bleeding through the arterial puncture site.

Conversion of an ischemic myocardial infarction into a hemorrhagic infarct as a complication of fibrinolytic therapy has been reported.[123] The relationship between lytic therapy and the few reported cases is unclear. Deterioration of cardiac function in the presence of an acute myocardial infarction during fibrinolytic therapy should lead the clinician to consider this possibility. Therapy should be discontinued until the cause of the cardiac decompensation is determined.

INTRAOPERATIVE THROMBOLYTIC THERAPY

Approximately 30% of lower extremity embolectomies are incomplete, with residual intravascular defects demonstrable by completion angiography.[145] Experimental studies suggest that the true incidence may be as high as 80%.[146] The idea of removing the bulk of thrombus surgically and lysing any remaining defects is attractive from a therapeutic standpoint. Alternatives include repeated embolectomy with the balloon catheter,[147] irrigation in an attempt to flush the residual clot,[148] passage of Dormia catheters,[149] and distal exploration. These alternatives will further injure the endothelium and thus increase its thrombogenicity. Certain endovascular procedures, such as endoscopy, atherectomy, or dilatation, may also temporarily increase the thrombogenicity of these vessels, leading to early thrombosis. Further mechanical manipulation is likely to result in further injury and thus is unlikely to solve the problem. For these reasons, controlled chemical intraoperative fibrinolysis may be a welcome alternative in the treatment of these complications. When dealing with delayed intervention in the presence of a thrombotic process, propagation of clot into the branches of the arterial tree may be problematic. After these clots lose their integrity with the parent thrombus, they are difficult to retrieve, and enzymatic dissolution may be the only alternative.

Bleeding complications secondary to intraarterial fibrinolytic therapy are the result of prolonged infusions necessary to lyse extensive thrombus. The potential for intraoperative or perioperative lytic therapy has been suggested by several investigators.[150-152] Common to all these observations was the lack of bleeding complications. There are several advantages to the intraoperative use of lytic agents when compared with the percutaneous method. First, the bulk of the thrombus has been surgically removed, so that less lysis is required. Second, a higher concentration of the agent, with control of inflow (and therefore circulation time), can be accomplished. Finally, infusion within the thrombus or adjacent to it is theoretically unnecessary, and repeated embolectomy with reassessment of the intervention can be done with repeated infusions, as necessary.

In 1985 Quiñones-Baldrich and colleagues[153] reported initial experience with five patients in whom intraoperative infusions of 20,000 to 100,000 units of streptokinase were successful in restoring adequate circulation to limbs still threatened after embolectomy. This experience has been expanded to 23 infusions in 22 patients.[154] In 17 of these patients, both preinfusion and postinfusion arteriograms were available; improvement following lytic therapy was seen in 13 patients (76%). Only one of these reconstructions rethrombosed in the postoperative period. All four patients without angiographic improvement suffered rethrombosis. Thus it appears that preinfusion and postinfusion arteriography has prognostic significance, implying that failure to improve after intraoperative infusion of the lytic agent suggests a high likelihood of failure; therefore alternative methods of reconstruction need to be considered at the time of surgery.

Clinical experience to date is summarized in Table 35.2.[119,153,155-157] Five additional clinical series have been reported since the initial report. Cohen and colleagues[119] performed 13 bolus infusions of 25,000 to 250,000 units of streptokinase. Eight (61%) of the infusions were successful. Five bleeding complications occurred, one of them resulting in death secondary to retroperitoneal bleeding during aortoiliac reconstruction. This result suggests that caution should be exercised when using lytic agents during major abdominal or retroperitoneal surgery. Norem and associates[156] reported their experience with 19 infusions of 50,000 to 200,000 units of streptokinase by bolus injection. They followed the infusion with repeated embolectomy and were able to retrieve additional thrombus in each instance. Two wound hematomas occurred in the postoperative period. Low doses of heparin (200 to 500 units/h) were maintained postoperatively. With this regimen, bleeding complications were minimized. In a report from Spain, investigators studied 66 femoropopliteal or distal acute arterial occlusions by means of arteriography and Doppler imaging before and after surgery. Patients were prospectively evaluated after either mechanical thromboembolectomy as a single technique ($n = 35$) or thromboembolectomy plus 250,000 IU of urokinase administered over 30 minutes intraarterially at completion of the operation ($n = 31$). Intraoperative angiography revealed residual thrombus in 30% of patients and unsuspected arterial lesions in 34%. Recurrence of thrombosis was associated with residual thrombus and amputation. Patients who received the intraoperative thrombolytic infusion had higher ankle-brachial indexes postoperatively than did those

TABLE 35.2 Results of Intraoperative Regional Fibrinolytic Therapy

Author	No. of Cases	Drug Dose and Method	Successful (%)	Complications	Remarks
Cohen and colleagues[119]	13	SK: 25,000–250,000 units by bolus	61	Five rethromboses; five bleeding complications; one death after retroperitoneal surgery	Two renal infusions, one partly successful; death related to retroperitoneal bleeding
Norem and colleagues[156]	19	SK: 50,000–200,000 units by bolus	100	Two wound hematomas	All patients underwent repeat embolectomy; postoperative heparin in low doses (200–500 units/h)
Parent and colleagues[157]	28	SK: 50,000–150,000 units by bolus UK: 35,000–150,000 units by bolus	88	Bleeding 11%; compartment syndrome 21%; two deaths	Deaths not related to lytic therapy; bleeding complications in two patients after retroperitoneal surgery
Comerota and colleagues[155]	38	SK: maximum 50,000 units UK: maximum 150,000 units by bolus in 2 patients; isolated limb, UK 1 million units	74	One wound hematoma; five deaths	Deaths not related to lytic agent
Quiñones-Baldrich and colleagues[153]	23	SK: 60,000–100,000 units UK: 250,000–375,000 units plus heparin 1–4 units/mL; gravity infusion over 30 min	74	Six rethromboses; five wound hematomas	All wound hematomas in patients fully heparinized postoperatively

SK, Streptokinase; *UK*, urokinase.

who underwent mechanical thromboembolectomy alone. Amputations and the need for distal revascularization were no different between the two groups, although quantitatively the results were better in the lytic group than in the thromboembolectomy-only group (failure rate, 9.68% vs. 22.86%, respectively). There were no bleeding complications with routine intraoperative use of lytic therapy after mechanical thromboembolectomy.

The preferred technique for intraoperative infusion of fibrinolytic agents consists of a drip infusion of the agent without occlusion of the inflow. Experimental evidence suggests that maintenance of blood flow in the system during administration of fibrinolytic agents enhances their effectiveness. This can be accomplished by insertion of a cannula distal to the arteriotomy after repair of the latter. Urokinase, 250,000 units dissolved in 100 mL of saline delivered over 30 minutes, is preferred. On the basis of an original experimental study, the addition of heparin to the infusate at 1 to 4 units/mL is recommended.[146] Preinfusion and postinfusion arteriography is recommended to document the effectiveness of the agent. Failure to show improvement in the postinfusion angiogram suggests a high likelihood of failure and that alternative management should be considered. More recently, the use of isolated limb perfusion with an extracorporeal pump has shown promise in further enhancing the effectiveness of the lytic agent.[158]

Urokinase appears to be a safer agent for intraoperative use. Allergic reactions are not seen. The mechanism of action is direct, and the risk of plasminogen depletion, which may occur with streptokinase, is eliminated. However, the best method of administration and the appropriate dosage have not been determined. The logistic advantages of bolus infusion are obvious. Nevertheless, a slow infusion has the theoretical advantage of providing a constant amount of the drug while plasminogen is being supplied by the collateral circulation. Bolus infusion, although achieving a high concentration of the agent rapidly, is likely to be washed out, resulting in a short-lived effect. An experimental study was performed to further elucidate the best method of infusion. In addition to bolus infusion and slow 30-minute infusion, the study included a group of animals in which the limb was isolated with a proximal tourniquet and the artery and vein connected to an extracorporeal pump. Angiographic results were significantly improved with use of the isolated limb perfusion technique with similar doses of urokinase.[158] In addition, maintenance of inflow during the slow infusion seemed to improve results compared with occluded inflow. However, these differences were not statistically significant, probably because of the number of animals studied. Thus isolated limb perfusion with extracorporeal pump support of the extremity during revascularization may enhance fibrinolytic activity and improve the efficacy of drug delivery. Clinical experience with this technique is promising but limited.

The high selectivity of t-PA for fibrin and the positive early results with relatively short-term infusion suggest that this agent is promising for intraoperative use. To date, there are no reports of intraoperative use of reteplase.

In summary, one can proceed with an intraoperative fibrinolytic infusion when faced with either residual thrombus inaccessible to the balloon catheter or persistent ischemia after restoration of flow. Although the best method of delivery and most appropriate dosage have not been fully determined, reported clinical experience has allowed guidelines that permit the clinician to obtain the benefits of fibrinolytic infusion in these difficult cases with both safety and efficacy.

REVIEW QUESTIONS

1. Streptokinase and urokinase have which of the following similarities: (1) both are bacterial products, (2) both are enzymes, (3) both are highly fibrin specific, or (4) both are direct fibrinolytic agents?
   a. 1, 2, 3
   b. 1, 3
   c. 2, 4
   d. 4
   e. None of the above
2. Which of the following statements about increasing the dose of streptokinase to decrease its lytic effect is true?
   a. It is indicated when bleeding occurs during therapy.
   b. It is a predictable response.
   c. It is scientifically correct but unnecessary.
   d. It increases the risk of bleeding.
   e. None of the above
3. Which of the following statements about tissue plasminogen activator is true?
   a. It is a nonenzymatic protein.
   b. It has fibrinolytic activity in plasminogen-free media.
   c. It is highly antigenic.
   d. It is mainly an exogenous fibrinolytic activator.
   e. None of the above
4. Which of the following statements is true of a patient with deep venous thrombosis of the femoral system: he or she (1) is a candidate for lytic therapy if the thrombosis is recent and it is the first episode, (2) may be treated with low-dose local lytic therapy, (3) has an approximately 50% to 60% chance of failure to clear the clot completely with lytic therapy, or (4) is at higher risk of pulmonary embolism with lytic therapy than with heparin?
   a. 1, 2, 3
   b. 1, 3
   c. 2, 4
   d. 4
   e. None of the above
5. Which of the following statements about intraarterial lytic therapy is true?
   a. It is initiated with a loading dose.
   b. It is highly effective in graft thrombosis.
   c. It is highly effective in postdilatation thrombosis.
   d. It can be safely administered in patients after a stroke.
   e. It usually prevents a systemic lytic state.
6. What is the dose of urokinase?
   a. Guided by plasminogen levels
   b. 2000 units/kg per hour without a loading dose
   c. 2000 units/kg per hour with a loading dose of 2000 units/kg over 10 minutes
   d. 2000 units/lb per hour
   e. None of the above
7. Which of the following statements about pulmonary emboli is true?
   a. They may be a complication of lytic therapy.
   b. They require at least 72 hours of systemic lytic therapy to completely resolve.
   c. They can be effectively treated by streptokinase 2000 units/kg per hour.
   d. They should always be treated with systemic thrombolytic therapy.
   e. None of the above
8. Which of the following statements is true of complications of thrombolytic therapy?
   a. They are caused by the antigenicity of the agent.
   b. They are caused by plasminemia.
   c. They are reduced by the avoidance of invasive procedures.
   d. They are sometimes treated by increasing the dose.
   e. All of the above
9. Which of the following statements is true of intraoperative thrombolytic therapy: it (1) is contraindicated because bleeding results from systemic absorption, (2) may improve the results of incomplete thrombectomy, (3) is done by intravenous administration of the agent, or (4) should include heparin in the infusate?
   a. 1, 2, 3
   b. 1, 3
   c. 2, 4
   d. 4
   e. None of the above
10. Which of the following statements about streptokinase administration is true?
   a. It results in a drop in plasminogen.
   b. It is contraindicated in patients who have received streptokinase any time in the past.
   c. It is more effective than urokinase when given intraarterially.
   d. It results in a predictable lytic response.
   e. None of the above

References available online at ExpertConsult.com.

36 CHAPTER

Descending Thoracic and Thoracoabdominal Aortic Aneurysms: General Principles and Open Surgical Repair

Kristofer M. Charlton-Ouw, Wande B. Pratt, Charles C. Miller III, Ali Azizzadeh, Anthony L. Estrera, Hazim J. Safi

The first reported repairs of descending thoracic aortic aneurysms were published in the early 1950s.[1,2] The first to successfully perform a thoracoabdominal aortic aneurysm repair were Samuel Etheredge and colleagues in 1955 in Oakland, California.[3] One year later, Michael DeBakey and colleagues performed a true thoracoabdominal repair using a homograft. Subsequently the same group devised an ingenious method of using a Dacron tube graft from the descending thoracic aorta to the infrarenal aorta, sequentially bypassing the celiac axis, superior mesenteric artery, and both renal arteries. This technique decreased the load on the heart and the ischemic time to the intestines and the kidneys. Stanley Crawford's contributions to thoracoabdominal aortic aneurysm repair incorporated three principles of vascular surgery: the Matas inclusion technique,[4] whereby the aneurysm sac is opened but not resected; the reattachment of the intercostal arteries to the graft, as described in an animal model by Spencer in 1950[5]; and the reattachment of the small arteries into a large artery, attributed to Carrel and Guthrie in 1906. Crawford accrued 28 cases by 1973 and published his results of a large group of aneurysm cases treated for the first time with the same clamp-and-sew technique.[6] This technique depended on expeditious repair with short aortic clamp times because the spine and viscera suffered ischemia during repair. Several adjunctive methods for spinal cord and visceral protection later emerged, including distal aortic perfusion,[7-9] cerebrospinal fluid (CSF) drainage,[10] and systemic or regional profound hypothermia.[11]

By the end of the 1980s the preferred method of treatment was still the clamp-and-sew technique, but it continued to be associated with high complication rates, predominantly because of spinal neurologic deficits and renal failure. Since 1992, supported by animal models and clinical experience, the clamp-and-sew technique has been largely abandoned in favor of distal aortic perfusion with the addition of perioperative CSF drainage and moderate passive hypothermia. This chapter provides a review of the authors' experience in the repair of descending thoracic and thoracoabdominal aortic aneurysms, including its natural history, pathology, diagnosis, open surgical treatment, postoperative complications, and management.

NATURAL HISTORY

The adjusted incidence of thoracic aortic aneurysms in population-based studies is 10 per 100,000 person-years.[12] The incidence appears equal in men and woman but increases with age. The goal of aneurysm repair is to prevent rupture, complications from dissection, and death. Open repair of descending thoracic and thoracoabdominal aortic aneurysms is one of the most technically demanding operations in vascular surgery. Adjunctive surgical techniques have led to significant reductions in morbidity, especially from spinal cord ischemia. These improvements underscore the importance of a multidisciplinary approach to this complex problem.

Nearly 10,000 people die annually from thoracic aortic aneurysm, making it the nineteenth leading cause of death in the United States.[13] Overall, aortic aneurysm and dissection accounted for 3.1 deaths per 100,000 people in the United States in 2013. This rate dramatically rises to 7.8 and 20.8 per 100,000 in the age groups of 65 to 74 and 75 to 84 years, respectively.[14] Death from thoracic aortic aneurysm is primarily due to rupture. The rate of rupture increases with aneurysm expansion.[15,16] The natural history of thoracic aortic aneurysm is expansion at a median 0.1 to 0.3 cm/year.[15,17] After 5 cm, growth and rupture can occur unpredictably.

In the Olmsted County study, no ruptures occurred in thoracic aneurysms less than 4 cm in size. The 5-year rupture risk increased to 16% for aneurysms less than 6 cm and was greater than 30% for aneurysms larger than 6 cm.[12] The risk of rupture or dissection occurs at nearly 7% per year.[17] After rupture, the mortality rate is greater than 90% in the first 24 hours.[18] Most patients die before reaching the emergency room. However, elective surgically repaired thoracic aortic aneurysms fare much better than those medically managed or after emergency surgery.[17]

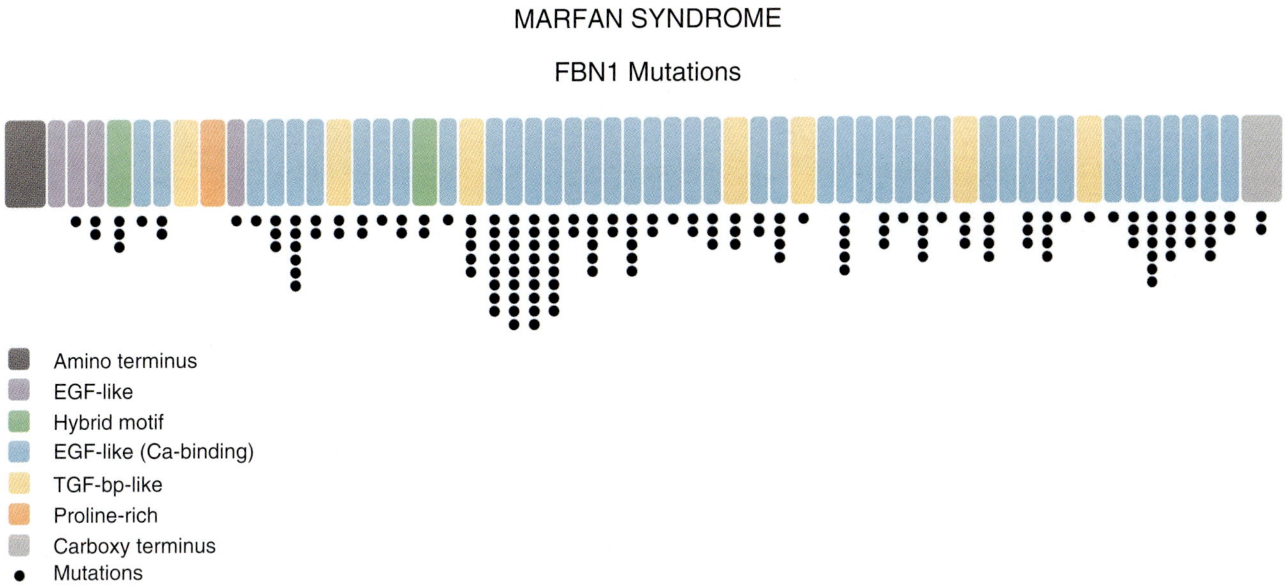

FIG 36.1 Marfan syndrome caused by a mutation in the *FBN1* gene. *EGF*, Endothelial growth factor; *TGF*, transforming growth factor.

The most common thoracic aneurysm occurs in the ascending aorta, but descending thoracic aortic aneurysms account for 45%, whereas thoracoabdominal aortic aneurysms account for approximately 5% of all thoracic aortic aneurysms.[19] Based on the natural history and risk of rupture, descending thoracic and thoracoabdominal aortic aneurysms are considered for repair when maximum diameter reaches 5 to 6 cm. Saccular aneurysms and those with growth greater than 5 mm in 6 months are also considered for repair, regardless of size. Aneurysms in patients with Turner syndrome, Marfan syndrome, and other connective tissue diseases are repaired at smaller diameters.

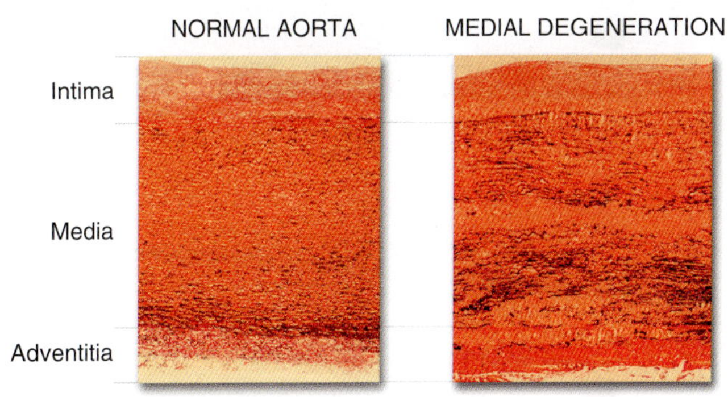

FIG 36.2 Medial degeneration of the aortic wall.

PATHOLOGY AND ETIOLOGY

An aneurysm is a localized or diffuse dilatation greater than 50% of the reference diameter. Most aneurysms are due to medial degeneration and appear to occur sporadically, but genetic factors are increasingly recognized. Up to 20% of individuals with thoracic aortic aneurysms and aortic dissections (TAADs) have a first-degree relative with thoracic aortic disease. Marfan syndrome is an inherited connective tissue disorder caused by any mutation—missense, nonsense, exon deletion or insertion—of fibrillin-1 protein that is encoded in the *FBN1* gene (Fig. 36.1). Other syndromes that predispose individuals to abdominal aortic aneurysms include Loeys-Dietz syndrome, variants of Ehlers-Danlos syndrome, and Turner syndrome. Mutations in α-actin, such as *ACTA2* and *FOXE3*, highlight the importance of vascular smooth muscle function in aortic aneurysm and dissection.[20,21] Familial TAAD is diagnosed based on three criteria: (1) the presence of dilatation and/or dissection of the thoracic aorta; (2) the absence of clinical features of Marfan syndrome, Loeys-Dietz syndrome, or vascular Ehlers-Danlos syndrome; and (3) the presence of a family history of TAAD. *TGFBR2*, *TGFBR1*, *MYH11*, *ACTA2*, *MYLK*, *SMAD3*, and two loci on other chromosomes, AAT1 (FAA1), and AAT2 (TAAD1) are associated with familial TAAD.[22] The recognition of genetic variants in the development of aortic aneurysm will surely increase because many patients report multiple family members with thoracic aortic disease despite a negative genetic workup.

Like atherosclerosis, aortic aneurysm pathophysiology includes a robust inflammatory component. However, unlike atherosclerosis, which primarily affects the intima and causes occlusive disease, the inflammation in aneurysms occurs in the media and adventitia. The histology of degenerative aortic aneurysms is characterized by thinning of the media with distraction of the smooth muscle and elastic tissue (elastin). There is infiltration of inflammatory cells, including mast cells, with neovascularization (Fig. 36.2).[23] There is also activation of proteolytic enzymes and their inhibitors within the aortic wall.[24]

A small percentage of aneurysms are related to infection, so-called mycotic infection, or to trauma, such as pseudoaneurysm. Bacteria or septic emboli may seed the atherosclerotic or ulcerated aortic wall. Infection may also spread from an adjacent empyema or lymph nodes. Organisms associated with aortic

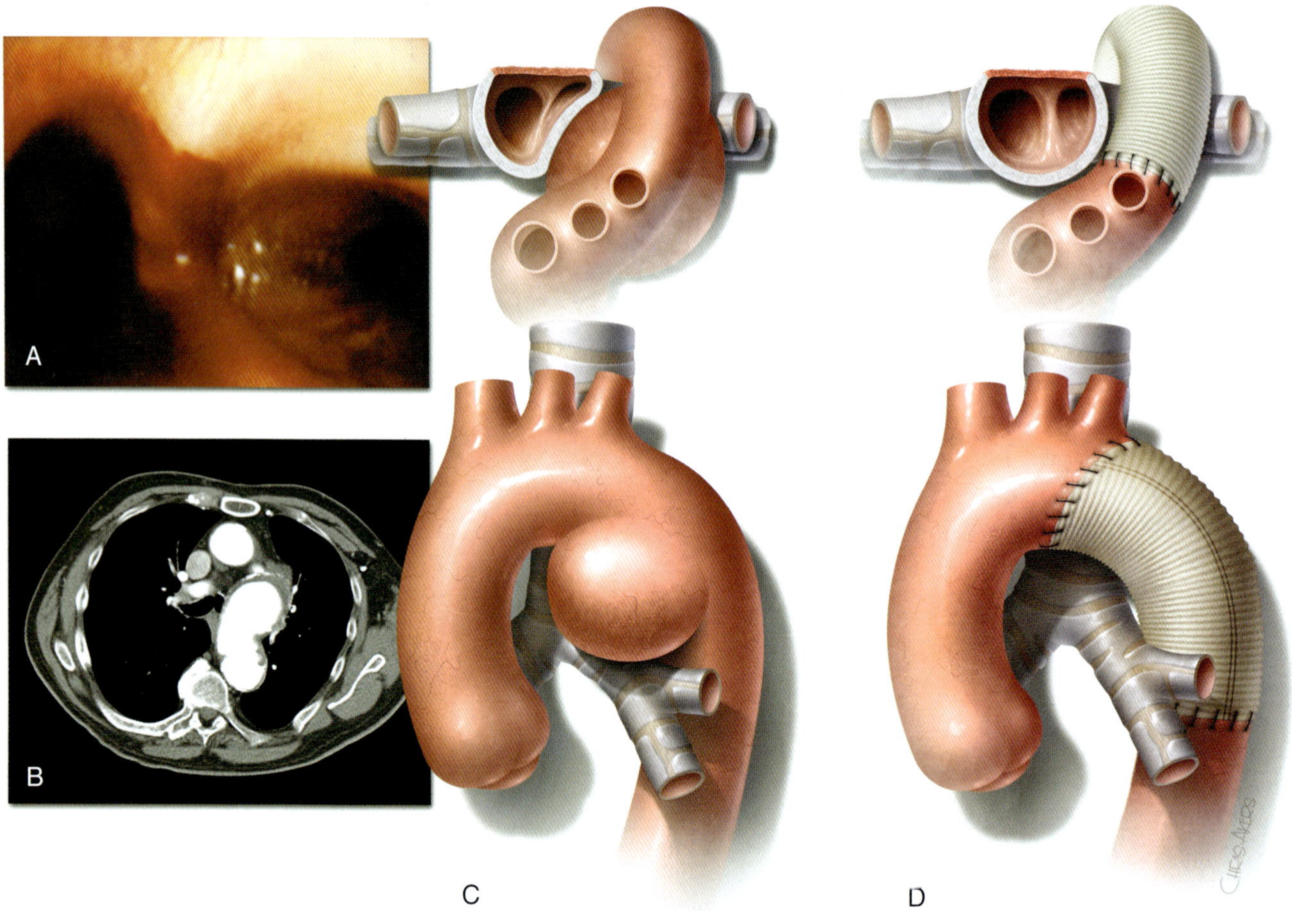

FIG 36.3 Saccular descending thoracic aortic aneurysm causing compression of the right main bronchus. (A) Endoscopic photo showing compression of the right mainstem bronchus. (B) Computed tomography image. (C) Preoperative illustration of aneurysm in caudal direction before repair. (D) Postoperative illustration after repair.

infection include *Salmonella* species, *Haemophilus influenzae*, *Staphylococcus* species, *Mycobacterium tuberculosis*, and *Treponema pallidum*. These aneurysms are usually saccular and carry a high risk of rupture.

Traumatic injuries of the thoracic aorta are also prone to rupture and should be repaired unless the injury is confined to the intima.[25-28] Consistent with consensus guidelines,[29-30] endovascular repair is commonly used for injuries of the distal aortic arch and descending thoracic aorta. Open repair is indicated when anatomy is not suitable for endovascular repair.

CLINICAL MANIFESTATION

Many thoracic and thoracoabdominal aneurysms are discovered incidentally and most often develop without symptoms. Indications for surgical intervention depend on the size of the aneurysm and the presence or absence of symptoms. Symptoms are usually due to sudden expansion of the aneurysm, which can cause a vague pain in the back or sometimes a sharp pain that may denote the presence of rupture or impending rupture. Other symptoms are related to pressure on adjacent structures, such as pressure on the bronchus, that can cause respiratory distress or pressure on the recurrent laryngeal nerve, causing vocal hoarseness (Fig. 36.3). Pressure on the esophagus can cause difficulty swallowing. On rare occasions, paraplegia and paraparesis can be caused by occlusion of critical intercostal arteries. There is also a risk of distal embolization causing "blue toe" syndrome (Fig. 36.4).

Certain manifestations of rupture in 10% to 20% of thoracoabdominal aortic aneurysms include the sudden onset of severe or sharp pain radiating to the back and causing a drop in hemoglobin and blood pressure. In a review of more than 100 ruptured descending thoracic and thoracoabdominal aortic aneurysms, the most common site of rupture was the pleural cavity.[31] Other sites of rupture occurred into the lung, esophagus, mediastinum, retroperitoneum, and peritoneal cavity. Thus, in addition to back, chest, or abdominal pain, patients may also have hemoptysis or hematemesis.

DIAGNOSIS

Computed tomography (CT) and magnetic resonance imaging (MRI) represent the preferred diagnostic modalities. CT allows for visualization of the aortic wall, the aneurysm size, the presence or absence of clot formation, intercostal arteries, and effects

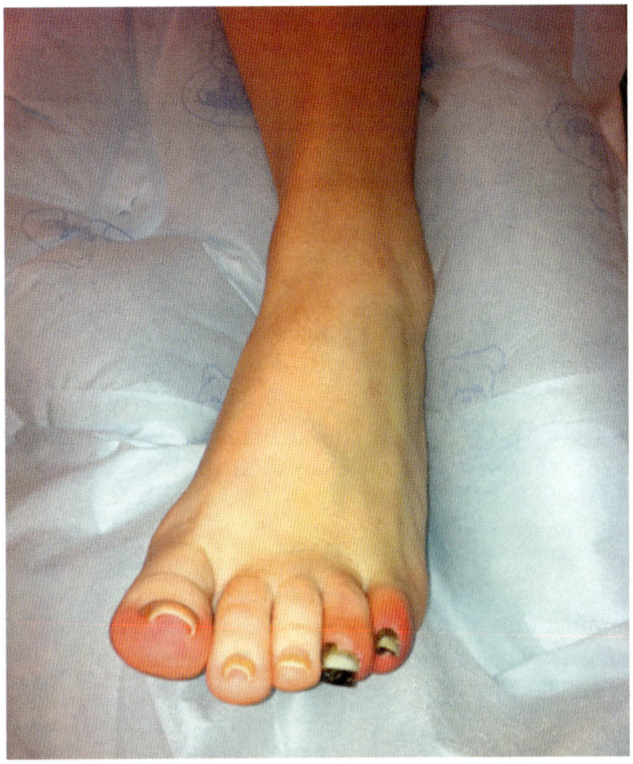

FIG 36.4 Example of blue toe syndrome.

on the surrounding tissues. The disadvantage of CT is the effect of ionizing radiation and the contrast media, which can exacerbate poor renal function. Three-dimensional reconstruction of axial imaging provides an additional view of thoracoabdominal aortic aneurysms (Fig. 36.5). MRI is now widely available and has the advantage of not using ionizing radiation or requiring an intravenous contrast agent. However, MRI has long acquisition times, provokes claustrophobia, and is contraindicated for patients with cerebral aneurysm clips, certain mechanical valves, or other internal metallic hardware. It is used less frequently because of these limitations.

Transesophageal echocardiography (TEE) provides excellent views of the ascending and descending aorta as well as heart function. TEE is an important tool in the diagnosis of acute aortic dissection. The limitation of TEE is that it is invasive, requires an expert echocardiographer, and does not provide adequate imaging of the aortic arch or areas below the level of the diaphragm.

Intravascular ultrasound (IVUS) is emerging as a useful adjunct, especially in circumstances of aortic dissection or when there is diagnostic uncertainty, as in traumatic aortic injury (Fig. 36.6). This modality allows for high-resolution imaging of the aortic wall, dynamic visualization of intimal lesions, and delineation of branch-vessel involvement.[32,33] The drawback is that it is operator-dependent, requires invasive intraarterial access, and adds additional cost.

THORACIC ANEURYSM CLASSIFICATION

Descending thoracic aortic aneurysms are divided into three extents (Fig. 36.7A).[34] Extent A designates an aortic aneurysm

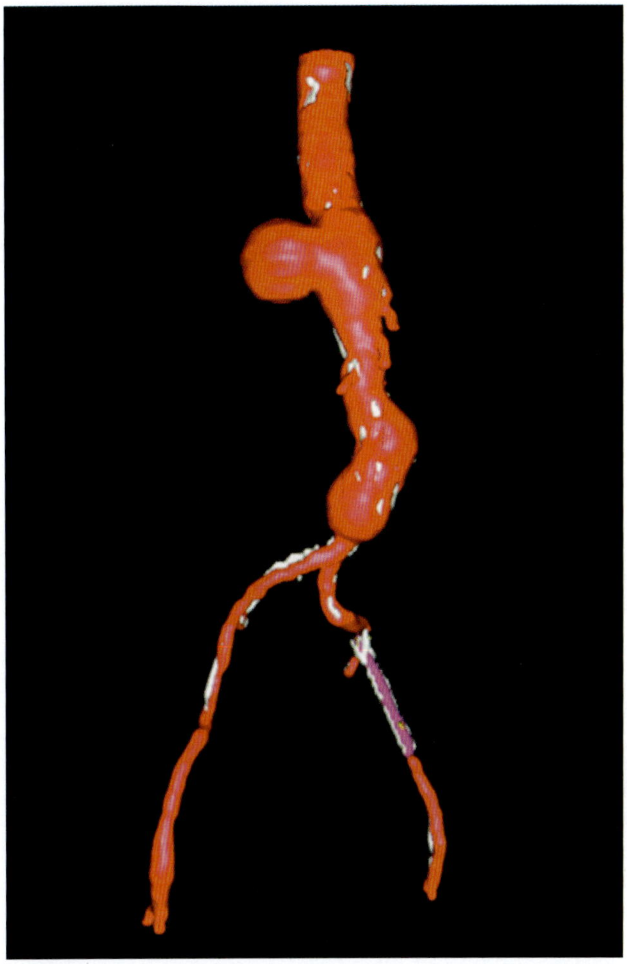

FIG 36.5 Three-dimensional reconstruction of a saccular thoracoabdominal aortic aneurysm extent V before repair. Note the proximity of the aneurysm to the celiac artery, the presence of a left iliac stent, and a synchronous infrarenal abdominal aortic aneurysm.

from the distal origin of the left subclavian artery to the level of the sixth thoracic intercostal space (T6). Extent B is from T6 to the 12th thoracic intercostal space (T12). Extent C denotes the entire descending thoracic aorta from the left subclavian artery to T12.

Thoracoabdominal aortic aneurysms are classified in five categories (see Fig. 36.7B). Extent I is from the left subclavian to above the most proximal renal artery. Extent II is from the left subclavian artery to below the renal arteries. Extent III is from the sixth intercostal space to below the renal arteries. Extent IV is from T12 to below the renal arteries. Extent V, which was introduced in the last 2 decades, is from T6 to just above the renal arteries. The importance of the classification scheme is that it correlated with the incidence of neurologic deficits and mortality. Currently we consider extents II and III to be higher risk for spinal ischemia and early mortality compared with the others.[35]

PREOPERATIVE EVALUATION

Preoperative evaluation of patients for elective thoracoabdominal aortic aneurysm should include a thorough history, physical

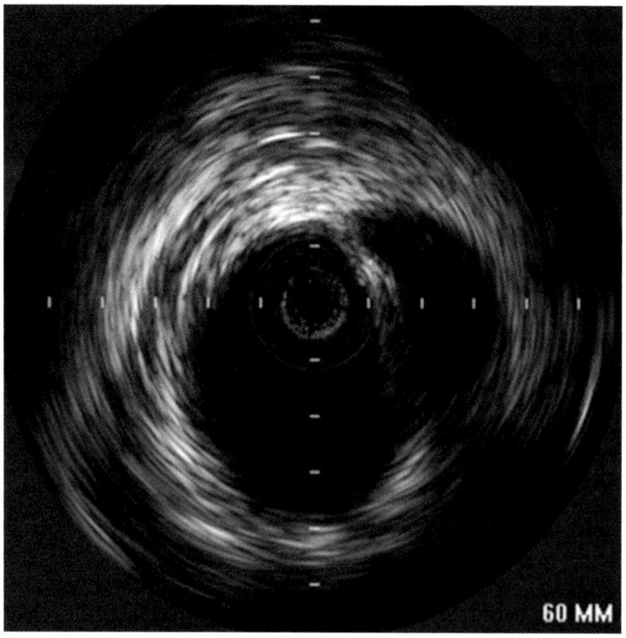

FIG 36.6 Intravascular ultrasound of traumatic injury to the descending thoracic aorta causing pseudoaneurysm (grade 3 injury).

examination, and determination of the presence of cardiovascular, pulmonary, and renal diseases. Pulmonary function testing and arterial blood gases, specifically $PaCO_2$, should be obtained, especially in those with a history of pulmonary disease. However, there is still controversy regarding optimal preoperative cardiac workup for noncardiac vascular disease despite published practice guidelines.[36,37] Preoperative left ventricular ejection fraction is a cardiac predictor of mortality,[38] and echocardiography assists in stratifying risk and helps determine the need for additional cardiac testing. Treatment of coronary artery disease can be with medical therapy, coronary artery angioplasty, or coronary artery bypass before thoracoabdominal repair. It is unclear whether preoperative coronary or carotid artery revascularization is beneficial in reducing perioperative heart attack and stroke.[39,40]

Renal function should be evaluated with estimation of the glomerular filtration rate (GFR). Normal values are greater than 60 mL/min per 1.73 m^2. GFR is easy to estimate by several methods (e.g., Cockcroft-Gault, modification of diet in renal disease, or Chronic Kidney Disease Epidemiology Collaboration formulas) and is a better predictor of risk than serum creatinine.[41] Many formulas are available in smart phone applications and can be calculated in seconds. The impact of preoperative renal function cannot be underestimated; 30-day mortality after open thoracoabdominal aortic aneurysm (TAAA) repair ranges from 5% for patients with a normal GFR to 27% for patients with a GFR less than 49 mL/min.

Axial imaging of the entire chest, abdomen, and pelvis is mandatory to determine the extent of the aneurysm as well as synchronous aneurysms (Fig. 36.8). Use of intravenous contrast is helpful in determining the presence of thrombus and atheromatous disease in the aortic wall. Echocardiography is also helpful to evaluate for atheromatous disease in the thoracic aorta. Imaging of the brain should be considered, since 12% of aortic aneurysm patients also harbor intracranial aneurysms.[42]

SURGICAL TECHNIQUE

General endotracheal anesthesia is induced with a double-lumen tube for selective ventilation of the single right lung. A pulmonary artery catheter and leads for motor-evoked and somatosensory evoked potentials are placed. The patient is positioned in the right lateral decubitus position for placement of the CSF drain (Fig. 36.9A). After the drain has been secured, the hips are tilted slightly posteriorly to gain access to the left common femoral artery. The shoulders are positioned perpendicular to the table. CSF pressure is kept at 10 mm Hg or less (see Fig. 36.9B). This pressure is maintained intraoperatively and for 3 days postoperatively.

A thoracoabdominal incision is tailored to fit the extent of the aneurysm. In descending thoracic aortic aneurysm (DTAA) TAAA extent I and V, a smaller modified thoracoabdominal incision is preferred (see Fig. 36.9C). The full thoracoabdominal incision begins posterior to the tip of the scapula and proceeds medially along T6. The incision is extended inferiorly at the midline toward the umbilicus. Next, the latissimus dorsi is divided and the serratus anterior muscle is mobilized. After the left lung is deflated, the left chest is entered. The sixth rib is resected or cut posteriorly and left in place, and a self-retaining retractor is used to aid in exposure.

The level of dissection depends on the extent of the aneurysm. For TAAA extent II, the dissection begins at the pulmonary hilum with opening of the pericardium to expose the left inferior pulmonary vein. The ligamentum arteriosum is divided after identification and preservation of the recurrent laryngeal nerve. This embryologic remnant is patent in approximately 20% of patients with inheritable connective tissue disorders. The aorta proximal to the aneurysm is circumferentially dissected free. The lateral muscular portion of the diaphragm may be divided and a retroperitoneal plane can be developed. The abdominal contents are retracted medially to the right of the abdominal aorta, including the left kidney (Fig. 36.10A).

Cannulas are placed for distal aortic perfusion. A purse-string suture is placed in the left inferior pulmonary vein and the vein is incised. Intravenous heparin is given at 1 mg/kg, and the left inferior pulmonary vein is then cannulated with the catheter tip directed toward the left atrium. The catheter is attached to a centrifugal pump with an in-line heat exchanger (see Fig. 36.10B). The left common femoral artery is exposed and an 8- or 10-mm woven Dacron tube graft is sewn in an end-to-side fashion to provide inflow. Instead of directly cannulating the femoral artery, a side-arm graft is used to preserve renal function and reduce extremity muscle ischemia.[43,44] Profound hypothermia, although seldom employed, is a useful adjunct for very large aneurysms, when severe atheromatous plaque at the distal arch or proximal descending thoracic aorta precludes proximal aortic control, or in cases of rupture at those locations.

A segmental clamp is applied to the proximal descending thoracic aorta and the midthoracic aorta before transecting the aorta (see Fig. 36.10C). In general, the inclusion technique

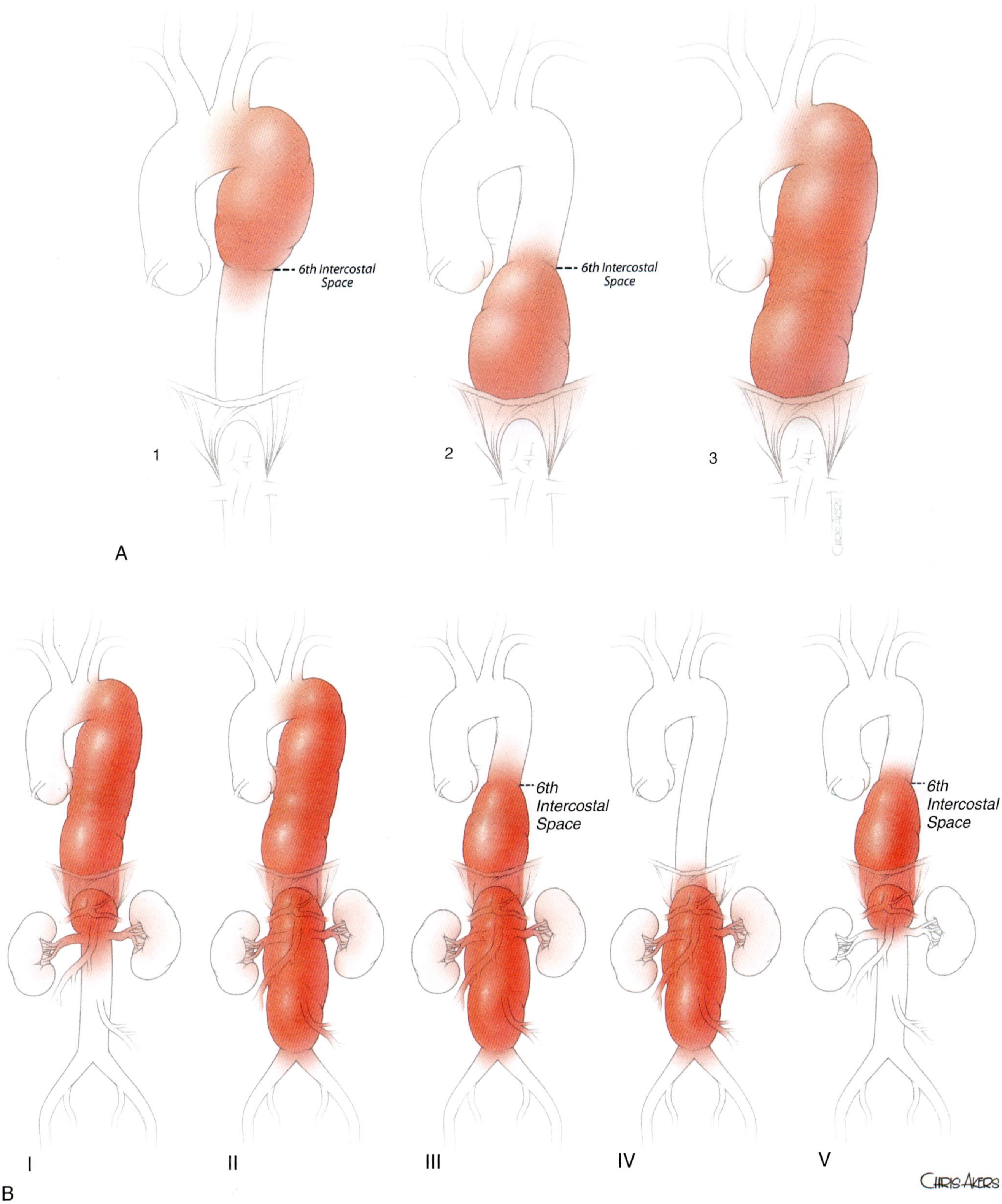

FIG 36.7 Classifications of thoracic aortic aneurysms. (A) Descending thoracic aortic aneurysms. (B) Thoracoabdominal aortic aneurysms with rates of postoperative neurologic deficit in the clamp-and-sew and current eras.

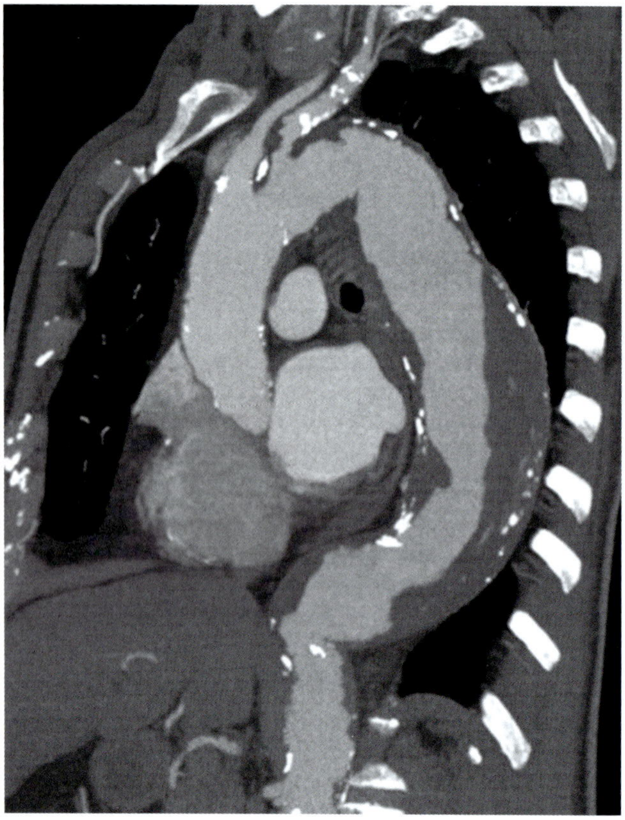

FIG 36.8 Parasagittal computed tomographic reconstruction of a thoracic aortic aneurysm with extensive thrombus and atheromatous disease in the aortic wall.

at the proximal anastomosis is no longer used. The proximal aorta is divided completely and separated from the underlying esophagus to mitigate the risk of graft-esophageal fistula (see Fig. 36.10D). A commercially available collagen- or gelatin-impregnated woven Dacron graft is sutured end to end with 2-0 or 3-0 polypropylene (see Fig. 36.10E). In cases of acute aortic dissection, 4-0 polypropylene sutures can be used. After completion of the proximal anastomosis, the clamp is moved distally to the celiac axis. The remaining thoracic aorta is opened, and upper intercostal arteries are ligated (see Fig. 36.10F). Lower thoracic intercostal arteries (i.e., T8 to T12) are temporarily occluded with balloon-tipped catheters.

The extent and timing of lower intercostal artery reattachment depend on intraoperative neuromonitoring results.[45] Patent intercostal arteries from T8 to T12 can be reattached, either as an opening in the graft or as an end-to-side loop graft (see Fig. 36.10G). The graft is tunneled from the chest to the abdomen through the aortic hiatus. The distal aortic clamp above the celiac artery is moved to the infrarenal abdominal aorta (see Fig. 36.10H). The upper abdominal aorta is opened, and the celiac and superior mesenteric arteries are perfused via balloon-tipped catheters with tepid blood (34°C) from the centrifugal pump (see Fig. 36.10I). The kidneys are similarly perfused with cool crystalloid to maintain renal temperature of 20°C. The patient's core temperature can passively drift to 33°C. The viscera are usually attached as a patch unless the patient is young or there is a known connective tissue disorder. Otherwise the viscera are reattached with a commercially available side-branched thoracoabdominal aortic graft (STAG; Figs. 36.10J and K).[46] The distal anastomosis can be performed either before or after pulsatile

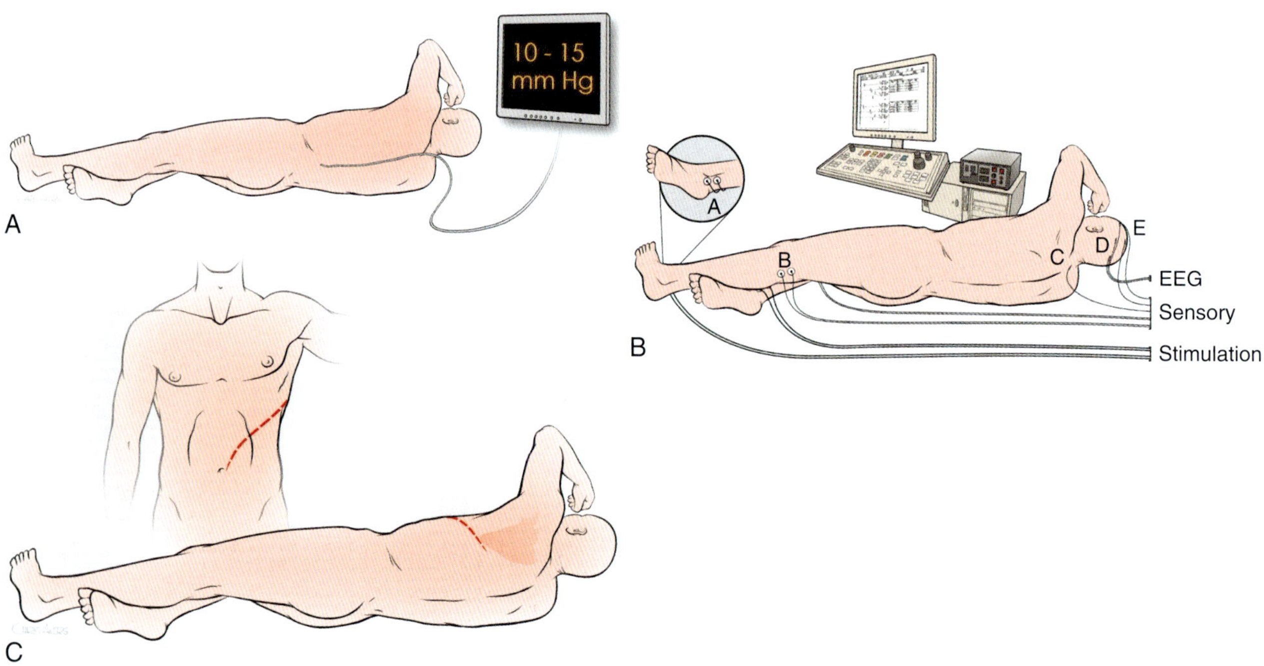

FIG 36.9 Right lateral decubitus position for (A) CSF drainage and (B) monitoring of motor and somatosensory evoked potentials. (C) Modified thoracoabdominal incision *(dashed line)*. *CSF*, Cerebrospinal fluid; *EEG*, electroencephalogram, electroencephalography.

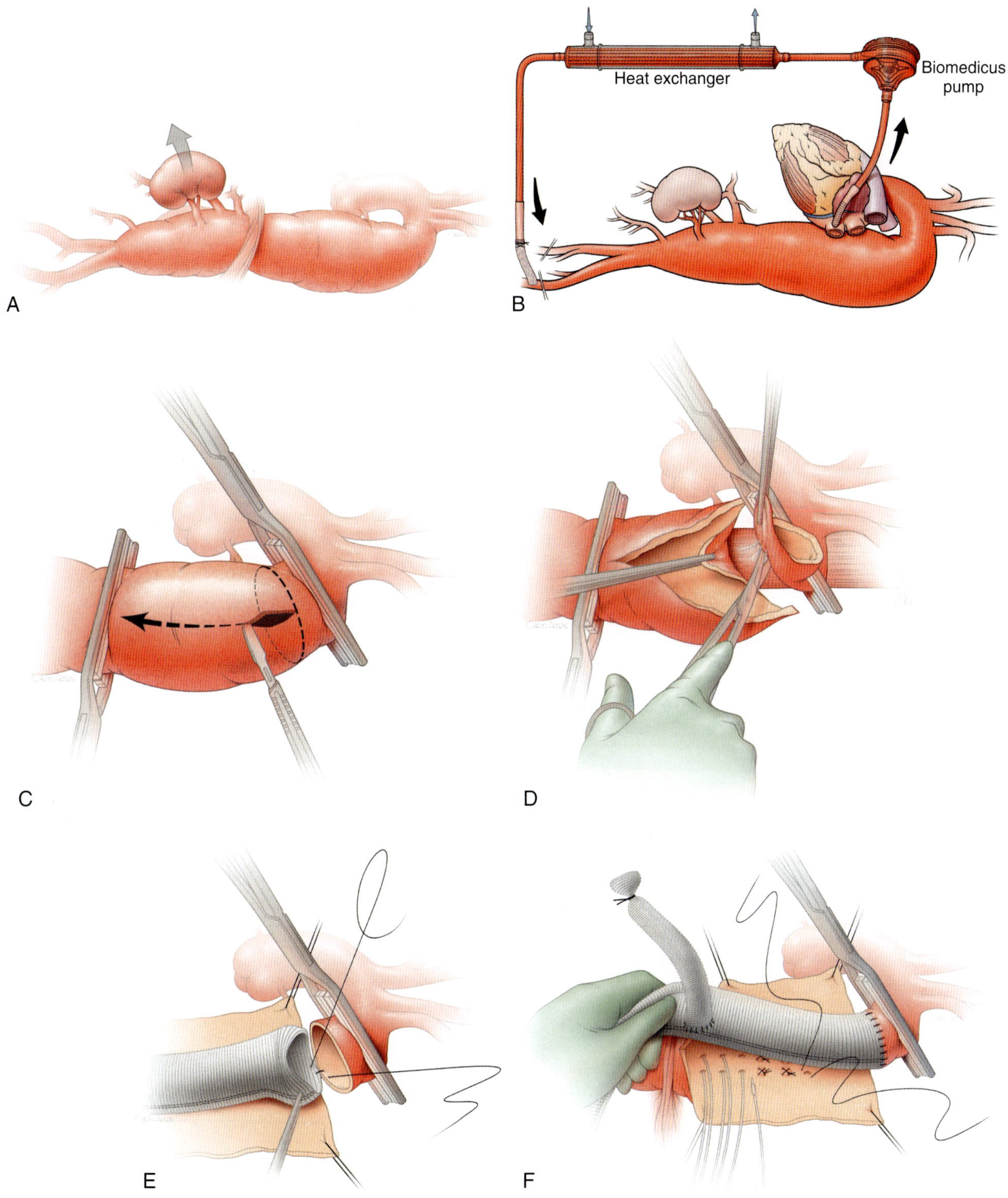

FIG 36.10 Technique of open thoracoabdominal aortic aneurysm repair. (A) Left medial visceral rotation, including mobilization of left kidney. (B) Left atriofemoral bypass. (C) Application of segmental clamp to proximal aorta. (D) Separation of the aorta from the underlying esophagus in preparation for the proximal anastomosis. (E) Construction of end-to-end proximal anastomosis. (F) Ligation of upper thoracic intercostal arteries and temporary balloon occlusion of lower thoracic intercostal arteries.

Continued

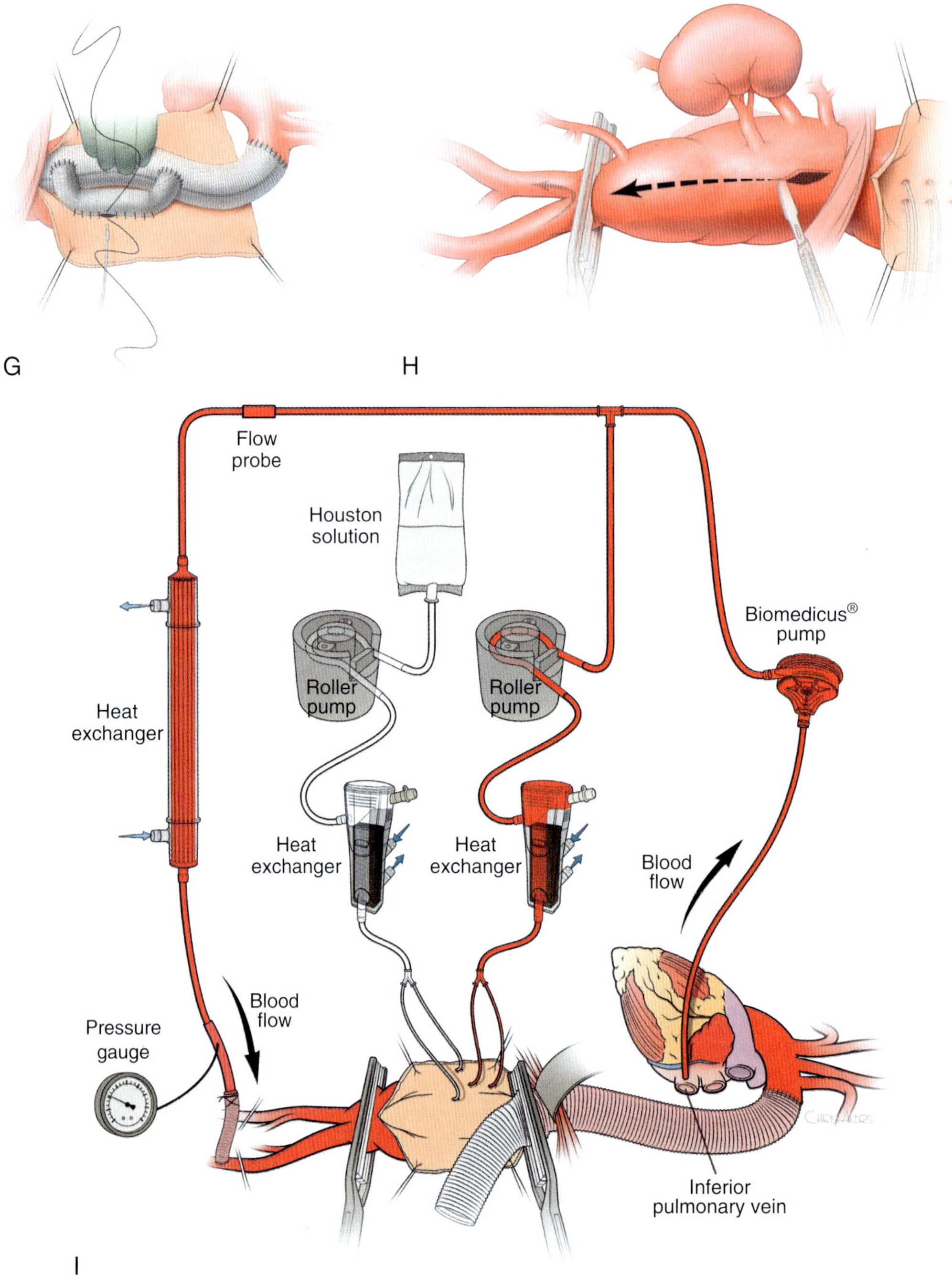

FIG 36.10, cont'd (G) Intercostal loop graft. (H) Application of clamp to infrarenal aorta. (I) Perfusion of mesenteric and renal arteries.

flow has been restored to the viscera and renal arteries (see Fig. 36.10L). After completion of the distal anastomosis, the graft is de-aired and clamps are released (see Fig. 36.10M).

The "distal-first approach," an alternative technique for the repair of DTAAs, is typically reserved for patients with severe aortoiliac occlusive disease, prior aortobifemoral bypass, or infrarenal aortic occlusion. The approach begins with attachment of a 10-mm Dacron side branch to the main body aortic graft. Alternatively, there is a commercially available woven, single-side-branched collagen- or gelatin-impregnated Dacron graft that can be used. The left inferior pulmonary vein is cannulated, as previously described. Depending on the extent of the aneurysm, a distal aortic clamp is applied at thoracic level 8 to 10. The distal aorta is opened and completely transected. The distal aortic anastomosis is then performed above the iliac bifurcation and below the celiac and superior mesenteric arteries, typically using a 3-0 running polyprolene suture. Once the distal aortic anastomosis had been completed, the aortic clamp is moved proximally onto the graft and distal aortic perfusion is initiated through the side branch or previously constructed side-arm graft. An aortic clamp is then placed proximally, either proximal or distal to the left subclavian artery. Subsequently the remaining

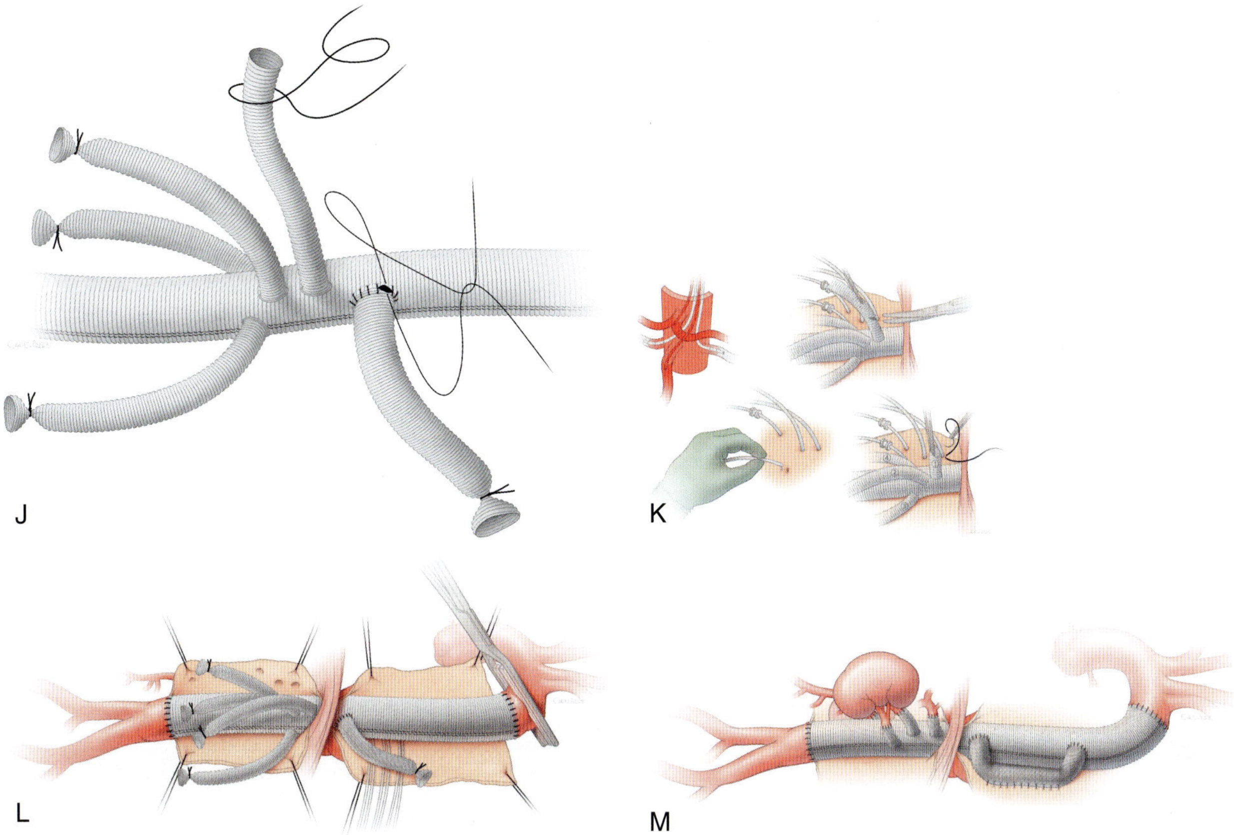

FIG 36.10, cont'd (J) Side-branched thoracoabdominal aortic graft (STAG). (K) Balloon-tipped perfusion cannulas are inserted into the origins of the visceral arteries. In patients with connective tissue disease or in young patients, visceral arteries are individually reattached using a presewn STAG technique. The celiac (1), superior mesenteric (2), left renal (3), and right renal (4) arteries are sequentially reattached. (L) Construction of end-to-end distal anastomosis. (M) Completed open repair of thoracoabdominal aortic aneurysm.

descending thoracic aorta is opened and the proximal anastomosis performed. Once these steps have been completed, the patient is placed in Trendelenburg, the graft is de-aired with an 18-gauge needle, the aortic clamps are removed, and distal pulsatile flow is reestablished.

The anastomoses are checked for hemostasis, and the distal aortic perfusion cannulas are removed once the nasopharyngeal temperature has reached 36°C. Anticoagulation is reversed with protamine sulfate and blood products as necessary. The muscular portion of the diaphragm is reapproximated with running no. 1 polypropylene suture. Two 36 French chest tubes are placed. The left lung is reinflated and the chest is closed with interrupted 2-0 polyglycolic acid sutures. The remainder of the chest and abdomen are closed in standard fashion. The double-lumen tube is usually exchanged for a single-lumen endotracheal tube before transfer unless there is significant airway edema.

IMMEDIATE SPINAL NEUROLOGIC DEFICIT

Spinal cord ischemia during thoracic aortic aneurysm repair occurs because of cessation of blood flow to intercostal arteries, distal embolization, inadequate collateral circulation, reperfusion injury, and decreased cerebrospinal perfusion pressure. Several techniques will minimize spinal ischemia during aortic clamping and after reconstruction. These include intercostal artery reattachment, distal aortic perfusion, cardiopulmonary bypass, regional[47] or systemic hypothermia,[48] and CSF drainage.

The proposed effect of CSF drainage is to lower spinal fluid pressure and thereby increase blood perfusion pressure.[49] A meta-analysis found that the use of CSF drainage in thoracic aortic aneurysm repair led to an absolute risk reduction in neurologic deficit of 9%.[50] It is possible that the risk reduction is even greater because the meta-analysis included older studies that limited CSF drainage to 50 mL intraoperatively.[51] It is typical to drain 400 to 500 mL over 3 days intraoperatively and postoperatively, with an incidence of subdural hematoma of less than 0.5%.[52] Cases of intracranial bleeding are rare with a strict postoperative CSF drain protocol.

In addition to CSF drainage, distal aortic perfusion from the left atrium via a cannula placed in the left inferior pulmonary vein can be performed as described previously. Blood flows through a roller pump with an inline heat exchanger into the left femoral artery graft. Despite the heat exchanger, the body is allowed to cool to 33°C passively. Other reported methods of distal perfusion include axillofemoral bypass[53] and aortoiliac bypass.[54]

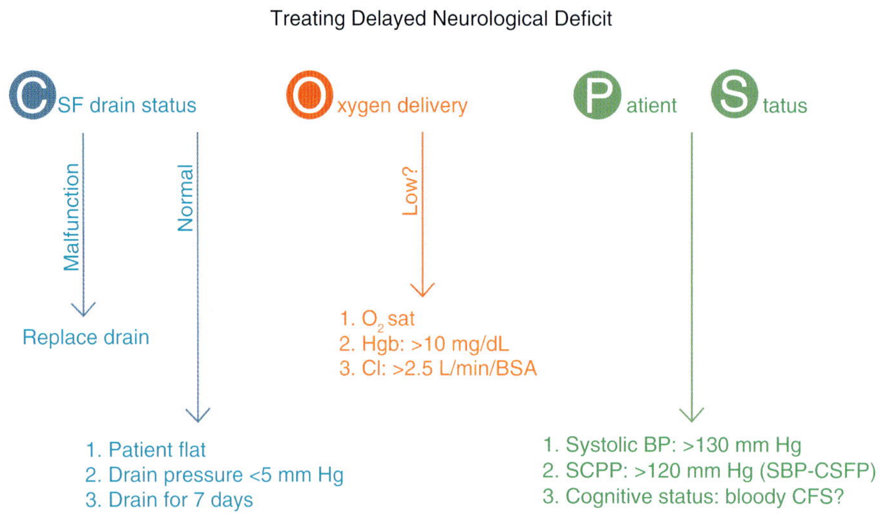

FIG 36.11 The cerebrospinal drain status/oxygen delivery/patient status (COPS) protocol for treatment of patients with delayed neurologic deficit: **c**erebrospinal fluid drainage, supplemental **o**xygen, maximizing patient **s**tatus (increasing blood pressure and spinal cord perfusion pressure). *CSF*, Cerebrospinal fluid.

Our spinal protective adjuncts are CSF drainage, mild to moderate passive hypothermia, and left atriofemoral bypass. With these techniques, recently published data for the repair of DTAAs showed immediate neurologic deficits in only 0.6%.[55] In the clamp-and-sew era, the rate was more than triple at 5% overall, but it increased to 9% in the highest-risk aneurysms.[56]

In the clamp-and-sew era, the incidence of neurologic deficits in TAAAs extent I was 15%; in extent II, 31%; in extent III, 7%; and in extent IV, 4%.[57] In addition to aneurysm extent, other predictors of neurologic deficit in the clamp-and-sew era included aortic clamp time and preoperative renal insufficiency. The use of adjuncts has mitigated aortic clamp time as a risk factor for immediate neurologic deficits. Currently, extents II and III are considered high risk for immediate postoperative spinal ischemia and occur in 8% of these procedures. Other groups report similar results, with neurologic deficits occurring in 6% to 22% of extent II and 2.6% to 8% in non–extent II cases.[58,59]

DELAYED SPINAL NEUROLOGIC DEFICIT AND CEREBROSPINAL FLUID DRAINAGE

Patients should be awakened as soon as possible postoperatively to ascertain neurologic status. The goal for mean arterial pressure is greater than 80 mm Hg (or systolic blood pressure greater than 130 mm Hg), and the CSF pressure goal is less than 10 mm Hg. A limit of 15 mL of CSF fluid is drained each hour to prevent intracranial hypotension and hemorrhage. If blood is noted in the effluent, the drain is capped and any coagulopathy corrected. The drain is usually removed on the third postoperative day if the patient is neurologically intact. Neurologic function is frequently assessed to detect delayed deficit.

Estrera and colleagues[45] report a rate of delayed neurologic deficit of 3% (3/105) in cases of descending thoracic and thoracoabdominal aortic aneurysm repair. Neurologic function recovered in two of those three patients before discharge. If delayed neurologic deficit occurs, several maneuvers—identified by the CSF drain status/oxygen delivery/patient status (the COPS acronym)—are performed with the goal of increasing the spinal oxygenation and perfusion pressure (Fig. 36.11).[52] Supplemental oxygen is given, and the patient is kept supine. The mean arterial pressure goal is raised to greater than 90 mm Hg, and the cardiac index is kept at greater than 2.5 L/min. Blood transfusions are given to keep the hemoglobin level greater than 12 g/dL. The CSF drain is opened to keep CSF pressure at less than 5 mm Hg regardless of the volume drained. The drain is kept in place for a total of 7 days in cases of delayed deficit.

Complications of CSF drainage are low but include CSF leak, headache, and intracranial hemorrhage (Table 36.1).[52] The overall complication rate was 1.5% in more than 1100 patients. Serious complications occurred in less than 1%. The most common complication was CSF leak with spinal headache. Most CSF leaks required hydration and blood patch but resolved without additional invasive management. Meningitis occurred in two patients (0.2%) who developed delayed neurologic deficit

TABLE 36.1 Complications of Cerebrospinal Fluid Drainage

Complication	Frequency (%)
CSF leak without spinal headache	0.1
CSF leak with spinal headache	0.54
Intracranial hemorrhage	0.45
Meningitis	0.2
Spinal headache without CSF leak	0.2
Fractured catheter	0.1

CSF, Cerebrospinal fluid.
Modified from Estrera AL, Sheinbaum R, Miller CC, et al: Cerebrospinal fluid drainage during thoracic aortic repair: safety and current management. *Ann Thorac Surg* 88:9–15, 2009.

with prolonged catheter insertion. The authors have not noted intracranial hemorrhage in recent cases since limiting the CSF drainage to 15 mL/h in neurologically intact patients.

POSTOPERATIVE RENAL FAILURE

Postoperative renal injury is defined according to the risk, injury, failure, loss, end stage (RIFLE) criteria[60] where there is an increase in creatinine of greater than 1 mg/dL per day over 2 consecutive days or a need for hemodialysis. In a review of the authors' experience in nearly 2000 open thoracoabdominal repairs since 1991, the strongest predictor of postoperative renal failure was low preoperative GFR. Other risk factors include aneurysm extents involving the renal arteries (extent II, III, and IV) and use of the clamp-and-sew technique.[35,61] The risk of postoperative renal failure was 17% in patients with normal preoperative GFR. In patients with a GFR of 40 or less, the risk of postoperative renal dysfunction was 38%.[43] Preoperative renal function inversely correlates with postoperative mortality (Fig. 36.12).

Miller and colleagues[43] showed that using a femoral artery end-to-side graft to provide distal perfusion inflow instead of direct artery cannulation decreased the risk of postoperative renal dysfunction. They speculated that avoiding occlusion of the femoral artery with the cannula would decrease skeletal muscle ischemia in the extremity, which in turn may decrease release of nephrotoxic factors and rhabdomyolysis.[62] The use of cold perfusate has also been shown to decrease the incidence of hospital mortality.[63] However, dramatic improvements in the rates of neurologic deficits have not yet been noted with renal failure.

POSTOPERATIVE GASTROINTESTINAL COMPLICATIONS

Gastrointestinal (GI) complications affect 7% of DTAA and TAAA repairs.[64] Overall mortality increased nearly threefold in patients with GI complications compared with the entire cohort, and even mild GI complications increased the risk of death. Involvement of the visceral aorta (extents II, III, and IV) and low preoperative GFR were risk factors. The pathophysiology is postulated to be release of atheromatous debris during aortic manipulation and visceral ischemia after aortic clamping. The manifestations include pancreatitis, ileus (>5 postoperative days), GI bleeding, peptic ulcers, liver dysfunction, bowel ischemia, and cholecystitis. The most common GI complication was bowel ischemia (2.5%), which was associated with 62% mortality. Interestingly, acalculous cholecystitis (0.3%) was the strongest harbinger of mortality risk at 75%.

SURVIVAL

Mortality for descending thoracic and thoracoabdominal aortic aneurysm repair primarily depends on comorbid conditions and the extent of the aneurysm. In 300 cases of open DTAA repair, 30-day mortality was 8%, with preoperative renal insufficiency and female sex emerging as risk factors.[34] Other groups have reported similar results, with rates of 30-day mortality ranging from 2.2% to 14% and rates of spinal neurologic deficit between 1% and 7.4%.[59,65-67] Risk factors for early mortality include age, GFR, extents II and III, history of coronary artery disease, and emergency presentation (Fig. 36.13).[35]

Published short-term mortality in TAAA repair ranges from 4% to 16%.[35,48,57,58,68,69] Long-term mortality reflects comorbid conditions, such as cerebrovascular and coronary disease. Nevertheless, TAAA repair is highly effective in reducing aneurysm-related death. Repair of thoracic aortic aneurysm nearly restores mortality to age-matched controls. In a study comparing untreated historical controls to patients receiving surgical repair, 5-year survival in the untreated group was only 13%, compared with 61% in the surgical treatment group.[70] Postoperative complications, such as acute renal failure and manifestations of GI ischemia, predict decreased survival.

For both DTAA and TAAA, the 5-, 10-, and 20-year survival is 58%, 43%, and 32%, respectively. Adjusted risk factors

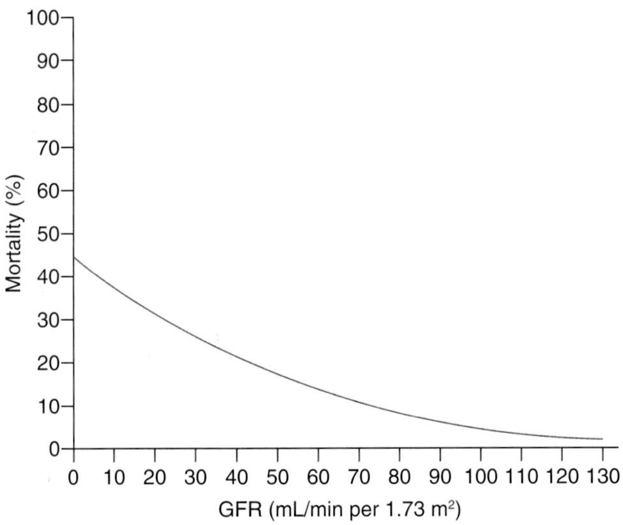

FIG 36.12 Graph showing postoperative mortality as a function of preoperative glomerular filtration rate.

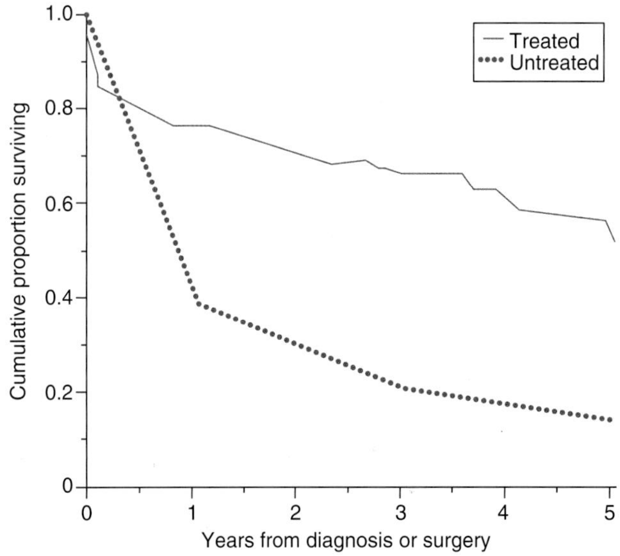

FIG 36.13 Kaplan-Meier survival graph of treated versus untreated thoracic aortic aneurysm from time of diagnosis.

affecting long-term survival include age, renal function, extent II or III, known connective tissue disorders, rupture, chronic obstructive pulmonary disease, tobacco smoking, and stroke history.[35]

ANEURYSMS ASSOCIATED WITH TYPE B AORTIC DISSECTION

There is evidence that rupture occurs at a smaller size in cases of aortic dissection. In a review of ruptured thoracic aortic aneurysms, 40% of ruptures in acute dissection occurred in patients with an aortic diameter less than 6 cm.[31] The median diameter at rupture in chronic dissection cases was 8 cm. Open repair of descending thoracic and thoracoabdominal aortic aneurysms in the setting of chronic dissection has shown excellent results with the use of surgical adjuncts. No increased risk compared with nondissected cases was noted in nearly 200 elective cases of chronic dissecting descending thoracic and TAAA.[71] However, thoracic aortic operations in cases of acute dissection are fraught with high morbidity and mortality. Medical management for acute uncomplicated type B dissection with strict blood pressure control is the treatment of choice. Surgery is reserved for complicated cases characterized by malperfusion syndromes, refractory hypertension, intractable pain, or rupture. The open surgical operative mortality rate in acute type B dissection is 14%, with spinal neurologic deficits in 32%.[72] The higher rate of spinal ischemia is multifactorial. Adjunctive spinal protection techniques, such as distal aortic perfusion and CSF drainage, are often not used because of the patient's hemodynamic instability. Critically, intercostal artery reimplantation is contraindicated because of the risk of bleeding. Several trials have demonstrated favorable long-term outcomes when stent grafts were used for acute complicated and subacute uncomplicated type B dissections.

RUPTURED THORACIC AORTIC ANEURYSMS

Most patients with a ruptured thoracic aortic aneurysm die before reaching the hospital.[18] Although elective repair of thoracic aneurysms restores actuarial survival to near normal, patients suffer increased morbidity and mortality even after successful repair of a ruptured aneurysm.[72] Thirty-day mortality was 24% in one early series, in which more than half the patients suffered cardiac arrest preoperatively.[31] Other reviews showed early mortality ranging from 12% to 54%, with neurologic deficits in 5% to 9%.[73-75] Since 2005, thoracic endovascular aortic repair (TEVAR) has become the primary modality for repair of traumatic aortic injury to the descending thoracic aorta.[76] Because early and late outcomes for open repair of ruptured thoracic aortic aneurysms are so dismal, we can expect a similar paradigm shift to TEVAR for ruptured DTAAs that meet anatomic criteria for endografting. However, until commercially available branched or fenestrated stent grafts become available, endovascular repair for ruptured TAAAs remains investigational.

CONCLUSION

DTAAs and TAAAs are fatal conditions, with the aneurysm size being the currently accepted factor in determining timing of elective repair. Open surgical repair offers durable and proven mortality benefits compared with nonoperative management. Current adjunctive techniques have successfully reduced the risk of spinal ischemia to acceptable levels, even in high-risk patients. Visceral ischemia and renal failure continue to be problematic, especially in more extensive thoracoabdominal aneurysms. The extent of the aneurysm and preoperative renal function are important risk predictors.

Endovascular repair offers an alternative method of repair. Approved devices for the descending thoracic aorta appear to have a lower short-term mortality but have higher reintervention rates and similar long-term mortality compared with open repair. Endovascular TAAA repair is a promising alternative to open surgical repair, but there is concern about neurologic deficits, especially in the more extensive aneurysms. Future endovascular techniques will likely have to allow revascularization of the critical lower thoracic intercostal arteries to maintain the improvement in rates of neurologic deficits found in open repairs.

REVIEW QUESTIONS

1. Increasing size correlates with risk of thoracic aortic aneurysm rupture. For thoracic aneurysms less than 6 cm, the 5-year risk of rupture is 16%. For thoracic aneurysms greater than 6 cm, the estimated 5-year risk of rupture is
   - **a.** Less than 15%
   - **b.** Between 15% and 30%
   - **c.** Between 31% and 90%
   - **d.** Greater than 90%
2. Signs and symptoms of thoracoabdominal aortic aneurysm rupture can include
   - **a.** Pain
   - **b.** Hypotension
   - **c.** Hemoptysis
   - **d.** Hematemesis
   - **e.** All of the above
3. The risk of spinal paralysis or paraparesis in open repair of extent II thoracoabdominal aortic aneurysm with spinal protective adjuncts is
   - **a.** Less than 5%
   - **b.** 5% to 10%
   - **c.** 11% to 15%
   - **d.** Greater than 15%
   - **e.** Not dependent on extent of aneurysm
4. A 58-year-old woman had an incidental finding on a CT scan of a 4.5-cm extent I thoracoabdominal aortic aneurysm. Your decision to operate is based on the genetic workup showing the presence of a mutation in
   - **a.** TGF beta receptor type II *(TGFBR2)*
   - **b.** *BRCA1*
   - **c.** *BCR-ABL*
   - **d.** Myosin heavy chain 11 smooth muscle *(MYH11)*
   - **e.** Tissue inhibitor of matrix metalloproteinase 9 *(MMP9)*

5. A 65-year-old woman had normal neurologic function immediately following open repair of her extent II thoracoabdominal aortic aneurysm. Nursing noted that she stopped moving her lower extremities in the ICU. The next best step in management is
   a. Steroid administration
   b. MRI of spine
   c. Cerebrospinal fluid (CSF) drainage
   d. Cardioversion
   e. Extubation as soon as possible
6. A 65-year-old man with an extent V thoracoabdominal aortic aneurysm has a serum creatinine of 0.8 mg/dL with an estimated glomerular filtration rate (GFR) of 90 mL/min per 1.73 m^2. His predicted mortality after open repair is
   a. 5%
   b. 10% to 15%
   c. 15% to 20%
   d. Greater than 25%
7. The most common complication of CSF drainage is
   a. Meningitis
   b. Intracranial hemorrhage
   c. CSF leak with headache
   d. Fractured catheter
   e. Spinal paralysis
8. A 40-year-old man with hypertension presents with acute type B aortic dissection. Medical management has begun, but open surgical repair is offered if there is
   a. Need for greater than three oral antihypertensive agents
   b. Visceral malperfusion
   c. Need for more than one intravenous antihypertensive agents
   d. Spinal headache
   e. Estimated GFR greater than 60 mL/min per 1.73 m^2
9. Patients with chronic thoracic aortic dissection and aneurysm are at no significantly increased risk of death or spinal neurologic deficits after open surgical repair.
   a. True
   b. False
10. Reattachment of intercostal arteries for prevention of spinal neurologic deficit is most important at the level of
    a. T1 to T4
    b. T4 to T8
    c. T8 to T12
    d. L1 to L4

References available online at ExpertConsult.com.

37 CHAPTER

Endovascular Repair of Thoracic Aortic Aneurysm

Michael J. Singh, Michel S. Makaroun

Thoracic aortic pathology is one of the leading causes of death in the world in those over the age of 65 and in the United States accounts for more than 11,000 deaths annually.[1] Thoracic aortic aneurysms (TAAs) occur less frequently than abdominal aortic aneurysms. The estimated incidence ranges from 5.6 to 10.4 cases per 100,000.[2,3] The incidence is difficult to discern because TAAs are relatively silent, and sudden fatalities are more often associated with alternative diagnoses. The prevalence of asymptomatic TAA, based on population studies, ranges between 0.16% and 0.34%.[4] With the aging population combined with advances in imaging technology, there has been a steady increase in the number of patients diagnosed with TAA. Epidemiologic data suggest an increasing incidence of TAAs, which may be related to the aging population, improved educational awareness of the general public and primary care pracitioners.[5] The natural history of TAAs is not well characterized, although it has been shown that approximately 70% of patients who forgo treatment will progress to rupture, with a fatality rate approaching 90%.[6]

Traditionally open surgical repair of TAAs was performed with or without distal aortic perfusion. These procedures carry significant morbidity and mortality, associated with the need for thoracotomy, single-lung ventilation, aortic cross clamping, and prolonged visceral or renal ischemia. Reported mortality rates of open TAA repair at centers of excellence range from 3% to 8% and are associated with paraplegia rates of 3% to 5%.[7,8] The first endovascular exclusion of a thoracic aorta was reported by Dake in 1994.[9] The US Food and Drug Administration (FDA) approved the first thoracic endograft in March 2005. after a nonrandomized trial showed that thoracic endovascular repair (TEVAR) compared favorably with the standard open surgical repair. Since then, there has been a paradigm shift in the treatment of descending thoracic aneurysms (DTAs), with most patients preferentially offered TEVAR, thus expanding the pool of patients that could undergo treatment. Despite the lack of randomized trial data, TEVAR has become the preferred method of treatment for all patients with DTAs who meet the anatomic criteria. A recent Cochrane Review of thoracic endograft use for the treatment of TAAs determined that there was a paucity of randomized control studies, but limited midterm data suggested clinical equipoise between TEVAR and open repair. However, numerous nonrandomized studies have shown that TEVAR is effective and durable in the short term, which may justify the paradigm shift.[10]

INDICATIONS FOR THORACIC ENDOVASCULAR REPAIR

The decision to repair a DTA depends on multiple factors; aortic diameter, anatomic location, expansion rate, underlying pathology, associated symptoms, and the patient's overall medical condition. The Society for Thoracic Surgeons Endovascular Task Force, in the absence of high-quality data, has recognized that thoracic aortic pathology is increasingly being treated with TEVAR.[11] The decision to treat a TAA with TEVAR or open repair must be made with the same rigor. Societal guidelines emphasize an individualized approach. Generally open repair of an asymptomatic TAA should be considered at a diameter greater than 5.5 to 6.0 cm and if the risk of rupture exceeds the risks associated with endovascular repair. Saccular, symptomatic aneurysms, those associated with connective tissue disorders, and select acute aortic emergencies may require repair at a smaller diameter. For genetically mediated conditions, a diameter greater than 5.0 cm is suggested. In addition, aneurysms that grow rapidly (>1.0 cm per year, or >0.5 cm in 6 months) should be considered for early repair.[12] Guidelines propose that TEVAR is beneficial for the treatment of a variety of thoracic pathology; acute type B dissection, blunt thoracic aortic injury, penetrating aortic ulcerations, embolizing aortic thrombus, and intramural hematomas (Box 37.1).[8,13-15] This chapter is limited to the treatment of TAAs.

PREOPERATIVE PLANNING: IMAGING

Anatomic considerations including aneurysm extent, availability of suitable landing zones and nature of the underlying pathology dictate repair options. The decision to proceed with TEVAR requires detailed imaging for procedural planning. Important anatomic characteristics, which require imaging assessment, include aortic arch anatomy, landing zones, aortic angulation, branch vessel location, and access vessel diameter and quality. Computed tomographic angiography (CTA) of the chest, abdomen, pelvis and femoral vessels has become the preferred imaging modality for the evaluation of aortic pathology and preoperative TEVAR planning. Multiplanar reconstructions in addition to three-dimensional modeling provide invaluable information regarding vessel sizes, angulation, length, and anatomic relationships as well as severity of calcification and presence

BOX 37.1 Indications for Thoracic Aortic Aneurysm Repair

- Thoracic aortic aneurysm diameter >5.5 to 6.0 cm
- Aneurysm growth >1.0 cm per year
- Aneurysm growth >0.5 cm in 6 months
- Blunt traumatic aortic injury
- Complicated or uncomplicated type B dissection
- Embolizing aortic wall thrombus
  - Intramural hematoma
  - Large penetrating aortic ulcers
  - Symptomatic descending thoracic aneurysm
- Ruptured descending thoracic aneurysm

of thrombus. The availability of advanced software such as Vitrea (Vital Images, Minnetonka, MN) and Aquarius (TeraRecon, San Mateo, CA) has empowered physicians, allowing them to determine accurate endograft sizing measurements and to perform predeployment planning. For patients who cannot undergo CTA due to contraindications for administration of intravenous iodinated contrast media, magnetic resonance angiography has been used successfully, although patients with renal failure are at risk for nephrogenic systemic fibrosis.[15]

ANATOMIC CONSIDERATIONS

Sizing

Accurate measurements of the proximal and distal seal zones and access vessel diameter are of critical importance in planning TEVAR. Thoracic aortic diameters vary according to gender, anatomic location, pathology, age, and body habitus.[16-18] According to industry-developed instructions for use (IFU), most thoracic aortic endografts require 10% to 20% oversizing in relation to the native aortic diameter. Overzealous endograft sizing has been associated with device infolding, gutter formation, endoleaks, and accelerated aneurysmal degeneration. Undersized endografts can lead to device migration and/or endoleak formation. Aortic diameters are most accurately measured in an orthogonal plane to the centerline of flow. Distal landing zone diameters are often smaller than the proximal landing zone, requiring the use of tapered endografts to compensate for the size discrepancy. Lengths of aortic coverage can be difficult to assess and are underestimated by centerline measurements because endografts are often positioned along the outer curvature of the aortic wall. The natural tortuosity of the aorta coupled with the large cavity of an aneurysm and the tendency of the endograft to locate against the greater aortic curvature usually results in a longer length for graft coverage. These factors must be taken into consideration during endograft sizing.

Access

The thoracic aortic diameter is typically larger than the abdominal aorta and requires larger devices and delivery systems. The largest devices are constrained in 24 to 26 French sheaths that require an iliac access greater than 8 mm for safe insertion and deployment. More recently, 46-mm low-profile Alpha thoracic stent-grafts (Cook Medical, Bloomington, IN) in 20 French sheaths have become available. Particular attention should be given to the proximal external iliac artery, as this area is prone to atherosclerotic narrowing and calcification. This is more important in women, who expectedly have smaller vessels. In situations where access is restricted, the common iliac artery can be directly accessed via a small retroperitoneal incision or an iliac conduit can be sewn in place. Conduit diameters measuring 10 mm are preferred and can be accessed via the retroperitoneal incision or tunneled to the femoral region to avoid angulation in large individuals. Occasionally this conduit serves as a bypass at the end of the procedure in cases of advanced external iliac artery occlusive disease. On rare occasions, the infrarenal aorta can be accessed at the time of exploratory laparotomy. The use of an internal endoconduit to address unfavorable iliac anatomy has been described. This technique requires the placement of covered stents or stent-grafts across the diseased iliac segment followed by aggressive balloon angioplasty for a controlled rupture that will facilitate insertion of the endograft.[19] The Terumo Solopath Balloon Expandable Transfemoral Access Sheaths (Terumo Medical Corporation, Somerset, NJ) provides an alternative approach to managing difficult iliac artery access. The Solopath Sheath is a 14 to 21 French hydrophilic sheath with an external noncompliant radially expanding balloon that gently dilates diseased vessels. The balloon decompresses before sheath removal, thus reducing the risk of iliac artery trauma.

Landing Zones

The tortuosity and high shear force in the thoracic aorta require a slightly longer seal zone than that employed in the infrarenal aneurysmal repair. A seal zone of at least 20 mm is recommended at each end of the endograft to prevent migration and minimize endoleak. The seal zones should be extended when endografts are placed in areas of severe angulation, conical aorta, calcified segments, or areas where mural thrombus is present. However, it is important to recognize the potential consequences of extending aortic endograft coverage, as the greater the number of excluded intercostal arteries and branch vessels impact the rate of paraplegia.

The proximal attachment zones are classified as zones 0 to 5 and the distal attachment zones as zones 5 to 11 (Fig. 37.1). Each zone is divided by a tangential line along the distal aspect of each great vessel; zone 0 is proximal the innominate artery origin, zone 1 is distal to the innominate and proximal to left common carotid artery (LCCA), zone 2 is distal to the LCCA and proximal to the origin of the left subclavian artery (LSCA), zone 3 is less than 20 mm from the LSCA without covering it, and zone 4 is greater than 20 mm from the LSCA and above the T6 vertebral body. The location of the proximal landing zone depends on aneurysmal morphology; however, the ideal location in terms of anatomic accommodation of the endograft is in the straight aortic segments (zones 3 and 4). An important consideration for the proximal seal zone is the angle of the aortic arch. Endografts placed within the aortic arch (zones 1, 2, and 3), especially those with acute angles, may fail to oppose to the inner curvature of the aortic arch (Fig. 37.2). These situations have occasionally resulted in untoward effects, such as device

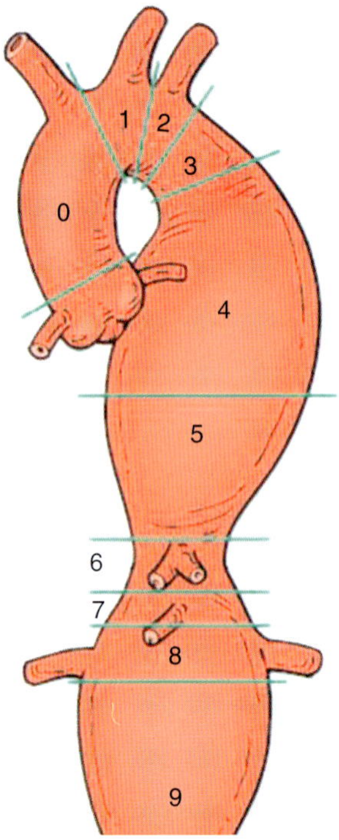

FIG 37.1 Classification of landing zones.

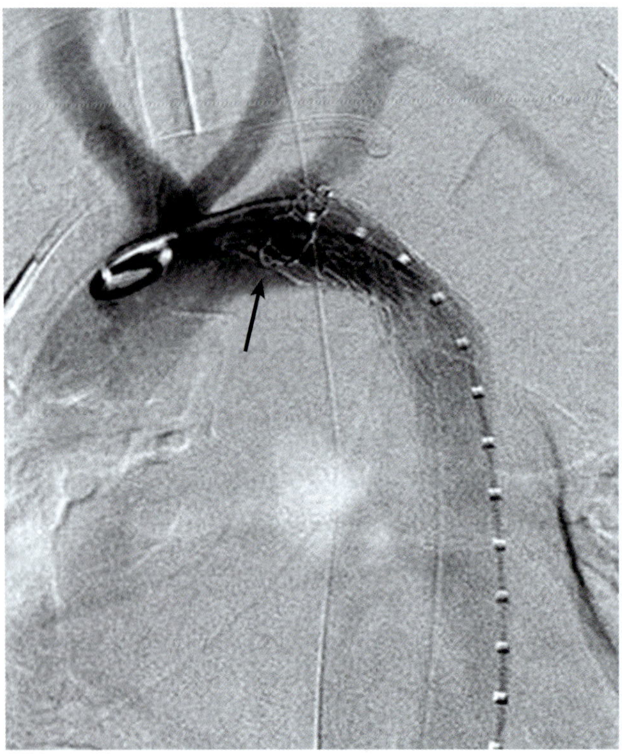

FIG 37.2 Angiogram showing "bird beaking" of the proximal endograft. The *arrow* shows proximal TEVAR "bird beaking" along the lesser curvature of the aortic arch.

migration and proximal endograft collapse, mostly in nonaneurysmal applications. Recent endograft modifications such as the Zenith Pro-Form and Alpha (Cook, Bloomington, IN) and the C-TAG (W. L. Gore, Flagstaff, AZ) have been designed to address this problem.

The distal attachment zones are classified as zones 5 to 11. Zone 5 starts in the distal half of the descending thoracic aorta but proximal to the celiac access, zone 6 extends from the celiac origin to the proximal aspect of the SMA, zone 7 is the SMA extending to the suprarenal aorta, zone 8 covers at least one renal artery, zone 9 covers the infrarenal aorta, zone 10 covers the common iliac artery, and zone 11 continues into the external iliac artery.

Management of the Left Subclavian Artery

Current practice guidelines from the Society for Vascular Surgery (SVS) recommend preoperative left SCA revascularization in elective TEVAR cases.[20] In approximately 20% of regulatory cases, adequate coverage required extending the endograft into zone 2, excluding the LSCA (Fig. 37.3).[21] The management strategy of the LSCA has evolved since the inception of TEVAR. Prophylactic revascularization of the LSCA with a carotid subclavian bypass or transposition is prescribed. The practice of LSCA coverage has come under severe scrutiny, with EUROSTAR data linking it to an increased risk of spinal cord ischemia (SCI) and brain stem strokes. Peterson and colleagues[22] observed a 63% (5/8) stroke and upper extremity ischemic symptom rate in patients who had LSCA coverage without revascularization. A review of the literature disclosed a 23% complication rate with LSA coverage, compared with a 3% rate when flow to the LSCA was maintained.[22,23] Additional reports of posterior circulation infarctions, arm ischemia, and SCI have reinforced the recommendations of preserving the LSCA. Intentional coverage without revascularization appears to be tolerated in some cases and can be performed in emergent settings in the presence of good collateral circulation. A review of 22 patients who underwent intentional coverage of the LSCA determined that almost 70% of patients remained asymptomatic, with 30% suffering mild symptoms of left arm claudication. Absolute contraindications to LSCA coverage include a dominant left vertebral artery, left internal mammary–to–coronary artery bypass, left arm hemodialysis access, aberrant right SCA, anomalous origin of the left SCA from the aortic arch, hypoplastic right vertebral artery, termination of the left vertebral artery in the posteroinferior cerebellar artery, and/or occluded internal iliac arteries. In addition, extended thoracic aortic coverage combined with prior abdominal aortic repair should be considered higher risk for SCI, and LSCA revascularization should be performed.[24-26] Current SVS guidelines recommend routine preoperative revascularization in elective TEVAR and expectant management in acute settings, excluding those with absolute contraindications.[26]

In order to precisely deploy an endograft at the level of the LSCA, it is often helpful to gain access to the aortic arch via the left brachial artery. This improves visualization of the junction between the subclavian and the aorta and allows for bailout stenting in the event of inadvertent coverage. Alternative techniques to maintain LSCA perfusion include endovascular debranching and in situ fenestration. Endovascular debranching with a chimney technique has been described for the left SCA and left common carotid artery. The goal for each is to extend the proximal landing zone and decrease operative morbidity.[26] In situ fenestration was first described by McWilliams in 2004. The transluminal

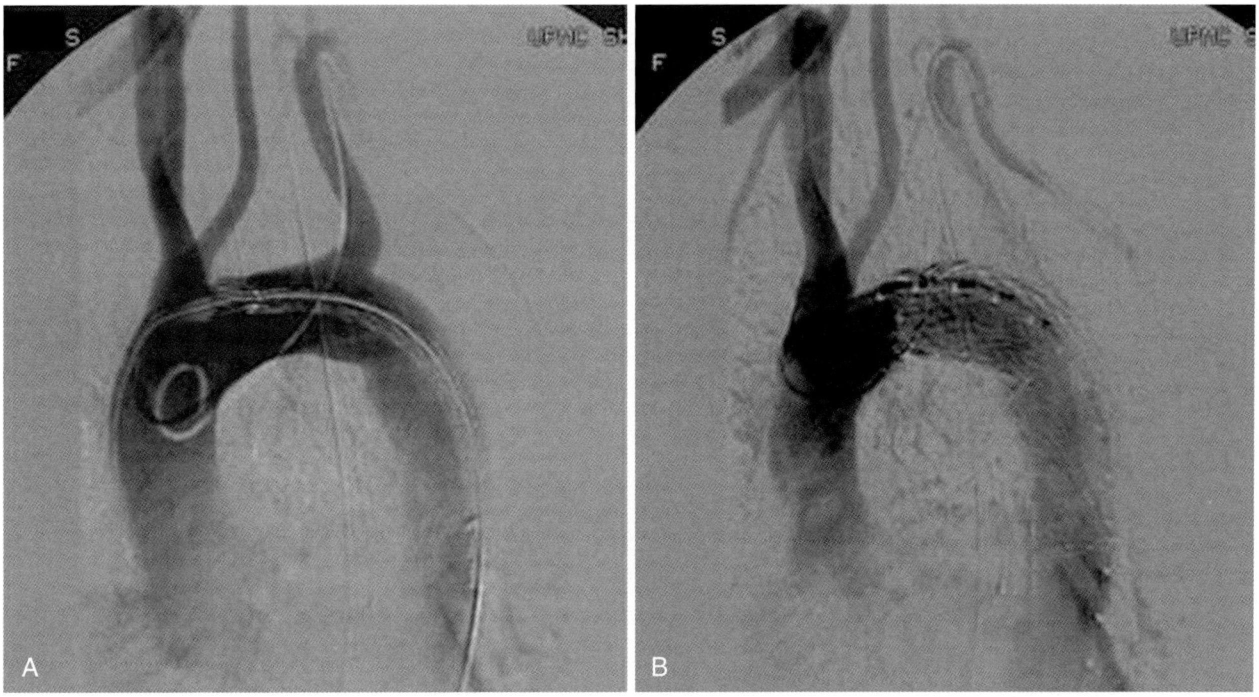

FIG 37.3 Angiogram—predeployment (A) and postdeployment (B). Note complete coverage of the left subclavian artery.

technique was performed using the back end of a stiff 0.018-inch guidewire and cutting balloons.[27] Since that time, reports of in situ laser fenestration (Turbo Elite Laser Catheter, Spectranetics, Colorado Springs, CO) have surfaced. The laser is similarly inserted via brachial access, juxtaposed to the endograft, a short laser energy burst is applied, and the fenestration is dilated with standard noncompliant balloons. Early technical reports and midterm follow-up were both favorable.[28]

Management of the Celiac Axis

The distal aortic landing zone places the endograft at least 2 cm cephalad to the celiac axis. When aneurysmal disease is more extensive, coverage of the celiac artery is an option, thus extending the distal seal zone. Visceral ischemia can occur, but reports suggest that adequate collateralization through the gastroduodenal and pancreaticoduodenal arcades minimize the physiologic insult.[29] A recent review reported selective coverage of the celiac axis in 31 patients during TEVAR.[30] Of these patients, two (6%) had bowel ischemia and five (16%) had an endoleak that required reintervention. A large review of worldwide data suggested a relatively low rate (6% to 8%) of foregut ischemia with celiac artery coverage and was associated with an overall mortality rate of 9%.[31] These findings illustrate that celiac coverage is feasible in most cases, but the variable and unpredictable arcade of collaterals between the celiac and SMA require an individualized approach. Tailoring patient care based on an assessment of preexisting comorbidities, operative morbidity of celiac revascularization, and physician skill set are all critically important. Patients with a prominent gastroduodenal artery arcade, replaced right hepatic artery, preexisting celiac stenosis, and/or well-developed SMA appear to have the most favorable results after covering the celiac origin. Open surgical or endovascular revascularization can be performed, if needed, with a relatively low morbidity. In the elective situations, open celiac debranching should be performed prior to TEVAR. Inflow may originate from a nondiseased segment of the infrarenal aorta or iliac artery. An end-to-end celiac artery anastomosis or end-to-side hepatic artery bypass should be considered. In the latter situation, ligation of the celiac origin should be performed to prevent a type II endoleak. Endovascular techniques are dictated by aneurysmal extent and anatomy, including parallel grafts (chimney, snorkel, sandwich, or periscope) and fenestrated or branched stent-grafts. Custom-made branch endografts are not FDA-approved for use in the United States.

STENT-GRAFT DESCRIPTION

Since FDA approval of the first TEVAR device in 2005, there has been a rapid increase in the number of stent-grafts available, with new modifications and designs along the way. In the past 2 decades, original TEVAR devices have undergone several rounds of modification: improved device materials, reduction of delivery size, advancement of device conformability, creation of longer lengths and tapered configurations, and development of larger diameter grafts. These developments have established TEVAR as the standard of care for most thoracic aortic pathology and increased the indications for use.

Gore C-TAG

The Conformable Gore TAG thoracic endoprosthesis (W.L. Gore, Flagstaff, AZ), the most recent advancement of the first FDA-approved endograft for the treatment of DTA (Fig. 37.4), has been the most widely implanted device in both on- and off-label use in the United States. The C-TAG endograft is an expanded

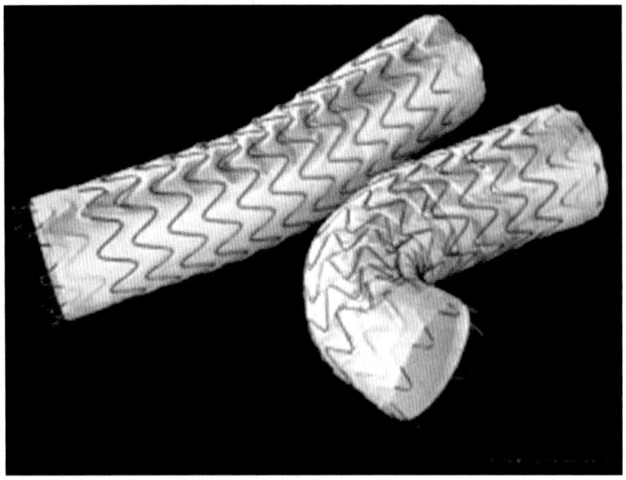

FIG 37.4 Conformable Gore TAG thoracic endoprosthesis. (Courtesy W.L. Gore & Associates.)

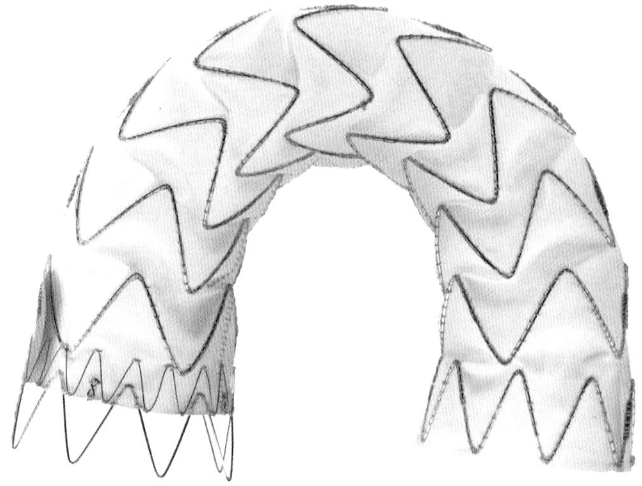

FIG 37.5 Medtronic Valiant device.

polytetrafluoroethylene (ePTFE) tubular graft reinforced with a layer of fluorinated ethylene propylene (FEP) and externally supported by Nitinol self-expanding stents. This endograft has lower porosity, which helps to avoid the sac enlargement associated with the earlier version of the device.[32,33] The FEP wrap has replaced the longitudinal deployment wire of the original device. Effective proximal and distal seals are achieved with flared edges of the graft as well as an additional ePTFE cuff. The graft has an inlaid gold band that marks the proximal and distal edges. The C-TAG device has been modified to increase conformability, especially on the lesser curvature of the aortic arch, by modifying the wire form's strength and pattern. The proximal covered scallops have also been replaced by short open bare metal stents ranging in length from 3 to 6.5 mm.

The C-TAG device is constrained in a sleeve of ePTFE/FEP film that is bound by a longitudinal seam running the entire length of the device. The device is deployed by pulling the string, which unzips the seam deploying the endograft from the middle to both ends. The device is available in diameters of 21 to 45 mm and lengths of 10, 15, or 20 cm. Two tapered devices (26 to 21 mm and 31 to 26 mm) are available and provide added flexibility in sizing. The device is delivered through an appropriately sized sheath with a pressurized hemostatic valve to minimize blood loss, these range in size from 18, 20, 22, or 24 French. The C-TAG device is designed to be oversized by 7% to 22%, incorporated in the IFU device sizing guide.

Advantages of the C-TAG device include a simple deployment mechanism and flexibility, which allows easy accommodation of tortuous anatomy. The endograft deploys from the middle of the graft out toward both ends. This design theoretically avoids the "wind sock" effect, which can occur if the proximal end is released first. Once the graft is deployed, the seal zones are ballooned with a trilobed balloon.

Medtronic Valiant

The Medtronic Valiant Thoracic Stent Graft on the Captiva delivery system device (Medtronic, Santa Rosa, CA) was approved for commercial use in the United States in January 2014. Prior to approval, the device was widely used outside the United States. Valiant, along with the Gore C-TAG, is approved for treating a variety of thoracic aortic pathology.

The Valiant stent-graft is composed of Nitinol sinusoidal springs attached to a woven polyester graft. There is a bare metal free-flow component at the proximal end to allow for extended fixation while maintaining flow to the branch vessels. Closed web designs are also available (Fig. 37.5). The Talent is available in a wide range of diameters, from 22 to 46 mm, and lengths of 10, 15, and 20 cm. There are a large number of tapered and nontapered configurations available. The device is oversized by 10% to 20% and constrained in a 22, 24, or 25 French sheath. The Valiant stent-graft uses the Captiva delivery system, which is said to have greater tractability for the tortuous aorta because of a hydrophilic outer coating and shorter tip on a braided sheath. Changes to the device were also introduced to improve flexibility and radial strength of the graft while reducing pressure points in the landing zones by increasing the number of shorter peaks on its uncovered stents from five to eight.

In June 2016, Medtronic announced the enrollment of the first patient in a clinical study assessing the Valiant EVO stent-graft system. Device modifications reduced the delivery sheath profile to 18 and 20 French. In addition, broader tapered endograft sizes and longer device lengths for anatomic customization are available. This system is not yet approved for commercial use in the United States.

Cook TX2 With Pro-Form and Zenith Alpha

The Cook TX2 stent-graft (Cook Medical, Bloomington, IN) was approved by the FDA for commercial use in the United States in 2008. This modular device consists of two components with active fixation. The Cook Zenith Alpha Thoracic Endograft received premarket approval from the FDA in September 2015 for vascular anatomy suitable for endovascular repair. The lower-profile endograft was developed to address vascular access issues associated with larger profile devices. Unlike the TX2 device, which is constructed of a stainless steel skeleton covered in woven Dacron, the Alpha device is composed of external Nitinol stents

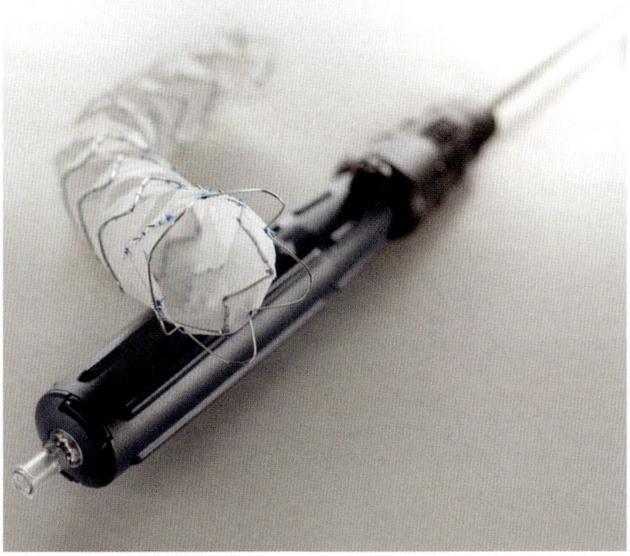

FIG 37.6 Cook Alpha device.

and woven polyester. The entire length of the polyester is supported by an exoskeleton except at the proximal end, where the stents line the inside. Similar to the TX2 device, the Alpha uses active fixation on both components in the form of proximal, caudally oriented barbs to prevent distal migration and distal, cranially oriented barbs to prevent proximal migration. The distal end is a bare stent designed to allow additional coverage of visceral vessels, if needed, while maintaining patency (Fig. 37.6).

There are gold radiopaque markers near the ends of the endograft, improving visualization and allowing precise placement of the endograft. The proximal Alpha device is available in diameters of 18 to 46 mm; distal extension components range from 22 to 46 mm. There are tapered proximal and distal endograft pieces that provide a 4-mm difference between the proximal and distal necks (diameter range: 26 to 46 mm). A large number of lengths are available—proximal 105 to 233 mm and distal 91 to 112 mm. The Alpha delivery system is constrained in a 16, 18, or 20 French delivery sheath, whereas the TX2 Pro-Form resides in a 20 or 22 French sheath. Cook recommends at least a 3-cm overlap of device components. The introduction of the Pro-Form mechanism allows the first stent to deploy at an angle to the second stent, thus facilitating apposition to the lesser curve in the arch.

Bolton Relay

The Bolton Relay thoracic stent-graft with plus delivery system (Bolton Medical, Sunrise, FL) has a skeleton of self-expanding Nitinol stents covered with a compliant polyester fabric (Fig. 37.7). The device received FDA approval in September 2012. The proximal portion of the device has an exposed bare metal stent that anchors the device in place while maintaining patency of branch vessels. The device is delivered via its transport system, which consists of a primary introduction braided hydrophilic outer sheath, curved flexible secondary delivery sheath, and a through lumen. The graft is released via the apex release mechanism and the coaxial system remains stationary during device deployment. There is a double S configuration of the support bar, which is designed to mimic the natural curve of the aorta while providing columnar strength. The conformable device has six unique performance zones, which are designed to absorb the hemodynamic effects of the thoracic aorta.

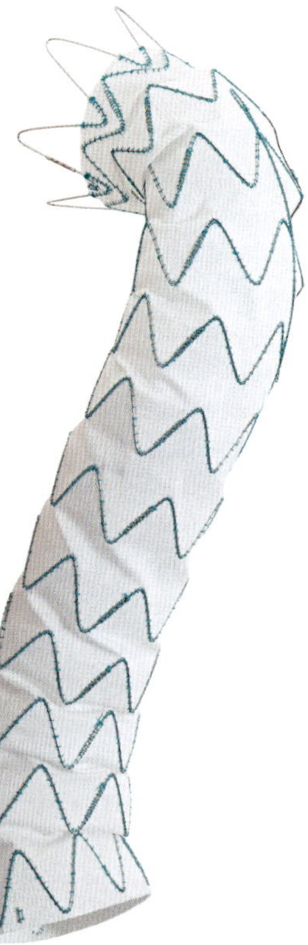

FIG 37.7 Bolton Relay device.

A number of platinum and iridium radiopaque markers are embedded in the graft to improve visualization. The device is available in both tapered and non-tapered configurations. The nontapered graft diameters range from 22 to 46 mm; their lengths range from 100 to 250 mm. The delivery system requires a primary introducer sheath of 22 to 26 French, depending on the device size. The tapered grafts are designed to gradually taper in 4-mm increments with recommended oversizing of 10% to 15%. The devices range in length from 150 to 250 mm. The Relay graft requires at least a 25-mm proximal and 30-mm distal landing zone. This device has the longest lengths; if multiple grafts are used, a minimum overlap of 50 mm is recommended. The four-step deployment and release mechanism is similar to that of the Cook Zenith TX2 device and entails a slow, controlled pullback of the outer sheath to allow expansion of the endograft. A separate mechanism is used to expand the proximal bare stents.

OPERATIVE TECHNIQUE AND DEPLOYMENT

The deployment of the four FDA approved thoracic stent-grafts differs slightly, but a series of general rules and tips are helpful for each. Once femoral access is obtained, a pigtail catheter is placed from the contralateral side for imaging while a Lunderquist stiff wire (Cook Medical, Bloomington, IN) is positioned in the ascending aorta from the ipsilateral access. Aortography is performed with the image intensifier rotated in an oblique projection to provide the optimal orthogonal view of the desired deployment zone. For proximal imaging near the LSCA, a left anterior oblique projection (30 to 60 degrees) is often needed, whereas the projection for distal endograft deployment most often is lateral. Angiography with a marker catheter serves to confirm device length and determine appropriate landing zones, but this step can be replaced by intravascular ultrasound in patients with compromised renal function.

The thoracic stent-graft is introduced and appropriate deployment steps followed based on the IFU. Usually the stent-graft is advanced beyond the proximal target and retracted to its desired landing zone, eliminating any stored forward energy. During endograft deployment, constant forward pressure is applied on the wire to buttress the endograft against the outer curve of the aortic wall, thus limiting the tendency for distal migration. Adjunctive techniques have been used to facilitate accurate proximal endograft deployment, such as the pharmacologic reduction of blood pressure, transient asystole induced by adenosine, and rapid ventricular pacing. These maneuvers reduce the blood pressure and shear force on the expanding endograft, thus preventing the wind-sock phenomenon. These maneuvers are not universally required but may be helpful in anatomically challenging cases.

If the extent of the aneurysm requires more than one endograft component for adequate coverage, the smaller device should be deployed first to allow for adequate seal between the two endografts. An acceptable overlap zone should greater than 5 cm in length. When the devices are the same size, longer overlap zones (7 to 10 cm) are recommended.

INVESTIGATIONAL DEVICES

As technology advances, a wider range of patients and aortic pathologies will benefit from device modifications that accommodate landing zones involving the ascending aorta, arch, or paravisceral aorta. Chuter was the first to successfully use a branched endograft for repair of a thoracoabdominal aortic aneurysm.[34] Since then, the Zenith T-branch thoracoabdominal endovascular graft (Cook Medical) and various patient-specific custom-modified Zenith devices have shown favorable results.[35,36] Three device manufacturers are attempting to develop commercially available devices. Cook Medical was the first to develop a multibranch endograft and currently has two device options: the multisize off-the-shelf T-branch device with four downward-facing external cuffs and a custom-modified device made to fit the patient's anatomy. The Gore Excluder (Gore and Associates) thoracoabdominal branch endograft is an off-the-shelf four-vessel branch device currently in clinical trial. Two design options are available, the first has four downward cuffs and the second possesses two upward renal cuffs and two downward branches. The device is designed to be used with the balloon-expandable Gore Viabahn Bx endoprothesis (Gore and Associates). Medtronic is developing a modular branched endograft based on the Valiant and Endurant platforms in order to treat thoracoabdominal aortic aneurysms. This device is currently under investigation in an investigational device exemption (IDE) study.

Extending indications for endograft repair of arch aneurysms requires the development of flexible, conformable modular devices specifically designed for deployment in zones 0, 1, or 2. All four thoracic endograft companies are developing arch endograft devices: the Cook Medical arch branch thoracic branch device, Bolton Relay NBS Plus, Medtronic Valiant Mona LSA stent-graft system, and Gore TAG Thoracic Branch Endoprosthesis (Figs. 37.8 and 37.9). Each of these devices is designed to eliminate the need for open surgical revascularization and extends the proximal landing zone into the ascending aorta. Device similarities include

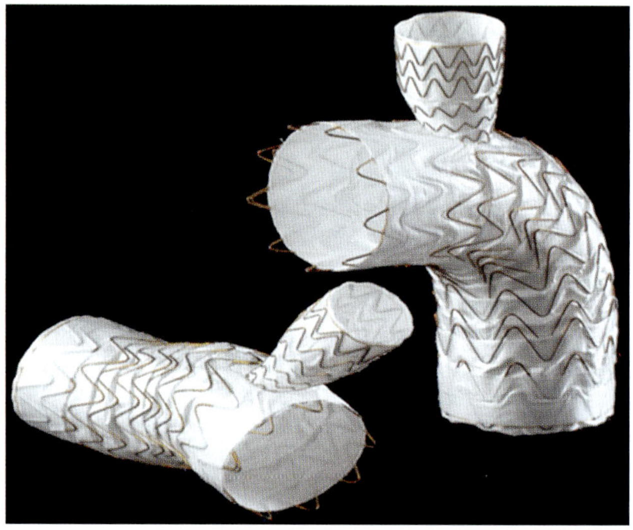

FIG 37.8 Gore TAG Thoracic Branch Endoprosthesis. (Courtesy W.L. Gore & Associates.)

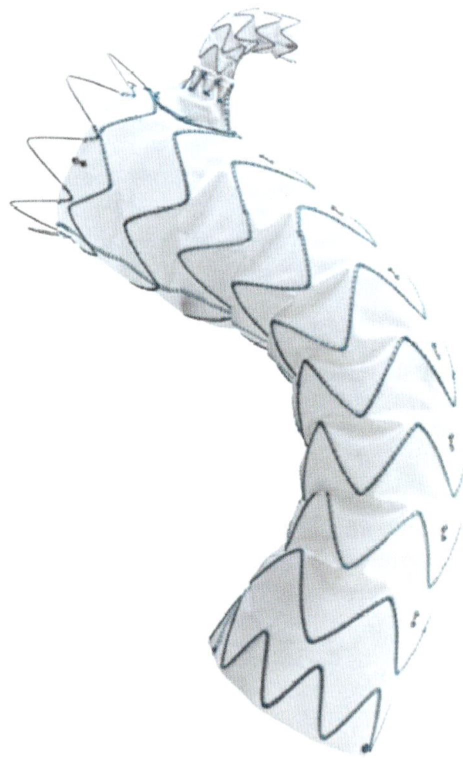

FIG 37.9 Medtronic Valiant Mona LSA stent graft. (Courtesy Medtronic.)

the use of a through-and-through wire, precannulated branches to facilitate device alignment, flexible bridging stent-grafts, and lower-profile delivery systems. Various commercial studies of these systems are under way in the United States.

RESULTS

Despite the introduction of TEVAR for thoracic aortic pathology nearly two decades ago, there remains intense debate regarding its indications for use, efficacy, and device durability. The Society for Thoracic Surgeons Endovascular Task Force acknowledged that thoracic aortic pathology is increasingly being treated by TEVAR without prospective randomized trial data comparing the two types of treatment.[37,28] It is important to recognize that the decision to treat DTA must be made with the same rigor for open and endovascular repair.[38,29] Although DTA appears to be a lethal disease process, it progresses slowly. Mortality rates after TEVAR vary widely (2% to 26%) and are dependent on the indication for intervention, comorbid conditions, and experience of the physician. However, an acceptable perioperative mortality (1.9% to 3.1%) has been found in elective TEVAR procedures using second-generation devices.[39,40] Limited data exist and despite the early effectiveness of TEVAR, long-term results are poorly described. Nonrandomized studies show a trend toward improved outcomes with regard to such issues as paraplegia, mortality, and hospital length of stay.[41] Midterm TEVAR results have demonstrated a shorter length of stay as well as lower in-hospital complication and mortality rates compared to open surgical repair.[42,30] Three industry-sponsored nonrandomized comparative trials have suggested clinical equipoise. In 2008, Makaroun and colleagues[40] described the benefits of TEVAR compared with open repair and recognized that it reduced early morbidity and mortality with similar long-term survival. Long-term follow-up from the Gore TAG trial documented no difference in all-cause mortality at 5 years (67% vs. 68%). In the TEVAR cohort, major adverse events were reduced significantly (57.9% vs. 78.7%, $P = .001$). It was recognized that late complications occurred more frequently with TEVAR requiring long-term surveillance and that rates of secondary interventions were higher in the TEVAR group.[43,31]

Open surgical repair of TAAs remains a morbid procedure that carries a combined paraplegia and mortality rate of greater than 20% in reports using national and regional databases.[44] Five- and 10-year survival rates following open TAA repair are somewhat limited at 60% and 38%, respectively.[7,8] Results comparing TEVAR with open repair are limited by the lack of prospective randomized trials. These data are often difficult to interpret because of the inclusion of a multitude of pathologies, different anatomic locations, varying device types, and patient comorbidities, which makes a direct comparison impossible. Premarket regulatory trials of devices still provide the best comparative information of TEVAR results to open repair because relatively similar groups are involved.

Early Results

Technical Success

Technical success in endograft deployment has been reported as high as 98% in all three FDA trials and the Talent thoracic registry.[33,45-47] Most failures were due to access problems preventing the delivery of the device. Interestingly, the EUROSTAR and United Kingdom thoracic registries report a lower deployment success rate, reflecting wider application of the technology in current clinical practice outside of trial guidelines.

Mortality

A significant operative survival benefit is observed with TEVAR when compared with open repair in the US trials (2% vs. 6%). The EUROSTAR registry of TEVAR reports a higher but still favorable mortality rate of 5.3%, likely because 52% of its patients were deemed to be at too high a risk for open repair and thus represented a sicker cohort.[48] A recent meta-analysis of published literature showed clear survival benefits with TEVAR compared with the open procedure.[24] In 2010, Cheng and colleagues published a meta-analysis of TEVAR versus open surgical repair for descending thoracic aortic disease.[30] Data from 39 comparative studies and 3 registries were combined and involved 5888 patients from 1998 to 2009. Patient characteristics were balanced except for age, TEVAR patients were 3 years older (54 ± 13 years for TEVAR vs. 51 ± 13 years for open surgery, $P = .0001$). Cumulative 30-day all-cause mortality was lower for TEVAR (OR: 0.44, 95% CI: 0.33 to 0.59) and cumulative all-cause mortality at 1 year (OR: 0.73, 95% CI: 0.53 to 1.02) and at 2 to 3 years did not differ between the two groups. Multicenter trials showed a reduction in all-cause 30-day mortality (OR: 0.24, 95% CI: 0.13 to 0.44) compared with single-center series (OR: 0.53, 95% CI: 0.38 to 0.74).[49]

Neurologic Complications

Neurologic complications are still among the most devastating complications after DTA repair. Advances in endograft technology have failed to improve stroke rates associated with DTA repair. Stroke rates for either open or endovascular repair range from 4% to 8% and are comparable with those following open repair.[22,33,45,50-52] Strokes are believed to occur during TEVAR because of instrumentation of the aortic arch, causing embolization and less frequently coverage of a critical arch branch vessel.[53] Deployment of thoracic endografts proximal to the LSCA have been associated with an increased risk of perioperative stroke. In the phase II TAG study, stroke occurred in 14% of patients with endografts deployed proximal to the LSCA compared with 1% when the endograft was deployed in zone 3. Similarly, the incidence of stroke in the VALOR high-risk trial was 26% when the endograft was deployed cephalad to zone 3.[54] In the STARZ trial, all four strokes occurred with stent-graft deployment distal to the LSCA.[45] These strokes may have been related to the recommended deployment sequence of the Cook TX2 device, which started proximal to the desired deployment zone and required a distal readjustment technique for device deployment.[12] Minimal manipulation and meticulous management of the wires, catheters, and delivery system as well as limiting the use of balloon molding to the inside of the graft cannot be overemphasized to minimize risk. Other independent predictors of stroke from the EUROSTAR data include female sex and prolonged procedure time (>2 hours 40 minutes).[52] Cheng and colleagues[55] determined that the overall risk of stroke was similar for both groups (OR: 0.75, 95% CI:

0.50 to 1.13) and paraplegia was significantly reduced for TEVAR (OR: 0.42, 95% CI: 0.28 to 0.63).

Paraplegia remains a catastrophic complication after TAA repair and is one of the most important predictors of death.[56] Data from the three FDA trials showed a cumulative advantage of TEVAR over open repair (6% vs. 10%). The incidence of paraplegia in the control groups, however, was significantly higher than rates reported from centers of excellence (3%), but they are similar to national data from administrative databases.[57,58] Part of the variance involves the inclusion of all SCI events in regulatory trials, whereas mild transient deficits are often overlooked in individual center series. The moderate protective effects of TEVAR against SCI may be due to avoidance of thoracic aortic clamping and reduced local hemodynamic disturbances at the level of the spinal cord secondary to lack of blood loss from intercostal back bleeding. A retrospective review of thoracic and thoracoabdominal aneurysm patients (724) who underwent TEVAR (352) or open repair (372) showed no significant difference in the rate of SCI (4.3% vs. 7.5%) between groups.[59] It should also be noted that SCI is not confined to the perioperative period, as delayed and recurrent SCI and paraplegia have also been reported after TEVAR.[60,61]

Several factors have been linked to an increased risk of SCI after TEVAR: concomitant or previous infrarenal aortic repair, lack of spinal fluid drainage, extensive thoracic aortic coverage (especially T9 to T12), renal insufficiency, intraoperative hypotension (systolic blood pressure <80 mm Hg), emergency surgery, and coverage of the hypogastric artery or LSCA or both.[22,52,53,62-66] Some of these risk factors are beyond the clinician's control, but coverage of the LSCA and hypogastric arteries should be avoided when possible. Occlusion of the LSCA has been associated with a significant increase in the incidence of paraplegia by the EUROSTAR collaborators, and recent reports suggest that LSCA revascularization may be required more frequently than previously recognized for either spinal cord protection or avoidance of symptoms of ischemia in the left upper extremity.[22,23,52,62,63] SVS Practice Guidelines recommend routine revascularization of the LSCA in elective cases where the LSCA must be sacrificed for effective proximal seal (grade 2, level C evidence).[26] It has been recognized that lumbar and pelvic collaterals account for 25% of the spinal cord's blood supply and that compromised hypogastric blood flow contributes to the development of SCI.[67] Preservation of internal iliac blood flow and a staged repair of synchronous TAA and abdominal aortic aneurysms (AAA) allow for the development of collaterals.[68]

The use of spinal cord protective techniques is at the discretion of the practitioner. Most operators optimize the mean arterial pressure and use cerebrospinal fluid (CSF) drainage to protect the spinal cord. The premise for CSF drainage is based on the principle that spinal perfusion pressure is equal to the mean arterial pressure minus the intrathecal pressure. Reducing CSF pressure through drainage helps to maintain better spinal perfusion. Although spinal drainage is used routinely in a few select centers, most operators use it selectively based on the estimated risk of paraplegia. The drain is inserted preoperatively and maintained for 48 to 72 hours, keeping the CSF pressure less than 10 cm H_2O. The efficacy of drainage has also been observed in reversing the delayed onset of paraplegia after TEVAR and open procedures. Although the practice can be associated with hemorrhagic complications from catheter placement, with a reported incidence of 0% to 3%, CSF drainage should be used when an elevated potential for SCI exists, such as extensive coverage of the thoracic aorta or with associated abdominal aortoiliac pathology.[56]

Vascular Complications

Access site vascular complications are less common with increasing experience and second- and third-generation TEVAR devices. These complications lead to deployment failure and significant early morbidity, which has been reported to be as high as 14% in some instances.[54] The size discrepancy between small iliac arteries and large sheaths accounted for most of these complications. This was especially apparent in women, who have smaller native arteries and constitute approximately 40% of patients with TAA. With increased awareness of this complication, the use of conduits, and development of smaller delivery profiles, the incidence in the confirmatory TAG trial decreased drastically from the previously reported 6%.[51]

Endoleaks

The overall incidence of endoleaks after TEVAR is 3.9% to 15.3%.[37,40,69-71] In a recent literature review of 3004 patients, Ricotta[72] reported the overall endoleak rate to be 10.4% at 30 days and 9.5% at 1 year, with the majority being type I or type II. Nearly half of the patients (46%) underwent a secondary procedure with technical success in nearly 86%.[73] Ongoing endograft surveillance is essential. The rate of secondary interventions due to endoleaks or migration is 3.6% to 24%. The indication for implantation and length of follow-up appear to impact the need for future intervention.[39,74,75]

Late Results

Late Survival

Aggregated 1 year data from the three published US trials show a clear aneurysm-related survival benefit for TEVAR over open repair (95% vs. 89%, respectively).[33,45,54] The VALOR trial reported a statistically significant aneurysm-related survival advantage over open repair (3.1% vs. 11.6%) at 1 year, whereas the STARZ Trial data noted no differences between groups.

The survival advantage persisted at the 5-year follow-up in the TAG study, which was the first to report long-term data. Although all-cause mortality was not different between groups (68% vs. 67%), aneurysm-related death rates remained significantly less for TEVAR than the open repair cohort, almost entirely because of the perioperative survival benefit.[54] There were a total of four aneurysm-related deaths in the TAG group (2.8%) compared with 11 in the open surgical cohort (11.7%; $P = .008$). Major adverse events occurred in 28% of TAG patients and 70% of surgical controls ($P < .001$) in the postoperative period; this advantage for the TAG patients persisted at 12 months (42% vs. 77%; $P < .001$) and 5 years (58% vs. 79%; $P = .001$).

The US Medicare database identified more than 10,000 TEVAR patients from 2005 to 2010. Isolated elective aneurysm patients had the lowest mortality compared with acute aortic syndromes patients. Of those who survived 6 months, 6% to 12% died annually thereafter.[40,76] For high-risk patient populations, studies from Stanford University have shown that late outcomes are poor, with an actuarial survival rate of 31% at 5 years.[73] This observation is akin to the findings of the EVAR-2 trial and of EUROSTAR data for patients with AAA and raises the question of the efficacy of such treatment in this patient cohort. There does appear to be subgroup of patients that are better candidates for TEVAR than for open surgical repair, especially if they are anatomically suitable. Older individuals (>75 years), those with ruptures, and those with significant pulmonary disease appear to benefit the most.[34,78,79] Patel and colleagues reviewed 46 patients who were considered at high-risk for open TAA surgical repair. TEVAR was performed in 21 patients with an all-cause mortality of 50% in the entire cohort.[79a] However, median actual time to mortality was 24.9 months for the TEVAR group and 9.2 months for the control group ($P = .01$). Improved survival was demonstrated in the high-risk group with TEVAR.[66]

Migration

Caudal device migration is a rare occurrence, with a reported incidence ranging from 1.2% to 3.9%. Graft migration greater than 10 mm occurred in 2.8% (3/107) of patients at 12 months with the Cook TX2, although there was no endoleak or need for reintervention in any case. All patients were noted to have implantation of the barbed endograft segment in an acutely angled aortic segment or within mural thrombus. In the Talent endograft study, the incidence of migration was 3.9%, resulting in one reintervention. Factors contributing to this included overzealous sizing and device implantation in angulated seal zones. Retrograde proximal migration can occur at the distal landing zone, with aortic remodeling. To prevent distal migration, some devices have distal fixation via bare metal uncovered stents with retrograde barbs.

Sac Behavior and Aortic Rupture

Aneurysmal sac enlargement has been reported in 7.1% to 14.5% of patients after TEVAR at 1 year.[48,79] The incidence did not differ between the three thoracic aortic endografts. In the TAG pivotal trial,[54] aneurysmal sac shrinkage of greater than 5 mm occurred in 50% of patients, whereas aortic sac enlargement was found in 19%. These results reflect data from the original, normal-porosity ePTFE grafts and do not represent the long-term performance of the currently available devices. Following the introduction of the low-porosity PTFE material, patients with sac enlargement (confirmatory TAG trial) decreased at 2 years from 12.9% to 2.9%.

Stent-Graft Collapse

Stent-graft collapse and acute aortic obstruction is a rare complication that has most frequently been reported in young trauma patients, especially those with overzealous endograft sizing and severe aortic angulation.[41,80] This phenomenon is extremely rare with aneurysmal disease. Poor endograft wall apposition along the lesser curvature of the aortic arch combined with high flow rates and pressure in the thoracic aorta appear to be the source of this potentially fatal complication.[81,82] Fortunately many of these situations can be treated urgently and repaired with either a balloon-expandable stent or an additional stent-graft component.[83,84]

CONCLUSION

When anatomically suitable, TEVAR is considered the treatment of choice and the standard of care for descending TAAs. TEVAR is a safe and effective therapeutic treatment modality, the results of which appear to be at the least comparable with those of open repair. Advancements in device modification and technology over the last 5 to 10 years have drastically improved endograft handling and performance. Disease-specific devices, modular branch endografts, and lower-profile devices will advance indications for the use of these procedures. As with all endovascular technology, close long-term follow-up is essential to ensure optimal outcomes.

REVIEW QUESTIONS

1. What are the indications for thoracic endovascular repair of descending thoracic aortic aneurysms?
2. How much should endografts be oversized to achieve adequate seal, and what are the problems with over- or undersizing the graft?
3. What are the landing zones of the thoracic aorta?
4. What is the current recommendation for the management of the left subclavian artery?
5. What is the current recommendation for management of the celiac axis?
6. What are the risk factors for paraplegia with (TEVAR)?
7. What is the risk of stroke with TEVAR and what is the primary cause believed to be?
8. What is the perioperative mortality of TEVAR?

BIBLIOGRAPHY

Bavaria JE, Appoo JJ, Makaroun M, et al. Endovascular stent grafting versus open surgical repair of descending thoracic aortic aneurysms in low-risk patients: a multicenter comparative trial. *J Thorac Cardiovasc Surg*. 2007;133:369–377.

Buth J, Harris PL, Hobo R, et al. Neurologic complications associated with endovascular repair of thoracic aortic pathology: incidence and risk factors. a study from the European Collaborators on Stent/Graft Techniques for Aortic Aneurysm Repair (EUROSTAR) registry. *J Vasc Surg*. 2007;46: 1103–1110.

Cheng D, Martin J, Shennib H, et al. Endovascular aortic repair versus open surgical repair for descending thoracic aortic disease a systematic review and meta-analysis of comparative studies. *J Am Coll Cardiol.* 2010;55:986–1001.

Cina CS, Safar HA, Lagana A, et al. Subclavian carotid transposition and bypass grafting: consecutive cohort study and systematic review. *J Vasc Surg.* 2002;35(3):422–429.

Elefteriades JA, Farkas EA. Thoracic aortic aneurysm clinically pertinent controversites and uncertainties. *J Am Coll Cardiol.* 2010;55:841.

Hiratzka LF, Bakris GL, Beckman JA, et al. 2010 ACCF/AHA/AATS/ACR/ASA/SCA/SCAI/SIR/STS/SVM guidelines for the diagnosis and management of patient s with thoracic aortic disease. *Circulation.* 2010;121:e266.

Lee WA, Matsumura JS, Mitchell RA, et al. Endovascular repair of traumatic thoracic aortic injury: clinical practice guideline of the SVS. *J Vasc Surg.* 2011;53(1):187–192.

Makaroun MS, Dillavou ED, Wheatley GH, et al. Five-year results of endovascular treatment with the Gore TAG device compared with open repair of thoracic aortic aneurysms. *J Vasc Surg.* 2008; 47:912.

Matsumura JS, Cambria RP, Dake MD, et al. International controlled clinical trial of thoracic endovascular aneurysm repair with the Zenith TX2 endovascular graft: 1-year results. *J Vasc Surg.* 2008; 47:247–257.

Matsumura JS, Rizvi AZ. Left subclavian artery revascularization: Society for Vascular Surgery Practice Guidelines. *J Vasc Surg.* 2010;52:65S–69S.

Olsson C, Thelin S, Stahle E, et al. Thoracic aortic aneurysm and dissesction increasing prevalence and improved outcomes reported in a nationwide population-based study of more than 14,000 cases from 1988 to 2002. *Circulation.* 2006;114:2611.

Svensson LG, Miller DC, Bavaria JE, et al. Expert consensus document on the treatment of descending thoracic aortic disease using endovascular stent-grafts. *Ann Thorac Surg.* 2008;85:S1–S41.

Svesson LG, Kouchoukos NT, Miller DC. Expert consensus document on the treatment of descending thoracic aortic disease using endovascular stent-grafts. *Ann Thorac Surg.* 2008;85:S1–S41.

References available online at ExpertConsult.com.

CHAPTER 38

Combined Endovascular and Surgical (Hybrid) Approach to Aortic Arch and Thoracoabdominal Aortic Pathology

Wesley Kwan Lew, William J. Quiñones-Baldrich

A hybrid aortic repair consists of an open surgical bypass to perfuse a single or multiple vessels so that a stent-graft can be deployed across their origin(s) to treat aortic pathology. This combined approach was first used at the University of California, Los Angeles to treat a type IV thoracoabdominal aneurysm in 1999 to minimize the morbidity and mortality of a complete open repair in a high-risk patient.[1] Because this technique has evolved, it is now used to treat more extensive pathology of the aortic arch and thoracoabdominal aorta (Fig. 38.1).

A hybrid repair of thoracoabdominal aneurysms avoids proximal aortic cross clamping, thoracotomy, and minimizes the visceral ischemia time. For the aortic arch, avoidance of hypothermic circulatory arrest makes a hybrid approach appealing. Use of thoracic stent-grafts in association with open surgical debranching is considered an "off-label" application of the device.[2]

This chapter focuses on patient selection for hybrid repairs and discusses the techniques of debranching and stent grafting for both the aortic arch and thoracoabdominal aortic pathology. Additional considerations such as use of spinal protection and postoperative management are discussed. The literature and outcomes from case series are also reviewed.

PATIENT SELECTION

Indications

The indications to treat an aortic aneurysm with a hybrid approach are no different than those used for open aneurysm repair. They include aneurysm diameter greater than 6 cm, growth greater than 0.5 cm/year, unusual aneurysm morphology suggesting a higher risk of rupture (pseudoaneurysm), or symptomatic aneurysm. The hybrid approach should be reserved for patients who are considered at high risk due to comorbidities and/or prior aortic or abdominal surgery.

Anatomy Considerations

Patients are considered for a hybrid repair if an appropriate proximal and distal landing zone is present, or can be created, allowing for exclusion of the aneurysm by a stent-graft. Partial or complete debranching of the aortic arch is performed to create additional proximal landing zones. For pathology involving the visceral aorta, critical vessels, such as the celiac artery, superior mesenteric artery (SMA), and renal arteries, can be covered by aortic stent grafts after a surgical bypass has been established. Distal landing zone must be present in the native aorta or a preexisting aortic graft. Open infrarenal aortic replacement may be necessary to create a distal landing zone in patients with an infrarenal aneurysm and a short segment of nonaneurysmal aorta.

In any hybrid repair case, planning is of utmost importance to assure that an adequate endograft seal will be obtained by an existing length of normal aorta or as a consequence of the open surgical intervention.

Open Versus Hybrid Approach

The choice of an open or hybrid approach is dependent on a combination of the patient's history, comorbidities, and overall condition. Patients considered high risk include those who cannot tolerate a thoracotomy given severe chronic obstructive pulmonary disease or previous left chest operations. Patients with severe renal insufficiency with an increased risk of renal failure after open repair are also candidates for a hybrid approach. Patients with significant cardiac conditions or an inability to tolerate proximal aortic clamping with increased afterload, should also be considered. Nonoperative, conservative management should be offered to patients with shortened life expectancies or those who are debilitated due to coexisting medical conditions.

Open aortic repair has been shown to be a durable procedure with acceptable results and is the treatment of choice in young patients and those with acceptable operative risk. The hybrid repair is currently reserved for high-risk patients who are considered poor candidates for an open repair.

Aortic Arch Aneurysm

Open repair of aortic arch aneurysms require a sternotomy, extracorporeal circulatory support often with deep hypothermic circulatory arrest, and hemiarch or total arch replacement.[3] In cases of concomitant descending thoracic aorta involvement, an "elephant trunk" technique can be utilized where a second intervention addresses the descending thoracic aorta component.[4,5] In high-risk patients, a hybrid approach is attractive because it avoids the need for hypothermic arrest, and in cases of descending thoracic involvement, the procedure can be done in one stage.

Safi and colleagues published one of the largest case series of open aortic arch aneurysm repair with thoracic or thoracoabdominal aortic involvement in 2004. They replaced the ascending

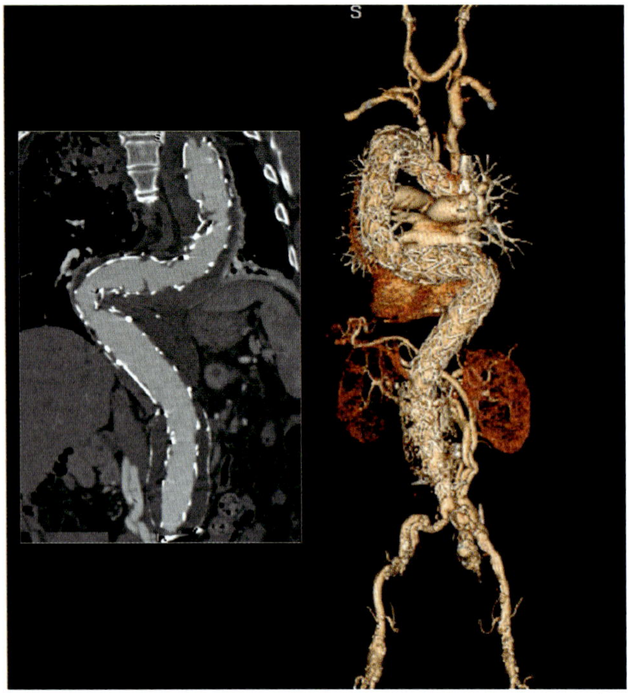

FIG 38.1 Type II thoracoabdominal aortic aneurysm with partial aortic arch debranching and visceral debranching. The aortic stent-graft spans nearly the entire aorta, from distal to the innominate artery to above the aortic bifurcation.

aorta and aortic arch, leaving an elephant trunk in the descending thoracic aorta in 218 patients. Strokes occurred in 2.7%, and 30-day mortality was 8.7%. Of the surviving 199 patients, 2% expired before returning for the second-stage thoracic or thoracoabdominal aortic repair completion. Of those completing the second surgery, 9.7% expired within 30 days of the second surgery.[6] Smaller case series of open arch repair in association with ascending or thoracoabdominal aortic aneurysms (TAA) involve heterogeneous populations, and report a wide range of perioperative mortality from 5.3% to 30.8%.[3]

There have been no randomized trials of hybrid versus open repair, but institutions have compared cohorts of open and hybrid repairs. The University of Florida in Gainesville identified 58 patients with aortic arch aneurysms and descending thoracic aortic involvement. An open cohort using a two-staged approach with aortic arch replacement and elephant trunk repair ($n = 21$) was compared to a cohort using a hybrid approach ($n = 37$). Rates of spinal cord ischemia (0% vs. 0%), stroke (10% vs. 11%), 30-day mortality (19% vs. 16%), and survival at 12 months (73% vs. 72%) were similar between the open and hybrid cases. These comparable results were present even though 68% of the hybrid cases still utilized cardiopulmonary bypass.[7]

In 2010, a more recent, single-institution study compared 27 hybrid arch procedures with a contemporary series of 45 cases of open arch repairs. The incidence of permanent cerebral neurologic deficit (4% vs. 9%) and in-hospital mortality (11% vs. 16%) were similar for the hybrid versus open cohort. In the open arch group, it was noted that patients older than 75 years of age had significantly higher mortality than those younger than 75 years of age (36% vs. 9%; $P = .05$).[8]

Two meta-analyses of hybrid case series have been published. Antoniou and colleagues reviewed 18 studies with a total of 195 patients. Complete arch debranching was performed in 122 patients (63%). The overall technical success rate was 86%. Overall perioperative morbidity and mortality rates were 21% and 9%, respectively. The stroke rate was 7%, and four aneurysm-related deaths were reported during follow-up (2%). No long-term data was reported.[9] The second meta-analysis identified 15 studies with 463 patients in studies published up to May 2008. Overall 30-day mortality was 8.3%, the stroke rate was 4.4%, the paraplegia rate was 3.9%, and the endoleak rate was 9.2%. Treatment on-pump or off-pump did not affect any of the endpoints.[10]

As increasing data on the hybrid approach emerge, the morbidity and mortality rates are comparable to open repair. Considering that hybrid series most often include higher-risk patients, a benefit of the hybrid approach may be implied.

Thoracoabdominal Aneurysm

Open repair of thoracoabdominal aneurysms involve a laparotomy, thoracotomy, proximal aortic cross clamp, and global visceral ischemia. Techniques to optimize open repairs have included left heart bypass and retrograde perfusion of the renal and mesenteric vessels. In high-volume centers, case series of open thoracoabdominal aneurysm repair demonstrate reasonable mortality of 5% to 8.3% with rates of spinal cord ischemia from 3.8% to 16%.[11-14] Late survival at 5, 10, and 15 years were 54% to 67%, 29%, and 21%, respectively.[13,14]

In a contemporary series of open thoracoabdominal aneurysm repair published in 2011, 305 patients were reviewed. Twenty percent underwent an urgent or emergent repair, and 57% were Crawford extents type I or II. The majority had cerebrospinal fluid drainage (97%) and left heart bypass (89%). Operative mortality was 8%, renal failure necessitating hemodialysis at discharge was 6%, and permanent paraplegia was 3%. Actuarial survival at 2 years was 79%.[15]

Despite these single-center outcomes, database outcomes find mortalities to be more dismal. In California, after open repair, patient mortality was 19% at 30 days and 31% at 1 year.[16] Nationwide, in-hospital mortality was found to be 22.3%. Higher mortality was seen when comparing low- versus high-volume hospitals (27.4% vs. 15.0%; $P < .001$) and low- versus high-volume surgeons (25.6% vs. 11.0%; $P < .001$).[17] Using NSQIP data from 2005 to 2010, Bensley and colleagues identified 450 patients (418 elective, 32 emergent) undergoing open surgical repair of TAA. Thirty-day mortality was better than the previous database studies at 10.0%. Complications included failure to wean from the ventilator (39.1%), pneumonia (23.1%), reintubation (13.8%), and acute renal failure requiring dialysis (10.7%). Multivariate analysis showed emergent repair, age over 70 years, preoperative dialysis, cardiac complication, and renal complications were predictive of mortality.[18]

There have been no randomized comparisons of open versus hybrid thoracoabdominal aneurysm repair. The Massachusetts General Hospital compared a contemporary cohort of open ($n = 77$) versus hybrid ($n = 23$) thoracoabdominal repairs. Of note, the hybrid patients were not open surgical candidates. Although not significant, the hybrid groups had a higher 30-day mortality

(17.4% vs. 7.8%; $P = .23$), in-hospital mortality (26.1% vs. 10.4%; $P = .27$), and reoperation rates (39.1% vs. 20.8%; $P = .03$). However paraplegia rates (hybrid, 4.3% vs. open, 3.9%; $P = .98$) and 1-year survival (hybrid, 68% vs. open, 73%) were similar for both groups.[19] Additional series of hybrid repairs are limited to small heterogeneous patient populations, with varying extents of type II and III thoracoabdominal aneurysms.

Thus far, the outcomes from hybrid thoracoabdominal and aortic arch aneurysm repair have not exceeded that of open surgery. It should be acknowledged that patients in hybrid case series are often high risk and do not qualify as candidates for open surgical repair. As experience and indications with the hybrid technique continue to grow, it may eventually prove to be an acceptable option for more than just high-risk patients.

Contraindications

An absolute contraindication to a hybrid aortic aneurysm repair is the lack of, or inability to create, a proximal and distal seal zone. Relative contraindications include the inability to safely perform debranching at the aortic arch and/or abdomen. The left carotid and left subclavian arteries require extraanatomic bypass for debranching. In hostile necks from previous surgery or radiation, exposure of the vessels and tunneling of grafts may not be feasible. The same applies in the abdomen. Exposure of the renal or visceral arteries may be difficult in a reoperative abdomen.

DEBRANCHING THE AORTIC ARCH

The surgical component of a hybrid repair to the aortic arch is used to create at least a 2-cm proximal seal zone for an endograft. A longer segment is preferred, particularly in an area of curvature or tortuosity. This is done to treat the proximal extent of thoracic or TAA or to treat isolated aortic arch aneurysms. The anatomy of the aneurysm will determine which vessels need to be addressed. A classification scheme separates the aortic arch into proximal seal zones and identifies which vessels will be affected (Fig. 38.2).[20] Zone 0 involves the origin of the innominate artery and a stent-graft landing here compromises blood flow to the left subclavian, left common carotid, and innominate arteries. Zone 1 involves the orifice of the left common carotid artery, and a stent-graft landing here compromises the left subclavian and left common carotid circulation. Zone 2 involves the origin of the left subclavian artery, and a stent-graft landing here affects only the left subclavian artery. Zones 3 and 4 are both distal to the left subclavian artery, within the descending thoracic aorta, leaving the arch vessels unaffected.

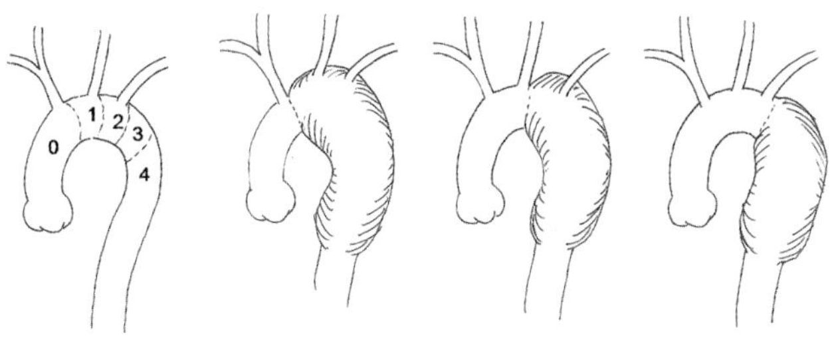

FIG 38.2 Thoracic landing zone diagram and aortic arch aneurysm configurations.

Left Subclavian Artery

Early in the endovascular treatment of thoracic aneurysms, coverage of the left subclavian artery (zone 2) was routinely done and appeared safe. It was assumed that a patent right vertebral artery would provide enough collateral circulation to both the basilar system and the left subclavian artery via retrograde flow from the left vertebral artery.[21,22] More recent data conflicts with this assumption. Meta-analysis suggests no neurological benefit from subclavian revascularization,[23] but in a registry from Europe, multivariate regression analysis found the risk of spinal cord ischemia to increase with left subclavian artery coverage.[24] Late development of subclavian steal and arm claudication was seen in 15% of patients in one series requiring further intervention.[25] We recommend revascularization of the left subclavian artery in all elective cases. In unstable patients, coverage of the left subclavian artery may be reasonable.

A left supraclavicular incision is used to perform either a left subclavian to carotid artery transposition or left common carotid to subclavian artery bypass. A left supraclavicular incision is made and platysmal flaps raised. The heads of the sternocleidomastoid are identified and the lateral head can be divided if needed. The internal jugular vein and common carotid artery are identified lateral to the sternocleidomastoid. The scalene fat pad is retracted laterally, taking care to ligate all lymphatic channels. The phrenic nerve and anterior scalene are identified. If needed, the anterior scalene can be divided for more lateral subclavian artery exposure. Exposure of the left subclavian artery proximal to the left vertebral artery will take the dissection into the mediastinum and the lymphatic duct will need to be ligated.

In a transposition, the subclavian artery is divided proximal to the left vertebral, the stump is ligated, and the subclavian artery sewn end to side onto the common carotid artery. In a bypass, the subclavian artery proximal to the left vertebral needs to be ligated surgically, or can be occluded by endovascular means to avoid a type II endoleak. Endovascular occlusion does not require the more proximal subclavian artery be exposed and can be performed with coils or an Amplatzer plug (ADA Medical Corporation, Plymouth, MN) deployed in a retrograde fashion though the distal anastomosis of the carotid–subclavian artery bypass or from a brachial approach (Fig. 38.3). This should be done after the aortic stent-graft is deployed to prevent developing thrombus on the Amplatzer plug from embolization while there is still antegrade flow through the subclavian artery. Alternatively, the patient can be maintained heparinized until the thoracic endograft covering the origin of the left subclavian artery is deployed.

In cases where a left internal mammary artery has been used for a coronary bypass graft, a transposition cannot be performed. In constructing the carotid–subclavian artery bypass, the subclavian anastomosis should be distal to the origin of the internal mammary artery, thereby maintaining native flow during sewing of the anastomosis. After the anastomosis and bypass are complete, the origin of the left subclavian artery is ligated and retrograde flow will fill the internal mammary artery.[26]

Partial Arch Debranching

Partial arch debranching involves revascularization of the left common carotid and left subclavian arteries using the right common carotid artery as inflow. This is in preparation for deploying an endograft just distal to the innominate artery origin (zone 1). This can be done with extraanatomic bypasses, without the need for a sternotomy or thoracotomy (Fig. 38.4).

The carotid bifurcation should be identified by ultrasound so that the incision is placed to expose the common carotid artery proximal and away from the bulb, thus avoiding the most common location of carotid plaque. The right common carotid artery is exposed anterior to the sternocleidomastoid muscle. The left common carotid can be exposed through a matching incision and exposure, or it can be exposed posterior to the sternocleidomastoid through the same incision used to expose the left subclavian artery.

A retropharyngeal tunnel is created between the two common carotid arteries staying just anterior to the anterior spinous ligament of the cervical spine. A bypass is performed with a 6-mm Dacron graft in an end side fashion. The tunnel is made with a gentle downward curve. Alternatively, the tunnel can be placed subcutaneously behind the manubrium for a better cosmetic result. Damage to this bypass can occur if a sternotomy is ever needed and patients should be so informed.[27]

The more proximal left common carotid artery is used to create the left subclavian artery transposition or bypass. The left common carotid artery is ligated proximally at the base of the neck.

Care is taken to avoid bilateral recurrent laryngeal or vagus nerve injury. The carotid arteries should be investigated preoperatively for stenosis. Intraoperative brain monitoring is usually not necessary when clamping is limited to the common carotid artery as external-to-internal carotid artery collaterals will maintain adequate flow to the affected internal system. Similarly, common carotid artery shunting has not been necessary.

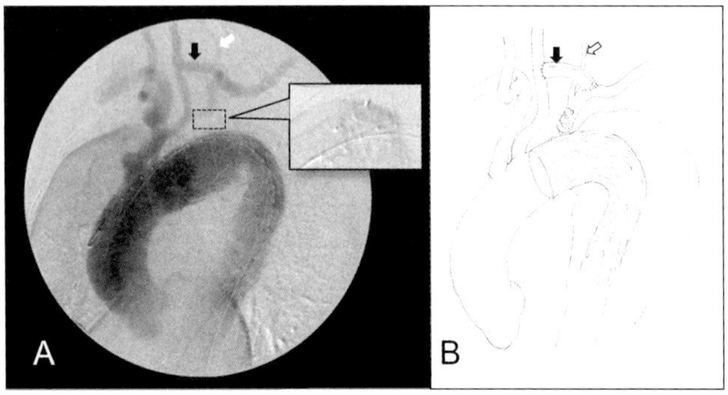

FIG 38.3 Left carotid–to–subclavian artery bypass. (A) Angiogram and (B) schematic of left carotid–to–subclavian artery bypass *(black arrow)* completed with Amplatzer plug placed at the left subclavian origin *(box)*. The left vertebral artery is preserved *(white arrow)*.

Complete Arch Debranching

Complete aortic arch debranching involves revascularization of the innominate, left carotid, and left subclavian arteries to create a landing zone in the ascending aorta proximal to the innominate artery (zone 0). This is done through a median sternotomy[28] and cardiopulmonary bypass is typically not necessary assuming the ascending aorta is not aneurysmal. A side biting clamp is placed on the ascending aorta and either a small bifurcated Dacron graft or preferably a larger tube graft (8 to 12 mm) with a side arm (6 to 8 mm) is fashioned to bypass the right innominate and left common carotid arteries, both in an end-to-end fashion (Figs. 38.5 and 38.6). The latter option is easier to configure than a bifurcated graft and avoids compression or kinking after sternotomy closure.

The left subclavian artery is extremely difficult to expose via a sternotomy and requires a separate left supraclavicular incision. This is best done prior to the sternotomy as a carotid-subclavian bypass or transposition. During innominate artery clamping,

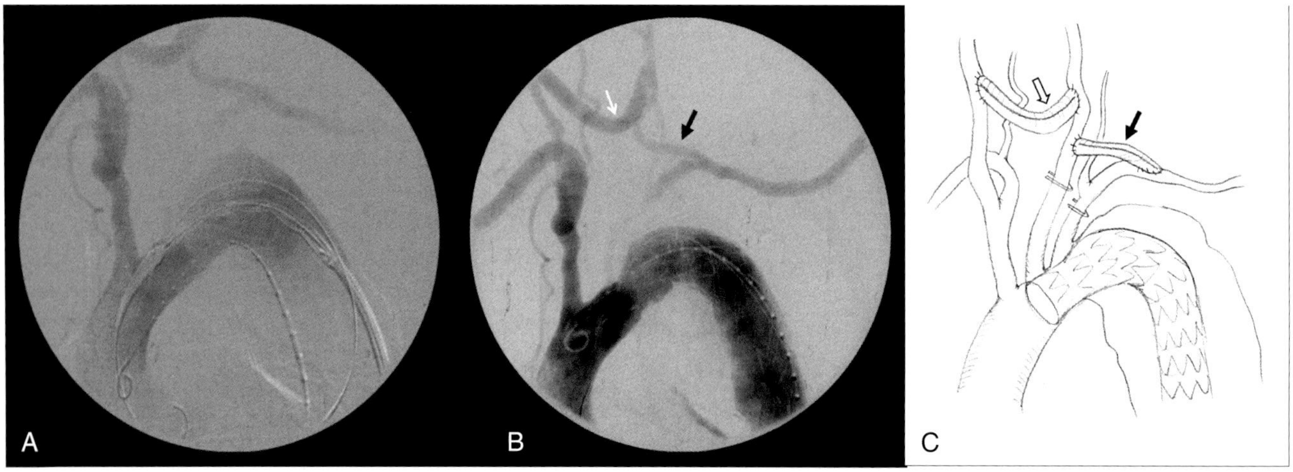

FIG 38.4 Partial arch debranching. Angiogram of the aortic arch (A) before and (B) after a stent-graft is deployed in zone 1 of the aortic arch. Partial arch debranching has been done with a right-to-left carotid artery bypass *(white arrow)* and left carotid–to–left subclavian artery bypass *(black arrow)*. (C) Schematic of the repair.

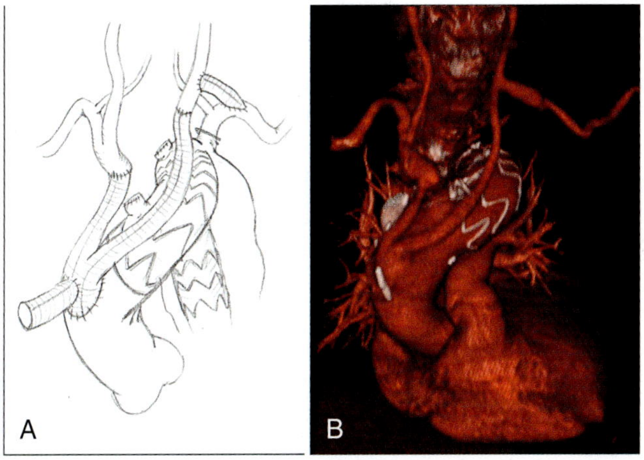

FIG 38.5 Complete arch debranching. (A) Schematic and (B) 3D reconstruction of a complete aortic arch debranching. The bypass graft originates off the ascending aorta to the right innominate and left carotid arteries. A left carotid–to–subclavian artery bypass can also be seen. In the schematic (A) there is a conduit off the ascending aortic graft.

the left subclavian artery will provide collateral flow through the vertebral-basilar pathway to the right subclavian and carotid systems. The origins of any bypassed vessel should be ligated or embolized to prevent a type II endoleak. Prior to sternotomy, patients should be screened for any cardiac pathology that should be addressed at the same intervention.

The tortuosity and distance from the femoral artery to the proximal aortic arch can make tracking an endovascular device difficult. Additionally, the endograft delivery system may not be long enough to reach the ascending aorta. The addition of a 10-mm Dacron graft onto the hood of the ascending aortic graft can serve as a conduit for antegrade deployment of the stent-graft (see Figs. 38.5 and 38.6).[29] Keep in mind that the device will be reversed in configuration. It is critical that the location of the conduit-to-graft anastomosis leads directly into the aorta. Tension at the heel of the ascending aortic graft anastomosis can develop during deployment due to the angle of entry of the deployment catheter. This risks a tear of the aorta and is to be avoided. Tunneling the conduit through an appropriately located stab wound can reduce this risk.[30]

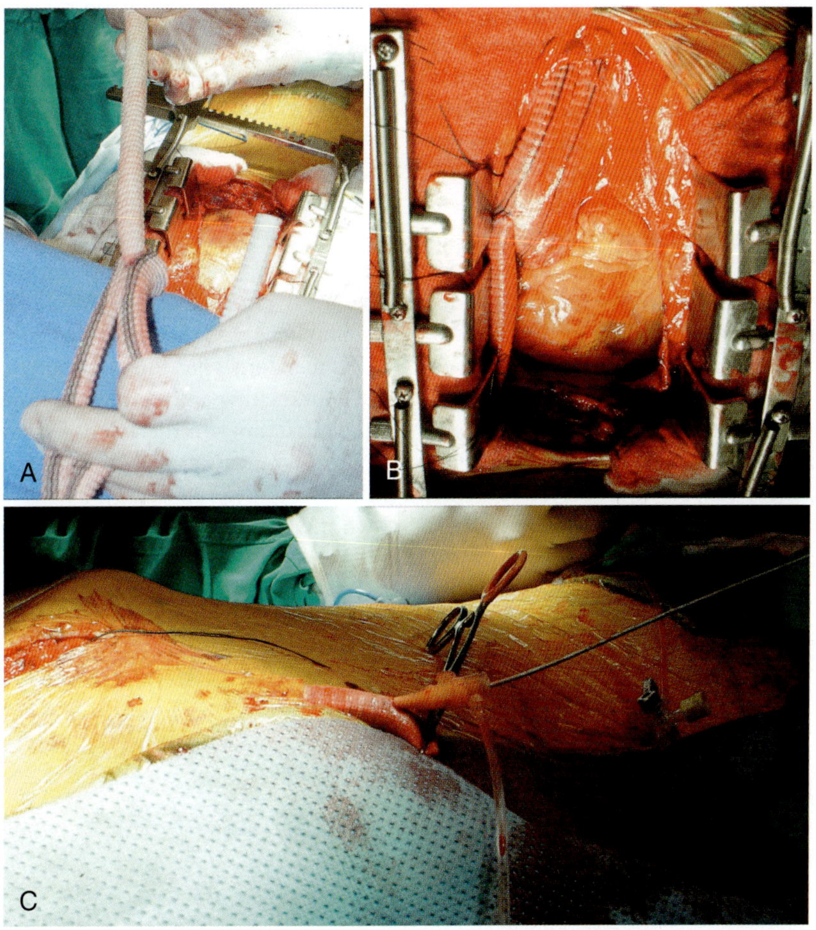

FIG 38.6 Operative images of a complete arch debranching. (A) Bifurcated Dacron graft with an additional limb sewn on as a conduit. (B) Bypass graft sewn onto the ascending aortic arch. (C) Conduit tunneled with a sheath in place for antegrade stent-graft deployment.

Ascending Aorta Replacement With Complete Arch Debranching

When aneurysms involve the aortic arch and ascending aorta there is no proximal landing zone for a stent-graft. To reconstruct these aneurysms, the ascending aorta can be replaced with a Dacron graft and the complete arch debranching done with a bypass taken off the ascending aortic graft to the innominate and left carotid arteries. There must be at least 2 cm of ascending aortic graft distal to the debranching graft to allow for endograft seal. This requires a sternotomy and cardiopulmonary bypass.[31]

There are variations of this technique including a frozen elephant trunk. Hypothermic cardiac arrest is required, hence the eponym "frozen." In these cases a modified Dacron graft with a stent attached distally is constrained in a sheath and deployed under fluoroscopy into a distal landing zone, usually the descending thoracic aorta. The proximal end of the modified Dacron graft is then sewn to the ascending aortic graft completing the reconstruction.[32-35]

Staging and Stent-Graft

Aortic arch debranching in combination with visceral debranching will be discussed later. Assuming the arch is debranched for aortic arch and/or thoracic aortic disease, then a single or two-stage approach is reasonable for partial arch debranching and/or left subclavian-carotid bypass or transposition. Both surgeries are extraanatomic operations, and can be done in a reasonable time with minimal surgical trauma making a single stage reasonable. If a single stage is chosen, the neck incisions should be left open until the endovascular portion is complete and there is no more heparinization.

Arterial access is through the common femoral artery (open or percutaneous). If a percutaneous arterial approach is chosen, two 6F Perclose ProGlide (Abbott Vascular, Redwood City, CA) devices are deployed prior to placement of the large sheath to allow for arteriotomy closure at the completion of the case.[36]

Given the large diameters of the thoracic aorta, the constrained diameters of endovascular grafts vary depending on the manufacturer and device, but in general the devices can be quite large. If the femoral or external iliac arteries are less than 8 mm and/or heavily calcified, the arteries can be injured. Additionally, tortuosity in the iliac system can create excess length and issues with pushability. To avoid these concerns, a conduit can be created. Through a retroperitoneal incision, the common iliac artery can be identified and a 10-mm Dacron graft is sewn in an end-to-side fashion. The 10-mm conduit is tunneled out of the skin at a smooth angle, and it can accommodate both the large endograft delivery sheath and the smaller (5F) sheath for the pigtail injection catheter (Fig. 38.7).

To track an endograft into the aortic arch via a retrograde approach, a stiff Lunderquist (Cook, Bloomington, IN) with a floppy "Q" tip is used. The tip of the wire can be positioned into the left ventricle or against the aortic valve to allow more wire support to help the device track. During deployment the wire is pushed to the outer curve of the aortic arch to minimize migration during deployment. We do not routinely use temporary rapid pacing or adenosine during deployment, but both can be an adjuvant to help precise delivery.[37] A "flossing" technique can also be used to help track devices by straightening tortuosity. This is done with a right brachial artery approach snaring the retrograde wire. Additionally, in cases of partial arch debranching, a right brachial access can allow for the pigtail to be placed in the innominate to serve as a marker for the proximal extent of the stent-graft.

Stent-grafts with uncovered struts allow for additional proximal aortic support, which can be helpful in the aortic arch curvature. Oversizing can also lead to bird beaking and should be avoided.[38] Additionally, landing within an acute angle within the arch is not recommended given the potential for poor apposition of the proximal graft to the inner curve of the aorta (bird beaking).[38] In these situations, debranching of additional arch vessels is recommended to extend the proximal landing beyond the acute angulation. With larger diameters in the ascending aorta and arch, care must be taken to assure the diameter of the aorta at the proximal landing zone can create a seal with the chosen stent-graft. Currently the largest US Food and Drug Administration (FDA)-approved thoracic stent-graft is 46 mm in diameter, which is appropriate to treat a 41- to 42-mm aorta.

As mentioned previously, in complete aortic arch debranching, the debranching and stent grafting should be done in one stage using a conduit on the ascending aorta bypass graft to deploy the endograft in an antegrade fashion. This avoids difficulties in tracking the graft from the femoral access, and length issues with the delivery system.

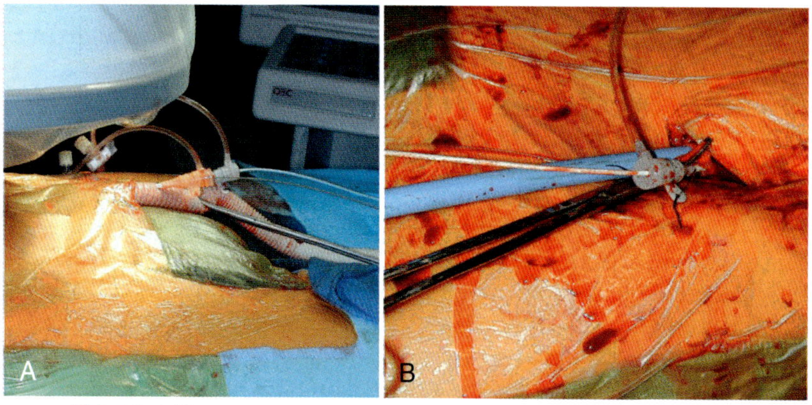

FIG 38.7 Iliac conduits used to accommodate multiple sheaths.

DEBRANCHING THORACOABDOMINAL ANEURYSMS

Given that the visceral vessels are in close proximity to one another, all four vessels (celiac, SMA, and bilateral renal arteries) will need to be bypassed in most hybrid thoracoabdominal aneurysm repairs. In pararenal aneurysms, debranching one or both renals may provide the needed seal zone for a hybrid repair.[39] In patients with preexisting renal failure, on hemodialysis, only the mesenteric arteries require debranching.

Origin of the Visceral Bypass Grafts

Case planning is the most critical step in debranching for TAA. At least 2 cm of healthy aorta or graft is required for endograft sealing distally. Selecting the optimal location of the visceral bypass origin will help determine how much distal seal is created. Additionally, the visceral bypass graft will provide all the flow to the viscera and must be based on a large-caliber vessel, ideally the aorta, common iliac artery, or an aortic or iliac graft. We prefer not to use the external iliac arteries given their small size and presence of atherosclerosis.

Occasionally patients will have had a prior aortic repair and this preexisting graft can serve as a takeoff for a retrograde visceral graft. If not, the anatomy of the aneurysm will dictate where a bypass graft can originate.

In a type I Crawford thoracoabdominal aneurysm, the native common iliac artery or infrarenal aorta is adequate for use as a graft origin. In a type II and III Crawford thoracoabdominal aneurysm, aneurysmal involvement of the infrarenal aorta and common iliac arteries makes this a more challenging hybrid repair. If the aneurysm is continuous throughout the aorta and iliacs, without a spared segment of nonaneurysmal aorta, a hybrid repair is not feasible and an open repair is the only option. Often there is a region of nonaneurysmal infrarenal aorta that can be clamped. In this case, an infrarenal replacement with a tube or bifurcated aortoiliac graft can be placed for a distal landing zone, and the debranching graft sewn onto the aortic graft (Fig. 38.8). The native aorta is reinforced with a strip of felt at the anastomosis given the aorta is not healthy (Fig. 38.9).

In a type IV thoracoabdominal aneurysm, open surgical repair is still preferred over a hybrid approach. Open repair can be accomplished via a retroperitoneal approach without a thoracotomy. Cross clamping of the supraceliac aorta is better tolerated than control at the proximal thoracic aorta. If a hybrid repair is undertaken, a debranching graft can originate from the descending thoracic aorta, infrarenal aorta, or common iliac artery.

Abdominal Debranching Techniques

A four-vessel visceral debranching is a lengthy operation. General endotracheal anesthesia, a line, central venous access, and a Foley catheter are all needed. Patients are placed supine and a midline transabdominal incision is preferred. A retroperitoneal approach can be used, but access to the right renal artery can be difficult (Fig. 38.10).

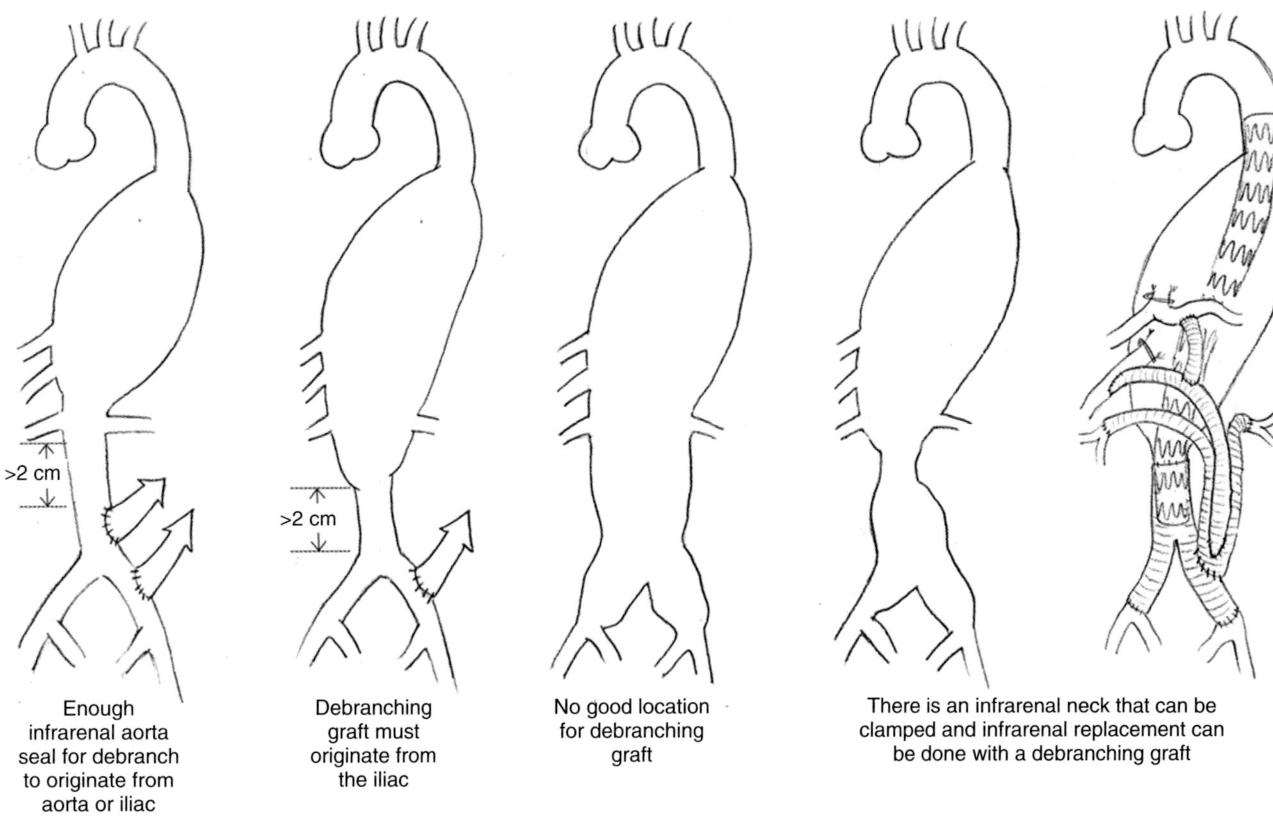

FIG 38.8 Diagrams demonstrating possible locations for the debranching bypass graft.

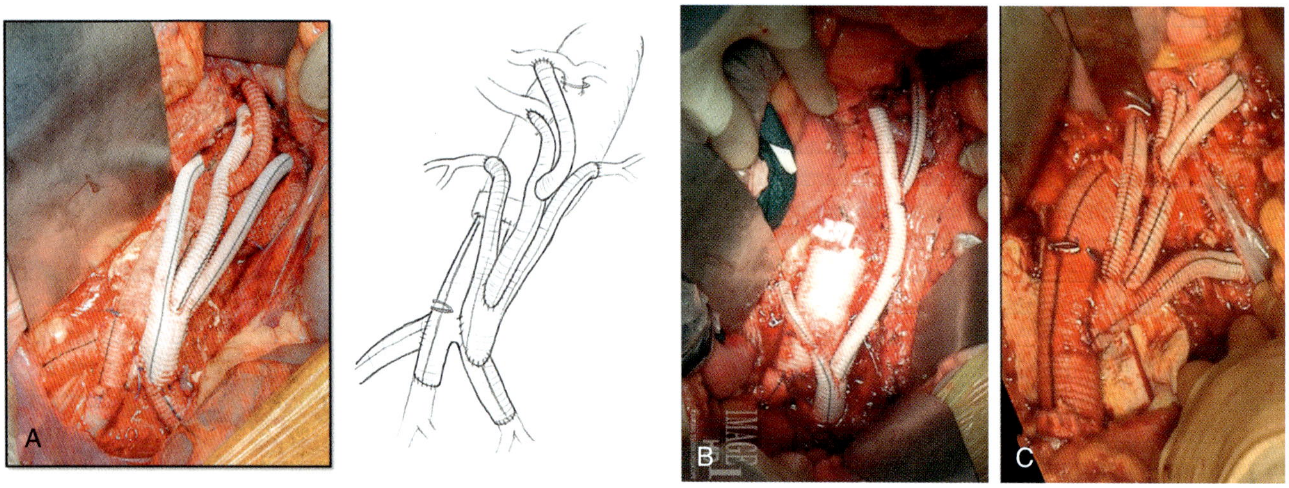

FIG 38.9 Completed four-vessel debranching with replacement of the infrarenal aorta. Note the felt strip used to reinforce the aortic anastomosis and marker clips above the debranching graft. If an aortoiliac graft is used, the debranch can be based off an iliac limb of the graft (A and B). If a tube graft is used, the debranch can come directly off the tube graft (C). In all cases, there must be at least 2 cm of aortic graft above the debranching for a distal endograft seal. In image (A) there is a conduit originating from the right iliac limb.

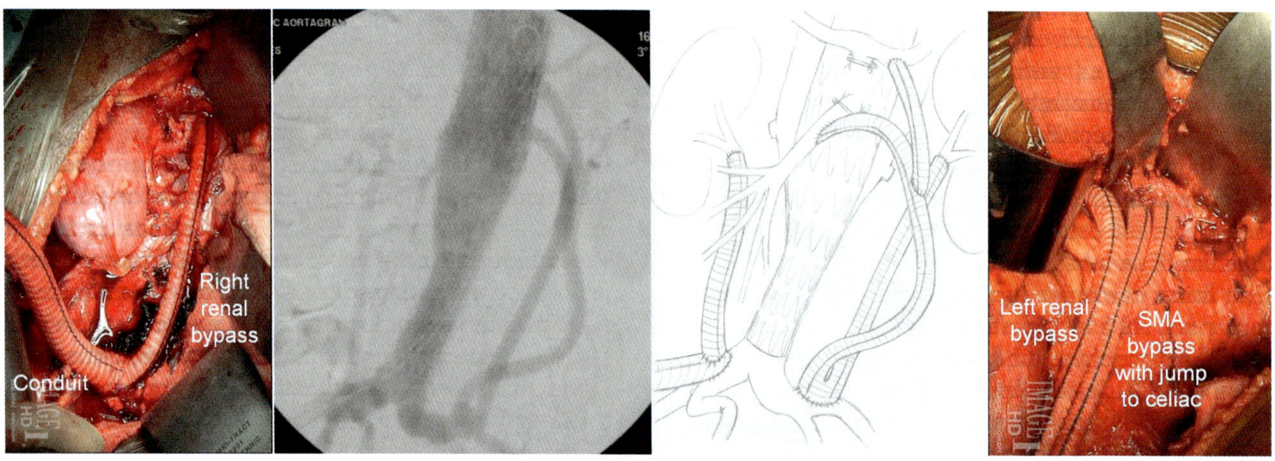

FIG 38.10 Patient with a hostile abdomen from previous surgery and chronic obstructive pulmonary disease. A staged repair was performed to avoid a midline laparotomy. A left retroperitoneal approach was used to debranch the superior mesenteric artery *(SMA)*, celiac, and left renal arteries off the left common iliac artery. In a second stage, a right retroperitoneal approach was used to place a conduit and right renal artery bypass from the right common iliac artery. A stent-graft was then deployed through the conduit sealing in the native aorta above the iliac bifurcation. Center images show the completion and schematic of the final repair.

Exposure of the Visceral Vessels

After entering the abdomen, the transverse colon is elevated, and the intestines are placed in a bag and retracted to the right. The peritoneum overlying the retroperitoneum is incised and the ligament of Trietz is mobilized medially. The aorta or iliac vessels serving as the debranching origin are isolated.

To expose the left renal artery, the left renal vein is identified and mobilized by ligation of the inferior mesenteric, gonadal, and adrenal veins. This allows access to the proximal left renal artery. If the proximal renal artery is heavily diseased, the bypass can go to the distal renal artery. On the left it is exposed by mobilizing the descending colon and rotating it medially. The bypass graft is tunneled through the mesentery of the descending colon for distal left renal artery bypass, otherwise no tunneling is needed to bypass the proximal left renal artery.

The proximal right renal artery is identified posterior to the confluence of the left renal vein and vena cava. A thin retractor on the veins can help expose the vessel. The distal right renal artery can be accessed by medial mobilization of the right colon, takedown of the hepatorenal ligament, and kocherization of the duodenum. The retrograde bypass graft is tunneled through the mesentery of the right colon anterior to the vena cava for more distal right renal artery revascularization.

Preoperative planning should identify if a proximal or distal renal anastomosis will be performed. If multiple renal arteries are present, they can be individually bypassed if large enough. In cases where the renal artery bifurcates very quickly, the branches can be controlled and sewn together to create a common orifice, which is then anastomosed to the bypass graft end to end. This can also be done to multiple renal arteries if they are close to each other and the anatomy allows.

The SMA is exposed with the third and fourth portions of the duodenum mobilized to the right. The base of the mesentery is identified and the SMA can be found inferior to the pancreas and superior to the left renal artery. Exposure of the vessel requires dissection of the surrounding fat with lymphatics and nerves that need to be divided and ligated.

The celiac artery is exposed by entering the lesser sac through the gastrohepatic ligament. A nasogastric tube will decompress the stomach and help identify the esophagogastric junction. Following the hepatic or the splenic artery, the bifurcation of the celiac artery is identified. To gain access to the main celiac branch, the dense celiac plexus is divided, and the coronary vein ligated. If more exposure is needed, the left gastric artery can also be ligated.

Constructing the Bypass

There are commercially available debranching grafts of Dacron or polytetrafluoroethylene (PTFE) with at least four limbs for a four-vessel debranch. We prefer to use a trifurcated graft (12 × 6,7,6) or create our own using a bifurcated Dacron aortobifemoral bypass (limbs are matched to the renal diameter, usually a 12- to 6-mm graft) with a third 8-mm Dacron tube graft sewn end to side on the main body of the graft. The two limbs are used to bypass the right and left renal arteries; the third limb is used for the SMA in an end-to-side fashion. A jump graft is then taken off the SMA graft to bypass the celiac artery.

The body of the graft is sewn to the aorta, common iliac artery, preexisting infrarenal graft, or in special cases the entire infrarenal is replaced as mentioned previously. Each visceral bypass is then constructed individually. The bypass will lie on top of the aorta. The anatomy will often dictate the location from which the bypass originates, but using the left iliac artery or the proximal left limb of an aortoiliac graft allows the best lay of the grafts.

The renal anastomoses are done end to end. There is usually not enough exposure for an end-to-side anastomosis. The stumps of the renal artery must be secured well with suture ligation. The bypass grafts should be pulled and trimmed to length. Too much redundancy in the grafts will lead to kinking.

The bypass to the SMA is placed in a lazy C configuration to prevent it from kinking. The anastomosis is done in an end-to-side fashion and the proximal SMA is ligated but not divided to keep the graft from kinking and to prevent a type II endoleak.

A jump graft is sewn to the apex of the SMA bypass and tunneled retropancreatic or through the transverse colon. We prefer the retropancreatic tunnel to shorten the graft and to minimize graft contact with the intestines. The graft is then anastomosed in an end-to-side manner to the hepatic or splenic artery. An anastomosis can be performed at the celiac bifurcation, but exposure is difficult and leaves little room for ligation of the main celiac artery, which is always done to prevent a type II endoleak. Clips can be used for ligation, but given the potential of clip dislodgement we add a silk ligature.[40]

To minimize contrast during stent graft placement, the origin of the retrograde bypass graft is marked. We prefer to use two partially closed clips that are sewn to the native aorta or aortic graft just proximal to the takeoff of the bypass graft, creating "a pair of eyes." This is easily seen under fluoroscopy and identifies the lowest point where the stent-graft can land to prevent covering the visceral bypass graft (Fig. 38.11).

Staging and Stent-Graft

Debranching the visceral vessels in a hybrid thoracoabdominal aneurysm repair can be a long operation, with periods of warm ischemia to the kidney and viscera during anastomosis. Before a contrast load, a compromised kidney may need time to recover. For these reasons, staging the procedures is preferred. The second endovascular stage should be performed as soon as the patient has recovered, preferably during the same admission.[28] Interval aneurysm rupture has been noted when patients are discharged from the hospital after debranching, awaiting stent-graft placement.[41,42]

Arterial access for the stent-graft can be from the common femoral artery, open or percutaneous. If the debranching bypass is off an iliac artery or graft, then the access should be contralateral to avoid limiting the flow through the debranching bypass while the sheaths are in place.

If the common femoral or iliac vessels are diseased, a conduit can easily be constructed beforehand during the visceral debranching. The conduit can be sewn to a contralateral common iliac artery, directly to the debranch graft, or in the case of infrarenal replacement, to the graft itself. A 10-mm Dacron tube is tunneled out of the skin, marked with clips, and then rolled up and left in the subcutaneous tissue. At the second stage, fluoroscopy can be used to identify the clips, and a small cutdown is made to expose the conduit. A thrombectomy is then done to clear the conduit for use (see Fig. 38.11). After the endovascular procedure is complete, the conduit is ligated as proximal as possible and buried in the subcutaneous tissue. It is important to maintain sterility when handling the conduit because any infection of the conduit can infect adjacent bypass grafts.

In the abdominal aorta, a stiff Amplatzer wire (Cook) can straighten tortuosity and facilitate device tracking. Ideally, stent-grafts are placed in a distal-to-proximal fashion. To minimize the amount of contrast used, the first device is deployed without contrast. The distal-most extent of the landing zone is identified by the "pair of eyes" previously placed just above the origin of the debranching graft. Without additional angiograms, the devices are deployed with the appropriate manufacturer required overlap, until the proximal landing zone is reached. The first aortogram is then performed with a power injector and the final device deployed (see Fig. 38.11).

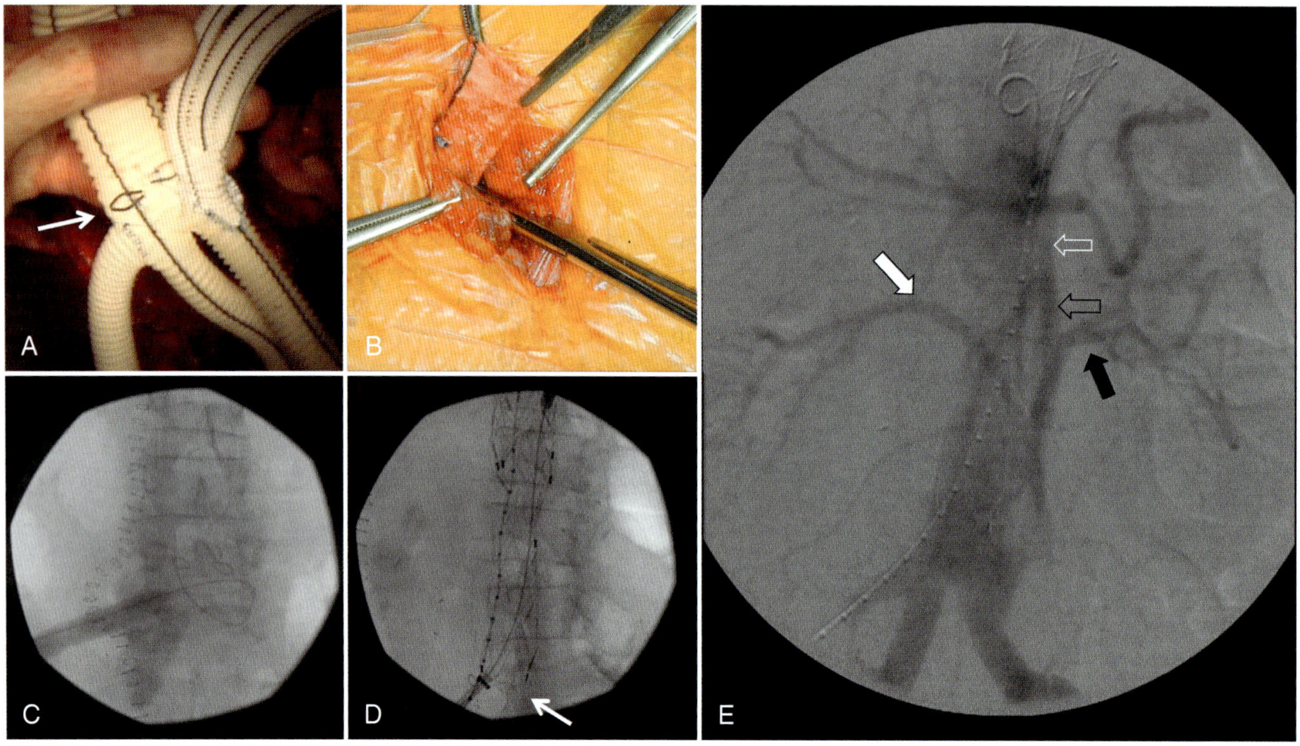

FIG 38.11 Deployment of a stent-graft through a conduit. (A) Infrarenal aortic graft with a conduit on the right iliac limb, and debranching on the left iliac limb. Note the partially closed clips sewn onto an aortobifemoral graft creating a "pair of eyes" *(arrow)*, indicating the lowest point at which the stent-graft can be landed to prevent covering the bypass graft. (B) Conduit identified in the subcutaneous tissue. (C) Angiogram of a conduit verifying clearance of the thrombus. (D) Stent-graft deployed through the conduit using the "pair of eyes" to identify the distal landing zone. (E) Completion angiogram with a pigtail placed through the conduit. Debranching graft seen with branches to the right kidney *(closed white arrow)*, left kidney *(closed black arrow)*, superior mesenteric artery *(open black arrow)*, and jump graft to the celiac artery *(open white arrow)*.

A completion angiogram is performed to identify endoleaks. A type I endoleak is treated with balloon inflation or additional stent-grafts if there is more aorta to cover. With proper planning and technique, bird beaking or inadequate seals should not be encountered, but if present, a Palmaz Stent (Johnson and Johnson, Warren, NJ) can help compensate as a last resort.[38] A type III endoleak can be treated with an interposition stent-graft component, and a type II endoleak is monitored at follow-up.

SPECIAL CONSIDERATIONS

Aortic Dissections

Aortic degeneration from dissections is a common cause of aortic aneurysms.

Repairs can be complicated, and are often staged to reduce the risk of paraplegia given the extent of aortic involvement. In most cases the thoracic aorta will dilate. Arch debranching and thoracic stent grafting is usually done in the true lumen just proximal to the celiac artery. Given the chronic nature of the dissections, the true lumen can be small and a stent-graft with good radial force should be used. In the thoracic aorta, the use of transesophageal echocardiogram can help identify which lumen the wires traverse. In the abdomen, endovascular ultrasound can be used (Fig. 38.12).

Often there is still flow in the false lumen of the chest from fenestrations below the graft causing a type IB endoleak. If the false lumen continues to expand and there is aneurysm growth, a visceral debranching can complete the repair and exclude the false lumen.

The origin of the debranch can be complicated if the dissection involves the infrarenal aorta and iliac arteries. There will be no healthy artery for the stent-graft to seal. In these cases a distal seal zone can be created by replacing the infrarenal aorta with a graft that can be used for the visceral debranch as well.

In a chronic aneurysmal dissection, the true lumen is often compressed and full expansion of a stent-graft can be limited. In patients who have had open interposition grafts in the proximal descending thoracic aorta as the initial treatment for their dissection, and the distal landing is in a normal nondissected segment of aorta or a surgically placed infrarenal graft, the false lumen can be used for placement of the endovascular graft. In this false lumen intentional placement (FLIP) technique, we cross from the true lumen (or graft) through the false lumen, then back into the true lumen (or graft). The false lumen is typically

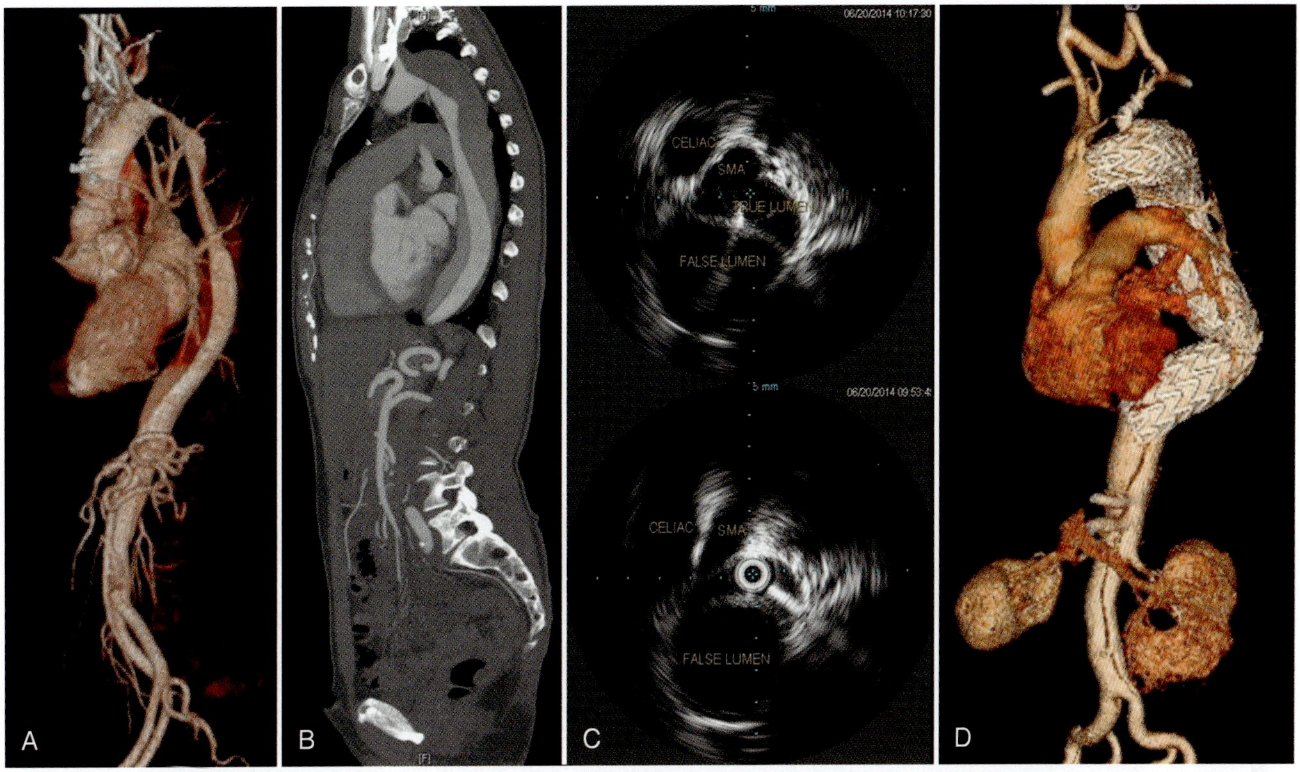

FIG 38.12 Partial arch debranching and endograft repair of a thoracic aneurysm after type B aortic dissection. (A) Preoperative 3D reconstruction and (B) maximum-intensity projection reconstruction. (C) Intravascular ultrasound used to navigate into the true lumen. (D) Completion of the repair with partial arch debranching for proximal seal zone. *SMA*, Superior mesenteric artery.

larger than the true lumen and allows the stent-graft to fully deploy (Fig. 38.13).

Combined Aortic Arch and Thoracoabdominal Aneurysm

In thoracoabdominal aneurysms that involve the aortic arch there are a number of ways to stage the procedure. To minimize the number of surgeries, the first stage would be abdominal debranching, followed by the second stage, which would include arch debranching and stent-graft deployment at the same time. Alternatively, a three-stage approach with arch debranching, then visceral debranching, then stent grafting can be considered (see Fig. 38.1).

Contained and Symptomatic Aneurysms

In a contained rupture or symptomatic aneurysm the debranching and stent grafting need to be completed in one stage. For a contained rupture in the thoracic aorta or arch, the debranchings are all extraanatomical and can be done without disturbing the aortic hematoma. In a thoracoabdominal aneurysm, assuming the hematoma is contained in the retroperitoneum, a debranching is still feasible. Dissection and bypass to the renals, SMA, and hepatic artery can be carried out distally away from the aorta and hematoma. After the stent-graft is placed, identification of the proximal SMA and main celiac trunk can then be done to ligate the origins and prevent the type II endoleak.

SPINAL PROTECTION

In open thoracoabdominal aneurysm repair, the use of spinal drainage has been shown to reduce postoperative paraplegia and paraparesis in a randomized trial (13.0% vs. 2.6%; $P = .03$).[43] Although the mechanism of paralysis and paraplegia in open and endovascular repair may differ,[44] use of spinal drainage has been shown to be beneficial and even to reverse cases of postoperative paraplegia in endovascular aortic repairs.[45]

Spinal drainage is recommend when there has been previous aortic surgery, a large coverage of aorta is planned, and/or collateral circulation from the internal iliac and subclavian arteries is compromised.[24,45] When the repair is limited to the aortic arch and proximal descending aorta, spinal drainage is not necessary.

Spinal catheters are placed a day prior to the endovascular portion to avoid delaying the case because of a bloody tap. If this happens, overnight observation usually resolves the issue, thus allowing safe heparinization. During the procedure and in the postoperative period, spinal catheters are allowed to drain continuously at 10 cm of water. To maximize the spinal perfusion pressure, the mean arterial pressure is maintained above 80 mm Hg using a phenylephrine drip if needed. After 48 to 72 hours, if the patient is hemodynamically stable and neurologically intact, the pressure of spinal drainage is increased to 20 cm of water for 6 hours, and then closed to assure no neurological changes prior to removal.[44,45]

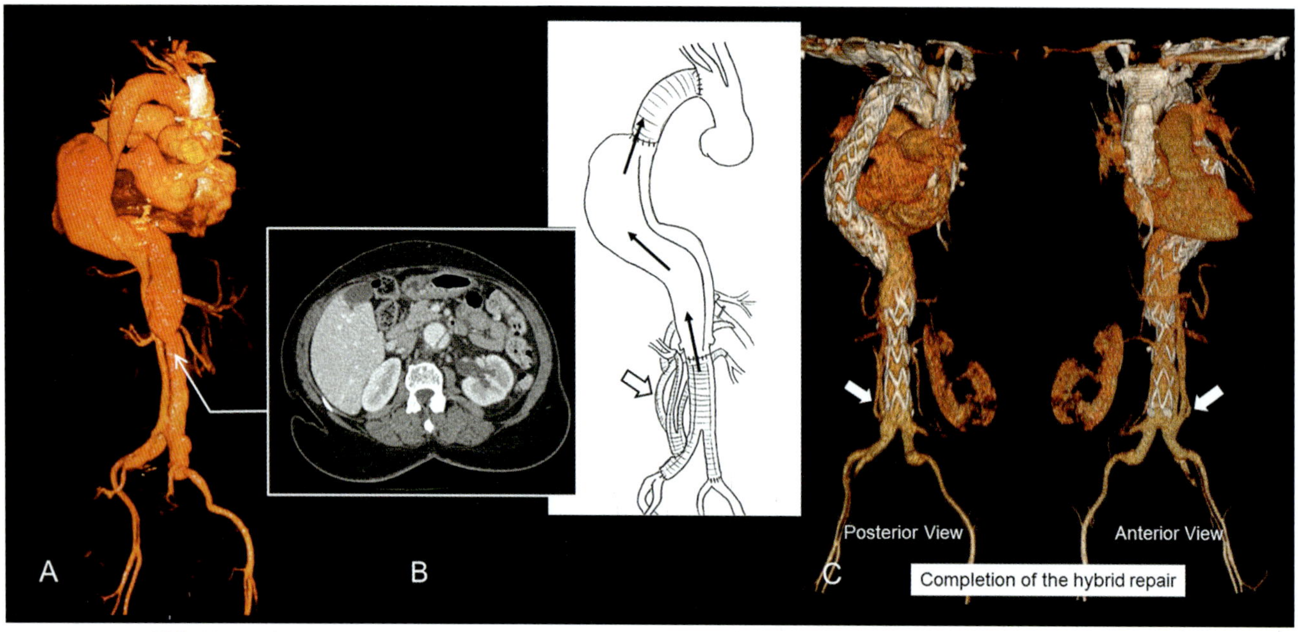

FIG 38.13 Aneurysmal degeneration of a type B dissection distal to a previous open descending thoracic aortic repair. (A) Preoperative 3D reconstruction showing that the dissected infrarenal aorta is suitable for clamping and replacement. (B) The schematic shows the previous open thoracic repair, and the infrarenal aorta replacement with four-vessel debranching *(open white arrow)*. A false lumen intentional placement can be done by placing the stent-graft in the false lumen *(arrow path)* to allow for full stent-graft expansion. (C) 3D reconstructions of the repair.

If the patient develops postoperative paraplegia, the spinal drain is assessed and replaced if malfunctioning. A magnetic resonance imaging (MRI) scan of the spine can be obtained to rule out reversible causes of paraplegia such as a spinal cord hematoma. The drainage pressure of the spinal drain can also be decreased to drain more spinal fluid to improve spinal perfusion. This must be weighed against the risk of draining too much spinal fluid and tearing the bridging veins with subsequent subdural hematoma. Blood in the spinal drain may come from the initial placement of the drain, but persistent blood is concerning for subdural hematoma and should be evaluated.

POSTOPERATIVE MANAGEMENT

After a visceral debranching, patients are given nothing by mouth until bowel function returns. Postoperatively, third spacing will occur given the laparotomy and lengthy operation. Proper fluid resuscitation with monitoring of urine output is important. Pancreatitis can occur from pancreas manipulation during graft tunneling. Death from pancreatitis has been reported and amylase and lipase should be monitored postoperatively.[46,47]

In various case series (Table 38.1) graft occlusions ranged from 0% to 14%. Although grafts can be occluded without clinical significance,[47] bowel ischemia and death,[46,48,49] as well as permanent renal failure requiring dialysis have been reported.[41] Renal graft patency is monitored with urine output and laboratories. Worsening renal function should be promptly evaluated with duplex ultrasound or computed tomography (CT) scan to check for patency. Celiac and SMA grafts are monitored clinically and by laboratories. If there is bowel ischemia the patient will become septic and imaging should be urgently performed. In cases of patent bypass grafts, embolic events during the bypass creation, or during wire and catheter manipulation can lead to bowel necrosis. If there is suspicion of bowel ischemia, laparotomy should be performed emergently.[49]

Management of an occluded bypass graft will depend largely on the patient's overall clinical condition. If patients are asymptomatic from the graft occlusion, then reintervention may not be warranted. With worsening renal failure or persistent sepsis, a decision to revise a graft should be considered.

In the aortic arch, transient ischemia attacks or permanent strokes can result from graft failures. Intervening for an occluded graft that has caused a significant stroke can worsen the patient's overall condition. Transient ischemia attacks should be promptly investigated with imaging of the grafts and revision if problems are identified. Embolic events from wire and catheter manipulation in the arch will present immediately after surgery and management is often supportive.

With any endovascular aneurysm repair, serial imaging is required to assure the aneurysm sac is decreasing in diameter and there are no endoleaks or problems with the stent-grafts. A CT scan is ordered in the first few weeks after surgery, then at 6 months, then every year if no issues are identified. If there is renal insufficiency, a magnetic resonance angiogram can be done using minimal gadolinium.

Type II leaks can be monitored if there is no aneurysm sac expansion, but type I and III endoleaks need to be addressed.

TABLE 38.1 Summary of Case Series (>10 Patients) on the Hybrid Repair of Thoracoabdominal Aortic Aneurysms

Primary Author	Year	Institute	Number of Patients	High Risk for Open Repair (%)	CRAWFORD CLASSIFICATION I	II	III	IV	V	Other	Emergent Cases (%)	30-Day Mortality	Paraplegia (%)	Morbidity (%)	Follow-Up (Months)	Overall Survival	Graft Occlusion (%) Based on Number of Bypass Created	Late Reintervention (%)
Fulton[39]	2005	UNC	10	80	—	—	—	4	3	Juxta -5	0	0%	0	60	Mean 8.7	100%	0/13 (0)	10
Resch[62]	2006	Cleveland Clinic	13	100	—	5	2	1	—	Dsxn-5	15	23%	9	NA	Mean 23	62%	NA	31
Black[40]	2006	St Marys- London, UK	29	80	3	18	7	1	—	3 Debranching aborted	10	24%	0	62[a]	Median 8	NA	2/94 (2%)	17
Zhou[63]	2006	Baylor	31	100	3	3	8	7	—	10 Arch aneurysms	NA	3%	0	19	Mean 16	90%	2/31 (6.4%)[b]	0
Lee[42]	2007	University of Florida	17	82	—	2	8	7	—	—	0	24%	0	24	Mean 8	NA	2/56 (3.5%)	6
Böckler[41]	2008	University of Heidelberg, Germany	28	96	2	8	4	1	—	Dsxn-7 Patch-1 Plaque-1 Missing-4?	22	14%	14	59	Mean 22	3 years, 70%	4/28 (14%)[b]	7
van de Mortel[48]	2008	Netherlands	16	50	1	1	1	4	6	Juxta-3	6	31%	0	56	Men 13	69%	7/58 (13%)	0
Patel[19]	2009	Mass General Hospital	23	100	9	5	9	—	—	—	9	23% in-hospital deaths	4	65	Mean 5.5	1 year, 68% 2 years, 34%	7/70 (10%)	17
Quinones[64]	2009	UCLA	20	100	—	3	8	4	1	Pararenal-1 Arch -3	0	0%	5	30	Mean 16.6	75%	0/20 (0%)[b]	5
Donas[65]	2009	Zurich Hosp, Switzerland	58	100	3	5	9	13	—	Pararenal-28 VORTEC used for debranching anastomosis	0	9%	3	NA	Mean 22.1	74%	3/113 (3%)	7
Drinkwater[66]	2009	Combined Series from Bockler, Wolfe, and Black	107	NA	1	45	32	1	1	Complex-17	0	15%	8	38[a]	NA	NA	14/107 (13%)	NA
Biasi[70]	2009	St George's Hosp, London, UK	18	NA	2	8	7	—	1	—	11	17%	6	17	Median 23	72%	1/54 (2%)	6
Wolf[47]	2010	Munich, Germany	20	75	1	11	7	—	1	—	10	10%	10	45	Median 5.8	75%	4/70 (5.7%)	10
Muehling[49]	2010	University of Ulm, Germany	16	100	3	3	1	9	—	—	38	31%	6	44	Median 12	81%	2/31 (6.5%)	13
Kabbani[71]	2010	University of Michigan	36	NA	1	10	12	10	—	Pararenal- 3	8	8%	0	47	Mean 6	6 months, 80%	9/123 (7%)	6
Ham[60]	2011	USC	24	100	—	3	—	12	—	Pararenal- 9	NA	4%	4	39	Mean 13.3	1 year, 84% 3 years, 54%	3/77 (3.9%)	NA
Hughes[67]	2012	Duke University	58	100	3	21	34	—	—	—	17	9%	4	19[a]	Mean 26	1 year, 78% 5 years, 62%	10/214 (4.7%)	3
Tshomba[68]	2012	Milan, Italy	52	100	20	6	10	6	—	10 Visceral patch aneurysms	2	14%	2	29	Median 24	63%[a]	11/151 (7.3%)	4[a]

[a]Calculated from available data in manuscript.
[b]Calculated per patient rather than per visceral bypass graft.

In case series, up to 17% of patients may require secondary interventions.[19,40]

RESULTS

Aortic Arch Debranching

Case series of hybrid aortic arch aneurysm repair are difficult to interpret given the heterogeneous patient populations and a lack of standardized reporting from individual studies. Table 38.2 summarizes the outcomes from series with more than 10 patients, focusing on aortic repairs with the proximal landing in zone 0 or zone 1. Patients with descending thoracic aorta aneurysms requiring coverage of the left subclavian artery (zone 2) are not the topic of this discussion. A benefit of the hybrid aortic arch repair is the lack of cardiopulmonary bypass, but in a number of series the ascending aorta was replaced in combination with complete arch debranching, thus requiring cardiopulmonary bypass. This further complicates analysis of outcomes and comparisons.

In one of the earliest case series by Saleh and colleagues from Egypt, 15 high-risk patients had complete arch debranching with zone 0 proximal landing. No cardiopulmonary bypass was utilized. Success was 100%, with no mortality, paraplegia, or stroke.[50]

These excellent results were not seen in another similar cohort of 26 patients in the series by Weigang and colleagues from the University of Mainz in Germany. All patients were high risk and had complete arch debranching without cardiopulmonary bypass. Their 30-day mortality was one of the highest of all case series at 15%. All deaths were from adverse cardiovascular events. There were no episodes of paraplegia or stroke.[30]

In two other series, all patients had complete arch debranching, but cardiopulmonary bypass was used in a subset of cases. The series by Bavaria and colleagues from the University of Pennsylvania included 27 patients, of which four were treated with a frozen elephant trunk. These four required cardiopulmonary bypass, as well as an additional 15 patients where a side-biting clamp could not be applied given the limited amount of aorta that existed between the sinotubular junction and the ascending aorta. Mortality was 11%, stroke 11%, and paraplegia 7%.[51] In a more recent series from the University of Pennsylvania, all of the 36 patients were treated with zone 0 landing. Fifty-six percent of the patients required cardiopulmonary bypass and ascending aorta replacement. Even these patients had reasonable outcomes: mortality (8%), stroke (8%), paraplegia (6%).[31]

Lee and colleagues compared patients who underwent open versus hybrid repairs. In the hybrid group of 37 patients, the 30-day mortality was 16%, stroke 11%, and paraplegia 0%. One-year survival was 72%. This series had one of the highest mortality rates, but 68% of the patients required cardiopulmonary bypass and 46% required an ascending aortic replacement. The indications for ascending aorta replacement were diameters greater than 36 mm, which would not have sealed a stent-graft.[7]

From Duke University, Hughes and colleagues published a series of 28 patients, 43% of whom required cardiopulmonary bypass at the time of hybrid repair. This included seven patients who had a modified frozen elephant trunk aortic reconstruction, four who required a concomitant cardiac procedure, and one with a pulmonary artery injury that required cardiopulmonary bypass to repair. Despite these challenging patients 30-day in-hospital rates of death, stroke, and permanent paraplegia/paresis were 0%, 0%, and 4%, respectively. Morbidity was limited to 21% and 3-year survival was 70%.[52]

Series that have treated patients emergently have had varying outcomes. In the series by Schumacher and colleagues from Heidelberg, Germany, 25 high-risk patients were reviewed. Nine patients had complete arch debranching, and 16 had partial debranching. The 30-day mortality and morbidity were quite high at 20% and 63%, respectively, but 32% of the patients were treated emergently for contained ruptures.[53] Another series from the University of Hong Kong treated 31% of the patients emergently. Sixteen patients (five complete debranching, eight partial debranching with carotid-carotid artery bypass, and three with carotid-to–left subclavian artery bypass) were identified. One patient also required cardiopulmonary bypass (6%), but in contrast to the previous series, there was no 30-day mortality. Of note, the morbidity was quite high at 67%, with 19% having strokes.[54]

Holt and colleagues also had a series with 26 patients. Complete debranching was done in 9 patients, and partial debranching was done in 17 patients. Mortality was 6%, stroke and paraplegia were 0% and 6%, respectively. They also treated 15% emergently, and none required cardiopulmonary bypass.[55] The series from St. Thomas Hospital in London, United Kingdom, also had a large emergent proportion (20%) with mortality at 10%.[57]

The remaining series were all elective operations without cardiopulmonary bypass use. These series include a combination of proximal landing in zone 0 or zone 1. From the University of Vienna, Austria, Gottardi and colleagues had one of the largest case series of 73 patients, but 24 (33%) had landing in zone 2, and 31 (42%) patients had other nonaneurysmal pathologies including acute dissections. The results of these patients were all combined, and in the entire cohort the 30-day mortality was 7% and stroke was 1%.[54]

A subgroup of patients in the series from Gottardi and colleagues was previously published by Czerny and colleagues 1 year earlier. There were 27 patients, with no zone 2 proximal landing. Ten had complete arch debranching and 17 had partial arch debranching. In-hospital mortality was 7% and there was no stroke or paralysis. One-year survival was 83% and 3-year survival was 72%.[58]

Bergeron and colleagues reported on 25 patients with a 30-day mortality of 8%, stroke 8%, and no paraplegia.[28] Over 10 years, Chiesa and colleagues at the Vita-Salute University in Milan, Italy, identified 52 patients with proximal zone 2 coverage and 51 patients with complete or partial arch debranching. Of the latter 51 patients, 24 required complete arch debranching (proximal zone 0), and 27 partial arch debranching (proximal zone 1). In these 51 patients, mortality, stroke, and paraplegia were 6%, 6%, and 0%, respectively. Thirty-day mortality in patients with complete and partial debranching were 13% and 0%, respectively.[59]

A single institution report from the University of Southern California reported the outcomes of both hybrid thoracoabdominal and aortic arch repairs. The subset of data from the

TABLE 38.2 Summary of Case Series (>10 Patients) on the Hybrid Approach to the Aortic Arch

Primary Author	Year	Institute	Number of Patients	High Risk for Open Repair (%)	Emergent Cases (%)	CPB/ Circulatory Arrest (%)	PROXIMAL LANDING ZONE: Zone 0	Zone 1	Zone 2	Mortality (%)	Morbidity (%)	Stroke (%)	Paraplegia (%)	Mean Follow-Up (months)	Overall Survival
Saleh[50]	2006	Ain Shams University, Cairo, Egypt	15	100	NA	0	15	0	0	0	26	0	0	18	93%
Bergeron[28]	2006	St Joseph Hosp, Marseille, France	25	100	NA	0	15	10	0	8	12	8	0	15	88%
Schumacher[53]	2006	Heidelberg, Germany	25	100	32	0	9	16	0	20	64	4	0	21	76%
Chan[54]	2008	University of Hong Kong	16	NA	31	6	5	8	3	0	67	19	0	14	100%
Gottardi[57a]	2008	University of Vienna, Austria	73	58	NA	0	13	36	24	7	NA	1	NA	37	1 year, 90% 3 years, 86% 5 years, 72%
Weigang[30]	2009	University Hosp Mainz, Germany	26	100	NA	0	26	0	0	15	13	0	0	NA	NA
Czerny[58a]	2007	University of Vienna, Austria	27	NA	NA	0	10	17	0	7	NA	0	0	15	1 year, 83% 3 years, 72%
Hughes[52]	2009	Duke	28	NA	0	43	19	9	0	0	21	0	4	14	3 years, 70%
Chiesa[59]	2010	Vita-Salute, Milan, Italy	51	NA	NA	0	24	27	0	6	16	6	0	23	NA
Holt[55]	2010	St George, London, UK	26	NA	15	0	9	17	0	6	NA	0	6	NA	NA
Lee[7]	2011	University of Florida, Gainesville	37	NA	NA	68	37	0	0	16	32	11	0	NA	1 year, 72%
Ham[60]	2011	USC	16	NA	NA	0	8	8	0	6	50	6	0	13	1 year, 83% 3 years, 80%
Ferrero[69]	2012	Mauriziano Umberto I Hospital, Turin, Italy	27	NA	19	11	11	4	12	11	52	0	4	17	78%
Vallabhajosyula[31]	2013	University of Pennsylvania	36	NA	NA	56	36	0	0	8	NA	8	6	30	1 year, 71% 3 years, 60% 5 years, 48%
Clough[56]	2013	St Thomas' Hospital, London, United Kingdom	51	100	20	0	4	31	16	10	NA	12	6	NA	NA
Metzger[61]	2014	Affiliated hospitals in Brazil	18	NA	NA	0	8	4	6	11	27	6	6	13	1 year, 90%

[a]Patients may be duplicated in these two studies.
CPB, Cardiopulmonary bypass.

hybrid approach to the aortic arch identified 16 patients. Eight had zone 0 proximal landing, and eight had zone 1 proximal landing. Mortality was 6%, but morbidity was 50%. Strokes occurred in 6% and none had paraplegia.[60] The latest series of 18 patients published in 2014 from affiliated hospitals in Brazil had a mixed proximal landing zone compilation with 44% in zone 0, 22% in zone 1, and 33% in zone 2. The outcomes were not much different from the previous series: mortality (11%), morbidity (27%), stroke (6%), paraplegia (6%).[61]

This discussion suggests that complete arch debranching has a higher mortality than partial arch debranching. This may be due to use of cardiopulmonary bypass when the ascending aorta has to be replaced in combination with complete arch debranching. As one would expect, emergent operations also had worse outcomes as compared to elective/urgent cases. Long-term data are limited for hybrid repair. Follow-up in the case series range from 1 to 3 years. One-year overall survival ranged from 70% to 100% (see Table 38.2).

Hybrid Thoracoabdominal Aneurysm Repair

Case series on hybrid repair of the thoracoabdominal aorta have been reported worldwide with increasing frequency since first described in 1999.[1] Defining outcomes from these cases series can be difficult given the heterogeneous groups of patients in these reports. In Table 38.1, factors such as the extent of aneurysmal involvement based on Crawford classification, emergent, and high-risk patients have been noted and should be kept in mind when examining outcomes. In general, reported mortalities range from 0% to 31%. These are based on 30-day or in-hospital mortalities. Morbidities range from 17% to 65%, but these values depend on how complications have been classified. Permanent paraplegia ranges from 0% to 14%.

One of the first series from the University of North Carolina at Chapel Hill, published in 2005, reviewed 10 patients. Their outcomes were quite impressive with no death or paraplegia, but there were no type I-II TAA in this series. Twenty percent of patients were type IV TAA, 30% were suprarenal abdominal aortic aneurysm (AAA), and 50% were juxtarenal AAA. The patients had an average of 1.3 bypasses per patient, and most did not involve clamping the aorta. Six patients had a single iliorenal bypass, three with a hepatorenal bypass, and one patient with complete visceral revascularization.[39] A more recent series ($n = 24$) from the University of Southern California also had a high proportion of type IV (50%) and pararenal AAA (38%). The remaining 12.5% of patients were Crawford type I, II, or III TAA. Their mortality and paraplegia rates were 4.2%.[60] The patients in both series were considered high risk for surgery.

Van de Mortel and colleagues looked at all hybrid procedures done in the Netherlands and identified 16 patients. This seemingly uncomplicated group, where only 50% were deemed unfit for open repair and only 19% were Crawford type I, II, or III TAA, had one of the highest mortality rates (31%) of any series. These patients also had a 13% graft occlusion rate (7/58 grafts), accounting for three of the deaths. Two patients expired from colonic ischemia secondary to an occluded SMA bypass graft, and the third patient expired from gallbladder necrosis, but also had renal failure requiring hemodialysis from a right renal artery graft occlusion.[48]

Another series of 16 patients from the University of Ulm in Germany also had a high mortality rate (31%) in a series of mainly type IV TAA (56%). This high mortality may be explained by the number of emergent operations (38%). All patients were considered high risk. Emergent mortality was 50% (3 of 6) compared to the elective/urgent mortality of 20% (2 of 10). Of the deaths, two were due to graft occlusion with bowel ischemia.[49]

Additional series with high mortalities had more patients with extensive Crawford types I-III TAA. From the Cleveland Clinic, 13 consecutive patients, all deemed unfit for conventional thoracoabdominal repair, had aortic dissections with aneurysmal degeneration ($n = 5$) or TAA aneurysms ($n = 8$). Mortality was 23%, and six patients required a proximal or distal aortic repair (two infrarenal reconstructions, three arch elephant trunk grafts, and one ascending aortic repair).[62] St. Mary's Hospital in London reported on 29 patients. The TAA distribution was Crawford type I in 3 cases, type II in 18, type III in 7, and type IV in 1. They had no paraplegia in their series, but overall mortality was 24% (7/29). Three patients had debranchings aborted. Two were secondary to intraoperative cardiac instability. These patients survived and were managed conservatively. The third patient had poor inflow for the debranching bypass due to an aortic dissection. This patient expired 10 days after the procedure. Of the completed hybrid repairs the mortality was 23% (6/26). Three patients treated emergently all expired. In three elective/urgent patients who died, one was from a pulmonary embolus, another from myocardial infarction (MI), and the last from emboli to the viscera. For emergent repairs, mortality was 100% (3/3) and for urgent and elective patients, mortality was 13% (3/23).[40]

At the University of Florida in Gainesville, 17 patients with TAA (Crawford extent: two type II, eight type III, and seven type IV) were reported. Perioperative mortality was 24%.[42] From Massachusetts General Hospital, 23 high-risk patients with TAA (Crawford extent: nine type I, five type II, nine type III) had a 30-day mortality of 17.4%, and in-hospital mortality of 23%. This series also had a total of 22% (5/23) endoleaks during the limited mean follow-up of 5.5 months. Three endoleaks were type I and two were type II. A total of three patients required endovascular reintervention. Of note, this series also compared the hybrid to a cohort of contemporary open TAA repairs (see earlier discussion).[19]

Of the series with the lowest mortalities, Zhou from Baylor reported on 31 patients with a mortality of 3% ($n = 1$). This series combined 21 TAAs with 10 cases of aortic arch aneurysms. In those with TAA, Crawford types were type I in three patients, type II in three patients, type III in eight patients, and type IV in seven patients. Aortic arch reconstructions were performed in 3 patients, supraaortic trunk debranching in 13 patients, and visceral vessel bypasses in 15 patients. Despite the complex patients, the outcomes were encouraging.[63]

From the University of California, Los Angeles, 20 patients were treated using a hybrid approach. Three had aortic arch aneurysm, but the remainder were TAA (Crawford type I-0, type II-3, III-8, IV-4), symptomatic supravisceral AAA (one), and contained pararenal pseudoaneurysm rupture (one). There was no mortality and only one patient with paraplegia. The latter patient had the entire aorta covered with a stent-graft from the left subclavian to aortic bifurcation treated in a single stage.[64]

In one of the largest series, Donas and colleagues, from Zurich Hospital in Switzerland, used a novel technique they described as the Viabahn Open Revascularization Technique (VORTEC). The bypass anastomoses were created using a Viabahn stent-graft (Gore, Flagstaff, AZ) deployed through one wall of the visceral vessel. The other end was directly sutured end to side with the main feeding bypass graft or fixed into an interposition branch graft off the main bypass. This technique avoided suturing an anastomosis and clamping of the visceral vessels with its associated warm ischemia time. In this series of 58 patients, all were treated electively. Thirty patients had TAA (Crawford types: I-3, II-5, III-9, IV-13, V-0) and 28 patients had pararenal AAA. Ninety-eight renal and 15 visceral vessels were revascularized using the VORTEC technique. The primary patency of the bypass was 97%, and the assisted primary patency rate was 98% because two occluded Viabahn grafts were reopened by thrombolysis and thrombus aspiration. The 30-day mortality rate was 8.6% and permanent paralysis occurred in 3.4%.[65]

In the largest case series report to date ($n = 107$), Drinkwater and colleagues used data from three major European Vascular Units: St. Mary's Hospital, London; University of Heidelberg, Germany; and University of Munich, Germany. Each of these three centers had already published individual case series, but this was a collaborative update on their patients.[40,41,47] There were no emergent cases. Long-term follow-up was not included. The Crawford type TAA distribution was 11 type I, 45 type II, 32 type III, 1 type IV, 1 type V, and 17 defined as complex. The 30-day mortality rate was 15%. Spinal cord ischemia was suffered by 12.1% of patients and in 8.4% it was complete and permanent. Long-term dialysis was required in 3.7% of patients and 2.8% of patients had bowel resection for an infarcted segment of bowel. The morbidity was not well defined, but was at least 38%. Three patients ruptured before the stenting procedure was undertaken.[66]

Two more recent series come from Duke and Milan Italy and are some of the larger single-institution series. At Duke there were 58 patients in the series. The results were quite good with mortality at 9%, and paraplegia at 4% despite the fact all patients had more extensive type I-III TAA (no type IV or pararenal), and 17% of the cases were emergent.[67]

The series from Milan, Italy, reported on 52 patients. They had a more diverse TAA spread (type I—38%, type II—11%, type III—19%, type IV—11%, visceral patch aneurysms—19%) with mortality at 14%, and a surprising low paraplegia rate of 2%.[68]

From the case series discussed, follow-up is difficult to interpret. A number of series report the outcomes based on median rather than mean months of follow-up, and range from 5.5 to 26 months. From Table 38.1, a rough estimate of survival appears to be about 80% at 1 year. The longest follow-up for any patient is now 14 years. This patient was treated in 1999[1] with the first hybrid procedure and continues to do well at the time of this writing, without additional interventions.

Examining outcomes of the hybrid approach to TAA is still limited by small case series compared with series on open TAA, in which there are thousands of patients and the outcomes by Crawford extent are well defined.[11-14] With the growing use of fenestrated and branched technologies, there will unlikely be case series of hybrid TAA repairs with thousands of patients. But from examining the data in these small case series, the outcomes of the hybrid TAA approach are still very reasonable in certain centers, especially considering that most of the patients were considered at high risk for open repair.

SUMMARY

The hybrid approach to aortic arch and thoracoabdominal aortic pathology is an alternative in properly selected patients. There have been no randomized trials comparing open to hybrid approaches, but based on prospective and retrospective case reports, morbidity and mortality seem comparable. Patient selection is critical and the success of a hybrid aortic repair depends on preoperative planning and execution. A hybrid approach to aortic arch and thoracoabdominal aortic pathology should be included in the armamentarium of vascular surgeons involved in the care of these complex, high-risk patients.

REVIEW QUESTIONS

1. In a debranching procedure for a type 3 thoracoabdominal aortic aneurysm (TAA), which artery should not be used as inflow for the bypass graft?
   a. Infrarenal aorta
   b. Common iliac artery
   c. External iliac artery
   d. Descending thoracic aorta
2. In an isolated arch aneurysm, which vessel is not debranched with a complete arch debranching?
   a. Celiac artery
   b. Innominate artery
   c. Left common carotid artery
   d. Left subclavian artery
3. True or false: Use of a stent-graft for a combined endovascular and surgical (hybrid) approach to treat aortic arch and TAA aneurysms is an **on-label** approved use of the device.
   a. True
   b. False
4. True or false: There have been randomized trials of hybrid versus conventional open repair that suggest a hybrid approach should be favored over open repair for patients with acceptable surgical risks.
   a. True
   b. False

5. Which procedure is not needed in a partial arch debranching where the proximal seal zone is expected to be in zone 1?
   a. Carotid to subclavian artery bypass
   b. Carotid to carotid artery bypass
   c. Sternotomy
   d. Placement of stent-graft from the a femoral approach
6. True or false: All hybrid procedures should be done in two stages.
   a. True
   b. False
7. What is a contraindication to a hybrid repair of a TAA aneurysm?
   a. Replaced right hepatic
   b. Inability to create a proximal or distal landing zone
   c. Previous infrarenal abdominal aortic aneurysm (AAA)
   d. Aneurysmal degeneration of an aortic dissection
8. Follow-up imaging after a hybrid repair should be:
   a. There is no additional imaging needed.
   b. The same as open surgery
   c. The same as any other endovascular aneurysm repair
   d. Done only if there are problems
9. Spinal drainage is not needed in a hybrid repair of the TAA in which of the following cases?
   a. A large amount of aorta is being covered.
   b. The bilateral internal iliacs were previously ligated.
   c. Spinal drainage is usually recommended.
   d. The patient has had a prior infrarenal AAA.
10. If a patient is undergoing complete aortic arch debranching with a sternotomy, which of the following is the least important to assess preoperatively?
   a. Coronary arteries
   b. Aortic valve
   c. Femoral arteries
   d. Ascending aorta

References available online at expertconsult.com.

CHAPTER 39

Fenestrated-Branched and Parallel Stent-Grafts for Endovascular Repair of Aortic Arch and Thoracoabdominal Aortic Aneurysms

Gustavo S. Oderich, Giuliano de A. Sandri

INTRODUCTION

Endovascular repair has become the first treatment option in most patients with abdominal and thoracic aortic aneurysms. Prospective randomized studies have shown that endovascular aortic repair (EVAR) is associated with lower morbidity, mortality, blood loss, and earlier recovery compared with open surgical repair.[1] For thoracic aneurysms and dissections, endovascular repair (TEVAR) has been shown to decrease mortality, morbidity, and risk of paraplegia compared with open surgical repair.[2] Anatomical factors such as short or angulated landing zones, side branch involvement, difficult access, tortuosity, and diffuse aortic disease have limited the widespread use of endovascular techniques to treat patients with more challenging anatomy. For these patients, innovative techniques have been developed to incorporate side branches with fenestrations, directional branches, and parallel stent-grafts. This chapter summarizes the indications, preoperative planning, techniques of implantation, and outcomes of fenestrated, branched, and parallel stent-grafts to treat thoracoabdominal aortic aneurysms (TAAAs) and aortic arch aneurysms.

HISTORICAL PERSPECTIVES

The first fenestrated endovascular repair was performed by Park and colleagues in 1996.[3] Subsequently, a group led by Michael Lawrence-Brown and David Hartley developed a novel fenestrated platform based on the Cook Zenith abdominal stent-graft (Brisbane, Australia). John Anderson from Adelaide, Australia, performed the first clinical implantation of a Cook Zenith fenestrated stent-graft for a juxta-renal aortic aneurysm in 1998.[4] In 2001, Tim Chuter from the University of California, San Francisco introduced the concept of multibranched endografts to treat TAAAs.[5] Concurrently, improvements in the design and delivery system have widened the applications of fenestrated and branched stent-grafts with significant contributions by Roy Greenberg (Cleveland, OH), Wolf Stelter (Frankfurt, Germany), Eric Verhoeven (Nuremberg, Germany), Stephan Haulon (Lille, France), Krassi Ivancev (Malmo, Sweden), Tim Resch (Malmo, Sweden), and multiple other investigators. These improvements included changes in the modular design, diameter reducing-ties, reinforcement of fenestrations, alignment stents, development of preloaded guidewires and catheters, and lower profile fabric. More than 20,000 patients have been treated worldwide by fenestrated and branched stent-grafts for arch, TAAA, and aortoiliac aneurysms. Other aortic device manufacturers have also embarked on the development of complex platforms to expand indications of EVAR to patients with complex anatomy.

Despite the increasing interest in these techniques, physician access has been limited by regulatory issues, cost, lack of specialized training, and time delay to manufacture devices. Other creative techniques have been introduced as a means to overcome the lack of widespread availability of manufactured devices. Roy Greenberg described the first use of parallel grafts to treat a pararenal aneurysm in 2003.[6] The technique was later disseminated by Criado, Lachat, Lobato, and other pioneers, who coined a variety of terms, including "chimney," "snorkel," "periscope," and "sandwich" grafts. These techniques had in common the use of aortic and bridging stent components deployed in parallel, side by side, to extend landing zones across side branches.[7–9] Device modifications were first described by Krassi Ivancev and Renan Uflacker in a report of three patients in 2006.[10] Ben Starnes coined the term "physician-modified endovascular graft" (PMEG) to describe modifications of manufactured devices by creation of fenestrations to incorporate branches.[11] Oderich has reported numerous technical refinements, including the addition of diameter-reducing ties, minicuffs, directional branches, and preloaded wire systems to facilitate the technique.[12–14]

INDICATIONS

The indications for endovascular repair using fenestrated, branched, and parallel stent-grafts are the same applied for open surgical or hybrid repair. Because these operations carry higher risks of morbidity and mortality, it is of paramount importance to carry out a balanced risk-benefit analysis, taking into consideration institutional experience and results. The risk of rupture should be analyzed in contrast to the risk of perioperative death or major disability, which should also consider the risks of paraplegia, major stroke, and dialysis. Treatment is recommended in patients with ruptured or symptomatic aneurysms, independent of the size. For elective repair, most patients have maximum aneurysm diameter greater than 6 cm. Analysis of body surface area helps optimize indications of repair based on size criteria.[15] Repair should be also considered in patients with rapid aneurysm enlargement (>5 mm growth in 6 months) and in those who develop dissection, intramural hematoma, or penetrating ulcers within the aneurysm. Saccular aneurysms have a poorly defined natural history, and therefore most experts agree that repair should be considered at smaller size diameter for saccular aneurysms. Finally, elective repair of a TAAA should only be considered when the risk of rupture outweighs the risks of the operation, given the patient's age, comorbidities, and anticipated long-term survival.

Endovascular repair of complex aneurysms is relatively contraindicated in patients with infectious etiology, systemic sepsis, connective tissue disorders (e.g., Marfan, Ehlers-Danlos, Loyes-Dietz syndrome), excessive amount of atherosclerotic debris, inadequate landing zones, unsuitable femoral access, and renal-mesenteric targets. Although endovascular repair can be applied in select patients with infected aneurysms and also for connective tissue disorders, studies are limited by small numbers of patients and short follow-up.[16–19] Endovascular repair is an alternative in patients with connective tissue disorders who have prior open surgical grafts that serve as landing zone for a new endograft, and in those with ruptured aneurysms as a bridge to definitive open surgical repair.

DEFINITIONS

The term *fenestrated endovascular repair* is applied when a fenestrated stent-graft is used to repair an aneurysm with inadequate or short infrarenal neck, yet the target vessels (e.g., renal arteries) originate from normal aorta. There is no gap between the fenestration and the target vessel. Alignment stents are typically used to prevent vessel occlusion or stenosis from misalignment between the fenestration and the origin of the target vessel. Examples of devices designed for fenestrated repair include the Zenith (ZFEN, Cook Medical Inc., Brisbane, Australia) and Vascutek Anaconda fenestrated stent-grafts.

A *branched endovascular repair* is indicated for aneurysms involving side branches. In these cases, the target vessel originates from the aneurysm, and there is a space gap between the main aortic stent-graft and the aortic wall. The branches can be constructed using one of two approaches. *Fenestrated-branches* are based on reinforced fenestrations, which are bridged by balloon-expandable covered stents that connect the fenestration to the target vessel, whereas *directional branches* are based on pre-sewn cuffs. The most commonly utilized branch configuration is a straight cuff or portal, which is accessed via the brachial approach. However, directional branches can be helical, upgoing (or retrograde), and can be internal or external to the main aortic device. Selection of bridging stent is more variable for directional branches, including self-expandable and balloon-expandable covered stents. Examples of thoracoabdominal multibranched stent-grafts include the Cook t-Branch and patient-specific stent-grafts, the Gore ThoracoAbdominal Multi-Branched Endograft (TAMBE), and recent developments using Bolton, Medtronic, and Jotec stent-grafts.

The term *parallel graft technique* refers to a wide range of techniques that use stent-grafts deployed alongside each other. The terms "chimney," "snorkel," "periscope," "octopus," and "sandwich" stent-grafts have all been coined to describe specific configurations of parallel grafts placed from proximal or distal landing zones. "Chimney grafts" consist of parallels grafts coming from the proximal landing zone and placed in parallel between a healthy aortic segment and the aortic stent-graft. These have been used to incorporate the renal-mesenteric arteries in patients with short-neck or pararenal aortic aneurysms. "Periscope grafts" utilize the same concept, but the side stents are placed in retrograde configuration and are based on the distal landing zone. "Sandwich grafts," a term coined by Armando Lobato from Sao Paulo,[7] Brazil, apply a "graft within graft" concept and can be combined with the previously mentioned techniques to treat more extensive aneurysms such as TAAAs, aortic arch, and aortoiliac aneurysms. The "octopus" technique was described by Kasijaran using abdominal bifurcated stent-grafts deployed in the thoracic aorta, coupled with parallel stent-grafts deployed within the iliac limbs to revascularize the renal-mesenteric arteries.[20]

PREOPERATIVE ASSESSMENT

Clinical Risk Evaluation

A comprehensive evaluation of cardiac, pulmonary, and renal performance is crucial to optimize patient selection. These operations are often indicated in the sickest patient, but clinical data suggest that prohibitively high-risk patients who have limited life expectancy are not ideal candidates for these procedures. The evaluation should include noninvasive cardiac stress tests, pulmonary function tests, and carotid ultrasound. Factors associated with increased risk include unstable angina, symptomatic or poorly controlled ectopy, recurrent CHF, ejection fraction <25%, myocardial infarction <6 months, vital capacity <1.8 L, FEV1 <800 mL, DLCO <30%, resting pO_2 <60 mm Hg and pCO_2 >50 mm Hg, and ongoing renal replacement therapy.

Medical Genetics Evaluation

Medical genetic evaluation should be considered in younger patients or in those with familial history or phenotypic features. These disorders are autosomal dominant and are strongest in the younger patient population affected by aortic dissection or aneurysm. Clinically relevant disorders include Marfan, Turner, Vascular Ehlers-Danlos, and Loeys-Dietz syndromes. The most common mutations are noted in the fibrillin *(FBN1)* or TGF-receptor 2 genes *(TGFBR2)* in Marfans and Loyes-Dietz syndromes, respectively. The most common nonsyndromic mutation associated with thoracic aneurysms and dissections is in the SMC actin gene *(ACTA2)*.

Imaging Evaluation

Computed tomography angiography (CTA) of the chest, abdomen, and pelvis is the single most important imaging modality to plan aortic repair (Fig. 39.1). Its utility relies on the accurate

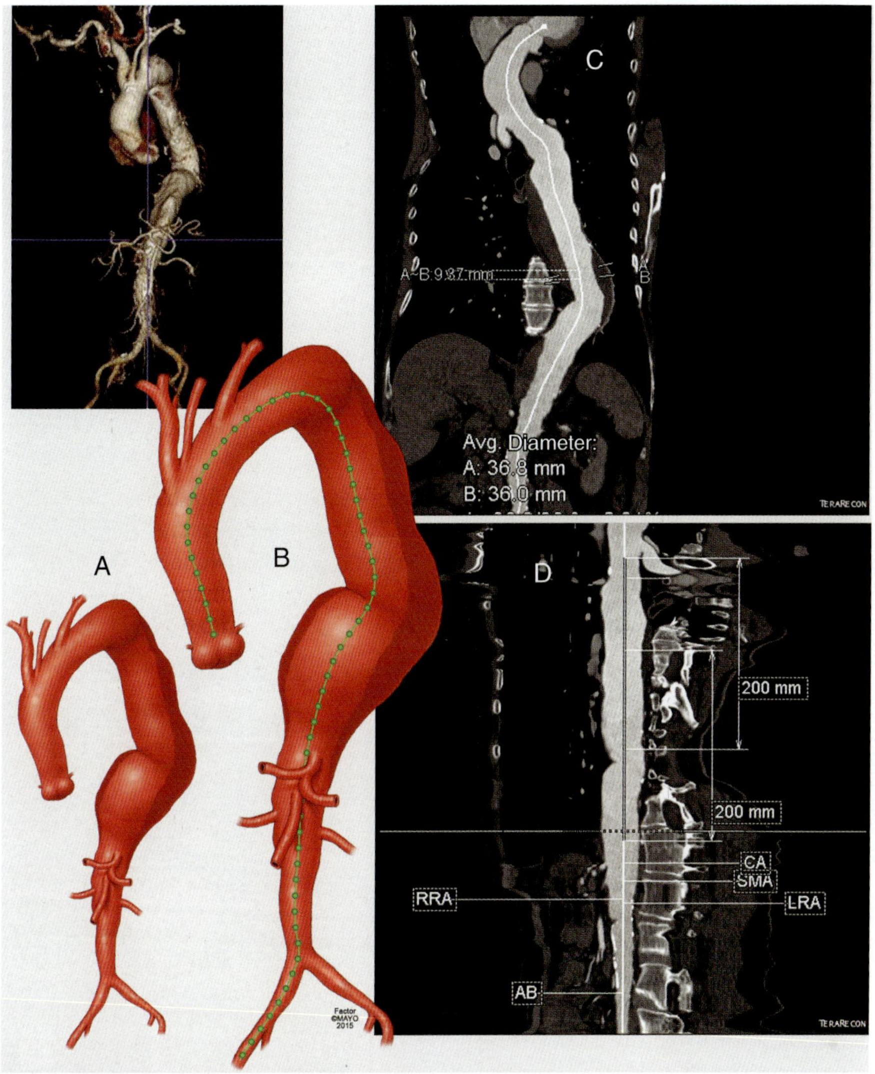

FIG 39.1 Analysis of a tortuous aorta with thoracoabdominal aortic aneurysm on three-dimensional computed tomography angiography (A) using centerline of flow (CLF, B). The curved multiplanar reformatting (MPR) image is created to analyze specific segments of the vessel (C). The straightened CLF is used for measurements of lengths and to assess the extent of aortic disease (D). *AB,* Aortic bifurcation; *CA,* celiac axis; *LRA,* left renal artery; *RRA,* right renal artery; *SMA,* superior mesenteric artery. (Used with permission of Mayo Foundation for Medical Education and Research. All rights reserved.)

assessment of etiology, extent of disease, involvement of side branches (Fig. 39.2), adequacy of access vessels, and presence of extravascular diseases that might affect treatment selection and approach. Imaging requires tailoring of the exam to a specific indication and established preexisting protocols in collaboration with radiologists. Communication among multiple specialties, including the radiologists performing the study, is critical to properly address specific issues.

Access

These procedures are most often performed using iliofemoral access. For complex repair, brachial or axillary access is often needed for directional branches or parallel grafts. Patients with small iliac arteries or severe calcification, stenosis, occlusion, excessive tortuosity, or dissections may require surgical or endovascular conduits to allow safe introduction of large delivery systems (>20 French). Conduits are needed in approximately 10% to 15% of patients. A staged permanent conduit can be performed using iliofemoral bypass via a retroperitoneal approach. Alternatively, an endoconduit offers an excellent alternative in patients who have occluded internal iliac arteries.

Sealing Zones

The proximal landing zone should be based on at least 2-cm length of "normal," noncalcified, parallel aorta to allow circumferential stent-graft apposition to the vessel wall (Fig. 39.3). Analysis of neck morphology determines the selection of "healthy aortic segments" for proximal and distal fixation. Regions that have extreme tortuosity or that appear conical or noncylindrical, and segments that contain atheromatous debris, thrombus, or

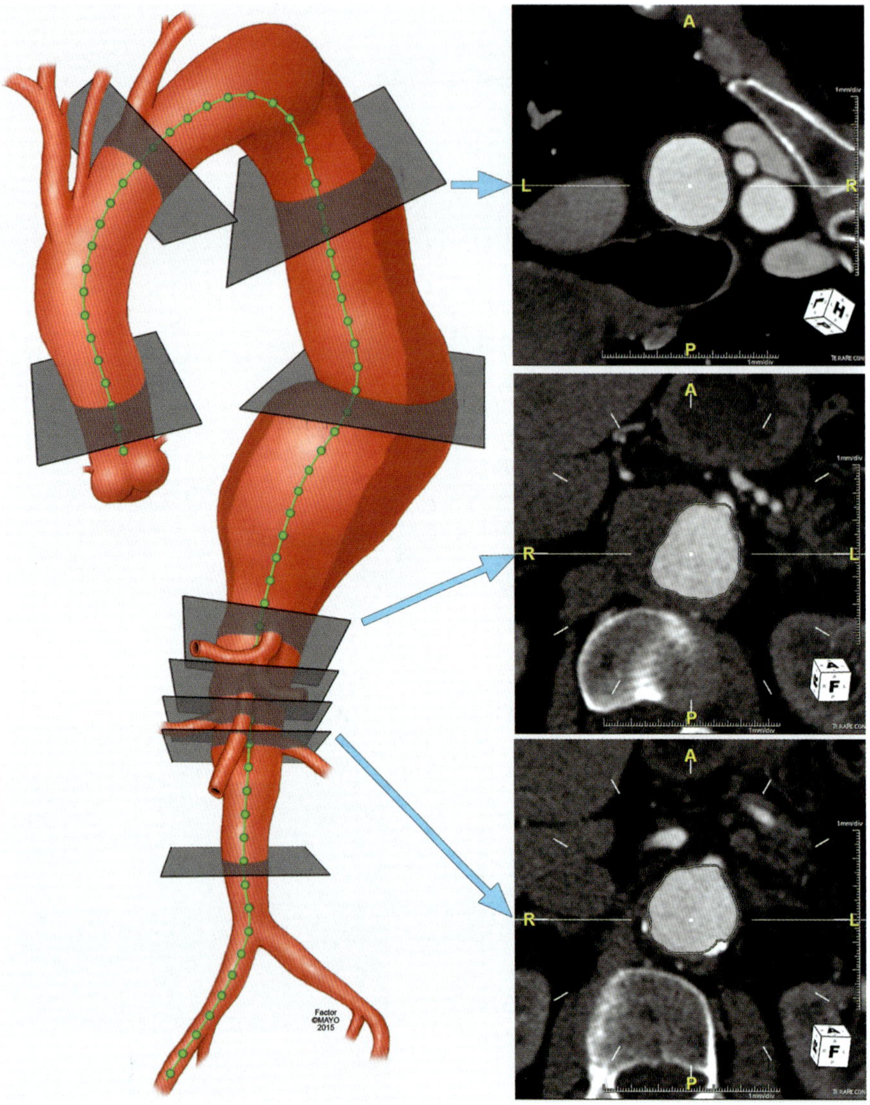

FIG 39.2 Centerline of flow is used to evaluate aortic diameters in each specific segment and the location of target vessels. (Used with permission of Mayo Foundation for Medical Education and Research. All rights reserved.)

calcification are not considered safe to fix and seal endovascular devices. Assessment of landing zones is performed using centerline of flow (CLF) projections. A parallel aortic segment with less than 10% variation in diameter is considered normal aorta for placement of endograft. Although the minimum recommended length for proximal landing zone is 20 to 25 mm, longer segments may be needed in patients with ectatic, thrombus-laden, or diseased aortas.

Side-Branch Involvement

The extent of repair is dictated by the involvement of side branches (see Fig. 39.2). In patients with pararenal or TAAAs, the celiac axis, superior mesenteric artery (SMA), renal arteries, and aberrant or unusual anatomy require meticulous analysis using CLF. The presence of concomitant occlusive or aneurysmal disease of the aortic branches should be noted to determine candidacy, stent design, and ideal approach. Minimum requirements are target vessel diameter between 4 and 11 mm and length to bifurcation greater than 12 mm. The presence of stents within the vessels or suprarenal fixation in patients with prior repair may increase technical difficulty. Independent of which technique is selected, anatomical factors may significantly impact technical difficulties and which method is selected to reconstruct the aorta. It is useful to illustrate in a template the patient's anatomy and measurements.

ENDOVASCULAR TECHNIQUES

Basic principles can be used to facilitate endovascular repair of complex aneurysms, independent of which technique is selected to incorporate side branches. Advanced endovascular skills and familiarity with branch vessel stenting and "bail-out" maneuvers are minimum requirements to achieve successful results with these complex procedures. A comprehensive endovascular inventory

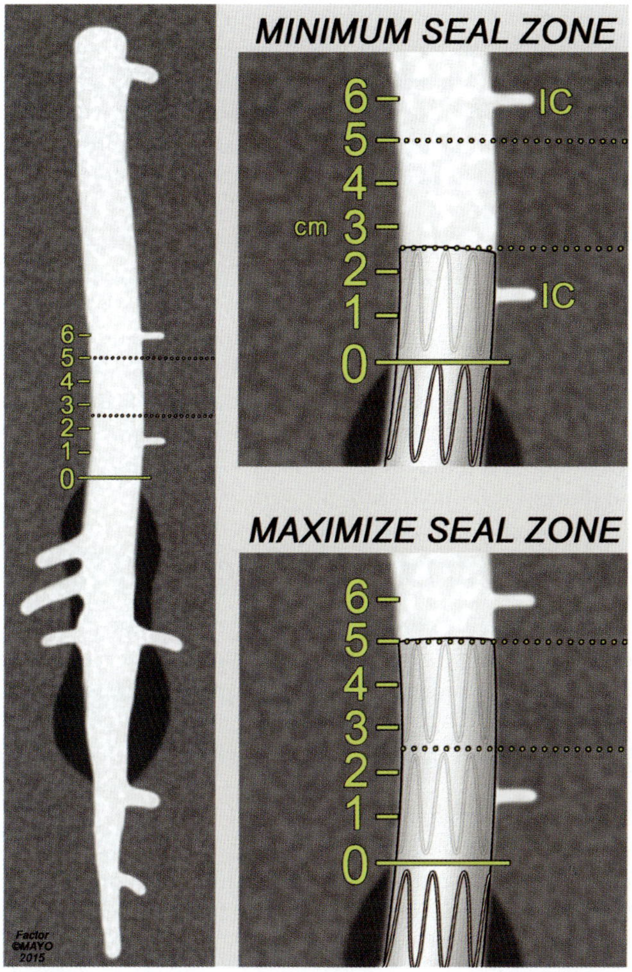

FIG 39.3 Selection of minimal proximal landing zone based on parallel aortic wall. Note a minimum landing zone of 2.5-cm is selected, but this is extended proximally just below the next intercostal arterial station to maximize seal at the proximal attachment site. (Used with permission of Mayo Foundation for Medical Education and Research. All rights reserved.)

with a wide range of catheters, balloons, and stents is required to perform these procedures.

Perioperative Measures

Hospital preadmission is recommended for patients with estimated glomerular filtration rate less than 60 mL/min or serum creatinine greater than 1.8 mg/dL, advanced age (>80 years), or multiple comorbidities. Oral acetyl-cysteine is administered to minimize the risk of renal function deterioration. Gentle bowel preparation (magnesium citrate) and intravenous hydration with sodium bicarbonate infusion is started several hours before the procedure. Acetyl-salicylic acid (325 mg/day) is used routinely, and clopidogrel is discontinued at least 10 days prior to the operation in patients who need placement of cerebrospinal fluid (CSF) drain. Beta-blockers and statins are continued on the day of the operation, but other vasodilator antihypertensive medications are decreased or discontinued. All patients are instructed to shower with Hibiclens liquid skin cleanser (chlorhexidine gluconate 4%) the day prior to the procedure to reduce bacterial counts. In the obese patient, the skin over the groin crease should be inspected several days prior to the procedure, and any fungal infection should be treated. Perioperative antibiotics are administrated intravenously prior to incision and up to 24 hours after the procedure.

Hybrid Endovascular Rooms

Optimal imaging with hybrid endovascular suite and fixed imaging unit is recommended. On-lay fusion imaging and cone bean computed tomography (CBCT) are ideal to facilitate device implantation, minimize radiation and contrast use, and immediately assess the technical result. Most procedures are performed using general endotracheal anesthesia, although local or regional anesthesia can also be used. Intraoperative blood salvage ("cell-saver") is recommended at the beginning of one's experience and for difficult cases with anticipated prolonged operating time. A useful tip is to create large pockets within the surgical drapes to allow for the blood to be collected with cell saver. EKG leads, urinary catheter, and other monitoring cables and lines should be taped or secured so that they are not in the path of the x-ray beam of the fluoroscopic unit or do not get caught during movement of the C-arm gantry.

Contrast Use and Radiation Safety

The use of iodinated contrast is minimized throughout all steps of the procedure using several maneuvers avoiding conventional contrast angiographies. Our preference has been to use small hand injections (3 mL of contrast in 7 mL of saline) to locate the side branches. A completion aortography is obtained after all the stents are placed using diluted contrast at 50%. Precatheterization to locate the target vessels is optional, but probably unnecessary if on-lay fusion imaging is available. Nonetheless, precatheterization can be beneficial to precisely locate a specific target and to facilitate deployment.

Radiation protection is critical when performing these procedures by following "as low as reasonably achievable" (ALARA) principles, which aim the lowest radiation exposure to complete the procedure. To achieve this, frame rates are reduced to the lowest possible (7.5 images/s), fluoroscopic pedal is left at the control of the most senior operating surgeon, and digital subtraction is avoided whenever possible. Gantry angulations are limited to greater than 30-degree anterior oblique views, and imaging is collimated with digital zoon instead of magnified views. Operator shielding is used to minimize scattered radiation, including protective garments, eye protection, lead hats, and protective surgical drapes.

Positioning

Patient position is dependent on access sites and specific stent design. This should be discussed with the anesthesia team and nursing staff prior to placement of monitoring lines. In general, patients are positioned supine with the left arm abducted or tucked to the side (Fig. 39.4), with the imaging unit oriented from the head of the table. Arterial access is obtained using femoral approach for pararenal aneurysms requiring up to three fenestrations. Brachial and femoral access is needed for nearly

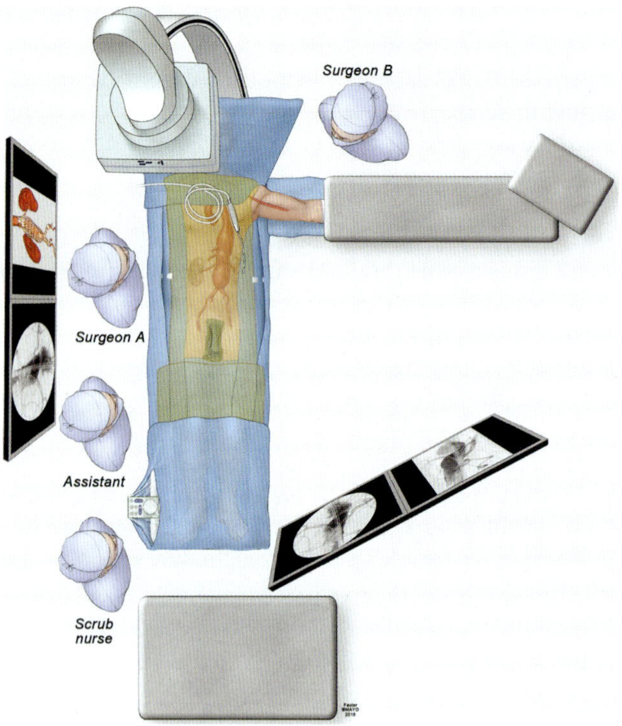

FIG 39.4 Endovascular suite setup for complex endovascular aortic repair with left arm prepped and abducted. The fixed imaging is positioned from the head of the table. Surgeon A stands at patient's right side for femoral access while Surgeon B stands in the left side and uses transbrachial access. (Used with permission of Mayo Foundation for Medical Education and Research. All rights reserved.)

patients treated for TAAAs with four-vessel designs or downgoing branches, unless there is a specific contraindication due to difficult arch or atherosclerotic debris.

Multibranched endografts require 12 French sheaths via brachial access. In these cases, the author's preference is to expose the brachial artery in the upper arm near the axillary hairline, provided the vessel measures ≥4 mm by duplex ultrasound. If the brachial artery is smaller, exposure is performed in the deltopectoral groove or infraclavicular fossa. If brachial access is needed for a single vessel using 7 to 8 French sheath, the distal brachial artery may be exposed above the elbow crease.

Arterial Access

Percutaneous femoral access is used whenever possible in patients with noncalcified or minimally calcified femoral arteries. This technique is avoided in patients with high femoral bifurcations, dense calcifications, or anterior plaque. A permanent or temporary iliac conduit is required in 10% to 20% of patients. Percutaneous femoral access is established using ultrasound guidance with a 0.018-inch micropuncture set. The femoral artery is accessed 1- to 2-cm proximal to the bifurcation (Fig. 39.5). A 6 French sheath is introduced over a 0.035-inch guidewire. A small oblique incision is made, and the subcutaneous tissue is circumferentially dissected to facilitate placement of the closure device. Each femoral puncture is preclosed using Perclose ProGlide closure devices (Abbott Vascular, Santa Clara, CA) deployed at the 1:30 and 10:30 o'clock position, prior to introduction of the larger diameter sheath (Fig. 39.6). At the end of the procedure, guidewire access should be maintained until adequate closure is confirmed. Open femoral artery exposure is performed in patients with contraindications to percutaneous closure. For arch devices, additional access is obtained in the carotid arteries.

Intraoperative Anticoagulation

The patient is systemically heparinized with intravenous bolus of heparin (80 to 100 units/kg), which is administered immediately after femoral and brachial access is obtained. It is important to communicate the heparin dose with the anesthesia team and to assure communication of therapeutic activated clotting time (ACT) greater than 250 seconds throughout the procedure every 30 minutes. A continuous drip of heparin (1000 units/h) is used, and diuresis is induced with intravenous mannitol.

THORACOABDOMINAL AORTIC ANEURYSMS

Device design and approach are tailored to the patient anatomy and take into consideration the orientation of target vessels, aortic diameter, and adequacy of access vessels. Manufactured fenestrated and branched stent-grafts can be tailored to fit the patient's anatomy or can be "off-the-shelf."

Specific Designs

The Zenith fenestrated stent-graft was approved by the US Food and Drug Administration (FDA) for commercial use in April of 2012 (Fig. 39.7). Design constraints for this device include the maximum of three fenestrations, two of the same type, and a minimum of 4 to 15 mm of infrarenal aortic landing zone. Other fenestrated and branched endografts are currently under clinical investigation. In general, fenestrations are ideal for narrow aortic diameter, but require precise deployment. Branches are preferred for vessels originating from larger aortic diameter and do not require the same degree of precision, but branched endografts tend to cover longer aortic segment (Fig. 39.8). These include patient-specific designs with any combination of fenestration and directional branches or multibranched off-the-shelf stent-grafts (e.g., p-Branch, t-Branch, and TAMBE).

Staging

Extent I–II TAAAs are usually staged in order to allow recovery of collateral circulation to the spine to decrease the risk of spinal cord injury (Fig. 39.9). In the first stage, the proximal thoracic aorta is covered to the level of the celiac axis. Cervical debranching and permanent iliac conduits are done as part of the first stage procedure if needed. Other methods of staged aortic repair include temporary aneurysm sac perfusion (TASP), incomplete repair, or intentional coil embolization of intercostal arteries. The second-stage procedure is completed with minimum of 5 days in between stages.

Fenestrated and Branched Stent-Grafts

Arterial access is obtained via femoral (20 to 22 French) and brachial approach (12 French). One of the renal arteries is catheterized to calibrate the on-lay fusion computed tomography

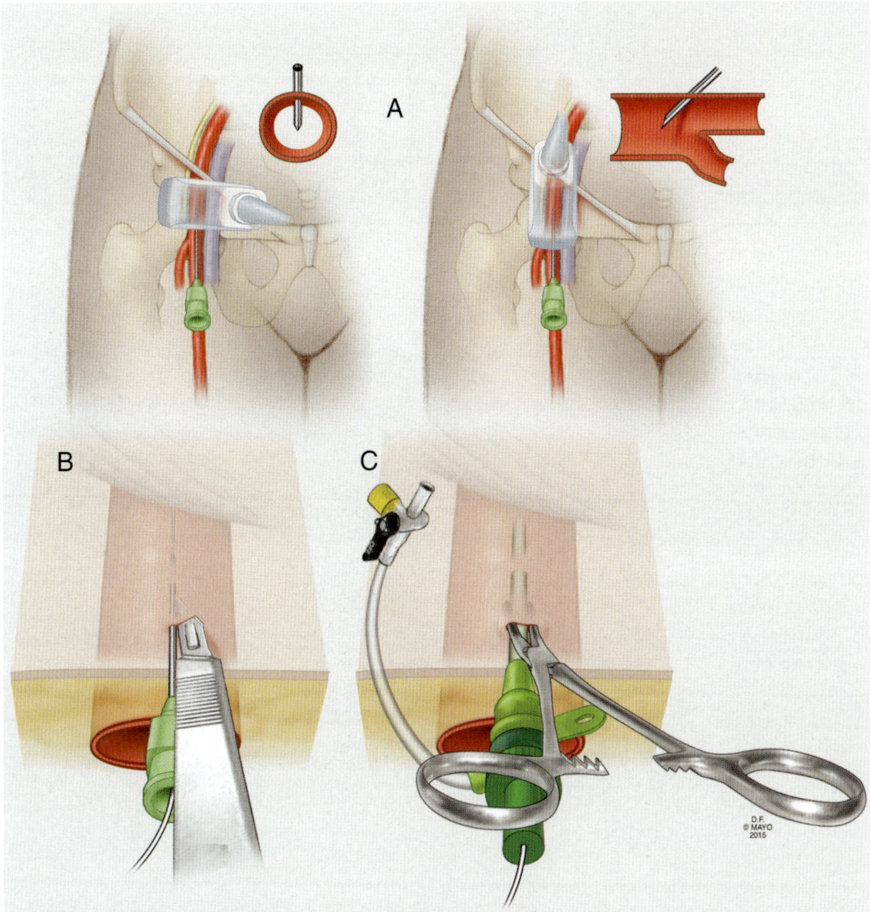

FIG 39.5 Percutaneous access is established using ultrasound guidance with a micro-puncture set (A). Note access is established just proximal to the origin of the profunda femoral artery. Once access is obtained, a small oblique incision is made with careful attention to avoid any dermal tissue within the entrance site (B). A 6 French sheath is advanced over a 0.035-inch guidewire and the soft tissue around the sheath is dilated with forceps (C). (Used with permission of Mayo Foundation for Medical Education and Research. All rights reserved.)

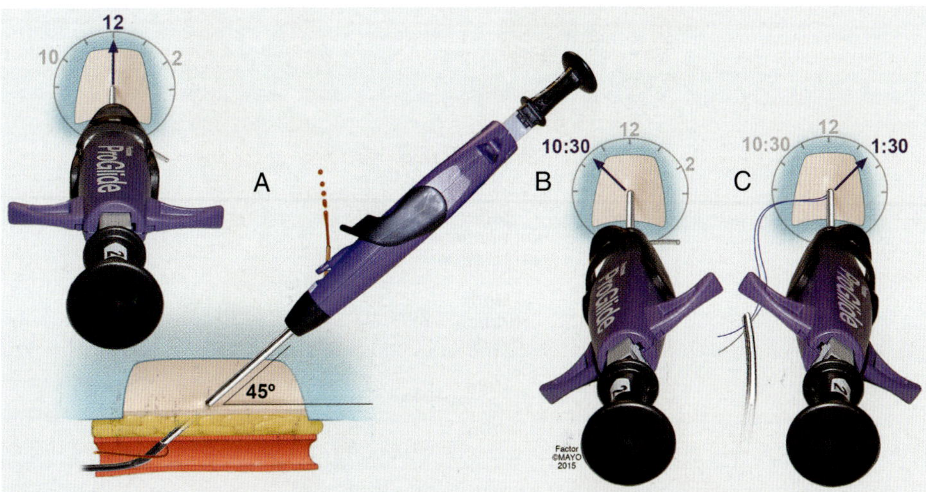

FIG 39.6 Standard preclosure technique is performed using the Perclose Proglide device. The device is introduced with a 45-degree angle to the skin entrance until there is pulsatile bleeding via the side port (A). Each of the percutaneous stitches are deployed at 10:30 (B) and 1:30 (C) o'clock positions. (Used with permission of Mayo Foundation for Medical Education and Research. All rights reserved.)

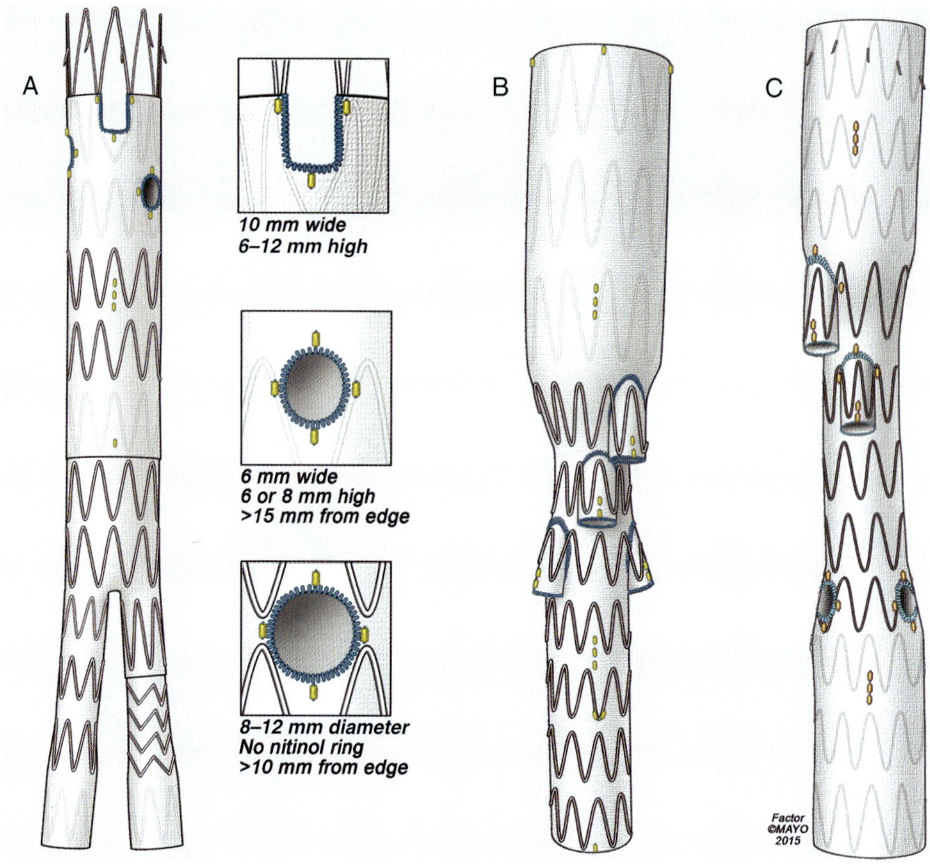

FIG 39.7 Different configurations of fenestrated and branched stent-grafts are depicted in this illustration. Patient specific stent-grafts are designed with a proximal fenestrated component and distal universal bifurcated component with iliac limb extensions (A). Three types of fenestrations are available including scallops, small fenestrations (6 × 6 or 6 × 8 mm), and large fenestrations (8 × 8 mm). The three most common designs described in this chapter include fenestrated stent-grafts (A), multibranched stent-grafts (B), and mixed designs with any combination of fenestrations and branches (C). (Used with permission of Mayo Foundation for Medical Education and Research. All rights reserved.)

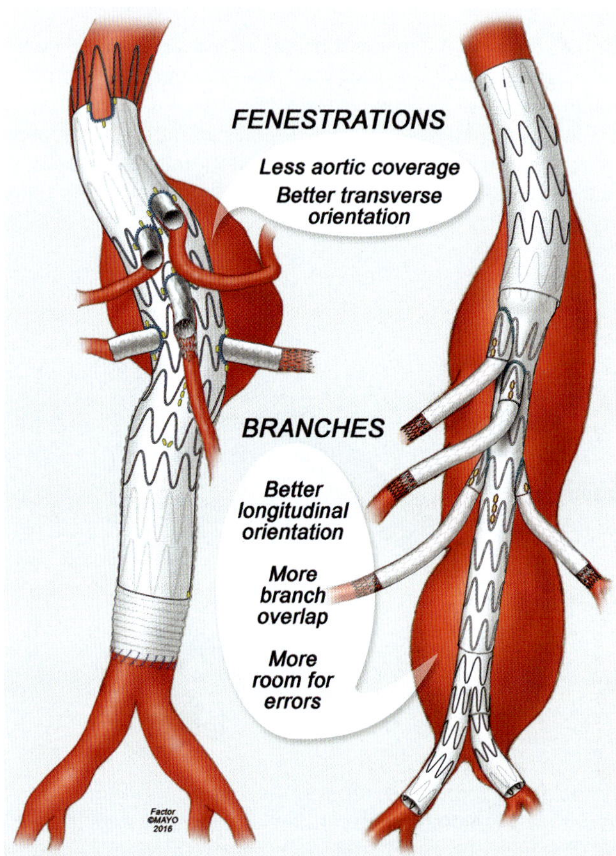

FIG 39.8 Illustration depicts Extent IV thoracoabdominal aneurysm and advantages and disadvantages of fenestrated versus branched stent-graft. (Used with permission of Mayo Foundation for Medical Education and Research. All rights reserved.)

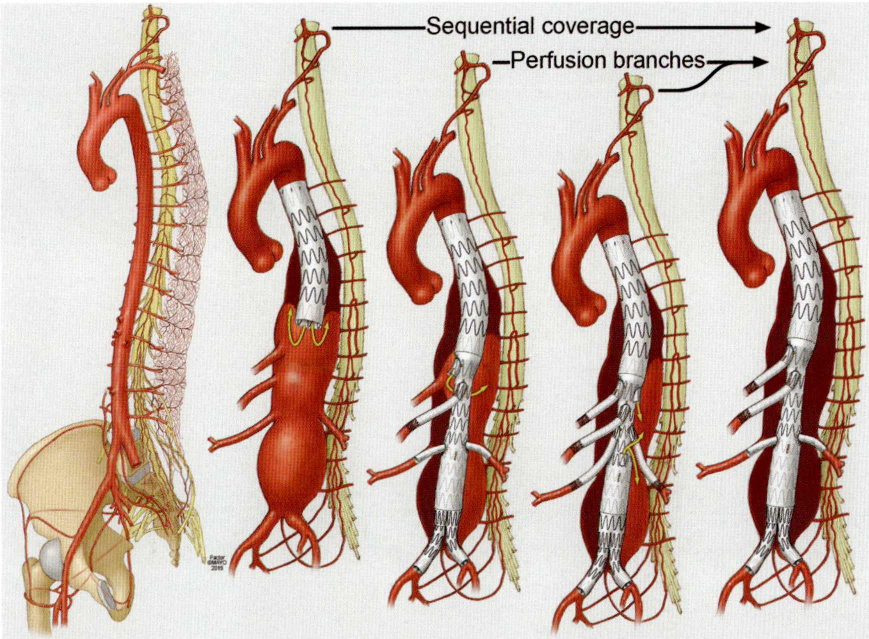

FIG 39.9 Optimization of the extensive spine collateral network including vertebral, intercostal, lumbar, and hypogastric arteries forms the basis for staged endovascular repair of complex aneurysms. Strategies include coverage of the proximal thoracic aorta up to the celiac axis, followed by visceral branch stenting in a second stage. Alternatively the sac can be perfused via perfusion branches or unstented celiac axis or contralateral iliac limb. (Used with permission of Mayo Foundation for Medical Education and Research. All rights reserved.)

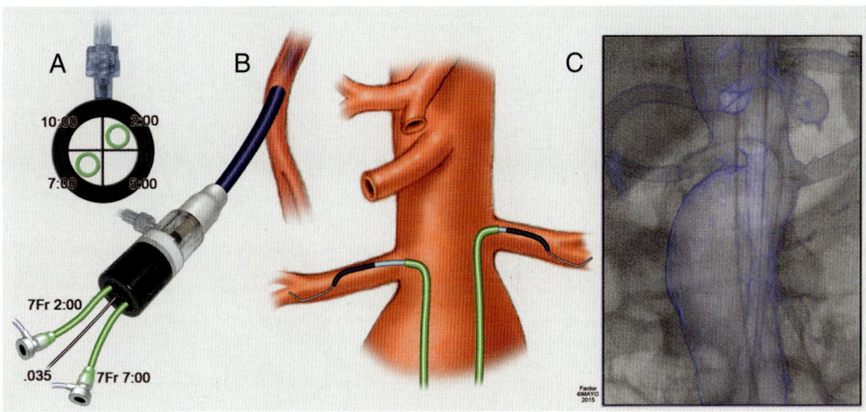

FIG 39.10 Right femoral multisheath access is established using a Check-Flo sheath (A). Technique of multisheath access (A) with placement of two 7 French *(Fr)* sheaths and guide-catheters for renal catheterization (B). On-lay fusion computed tomography (C) is used to locate the target vessels and minimize use of contrast. (Used with permission of Mayo Foundation for Medical Education and Research. All rights reserved.)

(CT; Fig. 39.10). Once the target vessels are located, the fenestrated-branched stent-graft is oriented extracorporeally and introduced over a stiff guidewire. The author's preference is to use preloaded catheters for the celiac and SMA, which exit in the top of the device. These catheters allow guidewires to be advanced and snared via the brachial approach prior to deployment of the aortic stent.

Fenestrations should be positioned precisely or slightly higher than the anticipated target. A diameter-reducing tie reduces graft diameter to allow minor repositioning of the device for optimal vessel alignment. This facilitates catheterization of target vessels. The proximal component is deployed only to the level of the SMA fenestration or branch, and use of the preloaded guidewire allows access the celiac and SMA from the brachial approach (Figs. 39.11 and 39.12). The preloaded catheters exit the device via an access scallop in the top part of the stent-graft. After guidewires are snared from the brachial approach, immediate access is obtained in the celiac and SMA fenestration or

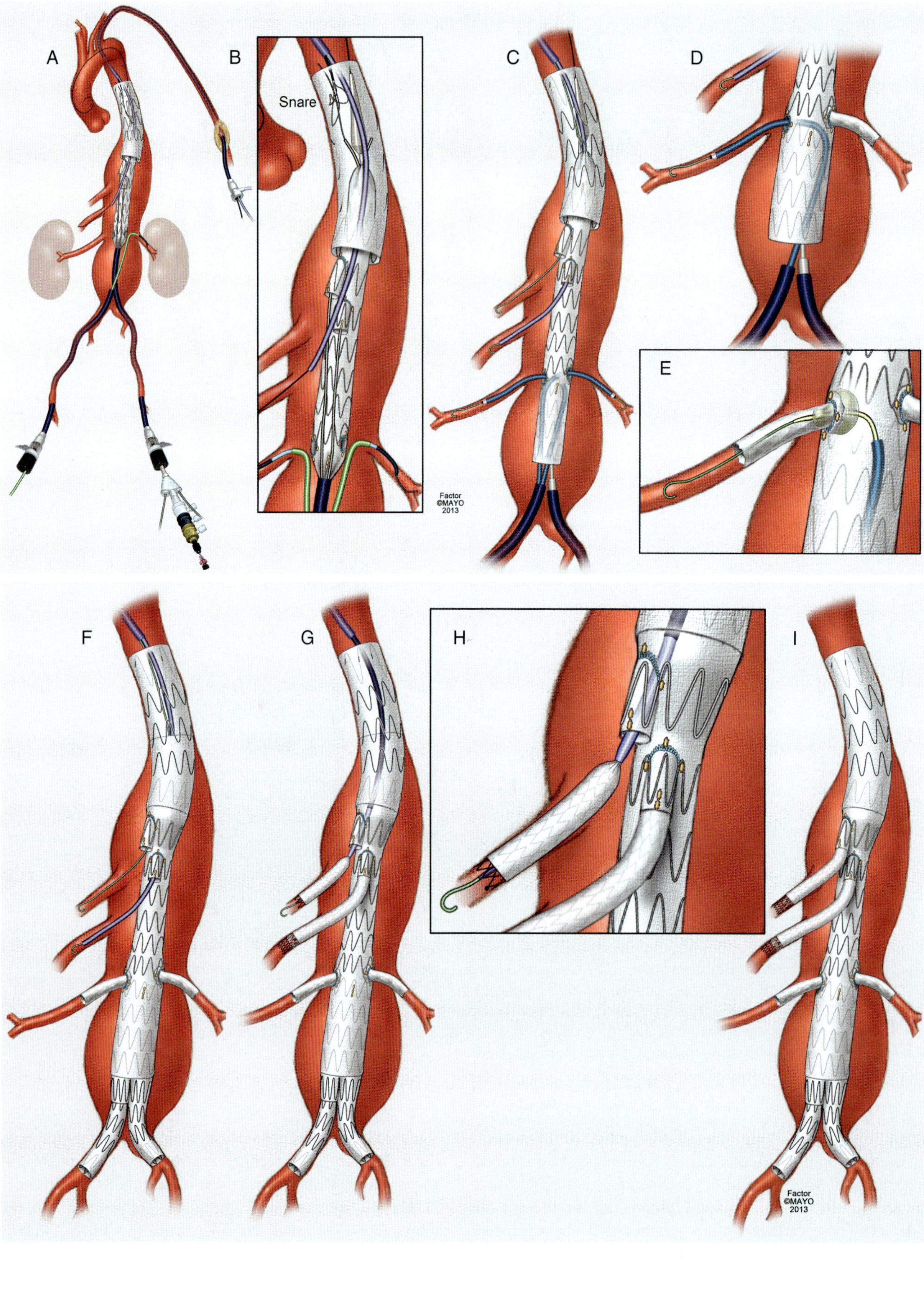
A
B
Snare
C
D
E
Factor
©MAYO
2013
F
G
H
I
Factor
©MAYO
2013

FIG 39.11 Technique of fenestrated-branched repair using design with two directional branches and two fenestrations stent-graft design has been used to treat complex thoracoabdominal aortic aneurysms. A proximal thoracic component is deployed first if needed (A). Precatheterization of at least one of the renal arteries is used to locate the target vessels using on-lay CT. The branched component is deployed up to the level of the renal fenestrations (A). Using preloaded catheters, guidewires are snared from the brachial approach (B), and the celiac axis and superior mesenteric artery (SMA) are catheterized from above. A sheath is typically placed into the SMA (C). The device is unsheathed completely (C) and the renal fenestrations and renal arteries are catheterized from the femoral approach. Hydrophilic sheaths are advanced into both renal arteries over 0.035-inch Rosen guidewires (C). Sequential renal artery stenting is performed using balloon-expandable covered stents (D), which are flared using a 10-mm angioplasty balloon (E). The bifurcated component and iliac limbs are deployed after placement of the renal stents (F). Flow is restored into both lower limbs. The procedure is completed by placement of the SMA and celiac self-expandable stents (G). Note that each stent is extended distally with a bare metal self-expandable stent (H). Final illustration depicts complete repair (I). (Used with permission of Mayo Foundation for Medical Education and Research. All rights reserved.)

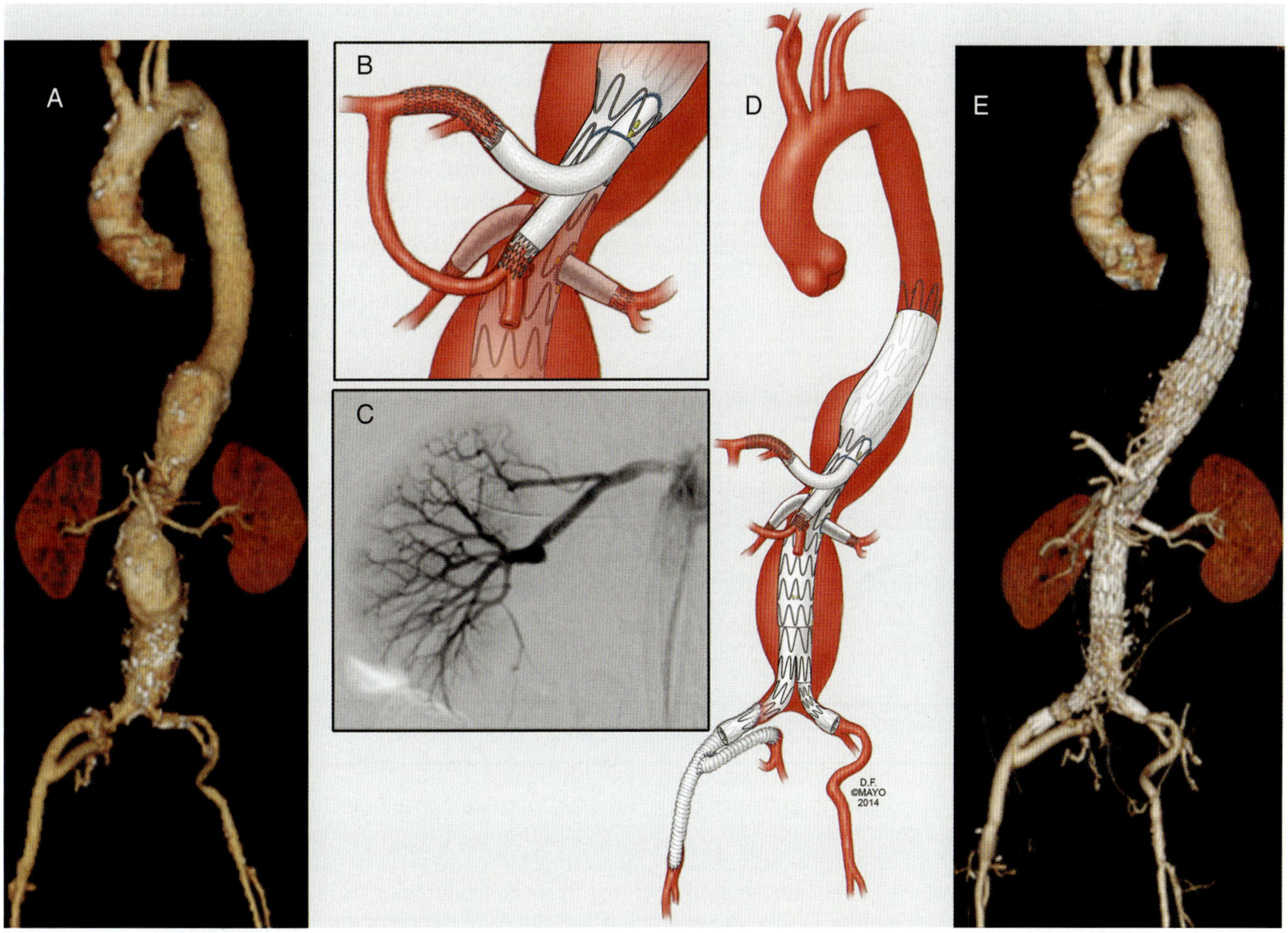

FIG 39.12 Computed tomography angiography (CTA) of a patient with type III thoracoabdominal aortic aneurysm (A). Note the renal arteries originate from narrow aortic segment and are transversely oriented. A design with two directional branches for the celiac and superior mesenteric artery and two renal fenestrations (B) allow optimal alignment with the target vessels. Renal angiography (C) confirms widely patent renal artery with no endoleak. Illustration depicts the complete repair (D), which is demonstrated on follow-up CTA (E). (Used with permission of Mayo Foundation for Medical Education and Research. All rights reserved.)

directional branch, and the vessel is catheterized with a "buddy" catheter. Stiff guidewires are positioned in the celiac axis and SMA, and a 7 French hydrophilic sheath is advanced into the SMA. The device is deployed distally, releasing the renal fenestrations. The renal artery fenestrations and renal arteries are catheterized from the femoral approach. Hydrophilic sheaths (7 French Ansel, Cook Medical Inc., Bloomington, IN) with flexible dilators are advanced into both renal arteries over Rosen guidewires.

The diameter-reducing tie is removed, allowing complete expansion of the device. The top cap is retrieved and the proximal landing zone is gently dilated using a compliable Coda balloon (Cook Medical Inc., Bloomington, IN). Alignment stents are sequentially advanced into the renal arteries and SMA under sheath protection. Deployment of side stents starts with the highest renal artery when using the femoral approach. For four-vessel designs with preloaded catheters, the renal arteries are done first, followed by placement of the bifurcated device while protecting both renal stents. After both iliac limb extensions are placed and the attachments are dilated with balloons, flow is restored to both lower extremities while guidewire access is maintained in the femoral arteries. The procedure is completed by placement of the SMA and celiac axis stents. In general, balloon expandable covered stents are used for fenestrations and self-expandable stent-grafts for directional branches. Prior to each stent deployment, the position of the stent is confirmed by hand injection and angiography is repeated after each stent is placed. For each fenestration, the stent is deployed 3 to 5 mm into the aorta and flared using a 10 mm × 2 cm balloon. Occasionally administration of 100 to 200 μg of nitroglycerin is used to minimize spasm.

Multibranched Stent-Grafts

Multibranched stent-grafts have down-going directional branches that are accessed via brachial approach using a 12-French sheath (Figs. 39.13 and 39.14). Device implantation does not require the same level of precision as described previously. Each cuff should be placed 1.5 to 2 cm above its intended target vessel. Once the target vessels are located, the multibranched stent-graft is deployed and the repair is extended distally using a bifurcated stent-graft and iliac limb extensions. The proximal and distal landing zones and attachment sites are gently dilated, and flow is restored to both lower extremities. The femoral arteries are closed and flow is restored into the lower extremities. Each directional branch and target vessel is sequentially catheterized, starting with the renal arteries, SMA, and celiac axis. Once the vessel is catheterized, the soft Glidewire is exchanged for a stiff guidewire, and a bridging self-expandable stent-graft is deployed from the target vessel to the directional branch cuff.

Fenestrations are typically aligned by balloon-expandable covered stents (Fig. 39.15). For directional branches, the author's preference is to use Gore Viabahn stent-grafts (WL Gore, Flagstaff, AZ) for the renal arteries because of excellent conformability and possible superior patency rates. For stenting of the celiac and SMA, Fluency stent-grafts (Bard Peripheral Vascular, Temple, AZ) are used because of smaller profile sheath with the larger diameter stents and greater availability of lengths. To prevent kinks in the transition of the stent-graft to the target artery, a self-expandable bare metal stent may be used. Each stent is balloon dilated to its profile, followed by a selective angiography. A completion angiography of the arch and thoracoabdominal aorta is obtained after all matting stent-grafts are deployed.

Physician-Modified Endovascular Grafts

Physician-modified fenestrated and branched stent-grafts have been widely utilized to treat high-risk patients who otherwise would not have access to manufactured stent-grafts, or those who cannot wait the time period required for device customization because of impending or contained ruptured, rapidly expanding, or excessively large aneurysm. Regulations on the use of device modifications are highly variable between centers and countries.

The same principles already described for manufactured devices should be used for PMEGs, including selection of landing zones, stent design, and implantation steps. Visceral artery incorporation is done using one of three types of modifications: reinforced fenestrations, mini-cuff fenestrations and directional branches (Figs. 39.16 and 39.17).

The author has used device modifications based on the Cook Zenith platform (Cook Medical Inc., Bloomington, IN), although others have reported modifications of any commercial devices. The Alpha thoracic low profile stent-graft (Cook Medical Inc.) is modified with fenestrations and/or directional branches to accommodate the renal-mesenteric arteries using the same

FIG 39.13 Multibranched stent-grafts are designed with four directional branches for the celiac axis, superior mesenteric artery (SMA), and both renal arteries. The procedure is done using bilateral femoral and left brachial access (A). One of the target vessels is catheterized (B) to guide deployment of the multibranched stent-graft (C). The distal bifurcated device and iliac limbs are added, and flow is restored to the lower limbs (D). Once all aortic components are deployed and blood flow is restored to the lower extremities, a small sheath is maintained in one of the femoral arteries for through-and-through access (E). Each branch is accessed via the brachial approach followed by placement of bridging stents into the target vessels (F), starting by the renal arteries, followed by SMA and celiac axis. A self-expandable bare-metal stent is added to avoid kink at the distal edge (G). The repair is completed by placement of all four side-branch stents (H). (Used with permission of Mayo Foundation for Medical Education and Research. All rights reserved.)

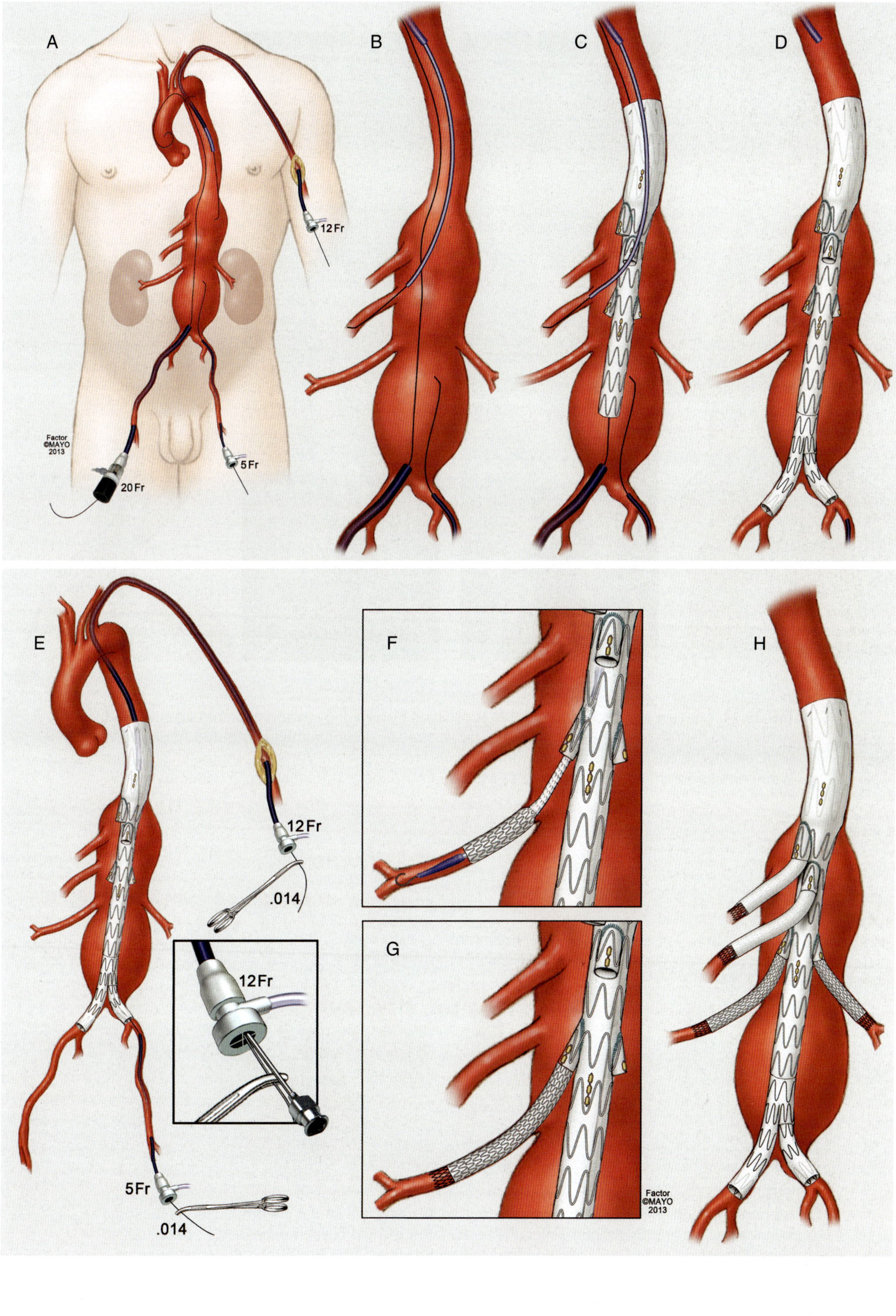
A
B
C
D
12 Fr
5 Fr
20 Fr
Factor
©MAYO
2013
E
F
G
H
12 Fr
.014
12 Fr
5 Fr
.014
Factor
©MAYO
2013

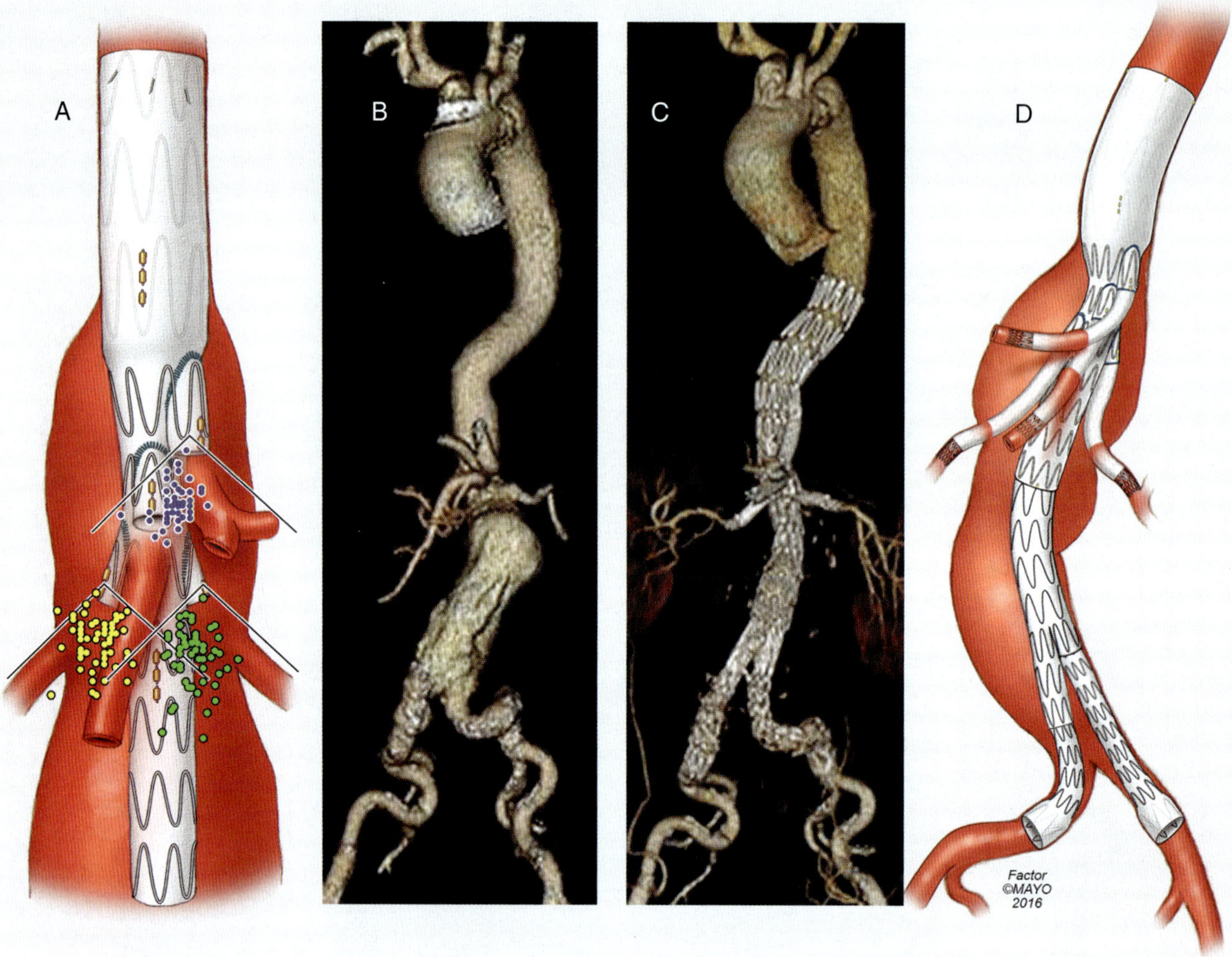

FIG 39.14 Directional branches have wide application by allowing incorporation of target vessels within a 90-degree angle from above (A). The illustration demonstrates computed tomography angiography before (B) and after (C) endovascular repair using t-Branch stent-graft (D). (Used with permission of Mayo Foundation for Medical Education and Research. All rights reserved.)

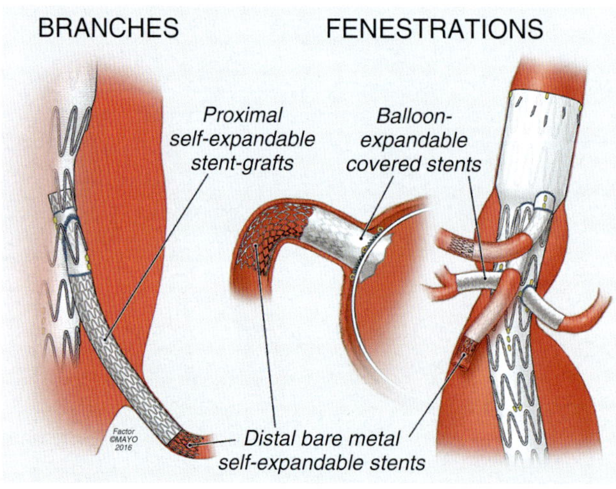

FIG 39.15 Selection of balloon-expandable covered stents for fenestrations and self-expandable stent-grafts for branches. Note that bare metal self-expandable stents are often used to reinforce distal branches and to prevent kinks after placement of rigid balloon expandable stents. (Used with permission of Mayo Foundation for Medical Education and Research. All rights reserved.)

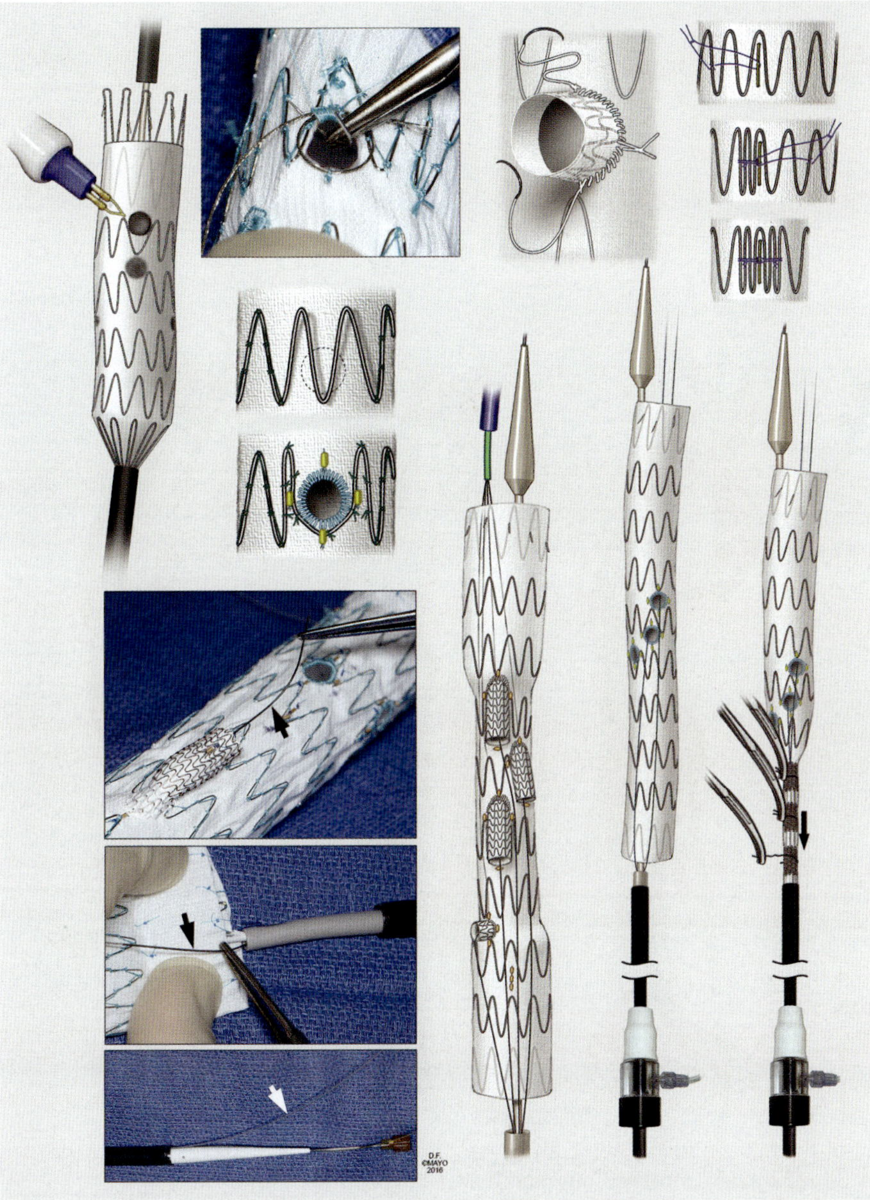

FIG 39.16 Modification of abdominal and thoracic aortic stent-grafts using ophthalmologic cautery to create fenestrations reinforced by nitinol ring. Directional branches and mini-cuffs are also used for target vessels that have origin from larger aortic diameter. The illustration also depicts the use of preloaded guidewires and resheathing of the device into the original delivery system. (Used with permission of Mayo Foundation for Medical Education and Research. All rights reserved.)

techniques already described for the TX2 stent-graft.[12] A Zenith abdominal stent-graft (Cook Medical Inc.) is modified by removing the uncovered stent to be used as a distal bifurcated device. Modifications such as reinforced fenestrations, mini-cuffs, directional branches, diameter-reducing wire, preloaded guidewires, and orientation markers can be made in the "back table." The stent-graft is resheathed into its original sheath by using 1-0 silk ties to sequentially collapse the Z stents. A large silastic vessel loop can be utilized to resheath branches and the proximal sealing stent, which contains barbs. The original sheath can accommodate four fenestrations or three fenestrations and one branch.

Parallel Grafts

Parallel grafts have been used as a bail-out for inadvertent coverage of side branches or to extent the proximal landing zone in patients with complex aneurysms (Fig. 39.18). Although several centers have used the technique electively, the author prefers fenestrated and branched stent-grafts for optimal sealing and reserves parallel grafts for exceptional situations in patients who are suitable candidates for fenestrated-branched grafts.

Parallel grafts have the advantage of wide availability by a combination of thoracic, abdominal, and bridging stent components as an off-label option to adapt to variable anatomical requirements. Ideally, a maximum of two parallel grafts should be used in single configuration to avoid "gutter" endoleaks. For pararenal aneurysms, two "chimney" stents can be placed in antegrade fashion via brachial access. In patients with TAAAs, most experts recommend two antegrade "chimney" or "sandwich" grafts for the celiac and SMA, while the renal arteries are incorporated using retrograde "periscope" grafts. Once bilateral femoral

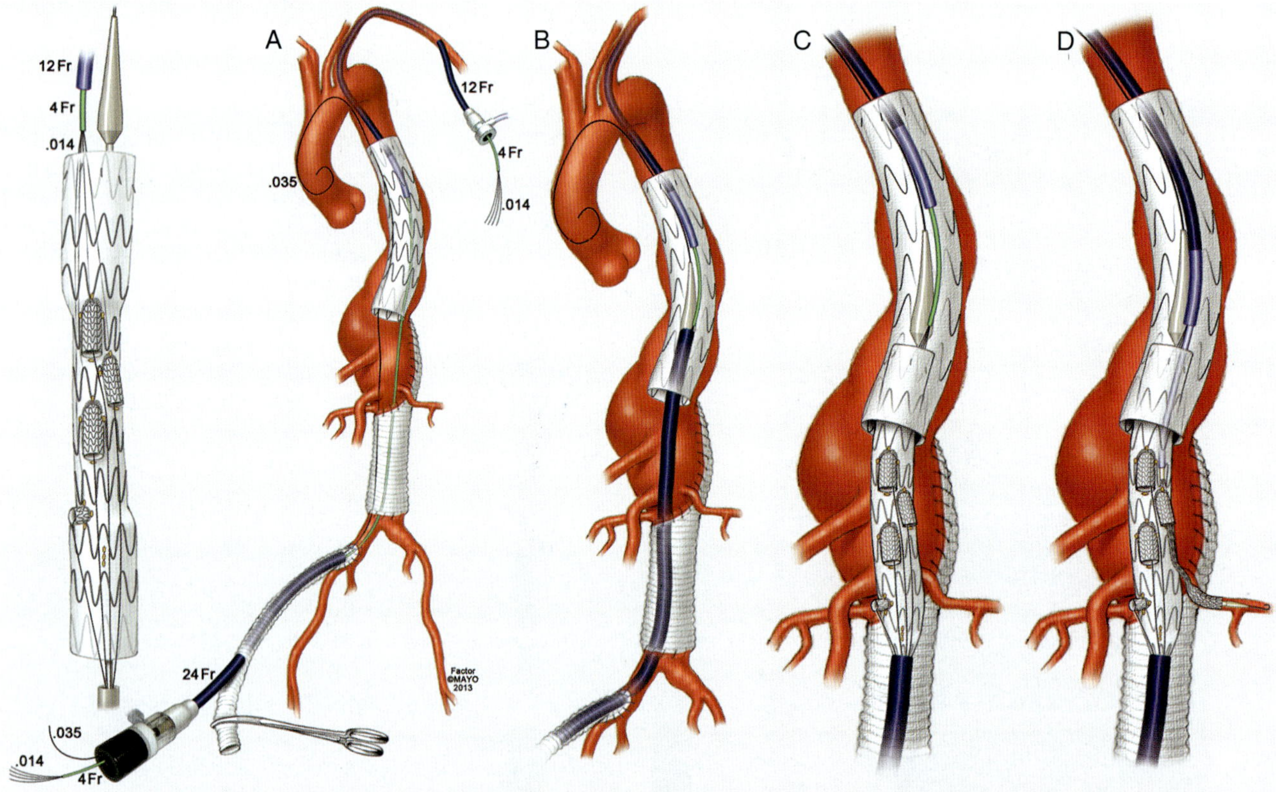

FIG 39.17 Endovascular repair of thoracoabdominal aortic aneurysm using directional branches with pre-loaded guidewires. A 36 × 32 × 157 mm TX2 stent-graft was deployed 6-cm proximal to the origin of the celiac axis (A). A 4 French *(Fr)* 110-cm sheath (Cook Medical Inc., Bloomington, IN) was introduced via the left brachial sheath and exteriorized via right iliac conduit (A). The branched TX2 stent-graft component was loaded over the Lunderquist wires, while the four preloaded 0.014-inch guidewires were loaded into the 4 Fr sheath (B). The TX2 stent-graft and the 4 Fr sheath were advanced to the visceral segment, and the stent-graft was deployed with the branches positioned 2 cm above each target vessel (C). The 4 Fr sheath was removed, and celiac axis, left renal artery, and superior mesenteric artery were sequentially catheterized using the preloaded guidewires (D). Each catheterization was facilitated by advancement of a 5 Fr shuttle sheath (Cook Medical Inc.) with a 0.018-inch dilator. (Used with permission of Mayo Foundation for Medical Education and Research. All rights reserved.)

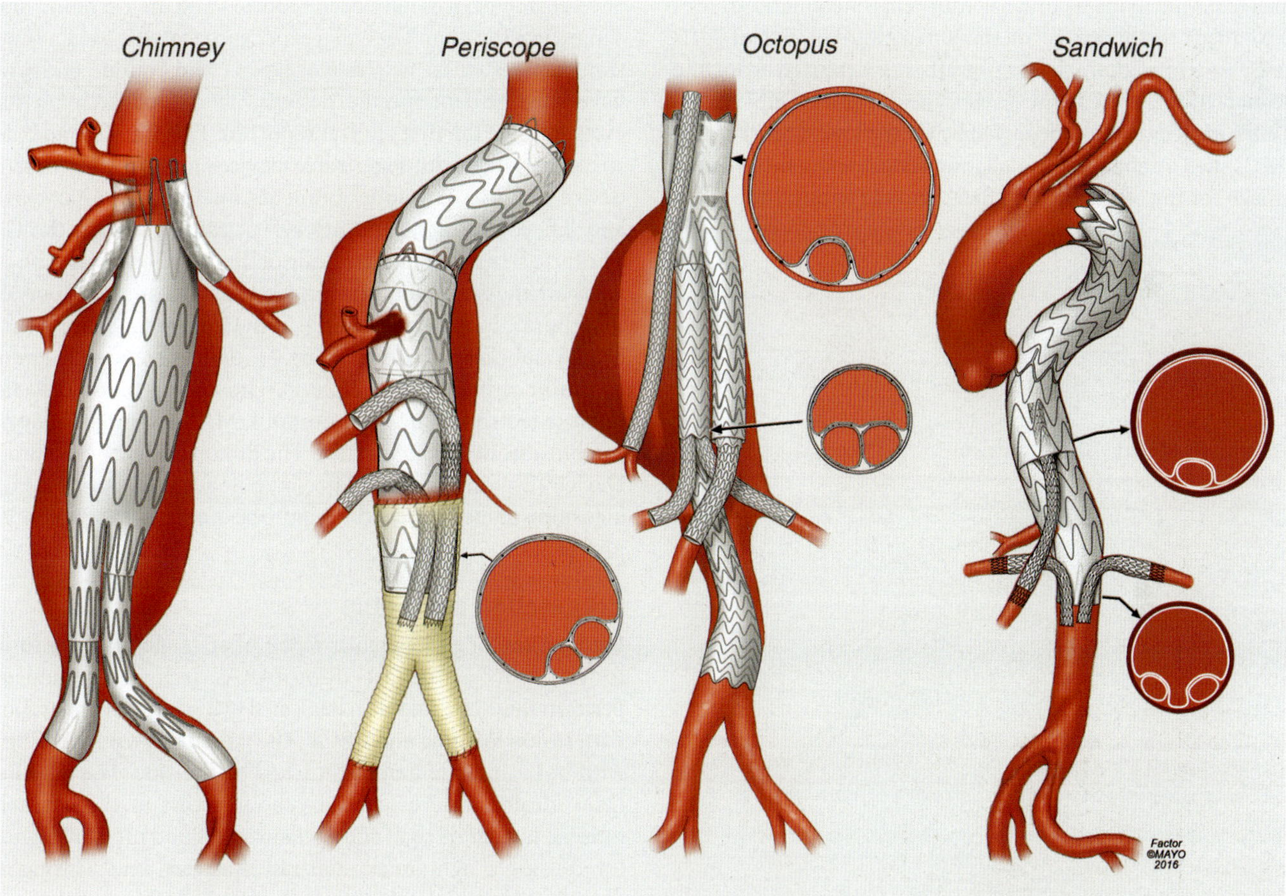

FIG 39.18 Parallel graft configurations for incorporation of renal-mesenteric arteries. (Used with permission of Mayo Foundation for Medical Education and Research.

and left axillary or brachial artery is established, each one of the target vessels is selectively catheterized and a 7 French hydrophilic sheath is advanced over a stiff guidewire. Covered self-expandable stents are positioned under protection of the sheath ready for deployment.

Pararenal aortic aneurysms or short-neck infrarenal aortic aneurysms are treated with one or two parallel grafts deployed from the brachial approach (Figs. 39.19 and 39.20). First the aortic stent-graft is deployed and gently dilated with a compliable balloon. Next both renal stents are sequentially deployed and dilated using a "kissing" balloon technique. Selective angiography of each renal artery is performed. The repair is extended distally using iliac limb extensions. TAAAs require a modification of the technique to incorporate all four renal-mesenteric arteries and to adapt to the extent of the aneurysm. For Extent I–III TAAAs, proximal thoracic stent-grafts are deployed from the proximal landing zone to the level of the celiac axis (Fig. 39.21), and a bifurcated device is deployed below the lowest renal artery. Access is then established into all four vessels, using the brachial approach for the celiac axis and SMA and the femoral approach for the renal arteries. Once the bridging stents are positioned into all four vessels ready for deployment, a thoracic stent-graft is placed between the proximal thoracic and distal abdominal stent-grafts, with minimum overlap of 5 cm with the parallel stents. Each parallel stent-graft is sequentially deployed. Any flow abnormalities to the renal-mesenteric branches should be aggressively treated by repeat angioplasty and reinforcement stents. In order to avoid gutters and endoleaks, 30% oversize is recommended for the aortic component.

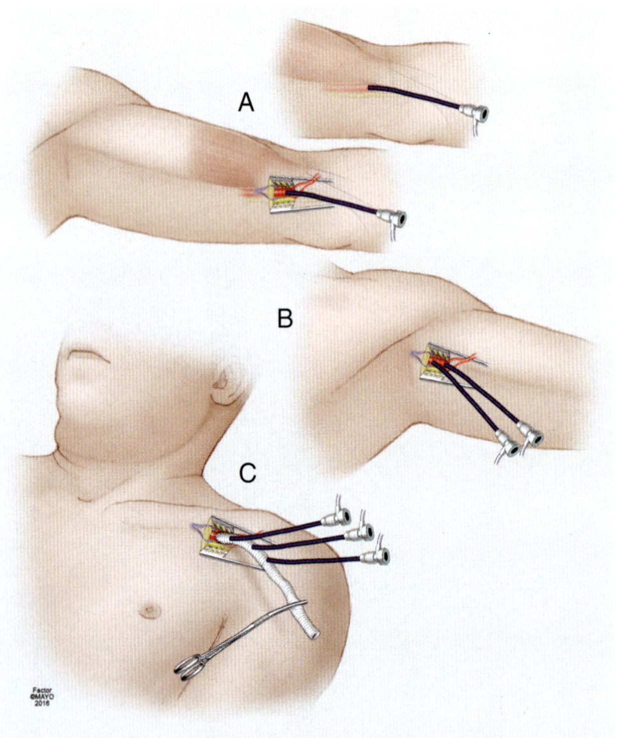

FIG 39.19 Small incision over palpable brachial artery near antecubital crease can be used when only single snorkel/chimney sheath is necessary (A). Skin incision via a high brachial incision near the axilla exposes the proximal brachial artery often giving adequate size for double puncture (B). Infraclavicular incision to expose the axillary artery necessary when three or four snorkel/chimney sheaths needed (C). A 10 mm or 12 mm Dacron conduit can be sewn into the axillary artery in this position. (Used with permission of Mayo Foundation for Medical Education and Research. All rights reserved.)

AORTIC ARCH ANEURYSMS

Specific Designs

Several arch devices have been reported and are currently under clinical investigation. The Asian experience with the Najuta (Kawasumi Laboratories Inc., Tokyo, Japan) and Innoue endografts have used patient-specific designs. The Cook arch platform evolved since the first clinical report by Tim Chuter and extensive experience with fenestrated devices to a newer generation device that uses two inner branches for the innominate artery and left common carotid artery.[21–23] More recently, the Gore Thoracic Branch Endoprosthesis (TBE, WL Gore, Flagstaff, AZ) is an off-the-shelf stent-graft designed with an inner portal to incorporate a single arch vessel, in the innominate artery (Zone 0), left subclavian artery (Zone 2), or less frequently the left common carotid artery (Zone 1). The Valiant Mona LSA Stent Graft (Medtronic, Inc., Minneapolis, MN) is a modular system modified from Valiant Captiva. The Bolton Medical Arch Branch Device (Bolton Medical, Barcelona, Spain, and Sunrise, FL) is a custom-made branched design based on the Relay NBS Plus platform.

Preparation and Setup

Preparation for endovascular repair of arch aneurysms is similar to what has been described for TAAAs. It is recommended to perform these operations in dedicated hybrid endovascular rooms with fusion imaging and CBCT. The patient is positioned supine with both upper extremities tucked by the side. The anesthetic team ideally achieves central venous access in the left upper internal jugular or right subclavian vein. Blood pressure is monitored using a right and/or left radial arterial line. Throughout the procedure, meticulous and thorough flushing of the endovascular equipment is performed to ensure that no air bubbles are introduced in to the aortic arch.

Subclavian Artery Revascularization

A left carotid to subclavian artery (LSA) transposition or bypass is performed prior to the arch branch graft repair. The revascularization can be done at the same time as the arch repair, or in a staged fashion. If a bypass is performed, the most proximal aspect of the LSA should be occluded proximal to the vertebral artery origin with coils or endovascular plug. If the procedure is done in a single stage, our preference is to leave the proximal subclavian artery open in case access to the internal branch from the left CCA is not possible, in which case we would switch to LSA access.

Text continued on p. 605

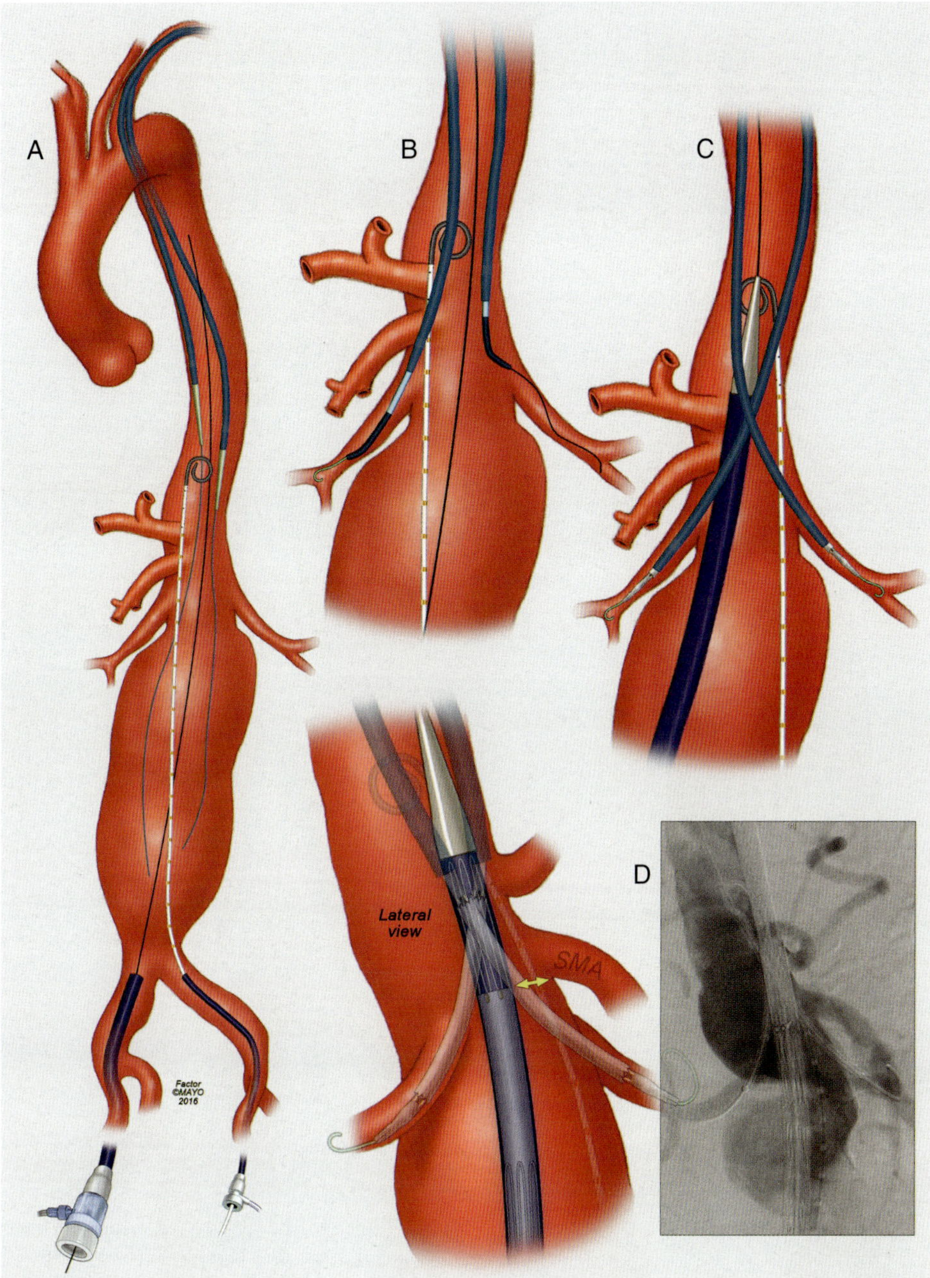

FIG 39.20 Technique of single or double snorkel grafts for treatment of juxta-renal abdominal aortic aneurysms. Two 7 French Terumo sheaths placed from arm access down descending thoracic aorta ready to be positioned near visceral aortic region (A). Right renal artery cannulated with glide wire and JB1 catheter (B). A flush catheter from below reveals in an angiogram the position of the left renal artery to be cannulated next. Both snorkel iCAST stents in position from arm approach along with main body endograft being put into position (C). Lateral view angiogram shows takeoff of superior mesenteric artery *(SMA; yellow arrow)* and positioning of the main body endograft fabric edge *(yellow arrow)* immediately below SMA (D). *Continued*

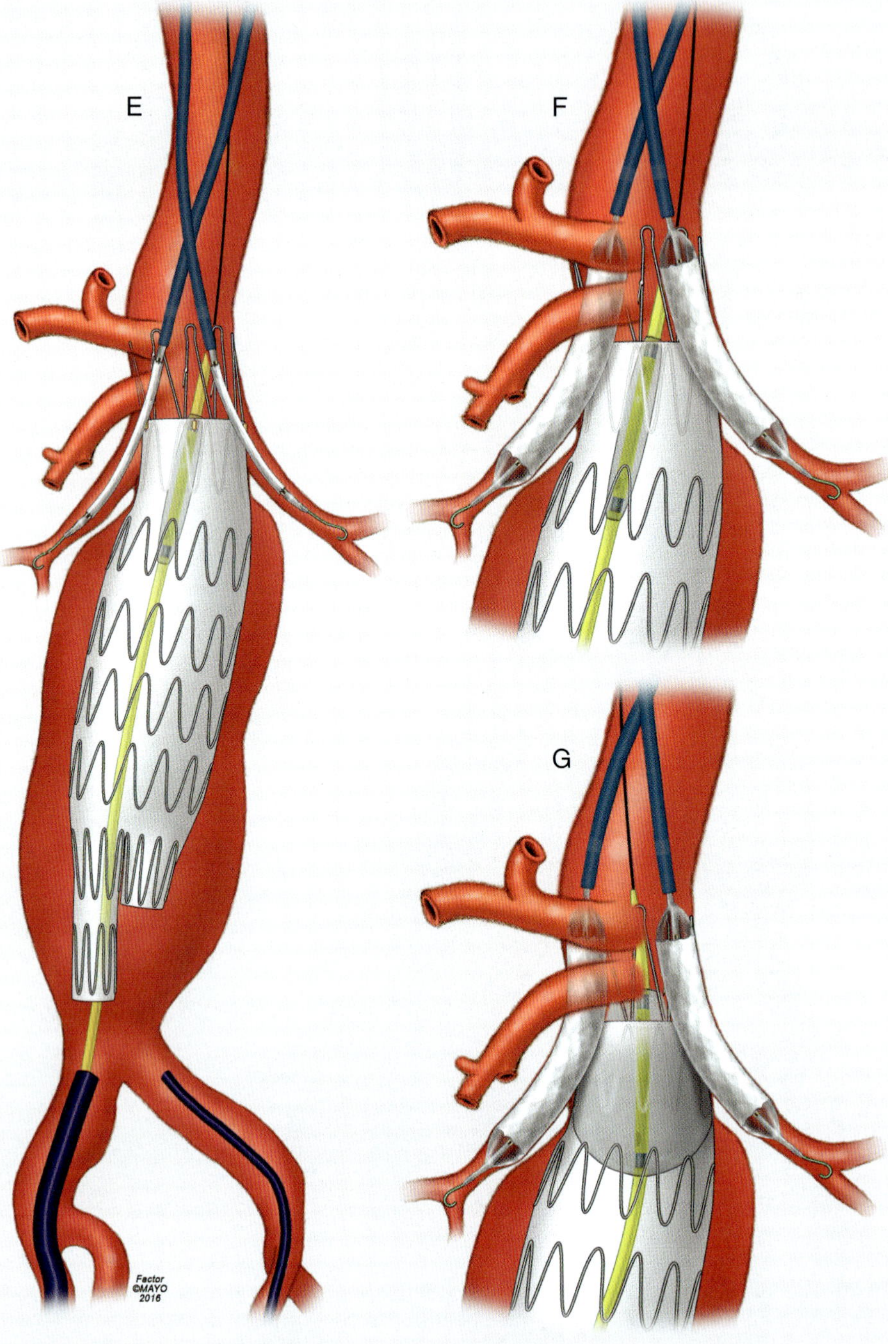

FIG 39.20, cont'd Main body endograft deployed in anteroposterior view with snorkel stents in position (E). After cannulation of contralateral gate and advancement of proximal molding balloon into aortic stent, the two snorkel stents are fully inflated (F).

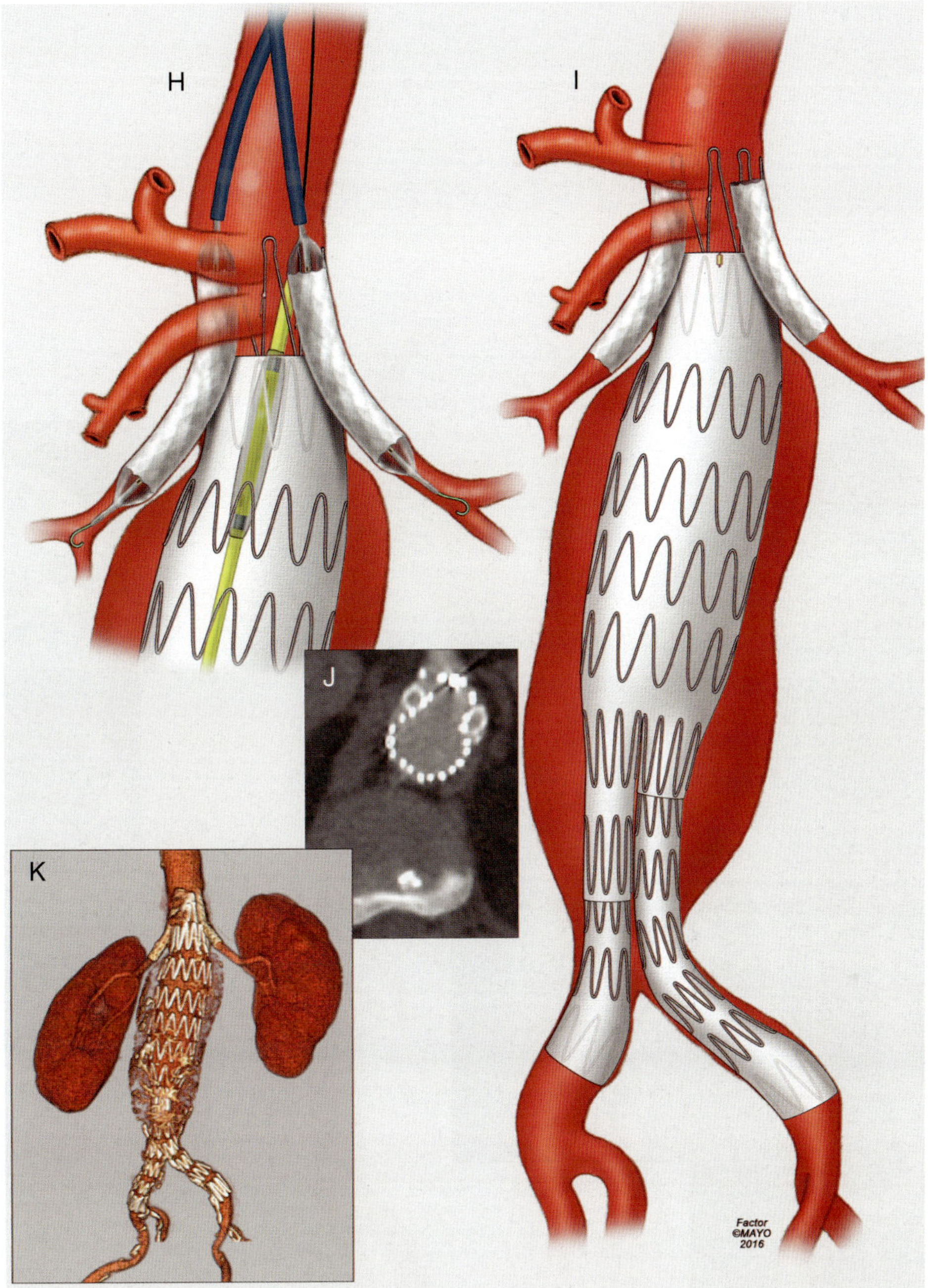

FIG 39.20, cont'd The molding balloon is then maximally inflated to profile and to minimize gutters (H). The molding balloon is completely deflated prior to snorkel stent balloon deflation (I). Postoperative computed tomography-A axial view showing molding of main body endograft around two widely patent snorkel stents (J). Three-dimensional reconstruction demonstrating excellent perfusion of both kidneys and no evidence of endoleak (K). (Used with permission of Mayo Foundation for Medical Education and Research. All rights reserved.)

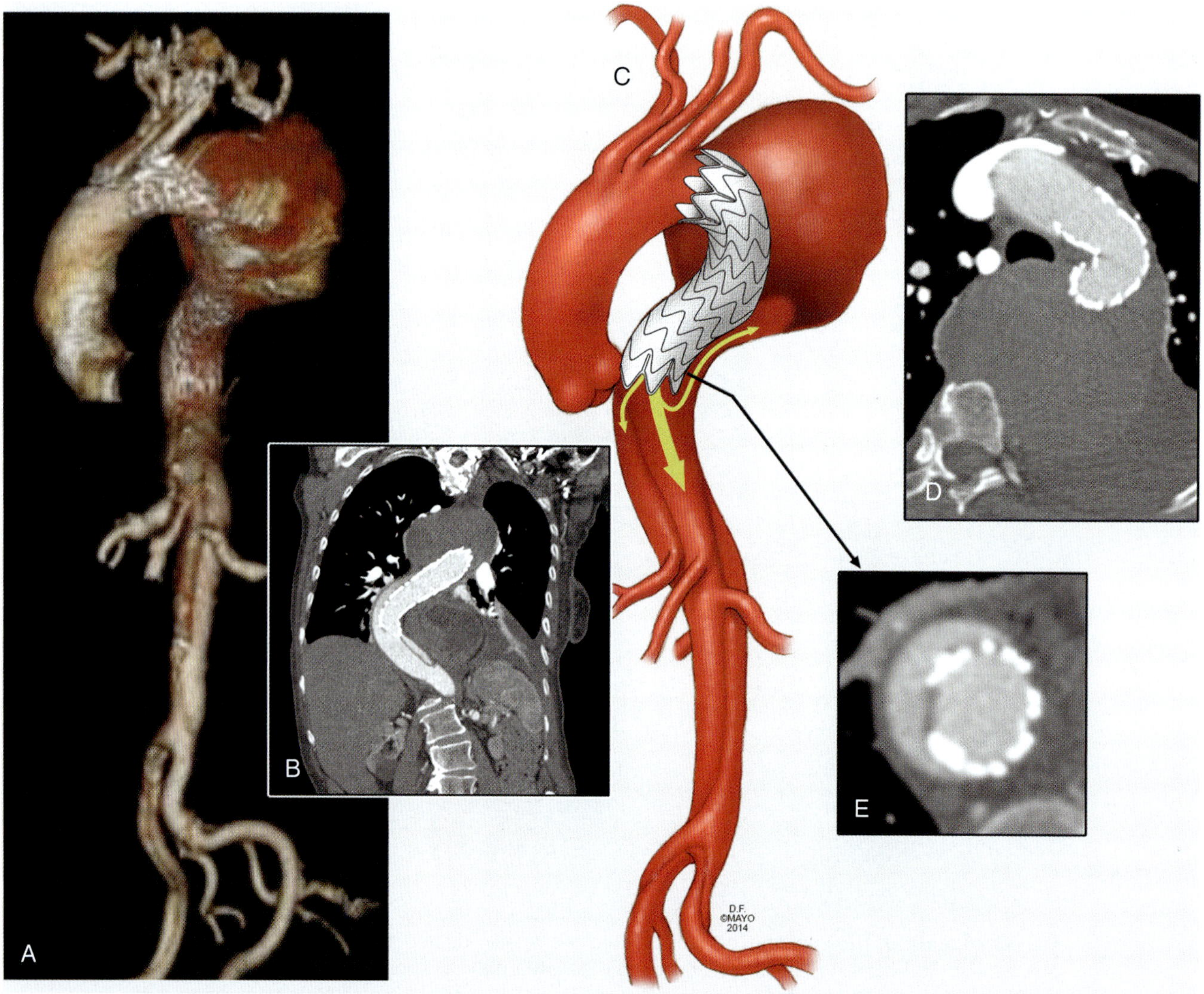

FIG 39.21 Computed tomography of a patient with contained rupture thoracoabdominal aneurysm and chronic dissection (A and B). Note the pressurized false lumen after thoracic aneurysms and dissections, endovascular repair (C and D), and mediastinal hematoma (E).

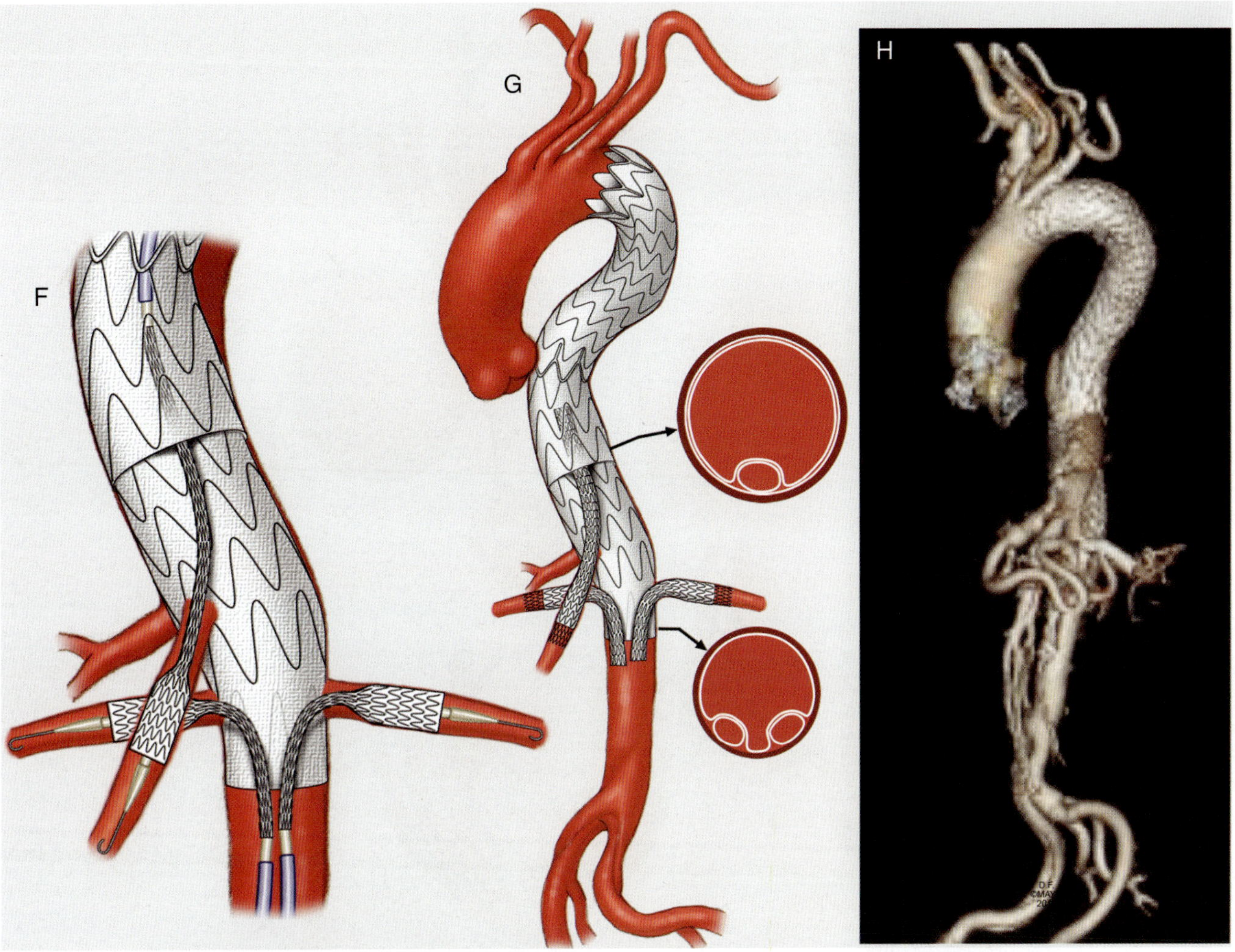

FIG 29.21, cont'd The patient was treated by sandwich graft to the superior mesenteric artery (F) and bilateral retrograde renal periscopes (G), resulting in successful exclusion of the ruptured aneurysm (H). (Used with permission of Mayo Foundation for Medical Education and Research. All rights reserved.)

Arterial Access

Arterial access is obtained in three locations: femoral (main device), right common carotid (innominate branch), and left brachial artery (left carotid branch). Reduction of cardiac-output is required during deployment of the aortic branch stent-graft, which is done using rapid ventricular pacing. After systemic heparin is administered, a target ACT greater than 300 seconds is maintained throughout the case. Right carotid access is obtained using a short 5 French sheath. Left axillary or upper brachial artery access is obtained using a short 10 French sheath, which is advanced through the LSA bypass. Using the femoral approach, a long 260 cm hydrophilic guidewire and 5 French 100 cm vertebral catheter are advanced and used to gently navigate through the aortic valve and into the left ventricle. The wire is exchanged for a curly (Curved or Extended Curved) Lunderquist Extra-Stiff Wire Guide (Cook Medical, Inc.).

Cook Inner Branch Arch Stent-Graft

The aortic arch device is advanced and positioned with the proximal sealing stent at the level of the proximal ascending aorta (Fig. 39.22). The tapered short tip of the delivery system must be advanced through the aortic valve and into the left ventricle. An angiogram is performed to check the position of the coronary arteries and supra-aortic trunks relative to the radiopaque markers, which should be positioned upstream of the innominate and left common carotid artery. The device is deployed under rapid pacing. The graft is unsheathed in its entirety, and normal cardiac output is resumed. The stiff guidewire and tapered delivery tip are then withdrawn from the left ventricle and positioned within the distal end of the endograft.

The right carotid artery is cross-clamped, and the first inner branch is cannulated in retrograde fashion using angled hydrophilic guidewire. The guidewire and catheter are positioned in the left ventricle, and exchanged for a 0.035 J-tipped Rosen wire. A useful maneuver is to inflate a 12-mm balloon in the inner branch to demonstrate catheterization. A modified Zenith iliac limb is advanced over the Rosen wire and deployed from the first inner branch to the innominate artery. Following balloon dilatation and angiography, flow is restored into the right common carotid artery, the sheath is removed, and the arteriotomy is closed. The second, more distal inner branch is catheterized

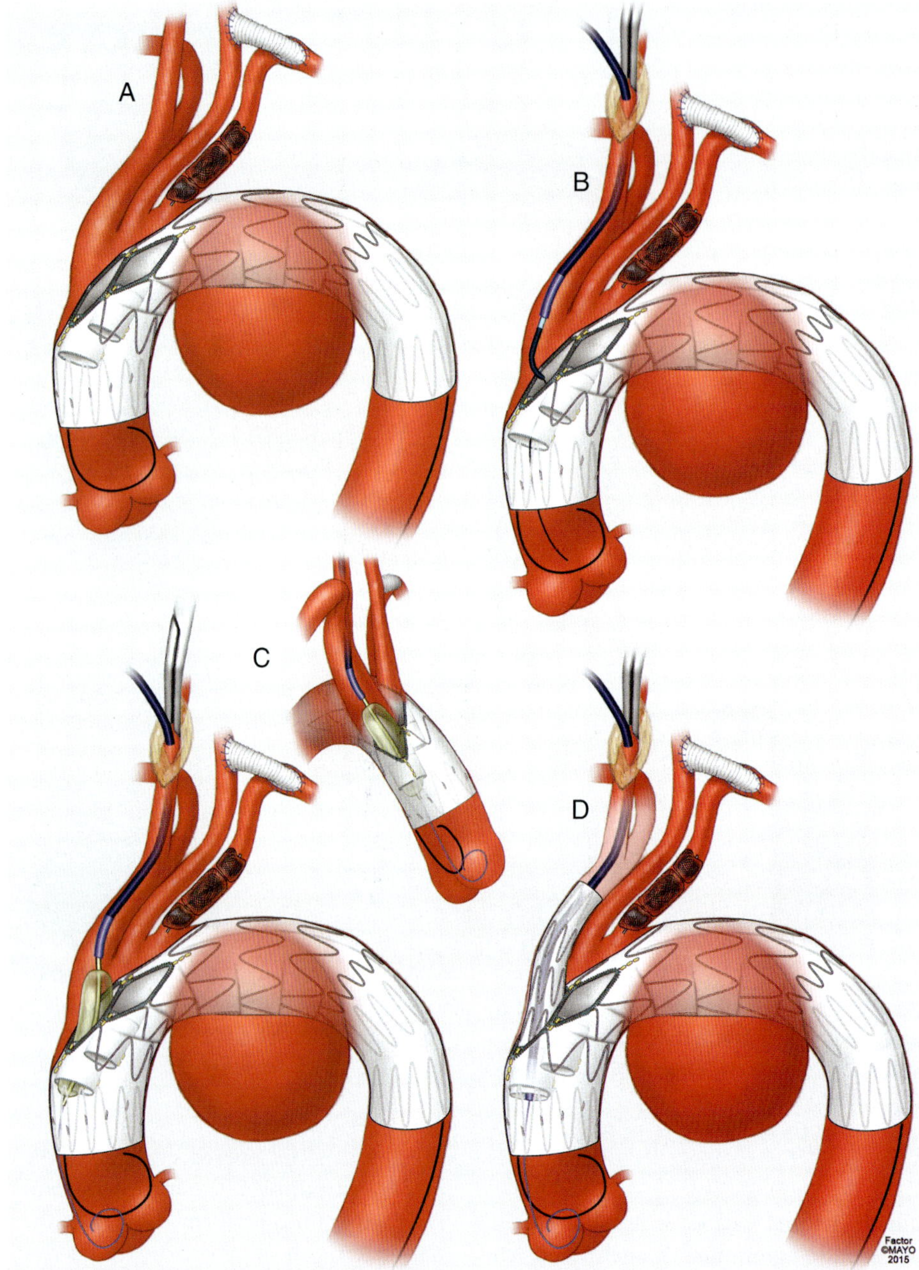

FIG 39.22 Deployment of the a-Branch stent-graft (A), followed by retrograde access of the right common carotid artery (CCA) via direct puncture (B). The innominate artery is catheterized using a soft-angled guidewire, which is exchanged for a Rosen wire. A balloon is inflated and the gantry is moved to right anterior oblique position to confirm that the correct inner branch has been cannulated (C). Stenting of the innominate artery is one using a modified iliac limb (D), noting that the right CCA is clamped during this portion of the procedure to avoid embolization. A completion angiography is done to document patency, the sheath is removed, and flow is restored to the right CCA.

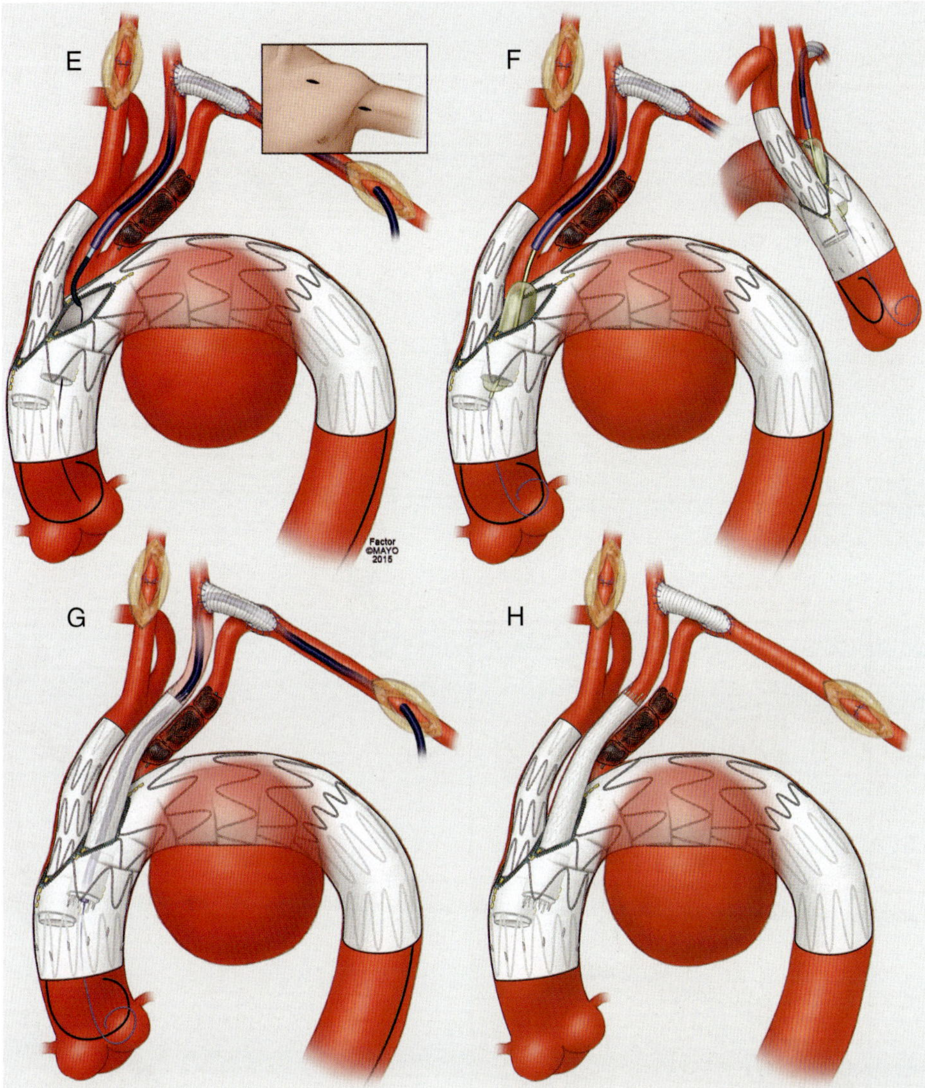

FIG 39.22, cont'd Access is established in the axillary artery using either an infra-clavicular or high upper brachial incision (E). A soft, angled Glidewire is used to catheterize the distal inner branch. The guidewire is exchanged for a Rosen wire, and an 8-mm balloon is inflated into the branch to confirm correct position in left anterior oblique position (F). A 10 French flexor sheath is advanced into the left common carotid artery and inner branch, followed by deployment of a self-expandable fluency stent-graft, which is reinforced by self-expandable bare metal stent (G). If needed, the repair is extended into the thoracic aorta, followed by completion angiography (H). (Used with permission of Mayo Foundation for Medical Education and Research. All rights reserved.)

from the left axillary artery access using guidewire and catheter as previously described. Balloon inflation maneuver is used to confirm correct cannulation, followed by placement of a bridging self-expandable covered stent-graft from the inner branch to the left common carotid artery. The distal end of the main body of the a-Branch stent-graft may need to be extended in to the descending thoracic aorta, depending on the extent of the aneurysm and location of the distal sealing zone.

Gore Thoracic Branch Endoprosthesis

The Gore TBE (Fig. 39.23) has been designed using the C-TAG platform and inner portals with a specially designed side branch stent-graft intended for the left subclavian (Zone 2) or innominate artery (Zone 0). Arterial access is established using bilateral femoral and left transbrachial approach for Zone 2 and right transbrachial approach for Zone 0. A 22 or 24 French DrySeal sheath (Gore, Flagstaff, AZ) is used for delivery of the TBE, and a contralateral 6 French femoral sheath is placed for diagnostic angiography. A curly Lunderquist wire is positioned in the ascending aorta using the technique previously described. The left brachial artery is surgically exposed just proximal to the antecubital crease and access is established. A catheter is advanced from the brachial approach to the descending thoracic aorta and snared from the femoral approach to establish brachial-femoral

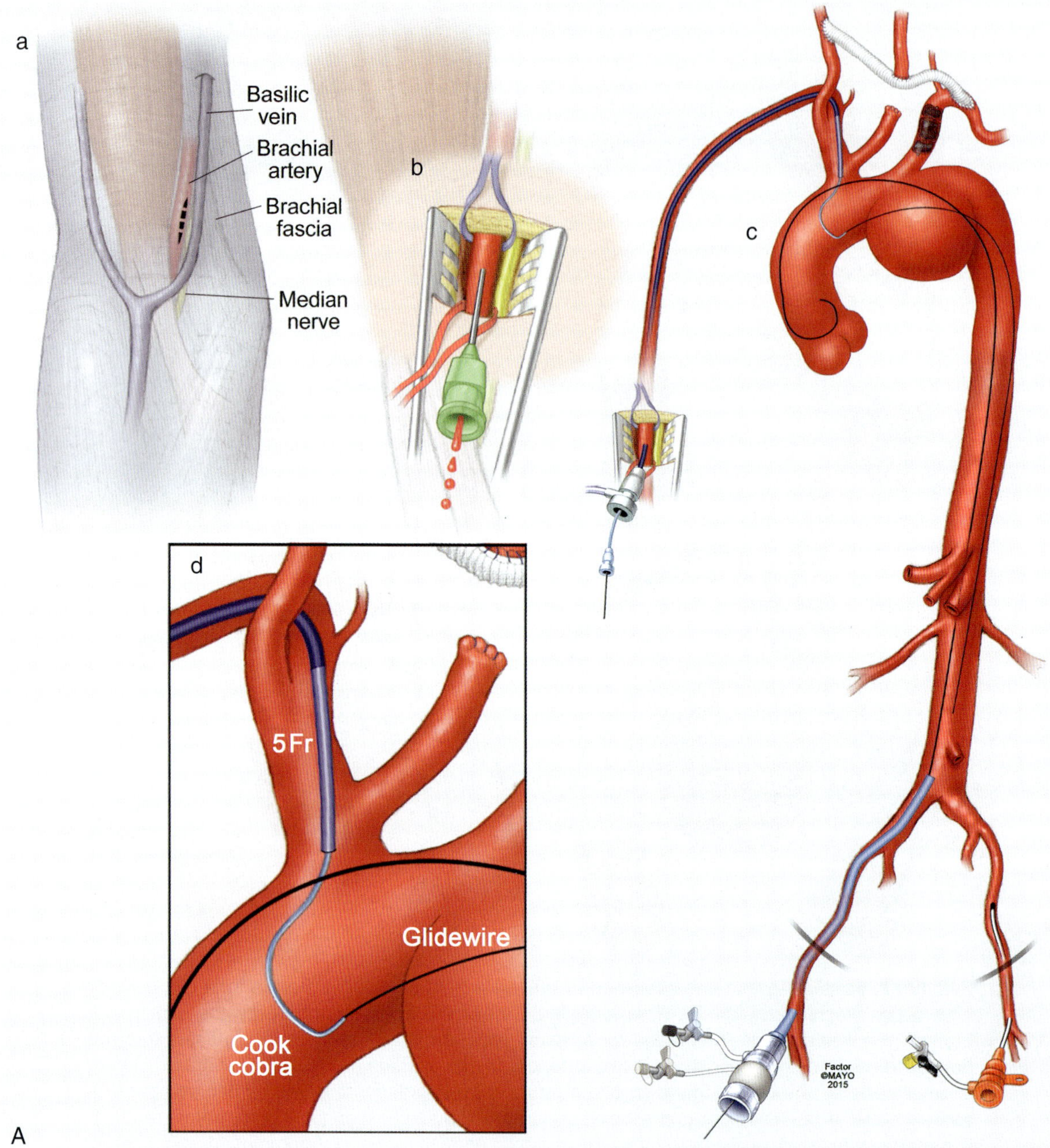

FIG 39.23 Technique of arch repair in Zone 0 using the the Gore Thoracic Branch Endoprosthesis. (A) The brachial artery is exposed in the lower arm via small incision (a) and access is established using micropunctured set (b). A C2 catheter is used to selectively catheterize the thoracic aorta (c and d).

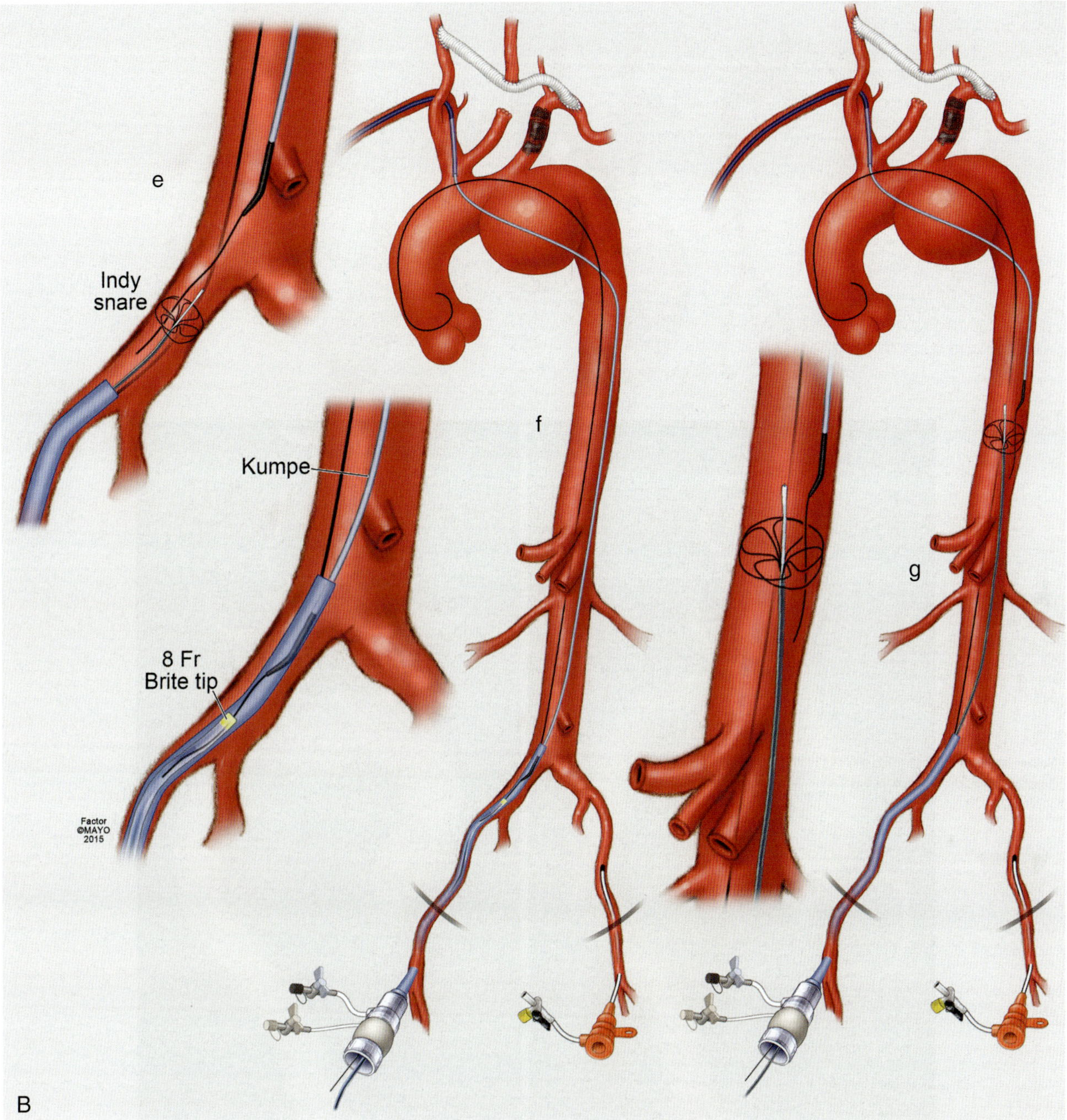

FIG 39.23, cont'd (B) The wire is snared in the iliac artery (e) or exteriorized via the sheath (f). Alternatively snaring can be done in the thoracic aorta (g). *Continued*

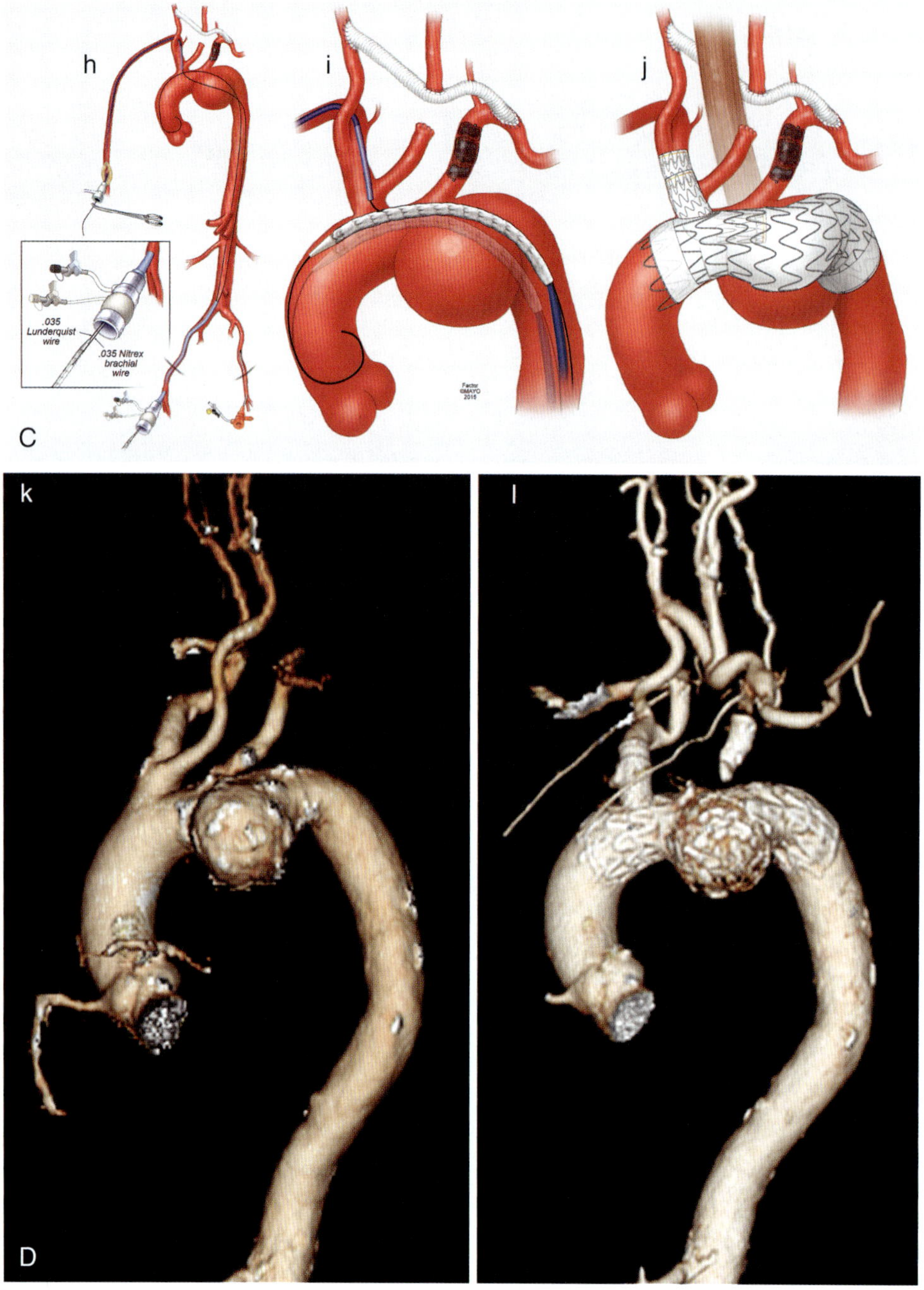

FIG 39.23, cont'd (C) The device is loaded in the aortic guidewire and in the brachial-femoral wire (h), advanced into position (i), and deployed. The bridging stent is deployed into the innominate artery (j). (D) Computed tomography angiography before (k) and after the repair (l). (Used with permission of Mayo Foundation for Medical Education and Research. All rights reserved.)

access. For Zone 2 repairs, a left brachial sheath is positioned in the LSA and can be used for small volume angiographies during deployment of the device. The TBE is advanced over the Lunderquist guidewire and deployed precisely with the inner side portal facing the LSA origin. The TBE delivery system is removed over the Lunderquist wire, allowing room in the femoral sheath for advancement of a 14 French DrySeal sheath through the portal and into the LSA. A bridging stent is positioned and deployed to extent the repair from the portal to the LSA without covering the left vertebral artery. A similar technique is used for Zone 0 TBE, except that staged carotid-carotid crossover bypass and left common carotid-subclavian bypass is needed. For deployment of the TBE device, right brachial approach is used for brachial-femoral guidewire access. The device is deployed with the portal under the origin of the innominate artery.

Parallel Arch Stent-Grafts

Parallel grafts for aortic arch aneurysms apply similar techniques already described for TAAAs and are dependent on the number of supraaortic trunks requiring revascularization and the configuration of the branch component (antegrade or retrograde). The author has used the technique mostly as a "bail-out" due to inadvertent coverage of one of the supra-aortic trunks or selectively to extend the landing zone across one of the branches using cervical debranching if more than one vessel requires coverage. For Zone 2 or Zone 1 arch deployment, access is established into the left upper extremity using the transbrachial approach (Fig. 39.24). A hydrophilic sheath is positioned across the target vessel alongside the aortic stent-graft. The thoracic endograft is advanced into position in the aortic arch and deployed just distal to the origin of the left common carotid artery (Zone 2) or innominate artery (Zone 1), covering the origin of the LSA or left common carotid artery, respectively. The sheath is withdrawn to expose the bridging stent, which is deployed into the target vessel. A short balloon-expandable covered stent (e.g., iCAST, Atrium Maquet, Hudson, NH) is preferred for short segments ("chimneys"). It is critical that the proximal intraaortic end of the chimney stent be positioned several greater than 10 mm proximal to the proximal-most fabric edge of the aortic stent-graft to ensure optimal intake of blood flow into the LSA branch.

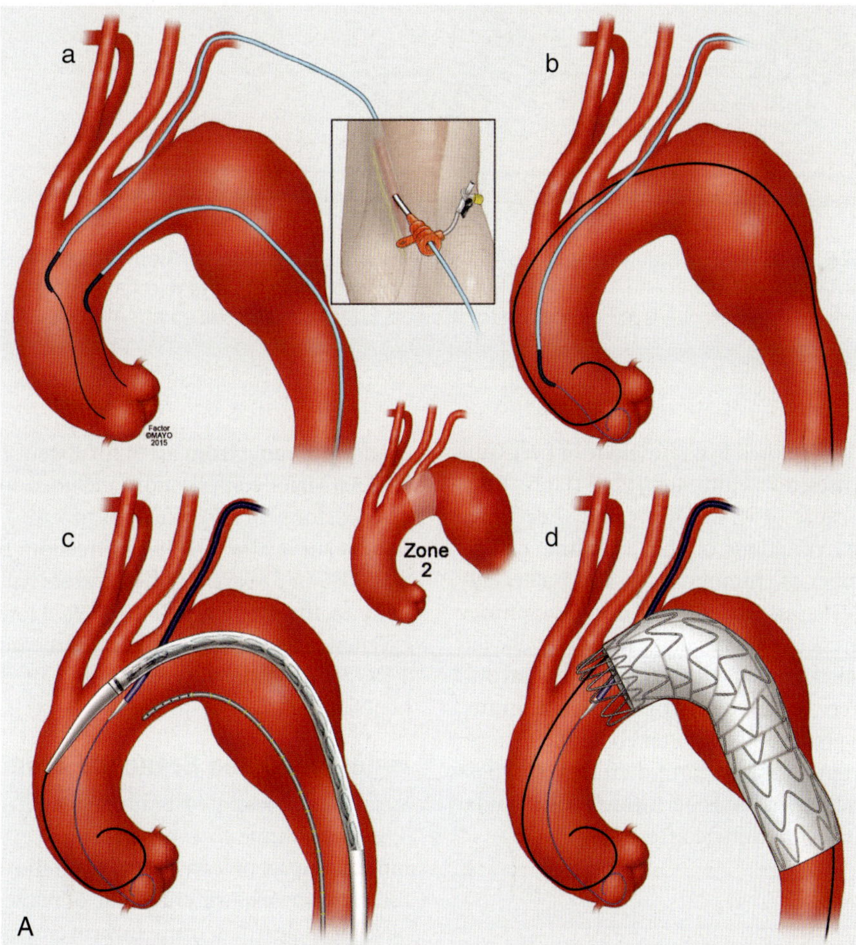

FIG 39.24 (A) Technique of parallel stent-graft for Zone 2 thoracic endovascular aortic repair. (a) Access is established using transbrachial percutaneous *(inset)* or surgical cut-down exposure. (b) Glidewire is exchanged for a 0.035-inch stiff wire for advancement of a thoracic stent-graft. (c) The thoracic endograft and left subclavian artery (LSA) chimney stent have been delivered to the target position, and (d) the thoracic device has been deployed. *Continued*

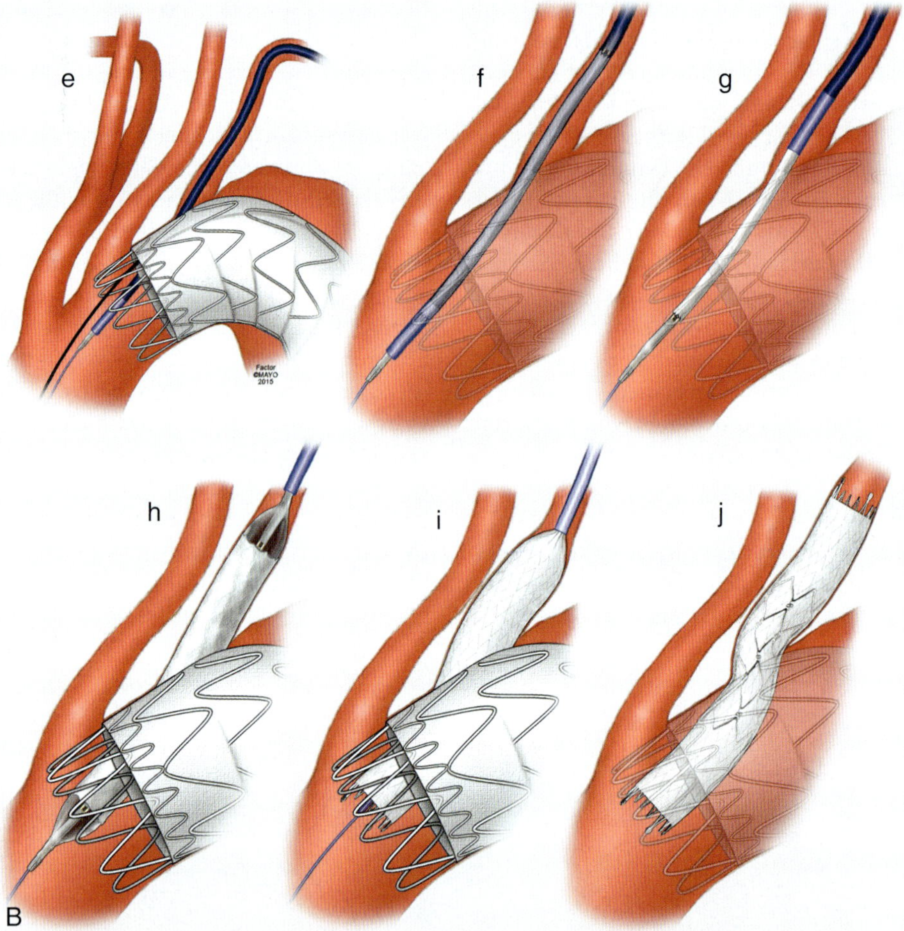

FIG 39.24, cont'd (B) Deployment of LSA chimney covered stent (e–h). Self-expanding stent is used for larger vessels (i) and should be reinforced with balloon expandable bare metal stent (j). (Used with permission of Mayo Foundation for Medical Education and Research. All rights reserved.)

Parallel grafts can also be deployed in a retrograde or periscope configuration. For these cases, a Viabahn stent-graft (Gore, Flagstaff, AZ) is preferred because of its flexibility and wide range of diameters and lengths. Variations of this technique can be used to decrease the number of chimney grafts and potentially the risk of gutter endoleaks associated with double chimney grafts. The author's preference is to use a left carotid-subclavian bypass and a single parallel graft to the left common carotid artery or innominate artery, rather than double parallel grafts, which are associated with greater risk of gutter endoleaks. Therefore, for Zone 0 deployment, a staged carotid crossover bypass with left subclavian revascularization is performed, followed by a single parallel graft to the innominate artery (Fig. 39.25).

RESULTS

Thoracoabdominal Aortic Aneurysms

Open surgical repair of TAAAs has been performed in large tertiary care centers with satisfactory results. Coselli and associates reported a landmark experience with 3309 open surgical TAAA repairs over 30 years. Operative mortality was 7.5% in 30-days, ranging from 5.1% for Extent IV to 8% for Extent I–III TAAAs. Major complications included spinal cord injury in 9.6%, tracheostomy in 8.5%, dialysis in 7.6%, and major stroke in 3%. Patient survival was 64% and freedom from aortic repair failure was 98% in 5 years.[24] Other centers have reported 30-day mortality in the range of 8% to 15%. However, outside centers of excellence results are dismal.[25] Rigberg and colleagues reported 19% 30-day mortality for repair of TAAA among Medicare beneficiaries.[26]

Fenestrated and Branched Stent-Grafts

Results of fenestrated-branched stent-grafts for pararenal and TAAAs continue to evolve. Clinical experience has shown significant impact of learning curve on mortality, morbidity, contrast use, radiation exposure, and rate of reinterventions. Several lessons have been learned from improvements in device design and delivery system. The technique can be performed with high technical success (>95%) and a mortality rate that averages 1% to 3% for pararenal and 3% to 10% for TAAAs.[27–32]

The Cleveland Clinic reported one of the first prospective studies in 119 patients treated by fenestrated endografts between

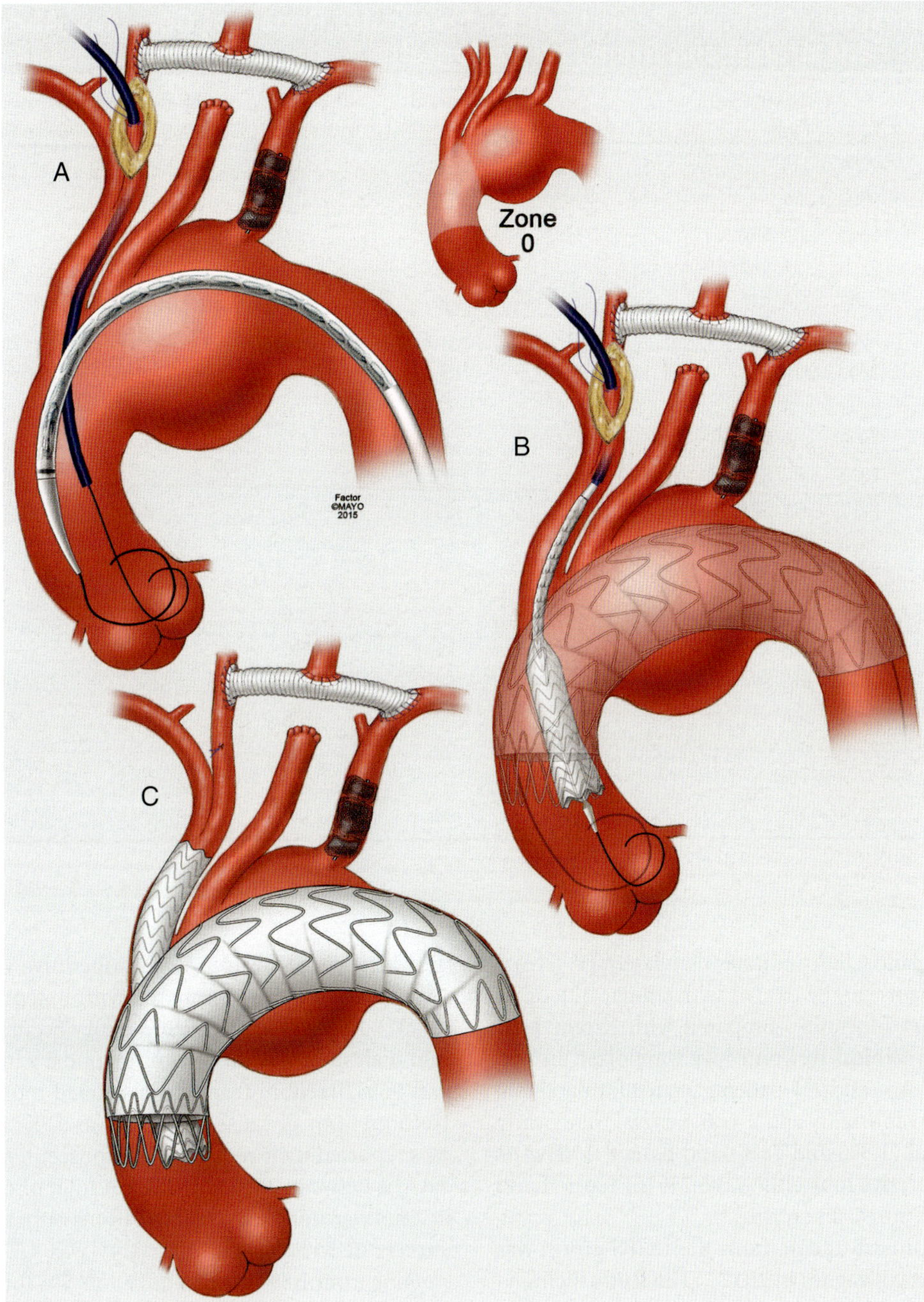

FIG 39.25 Surgical crossover bypass to the left common carotid artery (LCCA) and to the left subclavian artery (A). Deployment of the IA stent is completed (B). The right common carotid artery (RCCA) puncture is surgically repaired to reestablish normal antegrade flow immediately (C). (Used with permission of Mayo Foundation for Medical Education and Research. All rights reserved.)

2001 and 2005.[33] Procedural success was 100%, and 30-day mortality was 0.8%. The Western Australia group reported a series of 58 patients from seven centers with technical success of 91% and 30-day mortality of 3.4%.[34] Since these pioneering reports, several contemporary studies have shown 30-day mortality rates in the range of 0% to 3.5% for pararenal aortic aneurysms (Table 39.1).[11,30,32–44] Type I and III endoleaks are infrequent, and midterm target branch vessel patency is exceptionally high. The United States Zenith fenestrated trial included 67 patients treated by fenestrated stent-grafts for short neck infrarenal aneurysms with up to three fenestrations. Operative mortality was 1.5%, renal occlusion was 4%, and there was one type I endoleak at 3 years of follow-up.[45]

The complexity of an endovascular repair using fenestrated and branched endografts has been associated primarily with the extent of aortic coverage, the number of vessels requiring incorporation into the repair, and the difficulties imposed by the inability to access the aorta and target arteries. A recent clinical

TABLE 39.1 **Results of Clinical Reports of Endovascular Repair of Complex Abdominal Aortic Aneurysms With Fenestrated and Branched Endografts**

Author	Year	Aneurysm Type	*n*	Vessels	Technical Success (%)	30-Day Mortality (%)	Endoleaks (%)	Branch Patency (%)	Follow-Up (Months)
Greenberg et al.	2004	JRA	32	83	100	3.1	6.50	98	9.2
O'Neil et al.	2006	JRA	119	302	100	0.8	25	92	19
Semmens et al.	2006	JRA, SRA	58	116	91	3.4	7	95	24
Muhs et al.	2006	JRA, SRA	38	87	94	2.6	24	92	25
Ziegler et al.	2007	JRA, SRA	63	122	97	1.5	19	92	23
Scurr et al.	2008	JRA	45	117	—	2.0	0	97	24
Beck et al.	2009	JRA	18	56	100	0.0	—	95	23
Greenberg et al.	2009	JRA	30	54	100	0.0	60	94	24
Kristmundsson et al.	2009	JRA	54	134	98	3.7	31	96	25
Amiot et al.	2010	JRA, SRA	134	403	99	2.0	18	97	15
Haulon et al.	2010	JRA, SRA	80	237	99	2.5	11	95	10
Verhoeven et al.	2010	JRA	100	275	99	1.0	—	94	24
Tambyraja et al.	2011	JRA	29	79	—	0.0	21	—	20
GLOBALSTARCollaborators	2012	JRA, SRA	318	889	75	3.5	16	99	21
Starnes et al.	2012	JRA	47	82	98	2.0	13	—	20
Grimme et al.	2014	JRA, SRA	138	392	98	1.4	16	95	13
Oderich et al.	2014	JRA	67	178	100	1.5	—	97	37
Mastracci et al.	2015	JRA, Extent IV TAA	610	1463	97	2.3	10	96	96
Oderich et al.	2016	JRA, SRA	47	181	99	0	46	97	10

JRA, Juxtarenal aneurysm; *SRA*, suprarenal aneurysm; *TAA*, thoracoabdominal aneurysm.

update from the Cleveland Clinic indicates that Extent IV TAAAs and pararenal aneurysms can be treated with similar outcomes and significantly lower mortality compared with Extent I–III TAAA. In that study, clinical outcomes were reported in 406 patients treated for TAAAs and 227 patients treated for pararenal aneurysms. The 30-day mortality and 2-year survival were nearly identical for pararenal (1.8% and 78%) and Extent IV TAAAs (2.3% and 82%). Operative mortality was 5.2% for types II and III thoracoabdominal aortic aneurysms.[28]

The most recent clinical update from the UCFS group was reported by Reilly and colleagues in 2012.[46] The study included 81 patients with mean age of 73 years old treated by multibranched stent-grafts with 306 target renal-mesenteric arteries. Operative mortality was 6%, including three perioperative deaths (4%) and two late treatment related deaths. Spinal cord injury occurred in 24% of patients, including 5% paraplegia and 19% transient paraparesis. Four patients (5%) required dialysis, which was permanent in three. After a mean follow-up of 21 months, there were no aneurysm ruptures. Thirty-two patients (40%) required secondary interventions to treat endoleak or branch-related complications.

Results of contemporary reports of endovascular repair of TAAAs are summarized in Table 39.2. Thirty-day mortality ranges from 0% to 9% in the largest series, with spinal cord injury in 0% up to 17%. Eagleton and colleagues reported the largest experience, including 354 patients treated for Extent II–III TAAAs by fenestrated and branched endografts between 2004 and 2013. Technical success was 96%. Perioperative mortality was higher for Extent II (7.6%) compared with Extent III TAAAs (3.5%, $P < .001$). Permanent spinal cord injury occurred in 4% of patients and dialysis in 3%. At 3 years, secondary branch vessel patency was 96%, freedom from aortic-related mortality was 91%, and freedom from all-cause mortality was 51%.[47] Oderich and associates reported their results in 185 consecutive patients treated for TAAAs between 2007 and 2015. A total of 686 renal-mesenteric arteries were targeted by fenestrations or branches, with technical success of 94%. Overall mortality was 4.3% for entire cohort, ranging from 1.8% for Extent IV to 8.2% for Extent I–III TAAAs. Mortality decreased in the second half of experience from 7.5% to 1.2% ($P < .05$), including a decline in mortality from 3.3% to 0% for Extent IV and 16% to 2% for Extent I–III TAAAs. Spinal cord injury occurred in 2% of patients treated for Extent I–III TAAAs. At 5 years, patient survival was 59% and freedom from reintervention was 53%.[48]

The Mayo Clinic group reported the 1-year results of 127 patients enrolled in a prospective, nonrandomized study to evaluate four-vessel fenestrated and branched endografts for pararenal and TAAAs.[49] All patients had stents based on supra-celiac sealing zone with ≥4 vessels in 111 patients (89%). There were 47 pararenal, 42 Extent IV, and 38 Extent I–III TAAAs with a total of 496 renal-mesenteric arteries were incorporated (mean, 3.9 ± 0.5 vessels per patient). Technical success of target vessel incorporation was 99.6% (n = 493/496). There were no 30-day or in-hospital deaths, dialysis, ruptures, or conversions to open

TABLE 39.2 Clinical Results of Endovascular Repair of Thoracoabdominal Aortic Aneurysms Using Fenestrated and Branched Stent-Grafts

Author	Year	Aneurysm Type	*n*	Target Vessel	Technical Success	30-Day Mortality	30-Day Morbidity	Spinal Cord Injury *(%)*	Dialysis
Anderson et al.	2005	TAAA	4	13	92	25	25	0	0
Roselli et al.	2007	TAAA	73	—	93	5.5	14	2.7	1.4
Chuter et al.	2008	TAAA	22	81	100	9	41	—	—
Gilling-Smith et al.	2008	TAAA	6	—	100	0	16.7	0	0
Ferreira et al.	2008	TAAA	11	43	100	18	45	27	0
Bicknell et al.	2009	JRA, TAAA	15	40	98	0	33.4	6.7	6.7
Mohabbat et al.	2009	JRA, TAAA	287	518	98	4.2	—	—	3
Verhoeven et al.	2009	TAAA	30	97	93	6.7	43	16.7	3.3
Amiot et al.	2010	JRA, SRA, TAAA	134	403	99	2	12	0.7	4.5
Haulon et al.	2010	JRA, SRA, TAAA	80	237	99	2.5	11	1.3	4
Haulon et al.	2010	TAAA	33	116	98	9	—	12	9
Greenberg et al.	2010	JRA, TAAA	633	—	—	5.7	—	4.3	0.3
Metcalfe et al.	2012	JRA, SRA, TAAA	42	95	98	7	—	2	2
Guillou et al.	2012	TAAA	89	292	98	8.9	—	7.8	6.7
Ferreira et al.	2012	TAAA	48	—	—	—	—	2	8.5
Panuccio et al.	2015	JRA, TAAA	150	523	99	3	—	—	—
Eagleton et al.	2016	TAAA	354	1305	96	4.8	40	8.8	2.8
Oderich et al.	2016	TAAA	80	315	99	0	21	1.2	8.7

JRA, Juxtarenal aneurysm; *TAAA*, thoracoabdominal aortic aneurysms.

surgical repair. Major adverse events occurred in 27 patients (21%). Two patients had paraplegia, including one treated for Extent IV and one who had Extent II repair. There were no patients were lost to follow-up, which averaged 9 ± 7 months. Twenty-three patients (18%) had reinterventions (15 aortic, 8 non-aortic), seven renal artery stents were occluded, five patients had type Ia or III endoleaks, and none had aneurysm sac enlargement. Primary and secondary target vessel patency was 96 ± 1% and 98 ± 0.7% at 1 year. Freedom from any branch instability and any reintervention was 93 ± 2% and 81 ± 4% at 1 year, respectively. Patient survival was 96 ± 2% at 1 year for the entire cohort.

The choice of design and bridging stent is variable between investigators. In general, fenestrations are aligned by a balloon expandable covered stent, whereas branches are targeted by self-expandable stents. The use of a covered stent has the advantages of optimal seal, minimizing risk of endoleak, and improved patency rates, likely due to the occurrence of neointimal hyperplasia in the proximal aspect of bare metal stents.[50] Differences in angulation along with branch stent length have a direct impact on branch durability. In the study of Reilly and colleagues[46] (using down-going branches with self-expandable stents), occlusion rate was 9.5% for renal and 2% for mesenteric arteries. Mastracci and colleagues[51] reported a large experience with 650 patients treated by fenestrated-branched stent-grafts for TAAAs. In that study, 1679 visceral branches were evaluated. The most common stent-graft design consisted of two down-going branches for the celiac and SMA, and two fenestrations for the renal arteries. Whereas fenestrations rely on a nitinol ring and may be more prone to type III endoleak with large TAAAs, these allow a very short branch configuration, which is especially suited for renal arteries that have a neutral or up-going configuration. The renal artery occlusion rate was significantly lower at 1.7%, as compared with the rate reported by Reilly and colleagues[46] with no difference for mesenteric arteries. These two large single-center experiences demonstrate that there is not a single design that can be applied to all patients. Instead, individually adapting the best design to the patient anatomy, with directional branches and/or fenestrations, using custom-made or off-the-shelf designs, is likely the best strategy.

The most feared and vexing complication of TAAA repair is spinal cord injury. Regardless of the type of approach utilized, open or endovascular, paraplegia is a devastating complication for the patient, the family, and the medical team caring for these patients. Several factors have been demonstrated to affect rates of spinal cord injury. The single most important is the extent of aortic disease, with the highest rates observed for Extent II TAAAs. Greenberg and colleagues[52] compared rates of spinal cord injury among 724 patients treated by open or endovascular approach. In that study, there was a nonsignificant trend toward lower rates of spinal cord injury with endovascular (4.3%) as compared with open repair (7.8%). Extent of aneurysm was the most important independent predictor of spinal cord injury. For Extent II TAAAs, both open (22%) and endovascular (19%) were associated with high rates of spinal cord injury. Subsequently, Eagleton and colleagues[53] presented the results of 1251 patients enrolled in a physician-sponsored IDE protocol over the last 10 years, with an overall rate of spinal cord injury of 2.9%. Rates were 0.3% for abdominal, 0.5% for pararenal, 5.2% for thoracic, and 5% for TAAAs. The authors found that the presence of a single collateral bed occlusion (e.g., subclavian or iliac artery) predicted immediate onset of paraplegia and the lack of recovery. A reason for improved results may be the more frequent use of a staged approach to cover the intercostal arteries, along with better techniques of implantation.

The rationale for a staged coverage of the intercostal arteries has been supported by the concept that an extensive collateral network can be progressively recruited over a period of days to a few weeks.[54] In a chronic porcine model, staged segmental ligation of the intercostal arteries over a period of 1 week was associated with no occurrence of paraplegia.[55–57] Bischoff and colleagues reported a prospective, randomized study comparing single stage versus two-stage coverage or ligation of segmental intercostal arteries in a porcine model. In that study, 20 pigs had coverage of all thoracic intercostal arteries in one or two stages with monitoring of collateral network perfusion pressures. In the group treated in a single stage, collateral network pressure decreased to 34% of baseline values, as compared to 55% in the two-stage group. There was no paraplegia in the staged group, compared with 50% paraplegia rate in the single stage group.[54] Staged approaches to endovascular TAAA repair include the use of staged coverage of the thoracoabdominal aorta in two or more procedures, the use of perfusion branches, and the use of one of the visceral branches to perfuse the aneurysm sac. The Cleveland Clinic group has reported on the use of staged coverage of the thoracoabdominal aorta. The first stage includes placement of proximal stent-grafts from the subclavian to the celiac axis, depending on the extent of the aneurysm. After a period of 4 to 6 weeks, which is typically required for manufacturing of a custom-made device, the second stage is performed with the placement of a fenestrated-branched stent-graft and distal bifurcated device. Using this technique, Eagleton and colleagues reported a remarkably low spinal cord injury rate of 5% for TAAAs.[53]

Perfusion branches imply the use of additional directional branches directed to perfuse the aneurysm sac. Typically these devices include at least two branches positioned in the thoracic or abdominal component. The branches are left patent for 2 to 3 weeks, after which endovascular plugs are placed under local anesthesia to occlude the perfusion branch.[58] Based on current experience, endovascular repair of thoracoabdominal aortic aneurysms carries operative mortality in the range of 0% to 18% and results in spinal cord injury in 0% to 17% of patients.[28,50,59–67]

Parallel Stent-Grafts

The clinical data is scarce for parallel stent-grafts. Study limitations are relative small number of patients, short follow-up, and variations in techniques, extent of aneurysm, and types of stent-grafts used for parallel configurations. The largest collective worldwide experience, the PERICLES Registry, included 517 patients treated by parallel stent-grafts for complex abdominal aortic aneurysms.[68] An important difference from fenestrated-branched series is the lower average number of targeted vessels (1.7 vs. > vessels/patient), indicating that parallel grafts were indicated for less extensive aneurysms. Thirty-day elective mortality was 3.7%. Embolic stroke occurred in 1.7% and early type IA endoleak in 3.7%. After mean follow-up of 17 months, primary target vessel patency was 95%.[68]

The results of parallel grafts for pararenal aneurysms are summarized in Tables 39.3 and 39.4. The largest single-center series included from 14 up to 169 patients with mean of 1.4 up to 2.1 vessels per patient. Technical success was achieved in 94% to 100% of patients. Thirty-day mortality ranged from 1.7% to 10% of patients. A limitation of parallel grafts is the risk of "gutter" endoleaks, estimated in 10% in these reports, and potential risk of stroke from multiple transbrachial sheaths.

AORTIC ARCH ANEURYSMS

Fenestrated and Branched Stent-Grafts

The clinical experience in the Western world has been limited to a few centers with access to investigational branch devices. The first clinical experience with inner branches was reported by Lioupis and colleagues in 2012.[69] Recently, a multicenter analysis of the first 38 patients was published by Haulon and colleagues.[23] Technical success was 84%, with five (13%) 30-day

TABLE 39.3 Contemporary Results of Use Parallel Grafts for Aortic Disease

Author	Year	*n*	Branches	Technical Success (%)	30-Day Mortality (%)	Mean Follow-Up (Months) (%)	Branch Occlusion (%)
Larzon et al.	2008	14	14 (1.1)	94	0	6	—
Coscas et al.	2011	16	26 (1.6)	94	13	10	—
Bruen et al.	2011	21	37 (1.7)	97	5	—	0
Donas et al.	2012	72	137 (1.9)		0	—	—
Lachat et al.	2013	77	169 (2.1)	99	2.5	—	—
Lee et al.	2014	43	74 (1.7)	—	5	—	0
Scali et al.	2014	41	76 (1.8)	93	7	5	5
Banno et al.	2014	38	56 (1.6)	—	7.9	5	2.6
PERICLES	2015	517	898 (1.7)	97	4.9	1.7	3.1
Bin Jabr et al.	2016	51	73 (1.4)	—	90	10	23

TABLE 39.4 Outcomes of Endovascular Repair of Aortic Arch Disease

Author	Year	Patients (*n*)	Pathology (*n*)	Device/Method	Technical Success (%)	Mean F/U (Months)	Peri-Op Mortality (%)	Stroke (%)
Yunoki et al.	2014	13	Dissection (6), Aneurysm (4), Other (3)	Bolton Relay NBS Plus	100	22	0	0
Mangialardi et al.	2014	26	Aneurysm (10), dissection (27), other (5)	Parallel grafts (different devices)	100	37	4	12
Haulon et al.	2014	38	Aneurysm (28), dissection (10)	Custom Cook Medical Inner Branched Arch Endograft (Cook a-Branch)	84	12	13	16
O'Callaghan et al.	2014	33	Aneurysm (26), dissection (6), trauma (1)	Custom cook medical stent grafts (15) and non-custom grafts (18)	97	17	12	6
Kurimoto et al.	2015	37	Aneurysm (31), dissection (3), other (3)	Semi-custom handmade "Yokoi HIJ graft"	100	17	0	5
Zou et al.	2016	35	Aneurysm (3), dissection (27), other (5)	Parallel grafts (different devices)	94	29	0	0
Spear et al.	2016	27	Aneurysm (19), dissection (8)	Custom-made Cook Medical Inner Branched Arch Endograft (Cook a-Branch)	100	12	0	11
Tsilimparis et al.	2016	29	Dissection (11), Aneurysm (18)	Custom-made Cook Medical devices (fenestrated or branched)	97	9	10	10

deaths and six (16%) cerebrovascular complications. Mortality was higher in the first 10 patients (30% vs. 7%), although the difference was not statistically significant ($P = .066$). Spears and colleagues reported the experience with the subsequent 27 patients treated by the same authors. There was no 30-day mortality, and two patients (7%) had major strokes.[22]

Patel and colleagues reported the preliminary results of the US feasibility TBE multicenter clinical trial in the first 22 patients (mean age 74.1 ± 10.5 years, 54.5% male) undergoing branched thoracic endovascular aortic repair (B-TEVAR) in Ishimaru Zone 2.[70] The primary endpoint of device delivery and branch vessel patency was achieved in 100% of patients, without 30-day mortality, stroke, or permanent paraplegia. Median duration of hospitalization was 4.0 days. Type I endoleaks at completion angiography were observed in four patients, all resolving by 1 month without reintervention. All side branches were patent at 1 month. Kaplan-Meier survival at 6 months was 95%. The authors concluded that endovascular repair of distal Zone 2 arch aortic aneurysms can be safely achieved with the TBE.[70] Future studies will evaluate the feasibility of this approach for aneurysms encompassing the brachiocephalic trunk and left carotid artery.

CONCLUSION

Fenestrated and branched stent-graft techniques continue to evolve but have been widely applied to treat aortic arch, TAAA, and aortoiliac aneurysms. Clinical experience has shown the significant impact of the learning curve on perioperative mortality, morbidity, and rates of spinal cord injury. It is likely that these treatment methods will continue to expand the indications of EVAR and will significantly improve morbidity and mortality compared with the historical results of open surgical repair.

References available online at ExpertConsult.com.

40 CHAPTER

Acute and Chronic Aortic Dissection: Medical Management, Surgical Management, Endovascular Management, and Results

Sherene Shalhub, Benjamin W. Starnes

INTRODUCTION

Aortic dissection was first described in the autopsy of King George II of England in 1761, and later the term "dissecting aneurysm" was coined by Morgagni and Laennec in 1819: "aneurysme dissequant."[1] It is a life-threatening condition that is challenging to diagnose and one of the most complex clinical conditions encountered by vascular surgeons.

An aortic dissection is a tear in the intima of the aortic wall. Once an intimal tear occurs, propagation of the dissection is a dynamic process that can result in both antegrade and less commonly retrograde blood flow between the inner and outer layers of the media along the length of the aorta. This produces a *false lumen* separated from the true lumen by a septum composed of the aortic intimal and medial layers and creates a double-barreled aorta (Fig. 40.1). Fenestrations between the two channels connect the true and false lumen and usually occur at the origin of branch vessels. The most common location of the false lumen in descending thoracic aortic dissections is in the posterolateral aorta. Although significant variation occurs, the celiac trunk, the superior mesenteric artery, and the right renal artery most commonly arise from the true lumen, and the left renal artery often arises from the false lumen. Because the blood in the false lumen is contained by the thin outer third of the media and loose adventitial connective tissue, rupture of the aorta into the pericardial space, pleural space, or mediastinum is not uncommon.

CLASSIFICATION

Several classification systems have been used to describe aortic dissections. These are based on either the duration of symptoms or the anatomy of the aortic dissection. Treatment varies based on the age of the dissection and the anatomic location of the entry tear; therefore appropriate classification is crucial for initiation of proper therapy.

Temporal Classification

An aortic dissection has been classically classified as acute if the diagnosis is made within 2 weeks of the initial onset of symptoms, subacute if within 6 weeks of the initial dissection, and chronic if the diagnosis is beyond this time period. More recently, the International Registry of Aortic Dissection (IRAD) investigators proposed a more contemporary classification of: hyperacute (symptom onset up to 24 hours), acute (2 to 7 days), subacute (8 to 30 days), and chronic (>30 days).[2]

Anatomic Classification

Two distinct classification systems are currently used to classify aortic dissection based on the location of the intimal tear and the degree of distal extension (Fig. 40.2). Neither scheme addresses dissections originating in or limited to the aortic arch.

DeBakey Classification

The **DeBakey classification**, first developed in 1965, classifies aortic dissection into four types[3]:

- *Type I:* The entry tear originates in the ascending aorta and extends from the aortic arch into the descending or abdominal aorta for varying distances.
- *Type II:* The dissection originates and is confined to the ascending aorta.
- *Type IIIa:* The entry tear is just distal to the left subclavian artery, and the extent is limited to the descending thoracic aorta.
- *Type IIIb:* The dissection originates just distal to the left subclavian artery and extends for a variable distance of the abdominal aorta.

Stanford Classification

The **Stanford classification** categorizes the dissection primarily based on the location of the intimal tear[4]:

- *Stanford type A dissection*: originates in the ascending aorta and encompasses DeBakey types I and II.
- *Stanford type B dissection*: originates in the descending aorta and includes DeBakey types IIIa and IIIb.

The Stanford classification is the most widely adopted system for classification and management of the aortic dissection. The majority of patients with Stanford type A dissections require urgent surgical repair, because this disease entity is associated with high rates of mortality if left untreated. Conversely, patients with Stanford type B dissections do not usually require urgent surgical treatment and are treated with medical therapy. Certain indications for surgical treatment exist for these patients and will be discussed later in this chapter.

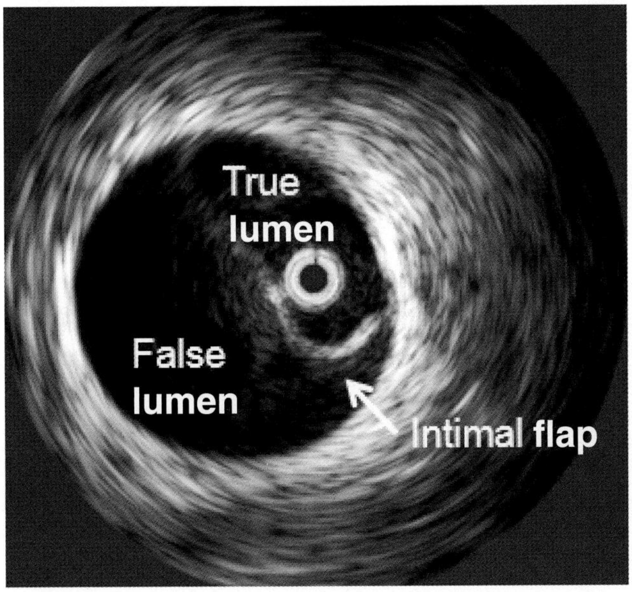

FIG 40.1 Cross-sectional imaging of an aortic dissection obtained with intravascular ultrasound showing the double-barreled aorta with a false lumen separated from the true lumen by a septum composed of the aortic intimal and medial layers.

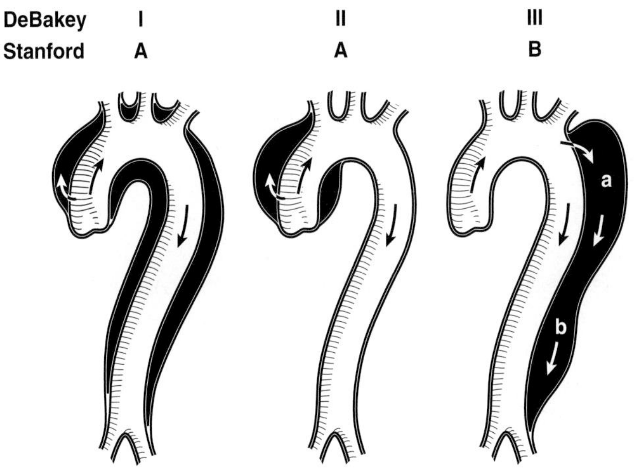

FIG 40.2 The DeBakey and Stanford classification systems for aortic dissection. (With permission from Erbel R, Alfonso F, Boileau C, et al: Diagnosis and management of aortic dissection. *Eur Heart J* 22:1642–1681, 2001.)

INCIDENCE AND SURVIVAL RATES OF AORTIC DISSECTION

The annual age- and sex-adjusted incidence of acute aortic dissection has been estimated at 2.9 to 3.5 per 100,000 persons. It is the thirteenth leading cause of death for individuals between the ages of 55 and 64 years. In the United States, it is estimated to affect 5 to 10 people per million per year with 43,000 to 47,000 deaths from involvement of the aorta and its branches.[1,5] Approximately 48.6% of patients with aortic dissection die before hospital admission.[6]

Aortic dissection is more common in males than females with a 4:1 ratio.[1] The entry tear originates in the ascending aorta in 65% of the cases, the arch in 10% of the cases, the descending aorta in 20% of cases, and the abdominal aorta in 5% of the cases.[7] In a report by the IRAD, a total of 67% (n = 2,952) of all patients enrolled in IRAD presented with type A aortic dissection, whereas the remaining 33% (n = 1476) presented with type B aortic dissection.[8]

The age at dissection ranges between 40 and 70 years, with dissections seen on the lower end of the spectrum in patients with heritable thoracic aortic disease (e.g., Marfan syndrome, Loeys-Dietz syndrome). In a report by the IRAD, the mean age of patients with type A aortic dissection was 62 ± 14.6 years, while the mean age of those with type B AAD was older, at 64 ± 14.1 years.[8]

Mortality of aortic dissection varies according to the entry tear location. The mortality associated with acute type A aortic dissection is estimated at 30% in the first 24 hours, 50% by 48 hours, and 90% at 1 year in a classic study by Hirst and colleagues in 1958.[9] Surgical mortality for acute type A dissections is 25.1% in IRAD.[10] The long-term survival rates for surgically treated type A aortic dissection patients who survive until hospital discharge range from 52% to 96% and 37% to 91% at 1 and 5 years, respectively.[11,12]

In contrast, early mortality for patients with acute uncomplicated type B aortic dissection ranges from 10% to 12%,[13] while operative mortality in patients with acute, complicated type B dissection approaches 25% to 50%.[14] The long-term survival of surgically treated patients with type B aortic dissections after discharge ranges from 56% to 96% and 48% to 83% at 1 and 5 years, respectively.[12,15]

PATHOPHYSIOLOGY OF AORTIC DISSECTION

Cystic Medial Degeneration

The pathogenesis of aortic dissection is complex. Our true understanding of aortic dissection pathology began with the dissertation by Shennan in 1934 describing cystic medial necrosis (degeneration) in autopsy results of patients with aortic dissections.[16] Cystic medial degeneration is a process that leads to loss of aortic wall smooth muscle cells, fragmentation of the elastic fibers, and accumulation of proteoglycans, effectively weakening the aortic wall.[17]

Aortic Wall Stress

Aortic dissection is believed to occur when intraluminal wall stress exceeds aortic wall strength.[18] Nathan and colleagues demonstrated, in a study using electrocardiogram-gated computed tomography angiography in 47 individuals with normal thoracic aortas, that peaks of aortic wall stress exist in the sinotubular junction and distal to the left subclavian artery ostium. These two locations are typically the entry point for aortic dissection: Ascending thoracic aorta dissections typically result from intimal tears above the sinotubular junction while descending thoracic aorta dissection originate distal to the left subclavian artery ostium.[18] These authors also found that the wall stress proximal to the sinotubular junction exceeded that of the area distal to

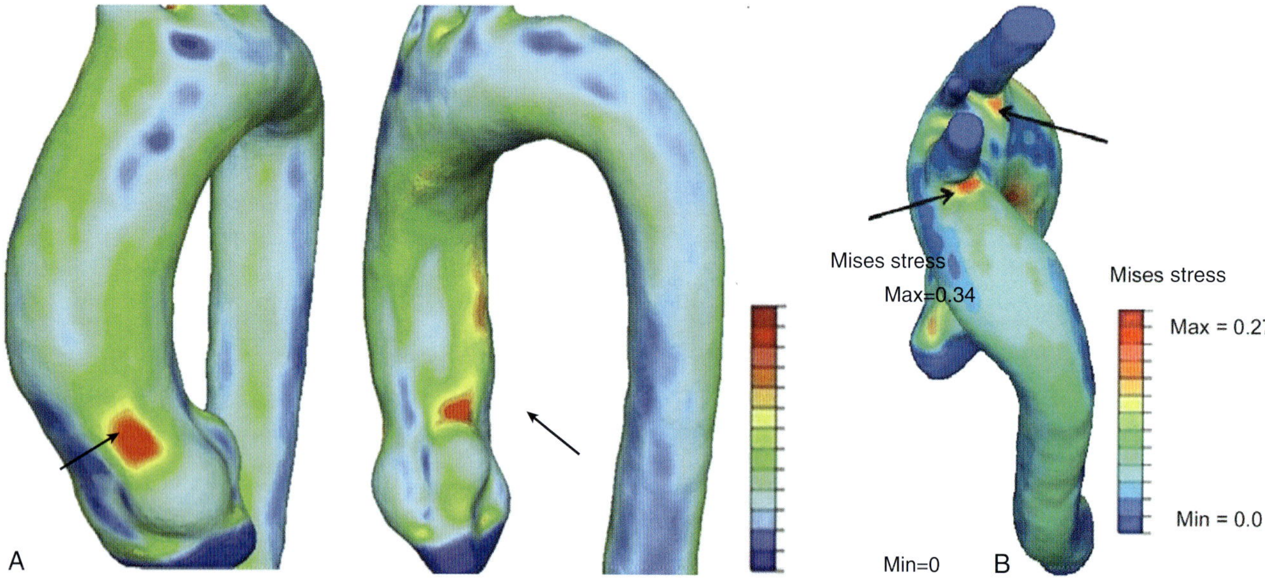

FIG 40.3 Three-dimensional wall stress distribution for the normal thoracic aorta. Stress in megapascals (MPa) is mapped, with the highest stress in *red* and the lowest stress in *blue*. The *black arrows* indicate maximal stress above the sinotubular junction in the ascending (A) and distal to left subclavian and innominate arteries in the descending thoracic aorta (B). (From Nathan DP, Xu C, Gorman III JH, et al: Pathogenesis of acute aortic dissection: a finite element stress analysis. *Ann Thorac Surg* 91:458–464, 2011.)

the left subclavian artery, thus supporting the increased prevalence of ascending thoracic aortic dissections compared with descending thoracic aortic dissections (Fig. 40.3). In contrast, significant atherosclerosis is relatively infrequent in patients with acute aortic dissection, and it has been hypothesized that the presence of atheromatous plaque may serve to terminate or limit the extent of the dissection. One potential theory is enhanced fusion of the aortic wall layers secondary to inflammatory aortic wall plaques.

Hypertension

Hypertension is a well-known risk factor for aortic dissection. More than 75% of patients with aortic dissection are hypertensive, although patients with type B aortic dissection are more likely to present with hypertension than those with type A aortic dissection.[8,19] Conditions associated with hypertension have also been associated with aortic dissection such as advanced age, pregnancy, especially with accompanying preeclampsia (rare), cocaine, and methamphetamine abuse.[8,20,21]

Other Risk Factors

An increase in aortic diameter has been implicated as a risk factor for type A dissection but not for type B dissection.[22] Structural abnormalities of the aortic wall, including bicuspid aortic valve, aortic coarctation, and chromosomal abnormalities (Turner syndrome and Noonan syndrome), have also been implicated. Seasonal variation has been observed in the development of aortic dissection, with more patients being seen in the winter months.[23] As with acute myocardial infarction or myocardial ischemia, physical and mental activities can also be triggers for acute aortic dissection.[24]

Genetics

Genetic risk factors are well described in association with type A aortic dissection. Syndromic (e.g., Marfan syndrome, Loeys-Dietz syndrome) and nonsyndromic heritable thoracic aortic diseases have been associated with aortic dissections. These mutations affect the TGF-β pathway (e.g., *FBN1, TGFb1, TGFb2, SMAD3*),[25] smooth muscle cell proteins (e.g., *ACTA2, MYH11*, and *PRKG1*), and adhesion molecules (e.g., *MFAP5, MAT2A*).[17] Collectively, these are called Heritable Thoracic Aortic Disease (H-TAD) gene mutations. Marfan syndrome is the most commonly described familial syndrome in patients with aortic dissection, occurring at an age younger than 40 years, and accounts for slightly more than 4% of the dissection cases enrolled in IRAD.[8,26] Table 40.1 summarizes the H-TAD gene mutations affected in syndromic and nonsyndromic aortic dissections. Sequencing of H-TAD genes may be considered in patients with a family history of aortic dissection to determine if gene mutations are responsible for the aortic pathology.[27] Genetic testing should only be performed in collaboration with medical geneticists and appropriate patient counseling.

NATURAL HISTORY OF AORTIC DISSECTION

The natural history of chronic aortic dissection is aneurysmal degeneration and dilation of the aorta. The aortic wall surrounding the false lumen is significantly weaker than that of the true lumen; thus in the majority of patients, the false lumen has the larger diameter (Fig. 40.4). In a recent series of 200 patients (61% men) with medically managed acute type B dissections, the mean rate of aortic growth was 12.3 mm/year for the total

TABLE 40.1 Heritable Thoracic Aortic Disease Gene Mutations Affected in Syndromic and Nonsyndromic Aortic Dissections

Mutation Effect	Gene	Protein	Associated Syndrome
Affects the TGF-β Pathway	*FBN1* [MIM 134797]	Fibrillin-1	**Marfan syndrome**. Ocular, skeletal involvement.
	TGFβR1 *TGFβR2* [MIM 190181] [MIM 190182]	TGF-β receptor type 1/type 2	**Loeys-Dietz syndrome**. Skeletal manifestations, craniofacial abnormalities, tortuous arteries, cutaneous anomalies
	TGFβ2 [MIM 190220]	Transforming growth factor β2	Intracranial aneurysms, subarachnoid hemorrhages
	SMAD3 [MIM 603109]	SMAD family member 3	**Aneurysm osteoarthritis syndrome**. Arterial aneurysms/tortuosity, mild craniofacial, skeletal, cutaneous anomalies, early onset osteoarthritis.
Alters smooth muscle cell contraction proteins and adhesion to the extracellular matrix	*ACTA2* [MIM 102620]	Smooth muscle α actin	
	MYH11 [MIM 160745]	Smooth muscle myosin heavy chain	
	MLCK [MIM 600922]	Myosin light chain kinase	
	PRKG1 [MIM 76894]	cGMP-dependent protein kinase type I	
Alters extracellular matrix structural proteins	*MFAP5* [MIM 601103]	Microfibrillar-associated protein 5	
	LOX [MIM 153455]	Lysyl oxidase	
Alters smooth muscle cells metabolism proteins	*MAT2A* [MIM 601468]	Methionine adenosyl transferase 2-α	
	FOXE3 [MIM 601094]	Forkhead box E3	

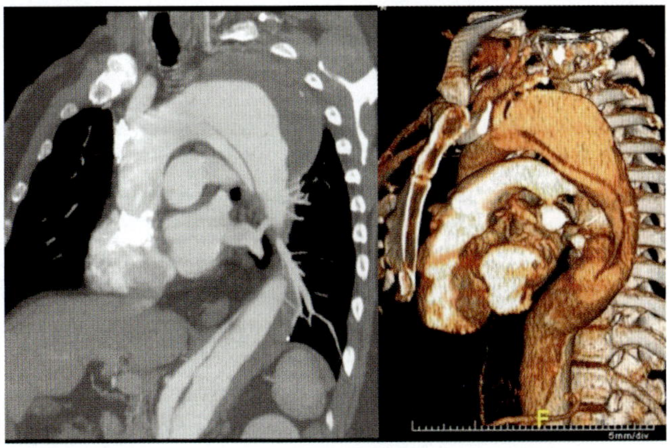

FIG 40.4 Oblique view of CTA imaging *(left panel)* and three-dimensional reconstruction *(right panel)* of the imaging showing aortic dissection of the descending thoracic aorta and delineates the aneurysmal degeneration and dilation of the false lumen.

aortic diameter. The only risk factor for future growth was aortic diameter at index presentation of greater than 3.5 cm, while complete thrombosis of the false lumen was protective against growth.[28] In a similar study, the presence of a patent false lumen and a maximum aortic diameter of greater than 4 cm upon initial presentation were found to be predictors of complications during long-term follow-up in a cohort of 76 patients treated medically for acute type B dissections.[29] A meta-analysis was performed investigating the long-term association between false lumen status patient outcomes. The analysis included 11 cohort studies with 2924 cases of aortic dissection. A patent residual false lumen was an independent predictor of long-term mortality in type A aortic dissection (HR, 1.71; 95% CI, 1.16 to 2.52; P = .007) and type B aortic dissection (HR, 2.79; 95% CI, 1.80 to 4.32; $P < .001$). The patent residual false lumen was associated with increased subsequent aortic events (HR, 5.43; 95% CI, 2.95 to 9.99; $P < .001$). In addition, partial false lumen thrombosis was independently associated with long-term mortality in type B aortic dissection (HR, 2.24; 95% CI, 1.37 to 3.65; $P = .001$).[30]

Several additional radiologic features as ascertained by CT scan have been shown to be predictors of dissection-related aneurysmal degeneration, including a large false lumen diameter relative to the size of the true lumen, lack of an outflow tear size of the primary tear (>10 mm), one entry tear, entry tear along the inner curvature, false lumen diameter greater than 22 mm, elliptic true lumen combined with saccular false lumen, and blood flow in the false lumen.[31–34] The latter phenomenon was demonstrated in an ex vivo model of chronic descending thoracic aortic dissection connected to a pulsatile pump with simultaneous pressures measured within the true and false lumen. Diastolic false lumen pressures were highest in the setting of smaller proximal tear size and the lack of a distal tear.[34]

While not directly correlated to dissection-related aneurysmal degeneration, augmented pressure within the false lumen may also contribute to significant compression of the true lumen and lead to increased dissection-related mortality. The proposed hypothesis for this increased risk is that thrombus within the false lumen occludes distal tears, resulting in restricted outflow with a subsequent increase in false lumen pressure.[35]

CLINICAL PRESENTATION

The most common symptom of acute aortic dissection is an abrupt onset of pain in the chest, back, and abdomen (83% in type A, 71% in type B).[8] This is typically associated with a "ripping or tearing" substernal chest pain when type A dissection is present and back and flank pain that may be migratory in nature when type B dissection is present. Symptoms associated with type A dissection include syncope (19%) due to cardiac tamponade and aortic valve dysfunction, and Horner syndrome from compression of the adjacent sympathetic ganglia (less common). Lower extremity paresthesias can occur from lumbar plexopathy, and severe limb pain can occur in the setting of acute arterial ischemia from malperfusion. Pulse deficit with or without extremity ischemia in a patient with severe chest or back pain should raise the suspicion of an acute aortic dissection. Spinal cord ischemia can occur in up to 10% of patients with dissection in the descending thoracic aorta.

Malperfusion Syndrome

Malperfusion following aortic dissection is defined as the loss of adequate blood supply to vital organs owing to aortic branch vessel obstruction, resulting in end-organ ischemia. Malperfusion syndrome is reported in about one-third of patients with type A dissection and 10% of patients with type B aortic dissection due to decreased perfusion of aortic branches (spinal, iliac, or visceral arteries) that typically leads to paraparesis or paraplegia, lower limb ischemia, abdominal pain, nausea, and diarrhea.[36,37] In a study by the IRAD investigators, 15% of all deaths following aortic dissection were related to mesenteric ischemia.[7] Malperfusion can be classified into two distinct categories based on the physiologic mechanism of obstruction: dynamic and static.

Dynamic occlusion of aortic branches occurs when the dissection flap intermittently obstructs the vessel origin, resulting in end-organ malperfusion. This process can occur with prolapse of the dissection flap into the vessel ostium, compression of the true aortic lumen resulting in inadequate blood flow to affected organs, or both. This type of malperfusion can vary with changes in hemodynamic forces influenced by blood pressure, cardiac output, heart rate, and peripheral vasoconstriction and resistance. The concept of dynamic obstruction is important to understand because patency of a branch on angiography or static imaging may not necessarily ensure vessel patency and adequate end-organ perfusion.

Static malperfusion occurs when the dissection flap extends directly into the vessel orifice, resulting in luminal narrowing or complete occlusion. This type of obstruction occurs less frequently than dynamic obstruction. Unlike dynamic malperfusion, this process is rarely improved upon despite optimal medical therapy or improved flow through the true arterial lumen. Thrombosis of the vessel distal to obstruction may exacerbate the degree of end-organ ischemia. Endovascular or surgical treatment, or both, are usually required for patients with continued malperfusion with static obstruction (Fig. 40.5).

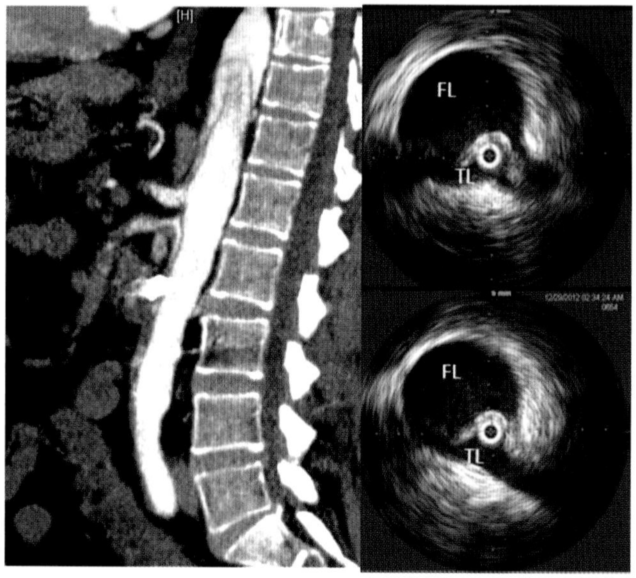

FIG 40.5. Descending thoracic aortic dissection with static mesenteric malperfusion of the celiac and superior mesenteric arteries. *Left panel:* Coronal section of a CT angiogram showing the dissection flap extending directly into the celiac and superior mesenteric arteries. *Right panel:* intravascular ultrasound of the celiac and superior mesenteric arteries showing the large false lumen *(FL)* and nearly obliterated true lumen *(TL)* due to dissection flap.

Diagnostic Pitfalls

Some patients present with few or no obvious symptoms or signs, which may cause an important delay in diagnosis.[2] In addition, common clinical signs and symptoms in patients with dissections are often attributed to various other clinical syndromes.[38] Acute chest pain is commonly associated with myocardial infarction and acute coronary syndrome, and delayed or incorrect diagnosis can occur if a high index of suspicion for dissection is not present. In addition, positive electrocardiogram and serologic markers for acute myocardial infarction do not rule out associated aortic dissection. Peripheral neurologic symptoms may also be mistakenly attributed to musculoskeletal pain, neuropathy, or radiculopathy. Chest pain in association with neurologic symptoms, murmur of aortic insufficiency, signs of arterial insufficiency, migratory nature, radiation to the back, association with severe abdominal pain, or a widened mediastinum on chest radiograph should prompt immediate imaging studies to confirm the diagnosis of aortic dissection as well as urgent surgical consultation.[39] With these scenarios, initiation of intravenous antihypertensive therapy is imperative to prevent propagation of the dissection as later discussed in this chapter

DIAGNOSTIC IMAGING

Chest Radiography

Chest radiography may reveal the presence of a widened mediastinum and aid in the diagnosis of aortic dissection. Widened mediastinum is documented in 54.3% of type A dissection patients and 43.1% of type B dissection patients. Notably, 29% to 36% of patients with aortic dissection have a normal chest radiograph.[8] Thus alternative diagnostic imaging modalities are necessary to establish the diagnosis.

Computed Tomography Angiography

This is currently the noninvasive imaging study of choice for aortic dissection diagnosis.[8] Improved spatial and temporal

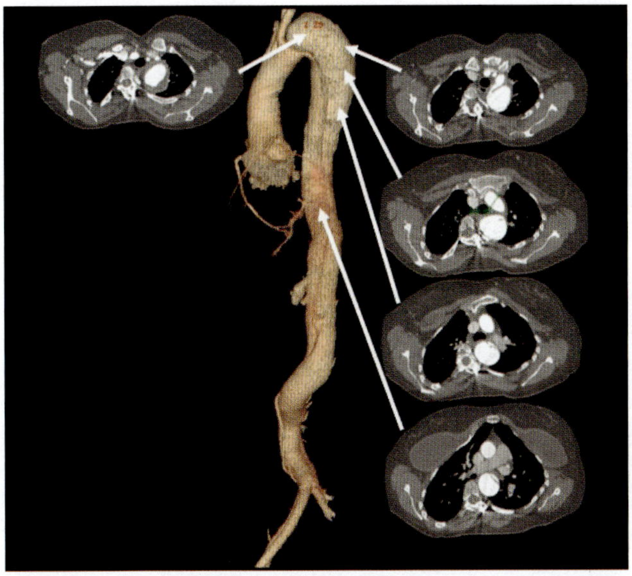

FIG 40.6 Computed tomography angiography images and three-dimensional reconstruction of aortic dissection delineates the complex anatomy of this disease process.

resolution, faster acquisition rates, algorithms to limit radiation dose, and reduced cost likely account for its increased rate of use. Computed Tomography Angiography (CTA) allows reliable imaging of both the true and false lumens, location of the intimal flap, fenestrations and branch vessel involvement, and three-dimensional reconstructions can be rendered and used for surgical planning (Fig. 40.6). Several studies have demonstrated a sensitivity and specificity for detection of aortic dissection and aortic intramural hematoma to be near 100%.[40,41] Multidetector CTA with electrocardiograph-gated synchronization improves diagnosis of type A aortic dissections by decreasing motion-related artifacts in the ascending aorta and aortic valve.[42] CTA is considered the first line imaging modality for type B aortic dissection. In type A aortic dissection, the frequency of using CTA as the initial diagnostic imaging modality has increased over the last 17 years from 46% to 73%.[8]

Echocardiography

Echocardiography provides information regarding the location of the intimal flap in the proximal ascending aorta, true and false lumens, coronary artery involvement, pericardial effusion, tamponade, aortic valve regurgitation, and flow within the false lumen. Transthoracic echocardiography (TTE) can be performed rapidly in the hemodynamically unstable patient, as it is portable and widely available. Sensitivity for TTE ranges from 78% to 90% for type A dissections, and 31% to 55% for type B dissections, while specificity ranges from 87% to 96% for type A dissections and 60% to 83% for type B dissections. It is important to note that a negative TTE result does not rule out aortic dissection, and additional imaging is required if there is a high degree of suspicion despite negative TTE results.[43,44] Transesophageal echocardiography (TEE) allows high resolution imaging from the aortic root to the descending thoracic aorta. The proximity of the esophagus to the aorta, as well as decreased interference from the chest wall and lung, allow high-quality images of the proximal aorta to be obtained, giving it a sensitivity of 86% to 100% and specificity of 90% to 100%.[43,44] Although echocardiography remains useful to rapidly evaluate the proximal thoracic aorta in type A aortic dissection, its use as the first diagnostic imaging study decreased over time from 50% to 23% in type A patients over the last 17 years as CTA use has increased.[8]

Magnetic Resonance Angiography

Contrast-enhanced (typically intravenous gadolinium) three-dimensional magnetic resonance angiography (MRA) offers anatomical and functional dissection information with excellent diagnostic sensitivity and specificity (95% to 100%).[45] Similar to CTA, MRA can accurately determine the presence or absence of intimal flaps and branch vessel involvement. Moreover, information regarding false lumen perfusion can also be readily obtained and may be helpful in the evaluation of visceral ischemia and impaired branch vessel perfusion. The delayed phase acquisitions with use of blood pool agents may improve visualization of the false lumen status, which may appear to be thrombosed on a first pass CTA study.[46] The technique of three-dimensional velocity-encoded cine magnetic resonance imaging offers visualization of pathophysiologic hemodynamics and geometrically triggered changes in blood flow characteristics within the dissected aortic lumens (Fig. 40.7).[47] Time resolved MR angiography (four-dimensional phase) provides an assessment of flow dynamics, which are potential dynamic predictors of complications such as branch malperfusion, helical blood flow in the false lumen, velocity, and false lumen stroke volume.[48] From a practical standpoint, the use of MRA in the acute setting remains limited due to long acquisition times. In addition, the technology has several limitations, including the inability to perform the study in patients with pacemakers or other metallic implants, long examination times, poor tolerance in claustrophobic patients, and the association with nephrogenic systemic fibrosis in patients with advanced chronic kidney disease.

Angiography

The routine use of angiography in patients with aortic dissection is no longer indicated because of its invasiveness and the evolution of the previously described noninvasive imaging modalities for diagnosing aortic dissection. The IRAD investigators reported an overall sensitivity of 87% with aortography for diagnosing aortic dissection.[49] Sensitivities for type A and type B dissections were 87% and 89%, respectively. False negatives may also occur in the presence of intramural hematoma and a thrombosed false lumen. The main indication for aortography is for endovascular treatment of aortic branches (e.g., angioplasty, stenting), the thoracic or abdominal aorta in association with stent-grafting, or fenestration. These techniques will be discussed later in this chapter.[49]

MANAGEMENT OF TYPE A AORTIC DISSECTION

Type A aortic dissection is a life-threatening emergency, and urgent surgical repair is indicated, given the overall mortality

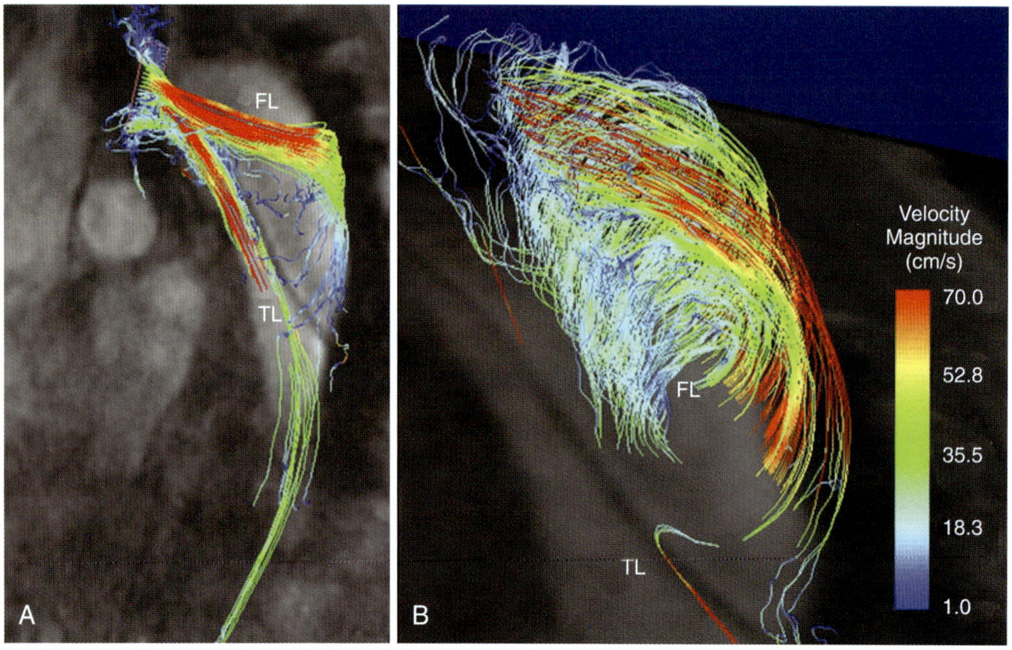

FIG 40.7 Streamline visualization shows (A) parasagittal view of blood flow in the true and false lumen and (B) a double-oblique view of blood flow in the false lumen distal to the primary entry. *FL*, False lumen; *TL*, true lumen. (From Müller-Eschner M, Rengier F, Partovi S, et al: Tridirectional phase-contrast magnetic resonance velocity mapping depicts severe hemodynamic alterations in a patient with aortic dissection type Stanford B. *J Vasc Surg* 54:559–562, 2011.)

of 57% for patients treated without surgical repair.[8] The majority of patients (86%) are managed surgically,[8] while medical therapy is reserved for those who are not candidates for surgical therapy. Potential complications of untreated type A dissections include intrapericardial rupture with cardiac tamponade, coronary artery obstruction, malperfusion of the great vessels resulting in end-organ ischemia, and extrapericardial rupture. Despite timely surgical intervention, perioperative mortality rates still remain significantly high.[10] The IRAD reported an 18% in-hospital mortality rate in 2552 patients who underwent surgical intervention for acute type A aortic dissection.[8] Among nonsurvivors, 41% of patients died within 48 hours after the beginning of the operation, and mortality in patients with surgical treatment delayed beyond 24 hours was 17.1%.[10] Independent preoperative predictors of operative mortality were a history of aortic valve replacement, migrating chest pain, hypotension, preoperative cardiac tamponade, and preoperative limb ischemia. A recent study by Sun reported significantly improved results compared with the IRAD registry, with a reported in-hospital mortality of 4.67% in 257 patients who underwent surgical treatment for type A disease. Fifteen patients developed postoperative respiratory failure, two patients experienced permanent paraplegia, and two patients had postoperative strokes.[50]

Open surgical repair is the standard of care for the treatment of type A aortic dissection. Several different techniques are generally used, depending on the presenting anatomic variation. A median sternotomy with total cardiopulmonary bypass is performed with selective use of hypothermic cardiopulmonary arrest and antegrade cerebral perfusion. Replacement of the ascending aorta with resection of the intimal tear can be used for most patients without involvement of the aortic root or aortic valve.[51] Detailed operative strategies for repair of acute type A dissection are beyond the scope of this chapter.

The role of endovascular repair for type A aortic dissection is in evolution. Fenestrated endografts for aortic arch repair are currently in development, and several "hybrid" techniques for managing acute aortic arch pathology have been described and are currently in use.[52] Pochettino and colleagues demonstrated comparable results to traditional open surgical repair following antegrade stent-graft deployment in the descending thoracic aortic dissection at the time of aortic arch replacement for acute type A dissection (Fig. 40.8). Both groups demonstrated equivalent cardiopulmonary bypass times, rates of malperfusion syndrome, rates of stroke, and in-hospital mortality. Resultant false-lumen thrombosis in the thoracic aorta was significantly higher in the stented group (63%) compared with the nonstented group (17%). In a follow-up study at the same institution by Desai and colleagues, 40 patients underwent similar repair of acute type A dissection with antegrade stent-graft placement. The occurrence of postoperative stroke and early mortality were both 15%, and none of the patients developed permanent paraplegia.[53] The long-term results of hybrid therapy for acute type A dissection are not yet known. Stent-graft manufacturers are currently developing prototypes for the complete endovascular management of type A dissection with devices tailored to covering the entry tear in the ascending aorta. These devices have been implanted on a limited and compassionate-use basis, but the technology is developing at a rapid pace.[54]

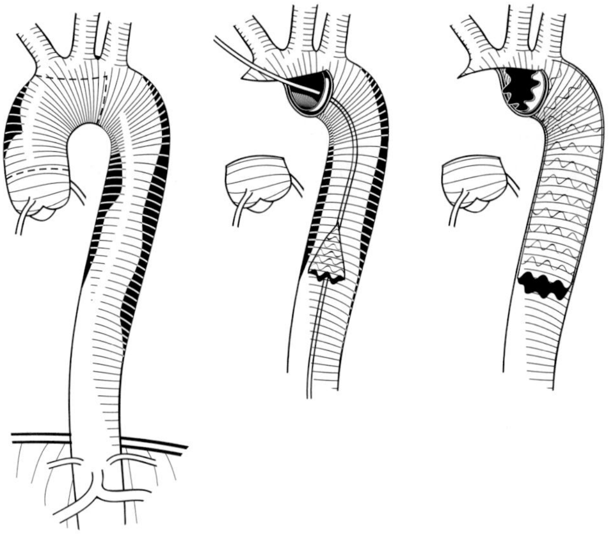

FIG 40.8 Antegrade deployment of a stent-graft during open repair of type A aortic dissection. (From Pochettino A, Brinkman WT, Moeller P, et al: Antegrade thoracic stent grafting during repair of acute DeBakey I dissection prevents development of thoracoabdominal aortic aneurysms. *Ann Thorac Surg* 88:482–490, 2009.)

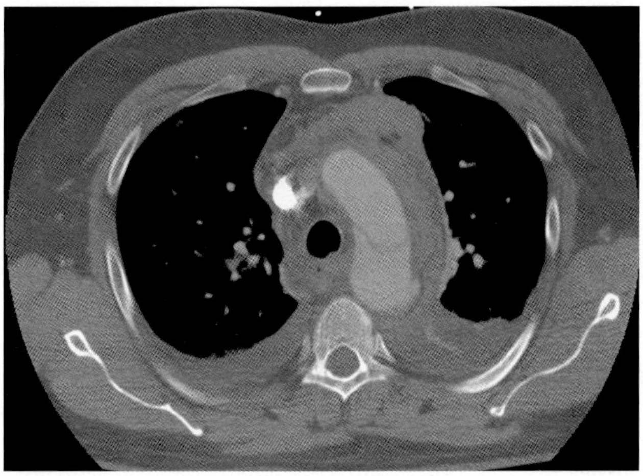

FIG 40.9 Computed tomography angiography demonstrating acute type B aortic dissection complicated by rupture.

MANAGEMENT OF ACUTE TYPE B AORTIC DISSECTION

Clinically, acute type B aortic dissection is subdivided into complicated and uncomplicated dissection, as the prognosis differs significantly. Complicated type B dissection is associated with "complications" such as aortic rupture (Fig. 40.9), hemodynamic instability (shock), malperfusion (neurological, visceral, acute renal failure, acute limb ischemia), recurrent or refractory pain, refractory hypertension, and/or early aortic aneurysmal degeneration or propagation of dissection. In comparison, uncomplicated type B aortic dissection patients are stable and lack these signs and symptoms at presentation and during their hospitalization.[55,56]

Approximately 25% of patients presenting with acute type B aortic dissection have complicated aortic dissection which carries an attendant high mortality risk.[55,56] In an IRAD review, the in-hospital mortality for patients requiring surgical treatment for acute type B dissection was 29.3%.[14] Preoperative malperfusion was present in 30% of patients, which included 14.5% of patients with mesenteric ischemia or infarction, and 16.9% with limb ischemia. Surgical intervention was indicated for aortic rupture in 23.1% of patients, for visceral ischemia in 23.9%, and for limb ischemia in 15.5%. Patients with severe hypotension and shock on admission or at the time of surgery had a mortality of 60%. The other independent predictor of surgical mortality was age greater than 70 years. Factors associated with favorable outcomes included radiating pain, normotension at the time of surgery, and reduced hypothermic circulatory arrest time.[14] In a more recent IRAD review, patients with visceral malperfusion had a 30-day mortality of 31% despite visceral patency after thoracic endovascular repair (TEVAR), compared with 9.1% in those without visceral malperfusion.[57]

Optimal Medical Treatment

Medical therapy has been the treatment of choice for uncomplicated type B aortic dissections since it was described in 1965 by Myron Wheat.[58] This was a result of the observation that type B dissection is associated with lower overall mortality compared with type A dissection, and surgical repair offered no substantial advantage over medical therapy.[59] Thus patients have been managed medically with favorable outcomes, and this has historically reduced the role of surgery to approximately 15% of the cases.

The cornerstone of medical therapy is "anti-impulse" treatment to diminish pulsatile flow and shear stress on the diseased aorta by reducing blood pressure and cardiac contractility (lower heart rate).[58] For this reason, all type B dissection patients should be managed with medical therapy to reduce hemodynamic forces on the aorta and mitigate the risk of rupture or further extension. In addition, medical management may improve the end-organ ischemia in patients with dynamic malperfusion. Patients who demonstrate clinical signs of persistent malperfusion despite optimal medical therapy will likely require endovascular or surgical treatment.

Optimal medical management requires inpatient admission to an intensive care unit for invasive arterial pressure monitoring and intravenous antihypertensive therapy to lower systolic blood pressure and pulse rate. First-line antihypertensive includes intravenous β-Blockers with the goal of reducing systolic blood pressure to less than 120 mm Hg and keeping the mean arterial pressure less than 80 mmHg. In cases not responsive to β-blockers or with poor tolerance to the medication, calcium channel blockers and/or renin-angiotensin inhibitors can be used as alternatives. In addition, vasodilators (nitroglycerin, sodium nitroprusside) can be used but never as first-line therapy, as a reflex tachycardia may be induced, potentially exacerbating the dissection. Pain should be relieved with intravenous opiates since emotional stress may increase blood pressure considerably, potentially further propagating the dissection.[60] The patient should remain in the intensive care unit until blood pressure and pain are adequately controlled, and changes in clinical condition should be strictly monitored. Aggressive pulmonary therapy, deep venous thrombosis prophylaxis, nutritional support, and patient mobilization should be undertaken. Prior to hospital discharge, all intravenous medication should be converted to oral agents and a baseline CTA confirming stability of the dissection should be obtained. Long-term blood pressure regulation and follow-up imaging (CTA or MRA) should be performed at 6 months. Chronic dissections that remain unchanged can be followed with yearly CTA or MRA.

Based on recent IRAD data, most patients with type B aortic dissection are managed medically with β-blockers (84.6%) and less commonly calcium channel blockers (36.1%).[8] Of interest, IRAD investigators also reported that calcium-channel blockers are associated with reduced aortic expansion and improved survival.[61]

Despite optimal medical therapy, in-hospital mortality for uncomplicated type B aortic dissection is 7.4%.[62] The IRAD investigators reported 8.7% overall in-hospital mortality for 923 patients with acute type B aortic dissections managed medically. Multivariable logistic regression analysis confirmed that recurrent or refractory pain or refractory hypertension following medical management was a strong predictor of in-hospital mortality.[63] In another review of 79 patients treated for acute type B aortic dissection, actuarial survival at 1 month and 8 years was 98.4% and 93.5%, respectively, in patients treated with medical therapy alone.[64]

Surgical Management of Complicated Acute Type B Aortic Dissection

Complicated type B dissections are accompanied by worsening clinical signs and conditions, which include rapid aneurysmal expansion, aortic rupture, hypotension, signs of malperfusion (visceral and/or limb ischemia), poorly controlled hypertension despite optimal medical treatment, and persistent intractable pain and rupture. Under these circumstances, surgical correction has been the mainstay of treatment.

Thoracic endovascular repair (TEVAR) is the first-line surgical therapy for complicated type B aortic dissection. The technique was first introduced by Dake in 1999[65] and subsequently supplanted open surgical repair as first-line therapy for complicated type B aortic dissections. Recent IRAD data published in 2015 have demonstrated an increase in use of TEVAR to treat type B aortic dissection from 7% to 31% over the last 17 years. In contrast, open surgical repair decreased from 17% to 8% in the same time period.[8] The goals of TEVAR in type B aortic dissection are to provide the following:

- Coverage of the entry tear
- Improved flow through the true lumen to improve organ perfusion (Fig. 40.10)
- Avoidance of aortic cross-clamping and thoracotomy
- Promotion of false lumen thrombosis and favorable remodeling of the true lumen (Fig. 40.11)
- Prevention of subsequent dissection-related aneurysmal degeneration

While there are no randomized controlled trials comparing TEVAR to open repairs, several studies have demonstrated the reduced morbidity and mortality associated with this technique. Three meta-analyses report an in-hospital mortality ranging from 7.3% to 11.5% and stroke rate from 1.9% to 6.3% in association with TEVAR for acute complicated type B aortic dissection.[66–68] In addition, two prospective studies support the use of TEVAR: the Virtue Registry and the trial using the PETTICOAT technique. The former is a prospective multicenter European clinical registry that showed a 30-day mortality of 8%, with 8% risk of stroke and 2% risk of spinal cord ischemia in 50 acute type B aortic dissection patients.[69] The latter is a single arm multicenter study for endovascular treatment of complicated type B aortic dissection using a composite device design (PETTICOAT technique—includes an uncovered infra-diaphragmatic aortic stent in addition to standard TEVAR), which showed a 1-year mortality of 10%. Stroke, transient ischemic attack, and progression of dissection were seen in 7.5%, 2.5%, and 5% of patients, respectively.[70]

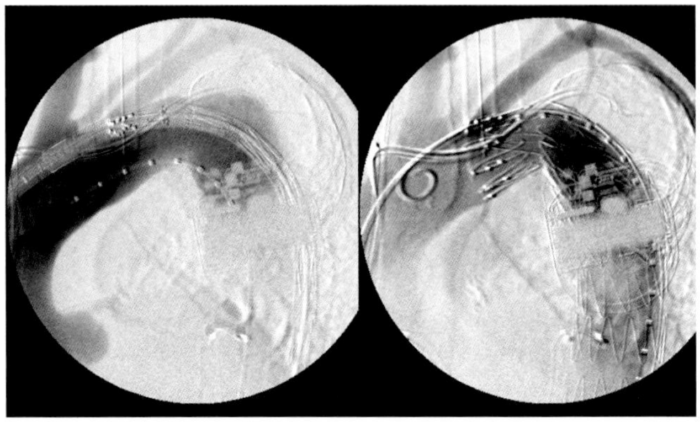

FIG 40.10 Intraoperative angiogram of pre *(left panel)* and post *(right panel)* thoracic endovascular repair deployment to expand a compressed true lumen in a case of complicated type B aortic dissection.

In addition to the survival advantages in the acute phase, there is evidence that aortic remodeling occurs following endograft coverage of the dissected true lumen and the proximal intimal tear, and this may decrease the risk of future aneurysmal degeneration.[71] Conrad and colleagues at the Massachusetts General Hospital reviewed their results following 33 thoracic endovascular repair (TEVAR) cases for complicated type B aortic dissection. Postoperative CT images demonstrated partial or complete false lumen thrombosis at 1 year in 88% of patients. Maximal aortic diameters and false-lumen diameters decreased significantly over time (P = .4 and .46, respectively), and true-lumen diameters increased over time (P = .02) in this patient cohort. Huptas and colleagues demonstrated similar results in their series of 27 patients who underwent TEVAR for type B dissection. In this study, true and false lumen volumes over the entire descending aorta were measured using contrast enhanced CT at baseline and at follow-up (mean, 14 ± 6 months). TEVAR resulted in a continued increase in total true-lumen volume compared with patients who underwent medical therapy alone. Total false-lumen volume also decreased significantly in the TEVAR group; however, no significant change in false-lumen volume was noted in the medical therapy patients.[72]

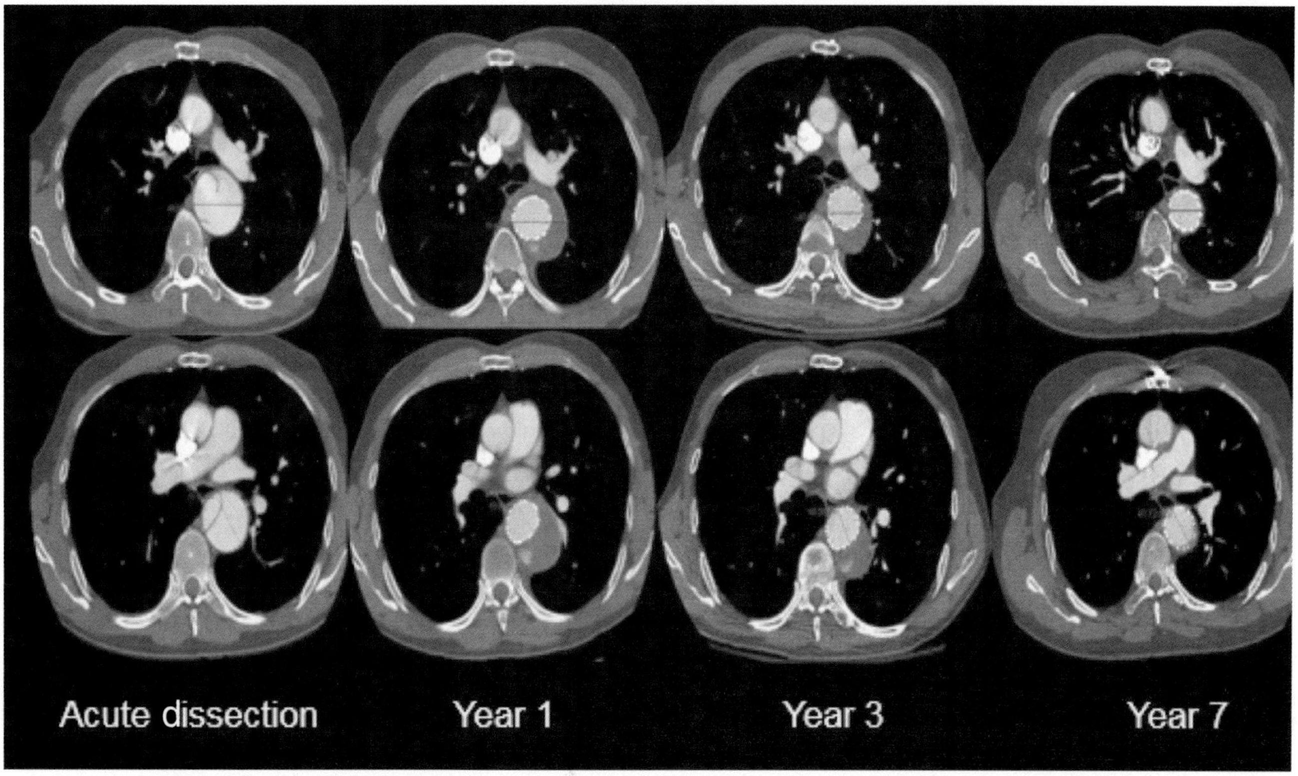

FIG 40.11 Computed tomography angiography imaging showing complicate aortic dissection in the acute phase treated with thoracic endovascular repair with subsequent false lumen thrombosis and favorable remodeling of the true lumen over 7 years of follow-up.

Techniques of Endovascular Repair

Access into the true lumen is usually achieved via the femoral artery either with cutdown or a percutaneous technique. Occasionally, iliac artery access with a conduit is required if the diameter of the access vessels are too small for device delivery. Transesophageal echocardiography and intravascular ultrasound (IVUS) can be used to verify placement of the guidewire in the true lumen and localize the location of the entry tear. Depending on which endovascular device is being used, sheath placement in the aortic arch may be required before endograft positioning. A marker pigtail flush catheter is placed into the ascending aorta through contralateral femoral or brachial access. A 260-cm stiff guidewire is then positioned in the ascending aorta and the endograft is advanced to the level of desired deployment. Ideally, 2 cm of seal zone proximal to the entry tear is required to minimize type I endoleak. Balloon molding of the endograft is generally avoided, especially in patients with acute dissection because the risk of retrograde dissection or rupture is thought to be high in these patients. Adequate device size should be based on the diameter of the aorta proximal to the dissected segment. Device oversizing should be no more than 0% to 10%, as oversizing is associated with stent-graft-induced new entry tears, retrograde type A dissection, and proximal neck dilatation with subsequent stent-graft migration.[73]

If coverage of the left subclavian artery is required, carotid-subclavian bypass prior to thoracic endovascular repair is performed in the presence of a dominant left vertebral artery, a patent left internal mammary artery to coronary artery bypass graft, or in patients with a history of arm ischemia. In the emergency setting, left carotid-subclavian bypass is not routinely required and can be performed postoperatively in symptomatic patients.[74]

Techniques of Endovascular Fenestration

In the setting of acute malperfusion syndrome, percutaneous fenestration of the dissection flap is an option for restoration of organ perfusion. The technique generally includes percutaneous catheterization of the true and false lumens with subsequent identification of entry tears and puncture through the dissection flap. Balloon angioplasty is used to enlarge the fenestration and provide improved end-organ perfusion through the true lumen. Aortic stents can be used to expand the true lumen if significant collapse persists following fenestration. If the organ bed perfused by aortic branch vessels is persistently impaired by extension of the dissection flap into the vessel origin, stenting of the orifice can be used to restore flow.

One early series of 40 patients treated with endovascular fenestration for complicated type B dissection demonstrated a successful revascularization rate of 93%. The 30-day mortality was 25%, and five late deaths were noted. At a mean follow-up of 29 months, the remaining 25 patients demonstrated persistent relief of ischemic symptoms.[75] Midulla and colleagues reported a 100% technical success rate in a more recent study following this procedure for 35 patients treated for malperfusion syndrome secondary to dynamic compression. A 34%, 30-day mortality was noted, and thoracic and abdominal aortic diameters were not significantly different after fenestration (mean follow-up, 48 ± 30 months).[76]

Limitations of endovascular fenestration compared with TEVAR include minimal stabilization of associated aneurysmal disease and no direct influence on false lumen thrombosis and aortic remodeling. Recent evidence demonstrate that TEVAR is associated with redirection of flow back into the true lumen, resulting in organ reperfusion, and may lead to false lumen thrombosis and prevention of aneurysmal degeneration.[77] Thus, primary stent-grafting followed by secondary fenestration is likely the treatment of choice for patients with acute malperfusion syndrome following aortic dissection.

Techniques of Open Surgical Repair

Since the introduction of TEVAR, open surgical repair is reserved for those who have contraindications to TEVAR (such as connective tissues disorders) or those in whom TEVAR has failed. A variety of surgical treatment options exist based on the anatomic variation of the dissection and the patients' clinical presentation.

When a proximal type B dissection is present, the goal is to close the intimal tear and eliminate flow through the false lumen in order to promote false lumen thrombosis and reestablish flow to compromised critical aortic branches. Open surgical repair involves exposure of the descending thoracic aorta through a left posterolateral thoracotomy. Total cardiopulmonary bypass and circulatory arrest are rarely required; however, in one study these techniques were used in 19.7% and 10.5% of patients, respectively.[78] The aortic cross-clamp is usually placed between the left common carotid artery and the left subclavian artery, and can sometimes be placed distal to the left subclavian artery if the intimal tear is more distal in the descending thoracic aorta. A short, woven Dacron graft can be used for central aortic replacement following resection of the intimal tear. Teflon strips in addition to glue aortoplasty are used to enhance anastomotic integrity. If the repair does not completely remove the entire length of dissected aorta, the septal flap is taken to the distal aortic wall to reperfuse the true lumen.

When malperfusion persists despite proximal surgical repair or when a more distal dissection is present with clinical evidence of malperfusion, surgical fenestration can be used to restore adequate organ perfusion. The goal of surgical fenestration is to provide free, unobstructed flow and equalization of pressures between the true and false lumen.[79] When the dissection involves the visceral aortic segment, external control of the renal and mesenteric branches is obtained through a left thoracoabdominal or retroperitoneal approach, depending on the extent of the dissection. Following supraceliac clamping, a longitudinal aortotomy can be used to resect the septum between the true and false lumen and inspect the orifices of the visceral and renal arteries. The clamp can be moved to the infrarenal aorta before reconstruction of the infrarenal aorta either with aortoiliac or aortofemoral bypass or primary closure (Fig. 40.12). Aortorenal

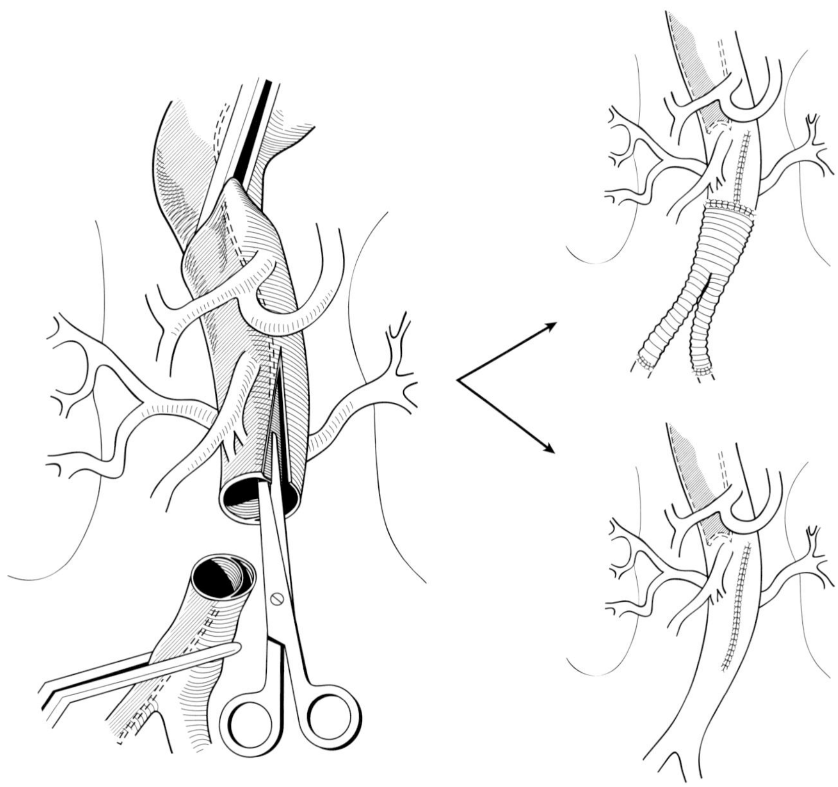

FIG 40.12 Different techniques for fenestration and reconstruction of the abdominal aorta following fenestration for dissection. (From Panneton JM, The SW, Cherry KJ, et al: Aortic fenestration for acute or chronic aortic dissection: an uncommon but effective procedure. *J Vasc Surg* 32:711–721, 2000.)

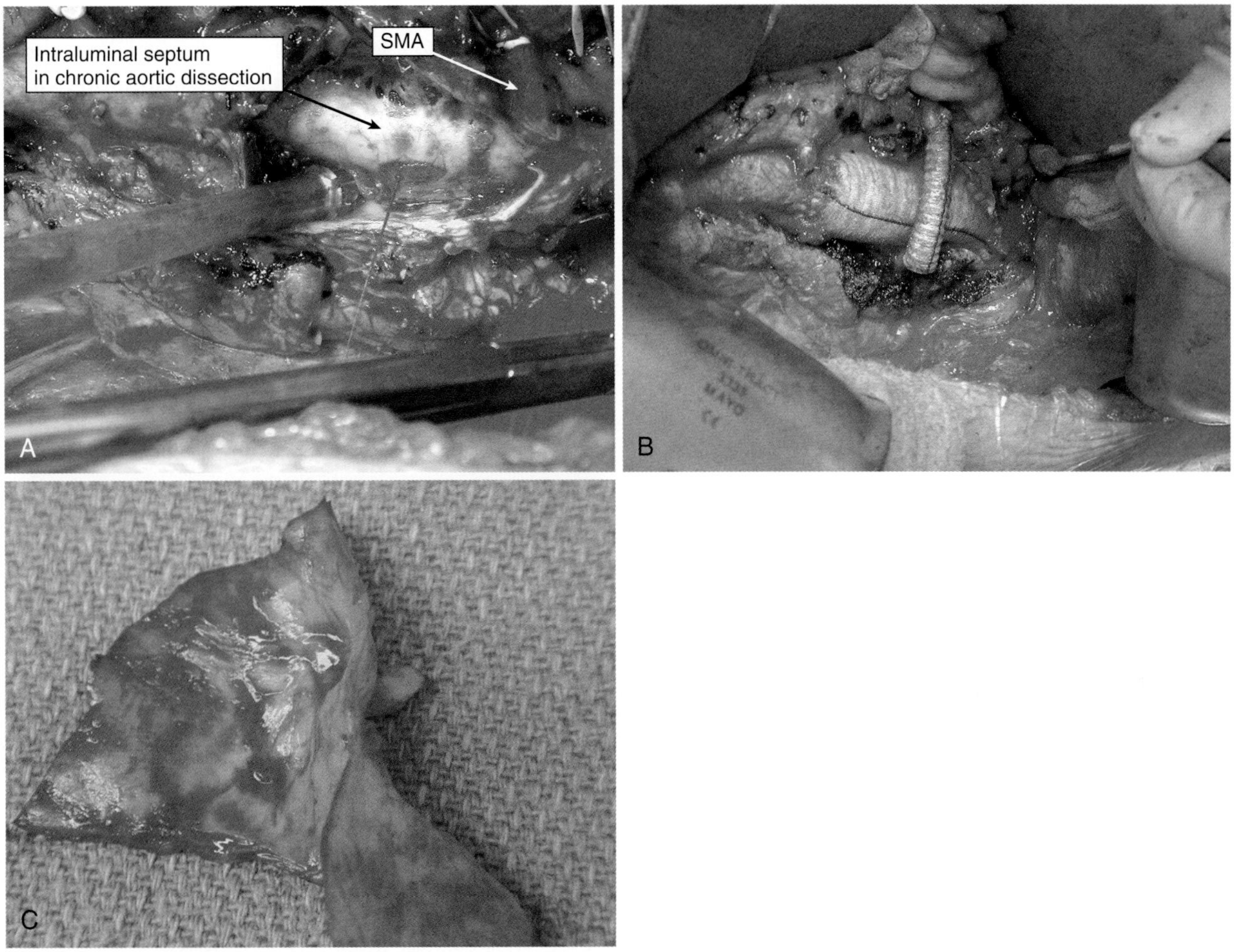

FIG 40.13 (A) Exposure of the septum between the true and false lumina following chronic dissection in the visceral aorta. (B) Reconstruction following aortic fenestration with interposition graft and renal artery bypass. (C) Septum removed following aortic fenestration in a chronic aortic dissection. *SMA*, Superior mesenteric artery. (Photographs courtesy William J. Quinones-Baldrich.)

or aortovisceral bypass may be used if static obstruction persists following aortic fenestration (Fig. 40.13).

MANAGEMENT OF CHRONIC DESCENDING THORACIC AORTIC DISSECTION

Medical Management

The goal of medical management in the chronic phase is to prevent dissection-related aneurysmal degeneration by slowing the rate of aortic expansion. The cornerstone for therapy is blood pressure control and lowering the heart rate using β-blockers.[80] While no large clinical trials specific to this indication have been undertaken, multiple studies have demonstrated that calcium-channel blockers, angiotensin receptor blockers, and statins are associated with reduced aortic growth and complications.[61,81] In patients with Marfan syndrome, β-blockers remain the first-line therapy, but angiotensin receptor blockers specifically appear to reduce aortic growth in this cohort.[80]

Endovascular Repair of Uncomplicated Type B Dissection

The optimal treatment of the uncomplicated type B aortic dissection remains under debate. The first randomized trial comparing TEVAR and medical therapy for uncomplicated type B dissection is the Investigation of Stent Grafts in Aortic Dissection (INSTEAD) trial.[82] Between 2002 and 2005, a total of 597 patients were screened, and 140 patients with stable, chronic (>14 days) type B dissection were randomized to optimal medical therapy plus stent-graft placement versus optimal medical therapy alone. Patients with acute and complicated type B dissections were excluded from this trial. The 5-year aorta-specific mortality was 6.9% ± 3.0% with TEVAR, and 19.3% ± 4.8% with optimal medical therapy alone ($P = .045$) with a survival benefit of TEVAR compared with optimal medical therapy between 2 and 5 years (100% vs. 83.1% ± 4.7%; $P = .0005$) rather than during the initial 2 years (93.1% ± 3.0% vs. 97.1% ± 2.0%; $P = .283$). Following TEVAR, 90.6% of patients demonstrated aortic remodeling with complete false lumen thrombosis in the thoracic aorta compared with 22% in the optimal medical therapy group. Moreover, the group managed with optimal medical therapy demonstrated continued expansion of maximum aortic diameter from 43.6 ± 9.2 to 56.4 ± 6.8 mm ($P < .0001$). This study thus recommended preemptive TEVAR in stable type B aortic dissection with suitable anatomy.

Endovascular Repair of Descending Thoracic Aortic Dissection-Related Aneurysmal Degeneration

The role of TEVAR for repair of descending thoracic aortic dissection-related aneurysmal degeneration is in evolution. Technical success rates of TEVAR for chronic type B aortic dissection range from 77.6% to 100% based on a systematic review of 17 studies with 567 patients.[83] Neurological complications included stroke and paraplegia in 1.5% and 0.45% of the cases, respectively. Retrograde type A aortic dissection occurred in 0.67% of the cases. Reintervention rates ranged from 0% to 60% in studies with a median follow-up of 31 months. Endoleaks (predominantly type I) developed in 8.1% of patients, while continued aneurysmal degeneration of the distal aorta or continued false lumen perfusion with aneurysmal degeneration developed in 7.8% of patients. The midterm mortality was 9.2%, and survival ranged from 59.1% to 100% in studies with a median follow-up of 24 months.[83] Chronic descending thoracic aortic dissections are frequently associated with a thickened and stiffened dissection flap,[84] which may be a risk factor for failure of aortic remodeling.

In a more recent series, 47 patients underwent TEVAR for descending thoracic aortic dissection-related aneurysmal degeneration (Fig. 40.14). The left subclavian artery was covered in 48.9%, and revascularization was performed in 87.0% of those. No retrograde aortic dissections occurred. Spinal cord ischemia developed in three cases (resolved in two and improved in one). False lumen thrombosis occurred in 87.3% of the cases. Secondary interventions were required in 38.3% of the cases. Subsequent 5-year survival was 89% ± 5%.[85]

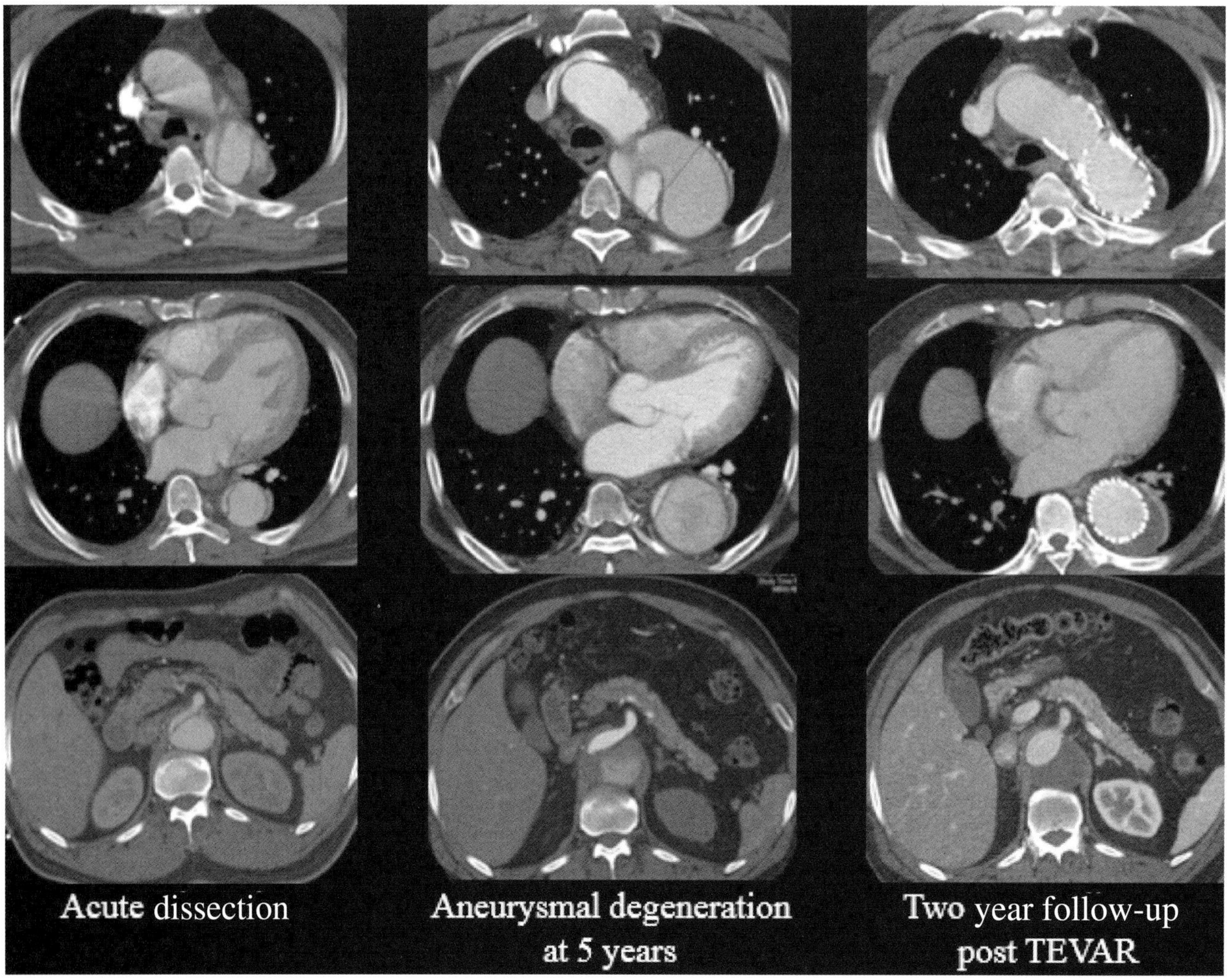

FIG 40.14 Computed tomography angiography imaging showing chronic type B aortic dissection with aneurysmal degeneration treated with thoracic endovascular repair *(TEVAR)* with subsequent false lumen thrombosis and favorable aortic remodeling at 2 years of follow-up.

Open Repair of Descending Thoracic Aorta Dissection-Related Aneurysmal Degeneration

The surgical approach includes aortic repair through a left thoracotomy or medium sternotomy using a frozen elephant trunk technique. In a recent series of 209 chronic distal aortic dissection-related aneurysms repaired between 1991 and 2011, the 30-day mortality was 8.6%, permanent neurologic deficit was 1.4%, and stroke rate was 2.4%. Survival at 5, 10, and 15 years was 72%, 60%, and 49%, respectively. Freedom from reoperation on the operated-on segment was 98% at 5 years.[86] In another series of 104 chronic distal aortic dissections repaired between 1994 and 2007, aneurysmal degeneration was the most common indication for surgical repair (73%). Other indications included rupture (11%), visceral malperfusion (6%), and intractable pain (6%). The reported in-hospital mortality in this series was 9.6%, with 4.8% of patients developing permanent paraplegia. Survival at 1, 5, and 10 years was 78%, 68%, and 59%, respectively. In this patient cohort, the presence of atheroma in the resected aorta and age were independent risk factors for long-term survival.[87]

Open repair remains the gold standard for patients with connective tissues disorders who have chronic aortic dissection such as Marfan syndrome and Loeys-Dietz syndrome.[88]

Hybrid Repairs

Surgical aortic arch replacement with antegrade stenting of the descending thoracic aorta was introduced in the mid-1990s as the "frozen elephant trunk" technique.[89,90] This approach is used for patients who present with both arch and distal aortic pathology where the risks of complete open surgery are high. Hybrid aortic repair has also been associated with promising outcomes for patients with connective tissue disorders (e.g., Marfan syndrome, Loeys-Dietz syndromes).[91]

REVIEW QUESTIONS

1. Which of the following is true regarding the incidence of aortic dissection?
   a. It occurs more commonly in women.
   b. Type B dissections are more common than type A.
   c. Patients with heritable thoracic disease generally present at an earlier age.
   d. Aortic dissection is more common in the elderly (>70 years of age).
   e. The majority of patients with type A dissection do not need intervention.
2. The following are recognized risk factors for aortic dissection:
   a. Uncontrolled hypertension
   b. Marfan syndrome
   c. Cystic medial degeneration of the aortic wall
   d. Methamphetamine abuse
   e. All of the above
3. Which of the following is true regarding the pathophysiology of aortic dissection?
   a. Acute type A dissections tend to occur in the mid ascending aorta.
   b. Acute type B dissections tend to occur just distal to the left common carotid artery.
   c. The aortic wall within the false lumen is significantly stronger than the true lumen.
   d. The true lumen is always larger than the false lumen.
   e. The celiac trunk and the superior mesenteric arteries always arise from the false lumen.
4. Regarding the clinical presentation of aortic dissection, which of the following is false?
   a. Pain in the chest, back, and abdomen is the most common presenting symptom of acute aortic dissection.
   b. Horner syndrome from compression of the adjacent sympathetic ganglia has been described.
   c. Spinal cord ischemia may occur as a result of type A aortic dissection.
   d. Pulse deficit with or without extremity ischemia in a patient with severe chest and back pain may be indicative of acute aortic dissection.
   e. All of the above
5. Which of the following is true?
   a. Magnetic resonance angiography is the most commonly indicated radiographic examination in patients with acute aortic dissection.
   b. Reliable imaging of both the true and false lumens is available with computed tomography angiography (CTA).
   c. Transthoracic echocardiography (TTE) is superior to transesophageal echocardiography (TEE) to image intimal tears in aortic dissection.
   d. Angiography should be obtained prior to CTA even in clinically stable patients.
   e. MRA has poor sensitivity and specificity for aortic dissection.
6. Optimal medical management for acute type B dissections includes all of the following except:
   a. Inpatient admission to an intensive care unit
   b. Pain control with opiates
   c. Arterial pressure monitoring
   d. First-line intravenous antihypertensive therapy is sodium nitroprusside
   e. Strict urine output monitoring with a Foley catheter
7. Indications for mandatory subclavian artery revascularization following endovascular repair of type B aortic dissections include:
   a. Patients younger than 30 years of age
   b. A dominant contralateral vertebral artery
   c. A patent left internal mammary artery to coronary artery bypass graft
   d. Patients without evidence of arm ischemia upon presentation
   e. All of the above

8. Which of the following is true regarding the Investigation of Stent Grafts in Aortic Dissection (INSTEAD) trial?
   a. This is the first randomized trial comparing TEVAR and optimal medical therapy for acute type B dissection.
   b. Patients with complicated type B dissections were included in the trial
   c. There was no significant difference aortic remodeling between the two treatment groups at 2 years.
   d. Dissection-related aneurysmal degeneration was mitigated in the TEVAR group but not the optimal medical therapy group at 5 years.
   e. There was no significant difference between aortic specific mortality between the two groups at 5 years.
9. Which of the following is FALSE regarding type A aortic dissection?
   a. The mid ascending thoracic aorta is the location of maximal shear stress, and most type A aortic dissections originate at this location.
   b. Nearly two-thirds of all aortic dissections are type A aortic dissection.
   c. Emergent surgical repair is usually required in patients with acute type A dissection.
   d. A preoperative predictor of operative mortality following type A dissections is preoperative cardiac tamponade.
   e. Endovascular repair with fenestrated stent-grafts is currently under investigation.
10. Which of the following is true regarding surgical repair of complicated acute type B dissection?
    a. The aortic cross clamp is usually placed between the left common carotid artery and the left subclavian artery.
    b. Circulatory arrest and cardiopulmonary bypass are not usually required.
    c. A woven Dacron graft may be used to replace the aorta following resection of the intimal tear.
    d. Teflon strips and glue aortoplasty are techniques that may be used to enhance anastomotic integrity.
    e. All of the above

References available online at ExpertConsult.com.

CHAPTER 41

Aneurysms of the Aorta and Iliac Arteries

Jerry Goldstone

Aneurysms of the abdominal aorta (AAAs) are common; the incidence (the number of new cases) and mortality increased steadily from the 1950s to the late 1990s in the United States and other Western countries. This was attributed to the aging of the population, improved diagnostic methods, and other less certain factors.[1-4] It is estimated, from large national health screening programs, that 1.1 million Americans have this condition—a prevalence of 1.4% in the 50- to 84-year-old general population.[5] Approximately 190,000 new AAA cases are diagnosed and more than 50,000 operations are performed annually. The incidence and prevalence vary, depending on a number of factors, including age, method of detection, and the population studied; it is lowest in unselected groups and higher in patient groups with known atherosclerotic risk factors and lesions (Table 41.1).[5-11] Prevalence rates of greater than 5% have been reported in men over 65 years of age who smoke. In a study at Massachusetts General Hospital, AAAs were found in 2% of 24,000 consecutive autopsies.[7] In a more recent autopsy series from Malmö, Sweden, AAAs were found in 4.3% of men and 2.1% of women.[12] This last study, as well as others, was performed on an almost entirely white population, and it is known that aneurysms are most common in white males. Aneurysms were found in 5.9% of male smokers older than 55 years in a US Department of Veterans Affairs screening program.[8] The prevalence in screening studies from Asian and African countries is much lower, as it is among African and Hispanic Americans (ratio of white to African American is 3.5:1). The male-to-female ratio is consistently 4:1 to 5:1 in the 60- to 70-year-old group, but beyond 80 years old the ratio approaches 1:1. The frequency of aneurysms increases steadily in men older than 55 years, reaching a peak of 5.9% at 80 to 85 years. In women, there is a continuous increase in prevalence after the age of 70 years, reaching a peak of 4.5% at age greater than 90 years. In community screening programs, the prevalence in men 65 to 74 years old ranges from 2.7% to 3.4%, whereas in elderly hypertensive men and women, the prevalence has been reported as high as 10.7% to 12%.[11-13] The incidence in patients with documented coronary disease is over 10%, at least twice that of the general population.[14]

The increased incidence and prevalence noted over the last decades of the 20th century occurred in both men and women during a time when the incidence of death from coronary artery and other forms of atherosclerosis was decreasing. More recent studies using data from the 21st century have shown a worldwide decrease in aortic aneurysm prevalence and mortality. Svensjo and colleagues reported a prevalence of only 1.7% in 65-year-old Swedish men.[15] Decreased mortality from aortic aneurysm has been reported in the United States, New Zealand, Australia, England and Wales, and The Netherlands by from 6.2% to 6.7% per year. These studies all suggest a real decline in incidence of aortic aneurysms. Several reasons for this unanticipated decline include better treatment of cardiovascular risk factors, decreased cigarette use, safer surgical treatment, and reduced incidence of rupture due to large screening programs. The decrease is not uniform among countries, however, and aortic aneurysm–related mortality continues to rise in some countries, including Hungary, Rumania, Austria, and Denmark and especially in countries where cigarette smoking is increasing.[16] In addition, the decreased mortality from aortic aneurysms is greater in men than women. These trends follow the worldwide trends of decreased smoking in men and increased smoking in women.

Untreated abdominal aortic aneurysms are highly lethal lesions. Their natural history is that of progressive growth and sudden rupture, leading to death. In the United States, approximately 15,000 deaths per year are due to AAA, making it the thirteenth leading cause of death but the tenth leading cause of death in men older than 65 years. It is the second most frequent cause of death from all emergency surgical conditions.[17] The importance of this condition is obvious: the proportion of elderly in the population is growing and there is no effective medical therapy, and rupture is a highly lethal event. Therefore, the only way to reduce the death rate is to identify and treat these lesions before rupture occurs.

There is disagreement about the definition of an aneurysm. The ad hoc committee on reporting standards of the Society for Vascular Surgery (SVS) defined an aneurysm as a permanent *localized* dilatation of an artery to an increase in diameter of greater than 50% (1.5-fold) of its normal diameter.[18] This ratio accounts for the normal variability in aortic diameter as a result of several factors, including age, sex, and blood pressure. The aortic diameter increases steadily with age. As a result, the infrarenal aortic diameter in a 75-year-old person can vary from 12.4 mm in a small woman to 27.6 mm in a large man.[19] An aortic diameter of 30 mm might not meet the definition of 50% increase in some people, but this value has been chosen as the definition for a number of studies on the natural history of small aneurysms and has been adopted by both the SVS and the European SVS because it is more than 2 standard deviations (SDs) above the mean for both men and women.[20,21] The normal average

TABLE 41.1 Incidence of Abdominal Aortic Aneurysms

Category	Incidence (%)
Autopsy	1.5–3.0
Unselected patients screened by ultrasonography	3.2–4.9
Selected patients with coronary artery disease	5.0–10
Selected patients with peripheral vascular disease	10.0
Patients with femoral or popliteal aneurysms	50.90

TABLE 41.2 Normal Diameter of Human Aorta[a]

Sex	11th Rib	Suprarenal Aorta	Infrarenal Aorta	Aortoiliac Bifurcation
Male	26.9 ± 3.9	23.9 ± 3.9	21.4 ± 3.6	18.7 ± 3.3
Female	24.4 ± 3.4	21.6 ± 3.1	18.7 ± 3.3	17.5 ± 2.5

[a]All measurements in millimeters, plus or minus standard error. Data from Steinberg CR, Morton A, Steinberg I: Measurement of the abdominal aorta after intravenous aortography in health and arteriosclerotic peripheral vascular disease. *Am J Roentgenol* 95:703, 1965.

sizes of the aorta in adult males and females are listed in Table 41.2.[18,19] Generalized dilatation of an arterial *segment* is frequently present in patients with aneurysms. This is termed *ectasia,* whereas *arteriomegaly* represents diffuse enlargement of the arterial tree, but not large enough to meet the definition of aneurysm.[22] *Arteriomegaly* is an interesting condition caused by a systemic alteration in the elastic components of the arterial wall. It was found in approximately 5% of nearly 6000 patients undergoing arteriography in one series, and there were discrete aneurysms in at least three different locations in about one-third of them. All were men who were approximately 5 years younger than those with solitary aortic aneurysms.[23,24]

Aneurysms of the infrarenal aorta are the most common arterial aneurysms encountered in clinical practice and men are affected more than women by a ratio of 4:1.[25] They occur 3 to 7 times more frequently than do thoracic aortic aneurysms. Other aneurysms frequently coexist in patients with AAA, including common or internal iliac aneurysms (in 20% to 30% of patients) and femoropopliteal aneurysms in approximately 4% to 5%. The converse is also true. Up to 85% of patients with femoral artery aneurysms have an aortic aneurysm. Popliteal aneurysms are also markers of AAA. Aortic aneurysms can be found in approximately 8% of patients with a unilateral popliteal aneurysm, but in up to 60% of patients who have bilateral popliteal aneurysms. In at least one group of patients with carotid atherosclerosis, there was a 10% incidence of abdominal aortic aneurysm, and a 40% incidence of aortic aneurysms was found in another group of patients with tortuous internal carotid arteries.[23,24] Overall, multiple aneurysms occur in from 3.4% to 13% of patients with AAA. Half of these are synchronous and are present when the AAA is discovered and the rest develop later (metachronous). Thoracic aneurysms occur in approximately 12% of patients with AAA.[26,27]

SCREENING

There have been several large ultrasound-based screening programs to detect aortic aneurysms that included over 200,000 persons.[23,24,30,31] Aortic aneurysms were found in 4.9% to 7.6% of ultrasound-screened British men older than 65 years, but only in 1.3% of women.[29] Similar data have been reported from Denmark, Australia, the Netherlands, and Norway. Although most screen-detected aneurysms are small (<4 cm), screening has been shown to decrease aneurysm rupture rate, decrease the number of emergency aneurysm operations and, most importantly, reduce aneurysm-related mortality in men.[29,32] A small reduction in all-cause mortality has also been attributed to large screening programs.[33] Screening has also been shown to be cost-effective, with cost of $10,754 per quality-adjusted life year (QALY), in 2001 dollars. This compares favorably with a value of $9500 for a three-vessel coronary bypass.[34,35] Because it is impractical and financially unfeasible to screen all adults, screening programs have been based on known aneurysm-related risk factors. Cigarette smoking is highly correlated with the presence of aortic aneurysms, with an 8:1 preponderance of aneurysms in smokers compared with nonsmokers.[36-38] The relationship between smoking and aortic aneurysm is linear and is several times stronger than the relationship between smoking and peripheral arterial occlusive disease. Aortic aneurysms have been detected by ultrasound screening in 8.8% of male smokers older than 65 years who have peripheral arterial vascular occlusive disease. There is also a well-recognized familial component to aortic aneurysms, present in 15% to 25% of first-degree relatives.[39-41] Documented coronary artery disease is associated with a greater than twofold increase in the prevalence of aortic aneurysms and future AAA-related events.[14] The current SVS Guidelines recommend ultrasound screening for all men 65 years of age or older and for women 65 years and older who have smoked or have a family history of AAA.[20] These recommendations are somewhat more inclusive than those of the United States Preventive Services Task Force, which did not include women without a family history or men who had never smoked, although it subsequently included men older than 65 years of age who never smoked. Their recommendations led to Medicare offering one ultrasound screening to men 65 to 75 years of age who have smoked at least 100 cigarettes and in both men and women of the same age with a family history of aneurysm. It is reasonable to also recommend screening for all first-degree relatives of any patient with an AAA diagnosis, based on the known genetic relationships.[39-41] Unfortunately, only 60% to 65% of those eligible have been screened in the large screening programs, and there has been no follow-up on about 35% of the patients whose aneurysms were first detected by the screening.

There has been considerable interest in the use of biomarkers as a means of identifying patients with or prone to develop aneurysms. Increased levels of matrix metalloproteinase-9 (MMP-9), tissue inhibitor of metalloproteinase 1 (TIMP-1), alpha 1-anti-trypsin, IL-6, D-dimer, apolipoprotein A, C-reactive protein

(CRP), and others have been found in the blood of patients with aneurysms, but so far none have sufficient sensitivity or specificity to be clinically useful.[42-44] It is also hoped that biomarkers will be able to identify aneurysms that are likely to grow rapidly or rupture.

PATHOGENESIS OF AORTIC ANEURYSMS

More than 90% of AAAs are associated with atherosclerosis, which, for many decades was considered the primary cause.[43] There are other well-known but uncommon causes of aneurysm of the abdominal aorta, including cystic medial necrosis, dissection, Ehlers-Danlos syndrome, HIV, and syphilis. Aneurysms and occlusive atherosclerosis share most of the same risk factors (e.g., aging, tobacco use, hypertension, male gender, hypercholesterolemia) and atherosclerosis is uniformly present in the wall of aortic aneurysms, but it is believed that several other factors, in addition to atherosclerosis, are involved in aneurysm development.[45-47] One observation that casts doubt on atherosclerosis being the sole or primary cause of aortic aneurysms is that most patients with aneurysmal disease do not have occlusive vascular disease involving the aorto-ilio-femoral segments. It has been estimated that no more than 25% of aortic aneurysms are associated with significant arterial occlusive disease. Another factor is the negative association of obesity and diabetes with aneurysms ("diabetic paradox") in contrast to its strong relationship with occlusive vascular disease. This may be an effect of taking the oral hypoglycemic agent metformin.[48] In addition, induction of aneurysms in animals fed an atherogenic diet has not been predictable, although regression of experimental atheromas has led to aneurysm formation in monkeys. Cigarette smoking is the only known modifiable risk factor associated with development, expansion, and rupture of AAA as well as being a causative association in an in vivo mouse aneurysm model.[16,32] These observations have led to the concept that atherosclerosis is either a coincidental or a facilitating process, rather than the primary cause of AAA and that other biological processes are responsible for the destruction of the media of the aortic wall that characterizes aneurysms.

Mature elastin and collagen are the major structural proteins responsible for the integrity of the aortic wall. Collagen composes approximately 25% of the wall of an atherosclerotic aorta, but only 6% to 18% of an aneurysmal aortic wall. Biochemical studies have shown decreased quantities of both elastin and collagen, but an increased ratio of collagen to elastin in the walls of aneurysms.[48-50] Elastin fragmentation is the initial structural event in *aneurysm formation*, and elastin depletion is complete early in aneurysm development.[51,52,57] This has been correlated with the histopathologic features of a thin, dilated wall with fragmentation of elastin in the media, its replacement by a much thinner layer of collagen (mostly types I and III), loss of smooth muscle cells, and remodeling of the extracellular matrix. This thinned wall usually contains calcium and atherosclerotic lesions, rendering the wall brittle. Laminated thrombus lines the lumen, often eccentrically, resulting in a nearly normal flow channel (Figs. 41.1 to 41.3; see color plate for Fig. 41.3C), but possibly making the inner layers of the aortic wall relatively hypoxic.

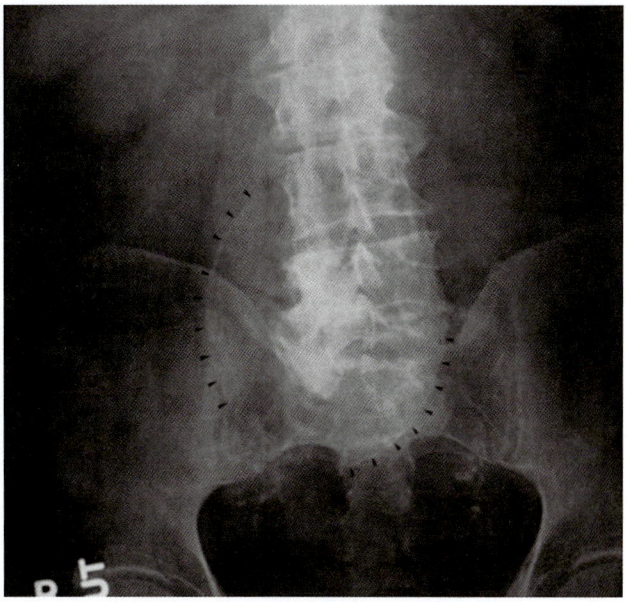

FIG 41.1 Plain abdominal radiograph showing large aortic aneurysm with calcified rim *(arrowheads).*

Aneurysms elongate as they dilate, causing them to become bowed and tortuous. It is believed that the weakening and fragmentation of the elastic lamellae is what permits vessels to lengthen excessively and become tortuous. As a result, the failure of elastin to provide sufficient retractive force in both the circumferential and longitudinal directions allows for increased aneurysm diameter and length, respectively.

The aortic wall is composed of lamellar units that consist of collagen (mainly types I and III) and elastin, as well as vascular smooth muscle cells. There are more lamellar units in the thoracic (58) than in the abdominal aorta (40), and there is a further abrupt decrease below the renal arteries (26). This structural factor is believed to have a role in the predilection for aneurysms to develop in the terminal portion of the aorta, combining with the fragmentation of the elastin and the overall thinning of the wall to contribute to its weakening. The large loss of elastin is one of the most consistent biochemical and histochemical findings in human aortic aneurysms.[50-52] A chronic inflammatory cell infiltrate is also prominent in the media and adventitia.[53-55] A key unresolved question is what triggers this inflammatory reaction and the subsequent chain of events. Many theories have been proposed, including a reaction to mural atherosclerotic plaque or a latent infectious process (e.g., *Chlamydia pneumoniae* or oral flora).[56]

These well-established histologic features have prompted a search for nonatherogenic mechanisms that disrupt collagen and elastin in the aortic wall. Several investigators have found excessive (upregulated) collagenase (MMP)-1, -2, -3 activity in the wall of aneurysmal aortas, and others have found increased elastase (MMP-9) activity. These are members of a family of MMPs that are believed to have an essential role in aneurysm formation. MMP-9 is found in abundance in medial smooth muscle cells as well as in inflammatory cells, and increased levels have been found in both the aortic wall and serum in up to 50%

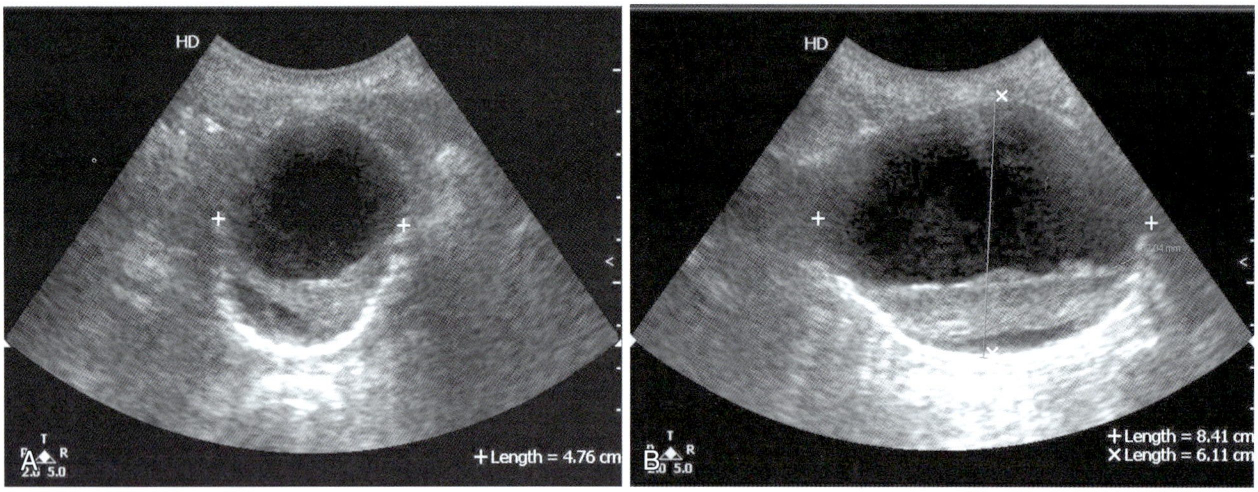

FIG 41.2 (A) B-mode ultrasound scan showing large aortic aneurysm measuring 47 mm in diameter and mural thrombus on posterior wall *(transverse view)*. (B) B-mode ultrasound scan in the same patient showing large aortic aneurysm (61 mm), mural thrombus, and enlarged flow channel *(sagittal view)*.

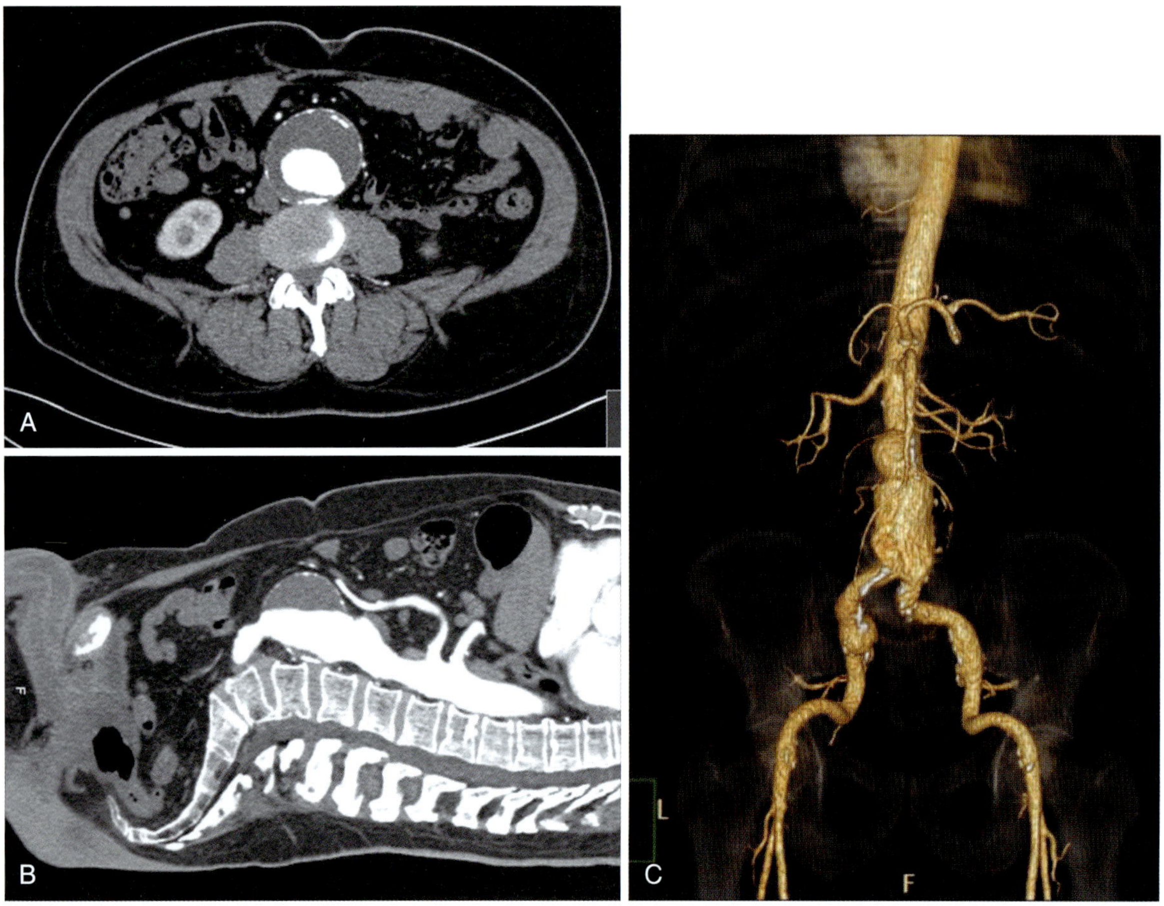

FIG 41.3 (A) Computed tomographic scan of the abdomen showing a large aortic aneurysm with partially calcified wall and abundant mural thrombus *(axial view)*. (B) Sagittal reconstruction showing the posterior flow channel, superior mesenteric artery, and celiac arteries. (C) Three-dimensional reconstruction, anteroposterior view, showing only the flow channel. Note the irregular aneurysm shape.

of patients with aortic aneurysms, but not in those with aortic occlusive disease. These increased serum levels decline to normal after aortic aneurysm repair. Increased activity of other matrix proteases in aneurysmal aortic tissue has also been reported, as has an increased leukocyte-derived elastase in the blood of smokers with aneurysms. Deficiencies in antiproteases, such as several tissue inhibitors of metalloprotease and α_1-antitrypsin, have also been described. α_1-Antitrypsin is one of the most important natural antagonists to elastase and is responsible for the association between chronic obstructive pulmonary disease (emphysema patients with reduced α_1-antitrypsin levels) and increased prevalence of aortic aneurysm and increased rate of rupture. Another factor is the chronic inflammatory infiltrate that occurs in the outer layers of aneurysmal aortas, consisting of macrophages and T and B lymphocytes. There are also increased levels of cytokines and immunoglobulin (IgG, and IgM) that are not seen in association with aging or with occlusive aortic lesions. These findings may be the explanation for the increased levels of serum inflammatory markers, such as IL-6, C-reactive protein, neutrophil elastase, and others found in patients with aneurysms but not in those with occlusive disease. These inflammatory cells and cytokines are believed to interact in some as yet unexplained way with the connective tissue cells and matrix proteins in the pathogenesis of aneurysms.[53,54] Most of the research has focused on the aortic media, but the role of the adventitia in aneurysm formation has recently received some interest. Normally, the adventitia, the strongest layer of the aortic wall, is thought to limit maximal aortic diameter. Topical application of elastase to the adventitia leads to aneurysm formation in experimental animals, solely as a result of elastin degradation.[52,57] Studies such as these have led to speculation about a possible adventitial role in aneurysm formation.

Although not all the studies are conclusive, it is generally agreed that an imbalance between aortic wall proteases and antiproteases is an important factor in the pathogenesis of human abdominal aortic aneurysms. This imbalance causes degradation of the extracellular matrix and loss of structural integrity of the aortic wall, and it is largely responsible for the extensive remodeling of the aorta that occurs during aneurysm formation.

There is also considerable evidence that there is a genetic susceptibility to aortic aneurysm formation.[58-62] Several investigators have discovered genetically linked enzyme deficiencies that are associated with aneurysms in experimental animals. For example, Tilson and Seashore[60,61,63] showed that a deficiency in the copper-containing enzyme lysyl oxidase is the cause of aortic aneurysms in a strain of mice. Lysyl oxidase is important in collagen and elastin cross-linking, and this enzyme defect is sex chromosome linked. In addition, several reports of familial clustering of abdominal aneurysms support the notion of a genetic predisposition to this disease. Approximately 20% to 29% of patients with abdominal aneurysms have a first- or second-degree relative with the same condition.[64-66] The age- and sex-adjusted increased risk of having an aneurysm is 11.6 times, according to one report. Female siblings are at particularly high risk in some studies, while males are more affected in others. The genetic pattern of increased susceptibility is yet to be completely worked out. Available evidence supports both X chromosome–linked and autosomal dominant patterns of inheritance. Among the mutant suspect genes are the type III collagen gene *(COL3A1)* and the fibrillin gene (on chromosome 15). Variations on chromosomes 4 and 19, as well as many other gene loci, have been identified in various patients and experimental animals. Many of these control the production of enzymes, enzyme inhibitors, cytokines, cell regulators, and signaling pathways. Each of these findings provides tantalizing clues; it seems likely that multiple gene variations will ultimately be linked to aortic aneurysm formation. So-called familial aneurysms do not appear to be anatomically or clinically distinguishable from those with no familial pattern, except that they develop earlier in life, have a decreased male-to-female ratio of 2 : 1, show more rapid growth, and appear to have an increased risk of rupture. In addition, there is an increased likelihood of developing aneurysmal disease proximal to the infrarenal aorta and an increased incidence of bilateral common iliac aneurysms.[66] The clinical implications of these genetic studies, as limited as they are, strongly support the screening of all first-degree relatives of patients with abdominal aortic aneurysms.

Hemodynamic (mechanical) factors may also contribute to aneurysm development. The abdominal aorta is subjected to large pulsatile stresses as a result of its tapering geometry, relatively increased stiffness distally, and the reflected pressure waves from the peripheral vessels. Reductions in the number of elastic lamellae and the virtual lack of vasa vasorum in the media of the distal abdominal aorta may also be factors favoring aneurysmal formation in this segment of the arterial tree, making the aorta structurally less capable of handling the increased hemodynamic stresses that occur there.

In summary, contemporary concepts of aortic aneurysm formation and growth incorporate two distinctly different pathophysiologic processes: (1) elastin fragmentation as the critical structural defect required for *initiation* of aneurysm formation; and (2) collagen deposition, degradation, and remodeling governing aneurysm *enlargement*. These two processes result in a complex remodeling of the aortic wall. The other factors described previously, including inflammation, smoking, biomechanical wall stress, and genetic predisposition, interact with these processes to produce the clinical features that are so well recognized. Clearly, aortic aneurysm formation is far more complex than passive arterial dilation because of age. Therefore, these aneurysms should be referred to as *degenerative* or *nonspecific* rather than *atherosclerotic aneurysms*. They account for more than 90% of aneurysms involving the abdominal aorta.

ANEURYSM ENLARGEMENT

Once an aneurysm develops, it tends to enlarge gradually yet progressively. The enlargement rate has been well studied and averages 0.2 to 0.3 cm/year for small aneurysms of 3 to 5 cm diameter to 0.3 to 0.5 cm/year for larger aneurysms.[67] In general, large aneurysms grow at a faster rate than smaller aneurysms. Unfortunately the growth rate is nonlinear, making it impossible to predict the rate of enlargement of any individual aneurysm. Some aneurysms remain the same size for many years, whereas others enlarge rapidly. Factors associated with more rapid growth include larger initial size, hypertension, increased pulse pressure, smoking, and cardiac or renal transplant. Smoking has been shown to increase the rate of enlargement by 35% and is the most important modifiable factor controlling aneurysm growth.[16,33] Interestingly, diabetes mellitus does not appear to be a factor in aneurysm development or growth. Once an aneurysm develops, regardless of the cause, its enlargement is governed by physical principles, especially Laplace's law, which describes the relationship between the tangential stress *(T)* tending to disrupt the wall of a sphere, the radius *(R)*, and the transmural pressure *(P)*: $T = PR$. Thus, for a given transmural pressure, the wall tension is proportional to the radius. Once dilatation of the aorta has started, Laplace's law explains why aortic enlargement progresses. It also explains why large aneurysms are more prone to rupture than small ones and why hypertension and pulse pressure are important risk factors for rupture. Using Laplace's law, tripling the aortic radius from 2 to 6 cm results in a more than threefold increase in wall tension, and when this tension exceeds the tensile strength of the collagen in the aortic wall, disruption occurs. Although Laplace's law has long been used as the sole explanation for aneurysm enlargement and rupture, it is at best an imperfect explanation because it was derived for perfect cylinders and spheres, and aortic aneurysms do not have uniform shape; it also does not consider the wall thickness, which can be highly variable. In addition, it does not explain why all aneurysms of the same diameter do not rupture or why some small aneurysms rupture and some large ones do not.

Aneurysms usually do not rupture at the point of greatest diameter, as would be predicted by Laplace's law. Recent studies using finite element analysis of computed tomography (CT) scan–derived data have measured peak wall stress and strain patterns and have shown that, in addition to decreased tensile strength, aneurysm walls have increased wall stress, an asymmetrical shape, and a complex radius (actually many radii) of curvature.[68-70] Wall stress varies with shape and thickness, and the points of maximal stress do not necessarily coincide with the location of maximal diameter. They do, however, correspond closely with the location of rupture. Wall stress data might also explain why eccentric and saccular aneurysms have a greater risk of rupture than those with smooth fusiform shapes. Inclusion of wall thickness in the analyses is reported to improve the predictability of these wall stress measurements on aneurysm expansion and rupture.[71] The influence of calcification and mural thrombus on stress patterns is uncertain but may be important. These stress analyses have been validated by several investigators but have not become widely used clinically for predicting risk of aneurysm rupture.

There has been wide interest in pharmacotherapy to reduce the rate of enlargement of small aortic aneurysms and thereby reduce rupture risk. β-Blockers have been studied in several randomized clinical trials, with disappointing negative results. Similar results have been found with doxycycline, roxithromycin, and angiotensin-converting enzyme (ACE) inhibitors. Both ACE inhibitors and angiotensin receptor antagonists (ARB) have been successful in reducing aneurysm growth in mice but not consistently in humans.[72] Statins, however, in nonrandomized trials, have been found to reduce expansion rate and rupture risk. Unfortunately most of the studies with these agents were not well designed or had insufficient statistical power to permit definitive conclusions, but it seems prudent for patients with small aortic aneurysms to be taking a statin drug for this purpose.[20,21,73]

CLINICAL MANIFESTATIONS

Seventy to 75% of all infrarenal AAAs are asymptomatic when first detected.[74] Detection of large aneurysms can occur during a routine physical examination, but overall only 50% are palpable. Diagnosis most often occurs during an imaging study performed for some other reason (e.g., upper gastrointestinal series, barium enema, intravenous pyelography, lumbosacral spine radiography, or abdominal CT or ultrasound examination). Occasionally, an aneurysm is first discovered during an unrelated abdominal operation.

AAAs can cause acute symptoms as a result of rupture or expansion, pressure on adjacent structures, embolization, dissection, or thrombosis. Chronic symptoms can be caused by compression of adjacent bowel leading to early satiety and even nausea and vomiting. Because the duodenum crosses in front of the aorta, it is the part of the bowel most frequently compressed. Virtually any type of abdominal, flank, or back pain can be aneurysm-related. This fact often leads to a delay in diagnosis. Chronic abdominal or back pain is the most common symptom, occurring in up to one-third of patients, but is not specific. Large aneurysms can actually erode the spine and cause severe back pain, even in the absence of rupture.

The abrupt onset of severe pain in the back, flank, or abdomen is characteristic of aneurysmal rupture or acute expansion. It is uncertain why pain is produced by an expanding but unruptured (intact) aneurysm. The best explanation is sudden stretching of the layers of the aortic wall, with pressure on adjacent somatic sensory nerves or overlying peritoneum. Tenderness of the palpated aneurysm suggests that abdominal symptoms are arising from the aneurysm, although tenderness by itself is not a reliable indicator of impending rupture. In most surgical series, symptomatic but unruptured aneurysms account for 6% to nearly 40% of cases (average of five series totaling 311 patients: 13.7%).[75] The increased morbidity and mortality for urgent operations on unruptured aneurysms is likely due to lack of patient optimization. The timing of surgical treatment is made more difficult in these cases. A good-quality CT scan may not show any sign of rupture but cannot predict when rupture might subsequently occur.

Ruptured aneurysms constitute between 20% and 25% of most series. The presence of an aneurysm is known in 25% to 33% of patients before rupture occurs. The nature of symptoms and their time course vary depending on the nature of the rupture.[76,77] Small tears of the aneurysmal sac can result in a small leak confined to the retroperitoneum that temporarily seals, with minimal blood loss; this is usually followed within a few hours by frank rupture, which produces a catastrophic medical emergency. Rupture most frequently occurs through the posterolateral aortic wall on the left side into the retroperitoneal space; less commonly, it occurs through the anterior wall into the free peritoneal cavity. The incidence of this latter type of rupture is higher than indicated in most surgical series, because most of these patients die before reaching the hospital. Rarely, an AAA ruptures into the inferior vena cava or one of the iliac veins, producing an *aortocaval (or aortoiliac) fistula*, or it ruptures into the gastrointestinal tract, producing a primary *aortoenteric fistula*.

The classic clinical manifestations of ruptured aortic aneurysm are severe mid or diffuse abdominal pain, shock, and a palpable, pulsatile abdominal mass. The pain may be more prominent in the back or flank, or it may radiate into the groin or thigh. Because the most frequent site of rupture is the left posterolateral wall, pain is more commonly felt on the left side. The pain tends to be severe and steady. The severity of the shock varies from mild to profound, depending on the amount of blood loss. Many patients feel light-headed, sweaty, or nauseated. Abdominal distention is common, often preventing palpation of the expected pulsatile abdominal mass. The duration of symptoms can vary from a few minutes to more than 24 hours. Although aneurysm rupture is usually an acute catastrophic event, it can be contained for prolonged periods. These chronic ruptures have masqueraded as radicular compression, symptomatic inguinal hernia, femoral neuropathy, and even obstructive jaundice. It is thought that chronic, contained ruptures eventually progress to free ruptures, and they should be treated surgically on an urgent basis.[78]

The pain of an expanding but intact aneurysm may closely mimic that of a ruptured one. It tends to be severe, constant, and unaffected by position. The signs of hypovolemia are absent because hypotension and shock do not usually occur in the absence of actual rupture.

The diverse and nonspecific nature of the pain caused by expanding and leaking aneurysms all too often leads to errors in diagnosis, delays in finally establishing the correct diagnosis, and catastrophic rupture in the midst of a diagnostic procedure. Occasionally, a patient with a contained rupture arrives in the emergency room with angina pectoris from blood loss and reflex tachycardia and is rapidly transported to a coronary care unit without the abdominal examination that would identify the true cause of the chest pain. A similar situation can occur with rupture into the vena cava, with the resulting aortocaval fistula presenting as congestive heart failure. Most diagnostic errors such as these are due to failure to palpate the expansile, pulsatile epigastric mass, or failure to consider ruptured aneurysm as a possibility.

DIAGNOSTIC METHODS

Aortic aneurysms lie against the thoracolumbar spine and project anteriorly in the midline in the epigastrium. Elongated tortuous aneurysms may be located to the right or left or even in the lower quadrants. Except in thin patients, an abdominal aortic aneurysm must be approximately 5 cm in diameter to be detectable on a routine physical examination. As a result, aneurysms are seldom palpated in obese patients unless they are large. The reported accuracy in establishing the correct diagnosis by physical examination alone ranges from 30% to 90% (average 55%), depending on aneurysm size, body habitus, and physician skill.[79] Obesity, ascites, and lack of patient cooperation can impair aneurysmal detection by physical examination. Conversely, tumors or cystic lesions adjacent to the aorta, unusual aortic tortuosity, and excessive lumbar lordosis can all lead to a diagnosis of abdominal aortic aneurysm when none is present. The expansile nature of a pulsatile mass is a key element in deciding whether it is an aneurysm or a transmitted pulsation from an adjacent tumor. However, even when an aneurysm is palpable, determination of its size by palpation is imprecise.

Although physical examination detects some large aneurysms, it is inadequate for diagnosis and planning treatment, so more objective methods are necessary in all AAA patients. Size determination is especially important because it is currently the most important predictor of rupture risk and is usually the basis of management decisions. Plain abdominal and lateral spine radiographs can establish the diagnosis of 67% to 75% of abdominal aortic aneurysms by detecting linear calcification of the aortic wall (see Fig. 41.1). Unfortunately, accurate determination of maximal aortic size is possible in only two-thirds of these cases.

IMAGING MODALITIES

Several imaging modalities are widely available to establish the presence of an aortic aneurysm and accurately determine its size. These modalities include ultrasound, CT, and magnetic resonance imaging (MRI).

Real-time B-mode ultrasound is available in most hospitals and clinics and is the imaging method used in the large aneurysm screening and surveillance studies.[80] It uses no ionizing radiation, provides physiologic data as well as structural detail of vessel walls and atherosclerotic plaques, and can accurately measure aneurysm size in longitudinal and cross-sectional directions (i.e., it is three dimensional [3D]; see Fig. 41.2). Compared with intraoperative aneurysm measurements, ultrasonic measurements are accurate to within ±5 mm. Many studies have documented the ability of ultrasound to establish the diagnosis (100% sensitivity, 95% to 99% specificity) and accurately determine the size of abdominal and peripheral aneurysms.[81] Transcutaneous ultrasound is not as useful for imaging the thoracic or suprarenal aorta because of the overlying air-containing lung and viscera. Similarly, it is less reliable in defining the relationship between abdominal aortic aneurysms and the renal arteries, although recent developments in 3D ultrasound may improve upon this limitation. Because ultrasonography can obtain images in longitudinal, transverse, and oblique projections, it can be especially helpful in differentiating a tortuous aorta from an aneurysm. Ultrasound imaging is degraded by obesity, intestinal gas, or barium in the bowel. The overlying bowel gas also interferes with evaluation of the iliac arteries. The major advantages of ultrasound are its wide availability, painlessness, absence of known side effects, lack of ionizing radiation, relatively low cost, and ability to image vessels in multiple planes. Most vascular surgery trainees are experienced in performing and interpreting ultrasound studies, which can be helpful in evaluating patients with acute symptoms due to suspected rupture. These factors make ultrasonography the modality of choice for the initial evaluation of pulsatile abdominal or peripheral masses and for follow-up surveillance of aneurysms to determine increases in size and for screening. In addition, the portability of ultrasound machines is advantageous for the emergency department, where it can quickly establish the presence of an aneurysm in most cases, although it is not nearly as accurate (approximately 50%) in demonstrating rupture.

CT uses ionizing radiation to obtain cross-sectional images of the aorta and other body structures. These images provide detailed information about the size of the entire aorta, including the thoracic portion, so that the extent and size of an aneurysm can be accurately measured. Modern multidetector CT scanners using helical (spiral) technology possess sufficient spatial resolution to allow precise identification of the celiac, superior mesenteric, renal, and iliac arteries and their branches, as well as their relationship to the aneurysm and adjacent organs.[82] Major venous structures, including anomalies, can also be identified.[83] The administration of intravenous contrast allows evaluation of the size of the aortic lumen, the location and status of aortic branch vessels, the amount and location of mural thrombus, and in cases of dissection, differentiation of the true lumen from the false lumen (see Fig. 41.3; see color plate for Fig. 41.3C). Contrast-enhanced CT scans are also useful for assessing the retroperitoneum and identifying retroperitoneal hematoma (aneurysmal rupture), renal abnormalities, and the periaortic fibrosis associated with inflammatory aneurysms (Fig. 41.4).[84,85] Metallic surgical clips and orthopedic hardware create artifacts that can interfere with CT interpretation. CT provides more information about other abdominal and retroperitoneal structures than ultrasound and has emerged as the most frequently used technique to image the abdominal aorta and its branches.[86] One of its most helpful features is the ability to define the often complex relationship of an aneurysm to the renal and other aortic branch vessels and demonstrate their patency. Multiplanar reconstructions are particularly useful in clarifying the true anatomic relationships when there is anterior or lateral displacement of the aorta. Scan times are extremely short, and slices as thin as 1.5 to 2.0 mm can be obtained, allowing 3D reconstruction of the overlapping cross-sectional images, producing a CT angiogram (CTA) (see Fig. 41.3C). The reconstructed 3D images can be rotated in space and viewed from any projection. CT scans require significant radiation exposure and a relatively large volume of intravenously administered contrast material, which limits their usefulness in the presence of severe renal functional impairment. Non–contrast-enhanced images can be used for determining aortic size and the degree and location of calcification in the aorta and its branch vessels. Overall, CT scans are currently the most useful imaging method for evaluating the abdominal aorta and have nearly obviated the need for catheter aortography in the evaluation of aneurysmal disease. It is also essential in the process of determining an aneurysm's suitability and device sizing for endograft treatment.

MRI is also a useful modality for the evaluation of aortic disease (Fig. 41.5).[86] MRI uses pulsed radiofrequency energy in a strong magnetic field to produce images in longitudinal, transverse, and coronal planes. MRI instruments are not as widely available as ultrasound or CT scanners, and the selection and interpretation of proper scan sequences and images require considerable experience and skill. The spatial resolution has significantly improved, but the presence of implanted metal-containing devices (artificial joints, cardiac pacemakers) or the need for monitoring equipment are contraindications to MRI. Most intravascular stents are MRI compatible. MRI studies are more expensive and require considerably more time than CT or ultrasound, which limits their use in emergency evaluation of possible ruptures. Nevertheless, MRI clearly distinguishes arteries and veins from viscera and other surrounding tissue, and there is excellent agreement between MRI and ultrasound or CT images in determining aortic diameter. MRI is better than ultrasound for demonstrating involvement of branch vessels, especially the renal

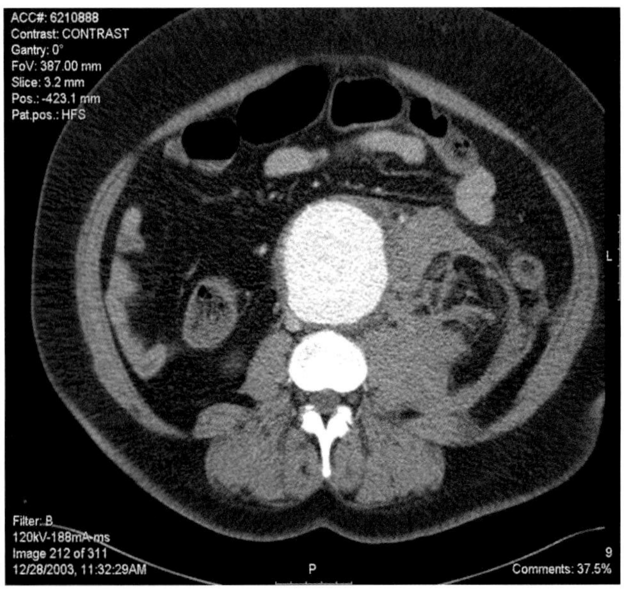

FIG 41.4 Computed tomographic scan showing contained rupture of aneurysm into the left retroperitoneal space *(axial view)*. Note the absence of mural thrombus.

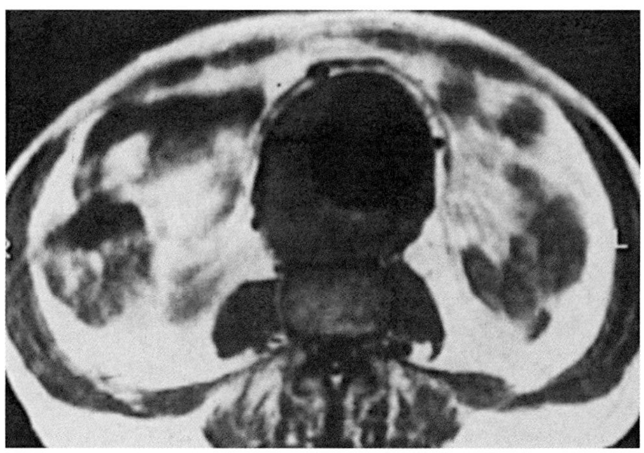

FIG 41.5 Magnetic resonance image of a large abdominal aortic aneurysm showing eccentric mural thrombus and flow channel.

arteries, with some authors reporting visualization of the renal arteries in more than 90% of cases. Other advantages of MRI over CT are the lack of ionizing radiation, and the relatively large image field. In addition, MRI does not require the use of nephrotoxic contrast agents to achieve intravascular enhancement. Instead, paramagnetic contrast agents, such as gadolinium, are routinely used to improve the imaging of vascular structures. This permits multiplanar image reformatting into MR angiograms (MRAs), similar to those of CT machines. The lack of need for iodinated contrast agents was initially thought to be a significant advantage of MR over CT in patients with abnormal renal function, but gadolinium can cause a severe and often fatal syndrome of nephrogenic systemic fibrosis in a small percentage these patients, which has limited its applicability. MRI machines are able to quantitate blood flow, although this feature is not commonly used clinically. However, adequate visualization of aortic branch arteries is not achieved as frequently with MRA as with CTA, and a significant number of patients cannot undergo MR scanning because of claustrophobia.

Objective documentation of the aortic size should be accomplished with one of these imaging modalities in all patients with suspected AAA. Each method can measure the diameter accurately. The initial scan can be used for comparison with subsequent scans to monitor aneurysmal enlargement. For most routine situations, ultrasonography is the method of choice because of its widespread availability, lower cost, and lack of ionizing radiation. When there is suspicion of suprarenal or thoracoabdominal aortic involvement or dissection, MRI or CT is preferable. For preoperative planning in these complex cases, a multiplanar study with 3D reconstruction (CTA, MRA) will delineate the aneurysm, aortic branch vessels, and neighboring structures. This is especially important if treatment by endografting is being considered. CT and MRI probably have equal capability to demonstrate unexpected features such as venous anomalies, perianeurysmal fibrosis, and horseshoe kidney, although the ureters are not easily identified by MRI. For symptomatic aneurysms, MRI and CT are also better than ultrasound in their ability to identify contained rupture.

Years ago, aortography was an essential step in the evaluation of patients with AAA. The limitations of catheter aortography for the diagnosis and evaluation of aortic aneurysms, like those of plain film radiography, are well known. Because the mural thrombus, which is nearly always present, tends to reduce the aneurysmal lumen size toward normal, aortography is not a reliable method to determine the diameter of an aneurysm or even to establish its presence. Aortography allowed the identification of frequent but unsuspected variations and abnormalities in renal and visceral vessels (Table 41.3). With better noninvasive imaging methods now routinely available, aortography has little use as a diagnostic method for AAA. Aortography is indicated as an initial step in the endovascular treatment of aortic aneurysms but should be performed very selectively in other patients with aneurysms for the following indications: (1) clinical suspicion of visceral ischemia, (2) occlusive iliofemoral vascular lesions, (3) severe hypertension or impaired renal function in a patient in whom a concomitant renal artery stenosis would be repaired if discovered, (4) suspicion of a horseshoe kidney to delineate renal artery anatomy, and (5) the presence of femoral or popliteal aneurysms. With the evolution and availability of CTA and MRA, it is usually possible to obtain this information with fewer risks. Newer CT scanners with large numbers of detectors (128 or more) perform even faster scans, with improved resolution and better 3D images. Sophisticated 3D reconstructions of CT scans are already available online from commercial vendors, making these sophisticated images available to any provider who can transfer the CT data onto a CD or transmit it electronically to the imaging facility.

TABLE 41.3 Angiographically Detected Lesions Associated With Abdominal Aortic Aneurysms

Findings	No. of Patients	Number (*n*)	Percent
Suprarenal extension	680	46	6.7
Renal stenosis or occlusion	763	138	18.0
Accessory or multiple renal arteries	680	92	13.5
Celiac or superior mesenteric artery stenosis	628	87	13.8
Iliofemoropopliteal stenosis or occlusion	680	298	43.8
Iliofemoropopliteal aneurysm	680	243	34.7

Collected data from Rich NM, Clagett GP, Salander JM, et al: Role of arteriography in the evaluation of aortic aneurysms. In Bergan JJ, Yao JST, editors: *Aneurysms: Diagnosis and Treatment*, New York, 1982, Grune and Stratton, pp 233–241; Gaspar MR: Role of arteriography in the evaluation of aortic aneurysms: the case against. In Bergan JJ, Yao JST, editors: *Aneurysms: Diagnosis and Treatment*, New York, 1982, Grune and Stratton, pp 243–254.

Molecular imaging is a rapidly developing modality that uses tracers aimed at physiologic processes attempting to provide functional information that is complimentary to the anatomical information of conventional scans. There are a variety of tracers and techniques being evaluated in experimental animals and humans, such as CVA-35, which labels collagen, and ^{15}F-labeled nanoparticles, targeting macrophages that may be able to predict which aneurysms are at high risk of rupture.[42]

RISK OF ANEURYSM RUPTURE

As noted earlier, the majority of AAAs are discovered in asymptomatic patients during an evaluation for an unrelated problem. Because of screening, aneurysms are being discovered at a smaller size than when the original studies in their natural history were first published by Estes, Wright, Szilagyi, and others.[87,88] Most aneurysms currently detected in screening programs are small (<4 cm), which has led to new concepts in the natural history of these lesions. Although aneurysms can cause symptoms and serious consequences from thrombosis and distal embolization, rupture is the most important risk, and aneurysm diameter is currently the most important factor that determines the risk of rupture. In general, the risk of rupture correlates directly with size: the larger the aneurysm, the greater the risk of rupture. For example, the yearly risk of rupture for abdominal aortic aneurysms,[5,89] between 4 and 5.4 cm in size is 0.5% to 1%; this increases to 6% to 10% for aneurysms between 6 and 7 cm and to 19% to 35% for aneurysms larger than 7 cm in diameter.[90] Calculated as 5-year rupture rates, these figures become 5%, 50%, and about 95%, respectively. The steepness of the curve plotting these data increases sharply at a diameter of approximately 5 cm, which is the basis for recommendations to defer elective aneurysm repair until a size of 5.0 to 5.5 cm is reached.[90,91] These data were derived from two randomized, controlled prospective clinical trials that studied survival in patients with asymptomatic small AAAs that were between 4 and 5.4 to 5.5 cm in diameter: the United Kingdom Small Aneurysm Trial, published in 1998, and the Veterans Administration–sponsored Aneurysm Detection and Management (ADAM) trial.[90,91] These two trials were similar in design, size, and results. The rupture rate for aneurysms in these trials was 0.5% to 1% per year, as noted previously, and neither trial showed a difference in long-term survival, which was the primary end point, between patients allocated to early operation or ultrasound or CT surveillance. The 6-year survival was similar in both trials, 64% in the UK trial and approximately 70% in the ADAM trial. Although 61% of those randomized to surveillance in both studies ultimately underwent aneurysm operation for enlargement or symptoms, long-term survival was not improved by early operation. Furthermore, delaying operation for these small aneurysms was not associated with increased operative or late mortality. These data are consistent with those from older, nonrandomized studies.[92,93] For example, population-based data from Rochester, Minnesota, showed a mean enlargement rate for aneurysms less than 5 cm in diameter of only 0.32 cm/year, and after 5 years of observation, no aneurysm smaller than 5 cm had ruptured.[92] The ADAM and UK trials enrolled mostly good-risk patients and rupture risk may be higher in high-surgical-risk patients. In both series, there was a higher rupture rate among the ineligible (i.e., high-risk) patients than in those randomized, suggesting that factors other than diameter influence rupture rate.

Other clinical features associated with increased risk of rupture include smoking, chronic obstructive lung disease, hypertension, female gender, transplant recipient, and rapid enlargement (defined as 1 cm/year or more). Cronenwett and associates[93] showed that chronic obstructive pulmonary disease and systolic hypertension are predictors of increased risk of rupture of small abdominal aneurysms. In a subsequent study, they confirmed that the rate of enlargement of small aneurysms was unpredictable, but either increased systolic or decreased diastolic pressure (i.e., increased pulse pressure) was associated with an increased rate of aneurysm expansion.[94] In this study, there was considerable variability in the rate of aneurysm enlargement, although the average rate of expansion was 0.4 cm/year in anteroposterior dimensions and 0.5 cm/year in lateral dimensions. Some clinical and experimental data suggest that the expansion rate of small aneurysms can be diminished by β-adrenergic blockade (propranolol), which should lead to a decreased rate of rupture.[95] Unfortunately, this theory was not supported in three randomized clinical trials. Other studies have shown that aneurysms are frequently elliptical rather than round and that aneurysmal expansion is initially more rapid in the lateral direction. It is interesting to recall that the most frequent site of aneurysm rupture is in the lateral wall. In a review of four series, including their own, Cronenwett and coworkers[93] described the outcome of 378 patients with small aortic aneurysms initially treated nonoperatively. After an average follow-up of 31 months, 27% of the patients were alive with intact aneurysms, 29% had died of other causes, 39% had elective aneurysm operations because the aneurysm diameter reached 5 to 6 cm, and 4% had suffered aneurysm rupture or acute expansion leading to emergency operation. Overall, there was a mean 5-year survival of 54% in these patients, somewhat less than the 6-year survival rates of 64% in the UK trial and 70% in the ADAM trial.[90,91] In light of these more recent studies, autopsy studies showing high rates of rupture of small aneurysms must be interpreted with caution.[7] Some have shown that 23.4% of aneurysms between 4.1 and 5 cm rupture, and the same is true for up to 10% of aneurysms less than 4 cm in diameter. Data such as these have led surgeons to recommend operation for almost all aortic aneurysms in good-risk patients. However, autopsy studies underestimate aneurysm size because of the lack of a distending blood pressure, and several more recent studies on living patients demonstrate a rupture rate of approximately 1% per year for aneurysms less than 5 cm in diameter, supporting the data from the ADAM and UK small aneurysm trials. In addition, two randomized trials comparing endovascular repair (EVAR) with open repair of small AAAs failed to demonstrate a survival benefit of early repair.[96,97]

There is little debate about the appropriateness of elective aneurysm surgery for patients with large aneurysms (>5.5 cm in diameter) because of the high risk of rupture and the associated mortality when rupture occurs. This is also valid in so-called high-risk patients because most of these patients will die from rupture and not from the conditions that caused them to be considered high risk. In addition, there is no agreement on what constitutes high risk. Patients who have a large AAA and are "unfit" for surgery constitute approximately 10% of AAA patients. Several reports dealing with these patients showed that rupture occurred in less than 50% and many of those survived emergency repair.[98,99] EVAR has early survival advantages compared with open repair in these patients. However, a recent report that included 1514 patients from 74 studies demonstrated lower than expected rupture rates ranging from 3.5% per year for 5.5 to 6.0 cm diameter AAAs to 6.3% per year for AAAs greater than 7.0 cm diameter and an overall risk of death from rupture of only 19% compared to 42% from all other causes; 32% were treated for rupture and 42% of these survived.[99] This study is one of many that suggest rupture rates overall are decreasing over time. Several cohort studies indicate that women have a greater risk of aneurysm rupture at a given size than men; therefore it has been suggested that women be offered definitive treatment at a smaller aneurysm size (i.e., 4.5 to 5.2 cm) than men.[25,100]

It must be emphasized that although the risk of aneurysm rupture correlates most closely with aneurysm size, and the average rate of aneurysmal enlargement is known (0.4 to 0.5 cm/

year), it is impossible to predict when a small aneurysm will rupture in a given patient. Perhaps the best explanation relates to the fact that aneurysms rupture at points of peak wall stress, as discussed earlier, and areas of peak wall stress do not necessarily coincide with areas of maximal diameter.[88,90] Clinical investigations of aneurysm wall stress using finite element analysis of CT-derived data may be better at predicting rupture but are not widely available. For now, diameter remains the best available predictor of risk of aneurysm rupture. The harmlessness of a small, asymptomatic abdominal aortic aneurysm is deceptive. Some do rupture, but still, coronary artery disease, and not rupture, is the most frequent cause of death in patients with small aneurysms.

RISKS OF SURGICAL TREATMENT

The natural history of untreated abdominal aortic aneurysms is well documented. This is especially true for those aneurysms measuring 5.5 cm or less in diameter. Since the first report of successful surgical resection and graft replacement of an infrarenal aortic aneurysm in 1952, many publications have documented the operative and long-term survival after surgical treatment. There has been a steady improvement in operative results for elective operations. Several large, contemporary series have reported operative mortality rates between 0.9% and 5% for large, single medical centers and only somewhat higher rates for community hospitals,[101-106] and the 1.8% operative mortality in the ADAM trial from selected Veterans Affairs (VA) medical centers compares favorably with these (Table 41.4). Higher mortality rates, ranging from 5% to 8%, have consistently been reported from analyses of large statewide or national data bases and lower operative mortality has been found to be associated with operations performed in high-volume institutions and by high-volume vascular surgeons, although the definitions of the term *high volume* are not uniform. The recently published SVS guidelines recommend that elective open surgical repair is best performed at high-volume centers with a documented in-hospital mortality of less than 5%.[20] Operative mortality in this range (<5%) justifies elective repair, even for relatively small aneurysms in good-risk patients.

The general improvement in surgical results has occurred despite the fact that more patients are being operated on who are older and have more comorbidities. Preoperative detection and treatment of significant cardiac disease have been important factors, as have improved anesthetic and critical care management and better perioperative drugs such as β-blockers, ACE inhibitors, ARBs, and statins.

Most of the deaths in elective operations occur in so-called "high-risk" patients; unfortunately, there is no consensus on what constitutes high risk. Chronologic age is not as important as physiologic age in assessing operative risk; therefore patients should not be denied elective operation based solely on age. Even octogenarians can undergo elective open aneurysm surgery with acceptable morbidity and mortality rates.[107,108] Most vascular surgeons have successfully treated ruptured aneurysms in patients previously rejected for elective operation because they were considered too old or too risky.

TABLE 41.4 Operative Mortality and Late Survival of Elective Open Surgical Treatment of Abdominal Aortic Aneurysm

Author (Year)	No. of Patients	Mean Age (Years)	Operative Mortality (%)	Cumulative 5-Year Survival (%)
Szilagyi et al. (1966)[88]	401	—	15	49
Hicks et al. (1975)[211]	225	67	8	60
O'Donnell et al. (1976)[212]	63	82	5	70
Crawford et al. (1981)[101]	860	66	5	63
Reigel et al. (1987)[112]	499	76	3	66
Bernstein and Chan (1984)[213]	123	71	1	72
UK trial (1998)[90]	563	69	5.8	64
Hertzer et al. (2002)[102]	1,293	71	1.2	75
ADAM trial (2002)[91]	569	68	1.8	70
Dream trial (2004)[214]	174	69	4.6	Not given
Schermerhorn et al. (2015)[105]	22,830	—	4.8	61
Lederle et al. (2004)[215]	441	70.5	3.0	75

The major risks for elective abdominal aortic aneurysm resection are similar to those for other major intraabdominal operations and include adequacy of cardiopulmonary and renal function. Recent studies have shown that decreased aerobic fitness and high frailty score both predicted increased morbidity and mortality after open aneurysm repair.[109,110] High-risk patients are those with unstable angina or angina at rest, cardiac ejection fraction less than 25% to 30%, congestive heart failure, serum creatinine level greater than 3 mg/dL, and pulmonary disease manifested by room air Po_2 of less than 50 mm Hg, elevated Pco_2, or both. A substantial percentage of these high-risk patients will die of a ruptured aneurysm and not from the disease that led to their categorization as high risk. With intensive perioperative monitoring and support, aneurysm resection can performed, even in these high-risk patients, with operative mortality of less than 6% as reported by Hollier and colleagues[111] and others.[112] Therefore, even high-risk patients with large abdominal aneurysms should be considered for elective treatment if the appropriate support facilities are available. It is in this group, however, that EVAR is the most attractive in anatomically suitable patients. However, a large number of randomized trials and cohort studies in low- and high-risk patients have shown only a small, statistically insignificant, advantage over open repair in early survival and this advantage disappears by the third postoperative year. Nevertheless, in the United States, 70% to 75% of abdominal aortic aneurysm repairs are now being treated with EVAR, driven largely by patient and physician preference. This has resulted in a higher proportion of open repairs being complex, including para- and juxta-renal aneurysms, which require suprarenal or supraceliac aortic clamping. The results have been quite good, with mortality only slightly higher than for infrarenal AAA, ranging from 0.8% to 6.1% in single-center series and 2.9% to 3.6% from larger databases like the Vascular Study Group of New England (VSGNE).[113,114] The incidence of renal dysfunction is also higher than for patients who do not require suprarenal clamping but permanent dialysis is uncommon. However, the increasing use of branched and fenestrated endografts has permitted endovascular treatment of juxtarenal, pararenal, and suprarenal aneurysms, which will decrease the need for open repair in a significant proportion of these cases. Nevertheless, there will always be some patients who require open repair, including those with failed EVAR and other uncommon situations. The consistent findings from clinical trials are that 70% to 80% of patients with AAAs are anatomically suitable for endoluminal repair with current commercially available devices (including fenestrated and branched), which can be accomplished with mortality rates equal to or slightly lower than those for open surgical repair.[116-118] Morbidity rates are clearly lower than those for open surgical repair, hospital stay is shortened, and patient satisfaction and surgeon enthusiasm are high; however, all aortic aneurysms can be treated by open repair. In addition, because of lingering uncertainties about long-term results of EVAR, with late mortality due to rupture being higher than for open repair, there is uncertainty regarding which patients and which aneurysms are best treated in this manner. For these reasons, the indications for endoluminal repair should be the same as those for open surgical repair in terms of aneurysm size and expected longevity. Endovascular aneurysm repair is covered in detail in Chapters 42 and 43.

Early detection and widespread elective aneurysm treatment programs have led to a decrease in the incidence of aneurysm rupture, but rupture is still highly lethal when it occurs. A substantial percentage (50%) of patients whose aneurysms rupture die before reaching a medical facility. An additional 24% arrive at a hospital alive but die before a definitive operation can be performed; therefore, operative mortality figures underestimate the true significance of aneurysmal rupture. The overall mortality from ruptured aneurysms, as reported in two large community-based studies, ranges from 74% to more than 90%.

The operative results for ruptured aneurysms are not nearly as favorable as those for elective aneurysm repair, but there has been a steady but limited decrease in operative mortality as documented in a 50-year review by Brown and colleagues.[119] They reported an average operative mortality of 47% in 171 studies published between 1950 and 2000, but mortality decreased from 55% at the beginning to 41% at the end of the study, an average decrease of 3.5% per 10 years. This occurred in spite of increasing age of the patients and before the impact of EVAR.[120]

Although there are a few series with better results, nearly 35% of patients die after being operated on for rupture. The nature of the rupture influences the results. Less than 10% of patients presenting in shock with free intraperitoneal rupture survive. Some reports indicate that preoperative cardiac arrest is uniformly fatal, and repair should not be attempted when this occurs. In contrast, patients in stable condition with small, contained leaks have a better than 80% survival rate. Several authors have reported improved mortality rates (30% to 35%) using endovascular treatment for ruptures, and others have reported no survival advantage.[121-123] There have been three randomized prospective trials (plus many observational studies) comparing open with endovascular treatment of ruptured aneurysms (AJAX [Dutch], ECAR [French], and IMPROVE [United Kingdom]).[124,125] All three reported no survival benefit of EVAR over open repair, but each of the studies had methodologic problems that have challenged the conclusions. Careful analysis of the data suggests that EVAR, when it can be done, is associated with decreased mortality (27% to 30%).[126] The operative mortality for open repair in some reports is as low as 27%, which is in the same range as most of the EVAR studies. Nevertheless the SVS guidelines give a strong recommendation for EVAR, when it can be done. In one study, endovascular treatment of ruptured aneurysms yielded worse outcomes in nonteaching and low-volume EVAR hospitals.[127]

The factors contributing to failure in the treatment of ruptured abdominal aortic aneurysm have been reviewed by Hiatt and associates.[128] The four most important factors were failure to perform elective aneurysmectomy in patients with known aneurysms; errors in diagnosing rupture when it occurred, leading to delay in operation; technical errors committed during the operation (all venous injuries); and undue delays in induction of anesthesia; these are all preventable. Other series have identified factors leading to death after aortic aneurysm rupture. Repeatedly, delays in performing surgery and the total volume of blood transfused are found to be important.[129,130] Preoperative cardiac arrest, female gender, age 80 years or older, massive blood loss, and ongoing major transfusion requirements were predictors of 90% to 100% mortality in the series by Johansen and colleagues,[120] which included a highly efficient transport and resuscitation response. Some of the differences in operative mortality among various reports are due in part to inconsistencies in patient categorization or considering all forms of rupture together. Many of these series also fail to separate patients with unruptured but symptomatic aneurysms who undergo emergency operations. The operative morbidity and mortality for symptomatic but not ruptured aneurysms is roughly double that of elective, asymptomatic patients.[130,131] It has been postulated that the reasons for this increased mortality is the omission of the usual preoperative optimization necessitated by the emergency operation as well as institution-based issues related to emergency procedures during nights and weekends.

LATE SURVIVAL

The most common cause of death among patients with large abdominal aortic aneurysm is rupture. The objectives of surgical repair are to prevent rupture and thereby prolong life. Without a doubt, surgical repair prevents rupture, and it does prolong life, but what is the long-term outlook for survivors? Several long-term studies using life-table methods have shown 5-year survival rates ranging from 49% to 75% (average, 61%; see Table 41.4).[131,132]

Although these data are far more encouraging than those for the survival of patients not undergoing operation, they do not equal the survival expected for the normal age-matched population. For example, Johnson and coworkers[133] reported a 50% survival of 7.4 years for patients after elective operative treatment for abdominal aneurysm, whereas the age-adjusted figure for the US general population was 15.7 years, and that for North Carolina citizens was 14.5 years. These authors could not identify an influence of age on operative mortality as did Hertzer and colleagues (5-year survival of 82% for ages 45 to 55 years vs. 60% for ages 76 and older),[102,134] although it affected late mortality as expected. Most of the excess late mortality could be attributed to coronary artery disease and cancer. This has led some centers to pursue an aggressive coronary evaluation and treatment protocol before elective aortic aneurysm operations.[135,136]

Several large surveys have shown that the safety of vascular surgical procedures in patients who have had previous coronary revascularization is comparable to that in patients with no evidence of ischemic cardiac disease, but this has not been evaluated by randomized clinical trials.[137,138] It has been estimated that, based on data from the Canadian Aneurysm Study, aggressive cardiac treatment increases the 5-year survival by only 5% to 10%.[139]

Dialysis-dependent renal failure is associated with high perioperative mortality in patients treated by EVAR or open repair and is also associated with significantly shorter survival after 1 and 3 years. This has led some authors to question whether the current recommendations for elective repair should be modified for patients on dialysis.[140]

Overall, aortic aneurysm repair is durable and approximately 70% of patients survive 5 years. Once they get beyond the perioperative period, the survival of those treated for rupture is similar to those with intact aneurysms. Interestingly, aneurysm size appears to be a factor in long-term survival; after treatment, larger aneurysms are associated with a shorter life span. Quality-of-life (QOL) studies have demonstrated that it is well maintained after either open or endovascular repair, although open repair has better QOL than EVAR after the first postoperative year.[141]

ASSESSMENT OF CARDIAC RISK

Approximately 30% to 40% of patients with aortic aneurysms do not have clinically evident coronary artery disease (e.g., no angina pectoris or history of myocardial infarction, normal electrocardiogram [ECG], normal exercise stress test result); however, 20% of these will have angiographically documented severe coronary artery disease, as will approximately 50% of those in whom coronary disease is clinically suspected (approximately 50% of the total).[135] Coronary artery disease is responsible for at least 50% to 60% of perioperative and late deaths after operations on the abdominal aorta.[142,143] The incidence of fatal myocardial infarction after elective abdominal aortic aneurysm surgery has been reported to be as high as 4.7%, and nonfatal infarction has been reported in up to 16% of patients and is associated with significant late cardiac morbidity. These data make it critical to minimize risk of periprocedural cardiac events. Comprehensive guidelines for perioperative cardiovascular evaluation and care for noncardiac surgery have been published by the American College of Cardiology and American Heart Association and endorsed by the SVS,[144] and the SVS has published its own guidelines dealing with this issue.[20] Readers are referred to these documents for details.

It is possible to identify high-risk cardiac patients using clinical assessment, exercise stress testing, radionuclide angiography, echocardiography, dipyridamole-thallium scanning, continuous portable electrocardiographic Holter monitoring, and coronary angiography. The challenge is deciding which patients need cardiac screening before aneurysm surgery. Patients with symptomatic cardiac disease require thorough cardiac evaluation and functional optimization before elective aneurysm repair. An ejection fraction less than 30% has been associated with increased cardiac complications in some series, but it does not predict postoperative myocardial infarction or death. Continuous portable ECG monitoring of vascular surgical patients for silent ischemia associated with ST-T segment changes has been shown to correlate with postoperative myocardial infarction in some series, but additional studies are needed to verify the value of this technique. Routine preoperative screening of all aortic aneurysm patients with coronary angiography is not feasible or prudent, even though Hertzer and colleagues[135-137] reported a nearly fivefold increase in operative mortality (5.1%) in aneurysm patients with suspected coronary disease, compared with those with no (1.1% mortality) or corrected (0.44% mortality) coronary artery disease. Late survival was also better in the groups with no or corrected coronary artery disease. Despite these data, no evidence has proved that there is decreased perioperative mortality or increased long-term survival among patients undergoing prophylactic coronary revascularization before aortic aneurysm repair. Furthermore, no single means exists to accurately predict perioperative cardiac risk after aortic aneurysmorrhaphy, but this is currently an area of intensive research.

Younger patients without overt cardiac disease with a normal 12-lead ECG and capable of at least moderate physical activity (MET >4) probably need no additional cardiac evaluation; in contrast, older patients with active coronary disease do need careful cardiac evaluation. The difficult decisions are in patients who fall between these two extremes (approximately 50% of the total), in whom unexpected coronary events still occur.[138] Because the ultimate objective of a cardiac evaluation is to identify and correct dangerous coronary artery lesions, the results of any subsequent intervention (e.g., coronary artery bypass grafting, percutaneous transluminal angioplasty/stenting) must be considered and balanced against the relatively low myocardial infarction rates that can be achieved in patients who do not undergo coronary revascularization. Overall, preliminary myocardial revascularization before aortic aneurysm repair is necessary in only 10% to 20% of patients and a significant number will already have had coronary revascularization prior to being seen for their aortic aneurysm.

Several other comorbid conditions are common in patients with aortic aneurysm, including renal, pulmonary, and hematologic diseases and diabetes mellitus. All can lead to morbidity and should be optimized before elective aneurysm repair. Perioperative use of beta blockers, statins, and ACE inhibitors are recommended for most patients.[20]

INDICATIONS FOR ANEURYSMS OF THE ABDOMINAL AORTA REPAIR

The objectives of surgical treatment are to relieve symptoms (if present) and prevent rupture (thereby prolonging life). These goals are best accomplished when operations are performed electively under optimal conditions. The natural history of unoperated abdominal aortic aneurysms and the excellent results currently achievable with conventional surgical treatment justify an aggressive diagnostic and therapeutic approach. Thus far, the only way to prevent or delay rupture is surgical treatment. The decision to recommend operation is often straightforward but can be difficult and must consider the rupture risk of the aneurysm, the life expectancy of the patient, and the operative risk of the procedure. Several scoring systems have been developed to aid decision making for individual patients as well as aid in making estimates regarding operative risks.[146,147]

Emergent operation is indicated for almost all patients with known or suspected rupture, regardless of the size of the aneurysm or age of the patient, but there are obvious exceptions to this recommendation. The coexistence of another fatal illness, such as metastatic cancer, or severe dementia with poor QOL may be sufficient reason for choosing a nonoperative approach. Some reports suggest that patients older than 85 years who are in shock or patients who present in cardiac arrest should be selected for nonoperative management because of the high operative mortality in this group; however, some do survive, so decisions must be individualized. Emergent or urgent operation is also indicated for symptomatic (abdominal or back pain) aneurysms in the absence of signs of rupture, because it is often impossible to determine whether an aneurysm has ruptured or is just expanding. Although CT and MRI scans can be relied on to detect the presence of periaortic blood in most cases, other more subtle findings, such as a break in the aortic calcium ring or stranding of retroperitoneal fat may provide clues to an impending rupture. The absence of these findings should not lead to unnecessary delays in operating, because actual rupture can occur at any time. Elective aneurysm repair should be recommended for asymptomatic patients with aneurysms 5.5 cm or larger in diameter, who are acceptable operative risks, and who have an estimated life expectancy of 2 years or more. Elective operation should also be considered for smaller aneurysms, between 5.0 and 5.4 cm in diameter, in good-risk patients, especially if they are hypertensive, active smokers, or live in remote areas where proper medical care would not be readily available should signs and symptoms of rupture develop. It is also appropriate to treat aneurysms between 4 and 5.5 cm in diameter that have shown documented rapid enlargement of more than 0.5 cm in less than 6 to 12 months by serial imaging studies. Enlargement at this rate has long been considered a sign of an unstable, changing aortic wall with an increased risk of rupture, but there are few if any published data supporting this concept. In the future, wall stress analyses will hopefully become readily available for use in making surgical decisions. Data from several studies have consistently showed that aneurysms in women rupture at a higher frequency and at a smaller size than in men; therefore it may be appropriate to recommend elective repair at 4.5 to 5.2 cm in women.[25]

There is considerable disagreement on what constitutes "high risk." High-risk patients include those who are very old or who have nonreconstructable coronary disease, poor left ventricular function with congestive heart failure, renal failure, or severe obstructive lung disease, and possibly other factors. Most recommend that such patients with small aneurysms should be observed until the aneurysm becomes symptomatic or large. High-risk patients with large aneurysms require thorough evaluation for the condition or conditions that put them in the high-risk category.[111] Frequently, such evaluations fail to substantiate the original degree of presumed risk, and it has been reported that less than 50% of "high-risk" patients die of the disease for which they were initially denied aneurysm repair. Unfortunately, there is lack of agreement on the definition of these various high-risk categories.

Before the introduction of EVAR, several groups advocated extraanatomic bypass in conjunction with induced thrombosis of the aneurysm in very high-risk patients with large abdominal aneurysms.[148] Thrombosis of the aneurysm, it was argued, would eliminate the risk of rupture, and the extraanatomic bypass would lower operative mortality by avoiding the risks of a major intra-abdominal operation and aortic cross-clamping. Unfortunately, nonresective therapy has not been as successful as originally hoped. Operative mortality exceeds 10%, and rupture still occurs in approximately 20% of patients so treated, which is higher than the mortality reported in similar but highly selected groups of patients subjected to conventional aneurysm operations.[149,150] Fortunately, this nonresective form of surgical therapy for abdominal aneurysms has been abandoned, even by some of its earlier proponents, and endoluminal stent-grafting has become the treatment of choice for these high-risk patients, when they have suitable anatomy.

Regardless of risk, a large majority of abdominal aortic aneurysms in all categories of risk are now treated with endovascular techniques as this is the recommended primary option.[20,151] About 20% of patients are anatomically unsuited for EVAR, according to the instructions for use (IFU) of the various endograft systems. Patients with short angulated necks, multiple renal arteries, inadequate access vessels, and infected graft/aneurysm are not suitable for EVAR. In addition, patients with failed EVAR (such as type I endoleak with enlarging aneurysm sac) may require conversion to open repair.[152] Fenestrated and branched endografts have been developed and there has now been a large experience with them in the treatment of complex aneurysms, including juxta-, para-, and suprarenal aneurysms. These complex aneurysms are technically more challenging for either open or endovascular treatment and the patients tend to have more comorbidities than those with just infrarenal involvement. Nevertheless, open surgical results are acceptable and this remains an appropriate option for some patients.[113,114]

There will probably always be some patients for whom there is not a good endovascular option, and these will require open surgical repair. Therefore this chapter focuses on open surgical treatment. EVAR is covered in detail in Chapter 42.

OPERATIVE TECHNIQUE

Incision and Exposure

There are three options for the incision for abdominal aortic aneurysm operations: full-length midline, wide transverse, and oblique.

The full-length midline incision is the most popular because it provides access to the entire abdominal cavity, including the supraceliac aorta and iliac arteries; it can be made and closed rapidly and has the fewest limitations. For the treatment of suprarenal or pararenal aneurysms, medial visceral rotation enables adequate exposure of the entire suprarenal segment of the abdominal aorta. This maneuver involves mobilization, from lateral to medial, of the left colon, spleen, and pancreas in what is normally an avascular plane. Splenic injury requiring splenectomy occurs approximately 25% of the time when this is done, and there is an increased risk of pancreatic injury. Midline incisional hernias occur more frequently after aneurysm repair than after other operations performed through midline incisions, possibly because of the same or similar connective tissue abnormality that is involved in the pathogenesis of aneurysms.

A wide transverse incision extending from flank to flank and curved either above or below the umbilicus, depending on the aortic and iliac pathology, also provides excellent transperitoneal exposure. It is more time-consuming to create and close than a midline incision, but is said to be stronger, although proof of superiority in terms of wound dehiscence is lacking. Transverse incisions are less painful and therefore interfere less with respiratory function postoperatively, because they cut across fewer intercostal nerves.

Both the midline and the transverse incisions offer wide access to the peritoneal cavity and retroperitoneum and its contents. These incisions permit a thorough abdominal exploration that should be performed as a preliminary step in all elective operations, because there is a significant incidence of coexisting intraabdominal pathology, including colon tumors and gallstones.

Retroperitoneal exposure of the aorta can be achieved through an oblique incision extending from the left 11th intercostal space or tip of the 12th rib to the edge of the rectus abdominis muscle.[152-154] The patient is placed in a semilateral position, but with the hips allowed to rotate back toward the supine position, which allows access to both femoral arteries. Through this retroperitoneal exposure, the suprarenal and supraceliac aorta can be controlled more easily, but access to the right iliac artery is often limited, especially if the aortic aneurysm is large or if there is a large right iliac aneurysm. Among the advantages of the retroperitoneal approach are less postoperative respiratory compromise, lower intravenous fluid requirements, less intraoperative hypothermia, a shorter period of postoperative ileus, and avoidance in many cases of the need for postoperative nasogastric intubation. Although the perception is that these patients generally fare better than those operated on through a midline incision, when the two approaches were compared in prospective studies, no significant differences were found.[153] One disadvantage of the retroperitoneal approach is that the contents of the peritoneal cavity are not visible for inspection, although an opening in the peritoneum can be made easily if necessary. Another is the occurrence of a postoperative flank bulge that can be particularly annoying to some patients. This is probably due to injury to the intercostal nerve in the line of the incision. The retroperitoneal approach loses most of its advantages when there is a retroaortic left renal vein or left-sided vena cava, because these structures are then in a vulnerable location. Nevertheless, many surgeons use this approach for all elective aneurysm operations, especially pararenal and suprarenal types. Some even use it for contained ruptured aneurysms because of the ability to achieve rapid control of the upper abdominal aorta.[155] The retroperitoneal approach is probably preferable in the presence of an inflammatory aneurysm or horseshoe kidney.

The choice of incision is a matter of surgeon preference and patient factors. Things to consider in making this choice include the extent of the aneurysm, the status of the iliac arteries, the degree of obesity and pulmonary disease, previous abdominal operations, the presence and location of stomas, the necessity to inspect intraperitoneal structures (especially in patients with atypical symptoms), and the speed with which aortic control must be attained. Surgeons should be familiar with all three approaches, so that they can take advantage of each when appropriate.

Transperitoneal or retroperitoneal exposure of the aorta through small incisions, with or without laparoscopic assistance, has been used successfully to treat aortic aneurysms by several surgical groups. The special instruments, vascular clamps, and retractors necessary to accomplish this have been developed and are being improved. Turnipseed[156] compared 50 patients who had aortic aneurysms or occlusive disease treated via minimal incisions with 50 similar patients treated using a long midline incision. The minimal incision technique was as safe and effective as the standard incision and was associated with shorter intensive care unit and total hospital stay, less morbidity, and reduced costs. It was more cost efficient than either the standard incision or endoluminal stent-grafting techniques. Completely laparoscopic aneurysm repair has also been performed, and several fairly large series have been reported, with improving results and reduced operative times.[157] Only a few groups have significant experience with the use of robotic devices for aneurysm replacement. With experience, the duration of the procedure has been reduced and the success rate is high.

When midline or transverse incisions are used, the aorta is exposed by an infracolic retroperitoneal incision that should be kept slightly to the right of the midline. The duodenum must be carefully reflected laterally, along with the rest of the small bowel; this requires division of the ligament of Treitz, which should be carefully reapproximated as part of the retroperitoneal closure. The left renal vein usually marks the cephalad extent of the dissection, unless the aneurysm extends to the renal arteries (juxtarenal aneurysm) or involves them (pararenal aneurysm; see Fig. 41.6). In either of these situations, suprarenal aortic clamping is necessary, and the left renal vein should be thoroughly mobilized so that it can be retracted cephalad or caudad to facilitate adequate exposure of the pararenal aorta.[158,159] It is

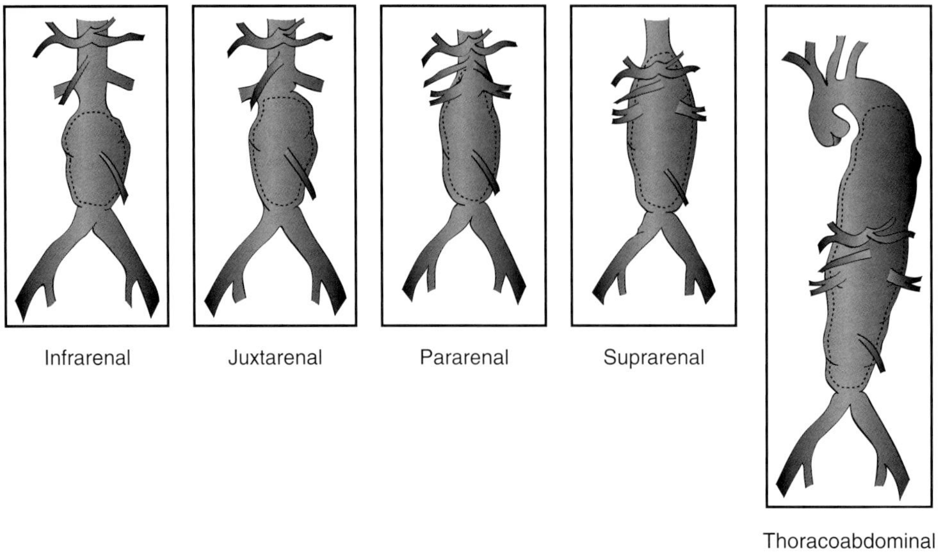

FIG 41.6 Morphologic classification of abdominal aortic aneurysms. Aneurysms can be classified according to their relationship to the renal arteries as infrarenal, juxtarenal, pararenal, and suprarenal.

sometimes necessary to divide the left renal vein; this is usually well tolerated if the left adrenal and gonadal veins are not ligated, but there is an increased risk of sustained elevation in the serum creatinine level, a temporary reduction of left renal function, and increased retroperitoneal bleeding.[160] Reanastomosis of the transected renal vein avoids these complications, but it is not always necessary.[144]

Distally, the dissection should avoid the fibroareolar tissue overlying the left common iliac artery in men because it contains branch vessels of the inferior mesenteric artery (IMA) and the autonomic nerves that control sexual function. If the common iliac arteries are relatively normal (i.e., not aneurysmal, stenotic, or heavily calcified), they can be clamped and a straight tube graft can be used for the aortic replacement. Significant disease at the aortic bifurcation or the common iliac arteries makes a bifurcated graft preferable. Control of the iliac arteries in these situations is best achieved by mobilizing the external and internal iliac arteries and controlling them individually. Particular care must be taken in this location to avoid injury to the accompanying posterior venous structures and to the ureters, which cross anterior to the common iliac bifurcation. Every effort should be made to ensure antegrade perfusion in at least one hypogastric artery, to minimize the risk of postoperative ischemia of the left colon as well as buttock claudication. Most reconstructions will require a bifurcated graft with distal anastomoses constructed to the transected common iliac artery. If this is not possible, the distal anastomosis can be made in an end-to-side fashion with the external iliac artery and the common iliac stump oversewn, thereby permitting hypogastric perfusion in a retrograde fashion. If this is not possible, hypogastric revascularization can be accomplished by a side-arm graft from the iliac limb of the bifurcation graft to the internal iliac artery. An easier technique is to perform an end-to-end anastomosis between the end of the iliac limb and the hypogastric and then place a graft from the iliac graft limb to the external iliac artery.

Extensive perioperative monitoring is indicated for patients undergoing abdominal aortic aneurysm repair.[161,162] This monitoring contributed significantly to the improved results reported in large series of electively treated patients. Monitoring usually includes continuous recording of the ECG, intraarterial pressure, body temperature, urine output, and central venous or pulmonary artery pressure. In high-risk patients, especially if the aorta will be cross-clamped above the renal arteries, transesophageal 2D echocardiographic monitoring of left ventricular function may be superior to measurements of pulmonary artery pressure for the evaluation of intravascular volume status.[162] Various blood components should be monitored as well, including arterial oxygen and carbon dioxide content and pH, plasma glucose, electrolytes, and coagulation factors. Monitoring the clotting system is especially important in ruptured aneurysms and in cases in which large volumes of blood and blood products have been infused or a supraceliac clamp has been used. The use of autotransfusion is routine in some institutions to minimize the need for homologous blood transfusion. Unfortunately, its use was not found to be cost effective in randomized trials. For elective operations, patients should be encouraged to donate their own blood for autologous transfusion in the perioperative period.

Aneurysm Repair

EVAR is covered in detail in Chapter 42. Therefore, the emphasis in this chapter is on open repair. Regardless of the extent of the aortic aneurysm, the proximal graft anastomosis should be made as close as possible to the renal arteries to prevent recurrent aortic pathology. The proximal aortic neck can be evaluated on the preoperative imaging studies to assess diameter, length, and wall characteristics, such as calcification, thrombus, and plaque. These features are important in determining where to place the proximal cross clamp, which in turn may influence the choice of incision. *Juxtarenal* aneurysms extend to the renal arteries but do not involve them. These aneurysms can be repaired with an infrarenal graft, but suprarenal cross clamping is required. In contrast, *pararenal* aneurysms involve the orifice of at least one of the renal arteries so that renal revascularization is required for at least one kidney. This procedure requires suprarenal and frequently supraceliac clamping to perform the aortic anastomosis and renal artery repair.[115] The degree of disease in the iliac arteries determines the distal extent of the graft. In some series, up to 80% of patients have been treated successfully with a straight tube graft, although in the experience of others, only approximately one-third of patients had suitable anatomy for this approach. There does not appear to be a significant incidence of subsequent iliac aneurysm formation when tube grafts are used in the presence of normal-sized or only slightly enlarged common iliac arteries (<2.5 cm diameter).

The choice of graft material—polyester (knitted or woven) or expanded polytetrafluoroethylene (ePTFE)—is a relatively unimportant issue; there is no proven superiority of either graft type, when used for aortic replacement. Polyester grafts are the most popular, and most surgeons prefer knitted grafts because they are easier to handle. Knitted grafts sealed with collagen or gelatin are not porous, do not require preclotting, can bind topically applied antibiotics, and have less bleeding through needle holes than ePTFE. For ruptured aneurysms, nonporous grafts are clearly preferable because of savings in time and interstitial blood loss.

Systemic heparin is administered almost universally during the occlusive phase of elective aneurysm operations, because most surgeons believe that its use provides added protection from distal thrombosis. It has been traditionally taught that distal clamps should be applied before the aortic clamp to prevent distal embolization, but recent evidence suggests otherwise because of the risk of renal embolization from reversed and turbulent flow produced by distal occlusion. It is probably best to clamp the most normal vessel first. The aorta is opened longitudinally and either partially or completely transected at the site of the proximal anastomosis. If there is a very short or no infrarenal neck (juxtarenal aneurysm), temporary proximal aortic clamping above the renal arteries is required to accomplish an adequate infrarenal anastomosis (see Fig. 41.2). This also requires control of the renal arteries to prevent the entrance of embolic debris. The proximal anastomosis can be done with a continuous or interrupted suture technique; the former is obviously quicker. If the aorta is especially weak or friable, the sutures can be supported with Teflon-felt pledgets or strips.

The distal anastomoses can be end to end or end to side, depending on their location and the status of the common and internal iliac arteries. All mural thrombus and atheroma should be debrided from the aneurysm wall. Several studies have shown a surprisingly high incidence of positive bacterial cultures of this material, ranging from 10% to 40% of patients. The significance of these positive cultures is unknown, but most of them have been due to coagulase-negative *Staphylococcus* species, an organism commonly found in aortic graft infections.[163] Back-bleeding lumbar vessels can be the source of significant blood loss and should be suture-ligated from within the aortic sac. If the IMA is patent and actively back-bleeding, it can also be ligated within the aneurysm sac, but if back-bleeding is meager, it should be preserved and reassessed after distal flow is reestablished, especially if internal iliac flow is compromised. Reimplantation of the IMA is relatively easy to perform, when necessary, with the use of the Carrel patch technique.

All anastomoses should be constructed with permanent synthetic sutures. Braided polyester and monofilament polypropylene or PTFE are the most commonly used. Theoretical fears about late fracture of polypropylene sutures have not been substantiated in clinical practice. If suprarenal clamping is necessary, the clamp should be moved onto the graft and below the renal arteries as soon as possible to minimize renal ischemia after ensuring that the proximal anastomosis is secure. The distal anastomoses can then be constructed as indicated by the iliac artery disease. If the iliacs are severely calcified, it is sometimes easier to control iliac artery back-bleeding by the use of intraluminal balloon catheters and to oversew the common iliac arteries from within the opened aortic or iliac aneurysms. In unusual circumstances, external iliac disease necessitates making the distal anastomosis to the common femoral artery.

Declamping hypotension is now an unusual event in elective aortic aneurysm surgery, but it is essential to maintain excellent communication with the anesthesiology team so that depth of anesthesia and blood and fluid replacement can be adjusted in anticipation of lower extremity reperfusion. Although the graft and native vessels are flushed and back-bled before reestablishing distal flow, it is preferable to reestablish flow first into one hypogastric artery to minimize the chance of distal embolization to the leg. Before abdominal closure, adequacy of lower extremity and left colon perfusion should be ensured by direct inspection or noninvasive instrumentation. The graft should be insulated from the overlying bowel by careful closure of the aneurysm sac over the graft. This is sometimes impossible when the aneurysm is small, and in these situations, rotation of a flap of the aneurysm wall or a vascularized omental pedicle can be used to separate the graft from the duodenum.

It is beyond the scope of this chapter to discuss all the technical details that might be encountered during the surgical treatment of an aortic aneurysm. The principles outlined here are generally applicable in most cases. It is generally unwise to perform concomitant procedures on the gastrointestinal (GI) or genitourinary (GU) tracts during AAA repair because of the risk of contaminating the newly implanted graft. But if additional vascular procedures are required, such as renal or visceral artery reconstruction, appropriate modifications in technique are obviously required.[164]

Repair of Ruptured Aneurysm

For ruptured aneurysms, the first priority is to control the hemorrhage by gaining proximal control of the aorta. Resuscitation is best done in the operating room rather than in the emergency department, and it is better to restore blood pressure only to levels sufficient to maintain vital organ function and cerebral perfusion before the induction of anesthesia (permissive hypotension). It is also better to have the patient prepared and draped, with the surgical team ready to make a rapid entry into the abdomen, before the induction of anesthesia. The induction of anesthesia in these circumstances is often associated with sudden and severe hypotension when the tamponade effects and reflex vasoconstriction are relieved by relaxation of the abdominal wall and the administered anesthetic agents. The practice of proximal aortic control by balloon occlusion (resuscitative endovascular balloon occlusion of the aorta [REBOA]) using a catheter inserted via a transbrachial or transfemoral approach has been repopularized largely to avoid this phenomenon. Most vascular surgeons now have sufficient experience with endovascular techniques that insertion of a femoral artery sheath and occlusion balloon can be done very quickly. The availability of high-quality digital fluoroscopy and endovascular supplies in the operating room makes this feasible. Surprisingly, this maneuver has been shown to reduce the number of intraoperative deaths but not 30-day mortality. Once proximal control is obtained, and if no preoperative CT was performed, an angiogram can be performed to determine suitability for EVAR and then proceed with that or open repair. For open repair, if the rupture is contained, proximal aortic control is best achieved at the level of the supraceliac aorta through the lesser omentum. This requires mobilization of the left lobe of the liver and can be far more difficult than anticipated when there is a large hematoma in the mesentery that pushes the transverse mesocolon and upper abdominal viscera cephalad (see Fig. 41.4). The hematoma can then be entered and the clamp repositioned distally after the aortic neck is identified. The hematoma usually makes this portion of the dissection relatively easy, but caution must be exercised to avoid injury to major venous structures, which is one of the most common causes of excessive hemorrhage and subsequent death. If there is free intraperitoneal rupture, the aorta can be quickly compressed against the spine at the diaphragm with an assistant's hand or a commercial compression device without formally dissecting this area. An infrarenal clamp or an intraluminal occluding balloon catheter should be substituted as soon as possible. After bleeding is controlled, adequate blood and volume replenishment should be achieved before attempting to restore flow to the lower extremities. Heparin is unnecessary and should be avoided in ruptured aneurysms because bleeding and coagulopathy are frequently associated with the shock, hypothermia, and massive blood loss and replacement that occur. The aggressive use of blood and blood products, including platelets and fresh frozen plasma, is essential for the survival of these patients.

COMPLICATIONS OF AORTIC ANEURYSM REPAIR

Survival after aortic aneurysm surgery was discussed earlier in this chapter. Operative mortality ranges from 0% to 3% for patients with uncomplicated aneurysms operated on electively to more than 80% for patients with rupture, hypotension, and oliguria. The most frequent cause of death is myocardial dysfunction, usually ischemic in origin.[137,143] Overall, 15% to 30% of patients have at least one complication after open surgical repair. Nonfatal myocardial infarction is fairly common, even after elective aortic aneurysm repair, occurring in 3.1% to 16% (average, 6.9%) of patients in reported series.[9] The varying incidence is due to different criteria used to define myocardial infarction (e.g., non-ST elevation, troponin leak) and possibly due to different protocols for evaluating and treating coronary artery disease preoperatively.[145]

Several other major complications can occur during or after aortic aneurysm operations. Hemorrhage is a constant threat, most often from injury to iliac or lumbar veins. It can be severe and extremely difficult to control, especially if it involves the left common iliac vein where it passes beneath the right common iliac artery. For this reason, extreme care must be taken when mobilizing and clamping the iliac arteries, especially if they are aneurysmal, in which case they are more likely to be adherent to the underlying veins. Injury to the left renal vein or one of its tributaries is also associated with brisk bleeding. This is particularly likely when there are venous anomalies such as a retroaortic left renal vein or a circumaortic venous collar. These venous anomalies can usually be identified preoperatively if a CT scan has been obtained. Intraoperatively, major venous anomalies should be suspected when, during cephalad dissection of the aortic neck, either a small or no left renal vein is encountered in its usual location crossing anterior to the aorta. Postoperative hemorrhage can occur in any patient, and hemodynamic instability and evidence of continued blood loss should lead to early reexploration of the abdomen. Nonsurgical bleeding can be minimized by careful monitoring of the coagulation system to provide the basis for administration of platelets, clotting factors, and protamine when appropriate.

Declamping hypotension is not as frequent or severe a problem as it once was. Better understanding of its physiology, more aggressive management of intravascular volume, and better monitoring and anesthetic techniques have all contributed to the reduction in the incidence and seriousness of this problem. The surgeon can help minimize this condition by giving the anesthesiologist advance notification of plans to restore distal perfusion and then doing it gradually. Instilling vasopressors down the leg before declamping is done rarely. Despite these precautions, declamping hypotension can still be a serious problem, especially in the setting of a ruptured aneurysm in a cold, hypovolemic patient with poor cardiac performance. Gradual restoration of distal flow can minimize the severity of declamping hypotension.

Renal failure is another serious but infrequent complication. At one time, 3% to 12% of deaths after elective abdominal aortic aneurysm operations and an even higher percentage after emergency operations for rupture were attributable to acute renal failure.[165,166] Renal failure or less severe degrees of renal impairment can occur even when there is no hypotension and the proximal aortic clamp was infrarenal in location. The cause of renal dysfunction in these situations is poorly understood but is believed to involve reflex renal vasoconstriction and intrarenal redistribution of blood flow. Atheromatous embolization from clamping or manipulation of the perirenal aorta is also a potential contributing factor, as is temporary suprarenal clamping when it is required. Sometimes, the large contrast load of an aortogram or CT scan obtained 1 or 2 days preoperatively can cause renal dysfunction that only becomes apparent postoperatively. Mannitol or loop diuretics are commonly administered before aortic cross-clamping to increase urine output and prevent renal failure. Although this seems reasonable, studies have shown that intraoperative urine volume does not predict postoperative renal function.[167] Renal failure because of acute tubular necrosis is much more common after operations for ruptured aortic aneurysms, occurring in 21% of survivors of operation in one series. Unfortunately, the mortality associated with this complication still ranges from 50% to 70%, despite the use of acute hemodialysis and adequate nutritional support.

Injury to the bowel or ureters can cause catastrophic infectious complications involving the newly implanted prosthetic graft. This is most likely to occur when there are adhesions from previous operations or the structures are in an unusual position (e.g., the ureters displaced anteriorly and laterally by the aneurysm). Such injuries should be meticulously repaired, and the area should be thoroughly irrigated with antibiotic solution. Ureteral injuries should be repaired and stented. In some situations, nephrectomy is the safest course to avoid possible graft contamination.

Gastrointestinal complications of a functional nature regularly occur after conventional aortic aneurysm surgery. Ileus is the rule for at least 2 to 3 days after transperitoneal surgery but earlier initiation of oral liquids is now the practice in many centers. Typically, gastric and colonic ileus persists longer than small bowel ileus. Nevertheless, the use of nasogastric tubes has not been shown to reduce the incidence of early gastrointestinal dysfunction, and they should be able to be removed by the first postoperative morning. Small amounts of liquids can often be safely administered orally beginning on postoperative day 1 or 2. Occasionally, duodenal obstruction persists for longer periods. The presence of hematoma and edema in the vicinity of the proximal anastomosis is thought to contribute to this problem as is improper reconstitution of the ligament of Treitz during the retroperitoneal closure. Postoperative pancreatitis is relatively common, as determined by elevation of the serum amylase and lipase levels, although clinically apparent pancreatitis is unusual. The pancreas can be injured by retractors, however, and a few patients have serious consequences from these seemingly minor injuries.

The most serious gastrointestinal complication is ischemia of the left side of the colon and the rectum. The incidence of ischemic colitis after aortic reconstruction is approximately 2% (range, 0.2% to 10%).[168] It is threefold to fourfold more common after operations for aortic aneurysm than after operations for occlusive disease, and the incidence is several times higher in patients studied prospectively with colonoscopy after sustaining a ruptured aneurysm. Ligation of a patent IMA in the presence of inadequate collateral circulation to the sigmoid colon and rectum is thought to be an important pathophysiologic mechanism, but the IMA is already occluded in 40% to 50% of patients with abdominal aneurysms. Improper ligation of the IMA too far away from the wall of the aneurysm can contribute to this complication by interfering with collateral blood supply to the rectosigmoid.[169] Postoperative hypotension and hemodynamic instability are significant contributory factors. Therefore, as noted earlier, it is important to maintain antegrade perfusion in at least one internal iliac artery after arterial reconstruction for aortic aneurysm.[170] Although most patients with occlusion of both internal iliac arteries and the IMA have adequate colonic perfusion, postoperative hypotension, bowel distention, and mesenteric vessel compression by hematoma can all contribute to postoperative colonic ischemia. The large experience with EVAR has shown that hypogastric artery occlusion is not as benign as was previously believed. There is a significant incidence of buttock claudication with unilateral occlusion, which can also limit collateral perfusion to the rectosigmoid and spinal cord. This emphasizes the importance of restoring direct flow into at least one hypogastric artery during the reconstructive phase of aneurysm repair.

Postoperative colonic ischemia can involve the mucosa only, which usually causes a transient, mild form of ischemic colitis, or it can involve mucosa and muscularis, which can result in fibrous healing and stricture formation. The most severe and dreaded form is transmural ischemia, which occurs in more than 60% of the reported cases. The clinical manifestations of bowel ischemia depend on its severity. Diarrhea, especially if it is bloody, is one of the earliest manifestations and usually begins within 48 hours of operation. It is an indication for colonoscopy to assess the status of the colonic mucosa. Other findings indicative of bowel gangrene and peritonitis may be present and demand prompt reoperation, resection of all compromised bowel, and creation of appropriate stomas. During bowel resection the underlying aortic prosthesis should be carefully isolated from the surgical field, although this is usually impossible, setting the stage for subsequent prosthetic infection. If the graft becomes grossly contaminated, the safest course is to remove it and restore lower extremity perfusion by axillofemoral bypass. Less severe degrees of colonic ischemia can be managed nonoperatively, although subsequent correction of a colonic stricture may be required. A high index of suspicion of this complication must be maintained to detect and treat it in a timely fashion. Some surgeons routinely perform flexible sigmoidoscopy on the first day after repair of a ruptured aortic aneurysm to establish early diagnosis of rectosigmoid ischemia.

The mortality for postoperative colonic ischemia following aortic aneurysm surgery is approximately 50% overall, but increases to 90% when full-thickness colonic gangrene and peritonitis occur. Preoperative evaluation of the blood supply to the colon and intraoperative assessment of colonic perfusion by Doppler or IMA back-pressure measurements may help to identify patients at highest risk for this disastrous complication so that preventive measures (i.e., IMA reimplantation) can be taken. Routine inferior mesenteric reimplantation is advocated by some surgeons, but there are no solid data on how often this is really necessary. The SVS guidelines recommend reimplantation of a patent IMA whenever there is an increased risk of colonic ischemia. Such circumstances include poor IMA back-bleeding, occlusive lesions of the celiac and superior mesenteric arteries, presence of a large meandering mesenteric artery, inability to restore hypogastric perfusion, and previous rectosigmoid colectomy. Intraoperative and postoperative hypotension, especially if vasopressors are used, exacerbates all these conditions. Even following these guidelines, IMA reimplantation should be necessary in only 5% to 10% of cases.

Paraplegia caused by spinal cord ischemia, a well-recognized complication of thoracoabdominal aneurysm repair, is a rare event after operations confined to the infrarenal aorta, with only slightly more than 50 cases reported. Szilagyi and coworkers[171] noted an incidence of 0.2% in more than 3000 aortic operations, and it occurred 10-fold more frequently in patients with ruptured aneurysms. This finding suggests that hypotension is a contributing factor in most cases, although injury to an unusually located arteria magna radicularis (artery of Adamkiewicz) to the spinal cord may be the primary event. Pelvic hypoperfusion associated with internal iliac artery occlusion is an important contributing factor in some patients; this reemphasizes the importance of maintaining perfusion of at least one hypogastric artery. Unfortunately, the paraplegia in this situation is not predictable or preventable. Treatment with spinal fluid drainage and high-dose steroids has been tried with limited success. Although the severity of the clinical manifestations varies and approximately 50% of affected survivors recover some neurologic function, there is a 50% mortality associated with this complication.

Ischemia of the lower extremities can also occur after aortic aneurysm surgery. This may be due to embolization of dislodged mural thrombus or atherosclerotic plaque from the aneurysm itself, thrombosis of a downstream vessel due to distal stasis, creation of an intimal flap, or crushed atherosclerotic plaque. The use of heparin during the occlusive phase of aneurysm repair does not prevent embolic events from occurring, but may limit the propagation of thrombus and should prevent the formation of stasis thrombi in the distal vascular beds. Before closing the abdomen, the surgeon must be satisfied with the perfusion status of the lower extremities.

Microembolization can also occur, resulting in small patchy areas of ischemia, usually on the plantar aspect of the feet. Pedal pulses are usually still palpable in this situation. Colloquially, this is known as *trash foot,* and if it is recognized intraoperatively, the passage of small balloon catheters can sometimes retrieve at least some of the atheromatous debris. Lumbar sympathectomy may also be beneficial in limiting or preventing full-thickness tissue loss.

Abdominal compartment syndrome has been recognized as an unusual but important cause of renal and respiratory failure, especially after operations for ruptured aneurysms. Manifested by massive abdominal distention, oliguria, and difficulty maintaining adequate ventilation, it is an indication for prompt reexploration of the abdomen to relieve the intraabdominal pressure. It can also occur after EVAR in cases of aneurysm rupture. Measurement of airway and urinary bladder pressures can be helpful in deciding to return a patient to the operating room for abdominal decompression. The usual finding is massive visceral edema and blood, and a deliberate abdominal wall hernia must be created, using a mesh-assisted delayed abdominal closure. Bladder pressure is a reasonable approximation of intraabdominal pressure and values greater than 30 cm H_2O indicate the need for abdominal decompression.

Infection involving the prosthetic graft used to restore aortic continuity is very unusual, occurring in 1% to 6% of patients. It is more common after treatment for ruptured than nonruptured aneurysms. It may be associated with graft-enteric fistula, which is more common after surgery for aortic aneurysm than after surgery for aortic occlusive disease. These infections usually become manifest months to years after graft implantation and are discussed in detail in Chapter 59.

UNUSUAL PROBLEMS ASSOCIATED WITH ABDOMINAL AORTIC ANEURYSMS

A number of anatomic and pathologic conditions can complicate the management of abdominal aortic aneurysms and adversely affect the outcome.

Saccular Aneurysms

Almost all AAAs are fusiform in shape, but they are often not uniform or round in cross-section and some have flattened areas, blebs, and other asymmetrical features. A small percentage are saccular in shape, involving only a portion of the aortic wall. These aneurysms typically have very thin walls and some are, in fact, pseudoaneurysms. Their etiology is variable, but infection is one of the most serious causes. Little is known about the relationship between size and rupture of saccular aneurysms, but there is consensus that these are more likely to rupture and should be treated regardless of size. Treatment must be individualized based upon location, etiology, and size. A saccular aneurysm arising from a normal caliber aorta may require aortic replacement, while others may be treated by focal excision and patch angioplasty or even endovascular coil-occlusion. Covered stents or stent-graft components are also useful to exclude saccular aneurysms from the hemodynamic forces of the circulation.

Venous Anomalies

There are several anomalies of the inferior vena cava and left renal vein that are important in aortic surgery. They were found in 2.8% of nearly 1400 aortic operations in one series and are potential sources of serious, unexpected hemorrhage. Most of these anomalies can be identified on preoperative CT scans.[172] The inferior vena cava may be present entirely on the left side (without situs inversus) or may be duplicated, with one on each side of the aorta. Double vena cava is estimated to occur in up to 3% of patients, but isolated left-sided vena cava occurs in only 0.2% to 0.5%.[173-175] An isolated left-sided vena cava usually crosses obliquely in front of the aorta and may be joined by a short, immobile right renal vein. It can also cross from left to right behind the aorta. These anomalies can be especially troublesome if the aorta is approached retroperitoneally from the patient's left side. Dissection near the neck of the aneurysm is when these anomalously positioned veins are most likely to be injured. Sometimes a crossing left inferior vena cava must be divided to enable satisfactory handling of the proximal aortic anastomosis. With a duplicated inferior vena cava, the left-sided one can be ligated if necessary, but care must be taken to ensure that adequate venous drainage of the adrenal gland and left kidney is maintained.

A retroaortic left renal vein, either alone or in association with an anterior vein in the usual location (circumaortic venous collar), is another rare anomaly that can lead to exsanguinating hemorrhage if it is injured during dissection or clamping of the aortic neck.[176] The incidence of this anomaly is 1.8% to 2.4% and is the most commonly encountered venous anomaly in some series. As mentioned earlier, when the surgeon cannot find the left renal vein in its usual preaortic location, he or she should assume that it is retroaortic and limit dissection in that area. Great care must be taken when applying the aortic cross-clamp to avoid tearing these posterior veins. If such a vein is injured, transection of the aorta is usually required to expose it well enough to control the bleeding.

Circumaortic venous collar is more common, occurring in up to 8.7% of cases.[173] This anomaly is even more prone to injury because the anterior component can be normal in size, leading the surgeon to disregard the possibility of a second, posterior renal vein.

Inflammatory Aneurysm

Nearly 5% of abdominal aortic aneurysms are associated with a dense, inflammatory, fibrotic reaction involving the aortic wall and the retroperitoneum that incorporates adjacent structures.[177-180] This appears to be a distinct clinicopathologic entity of uncertain cause, although an autoimmune process has been proposed. It is characterized histologically by marked thickening of the adventitia and media (in contrast to other aortic aneurysms, which have a thinned, attenuated medial layer). Both layers are infiltrated with a prominent acute and chronic inflammatory reaction that includes giant cells. The majority of the inflammatory cells are activated T lymphocytes. The desmoplastic inflammatory reaction involves the duodenum in 90% of cases, the inferior vena cava and left renal vein in more than 50%, and the ureters in approximately 25%; it can extend above the renal arteries and to the iliac arteries. These aneurysms tend to be large, and most patients are symptomatic (i.e., pain) in the absence of rupture. Despite the extremely thickened wall, these aneurysms can and do rupture. A majority of patients have an elevated erythrocyte sedimentation rate of uncertain significance, and many have elevated C-reactive protein levels and have lost weight. The diagnosis can be suggested based on the CT scan, where the periaortic fibrous tissue can easily be seen obliterating the normal tissue planes around the aorta, and a typical halo effect of this tissue appears after intravenous contrast administration. MRI also shows a characteristic appearance of inflammatory aneurysm consisting of several concentric rings surrounding the aortic lumen. This contrast-enhancing halo represents the highly vascular nature of the inflammatory fibrous tissue. Either of these imaging techniques can establish the presence of an inflammatory aneurysm in a high percentage of cases.

Published reports have pointed out several advantages of the left-sided retroperitoneal approach for these lesions, as discussed earlier, and establishing this diagnosis preoperatively permits the selection of this technique. In cases of ureteric involvement, the ureters are typically pulled medially by the fibrotic process and may be obstructed (again, in contrast to other large aneurysms, which tend to push the ureters laterally). At laparotomy, the diagnosis is usually immediately obvious by the unmistakable appearance of a dense, shiny, white, highly vascular reaction in the retroperitoneum, centered over the aortic aneurysm. Once this is recognized, the usual maneuvers of aneurysmorrhaphy should be modified to avoid injury to adherent structures, especially the duodenum. The aorta should be exposed cephalad to the renal vein or at the diaphragm and opened without dissecting the duodenum off the wall. The advantage of the retroperitoneal technique in this condition is that the aorta is approached from a lateral direction and the left kidney and renal vein are displaced anteriorly, out of harm's way. The duodenum does not have to be mobilized, and the inflammatory tissue, which is mostly anterior, can mostly be avoided. There have been several reports of successful EVAR of inflammatory aneurysm using standard patient selection criteria. With either approach, concomitant ureterolysis is seldom necessary because the inflammatory reaction usually resolves postoperatively. Ureteral catheterization can be a useful adjunct, however, and can help to avoid intraoperative ureteral injury. Although the transfusion requirements and operative mortality are slightly higher than for noninflammatory aneurysms, the long-term outlook for these patients is comparable to that for patients with ordinary abdominal aortic aneurysms, and the usual criteria for recommending elective operation should be applied, because these aneurysms can rupture despite their thick anterior wall.[179,180] Numerous reports exist of successful treatment of inflammatory aneurysms by EVAR, using the standard criteria.

Horseshoe Kidney

Horseshoe kidney is another rare problem that occurs in 1 in 400 to 1 in 1000 of the general population. Its association with abdominal aortic aneurysm is rare, but it complicates graft replacement because the kidney mass is usually fused anterior to the aorta, the collecting system and ureters are medially displaced, and there are frequently multiple renal arteries arising from the aorta (including the aneurysmal part), the iliac arteries, or both.[181,182] The renal blood supply is anomalous in 80% of cases and may require some form of surgical correction in most of them.[183] The anomalous fused renal mass is readily apparent on diagnostic imaging studies (CT, MRI, ultrasonography), but if the renal arterial anatomy is not well defined by CTA, preoperative arteriography may be necessary for its proper evaluation. The isthmus of a horseshoe kidney seldom needs to be divided (nor should it be), because the aortic graft can be tunneled behind it. If renal arteries arise from the aneurysm, they can be bypassed or reimplanted into the graft as a Carrel patch. The presence of a horseshoe kidney is another situation in which a left retroperitoneal approach is preferable, because it allows easier management of the multiple and accessory renal arteries. There have been recent reports of successful EVARs of aortic aneurysms in association with horseshoe kidney and favorable renal artery anatomy.

Associated Intraabdominal Pathology and Concomitant Surgical Procedures

Occasionally, there are stenotic atherosclerotic lesions in aortic branches that require surgical correction at the time of aortic aneurysm repair. This most often involves the renal arteries in patients with renovascular hypertension or impaired renal function.[184,185] Rarely, chronic visceral ischemia necessitates concomitant aortic aneurysm and visceral artery repair. In most series, the morbidity and mortality of combined procedures exceed those of elective aneurysm repair alone; therefore, caution is urged in the performance of purely prophylactic procedures in this setting.

Malignant tumors, most of them colonic, are unexpectedly found in 4% to 5% of patients undergoing operation for abdominal aneurysm. They are much more common in patients with aortic aneurysms than in those with aortic occlusive disease. Because operating on the colon converts a clean procedure into a contaminated one, with the potential for prosthetic graft infection, the decision regarding how to treat each lesion (aneurysm, colon mass) and the sequence is not easy. It is sometimes difficult to distinguish colon cancer from inflammatory lesions intraoperatively by palpation. In addition, most vascular surgeons do not use a formal bowel preparation for patients undergoing elective aortic aneurysm surgery. For these reasons, unless there are compelling reasons for treating the colon lesion (perforation, obstruction, hemorrhage), the aneurysm procedure should be completed and the colon left alone. The colon lesion can then be properly evaluated and treated postoperatively. Generally, it is possible to perform an elective colon operation sooner after an aortic aneurysm repair than vice versa, especially if there has been a septic complication (common after colon surgery but rare after aortic surgery). This is another situation for which EVAR can provide an excellent option for both surgeon and patient.

The presence of asymptomatic gallstones is a far more common condition that is found unexpectedly in 5% to 20% of patients undergoing aortic surgery. Several series have been published attesting to the safety of concomitant cholecystectomy and aortic repair.[186,187] A major impetus for this philosophy is the purported high incidence of postoperative cholecystitis in patients in whom only the aortic pathology is treated. In the series reported by String,[186] there was only one documented late graft infection in 34 patients who underwent combined procedures. However, the follow-up was rather short, especially considering the usual long interval between aortic grafting and the first manifestations of graft infection. In addition, the incidence of positive cultures from the bile of patients with cholelithiasis is as high as 33%. As with colon lesions, performance of elective cholecystectomy, which could lead to contamination of a newly implanted aortic prosthesis, should not be performed in conjunction with vascular grafting operations.[188] The consequences of infection of the aortic graft are so grave that the risk of performing elective cholecystectomy is unjustified. The advent of laparoscopic cholecystectomy has made this less of an issue because of the relatively benign nature of this procedure, which can be performed safely either shortly before or after aortic aneurysm repair, if necessary.

Aortocaval Fistula

Abdominal aortic aneurysms can erode into the inferior vena cava or iliac veins, producing an arteriovenous (aortocaval) fistula. This occurs in 0.2% to 1.3% of patients with typical, nonspecific abdominal aortic aneurysms.[189,190] The incidence is at least twice as high in cases of ruptured aneurysm. Approximately 5% to 10% of spontaneous aortocaval fistulas occur in conjunction with other entities, such as mycotic aneurysm, Ehlers-Danlos syndrome, and Marfan syndrome. The most frequent site of fistulization is the distal aorta at or just above the confluence of the iliac veins. Almost all aortocaval fistulas are symptomatic, and impaired renal function is common. Hemodynamically, there is typically a hyperdynamic, high-output state (tachycardia, decreased diastolic blood pressure, and cardiac dilatation) that can quickly progress to medically refractory congestive heart failure. Abdominal or back pain is present in more than 80% of patients, and most have a palpable mass; 75% have an audible continuous bruit, but only about 25% have a palpable thrill. Venous hypertension can affect the gastrointestinal and urinary tracts as well as the lower extremities, and this is why swollen legs, lower gastrointestinal tract bleeding, and hematuria are common.

Despite these protean manifestations, the diagnosis of aortocaval fistula is usually not initially considered, resulting in a multitude of diagnostic tests being performed. Aortography has been the most accurate diagnostic modality, but the fistulas can usually be documented by contrast-enhanced CT, MRI, or even ultrasound scans. The inferior vena cava (IVC) and iliac veins are usually large and the fistula demonstrated by early appearance of contrast in the venous system. The natural history of aortocaval fistula is progressive cardiac decompensation and death. Surgical correction offers the only hope for survival and should be undertaken promptly. A conventional infrarenal aortic aneurysm operation with oversewing of the fistula from within the opened aneurysm sac cures the fistula. EVAR has been successful in treating a significant number of these lesions and is preferable in anatomically suitable patients. Hemodynamic improvement is immediate, and renal function usually recovers rapidly. Nevertheless, reported mortality rates are between 22% and 51%, largely a result of blood loss, cardiac decompensation, and pulmonary embolism.[190]

MYCOTIC AORTIC ANEURYSMS

A mycotic aneurysm is one of infectious but not necessarily fungal origin. The term *mycotic* is derived from the typically mushroom-shaped false aneurysm of the arterial wall. These aneurysms usually occur when a sufficient quantity of bacteria or septic emboli lodges at a point on the intimal surface of an artery to produce a locally invasive infection that becomes a transmural arteritis. Although this can occur in normal arteries, it more commonly affects large atherosclerotic vessels and their branches. Septic emboli can also lodge in the vasa vasorum and initiate the infectious necrotizing process in the arterial wall. A third mechanism is arterial invasion from a septic focus adjacent to a major artery, osteomyelitis of the spine being one example (see Fig. 41.7). Traumatic contamination of an artery has replaced endocarditis as the most common cause, often as a result of drug abuse or even arterial catheterization procedures.[191]

In the largest collective review of mycotic aneurysms, the abdominal aorta was the second most frequent site of involvement (31%), exceeded only by the femoral artery (38%).[172] Chan and associates reported 22 mycotic aortic aneurysms in a series of 2585 patients, an incidence of 0.85%.[192] Coincident with the change in causation, there has been a change in the bacteriology of mycotic aneurysms, with *Salmonella* species declining and *Staphylococcus* species increasing. Together, these are still the most frequently cultured organisms from mycotic aortic

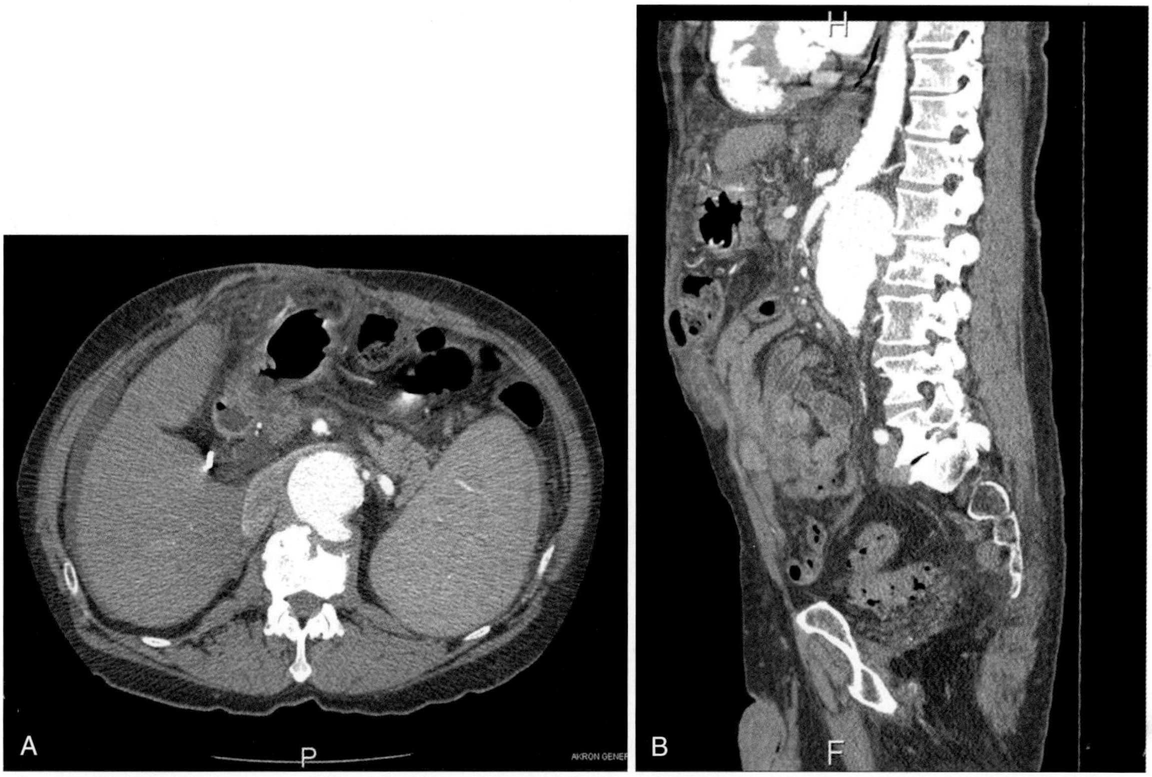

FIG 41.7 Computed tomographic scan showing large mycotic aneurysm adjacent to septic process in lumbar vertebral body. (A) Axial view showing erosion of lumbar vertebral body. (B) Sagittal reconstruction showing relationship of aneurysm to the superior mesenteric artery.

aneurysms.[193-195] The predilection for the infrarenal abdominal aorta probably relates to the frequent occurrence of atherosclerotic plaques in this location.

The triad of abdominal pain, fever, and a pulsatile abdominal mass should suggest the diagnosis of mycotic aneurysm. However, many of these aneurysms are small or saccular and not palpable. Usually there is an initial diagnosis of a nonspecific febrile illness of variable duration. Approximately one-third have abdominal pain. Leukocytosis is a common finding, but only approximately 50% have positive blood cultures. Mycotic aneurysms are often detected by CT scans performed for the evaluation of undiagnosed fever; they appear as a mass located on one side of the aorta rather than a circumferential enlargement. These aneurysms enhance with intravenously administered contrast, but the significance of this can be difficult to appreciate. Both CT and catheter angiography demonstrate the characteristic lobulated saccular aneurysm, which may be multiple and contiguous. These are false aneurysms, contained by compressed periaortic tissue. The aneurysm wall tends to be thin and friable and is associated with contiguous lymphadenopathy and obvious inflammation. Blood clot of varying age is present both within and outside the aneurysmal sac, because there is a high incidence of rupture, although it is usually contained. Periaortic abscess may also be present. The opening between the aorta and the aneurysm tends to be irregular or ragged.

Mycotic aneurysms are a fulminant infectious process and must be treated vigorously and promptly.[191-195] Control of clinical sepsis does not appear to be necessary before surgical treatment, and delays in operative intervention are associated with aneurysmal rupture. Proper antibiotic therapy must be combined with resection of the infected arterial segments, debridement of all adjacent necrotic tissue, and arterial reconstruction. Control of infection by antibiotics does not prevent rupture of the aneurysm, and excision is mandatory and should be carried out promptly. Many of these aneurysms involve the upper abdominal aorta, where it is not always possible to avoid aortic and branch vessel reconstruction. In situ replacement using femoral veins as the conduit is the safest but most challenging approach when renal or visceral perfusion would be compromised by aortic excision. In situ replacement with an antibiotic-soaked graft has been used successfully if the intraoperative Gram stains are negative and there is no periaortic purulence. It should be followed with at least 6 to 8 weeks of intravenous culture-specific antibiotic therapy and, in the case of *Salmonella* infections, probably lifelong antibiotics. When there is frank periaortic pus or a positive Gram stain of an infrarenal mycotic aneurysm, the safest approach is aortic debridement and ligation and extraanatomic bypass or, for nonvirulent organisms, in situ grafting with femoral veins. Recent data indicate that the in situ method is becoming more popular.[195,196] Using these principles, Chan's group reported an operative survival rate of 86%, with only one recurrent infection.[192] There have been isolated reports of early success with endovascular treatment combined with suppressive antibiotics, but long-term follow-up is not yet available.

ILIAC ARTERY ANEURYSMS

Common iliac artery aneurysms occur in continuity or association with abdominal aortic aneurysms in 16% to 20% of patients, but as isolated lesions they are uncommon, accounting for only 1% to 2% of all aneurysms involving the aortoiliac segments and being identified in only 0.03% of autopsies (see Fig. 41.8).[178-180] The cause in the vast majority of cases is the same as that for nonspecific or multifactorial aortic aneurysms; therefore they occur in association with atherosclerosis in the atherosclerosis-prone age group. However, iliac artery aneurysms can develop during pregnancy in the absence of atherosclerosis, and several other causes have been recognized. Mycotic and traumatic iliac artery aneurysms have been reported, the latter usually after lumbar disk or hip surgery. Other less frequent causes include cystic medial necrosis, dissection, Takayasu disease, Marfan and Ehlers-Danlos syndromes, and Kawasaki disease.

Most isolated iliac aneurysms involve the common iliac (70%) or internal iliac (20%) arteries.[182,183] Isolated external iliac artery aneurysms are extremely rare. Multiple iliac aneurysms occur in the majority of patients, and they are bilateral in approximately 33%. In the series by Richardson and Greenfield,[203] two or more vessels were involved in 67% of patients. Internal iliac aneurysms are found in association with aortic and common iliac aneurysms in 5% and 29% respectively. Because most of these aneurysms occur in association with atherosclerosis, the average age at diagnosis is around 69 years, and the male-to-female ratio is 7 : 1. The left and right sides are involved equally.

The clinical presentation of iliac aneurysms is variable and often obscure. Because they are in the pelvis, they are difficult to palpate on physical examination unless they are large. The majority, 50% to 67% in older reviews, were symptomatic, even in the absence of rupture. Symptoms are caused mainly by pressure on adjacent pelvic structures (e.g., urinary tract, lower gastrointestinal tract, lumbosacral nerves, pelvic veins).[185] Thus, lower abdominal, flank, and groin pain is common. Because these are not usually symptoms attributable to the arterial system, delays in diagnosis occur frequently. With the widespread use of CT and other imaging modalities in contemporary medical practice, the majority of isolated iliac aneurysms are detected on unrelated imaging studies. Both CT and ultrasonography are highly reliable for these lesions, and there is excellent correlation between CT and ultrasound measurements.

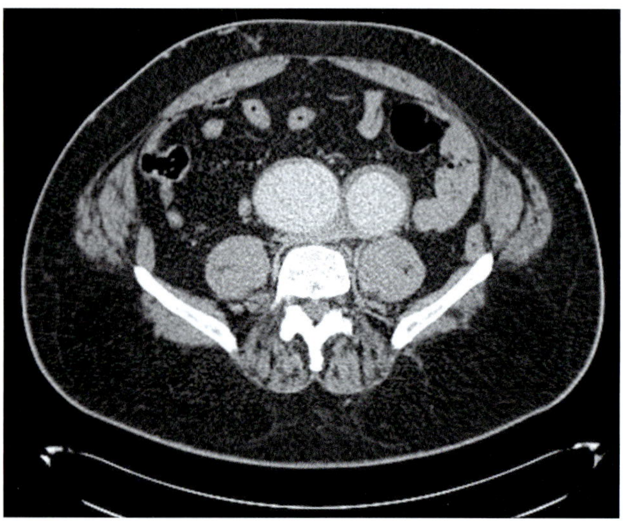

FIG 41.8 Computed tomographic scan showing bilateral common iliac aneurysms *(axial view)*.

Many are diagnosed during cardiac catheterization but, as with aortic aneurysms, arteriography identifies the presence of iliac aneurysms but frequently underestimates their size, because of the presence of laminated thrombus. Other studies that occasionally suggest the diagnosis are barium enema, proctosigmoidoscopy, cystoscopy, and plain radiographs.

Although iliac artery aneurysms are difficult to detect by routine physical examination, large ones can be palpated on abdominal, rectal, or pelvic examination. Common iliac aneurysms are generally more easily felt abdominally, whereas internal iliac aneurysms are more easily felt rectally.

In older reports, iliac aneurysms tended to be large when diagnosed, which probably accounted for the high incidence of symptoms and rupture. In Schuler and Flanigan's collected review, the average size was 8.5 cm, and the incidence of rupture was 51%.[200] In Krupski and coworkers' later report, the average size was 5.6 cm, with a 29% rupture rate.[205]

There are no prospective studies of isolated common iliac artery aneurysms, but the natural history of large ones appears to be unfavorable. The reported high rate of rupture within a few months of diagnosis probably reflects the aneurysms' large size at the time of discovery. Not surprisingly, operative mortality in patients with ruptured aneurysms ranges from 25% to 56%, with an average of 40%. In contrast, the operative mortality for elective operations is much better, averaging 10% to 11%. The adoption of endovascular treatment has resulted in more patients being treated with better results. More iliac aneurysms are being detected and at smaller sizes. A recent review involving 33,161 patients (National Inpatient Sample) covering the years 1988 to 2011 revealed that the number of cases treated has increased and in-hospital mortality has decreased.[187,204,207] Endovascular treatment now involves 65% of cases. Mortality for elective and urgent repair has decreased to 0.5% and 1.1% for endovascular and 7.5% and 1.8% respectively for open repair. Overall morbidity was higher for open repair.[188,210]

The outlook for smaller iliac aneurysms is better than for large ones. In Santilli and associates' series of 47 isolated iliac aneurysms, the average size was 2.3 cm, and the only rupture was an aneurysm larger than 5 cm.[206] The average rate of enlargement in that series was 0.12 to 0.26 cm/year, with larger aneurysms expanding at a greater rate than smaller ones. No patient developed symptoms with an aneurysm smaller than 4 cm. These and other data suggest that isolated common iliac aneurysms smaller than 3 cm can be followed with semiannual ultrasound or CT scans, with minimal risk of symptom development or rupture. Aneurysms 3.5 to 4 cm or larger should be repaired, even if asymptomatic. Symptomatic iliac aneurysms should be repaired regardless of size. The same size guidelines should be used for internal and external iliac aneurysms because so few data are available regarding these uncommon lesions. Common iliac aneurysms associated with aortic aneurysms appear to have the same rupture potential as isolated ones. It is prudent to deal with contiguous common iliac aneurysms larger than 2 to 2.5 cm at the time of aortic aneurysm repair using a bifurcated graft. Smaller-sized iliac arteries can be left in place, allowing tube graft replacement of the aorta, with a very low probability that they will ever enlarge enough to become clinically significant.

The standard open surgical treatment for isolated common iliac aneurysms is graft replacement, and because the external iliac artery is almost never aneurysmal, the operation can be confined to the abdomen. Bilateral common iliac aneurysms necessitate the use of an aortoiliac graft configuration. EVAR has become the procedure of choice as it has with aortic aneurysms and has largely replaced open repair but has demonstrated the importance of maintaining internal iliac perfusion. Occlusion of one internal iliac artery is associated with buttock claudication in 28% of patients. Bilateral internal iliac occlusion is associated with 42% incidence of buttock claudication as well as a small risk of spinal cord and colonic ischemia. Techniques employing newly available branched stent-grafts designed specifically for the iliac system can limit the occurrence of these complications. Small internal iliac aneurysms have been treated with catheter-based techniques by injecting coils, plugs, and other thrombogenic materials into the aneurysm and its branches. Alternatively, they can be treated by open endoaneurysmorrhaphy and grafting, which can be challenging for large lesions deep in the male pelvis because of difficulty obtaining distal control and controlling back-bleeding. These aneurysms should not be treated by simple ligation of the neck because they will remain pressurized via collaterals, enabling further enlargement and potential rupture.[191]

The long-term prognosis of isolated iliac aneurysms after treatment has not been well documented. Nachbur and colleagues[208] reported a 55% 5-year survival rate for patients with ruptured iliac aneurysms. It is reasonable to expect the survival rates to be similar to those for the treatment of aortic aneurysms.

OPEN VERSUS ENDOVASCULAR REPAIR

EVAR now accounts for approximately 70% to 80% of elective abdominal aortic aneurysm repairs and 65% of iliac aneurysm repairs in the United States and many other countries.[207] Most studies have shown a small early survival benefit for EVAR, but this disappears after 1 to 3 years; from then on, survival is better after open repair.[209,210] The same is true for QOL: EVAR is better up to about 6 months after which open repair is better, because patients do not need to worry about future CT scans and endoleaks. As noted earlier, there are a number of situations when open repair is necessary including: (1) anatomically unsuited for EVAR; (2) failed EVAR; (3) Type 1 endoleak with enlarging aneurysm; (4) inadequate access for EVAR; (5) infected EVAR/graft. Advances in stent-graft technology with fenestrated and branched endografts have enabled FEVAR (fenestrated endovascular aortic aneurysm repair) to be used to treat most but not all of these complex aneurysms. In one recently published series comparing FEVAR and open repair in propensity-matched patients, FEVAR was found to have higher morbidity and mortality than open repair. In another series, there was no survival advantage of FEVAR, but late survival and renal function was better in the open surgery group.[114,118] This and other studies indicate that there will always be a need for open surgical treatment of complex abdominal aortic problems, and this has profound implications for vascular surgery training.

REVIEW QUESTIONS

1. All the following are thought to be involved in the pathogenesis of abdominal aortic aneurysms except:
   - **a.** Heredity
   - **b.** Atherosclerosis
   - **c.** Enzyme imbalance
   - **d.** Smoking
   - **e.** Diabetes mellitus
2. The incidence of abdominal aortic aneurysm is highest among patients with which of the following?
   - **a.** Intracerebral aneurysm
   - **b.** Aortoiliac occlusive disease
   - **c.** Thoracic aortic aneurysm
   - **d.** Popliteal aneurysm
   - **e.** Isolated iliac artery aneurysm
3. Which of the following statements about the risk of rupture of infrarenal abdominal aortic aneurysms is true?
   - **a.** It increases with increasing size of the aneurysm.
   - **b.** It is reduced in patients taking beta-blockers.
   - **c.** It is negligible for aneurysms less than 6 cm in diameter.
   - **d.** It is not affected by blood pressure.
   - **e.** It is related to plasma lipoprotein levels.
4. Which of the following is true regarding screening for abdominal aortic aneurysms?
   - **a.** Reduces aneurysm ruptures
   - **b.** Identifies aneurysms but does not reduce mortality
   - **c.** Identifies aneurysms but is not cost-effective
   - **d.** Is prudent in non-smoking women
   - **e.** A screen-detected 4.0 cm AAA should have follow-up scans every 6 months
5. Which of the following is true about abdominal aortic aneurysms in women compared with men?
   - **a.** Weaker relationship with smoking
   - **b.** Rupture more frequently
   - **c.** Occur at a younger age
   - **d.** More commonly associated with femoral or popliteal aneurysm
   - **e.** Lower operative mortality

6. During the course of an aortic aneurysm operation from a transperitoneal approach, the surgeon does not expose the left renal vein crossing anterior to the aorta. The surgeon should do which of the following?
   a. Extend the dissection farther cephalad to the superior mesenteric artery.
   b. Thoroughly mobilize the neck of the aneurysm.
   c. Carefully preserve the adrenal and inferior mesenteric veins.
   d. Assume the left renal vein is probably congenitally absent.
   e. Take extra care during application of the aortic cross-clamp.
7. Which of the following statements about aortocaval fistulas is true?
   a. They are usually infectious in origin.
   b. They are usually symptomatic.
   c. They usually occur just below the left renal vein.
   d. All of the above
   e. None of the above
8. Which of the following statements about complications of aortic aneurysm repair is true?
   a. Colon ischemia is associated with a mortality rate of about 50%.
   b. Renal failure does not occur if the aortic cross-clamp is totally infrarenal.
   c. Paraplegia occurs only with suprarenal clamping.
   d. Myocardial dysfunction is now an uncommon cause of postoperative death.
   e. The use of autotransfusion devices has greatly reduced the degree of postoperative hemorrhage.
9. All the following statements about inflammatory aneurysms are true except:
   a. They have thick fibrous walls.
   b. They are frequently associated with abdominal tenderness in the area of the aneurysm.
   c. They require CT scanning for definitive preoperative diagnosis.
   d. They frequently rupture.
   e. They are frequently associated with ureteral obstruction.
10. All the following statements about iliac artery aneurysms are true except:
   a. Asymptomatic aneurysms should be at least 2.5 cm in diameter for repair to be indicated.
   b. Most are associated with or are an extension of infrarenal abdominal aortic aneurysms.
   c. Most isolated iliac aneurysms manifest symptoms before rupture.
   d. They may be diagnosed by digital examination of the vagina and rectum.
   e. They are commonly bilateral.

BIBLIOGRAPHY

Brown MJ, Sutton AJ, Bell PRF, Sayers RD. A meta-analysis of 50 years of ruptured abdominal aortic aneurysm repair. *Brit J Surg*.2002; 89:714-730.

Buck DB, Bebsley RP, Darling J, et al. The effect of endovascular treatment of isolated iliac artery aneurysm treatment and mortality. *J Vasc Surg*. 2015;62: 331-335.

Chaikof EL, Dalman RL, Eskanderi M, et al. The care of patients with an abdominal aortic aneurysm: the Society for Vascular Surgery practice guidelines. *J Vasc Surg*. 2016.

Kent KC, Zwolak RM, Egorova NN, et al. Analysis of risk factors for abdominal aortic aneurysm in a cohort of more than 3 million individuals. *J Vasc Surg*. 2010;52:539–548.

Kokje VBC, Hamming JF, Linderman JHN, et al. Pharmacologic management of small abdominal aortic aneurysms: review of the clinical evidence. *Eur J Vasc Endovasc Surg*. 2015;50:699-710.

Lederle FA, Wilson SE, Johnson GR, et al. Immediate repair compared with surveillance of small abdominal aortic aneurysms. *N Engl J Med*. 2002;346:1437.

Lo RC, Schermerhorn ML. Abdominal aortic aneurysms in women. *J Vasc Surg*. 2016;63:839-844.

Multicentre Aneurysm Screening Study (MASS): cost effectiveness analysis of screening for abdominal aortic aneurysms based on four year results from randomised controlled trial. *BMJ*. 2002; 325:1135.

Parkinson F, Ferguson S, Lewis P, et al. Rupture rates of untreated large abdominal aortic aneurysms in patients unfit for elective repair. *J Vasc Surg*. 2015;61: 1606-1612

Sidloff D, Stather P, Dattani N. Aneurysm global epidemiology study. Public health measures can further reduce abdominal aortic aneurysm mortality. *Circulation*. 2014;129:747-753.

Stather PW, Sidloff D, Dattani N, et al. Systematic review and meta-analysis of the early and late outcomes of open and endovascular repair of abdominal aortic aneurysms. *Brit J Surg*. 2013;100:863-872.

References available online at ExpertConsult.com.

CHAPTER 42

Endovascular Repair of Juxtarenal (Chimney), Infrarenal, and Iliac Artery Aneurysms

Grace J. Wang, Ronald M. Fairman

In 1991, Parodi and colleagues[1] published a seminal study of patients who underwent abdominal aortic aneurysm (AAA) repair using an intraluminal, stent-anchored polyester prosthetic graft delivered retrograde from the common femoral artery and revolutionized the field of vascular surgery. Although initially considered the preferred modality for patients deemed unfit for open surgery, endovascular aneurysm repair (EVAR) has rapidly evolved as an important alternative, less invasive, and frequently preferred treatment for patients with AAAs. The technology has significantly reduced perioperative morbidity and mortality resulting in expanded application, and the wide acceptance by physicians has been the impetus for subsequent device evolution. Since its inception, the technology has undergone multiple iterations, with earlier-generation grafts having been abandoned in favor of current endografts with their superior radial force, columnar support, and additional modes of fixation. There are currently six endografts approved by the US Food and Drug Administration (FDA) and on the market for the treatment of infrarenal AAAs (Table 42.1). The endograft consists of a metal stent attached to prosthetic graft material, which is housed in a sheath to allow for intraarterial delivery of the device. Most bifurcated stent-grafts use a modular design, the exception being the Endologix device in which the bifurcated component is deployed in a unibody fashion. The basic differences in construct are outlined in Table 42.1.

PATIENT SELECTION

The introduction of EVAR as a lesser invasive alternative to open aortic aneurysm repair has not changed the indications for repair. Repair is undertaken when AAAs reach 5 to 5.5 cm in diameter; however, certain anatomic criteria need to be met for successful EVAR to occur. The most important area of interest is the proximal aortic neck. A cylindrical neck of at least 15 mm in length measured from the renal arteries, with a diameter of 33 mm or less is preferred. In addition, the neck should be relatively free of thrombus and calcification because these interfere with apposition of the stent-graft against the aortic luminal surface. Neck angulation, defined as the angle between the infrarenal aorta and the neck of the aneurysm, of greater than 60 degrees can also interfere with the ability to achieve a proximal seal. The distal landing zone has several elements that require evaluation. The aortic bifurcation should be large enough to accommodate both limbs of the bifurcated stent-graft, preferably greater than 22 mm in diameter. The maximal iliac artery diameter must be at least 2 mm smaller than the largest limb size available. Several manufacturers produce iliac limbs with flared diameters, allowing for preservation of the internal iliac artery, and this is referred to as the bell-bottom technique. If the common iliac artery is short or aneurysmal and external iliac artery landing is required, internal iliac artery embolization is performed to prevent an endoleak. Typically, unilateral hypogastric artery occlusion is well tolerated. If a patient has bilateral common iliac artery aneurysms, repair should be staged to avoid complications with pelvic ischemia. In practice, discussions with patients about potential hip and buttock claudication, as well as erectile dysfunction, should be undertaken preoperatively. Access for delivery of the device is another important consideration. The diameter of the femoral and iliac vessels must be of sufficient size for traversal of the sheath delivery system. Preoperative assessment of the patient's imaging, as well as careful consideration of the device manufacturer's specifications in regard to outer diameter of the delivery system, will allow the formulation of an access strategy. Alternatively, iliac conduits and retroperitoneal approaches have expanded the application of EVAR beyond traditional femoral approaches; that is, iliac artery tortuosity should be routinely assessed because severe degrees may necessitate adjunctive maneuvers such as brachiofemoral access techniques to straighten and "rail" the system. The ability to navigate difficult anatomy has been greatly improved by modern stiff wires. Any patient whose intestinal circulation is based on the inferior mesenteric artery (in the instance of celiac and superior mesenteric artery [SMA] occlusions) should also not undergo EVAR. Patients who have accessory renal arteries are not routinely disqualified from EVAR consideration, unless their coverage would likely affect renal function. In patients who have diabetes mellitus and an elevation of their baseline creatinine, covering even small accessory renals may result in deterioration of renal function. Patients who are reluctant to undergo the surveillance protocol should not be considered for EVAR, because the need for secondary intervention following EVAR is not insignificant.

ENDOVASCULAR TREATMENT OF JUXTARENAL AORTIC ANEURYSMS

Juxtarenal refers to AAAs extending up to the renal arteries with an infrarenal neck less than or equal to 1 cm in length. *Pararenal* is sometimes used interchangeably with juxtarenal and refers to AAAs that involve the origins of the renal arteries. In contrast, *suprarenal* AAAs extend above the renal arteries, and *paravisceral*

TABLE 42.1 **Current Commercially Available Abdominal Aortic Stent-Grafts**

Device Name	Company	Configuration	Max Device Diameter	Min Device Diameter	Fabric	Metal	Active Fixation	Anatomic Fixation
Zenith	Cook	Trimodular	36	22	Woven polyester	Stainless steel	Suprarenal stent with barbs	
Aorfix	Lombard	Bimodular	31	24	Woven polyester	Nitinol	Hooks	
Endurant	Medtronic	Bimodular	36	23	Woven polyester	Nitinol	Suprarenal stent with barbs	
Excluder	Gore	Bimodular	35	23	ePTFE	Nitinol	Barbs	
AFX	Endologix	Unibody	34 (Cuff)	22	ePTFE	Cobalt chromium	Suprarenal stent on aortic cuff	Deployment at aortic bifurcation
Ovation	Trivascular	Trimodular	34	20	ePTFE	Nitinol	Suprarenal stent with barbs and infrarenal sealing rings	

ePTFE, Expanded polytetrafluoroethylene.

aneurysms involve the SMA and/or the celiac artery. Although these aneurysms historically required an open approach, the drive of industry and technology, as well as a comorbid patient population, have motivated the expansion and use of endovascular approaches for repair. This chapter discusses treatment of juxtarenal and pararenal aneurysms using off-the-shelf components to extend the seal zone, with so-called "chimney" or "snorkel" stents. Fenestrated grafts also offer a "totally endovascular" solution, but require time (weeks) to manufacture. Branched grafts are only available to patients enrolled in a clinical trial, or as part of investigational device exemption, and take 6 to 8 weeks to manufacture, provided the patient meets protocol-defined anatomic and clinical constraints. The latter endografts are discussed in a separate chapter.

Renal artery stenting via the encroachment or snorkel (or chimney) technique allows preservation of renal blood flow when treating juxtarenal aneurysms with traditional infrarenal stent-grafts. This chapter outlines these endovascular approaches to treating juxtarenal aneurysms.

SETTING

Endovascular AAA repair can be done in a hybrid operating room with fixed C-arm positioning, in an operating room using a portable C-arm, or in an interventional or cardiac catheterization suite. EVAR has been described with regional block, local anesthesia, and general anesthesia. Although traditionally performed through either one or two femoral artery cutdowns, the advent of smaller delivery systems have allowed percutaneous technique to be increasingly employed, decreasing the morbidity of the procedure even further.

Although EVAR is being performed increasingly using a percutaneous technique, having immediate access to an open vascular set is paramount and at times lifesaving, should intraoperative issues arise, and where open conversion is required. General anesthetic is also preferred when attendant open adjunctive procedures such as femoral-femoral artery bypass grafting, iliac conduit, or local femoral endarterectomy is planned. Because EVAR is being performed increasingly in much older comorbid patients with less than ideal anatomy, the need for sophisticated operative imaging to optimize precision deployment, as well as a surgical preparedness for potentially catastrophic access issues, underscores the importance of the operating room or hybrid suite in performing these procedures. The outcomes of EVAR for ruptured AAA have also been favorable, particularly in institutions where a systematic algorithm ensures that the appropriate endovascular team is alerted when a ruptured aneurysm is identified in the emergency room.[2,3] It is clear that, in this subset of patients, having the ability to convert from an endovascular to an open approach should the patient rapidly deteriorate, is an important consideration. Of paramount importance to the success of every aortic endovascular program is identifying and training a dedicated endovascular team of nurses, operating room scrub technicians, and radiology technologists.

ENDOVASCULAR STENT-GRAFT PLANNING AND PLACEMENT FOR INFRARENAL AORTIC ANEURYSMS

Axial imaging is obtained via computed tomography (CT) angiography or magnetic resonance angiography provided that the patient does not have renal insufficiency. Three-dimensional reconstructions performed by Terra Recon (Foster City, CA), Vitrea (Vital Images), Leonardo (Siemens), or M2S (Lebanon, NH) have become the standard and are used to measure the distance from the lowest renal artery to the aortic bifurcation, the lowest renal artery to the ipsilateral hypogastric artery, and the lowest renal artery to the contralateral hypogastric artery (Figs. 42.1 and 42.2). Diameter measurements of the neck and of the common iliac arteries are then performed. It is important at this time to note the extent of neck angulation and rotation of the juxtarenal aorta to optimize accurate endograft deployment. Broeders and Blankensteijn[4] describe a simple technique to optimize imaging prior to endograft deployment. The juxtarenal aorta should be visualized in the sagittal plane to measure

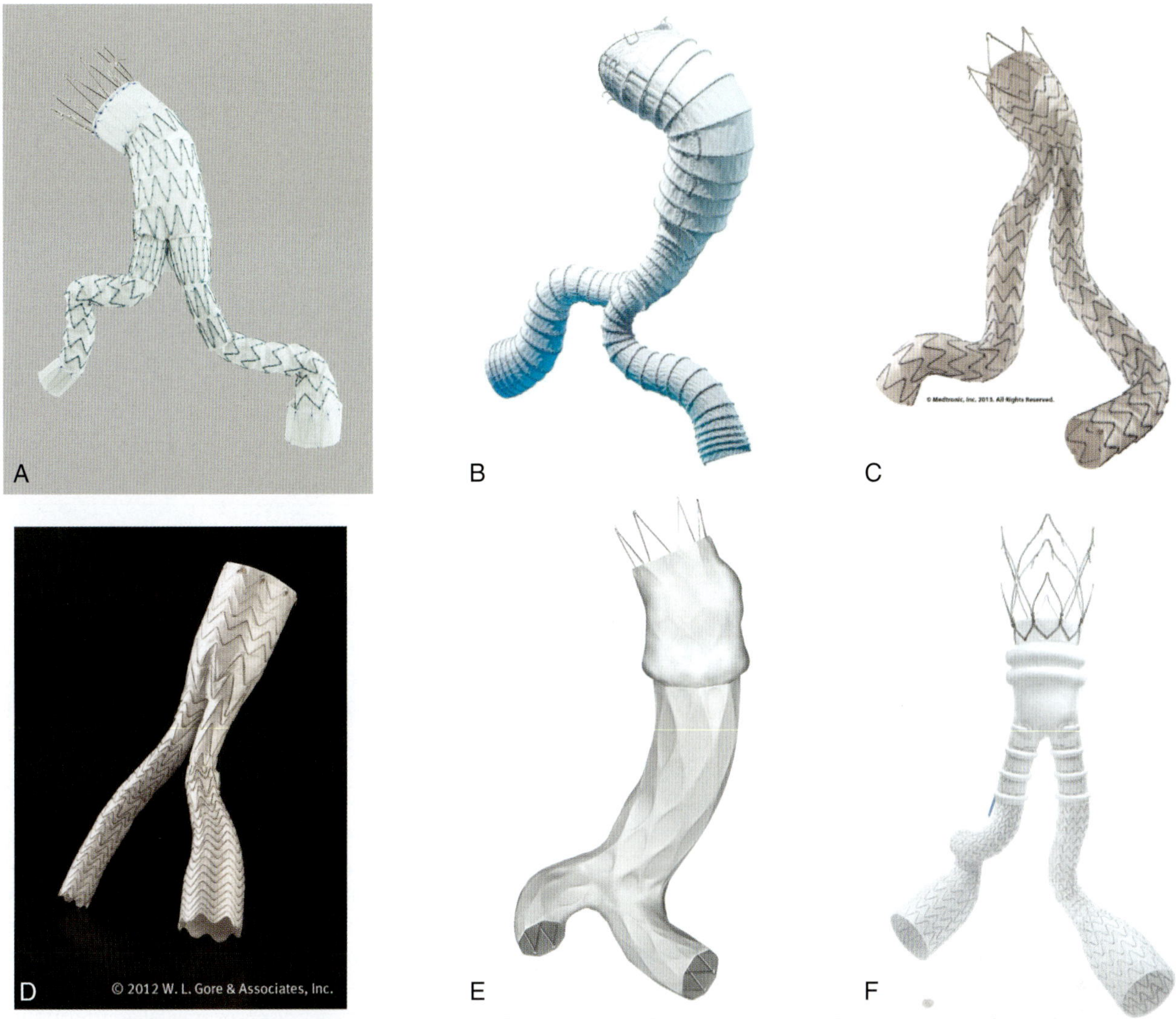

FIG 42.1 (A) Cook Zenith stent-graft (Cook Medical, Bloomington, IN). (B) Lombard Aorfix graft (Lombard Medical, Oxfordshire, UK). (C) Medtronic Endurant stent-graft (Meditronic, Santa Rosa, CA). (D) Gore Excluder stent-graft (Gore, Flagstaff, AZ). (E) Endologix AFX stent-graft (Endologix, Irvine, CA). (F) Trivascular Ovation stent-graft (Endologix, Irvine, CA).

the degree of craniocaudad angulation (Fig. 42.3). The axial sections are then used to measure the degree of aortic neck rotation (Fig. 42.4). These angle calculations should be noted to ensure that the C-arm is orthogonal to the takeoff of the lowest renal artery. The tortuosity of the vessels, the degree of calcification, and any thrombus is also noted. Circumferential thrombus or calcification will prevent complete apposition of the stent-graft to the aortic wall and thus compromise the ability to achieve a proximal seal. Using 10% to 20% proximal graft oversizing, the stent-graft devices are housed in relatively large sheaths that require bilateral groin incisions and femoral artery repair or percutaneous access that is closed with vascular closure devices. After introduction of the delivery system over a stiff wire to the juxtarenal aorta, an aortogram is performed, and under "roadmap" guidance, the main body of the stent-graft is positioned and deployed just under the lowest renal artery. With modular bifurcated grafts, care is taken to insert and deploy the main body of the graft with the contralateral gate deployed in an anterolateral position, which is optimal for subsequent retrograde cannulation. Once the contralateral gate is deployed, it is cannulated, and efforts are made to ensure that the catheter is indeed within the stent-graft and not behind the graft in the aneurysm sac. When deploying devices with separate suprarenal fixation, a magnified aortogram is performed at this time to confirm the location and position of the renal arteries. Cranial obliquity is usually required to ensure that the origin of the lowest renal artery is seen in an orthogonal orientation. Once the suprarenal stent is deployed, the stiff wire is placed up the contralateral limb and a pelvic arteriogram with the C-arm at an oblique angle of 15 to 20 degrees to the other side is performed to demonstrate the origin of the contralateral hypogastric artery. The contralateral iliac limb is then deployed taking care to preserve flow to the internal iliac artery. The remainder of the main body or ipsilateral limb is deployed. In an obligate three-piece

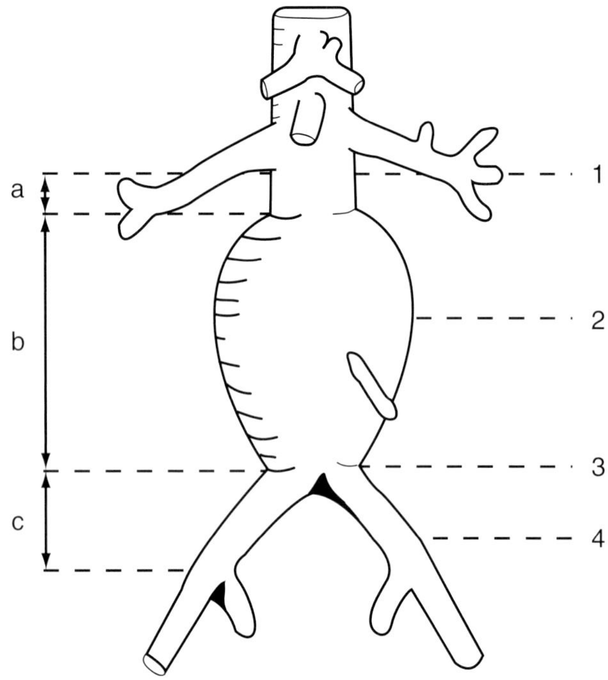

FIG 42.2 Schematic of abdominal aortic aneurysm measurements for stent-graft sizing. *a,* Length of neck; *b,* length of aneurysm; *c,* length of common iliac artery; $a + b + c$ = distance from lowest renal artery to ipsilateral internal iliac artery; *1,* diameter of aortic neck; *2,* maximal diameter of aneurysm; *3,* diameter of aortic bifurcation; *4,* diameter of common iliac artery.

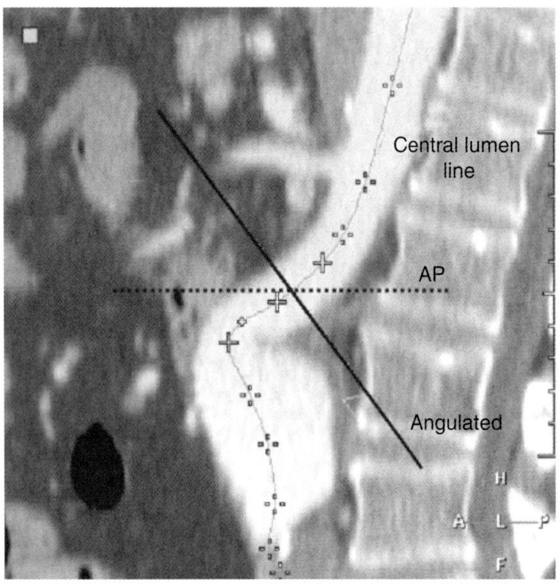

FIG 42.3 Sagittal computed tomographic angiography reconstruction demonstrating the central lumen line and the axes relative to the aorta in the anteroposterior *(AP)* and angulated projections. Note that the angulated line is perpendicular to the aortic center line axis. (From Broeders IA, Blankensteijn JD: A simple technique to improve the accuracy of proximal AAA endograft deployment. *J Endovasc Ther* 7:389–393, 2000.)

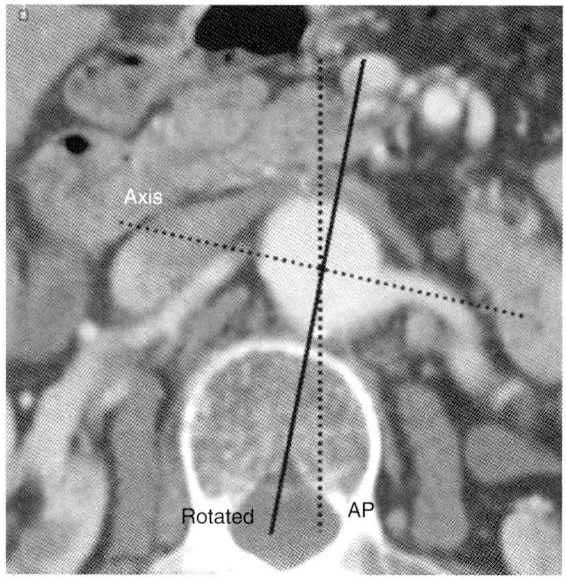

FIG 42.4 Axial computed tomographic angiography image demonstrating the axes relative to the aorta in the anteroposterior *(AP)* and rotated projections relative to the axis between the lowest renal artery orifice and the center of the aorta. (From Broeders IA, Blankensteijn JD: A simple technique to improve the accuracy of proximal AAA endograft deployment. *J Endovasc Ther* 7:389–393, 2000.)

system, another pelvic arteriogram is performed in the opposite obliquity to demonstrate the takeoff of the ipsilateral internal iliac artery. The junctions are ballooned, and stiff wires are removed before the completion of arteriography to ensure that limb kinking is not a concern. Graft limb kinking is of particular concern in individuals with external iliac landing because of concomitant iliac artery aneurysms or small iliac artery diameters. Any type I or III endoleaks should be addressed in the operating room. Type I endoleaks can be addressed with proximal extensions, large-diameter bare stents, or simple ballooning. Type III endoleaks can be addressed with bridging pieces or repeated ballooning. Type II endoleaks can be observed, as the majority of them resolve with conservative management within 6 to 12 months. Completion arteriography should demonstrate both renal and hypogastric artery patency and good flow down both iliac limbs. In the setting of small calcified aortic bifurcations (<20 mm diameter), adjunctive bilateral kissing balloon angioplasty should be a consideration.

ENDOVASCULAR REPAIR OF COMMON AND INTERNAL ILIAC ARTERY ANEURYSMS

The relationship between aneurysm diameter and rupture risk is not as well delineated for iliac aneurysms as it is for the abdominal aorta. However, it is generally agreed that repair should be undertaken when the diameter reaches 3.0 to 4.0 cm in size.[5,6]

Common Iliac Artery Aneurysms

Endovascular repair of isolated common iliac artery aneurysms require suitable proximal and distal landing zones. Lack of a proximal landing zone in the common iliac artery would necessitate concomitant stent-grafting of the abdominal aorta to achieve a seal. Current stent-graft technology allows treatment of iliac artery aneurysms with a seal zone diameter of up to 25 mm at the common iliac artery bifurcation. The largest iliac limb diameter is 28 mm, provided by the Endurant endograft (Medtronic Inc., Minneapolis, MN). When the diameter of the seal zone is greater than 25 mm or the aneurysmal disease extends into the external iliac artery, the endograft can be extended into the external iliac artery, with coil embolization or plug occlusion (Amplatzer vascular plug, St. Jude Medical, Inc., St. Paul, MN) of the proximal internal iliac artery to prevent a type II endoleak. In some patients with contralateral internal iliac artery occlusion or bilateral common iliac artery aneurysms who are perceived to be at high risk for spinal cord ischemia, it is essential to preserve internal iliac artery flow.[47,48] In these patients, an external-to-internal iliac artery bypass can be performed with proximal ligation of the internal iliac artery to effectively "move" the iliac bifurcation more distally. In one series of 22 patients, all bypasses remained patent at a mean follow-up of 15 months, with only mild buttock claudication occurring in two patients ipsilateral to the site of coil embolization.[7] Another series showed similar excellent internal iliac bypass patency rates of 91%, as well as freedom from ischemic symptoms.[8]

Iliac Branch Devices

The iliac-branched device (IBD) designed by Cook (Cook Medical, Bloomington, IN) was the first to be developed, is currently in trial in the United States, and has already been used with success outside the United States (Fig. 42.5).[49] The delivery system comes with a preloaded, curved catheter, which simplifies cannulation of the internal iliac artery from the contralateral groin. The IBD is passed over a stiff wire in typical fashion. Wire passage through the curved catheter is snared from the contralateral femoral artery. Following stiff wire exchange and partial deployment of the IBD, a sheath is then introduced from the contralateral femoral artery into the internal iliac artery branch. A covered bridging stent is then deployed after fully unsheathing the IBD (Fig. 42.6A–D). In a single institution study of 46 patients, IBD side-branch patency was 87% at 5 years.[9] In another series with 100 patients, internal iliac artery patency was 91.4% at 5 years.[10] Despite these high technical success rates, initial results from

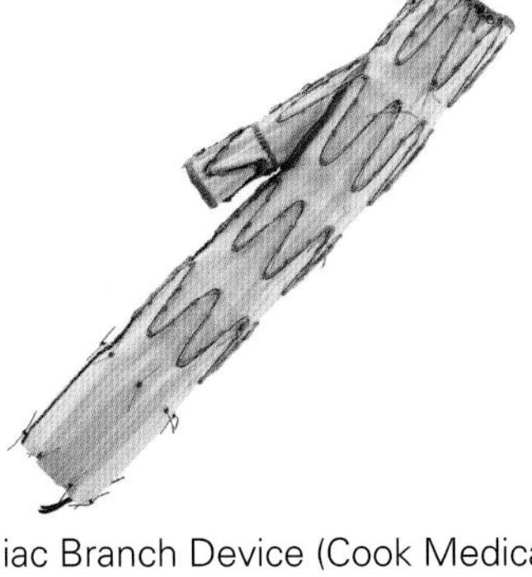

FIG 42.5 Cook Iliac Branch Device (Cook Medical, Bloomington, IN).

the trial in the United States revealed a stent fracture in the connecting stent causing a type III endoleak, which has been treated with relining. Further follow-up is needed regarding the long-term efficacy of this device. The recent FDA approval of the Gore Excluder Iliac Branch Prosthesis in the United States will likely herald a new era in the use of iliac branched devices to achieve a more stable seal in patients with ectatic iliac arteries. This prosthesis will also preserve important pelvic collaterals to decrease the troublesome complication of buttock claudication and reduce the complications of spinal cord ischemia should further aortic repair be required (Fig. 42.7). In a study of 10 patients evaluating the safety and short-term efficacy of this device in the treatment of iliac artery aneurysms, there was a 100% technical success rate, with 100% branch patency at 1 month, and 90% branch patency at 6 months.[11] FDA approval was based on the results from a prospective, multicenter trial of 62 patients that completed enrollment in February 2015. Additional patients were enrolled through continued access to evaluate its safety and efficacy in cases of bilateral iliac branch device implantation. Again, longer-term follow-up is essential to determine the durability of repair using this device.

Internal Iliac Artery Aneurysms

Internal iliac artery aneurysms are typically managed with endovascular coiling/plug occlusion with stent-graft coverage of the origin. Because of the multiple branches that emanate from the internal iliac artery, preservation of flow in the presence of an internal iliac artery aneurysm is challenging. In the patient in whom internal iliac flow is desired because of contralateral occlusion, stent-graft repair is possible provided proximal and distal landing zones are present, and an iliac branch device solution could be considered, anatomy permitting. This may require landing the stent in the largest branch available following coil embolization of smaller branches feeding into the aneurysm sac. If the proximal landing zone is compromised, a chimney/snorkel can be deployed extending into either the common or external iliac artery,[12] or the sandwich technique may be employed.[13] In the latter technique, the covered stent within the internal iliac artery lies side by side with the iliac limb extender within the common iliac limb. A hybrid technique has also been described. An aortouniiliac endograft with a femoral-to-femoral artery bypass can be performed with a covered stent deployed from the contralateral external to the internal iliac artery in a "reverse U" fashion. This would allow for preservation of pelvic blood flow without the need for retroperitoneal exposure.[14] As above, if both internal iliac arteries are large and are not amenable to preservation, coil embolization of the aneurysms can be staged by one to several weeks to ameliorate the sequelae of pelvic ischemia.

ENDOVASCULAR REPAIR OF JUXTARENAL AORTIC ANEURYSMS

For some patients with a proximal infrarenal neck length less than 15 mm (the traditional desired neck length for endovascular aortic aneurysm repair), partial renal artery coverage with adjunctive renal artery stenting can be performed.[15] Using either the

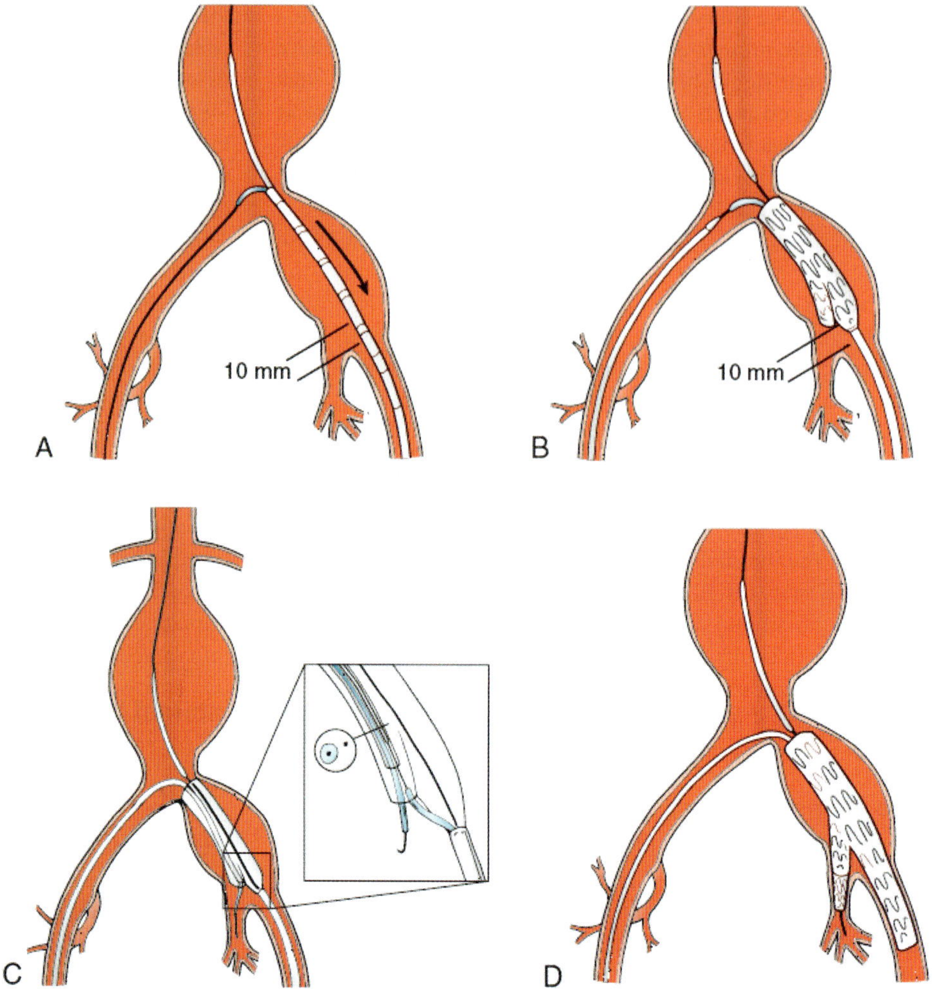

FIG 42.6 Deployment of Cook Iliac Branch Device. (A) The guidewire is passed through the curved catheter and snared from the contralateral groin. (B) The IBD is partially deployed, and the sheath is advanced from the contralateral groin into the side branch of the IBD. (C) The wire is advanced into the internal iliac artery. (D) Following stiff-wire exchange, the covered stents are deployed after fully unsheathing the IBD. (From Serracino-Inglott F, Bray AE, Myers P: Endovascular abdominal aortic aneurysm repair in patients with common iliac artery aneurysms: initial experience with the Zenith bifurcated iliac side branch device. *J Vasc Surg* 46:211–217, 2007.)

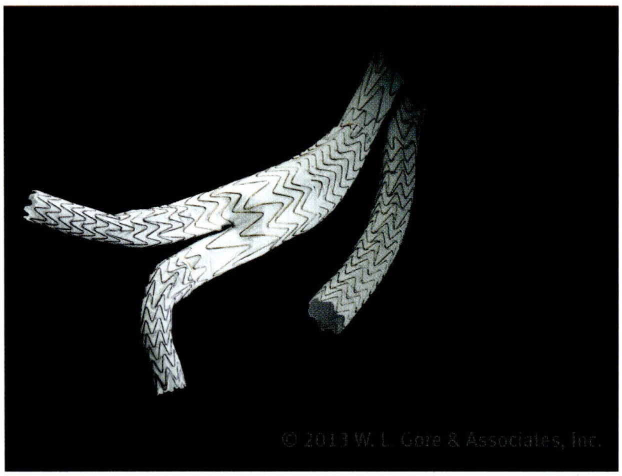

FIG 42.7 Gore Iliac Branch Device (Gore, Flagstaff, AZ).

encroachment technique, where the superior margin of the stent-graft is pushed inferiorly by the renal stent, or the snorkel technique, where the stent-graft is pushed inward by the renal stent (Figs. 42.8 and 42.9), a case series showed that sealing of the aneurysm was possible (no type I endoleak at 1 month follow-up) with a primary assisted patency of renal artery stents of 100%. Transbrachial access is key for the snorkel maneuver, because it is often used when more extensive coverage of the renal artery is required, and the stent is required to run alongside the stent-graft before entering the orifice of the artery. The encroachment methods, however, can usually be effectively approached transfemorally. Both techniques allow for extension of the proximal landing zone while preserving blood flow to the renal arteries using common, off-the-shelf devices.

Encroachment Technique

This technique is used when partial renal artery coverage is needed to achieve a seal. The aortic stent-graft is deployed in the usual fashion, with careful attention paid to the relationship between the top of the stent-graft fabric and the lowest renal artery. The optimal degree of angulation and rotation for visualizing the takeoff of the renal artery is then determined. Catheter and wire access of the renal artery is obtained. If a device with a suprarenal stent is used, care is taken to access the base of the triangular stent rather than in between the triangular stents. One recommendation is the use of a combination of a Rosen wire (Cook Medical, Bloomington, IN) and a guide catheter system to serve as a platform for performing the renal stent. Balloon-expandable

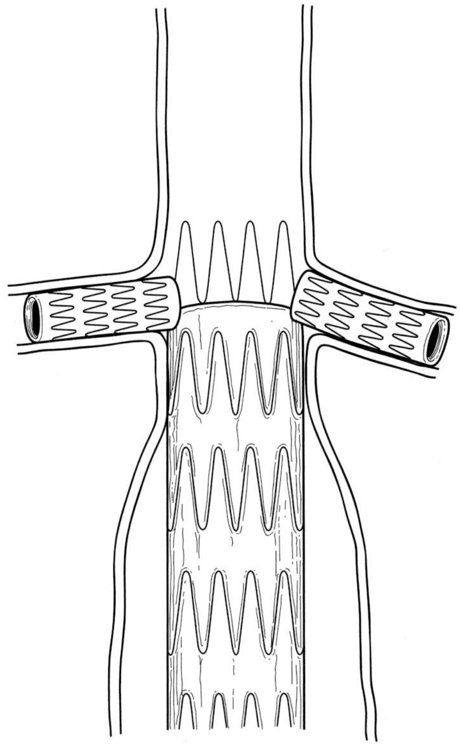

FIG 42.8 The encroachment technique during endovascular aneurysm repair. (From Chaikof E, Cambria R: *Atlas of vascular surgery and endovascular therapy,* Philadelphia, 2013, Elsevier.)

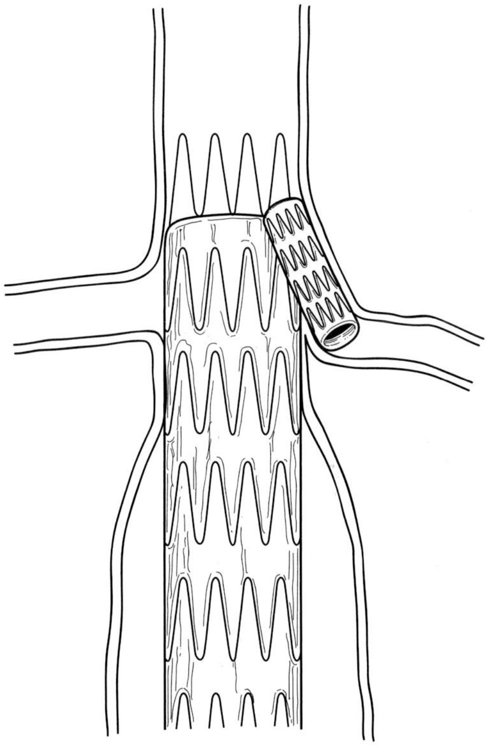

FIG 42.9 The chimney technique during endovascular aneurysm repair. (From Chaikof E, Cambria R: *Atlas of vascular surgery and endovascular therapy,* Philadelphia, 2012, Elsevier.)

stents are favored in this location because the increased radial force is essential to push the superior margin of the stent-graft inferiorly to preserve renal artery flow.

Snorkel Technique

The snorkel technique is used when complete coverage of the renal artery origin is required to achieve a seal. Axillary or brachial access to the renal is performed before stent-graft deployment. A combination of a Rosen wire and a long Destination sheath (Terumo, Somerset, NJ) as a platform is recommended. The renal stent comes to lie entirely outside the aortic stent-graft, parallel to it until it enters the renal artery orifice. Both balloon-expandable and self-expanding covered stents[16,17] have been used for this purpose with excellent success. In a recent metaanalysis of the endovascular chimney technique for the treatment of juxtarenal AAAs, in a total of 236 patients treated with a total of 35 chimney grafts, perioperative mortality was only 3.8% and chimney patency at 6 months was 96.6%.[18] The length(s) of the stents need to be long enough to account for the distance along the aortic stent-graft, which needs to be traversed before reaching the origin of the renal artery. If the renal stent is deployed prior to the aortic stent, it is essential to maintain wire and/or balloon support of the renal stent while ballooning the aortic graft, because compression of the stent can occur with this maneuver, and repeat angioplasty of the renal stent is required to maintain patency.

Although the authors admit that the long-term durability of these methods are not known, both techniques effectively lengthen the seal zone while preserving renal blood flow, allowing the use of off-the-shelf stent-grafts for pararenal aneurysm repair. In addition, the authors have been more enthusiastic and aggressive in the use of these endovascular opportunities in much older and frail patients with significant comorbidities.

POSTOPERATIVE COMPLICATIONS

Local

Groin wound complications include hematoma, pseudoaneurysm formation, seromas, and cellulitis. Attention to detail in closing the arteriotomy sites and reapproximating the subcutaneous tissues in multiple layers, including the oversewing of lymphatics, can help to avoid the majority of these local wound complications. We and others have endorsed the use of transverse groin incisions.

Systemic

Renal insufficiency can be exacerbated in patients with underlying chronic renal insufficiency and can be overcome with adequate preoperative and perioperative hydration with a bicarbonate solution and judicious use of diluted contrast agents in the operating suite. Thromboembolic complications from thrombus-laden aortic necks to the renal arteries following EVAR have been described, but are surprisingly less frequent than anticipated when these procedures are performed with regularity. Patients with short, angulated necks and challenging proximal seal zones who may require adjunctive renal stenting for preservation should be closely monitored for any drop in urine output. If there is any doubt as to whether renal artery flow is compromised, urgent interrogation via duplex or arteriography is required.

Postimplantation syndrome is characterized by low-grade fever and an elevated white blood count without an obvious infectious source and is believed to be secondary to cytokine release following thrombosis of the aneurysm sac. It is important in these patients to rule out an infectious source as an etiology for these fevers. This syndrome is typically self-limiting and lasts 7 to 10 days.

LATE COMPLICATIONS

Late complications following EVAR are largely attributable to endoleak. Fig. 42.10 depicts the different types of endoleak. The need for secondary intervention following EVAR is not insignificant, with a reported frequency of 10% to 18%.[19] The majority of these interventions can be performed endovascularly (76%), underscoring the importance of regular surveillance for maintenance of successful endovascular repair. Late failure can be categorized as secondary to a change in structure or position of the stent-graft, resulting in endoleak or graft thrombosis, or due to a change in aortic anatomy.

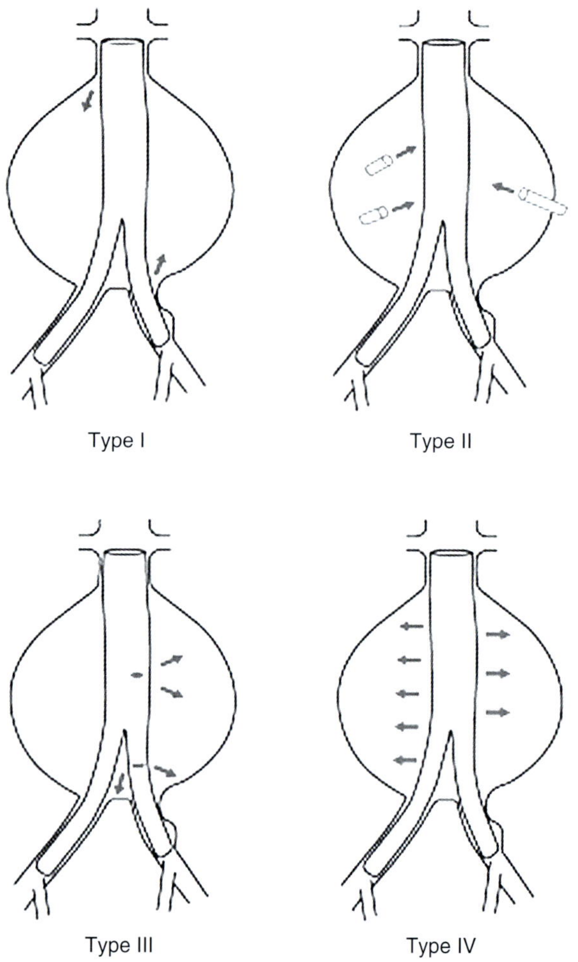

FIG 42.10 Diagram of the different types of endoleak. Type I endoleaks occur at the proximal (Ia) or distal (Ib) seal zones. Type II endoleaks occur because of back-bleeding from branch vessels such as the lumbar arteries or inferior mesenteric artery. Type III endoleaks are the result of a defect in the graft fabric or lack of intercomponent seal. Type IV endoleaks are due to graft fabric porosity.

Migration is defined as caudal migration of the stent-graft by more than 1 cm; this can result in a proximal type I endoleak, which can result in sac pressurization, growth, and rupture if not treated. Proximal device extension, bare-metal stent deployment to buttress radial support in the area, or renal artery snorkel or encroachment techniques can be used to achieve a proximal seal again. If the main body of the prior stent-graft is too short for the deployment of a proximal extension, an aortouniiliac device can be used, necessitating a femoral-femoral artery bypass and embolization of the contralateral proximal iliac artery with an occlusion device. Type III endoleak from fabric erosion is effectively treated with stent-graft relining or bridging of components to effectively seal the hole. Component separation is likewise treated with relining. When the device pieces are particularly separated in space due to excessive tortuosity, obtaining wire access through both components may be challenging; transbrachial access with a snare may be useful in this situation. Stent fracture has been noted in follow-up and for the most part is not associated with untoward effects. Proximal extension or relining may be appropriate if fracture results in concomitant migration and endoleak.

Aortic neck dilation may be another mode of failure following EVAR. Provided that there is a commercial device available to seal the dilated aortic neck, a proximal extension may be deployed to achieve a proximal seal. Distal common iliac artery dilation with a type IB endoleak is retreated with hypogastric artery occlusion and extension to the external iliac artery.

There is consensus that type II endoleaks in the presence of an enlarging aneurysm sac require intervention; these are typically due to a patent inferior mesenteric artery or iliolumbar arteries. Embolization can be performed using coils or *N*-butyl cyanoacrylate glue. The transarterial approach can be used to embolize the inferior mesenteric artery through the SMA from the marginal artery of Drummond. The translumbar approach uses a direct aneurysm sac puncture technique. Regardless of the approach, these endoleaks physiologically behave like arteriovenous malformations, and embolization of the nidus of the endoleak including the inflow and outflow vessels is the optimal approach. Retroperitoneal endoscopic ligation of the lumbar arteries has also been described. Type IV endoleaks are related to porosity of the graft fabric, occur less frequently with current-generation stent-grafts, and are noted within 30 days of graft implantation. These endoleaks are most commonly observed as a blush of contrast coming through the fabric of the stent-graft on the completion arteriogram before heparin reversal; they usually resolve once graft interstices thrombose. Endotension, or type V endoleak, is defined as elevated sac aneurysm pressure without a clearly defined endoleak. It is generally believed that the etiology is an undetected endoleak or transmission of systemic pressure through thrombus. Endotension is typically detected as continued sac enlargement on CT scan, but can also be detected by direct aneurysm sac pressure sensors (Cardiomems, Atlanta, GA).

TABLE 42.2 Types of Endoleaks and Management Strategies

Classification	Causes of Perigraft Flow	Therapeutic Options
Type I	Inadequate seal of proximal or distal end of endograft Inadequate seal of iliac occluder plug	Proximal or distal extension or cuff Overstenting, embolization, or glue conversion
Type II	Flow from patent lumbar, middle sacral, or inferior mesenteric artery; hypogastric, accessory renal, or other visceral vessel	Observation, coil embolization, or glue Laparoscopic ligation conversion
Type III	Fabric disruption or tear Module disconnection	Secondary endograft or cuff conversion
Type IV	Flow from fabric porosity, suture holes (<30 days after graft placement)	Observation
Endoleak of undefined origin	Flow visualized from unidentified source	Observation Angiographic investigation

A summary of the types of endoleaks and how they are managed is provided in Table 42.2. Should the methods discussed here prove unsuccessful in managing EVAR failure, open conversion and explant should be performed. This has been shown to be possible with acceptable morbidity and mortality in both the elective and emergent setting.[20]

Graft limb occlusion has been estimated between 3% and 7%,[21,22] usually occurs within the first 6 months following EVAR, and is more frequent in patients with aortoiliac occlusive disease, with a small distal aorta (<14 mm), who have tortuous iliacs, or who require external iliac artery landing. Earlier-generation stent-grafts with unsupported limbs are also at risk for limb kinking.[23,24] Most patients exhibit buttock, thigh, or calf claudication. In the majority of instances, the limb can be recanalized with thrombolysis or surgical thrombectomy techniques, with adjunctive iliac stenting as needed. It is of utmost importance that the etiology and site of the limb kink be identified. Arteriography with oblique orientation can be helpful in providing the views to help identify the problem. In addition, intravascular ultrasound and measurement of pullback pressures may help to identify graft infolding, which might not be noted on arteriography.[25] In patients in whom the limb cannot be reopened, femoral-femoral bypass is performed to revascularize the contralateral leg.

Infection of the aortic stent-graft is a rare event, with small case series reporting an incidence of 0.2% to 0.7%.[26] In the largest case series to date, nine patients presented with infected EVAR at a tertiary referral center.[27] All patients underwent complete explants of the stent-graft with preemptive revascularization (axillary femoral–to–femoral artery bypass) in five patients or in situ reconstruction with Rifampin-soaked polyester in the other four. Seven of the patients survived to discharge, and the mean follow-up of the surviving patients was 11 months. In this series, the presence of a concomitant aortoenteric fistula was particularly virulent. Two of the three patients with aortoenteric fistula died before discharge. Although generally considered a highly morbid condition with mortality rates estimated at 36%,[28] the findings from this study suggest that explantation of infected grafts can be performed with an acceptable mortality rate.

POSTOPERATIVE SURVEILLANCE

Postoperative surveillance following EVAR is essential for ensuring success. Postoperative surveillance allows the detection of endoleaks, aneurysm sac expansion, stent fracture, limb kinking, and material fatigue. Initial protocols were adopted from the initial FDA-sponsored trials that recommended CT scans at 1-, 6-, and 12-month intervals and annually thereafter.[29] The frequent use of CT scanning has raised concerns related to the added cost of these studies, cumulative radiation exposure,[30,31] and use of nephrotoxic agents. Although ultrasound duplex avoids radiation exposure and the use of contrast dye, concerns have been raised in the past regarding its variable sensitivity in detecting endoleaks.[32] The utility of ultrasound is also limited in obese patients or those with substantial bowel gas. Based on these recent reports, some investigators have proposed that follow-up with duplex as the sole imaging modality is appropriate, provided there is no endoleak or sac enlargement documented on the first annual CT scan.[33] A significant increase in sac size or a newly diagnosed endoleak would then prompt CT imaging.[34] Omitting the 6-month scan has also been recommended if CT imaging at 1 month does not identify an endoleak.[33,35] These protocols have been shown to be safe, with minimal risk of a clinical adverse event.[36] The Society for Vascular Surgery practice guidelines currently recommend contrast-enhanced CT scanning at 1 and 12 months during the first year after EVAR.[29] Detection of an endoleak at 1 month would prompt another CT scan at 6 months to evaluate the need for intervention. If neither endoleak nor aneurysm expansion is detected during the first year after EVAR, duplex may be a reasonable alternative. In patients with renal insufficiency, duplex ultrasound in combination with a noncontrast CT scan is a reasonable surveillance strategy. A summary of this management strategy is provided in Fig. 42.11. Although the risk of endoleak declines with each negative surveillance CT scan, new endoleaks have been identified as late as 7 years after EVAR,[37] underscoring the importance of lifelong surveillance. The long-term (>20 years) outcome of stent-grafts has not been established, and multiple studies reporting the midterm results of EVAR using various devices cite a need for secondary intervention. From the EVAR-1 and EVAR-2 trials, the secondary intervention rates were 7.0% for the Zenith and 9.4% for the Talent grafts at approximately 4 years of follow-up.[38] In the 5-year follow-up study of the patients who underwent Zenith stent-graft repair as part of the pivotal trial, the cumulative risk of conversion, limb occlusion, migration greater than 10 mm, or component separation was 3% or less at 5 years. The cumulative risk of late endoleak was 12% to 15%, accounting for the majority of secondary interventions, and underscoring the importance

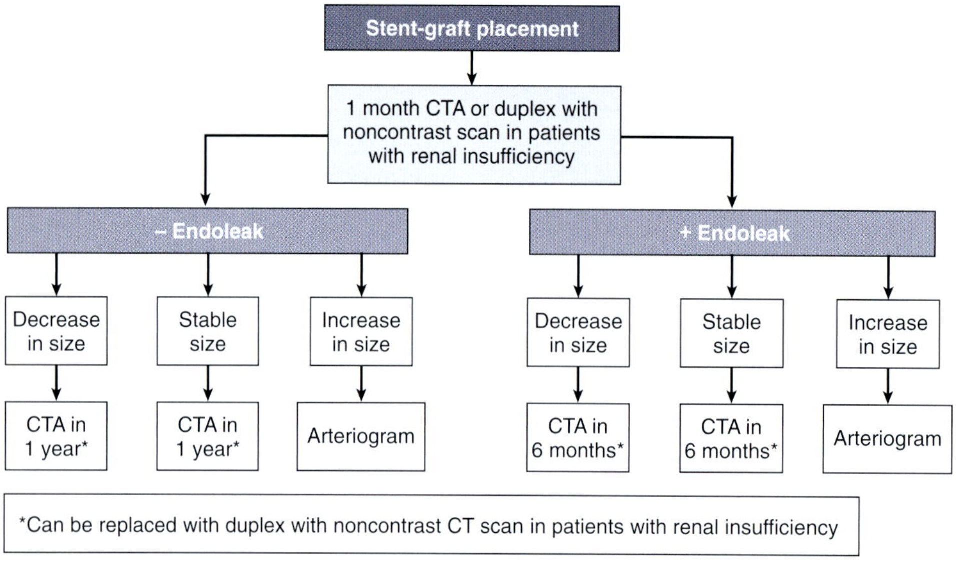

FIG 42.11 Surveillance following endovascular repair of abdominal aortic aneurysm. *CT,* Computed tomography; *CTA,* computed tomographic angiography.

of continued long-term surveillance.[39] Although most of these secondary interventions can be performed by endovascular means, a minority of patients will require explant of the graft and formal open repair of their aneurysm.

MIDTERM OUTCOMES

Despite the early perioperative benefits noted with EVAR,[40] randomized trials and population-based studies have shown similar late survival after endovascular and open AAA repair.[41–45] In the DREAM and EVAR-1 trials, there was a 3% reduction in aneurysm-related mortality throughout the follow-up period, but the initial reduction in all-cause mortality was eliminated within 1 to 2 years. The survival curves overlapped by 18 months in randomized controlled trials and at 3 years in Medicare beneficiaries.[41-43] In addition, EVAR was associated with a greater number of late complications and secondary reinterventions. In the EVAR-1 trial, reinterventions occurred at a rate of 20% at 4 years, compared with 6% for open surgical repair.[42] The DREAM trial showed a higher reintervention rate in the EVAR group at 9 months compared with the open surgical group (hazard ratio, 2.9; 95% confidence interval, 1.1 to 6.2). In a population-based study of 45,660 Medicare beneficiaries, AAA-related intervention was 9.0% following EVAR compared with 1.7% after open repair. AAA rupture was also slightly higher after EVAR at 1.8% versus 0.5% after open repair. As expected, laparotomy-related complications were more likely in the open repair group (9.7% vs. 4.1%). Giles and colleagues[46] conducted a study in Medicare beneficiaries in an attempt to discern the effect of reintervention on survival. Reintervention and readmission rates were slightly higher after EVAR (7.6% vs. 7.0%). They also found that reinterventions or readmissions accounted for 9.6% of all EVAR deaths and 7.6% of all open repair deaths in the follow-up period. These findings indicate that survival is negatively affected by reintervention or readmission after EVAR and open surgery, which could account for the lack of survival benefit of EVAR over time.

In summary, EVAR has been associated with reduced morbidity, reduced intensive care unit and hospital length of stay, and lower perioperative mortality rates; however, further research is needed to optimize the risk-to-benefit ratio in the long term. Continued improvements in device design, favorable patient and anatomic selection, and imaging capabilities will surely advance this technology and lead to durable endovascular AAA repair.

REVIEW QUESTIONS

1. What is the most important anatomic variable for determining a patient's suitability for EVAR?
   a. Proximal aortic neck
   b. Size of iliac vessels
   c. Tortuosity of iliac vessels
   d. Degree of calcification in the aneurysm sac
2. Which type of endoleak is initially managed with continued monitoring?
   a. Type I
   b. Type II with stable or decreased aneurysm sac size
   c. Type II with increased aneurysm sac size
   d. Type III

3. True or false: Patients undergoing EVAR exhibit decreased perioperative morbidity and mortality rates but equivalent long-term survival rates compared with patients undergoing open surgical repair.
4. Which of the following device characteristics can prevent graft migration?
   a. Radial force
   b. Suprarenal fixation
   c. Hooks or barbs
   d. All of the above
5. True or false: Patients with juxtarenal abdominal aortic aneurysms can be treated with EVAR and renal stenting via the encroachment or chimney maneuvers.
6. True or false: Patients undergoing EVAR have a lower rate of secondary intervention compared with the open surgical repair group.
7. Which of the following is the most appropriate postoperative surveillance study?
   a. Arteriogram
   b. Computed tomographic angiography
   c. Abdominal radiograph
   d. Serum creatinine level
8. All the following endografts use a modular system except:
   a. AneuRx
   b. Zenith
   c. Powerlink
   d. Excluder
9. True or false: Most type I endoleaks are treated with immediate surgical conversion.
10. True or false: An occluded superior mesenteric artery and an enlarged inferior mesenteric artery and marginal artery of Drummond preclude endovascular stent-graft repair.

References available online at ExpertConsult.com.

43 CHAPTER

Open Surgical and Endovascular Management of Ruptured Abdominal Aortic Aneurysm

Frank J. Veith, Neal S. Cayne, Dieter Mayer, Mario Lachat

A ruptured abdominal aortic aneurysm (AAA) is a relatively common but catastrophic problem that, if untreated, will almost always result in the death of a patient. However, with treatment, which can consist of open surgical repair or endovascular graft exclusion of the ruptured AAA (RAAA), many patients will survive and go on to live out their normal lifespan. This chapter discusses important aspects of the open surgical and endovascular graft repair of RAAAs that have a rupture site in the aorta or common iliac arteries. Because the preoperative, intraoperative, and postoperative management associated with open surgical repair is well known and well standardized, this chapter stresses only crucial and less well-known aspects of these areas of open repair (OR). The remainder of this chapter deals with the history and current status of endovascular treatment of RAAAs, with an emphasis on endovascular aneurysm repair (EVAR) by endograft exclusion of the RAAA. It will also emphasize key management strategies, technical maneuvers, and adjuncts that are important in achieving optimal outcomes in the very sick patient group with a RAAA.

OPEN SURGICAL MANAGEMENT—KEY POINTS

Crucial Diagnostic Triad

Pain, syncope, and a known or palpable AAA form a crucial diagnostic triad. If a patient has all three elements, he or she should be considered to have a presumptive diagnosis of an RAAA. If open surgical treatment is planned, such a patient should be taken immediately to the operating room and prepared for operation. No further diagnostic evaluation is necessary. Although an occasional patient will have another catastrophic problem, most of these patients require a laparotomy anyhow. The only exceptions are an acute myocardial infarction and pancreatitis. The former can be suspected because of EKG findings, the latter because of a high hematocrit and an elevated amylase.

The history of syncope is usually a manifestation of hypovolemia if cardiac courses can be excluded. The known AAA may be confirmed by history or the presence of a palpable pulsatile mass on physical examination. Although the pain element of the triad is usually in the mid-abdomen or back, it may be in the chest, the lower abdomen, the flank, or the groin. These unusual locations are caused by the pressure of the hematoma, which may not be centrally located and therefore producing unusual pain patterns. One example would be flank and groin pain mimicking a renal or ureteral stone. Another would be left lower quadrant pain and a mass mimicking diverticulitis.

If a patient has only two elements of the triad, further emergent diagnostic studies with ultrasound or computed tomography (CT) scanning are justified. However, a member of the surgical team should be with the patient during these urgent studies in case hemodynamic collapse occurs. The main purpose of these studies is usually to confirm the presence of an AAA, although occasionally blood can be seen outside the wall of the AAA or other important information can be provided.

Other Diagnoses That Can Be Mimicked by a Ruptured Abdominal Aortic Aneurysm

These diagnoses include most commonly a ureteral stone or diverticulitis. Other intraabdominal acute entities such as a perforated ulcer, a small bowel problem, or a pancreatic lesion can be mimicked by an RAAA and its associated hypovolemic shock and abdominal pain. Finally, an RAAA may present as a myocardial infarction with lower chest pain and nonspecific EKG changes because of the hypovolemic shock. One of the aspects of an RAAA that can contribute to this diagnostic confusion is the variable time course of the process depending on the variable containment of the rupture by adjacent structures. Another is the variable location of the rupture site and its associated hematoma.

Strategies in Planning Operative Treatment

When the diagnosis of an RAAA is presumed (three elements of the triad) or confirmed if two elements are present initially, a decision can be made to proceed with operative treatment. Although the patient should be taken immediately to the operating room, other elements or strategies in the treatment are important. The team must be assembled. This includes junior and senior surgeons, nurses, and anesthesiologists. Because these RAAA emergencies often occur at night or on weekends, assembling the team needed to treat them can take some time and organization. However, most operative procedures should not begin and the patient should not be anesthetized until all members of the team are present. While the team is gathering, lines and nasogastric and bladder tubes can be placed, instruments set up, and the abdomen prepared and draped. Only when all personnel are present should the patient be anesthetized because circulatory collapse is prone to occur when anesthesia removes the sympathetic compensation, which maintains the circulation in the hypovolemic state. Only if the patient's circulation collapses completely should a junior member of the team begin the operation before the whole team is fully assembled and operative preparations are completed. The strategic principle should be to rapidly get the patient to the operating room, but then proceed deliberately and only anesthetize the patient and begin the operation when everyone and everything is set up and in place.

One final strategy that is as effective in OR management as it is in endovascular treatment, is the use of hypotensive hemostasis or restricted fluid resuscitation. This means that bleeding is limited by allowing the patient to be hypotensive throughout the pre- and intraoperative phases of treatment. This will be discussed in greater detail in the endovascular treatment section.

Key Technical Points for Open Repair of Ruptured Abdominal Aortic Aneurysms

Once the abdomen is opened through a short midline incision, the base of the mesentery is inspected, and if blood is seen, the diagnosis of rupture is confirmed. The incision is then extended from xiphoid to pubis.

If the area of the infrarenal neck of the AAA is involved with hematoma, supraceliac aortic control should be obtained as shown in Figs. 43.1A–H.[1] This is done without direct vision by tearing the lesser omentum with a finger (Fig. 43.1A). This exposes the retroperitoneum above the celiac axis and pancreas (Fig. 43.1B). Then, using the gloved index finger and its nail, the posterior peritoneum over the diaphragmatic crura is torn as indicated by the line in Fig. 43.1C and the fingertip pushed through the muscle fibers until the periadventitial space of the aorta is encountered (Fig. 43.1D). Then the finger bluntly dissects medially and laterally in the same plane creating a potential space on both sides of the aorta (Figs. 43.1E–G). Then two fingers are placed in the potential space and pulled caudally (Fig. 43.1G). A large covered DeBakey clamp is then placed vertically above the fingers into the space to occlude the aorta (Fig. 43.1H). Only if the aorta is freed from the crural fibers anteriorly, medially, and laterally will the clamp be occlusive. It is also crucial to have a nasogastric tube in the esophagus during these maneuvers so that this structure can be identified and protected from injury.

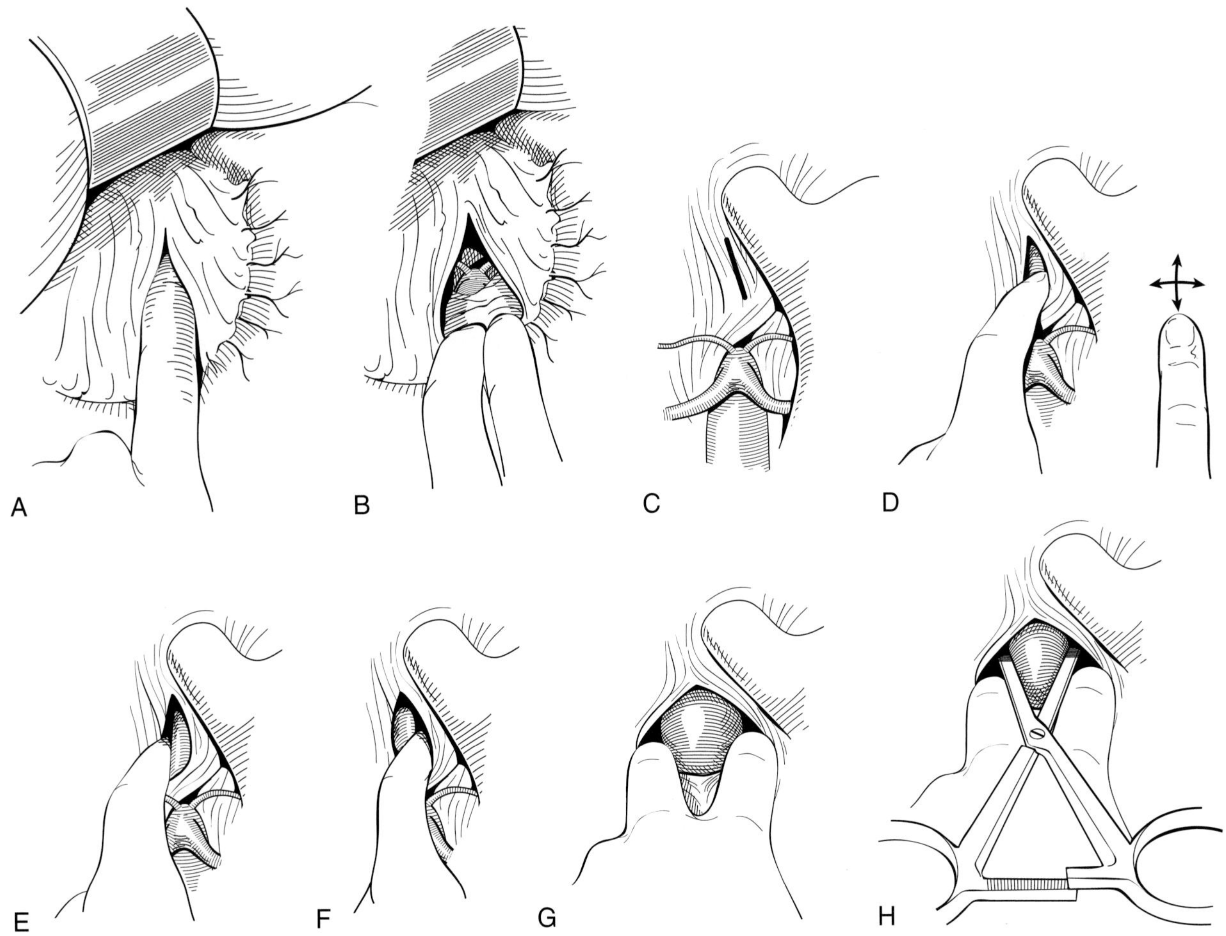

FIG 43.1 (A–H) Technique for occluding the supraceliac aorta without visualization of the structures dissected. (From Veith FJ, Gupta S, Daly V. Technique for occluding the supraceliac aorta through the abdomen. *Surg Gynecol Obstet* 151:648–650, 1980.)

Following placement of this clamp, it is essential to minimize the time of supraceliac aortic occlusion (15 to 20 minutes is tolerable) to minimize liver and gut ischemia. To do this, the anterior wall of the AAA is exposed in its most prominent portion away from all venous and other structures. The anterior wall of the AAA is incised and a finger is placed within the AAA sac to identify the aortic neck. This may be deviated sharply to the right, left, or anteriorly because of aortic tortuosity associated with AAAs. With a finger inside to identify the position of the neck, it can gently be dissected bluntly from adjacent structures in the periadventitial plane without injuring major veins. Once dissected anteriorly, medially, and laterally, an infrarenal aortic clamp can be placed and the suprarenal clamp removed.

The iliac arteries can then be identified from without and clamped with gently placed atraumatic clamps. If they cannot be easily identified by palpation from without, they can be identified from within the lumen by a finger within the AAA sac. Clamps can then be placed on them without further dissection or with minimal dissection.

Clots are then removed from the interior of the AAA. Bleeding lumbar and any other branches are identified and controlled with sutures from within. A prosthetic graft is sutured in place from within the lumen of the AAA. The posterior walls of the aortic and iliac arteries should never be dissected, to prevent damage to other vascular structures. The posterior walls of the aorta and iliac arteries should not be transected, to avoid injuries to adherent major veins and minimize bleeding from other vascular structures.

Although it is controversial, heparin should be administered as soon as aortic clamp control is obtained. All dissection should be minimized in these RAAA repairs to minimize injury to other structures and blood vessels, the position of which can be distorted by the AAA and the hematoma. Otherwise, the repair should be as much like a standard AAA repair as possible. Care should be taken to monitor and treat hypothermia and coagulation defects. Finally, care should be taken to diagnose and treat abdominal compartment syndrome as detailed in the endovascular section later in this chapter.

ENDOVASCULAR MANAGEMENT

History

Endovascular repair of an RAAA was first performed successfully by Marin et al. on April 21, 1994.[2] Another case was first reported by Yusuf et al. in 1994.[3] Since then, many centers have employed endovascular aneurysm repair (EVAR) to treat RAAAs, with varying results.[4–15] Several groups have developed standardized systems of management in the RAAA setting, have used EVAR whenever possible, and have achieved good results with EVAR.[4–10] In contrast, other authors have used EVAR for RAAAs more selectively and have reported no better results with EVAR than with traditional OR.[11–15]

On the basis of these many reports, it is reasonable to say that the comparative efficacy of EVAR and OR for RAAAs is controversial, and some have advocated randomized, prospective, comparative trials of the two treatment methods with this entity. Three such randomized controlled trials (RCTs) were recently published and presented their results: the AJAX or Amsterdam (Dutch) trial,[16] the ECAR or French trial,[17] and the IMPROVE or UK trial.[18] All three trials concluded that 30-day mortality outcomes after EVAR for RAAA are no better than those after OR. However, all three of these trials have serious flaws that render their results and conclusions misleading. These flaws are summarized in a recent publication.[19] Because these RCTs are potentially misleading, the comparative efficacy of EVAR and OR in the RAAA setting remains controversial. We and many others believe that other evidence supports the superiority of EVAR when it can be performed. This view is also supported by a two-center study from Zurich, Switzerland and Orebro, Sweden in which all 70 RAAA patients seen over a 2-year period were treated by EVAR, although 24% required a chimney graft or other adjunct.[20] The 30-day mortality for all these patients was only 24% and the turn-down rate for these RAAA patients was a remarkably low 4%.

In this chapter, we summarize other reasons that support the superiority of EVAR for RAAAs when the anatomy is suitable and suitable facilities, equipment, and skills are available.

Theoretical Considerations

EVAR has been used increasingly to treat RAAA and offers many theoretical advantages over OR. It is less invasive, eliminates damage to periaortic and abdominal structures, decreases bleeding from surgical dissection, minimizes hypothermia, and lessens the requirement for deep anesthesia. Because of these potential advantages, together with single-center reports of lower procedural mortality, EVAR has been deemed superior to OR for the treatment of RAAA.[4–10]

A Single-Center Experience

Between April 22, 1994 and January 15, 2008, 57 patients with RAAAs were treated at Montefiore Medical Center in New York.[21] Much of this experience has been reported previously.[5] Briefly, after an initial experience of EVAR in 12 patients with RAAA (who were deemed unsuitable for OR) showed only a 17% 30-day mortality, we adopted a policy of using EVAR to treat all RAAA patients with suitable anatomy if appropriate staffing and endografts were available.[5,21] A total of 45 patients were treated with endografts and 12 with OR. In the patients who underwent EVAR, 25 received surgeon-made endografts and 20 received industry-made modular endografts. The surgeon-made endografts were constructed from a large balloon-expandable stent and a tulip-shaped polytetrafluoroethylene (PTFE) graft, placed in an aortounifemoral position with contralateral iliac artery occlusion and a femorofemoral bypass.[5] Twelve of the 57 patients with RAAA underwent OR: 10 because their anatomy was unsuitable for EVAR and two because appropriate staff or grafts were not available. Many of the patients treated with EVAR were prohibitive risks for OR, yet many of these survived exclusion of their RAAA by an EVAR procedure.

EVAR was performed without a preprocedural CT scan in 17 patients. In these patients, intraoperative arteriography using calibrated catheters was used to determine suitability for EVAR and to make measurements for graft sizing. A preprocedural CT scan was obtained in the other 28 patients because of uncertainty in the diagnosis or because the patient was initially admitted to another hospital or service. No differences in outcomes were observed between these two small groups.

Fluids were aggressively restricted and the patient's blood pressure was allowed to fall to 50 mm Hg without fluid administration, or lower if the patient was moving or talking.[5] Although local anesthesia was used in the early phases of most EVAR procedures (placement of catheters, guidewires, and sheaths), general anesthesia was used to prevent motion to optimize imaging and allow precise endograft deployment. Large sheath placement and balloon occlusion were used only in the case of cardiovascular collapse, and were required in 10 of 45 patients undergoing EVAR and 3 of 12 undergoing OR.[21] The technique for continuous balloon control of the aorta while deploying a modular endograft has been described by Malina and colleagues.[22] Abdominal compartment syndrome (ACS) was detected in only three of the 45 patients undergoing EVAR when they became hypotensive and difficult to ventilate. Laparotomy and evacuation of the hematoma relieved the problem. However, unrecognized ACS probably contributed to fatal multiorgan failure in some patients. Six of the 45 patients treated by EVAR and one of the 12 patients treated by OR died within 30 days.[21]

Collected World Experience

Data from 49 centers around the world that perform EVAR for RAAAs were collected between July 1, 2002 and January 15, 2009. Data from the 13 centers that were committed to EVAR and performed this procedure on all or almost all patients with RAAA who had suitable aortic neck and iliac artery anatomy were updated to January 15, 2009. These updated data, as well as all the data from the other centers, were reported in November 2009.[21]

Data from 1037 patients with an RAAA or a ruptured aortoiliac aneurysm treated with EVAR show an overall 30-day mortality of 21.2%, which is clearly lower than the rates of 35% to 55% with OR for RAAAs reported in multiple studies.[23] However, many of the centers in the collected experience limited the use of EVAR to "stable" patients with RAAA or even those with "contained" ruptures. Because hemodynamic instability is associated with a higher risk of procedural mortality,[6,8,23] it is invalid to compare procedural mortality with EVAR and OR in this way.

Because of this, the updated outcomes for EVAR were examined in the selected group of 13 centers that were committed to performing EVAR to treat RAAA in all patients with anatomy suitable for endograft treatment, including those who were hemodynamically unstable and those in profound shock.[21] These centers were usually the ones with the greatest experience. Although there was some variability in the approach used in these centers to the treatment of patients with RAAA, most had some degree of standardization and many had a defined protocol. All were experienced in the use of EVAR and endovascular adjuncts for elective treatment of abdominal aneurysm, and all had dedicated endovascular facilities and imaging equipment. The use of EVAR to treat all possible patients with RAAA and suitable anatomy was associated with a favorable 30-day mortality of 19.7% in 680 patients (range 0% to 32%).[21] During this same period, these same 13 centers performed OR for RAAAs in 763 patients whose anatomy was thought to be unsuitable for EVAR. The 30-day mortality for OR was 36.3% (range 8% to 49%; $P < .0001$ for EVAR vs. OR).[21]

These updated comparative outcome results (30-day mortality 19.7% for EVAR vs. 36.3% for OR from the 13 centers committed to EVAR of as many RAAAs as possible) strongly suggest that EVAR is a superior way to treat RAAAs in patients whose aortic neck and iliac anatomy is suitable for endovascular graft treatment. Additional proof that EVAR is a better treatment for some patients with RAAA is that many patients (~15%) in this collected experience who were categorically unsuitable or prohibitively high risk for OR survived for many years after EVAR.

Why Are Results Variable?

Several possible reasons might explain the discordant results reported by different authors for treatment of RAAA by EVAR.[4–15] These include strategies, adjuncts, and technical factors that are thought to influence the outcome of EVAR for RAAAs, and probably account for the favorable outcomes with EVAR in the 13 centers in the collected experience.[21] Some of the key reasons are described below.

Standard Approach or Protocol

The use of a protocol allows the most effective decision making and treatment of patients in circumstances that are often confusing and stressful.[9,10] Protocols are also important to facilitate education of generalists, emergency room personnel, and others to recognize RAAAs, and to enable early diagnosis and mobilization of the specialized care givers best trained to optimize treatment.

Fluid Restriction (Hypotensive Hemostasis)

Fluid resuscitation should be restricted even if the patient becomes hypotensive. Experience has shown that systolic arterial pressures of 50 to 70 mm Hg are well tolerated for short periods and limit internal bleeding and associated loss of platelets and clotting factors.[5,6,10,21,24] Whether pharmacological lowering of blood pressure is beneficial remains to be shown conclusively, however.[6,10]

Treatment Site

EVAR procedures are optimally performed in a site equipped for excellent fluoroscopic imaging and open surgery, because some patients will require OR or open adjuncts to EVAR.

Anesthesia and Catheter-Guidewire Placement

Guidewire placement should be done percutaneously under local anesthesia. This permits arteriography to define aortic and arterial anatomy, facilitates large sheath and supraceliac balloon placement if needed, and prevents circulatory collapse caused by the induction of general anesthesia. Whether general anesthesia is subsequently required to eliminate motion and improve fluoroscopic imaging to permit precise graft deployment remains controversial. Some groups have successfully used local anesthesia supplemented by sedation throughout as an alternative.[4,6,10]

Supraceliac Aortic Sheath Placement and Balloon Control

Most groups use these techniques only when there is severe circulatory collapse. However, in such cases, deflation of the balloon before sealing of the rupture site will result in immediate recurrence of the circulatory collapse. Techniques have therefore been developed to maintain continuous aortic control until the endograft has sealed the leak.[5,6,22,25,26] Renal and visceral ischemia is minimized by placing secondary balloons within the endograft as the supraceliac balloon is deflated and removed though its supporting sheath. One technique for accomplishing this has recently been described and illustrated.[26]

Endograft Type and Configuration

Both bifurcated and aortouni-iliac (or femoral) grafts can be used successfully, although some patients have unilateral iliac disease, which mandates a unilateral configuration. Modular and unibody grafts have been used successfully in both configurations. An appropriate inventory of suitable grafts and accessories must be stocked sterile in the treatment site and must be available for the procedure and unexpected contingencies.

Abdominal Compartment Syndrome

Abdominal compartment syndrome (ACS) is a major cause of morbidity and mortality after EVAR for RAAA, and a high index of suspicion for this entity should be maintained. Monitoring of bladder pressure has been helpful in early detection of ACS.[6,10] Conservative measures (diuretics, colloid administration, and neuromuscular blockade) may be helpful for minimal elevations in intraabdominal pressure. However, laparotomy and open abdomen treatment (OAT) are required to alleviate the hypotension, high ventilatory compliance, and oliguria that occur with full-blown ACS. Early laparotomy with OAT and suction/sponge dressings may allow survival in otherwise hopeless circumstances when small-bowel and mesenteric edema causes loss of domain for the abdominal viscera.[10] Contrary to general belief, evacuation of the retroperitoneal hematoma is usually not needed with OAT and should usually be avoided to prevent further bleeding and damage to the adjacent structures.

Endovascular Aneurysm Repair for Highest-Risk Patients

EVAR is probably most beneficial in augmenting survival when it is used in the highest-risk patients who are unlikely to survive an OR. This category includes patients who are hemodynamically unstable or in profound circulatory collapse, those who have a hostile abdomen, and those unable to receive transfusion. If such patients, particularly those who are hemodynamically unstable, are excluded from EVAR, it is likely that the improved survival that can accrue from this form of treatment would be diminished.[21]

Are Further Randomized Controlled Comparisons of Endovascular Aneurysm Repair Needed?

The reduced 30-day mortality after EVAR compared with OR (19.7% vs. 36.3%), together with the survival of many RAAA patients who are prohibitive risks for OR, constitute strong evidence that EVAR is a better way to treat RAAAs in at least some patients, provided that the described strategies, adjuncts, and techniques are employed. Accordingly, many believe that there is no need for a randomized controlled comparison of EVAR and OR in patients with RAAA, given the data from the collected experience and other evidence.[21] Moreover, as demonstrated by the three existing randomized controlled trials, such studies are difficult to perform in this setting, subject to methodological problems, and may lead to conclusions that are not generally applicable.[16-19] Thus, at present, it is reasonable to conclude that EVAR is the best treatment for patients with an RAAA if the anatomy is suitable and the equipment and skilled personnel are available to do it.

REVIEW QUESTIONS

1. True or False. RAAAs can have a variable time course.
2. True or False. The variability in the time course of an RAAA depends on the previous health of the patient.
3. True or False. When performing a laparotomy for an RAAA, the initial incision should be very long.
4. True or False. Supraceliac aortic control can be achieved rapidly without visualizing all involved structures.
5. True or False. Supraceliac aortic control can be achieved by placing the clamp on the aorta with minimal dissection of diaphragmatic fibers.
6. True or False. Abdominal compartment syndrome can occur after open RAAA repair.
7. True or False. Supraceliac aortic balloon control must always be obtained during an EVAR procedure for an RAAA.
8. True or False. Having an established protocol is crucial to achieving optimal results with EVAR for RAAAs.
9. True or False. During open repair of an RAAA, isolation of the proximal neck is often facilitated by opening the aneurysm and inserting a finger in the lumen rather than by dissection of the neck from surrounding structures.
10. What is the best way to detect abdominal compartment syndrome after EVAR for RAAA?
    - **a.** By symptoms of hypotension, difficulty in ventilation, and organ dysfunction.
    - **b.** By feeling abdominal distension.
    - **c.** By measuring intragastric pressure.
    - **d.** By monitoring bladder pressure.
    - **e.** By observing the colonic mucosa.

References available online at ExpertConsult.com.

CHAPTER 44

Laparoscopic Aortic Surgery for Aneurysm and Occlusive Disease: Technique and Results

Ralf R. Kolvenbach, Catherine Cagiannos

INTRODUCTION

Today the vast majority of aortic and iliac vascular procedures can be performed by endovascular techniques, yet there are still some indications where open surgical repair or a less invasive technique is indicated. Some of these procedures can be performed using video endoscopic approaches.

Currently two laparoscopic approaches are available for abdominal vascular surgery: total laparoscopic aortic surgery in patients with occlusive disease and hybrid techniques that combine laparoscopy with endovascular techniques to treat failing endografts. We also have to distinguish between a total laparoscopic approach versus a laparoscopic assisted procedure.

The role that laparoscopic surgery will play in vascular surgery must be determined in the context of randomized controlled trials (RCTs). At present it is not realistic to believe that laparoscopic surgery will be widely adopted and implemented by the vascular surgical community because of alternative procedures that are easier to perform and have low morbidity. Although the potential to avoid the cost and inconvenience of lifelong surveillance that is required to monitor and address complications that develop following endovascular interventions is enticing, new laparoscopic instruments and technology that make intracorporeal suturing, hemostasis, and clamping easier are needed to help spur continued interest in laparoscopic vascular surgery and facilitate the performance of these techniques by more vascular surgeons.

Laparoscopy has played a crucial role in the development of abdominal surgery over the past three decades as it is generally perceived as a less invasive treatment modality. Advances in catheter-based interventions have similarly raised an overall level of enthusiasm in minimally invasive vascular treatment strategies. Although endovascular intervention is commonly regarded as the less invasive treatment modality in the treatment of occlusive and aneurysm conditions, laparoscopic intervention has played an increasingly important role in the contemporary treatment paradigm of vascular disease management. Laparoscopy can be incorporated into vascular surgery in several ways, including (1) hand-assisted laparoscopic surgery (HALS), where the nondominant hand is placed intracorporeally to assist with dissection and anastomosis; (2) laparoscopically assisted dissection with mini-incision, where the vascular anastomosis is performed using open surgical techniques; and (3) total laparoscopic surgery, where the dissection and vascular anastomosis are performed under pneumoperitoneum.

Just as there are many ways in which the aorta can be exposed during open surgery, aortic exposure can also be accomplished in several ways laparoscopically. Several examples of these approaches include (1) a direct midline transperitoneal approach,[1–3] (2) a retrocolic intraperitoneal approach,[4–7] (3) a retrorenal intraperitoneal approach,[8] and (4) a retroperitoneal approach.[9] The advantages and disadvantages of each of these techniques are published in the literature and are not the focus of this chapter; suffice it to say that there are proponents and opponents of laparoscopically assisted procedures, hand-assisted procedures, and totally laparoscopic procedures and of the various exposures. To date, the majority of the vascular community does not accept that the acquisition of laparoscopic skills is warranted because unless there are dramatic advances in the ease with which laparoscopic suturing, clamping, control of bleeding, and hemostasis can be accomplished, it is unlikely that laparoscopic procedures will gain the widespread popularity that endovascular interventions enjoy. However, not all patients are amenable to endovascular repair, and laparoscopic aortic repair may have a niche indication in select cases. Anatomic limitations are the impetus behind the pursuit of other minimally invasive therapeutic alternatives in vascular surgery.

TECHNIQUES

Laparoscopic Aortobifemoral Bypass

Laparoscopic procedures are best performed in designated minimally invasive operating suites with monitors placed enabling the entire team to follow the case. Our preference is for the surgeon and two assistants to stand on the patient's right side. The patient is placed on a vacuum bag to maintain him or her in the right lateral decubitus position during the procedure. To optimize displacement of the viscera, the table is also tilted to achieve a right-sided 70-degree rotation. Six or seven laparoscopic ports are used, depending on the size of the patient (Fig. 44.1). The first 11-mm trocar is placed through a left paramedian incision, two finger widths from the umbilicus, and is used to establish the pneumoperitoneum (12 mm Hg). A 45-degree optic (Storz Endoscopy, Tuttlingen, Germany) is the preferred camera system. Three or four more trocars are placed four finger widths apart from each other along this line. The trocars are used for passage

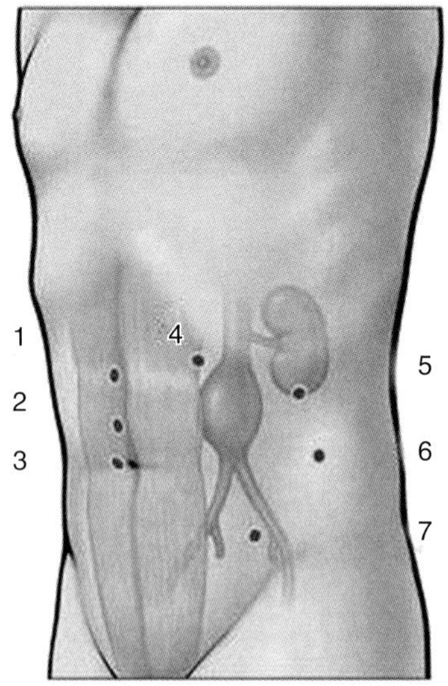

FIG 44.1 Port placement for a total laparoscopic procedure. *Ports 1 to 3:* needle holders and/or graspers; *port 4:* aortic cross-clamp; *port 5:* camera port; *port 6:* table-mounted retractor for kidney; *port 7:* iliac clamp and/or suction-irrigation apparatus.

of the optic, dissection instruments, laparoscopic sponge sticks, and needle drivers. During the initial retrorenal or retrocolic dissection, the optic is placed in one of the upper paramedian ports. Another trocar is placed in the left subcostal position in the midclavicular line for passage of the optic during dissection of the aorta and performance of the proximal anastomosis. Trocars are also placed paralleling the left inguinal ligament for passage of the distal aortic or iliac clamps and the suction-irrigation apparatus. A trocar placed laterally in the left flank is used for the kidney retractor to facilitate exposure during the proximal anastomosis. A subxiphoid trocar serves for placement of the proximal aortic clamp (Storz Endoscopy).

The left hemicolon, including the splenic flexure, is mobilized medially. The technique of medial mobilization to separate the abdominal contents from the retroperitoneal space was originally described by Dion and colleagues.[4,10] The line of Toldt is used as a landmark when the lateral attachments of the sigmoid colon are being incised. Incomplete mobilization of the splenic flexure may result in splenic injury during retraction, particularly in cases with adhesions from previous surgery. We use a left hemicolic retrorenal approach in most patients. This approach permits expeditious exposure of the aorta while avoiding mobilization and potential devascularization of the ureter. This approach also provides access to the suprarenal aorta. A special table-mounted laparoscopic holding system and fan retractor (Storz) are sufficient to maintain aortic exposure, even in obese patients. A large lumbar branch tethering the left renal vein on the lateral surface of the aorta is sectioned to allow complete retraction of the kidney. If thromboendarterectomy of the juxtarenal aortic stump is necessary, it is prudent to have suprarenal control; thus dissection is extended proximally. In patients with aortoiliac occlusive disease (AIOD), only the aorta proximal to the origin of the inferior mesenteric artery (IMA) is dissected to avoid damaging the lumbosacral nerves adjacent to the aortic bifurcation.

Deployable clamps (Storz Endoscopy) can be used to occlude the distal aorta; in this way, only the port for the proximal aortic clamp is obstructed with an instrument.[11] The first assistant holds the camera and also helps put the tissue on tension with a grasping clamp. Alternatively, the first assistant provides suction and retraction while the second assistant folds the optic.

Lumbar arteries are controlled extraluminally from the left side using a laparoscopic clip applier (Tyco Healthcare, Mechelen, Belgium). After the left-sided lumbar arteries are clipped and divided, the adjacent right-sided lumbar arteries can be clipped. The limbs of a bifurcated graft are ligated with number 2 silk, the graft body is cut short in the appropriate configuration for the proximal anastomosis, and the prosthesis is passed intracorporeally. The right limb of the bifurcated graft is tunneled to the right groin to achieve a certain degree of stabilization of the prosthesis. Alternatively, the first assistant stabilizes the graft with a grasper. Tunneling to the left groin is not performed initially to minimize loss of pneumoperitoneum. In case of end-to-end aortic anastomosis, closure of the distal aortic stump is performed with a running polypropylene (Prolene) suture with pledgets. Coggia and colleagues have described fixing pledgets to 3-0 Prolene sutures to avoid the need for tedious laparoscopic knot tying.[6] Stapled closure of the distal aortic stump is possible, but hemostasis is usually unsatisfactory. In patients with an end-to-side anastomosis, an aortotomy is performed and the anastomosis is started posteriorly with a 12-cm 3-0 Prolene suture. A second suture is taken anteriorly, and both are tied together intracorporeally. A laparoscopic nerve hook is useful to put the suture line on tension. The first assistant can follow the suture with an atraumatic DeBakey clamp (Storz) and suction blood that may be obscuring the operating field.

Laparoscopic Repair of an Abdominal Aortic Aneurysm

The initial retrorenal dissection is similar to that for laparoscopic aortobifemoral bypass (ABF). Dissection of the infrarenal aorta proceeds from the left iliac to the left renal artery. If needed, dissection of the juxtarenal aorta is possible from a retrorenal approach.[8]

Lumbar arteries are clipped extraluminally either before cross clamping or after the aneurysm is clamped and the sac is decompressed. The ostia of arteries that are still bleeding after incision of the aneurysm sac are stitched with pledgeted laparoscopic 2-0 polyglactin 910 (Vicryl) sutures and secured with a titanium clip. The IMA is identified and, depending on the extent of backflow or the need for better exposure of the right iliac artery, can be ligated with a 12-mm endovascular GIA stapler (TSW 35, Autosuture, United Kingdom) or reimplanted. For an end-to-end anastomosis, the aorta is completely transected. Transection is carefully performed under laparoscopic visualization with a 45-degree-angled laparoscope to avoid any injury to lumbar arteries or veins. If anatomically suitable, tube grafts are inserted. When the iliac arteries are too calcified to permit stapling, the ostium of the common iliac artery (CIA) can be oversewn with a running 3-0 Prolene suture.[12] Alternatively the common iliac artery can be blocked with a balloon catheter.[13]

Hybrid Remodeling Techniques Post–Endovascular Aneurysm Repair

Laparoscopic techniques can be used after endovascular aneurysm repair (EVAR) to treat patients with type II endoleaks and graft migration. Considering that thrombus is not an inert substance, laparoscopic removal of thrombus material can potentially enhance endograft incorporation.[14] Using suturing techniques or banding to enlarge the landing zone, the endoprosthesis can be anchored to the aortic wall, thus preventing graft migration and neck dilation (Fig. 44.2). Depending on the degree of retroperitoneal inflammation, a direct transperitoneal or left retrocolic approach is chosen. The aneurysm and aortic neck are carefully dissected to establish proximal control. The origin of the IMA is identified and the artery is divided to facilitate further mobilization of the aorta and prevent endoleak. Similarly, patent lumbars are identified and clipped. These steps are performed without clamping the aorta, as this can damage the endograft; instead, an aortic occlusion balloon is introduced transfemorally through a hemostatic sheath and advanced proximally under fluoroscopic guidance. After systemic heparinization, the balloon is inflated and the aneurysmal sac incised. This stabilizes the endograft inside the aorta and prevents dislodgment during evacuation of the thrombus. The sac is incised and opened with laparoscopic scissors in an H-shaped configuration (Fig. 44.3). The aneurysm sac thrombus is removed, and the graft is inspected using laparoscopic magnification to exclude defects in the endograft fabric. Bleeding lumbar arteries are stitched with a pledgeted 2-0 Vicryl suture. Using a running 2-0 Prolene suture, the sac of the aneurysm is wrapped tightly around the endograft to decrease the risk of migration. A circumferential band can be placed around the neck of the aneurysm to prevent neck dilatation. Using a curved grasping instrument originally designed for laparoscopic fundoplication, a band of polytetrafluoroethylene is wrapped around the aortic neck (Fig. 44.4). The band is put on tension and secured with interrupted Prolene sutures. Additionally, sutures placed from the endograft into the aortic wall can further stabilize the graft and prevent migration. Fluoroscopy is used to identify the bare stent of the endograft so that the stitches can be placed in the fabric-covered portion. The technique described should be avoided in case of extensive graft migration because free rupture is possible even with the occlusion balloon in place.

Laparoscopic remodeling can be used with concurrent endovascular interventions such as placement of extension cuffs, angioplasty, or graft limb thrombectomy to salvage failed or failing endografts. Laparoscopic hybrid approaches can improve the long-term performance of endografts, thus reducing the need for conversion to open surgery and decreasing the expense of repeat interventions.

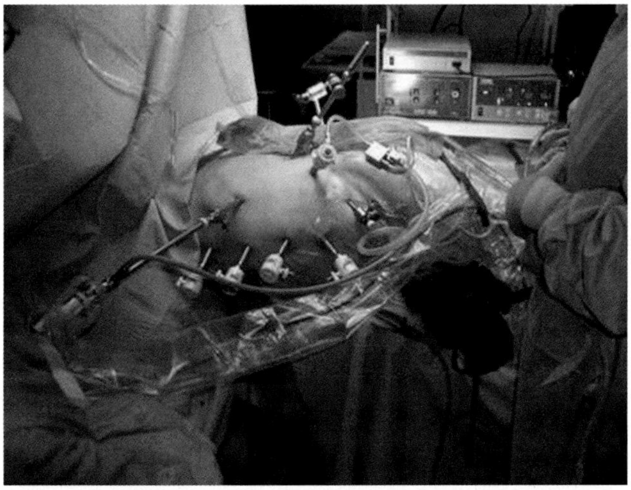

FIG 44.2 Adjunctive laparoscopic measures that can be performed following endovascular aneurysm repair include clipping the inferior mesenteric and lumbar arteries, intrasac thrombus evacuation, closure of the aneurysmal sac and banding of the aneurysmal neck, or endograft suture fixation to stabilize the endoprosthesis.

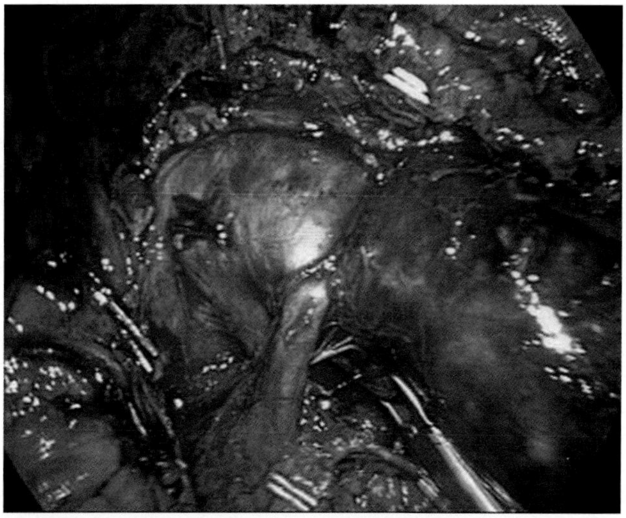

FIG 44.3 An H-shaped incision is made laparoscopically in the sac of the aneurysm to remove thrombus and oversew any bleeding lumbar arteries that might account for type II endoleaks.

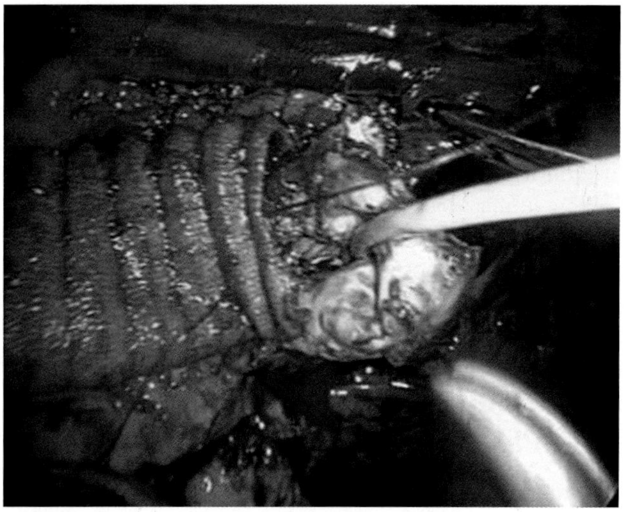

FIG 44.4 Proximal and distal banding to laparoscopically increase the landing zone for aortic endografts.

ADVANTAGES OF LAPAROSCOPIC PROCEDURES

Patients having a total laparoscopic procedure require less analgesia and ambulate sooner compared with those who have a minilaparotomy to convert to a laparoscopically assisted procedure.[12,15] A lower incidence and duration of pulmonary complications and ileus is expected following laparoscopy because of decreased analgesic requirements.[16] Abdominal wall dehiscence occurs in 10% to 15% of patients undergoing open aortofemoral bypass (AFB) surgery.[17–19] A midline mini-incision has the same propensity as the standard laparotomy to develop incisional hernias, whereas there is a 3.9% incisional hernia rate at the trocar sites after total laparoscopic treatment.[20,21]

EXCLUSION CRITERIA AND DISADVANTAGES OF THE LAPAROSCOPIC APPROACH

Patients with hostile abdomen from previous aortoiliac surgery, inflammatory aneurysms, and ruptured aneurysms should not undergo laparoscopic aortic surgery. In the past, aneurysms requiring suprarenal cross clamping were excluded, but with increasing experience, laparoscopic surgeons are now also treating pararenal aneurysms.[22] Patients with AIOD, extensive calcification, and porcelain aorta are excluded because a lack of tactile feedback precludes safe cross clamping.[23]

Physiologic comorbidities accounting for unsafe aortic cross clamping, such as severe cardiac insufficiency, are also contraindications. Patients with an American Society of Anesthesiologists' physical status classification of II and III are acceptable for laparoscopic procedures because the hemodynamic consequences of infrarenal aortic clamping in good-risk surgical patients are low despite the fact that pneumoperitoneum and placement of the patient in the right lateral decubitus position impair myocardial perfusion.[8,23–26]

Higher blood loss has been reported by some during laparoscopy. Uncontrolled bleeding is a criterion for conversion to open surgery. Experts, however, emphasize that there is an inherent bias in the literature because blood in compresses is not quantified during open repair, since data collection is retrospective, whereas all blood lost is collected and quantified during laparoscopy.[23] Nevertheless it may be harder to achieve effective tamponade and hemostasis during laparoscopy because vigorous suction evacuates the pneumoperitoneum and decreases visualization in the operative cavity.[23] Laparoscopic control of the bleeding lumbar arteries can be challenging. Development of a high-flow insufflation device and further instrumentation specific to laparoscopic hemostasis is warranted.[26]

LAPAROSCOPY IN THE CONTEXT OF ENDOVASCULAR ANEURYSM REPAIR AND OPEN SURGERY

Simply showing that laparoscopic surgery is feasible and no worse than open surgery is not sufficient to convince vascular surgeons to perform laparoscopic procedures, especially when there are concerns that they are longer, more technically demanding, and associated with greater blood loss.[23,27] Minimizing access trauma is only part of the problem. Avoiding ischemia-reperfusion injury and bleeding complications is equally important. One solution is to combine laparoscopic and endovascular techniques to reduce ischemia and the need for nephrotoxic agents while optimizing durability and decreasing the need for reintervention.[28–30] Hybrid procedures can be used following EVAR to correct endoleaks, graft migration, and thrombosis as well as to facilitate visceral artery revascularization and expand the applicability of endografts in patients with anatomy of the neck and aneurysm that would have precluded endovascular repair.[28–33]

Laparoscopic interventions must be evaluated in the context of the strengths and weaknesses of well-established open and endovascular interventions. Open ABF bypass has better long-term patency for diffuse AOID than endovascular interventions.[34,35] The Trans-Atlantic Inter-Society Consensus (TASC) document recommends open surgery for complex iliac disease (type D) and for patients who have failed endovascular interventions.[36]

EVAR is less invasive than open surgery because smaller incisions are used and the avoidance of aortic cross-clamp reduces cardiac stress. There is no doubt whatsoever that EVAR will replace aortic aneurysm surgery in almost all cases in spite of a higher need for secondary procedures.[37,38] Significantly reduced morbidity and mortality is a good justification for the lifelong radiographic surveillance that is mandatory after EVAR.[35,39,40]

Two randomized European trials comparing EVAR with open surgery have been published.[41,42–46] One problem remaining is that even after initial successful exclusion of the abdominal aortic aneurysm (AAA), patent lumbar arteries or the IMA can result in endoleaks—a problem that we do not see with open surgical procedures.[30]

Laparoscopic surgery can be used as an adjunct to improve outcomes following EVAR and to salvage failing endografts without resorting to open conversion. Several approaches are used to manage type II endoleaks, including endovascular interventions such as transarterial collateral embolization, translumbar embolization, and intrasac thrombin injection. A wide discrepancy in the efficacy of these methods has been observed, and the results for the techniques are highly operator-dependent.[47,48] Alternatively, vessels responsible for endoleaks after EVAR can be clipped directly by open surgery or laparoscopy.[49,50] By ligating vessels laparoscopically, surgeons can address endoleaks definitively without the long, painful incisions used in standard open procedures. Laparoscopic ligation is expeditious, whereas endovascular techniques of sac exclusion can be cumbersome.[27]

There are further potential applications for laparoscopy in vascular surgery. As described earlier, a hybrid laparoscopic technique has been developed to help remodel aneurysms, facilitate graft incorporation, and prevent neck dilation and graft migration after EVAR.[27] In patients with renal insufficiency, placement of radiopaque metal markers at the level of the renal and hypogastric arteries can permit the insertion of endografts without the need for dye administration.[27] Hybrid techniques that incorporate both laparoscopic and endovascular interventions can be used to explant failed endografts or repair aortoiliac aneurysms.[13,30,51] After the outflow vessels have been occluded with intraarterial balloon occlusion catheters to minimize difficult dissection and avoid clamping calcified vessels, the endograft can be explanted laparoscopically and the proximal anastomosis performed using a Dacron graft. The distal limbs of the Dacron graft can be cannulated with stent-grafts, which are then deployed into the iliac vessels, thus decreasing prolonged clamp times by avoiding laparoscopic suturing of the distal anastomoses.[30] Additionally, when guidewire traversal in not possible owing to difficult vascular anatomy, endografts can be placed laparoscopically to facilitate rapid revascularization of the renal and mesenteric vasculature.[31,52]

LEARNING CURVE

It is reported that 25 to 30 cases are needed to overcome the learning curve. Fourneau and colleagues analyzed the first 50 patients with AIOD whom they treated with totally laparoscopic aortofemoral bypass. These authors observed improvement in specific operative parameters—such as morbidity, aortic clamp time, and blood loss—between the twentieth and thirtieth patients.[53] These improvements occurred despite the fact that the difficulty of cases increased during the course of the study. They also noted a decrease in the rate of conversion from laparoscopic to open surgery. Conversion was 32% for the first 25 patients but only 12% for the last 25 patients. The authors commented that during the learning curve, the morbidity and mortality of laparoscopic aortic surgery were not higher than for open surgery. A meta-analysis by de Vries and Hunink that examined the morbidity and mortality of open ABF for AIOD showed 3.3% (range 0 to 7.7) mortality, 8.3% (range 3.8 to 13) systemic morbidity, and 11.4% (range 9.9 to 22) local morbidity.[54] Even including patients in the learning curve, Fourneau and colleagues observed local morbidity of 10% and a systemic morbidity of 12%.[53]

Laparoscopic suturing is a major component of the learning curve and a major obstacle to widespread acceptance of laparoscopic vascular surgery. Other than training on pelvic trainers to decrease operative times and increase dexterity, a solution may involve the use of laparoscopic staplers. It is expected that the ability to perform a rapid mechanical anastomosis in combination with minimal tissue manipulation will yield morbidity results comparable to those with endovascular grafting, with durability comparable to that of open surgical repair. Laparoscopic staplers are in development and undergoing design modifications.[55–56]

LACK OF RANDOMIZED CONTROLLED TRIALS

There is a lack of prospective RCTs evaluating the role of laparoscopic surgery, making it hard to comment on the cost-benefit ratio of laparoscopic interventions in a nonbiased manner. There are no RCTs comparing totally laparoscopic vascular surgery with conventional open surgical interventions or with endovascular interventions to definitively determine if the claims made by laparoscopic surgeons of decreased trauma and comparable durability are indeed true. A 2006 systematic review highlighted this lack of RCTs. Thirty selected studies were included in the systematic review.

Most of the studies were observational and included comparisons between contemporary series and endovascular repair. A total of 1044 patients underwent surgery, 630 for AIOD and 414 for aneurysmal disease.[57] The few comparative studies included in the systematic review revealed trends of longer operative time and shorter hospital stay when laparoscopic interventions were compared with open surgery.[57]

Hand-assisted procedures have the shortest cross-clamping times (all <1 hour) as compared with both laparoscopically assisted and totally laparoscopic procedures. Both clamping and operative times were shorter for AIOD than for aneurysmal disease. The mortality rate was 2% with mortality after aneurysm repair, being higher than in AIOD.[57] Although laparoscopic procedures are longer, they were not associated with increased morbidity or mortality as compared with open procedures or endovascular procedures. Short-term patency following laparoscopic ABF approaches that of open surgery.[17,21,58] Recently Di Centa and colleagues reported 3-year primary and secondary patency rates of 93% and 95.6%, respectively, following totally laparoscopic ABF; these rates are comparable to those with open surgical reconstruction.[17]

To date, only one RCT has compared HALS with open AFB surgery in the management of AIOD.[59] This study showed that diet was tolerated earlier, the epidural was removed sooner, and in-hospital stay was shorter in the HALS group. The assisted primary graft patency was 97.5% at 1 and 2 years in the HALS group and 100% and 95% in the conventional open group. The authors found a comparable incidence of hernia formation and patency in the HALS and open AFB groups.[59]

CONCLUSION

Compared with laparoscopic repair of AIOD, laparoscopic repair of aneurysms is more involved and technically demanding. Some patients, however, are unsuitable for EVAR owing to neck anatomy and vascular access limitations. These patients can benefit from the minimally invasive aspect and durable results of laparoscopic repair.

Questions remain despite the demonstrated safety and feasibility of laparoscopic surgery. The reports in the literature are from centers and surgeons with a dedicated interest in laparoscopic surgery and, for the most part, patients are carefully selected. The data are observational, noncomparative, and prone to selection bias. Although there are reports of reduced hospital stays, decreased analgesia, and earlier ambulation and resumption of diet, there are technical difficulties that must be overcome and a need for reliable data before wide implementation of these techniques can be justified by the majority of vascular surgeons.

The role that laparoscopic surgery will play in vascular surgery must be determined in the context of RCTs. At present, it is not realistic to believe that laparoscopic surgery will be widely adopted and implemented by the vascular surgical community because of other alternatives that are easier to perform and have low morbidity.

REVIEW QUESTIONS

1. Choose the correct answer.
   a. The outcome of laparoscopic aortic procedures is different from open surgery.
   b. The outcome of laparoscopic aortic procedures is similar to conventional aortic surgery.
2. The most common used approach to the aorta is
   a. transperitoneal.
   b. retroperitoneal.
   c. transperitoneal, left hemicolic.
3. Choose the correct answer.
   a. The left kidney is always mobilized medially.
   b. The left kidney always stays in situ.
4. A combination of laparoscopic and endovascular procedures is most commonly used in
   a. patients with occlusive disease.
   b. patients with iliac artery aneurysms.
5. Several answers are correct. Hand-assisted aortic surgery is
   a. a laparoscopic procedure.
   b. a laparoscopic-assisted procedure.
   c. a total laparoscopic operation.
6. Only one answer is correct. Most laparoscopic aortic operations are performed
   a. with mechanical elevation of the abdominal wall.
   b. with the help of pneumoperitoneum.
7. Choose the correct answer.
   a. An aortic anastomosis requires a minilapartomy.
   b. An aortic anastomosis can be performed entirely laparoscopically.
8. Choose the correct answer.
   a. Conversion is always a major complication.
   b. Conversion should be performed at any stage if necessary to avoid complications.
9. Choose the correct answer.
   a. Laparoscopic aortic surgery should always be started with total laparoscopic procedures.
   b. A laparoscopic aortic program should be started with a hand-assisted approach.
10. Choose the correct answer.
    a. Staplers can never replace a hand-sewn aortic anastomosis.
    b. Without staplers, total laparoscopic procedures will be performed in a few centers only.

References available online at ExpertConsult.com.

CHAPTER 45

Building a Hybrid Operating Suite Including Robotic Capability

Alan B. Lumsden

One of the fastest-growing developments in interventional cardiovascular medicine is the development of the hybrid suite.[1-4] These are constructed either in a traditional operating room or catheterization laboratory ("cath lab") environment, thereby permitting a combination of both open and catheter-based procedures. Although hybrid rooms were developed largely to support vascular surgeons, there has been rapid expansion of hybrid room use into other cardiovascular services.[5-8] Some rooms are now designed by surgeons, others by cardiologists; some, as is most appropriate, are designed by both. For example, the first hybrid room was built at Houston Methodist Hospital in 2008 to support the development of advanced vascular procedures, especially hybrid aortic procedures. However, the hospital's most recently constructed room has designated days for dealing with percutaneous aortic valves and has been used extensively for hybrid coronary revascularization, atrial appendage ligation, laser lead extraction, and an increasing variety of vascular procedures. Furthermore, the advanced imaging capabilities of these new rooms, especially cone-beam computed tomography (CT) and image fusion capabilities,[9-12] promise to revolutionize how all of these procedures are performed.

In reality, it makes no sense not to be able to switch between open and endovascular therapies. The primary limitations have been traditional turf issues, meaning that cath labs and interventional suites "belonged" in cardiology and radiology, respectively. Those barriers are rapidly being broken down, with renewed emphasis on the most minimally invasive but appropriate approach for the benefit of the patient. We believe that the cone-beam CT capabilities of modern imaging systems can transform surgery and are now performing lung nodule localization for thoracic surgeons using techniques developed for translumbar embolization. A "CT scanner" in the operating room is as empowering as the initial angio-equipped portable C-arm, which led vascular surgeons into the minimally invasive world.

However, hybrid suites should best be defined by their purpose. That purpose, we submit, is to provide a seamless transition from open to endoluminal procedures and, most importantly, to select the most appropriate therapy for the disease process being treated. Consequently, when defining the hybrid suite concept, clear agreement on the proposed role of the suite, appropriate consultation for adjunctive equipment, and a rigorous planning process are necessary to avoid disenfranchisement and costly construction mistakes. There are no established guidelines for the development of a hybrid suite. In this chapter, we review the roles of such a suite, the planning process, financial models, and appropriate case selection.

PLANNING A HYBRID ROOM

Planning and construction of a hybrid room is a complex process, governed by regulatory requirements, room dimensions, power availability, heat dispersal capabilities, and structural requirements to support the heavy imaging apparatus. This all must occur before construction and installation of the imaging system even begins. Mistakes are expensive and difficult to remedy. Having worked through this process now on several occasions, we are able to provide a guide for those planning to place an interventional suite within an operating suite. This is meant to be a very practical guide, with checklists, financial estimates, and a discussion of the problems we have encountered. We have tried to do the following:

1. Define the concept of a hybrid suite and describe the major components and equipment capabilities of a successful suite.
2. Document the construction steps and permissions necessary to proceed with the suite.
3. Explain costs and reimbursement potential of a hybrid suite and utilization requirements.
4. Present aortic, coronary, and ablation cases that can most appropriately benefit from a hybrid approach.

Do You Need a Hybrid Room?

First you must ask whether you really want to do this. What are the advantages and disadvantages? In our opinion, a hybrid room is absolutely necessary for a modern cardiovascular service line. It is necessary for the performance of cutting-edge procedures, which rapidly become contemporary procedures, and to recruit and retain the best interventionalists (a word we use in its broadest terms).[1] However, all hybrid rooms are not the same, and the very word *hybrid* conjures up a variety of interpretations to cardiologists, surgeons, and administrators alike. At present it is clear that the renewed wave of enthusiasm for hybrid room has been engendered by the approval of percutaneous aortic valves. In Europe, many of these procedures are conducted in a cath lab that has been upgraded to permit surgical interventions if they are absolutely necessary. This is hardly ideal for performing an emergency surgical procedure.

In our opinion, the ideal setting is a cath lab. What we describe here is a room that can easily accommodate major open cardiac and vascular procedures in addition to endovascular interventions. There is no doubt that an institution can "make do"; indeed, finances and physical plant may dictate that. What we are describing is the optimal situation, which provides the best environment regardless of approach. The hybrid room in our organization is where imaging, navigation, and robotics all come together. Many of the interventions currently requiring surgical access or a surgical component may well evolve to be totally percutaneous. That is the natural history of an endovascular procedure. However, interventions not yet even imagined will be introduced, and many of these early-phase procedures will be most appropriately performed in a hybrid room. Thus hospitals will need an increasing number of hybrid rooms for the foreseeable future.

Where Should You Build the Hybrid Room?

The issue then is not so much whether you need a hybrid room, but whether you want it to be in the operating room or the cath lab. There are clearly many advantages and disadvantages to both (Table 45.1).[2] Ultimately the ideal setup is to colocalize the cath labs, operating rooms, and the hybrid rooms. For new facility construction, we believe this is the optimal arrangement for a cardiovascular service line. However, for most organizations, this is not feasible and a decision on where to place the hybrid room must be made. The first question often asked is, "Can I easily convert a preexisting operating room or cath lab?" The answer is probably not, and certainly not easily. Creation of such a space in an established operating room can present considerable challenges. Preexisting rooms are often too small, may not be lead-lined, or may have inadequate air-handling capabilities. However, a combination of two rooms or operating rooms with adjacent storage space for a control room can be considered.

The second and more common question is, "Should this be built in an operating room suite or a cath lab suite?"[3] Typically, for the reasons outlined in Table 45.1, the operating room is the preferable environment. In our experience, this then sets in motion a series of issues that must be addressed. First is the understanding that this room does not "belong" to the surgeons. Procedures should be prioritized based on the most appropriate use of the facility, with no particular preference to any specific user group (Box 45.1). In our organization, we have set aside Wednesdays for percutaneous aortic valve procedures with the expectation that this need will increase. This is an organizational decision based on strategic priorities for the heart and vascular center. All other days have an open booking system wherein cardiologists and surgeons are treated equally. Although the hybrid room is located within the operating suite, it is extremely important that the cardiologist and the cath lab staff are welcomed, empowered, and not treated as second-class citizens. That message must come from surgical and cardiology leadership combined. The room is part of our heart and vascular center and is not owned by any particular group.

Understanding the Finances

In making the case for construction of a hybrid room there are several ways in which the new and potentially costly space can

TABLE 45.1 Pros and Cons of Planning a Hybrid Room in a Cath Lab Versus the Operating Room

Cardiac Catheterization Lab	Operating Room
Staff familiar with fixed C-arm imaging system	Staff less familiar with imaging, perhaps mobile C-arms
Staff less familiar with open surgical procedures	Staff familiar with open surgical procedures
Rapid turnover, more conscious sedation procedures	Relatively slow turnover, more general anesthesia procedures
Lead-lined walls	May or may not have lead-lined walls
Staff aware of radiation safety measures	Relatively less radiation safety aware
With or without anesthesia gas support	With anesthesia gas support, mechanical circulatory support
Layout designed for catheter angiography	Layout designed for open surgery (HVAC)
Ceiling struts in place, may not have laminar airflow	Located in sterile core with laminar airflow
Smaller rooms (not necessarily close to PACU)	Relatively larger rooms (with proximity to PACU)
Availability and staff familiarity with endovascular devices	Staff more familiar with open surgical instruments
Staff familiar with cardiac hemodynamic monitoring systems	Patient monitoring by anesthesiologists

HVAC, Heating/ventilating/air-conditioning; *PACU*, perioperative anesthetic care unit.

BOX 45.1 Procedures Performed in the Hybrid Room

Highly Appropriate

True hybrid procedures (open surgical and endovascular)

- Aortic debranching and endografts
- Retroperitoneal access and conduit for endograft delivery
- MICS CABG with completion coronary angiogram or intervention
- MICS AFib—combined transpericardial and endovascular approach
- Left atrial appendage exclusion
- TAVR with transapical, direct aortic, or minithoracotomy access
- Remote live-case broadcasting
- Complex endograft (FEVAR, ChEVAR) procedures

Moderately Appropriate

Abdominal endografts (EVAR)
Thoracic endografts (TEVAR)
Total occlusions (iliofemoral, venous)
Percutaneous valve procedures (TAVR, TMVR)
Venus recanalization procedures

Less Appropriate

Percutaneous diagnostic angiograms and interventions
Laser lead extraction procedures

AFib, Atrial fibrillation; *CAB*, coronary artery bypass; *ChEVAR*, chimney endovascular aortic repair; *FEVAR*, fenestrated endovascular aortic repair; *MICS*, minimally invasive cardiac surgery; *TAVI*, transcatheter aortic valve implantation; *TAVR*, transcatheter aortic valve replacement; *TEVAR*, thoracic endovascular aortic repair; *TMVR*, transcatheter mitral valve repair.

BOX 45.2 Making the Case for a Multimillion-Dollar Investment in a Hybrid Operating Room

Recruit physicians and other personnel
Retain and augment volume
- Is there additional revenue?
- Incremental volume?

Attract new technologies/patients
Remain competitive

BOX 45.3 Overriding Factors That Can Determine Location Suitability

Age of the operating room
- Asbestos abatement
- Power capabilities
- Floor and ceiling structures (in terms of load bearing)

Impact of construction on daily operating room work flow
Need for "after hours" construction

benefit the organization (Box 45.2). Numerous factors can markedly affect construction costs, and some of these may be financial "deal breakers" (Box 45.3). These issues must be identified very early so that a great deal of time and effort will not be expended on planning a room in a cost-prohibitive location. For example, if the only suitable room is in the center of an operating room corridor where construction would prevent utilization of the other rooms during the construction period, the idea of a hybrid room may be impractical for the facility.

Typically the facility's management will coordinate the process to establish realistic demolition, construction, and lost revenue costs. Table 45.2 provides an example of a pro forma calculation of the cost of building a typical hybrid room. Table 45.3 breaks down the estimated revenue stream for the hybrid room. All of these pro formas demonstrate that with moderate utilization, hybrid suites can be highly profitable.

Planning for Construction

Prior to assembling all of the physician stakeholders (Box 45.4), it is important to establish the specific uses for the room.[13-20] It is not realistic to create a room that can provide for highly disparate services such as neurosurgery and thoracic surgery. Indeed, it can be challenging to have a fully functional electrophysiology room because of the complexity and quantity of the needed equipment. However, hybrid rooms readily accommodate cardiac and vascular surgeons as well as interventional cardiologists. At the kick-off stakeholders' meeting, a nonphysician project leader/coordinator should be appointed whose job would be to coordinate future meetings, develop the project time lines, and interface with building contractors and architects.

Learning From Experience

The first hybrid room was built at Houston Methodist Hospital in 2005. It featured a floor-mounted system in an 800-square-foot operating room. A control room was built from an adjacent

TABLE 45.2 Breakdown of the Investment Costs for a Hybrid Room

	Estimated Cost
Construction	
Ceiling reinforcement	$75,000
Lead shielding	$100,000
Heating/ventilating/air-conditioning	$250,000
Plumbing	$10,000
Cabinets/room storage	$7,500
Cost for space	$320,000
Medical gases	$50,000
Demolition and miscellaneous construction	$500,000
Total construction	$1,312,500
Equipment	
Angiography (single-plane panel detector)	$1,500,000
Angiography equipment/software	$50,000
Radiolucent tables	$50,000
Heart-lung machine	$100,000
General equipment	$200,000
Integrated booms	$175,000
Total equipment	$2,075,000
Total (equipment + construction)	$3,387,500

Source: Advisory board research and analysis.

TABLE 45.3 Expense and Revenue Considerations for a Hybrid Room

Incremental admissions	150
Gross patient revenue	$6,187,693
Net patient revenue	$2,442,278
Total expenses	
Salaries	$397,634
Supplies	$304,950
Other	$145,191
Excess of revenue over expenses	$1,594,503
Net present value	
2010	$776,443
2015	$5,390,988
Internal rate of return	
2010	184.6%
2015	284.6%

BOX 45.4 Hybrid Room Stakeholders

Presentation input:
Surgeons: vascular, cardiac, thoracic
Cardiologists
Interventionists
Anesthesiologists
Supply chain
Facility planning
Administrators
Architects

store room with access only through the hybrid room itself. Although this room remains in use today, it was created primarily to support a rapidly evolving vascular surgery service and is in many ways inadequate for today's more complex cardiac and vascular procedures. Since 2005, we have built three other hybrid rooms throughout our system and are currently planning to add five more. During this process, we have learned many valuable lessons in both process and room design. For the pending rooms, we created a task force that will develop an optimal hybrid room template built on our previous experience. This standardized template will be used to build all the hybrid rooms in our system with a view to developing consistent training and procedural protocols.

DESIGNING THE HYBRID ROOM

In reality, the hybrid room is a suite of components including (1) an operating and imaging suite, (2) control room, (3) equipment room, (4) storage room, and (5) integrated audiovisual equipment. In planning gross space requirements, we recommend allotting 1038 sq ft to the operating room, 150 sq ft to the control room, 117 sq ft to imaging equipment, and 235 sq ft to storage. The total footprint for this hybrid suite comes to 1540 sq ft.

When designing the room, look for creative ways to visualize and experiment with the end product. For instance, consider visiting another site with an operational hybrid room similar to the one you are planning. This should include an opportunity to discuss pros and cons with nursing staff, technologists, and physicians. Another option is to mock up the room with models, including movable booms and a cardboard imaging system. This can be specifically designed to simulate the exact room under consideration. Many imaging companies also have the ability to create a virtual room in which equipment interactions can be evaluated.

These extra steps—particularly the virtual rooms—are good opportunities to test overhead boom conflicts, which are among the more common problems we have encountered. Overhead structures include anesthesia gas columns, surgical lights, monitors for the imaging system and video feed, cameras, and radiation shields. Care must be taken to avoid collision of the ceiling-mounted displays with operating lights or other ceiling-mounted equipment. Ceiling-mounted systems with running parts above the operating field can be difficult to clean and may interfere with the airflow by causing turbulence.[4]

The Imaging System

It is important that an imaging system have enough mobility to be able to evaluate patients from the top of head to the tips of toes. Increasingly, procedures demand that rotational angiographic and three-dimensional (3D) reconstruction be enabled throughout this range. Imaging companies have developed innovative techniques to accommodate this need. For instance, Siemens created the robotic Artis zeego system and Phillips recently introduced its FlexMove in which the C-arm can be swung on a gantry from left to right. GE created the Discovery system to maximize space utilization and ease of use. Although electrophysiologists often use a biplanar system, such a limitation is impractical in the hybrid room environment; there are too many conflicts with other necessary pieces of equipment for the lateral C-arm to be accommodated.

An additional area of disagreement in cardiology versus surgery centers around the size of the image intensifier. Whereas interventional cardiologists prefer the higher resolution and viewing angles that can be achieved with a 9- to 12-in flat-panel detector, surgeons prefer a 16-in field. Generally a multitude of different procedures may have to be hosted in hybrid rooms; therefore most planners select the 16-in detector.

The anesthesia team should be involved throughout the planning process, as we have found that they are greatly affected by the imaging system. One specific anesthesiologist should act as the point person for helping to design the room. There should be two anesthesia booms—right and left side—which enable the entire anesthesia setup to be flipped and the imaging system moved to either side of the patient. There are many other nuances that need a vested anesthesiologist: Managing the gas lines, monitoring lines, and arterial lines, and minimizing the real risk of inadvertent extubation during rotational acquisition are extremely important.

Table Considerations

Traditional surgical tables can break in the middle, the head can be flexed or extended, and they have Trendelenburg, reversed Trendelenburg, and lateral roll capability. They frequently have radiopaque hinges and rails and are typically supported on a central pedestal. On the other hand, the traditional fluoroscopy table is a single nonbreakable carbon-fiber piece that floats from a support at one end. It provides a radiolucent field to allow fluoroscopic imaging of the entire length of the patient. Most incorporate Trendelenburg, reverse Trendelenburg, and lateral role positions. However, this is not universal; indeed, some "hybrid" room tables do not have this capability and instead use inflatable cushions for positioning. Such systems should be completely avoided as they significantly impede optimal surgical access.

Special rails for mounting self-retaining retractor systems can be attached. The fluoroscopy table should be regarded as part of the imaging system. Stepwise programmed table motion allows digital subtraction runoff, which is necessary for peripheral vascular interventions. In order to perform 3D imaging with the operating table, the C-arm has to be fully integrated with the table to allow fast and precise rotation around the patient lying in the isocenter. More recently, several imaging vendors have incorporated surgical tables into their imaging system. Although these lack some of the imaging functionalities (i.e., they do not pan and do not provide stepped runoff), they nevertheless have a role where there is not enough institutional volume to completely occupy a hybrid room full time. In this situation, the C-arm can be parked out of the way, leaving a fully functional operating room.

Staffing

Staff calculations for hybrid procedures require a team of 8 to 20 people including anesthesiologists, surgeons, nurses, technicians, perfusionists, experts from device companies, and so forth.[5] Table 45.4 provides basic staffing recommendations.

TABLE 45.4 Staffing the Hybrid Suite

Typical Staffing Recommendations	FTE	Coverage Options
Radiology/cath lab technicians	2	Integrate with cath lab coverage
Nursing staff (1 RN should be lead nurse in the room)	4	Integrate with OR coverage
Perfusionist	0.25	Integrate with OR coverage
Anesthesiologist	1	

FTE, Full-time equivalent; *RN*, registered nurse; *OR*, operating room.

There are numerous variations in operating room staffing depending on the type of procedure to be performed. For example:

1. Hybrid coronary procedures need a cardiovascular anesthesiologist and a perfusionist.
2. Hybrid electrophysiology procedures may need echocardiography and an echocardiographer, as well as catheter ablation of cardiac arrhythmias guided by electroanatomic imaging (CARTO) support.
3. Hybrid robotic procedures need an additional level of nursing expertise for setup.
4. Hybrid aortic procedures will need cell-saver support.
5. Transcatheter aortic valve implantation (TAVI) procedures also need an echocardiographer or cardiovascular anesthesiologist with these skills.

A dedicated nursing leader who is responsible for the room and evolving case support and instrumentation is very important. The optimal candidate would be a nurse who has both operating room and cath lab experience, although such a leader may be difficult to find. A great deal of cross-training is necessary, particularly for call coverage. Also, there tends to be nothing standard about these procedures; each case can represent a learning environment and a lead nurse who has been intimately involved in the development of the room and its procedures is very beneficial. For example, rotational angiographic acquisition to create a CT-fluoroscopy overlay necessitates wrapping the patient with sterile barriers circumferentially in order to accommodate the rotating C-arm.

Similarly a vested anesthesiologist is absolutely necessary. The anesthesiologist may have the most difficult challenge in learning how to work in this environment, especially minimizing risk from large moving imaging systems. It is also important that the anesthesiologist learns to flex the level of anesthesia mandated for each case. This means understanding the case and providing minimal anesthesia and monitoring consistent with a safe environment. When we deal with percutaneous valves at our institution, the entire team reviews the game plan in advance and debriefs after the procedure. This is a discipline we will introduce into other complex procedures as they are introduced.

The Control Room

The control room should house the image control and postprocessing equipment, picture archive and communication system (PACS) terminals, printers and video- and flow-control stations, and work stations. There are certain criteria for creation of the optimal control room:

1. Independent access from corridor without passing through hybrid room
2. Large viewing window into hybrid room
3. Recommended size: 160 to 230 sq ft
4. Separate imaging equipment storage room (120 to 140 sq ft) attached to control room

Video Transmission

Although video transmission is not mandatory to create a fully functional hybrid room, the optimal time to install a video recording and streaming system is during room construction. In addition to the selection of a vendor, initial decisions include camera placement, number of video streams that can be recorded, storage and editing locations, security, and recording policies. Assuring the security of remote viewing should be a prime consideration.

Utilization

Hybrid suites are expensive and come with a clear expectation of return on investment. However, they are very flexible in terms of the types of cases that can be performed. Our approach, in general, is the right case in the right facility. Neither our operating room suites nor cath lab suites are regarded as the province of one service alone. With appropriate credentialing,[a] any physician can post a case in either facility. We have included a sample list of cases that we consider least to most appropriate for the hybrid room (see Box 45.1). However, filling the room is the most important criterion for us. In a faculty where there are not enough of the "most appropriate" cases to fill the schedule, clearly room utilization can be kept high with the less invasive cases.

Robotics in the Hybrid Room

Fig. 45.1 is from a presentation at the Massachusetts Institute of Technology on robotics in the cardiovascular operating room. There are three robots, all being utilized frequently. The imaging arm is a robot derived from car assembly lines; it provides flexibility in movement of the imaging system and allows a higher rate of rotation to minimize motion artifact.

The Intouch Visitor 1 is a remote viewing robot, which permits remote viewing, remote proctoring, and case support.

The Hansen robot is a catheter robot designed for endoluminal navigation. We have published extensively on use of this robot and believe that its use will be especially effective when combined with 3D imaging, image fusion, and autonomous motion. We have used the robot for carotid stenting, crossing iliac occlusions, and fenestration of dissections, among others.[21-23]

FUTURE DIRECTIONS

The modern hybrid room is a remarkable technologic environment. The DICOM 3D dataset, created during the acquisition of CT/magnetic resonance imaging (MRI), is now portable and empowering. Our workflow for aortic endografts includes importing the previously acquired CT angiography data set,

[a]Regarding credentialing for the hybrid room, we mandate that a training program be completed for that room before a physician is allowed to post cases.

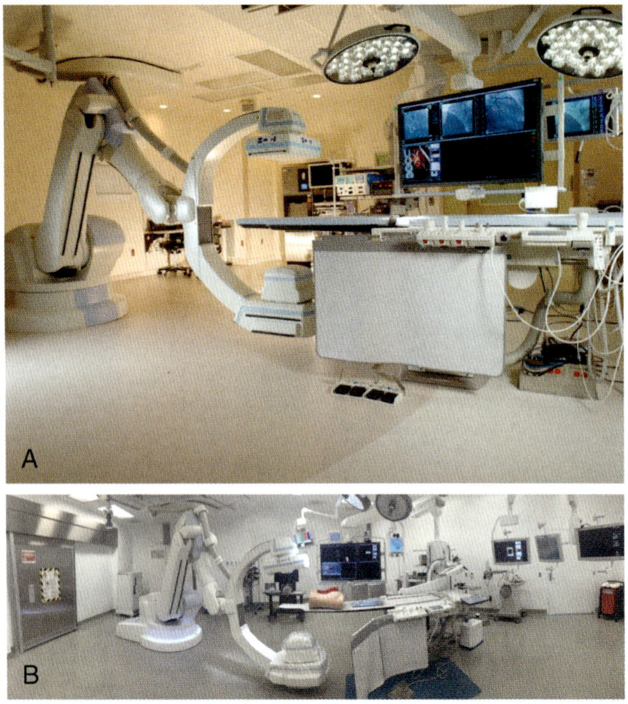

FIG 45.1 Hybrid rooms at (A) the Houston Methodist DeBakey Heart & Vascular Center and (B) Methodist Institute of Technology, Innovation & Education.

performing an on-table noncontrast cone-beam CT, and fusing these data sets together. This fusion is based on fusion of vascular wall calcification patterns. This permits highly accurate vascular fusion. Automatic algorithms trace the aorta, draw a center line, and mark the appropriate landmarks. Our catheter robots have recently demonstrated autonomous movement to these "pre-flighted" vascular orifices. It is indeed an exciting experience to work in the hybrid room.

CONCLUSION

Hybrid operating rooms are being built in most cardiovascular centers, often with little guidance in how to optimally plan this expensive resource. In this article we share our expertise in the planning, construction, and utilization of these rooms. The types of procedures that can be performed continue to evolve rapidly. New imaging systems come loaded with previously unimagined capabilities: CT fluoroscopy scanning, 3D reconstruction, image import, and fusion. These postprocessing capabilities will become mainstream imaging requirements, much like fluoroscopy, digital subtraction, and road mapping. It is the placement of these advanced imaging capabilities in the hands of innovative interventionalists that will herald even more exciting interventions in a more minimally invasive fashion for our patients. This will fundamentally alter all aspects of interventional cardiovascular therapy.

REVIEW QUESTIONS

1. The primary purpose of a hybrid room is to:
   a. Increase referrals for complex cases
   b. Permit cone-beam CT acquisition
   c. Allow seamless integration between open and catheter-based cases
   d. Enhance radiation safety for complex procedures
   e. Increase billing based on imaging codes
2. Which of the following pieces of equipment can be found in hybrid operating rooms?
   a. Flat plate detectors
   b. Fluoroscopic table
   c. Intravascular ultrasound
   d. Audiovisual integration
   e. All of the above
3. Which of the following are optimal criteria for creation of the control room?
   a. Independent access from corridor, without passing through hybrid room
   b. Nurse charting station
   c. Image control terminals and post-processing work station.
   d. a and b
   e. a and c
4. Cone-beam CT refers to:
   a. Importing and fusing a CT scan
   b. Presence of a multislice CT scan in the hybrid room
   c. Importing and fusing an MRI scan
   d. Creating a CT dataset using the fluoroscopic arm
   e. Rotational angiography
5. Which of the following procedures are appropriate for a hybrid room?
   a. LIMA to LAD bypass and right coronary stenting
   b. Laser lead extraction
   c. Arch debranching and aortic stent grafting
   d. TAVR
   e. All of the above
6. Necessary staff for a hybrid operating room include:
   a. Perfusionist and radiation safety officer
   b. Anesthesiologist and nurse manager
   c. Radiology (cath lab) technician and dedicated nursing staff
   d. Audiovisual technician and catheter manager
   e. Endovascular surgeon and interventional cardiologist

References available online at ExpertConsult.com.

CHAPTER 46

Splanchnic and Renal Artery Aneurysms

James C. Stanley, Dawn M. Coleman, Jonathan L. Eliason

Aneurysms of the visceral branches of the abdominal aorta are being recognized with increasing frequency. More than half of the splanchnic and renal artery aneurysms described in the English-language literature have been reported in the past 25 years. Splanchnic aneurysms are approximately threefold more common than renal aneurysms. Both aneurysm types are best addressed individually because of the marked variability in their biologic character and clinical importance.

SPLANCHNIC ARTERY ANEURYSMS

Splanchnic artery aneurysms are an uncommon but important vascular disease (Table 46.1). Nearly 22% of these aneurysms appear as surgical emergencies, including 8.5% eventuating in the patient's death. The major splanchnic vessels involved with these macroaneurysms, in decreasing order of frequency, are the splenic; hepatic; superior mesenteric; celiac; gastric and gastroepiploic; jejunal, ileal, and colic; pancreaticoduodenal; and gastroduodenal arteries.

The clinical manifestations of splanchnic artery aneurysms have become relatively well defined. Rupture is the most serious complication of these aneurysms (Table 46.2). Endovascular therapy has proven in recent years to have distinct advantages over conventional open surgical therapy.[1-15] Nevertheless appropriate treatment of certain splanchnic artery aneurysms is an open operation.[16-21] The cause, presentation, and management of aneurysms affecting each of the splanchnic arteries deserve separate comment and are reviewed in the following text.

Splenic Artery Aneurysms

Splenic artery aneurysms account for 60% of all reported splanchnic artery aneurysms. The frequency of these aneurysms in the general population approaches the 0.78% incidence noted in nearly 3600 consecutive abdominal arteriographic studies performed for reasons other than suspected aneurysmal disease.[19] Historically, women appeared nearly fourfold more likely than men to have these aneurysms,[22,23] although in more contemporary times this female predilection appears to be less.[24]

Four distinct, preexisting conditions are suspected to contribute to the development of splenic artery aneurysms. First is medial fibrodysplasia, a subset of fibromuscular dysplasia (FMD), with its derangements and thinning of the vessel's medial smooth muscle, which is more commonly recognized as a cause of hypertension secondary to its renal artery involvement. Approximately 2% of patients exhibiting this form of renal artery disease have splenic artery aneurysms.[19] Blood pressure elevations in these patients may also contribute to aneurysm development. Coexistence of renal artery medial fibrodysplasia and splenic artery aneurysms has been identified only in women.

Second are the effects of excessive splenic blood flow and the increase in reproductive hormones accompanying pregnancy. Both cause changes in elastin and other matrix proteins within the splenic artery wall. In past decades, approximately 40% of women harboring these aneurysms had completed six or more pregnancies.[19] In contemporary times, fewer children are being born to women in Western societies, and the frequency of multiparous individuals exhibiting these aneurysms has declined to approximately 10%.[24]

Third, portal hypertension with splenomegaly is associated with splenic artery macroaneurysms in 10% to 15% of patients.[25-28] The resistance encountered by the effluent from the spleen through the portosystemic venous channels of these patients is low compared with the relative high resistance of the liver's hepatic sinusoids. This results in higher velocities in splenic artery blood flow, dilation of the artery, and the evolution of aneurysms.[29-31] Increased estrogen activity associated with advanced cirrhosis may also affect arterial walls and contribute to aneurysmal development. This accounts for the increased presence of these aneurysms in patients subjected to orthotopic liver transplantation.[25,27,32,33] Aneurysms are more common in female than male liver transplant recipients, and they appear to be directly related to the severity of the patient's portal hypertension.[34,35]

Fourth, inflammatory disease, such as chronic pancreatitis with pseudocyst erosion into an adjacent splenic artery, is a less common but important cause of these aneurysms. In contrast, microaneurysms within the splenic parenchyma, most often associated with a generalized inflammatory vasculitis such as polyarteritis nodosa, are of less clinical relevance than extraparenchymal macroaneurysms.

Penetrating trauma and iatrogenic injury following abdominal operations are well-recognized causes of splenic artery pseudoaneurysms. Blunt injury is a less frequently encountered etiology,[36] although small intraparenchymal aneurysms may commonly accompany the arterial disruptions within a fractured spleen.

Most splenic artery aneurysms also exhibit elements of arteriosclerosis, although this is considered a secondary event rather than an etiologic process (Fig. 46.1). Nevertheless, arteriosclerotic-mediated inflammation may contribute to further aneurysmal degeneration.

TABLE 46.1 **Distribution and Etiology of Splanchnic Artery Macroaneurysms**

Aneurysm Location	Frequency Within Splanchnic Circulation (%)	Male:Female Ratio	Common Contributing Factors
Splenic artery	60	1:2	Medial degeneration, arterial fibrodysplasia, multiple pregnancies, portal hypertension, pancreatitis with arterial erosion by pseudocysts, trauma
Hepatic artery	20	2:1	Blunt and penetrating liver trauma, iatrogenic trauma during hepatobiliary procedures, medial degeneration
Superior mesenteric artery	5.5	2:1	Infection related to bacterial endocarditis, often associated with nonhemolytic streptococci; medial degeneration
Celiac artery	4.0	1:1	Medial degeneration
Gastric and gastroepiploic arteries	4.0	2:1	Periarterial inflammation, medial degeneration
Jejunal, ileal, and colic arteries	3.0	1:1	Medial degeneration, infection, connective tissue diseases
Pancreaticoduodenal and gastroduodenal arteries	1.5	2:1 (1:1 in flow-related aneurysms)	Secondary to excessive blood flow as a collateral vessel, pancreatitis-related inflammation, medial degeneration

TABLE 46.2 **Rupture and Treatment of Splanchnic Artery Macroaneurysms**

Aneurysm Location	Frequency of Reported Rupture	Site of Bleeding	Mortality With Rupture	Usual Treatment Options
Splenic artery	2% bland, 5% inflammatory	Intraperitoneal within lesser sac, intragastric with pancreatitis-related inflammatory aneurysms	25% bland and unassociated with pregnancy; during pregnancy, 70% maternal, 75% fetal	Endovascular aneurysm obliteration, open aneurysm exclusion or excision without splenectomy, splenectomy
Hepatic artery	25%	Intraperitoneal and biliary tract with equal frequency	40%	Endovascular aneurysm exclusion with stent graft or obliteration, open aneurysmectomy with and without hepatic artery reconstruction
Superior mesenteric artery	10%; thrombosis with dissections relatively common	Intraperitoneal and retroperitoneal, intestinal ischemia with thrombosis	50%	Endovascular occlusion or stenting in select cases, open aneurysmectomy with superior mesenteric artery reconstruction, ligation if collateral circulation is adequate
Celiac artery	13%	Intraperitoneal	50%	Open aneurysmectomy with celiac artery reconstruction, ligation if circulation is adequate, endovascular stenting
Gastric and gastroepiploic arteries	90%	Intraperitoneal (30%), intestinal tract (70%)	70%	Endovascular aneurysm obliteration, open aneurysm excision with involved gastric tissue or ligation if extramural
Jejunal, ileal, and colic arteries	30%	Intestinal tract, intramesenteric and intraperitoneal with equal frequency	20%	Open aneurysm excision with involved intestine if intramural, ligation if extramural, Endovascular aneurysm obliteration
Pancreaticoduodenal and gastroduodenal arteries	20%–40% bland; 10% pancreatitis-related	Retroperiteonal and intraperitoneal, intestinal tract with pancreatitis-related	30% bland (10% with flow related and 20% pancreatitis-related aneurysms)	Endovascular aneurysm obliteration, open aneurysm ligation within false aneurysms (pseudocyst-related), ligation if extrapancreatic, pancreatic resection

Splenic artery aneurysms associated with arterial fibrodysplasia and those associated with the flow and hormonal changes of pregnancy as well as portal hypertension evolve in arteries that often exhibit considerable tortuosity (Fig. 46.2). Discontinuities exist in the internal elastic lamina of normal vessels at branchings, and subsequent alterations in elastic tissue likely favor aneurysmal changes at these sites. These are true aneurysms, not false aneurysms. Aneurysms unrelated to portal hypertension are multiple 20% of the time. Among patients with portal hypertension and cirrhosis undergoing liver transplantation, multiple aneurysms are even more common.[27,34] In contrast, false aneurysms associated with pancreatitis usually involve the main splenic artery and tend to be solitary (Fig. 46.3).

Curvilinear or signet-ring dystrophic calcifications in the left upper quadrant on radiographs may often be the first evidence of a splenic artery aneurysm. However, in contemporary practice, these aneurysms are recognized most often during imaging undertaken for other disease states. Conventional arteriography, ultrasonography, computed tomography (CT), CT arteriography, and magnetic resonance arteriography (MRA) are useful not only in recognizing these lesions but are often helpful in identifying ruptured or leaking aneurysms.

Abdominal discomfort has been reported in approximately 20% of these patients,[13] although left-upper-quadrant or epigastric pain directly attributable to an intact splenic artery aneurysm is rare.[24] In contrast, a 1996 review of 83 cases, which included many single individuals, reported that 46% of patients had abdominal pain and 25% were in shock.[37] The disparity in these publications is attributed to the fact that reviews often summarize spectacular individual case reports that are unlikely to be representative of the usual clinical course in the general population.

True rupture of a splenic artery aneurysm may cause bleeding that is initially contained within the lesser sac. Eventually free hemorrhage into the peritoneal cavity occurs, causing vascular collapse. This "double rupture" phenomenon is often referred to in discussions of splenic artery aneurysms, but its occurrence is exceedingly uncommon. Pseudoaneurysms due to pseudocyst erosion into the adjacent splenic artery and subsequently into the stomach or pancreatic ductal system are often a source of gastrointestinal hemorrhage.[37-41] Arteriovenous fistula formation is a rare complication of splenic artery aneurysm rupture into the adjacent splenic vein. This is a recognized cause of left-sided portal hypertension and gastrointestinal bleeding from esophageal varices.[42]

The risk of splenic artery aneurysmal rupture is related to its cause. Rupture of bland asymptomatic aneurysms has been reported to be approximately 2%.[19] However, reported rupture rates may be overstated. In fact, a recent review of 168 patients with these aneurysms reported a rupture rate of zero among those not subjected to surgical therapy.[22] Contrary to earlier misconceptions, rupture is just as likely to affect a calcified aneurysm in a normotensive elderly patient as in a hypertensive young

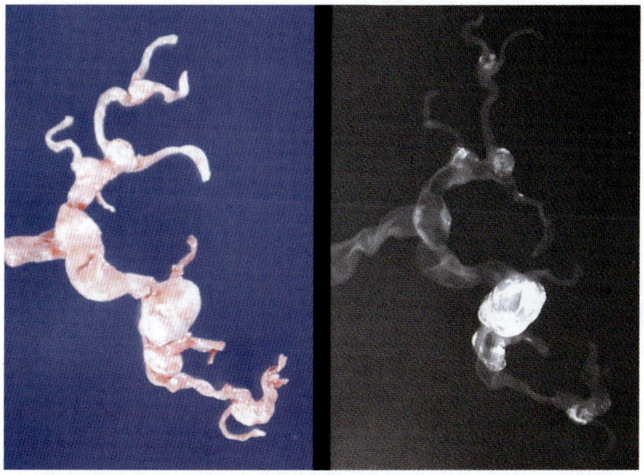

FIG 46.1 Multiple splenic artery aneurysms occurring at bifurcations of the distal artery (gross specimen). Calcific arteriosclerosis apparent within the aneurysms and not the intervening splenic artery (radiographic specimen).

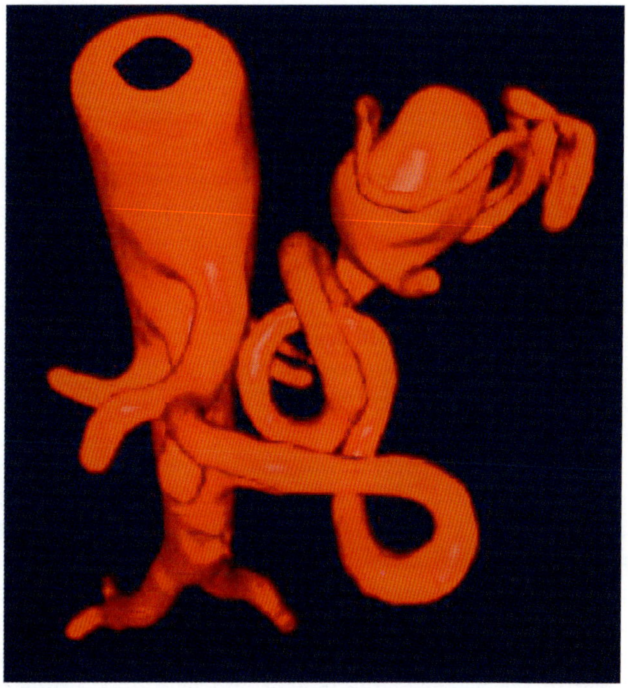

FIG 46.2 Splenic artery aneurysm. Characteristic tortuous-coiled main splenic artery most often observed in women having completed numerous pregnancies (computed tomographic arteriogram).

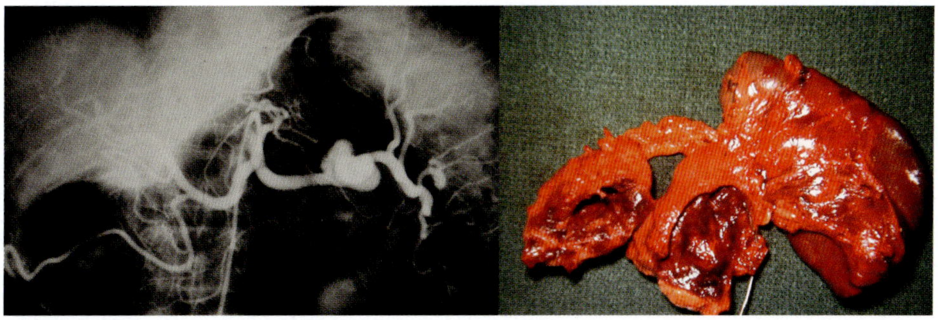

FIG 46.3 Solitary splenic artery pseudoaneurysm affecting the midportion of the vessel (arteriogram) caused by pancreatic pseudocyst erosion into the artery; aneurysm excision with a distal pancreatectomy and splenectomy (gross specimen).

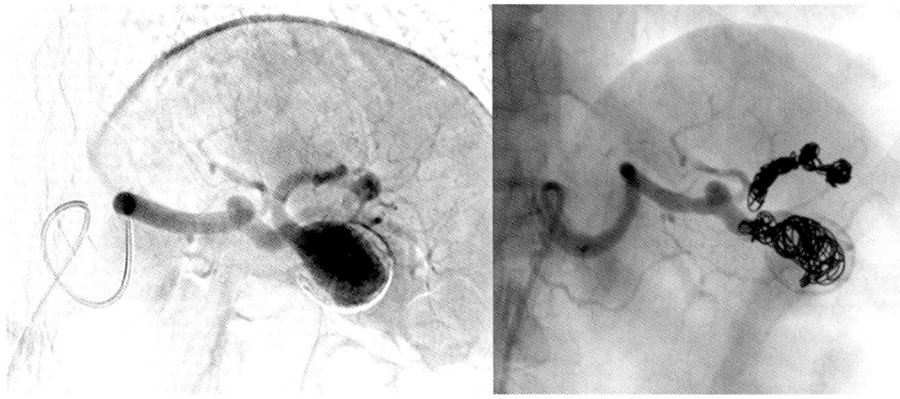

FIG 46.4 Splenic artery aneurysm treated by endovascular coil embolization.

patient with a noncalcified aneurysm. Giant aneurysms (> 5 cm in diameter) have a reported overt and covert rupture rate totaling 30%.[43] In the past, the mortality accompanying rupture of a bland splenic artery aneurysm in a nonpregnant patient has been reported to be 25%.[23]

Bland aneurysms in liver transplant recipients appear to be nearly twice as likely to rupture as those in other patients.[32,34] Rupture is most likely to occur early in the period after transplantation.[25,27] The mortality following rupture of a splenic artery aneurysm in a liver transplant patient exceeds 50%.[26] Nevertheless, aneurysmal rupture in this setting is uncommon.[44] Inflammatory pancreatitis-related splenic artery aneurysmal rupture occurs more often than rupture in bland aneurysms, affecting approximately 5% of aneurysms and resulting in death in 40% of cases.

Nearly 95% of reported aneurysms recognized during pregnancy have ruptured.[45-48] However, this figure may be misleading, since few splenic artery aneurysms actually rupture during pregnancy.[49] It is hypothesized that although women may develop splenic artery aneurysms during the course of repeated pregnancies, they are rarely diagnosed unless they rupture. Nevertheless, aneurysmal rupture during pregnancy does represent a serious threat to the health of the mother and fetus. Two-thirds of reported ruptures have occurred during the third trimester and nearly one-fifth rupture at parturition or in the early postpartum period. Overall reported maternal and fetal mortality in these cases approaches 75% and 95%, respectively.[50] Rupture in pregnancy, when recognized early enough to allow for operative intervention, still carries a reported maternal mortality of 22% and fetal mortality of 16%.[45]

It would seem reasonable to consider elective operative intervention for asymptomatic (bland) splenic artery aneurysms greater than 2 cm in diameter, when the risk of operative death is less than 0.5%. The latter figure represents the product of the 25% open operative mortality and the 2% rupture rate of bland aneurysms. However, in more contemporary times, the mortality rate accompanying operation for rupture may be less. Therefore any elective open surgical or endovascular intervention should be undertaken only when the operative risk is exceedingly low. In certain elderly patients the cost-effectiveness of an intervention is minimal and a conservative nonoperative approach seems prudent.[51]

Percutaneous transcatheter embolization using various agents—including differing types of particulate matter, coils, and glue (acrylate derivatives)—is preferred over open operative interventions in the treatment of most splenic artery aneurysms (Fig. 46.4).[a] Endovascular interventions may be particularly useful in high-risk patients with liver cirrhosis.[56] Nevertheless, recanalization, splenic infarction, delayed rupture of the spleen, inconsistent obliteration of the aneurysm, as well as migration and erosion with stricture of adjacent viscera are all recognized complications of endovascular therapy.[7,12,24,57-60] Thus close follow-up of endovascular-treated patients becomes mandatory. Stent-graft and multilayer stent exclusion of an aneurysm with maintenance of splenic artery flow may avoid certain complications of embolic interventions.[61-65]

Splenectomy was the most commonly reported open surgical intervention undertaken for the treatment of bland splenic artery aneurysms prior to the introduction of endovascular therapies.[19,37] Given the immunologic benefits of splenic preservation, even in the aged, simple ligature obliteration or excision of these aneurysms unaccompanied by a splenectomy is preferred when an open surgical procedure is required.[66] In select cases, a laparoscopic or robotic approach is favored.[67-71]

Inflammatory splenic artery aneurysms embedded in the pancreas may require distal pancreatectomy. Large pseudoaneurysms associated with pseudocyst erosion into the adjacent artery may be treated initially by incising the aneurysmal sac and ligating the entering and exiting vessels.[40] Pancreatic resection in the former cases depends on the degree of associated pancreatic inflammation and the general condition of the patient.[72]

Hepatic Artery Aneurysms

Hepatic artery aneurysms account for 20% of all reported splanchnic artery aneurysms[73-76] and are most often discovered during the sixth decade of life. Men are affected twice as often as women, although gender differences appear to be less in recent times. More than one-third of patients with these aneurysms have other splanchnic artery aneurysms.[6,73]

Blunt liver injuries have led to a marked increase in the number of reported hepatic artery aneurysms, being recognized as small pseudoaneurysms on CT studies performed for major abdominal

[a]References 1, 7, 9, 12–15, 24, 52–55

trauma. Such traumatic etiologies are a likely reason that almost half of the reported hepatic artery aneurysms affect the intrahepatic arterial branches. Penetrating trauma and percutaneous and therapeutic hepatobiliary injuries are well recognized additional causes of hepatic artery pseudoaneurysms.[7,37,77]

Connective tissue arteriopathies, such as periarteritis nodosa, have also been incriminated as a cause of occasional macroaneurysms involving the hepatic arteries. Mycotic aneurysms associated with sepsis, often related to intravenous drug abuse and endocarditis, are relatively uncommon in contemporary practice.

Hepatic artery aneurysms are usually solitary; they are extrahepatic in nearly 80% of cases and intrahepatic in 20% (Fig. 46.5). Arteriosclerosis is considered a secondary event rather than an initiating cause of hepatic artery aneurysms.

Most hepatic artery aneurysms are asymptomatic and are discovered incidentally during imaging for other illnesses.[37,75,76] A minority of aneurysms are symptomatic, characteristically causing right-upper-quadrant and epigastric pain. Acute expansion of hepatic artery aneurysms can cause severe abdominal discomfort, similar to that of pancreatitis. Large aneurysms may cause obstructive jaundice.[78]

The incidence of hepatic artery aneurysmal rupture remains ill-defined, but the reported rupture rate in contemporary times approaches 25%.[6,73,79] However, bleeding occurred in more than half of the aneurysms reported from experiences having a predominance of iatrogenic intrahepatic aneurysms.[7]

Bleeding from ruptured hepatic artery aneurysms occurs equally into the biliary tract and into the peritoneal cavity. In the case of the former, hemobilia is often evident, manifested by biliary colic, hematemesis, and jaundice.[80,81] Chronic gastrointestinal hemorrhage is a very uncommon but recognized sequela of this form of rupture. Intraperitoneal bleeding is usually associated with inflammatory pseudoaneurysms. Multiple nonarteriosclerotic aneurysms have an apparent greater risk of eventual rupture.[73] The reported mortality rate attending aneurysmal rupture approaches 40%.[6]

Interventional therapy is recommended for all symptomatic aneurysms and all asymptomatic saccular hepatic aneurysms exceeding 2 cm in diameter. Smaller intrahepatic aneurysms that appear to be expanding and pseudoaneurysms of the extrahepatic arteries warrant earlier treatment.

Percutaneous transcatheter obliteration of hepatic artery aneurysms with balloons, coils, various types of particulate matter, and even thrombin is preferred over an open surgical intervention by many interventionists (Fig. 46.6).[7,14,77,83-85] Long-term

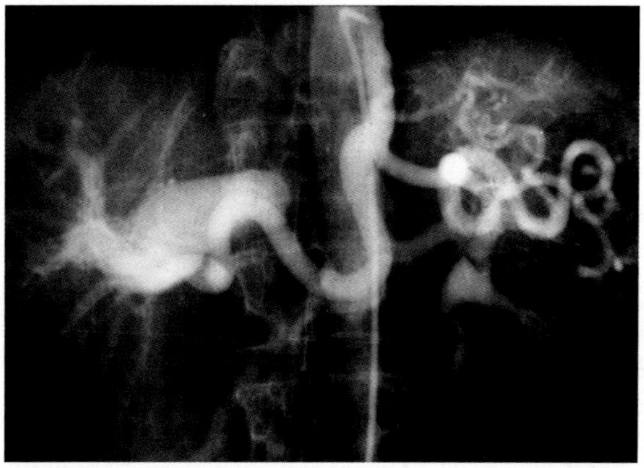

FIG 46.5 Large common hepatic artery aneurysm affecting the distal artery at the origin of the proper hepatic artery. (From Rectenwald JR, Stanley JC: Celiac, hepatic, and splenic artery aneurysms. In Stanley JC, Veith FJ, Wakefield TW, editors: *Current Therapy in Vascular and Endovascular Surgery*, ed 5, Philadelphia, 2014, Elsevier, p 744.)

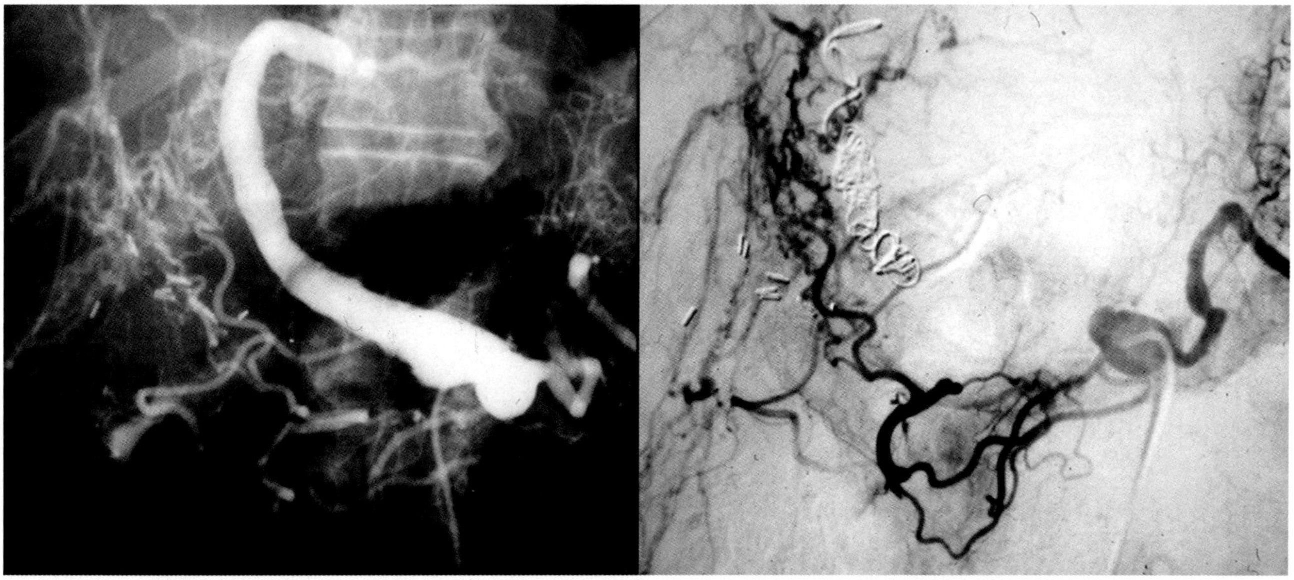

FIG 46.6 Hepatic artery aneurysm with extensive thrombus surrounding the patent channel in the common hepatic artery treated by endovascular means with reconstitution of distal collateral vessels entering the liver parenchyma. (From Upchurch GR, Jr, Zelenock GB, Stanley JC: Splenic artery aneurysms. In Rutherford RB, editor: *Vascular Surgery*, ed 6, Philadelphia, 2005, Elsevier-Saunders, p 1572.)

follow-up is required, since transcatheter embolization may be only transiently successful and repeated embolization or eventual surgical therapy may be required in some patients. The most serious complication of endovascular embolization is liver necrosis and death.[82] Endovascular stent-graft exclusion of select aneurysms avoids some of the limitations accompanying embolization alone.[86-90]

Open surgical treatment of hepatic artery aneurysms—including ligation, aneurysmectomy, or aneurysm exclusion with or without arterial reconstruction—is favored by some.[3,6,24,37,91] In this setting, if liver blood flow appears compromised on temporary hepatic artery occlusion, a direct vascular reconstruction should be undertaken with a prosthetic or autologous graft.[3,12,17,73] Hepatic ischemia is most likely to accompany exclusion of aneurysms involving the proper hepatic artery. Simple ligation of extrahepatic branches on rare occasions may cause liver necrosis and necessitate hepatic territory resection.[75]

Superior Mesenteric Artery Aneurysms

Aneurysms of the proximal superior mesenteric artery are the third most common splanchnic artery aneurysm, accounting for 5.5% of these lesions (Fig. 46.7). Men are affected nearly twice as often as women.[92] An infectious etiology associated with bacterial endocarditis was more common in the distant past.[93-95] Nonhemolytic streptococci account for the majority of mycotic lesions encountered in contemporary practice, although these aneurysms are relatively rare.[96] Superior mesenteric artery (SMA) aneurysms may also be related to medial degeneration, spontaneous SMA dissection, periarterial inflammation, and trauma. Arteriosclerosis, when present, is considered a secondary event rather than an etiologic process.

SMA aneurysms are usually recognized during imaging studies for other diseases. The majority of these aneurysms are asymptomatic. When they are symptomatic, there is usually an acute expansion, dissection, or rupture of the aneurysm. Rupture occurred in a little more than one-third of cases recently reported from a large health care system.[92] However, a rupture rate of less than 10% is more representative of contemporary practice; mortality approaches 50% with rupture.

SMA dissections with mural aneurysms (Fig. 46.8) are believed to be more common than simple aneurysms.[97-100] The unique location of dissecting aneurysms near the origins of the inferior pancreaticoduodenal and middle colic arteries place the intestine of the distal mesenteric circulation at risk for ischemia if these branches become occluded. In such cases a loss of the usual collateral networks from the adjacent celiac and inferior mesenteric arterial circulations may result in bowel ischemia. Occasionally the latter is responsible for postprandial abdominal pain suggestive of intestinal angina. Symptomatic, expanding aneurysms and those greater than 2 cm in diameter warrant interventional therapy.

Endovascular stent-graft placement is an appealing treatment option for selected SMA aneurysms.[101-104] Although late complications of thrombosis and infection may accompany endovascular stent-graft therapy, the early morbidity and mortality are much less than those accompanying an open surgical procedure. Obliteration of these aneurysms by coils or direct thrombin injection is preferred in high-risk patients with discrete aneurysm necks.[92,105] This assumes that the distal mesenteric circulation will be preserved by the collateral circulation.

Similarly, open surgical ligation of superior mesenteric artery aneurysms without arterial reconstruction has proved efficacious in certain cases, especially for aneurysms associated with prior arterial obstruction and the development of an adequate collateral circulation to the midgut structures.[92,106] In fact, ligation has been the most common reported surgical means of managing

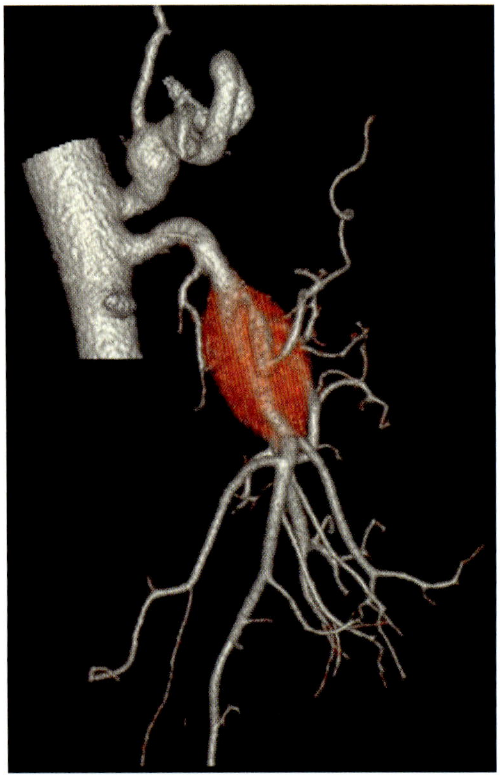

FIG 46.7 Fusiform thrombus-containing superior mesenteric artery aneurysm involving the artery's proximal branches.

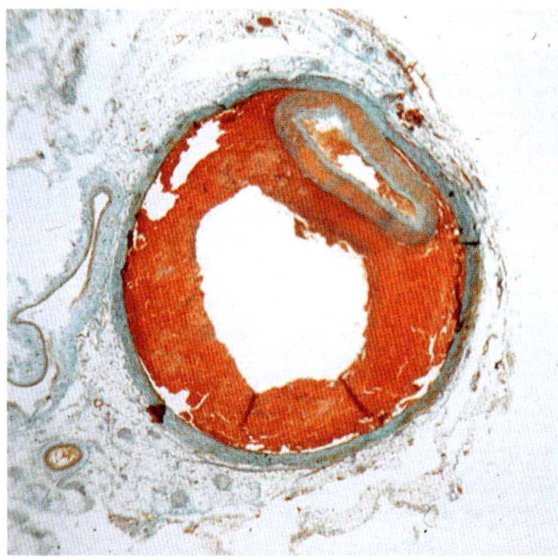

FIG 46.8 Superior mesenteric artery aneurysm associated with a dissection-related mural hematoma compressing the arterial lumen (Movat stain, original magnification 10×).

these lesions. If trial clamping results in bowel ischemia in this setting, then intestinal revascularization is required.

Celiac Artery Aneurysms

Celiac artery aneurysms account for 4% of all splanchnic artery aneurysms, and men and women appear to be equally affected. Half the celiac artery aneurysms encountered before 1950 were mycotic, although infectious lesions have become rare in recent years.[107] Most of these aneurysms are associated with medial degeneration. Aortic aneurysms occur simultaneously in nearly 20% of these patients, and 40% have other splanchnic aneurysms.

These aneurysms are usually recognized as incidental findings during imaging for other diseases, most often in patients in their seventh decade. Arteriosclerosis is a frequent finding, but as in the case of other splanchnic artery aneurysms, it is considered a secondary process. Celiac artery aneurysms are usually saccular, affecting the distal trunk of this vessel (Fig. 46.9), with some evolving from poststenotic dilatations associated with median arcuate ligament entrapment or arteriosclerotic occlusive disease affecting the proximal celiac artery.

Most celiac artery aneurysms are asymptomatic or are associated with vague abdominal discomfort.[37,107,108] Rupture reportedly occurs in 13% of these aneurysms, is usually intraperitoneal, and carries a mortality of 50%.[107] Aneurysmal rupture rarely occurs into the gastrointestinal tract. Intervention is warranted for all symptomatic celiac artery aneurysms and those exceeding 2 cm in size.

Endovascular treatment of celiac artery aneurysms is challenging because of the need to occlude the hepatic, splenic, and left gastric arteries and in some cases the inferior phrenic arteries. Nevertheless, conventional endovascular therapy, as well as that using multilayer stents, has been successful and has a role, especially in patients at high risk for open surgery.[7,14,109-113] Celiac artery dissections may be associated with mural aneurysms, and those not resolving spontaneously are appropriately treated by stenting or open repair.[114,115]

Open surgical procedures historically have been the most common reported interventions for celiac artery aneurysms and may be performed unless prohibitive operative risks exist. Most nonruptured aneurysms can be treated through an abdominal approach, although in the presence of acute expansion or rupture, a thoracoabdominal incision may be favored. Arterial reconstruction of the celiac trunk is preferred following aneurysmectomy,[107,116] but simple aneurysmal exclusion with ligation of entering and exiting branches may be performed in selected patients.[37,107,117,118] If the latter is undertaken, the foregut collateral blood flow to the liver must be sufficient to prevent severe hepatic ischemia. When such is not the case, an aortoceliac or aortohepatic artery bypass is usually undertaken. Occasionally the aneurysm is resected and an end-to-end anastomosis of the hepatic artery to the splenic artery is performed. Successful outcomes of open surgical therapy are greater than 90%.[107]

Gastric and Gastroepiploic Artery Aneurysms

Gastric and gastroepiploic artery aneurysms account for 4% of splanchnic artery aneurysms (Fig. 46.10). Gastric artery aneurysms are tenfold more common than gastroepiploic artery aneurysms, and men are twice as likely as women to have these aneurysms. The majority of these lesions are solitary, acquired as a result of periarterial inflammation, postgastrectomy arterial injury, or medial degeneration suggestive of segmental arterial mediolysis.[119] Most aneurysms have occurred in patients older than 50 years. Arteriosclerosis, when present, is invariably a secondary accompaniment of these lesions. These aneurysms are usually very small, and an intraoperative search for them is often tedious if they have not been localized preoperatively by detailed imaging.

Most reported gastric or gastroepiploic artery aneurysms have been symptomatic when initially recognized. In fact, these perigastric aneurysms usually appear as emergencies with few antecedent symptoms.[120-122] Rupture has occurred in more than 90% of reported cases, with gastrointestinal bleeding occurring twice as often as intraperitoneal hemorrhage. Postgastrectomy intestinal hemorrhage has frequently been associated with ruptured pseudoaneurysms.[123] Aneurysmal rupture may be catastrophic, as

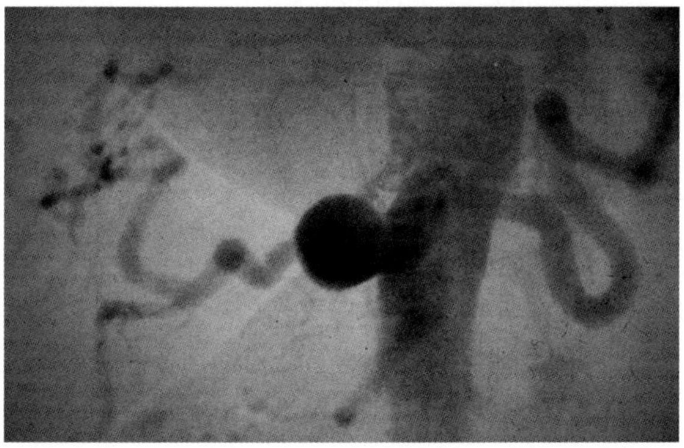

FIG 46.9 Celiac artery aneurysm affecting the distal trunk of the vessel. (From Rectenwald JR, Stanley JC: Celiac, hepatic, and splenic artery aneurysms. In Stanley JC, Veith FJ, Wakefield TW, editors: *Current Therapy in Vascular and Endovascular Surgery*, ed 5, Philadelphia, 2014, Elsevier, p 743.)

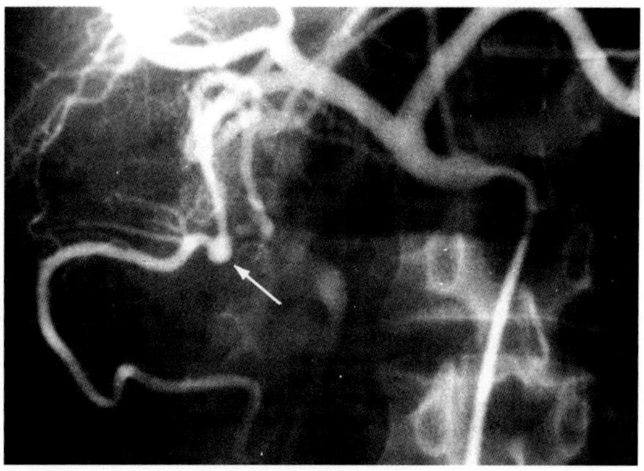

FIG 46.10 Gastroepiploic artery aneurysm. Selective celiac arteriogram documenting small saccular aneurysm. (From Zelenock GB, Stanley JC: Splanchnic artery aneurysms. In Rutherford RB, editor: *Vascular Surgery*, ed 5, Philadelphia, 2000, WB Saunders, p 1378.)

emphasized by the reported 70% mortality after such an event.[23] Given the life-threatening risk of these aneurysms, it is recommended that most be treated once the diagnosis is established.

Surgical treatment of gastric and gastroepiploic artery aneurysms does not involve vascular reconstructive surgery. Intramural gastric aneurysms, especially those having ruptured, usually require excision with the involved portion of the stomach. Extramural aneurysms may be treated by arterial ligation alone, with or without aneurysm excision. In contemporary practice endovascular exclusion of intact aneurysms in hemodynamically stable patients is favored over open surgery.[7,14,124,125]

Jejunal, Ileal, and Colic Artery Aneurysms

Aneurysms of the jejunal, ileal, and colic arteries account for 3% of splanchnic artery aneurysms (Fig. 46.11). They are usually recognized in patients older than 60 years, with men and women affected equally. Solitary aneurysms are reported in 50% of cases. Multiple aneurysms tend to evolve as a result of emboli associated with subacute bacterial endocarditis[126] or from an underlying arteriopathy.[127] Isolated aneurysms affecting the proximal inferior mesenteric artery often result when this vessel has been subjected to markedly high flow in patients having celiac and SMA occlusive disease.[128] Middle colic artery aneurysms are most often of an undetermined etiology, although some exhibit segmental arterial mediolysis.[129] Arteriosclerosis, present in 20% of these aneurysms, is considered a secondary event, not a causative process.

Most reported aneurysms affecting these small arteries have been symptomatic, with the majority exhibiting abdominal pain.[128-132] Nevertheless, many aneurysms likely go unreported, being recognized as incidental findings during arteriography for other diseases. Reported intestinal branch aneurysm rupture rates approach 30%, with ileal branch rupture occurring most often and jejunal aneurysm rupture being relatively rare. Rupture occurs with nearly equal frequency into the intestinal tract, mesentery, or mesocolon as well as the peritoneal cavity and carries a mortality risk of approximately 20%.

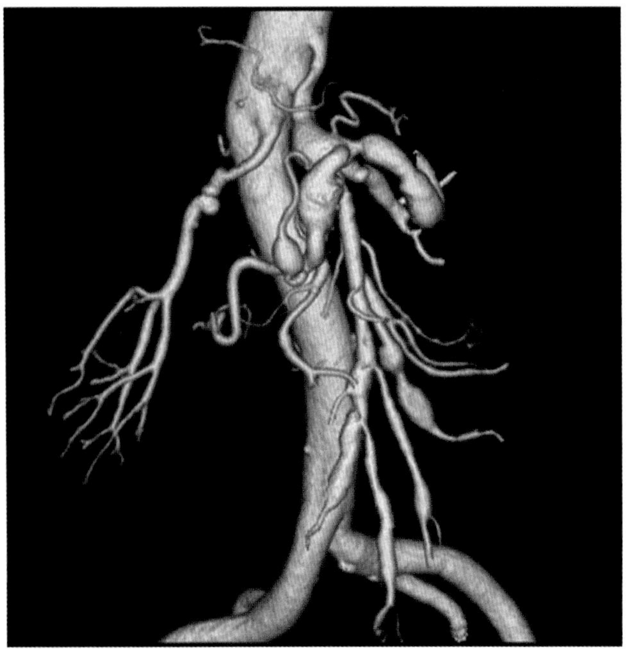

FIG 46.11 Ileal artery branch aneurysms in a patient with a systemic arteriopathy of undetermined cause. (From Stanley JC, Escobar GA: Mesenteric artery aneurysms. In Stanley JC, Veith FJ, Wakefield TW, editors: *Current Therapy in Vascular and Endovascular Surgery*, ed 5, Philadelphia, 2014, Elsevier, p 748.)

Operations for extraintestinal aneurysms usually entail arterial ligation with or without aneurysmectomy. Intramural aneurysms or those associated with bowel infarction usually necessitate resection of the involved segment of intestine. In select patients, transcatheter embolization may be undertaken, but intestinal necrosis with acute perforation or late stricture formation is a recognized complication of such therapy.[133-136] Occasionally aneurysms may require an arterial reconstruction, such as those of the inferior mesenteric artery in patients having occlusive disease of the superior mesenteric and celiac arteries, when the inferior mesenteric artery provides critical flow to the intestines.[137]

Pancreaticoduodenal and Gastroduodenal Artery Aneurysms

Pancreatic and pancreaticoduodenal artery aneurysms account for 2% of splanchnic aneurysms and gastroduodenal artery aneurysms for 1.5% of all splanchnic artery aneurysms, respectively. Men are twice as likely as women to have these aneurysms, a reflection of the greater frequency of pancreatitis in the former. Most of these aneurysms affect patients older than 45 years. There are two types of these lesions: pseudoaneurysms, associated most often with pancreatitis and true aneurysms. Arteriosclerosis is often present in both aneurysmal types and is considered a secondary process.

True aneurysms of these arteries exhibit medial thinning and disruption of elastic tissue. It appears that the majority evolve as a consequence of excessive blood flow within the pancreaticoduodenal and gastroduodenal arteries, which are functioning as collaterals to the foregut in patients having severe stenoses or occlusions of the celiac artery (Fig. 46.12).[138-144] There is no gender predilection in the subgroup of aneurysms associated with celiac artery narrowings.[141] Among the latter individuals, pancreaticoduodenal artery aneurysms are tenfold more common than those affecting the gastroduodenal arteries. Although less well recognized, similar aneurysms may develop in the presence of a SMA stenosis.[145]

Approximately one-quarter of patients with true aneurysms experience abdominal pain. Rupture of true aneurysms has been reported to affect 20% to 40% of these lesions, with bleeding occurring most often into the retroperitoneum. Small size does not negate the risk of rupture. The overall mortality following rupture of true gastroduodenal aneurysms approaches 20%, but the mortality following aneurysmal rupture in patients with celiac artery stenoses or occlusions is less than 10%.[140]

Approximately 50% of gastroduodenal and 30% of pancreaticoduodenal artery aneurysms are pancreatitis-related (Fig. 46.13). These are pseudoaneurysms, developing as a consequence of pancreatitis-associated vascular necrosis or vessel erosion by an adjacent pancreatic pseudocyst. Trauma, especially iatrogenic injury, is another but very uncommon cause of pseudoaneurysms, most frequently involving the gastroduodenal artery.[146] Most

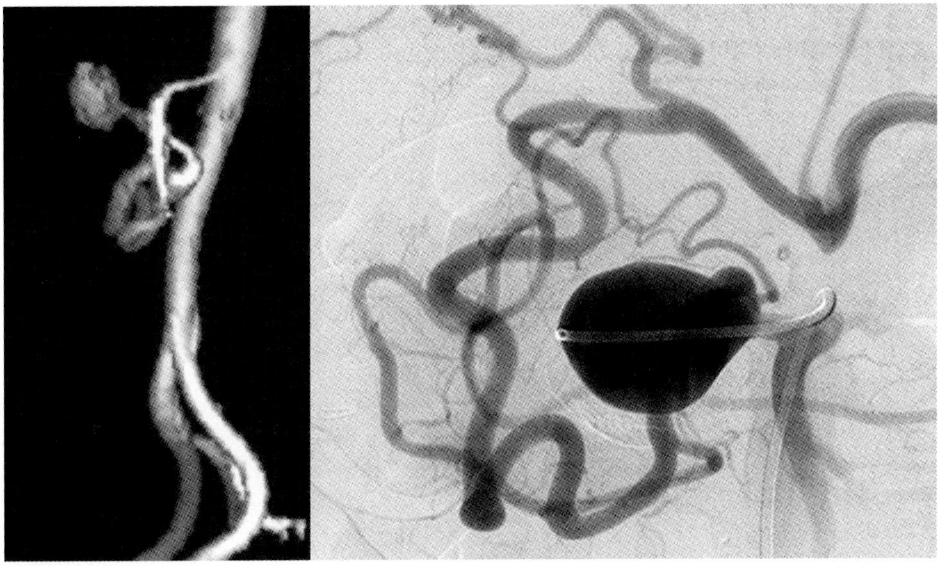

FIG 46.12 Gastroduodenal aneurysm (computed arteriographic tomogram) and pancreaticoduodenal artery aneurysm (arteriogram) associated with celiac artery occlusion. (From Vandy FC, Stanley JC: Gastroduodenal and pancreaticoduodenal artery aneurysms. In Stanley JC, Veith FJ, Wakefield TW, editors: *Current Therapy in Vascular and Endovascular Surgery*, ed 5, Philadelphia, 2014, Elsevier, p 751.)

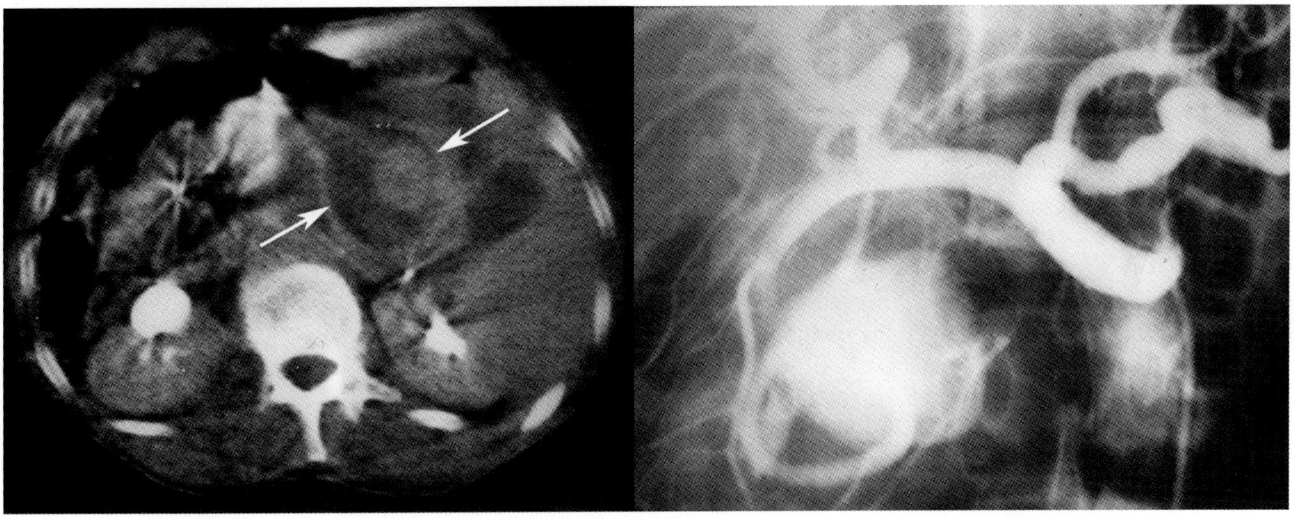

FIG 46.13 Gastroduodenal artery aneurysm *(arrows)* associated with arterial erosion by a pancreatic pseudocyst in a patient with pancreatitis. (From Eckhauser FE, Stanley JC, Zelenock GB, et al: Gastroduodenal and pancreaticoduodenal artery aneurysms. A complication of pancreatitis causing spontaneous gastroduodenal hemorrhage. *Surgery* 88:335–344, 1980.)

patients with pseudoaneurysms experience abdominal pain, often associated with their underlying pancreatic disease. Rupture is the most serious complication of these pseudoaneurysms, occurring in 10% of cases. Bleeding of ruptured pseudoaneurysms occurs into the intestinal tract more often than into the peritoneal cavity or retroperitoneum. Rupture carries a mortality of 20%.

Despite the fact that some have considered the natural history of true aneurysms to be relatively benign,[147] most clinicians favor early treatment of gastroduodenal and pancreaticoduodenal arterial aneurysms. Endovascular or open operative interventions have been proposed for all but the highest-risk patients with these lesions.[5,148-151] Endovascular embolization is favored as the initial treatment of most aneurysms in patients stable enough to be treated electively or semiurgently.[b] In some cases, stent-graft placement may prove advantageous.[156] Even in critically ill patients, endovascular occlusion of a bleeding aneurysm may be a lifesaving measure. In patients with pancreatitis-related pseudocyst erosions into an artery, exclusion or excision of the aneurysm may require a later definitive open operation or an endoscopic transpapillary drainage procedure.[138,155,157,158] Infection or even

[b]References 5, 7, 9, 39, 124, 139, 143, 152–155.

late aneurysmal rupture may follow endovascular therapies and justifies careful long-term follow-up.

Open surgical treatment is most often pursued when endovascular therapy is not technically feasible, when it might result in ischemic organ injury, or when bleeding from a ruptured aneurysm persists. Among patients having pancreaticoduodenal artery aneurysms and coexistent celiac artery occlusions or stenoses, the affected artery may be part of an essential collateral network. Transcatheter embolic occlusion of such an aneurysm may be accompanied by thrombus spillover into the SMA and result in profound foregut ischemia. In these circumstances, open surgery and revascularization of the celiac circulation should be considered.[7,138,139,143,159]

Large pancreatitis-related pseudoaneurysms associated with pseudocysts are often treated by open arterial ligation from within the aneurysmal sac rather than by extraaneurysmal arterial ligation. Extensive dissection around the pancreas in this setting is hazardous and some form of pseudocyst drainage is often needed. Concurrent or later pancreatic resection to address the underlying pancreatic disease may include distal pancreatectomy or even pancreaticoduodenectomy.[160]

RENAL ARTERY ANEURYSMS

Renal artery aneurysms constitute an uncommon vascular disease (Table 46.3). It is likely that the complications and clinical importance of these aneurysms have been overestimated in reports of spectacular cases and small series rather than relying on population-based experiences.[161-165] Discussion of these lesions requires an understanding of the difference between true and dissecting renal artery aneurysms.

True Renal Artery Aneurysms

The incidence of true renal artery aneurysms approaches 0.1%, a figure derived from arteriographic exams in approximately 8500 patients being studied for nonrenal disease.[166] Women are nearly twice as likely as men to have renal artery aneurysms.[168] Most renal artery aneurysms are saccular, including 75% located at first-order or second-order renal artery bifurcations (Fig. 46.14).[165,167] Intraparenchymal aneurysms occur in less than 10% of cases.

True renal artery aneurysms may reflect an acquired medial degenerative process or a preexisting congenital defect. Medial arterial fibrodysplasia may underlie other aneurysms. The fact that the right renal artery is more likely than the left to develop aneurysms may be due to fibrodysplastic disease affecting the right more than the left renal artery. Other arteriopathies, such as Ehlers-Danlos syndrome, are relatively uncommon causes of these aneurysms. Necrotizing arteritides, such as polyarteritis nodosa, are a cause of microaneurysms and an occasional macroaneurysm.[167] Arteriosclerosis affects one-third of true aneurysms and is thought to represent a secondary event.

Most true renal artery aneurysms are asymptomatic.[167] Nevertheless aneurysmal expansion or renal infarction from dislodged thrombus may occasionally account for flank and abdominal pain that may mimic renal colic. An ill-defined relation exists between renal artery aneurysms and elevated arterial blood pressure.[167,169] In certain instances aneurysmal thrombus may embolize

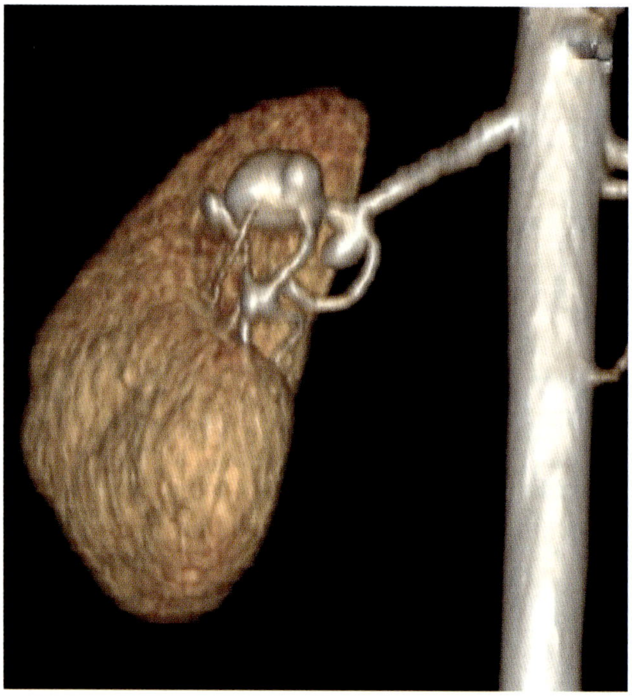

FIG 46.14 Saccular renal artery aneurysms (computed tomographic arteriogram) occurring at multiple branchings. (From Coleman DM, Stanley JC: Renal artery aneurysms. *J Vasc Surg* 62:779–784, 2015.)

TABLE 46.3 Renal Artery Aneurysms

Lesion	Male:Female Ratio	Common Contributing Factors	Frequency of Reported Rupture	Mortality With Rupture	Usual Treatment Options
Renal artery aneurysm	1:2	Medial degeneration, arterial fibrodysplasia, hypertension	3% bland (overt and covert combined)	10% bland; during pregnancy 50% maternal, 75% fetal	Aneurysmectomy with renal artery reconstruction, endovascular aneurysm obliteration, nephrectomy for ruptured aneurysms
Renal artery dissection	10:1	Deacceleration arterial stretching, medial defect with arteriosclerosis and fibrodysplasia, connective tissue diseases	Uncommon (thrombosis more common)	Very uncommon	Renal artery reconstruction, nephrectomy for irreparable renal ischemia

or propagate and occlude a distal renal artery, thereby producing renal ischemia and renovascular hypertension.[166,170] Computational modeling suggests that deformation of branches adjacent to aneurysms at bifurcations may produce a pressure gradient in these instances and contribute to renin-mediated renovascular hypertension.[171] It has also been hypothesized that energy dissipation in large aneurysms causes a similar drop in distal renal blood pressure, increased renin release, and systematic blood pressure increases. However, intrinsic stenotic disease adjacent to an aneurysm, not always evident on imaging studies, is a more likely cause of secondary hypertension, especially in patients with renal arterial fibrodysplasia.

Rupture represents the most serious complication of true renal artery aneurysms. It has been suggested that aneurysms less than 1.5 cm in diameter, calcified aneurysms, and those occurring in normotensive patients are not likely to rupture, but this has not proved to be the case. Rupture may be overt into the retroperitoneal and abdominal cavity or covert into an adjacent renal vein. Such events affect less than 3% of these aneurysms.[167]

Overt rupture causes flank pain and often hypovolemic hypotension, which carries a reported mortality of approximately 10%, although that figure appears less in contemporary practice. Loss of the kidney is greater than 90% with overt aneurysmal rupture. Renal artery aneurysmal rupture surrounding pregnancy does not appear to be related to patient age, presence of hypertension, or parity. Rupture in the latter individuals is associated with a fetal mortality rate of nearly 75% and 50% maternal mortality.[172]

Symptomatic patients thought to be due to aneurysmal expansion should be treated. Intervention is also recommended for aneurysms coexisting with functionally important renal artery stenoses. Asymptomatic aneurysms greater than 3 cm in diameter, especially those associated with hypertension, justify treatment by experienced interventionists. Smaller aneurysms provide a relative indication for elective treatment only when a high degree of suspicion exists that they are the cause of refractory renovascular hypertension. Treatment is recommended for all aneurysms in women of childbearing age who might conceive in the future because of the catastrophic outcomes accompanying rupture in pregnancy.[173]

Endovascular therapy of true renal artery aneurysms offers an important alternative to open aneurysmectomy.[174-178] However, endovascular embolic or stent-graft exclusion of extraparenchymal renal artery aneurysms without segmental renal artery occlusion is difficult because of the aneurysm's usual location at an arterial bifurcation. Nevertheless newer multilayered stents and coil embolization facilitated by prior stent placement by experienced interventionists may entail less risks than open procedures. Certain intraparenchymal aneurysms may be ablated by embolization and the kidney substance beyond them infarcted with alcohol administered through an endovascular catheter.

Open surgical therapy of nonruptured renal artery aneurysms is directed at eliminating the aneurysm without loss of kidney substance or compromise of normal renal blood flow.[179-188] Large aneurysms of the main renal artery or its bifurcation can often be excised with a simple angioplastic closure of the artery. Excision of some aneurysms may necessitate a vein patch closure or implantation of the involved artery into an adjacent uninvolved artery. In selected cases, especially involving small noncalcified aneurysms, closed aneurysmorrhaphy may be appropriate. Renal artery reconstructions with autogenous saphenous vein or internal iliac artery aortorenal bypass grafts are preferred for most aneurysms coexisting with functionally important stenoses. In certain complex cases, ex vivo repairs may be appropriate.[189] Robotic treatment of renal aneurysms has been undertaken by some, but this approach has not been widely adopted. Open surgical treatment of true renal artery aneurysms is successful in more than 90% of cases and results in improved blood pressure control in nearly 50% of patients.[167,181,185,188]

Renal Artery Dissection

Isolated dissection of the renal arteries, excluding those associated with aortic dissection and iatrogenic endocatheter-related dissection, are due to blunt or penetrating trauma or occur spontaneously.[190-195] All forms of dissection may be associated with the formation of false aneurysms (Fig. 46.15). Men are nearly tenfold more likely than women to exhibit these dissections.[190]

Traumatic dissections affect the left more than the right renal artery. These are most often associated with renal artery stretching accompanying rapid deceleration events, as occurring in motor vehicle accidents. Lesser trauma—such as repeated forceful ptosis of the kidney and stretching of the renal artery in long-distance runners—has also been reported to cause these dissections.[196]

Spontaneous dissections affect the renal arteries more than any other muscular artery. Nearly one-third of these dissections

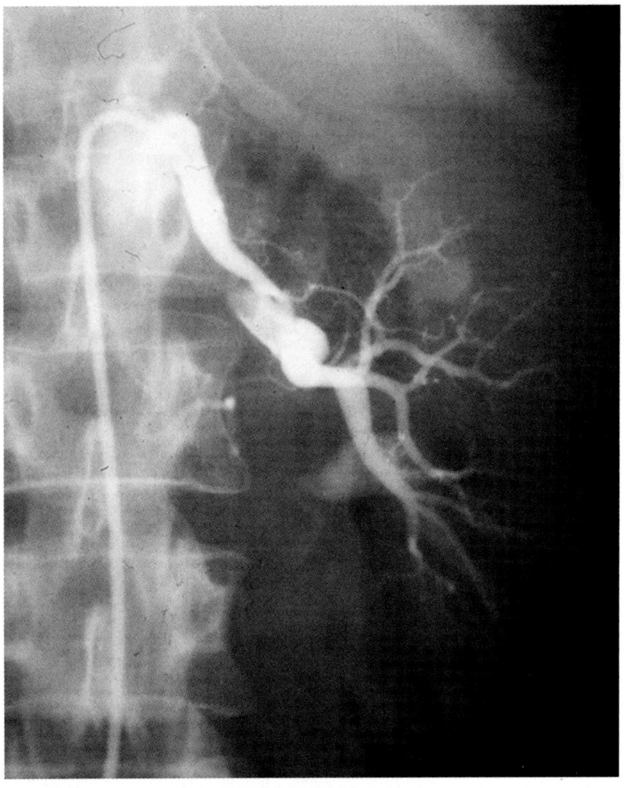

FIG 46.15 Renal artery dissection with contrast in the false lumen and a narrowing of the adjacent renal artery. (From Gewerty BL, Stanley JC, Fry WJ: Renal artery dissections. *Arch Surg* 112:409–414, 1977.)

have been preceded or are followed by a dissection involving the contralateral renal artery. These dissections are usually related to an underlying unstable arteriosclerotic plaque or fibrodysplastic renovascular disease. They have been reported in 0.5% of patients exhibiting renal artery fibrodysplasia.[191] Spontaneous dissections usually extend within the outer media, in contrast to the subintimal and inner medial location of traumatic dissections. Aneurysms are occasionally associated with a systemic arteriopathy such as Ehlers-Danlos or Marfan syndrome. Spontaneous renal artery dissections most often originate in the middle of the main renal artery and terminate at a first-order branching.

Flank pain, hematuria, and elevated blood pressure are common manifestations of both acute spontaneous and traumatic renal artery dissections. Frank rupture is uncommon. Chronic dissections may be silent, although some patients develop renovascular hypertension and impaired renal function. Loss of life accompanying an isolated renal artery dissection is very uncommon.

The initial clinical diagnosis is incorrect in more than half the acute renal artery dissections; this contributes to treatment delays and poor clinical outcomes. Prompt diagnosis may improve therapeutic results, justifying early imaging studies. Criteria for the arteriographic diagnosis of renal artery dissection include luminal irregularities with aneurysmal dilation or saccular dissections associated with segmental stenosis; the predilection of dissections to extend distally to the first renal artery bifurcation; cuffing at branchings, or a "rolled-down sock" appearance; and variable degrees of reversibility documented by serial studies.

Acute spontaneous dissections involving the distal main renal artery warrant operative intervention if hemodynamically significant stenoses or occlusions appear responsible for refractory hypertension or a deterioration in renal function. Some isolated dissections, especially branch lesions, may be managed without surgical intervention.[197-199] Kidney parenchymal preservation is of prime importance in patients having spontaneous dissections given the frequent presence of contralateral renal artery occlusive disease.

Acute traumatic renal artery dissections associated with blunt injuries usually necessitate emergent arterial reconstruction for kidney salvage, with delayed repairs for chronic dissections being undertaken in the presence of renovascular hypertension or deterioration in renal function. Open arterial reconstruction or nephrectomy in selected patients results in improved or cured hypertension in 85% to 90% of cases.[193,194,199] Treatment using endovascular coils and stents has appeal in managing both acute and chronic dissections but is technically challenging and is still an evolving therapy.[200-203]

REVIEW QUESTIONS

1. Which of the following represents the reported ranking of splanchnic artery aneurysms in order of decreasing frequency?
   - **a.** Splenic, hepatic, superior mesenteric, celiac
   - **b.** Hepatic, splenic, celiac, superior mesenteric
   - **c.** Jejunal, celiac, hepatic, splenic
   - **d.** Splenic, hepatic, celiac, superior mesenteric
2. Which of the following statements about splenic artery aneurysms is true?
   - **a.** They are more common in women than men.
   - **b.** They tend to be saccular and occur at vessel branchings.
   - **c.** They may exhibit a "double-rupture" phenomenon.
   - **d.** All of the above
3. Which of the following statements about hepatic artery aneurysms is true?
   - **a.** They account for 20% of reported splanchnic artery aneurysms.
   - **b.** They often present with obstructive jaundice.
   - **c.** Rupture has occurred in 50% of reported cases, with a 50% mortality rate.
   - **d.** They are fourfold more likely to rupture into the biliary tract as into the peritoneal cavity.
4. Which of the following statements about aneurysms of the superior mesenteric artery is true?
   - **a.** They are the fifth most common splanchnic artery aneurysm, accounting for 2.5% of all such aneurysms.
   - **b.** They are frequently mycotic in origin.
   - **c.** They affect women four times more often than men.
   - **d.** Rupture has occurred in 20% of reported cases.
5. Which of the following statements about celiac artery aneurysms is true?
   - **a.** They are best treated by simple ligation with or without aneurysmectomy.
   - **b.** They are rarely diagnosed before rupture in contemporary practice.
   - **c.** Mortality is 70% when they rupture.
   - **d.** They affect women four times more often than men.
6. Which of the following statements about jejunal, ileal, and colic artery aneurysms is true?
   - **a.** They are most commonly caused by atherosclerosis.
   - **b.** They affect men nearly 10 times more often than women.
   - **c.** When multiple, they tend to be associated with subacute bacterial endocarditis or or a systemic arteriopathy.
   - **d.** They carry an 80% risk of rupture.
7. Which of the following statements about pancreatiocoduodenal and gastroduodenal artery aneurysms is true?
   - **a.** Men are affected 5 times more often than women.
   - **b.** Those associated with celiac artery narrowings are pseudoaneurysms.
   - **c.** Inferior pancreaticoduodenal artery aneurysms are more common than gastroduodenal artery aneurysms.
   - **d.** Pancreatitis-related gastroduodenal artery aneurysms are best treated by endovascular stent-graft exclusion.

8. Which of the following statements about renal artery aneurysms is true?
   a. They are demonstrated in 10% of patients undergoing angiography for nonrenal indications.
   b. Most are saccular and the majority occur at arterial branchings.
   c. They are usually caused by atherosclerosis.
   d. They cause hypertension in approximately 80% of cases.
9. Renal artery aneurysms may be associated with hypertension due to which one of the following?
   a. Obstruction of urine flow in the collecting system.
   b. Compression of adjacent renal veins.
   c. Intrinsic renal artery stenotic disease adjacent to the aneurysm.
   d. Contralateral release of renal renin.
10. Which of the following statements about spontaneous dissection of the renal artery is true?
   a. It is a common form of renal artery disease.
   b. It occurs most often in women.
   c. It is bilateral in one-third of cases.
   d. It rarely requires surgical therapy.

BIBLIOGRAPHY

Batagini NC, El-Arousy H, Clair DG, et al. Open versus endovascular treatment of visceral artery aneurysms and pseudoaneurysms. *Ann Vasc Surg.* 2016;51:1–7.

Brocker JA, Maher JL, Smith RW. True pancreaticoduodenal aneurysms with celiac stenosis or occlusion. *Am J Surg.* 2012; 204:762–768.

Corey MR, Ergul EA, Cambria RP, et al. The natural history of splanchnic artery aneurysms and outcomes arter operative intervention. *J Vasc Surg.* 2016;63:949–957.

Erben Y, De Martino RR, Bjarnason H. Operative management of hepatic artery aneurysms. *J Vasc Surg.* 2015;62:610–615.

Ha JF, Phillips M, Faulkner K. Splenic artery aneurysm rupture in pregnancy. *Eur J Obstet Gynecol Reprod Biol.* 2009;146: 133–137.

Henke PK, Cardneau JD, Welling TH, et al. Renal artery aneurysms: a 35-year clinical experience with 252 aneurysms in 168 patients. *Ann Surg.* 2001;234:454–463.

Hogendoorn W, Lavida A, Hunink MGM, et al. Cost-effectiveness of endovascular repair, open repair, and conservative management of splenic artery aneurysms. *J Vasc Surg.* 2015;61:1432–1440.

Shukla AJ, Eid R, Fish L. Contemporary outcomes of intact and ruptured visceral artery aneurysms. *J Vasc Surg.* 2015;61: 1442–1448.

Stanley JC, Fry WJ. Pathogenesis and clinical significance of splenic artery aneurysms. *Surgery.* 1974;76:889–909.

Stone WM, Abbas M, Cherry KJ, et al. Superior mesenteric artery aneurysms: is presence an indication for intervention? *J Vasc Surg.* 2002;36:234–237.

References available online at ExpertConsult.com.

47 CHAPTER

Aneurysms of the Peripheral Arteries

Sarah Michelle Wartman, Fred A. Weaver

Peripheral arterial aneurysms are less common than aortic aneurysms, but can cause significant morbidity and occasionally lead to death; however, the most common serious complication is end-organ loss or dysfunction. The peripheral aneurysms discussed in this chapter will be the most common ones, including those of the lower extremity arteries below the inguinal ligament, including the femoral artery, as well as the extracranial carotid arteries, and the upper extremity arteries distal to and including the subclavian artery. The focus will be on true peripheral artery aneurysms, although the diagnosis and techniques used to manage them can be applied to the treatment of false aneurysms as well. Iatrogenic and mycotic peripheral aneurysms are discussed separately at the end of the chapter, with a focus on management and traumatic peripheral aneurysms are discussed in Chapter 48.

PERIPHERAL ANEURYSMS

The most common cause of nonmycotic peripheral arterial aneurysms is atherosclerosis and all peripheral aneurysms are uncommon when compared to aortic aneurysms. In descending order, the relative frequency of these aneurysms is popliteal, femoral, subclavian or axillary, and carotid. Atherosclerotic peripheral aneurysms are frequently associated with synchronous aortic, iliac, or splanchnic aneurysms. Reports on distal aneurysms involving the brachial, radial, ulnar, deep femoral, and tibial or peroneal arteries are limited to small series or case reports. Although true aneurysms have been reported in these areas, for the most part, forearm, hand, tibial, and peroneal aneurysms are secondary to trauma or are mycotic in origin.[1-3]

Age and sex distribution of peripheral aneurysms are dependent on cause. Atherosclerotic aneurysms tend to occur primarily in men older than 50 years of age, and aneurysms caused by trauma are also more common in men, but occur at a younger age. Aneurysms secondary to thoracic outlet syndrome are most commonly seen in middle-aged women (75%). The etiologies of peripheral aneurysms are listed in Table 47.1.

As with aortic aneurysms, peripheral aneurysms can be asymptomatic or lead to significant complications. Unlike aortic aneurysms, which tend to rupture, peripheral aneurysms most commonly thrombose or give rise to distal arterial emboli and since there are rarely warning signs before embolization, the mere presence of a peripheral aneurysm often suggests the need for repair. The decision to repair must be tempered by the patient's overall medical condition, and the risk of repair must be less than the risk of the natural history of the disease. The two primary objectives of treatment are exclusion of the aneurysm and restoration of arterial continuity, and in most cases, both objectives can be achieved. In the rare aneurysm that is not surgically accessible, exclusion alone may be required in this situation. Additional considerations include relieving associated compressive symptoms from the aneurysm and minimizing the risk of late aneurysm expansion.

Because most patients with peripheral aneurysms do not often have extensive atherosclerotic occlusive disease, the results of reconstructive vascular procedures are usually excellent. In some cases, however, prior embolization from the aneurysm can lead to obliteration of some, or all, of the distal arterial bed, leading to less satisfactory results.

Femoral Artery Aneurysms

Incidence and Cause

A common femoral artery (CFA) aneurysm is defined as a localized dilatation of 1.5 times the expected size of a normal adjacent segment of artery. According to the reporting standards for the Society for Vascular Surgery, the normal diameter of the CFA is 0.78 to 1.12 in men and 0.78 to 0.85 in women. Cutler and Darling[4] classified CFA aneurysms into two categories: type 1 which involved the CFA up to the femoral bifurcation; and type 2 which extended into the profunda femoris. Type 1 represent the majority, with 44% to 85%.[5] CFA aneurysms are the most common, but occasionally these aneurysms are located only in the deep or superficial femoral artery.

Dent and colleagues showed an association between femoral and popliteal aneurysms and other aneurysms of atherosclerotic origin.[6] Most commonly, these associated aneurysms are located in aorta-iliac vessels, but more rarely can involve the renal, splanchnic, and brachiocephalic vessels. Among patients with at least one peripheral aneurysm, 83% had multiple aneurysms. Among patients with a common femoral aneurysm, 95% had a second aneurysm, 92% had an aorta-iliac aneurysm, and 59% had bilateral femoral aneurysms.

Natural History

The natural history of femoral aneurysms, like popliteal aneurysms, is associated with a significant incidence of thromboembolic events. Hall and colleagues[5] reported that approximately 30% to 40% of patients with CFA aneurysms are asymptomatic

TABLE 47.1 Etiology of Peripheral Artery Aneurysms
Atherosclerotic/Degenerative
Inflammatory
Dissection
Developmental
Infectious (Mycotic)
Congenital
Iatrogenic
Traumatic
Anastomotic

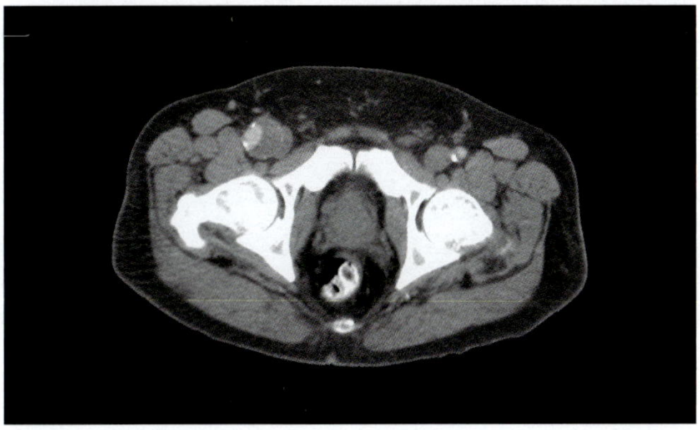

FIG 47.1 CT angiography showing a right femoral artery aneurysm.

at initial presentation, while anywhere from 10% to 65% present with ischemic complications due to either thrombosis or distal embolization. Symptoms can vary from claudication to critical limb ischemia. Tolstedt and associates[7] reported a 43% rate of thrombosis in conservatively managed femoral aneurysms, and in Cutler and Darling's series,[4] 47% exhibited major complications. Rupture of femoral aneurysms is rare. Deep femoral aneurysms, however, are thought to be particularly prone to rupture, with reported rates of 13% to 45%. While the incidence of deep femoral aneurysms is much lower, more than half will present with complications and greater than 80% will have associated aneurysms in other vascular beds.[5]

Diagnosis

Diagnosis is most often made by palpation because of the femoral artery's relatively superficial location. Femoral aneurysms should be considered in any patient with an acute lower extremity arterial occlusion or with evidence of embolic disease affecting the foot and leg. Femoral aneurysms are easily diagnosed by ultrasonography and some authors have suggested the routine use of ultrasonography to look for femoral and popliteal aneurysms in men with aortic aneurysms.[13] Computed tomography angiography (CTA) is particularly accurate in making the diagnosis and is helpful in planning open and endovascular repair (Fig. 47.1). Arteriography is usually not required when a high-quality CTA is available.

Indications for Aneurysm Repair

Conventional recommendations for the treatment of femoral aneurysms include all symptomatic aneurysms of any size, aneurysms with intramural thrombus, aneurysms greater than 2.5 cm, aneurysms that show growth with surveillance, and those that change their baseline pulse exam, indicating embolization.[5,8] This recommendation is based on the high incidence of thromboembolic complications associated with these lesions, as detailed earlier, and the low morbidity and mortality associated with repair.

A more recent study by Lawrence and the Vascular Low-Frequency Disease Consortium[8] has brought into question the current recommendations for repair based on a size of 2.5 cm. In their multivariate analysis they found that size 4 cm or greater and intraluminal thrombus were indications for repair and significantly associated with complications in patients managed nonoperatively ($P = .001$), as was age less than 60 years ($P = .004$). Location of the femoral aneurysm (common, profunda, superficial) was not significantly associated with complications. This analysis indicates that the current recommendation of greater than 2.5 cm as an indication for repair of asymptomatic common femoral, superficial femoral, and profunda aneurysms without thrombus may be too liberal and should be changed to 3.5 cm or more. One caveat to this recommendation is that the presence of thrombus was a predictor of symptomatic progression and an indication for repair at a smaller size.

Treatment

The treatment of degenerative femoral artery aneurysms is usually resection and graft interposition (Fig. 47.2). Because of the size of the CFA, a prosthetic graft is preferred. When the deep femoral artery is involved, the graft may be sewn end to end to the superficial femoral artery, and the origin of the deep femoral artery implanted into the side of the graft. When femoral aneurysms are being treated concomitantly with an inflow or outflow procedure, it is preferable to replace the CFA with an interposition graft with inflow or outflow grafts anastomosed to the interposition graft in an end-to-side fashion. Releasing the inferior border of the inguinal ligament, dividing the inguinal ligament, or making a separate retroperitoneal incision can assist in gaining proximal control of the external iliac artery. Additionally, proximal endovascular balloon control from a contralateral femoral access can help in selected cases. Stent-grafting for common femoral aneurysms is rarely if ever indicated. Stents and stent-grafts in the CFA are subjected to significant flexion forces as a result of hip flexion, and there is concern regarding stent fracture and compression. In addition, stents and stent-grafts in this area may complicate future arterial access. Furthermore, coverage of the profunda femoris orifice by the stent-graft excludes a critical thigh vessel from antegrade flow.

Repair of a deep femoral artery aneurysm is dictated by the patency of the superficial femoral artery and the distal extent of the aneurysm. Although, approximately 50% of deep femoral aneurysms can be safely ligated, in-line repair should be performed when technically feasible.[3] Exposure for the profunda femoris artery requires reflecting the sartorius and rectus femoris

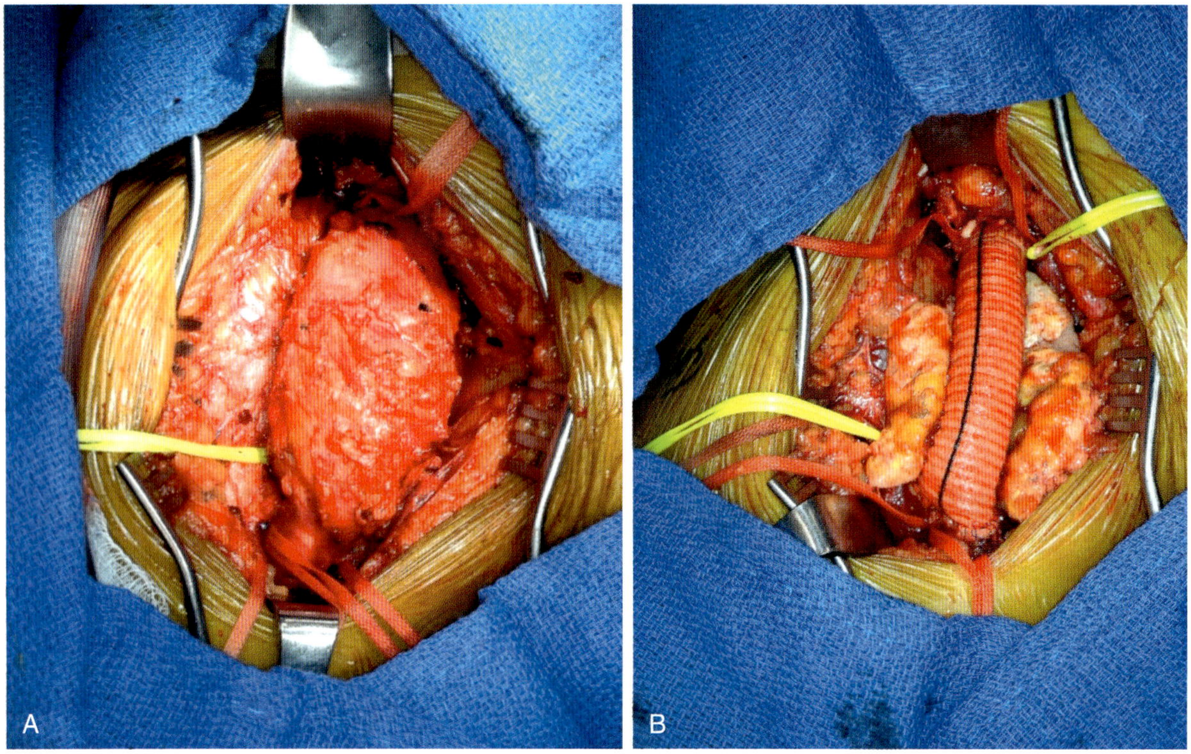

FIG 47.2 Femoral artery aneurysm before (A) and after (B) interposition graft with Dacron.

muscles laterally. Division of deep femoral vein branches is often required, and associated femoral nerve branches should be identified and protected. Repair can be accomplished with an interposition graft of saphenous vein, but prosthetic grafts are also acceptable in the absence of vein conduit.

Usually, superficial femoral artery aneurysms are an extension of a popliteal aneurysm. Treatment of isolated superficial femoral artery aneurysms can be performed by either open surgical repair or endovascular techniques. Open repair can be accomplished by either aneurysm resection and interposition grafting or aneurysm ligation and bypass. Stent-grafting can be applied anywhere along the superficial femoral artery as long as there are adequate landing zones. As with popliteal artery aneurysms, superficial femoral artery aneurysms treated with ligation or a stent-graft may be subject to enlargement secondary to type II branch endoleaks.

Outcomes

When femoral aneurysms are treated before complications arise, the results are excellent. The 18 asymptomatic patients with femoral aneurysms in the series by Cutler and Darling all had excellent early and late results (no graft occlusions).[4] However, of the 45 symptomatic patients with femoral aneurysms, 4 had amputations, and 17 remained symptomatic despite therapy.

Harbuzariu and colleagues[9] followed 17 patients with profunda femoris aneurysms, 11 of which were asymptomatic. Fifteen of the profunda femoris aneurysms were treated with bypass grafting. There was no 30-day death, graft thrombosis, or limb loss. Long-term graft patency was 100%.

As mentioned previously, Lawrence and colleagues collected a series of 236 femoral artery aneurysms (191 CFA, 11 PFA, 34 SFA) in 182 patients. One hundred fourteen patients were initially managed nonoperatively, and 64% of these patients later required repair. Of these patients, the most common indication for repair was development of intraluminal thrombus, followed by increase in diameter to greater than 2.5. In addition, acute complications occurred in 12 and rapid enlargement in 7. Of the patients treated surgically, 98% were treated with open repair, 80% interposition graft, and 20% bypass. Major postoperative complications occurred in 20%. Five-year survival was 61%, and none of the patients developed critical limb ischemia or required amputation during the follow-up period (range 1 to 93 months), providing a 100% limb salvage rate at 5 years.

Popliteal Artery Aneurysms

Incidence and Cause

Aside from trauma and rare degenerative and congenital disorders, popliteal aneurysms are almost exclusively atherosclerotic in origin.[10,11] These aneurysms account for about 70% of peripheral aneurysms, occurring in about 1% of men aged 65 to 80 years old, with a 20-to-1 male-to-female ratio.[5,12]

Among patients with a popliteal aneurysm, 78% have a second aneurysm, 64% have an aorta-iliac aneurysm, and 47% have bilateral popliteal artery aneurysms.[6] In a recent study, the incidence of femoral and popliteal aneurysms in men with a known abdominal aortic aneurysm was 14% (0% in women).[13] Of importance is that most of the femoral and popliteal artery aneurysms were undetectable by physical examination, emphasizing the need for ultrasound screening for femoral and popliteal aneurysms in men with an abdominal aortic aneurysm. Patients with peripheral aneurysms are also at high risk for the development of future peripheral aneurysms. Dawson showed that in patients with a popliteal artery aneurysm, new peripheral aneurysms were detected in 32% of these patients after 5 years and in 49% of these patients after 10 years.[14]

Natural History

The natural history of popliteal aneurysms is associated with a high incidence of thromboembolic events, both acute and chronic. Szilagyi and colleagues[10] reported that only 32% of patients with popliteal aneurysms managed conservatively remained without complications at 5 years. Dawson and colleagues[14] compared operative and nonoperative approaches in 50 patients with 71 popliteal artery aneurysms. Thromboembolic complications developed in 57% of patients over a mean follow-up period of 5 years. In patients followed for a full 5 years, the complication rate was 74%. Up to three-quarters of patients with popliteal aneurysms present with symptoms, including claudication, chronic embolization with ischemia, acute limb ischemia from embolism or thrombosis, or swelling and pain from aneurysm expansion and compression.[5,12] Rupture of a popliteal aneurysm is rare. Rupture can occur into the popliteal vein and is associated with a high rate of limb loss.[5,12,15] Less catastrophic complications include pain secondary to tibial nerve compression and popliteal vein thrombosis secondary to popliteal vein compression.

Diagnosis

A popliteal aneurysm should be suspected in any patient in whom the popliteal pulse is widened and easily palpated, in any patient with an acutely ischemic limb despite a femoral pulse, or in any patient with evidence of distal embolic occlusion of the infrapopliteal arterial tree. Many popliteal aneurysms are calcified on plain radiographs of the popliteal fossa. The diagnosis of a popliteal aneurysm is most expeditiously made by ultrasonography. CTA is particularly helpful in confirming the diagnosis and planning open or endovascular treatment (Fig. 47.3). Arteriography is currently rarely necessary for elective operative repairs, but is essential for patients with acute thrombosis and limb threatening ischemia. The status of the infra-popliteal arterial tree demonstrated on either CTA or arteriography is particularly important, since the patency of runoff vessels directly correlates with early and late graft patency for both open and endovascular approaches (Fig. 47.4A to D).[16]

Indications for Aneurysm Repair

Current recommendations for repair of popliteal aneurysms include aneurysm size 1.5 to 2.0 cm with thrombus, all aneurysms of 2 cm or greater in size, all symptomatic aneurysms, and those with evidence of occult distal embolization. This recommendation is based on the high incidence of thromboembolic complications associated with these lesions, as detailed earlier, and the low morbidity and mortality associated with repair.[17] The indications for revascularization in the patient with a chronically thrombosed popliteal aneurysm are the same as those used for patients with peripheral arterial occlusive disease.

Treatment

Repair of a popliteal artery aneurysm can be accomplished by either open or endovascular repair. Which approach is used depends on a number of factors including patient comorbidities, runoff vessel patency, popliteal artery tortuosity and length of vessel involvement.

Open repair of popliteal artery aneurysms was first accomplished by aneurysm ligation with above-knee to below-knee bypass through a medial approach.[18] More contemporary series have described a posterior approach with aneurysm resection and interposition graft replacement. Since both approaches are effective, which one is employed for a given patient is dependent on surgeon experience, aneurysm size, and proximal and distal extent of the aneurysm. Extension of aneurysmal degeneration into the superficial femoral artery or infra-geniculate arterial tree precludes a posterior open approach. In this anatomic situation, the proximal and/or distal anastomoses of the arterial reconstruction are best approached medially. When popliteal aneurysms are large enough to cause symptomatic compression of the surrounding tibial nerve and popliteal vein, resection of the aneurysm with interposition grafting through a posterior approach is preferred, as long as the aneurysm extent does not preclude a posterior approach. The posterior approach has the benefit of complete aneurysm decompression, which does not always occur with medial ligation and bypass. There have been reports of higher rates of nerve damage from a posterior approach, particularly with large extensive aneurysms; however, a recent meta-analysis found no statistically significant difference between the two approaches with respect to nerve damage.[19]

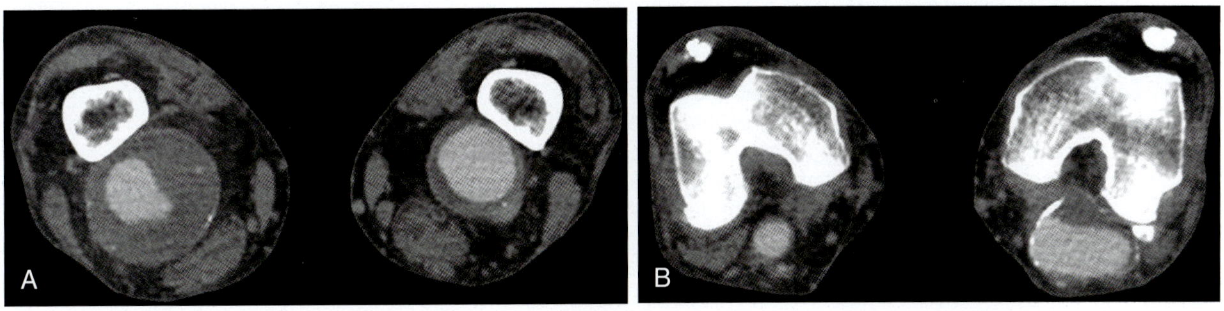

FIG 47.3 CT Angiography of bilateral lower extremities. Axial images demonstrate bilateral popliteal artery aneurysms (A and B).

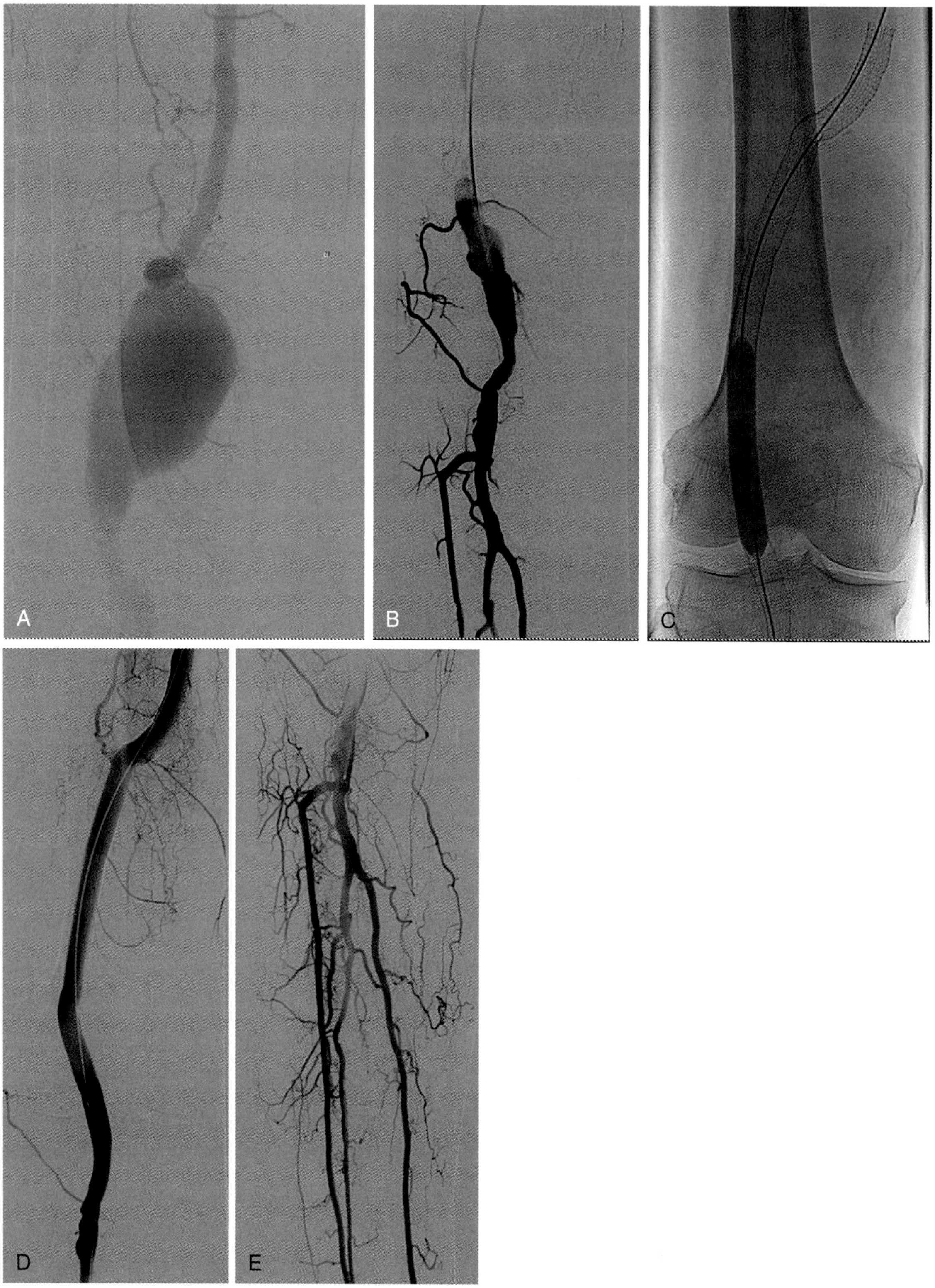

FIG 47.4 Endovascular repair of popliteal artery aneurysm with covered stent. (A) Angiogram demonstrating aneurysm of the above-knee popliteal artery. (B) Angiogram demonstrating three-vessel runoff. (C) Image of the popliteal artery poststent deployment; the calcified, excluded aneurysm is visualized. (D) Angiogram demonstrating exclusion of the popliteal artery aneurysm. (E) Angiogram demonstrating preservation of three-vessel runoff after repair.

Results of surgery are generally better when autogenous vein is used for surgical repair, when compared to polytetrafluoroethylene (PTFE) grafts, with superior patency in long-term follow-up.[20] PTFE, when used, provides reasonable results for focal aneurysms with good vessel runoff.[21,22] When chronic embolization leads to obliteration of the outflow tract of the popliteal artery, bypass to the tibial or peroneal arteries is required, and these bypasses should always be performed using autogenous vein.

When patients develop acute thromboembolic complications of popliteal artery aneurysms, the degree of arterial occlusion is often so great that no outflow vessel is visualized by CTA or arteriography. Many of these patients also have thrombosis of the microcirculation. In such patients, bypass is often not possible or is subject to a high failure rate, due to poor runoff. In this situation, the use of pre-repair thrombolytic therapy can frequently establish patent runoff and improve the microcirculation, thereby allowing for successful bypass or stent-grafting. Following acute thrombosis of a popliteal artery, graft patency and limb salvage rates after initial thrombolysis have been reported to be superior to early operative intervention alone.[23,24]

Endovascular stent-graft repair of a popliteal artery aneurysm was first reported in 1994 by Marin and colleagues. Since then, numerous reports have been published on the use of stent-grafts in this arterial location. These studies report shorter operative time and hospital stay and less perioperative morbidity.[12,25-32] For endovascular stent-graft repair, it is clear that patients with two to three vessel runoff and proximal and distal landing zones, ideally 2 cm, but at a minimum 1.5 cm, are the best candidates. Stent-grafts have also been used successfully in the treatment of ruptured popliteal aneurysms.[33] Relative contraindications to endovascular repair of popliteal artery aneurysms include extension of aneurysmal disease to the superficial femoral artery proximally or distally into the anterior tibial, tibioperoneal trunk origin, as well as tortuosity, single vessel runoff, and large aneurysms with compression symptoms.[34]

Outcomes

Open repair of popliteal aneurysms has been extensively studied; outcomes are influenced by acuity, symptom status, and runoff vessel patency. In a study of 48 popliteal aneurysms, the 5-year patency for reconstructions of asymptomatic lesions was 91%, compared with 54% for symptomatic lesions,[35] and results were directly related to the status of the tibial runoff vessels. In a series of 51 popliteal aneurysms reported by Shortell and colleagues,[36] results were dependent on the clinical presentation and the status of the runoff vessels. Patients with limb-threatening ischemia had a graft patency of 69% at 1 year, whereas all electively performed grafts in asymptomatic patients were patent at 1 year. After 3 years, runoff dictated patency; grafts with good runoff had a patency rate of 89%, whereas poor runoff was associated with a 3-year patency rate of only 30%. Numerous, more recent reports of large series of popliteal aneurysms have confirmed these earlier results.[37-41] Huang and colleagues[42] reported on 358 popliteal aneurysms treated with open surgical approaches. Forty percent were asymptomatic, 39% had chronic ischemia, and 21% had acute ischemia. The 30-day thrombosis rate was 1% in asymptomatic limbs, 4% in limbs with chronic ischemia, and 9% in limbs with acute ischemia. There were three deaths and six early amputations, all in the acute ischemia group. Five-year primary and secondary patency rates were 76% and 87%, respectively, with saphenous vein patency being significantly higher than PTFE patency (94% vs. 85%). The 5-year limb salvage rate was 97%, but only 85% in the acute ischemia group. Within that group, limbs treated with preoperative thrombolysis had better limb salvage (96%) than those limbs treated with surgery alone (69%). Two percent of aneurysms required reintervention for aneurysm enlargement, and all these limbs had been treated with ligation and bypass. In 2015, a retrospective review of 234 open popliteal artery aneurysm repairs in 196 patients evaluated long-term patency. This study found primary patency rates of 65.5%, 58%, and 55% at 5 years, 10 years, and 13 years, respectively. Secondary patency rates were reported to be 75.7% at 5 years, 69.5% at 10 years, and 68% at 13 years.[41]

Since Edwards[18] first described the technique of bypass with aneurysm ligation through a medial approach, it has been the preferred open method of repair. In the vast majority of surgical series described above, the Edwards technique was used. However, as experience has accumulated, it became evident that late aneurysm expansion and even rupture can occur. In 2003, Ebaugh and colleagues[43] reported the Northwestern experience with 57 popliteal aneurysms treated with aneurysm ligation and bypass. At a mean follow-up of 4.3 years, 32% of aneurysms treated in this manner had expanded. The authors hypothesized that type II endoleaks were the cause, but neither graft patency nor contrast filling of the aneurysms on contrast CT scans could be found to correlate with aneurysm expansion. Bellosta and colleagues[44] also assessed late aneurysm expansion after the ligation–bypass technique and found an 8% incidence of postoperative aneurysm expansion in 53 aneurysms followed for a mean of 35 months.

Beseth and Moore[22] reported on 30 popliteal aneurysms that were treated through a posterior approach using a short prosthetic interposition graft repair. Mean follow-up was 21.5 months. Primary patency, primary assisted patency, and secondary patency were 92.2%, 95.8%, and 95.8% at 1 and 2 years. Limb salvage was 100%. Aneurysms that extended proximal to the adductor canal were excluded from the posterior approach, and all aneurysms had one or more patent tibial artery runoff vessels. The authors noted that their results were comparable to the exclusion–bypass technique, but had the added advantage of allowing aneurysm resection or aneurysmorrhaphy with oversewing of popliteal perigeniculate branches with the elimination of risk for postoperative aneurysm expansion. Ravn and colleagues[24] analyzed the Swedish Vascular Registry which contained 717 popliteal aneurysms. Mean follow-up was 7.2 years. The medial approach was used in 87%, the posterior approach in 8.4%, and an endovascular approach in 3.6%. There was no difference in patency between vein and prosthetic graft when the posterior approach was used, but there was better patency with vein using the medial approach (90% vs. 72%). Emergency procedures and the use of prosthetic graft were associated with higher amputation rates. Postoperative aneurysm expansion was demonstrated in 33% when the medial approach was used, but in only 8.3%

when the posterior approach was used. Zaraca and colleagues[45] found that the posterior approach was possible in 78% of aneurysms using proximal extension above the adductor canal as the primary contraindication to posterior repair.

A 2016 meta-analysis by Phair and colleagues[19] compared the posterior and medial approach for open repair. Primary outcomes were major perioperative complications, primary patency, secondary patency, and limb loss. A total of seven studies from 2007 to 2015 with a total of 1427 patients were evaluated. There were 338 that underwent a posterior approach and 1089 that underwent a medial approach. Use of preoperative or perioperative thrombolysis was not consistently reported. There was no statistical difference in nerve damage, 30-day complications, 30-day limb loss, or 30-day primary patency. When looking at 30-day secondary patency, results suggested superiority of the posterior approach (risk difference [RD], 0.05; 95% confidence interval [CI], 0.02 to 0.07; $P = .002$). Follow-up ranged from 46 to 96 months (217 posterior, 740 medial) with long-term primary patency favoring the posterior approach (odds ratio [OR], 1.61; 95% CI, 1.06 to 2.43; $P = .02$). Successful aneurysm exclusion (138 and 107 posterior and medial approaches, respectively) and reoperation (122 posterior and 683 medial) confirmed posterior approach superiority with OR 4.2 (95% CI, 1.4 to 12.6; $P = .01$) and OR 0.26 (95% CI, 0.09 to 0.72; $P = .01$), respectively. Limb loss at the study end point was not significantly different between the two groups. Based on these findings they concluded that the posterior approach should be considered as the preferred approach for popliteal artery aneurysm (PAA) not extending above the adductor hiatus.

Because of the inferior results of endovascular or open repair once acute thromboembolic complications have occurred, attention has focused on the reestablishment of runoff preoperatively through the use of thrombolytic therapy. Most reports indicate good success in improving runoff and suggest improved limb salvage when preoperative thrombolytic therapy is used.[5,24] Varga and coworkers[23] performed a retrospective, multicenter study of 200 popliteal aneurysms and concluded that intra-arterial thrombolytic therapy clearly improves preoperative runoff in patients with acute limb-threatening ischemia. Hoelting and associates[46] described 24 patients with acute ischemia secondary to popliteal artery aneurysm thrombosis. Nine patients were treated with preoperative thrombolysis and underwent successful bypass. Six of these patients achieved complete lysis. For three patients, lysis was incomplete but established sufficient runoff so that successful bypass could be performed. These authors also reviewed the literature and reported an amputation rate of approximately 27% in 455 patients treated with bypass alone, compared with approximately 20% in 14 patients in whom only thrombolytic therapy was used. In 30 patients in whom thrombolytic therapy was combined with bypass, no limb was lost. Varga and colleagues suggested that thrombolysis is of value in restoring distal runoff before bypass in the presence of limb-threatening ischemia. Carpenter[16] reported on seven limbs with popliteal aneurysm thrombosis and complete thrombosis of all runoff vessels. These patients were treated with preoperative thrombolysis, with 100% limb salvage and superior graft patency compared to similar patients not treated with preoperative thrombolysis.

Early experience of popliteal artery aneurysms with stent-grafts demonstrated technical success, but patency was considerably lower than that achieved with aneurysm ligation and bypass. However, Tielliu[47] in 2005 reported on 57 popliteal aneurysms treated (five emergently) with stent-grafting. Primary and secondary patency rates were 80% and 90% at 1 year and 77% and 87% at 2 years; use of postoperative clopidogrel was predictive of success.

More recent analyses comparing open and endovascular repair have demonstrated inferior patency with endovascular repair in the early postoperative period.[40,48] In a review of the Vascular Quality Initiative from 2015, open repair demonstrated superior 1 year primary patency, with hazard ratio (HR) of 0.25 (95% CI, 0.10 to 0.58).[48] A similar review of a prospectively collected database in Sweden with 592 repairs reported inferior primary and secondary patency at 1 year with endovascular repair.[40] This difference was most pronounced in patients presenting with acute limb ischemia with primary and secondary patency for endovascular repair being 42% and 48%, respectively, compared to 78% and 87% for open repair. With regard to patients with asymptomatic aneurysms, there was a significantly better primary patency and secondary patency at 1 year ($P < .001$; $P = .026$) following open repair.

Golchehr and colleagues[20] reported their experience with a placement of heparin bonded ePTFE stent-grafts in a smaller cohort of patients with follow-up over a 5-year period. Published in 2016, they retrospectively reviewed a prospectively collected database and identified a total of 72 aneurysms treated in 70 patients. All patients had aneurysms greater than 2 cm, with two or more outflow vessels, and greater than 1.5 cm proximal and distal landing zones. Patients with below knee popliteal arteries of less than 4 mm were excluded, and maximum oversizing of stent-grafts was 15%. All patients received dual antiplatelet therapy for 6 months, followed by single agent long-term. Of these patients, 78% were initially asymptomatic and only 9% had acute limb ischemia on presentation. There were no significant factors identified that were associated with loss of patency. Primary patency at 1, 2, and 3 years was 83%, 69%, and 69%, respectively. Secondary patency was 88%, 81%, and 76% at 1, 2, and 3 years, respectively, and there were no major amputations during the follow-up period of 0 to 63 months (median 13). The authors concluded that mid-term outcomes with stent-grafts were promising and this approach deserved consideration.

In 2015, the largest meta-analysis to date was published comparing endovascular to open repair. A total of 652 repairs were evaluated across five studies (236 endovascular, 416 open).[12] Endovascular patients were significantly older (75 ± 6 years vs. 68 ± 3 years mean diff [MD], 6.95; 95% CI, 4.04 to 9.86; $P < .001$) and had fewer symptoms (OR, .38; 95% CI, 0.26 to 0.54; $P < .001$). No difference in emergency cases or poor vessel runoff was found. All patients were treated postoperatively with dual antiplatelet for at least 1 month, or oral anticoagulation plus one antiplatelet agent. Thirty-day graft occlusion rates (9% vs. 2%; OR, 3.16; 95% CI, 1.31 to 7.62; $P = .01$) and reintervention rates (9% vs. 4%; OR, 2.15; 95% CI, 1.02 to 4.55; $P = .04$) were significantly higher for endovascular repair. Length of procedure and length of hospital stay (3.5 vs. 7.3 days; $P < .001$) were significantly less for endovascular repair, consistent with nearly all studies comparing the two treatment modalities. There were no significant differences in survival, limb loss, and primary patency, and 4-year cumulative primary patency rates were 54% to 86% for endovascular versus 63% to 88% for open. They concluded that dual antiplatelet therapy appeared to assist with improved early patency rates as compared to earlier studies and reported that midterm patency rates are comparable to open repair.

These recent reports suggest that an endovascular approach to patients who have certain anatomic prerequisites is reasonable, particularly in elderly patients with comorbidities or in patients lacking autogenous vein. Anatomic prerequisites include 1.5 to 2 cm proximal and distal landing zones in the popliteal artery and at least two-vessel runoff. Dual antiplatelet therapy is also critical and required for a durable repair.

Infrapopliteal Aneurysm

Incidence and Cause

Infrapopliteal, or tibial artery, aneurysms are uncommon, and true aneurysms are exceedingly rare. The majority of reported cases of aneurysms of the infrapopliteal arteries are secondary to trauma or infection.[49-51] Data in the literature on true aneurysms consist of individual cases or small case series.[49,50,52]

Natural History

Patients may be asymptomatic, complain of intermittent claudication, painful pulsatile mass, or neurologic symptoms from nerve compression. Alternatively, patients may present with acute or chronic critical limb ischemia from distal embolization or thrombosis of the aneurysm, or rarely of rupture.

Diagnosis

Tibial aneurysms are readily diagnosed by both ultrasound and CT. Nonpalpable aneurysms are generally found on CT or arteriography in patients being studied for evidence of distal artery occlusion and ischemia.[50]

Indications for Aneurysm Repair

Repair is indicated for aneurysms two times the size of normal, adjacent artery, or for any symptomatic aneurysms, particularly those associated with pain and ischemic symptoms.

Treatment

Aneurysms of the tibial arteries can be treated by ligation or coil embolization if the remaining infra-popliteal arteries provide adequate collateral circulation to the foot. In the absence of adequate collateral circulation, primary repair, vein interposition grafting, or ligation and bypass is required.

Outcomes

Both ligation in the presence of adequate collateral circulation and repair are successful in the treatment of tibial aneurysms.[50]

Extra-Cranial Carotid Artery Aneurysms

Incidence and Cause

Extra-cranial carotid artery aneurysms (ECAA) are rare, comprising only 0.4% to 4% of all peripheral aneurysms and making up anywhere from 0.1% to 2% of all carotid interventions.[53,54] The common carotid artery, near the carotid bulb, is affected most often, followed closely by the internal carotid artery. The external carotid artery is rarely involved.[55] Of 2300 aneurysms reported from Baylor University, only seven were extra-cranial carotid aneurysms.[56] The largest single series of patients with true extra-cranial carotid aneurysms was reported by McCollum and coworkers,[57] who saw 37 such aneurysms over a 21-year period. Zhang and associates[58] reported 66 extra-cranial carotid aneurysms, 28 of which were true, nonmycotic aneurysms.

These aneurysms tend to be atherosclerotic and fusiform, and are almost always found in patients with hypertension.[55] A recent review of the literature reports hypertension in 20% to 83.5%, associated vascular pathology in 14% to 22%, and coronary artery disease in 20% to 74% of patients with ECAA.[53] Other causes of carotid aneurysms are trauma, both blunt and penetrating, and carotid dissection. False aneurysms of the carotid artery also occur after carotid endarterectomy.[59] Rarer causes include cystic medial necrosis, Marfan syndrome, fibromuscular dysplasia, medial arteriopathy, granulomatous disease, radiation, and congenital defects. El-Sabrout reviewed the literature from 1950 through 1995 and found that of 392 carotid aneurysms, reported etiology was as follows: 40% atherosclerotic, 21% false aneurysm, 14% trauma, 12% dissection, 8% fibromuscular disease, 2% infection, and 3% other.[60]

Natural History

Central neurologic events are common in patients with ECAA, with approximately 14% to 43% initially presenting with neurologic symptoms including amaurosis fugax, transient ischemic attacks, and stroke.[60,61] Rhodes and coauthors[55] reported that 13 of the 19 patients with carotid aneurysms reported in the University of Michigan series had amaurosis fugax, transient ischemic attacks, stroke, or vague neurologic symptoms such as dizziness. Most of these symptoms are thought to be secondary to embolization. Cranial nerve compression can cause facial pain (cranial nerve V), oculomotor palsies (cranial nerve VI), auricular pain (cranial nerve IX), and hoarseness (cranial nerve X). Horner syndrome can also occur from compression of the sympathetic chain. As cervical carotid aneurysms enlarge they can cause dysphagia, and hemorrhage has also been seen as a complication of these aneurysms; however, rupture is uncommon.

Diagnosis

Excluding neurologic findings, the most common physical finding in patients is a palpable pulsatile, submandibular, lateral neck mass or a mass in the tonsillar fossa. The former presentation is most often seen with common carotid aneurysms, whereas presentation in the tonsillar fossa is more often due to an internal carotid artery aneurysm. Because of the variability in the location of the carotid bifurcation, the presentation is only a rough guide to the segment of the carotid artery involved. The differential diagnosis includes kinked or redundant carotid arteries, enlarged lymph nodes, salivary gland tumors, branchial cleft cysts, cystic hygromas, and carotid body tumors. When the diagnosis is not clear, carotid duplex scanning and CTA or magnetic resonance angiography (MRA) are usually diagnostic and help with preoperative planning.

Indications for Aneurysm Repair

The indication for repair is usually the presence of the aneurysm. Because patients with this condition are rarely seen when asymptomatic, most patients are treated for symptomatic relief or for prevention of symptoms. The high incidence of cranial nerve compression and central nervous system events in untreated patients (68%) justifies treatment for asymptomatic carotid aneurysms.[55] These indications are common in nearly all reported studies.[62-64]

Treatment

The techniques applied to the management of extra-cranial carotid aneurysms are ligation (or angiographic occlusion), endoaneurysmorrhaphy, resection with primary anastomosis, resection with interposition graft placement, and stent-grafting.

The preferred treatment is resection with primary anastomosis or interposition graft. Redundancy of the carotid artery is not uncommon when an aneurysm is present. In such cases, resection of the aneurysm with mobilization of the carotid artery and primary anastomosis is sometimes possible. This technique is most applicable to internal carotid artery aneurysms. An alternative technique for flow restoration after resection of an internal carotid artery aneurysm is to divide the distal external carotid artery and perform an end-to-end anastomosis between the proximal external carotid and the distal internal carotid arteries. Aneurysms of the external carotid artery are rare and can be resected without the need to restore arterial continuity. Aneurysms of the carotid bifurcation usually require resection with graft placement between the common and internal carotid arteries. When the internal carotid is redundant, it can occasionally be mobilized and anastomosed end to end to the common carotid artery. In both these cases, the external carotid is usually ligated. Aneurysms involving the common carotid artery can usually be treated by resection and primary anastomosis or interposition graft. All these procedures can be performed through the standard neck incision used for carotid endarterectomy.

The need for an indwelling carotid artery shunt is no better understood for aneurysm patients than for patients undergoing carotid endarterectomy. If shunting is desired, it can be accomplished in most patients. In patients undergoing resection with primary anastomosis, a shunt can be inserted into the open ends of the arteries after opening of the aneurysm. If a graft is to be used, the shunt is placed through the graft before performing the anastomosis and is inserted into the proximal and distal arterial ends after opening of the aneurysm.

Aneurysms that involve the distal cervical internal carotid artery are often inaccessible using standard surgical techniques. Alternative approaches are often required for high internal carotid lesions. Some techniques described in the carotid endarterectomy literature that allow for exposure of distal internal carotid artery (ICA) are highly morbid procedures—division of styloid process, lateral mandibulotomy, mastoidectomy. Mandibular advancement, however, can be accomplished with significantly less morbidity by wiring the jaw or, as described by Yoshino and colleagues,[65] by creating a dental mold of a patient with the mandible positioned anteriorly. This allows for up to 1 to 2 cm of additional exposure with less morbidity and minimal addition of operative time. In some patients, high-fusiform aneurysms can be treated with aneurysmorrhaphy using an indwelling shunt for flow continuity and as a method of distal arterial control, while in others, distal lesions must be treated by ligation. Unfortunately, acute occlusion of the internal carotid artery in these patients is associated with high neurologic morbidity. Stroke rates from 30% to 60% have been reported, with half of those patients dying as a result of the stroke. The high degree of morbidity and mortality associated with ligation clearly approaches that associated with the natural history of the disease.

One way to select patients who may safely undergo carotid ligation is to measure intraoperative carotid stump pressure. The carotid stump pressure can also be measured by temporary balloon occlusion using preoperative arteriography, with an end-hole balloon catheter.[66] Stump pressures greater than 70 mm Hg appear to be safe for patients undergoing carotid ligation. The balloon occlusion test can also be used to determine if embolization or surgical ligation will lead to neurologic deficit. Because strokes that occur after carotid ligation may manifest hours to days after the procedure, these patients should be fully anticoagulated perioperatively and preferably for at least 3 to 6 months.

When stump pressure measurements indicate that carotid ligation is not safe, the performance of an extra-cranial-to-intra-cranial bypass using ipsilateral superficial temporal artery, radial artery graft, or vein graft has been suggested. Because this procedure is generally only necessary for high internal carotid lesions, the ipsilateral external carotid artery is usually preserved, thus allowing for adequate inflow into the superficial temporal artery.

Endovascular treatment modalities have become commonplace in some centers.[61,66-68] Zhou looked at the Baylor experience from 1985 to 1994 and compared it to the experience from 1995 to 2004.[61] All procedures were surgical during the early period, whereas during the later period 70% of procedures were endovascular, consisting of stent-grafts, stents combined with coil embolization, and endovascular occlusion. In some cases, coil embolization of the external carotid artery may be necessary to allow coverage of the entire aneurysm and to prevent endoleak.[69] Endovascular interventions reduce the risk of cranial nerve injury, can be done without general anesthesia, are useful for distal lesions where surgical exposure is difficult, are associated with shorter hospital stays, and have lower morbidity and mortality rates.[61]

Outcomes

The small number of patients included in reports assessing the results of surgical therapy for carotid aneurysms hampers an accurate determination of morbidity and mortality. Most reports indicate that these procedures can be performed safely. In a study from Michigan that included only atherosclerotic aneurysms, 1 of 19 aneurysm operations resulted in a stroke, which was thought to be due to intraoperative embolization.[55] No operative death occurred but excision of large and distal aneurysms was associated with an increased incidence of cranial nerve injury. El-Sabrout and Cooley found a similar incidence of 30-day stroke at the Texas Heart Institute for atherosclerotic aneurysms, but the incidence of 30-day stroke was higher (11%) for false aneurysms.[60] Overall, in the Texas Heart Institute experience, the 30-day stroke–death rate was 9%. Long-term results of treatment showed that at a mean follow-up of 5.9 years (1.5 months to 30 years), 30% of patients died, but none were procedure-related deaths and no late strokes were reported. Lauder and colleagues[70] followed 50 patients who had carotid bypass grafting with saphenous vein for pathologies postendarterectomy, including thin endarterectomy zone, penetrating atheroma, and patch infection. Patients with primary carotid aneurysms were not included in this study. Cumulative freedom from recurrent stenosis greater than 70% was 86% at 1 year and 83% at 3 years. Most investigators agree that the results of surgery are vastly superior to the natural history of the disease.[55,60,62-64]

Long-term results for carotid aneurysm repair using stent-grafts are not well established. However, Zhou and colleagues showed a decrease in the 30-day stroke–death rate from 14% (1985 to 1994, all treated surgically) to 5% (1995 to 2004, 70% treated with endovascular techniques). A more recent study by Welleweerd and colleagues[71] looked at seven consecutive patients with symptomatic extra-cranial internal carotid aneurysms who underwent placement of bare metal stents to exclude the aneurysms. With a mean follow-up of 57 months, only one patient required a return to operating room for coil embolization for residual flow into aneurysm. All patients remained free of local or central neurologic symptoms during the study period and all stents were patent, with complete thrombosis of the aneurysms at follow-up. Of note, all patients received Plavix for 3 months postoperatively and then aspirin for life.

A review of the literature from 2015 reporting papers with 10 or greater patients identified 39 articles with a total of 1239 patients with extra-cranial carotid aneurysms. Of the patients in these studies, 89% were intervened upon. Of these, 94% underwent open surgery, 5% underwent endovascular intervention, and 1% had a combined approach. Twenty-four patients died within 30 days of surgery, 13 of whom had a stroke. Thirty-four patients had a nonfatal stroke within 30 days. Cranial nerve deficit was reported in 12% of open surgical patients. The majority of long-term mortality (83%) was unrelated to stroke; however, eight patients experienced a fatal stroke, and eleven a nonfatal stroke. While early and long-term outcomes of invasive treatment appear favorable, the authors were not able to provide evidence-based recommendations.[72]

Subclavian and Axillary Artery Aneurysms

Incidence and Cause

True aneurysms of the subclavian and axillary arteries are rare. In 1982, Hobson and colleagues[73] reviewed the literature on the subject and found only 195 aneurysms, accounting for only 1% of all peripheral aneurysms. Of the 195 cases, 88% involved the subclavian artery. Subclavian and axillary aneurysms are rarely associated with atherosclerosis, with this finding present in only 15% of the aneurysms. Thoracic outlet syndrome is responsible for the majority of subclavian artery aneurysms (74%) (Chapter 33), whereas trauma accounts for most axillary artery aneurysms (54%) (Chapter 48) and other rare causes have also been reported (Table 47.2). Subclavian aneurysms can be categorized based on location of vessel and the aneurysm, with proximal aneurysms more likely to be atherosclerotic and distal ones likely due to thoracic outlet syndrome.[74,75] Additionally, there are those associated with an aberrant subclavian artery.[74] Isolated axillary artery aneurysms are rare and usually occur following trauma, using crutches, or from repetitive motion.[76,77]

TABLE 47.2 Causes of Subclavian and Axillary Artery Aneurysms

Cause	Subclavian	Axillary	Total
Thoracic outlet syndrome	127	1	128
Crutch trauma	—	13	13
Atherosclerosis	24	5	29
Pseudoaneurysm	5	2	7
Blunt trauma	2	—	2
Fibromuscular dysplasia	—	2	2
Dissection	—	1	1
Other	13	—	13
Total	171	24	195

Data from Hobson RW II, Isreal MR, Lynch TO: Axillo-subclavian arterial aneurysms. In Bergan JJ, Vito JST, editors: *Aneurysms*, New York, 1982, Grune and Stratton, pp 435–447.

TABLE 47.3 Clinical Findings in Subclavian and Axillary Artery Aneurysms

Finding	Number	Percent
Asymptomatic	20	10
Claudication	9	5
Pain	36	18
Brachial plexus palsy	24	12
Tissue loss	20	10
Embolization	136	68

Natural History

Only 10% of patients with known subclavian or axillary aneurysms are asymptomatic. Good natural history studies are not available, probably because of the small number of patients with this problem. Because 90% of patients are symptomatic at the time of presentation, the likelihood of complications eventually occurring in asymptomatic aneurysms appears to be great. The primary complication seen with subclavian and axillary aneurysms is embolization (68%). Thrombosis and rupture are rare but have been reported.[73]

Diagnosis

The most common presenting signs and symptoms of subclavian and axillary aneurysms are secondary to distal embolization (68%; Table 47.3). Small, punctate, cyanotic lesions affecting the fingers and palm occur suddenly are often present due to distal emboli. Other signs and symptoms include tissue loss, claudication, pain, pulsatile mass, and arm swelling from venous compression. Additionally, nerve compression can lead to different symptoms, depending on location, including brachial plexus neuropathy, Horner syndrome, stridor, and hoarse voice.[74,78] Aneurysms secondary to atherosclerosis tend to be larger and are palpable in two-thirds of patients, as opposed to those secondary to thoracic outlet, which are often not palpable.[78] When all types of subclavian and axillary aneurysms are considered, only 16% can be palpated.[73] A bruit may be present in the subclavian fossa or in the axilla. Rarely, embolization causes downstream large artery occlusion. This event usually requires immediate embolectomy, but can lead to claudication if the initial ischemia does not precipitate the need for immediate medical attention. With chronic small emboli, the distal radial and ulnar pulses may not be palpable. Repeated embolization may be associated with distal digital ulceration or tissue loss and severe pain. Many patients complain of vague shoulder pain. Rupture produces severe shoulder pain radiating into the upper arm and lower neck.

Duplex ultrasound is useful to diagnose subclavian and axillary artery aneurysms, but the bony cage of the thoracic outlet may preclude adequate insonation of the proximal subclavian artery. CTA and MRA are very helpful in demonstrating subclavian and axillary aneurysms.

Indications for Aneurysm Repair

The presence of a subclavian or axillary aneurysm is an indication for repair since the natural history suggests that these lesions are both life threatening and limb threatening. As is the case with carotid aneurysms, most patients are symptomatic at the time of presentation and have clear indications for intervention. Some controversy exists regarding the small, fusiform, poststenotic subclavian dilatation seen with thoracic outlet compression of the subclavian artery. The natural history of this lesion, if not resected at the time of thoracic outlet decompression, is not well established. In one report on four patients with subclavian artery aneurysms who had only thoracic outlet decompression, no subsequent thromboembolic events occurred during follow-up.[78]

Treatment

The surgical approach to subclavian and axillary artery aneurysms depends on the cause, size, and location of the aneurysm and the status of the distal circulation. Except in cases of small, asymptomatic subclavian artery aneurysms secondary to thoracic outlet (for which thoracic outlet decompression alone may be adequate), the aneurysm should be excluded and arterial continuity restored with either a bypass or interposition graft. Proximal and distal ligation alone has been reported and although tissue loss does not usually occur, exercise-induced arm pain is common.[78]

When a symptomatic or large asymptomatic subclavian aneurysm is present due to a cervical rib, repair of the aneurysm should be accompanied by cervical rib resection. Full thoracic outlet decompression (first rib resection and scalenectomy) should also be considered if concomitant neurogenic thoracic outlet symptoms exist. (Discussion of this issue can be found in Chapter 33.) Although this combined technique has been reported through an axillary approach, the supraclavicular approach is generally preferred since this allows for safe control of the artery and excellent exposure for repair.

Atherosclerotic and traumatic distal subclavian artery aneurysms or false aneurysms can be managed with a supraclavicular approach. When the aneurysm is proximal enough that proximal control cannot be safely obtained through this approach, a median sternotomy (right side) or thoracotomy (left side) is used, usually in combination with the supraclavicular approach. Mid-subclavian lesions can usually be managed through a supraclavicular approach with either a medial clavicular resection or a trapdoor mini-sternotomy required in a small subsegment of patients with large aneurysms.

Primary anastomosis is usually not possible, and graft replacement is the routine. This is most commonly performed as an interposition graft using either saphenous vein or prosthetic graft. Prosthetic grafts are more commonly used because of the size match with the subclavian artery. The vertebral artery should be preserved when possible, particularly if the ipsilateral vertebral artery is dominant. High-risk patients with proximal aneurysms who are considered too frail to undergo a major procedure can be treated with distal ligation and axillary-axillary bypass or endovascular stent-grafts.

More recently, stent-grafting has been applied to carefully selected patients with subclavian aneurysms, but long-term results are not yet known.[79-81] Stent-grafting of the subclavian artery can avoid a major surgical procedure particularly in high-risk patients. Stent-grafts have been used in the treatment of true and false subclavian artery aneurysms and traumatic subclavian arteriovenous fistulae. Limitations of stent-grafting include short fixation zones and the risk of covering important vessel origins such as the right carotid, the vertebral artery, and the internal mammary artery. Concern has also been raised regarding stent compression in the area of the thoracic outlet. Stent-related complications that have been reported to include strut dislocation and stent fracture, stent compression, false aneurysm, and in-stent stenosis. Morbidity due to stent complications has been reported as high as 28%.[75]

Management of axillary artery aneurysms can often be accomplished through the axillary approach. In most patients, proximal control can be obtained through an infra-clavicular approach, but with more proximal aneurysms or aneurysms involving both the subclavian and the axillary arteries, a combined supraclavicular and infra-clavicular approach is necessary. Aneurysms involving the axillary artery are often intimately involved with the cords of the brachial plexus, and resection may be hazardous. When symptoms of brachial plexus compression are present, resection and interposition grafting is required. For smaller and more complex lesions without symptoms of compression, proximal and distal ligation combined with saphenous vein bypass can be performed, avoiding dissection and potential injury to the brachial plexus. Stent-grafting of the axillary artery has been performed most commonly for traumatic hemorrhage and false aneurysms. Although there are individual case reports of endovascular management of axillary artery aneurysms, no significant series of axillary artery stent-grafting was found in a review of the literature.

When subclavian and axillary aneurysms are complicated by downstream embolization and ischemia, revascularization of the arm may be required in combination with aneurysm repair. This is usually accomplished by autogenous vein bypass from a site proximal to the aneurysm to the most appropriate distal artery. In this situation, the aneurysm can be either ligated or resected. Alternatively, stent-grafting of the aneurysm, followed by local bypass of the occluded segments, can be considered.

Outcomes

The results of surgery for subclavian and axillary aneurysms are similar to those for upper extremity reconstruction for occlusive disease. Pairolero and colleagues[78] reported on 31 patients with aneurysms in this location, and 19 of them underwent surgical repair. The repair in 11 aneurysms was by resection with graft interposition and in eight by aneurysmorrhaphy. Patent reconstructions without complication or aneurysm recurrence were documented in all during an average of 9.2 years of follow-up. However, patients with obliteration of the radial and ulnar arteries have a high failure rate following arm revascularization.[82] This latter point further emphasizes the need for early surgical intervention. Primary and secondary patency rates as high as 89% and 100% have been reported at 29 months for stent-graft repair of subclavian artery aneurysms.[80]

Forearm and Hand Aneurysms

Incidence and Cause

True aneurysms in the forearm and hand are extremely rare. During a 10-year period, only 10 such patients were treated at the University of Chicago.[1] Half of the true aneurysms in these areas are associated with occupational or recreational trauma. Most forearm and hand aneurysms are false aneurysms secondary to penetrating trauma[2]; most true aneurysms in these locations are secondary to blunt trauma.[83] Aneurysms involving the palmar arch of the ulnar artery can occur due to occupational use of vibrating tools such as a jackhammer, which causes repetitive compression of the palmar arcade against the hamate bone. This is referred to as hypothenar hammer syndrome.[84]

Natural History

The most common presenting signs and symptoms of aneurysms in the forearm and hand are mass and pain. Paresthesia may be present from compression of the median nerve and rapid expansion or bleeding may lead to compartment syndrome. Distal embolization occurs in approximately one third of patients.[1]

Diagnosis

Forearm, and especially hand, aneurysms are most often diagnosed by palpation of a pulsatile mass. These aneurysms are readily diagnosed by either ultrasound or CTA, but nonpalpable aneurysms are generally found on arteriography in patients being studied for evidence of digital artery occlusion and ischemia.

Indications for Aneurysm Repair

Repair is indicated for aneurysms two times the size of normal, adjacent artery, or for any symptomatic aneurysms, particularly those associated with pain and tissue necrosis, and those with intraluminal thrombus.

Treatment

Aneurysms of the forearm arteries can be treated by ligation if the remaining vessels provide adequate collateral circulation to the hand. In the absence of adequate collateral circulation, as evidenced by an abnormal Allen's test, primary repair or vein interposition grafting is required. Aneurysms of vessels in the hand tend to be less well collateralized, and vein graft repair is usually necessary.[1]

Outcomes

Both ligation in the presence of adequate collateral circulation and vein graft repair are successful in the treatment of forearm and hand aneurysms. Clark and associates[1] reported 100% patency at 7 years for vein graft repairs in the forearm and hand.

IATROGENIC PERIPHERAL ARTERIAL ANEURYSMS

Femoral artery false aneurysms following femoral artery puncture for catheterization procedures occurs in approximately 0.5% to 2% of diagnostic procedures and up to 2% to 8% of interventional procedures.[85,86] Management options for femoral false aneurysms include observation, ultrasound guided compression, ultrasound guided thrombin injection, or open surgical repair.

Reported rates of success for compression and thrombin inject range from 71% to 99% and 90% to 100%, respectively.[85,86] Taylor compared these two approaches and found that compression was successful in 63% of patients, whereas thrombin injection was successful in 93% of patients.[87] Not only was thrombin injection more often successful, but it was associated with less pain and less need for sedation. Neither treatment was associated with complications in Taylor's series; however, iatrogenic arterial thrombosis has been reported with thrombin injection. Taylor attributed the lack of iatrogenic thrombosis in his series to the use of more dilute thrombin (100 U/mL) and slow injection with immediate cessation of the injection once thrombus was seen. Taylor advised observation for false aneurysms less than 2 cm, as spontaneous thrombosis often occurs.

Kresowik and colleagues[88] found the incidence of femoral false aneurysm after femoral artery puncture for coronary angioplasty to be 6%. The false aneurysms ranged in size from 1.3 to 3.5 cm and 88% of these thrombosed spontaneously within 4 weeks, without the need for further treatment. Dzijan-Horn[85] reported an incidence of false aneurysm of 1.5% (432 patients) of all femoral artery catheterizations (29,000 patients). They managed all patients with either manual or ultrasound guided compression or thrombin injection. All false aneurysms which were smaller than 2 cm, without a definable neck, that were directly adjacent to vessels, or had a concomitant arteriovenous fistula were managed with compression (145 patients); the remainder (287 patients) underwent thrombin injection. They did not discontinue any anticoagulation during the time of treatment. Of patients treated with compression 77% were successfully thrombosed on the first attempt and 7% were treated with more than one attempt. Of the thrombin-injected false aneurysms, 74% were successfully treated on the first attempt and an additional 14% were treated with multiple injections. Of note, 12 of patients crossed over from thrombin injection to compression and were successfully treated, and 28 patients crossed over from compression to thrombin injection, giving an overall success rate with combined treatment of 97%. Of the 12 patients that did achieve success with these two approaches, two had covered stent placement and 10 underwent surgical repair. Complication rates for both modalities were 1.5% and included deep venous thrombosis (DVT), infection, and rupture in the compression group and embolization, DVT, and infection in the injection group.

Femoral false aneurysms that are rapidly expanding, ruptured, infected, or cause mass effect with ischemia of the overlying skin, or those that fail compression and thrombin injection should be surgically corrected. Morbidity was reported to occur in 30% among patients requiring surgery; other studies have demonstrated similarly high morbidity.[86]

MYCOTIC PERIPHERAL ARTERIAL ANEURYSMS

Mycotic aneurysms are considered separately because they generally have a different cause, affect arteries in a different distribution, require different treatment, and have worse outcomes than bland aneurysms. Despite the term "mycotic," any aneurysm is considered to be mycotic that is infected.

Incidence and Cause

Numerous classifications for mycotic aneurysms have been proposed and are nicely described by Moore[89] and Wilson and colleagues.[90] Often, infected aneurysms are divided according to etiology: (1) microbial arteritis with aneurysm formation due to bacteremia and septic microemboli; (2) contiguous spread of localized infection; (3) posttraumatic infected pseudoaneurysm; and (4) infection of a preexisting atherosclerotic aneurysm.[91,92] Patel and Johnston[93] indicated that the source of infection must be either endogenous or exogenous. Endogenous sources include embolism, septicemia, or direct extension; exogenous sources include trauma and iatrogenic injury. They further suggested that classifications be based on the preexisting status of the artery: normal, atherosclerotic, aneurysmal, or prosthetic. Any classification must consider these factors.

Normal axial arteries are seldom infected primarily, but clumps of bacteria or fungi may lodge in smaller vessels and cause transmural necrosis and aneurysm formation. Normal larger arteries can be infected by organisms that lodge in the vasa vasorum. Arteries with atherosclerosis or aneurysmal degeneration, as well as prosthetic grafts, are subject to local invasion by exogenous contamination in the operating room and by circulating organisms. The process is similar to that described earlier, in that infection leads to arterial wall weakening and subsequent aneurysm formation. Infection may spread to arterial walls from outside the vessel through direct contact with abscesses, wound infections, salivary glands, etc. Exogenous sources of arterial infections include diagnostic and therapeutic catheterizations, penetrating trauma, and drug abuse. Graft infections may also lead to infected false aneurysm formation, usually as a result of disruption of an anastomosis.

Mycotic aneurysms have been reported in essentially all arteries, and their location is determined primarily by their cause. In general, the aorta, peripheral arteries, cerebral arteries, and visceral arteries are involved in descending order of frequency.[92] Those secondary to bacterial endocarditis favor the superior mesenteric artery, followed by the aorta and femoral arteries. Mycotic aneurysms that occur after trauma most commonly involve the extremities, whereas those caused by infection of preexisting aneurysms commonly affect the aorta and the femoral and popliteal arteries. Those secondary to atherosclerosis alone involve the aorta and superficial femoral arteries as well as other common atherosclerotic sites. Those secondary to catheters and drug abuse involve the brachial, radial, and, most commonly, femoral arteries.

The organisms most commonly involved in mycotic aneurysms differ, depending on the source of the organism. When bacterial endocarditis is the source, *Streptococcus* and *Staphylococcus* species prevail. *Salmonella* species, *Staphylococcus* species, and *Escherichia coli* are the most common organisms causing mycotic aneurysms secondary to bacteremia. Mycotic aneurysms secondary to direct extension of infections are predominantly caused by *Salmonella, Staphylococcus,* and *Mycobacterium* species and fungi.[89] *Staphylococcus aureus* and *E. coli* are the most common organisms seen in mycotic aneurysms secondary to trauma (all types).[91,92,94] Currently, *Staphylococcus* species are the most common pathogens causing any mycotic arterial infection; many of which are methicillin resistant *Staphylococcus aureus*.[92,95,96]

In the era preceding antibiotic drugs, most mycotic aneurysms were secondary to bacterial endocarditis and syphilis. Today, most mycotic aneurysms are secondary to trauma (including drug abuse, surgery, and arterial catheterization) and/or associated with immunosuppression in patients with chronic illnesses, diabetes, or malignancies.[92] This change is most likely due to the use of antibiotic therapy for endocarditis, the significant decrease in the prevalence of syphilis, the increasing use of diagnostic catheterization, the increase in major trauma, and widespread drug abuse. These forces have made CFA mycotic aneurysms the most common peripheral arterial mycotic aneurysm currently encountered.

Natural History

Once established, the natural course of a mycotic aneurysm is to enlarge and eventually rupture. Occasionally, spontaneous thrombosis may occur, with resolution of the septic process; however, the thrombosed aneurysm may serve as a continuing septic focus. Septic emboli arising from aneurysms are not uncommon and can lead to miliary abscesses and septic arthritis. Peripheral mycotic aneurysms are associated with a mortality ranging from 0% to 15%, likely due to their superficial location; prompt diagnosis significantly impacts prognosis.[47]

Diagnosis

Patients with mycotic aneurysms manifest a clinical spectrum of findings from acute catastrophic sepsis, to insidious, indolent infection. Most patients have some combination of fever, malaise, weight loss, chills, night sweats, pain, leukocytosis, positive blood cultures, and elevated erythrocyte sedimentation rate. A history of trauma or a recent infectious disease usually exists. Patients will have sterile blood cultures in 18% to 50% of cases.[92] When the aneurysm is superficial, as most peripheral aneurysms are, it can be palpated in the majority of patients. The aneurysm may appear bland, but more commonly shows signs of erythema, warmth, and tenderness. Particularly large aneurysms may also show skin necrosis and are at risk of imminent rupture. Petechial lesions in the skin may be seen distal to the aneurysm when embolization has occurred. Many patients have a ruptured aneurysm on presentation.

The diagnosis is often deduced by combining the history and physical examination with confirmatory laboratory tests and imaging. In some patients, the history and physical examination may be sufficient. In other patients, the diagnosis is made by a positive blood culture in a patient with an aneurysm in whom no other septic focus can be documented.

Ultrasound and CT scans can be used to visualize mycotic aneurysms (Fig. 47.5). CT scans have the advantage of being able to clearly demonstrate surrounding inflammation, fluid, or gas, a finding consistent with infection. Gallium scans and radioactively tagged white cell scans are rarely required for diagnosis but are reliably positive when utilized. Arteriography is often required for preoperative planning, and usually demonstrates a saccular aneurysm or false aneurysm as well as the quality of the proximal and distal runoff vessels (Fig. 47.6).

Treatment

The indication for treatment of a mycotic aneurysm is its presence. Antibiotic therapy, guided by culture results when available, should be used in all patients. Antibiotics alone are not sufficient, and surgical removal of the mycotic aneurysm is required in nearly all cases. Basic surgical principles dictate that all infected tissue must be removed and that adequate circulation to the extremities preserved. The availability of cryopreserved femoral-popliteal arterial segments offers an alternative conduit in the setting of infected aneurysms in these locations or in similarly sized arteries where autogenous vein is not available or is not a suitable size-match, or when extra-anatomic reconstruction is not possible or not felt to be necessary (Fig. 47.7).

Lower Extremity Mycotic Aneurysms

The femoral artery is the most frequently infected peripheral artery and the treatment of infected femoral aneurysms has evolved. Although most of these lesions are secondary to trauma or drug abuse, the same management principles apply to mycotic femoral aneurysms from other causes. Several options are available, including remote bypass followed by aneurysm resection, aneurysm resection followed by remote bypass, aneurysm resection alone, or aneurysm resection with in situ reconstruction.

The option of an obturator bypass followed by aneurysm resection usually requires the use of prosthetic material, and since most of these patients are drug addicts whose saphenous veins have been destroyed, Reddy[94] showed that this approach was associated with a 100% graft infection rate in drug addicts. However, in patients in whom vein is available, this approach is a reasonable option. Reddy and colleagues reported an amputation rate (19%) with excision and ligation. They reported that excision and ligation of only one of the three femoral arteries in the groin can be performed without limb loss, but that when the CFA is involved, thus necessitating the ligation of all three

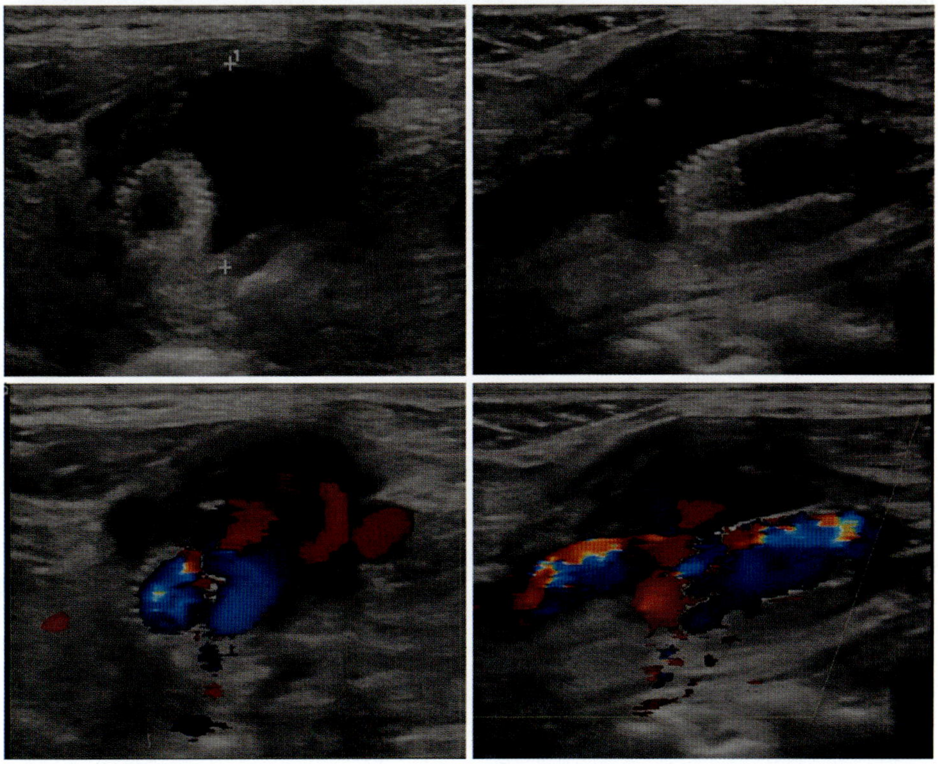

FIG 47.5 Duplex ultrasound demonstrating mycotic false aneurysm.

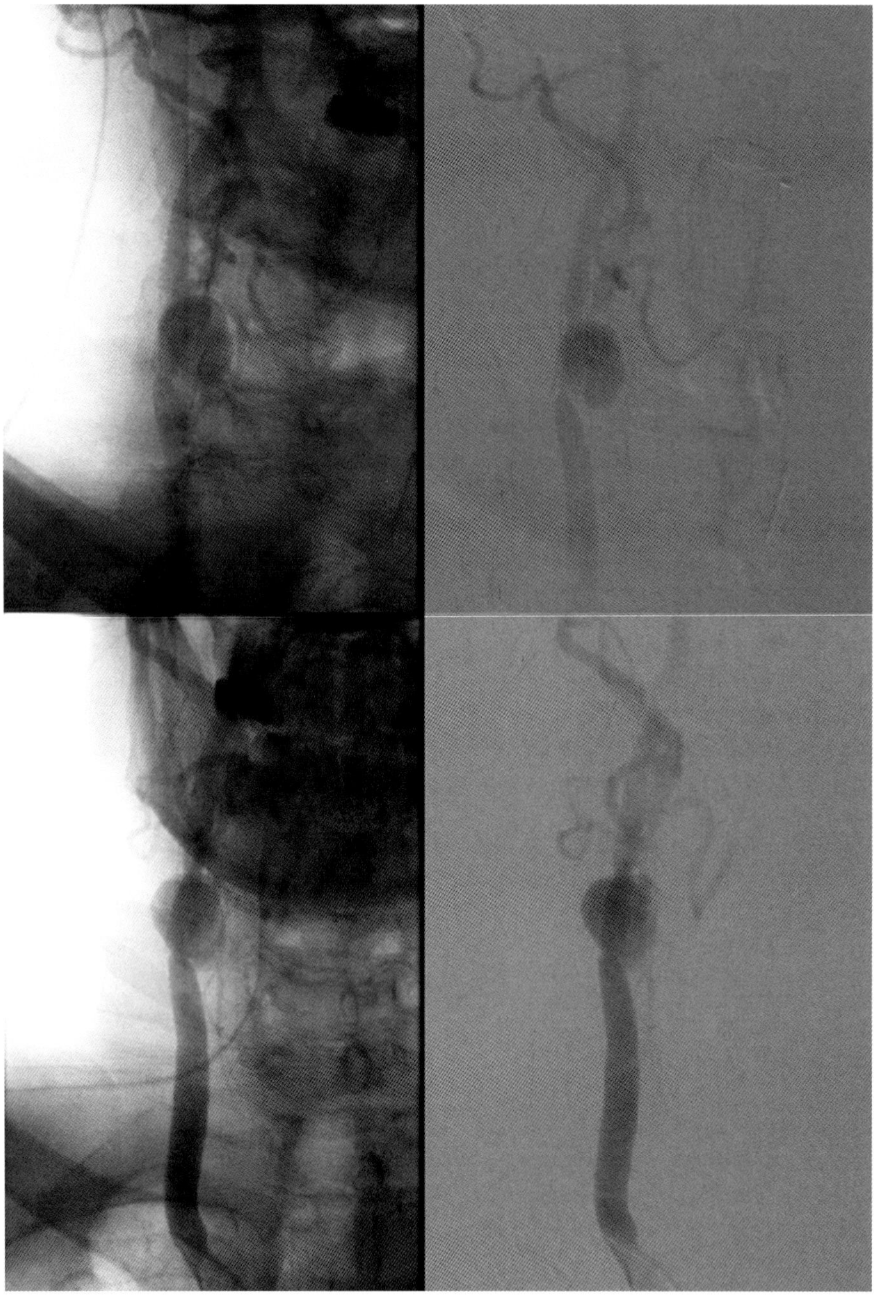

FIG 47.6 Arteriogram of a mycotic carotid artery false aneurysm

vessels, the amputation rate is high. As an alternative in these latter patients, they suggested that immediate autogenous vein reconstruction with sartorius muscle flap coverage be used when adequate debridement can be performed to control sepsis. Using this approach, they reported a 9% amputation rate without mortality. They found that even in drug addicts, satisfactory saphenous vein usually exists in the thigh for femoral artery reconstruction. Benjamin and coworkers[97] reported successful treatment of mycotic aneurysms using deep leg veins when larger-sized conduits were required.

Mycotic aneurysms involving the popliteal artery are uncommon, and few guidelines are provided in the vascular literature. In general, aneurysm excision with in situ autogenous interposition grafting or cryopreserved artery works well. Most of these patients have normal tibial artery runoff, facilitating long-term patency, and the readily available soft tissue coverage afforded by the muscles in the popliteal space facilitates healing of the surgical wound without complications. Infected aneurysms below the popliteal artery are uncommon and often times can be ligated and excised if isolated to a single tibial artery.

Extracranial Carotid Artery Mycotic Aneurysms

As noted earlier, cervical carotid aneurysms are rare, and cervical carotid mycotic aneurysms extremely rare. In 1988, Jones and Frusha[98] reviewed the English-language literature and found only 23 bacteriologically proven cases. In 1991, Jebara and colleagues[99] reported an additional four cases. When evaluating an extracranial carotid aneurysm on CTA, findings suggestive of infection include

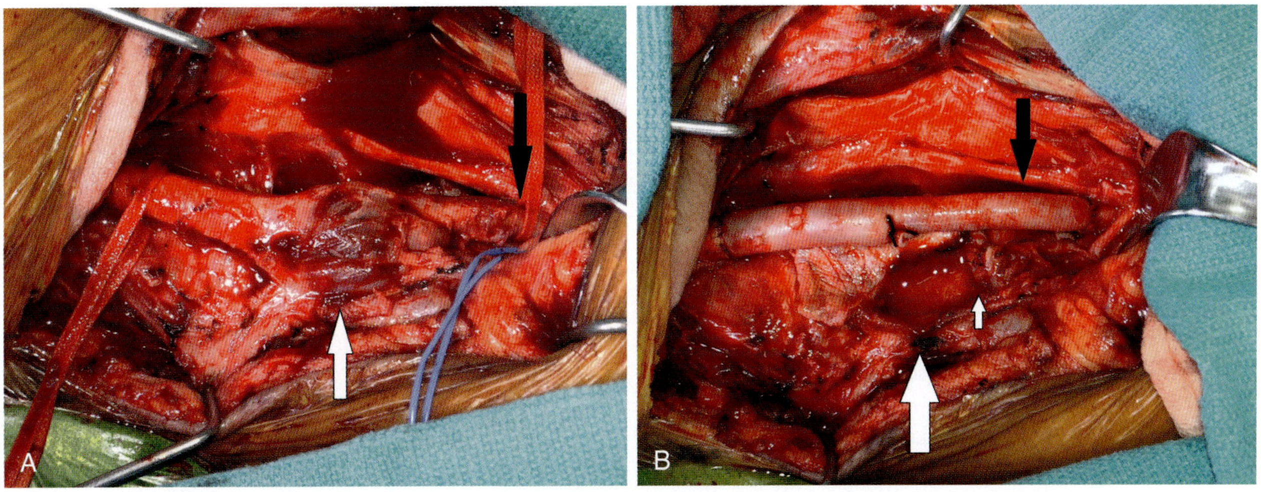

FIG 47.7 Carotid artery false aneurysm repair. (A) Thrombosed false aneurysm *(white arrow)* arising from the distal common carotid artery (*black arrow* indicates distal internal carotid). (B) Common carotid artery to internal carotid artery interposition graft *(black arrow)* with cryopreserved superficial femoral artery (*large white arrow* identifies false aneurysm cavity; *small white arrow* identifies ligated external carotid artery).

soft tissue inflammation and eccentrically configured aneurysms (saccular, multilobulated, narrow neck).[100]

Treatment of these lesions requires complete excision of the artery under antibiotic coverage and debridement of all infected tissue. Concomitant vascular reconstruction is controversial. Some authors suggest avoiding reconstruction in the setting of infection, due to the risk of graft sepsis with blowout or embolization; however, this comes with risk of neurologic morbidity and mortality.[100] Alternatively, some authors suggest in situ reconstruction with tissue debridement and use of a muscle flap. Patients may be selected for arterial ligation based on carotid stump pressure as described earlier. Intravenous antibiotics should be continued for at least 6 weeks, followed by an additional 6 weeks of oral antibiotics.[100] Anticoagulation should be continued for 3 to 6 months postoperatively when ligation is used. If ligation is not safe, reconstruction using autogenous vein is the treatment of choice. In the review by Jones and Frusha,[98] the overall mortality was 23% and the mortality was 27% in the ligation group, compared with 11% in the grafted group.

Upper Extremity Mycotic Aneurysms

Mycotic aneurysms in this area are also rare and are usually the result of trauma or drug abuse. The approach to the subclavian artery depends on the size and the distal and proximal extent of the aneurysm. Complete excision of the aneurysm may be too risky in view of the proximity of the brachial plexus and subclavian vein. Successful treatment with arterial ligation and incision and drainage of the aneurysm has been reported.[101] Proximal subclavian artery ligation usually does not require revascularization.

Axillary mycotic aneurysms are usually palpable. The management principles for subclavian mycotic aneurysms generally apply to axillary lesions as well. Axillary artery ligation may be associated with a greater risk of ischemia; however, an extraanatomic bypass may be required. This can usually be performed in separate clean tissue planes around the shoulder, using autogenous vein.

The brachial artery is the most commonly infected aneurysm of the upper limb, often associated with intravenous drug abuse, catheterization procedures, and endocarditis. Distal arm mycotic aneurysms are rare and are often encountered after arterial line cannulation.[91,92] Treatment of mycotic aneurysms in these areas follows the general guidelines for other mycotic aneurysms. Arterial ligation with aneurysm excision is often all that is required, particularly when the profunda brachial artery is patent, but occasionally autogenous revascularization in a clean plane is required.

REVIEW QUESTIONS

1. Subclavian artery aneurysms are most commonly caused by which of the following?
   a. Atherosclerosis
   b. Thoracic outlet syndrome
   c. Fibromuscular dysplasia
   d. Trauma
2. What is the most common complication of subclavian artery aneurysms?
   a. Rupture
   b. Pain secondary to nerve compression
   c. Embolization
   d. Thrombosis

3. Most carotid artery aneurysms are identified because of which of the following?
   a. Rupture of the aneurysm
   b. Mass in the neck
   c. Neurologic complications
   d. Swishing sound heard in the patient's ipsilateral ear
4. Which of the following statements is true regarding femoral and popliteal artery aneurysms?
   a. These aneurysms should be repaired only when they become very large and cause pain from adjacent nerve compression.
   b. These aneurysms are rarely associated with other peripheral aneurysms.
   c. These aneurysms are particularly dangerous because of a high incidence of distal embolization or aneurysm thrombosis.
   d. Long-term results of the surgical treatment of these aneurysms are not dependent on the degree of arterial occlusive disease distal to the aneurysm.
5. What is the most common cause of peripheral aneurysms?
   a. Atherosclerosis
   b. Infection
   c. Trauma
   d. Connective tissue disorders
6. Which of the following peripheral aneurysms is most likely to rupture?
   a. Popliteal
   b. Carotid
   c. Deep femoral
   d. Axillary
7. For a patient with ischemia secondary to thrombosis of a popliteal artery aneurysm and occlusion of the popliteal outflow tract, what is the best initial treatment?
   a. Thrombolytic therapy
   b. Thrombectomy and bypass
   c. Observation
   d. Sympathectomy
8. What is the most common cause of mycotic aneurysms?
   a. Trauma
   b. Bacterial endocarditis
   c. Direct extension of adjacent infection
   d. Food poisoning
9. Which of the following statements about popliteal aneurysms is true?
   a. They are frequently bilateral.
   b. They are commonly associated with abdominal aortic aneurysms.
   c. They rarely rupture.
   d. All of the above.
10. A 64-year-old man has a 3.4-cm-diameter left popliteal artery aneurysm. The proximal portion of the aneurysm ends 3 cm distal to the adductor tendon. There is 2.5 cm of uninvolved distal popliteal artery. He has three-vessel runoff. He is an acceptable surgical candidate. Which of the following treatments is most likely to successfully treat the aneurysm and result in no need for future treatment of the same aneurysm?
   a. Stent-graft placement
   b. Above-knee to below-knee popliteal to popliteal bypass using saphenous vein coupled with aneurysm ligation through a medial approach
   c. Posterior approach with aneurysm resection and interposition graft using either polytetrafluoroethylene or saphenous vein
   d. Above-knee to below-knee popliteal to popliteal bypass with aneurysm ligation using PTFE

BIBLIOGRAPHY

Beseth BD, Moore WS. The posterior approach for repair of popliteal artery aneurysms. *J Vasc Surg*. 2006;43(5):940–944, discussion 4–5.

Cutler BS, Darling RC. Surgical management of arteriosclerotic femoral aneurysms. *Surgery*. 1973;74(5):764–773.

Dzijan-Horn M, Langwieser N, Groha P, et al. Safety and efficacy of a potential treatment algorithm by using manual compression repair and ultrasound-guided thrombin injection for the management of iatrogenic femoral artery pseudoaneurysm in a large patient cohort. *Circ Cardiovasc Interv*. 2014;7(2):207–215.

Golchehr B, Tielliu IF, Verhoeven EL, et al. Clinical Outcome of Isolated Popliteal Artery Aneurysms Treated with a Heparin-bonded Stent Graft. *Eur J Vasc Endovasc Surg*. 2016;52(1):99–104.

Hall HA, Minc S, Babrowski T. Peripheral artery aneurysm. *Surg Clin North Am*. 2013;93(4):911–923, ix.

Lawrence PF, Harlander-Locke MP, Oderich GS, et al. The current management of isolated degenerative femoral artery aneurysms is too aggressive for their natural history. *J Vasc Surg*. 2014;59(2): 343–349.

Phair A, Hajibandeh S, Kelleher D, et al. Meta-analysis of posterior versus medial approach for popliteal artery aneurysm repair. *J Vasc Surg*. 2016.

Ravn H, Bjorck M. Popliteal artery aneurysm with acute ischemia in 229 patients. Outcome after thrombolytic and surgical therapy. *Eur J Vasc Endovasc Surg*. 2007;33(6):690–695.

von Stumm M, Teufelsbauer H, Reichenspurner H, et al. Two Decades of Endovascular Repair of Popliteal Artery Aneurysm—A Meta-analysis. *Eur J Vasc Endovasc Surg*. 2015;50(3):351–359.

Zhou W, Lin PH, Bush RL, et al. Carotid artery aneurysm: evolution of management over two decades. *J Vasc Surg*. 2006;43(3):493–496, discussion 7.

References available online at ExpertConsult.com.

CHAPTER 48

Surgical and Endovascular Management of Vascular Trauma Including Aortic Transection

Micheal T. Ayad, David L. Gillespie

The origins and development of current vascular surgical trauma care are largely based on experiences from wartime casualties and practice. Care for this segment of the population has always presented challenges for physicians to improve medical and surgical practices. Advances in limb salvage were achieved in the mobile surgical hospitals and vascular specialty centers of the Korean and Vietnam Wars. Arterial repairs and vein bypass grafting performed far forward in these wars resulted in a decrease in amputation rates from 50% with arterial ligation to 13%. In the Vietnam Vascular Registry, data was collected and analyzed to develop best practices for vascular trauma management. As such, lessons learned about the management of vascular trauma in combat and war zones were disseminated to the civilian sector.[1] In this day-and-age, civilian trauma algorithms are deeply rooted in these lessons learned from our military heritage.

The application of endovascular techniques has revolutionized the modern management of vascular trauma. A 9-year analysis of 23,105 patients in the National Trauma Data Bank demonstrated a marked increase in the use of these techniques. During this 9-year period, the prevalence of using endovascular techniques increased from 0.3% in 2002 to 9.0% in 2010. This was particularly true among blunt trauma patients (from 0.4% in 2002 to 13.2% in 2010; $P < .001$), and injuries of the internal iliac artery (from 8.0% in 2002 to 40.3% in 2010; $P < .001$), thoracic aorta (from 0.5% in 2002 to 21.9% in 2010; $P < .001$), and common/external iliac arteries (from 0.4% in 2002 to 20.4% in 2010; $P < .001$).[2]

The pivotal step in performing vascular surgery is to have control of the vessel being operated on. In open surgery, the operator needs to have proximal and distal control before any intervention is performed. In endovascular surgery, the operator needs to have a wire across the lesion before any intervention is performed. These basic tenets are the same in the management of traumatic vascular injuries but are much more challenging to achieve. The vascular trauma patient is unique due to the severe physiologic derangements secondary to massive hemorrhage and concomitant injuries. These hurdles can be compounded by limited resources, which are sometimes encountered in the battlefield or in small community hospitals.

Mean 1-year cost per patient of trauma care in our population was $75,210. On average, 58% of cost was accounted for by the index hospitalization. Total 1-year treatment cost of adult major trauma in the United States was conservatively estimated to be US$27 billion annually in 2005. In 2013, the CDC estimated the total lifetime medical and work loss costs of injuries and violence at $671 billion.[3] In both civilian and combat settings, the incidence of vascular injury is approximately 0.2% to 7% of all injured patients.[4–8] The social impact of trauma goes beyond the cost of health care for trauma victims. It extends to the lost lifetime productivity, lost wages, and the need for social support such as unemployment wages and workers compensation. Trauma is the leading cause of death in the 1- to 44-year-old age group in the United States, as a consequence of unintentional injury, assault, homicide, and suicide.[9] Iatrogenic vascular injury has also been increasing in prevalence as the number of invasive procedures increases. In fact, it has been described as high as 33% of all vascular trauma at a Level I trauma center.[10]

Hippocrates was credited with saying, "War is the only proper school for a surgeon." Vascular trauma management is no exception. As we already mentioned in the onset of this chapter, many of the trauma management paradigms used in the civilian society are extension of the experiences encountered by surgeons in combat during war. Similarities exist between civilian and military vascular trauma that allows us to extrapolate on our military experience and utilize the acquired knowledge to guide trauma management in the civilian setting. Nonetheless, it is important to point out that there are many differences between patterns of military versus civilian vascular trauma.

Among civilian victims, gunshot wounds are responsible for the majority of peripheral vascular injury, stab wounds for a smaller percentage, and the remainder is due to blunt trauma.[11,12] As such, most civilian gunshot wounds are generally due to low-velocity projectiles. This is in contradistinction to military trauma where arterial injury usually occurs in the setting of massive extremity involvement, where orthopedic fractures, large soft tissue defects, nerve injury, and vein injury are common. This pattern is seen in one-third of patients presenting with vascular injury to combat trauma-receiving centers; it can also be seen in civilian close-range shotgun blasts. The majority of military traumatic injuries are due to explosive devices (74%) with high-velocity gunshot wounds responsible for most of the remainder (17%); blunt injury is infrequent.[6,13]

Vascular trauma, whether in the civilian or military setting, most commonly causes the patient's demise due to uncontrolled hemorrhage. If the patient survives the initial physiologic insult, it can still lead to death if the lethal triad of hypothermia, coagulopathy, and acidosis sets in and takes control of the victim. Care of vascular trauma patients should first aim at hemorrhage control and managing the trauma and hemorrhagic homeostatic derangement consequences. If repair can be done in a safe and expedited fashion without further compromising the patient's homeostasis, then it should be performed. Otherwise, damage control resuscitation approach for reversal of the lethal triad and stabilizing the patient might be the best chance at survival. The principle of live to fight another day is based on immediate control rather than immediate repair. The basic tenet of damage control surgery is to stop ongoing contamination and hemorrhage, transfer the patient as rapidly as possible to an intensive resuscitative care unit, and employ all medical resources at hand to halt the progression of the lethal triad.

In order to address concerns that damage control resuscitation (DCR) might have a deleterious effect on vascular reconstructions, Fox and colleagues performed a case-control study of battlefield casualties who underwent vascular repair and compared patients treated by a rigorous DCR protocol versus conventional crystalloid and nonmatched erythrocyte resuscitation. There was no worse outcome among patients when the coagulopathy was treated. The author's admonition was to "fix the injury, fix it well, and trust that your patient doesn't need to be coagulopathic for the graft to work."[14] Damage control options for vascular trauma include tourniquet use, temporary vascular shunting (TVS), ligation, or balloon tamponade.[15–18] None of these technique has proven superior to the others in temporizing vascular injury. Taken as a whole, however, damage control for major trauma is associated with improved physiology, increased limb salvage, and decreased mortality.[14,15,19,20]

DIAGNOSING VASCULAR TRAUMA

Initial Assessment

Initial management of vascular trauma should follow the guidelines of advanced Trauma Life Support (ATLS) with attention to the airway, ventilation, external hemorrhage control, and restoring circulating blood volume. Once the initial survey of the trauma patient is complete, the secondary and tertiary assessment of the trauma patient with a detailed history and physical exam followed by the necessary diagnostic imaging.

Trauma victims usually have multisystem injuries. Before embarking on a complex and potentially lengthy vascular repair, the provider must ensure there are no missed and more life threatening injuries which need to be addressed first. Unrecognized severe intraabdominal or intracranial injuries can lead to disastrous outcomes if not addressed early.

Hard signs, such as active arterial hemorrhage, expanding hematoma, loss of distal pulse, signs of ischemia, and a bruit or thrill are highly suggestive of arterial injury. Profound signs of acute ischemia include the classic 6 "Ps": paresthesia, paralysis, pulselessness, pain, pallor, and poikilothermia. With such findings, no diagnostic imaging is usually required before surgical exploration of extremity vessels. Soft signs raise the suspicion of arterial injury and include moderate-sized hematoma, history of significant blood loss or hypotension at the prehospital scene, diminished distal pulses, and ipsilateral neurologic deficits. Soft signs warrant additional diagnostic imaging (Table 48.1).

TABLE 48.1 Clinical Manifestations and Signs of Arterial Injury

Hard Signs[a]	Soft Signs[a]
• Arterial bleeding	• History of prehospital blood loss
• Loss of pulse	• Diminished pulse
• Expanding hematoma	• Moderate hematoma
• Bruit or thrill	• Proximity to large vessel or bony injury
• Signs of ischemia (6 Ps[b])	• Ipsilateral neurologic deficit

[a]Hard signs require surgical exploration and control while soft signs provide time for further diagnostic workup.
[b]Paresthesia, paralysis, pulselessness, pain, pallor, and poikilothermia.

Diagnostic Studies

Diagnostic evaluation of the trauma patient starts with the primary survey on presentation. An unstable patient would need to go directly to the OR for either operative repair or damage control surgery. Once the primary and secondary surveys have been completed, further investigation would assist in localizing the injury if not obvious. Ankle-brachial index (ABI) is a diagnostic exam that is instrumental in the management of lower-extremity trauma patient and is feasible to perform at bedside. An ABI of <0.9 may suggest arterial injury and need for further diagnostic imaging.[6] A good H&P and examination of the uninjured contralateral limb is paramount to appropriately interpret the ABI exam. Older patients with peripheral arterial disease may present with diminished ABIs, confounding the exam. In general, young healthy patients with lower extremity injuries in proximity to major vascular structures but with an ipsilateral ABI of greater than 0.9 can be observed.

Duplex Ultrasonography

In the stable trauma patient without moderate to severe soft tissue damage, an ultrasonography evaluation might provide valuable information to the presence or absence of blood flow, intimal flap, vessel transection, and vessel thrombosis. Albeit operator-dependent, ultrasound imaging provides high quality vascular images. This allows assessments, which are reproducible low cost, and few if any side effects. This modality is particularly helpful in extremity trauma. Wani and colleagues showed that Doppler had a sensitivity of 94% and specificity of 82.5% in diagnosis of vascular injury.[21]

Computer Tomography

CAT scans have become a main stay diagnostic modality in many if not all trauma centers and emergency departments. Many trauma victims will undergo CAT scan evaluation of various body parts, depending on the nature of the injury. CT angiography is so sensitive and specific to detecting and localizing vascular injuries that it has become the gold standard. In their meta-analysis of 11 studies, Jens and colleagues estimated the sensitivity and specificity of CTA were 96.2% (95% CI 93.5% to 97.8%) and 99.2% (95% CI 96.8% to 99.8%), respectively.[22]

In patients where extremity vascular injury is suspected by mechanism or physical findings, angiography has been the gold standard diagnostic test. However, new research is suggesting that multislice (32 or 64) CT angiography may have sufficient sensitivity to detect these injuries. A prospective study of 21 patients with potential extremity vascular injuries, primarily due to gunshot wounds, and abnormal ankle brachial indices underwent CT angiography followed by either conventional angiography or operative exploration. CTA had 100% sensitivity for clinically relevant findings. Fifty percent of patients had concomitant orthopedic injuries as well.[163] Vascular surgeons at Walter Reed Army Medical Center evaluated the use of CTA to detect vascular injuries and found that it performed well even in the presence of metallic fragments or external fixators.[164]

Magnetic Resonance Imaging

MRI and MRA long acquisition time has been the limiting factor in utilizing these modalities in the setting of acute trauma. Other shortcomings include the high cost, noncompatibility in trauma patients with potential for metallic fragments, whether in civilian or military settings from gunshot wounds, improvised explosive devices, and so on. There is also the potential for nephrogenic systemic fibrosis in patients with advanced renal insufficiency.

Angiography

Historically speaking, angiography has always been the gold standard for diagnosing vascular injury. In this day and age, high resolution, multidetector CT angiography had largely replaced angiography for diagnostic purposes, as it provides similar quality imaging while bypassing the risk of the invasive nature of angiography. Endovascular techniques are largely reserved nowadays for intervention. Nonetheless, it remains as another diagnostic modality in the armamentarium of the vascular surgeon or interventionalist.

BASIC TENETS OF OPEN MANAGEMENT OF VASCULAR TRAUMA

As mentioned earlier in the chapter, once operative repair is deemed necessary, basic principles for management of vascular surgery apply irrespective of types and location of injury. Before exploring the injured vessel, proximal and distal control must be obtained. Vessel control can be obtained by various methods, such as vascular tapes or loops, vascular clamps, manual direct pressure with a finger or sponge stick, or balloon occlusive devices. Debridement of the injured segment of vessel is the initial step in vascular repair. Damaged intima, if unattended to, increases the risk of postrepair thrombosis significantly. Resection and debridement of the vessel might need to be extended beyond the site of obvious injury to include the total zone of damaged artery. External examination of the artery alone might not permit proper assessment of the extent of injury. If a simple laceration of large vessels is encountered, lateral suture repair can suffice as long as the vessel is large enough and the laceration is less than 50% of the circumference. Larger lacerations (over 50% of the vessel diameter) or smaller vessels may require a patch angioplasty to prevent stenosis. Autogenous vein is the preferred patch material. Also, segmental resection with an end-to-end anastomosis can be performed for more complex injuries spanning a distance of less than or equal to 1 cm. The vessel ends should be spatulated to avoid anastomotic stricture. The goal of the repair is to produce a tension-free anastomotic repair. Generally, 3 cm of artery need to be mobilized for every 1 cm resected. For injuries greater than 1 cm in length, an interposition graft is usually required. Ideally, the contralateral saphenous vein, if available, should serve as the conduit of choice. The ipsilateral saphenous vein should not be sacrificed if there is any concern for concomitant ipsilateral venous injury, as it is an important collateral venous return pathway. If the autogenous vein is unavailable, prosthetic graft is an alternative, and polytetraflouroethylene (PTFE) is most commonly used. In multiply injured extremities, finding adequate conduit may be challenging. PTFE provides a rapidly accessible option and can be used if the autologous vein is not available or if the patient will not tolerate a long vein harvest; this latter scenario may also argue for TVS. One major concern with prosthetic graft is its use in infected surgical beds. Vertrees and colleagues demonstrated that in patients with limited autologous vein, prosthetic graft can be used temporarily in contaminated wounds in multiple anatomic locations with acceptable short-term patency and an opportunity for later revision.[122]

CERVICAL VASCULAR INJURY

Cervical trauma poses a diagnostic and therapeutic dilemma, as the neck houses numerous vital structures in a very limited space. Anatomically, this spans the area from the base of the skull to the thoracic outlet. The aerodigestive tract, brachial plexus, and nerves, as well as the carotid sheath, subclavian, and vertebral vessels, are all at risk.

Blunt Cervical Vascular Trauma

During the 1990s, work from trauma groups in Memphis and Denver uncovered a much larger incidence of this type of injury that had been previously suspected. One of the initial reports evaluated 20,349 trauma admissions at the Presley Regional Trauma Center; 67 patients (0.33%) were found to have 87 blunt cerebrovascular injury (BCVI).[23] In a pilot study of all patients undergoing post-injury thoracic aortograms performed at the University of Colorado, 3.5% of patients were found to have a documented BCVI, only half of whom manifested symptoms.[24] Disconcerted by these findings, the trauma surgeons in Denver undertook a prospective study in 249 patients, 40 with symptoms consistent with BCVI and 209 with high-risk features (Table 48.2).[25] This report documented BCVI in 28 (70%) of the symptomatic patients and 57 (27%) of the asymptomatic patients. Injuries included 65 isolated carotid artery injuries, 10 isolated vertebral artery injuries, and 10 combined carotid and vertebral artery injuries.[25] In another report from the same year, their overall incidence was reported at 0.38% of trauma admissions, but was 1.07% among admissions during the time they performed aggressive screening.[26] Contemporary estimates of BCVI incidence is 0.4% to 1.0% of blunt trauma admissions.[27,28] The mechanism of the majority of these injuries is motor vehicle crash, reported in 45% to 82% of series, followed by pedestrian trauma (12%), motorcycle crash (11%), falls (9% to 10%), and assaults (5% to 6%).[23,25] Nowadays BCVI is estimated to occur in 3% to 10% of blunt trauma victims, with a stroke rate up to 25%. Guidelines

TABLE 48.2 Criteria for Screening for Blunt Cerebrovascular Injury

Hard Signs of BCVI	Signs Suggestive of Occult BCVI
Hemorrhage from the mouth, ears, nose, or wounds	Severe cervical hyperextension and rotation or hyperflexion if associated with displaced midface or complex mandibular fracture or closed head injury consistent with diffuse axonal injury
Expanding cervical hematoma	Near hanging resulting in anoxic brain injury
Cervical bruit in a patient <50 years old	Seat belt abrasion or other soft tissue injury of the anterior neck resulting in significant swelling or altered mental status
Evidence of cerebral infarction on computed tomography scan	Basilar skull fracture
Unexplained or incongruous neurologic deficit, transient ischemic attack, amaurosis fugax, or Horner syndrome	Cervical vertebral body fracture

BCVI, Blunt cerebrovascular injury.

TABLE 48.3 Grading Scale for Blunt Carotid Injury

Injury Grade	Description
I	Luminal irregularity or dissection with <25% luminal narrowing
II	Dissection or intramural hematoma with ≥25% luminal narrowing, intramural thrombus, or raised intimal flap
III	Pseudoaneurysm
IV	Occlusion
V	Transection with free extravasation

for BCVI screening are based on clinical and radiographic findings, as noted in Table 48.2.[29,30]

The grading system proposed by the Denver group in 1999 is still in use today to guide the management of BCVI (Table 48.3).[25] This system correlates well with mortality and stroke risk, and has been used as the basis for treatment recommendations. In a recent report, the overall stroke risk for patients with BCVI was 14% and the in-hospital mortality was 10%.[28] Another report cited a 26% in-hospital mortality. Among those who survived to discharge, only 31% were discharged home, whereas 43% were transferred to another inpatient facility such as rehabilitation or skilled nursing.[31] By injury grade, mortality was 0 % to 33% for grade I to III lesions, 11% to 60% for grade IV, and 100% for grade V; stroke risk was 3% for grade I, 11% for grade II, 33% for grade III, 44% for grade IV, and 100% for grade V.[32]

Management of Blunt Cervical Vascular Injury

There are no level I evidence to guide management recommendations. EAST (Eastern Association for the Surgery of Trauma) statement recommends diagnostic evaluation should be pursued for the screening and diagnosing of DCVI based on level II evidence in patients presenting with any neurologic abnormality that is unexplained by an already diagnosed injury; blunt trauma patients presenting with epistaxis from a suspected arterial source after trauma should be evaluated for BCVI. EAST also recommends considering diagnostic evaluation based on level III evidence in asymptomatic patients with significant blunt head trauma are at significantly increased risk for BCVI, and screening should be considered.[33] Risk factors are as follows:

- Glasgow Coma Scale score ≤8
- Petrous bone fracture
- Diffuse axonal injury
- Cervical spine fractures particularly those with
  - Fracture of C1 to C3 and
  - Fracture through the foramen transversarium
- Cervical spine fracture with subluxation or rotational component
- Lefort II or III facial fractures

Based on level II evidence, diagnostic four-vessel cerebral angiography (FVCA) remains the gold standard for the diagnosis of BCVI. Nonetheless, multislice (eight or greater), multidetector CTA has a similar rate of detection for BCVI when compared with historic control rates of diagnosis with FVCA and may be considered as a screening modality in place of FVCA.

Once diagnosed, management of BCVI is based on the grade of injury sustained.[33] Based on level II evidence, in the absence of contraindications, grade I and II injuries are treated with antithrombotic agents. Based on level III evidence, either antiplatelet or anticoagulation therapy can be used with seemingly similar outcomes. If anticoagulation is selected for treatment, the infusion should be started without a bolus and continued till an oral agent is started and therapeutic levels are achieved. Therapy for 3 to 6 months is recommended. In grade III injuries, pseudoaneurysms rarely resolve with observation or heparinization, and invasive therapy (open or endovascular approach) should be considered. If carotid stents are placed without subsequent antiplatelet therapy, a high rate of thrombosis was noted in this population.[34] If the patient is presenting with early neurologic deficit and an anatomically accessible carotid lesion, operative (open or endovascular) repair should be considered to restore flow. Grades IV and V are highly morbid and lethal injuries. Some authors feel that outcomes are generally independent of treatment efforts, although others have suggested decreased stroke risk with heparin therapy for grade IV lesions.[26] Interestingly, one center reported treating occlusion of the internal carotid artery in asymptomatic patients after penetrating trauma with embolization to prevent an occluded artery "reopening" and providing a substrate for distal embolization after vasospasm dissipates.[35] Grade V transections require obtaining proximal and distal control, which can be extremely challenging depending on the location of the injury. Outcomes are miserable; one series reported 100% mortality from this injury.[26]

Penetrating Cervical Vascular Trauma

Penetrating cervical injuries are inherently differently than BCVI, due to differences in pathophysiology, diagnosis, treatment, and outcomes. The mechanism of injury is different between military and civilian population. In a series of 63 combat-trauma-related penetrating cervical injuries, 33 (53%) had positive findings. A total of 25 patients were explored in-theater, and eight had findings detected after evacuation to the United States and underwent repair in a delayed fashion. Blast fragments were responsible for the majority of these wounds (79%), with high-velocity gunshot wounds being responsible for the remainder.[36] This incidence did not change much over the years. Brennan and colleagues reported 98% of these neck injuries were due to high-velocity projectiles.[37] In civilian trauma, the most common mechanism is gunshot wounds. In a series of 38 civilian gunshot wounds to the internal carotid artery (ICA), 89% of patients had symptoms including neck hematoma (84%), active hemorrhage (32%), and neurologic deficits (26%).[38] The current mortality rate in civilians with penetrating neck injuries ranges from 3% to 6%.[39–40]

Traditionally, the cervical area was divided into three zones progressing from caudal to cephalad. This is based on the classification proposed by Monson and colleagues in 1969.[41]

Zone I extends from the thoracic outlet to the cricoid cartilage; Zone II extends from cricoid cartilage to the angle of the mandible; and Zone III extends from angle of the mandible to the base of the skull. Knowledge of vascular structures that commonly traverse each zone is paramount as initial triage and management of the cervical trauma is dependent on the zone and type of injury incurred (Table 48.4).

In a hemodynamically stable patient, diagnostic evaluation would be considered. Sclafani and colleagues found that the presence of nearby fragments decreased the sensitivity of this modality in military trauma situations and recommended checking a plain film first if MDCT-A is planned.[36] The gold standard remains FVCA. In civilian trauma, the current practice trend is to rely on MD-CTA evaluation and resort to angiography if intervention in planned or if the CTA images are suboptimal. Duplex examination is often limited by the wound, dressing, or injuries to the cervical spine.

TABLE 48.4 Three Zones of the Cervical Region and the Vascular Structures in Each Zone

Zone I: Thoracic Outlet to Cricoid Cartilage	Zone II: Cricoid Cartilage to Angle of Mandible	Zone III: Angle of Mandible to Base of Skull
• Common carotid artery • Innominate artery (on the right) • Subclavian artery and vein • Internal jugular vein • Aortic arch • Innominate vein • Thoracic duct (on the left)	• Common, external, and internal carotid artery • Vertebral artery (V1 and V2 segments) • Internal jugular vein	• Internal and external carotid artery • Vertebral artery (V3 and V4 segments) • Internal jugular vein

Hemodynamic instability would mandate immediate exploration in the operating room regardless of the zone of injury without further imaging beyond cervical plain films. In this day and age, endovascular techniques would provide the advantage of obtaining further diagnostic imaging intraoperatively, with the ability of vascular control and possibly intervention. This is particularly important for vascular injury in Zones I and III where anatomical restraints makes it difficult to obtain vascular control and intervention.

Approach for Open Surgical Exposure by Cervical Zone

Zone I. Proximal control is obtained via a median sternotomy incision with extension of the incision on to the neck as necessary. The aortic arch, innominate, and left common carotid artery can be controlled through this incision. If injury is suspected to the left proximal subclavian artery, a second or third left intercostal space anterolateral thoracotomy would be the preferred approach for control and intervention.

Zone II. A cervical incision along the anterior border of the sternocleidomastoid muscle is required for Zone II injury (a generous version of a carotid endarterectomy incision). If the bleeding is then noted to be coming from a more proximal source, then the cervical incision can be extended into a median sternotomy. If bilateral cervical vascular injuries are present, either a transverse Kocher incision or bilateral cervical incisions will gain exposure to both carotid sheathes. If the arterial injury is known to involve only the left subclavian artery, a supraclavicular incision can be utilized for exposure of the mid to distal left subclavian artery. An infraclavicular incision can be utilized for exposure of the distal right and left subclavian arteries and the proximal axillary arteries.

Zone III. For Zone III arterial injury, subluxation or resection of the angle of the mandible and resection of the posterior belly of the digastric muscle may be needed. In this zone, control of the distal internal carotid artery is particular difficult due to the anatomic constraints. Other methods to gain distal control are balloon occlusive devices with access through the common carotid artery or site of injury. Due to the difficulty in exposure and control of Zone III injuries, endovascular approach is the preferred option when possible.

Management of Penetrating Cervical Vascular Injury

There are several damage control options available in the cervical region. Rapid insertion of a balloon catheter such as a Foley into the wound tract, inflation, and outward traction may provide tamponade and temporize bleeding. In Zone III, exposure is generally difficult and the ICA may be difficult to compress. One option is to perform an arteriotomy on the common carotid after controlling it with vessel loops, insert a number 3 or 4 Fogarty embolectomy catheter, and advance and inflate in a serial fashion until bleeding from the distal ICA abates. This may also be done under angiographic guidance if the patient is in the fluoroscopy suite. An additional advantage of intramural balloon occlusion is that a determination of patient tolerance to ligation can be determined; if the patient manifests a focal neurologic deficit with occlusion, some form of repair should be attempted if at all possible. Finally, for resistant bleeding high in Zone III, packing of the carotid canal with bone wax may allow tamponade for life-saving purposes.[35,42] After hemostasis is achieved with a damage control strategy, the options include formal high cervical exploration for repair or ligation; arteriographic embolization or/and stenting; or 48 hour balloon occlusion. The Fogarty balloon is filled with contrast and the patient is monitored for signs of cerebral ischemia. If there is no sign of ischemia, the balloon remains in place until 48 to 72 hours postplacement, at which time it is deflated and removed. The patient should be imaged with a crossover angiogram to rule out a pseudoaneurysm above the occlusion. If the patient manifests signs of ischemia, a bypass from the cervical ICA to the petrous ICA is necessary and will require the assistance of a neurosurgeon.[43]

The types of injuries that can be present with penetrating trauma are very similar in type and recommended treatment to those for BCVI, although major wall disruption is much more likely. For intramural hematomas, intimal defects, or dissection with preserved distal flow, treatment similar to grades I and II BCVI is appropriate—namely heparinization. Stenting may be appropriate to tack down the intima for major dissections. Patients should undergo repeat imaging in 1 to 2 weeks. Pseudoaneurysm with contrast extravasation should be either observed (for small aneurysms) or stented with or without coil embolization. According to Feliciano, heparin is risky in this situation given the possibility of rupture.[42] Antiplatelet therapy should be used if a stent is placed, however. For occlusions, anticoagulation is recommended to prevent distal propagation or embolization. As previously mentioned, Sclafani and colleagues recommend embolization of the thrombosed ICA.[35] Finally, carotid-jugular arteriovenous fistulae may be asymptomatic if small, but if sufficiently large may produce high-output heart failure or coma secondary to elevated intracranial pressure. Treatment is with operative repair for lesions in Zone II and embolization in Zone III.[35,42]

There has historically been controversy regarding the surgical management of the patient with a cervical vascular wound and a neurologic deficit, with concern that revascularization would convert an area of ischemia into hemorrhage. This issue was addressed in an article in 1978 by Liekweg and Greenfield. Among noncomatose patients, 85% of patients with neurologic deficits who are revascularized have positive outcomes versus 50% of those ligated ($P < .05$). However, among comatose patients, favorable outcome with repair was seen in 27% versus 25% of patients undergoing ligation ($P = \text{NS}$).[44] Current practice is to revascularize all patients with penetrating injury regardless of neurologic deficits except for coma. Patients with GCS less than 8 not related to hypovolemia, hypothermia, or intoxication are likely to have an adverse outcome regardless of management. If the presentation is delayed more than 3 to 4 hours postinjury, a CT scan should be obtained; if there an ischemic stroke is present, revascularization is contraindicated, as this may convert to a hemorrhagic infarct.[42]

Surgical options include ligation, primary repair, bypass graft with autogenous vein or prosthetic graft, patch graft, or external carotid to internal (Figs. 48.1 and 48.2) for injuries near the carotid bulb. As previously mentioned, Liekweg and colleagues demonstrated improved outcomes for revascularization over ligation for noncomatose patients. For comatose patients, they recommend repair only if there is evidence of prograde flow.[44] If bypass grafting is performed, PTFE is appropriate for common carotid injuries; autogenous vein should be used for ICA repairs, given the improved patency rates.[42] As always, prosthetic grafts should be avoided if possible in contaminated wounds.[36] If surgical repair is performed, a careful search for injury to other structures, especially the aerodigestive tract. If such an injury is encountered, in addition to repairing it appropriately, the vascular suture line should be isolated by means of interposition of vascularized tissue. The sternocleidomastoid muscle can be detached from its sternal head and rotated to cover the repair. Nonoperative therapy options include angioplasty to tack down intimal flaps and coil embolization and stents for pseudoaneurysms. In patients where observation is selected as the treatment plan, repeat imaging is necessary to ensure the resolution of the lesion. In the series by Fox, vertebral artery occlusions were safely observed.[37]

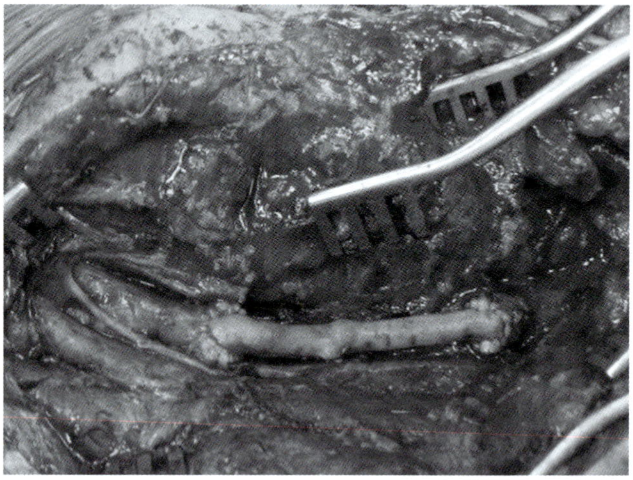

FIG 48.1 Repair of a penetrating carotid injury with autogenous vein.

THORACIC VASCULAR INJURY

Trauma victims sustaining thoracic vascular trauma are generally divided into three categories. The first group dies immediately at the scene of trauma due to rapid exsanguination. The second group becomes unstable en route to medical care, and the majority of this group (>96%) die secondary to multisystem trauma. The third group represents those who survive the initial trauma and remain relatively stable till their arrival to a medical care; their chance of survival goes up substantially to approximately 70% to 95%, with deaths in this group often being secondary to neurologic injury.[45]

On presentation at the trauma bay, there are several findings, which should raise the clinician's index of suspicion for a thoracic vascular injury. These include hypotension, upper extremity hypertension, intermittent paralysis or focal neurologic findings, inequality of blood pressure or pulses between extremities, external evidence of chest trauma, an expanding hematoma at the thoracic outlet, an intrascapular murmur, a palpable fracture of

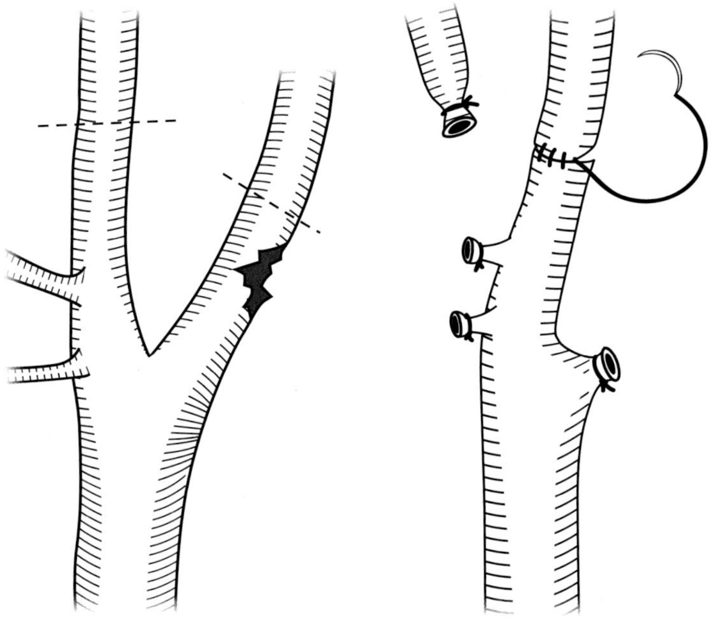

FIG 48.2 External to internal carotid artery bypass. The proximal internal and distal external carotid arteries are ligated and the proximal external carotid artery is swung over and anastomosed to the internal carotid artery.

the sternum or the thoracic spine, or a left-sided flail chest.[45] If the patient is suspected of having a hemothorax based on physical exam and chest x-ray, we recommend placing a 36 to 40 French chest tube in, as a large bore chest tube might serve better in draining a hemothorax without clotting which can happen with a smaller (e.g., 20 French) chest tube. Once chest tubes are placed as indicated, output greater than 1500 mL initially or ongoing hemorrhage at or over 200 to 250 mL/h are indications for thoracotomy.

Initially, care for these patients should be no different than any other trauma patients following the guidelines of Advanced Trauma Life Support (ATLS) protocol. The one lesson to keep in mind in these patients is that fluid resuscitation should be minimized for several reasons. Permissive hypotension will help stabilize early soft platelet plugs. Any patients presenting with military antishock trousers (MAST) in place and the suspicion of a proximal vascular injury should have them removed immediately, as this is effectively a "distal cross-clamp" and can lead to instability of clots and worsened bleeding.[63] If there is blunt injury, aggressive prevention of hypotension helps avoid propagation of the injury. Finally, concomitant pulmonary contusions or other injuries are commonly associated with thoracic vascular injury, and minimizing fluid resuscitation can avoid iatrogenic worsening of respiratory status.

Traditional open repair, while effective in the long-term, is associated with periprocedural mortality between 10% and 20%, along with a 5% risk of stroke and up to a 5% risk of spinal cord ischemia. The advent of endovascular stent-graft repair has allowed single centers to cut periprocedural mortality in half and decrease the risk of major neurologic events to less than 2%.[46]

Blunt Thoracic Aortic Injury

Historically, aortic injury (predominantly located at the isthmus) is the second most common cause of death in blunt trauma.[47] Despite the advances in the management of these patient, these injuries remain the second most lethal condition in blunt trauma patients, after head trauma.[48] Parmley and colleagues first described thoracic blunt aortic injury in his series in 1958. He advocated for urgent surgical intervention in these patients due to the high mortality rate in his series, a 61% mortality rate at 7 days.[49] Operative mortality has historically ranged from 15% to 28%,[50] and paraplegia has complicated nearly 9% of cases[47] prior to the advent of alternative treatment modalities. In Parmley's initial report, 57% of cases of BAI were secondary to automobile crashes and 16% were due to airplane crashes. This remains true today; more than 80% of BAI is due to automobile accidents.[51]

On plain film chest radiography, findings associated with blunt aortic injury vary dramatically. Most commonly, there is a widened mediastinum, seen in 85% of cases. Other findings include an indistinct aortic knob (24%), a left pleural effusion (19%), an apical cap (19%); uncommon findings include fracture of the first or second rib, tracheal deviation, a depressed left bronchus, and nasogastric tube deviation. A completely negative film is seen, however, in 7% of patients.[47] Historically, aortography was the most common diagnostic modality, with transesophageal echocardiography being a distant second. However, both of these modalities have been supplanted by MDCTA in the updated report by the American Association for the Surgery of Trauma multicenter trial (AAST), known as the AAST II study. Aortography decreased from 87% to 8% of cases, echocardiography

TABLE 48.5 Grading System Used for Assessing Thoracic Blunt Aortic Injury

Injury Grade	Description
I	Intimal tear
II	Intramural hematoma
III	Pseudoaneurysm
IV	Rupture

from 12% to 1%, with CT angiography increasing from 35% to 93% of cases.[71] MDCTA now stands as the modern gold-standard diagnostic modality for BAI.[52]

Table 48.5 reflects the currently accepted grading system of blunt thoracic aortic injury, which was adopted by the SVS in their statement regarding clinical practice guidelines for thoracic BAI management.[53]

BOX 48.1 Recommended Indications for Selective Left Subclavian Artery Revascularization During TEVAR With Left Subclavian Artery Origin Coverage

- Presence of a patent left internal mammary artery to coronary artery bypass graft
- Termination of the left vertebral artery at the posterior inferior cerebellar artery or other discontinuity of the vertebrobasilar collaterals
- Absent or diminutive or occluded right vertebral artery
- A functioning arteriovenous shunt in the left arm
- Prior infrarenal aortic repair with ligation of lumbar and middle sacral arteries
- Planned long-segment (≥20 cm) coverage of the descending thoracic aorta where critical intercostal arteries originate,
- Hypogastric artery occlusion
- Presence of early aneurysmal changes that may require subsequent therapy involving the distal thoracic aorta

TEVAR, Thoracic endovascular aortic repair.

Management of Blunt Thoracic Aortic Injury

Modern treatment strategies of BAI follow three principles. The first is aggressive pharmacologic blood pressure control, the second is appropriate selection and prioritization of repair, and the final is the utilization of endovascular techniques in an increasingly broad set of indications.

Antihypertensive therapy has been shown to decrease the rate of in-hospital aortic rupture from 12% to less than 2%.[47,54] Intravenous esmolol or labetalol is used to titrate systolic blood pressure to approximately 100 mm Hg with a relative bradycardia. Nitroprusside can be added if additional blood pressure control is needed. It is important to keep in mind that these patients frequently suffer from multisystem trauma; thus their management has to be balanced between all their organ-systems as not to deteriorate one while trying to save the other. Patients with more significant injuries should undergo repair, but their intervention can be delayed if aggressive antihypertensive therapy is instituted. Hemmila and colleagues showed that surgical delays beyond 16 hours did not increase mortality if a strict antihypertensive regimen was followed, but the price was increased ICU and ventilator days.[54] Prioritization of repair requires a balancing of the degree of injury, the risk of rupture, the ability to aggressively control blood pressure, and the risk to the patient of an intervention.

The clinical practice guidelines published by the Society of Vascular Surgery (SVS) are based on a systematic review from 139 studies, which included 7768 patients. The mortality rate was significantly lower in patients who underwent endovascular repair, followed by open repair, and nonoperative management (9%, 19%, and 46%, respectively, $P < .01$). Based on the overall very low quality of evidence (grade 2, level C), the SVS committee suggests that thoracic endovascular aortic repair (TEVAR) of thoracic aortic transection is associated with decreased risk of spinal cord ischemia, renal injury, graft, and systemic infections, as well as better survival compared with open repair or nonoperative management. The committee also recommended operative repair for all but grade I blunt thoracic aortic injuries. These can be followed with serial imaging. The SVS committee's majority opinion suggests urgent repair after stabilization of other injuries and selective versus routine revascularization in cases of left subclavian artery coverage (Box 48.1). Spinal drainage is not routinely required in these cases.[53]

Descending thoracic aortic open repair (DTAR) of BAI is still needed in some cases. Historically, a rapid clamp and sew repair has been promoted as the most straightforward repair. If open surgical approach is utilized for aortic repair, the thoracic aorta is approached through a postereolateral thoracotomy incision in the fourth intercostal space. Proximally, the arch can be clamped between the left common carotid and the left subclavian arteries. Distally, the descending thoracic aorta is controlled just distal to the level of the traumatic injury. The repair can be achieved with direct suturing or graft interposition. Some of the major drawbacks for this approach are the need for systemic anticoagulation in a patient population with multisystem injuries, and the need for single lung ventilation in patients who usually have associating pulmonary contusions. Also, multivariate analysis of risk factors for paraplegia found cross-clamp times greater than 30 minutes and the clamp and sew technique to be independently predictive of paraplegia postoperatively.[47] One group proposes the following principles to avoid this dreaded complication: preservation of intercostal vessels interoperatively when possible, avoidance of clamp and sew technique, use of permissive hypertension postoperatively to improve spinal blood flow, and the use of spinal drains only in highly selected patients.[55]

Penetrating Thoracic Aortic and Great Vessels Injury

The most common mechanism of injury to thoracic great vessels is penetrating trauma, responsible for 90% of injuries. In a series of 3823 gunshot wounds or stab wounds to the chest or abdomen, the aorta was injured in 1.6%. Most of these injuries were due to gunshot wounds (69%), with stab wounds (18%) and shotgun wounds (12%) making up the remainder of penetrating thoracic injuries. Whereas thoracic aortic injury was less common than abdominal aortic injury (28% vs. 72%), it was associated with a decreased likelihood of having a recordable blood pressure (27% vs. 71%), increased need for emergency department thoracotomy (EDT, 77% vs. 21%), and decreased survival (8% vs. 24%). Most patients with penetrating injury to the thoracic aorta arrived in shock (83%), with half of these patients demonstrating no recordable blood pressure. Mortality was 81% overall in this cohort, with gunshot wounds having a higher associated mortality (88%) than stab wounds (65%). Predictors of mortality in this series were gunshot wounds, injury to the thoracic aorta as opposed to the abdominal aorta, an unrecordable blood pressure on admission, and the need for an EDT. While concomitant injury to other structures occurred in 81% of patients, most commonly the lung, there was no association with mortality.[56] A recent retrospective analysis of more than 3000 patients registered in the National Trauma Data Bank reported concomitant head injury in 31%, as well as major abdominal (29%) and pelvic injuries (15%).[57]

Plain film radiography in these patients may reveal findings suggestive of great vessel injury, such as mediastinal widening, a foreign body out of focus with other structures indicating possible intracardiac location, a foreign body in close proximity to vascular structures, a confusing missile trajectory suggesting possible missile embolism, or a missile that is altogether missing, which suggests possible distal embolism. Radiopaque markers should be placed at the entrance and exit wounds in order to help delineate missile trajectories.[45]

Management of Penetrating Thoracic Aortic and Great Vessels Injury

If the patient is a candidate for an ED thoracotomy, it is performed by making a left anterolateral thoracotomy in the fourth interspace. A Finochietto rib spreader is placed, oriented with the handle toward the lateral aspect of the wound in case the incision needs to be extended across the midline, and the lung is examined. If there is evidence of lung bleeding, it is either clamped or, if it is central or hilar, the inferior pulmonary ligament is divided and a hilar clamp placed. Alternatively, the lung can be twisted 180 degrees on its hilum to temporarily control bleeding. The pericardium is then grasped anterior to the phrenic nerve and opened longitudinally, delivering the heart. Any obvious injury is sutured with 3-0 polypropylene pledgeted sutures or stapled. Open cardiac massage is then initiated. Finally, a cross-clamp is placed on the aorta. A nasogastric tube should be inserted to assist in differentiation of the aorta from the esophagus, not always an easy task in the exsanguinated patient. Any additional sources of bleeding should be controlled with finger tamponade, clamps, or packing, and the patient taken immediately to the operating room.

Anatomically the aortic arch is oriented in an anterior posterior direction. As such, the left subclavian artery originates off of the aorta in the posterior mediastinum. Thus it is nearly impossible to obtain rapid proximal control of this artery through a median sternotomy. In a patient with a penetrating injury above or below the left clavicle, the best approach to control the left subclavian artery is through an incision in the third interspace of the left chest. This high anterolateral thoracotomy will allow adequate visualization of the root of the left subclavian artery to gain vascular control. Once controlled, the surgeon can explore the injured subclavian artery through standard supraclavicular incision (Fig. 48.3).

The most versatile exposure for penetrating thoracic trauma is a left anterolateral thoracotomy through the fourth interspace. It is not an accident that this is the same incision used for the EDT. The left side of the mediastinum, including the pericardium and the descending aorta, can be accessed through this incision. If this does not provide sufficient access, the incision is extended across the midline via a transverse sternotomy and can be continued into a right anterolateral thoracotomy in the third interspace. This is known as the "clamshell" incision. It is a highly morbid procedure, but if it is necessary, the patient is near death and all maneuvers are considered heroic at this point.

In the patient with a known site of injury, alternative incisions may be used. One of the most common approaches to the thoracic cavity is the midline sternotomy. An incision is made vertically from the sternal notch to the xiphoid process down to the sternum. Using blunt dissection, a retrosternal space is established and a sternal saw is used to divide the sternum longitudinally. The Finochietto retractor is then placed and the thoracic cavity is opened. This affords access to the ascending aorta, the brachiocephalic vein, and the pulmonary artery. The transverse aortic arch may be reached through this incision, although it may require a cervical extension. In order to fully control the innominate artery or the right subclavian artery or vein, the median sternotomy is extended to include a right cervical incision. Extension of the sternotomy into a left cervical incision will provide access to the left common carotid artery. The mid- and distal left subclavian artery and vein are more challenging to access and require a left anterolateral thoracotomy in the third or fourth interspace, coupled with a left supraclavicular incision. Connecting these incisions with a vertical sternotomy is the "trapdoor" incision, much talked about but associated with significant morbidity and risk of causalgia. The descending aorta can be reached, as previously mentioned, through a left fourth interspace anterolateral thoracotomy, but preferentially should be exposed through a posterolateral thoracotomy in the same interspace. Finally, the distal pulmonary veins or the pulmonary hilum can be reached through a posterolateral thoracotomy on the appropriate side.

Penetrating injuries of the anterior wall of the ascending aorta can be repaired with simple interrupted sutures. However, posterior wall or through-and-through injuries of this segment of the aorta will require bypass to correct. Injury in the transverse arch requires extension of the sternotomy into cervical incisions to control the branch vessels. The brachiocephalic vein can be ligated and divided if necessary to improve exposure. Again, if complex repairs are necessary, cardiopulmonary bypass is required.

Injury to the innominate artery from penetrating trauma can occur anywhere along its length. If possible, proximal and distal control through appropriate incisions should be secured, and then debridement and repair versus interposition grafting can be accomplished. A special situation is injury to the proximal innominate artery near its origin; this is also the most common site of injury for blunt innominate artery trauma. This

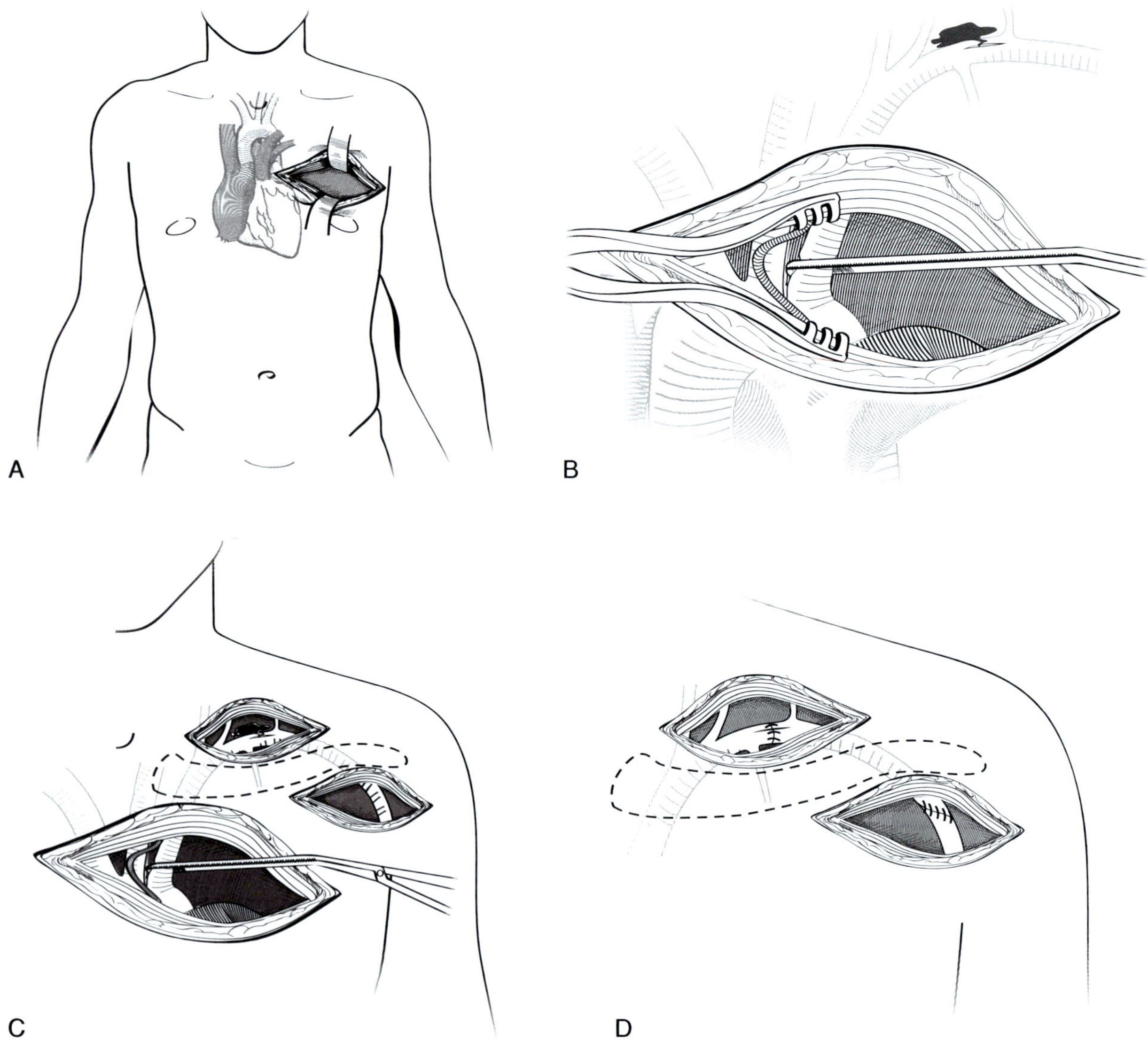

FIG 48.3 (A and B) Proximal control of the left subclavian artery is obtained through a left third space anterolateral thoracotomy. (C) Once proximal control is achieved, distal control can be obtained through an infraclavicular incision, and the wound is exposed through a supraclavicular incision. (D) The subclavian artery is repaired via the supraclavicular and infraclavicular incisions.

is essentially an ascending aortic injury. The bypass and exclusion technique is useful in this scenario. Prior to entering the hematoma, the distal innominate artery just proximal to the bifurcation is controlled, clamped, and divided; collateral flow to the right carotid is maintained via the subclavian artery. A prosthetic graft is anastomosed to the distal innominate artery. A side-biting Satinsky clamp is placed on the aorta proximal to the origin of the innominate artery, and the graft is anastomosed to the aorta. Finally, the hematoma is entered, the injury identified, and the proximal innominate artery is divided and the side hole in the aorta is oversewn. If there is a concomitant venous injury, a pericardial patch should be placed between the graft and the venous repair to avoid erosion and fistula formation.

ABDOMINAL VASCULAR TRAUMA

Almost all cases of abdominal vascular injury are caused by penetrating trauma, usually from a gunshot wound. The aorta is the most commonly injured vessel in the abdomen. Among the approximately 10% of aortic injury due to blunt trauma, motor vehicle collisions are the usual mechanism.[11,58,59]

Aortic injury represents 10% to 38% of intraabdominal vascular injuries in trauma series in recent decades. Of these injuries, 62% involve the pararenal or suprarenal segments of the aorta, which are associated with 92% mortality, compared with 66% in the infrarenal segment.[60,61]

One of the problems leading to a high mortality rate is that the symptoms are often not specific, and they are often associated with other injuries. Associated damage to gastrointestinal organs is very common, yielding a lethal combination with an associated mortality rate over 50%. Heuer and colleagues analyzed 10,530 trauma patients with abdominal trauma. A total of 760 (7.2 %) of these patients showed abdominal vascular injury (AIS abdomen ≥2, AIS vascular 2 to 5) and were analyzed based on the classification of the American Association for Surgery of Trauma (AAST) organ severity score (AAST vascular injury grade: II, 2.4%; III, 2.7%; IV, 1.8%; V, 0.2%). Patients with high-grade abdominal vascular injury (grades IV and V) showed a significant increase in mortality (IV, 44.6%; V, 60%).[62] Hypotension and abdominal distension are commonly seen, and distal pulse deficits may be appreciated. Patients with abdominal aortic injury generally present in hypovolemic shock; the lethal triad of hypothermia, acidosis, and coagulopathy is commonly seen. While some authors are aggressive with emergency department thoracotomy (EDT) in these patients, the results are very poor, and others recommend avoiding EDT in patients with abdominal vascular injury.[58] Clues to the location of injury can be gleaned from the physical examination. Injury above or involving the superior mesenteric artery will produce abdominal pain, pararenal involvement may lead to hematuria, or injury to the infrarenal aorta may manifest as unilateral or bilateral lower extremity ischemia.

Generally from the trauma prospective, the abdomen is divided into three retroperitoneal zones. Zone I represents the midline, which includes the abdominal aorta, celiac trunk, superior mesenteric artery, renal arteries, inferior vena cava (IVC), and its branches. Zone I is divided to Ia (supramesocolic region) and Ib (inframesocolic region). Zone II is the perinephric (lateral to the psoas muscles) region bilaterally. Zone III is the pelvic region, which includes the iliac vessels.[63] Management of abdominal vascular trauma depends on the location and type (penetrating vs. blunt) of injury.

The AAST adopted a grading system for abdominal vascular injury devised by Moore and colleagues (Table 48.6).[64]

TABLE 48.6 American Association for the Surgery of Trauma Multicenter Trial Abdominal Vascular Injury Grading Scale[a]

Injury Grade	Abdominal Vascular Injury
I	Nonnamed superior mesenteric artery or superior mesenteric vein branches. Nonnamed inferior mesenteric artery or inferior mesenteric vein branches. Phrenic artery/vein. Lumbar artery/vein. Gonadal artery/vein. Ovarian artery/vein. Other unnamed small arterial or venous structures requiring ligation.
II	Right, left, or common hepatic artery. Splenic artery/vein. Right or left gastric arteries. Gastroduodenal artery. Inferior mesenteric artery, trunk, or inferior mesenteric vein, trunk. Primary named branches of mesenteric artery (e.g., ileocolic artery) or mesenteric vein. Other named abdominal vessels requiring ligation or repair
III	Superior mesenteric vein, trunk. Renal artery/vein. Iliac artery/vein. Hypogastric artery/vein. Vena cava, infrarenal.
IV	Superior mesenteric artery, trunk. Celiac axis proper. Vena cava, suprarenal and infrahepatic. Aorta, infrarenal.
V	Portal vein. Extraparenchymal hepatic vein. Vena cava, retrohepatic or suprahepatic, aorta, suprarenal, subdiaphragmatic.

[a]This classification system is applicable for extraparenchymal vascular injuries. If the vessel injury is within 2 cm of the organ parenchyma, refer to specific organ injury scale. Increase one grade if multiple grade III or IV injuries involving >50% vessel circumference. Downgrade one grade if 25% vessel circumference laceration for grades IV or V.

Management of Abdominal Aortic Trauma

Surgical Exposure

Exposure of the suprarenal aorta can be significantly challenging, especially in a patient with multiple organ injury. The most versatile option is the anterior approach. Temporary proximal control is achieved by compression of the aorta against the vertebral bodies at the diaphragmatic hiatus. This can be accomplished most expeditiously with the surgeon's hand; this task should then be given to the assistant so that the surgeon can proceed with dissection. The lesser omentum is then opened through the bare space, the stomach and esophagus are retracted to the left, and the aorta is identified and compressed behind the esophagus. Once further dissection is completed, a clamp may be applied. If additional exposure is required, the celiac axis can be ligated and divided in a young patient; this vessel should be preserved in older patients, however, as the status of the SMA orifice is unknown.

Exposure of the infrarenal aorta is best achieved via an anterior approach unless the abdomen is rather hostile; the transverse colon is elevated, the small bowel is eviscerated to the right, and the ligament of Treitz is divided. The retroperitoneum covering the aorta is then opened and the left renal vein identified. The left and right renal arteries are then identified after the left renal vein is retracted superiorly; great care must be taken to ensure that there is no circumaortic or retroaortic left renal vein prior to the application of an aortic clamp.

Another option for exposure of the supramesocolic Zone I requires mobilization and medial rotation the left colon, spleen, tail of pancreas, stomach along the white line of Toldt (a Mattox maneuver), and possibly left kidney. This will allow visualization and control of the aorta, celiac and superior mesenteric arteries, and left renal artery. Mobilization and medial rotation of the right colon, kocherization of the duodenum, and head of pancreas along with the root of the mesentery (a Cattell and Braasch maneuver) will expose the right renal artery and supramesocolic IVC. Retracting the mesocolon cephalad and small bowel to the right and dividing the parietal peritoneum overlying the aorta or IVC expose the inframesocolic Zone I. If additional proximal exposure is needed, the left crus of the aortic hiatus can be divided radially at the 2-o'clock position to expose the distal descending aorta. It is important to realize that this approach will allow exposure of the proximal portion of the celiac and SMA arteries. Access to their branches will be difficult and limited.

Management

Among patients who survive the initial operation, primary suturing is the most common repair technique (69% to 86%), followed by prosthetic graft in 14% to 23%. Between 17% and 32% of patients do not survive the operation.[58,59,61] Small wounds of the aorta can be closed primarily with 3-0 or 4-0 polypropylene sutures. If there are multiple aortic wounds in close proximity, they can be connected surgically to allow for a single closure. If possible, the wound should be closed transversely to prevent stenosis, although up to a 50% luminal narrowing is generally well tolerated and may be dealt with at a later date. If there is significant tissue loss to the aortic wall, patch aortoplasty with PTFE or interposition grafting with 12 to 16 mm Dacron woven grafts may be necessary.

One common problem in the management of significant aortic injury is concomitant hollow viscus injury and field contamination.[62,63] One technique for managing this injury is to use a Dacron graft, as the literature does not support a high-risk of graft infection in young trauma patients. It is wise to thoroughly irrigate the abdomen and protect the graft with an omental pedicle if interposition grafting is performed. The alternative is ligation and delayed extra-anatomic bypass.[60] The obvious downside of this approach is the need for two general anesthetic cases, as well as an iatrogenic ischemia-reperfusion insult.

In cases of blunt aortic injury, endovascular strategies may be useful. Chronic dissections are best treated by rigid, balloon-expandable stents, whereas self-expanding stents are better tolerated for acute dissections. The obvious advantages of this approach are the avoidance of a retroperitoneal dissection, aortic cross-clamping, and the prevention of contamination of vascular graft materials in cases of contaminated fields. Yeh and colleagues describe a case report of a ruptured mycotic pseudoaneurysm treated successfully with endovascular exclusion 14 days after the initial injury and primary aortic repair. The field had been contaminated due to multiple enterotomies, leading to the mycotic pseudoaneurysm. This approach avoided a tedious, dangerous dissection through a hostile abdomen in a hemorrhaging patient; the patient survived.[65]

Management of Abdominal Nonaortic Vascular Trauma

Surgical Exposure

Zone Ia. Access to these structures is gained by dividing the avascular portion of the gastrohepatic ligament and entering the lesser sac. The esophagus is swept laterally away from the liver to allow the diaphragmatic crus to be isolated and divided, yielding access to the supradiaphragmatic aorta. A clamp is then placed on the aorta in this location. The infrarenal aorta is then exposed in the usual fashion and clamped to isolate the Zone Ia arterial system. This allows exploration of this region of the retroperitoneum under relative vascular control.

Zone Ib. An infracolic hematoma should be approached proximally through the root of the mesocolon to obtain proximal control. These injuries often involve the pancreas, duodenum, liver, and portal venous system. A left medial visceral rotation (Mattox maneuver) can be used to expose the aorta from the diaphragm to the bifurcation, all the visceral branches, and the left renal branch. Access to the right renal branch and the right common iliac artery is challenging from this exposure.

Zone II. Left-sided Zone II structures include the left kidney and its associated artery, vein, and ureter. Access to this area requires a left medial visceral rotation (a Mattox maneuver, as described previously). The kidney may be elevated into the field or left in situ. Access to Zone II on the right medial visceral rotation (a Cattell-Braasch maneuver, as described previously) and exposes Zone II on the right and the entire infrarenal vena cava as well as the majority of the aorta from the superior mesenteric artery inferiorly.

Management

Open surgical management of abdominal vascular injuries follows the same principles of vascular surgery in general. Lateral arteriorrhaphy or end-to-end anastomosis can be utilized for primary repair if possible. If not, the surgeon can utilize a patch angioplasty or a bypass conduit, preferably using vein, as concomitant injuries are common in these patients and the field of operation is complicated with enteric contaminates. If the vein is not available, polytetrafluoroethylene conduits for patching or as a bypass graft are permissible to use in life-saving situations, albeit undesirable. If that is the route for repair, copious irrigation and anastomotic coverage with omentum pedicle is paramount.

In younger patients, ligation of the celiac trunk (or its branches) or the inferior mesenteric artery is usually well tolerated. The authors would advise caution in doing so in other patients, as the status of the atherosclerotic disease in the superior mesenteric artery are not known and collateral vasculature might not be available to provide collateral blood supply to the gut. If ligation of these vessels is needed, a second look laparotomy is advised at 24 to 48 hours to assess for any ischemic consequences. Also, ligation is not an option if at all possible for the superior mesenteric artery in any age group. This would carry a significant risk for extensive gut ischemia.

It is not uncommon to encounter hematomas during the abdominal exploration for vascular trauma patients. Management of these hematomas is dictated by the location of the hematoma and the patient's condition.

Zone I. Zone I hematoma need to be explored and the injury managed accordingly. Aortic injuries are managed according to the discussion noted previously.

Injury to the celiac artery is extremely rare. In a series of 2357 patients who underwent laparotomy for trauma, 13 cases of celiac artery injury were identified for a rate of 0.01%.[66] Almost all celiac artery traumatic injuries have been secondary to penetrating trauma (97.8%). Among the cases where the type of repair was documented, ligation was the most common procedure (63.9% of cases); there was an associated mortality of 56.3% among the 16 cases where outcome was given.[66-68]

Similar to other retroperitoneal artery injuries, the approach to these injuries usually requires either a left or right medial visceral rotation. Dissection of the vessel is challenging due to the dense neurolymphatic plexus surrounding the takeoff of the celiac artery. Once vascular control is established, a decision between ligation and attempted repair is required. The celiac trunk has a rich collateral circulation, and therefore ligation of the splenic and left gastric arteries may be performed without hesitation. Ligation of the common hepatic is relatively safe if the gastroduodenal artery remains patent. Ligation of the proper hepatic artery is higher risk and should not be performed concomitantly with portal vein ligation; an alternative would be to consider a small intraluminal shunt in this position.

Injury to the superior mesenteric artery (SMA) is a highly lethal injury, due to several factors. It is difficult to access, it supplies a large portion of the gastrointestinal tract, and injury to the SMA is often associated with severe injury to surrounding structures such as small bowel, colon, liver, and pancreaticoduodenal complex. Operative findings include hemoperitoneum, a mesenteric hematoma around the superior mesenteric artery, and bowel ischemia. The management of this injury begins with direct compression of the likely site of trauma, followed by cross-clamping of the aorta proximal to the origin of the SMA. If the injury is retropancreatic, either a left medial visceral rotation or a direct approach by dividing the neck of the pancreas can be used to access the artery. The infrapancreatic SMA can be isolated by direct dissection. It is generally wise to avoid exploration of stable hematomas or those found in blunt trauma cases in the absence of bowel ischemia. Angiography or color-flow Doppler interrogation is helpful to delineate the nature of the injury in questionable cases. The grade of injury can be classified according to the AAST system shown in Table 48.6.

The most extensive series of patients with SMA injuries in the literature was reported by Asensio and colleagues in 2001.[69] In this study, 13 institutions contributed retrospective data on patients with SMA injuries between 1990 and 1999. A total of 250 patients were reviewed, and many interesting observations were made. First, and not surprisingly, there was a very high mortality rate (39%). The majority of deaths (71%) occurred in the operating room or within the first 24 hours. Contrary to expectations, there was an even proportion of blunt and penetrating trauma in this series.

Ligation was the most frequent repair option (72%), followed by primary repair (22%). The remainder of patients underwent attempted grafting with either saphenous vein or PTFE. There was only one shunt used in this series. Heparinization was infrequent. There was a high likelihood of associated injuries. Nonvascular injuries included the small bowel (64%), colon (43%), liver (28%), duodenum (24%), and pancreas (22%). Other abdominal organs were injured approximately 15% of the time. The biliary tree proper was only injured in 3% of cases.

The most common associated vascular injury was to the superior mesenteric vein (SMV), in 33% of cases. Interestingly, there was no mortality difference whether the vein was ligated or repaired (44.2% vs. 40.0%, $P = .916$). In approximately 5% to 10% of cases, other vascular structures were injured. Not surprisingly, the lethal triad of metabolic acidosis, hypothermia, and coagulopathy was frequent, seen in approximately 50% of cases. The most frequent injury-specific complications were gut ischemia (20%) and infarction (15%). Out of 16 attempted graft repairs (10 with vein graft and 6 with PTFE), three failed (19%).

In terms of SMA injury management, plan to move early to damage control measures. Any evidence of massive blood loss, coagulopathy, shock, or acidosis should suggest abandonment of attempts and vascular repair and lead to temporizing measures or ligation. Likewise, ligation of the SMV should be considered if the alternative is a lengthy or challenging repair. Be thorough and search for associated injuries, as isolated SMA injuries are extremely rare. Expect that heparinization will be contraindicated due to the nature of the patient's injuries. Given the high likelihood of associated pancreatic injury, it is critical to isolate the vascular anastomosis from a ductal disruption by a pancreatic leak using omentum or other surrounding soft tissues. If a graft to the SMA is planned, it should be taken off the distal aorta to move the anastomosis from the region of the pancreas. And finally, plan for a second look operation within 24 hours if the patient is stable.[63,69]

Caval injury is secondary to penetrating trauma in 68% to 96% of cases and is associated with 48% mortality. Of these, gunshot wounds are the most prevalent (75% to 94%). Knife wounds are less prevalent (2% to 20%) and are associated with infrequent mortality. Shotgun wounds are generally devastating; Rosengart and colleagues cited a 14% incidence in their series of shotgun wounds for penetrating caval injuries, with an associated 100% mortality.[70] Blunt injuries are less frequent than penetrating injuries, ranging from 7% to 22% but associated with higher mortality, 63% in the Rosengart series.[70–73] The most common preoperative factor associated with mortality is severe or refractory hypotension. Vena cava injury management and outcome is largely dependent on its location and extent. Exposure can be obtained with a Cattell and Braasch maneuver. Control of the IVC can be done with sponge sticks proximally and distally, a side biting Satinsky clamp or balloon occlusion. Generally speaking, vena cava injury is usually repaired with either lateral venorrhaphy or patch angioplasty. If needed, polytetrafluoroethylene or rifampin soaked Dacron interposition graft can be used. The decision regarding which kind of repair depends on the patient's condition and the surgeon's decision, with the goal of maintaining luminal diameter as close to normal as possible to avoid thrombosis or embolism, which can be associated with stenotic repair.[63] A consideration for placement a temporary IVC filter can be evaluated at the time of repair. In an unstable patient with an infrarenal IVC injury, ligation may be tolerated and necessary in a damage control approach to the patient's care. This is not the case for suprarenal IVC injuries. All suprarenal IVC injuries must be repaired or temporarily shunted if the patient is too unstable for repair. Ligation of suprarenal IVC is not well tolerated and would complicate the patient's instability due to the drop in preload and significant risk of renal failure with ligation.[74] Exposure of the retrohepatic vena cava is very difficult, which would complicate management of a suprarenal IVC injury. A retrohepatic hematoma is the only exception to mandatory exploration of all penetrating trauma hematoma. Perihepatic packing is utilized as the first-line treatment. It can be changed every 24 to 48 hours with a second-look operation. If all else fails, total hepatic vascular isolation, an atriocaval shunt or division of the liver to gain exposure, can be attempted for hemorrhage control. Hepatic isolation is performed by placing a supraceliac aortic clamp, followed by a clamp on the proximal and distal IVC, and finally portal triad occlusion with a Pringle maneuver. This technique was originally described by Waltuck and colleagues and Yellin and colleagues.[75,76] This maneuver may be tolerated if the patient is volume resuscitated (a rare occurrence in retrohepatic caval trauma). If the decrease in venous return causes the patient to become unstable, as it will in hypovolemic patients, consider atriocaval shunt at this point. The atriocaval shunt was first described by Schrock and colleagues in 1968.[77] After sternotomy or right thoracotomy, the right atrium is grasped with a clamp, a purse string suture placed in the right atrial appendage, a cardiotomy is performed in the middle of the stitch, and a chest tube, at least 32 French in size, or a 9-mm endotracheal tube is placed into the right atrium through the purse-string suture. The tube should be prepared ahead of time with side holes cut to allow adequate blood flow proximal and distal. Rummel tourniquets are used at both ends to secure the shunt in place; alternatively, for the endotracheal tube, the balloon may be inflated to exclude the inferior cava.

Over the past decade or so, reports had emerged regarding utilizing endovascular techniques for vena cava injury repair. Burket and colleagues, Azizzadeh and colleagues, and Anaya-Ayala and colleagues have all reports utilization of aortic endografts for repair of vena caval tear.[78–80] Watarida and colleagues reported using a fenestrated endograft for repair of a juxtahepatic IVC injury.[81]

Zone II. Renovascular trauma as a result of blunt injury occurs in approximately 0.08% of all abdominal blunt traumas. This is often the result of rapid deceleration that causes the disruption of the inelastic intimal layer. Penetrating trauma causes renovascular injury in 0.5% of cases.[82] Workup of the patient with a renovascular injury is challenging. Physical examination is rarely helpful in diagnosis, and delayed presentation is common, as the focus is generally on other more apparent life-threatening injuries.[83] One major indicator that renal injury may be present is hematuria, either gross or microscopic. Microscopic hematuria was seen in 54% to 89% of patients with renal vascular trauma.[84–87] CT scans are quite useful for the diagnosis of renal vascular trauma; they are able to demonstrate regional or global renal perfusion deficits, perirenal hematomas, or extravasation of contrast. They are both sensitive and specific for delineating renovascular, collecting system, and parenchymal injuries, as well as associated intra-abdominal trauma.[88,89] One drawback is that they tend to miss intimal flaps, however.[90] Intravenous pyelography has been the traditional mainstay of diagnosis prior to the advent of multislice CT scanners. It remains a useful adjunct in that it is portable and can be performed interoperatively. The absence of the kidney on the image is a sign of severe injury. It is rather nonspecific, however, which is its major drawback.[83] The other major diagnostic modality is arteriography, which is very sensitive for injuries including intimal flaps, and is also therapeutic. The drawback is that arteriography is invasive, labor intensive, and in some places cannot be performed intraoperatively. Computed tomography angiography has largely replaced catheter-based arteriography, which had been reserved for therapeutic management of ongoing or delayed bleeding, for which selective angiography and embolization can be used.[89]

Renal vascular injury can occur in several different ways. Vascular stretch and intimal disruption can occur during a deceleration injury, leading to intimal flaps and thrombosis. Vascular compression against vertebral bodies can be caused by compressive injuries, causing thrombosis, avulsion, or spasm.[83] The extent of injury can be graded according to the AAST grading system, as noted in Table 48.7. Penetrating injuries account for 4% to 24% of all renovascular trauma and leads to direct disruption of the vascular wall.[86] Overall, 44% of renal vascular injuries are due to thrombosis, 12% avulsion, 7% intimal flaps, 4% lacerations, and 4% vascular spasm.[89,91]

TABLE 48.7 American Association for the Surgery of Trauma Multicenter Trial Renal Injury Grading Scale

Injury Grade	Renal Injury
I	Renal contusion or nonexpanding subcapsular hematoma without a parenchymal laceration
II	Nonexpanding perirenal hematoma or a renal cortex laceration (<1 cm) without urinary extravasation
III	Renal cortex laceration (>1 cm) and no urinary extravasation
IV	Renal cortical laceration extending into the collecting system Segmental renal artery or vein injury Main renal artery or vein injury with a contained hematoma
V	Avulsion of the renal pedicle, or thrombosis of the main renal artery

In blunt trauma, a Zone II hematoma should not be explored unless it is expanding. All penetrating trauma Zone II hematomas should be explored. Proximal vascular control should be secured first via transperitoneal exposure of the perirenal aortic segment. The left renal vein is identified and retracted superiorly to expose the origins of the renal arteries. Once proximal control is secured, a Mattox maneuver is performed to access the left kidney or a Cattell-Braasch maneuver is used to access the right kidney. Distal vascular control can be achieved with fingertip pressure or a balloon catheter. The arterial wall should be gently debrided. Frequent irrigation with heparinized saline to prevent distal embolization is critical. The kidney should be perfused intermittently with iced heparinized saline to maintain viability. Just prior to completion of the repair, a thrombectomy catheter should be gently passed along the proximal and distal vessel. An associated renal vein injury on the right should be repaired if at all possible; otherwise, the kidney should be removed. Ligation of the right renal vein is incompatible with the function of the right kidney. Distal (near the IVC) injuries of the left renal vein can be safely ligated if repair is complex, as venous drainage will occur through the adrenal, gonadal, and posterior lumbar vessels.[63,89]

Treatment options vary depending on the extent of the injury and the patient's hemodynamic status. They include nonoperative management, revascularization, or nephrectomy. An occluded renal artery should not be re-vascularized unless ischemia time is less than 6 hours, there are bilateral renal injuries, or there is injury to a solitary kidney.[83]

Renal salvage is only effective in 25% to 35% of cases. The length of time between injury and reperfusion is a major factor in the outcome of the kidney. Irreversible damage begins, occurring at 30 to 90 minutes of warm ischemia time.[89,92] Relative contraindications to attempted repair include the following: multiple injuries, prolonged ischemic time, hilar injuries, extensive associated arterial injury, and a normal contralateral kidney.[93] The presence of two or more of the listed factors suggests that nephrectomy may be preferable for the patient, especially if there is a normal contralateral kidney. In the case that the injury is bilateral or the patient has only one functional kidney, efforts at repair should be undertaken at longer ischemia times—up to 18 hours. Lock reported a 42% success rate with repair; the mean ischemic time for successful repair was 12.3 hours, compared to 26 hours for unsuccessful repairs.[92] The final option is nephrectomy. There is controversy over the use of early nephrectomy. Proponents recommend it for all injuries not diagnosed early or amenable to repair, whereas others recommend waiting and performing nephrectomy only in the subset of patients who develop hypertension.[94] Renovascular hypertension develops in 4% to 50% of nonoperatively treated and 35% of operatively treated patients; most cases present within the first year.[94]

Endovascular stenting in renal trauma is still relatively rare. One of the major disadvantages to using endovascular intervention in the polytrauma patient is the inability to anticoagulate patients. Lopera and colleagues reported on eight cases with traumatic main renal artery occlusion or dissection, who were managed endovascularly. Successful recanalization of the occlusion with stent placement occurred in six of the eight patients. Two of the eight patients underwent embolization secondary to contrast extravasation during the procedure. Of those with successful treatment, four developed renal atrophy.[95]

Despite the relatively small amount of literature on endovascular repair in blunt renovascular trauma, there is agreement on the following: ischemia time is very important; intervention before 3 hours of complete and 6 hours of incomplete occlusion is associated with a higher incidence of positive outcomes; and in order to increase the rate of renal preservation, the longevity of repair, and to decrease renal hypertension, you must be able to anticoagulate the patient post intervention. Renovascular trauma must be triaged appropriately. If the patient requires exploratory laparotomy for other injuries, endovascular intervention should not delay treatment for other life-threatening injuries.[89]

Zone III. Patients who present in shock from pelvic hemorrhage have a high mortality. This owes to the large volume of blood the pelvis can accommodate and the difficulty of open surgical exposure to adequately and expeditiously control the source of hemorrhage. Initial control aims at tamponading the pelvic region with a pelvic binder, MAST, or a bed sheet wrapped around the pelvis. Endovascular intervention has revolutionized the ability to manage and treat pelvic bleeding with angiography and embolization of balloon tamponade for hemorrhage control. Overall the mortality of pelvic trauma patients has decreased in recent years. In their 13-year experience report, Sheena and colleagues reported that age, shock, head injury, increasing ISS (injury severity score), and earlier period were significantly associated with increased mortality.[96]

In blunt trauma, a Zone III hematoma should not be explored unless it is expanding or there is an abnormal femoral pulse. All penetrating trauma Zone III hematomas should be explored. Today, the endovascular approach is the first-line treatment of Zone III hematomas in a stable patient. The surgeon can pack the pelvis and perform an on-table angiogram or take the patient to the angiography suite and perform a dye study. This can help identify bleeding from external iliac or hypogastric branches, which can be managed with coil embolization. Injury of the common or external iliac arteries can also be managed with covered stent-graft deployment. Ligation of common or external iliac arteries is not well tolerated, and all injuries should be repaired if at all possible. In damage-control surgery, intraluminal shunting is good technique to temporize the patients' injury till they are hemodynamically fit to undergo an operative repair. As with extremity vascular injuries, development of compartment syndrome should be monitored and the surgeon should have a low threshold for fasciotomy. Venous bleeding can be managed with packing or ligation. If the patient is stable enough, repair of the major pelvic venous structures should be attempted.

Special Consideration: Portal and Mesenteric Venous Injury

Injury to the portal and mesenteric venous system is an uncommon and devastating injury. It occurs in approximately 1 in 1000 trauma admissions, and in approximately 1% of patients requiring laparotomy for trauma.[97,98] Due to its rarity, few surgeons develop familiarity with the management of this condition, and multiinstitutional retrospective reviews are generally required to study the management of this problem.[18] Mortality ranges from 40% to 72%, behind aortic injury and retrohepatic caval injuries for lethality.[60,97–101] Interoperative uncontrolled hemorrhage is the primary cause of death in these patients, responsible for 38% to 92% of deaths.[99,100,102] Fraga and colleagues evaluated the trend in mortality versus time and found worse mortality in the recent era, leading to the concern that this injury may be "too lethal" for our current management strategies.[98] The major predictor of mortality, unsurprisingly, is shock, with hemodynamically stable patients sustaining 17% to 43% mortality versus 55% to 91% for patients presenting in shock.[98,100] The degree of injury to the vessel also predicts outcome. Associated injuries, especially vascular injuries, is another significant predictor of outcome.[100,102] The inferior vena cava and the superior mesenteric artery are the most common additional vascular injuries in these patients,[99,100] whereas there is a broad range of associated hollow and solid organ injuries. Jurkovich described the most common location of portal vein injuries as being in the hepatoduodenal ligament (in 68% of injuries), facilitating a double Pringle maneuver for isolation.[102] Exploration of these patients is almost always notable for a retroperitoneal hematoma, although its location may be misleading; while 73% of hematomas are the midline (Zone I), 18% are in Zone II and 9% in Zone III.[99]

There are a variety of surgical options described in the literature for this complex of injuries. The safest approach, however, is to rapidly assess whether there is a straightforward repair option available and whether the patient will tolerate the attempt. If the answer to either question is no, the best option is ligation. Child performed a series of experiments in 1950, which led to his belief that 80% of humans would tolerate ligation of the portal vein, although it is notable that these experiments did not take into account the massive physiologic derangements of multisystem trauma.[103] It is clearly the best option, however, in the unstable patient. Patients may develop systemic hypotension and portal hypertension, which resolves over the next week in most patients. These patients tend to require aggressive fluid resuscitation, however, to compensate for 50% reduction in sequestered blood volume.[100] Asensio reported an incidence of this syndrome of approximately 5% in patients undergoing SMV ligation. However, if the patient should not develop collateral circulation, another option may become necessary. There is a case report of a delayed interposition graft at 15 hours after initial exploration where the SMV was oversewn, likely with many of the collaterals including the middle colic vein, with a good outcome.[104] It is also recommended that all patients with ligated portomesenteric venous vessels undergo a second look operation at 24 to 48 hours postoperatively. Portal vein ligation has been performed in 0% to 50% of injuries in several major series, with mortality rates ranging from 27% to 100%.[98,100–101] Stone and colleagues discovered that when they performed PV ligation as a last-ditch effort after a failed attempt at reconstruction the mortality was approximately 60%, whereas when they went to ligation early for clearly nonreconstructible damage, the mortality fell to 15%.[101] Similarly, SMV ligation has been performed in 17% to 60% of cases, with mortality ranging from 15% to 50%.[98–101] It is crucial to note that if the hepatic artery is concomitantly injured, patency must be restored to either the portomesenteric circulation or the hepatic artery, as occlusion of both is incompatible with life.

Primary repair of the portal vein and superior mesenteric vein has been successful in 38% to 100% and 31% to 64% of series, respectively, with mortality rates of 14% to 67% and 29% to 45%, respectively.[98–101] Complex repairs such as end-to-end anastomosis, interposition grafts, saphenous vein patches, and portocaval shunts have been attempted with poor outcomes. At present, there are no reports of the use of shunts in the portomesenteric circulation for trauma.

The operative approach to the portomesenteric system is through a right medial visceral rotation, which can be extended to a Cattell-Braasch maneuver to achieve full exposure of the retroperitoneum. The top priority is to identify and control the source of hemorrhage. Once exposure is obtained, pressure from packs or the operator's hand should be used to obtain initial control. In most cases, a Pringle maneuver will control vascular inflow, and in the majority of portal venous injuries, a double Pringle maneuver will isolate the injury and may allow for a lateral venorrhaphy. Access to the portal-SMV confluence may require division of the neck of the pancreas. Finally, as previously stated, all patients with trauma to this system should be considered for a second look laparotomy in 24 to 48 hours, postoperatively.

In recent years reports have surfaced regarding endovascular techniques being utilized for managing mesenteric and porta venous injuries. In 2013, Sundarakumar and colleagues reported two cases where they used coil embolization techniques and stent-graft endoprosthesis to control portal venous bleeding in patients with portal venous bleeding complicated by portal hypertension.[105]

A variety of postoperative complications have been described. Aside from the previously described sequestration syndrome, other documented complications include sepsis and wound infection in nearly 80%, intraabdominal abscess, pancreatitis, thrombosis of the portomesenteric system, hemorrhage, and respiratory failure. This is a challenging patient population to manage, both due to the initial physiologic insult as well as the commonly associated multiple organ and vascular injuries.

EXTREMITY VASCULAR TRAUMA

Injury to the arterial and venous systems of the extremities is commonly encountered in both military and civilian trauma, secondary to both blunt and penetrating mechanisms.

The incidence of combat vascular trauma overall has increased over the past decades. Debakey and colleagues reported an incidence of 0.96%.[4] This incidence increased to 2% to 3% during the Korean and Vietnam wars.[106,107] A more recent report by White and colleagues analyzed the US Joint Theater Trauma Registry (JTTR) from 2002 to 2009 and reported an incidence of 12%, with 75% of this group requiring operative intervention for the vascular trauma.[108] Vascular traumatic injury is also encountered in patients with mangled extremities whose management is specially challenging, as they are often associated with severe soft tissue damage along with orthopedic trauma, nerve injury, and contaminated field. The Mangled Extremity Severity Score (MESS) can help predict the patient's outcome, with scores greater than 7 being predictive of amputation (Table 48.8).

In the civilian population, the impact of vascular trauma is largely unknown due to the paucity of large-scale population-based

TABLE 48.8 The Mangled Extremity Severity Score

Category	Points
Skeletal and Soft Tissue Injury	
Low energy (stab wound, low-velocity GSW, simple fracture)	1
Med energy (open or multiple fracture or fracture with dislocation)	2
High energy (high-speed deceleration, high-velocity GSW)	3
Very high energy (high-speed trauma with gross contamination)	4
Ischemia (Double for Ischemia Time >6 h)	
Pulse reduced or absent, normal perfusion and capillary refill	1
Pulseless, paresthesias, diminished capillary refill	2
Cool, paralyzed, insensate, numb	3
Shock	
Normotension	0
Transient hypotension <90 mm Hg	1
Persistent hypotension <90 mm Hg	2
Age	
<30 years	0
30–50 years	1
>50 years	2

GSW, Gun shot wound.

studies to accurately assess its incidence. In 2014, a study by Branco and colleagues evaluated 23,105 patients in the National Trauma Data Bank and reported a 2.2% incidence of vascular trauma.[2] In civilian arterial trauma, the extremities are the most common location of injury. Among arteries in the extremities, 50% to 60% of injuries occur in the femoral or popliteal arteries and 30% in the brachial artery.[109–111]

Initial Management of Extremity Vascular Trauma

Hemorrhage Control

Vascular injuries of the extremities often present with massive bleeding. The source might be arterial, venous, or both. The first step in the patient's management is to immediately control the bleeding. There are several factors that dictate the most effective method for bleeding control. This depends on the location/site of the injury, expertise level of the health care provider, and the resources available at the site.

The most basic maneuver of direct digital compression works extremely well in most injuries and does not require any sophisticated tools. In the prehospital setting, more secure control can be obtained by prompt and proper application of tourniquets. A review from a military registry showed that 30% of the victims underwent application of tourniquets for vascular control. Over a period of 10 years, tourniquet use increased by 10-fold, and survival rates improved markedly for casualties that had injuries amenable for tourniquets. Once the patient reaches a facility where surgical expertise is available, additional maneuvers can be performed (if needed) to control the source of hemorrhage, including application of vascular clamps to the injured vessels or deployment of intraluminal occlusive balloons. In the most extreme situations, the aorta (thoracic or abdominal) can be controlled with the bedside application of the resuscitative endovascular balloon occlusion of the aorta (REBOA). The balloon-carrying catheter can be inserted using percutaneous techniques via the femoral artery and advanced, without fluoroscopy, into the aorta. It is then inflated to achieve interruption of blood flow through the aortic below the balloon. This technique is usually used for damage control resuscitation of patients with severe injuries but who are too unstable to undergo surgical intervention.

Tourniquet Use

There has been a resurgence of interest in the use of tourniquets in the combat setting. The Romans first developed tourniquets between 200 and 500 AD, but the modern design of collar and windlass was introduced by Jean Louis Petit in 1718. Historically, there has been concern that tourniquet use for the control of extremity hemorrhage would lead to limb dysfunction or loss with prolonged ischemic times. However, there has been a clear documentation that uncontrolled bleeding from extremity vascular injuries is one of the leading causes of preventable trauma deaths.[112] This led the US military as well as other countries to supply tourniquets to combat medics and troops. The evaluation of recent outcomes of tourniquet use has documented several critical points. First, there is a clear decrease in mortality with the early use of tourniquets, especially when applied prior to the onset of shock.[113–115] Even in cases where the wound was too proximal for the proper placing of the tourniquet (5 cm proximal to the most proximal wound, placed on bare skin), there was a 75% survival rate. In addition, morbidity directly attributable to the tourniquet was rare and reversible. In a series of 232 patients treated with 428 tourniquets on 309 limbs, there were only four (1.7%) transient nerve palsies at the level of the tourniquet, all of which resolved subsequently.[115] There was no association of tourniquet duration with other morbidities such as vascular clots, myonecrosis, rigor, pain, fasciotomy, or renal failure.

It is critical that those responsible for placing tourniquets are trained in their use. Proper application of the tourniquet is indicated by both the cessation of bleeding and the absence of a distal pulse. Misplacement of the tourniquet is associated with a 44% mortality. There was an identifiable pattern of clinical deterioration with ineffective tourniquet application: persistent pulse, venous congestion, venous distension, rebleeding after a period of hemorrhage control, expanding hematomas, compartment syndrome, fasciotomy, and death. This pattern was seen in 61% of cases where there was continued bleeding, despite application of the tourniquet, and in 51% of cases where there was a persistent distal pulse.[115]

It is also critical to use correctly designed tourniquets. The three most commonly used tourniquets in the American military are the Emergency Medical Tourniquet (EMT, Delfi Medical Innovations, Inc., Vancouver, British Columbia), the Combat Application Tourniquet (CAT, North American Rescue Products, Inc., Greer, SC), and the Special Operations Forces Tactical Tourniquet (SOFTT, Tactical Medical Solutions, LLC, Anderson, SC). All three designs were 100% effective in laboratory self-application use,[116] but among actual casualties, the EMT was shown to be 92% effective, the CAT to be 79% effective, and the SOFTT to be 66% effective.[115] The EMT, however, is not a prehospital tourniquet, and therefore the US Army issues CAT tourniquets for medics and troops and supplies EMTs for aid stations and higher levels of care. The width of the tourniquet seems to be related to its effectiveness.

A final critical point to effective tourniquet use is maintenance of vigilance. Slippery skin, underlying clothing or padding, or gradual decrease in limb diameter due to exsanguination can lead to a loose tourniquet and rebleeding. Initial inappropriate application due to occult wounds may also put the casualty at risk. Frequent checks of the tourniquet with application of additional tourniquets if necessary are critical for optimal outcomes.

Tourniquet use in civilian trauma has been less uniform. Most reports and evaluations have been in the military setting. Inaba and colleagues retrospectively evaluated the outcome in 87 civilian trauma patients who required tourniquet use. They concluded that the use in civilian setting is associated with a low rate of complications.

EVALUATION AND DIAGNOSTIC TESTS

Patients presenting with extremity vascular trauma must be assessed using the standard protocols for trauma patients. A rapid assessment of airway and breathing are followed by the evaluation of circulation. Any hemorrhage is controlled, ideally, with point pressure on the vascular injury, or if that is not possible, tourniquet application. The patient is fully examined while appropriate resuscitation is being performed. A distal pulse physical examination is documented; the Doppler ultrasound probe can augment this physical examination. A thorough physical examination is critical in the management of these injuries. In a study of 99 military trauma patients, 36 of 73 (49%) patients with normal physical examinations had angiographic abnormalities, yet only 6 (8%) required intervention. Among 26 patients with abnormal physical examinations, 22 (85%) had angiographic findings and 19 (73%) required intervention. While a normal physical exam does not rule out an injury requiring treatment, it does a good job of picking up the majority of clinically significant vascular injuries.[158] Physical examination findings are classically divided into "hard signs" and "soft signs" (see Box 48.1). Patients with hard signs should undergo operative exploration if the mechanism is penetrating and the location of injury is apparent. When the site of injury is unclear (e.g., a shotgun blast with multiple entry injuries, blunt trauma), preoperative or interoperative angiography is appropriate. The presence of physical findings suggestive of injury allowed Asensio and colleagues to decrease preoperative angiography to 15% and proceed with expeditious repairs.

Both the Eastern and Western Associations for the Surgery of Trauma issued guidelines for managing patients with extremity trauma. Penetrating trauma patients that have hard signs of arterial injury (see Table 48.1) do not need any vascular imaging studies. These patients should be surgically explored as soon as possible (within 6 hours) to maximize the chances of limb salvage. In the vast majority of patients, the level of vascular injury matches the site of penetrating trauma, except in rare cases of multiple gunshot wounds or shotgun injuries.[118]

If needed, an on-table angiogram can always be performed during the operation. In patients with blunt trauma (or penetrating trauma with long bone fracture), reduction of the fracture with reassessment should be performed first, as the pulse loss could be due to arterial entrapment, which may resolve with the reduction of fracture. Patients with soft signs (history of prehospital blood loss, diminished pulses, moderate hematoma, proximity to vessels, high risk fractures/dislocations, ipsilateral neurologic deficit) or ankle-brachial index (ABI) less than 0.9 are suitable candidates for imaging studies to rule out a vascular injury, with computed tomographic angiography (CTA) being the test of choice. Finally, patients with normal exam (and no hard or soft signs) and ABI greater than 0.9 do not need any additional workup for vascular injuries. Data from high-volume trauma centers support these recommendations. As it is a noninvasive test that does not require the presence of an interventional radiologist, CTA is rapidly replacing conventional angiograms as the diagnostic test of choice. Currently the role of Doppler pressure monitoring and duplex ultrasonography in diagnosing or excluding vascular injuries is not well defined.

Temporary Vascular Shunting

The use of temporary vascular shunting (TVS) has been used routinely for carotid surgery and has been studied extensively in the past 2 decades for traumatic injuries. In patients requiring damage control surgery, shunts can rapidly provide temporary blood flow to a vascular bed distal to an injury (Fig. 48.4A and B). Both Javid and Sundt shunts work well in the setting of complex vascular injury, yet many tubular devices can be made to work in austere environments. The duration of shunting should be minimized, but they are adequate for up to 24 hours without systemic heparinization of the patient. One report documented the experience of a US Navy surgical unit in Operation Iraqi Freedom. A total of 27 vascular shunts were placed in patients with a mean ISS score of 18 (range 9 to 34) and a mangled extremity severity score (MESS) of 9 (range 6 to 11). All patients survived, although three (15%) ultimately required amputation. Six (22%) of the shunts clotted during transport, but they provided an effective perfusion window, which allowed the majority

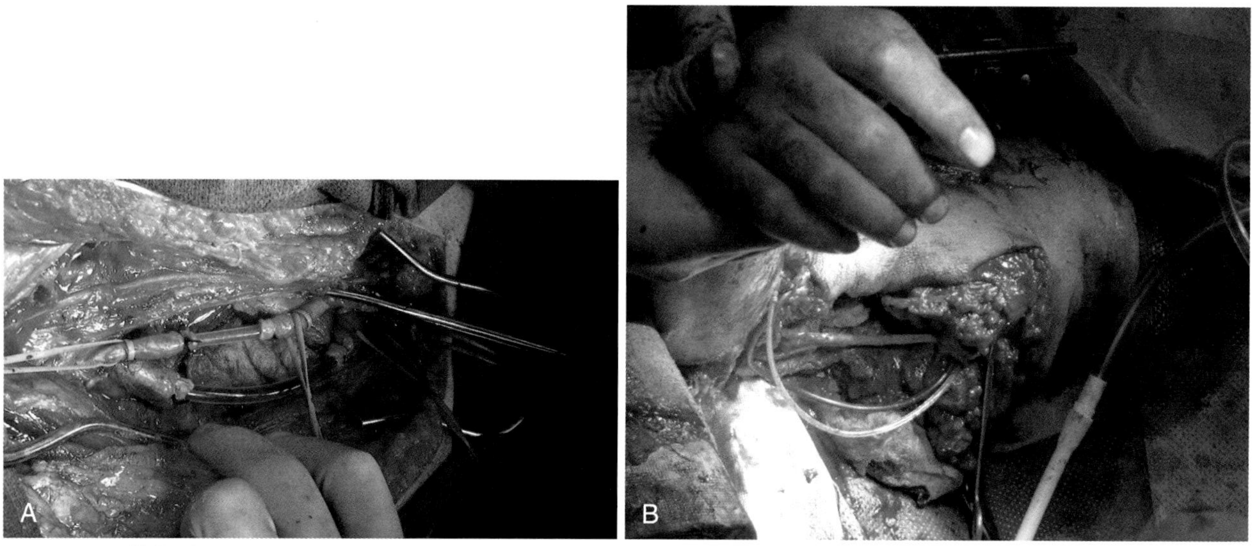

FIG 48.4 (A) Temporary arterial and venous shunts. (B) A Morgan Lens ocular irrigation catheter (MorTan, Inc., Missoula, MT) was modified to use as a vascular shunt in this patient. (Courtesy Jonathan Eliason and Sandra Halterman. Used with permission.)

of limbs to be salvaged.[119] Other reports from military investigators have documented that 50% to 60% of patients being treated for vascular trauma at forward surgical units have shunts placed; patency rates range from 86% to 96% when the patients arrived at the next echelon of care for definitive surgery.[120] Air Force investigators at Balad found that the patency rates for proximal arterial shunts was 86% and 100% for venous shunts; distal shunts (e.g., infrapopliteal) had a very poor patency rate of 12%.[117] While there is no level I data demonstrating improved survival or limb salvage, research by Gifford and colleagues demonstrated a trend toward a decreased amputation rate with TVS in a case control study using propensity adjustment.[17]

Principles for Open and Endovascular Repair

For open repair, the four basic principles include obtaining adequate exposure, obtaining proximal and distal control before exploring the site of injury, preparing the potential vein harvest site, and finally performing the repair procedure. After exposing the injured vessel, assessment should be made regarding the extent of damage. Simple arterial repairs fair better than grafts and should be considered if technically possible. If there is concern about stenosing the diameter of the injured vessel, then a vein patch should be considered. However, blunt injuries, crush, gunshot wounds, and so on cause significant damage to the vessel wall. The vessel should be opened past the area of injury to examine the intima, which should be trimmed back to healthy tissues before proceeding with the repair. If the missing segment is short, a primary repair should be performed by anastomosing the spatulated edges of the vessel. This usually requires mobilizing the vessel for a long segment to allow primary repair of the artery. However, larger segment vascular injuries should be replaced with reversed saphenous vein grafts.

If an autologous conduit is not an option due to injury or due to size of the venous conduit, prosthetic grafts can be used for limb salvage even in contaminated wounds.[121] Before the repair, good inflow and outflow should be ensured by removing any thrombus, and after the repair, good distal flow must be confirmed with either ultrasound assessment or a completion angiography. In most cases, systemic anticoagulation is not an option, due to the multitrauma nature of the patient. Early four-compartment lower leg fasciotomy should be whenever possible considered when the total ischemia time is more than 4 hours or if there are associated injuries, particularly in combined arterial and venous injuries.[122] However, fasciotomy is not without complications, and the decision has to be made judiciously based on case-by-case evaluation. If prophylactic fasciotomy is not performed, serial physical exams are required, and if possible, measuring serial compartment pressure is advised.

Management of Upper Extremity Vascular Trauma

Subclavian Artery

Please refer to the Management of Penetrating Thoracic Aortic and Great Vessels Injury section.

Axillary Artery

Injury to the axillary artery represents approximately 5% to 23% of arterial trauma in most civilian and military series.[123–125] A total of 95% of these injuries are due to penetrating mechanisms; blunt trauma is uncommon, given the high degree of protection by overlying tissues in this anatomic location; likewise, presentation in hypovolemic shock is rare due to trauma to this artery. The axillary vein is in very close proximity to the artery in this location, however, and there is a fairly high risk of arteriovenous fistula, which can develop from minor vascular trauma in this location. The artery and vein are also in intimate communication the brachial plexus, especially at the distal extent, making concomitant neurologic injury the rule rather than the exception.

Injury to the axillary artery should be suspected if there is a palpable subclavian pulse felt in the supraclavicular fossa, a weak or absent pulse distally in the brachial artery, and a discrepancy between the blood pressure measurements between the bilateral upper extremities.

Exposure of the axillary artery for trauma can be achieved with the deltopectoral approach. The arm is abducted 30 degrees and externally rotated. An incision is made from the midpoint of the clavicle 5 to 7 cm along the anterior border of the deltoid muscle. This incision is carried down to the intermuscular groove between the pectoralis and deltoid muscles, containing the cephalic vein. The pectoralis muscle is then retracted medially and the underlying clavipectoral fascia divided. The cephalic vein and deltoid muscle are retracted laterally. The third part of the axillary artery is then encountered with the brachial plexus cords surrounding it. Division of the thoracoacromial trunk and the pectoralis minor muscles permits access to the second and first parts of the axillary artery.

Brachial Artery

The brachial artery is the most commonly injured artery in the upper extremity, occurring in 40% to 50% of cases.[123–125] The most common mechanism is penetrating injury (92%).

On examination, the absence of an arterial pulse is the most common presentation (88%); weakness of the brachial pulse is found in 12%. Using brachial-brachial indices (BBI, with <0.85 being considered abnormal), preoperative BBI was found to be 0.43 ± 0.5 (range 0.23 to 0.48) in patients with brachial artery injuries. This increased to 0.89 ± 0.03 (range 0.83 to 0.93) postoperatively.[126]

Exposure of the brachial artery is very straightforward. With the arm abducted 90 degrees and supported on an arm board, an incision is made in the groove between the biceps and triceps muscle on the medial aspect of the arm. This incision is considered extensile, and can be extended proximally or distally as needed. It is important to avoid the basilic vein as the brachial artery is approached; it courses through the subcutaneous tissues just posterior to the brachial groove to the midpoint of the upper arm, where it penetrates the fascia and then runs near the brachial structures. The deep fascia at the inferior border of the biceps muscle is incised and the biceps retracted anteriorly. The basilic vein is then retracted posteriorly and the brachial sheath is opened. The median nerve is the most superficial structure. It is widely mobilized and gently retracted anteriorly. The artery is then found deep to the median nerve with two veins on either side. The deepest structure in this sheath is the ulnar nerve. Occasionally two arteries may be encountered in the sheath; this represents a high bifurcation of the artery, and they represent the radial and ulnar arteries.

Exposure of the distal brachial artery in cases of trauma should be performed through a lazy–S shaped incision placed over the antecubital fossa. The superior longitudinal portion is located along the medial border of the biceps muscle, and the inferior portion is lateral to the midpoint of the volar forearm for 4 to 6 cm. Identify and protect the basilic vein and the medial antecubital nerve which should be retracted medially. The bicipital aponeurosis is then divided, exposing the brachial artery. Ligation of two crossing vein branches permits wider exposure of this artery and its bifurcation into the radial and ulnar arteries.

Radial and Ulnar Arteries

Forearm vascular injuries occur in 10% to 50% of cases.[123–125] Control of the radial artery at midforearm can be accomplished through an incision over the medial border of the brachioradialis muscle, located on a line between the midpoint of the antecubital fossa and the styloid process of the radius. The antebrachial fascia is divided and the brachioradialis muscle retracted laterally to expose the radial artery. Exposure of the radial artery at the wrist is accomplished by making a longitudinal incision over the radial pulse if one exists, or just lateral to the flexor carpi radialis tendon and extending proximally 3 to 4 cm. The cephalic vein is lateral to the artery and should be preserved in the subcutaneous tissues if possible and retracted laterally. The antebrachial fascia is then incised and the artery exposed. Exposure of the ulnar artery in the wrist is accomplished through a longitudinal incision lateral to the flexor carpi ulnaris tendon. Division of the antebrachial fascia exposes the artery.

Upper Extremity Fasciotomy

The forearm fasciotomy is performed by making a long S-type incision on the volar aspect of the forearm (Fig. 48.5). The incision starts distally along the base of the thenar eminence, bends slightly radially at the proximal thenar eminence, then moves directly transverse from radial to ulnar across the wrist, releasing the carpal tunnel. This is complete when the median nerve is visualized. The incision then continues along the ulnar aspect of the forearm, looping back radially in the midportion of the forearm (which allows a flap to be created to cover the median nerve if necessary) and again moving in an ulnar direction behind the medial epicondyle. The incision then moves somewhat to in the radial direction and finally follows the medial border of the biceps muscle. If the incision has not decompressed the mobile wad on the medial aspect of the flexor compartment, a separate longitudinal incision over this compartment will release it. On the dorsal surface, a longitudinal incision is made over the forearm

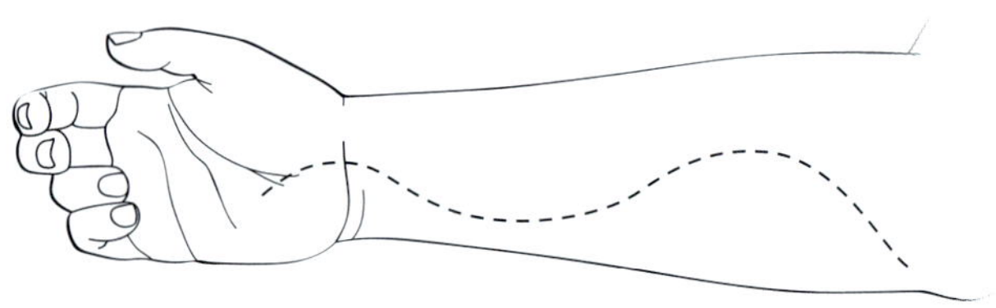

FIG 48.5 Forearm fasciotomy incision.

flexor compartment. The dorsal surface of the hand should be decompressed with linear incisions between the extensor digitorum tendons of the second and third and the third and fourth digits. The interossei can then be detached from the metacarpals, if necessary, to further decompress the hand.[127]

Dente and colleagues reported a series of 37 upper extremity fasciotomies performed in 27 patients. The mechanisms were distributed between penetrating trauma (35%), blunt trauma (24%), and burn injury (14%), of which 80% were due to electrical injuries. Most fasciotomies (89%) were performed at the initial operation and usually were based on clinical assessment. Of the 22% of cases where compartment pressures were checked, the mean pressure was 52 mm Hg, with a range of 40 to 87. In this series, no amputations were required because of failure to perform fasciotomy.[128] Risk factors for compartment syndrome of the forearm in cases of brachial artery injury include combined arterial injuries, concomitant nerve injury, motor deficits, fractures, and significant blood loss interoperatively.[129]

Endovascular Intervention for Upper Extremity Trauma

Just as is the case for most vascular interventions, cases of successful endovascular repair of suitable lesions in the upper and lower extremities have been increasingly reported. Valentin and colleagues present a case of a traumatic subclavian artery dissection treated successfully with a self-expanding stent.[130] Desai and colleagues reported on outcomes after endovascular repair of arterial trauma in upper and lower extremities in 28 patients. They were able to successfully treat all 28 patients utilizing endovascular techniques. They concluded that the inclusion of endovascular modalities in algorithms of trauma care holds considerable promise.[131] Strict contraindications included long segmental injuries, lack of fixation points, and arterial transection. They reported that approximately 50% of the lesions they evaluated would be amenable to endovascular repair.[132] The authors would encourage the surgeon to assess the patients on a case-by-case basis, as many of the trauma patients are young, and despite the initial success of endovascular technique in this population, we simply do not have the knowledge regarding the long-term durability of the repair in these circumstances.

Outcomes

The overall limb salvage rate in upper extremity arterial injury has been reported to range from 96% to 98% with little or no mortality related to the extremity injury. Frech and colleagues re-examined 65 patients who had repairs for upper extremity trauma and found the patency rate to be 97% at median follow-up of 5.3 years.[133] In the uncommon cases of amputation, early graft failure, compartment syndrome, and associated skeletal and brachial plexus injury were found to be significant predictors of limb loss. Military mechanisms are also significantly associated with risk of amputation.[123–125] However, despite maintenance of limb viability, neurologic injury has been found to be the most significant predictor of functional outcome.[134]

The outcome after upper extremity trauma is a multifactorial goal which extends beyond the success of operative repair. Given the importance of the hand in all aspects of life, individuals with upper extremity and hand injuries may experience significant consequences in their physical, psychological and social wellbeing. Galanakos and colleagues noted that psychological morbidity is an important part of patients' perceived general health. The role played by these issues plays a paramount part in the final functional outcome of their therapy. Therefore, early identification and treatment of trauma-related distress in this patient population could prevent progression of psychological pathology.[135]

Management of Lower Extremity Vascular Trauma

Femoral artery. The femoral artery is the most commonly injured vessel in the lower extremity. This holds true for both military and civilian trauma. In a report of nearly 2500 wartime vascular injuries from World War II, Debakey and Simeone reported 517 (21%) injuries to the femoral artery.[4] Reports from the Korean War and Vietnam vascular registry showed similar incidence rates.[5,106] Civilian series cite rates of approximately 70%.[118] Injury at this site is generally considered nonlethal, although postoperative morbidity is high; the complication rate is 23% and the wound infection rate is 15%. The mechanism is primarily penetrating, with gunshot wounds being the most common cause. Associated injuries are frequent: combined arteriovenous trauma is seen in 46%, orthopedic injuries are seen in 22% (generally femur fractures), femoral nerve injuries in 10%. Distal ischemia is present in 48% of cases; pulses are weak or absent in 43%, and an expanding hematoma is seen in 29%. Soft signs such as delayed capillary refill are less common. The ankle-brachial index averages 0.92 in these injuries, which is very misleading.[118]

Surgical treatment of these lesions is similar to other areas. A total of 145 combat-related femoral and popliteal injuries were treated primarily with autogenous vein graft (88%). Ligation was rare (5%).[8] In a series of 204 civilian femoral injuries, a reversed saphenous graft was used in 53%, primary repair in 26%, PTFE interposition in 10%, and ligation in 6%, and vein patch in 4%.[118]

The surgical approach to the femoral artery should follow the same principles discussed previously. The incision should be made longitudinally to allow for extension proximally and distally. An obvious wound or hematoma should be avoided initially until proximal and distal control is achieved. The proximal approach to the femoral artery begins just inferior to the inguinal ligament at approximately midway between the anterior iliac spine and the pubic tubercle. Once the vessel is isolated proximally, it is controlled with a double-looped vessel loop or a clamp. Prior to occlusion, the patient should be heparinized if possible, given the catalog of injuries. If necessary, the inguinal ligament can be divided to achieve more proximal control of the vessel for high injuries. If this maneuver is insufficient to gain control, a low midline laparotomy and intra-abdominal control should be secured. Once high proximal control is established, clamps can be moved distally in a serial fashion known as "walking the clamps." Distal control of the vessel should occur similarly. Begin by avoiding the zone of injury and moving more proximally. Back bleeding is rarely as problematic as forward bleeding, however, and entry into the wound to achieve distal control can work if necessary. Another option for control of vessels is balloon occlusion, either endovascularly from a remote access site or directly through the wound using balloon catheters.

Popliteal artery. These injuries occur less frequently than femoral artery injuries, yet there is a particular injury pattern associated with the popliteal artery, which can be subtle yet devastating. After blunt injury, especially following posterior knee dislocations, the rate of vascular injury is substantial. Of 18 patients in one study with posterior knee dislocations and popliteal artery injury, there were 4 (22%) amputations.[136] Among 1395 popliteal injuries in the National Trauma Data Bank, the incidence was 0.2% of all traumas. Blunt trauma was the mechanism in 61% of cases. The overall rate of amputation was 15%; risk factors for amputation were fracture, complex soft tissue injury, nerve injury, and elevated Abbreviated Injury Scale.[137] Using a protocol of performing angiography in the operating room, investigators at the University of Wisconsin have demonstrated improvement in limb salvage, 100% versus 70%, if angiography is performed in the operating room versus the radiology suite, likely due to the decrease in ischemic time.

Approach to the popliteal artery is best done through a large medial incision. The posterior margin of the femur and the tibia are the major landmarks. The saphenous vein should be protected during exposure. An incision is placed along the anterior border of the sartorius muscle. The fascia is incised and the muscle retracted posteriorly. The vastus medialis is then retracted anteriorly. The fascial bridge connecting the adductor magnus tendon and the semimembranosus muscle is divided, and the neurovascular bundle is exposed. If additional exposure is necessary, the adductor magnus tendon can be divided, allowing more proximal control of the artery. The artery is then controlled below the knee through an incision placed 1 cm behind the posterior border of the tibia. The crural fascia is incised 1 cm posterior to the tibia and opened to the semitendinosus proximally. The medial head of the gastrocnemius is then retracted posteriorly; allow the neurovascular bundle to be approached. If necessary, the semitendinosus, gracilis, and sartorius muscles can be divided for further exposure, but should be repaired at the end of the case for maintenance of knee stability.

Lower Extremity Fasciotomy

In patients with concern of compartment syndrome, fasciotomy should be performed in an expeditious fashion to avoid permanent nerve damage.

The thigh has three compartments. A lateral incision made from greater trochanter to lateral condyle of femur. The iliotibial band incised and vastus lateralis reflected off intermuscular septum bluntly, releasing anterior compartment. Next, the intermuscular septum is incised the length of the incision, releasing posterior compartment. (This release of intermuscular septum should not be made close to femur because there are a series of perforating arteries passing through septum from posterior to anterior near bone.) Lastly, the medial adductor compartment is released through separate anteromedial incision

In the lower leg, a four-compartment below-knee fasciotomy should be performed. The two-incision technique is technically the easiest and safest approach. A longitudinal incision is made on the lateral leg two fingerbreadths laterally to the tibia. This incision is carried down to the fascia of the muscular compartment. Care is taken to avoid the superficial peroneal nerve. An incision is then made in the fascia of the muscular compartment and the incision is carried proximally to the tibial tuberosity and distally to 3 to 4 cm from the lateral malleolus. It is vital that once either the anterior or lateral compartment is entered, the intermuscular septum is identified to ensure that the other compartment is then decompressed in the same way; a critical mistake is to decompress the same compartment twice, leaving the remaining compartment at high pressure and high risk of myonecrosis, nerve loss, and dysfunction. The second incision is made 2 fingerbreadths medial to the tibia. In this case, the saphenous vein should be avoided. Both the deep and superficial posterior compartments can be reached easily through this incision. Again, ensure that both compartments are fully released.

Gonzalez studied 321 patients with 393 lower extremity-penetrating injuries and found that the most common cause of lower extremity compartment syndrome was due to penetrating injury to the proximal infra-geniculate leg. Development of compartment syndrome secondary to thigh injuries occurred only in the presence of surgically significant vascular injury, including injury-requiring ligation of the femoral vein.[138] Asensio and colleagues documented a 12% rate of fasciotomy; their indications were the presence of shock, combined arteriovenous injury, or associated fracture requiring external fixators or internal fixation.[118]

Endovascular Intervention for Lower Extremity Trauma

Reports regarding the routine use of endovascular techniques following lower extremity penetrating arterial trauma are limited. Endovascular interventions techniques range from temporary vascular control with a balloon, to embolization of a bleeding vessel, and covered stent repair of an injury. Theoretically, endovascular approach to a peripheral vascular injury for trauma patients has the advantage of remote access to the injured vessel, which can prove to be crucial in difficult-to-expose anatomic areas, reduces the risk of injury to nearby structures (nerves), and avoids the need for surgically traversing already injured and, sometimes, devitalized tissue. Victims undergoing endovascular interventions can have decreased operative time and reduced blood loss.[139] Nonetheless, there are no large series to prove the advantage of endovascular intervention over open repair in trauma patients. Thus a decision to use these techniques would have to be made on an individual case-by-case basis.

Arterial embolization is generally reserved for branch vessel occlusions. This is most commonly used for internal iliac, profunda femoris, or tibial branch bleeding. Three small series described arterial embolization of bleeding lower extremity branches following penetrating trauma. Thirty patients were treated with coils, *N*-butyl 2-cyanoacrylate (NBCA), or thrombin. Target vessels included branches of the internal iliac, profunda femoris, and tibial arteries. Hemostasis was successful in all cases, and nontarget embolization was reported in two patients.[140–142]

Covered stent-graft utilization for arterial traumatic injury repair has also been reported in the literature. White and colleagues reported a series of 62 patients with upper and lower extremity arterial trauma treated with a covered stent. Thirty-three patients had iliac artery injury, while 11 involved the femoral artery.[143] The 1-year exclusion rate for iliac lesions was 91% but only 62% for femoral intervention. The 1-year primary patency rates for the stent-grafts in the iliac artery were 76% and in the femoral artery were 86%. The most common adverse events were stenosis in 4.8% of the entire cohort and stent-graft occlusion, which occurred early in 6.5%. Fifteen percent required surgical bypass within 1 year for various indications. Another technique is to utilize stent-grafts as an intravascular shunt prior to orthopedic repair. Simmons and colleagues reported on using this technique in patients with lower extremity arterial injury with combined skeletal injury for vascular intervention prior to orthopedic with later open surgical repair after bony fixation.[144] Other reports confirm that both bare metal and covered stents can be used to treat arterial trauma (disruptions, dissections, and pseudoaneurysms) of the iliac, superficial femoral, popliteal, and even the tibial arteries.[145,146]

It is important to acknowledge that the lack of large series regarding endovascular intervention in this patient population, especially given that most trauma patients are younger than the usual vasculopathy patient we deal with on an everyday basis. Also, long-term data on patency and success of these techniques are lacking. Both the Western Trauma Association and the Eastern Association for the Surgery of Trauma guidelines on the management of lower extremity arterial trauma acknowledge data in this field is scarce, and that there are no data to support routine utilization of endovascular interventions following femoral-popliteal trauma. Nonetheless, both guidelines recommend embolization of profunda femoris branches or tibial vessels in appropriate patients.

EXTREMITY VENOUS INJURY

The first successful lateral repair of a lacerated femoral vein was performed by Schede in 1882.[6] Also, Goodman is reported to have performed one of the first wartime venous repairs in 1918.[147] However, ligation of venous injuries was the accepted standard of care during World War I. In an attempt to improve limb salvage, Makins in 1919 recommended ligation of the uninjured vein when an arterial injury was treated by ligation.[148] It was not until the Korean War that a more concerted effort was made at perfecting the repair of venous injuries. Work by Hughes and Rich observations in 1957 and 1970 respectively showed that repair of military venous injuries could be performed safely.[148,149] Quan and colleagues reported only 25% of patients with extremity vascular trauma who had isolated venous injuries.[148] This current report is similar to historical reports on the incidence of venous injuries occurring during wartime. Despite dramatic differences in magnitude of injury, reports on civilian vascular trauma report that the majority (75%) of venous injuries also occur in association with arterial injuries.[150–152]

A review of the recent literature shows that nearly 90% of civilian venous trauma occurs in the extremities, with a near equal distribution between upper and lower extremities.[153] Gaspar and Trieman[154] documented the incidence of civilian venous injuries as 17% superficial femoral vein, 15% inferior vena cava,

15% internal jugular vein, 14% brachial vein, and 8% popliteal vein. In a report from Louisiana State University, Smith and colleagues[155] reported 25% of venous injuries involved the iliac veins, 45% femoral, 20% popliteal, and 10% basilic veins.

Recognition of injured venous structures in patients with non-life-threatening or non-limb-threatening trauma can be more of a challenge. Ultrasonography is the initial technique of choice for the detection and evaluation of venous thromboses associated with trauma. The loss of spontaneous venous flow, respiratory variation, and compressibility confirm venous thrombosis. Gagne and colleagues[156] reported that color-flow duplex ultrasonography (CFD) detected seven of eight (88%) venous injuries in 37 civilian patients with penetrating proximity extremity trauma.

In suspected venous injuries, which involve the vena cava, any of the mesenteric veins (portal vein, superior mesenteric vein, splenic vein, and inferior mesenteric vein) and the iliac veins, ultrasound studies have limited utility, owing to the difficulty of visualizing these structures in a nonfasting patient and due to the body habitus of some patients. Venography would remain the gold standard for diagnosing, and it adds the potential of being able to intervene endovascularly for repair or vascular control, but it also carries the risk of being an invasive procedure. In a hemodynamically stable patient, CT scan with delayed images to assess the venous phase is generally the test of choice for assessing such injuries.

Management options range from ligation to primary repair and interposition grafting. Over the past 10 to 15 years, many reports have emerged to support the utilization of endovascular techniques in management of venous trauma, which ranged from endovascular assistance for open repair to complex endovascular reconstructive techniques.[157–161]

The management of traumatic venous injuries should be performed with consideration for the overall physiologic status of the patient. For patients with multisystem injury and hemodynamic instability, ligation of the venous injury, even if caval, iliac, common femoral, or popliteal, would be prudent. In stable trauma patients with single-system injuries, however, major venous injuries should be repaired, if possible. Specifically, the axillary, subclavian, common iliac, external iliac, common femoral, popliteal veins, and vena cava should be repaired. Even short-term patency of these veins in the acute trauma patient will help avoid massive swelling distal to these injuries in the extremities and the possibility of developing a compartment syndrome.

REVIEW QUESTIONS

1. Based on the Eastern Association for the Surgery of Trauma (EAST), diagnostic evaluation for blunt cervical vascular injury in an asymptomatic patient is recommended in all the following patients *except:*
   a. Petrous bone fracture
   b. Diffuse axonal injury
   c. Le Fort III facial fracture
   d. GCS greater than or equal 14
   e. Cervical spine fracture through the transversarium
2. A patient presents to the trauma bay with a gunshot wound to the thigh. On exploration, you find a superficial femoral artery injury with a 3-cm defect. He is hemodynamically stable. What is the best approach to managing this kind of injury?
   a. Primary repair of the arterial injury
   b. Replace the missing segment with an interposition PTFE graft
   c. Replace the missing segment with an interposition ipsilateral GSV graft
   d. Replace the missing segment with an interposition contralateral GSV graft
   e. Ligate the artery proximally and distally
3. A 17-year-old high school football player was brought to the trauma bay after suffering being hit on a play and falling down while grabbing his right leg. Which orthopedic injury should raise suspicion for a possible associated vascular injury?
   a. A medial meniscus tear
   b. A midfemur shaft fracture
   c. A posterior knee dislocation
   d. An anterior cruciate ligament tear
4. The lethal triad of trauma includes all of the following *except:*
   a. Tachycardia
   b. Acidosis
   c. Coagulopathy
   d. Hypothermia
5. Presence of pulse is a reliable method to rule out the presence of extremity compartment syndrome:
   a. True
   b. False
6. Which of the following statements is false?
   a. All suprarenal vena cava injury must be repaired or temporarily shunted.
   b. A blunt Zone I hematoma can be observed and managed conservatively.
   c. Injury to the portal vein is very common and can be readily repaired with low mortality.
   d. Fasciotomy of the upper extremity is performed by making a long "S"-type incision on the volar aspect of the forearm.
7. What is the most commonly injured artery in the upper extremity?
   a. Axillary artery
   b. Brachial artery
   c. Radial artery
   d. Ulnar artery

References available online at ExpertConsult.com.

49 CHAPTER

Venous Thromboembolic Disease

Dawn M. Coleman, Peter K. Henke, Benjamin Jacobs, Andrew Kimball, Jordan Knepper, Andrea Obi, Scott T. Robinson, Thomas Wakefield

Venous thromboembolism (VTE), which includes both deep venous thrombosis (DVT) and pulmonary embolism (PE), is very common. Although the etiology of acute venous thrombosis (VT) is defined by Virchow triad of hypercoagulability, stasis, and endothelial injury, it is clearly a multifactorial process influenced by many other conditions. The acute thrombotic process must be managed appropriately to relieve edema and pain, to prevent death from PE, and to avoid reoccurrence and the long-term sequelae of postthrombotic syndrome (PTS), which is estimated to occur in 30% of patients older than 8 years, although it may be higher, especially with iliofemoral DVT. In addition to compression and ambulation, there are a number of pharmacologic treatment options: unfractionated heparin (UFH), low-molecular-weight heparin (LMWH), and vitamin K antagonists (VKAs), such as warfarin (Coumadin). Many new and alternative agents are becoming available and may require less rigorous monitoring. Length of anticoagulation typically ranges from 3 months for a first-time event, although certain conditions may warrant lifelong therapy. In other cases, surgical placement of inferior vena cava (IVC) filters may be indicated to prevent further propagation of PE. The present chapter is divided into sections encompassing discussions on all of these topics, including pathophysiology of VT, epidemiology of thrombosis, biomarkers, risk factors, anticoagulants (including the new agents), length of anticoagulation for VTE treatment, thrombolysis and vein wall abnormalities after DVT, diagnosis and treatment of superficial thrombophlebitis, and a discussion about inferior vena caval interruption.

PATHOPHYSIOLOGY OF VENOUS THROMBOSIS

VT is governed by the three principles of the Virchow triad: hypercoagulability, stasis, and endothelial injury. Activation of coagulation is critical in the pathogenesis of DVT. Although the hemostatic system is continuously active, thrombus formation is ordinarily confined to sites of local injury by a precise balance between activators and inhibitors of coagulation and fibrinolysis. A prothrombotic state may result either from imbalances in the regulatory and inhibitory systems or from activation exceeding antithrombotic capacity.[1] Regardless of etiology, most venous thrombi originate in areas of static, low blood flow, often behind valve pockets.[2] Furthermore, many risk factors for acute DVT are associated with immobilization and slow venous flow, and these mechanisms have been advanced to explain the role of stasis in thrombogenesis. For example, in comparison to pulsatile flow, static streamline flow is associated with significant hypoxia at the depths of the venous valve cusps and may induce endothelial injury.[3] Under basal conditions, the endothelium provides a vasodilatory and local fibrinolytic environment via plasminogen activators, such as tissue plasminogen activator and urokinase plasminogen activator. In this setting, coagulation, platelet adhesion, platelet activation, inflammation, and leukocyte activation are inhibited.[4] After a disturbance of the endothelium, a prothrombotic and proinflammatory state occurs and is defined by vasoconstriction, activated platelets, and upregulation of cellular mediators to recruit inflammatory cells to the site of endothelial damage.[5] Indeed, experimental evidence suggests that platelets may be involved with early VT.[6]

Individually, stasis, endothelial injury, and activated coagulation factors may be insufficient to provoke thrombosis.[7] However, when localized in regions of stasis and incited by endothelial disruption, the coagulation cascade allows activated factors to rapidly intensify the thrombotic stimulus, leading to platelet aggregation, coagulation factor localization, and fibrin formation.[8] Thus thrombosis appears to be a multifactorial phenomenon, with convergence of several pathologic factors often required to produce a thrombotic event.[9] A good example of this clinically is the postoperative patient who suffers an infectious complication.[10]

The pathophysiology of VT is a cyclic event, amplified by the associated inflammatory process.[11] With inflammation, there is an increase in tissue factor, platelet reactivity, fibrinogen, phosphatidylserine expression on membrane surfaces, and PAI-1 (inhibiting fibrinolysis) and a decrease in thrombomodulin (and thus a decrease in the activity of protein C).[12] Cell adhesion molecules, such as selectins, allow leukocyte transmigration and are intimately involved in this process. Venous stasis and ischemia result in upregulation of P-selectin, and this localizes microparticles, which are prothrombotic, to the area of evolving thrombosis.[13,14] The role of the inflammatory cell adhesion molecule P-selectin in thrombosis is critical. Data suggest that elevated levels of soluble P-selectin combined with a clinical examination favoring DVT has a positive predictive value for diagnosing DVT far exceeding that of D dimer.[15,16] More in-depth reviews highlight this interesting area for research.[1,17,18]

Epidemiology

The incidence of recurrent, fatal, and nonfatal VTE has been estimated to be 300,000 to 600,000 cases annually in the United States.[19] VTE has been estimated to occur with an incidence of approximately 1 per 1000 adult patients annually.[20] This figure is supported by the 35-year population-based Rochester Epidemiology Project database of Olmstead County, Minnesota, which demonstrated an overall average age- and sex-adjusted annual incidence of VTE of 122 per 1,000,000 person-years.[21] This landmark study also demonstrated higher age-adjusted rates in men compared with women (134 vs. 115 per 100,000 patients, respectively). First-time, or incident, VTE cases are estimated to occur in approximately 250,000 individuals annually in the United States.[22] However, there is a difference in ethnic groups diagnosed with VTE. African Americans demonstrate greater than a 25% increased incidence in first-time VTE compared with whites (103 vs. 141 per 100,000 patients). Conversely, the incidence of first-time VTE in both Hispanic and Asian or Pacific Islanders is significantly lower than in whites (62 vs. 104 per 100,000 patients; 29 vs. 104 per 100,000 patients, respectively).[23,24] Nevertheless, the issue of VTE is not isolated to the United States. Recent estimates across the European Union have totaled nearly 700,000 cases of DVT, 435,000 cases of PE, and 543,000 fatalities.[25]

Although estimated incidences of VTE in both the community and hospital have been well documented, individuals at risk for VTE have been less well studied. Substantial differences have been noted in the distribution of risk factors between inpatients and outpatients. Extrapolating hospital inpatient data on the estimated 38 million patients discharged in 2003, 31% were considered to be at risk for VTE secondary to either major surgery or a medical illness.[26] Although the incidence of VTE varies with the population studied, use of thromboprophylaxis, the intensity of screening, and the diagnostic test used, specific risk factors have been significantly associated with increasing VTE. Patients at highest risk are exemplified in the critically ill and trauma patients in whom bleeding risks prohibit thromboprophylaxis, and immobility contribute up to a greater than 80% DVT rate in specific populations.[27] Risk stratification for VTE based on a number of individualized patient-specific clinical attributes was initially proposed by Caprini.[28] In a large, single-center validation study, a modified Caprini risk assessment tool was applied to patients undergoing general surgery, associating higher scores with an increased incidence of VTE.[29] Currently, electronic order entry to mandate a modified Caprini risk assessment tool is recommended for all hospitalized patients (Fig. 49.1).[30] Recognition of patients at high risk for VTE is a critical part in its prevention. In the next section, risk factors for VTE will be discussed in detail.

Biomarkers

The "gold standard" for diagnosis of DVT remains duplex ultrasound.[31] However, there has been research directed toward the development of a simple, reliable, and accurate serum biomarker for the presence of DVT. Given that ultrasound can be both operator dependent and, in some institutions, unavailable at off-hours, a serum biomarker that speeds and simplifies diagnosis would be of great benefit to patients; moreover, the ability to obviate the need for ultrasound would represent a significant cost savings to the health care system.

Currently, the most well-validated and widely used serum biomarker is D dimer, a fibrin-degradation product.[32,33] D dimer is evaluated by a blood test using one of a variety of enzyme-linked immunosorbent assays (ELISAs). Pretest probability of VTE is determined based on a clinical score, most commonly the Wells score. VTE can be excluded safely in patients in whom there is a low pretest probability and a negative D dimer.[31] When combined with Wells score, D dimer performs excellently in a number of patient populations, including outpatients,[33] emergency department patients,[34] pregnant patients,[35] and cancer patients.[36] Concerns remain regarding the specificity of the test, which can be elevated in numerous other states, such as postoperatively and in postpartum individuals; these states also represent risk factors for VTE.[37,38] D dimer appears to be less effective for diagnosis in certain patient populations, including the elderly[39] and orthopedic surgery patients.[40,41] Age adjustment of cutoff values may increase the diagnostic performance of the test in elderly individuals.[42]

Soluble P-selectin, a cell adhesion and signaling molecule released with endothelial injury, has been evaluated as a biomarker for DVT. Elevated P-selectin is associated with increased risk of VTE in cancer patients.[43] Vandy and colleagues[44] demonstrated good rule-in performance for soluble P-selectin, with a positive predictive value of 91%—significantly more accurate at ruling in than D dimer with a positive predictive value of 69%. Although not yet widely available clinically, the literature suggests that a combination of Wells score, D dimer, and P-selectin may provide the greatest diagnostic performance by alleviating the low specificity of D dimer alone.

Risk Factors

Age

A higher incidence of VTE has consistently been associated with advanced age. In a community-based study of phlebographically documented DVT, the yearly incidence of DVT increased progressively from almost 0 in childhood to 7.65 cases per 1000 in men and 8.22 cases per 1000 in women by age 80.[45] Similarly, in a more recent study reevaluating the Framingham Heart Cohort, age was significantly associated with VTE, with a hazard ratio per increase in 10 years of age of 1.69 (95% confidence interval [CI] 1.48 to 1.92).[46]

Immobilization

Immobilization promotes venous stasis and is a major risk factor for VTE. The prevalence of lower extremity DVT in autopsy studies parallels the duration of bed rest, with DVT occurring

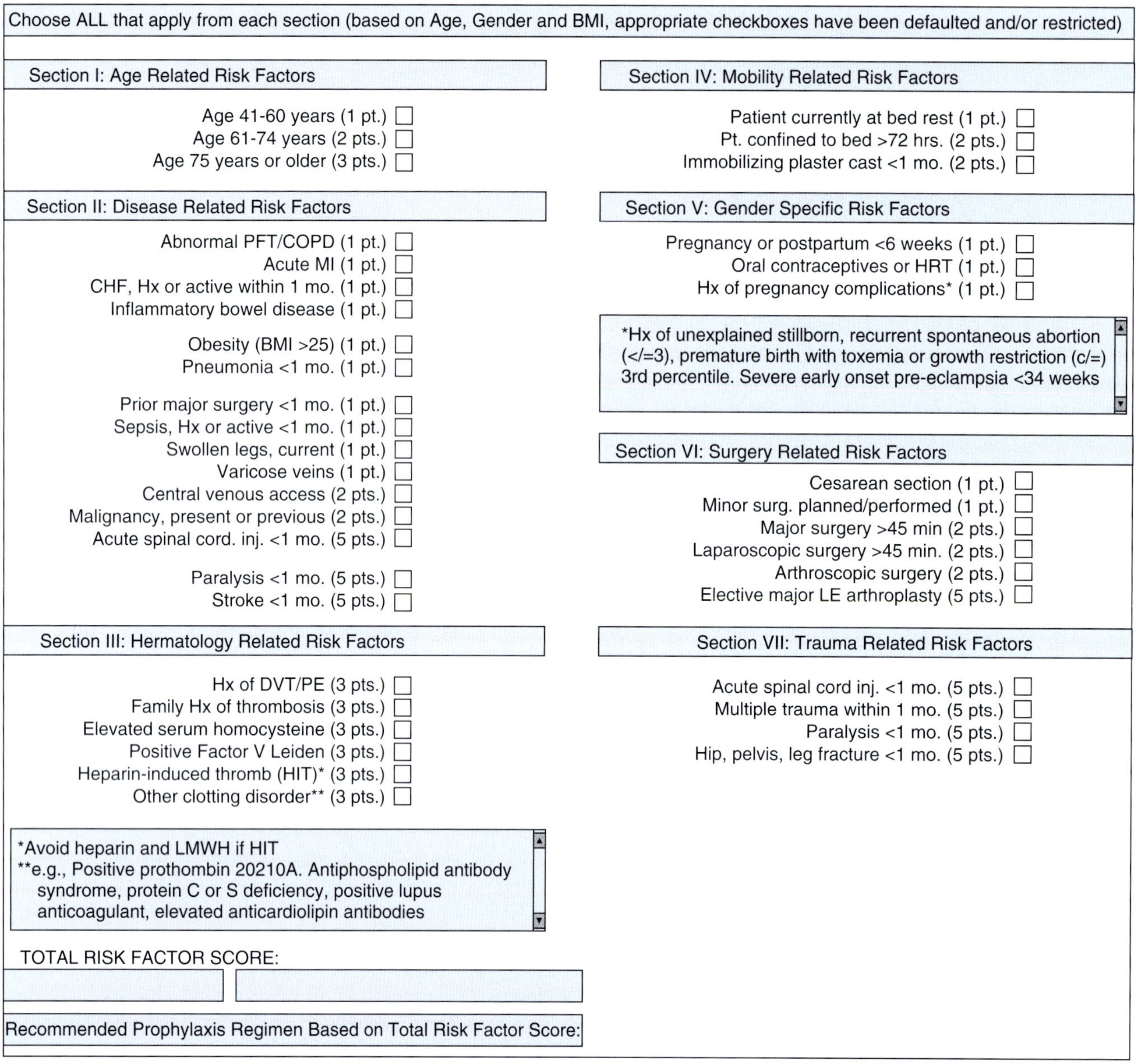

Choose ALL that apply from each section (based on Age, Gender and BMI, appropriate checkboxes have been defaulted and/or restricted)

Section I: Age Related Risk Factors

- Age 41-60 years (1 pt.) ☐
- Age 61-74 years (2 pts.) ☐
- Age 75 years or older (3 pts.) ☐

Section II: Disease Related Risk Factors

- Abnormal PFT/COPD (1 pt.) ☐
- Acute MI (1 pt.) ☐
- CHF, Hx or active within 1 mo. (1 pt.) ☐
- Inflammatory bowel disease (1 pt.) ☐
- Obesity (BMI >25) (1 pt.) ☐
- Pneumonia <1 mo. (1 pt.) ☐
- Prior major surgery <1 mo. (1 pt.) ☐
- Sepsis, Hx or active <1 mo. (1 pt.) ☐
- Swollen legs, current (1 pt.) ☐
- Varicose veins (1 pt.) ☐
- Central venous access (2 pts.) ☐
- Malignancy, present or previous (2 pts.) ☐
- Acute spinal cord. inj. <1 mo. (5 pts.) ☐
- Paralysis <1 mo. (5 pts.) ☐
- Stroke <1 mo. (5 pts.) ☐

Section III: Hermatology Related Risk Factors

- Hx of DVT/PE (3 pts.) ☐
- Family Hx of thrombosis (3 pts.) ☐
- Elevated serum homocysteine (3 pts.) ☐
- Positive Factor V Leiden (3 pts.) ☐
- Heparin-induced thromb (HIT)* (3 pts.) ☐
- Other clotting disorder** (3 pts.) ☐

*Avoid heparin and LMWH if HIT
**e.g., Positive prothombin 20210A. Antiphospholipid antibody syndrome, protein C or S deficiency, positive lupus anticoagulant, elevated anticardiolipin antibodies

Section IV: Mobility Related Risk Factors

- Patient currently at bed rest (1 pt.) ☐
- Pt. confined to bed >72 hrs. (2 pts.) ☐
- Immobilizing plaster cast <1 mo. (2 pts.) ☐

Section V: Gender Specific Risk Factors

- Pregnancy or postpartum <6 weeks (1 pt.) ☐
- Oral contraceptives or HRT (1 pt.) ☐
- Hx of pregnancy complications* (1 pt.) ☐

*Hx of unexplained stillborn, recurrent spontaneous abortion (</=3), premature birth with toxemia or growth restriction (c/=) 3rd percentile. Severe early onset pre-eclampsia <34 weeks

Section VI: Surgery Related Risk Factors

- Cesarean section (1 pt.) ☐
- Minor surg. planned/performed (1 pt.) ☐
- Major surgery >45 min (2 pts.) ☐
- Laparoscopic surgery >45 min. (2 pts.) ☐
- Arthroscopic surgery (2 pts.) ☐
- Elective major LE arthroplasty (5 pts.) ☐

Section VII: Trauma Related Risk Factors

- Acute spinal cord inj. <1 mo. (5 pts.) ☐
- Multiple trauma within 1 mo. (5 pts.) ☐
- Paralysis <1 mo. (5 pts.) ☐
- Hip, pelvis, leg fracture <1 mo. (5 pts.) ☐

TOTAL RISK FACTOR SCORE:

Recommended Prophylaxis Regimen Based on Total Risk Factor Score:

FIG 49.1 The mandated electronic order entry associated venous thromboembolism risk assessment that must be completed on each patient before additional order entry.

in 15% of patients dying after 0 to 7 days of bed rest as opposed to 79% to 94% of those dying after 2 to 12 weeks.[47] Preoperative immobilization is associated with postoperative DVT, contributing a twofold higher risk.[48] Patients with extremity paresis have a threefold higher risk for DVT and PE independent of hospital confinement, and with no significant differences in platelet counts, fibrinogen levels, von Willebrand factor (vWF), platelet factor-4, or beta thromboglobulin levels between patients with or without DVT—signifying immobilization is the major contributing factor.[49,50]

Travel

Despite the questionable importance of prolonged travel as a risk factor for VTE, in 2001 the World Health Organization acknowledged an association between air travel and VTE.[51] Lapostolle and coworkers observed that over an 86-month period, 56 of 135.3 million airline passengers had severe PE. The frequency of PE in those who traveled more than 5000 km was 150-fold higher than those who traveled less than 5000 km.[52] Paganin and associates observed a high incidence of VTE in patients with risk factors for DVT who traveled long distances. These investigators concluded that low mobility during flight was a modifiable risk factor for PE and that those with additional risk factors should increase their mobility.[53] Most recent estimates stipulate a risk of DVT of 1/600 for flights longer than 4 hours and 1/500 for flights longer than 12 hours.[54]

History of Venous Thromboembolism

Approximately 23% to 26% of patients with acute DVT have a previous history of DVT, and histologic studies confirm that acute thrombi are often associated with fibrous remnants of previous thrombi in the same or nearby veins.[55-57] Depending on sex and age, population-based studies have demonstrated that recurrent thromboembolism develops in 1 of every 11 to 50 persons with a previous episode of thromboembolism, with the risk for recurrent thromboembolism being higher in patients with idiopathic DVT.[58,59]

Obesity

The evidence supporting obesity as a risk factor for DVT has been controversial. In postmenopausal women, a body mass index of greater than 25 to 30 kg/m^2 has been associated with significantly increased risk.[60,61] Some investigators have reported obesity to be associated with a twofold greater risk for postoperative DVT,[62] but multifactorial analysis by others has not shown obesity to constitute an independent risk.[63] However, more recently a review of the Framingham Heart cohort revealed in multivariate analysis a body mass index [BMI] ≥ 30 afforded a hazard ratio of 1.88 (95% CI 1.44 to 2.45) for VTE.[46] Similarly, in other studies, obesity has been found to be a risk factor for recurrent DVT.[64,65]

Malignancy

Approximately 20% of all first-time VTE events are associated with malignancy.[66] Either DVT or PE will develop in an estimated 1 in 200 individuals with malignancy, a fourfold higher risk than in those without malignancy.[49] Considering all-cause in-hospital mortality for cancer patients, one in seven will die of PE.[67] Correlation with location of the tumor reveals that the highest rates of VTE are associated with pancreatic malignancies, followed by kidney, ovary, lung, and stomach malignancies.[68] Venous compression secondary to tumor growth, cancer-associated thrombocytosis, immobility, indwelling central lines, and chemotherapy or radiation therapy are all risk factors that increase the likelihood of developing VTE.[69] Furthermore, as many as 90% of patients with cancer have abnormal coagulation parameters, including increased levels of coagulation factors, elevated fibrinogen or fibrin degradation products, thrombocytosis, and elevated levels of circulating prothrombotic microparticles.[70-72]

Surgery

All components of the Virchow triad may be present in surgical patients: perioperative immobilization, transient changes in coagulation and fibrinolysis, and the potential for gross venous injury. In addition, surgery constitutes a spectrum of risk that is influenced by patient age, coexistent thrombotic risk factors, type of procedure, extent of surgical trauma, length of the procedure, and duration of postoperative immobilization.[73,74] Approximately half of postoperative lower extremity thrombi detected by ^{125}I-labeled fibrinogen scanning develop in the operating room, and the remainder occur over the next 3 to 5 days.[75] However, the risk for development of DVT does not end uniformly at hospital discharge. In one study, 51% of the thromboembolic events that occurred in patients undergoing gynecologic surgical procedures occurred after initial discharge.[76] One of the most at risk groups for VTE are those patients undergoing bariatric surgery, in which VTE was identified in 1% to 6% of patients, with a mean time to diagnosis of 24 days post operation.[77] Consequently, many bariatric surgery programs have begun prophylactic LMWH administration for the first month following the procedure.

Trauma

Despite improvements in trauma care and thromboembolism prophylaxis, DVT remains a significant source of morbidity and mortality in injured patients. In modern venographic series the incidence of DVT in the trauma patient is as high as 58%.[27] Recent trauma was the second most common risk factor for thromboembolism in the Olmsted County study by Heit and associates[78] and was associated with a nearly 13-fold increase in risk. As with postoperative DVT, several pathophysiologic elements may be responsible for the high incidence of DVT in trauma patients. Immobilization by skeletal fixation, paralysis, and critical illness are obviously associated with venous stasis, whereas mechanical injury is important after direct venous trauma and central venous cannulation. Less appreciated is the hypercoagulable state after depletion of coagulation inhibitors and components of the fibrinolytic system.[79,80] Finally, more recently, acute trauma has also been linked to neutrophil activation with the formation of intravascular neutrophil extracellular traps or "NETs" that have a clear link with activation of the coagulation cascade and VTE.[81]

Inherited Thrombophilia

Resistance to activated protein C was initially described by Dahlbach and associates[82] in 1993. Subsequent studies from the Leiden University Hospital in the Netherlands revealed a mutation in the gene for factor V conferring resistant to cleavage by activated protein C.[83,84] The factor V Leiden mutation has an autosomal dominant mode of inheritance and is at least tenfold more common than other inheritable defects.[85,86] The relative risk for first-time DVT is increased sevenfold in those who are heterozygous for the factor V Leiden mutation. However, the relative risk is increased eightyfold in individuals who are homozygous for the mutation.[87]

The prothrombin G20210A mutation, first described by Poort and associates[88] in 1996, was demonstrated in 28 families with a documented history of VTE. The mutation is characterized by a transition from guanine to adenine at the 20210 nucleotide on the prothrombin gene, and the mechanism of increased risk of thrombogenesis is unknown. The risk for VTE in the presence of the prothrombin G20210A mutation is threefold higher in heterozygotes than in wild type, and the presence of homozygosity further increases this risk.[89] Although prothrombin G20210A is rare in individuals of Asian or African descent, additional investigations have shown that in those with spontaneous DVT, the incidence of the mutation may range from 7% to 16%.[90,91]

Protein C is a vitamin K–dependent serine protease that inhibits the coagulation system by inactivating factors Va and VIIIa.[92] In a study of 10,000 healthy blood donors the observed prevalence of inherited protein C deficiency was 1.45 per 1000.[93] In a study of 2132 patients with VTE, 3.2% were found to have protein C deficiency.[94] It is estimated that individuals who are heterozygous for protein C deficiency have a sevenfold higher risk for the development of VTE than the general population.[95]

Protein S is a vitamin K–dependent cofactor for the protein C–mediated inactivation of factors Va and VIIIa. Inheritance of protein S deficiency is autosomal dominant, and it is more common than protein C deficiency. The incidence of protein S–associated VTE has been reported to be 5% to 7%, with the prevalence in the general population being 0.13%.[94,96,97] It is estimated that individuals who are heterozygous for protein S deficiency have an 8.5-fold higher risk for the development of VTE than the general population.[98]

Antithrombin inhibits thrombin as well as factors Xa, IXa, XIa, and XIIa.[99] Antithrombin deficiency is inherited in an autosomal dominant fashion. The majority of patients are heterozygous because homozygote patients usually die in utero. The incidence of VTE associated with antithrombin deficiency has been reported to be 0.5% to 3%, with a prevalence in the general population of 0.2%.[94,99] However, it is estimated that individuals who are heterozygous for antithrombin deficiency have a twentyfold higher risk for the development of VTE than in the general population.[100]

Pregnancy

The incidence of VTE in the pregnant population is fivefold to tenfold greater than in nonpregnant, age-matched controls.[101] VTE accounts for approximately 10% of all maternal deaths.[102] The risk for VTE is highest in the postpartum period, with greatest risk occurring at 3 to 6 weeks post partum and in those patients whom underwent cesarean section.[103-105] DVT in pregnancy has been attributed to impaired venous outflow secondary to uterine compression, and up to 97% of reported thromboses have been isolated to the left leg.[106] Furthermore, pregnancy is associated with a transient hypercoagulable state because of increases in levels of fibrinogen; vWF; and factors II, VII, VIII, and X.[107]

Oral Contraceptives and Hormonal Therapy

Case-control and population-based studies have established the use of oral contraceptives as an independent risk factor for the development of DVT. Most studies have reported odds ratios of 3.8 to 11.0 for idiopathic thrombosis,[108-112] with an unweighted summary relative risk of 2.9 in 18 controlled studies.[109] Approximately one-quarter of idiopathic thromboembolic events in women of childbearing age have been attributed to oral contraceptives.[110] The risk of hospital admission for a thromboembolic event, including cerebral thrombosis, has been estimated to be 0.4 to 0.6 per 1000 for oral contraceptive users versus 0.05 to 0.06 for nonusers.[108,113,114] Estrogenic compounds also increase the risk for VTE when used for suppression of lactation,[115] in the treatment of carcinoma of the prostate, and as postmenopausal replacement therapy.[116] Several studies have now reported a twofold to fourfold higher risk in women taking hormone replacement therapy.[60,61,116-118] This increased risk is greatest during the first year of treatment.[60,118]

Central Venous Catheters

The use of peripherally inserted central catheters (PICCs) and centrally inserted central catheters (CICCs) for hemodynamic monitoring, infusion, antibiosis, and supplementation of alimentation have been associated with an increased risk of DVT. This is particularly true for upper-extremity thrombus, with as many as 65% being related to central venous cannulation.[119] Although the incidence of symptomatic thrombosis may be low, studies using objective surveillance have reported thrombosis to occur at a mean incidence of 28% after subclavian cannulation.[120] This risk also extends to femoral venous catheters, where ipsilateral thrombosis develops in 12% of patients undergoing placement of large-bore catheters for trauma resuscitation.[121] In a single institution study of 64,000 admissions, central venous catheters of any type were associated with a 14-fold increased risk of upper-extremity DVT (UEDVT), with PICC lines having a fourfold increased risk of UEDVT compared with CICC lines.[122]

Inflammatory Bowel Disease

Clinical series have reported VTE to complicate inflammatory bowel disease (IBD) in 3.9% of all cases. Specifically, in one series, with 2284 admitted patients with IBD, 3.4% of Crohn disease (CD) patients developed VTE (2.4% DVT, 1.5% PE), whereas 4.7% of ulcerative colitis (UC) patients developed VTE (3.2% DVT, 2.4% PE). Overall, IBD patients have an approximately threefold increased risk of VTE compared with the general population.[123,124] Patients with CD have incidence rates of 31.4 and 10.3 per 10,000 person-years for DVT and PE, respectively. Meanwhile, UC patients are reported as having incidence rates of 30.0 and 19.8 per 10,000 person-years for DVT and PE, respectively. Such thrombosis events occur more frequently in patients with active disease and may affect unusual sites such as the cerebral veins.[125,126] IBD has been linked to intravascular neutrophil activation and subsequent release of NETs, which may explain this systemic prothrombotic diathesis.[81]

Systemic Lupus Erythematosus

In patients with systemic lupus erythematosus (SLE), the incidence rates of DVT, PE, and VTE are estimated at 3.33, 2.58, and 5.32 per 1000 person-years, respectively. In comparison to normal controls, patients with SLE have adjusted hazard ratios for DVT, PE, and VTE of 4.46, 3.04, and 3.55, respectively.[127] Among patients with SLE, those with lupus anticoagulant have a sixfold higher risk for VTE, whereas those with anticardiolipin antibodies have a twofold greater risk.[128] As earlier, SLE has also been linked to systemic neutrophil activation and NET formation, which offers explanation for the increased rates of VTE.[81]

INITIAL ANTICOAGULATION FOR VENOUS THROMBOEMBOLIC DISEASE TREATMENT

Therapy for DVT is undertaken with the goals of reducing the risk of thrombus extension, thrombus recurrence, and ultimately reducing the risk of PE. Immediate systemic anticoagulation should be administered for proximal DVT (tibial veins and above) because the risk of extension or recurrent venous thromboembolism is significantly increased if anticoagulation is not therapeutic within the first 24 hours.[129,130] In cases of suspected PE, this may necessitate heparinization before completion of diagnostic testing. Confirmation of DVT with duplex imaging is rapid and, as a result, usually precedes anticoagulation.[129,131]

Historically, initial systemic anticoagulation has been undertaken with UFH with a loading dose of 80 U/kg and infusion rate adjusted to achieve activated partial thromboplastin time to 2 to 2.5 times normal. However, because of decreased rates of thrombotic events, decreased bleeding complications, decreased mortality (in cancer patients), and improved pharmacokinetic profile, LMWH is preferred over UFH for the initial treatment of acute DVT in most cases.[131] LMWHs are dosed in a weight-based fashion and rarely require monitoring, except in circumstances such as renal failure, pregnancy, and morbid obesity. LMWH can be given subcutaneously once or twice daily with equal efficacy on an outpatient basis. Following initial anticoagulation with UFH or LMWH, most patients are switched to an oral agent for either short-term (3, 6, or 12 months) or indefinite anticoagulation.[130]

Low-Molecular-Weight Heparins

There are many LMWHs in clinical use; enoxaparin, dalteparin, and tinzaparin are approved for use in the United States.[132] The class of LMWHs are defined most notably as being a more specific inhibitor to factor Xa than factor IIa, and the average molecular weight of the compound is 30% less than UFH. Clinical trial data have nearly unanimously revealed that LMWHs are as effective if not more effective than UFH, with their safety profile at least equivalent.[133]

A limitation to LMWH use is in those patients with renal dysfunction (creatinine clearance less than 30 mL/min). In these cases, effects are not predictable and safe dosing is difficult because LMWHs have the majority of their elimination by the kidneys.[132] In addition, in an obese patient or another patient whose dosing appears complicated, anti-Xa activity can be measured to titrate therapeutic effect.[132] The half-life of LMWH is longer and as such may not be ideal for a high-risk patient with bleeding concerns, but in most other patient groups the LMWHs are viable and in many cases the current preferred method of anticoagulation for VTE.

Vitamin K Antagonists

Oral administration of VKAs (warfarin being most common) is begun shortly after initiation of heparin therapy, because several days are usually required to bring the prothrombin time to an internal normalized ratio (INR) of 2.0 to 3.0. When initiating warfarin therapy, patients should be continued on heparin-based anticoagulation to avoid the transient, paradoxical, prothrombotic effect of warfarin by its early suppression of protein C, prior to its suppression of the vitamin K–dependent clotting factors. Nonhemorrhagic side effects are uncommon but include skin necrosis, dermatitis, and a syndrome of painful erythema in areas with large amounts of subcutaneous fat. VKAs block the γ-carboxylation of several clotting factors, and prolongation of the prothrombin time beyond the range suggested is associated with a high incidence of bleeding complications. Most changes are reversible if the drug is stopped, and the administration of fresh frozen plasma usually restores the prothrombin time. After an episode of acute DVT, anticoagulation should be maintained for a minimum of 3 months; some investigators favor 6 months for thrombi in the larger veins or after a second thromboembolic event (see duration of therapy later).[130] Many drugs alter the pharmacodynamics of warfarin by altering its metabolic clearance, rate of absorption, or inhibition of vitamin K–dependent coagulation factor synthesis or by altering other hemostatic factors. Phenylbutazone, sulfinpyrazone, disulfiram, metronidazole, and trimethoprim-sulfamethoxazole all potentiate the action of warfarin.[134] Therefore regular monitoring of prothrombin time is essential. In addition, levels of concurrent medications should be monitored because warfarin may compete for binding sites, thus altering plasma levels of these drugs. Some foods that have high levels of vitamin K, such as broccoli, green leafy vegetables, and green teas, are also known to alter the effects of warfarin. Oral anticoagulants are teratogenic and should not be used during established or planned pregnancy. In a pregnant patient, LMWH is the drug of choice, and for long-term management, subcutaneous self-administration should be taught. This regimen allows a normal delivery and can be continued postpartum. There are many new agents coming for the prophylaxis and treatment of thrombosis (Table 49.1).

Fondaparinux

Fondaparinux is a pentasaccharide that is in current use for the prevention and treatment of VTE with a subcutaneous delivery. Similar to LMWHs, fondaparinux is derived from UFH. It is

TABLE 49.1 Characteristics of Traditional and New Anticoagulants

	VKA	LMWH	Heparin	Fondaparinux	Apixaban	Rivaroxaban	Dabigatran
Route	PO	SQ	IV/SQ	SQ	PO	PO	PO
Frequency	QD	bid or qid	Infusion bid or tid	bid or qid	bid	qd	bid or qd
VTE prophylaxis data	Yes	Yes	Yes	Yes	Yes	Yes	Yes
VTE treatment data	Yes	Yes	Yes	Yes	Yes	Yes	Yes
Reversibility	Vitamin K, FFP	Partially with protamine	Protamine, short half-life	No	In development	In development	praxbind
Food interactions	Many	No	No	No	None apparent	None apparent	None apparent/needs to be taken with food

bid, Twice per day; *FFP,* fresh frozen plasma; *IV,* intravenously; *LMWH,* low-molecular-weight heparin; *PO,* by mouth; *qd,* 1 time per day; *SQ,* subcutaneously; *tid,* 3 times per day; *VKA,* Vitamin K antagonists; *VTE,* venous thromboembolism.

based on the pentasaccharide moiety of the heparin molecule that selectively inhibits factor Xa via antithrombin, and it exhibits no endothelial or protein binding and is not thought to produce thrombocytopenia.[132] Fondaparinux has been approved for VTE prophylaxis in total hip, total knee, and hip fracture patients, in extended prophylaxis of hip fracture patients, in abdominal surgery patients, and for the treatment of DVT and PE.[135,136] As seen later in this chapter, it is also recommended for complicated superficial thrombophlebitis.

Dabigatran

Dabigatran is an oral, direct thrombin inhibitor introduced by Boehringer Ingelheim.[137] Uniquely, dabigatran has some reversal with recombinant activated factor VII.[137]

The RE-MODEL trial was a VTE prophylaxis trial following total knee replacement. The trial showed that dabigatran was not inferior to daily enoxaparin at 40 mg once per day.[138] The RE-NOVATE trial in a hip replacement population also showed noninferiority.[139] The RE-MOBILIZE trial showed dabigatran was inferior to 30 mg enoxaparin twice daily for postoperative VTE prophylaxis.

The RE-COVER trial compared dabigatran with therapeutic anticoagulation VKAs (INR 2.0 to 3.0) in the treatment of acute VTE for 6 months. Dabigatran was not inferior in the 6-month rate of VTE recurrence and with similar bleeding rates. This important study showed that dabigatran can be effective in longer-term anticoagulation and had a similar safety profile to warfarin without the need for laboratory monitoring.[140] Dabigatran is US Food and Drug Administration (FDA) approved for stroke and thromboembolism prevention in atrial fibrillation patents after similar effectiveness to warfarin was seen in the RE-LY trial.[141] Thus dabigatran is approved for the treatment of DVT, for DVT prophylaxis, and for prevention of embolic events in atrial fibrillation.

Lastly and most importantly, dabigatran is the first direct oral anticoagulant (DOAC) to have a reversal agent. Praxbind (idarucizumab) was approved and found to have an adequate safety profile.[142]

Apixaban

Apixaban is an oral, direct factor Xa inhibitor by Bristol-Myers Squibb. The ADVANCE-1 study compared apixaban with a prophylactic dose twice daily of enoxaparin in total knee replacement patients. The bleeding rates were significantly lower in the apixaban group, but major bleeding rates were similar between compounds and they did not show noninferiority.[143] The ADVANCE-2 trial compared apixaban with 40 mg daily of enoxaparin in the same population, concluding that apixaban was not inferior to the 40 mg daily of enoxaparin in VTE prophylaxis.[144] ADVANCE-3 showed that apixaban compared with 40 mg daily of enoxaparin in hip replacement patients was not inferior in VTE prevention, and the bleeding events were not significantly different.[145] Apixaban was further trialed in symptomatic DVT patients in the AMPLIFY study and showed noninteriority to standard therapy.[146] Thus apixaban is FDA approved for the treatment of DVT, for DVT prophylaxis, and for prevention of embolic events in atrial fibrillation.

Rivaroxaban

Rivaroxaban is an oral, direct factor Xa inhibitor by Bayer.[147] RECORD-1 showed superiority of rivaroxaban and nonsignificantly different major bleeding events when comparing extended duration anticoagulation to 30 days for VTE prohpylaxis.[147,148] The RECORD-2 trial examined extended duration rivaroxaban compared with standard short-term enoxaparin at 40 mg daily in patients undergoing hip replacement and again showed rivaroxaban to be superior.[149] The RECORD-3 trial studied the same dosages, but both treatments were 14 days in duration in patients who had undergone knee replacements. This trial showed noninferiority of rivaroxaban, with a similar safety profile.[150] The RECORD-4 trial compared rivaroxaban (10 mg daily) with enoxaparin (30 mg twice per day) in patients with knee replacements and again showed noninferiority with rivaroxaban, with no statistical significant increase in bleeding.[151]

The EINSTEIN trial evaluated rivaroxaban versus standard anticoagulation in the treatment of acute DVT for standard duration.[152] The primary outcome was recurrent VTE. The results indicated that rivaroxaban is statically not inferior to standard therapy in the treatment of acute DVT, without increased bleeding risk. The EINSTEIN group also added a continued treatment group to compare rivaroxaban with placebo for an additional 6 to 12 months after completion of their prescribed anticoagulation course. This study demonstrated a significant decrease in recurrent VTE, but there were four clinically significant bleeds in the treatment group and none in the placebo group, which did not reach statistical significance.[152] Thus rivaroxaban is FDA approved for the treatment of DVT, DVT prophylaxis, extended DVT prophylaxis, and prevention of embolic events in atrial fibrillation.

Edoxaban

Edoxaban is another oral factor Xa inhibitor that has been developed by Daiichi Sankyo (Tokyo, Japan). Edoxaban is currently FDA approved for prevention of atrial fibrillation–related embolization and treatment of VTE.

The three direct Xa inhibitors do not yet have an approved reversal agent. However, andexanet alfa has completed phase III trials with promising results and seems to be a likely option to improve the safety profile, and other similar agents are also under development.[142]

Future Anticoagulants

In addition to these anticoagulants, there are other promising compounds currently in preclinical development. One such example is soluble P-selectin/PSGL-1 inhibitors. In a series of nonhuman primate studies using a model of proximal VT, inhibition of P-selectin or its ligand PSGL-1 was similar to LMWH in preventing and treating DVT.[153] The P-selectin inhibitors reduce inflammation and therefore reduce thrombosis without inhibition of the coagulation cascade, with less bleeding risk. Future clinical trials with these compounds are likely.

Duration of Anticoagulation

Anticoagulation following an episode of VTE should be continued until the benefits of preventing recurrent VTE no longer outweigh the risks of bleeding.[154] The major risks of recurrence of VTE depend upon whether the initial episode was provoked or unprovoked, if the patient has unmodifiable risk factors, and whether the initial episode was appropriately treated.[130] An unprovoked DVT occurs when there is no identifiable provoking environmental event evident.[155] On the other hand, a provoked DVT is associated with some modifiable risk factor, such as the following major and minor risk factors: recent major or minor surgery, inpatient hospitalization or immobility greater than 3 days, pregnancy, estrogen therapy, reduced mobility greater than 3 days, and leg injury associated with immobility. Other unmodifiable risk factors for DVT include active IBD, active SLE, untreated cancer, and hereditary thrombophilias. In general, the greater the provoking risk factor, without unmodifiable risk factors, the lower the risk of recurrent DVT once anticoagulation therapy is stopped.[156] Patients with provoked DVT should be treated for 3 months for a proximal (iliofemoral) DVT and for a distal DVT.[130] Shorter durations of therapy are associated with double the risk for recurrent DVT or PE within the next year.[157-159]

In those patients who receive short-term anticoagulation, 3 months of anticoagulation therapy is sufficient to decrease the risk of recurrent thrombosis related to the initial DVT. However, after therapy is discontinued, the risk for recurrence rises dramatically, with 30% to 50% of patients experiencing a recurrence at 10 years.[160,161] Male gender, elevated D dimer, incomplete resolution of DVT, body mass index of 30 kg/m^2 or greater, PTS, and importantly idiopathic etiology are all associated with increased likelihood of recurrence.[162] Additional anticoagulation therapy beyond 3 months is useful at preventing further episodes of recurrence not related to the initial event. Following the initial 3 months of therapy, all patients should be evaluated for indefinite anticoagulation therapy.[130,163] Similarly, patients with a recurrent VTE are at increased risk of additional episodes. In patients with a second DVT who were treated with 6 months of therapy, 20.7% experienced recurrent thrombosis, compared with 2.6% of patients treated indefinitely with anticoagulation.[164] In high-risk patients the risks of major bleeding during prolonged therapy (1.1% per patient-year) should be periodically weighed against the benefits of continuing anticoagulation. Advanced age (older than 75 years), history of gastrointestinal hemorrhage, noncardioembolic stroke, renal or hepatic disease, concomitant antiplatelet therapy, and poor control of anticoagulation increase the risk of bleeding complications.[130]

Two additional tests may be used to guide length of anticoagulation in selected patients. Follow-up duplex ultrasound screening identifies patients with residual thrombus. These patients have a twenty-five-fold greater risk of recurrence compared with patients who demonstrated recanalization of veins.[161] A study demonstrated a 35% decrease in recurrent VTE events when duration of anticoagulation was guided by ultrasound evidence without any increase in bleeding complications.[165] A second, better-validated parameter is the D-dimer level, measured 1 month after completion of a standard oral VKA course. Patients with elevated D-dimer levels are prothrombotic and should continue to receive anticoagulation therapy until the D-dimer level normalizes.[166]

For patients with unmodifiable risk factors, including those with IBD, SLE, and active cancer, the consideration for utility of anticoagulation should be carefully weighed against the risks of bleeding. Patients with cancer have a greater risk of recurrence and major bleeding complications compared with all other causes of DVT.[167] Vomiting, malnutrition, and liver dysfunction, common among cancer patients, make achieving consistent anticoagulation goals with oral VKA therapy challenging. Several randomized studies have been conducted comparing LMWH to oral VKA in this particular subset of patients; because of decreased mortality from bleeding complications and decreased risk of recurrence, initial treatment with LMWH is recommended with grade 1A evidence.[168-170] Baring significant bleeding risks, these patients should be maintained on LMWH for the first 3 to 6 months and continued on anticoagulation until the cancer resolves. For patients with inflammatory diseases such as IBD and SLE, there remains controversy as to the appropriate setting for thromboprophylaxis and therapeutic anticoagulation, but recent guidelines in the IBD literature have suggested thromboprophylaxis for all inpatients with flares of their disease and indefinite anticoagulation following the first episode of VTE, at least until the flare has resolved.[123]

Among patients with a thrombosis at an age younger than 40 years, a strong family history of VTE (two or more symptomatic relatives), or thrombosis at unusual locations, screening for hereditary thrombophilias is indicated.[171] Screening of unselected individuals is not useful in predicting recurrence and should not guide therapy.[156,172] Selected patients with clinically significant thrombosis and genetic defect may be maintained on anticoagulation indefinitely with periodic reassessments of the risk-to-benefit ratio of continuing anticoagulation. Heterozygote carriers of factor V Leiden and prothrombin G20210A gene mutations have only a modest risk of recurrence and should be treated according to standard recommendations.[92] However, an individual who is a heterozygote carrier of both traits has an increased risk of VTE events and should be considered for lifetime anticoagulation.[173]

Patients with DVT in the absence of any identifiable risk factor are said to have an idiopathic DVT or unprovoked DVT. Compared with patients with a reversible risk factors, recurrent VTE events are much more common in this patient population ($\leq$3% vs. 10% at 1 year).[174] Kearon and colleagues[163] studied patients with unprovoked DVT, comparing 3 months of anticoagulation with indefinite anticoagulation. They demonstrated a 95% relative risk reduction in recurrence in patients receiving indefinite anticoagulation, but with a trend toward an increased risk of nonfatal major bleeding ($P = .09$). Because longer durations of anticoagulation reduced DVT recurrence but were associated with increased bleeding risk, Ridker and colleagues[175] studied long-term subtherapeutic anticoagulation. The PREVENT investigators randomized patients after completing their full course of VKA anticoagulation (3 to 6 months) to either placebo or subtherapeutic VKA therapy (target INR of 1.5 to 1.9). At 2.1 years of follow-up, patients receiving indefinite subtherapeutic anticoagulation had a 62% relative risk reduction of recurrent DVT (14.6 vs. 5.5%; $P < .001$). Although this study is enticing, for now and for most patients, the current standard practice remains to treat them with full therapeutic anticoagulation.

VEIN WALL ABNORMALITIES AFTER DEEP VENOUS THROMBOSIS

Chronic venous disease (CVD) encompasses mild varicosities to disabling ulcers, which occasionally can progress to limb loss.[176,177] The underlying pathophysiology is related to venous injury, valve damage, and obstruction; all of which culminate as venous hypertension when in the upright position. Venous hypertension leads to end-organ damage, namely the skin and dermis. The sine qua non is hyperpigmentation, corona phlebectatica, lipodermatosclerosis, or frank ulceration of the limb.[178] Once skin changes occur, dermal fibrosis and inflammation are present histologically.[177] Factors involved include leukocyte activation with adhesion and emigration through the basement membrane with release of fibrotic growth factors and proteases. Dysregulation of iron may exacerbate this process.[179]

PTS is a chronic sequelae of DVT, and typical symptoms include pain, heaviness, swelling, and cramping of the leg, which are generally worsened by standing and exercising.[180] In advanced cases, venous ulceration occurs, causing additional pain and disability and increasing the cost of treatment.[181,182] Postthrombotic morbidity has been reported to occur in 25% to 46% of patients following anticoagulation alone for acute DVT.[11,180] The severity of PTS manifests relatively early after DVT and usually neither worsens nor improves, highlighted by a prospective multicenter cohort of 387 patients with acute DVT.[12,183] Variables that predicted more severe postthrombotic morbidity include severity of venous symptoms at 1 month, iliofemoral location, recurrent ipsilateral DVT, high body mass index, older age, and female gender.[183] Calf vein thrombosis is less often associated with PTS. Vein valve reflux plays a role in PTS, both in the affected deep segments and the superficial system.[184]

Definition of Postthrombotic Syndrome and Diagnosis

Unlike arterial diseases, PTS is more difficult to quantify. Expert consensus for PTS definition is the Villalta score, combining patient limb symptoms and signs in a graded scoring system (Box 49.1).[185] The higher the score, the greater the severity of PTS (e.g., a score of greater than 15 suggests severe PTS). This system also allows for an evaluation of change in severity of disease over time.

The Clinical Etiologic Anatomic Pathophysiology (CEAP) score is used for objectively characterizing CVD (see Box 49.1).[186] The parameters in this system include clinical features of the limb, etiology, anatomy, and pathophysiology. Although useful, this static measure does not reflect quality-of-life issues or functional status. The Venous Clinical Severity Score (VCSS) is also useful to capture the disability and functional aspects of PTS

BOX 49.1 Villalta Scale and CEAP: Classification Scales for Postthrombotic Syndrome

Villalta Scale

Symptoms

- Heaviness
- Pain
- Cramps
- Pruritus
- Paresthesias

Signs

- Pretibial edema
- Induration
- Hyperpigmentation
- New venous ectasia
- Redness
- Pain of calf compression
- Ulceration (receives a score of 15)

Each Factor Receives a Range of 0–3 (0 = None; 3 = Severe)

- Mild: 5–9
- Moderate: 10–14
- Severe: 15 or greater

CEAP

Clinical

- 0 = None
- 1 = Telangiectasis
- 2 = Varicosities
- 3 = Edema
- 4 = Pigmentation, lipodermatosclerosis
- 5 = Healed ulceration
- 6 = Ulcer

Etiology

- Congenital
- Primary
- Secondary

Anatomic Distribution

- Superficial
- Deep
- Perforator
- Combination

Pathophysiology

- Reflux
- Obstruction
- Combination

Severe: > (CEAP Class)

CEAP, Clinical etiologic anatomic pathophysiology.

Modified from Kahn SR, Partsch H, Vedantham S, et al: Definition of post-thrombotic syndrome of the leg for use in clinical investigations: a recommendation for standardization. *J Thromb Haemost* 7:879–883, 2009; and Eklof B, Rutherford RB, Bergan JJ, et al: Revision of the CEAP classification for chronic venous disorders: consensus statement. *J Vasc Surg* 40:1248–1252, 2004.

over time. The VCSS is composed of 10 variables: pain, varicose veins, venous edema, skin pigmentation, inflammation, induration, active ulcer number, active ulcer duration, active ulcer size, and use of compression therapy, with a higher score representing more severe disease.[187]

Duplex ultrasound is the standard for quantifying venous reflux and location, as well as documenting thrombotic obstruction, but imaging per se is neither part of the definition of PTS nor correlated with severity. Similarly, computed tomography (CT) venography and magnetic resonance venography can delineate thrombotic obstruction but are not routinely used outside of planning for interventions or defining proximal iliac or IVC thrombosis.[188]

Prevention of Postthrombotic Syndrome by Preventing Deep Venous Thrombosis

Primary Deep Venous Thrombosis

The most effective way to decrease PTS occurrence is to prevent DVT. When DVT occurs, rapid treatment with evidence-based therapies is indicated. It is clear that surgical patients are at high risk for VTE and prophylaxis is often underprescribed.[189] All surgical patients should have a VTE risk assessment, and excellent guidelines exist.[190] Several studies have shown the utility of the Caprini risk assessment tool among a wide variety of postsurgical patients.[29,191-193] Among vascular patients, those undergoing aortic surgery have a risk of VTE ranging from 2% to 8%,[194] and there is increased risk among those with preoperative dyspnea, obesity, chronic steroid use, postoperative pneumonia, or return to the operating room (OR) and ventilation greater than 48 hours. VTE is similarly common, approximating 10%, among lower extremity amputation patients.[195,196] Among patients undergoing outpatient surgery, those undergoing a venous procedure have the highest rate of VTE.[197] Patients at high risk (e.g., prior VTE, family history, active malignancy) should receive both pharmacologic and mechanical prophylaxis. For others with expected length of stay less than 24 hours, such as carotid surgery, no prophylaxis outside of ambulation is usually needed.[198]

Recurrent Deep Venous Thrombosis

Recurrent DVT is both etiologic and a consequence of the damaged vein wall, and it is a major factor for PTS.[180,183] The quality of early anticoagulation for acute DVT significantly affects the likelihood of recurrence. Hull and colleagues[199] reported that subtherapeutic anticoagulation early in the course of patient management (the first 24 hours) increased the risk of recurrent venous thromboembolic events 15-fold (24.5% vs. 1.6%; $P < .001$).

Anticoagulation is typically LMWH or factor Xa inhibition followed by oral VKAs (e.g., sodium warfarin [Coumadin]).[190] A reduction in postthrombotic morbidity (including reduction of venous ulcers) with the use of LMWH was published by Hull and colleagues,[200] supporting the advantage of LMWH in the early management of acute DVT. Similarly, LMWH as compared with warfarin showed benefit in deep vein recanalization and a trend toward less PTS.[201] How the newer anticoagulants will factor into PTS prevention requires study.

Identifying Patients at Risk of Recurrent Deep Venous Thrombosis

Determining who is at increased risk of recurrent DVT (and hence PTS) is important for balancing prevention of recurrent DVT (and decreased PTS risk) against bleeding. New management paradigms may help to determine who is at risk for recurrent DVT after incident DVT, including imaging the deep venous system for residual thrombus (or wall abnormality) and identifying patients with elevated D-dimer levels, which reflect active thrombus metabolism.

Prandoni and colleagues[164] evaluated patients with venous duplex imaging for residual thrombus (abnormal vein wall) at the time anticoagulation was discontinued. They demonstrated a nearly threefold increase in recurrent DVT in patients with residual abnormality compared with those with a normal venous duplex. However, these criteria need further study because others have not replicated the findings.[202] Using D dimer as a blood test to evaluate thrombus activity, Eichinger and colleagues[203] and Palareti and colleagues[204] demonstrated that elevated D-dimer levels following termination of oral anticoagulation identified patients who faced a threefold increased risk of recurrence during the next 2 years. Furthermore, extending anticoagulation in those with a significantly elevated d-dimer was associated with a marked reduction in recurrence. Extended anticoagulation in those patients with elevated D dimer and idiopathic first-time proximal DVT is currently endorsed by the American College of Chest Physicians (ACCP) with a grade 2B recommendations.[130] Future studies are needed to define the role of duplex in DVT recurrence management.

Compression and Ambulation for Acute Deep Venous Thrombosis to Decrease Postthrombotic Syndrome

Initial treatment of acute DVT with effective leg compression and ambulation is essential. Initial small randomized trials have demonstrated the value of 30 to 40 mm Hg ankle-gradient stockings in the management of acute DVT.[205,206] Randomized trials with applied compression and ambulation early in the course of treatment have shown significantly reduced progression of thrombus length and volume, reduced pain, and reduced edema.[207,208] The largest double blind, randomized trial to date, the SOX trial determined no difference in development of PTS in patients wearing 30 to 40 mm Hg stockings (52%) compared with a control group (52%).[209] Early data also suggest that structured exercise may decrease PTS.[210] These data highlight the need for new therapies to prevent development of PTS. It is of the authors' belief that although stockings may not decrease incidence of PTS, they are still a valuable method of controlling early symptoms of pain and swelling.

Active Thrombus Removal to Decrease Postthrombotic Syndrome

Although anticoagulation reduces thrombus propagation, the risk of PE, and the risk of recurrent DVT, it does not affect the natural consequences of venous obstruction and valvular destruction that result in ambulatory venous hypertension. Patients with extensive DVT, defined as those with iliofemoral venous occlusion, are at increased risk of PTS.[183,211,212] The quantity of remaining thrombus burden has been shown to directly correlate with the Villalta score and C classification.[213,214] Therefore removing thrombus has been advocated to decrease development of PTS and potentially reduce the risk of recurrence. The CaVent trial randomized 102 patients to catheter-directed thrombolysis (CDT) with conventional therapy or conventional therapy alone. Patients in the CDT demonstrated improved iliofemoral patency at 6 months (64% vs. 36%, $P = .004$)[215] and PTS at 2 years (41% vs. 56%, $P = .0047$).[216] To more fully determine the role of aggressive therapies, the ATTRACT Trial randomized 692 patients with acute proximal DVT to either pharmacomechanical thromobolysis plus anticoaguation or anticoagulation alone. The authors found that more aggressive therapy did not decrease PTS measured by Villalta score, but did result in more bleeding. However, the severity of PTS seemed to be lessened by pharmacomechanical thrombolysis for iliofemoral DVT, suggesting that more aggressive therapies may still be indicated in patients with significant iliofemoral DVT who do not respond to a course of therapeutic anticoagulation.[216a] A suggested treatment algorithm is shown in Fig. 49.2.

Other Consideration for Postthrombotic Syndrome

Pharmacologic Interventions

Although no pharmacologic agents specifically treat PTS, several agents may have potential benefit. Daflon (micronized purified flavanoid fraction) is available in Europe and is effective for chronic venous insufficiency.[217] Pentoxifylline has been shown to be of benefit for chronic venous insufficiency (CVI) symptoms and venous ulcer healing.

Deep System Reconstruction

Native valve reconstruction procedures are less effective in patients with PTS compared with those with primary venous insufficiency.[177] Prosthetic valves for the venous system have undergone limited experimental evaluation.[218] The risk of thrombosis and durability of these bioprosthesis is still uncertain. Furthermore, whether valves can reduce venous hypertension in the setting of long-segment postthrombotic vein wall damage is not clear.

Biomarkers

An active area of research involves biomarkers to stratify patients at risk of PTS after DVT. Interleukin-6 and C-reactive protein correlate with anatomic extent of DVT and severity of venous

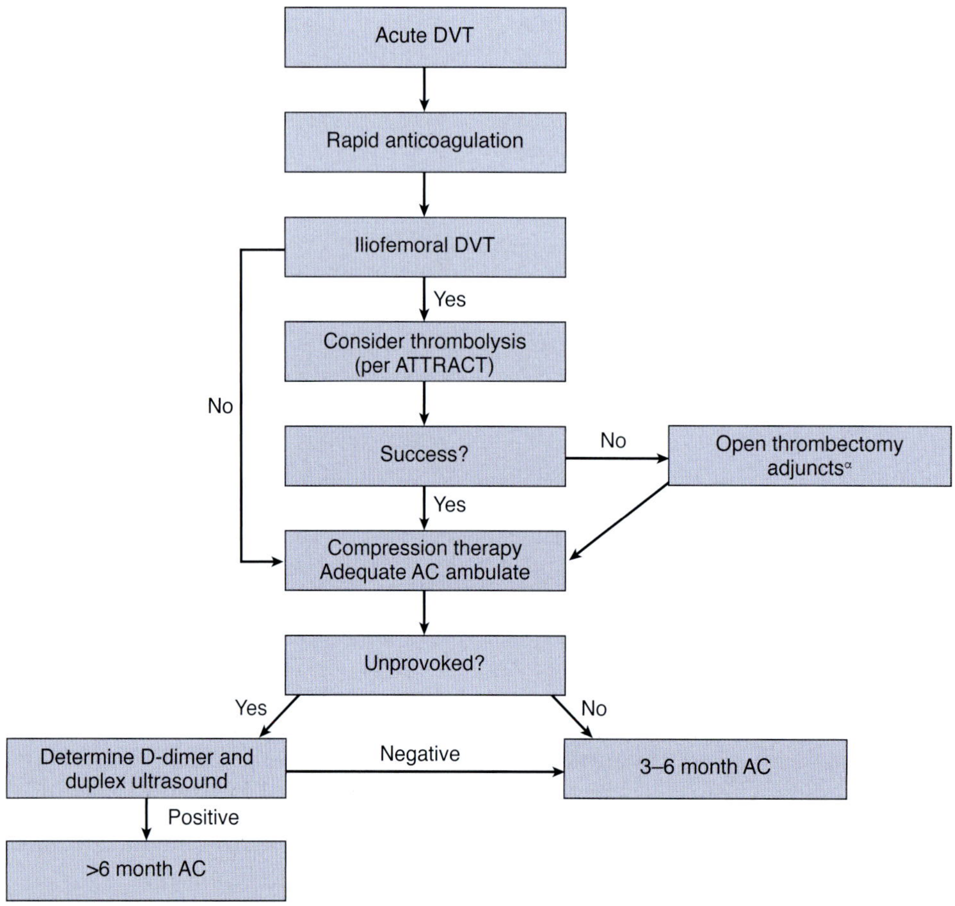

FIG 49.2 Algorithm of recommended therapy for acute venous thromboembolism to decrease postthrombotic syndrome. [a]Adjuncts = webectomy; venoplasty; AV fistula. *AC*, Anticoagulation; *DVT*, deep venous thrombosis.

signs and symptoms.[219] Preliminary studies on humans also suggest alteration in matrix metalloproteinase (MMP) levels in acute DVT and nonresolution a risk for PTS.[220] Larger studies will be necessary to determine their sensitivity and specificity in relation to clinical PTS. Ideally, a biomarker panel could be drawn at the time of diagnosis of DVT, and if predictive of PTS, these patients might be best served by active thrombus removal and increased compression strength and duration.

Endothelial Protection

In humans, it is likely that the endothelium is damaged after DVT, and the healing response and function of the endothelium is critical to prevent rethrombosis. The JUPITER trial suggests a benefit of hydroxymethylglutaryl coenzyme A (HMG-CoA) reductase inhibitors (statins) in patients at modest cardiac risk also reducing incident VTE.[221] It is interesting that the risk reduction for DVT (but not PE) was of similar magnitude to the reduction in arterial cardiovascular events. It is still unknown whether statins may decrease PTS in the long term. Statins may reduce perioperative DVT risk and will be addressed by the ongoing STOP-DVT trial.[222]

DIAGNOSIS AND TREATMENT OF SUPERFICIAL THROMBOPHLEBITIS

Superficial vein thrombophlebitis (SVT) is characterized by a painful erythematous and palpable cordlike structure, usually involving the lower extremities but capable of affecting any superficial vein in the body. SVT has historically been managed with compression support, nonsteroidal antiinflammatory drugs (NSAIDs), and lower extremity elevation. However, SVT may coexist with DVT, propagate, and rarely cause PE.[223-226] Although this approach may still be appropriate for mild cases of SVT, data now support a role for more aggressive treatment of select cases of SVT.

In a prospective epidemiologic study including 844 patients with symptomatic SVT, 210 (24.9%) had concomitant DVT upon enrollment. Of the 600 patients without DVT followed for 3 months, 58 (10.2%) developed thromboembolic complications, including 3 (0.5%) with PE, 15 (2.8%) with DVT, 18 (3.3%) with extension, and 10 (1.9%) with recurrence of SVT. These events occurred despite the use of anticoagulant treatment with LMWH 374 (62.9%) at therapeutic and 216 (36.7%) at prophylactic dose for 10 to 17 days. Almost all patients (584, 97.7%) received elastic compression stockings. Risk factors for complications at 3 months were male sex, history of DVT or PE, previous cancer, and absence of varicose veins.[227]

The incidence of SVT has been reported to occur in approximately 125,000 people per year in the United States.[228] Others estimate that this number could be even higher than that of DVT, which has been reported at 56 to 160 per 100,000 people per year.[229] Lower extremity veins are most commonly involved, followed by upper extremity veins.[230] Approximately 54% to 65% of the reported cases affect females, with an average age 58 to 65 years.[45,227,231] The presence of varicose veins is the most frequent predisposing risk factor for SVT, being seen in approximately two-thirds of patients.[227] Other risk factors associated with nonintravenous line–associated SVT include immobilization, trauma, postoperative states, older age (>60 years), obesity, tobacco use, history of DVT or SVT, pregnancy and the puerperium, autoimmune disease, use of oral contraceptives or hormonal replacement therapy, and hypercoagulability.[45,227,231,232] Thrombophilic disorders may be associated with SVT as a significant or presenting clinical sign.[233] In patients with ascending or worsening thrombosis despite initial treatment, hypercoagulable testing should be considered.[234,235] Malignancy is a risk factor for SVT, affecting 13% to 18% of patients.[225,236] Although lower in frequency, SVT developing in nonvaricose veins may be associated with a risk of malignancy (4.8% of 42 cases), nonneoplastic disease (9.5% of 42 cases), or thrombophilia (48% of 42 cases).[237] The overall recurrence of SVT is 18% over an average observation period of 15 months and is equally frequent in varicose and nonvaricose veins. Deep venous reflux increases the recurrence to 33%, and hypercoagulable states increase recurrence rates to 42% over the same time period.[238]

The clinical diagnosis of SVT usually involves pain, a firm palpable cord with inflammation, tenderness, surrounding erythema, and edema.[239,240] Low-grade fever or malaise may be present. The superficial veins of the upper or lower extremities, the breast in the case of Mondor disease, or the dorsal veins of the penis may all be affected by SVT. The most common locations affected by SVT include the great saphenous vein and its tributaries, followed by the cephalic and basilic veins of the upper extremity.[230] Duplex ultrasound remains the diagnostic modality of choice for SVT; study of bilateral extremities should be performed to rule out extension into the deep venous system or concomitant DVT.[234,239] Complete thrombophilia workup, although not routinely supported by current guidelines, may be indicated in select patients with recurrent primary thrombophlebitis or a strong family history. Notably, patients with SVT exclusive of lower extremity varicose veins are more likely to have a hypercoaguable state, and an increased risk of SVT has been identified in patients with inherited coagulopathies.[231,241] The workup is similar to that obtained for patients with DVT. Screening for underlying diseases, including malignancy or vasculitis, should be performed if indicated, including mammography and colonoscopy, and chest radiograph if the patient is a smoker.[239]

Treatment for SVT should be tailored accordingly to thrombus location, the extent of thrombus burden, and the presence of concomitant DVT. Historically, the treatment for primary SVT localized in tributary veins and the distal great saphenous vein included simply ambulation, warm soaks, elastic compression, and NSAIDs.[233,242] Those patients with SVT and concomitant DVT benefit from therapeutic anticoagulation. Most recent guidelines support daily treatment for 45 days for those patients with symptomatic superficial thrombophlebitis of at least 5 cm length and at least 3 cm distal to the saphenofemoral junction at a (prophylactic) dose of 2.5 mg/day subcutaneously of fondaparinux or LMWH.

Studies are prolific comparing different approaches for the medial treatment of SVT. Compared with NSAIDs, LMWH over a 7-day period has been found to decrease the persistence of signs and symptoms of SVT at both 1 week and 2 months after diagnosis.[243] In a second study of patients with documented acute symptomatic superficial vein thrombosis of the legs, the incidence of deep and superficial venous thromboembolism by day 12 was significantly reduced in all active treatment groups (LMWH and NSAIDs) compared with placebo, with a trend that remained in favor of the active treatments for DVT and SVT combination at 3 months of follow-up.[244] No major bleeding or heparin-induced thrombocytopenia was observed in any treatment group. There was a trend in favor of LMWH relative to NSAIDs. Prophylactic LMWH was equivalent to bodyweight therapeutic LMWH once daily for 1 month in another study, in which the cumulative rate of SVT progression and venous thromboembolism complications did not differ between groups after 3 months of follow-up.[245]

Prophylactic intravenous UFH was used as a comparator treatment in two studies. The first study in 562 patients with SVT with large varicose veins without systematic disorders treated patients with elastic compression alone, compression plus early surgery (flush ligation or complete stripping), compression plus standard heparin or LMWH, or compression plus warfarin only.[246] At 3 to 6 months, the incidence of superficial thrombus extension was greater in the elastic compression and saphenous vein ligation groups ($P < .05$), with no significant differences in DVT incidence at 3 months. A second study compared high- versus low-dose intravenous UFH.[247] With 6-month follow-up, patients with high-dose UFH had better results than those with low-dose UFH.[247] There was no major bleeding or heparin-induced thrombocytopenia in either group.

LMWH has been compared with saphenofemoral disconnection for the treatment of proximal great saphenous vein thrombophlebitis in a prospective, randomized clinical study.[248] In this study, 84 consecutive patients with a diagnosis of proximal thrombophlebitis alone were divided into two comparable groups treated with saphenofemoral disconnection under local anesthesia with a short hospital stay ($n = 45$) or enoxaparin (1 mg/kg bid) on an outpatient basis for 4 weeks ($n = 39$). Thirty patients in each group completed the study requirements. Follow-up was at 1, 3, and 6 months. In the surgical group, two patients (6.7%) presented complications of the surgical wound, one (3.3%) had thrombophlebitis recurrence, and two (6.7%) developed nonfatal PE over 6 months. In the medical group, there was no progression of the thrombosis to the deep venous system or PE; there were two cases (6.7%) of minor bleeding and three cases (10%) of thrombophlebitis recurrence. Although the study found no statistically significant difference between the two groups, the LMWH group had a significant socioeconomic advantage and confirmed the efficacy of LMWH treatment in resolving symptoms and signs and preventing DVT and PE.

Finally, in the CALISTO study, fondaparinux was given over 31 to 45 days (along with graduated compression stockings) to patients with SVT of at least 5 cm length.[249] There was a significant improvement in those treated with fondaparinux compared with placebo in composite end points of death, PE, DVT, and extension or recurrence by both days 47 and 77, suggesting that this therapy should be considered in these patients. The 2012 ACCP CHEST guidelines advocate medical treatment with a prophylactic dose of fondaparinux or LMWH for 45 days over no anticoagulation (grade 2B) for patients with SVT of the lower limb that measures at least 5 cm in length, with grade 2C evidence favoring a daily dose of fondaparinux (2.5 mg) over a prophylactic dose of LMWH for patients with SVT being treated with anticoagulation.[250] A recent Cochrane review that included 30 randomized controlled trials and 6507 total patients identified that both LMWH and NSAIDs reduce SVT extension and recurrence without any effect on symptomatic VTE; topical treatments relieve local symptoms; surgical treatment and elastic stockings offer a lower rate of VTE and SVT progression over elastic stockings alone; and fondaparinux appears to be adequate in reducing symptomatic VTE and SVT extension and recurrence.[251] Finally, the potential role for the use of novel and DOACs remains unclear for the treatment of SVT but certainly warrants investigation.

In conclusion, SVT is common, and in light of the risk of progression to DVT and PE, treatment must be individualized. Although milder forms of SVT may be successfully managed with NSAIDs, compression, and warm compresses, those with thrombus burden of at least 5 cm length and located at least 3 cm distal to the saphenofemoral junction should be managed more aggressively with either prophylactic fondaparinux or LMWH. Therapeutic anticoagulation should still be considered for any patient who develops VTE. For those patients with contraindication to anticoagulation and moderate thrombus burden, consider great saphenous vein (GSV) disconnection and ligation at the saphenofemoral junction (SFJ). Finally, surgical treatment with saphenous ablation and phlebectomy of involved branch varicosities should be considered for those patients with symptomatic SVT and evidence of complicated venous insufficiency, especially after the acute episode of SVT has resolved.

INFERIOR VENA CAVAL INTERRUPTION

Because of the general lack of prospective, randomized data for IVC filter use, the use of IVC filters has been driven primarily by their relatively low complication rate, ease of placement, and the fact that a mechanical barrier to prevent PE makes intuitive sense. However, adequate anticoagulation whenever possible is the cornerstone of effective treatment of DVT and PE, and physicians must remember that an IVC filter does not treat existing DVT and PE but only prevents further significant PE. Unfortunately, not all patients can be safely or effectively anticoagulated, and it is this patient population that benefits from placement of IVC filters. The indications for IVC filter placement have historically been classified into three types: absolute or classic indications, relative indications, and extended indications for IVC filter placement (Box 49.2). Classic indications require the presence of DVT or PE and either a significant bleeding complication directly related to anticoagulation, an underlying contraindication to anticoagulation, or a failure of anticoagulation to prevent PE or DVT. Relative indications for IVC filter placement also require the presence of DVT or PE in patients with high risk of morbidity and mortality with further PE. Extended indications for the use of IVC filters remain the most controversial and least supported by the medical literature. In contrast to the absolute and relative indications for IVC filter placement, the extended indications do not require the presence of DVT

BOX 49.2 Indications for IVC Filter Placement

Absolute (Classic)

Presence of DVT or PE plus one of the following:

- Bleeding complication related to anticoagulation
- Contraindication to anticoagulation
- Failure of anticoagulation to prevent DVT or PE

Accepted (Relative)

Presence of DVT or PE plus one of the following:

- Chronic PE with residual DVT and no cardiopulmonary reserve
- Previous pulmonary thrombectomy for PE
- Preexisting severe pulmonary hypertension or right heart failure
- Free-floating iliocaval thrombus
- Significant fall risk

Extended

Does not require the presence of DVT or PE:

- Prophylactic (prevention of PE; e.g., trauma, long bone or pelvic fractures)
- High-risk immobilized patient (e.g., paraplegia)
- Preoperative patient with multiple risk factors for DVT

DVT, Deep venous thrombosis; *IVC,* inferior vena cava; *PE,* pulmonary embolism.

or PE and encompass the placement of IVC filters for prophylactic purposes (prevention of PE).

There is a growing body of evidence to suggest that prophylactic IVC filter placement provides no protection from PE. Studies in patient populations with elevated risk for PE, including trauma patients[252] and bariatric surgery patients,[253] have demonstrated no benefit of prophylactic IVC filter placement for prevention of PE. In fact, guidelines from the American Heart Association (AHA) and ACCP recommend against the use of IVC filters for extended indications. The most recent guidelines from the Society of Interventional Radiology (SIR) support more liberal use of IVC filters; however, future recommendations may exclude these extended indications, due to a lack of evidence establishing a clear benefit for PE prevention.

Inferior Vena Cava Filter Devices

The Greenfield filter remains the standard with which all other filters are compared. The cone-shaped Greenfield filter was developed more than 30 years ago to prevent PE while maintaining caval patency. Currently there are 14 commercially available IVC filters. The complications of filter insertion range in severity from minor wound hematoma resulting from early resumption of anticoagulation to potentially lethal migration of the device into the pulmonary artery or right ventricle, as documented initially with the bird's nest filter and with the Recovery nitinol filter (Bard). Filter fracture and embolization of the device or fragments of the device have been problematic for some filters, despite several generations of redesign.[254] As a result of device complications, the FDA delivered an Alert letter in 2010, indicating they had received 921 adverse event reports, and as a result suggested that "implanting physicians and clinicians responsible for the ongoing care of patients with retrievable IVC filter consider removing the filter as soon as protection from PE is no longer needed."[255] The FDA updated these recommendations in 2014, indicating that filters should be removed between 25 and 54 days after implantation. The Predicting the Safety and Effectiveness of Inferior Vena Cava Filters (PRESERVE) trial is designed as a multicenter nonrandomized open-label study to determine the safety and effectiveness of the various types of IVC filters. With expected completion in 2019, the PRESERVE trial (NCT02381509) may help to evaluate whether certain filter types are prone to failure.

When obesity precludes fluoroscopy, intravascular ultrasonography can be used to identify the renal veins and guide filter placement. Bedside placement using either surface or intravascular ultrasonography has also been recommended for patients at risk during transport to the radiology suite, such as severely injured trauma patients. PE has occurred in 2% to 4% of cases after filter placement and may be caused by a source of thrombus outside of the filtered flow, such as the upper body veins or the right atrium. Recurrent embolism is an indication for inferior venacavography to evaluate the filter for possible attached thrombus. This finding is rare and can be managed either by thrombolytic therapy if the amount of thrombus is small or by placement of a second filter in the suprarenal vena cava. The capture of a very large embolus within a filter may suddenly occlude the vena cava, with a precipitous fall in blood pressure. In a patient with known prior PE, this event can be mistaken for recurrent PE, with disastrous results if vasopressor therapy is administered. The basic distinction between functional hypervolemia of caval occlusion and right ventricular overload from recurrent PE can be made at the bedside by measuring the central venous pressure and arterial oxygen tension and observing for jugular venous distension. The response to volume resuscitation for a patient with sudden vena caval occlusion should be dramatic improvement.

Retrievable Optional Filters

It is important to realize that the basis for the retrievable filter design has been driven by the publication of the 2- and 8-year results of the PREPIC trial.[256,257] The PREPIC study, the first of two long-term randomized studies of caval filter placement in the prevention of PE, had its 2-year results published in 1998. In this multiinstitutional trial, 400 patients with venographically confirmed acute proximal DVT were randomized to treatment with anticoagulation (LMWH for 8 to 12 days and a VKA for at least 3 months) alone versus anticoagulation and a permanent caval filter. At 12 days, there were two PEs in the filter group (1.1%) versus nine PEs in the nonfilter group (4.8%; $P = .03$). At 2 years, there were 6 PEs in the filter group (3.4%) and 12 PEs in the nonfilter group (6.3%; $P = .16$). The incidence of recurrent DVT was 37 (20.8%) in the filter group and 21 (11.6%) in the nonfilter group ($P = .02$).[256] These 2-year results suggested that caval filters provided significant additional short-term protection from PE compared with anticoagulation and that this benefit seemed to wane over time and was associated with an increased risk of recurrent DVT. The 8-year results of the PREPIC trial, published in 2005, showed that there were 9 PEs in the filter group (6.2%) versus 24 PEs in the nonfilter group (15.1%; $P = .08$). The filter group had 57 patients with DVT (35.7%) versus 41 (27.5%) in the nonfilter group ($P = .042$). The incidence of PTS was similar: it was observed in 109 (70.3%) filter patients and 107 (69.7%) nonfilter patients at 8 years. Mortality was also similar: 103 filter patients had died, compared with 98 nonfilter patients.[257] These results showed that, at 8 years, vena cava filters reduced the risk of PE while increasing the incidence of DVT and without effect on the incidence of the PTS or on survival.

Although the PREPIC trial is notable for being the first randomized control trial to evaluate IVC filter effectiveness, it had several notable weaknesses. The study included a 2 × 2 factorial design which also compared UFH with LMWH in addition to comparing IVC filter with anticoagulation with anticoagulation alone. The trial was underpowered for such an analysis. In addition, no standardization for device type was used, so four different IVC filters were used at the discretion of the physician during the trial. The recently published PREPIC2 trial[258] attempted to address some of these weaknesses. In this study, 398 patients were randomized to receive either 6 months of anticoagulation alone or anticoagulation with and IVC filter. Patients randomized into the filter group received an ALN filter, had the filter retrieved after 3 months, and then received an additional 6 months of anticoagulation following retrieval. There was no significant difference in incidence of PE at 3 months (3% filter vs. 1.5% no filter, $P = .5$) and no difference in mortality, PE, or recurrent DVT at 6 months. The authors concluded that IVC filters in combination with anticoagulation provided no benefit over anticoagulation alone. However, both the PREPIC and PREPIC2 trials failed to assess the use of IVC filters in the target population that would potentially benefit most: patients who cannot be anticoagulated or who have failed anticoagulation.

Since the initial publication of the PREPIC trial in 1998, there has been increased interest in filters designed to provide the option of retrieval. In fact, the majority of filters recently introduced into the market have been retrievable optional filters: the G2, Eclipse and Denali filters (Bard Peripheral Vascular), Gunther Tulip and Celect filters (Cook), OptEase (Cordis, Miami, FL), the Option filter (Argon Medical, Athens, TX; Fig. 49.3), the ALN Optional Filter (ALN), and the Crux filter (Volcano). Interestingly, the Recovery filter was taken off the market in 2005 for problems with filter fracture and embolization. Filter migration was also problematic for this particular filter. Since 2005, this filter has gone through multiple additional adaptations, the G2 (Generation 2), the Eclipse, and was most recently redesigned

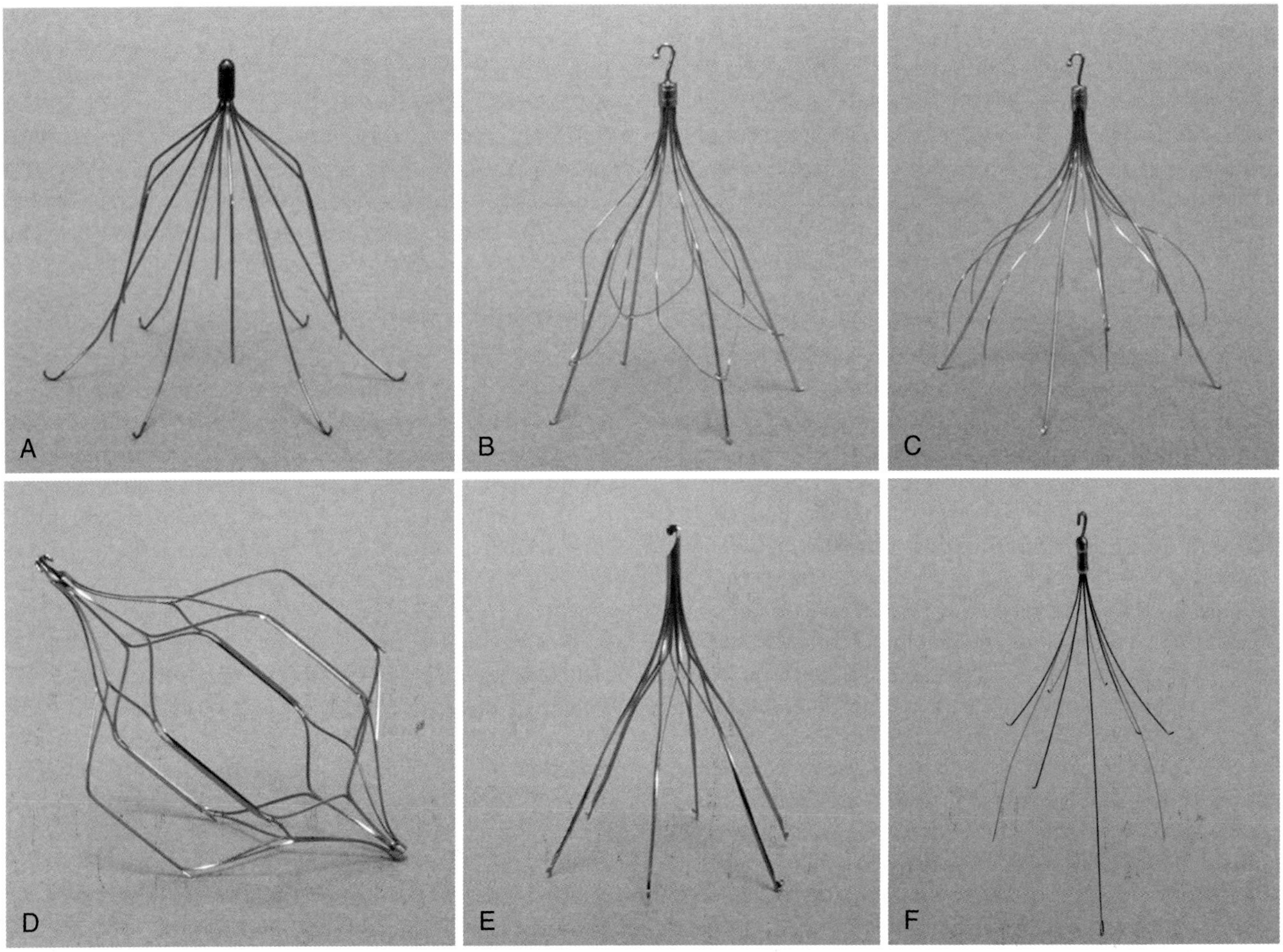

FIG 49.3 Retrievable optional inferior vena cava filters. (A) G2 Filter (Bard Peripheral Vascular, Tempe, AZ). (B) Gunther Tulip Filter (Cook, Bloomington, IN). (C) Celect Filter (Cook). (D) OptEase Filter (Cordis, Miami, FL). (E) Option Filter (Argon Medical, Athens, TX). (F) ALN Filter (ALN International, Miami, FL).

as the Denali. Most of the commercially available retrievable IVC filters have a conical design similar to that of the original Greenfield filter. The lone exception is the Crux filter, which is a significant departure from the traditional conical filter design and consists of a nitinol frame with two sinusoidal wave forms connected to form a figure of eight when deployed. One of the "loops" contains an expanded polytetrafluoroethylene (ePTFE) net to entrap emboli.

The features that make a device retrievable—lack of endothelial incorporation and flexible hooks—are also the features that make it less secure as a permanent device. More information on patient outcomes after filter removal is necessary to determine whether the concept of retrieval, with its added risk and cost, is appropriate. Classical indications for the use of IVC filters are unlikely to be altered, but further study to determine the most appropriate indications for filter placement, especially in the case of relative and extended indications, is warranted. The current trend in IVC filters is clearly weighted in favor of further development of retrievable IVC filters despite the limited data to support their use. Regardless of the current questions surrounding the use of retrievable filters, it is clear that the use of IVC filters in appropriately selected patients saves lives and will remain an important tool in the armamentarium of clinicians in the treatment of DVT and PE.

REVIEW QUESTIONS

1. Which of the following are significant risk factors for venous thromboembolism?
   - **a.** Age, immobilization, Caucasian race
   - **b.** History of DVT, malignancy, malnutrition
   - **c.** Surgery, obesity, malignancy, inflammatory bowel disease
   - **d.** Central venous catheters, hypertension, hyperlipidemia, pregnancy
2. In the treatment algorithm for VTE, which of the following would be appropriate?
   - **a.** Rapid anticoagulation should be considered for only iliofemoral DVT.
   - **b.** Catheter-directed thrombolytic therapy should be considered for an acute extensive iliofemoral DVT.
   - **c.** Rapid anticoagulation is initiated not only to prevent further extension of clot but also to help break down any existing thrombus.
   - **d.** Open thrombectomy should be considered before thrombolysis.
3. A limitation of LMWH is that:
   - **a.** LMWH is eliminated by the kidneys, making safe dosing difficult with renal dysfunction (defined at CrCl <30 mL/min)
   - **b.** LMWH is as effective as unfractionated heparin, but the safety profile is not well defined.
   - **c.** LMWH is a more specific inhibitor of factor Xa, which cannot be measured and titrated to therapeutic effect.
   - **d.** LMWH has a shorter half-life and is not ideal for high-risk patients with bleeding concerns.
4. Which of the following inherited thrombophilias is associated with the greatest increase in risk for VTE (in the heterozygous form)?
   - **a.** Factor V Leiden
   - **b.** Prothrombin G20210A
   - **c.** Protein C deficiency
   - **d.** Antithrombin deficiency
5. After an episode of acute DVT, anticoagulation should be initiated for:
   - **a.** 6 weeks
   - **b.** 3 months
   - **c.** Indefinitely
   - **d.** Until the etiology of the DVT can be determined and reversed
6. New management paradigms in determining who is at increased risk of recurrence (and PTS) at 3 to 6 months after incident DVT include which of the following?
   - **a.** Imaging of the deep venous system for evidence of residual thrombus
   - **b.** Identifying patients with elevated C-reactive protein
   - **c.** Identifying patients with elevated D-dimer levels
   - **d.** Both *a* and *c*
7. Which of the following is true regarding superficial vein thrombophlebitis (SVT)?
   - **a.** Duplex ultrasound of the affected extremity to rule out extension to the deep venous system is not indicated.
   - **b.** A complete thrombophilia workup is almost always indicated.
   - **c.** Regardless of location, SVT never warrants treatment with therapeutic doses of LMWH, although treatment with a 30- to 45-day course of fondaparinux may be beneficial if the lesion is greater than 7 cm in length.
   - **d.** The clinical diagnosis usually involves pain, a firm palpable cord with inflammation, tenderness, surrounding erythema, and edema.
8. PTS is chronic sequelae of DVT with typical symptoms including pain, heaviness, swelling, and cramping of the leg, worsened by standing and exercising. Which of the following are true regarding PTS?
   - **a.** It is defined by the CEAP score, with parameters including clinical features of the involved limb, etiology, anatomy, and pathophysiology.
   - **b.** PTS is defined by duplex ultrasound imaging, with resulting imaging that correlates to disease severity.
   - **c.** PTS is defined by the Villalta score, combining patient limb symptoms and signs into a graded scoring system, with a score greater than 15 suggesting severe disease.
   - **d.** Severity of disease is inversely related to body mass index, female gender, older age, iliofemoral location, or recurrent ipsilateral DVT.

9. In addition to anticoagulation, the initial management of acute DVT includes early ambulation and effective leg compression with 30 to 40 mm Hg ankle-gradient stockings. A recent double blind randomized trial regarding stockings suggested:
   a. Significant reduction in PTS.
   b. There is some evidence of increased incidence of PE with lower extremity compression.
   c. There is no randomized prospective evidence that PTS is significantly reduced with stockings.
   d. These therapies are minimally effective at reducing thrombus length and volume but may improve the patient's subjective evaluation of pain.

10. In what percentage of patients does a PE occur with an IVC filter in place?
   a. Less than 1%
   b. 2% to 4%
   c. 6% to 8%
   d. Greater than 10%

BIBLIOGRAPHY

Decousus H, Prandoni P, Mismetti P, et al. Fondaparinux for the treatment of superficial-vein thrombosis in the legs. *N Engl J Med.* 2010;363:1222–1232.

Eklof B, Rutherford RB, Bergan JJ, et al. Revision of the ceap classification for chronic venous disorders: Consensus statement. *J Vasc Surg.* 2004;40:1248–1252.

Enden T, Haig Y, Klow NE, et al. Long-term outcome after additional catheter-directed thrombolysis versus standard treatment for acute iliofemoral deep vein thrombosis (the cavent study): A randomised controlled trial. *Lancet.* 2012;379:31–38.

Esmon CT. Inflammation and thrombosis. *J Thromb Haemost.* 2003;1:1343–1348.

Heit JA. The epidemiology of venous thromboembolism in the community. *Arterioscler Thromb Vasc Biol.* 2008;28:370–372.

Kahn SR, Shapiro S, Wells PS, et al. Compression stockings to prevent post-thrombotic syndrome: A randomised placebo-controlled trial. *Lancet.* 2014;383:880–888.

Kearon C, Akl EA, Ornelas J, et al. Antithrombotic therapy for vte disease: Chest guideline and expert panel report. *Chest.* 2016;149: 315–352.

Mismetti P, Laporte S, Pellerin O, et al. Effect of a retrievable inferior vena cava filter plus anticoagulation vs anticoagulation alone on risk of recurrent pulmonary embolism: A randomized clinical trial. *JAMA.* 2015;313:1627–1635.

Palareti G, Cosmi B, Legnani C, et al. D-dimer testing to determine the duration of anticoagulation therapy. *N Engl J Med.* 2006;355: 1780–1789.

Wakefield TW, Myers DD, Henke PK. Mechanisms of venous thrombosis and resolution. *Arterioscler Thromb Vasc Biol.* 2008;28: 387–391.

References available online at ExpertConsult.com.

CHAPTER 50

Thrombolysis and Mechanical Thrombectomy for Deep Venous Thrombosis and Pulmonary Embolism

Anthony J. Comerota, Maxim E. Shaydakov

INTRODUCTION

Thrombolytic therapy for venous thromboembolism is an increasingly important option for the management of patients with extensive venous thromboembolic disease, namely iliofemoral venous thrombosis and pulmonary embolism (PE), which alter venous and cardiopulmonary hemodynamics and cause pathologic myocardial stretch or cellular damage. This chapter addresses those patients. Specifically, in patients with deep venous thrombosis (DVT), iliofemoral DVT (IFDVT) is associated with the most severe acute and long-term postthrombotic sequelae.

Patients with massive PE defined by sustained hypotension and those with submassive PE characterized by right heart strain are those who would benefit most by eliminating the acute obstruction of right ventricular outflow.

There is a common theme in treating both extensive venous thrombosis and large pulmonary emboli, and that is restoring hemodynamics. In the lower extremity the goal is to avoid venous hypertension (ambulatory venous hypertension), and in the cardiopulmonary circulation the goal is to correct cardiopulmonary hemodynamics and avoid chronic thromboembolic pulmonary hypertension.

ACUTE ILIOFEMORAL VENOUS THROMBOSIS

The postthrombotic morbidity of IFDVT treated with anticoagulation is illustrated by a 22-year-old woman who was referred with severe venous claudication. As a high school student, this patient was the state champion in the 400-m and 800-m run. She was awarded a full college scholarship as a member of a Big Ten women's track team. Three months after starting birth control pills, she developed an extensive iliofemoral venous thrombosis. She was hospitalized, treated with low-molecular-weight heparin (LMWH) and converted to warfarin. Her leg remained swollen and her venous claudication persisted. Her symptoms limited her activity; she could no longer participate as a member of the track team and had difficulty with sustained walking. She lost her athletic scholarship and, because of family finances, could not remain in college. The result was a part-time job paying minimum wage. Her IFDVT with its postthrombotic sequelae irrevocably changed her life and the life of her future family.

Acute obstruction of the single channel outflow from the lower extremity (common femoral, external iliac, and common iliac veins) leads to high compartment and venous pressures. Qvarford and colleagues[1] reported compartment pressures in patients presenting with IFDVT who subsequently underwent venous thrombectomy. Upon presentation, these patients had high compartment pressures, which is a surrogate for venous pressure. Following thrombus removal and restoration of venous outflow, compartment pressures significantly decreased and returned to normal in many.

The pathophysiology of chronic venous disease is venous hypertension, specifically ambulatory venous hypertension. Venous valve function and luminal obstruction are the two main components leading to ambulatory venous hypertension. However, it is this author's opinion that obstruction is far more important than valvular dysfunction in producing severe venous hypertension and the most debilitating form of chronic venous disease.

Labropoulos and colleagues[2] measured venous pressure and calculated the arm-foot pressure differential in patients with the spectrum of postthrombotic venous disease; they showed that patients with postthrombotic obstruction of the iliofemoral venous system had the highest venous pressures (highest arm-foot pressure differential), which translates into clinical morbidity.

Anticoagulation alone for IFDVT reduces the risk of pulmonary embolization and reduces the extension of thrombus. Unfortunately, obstruction of the venous outflow channel remains, producing significant venous hypertension. Fig. 50.1 is a photograph of a man who had IFDVT treated with anticoagulation alone 3 months earlier. Despite therapeutic anticoagulation and wearing 30- to 40-mm ankle-gradient compression stockings, he suffered with venous claudication, swelling of the lower extremity, and skin discoloration in the lower leg, with the ascending phlebogram showing extensive deep venous obstruction. Another ascending phlebogram (Fig. 50.2) of a patient with severe postthrombotic morbidity and venous ulceration 10 years after anticoagulation alone for IFDVT shows chronic recanalization but understates his venous obstruction. The day following the phlebogram, the patient underwent a classic Linton procedure. The operative photograph of a cross section of his postthrombotic femoral vein demonstrates the fibrotic obstruction with multiple, small channel recanalization which occur in these patients, causing much more obstruction to venous return than can be appreciated on the phlebogram.

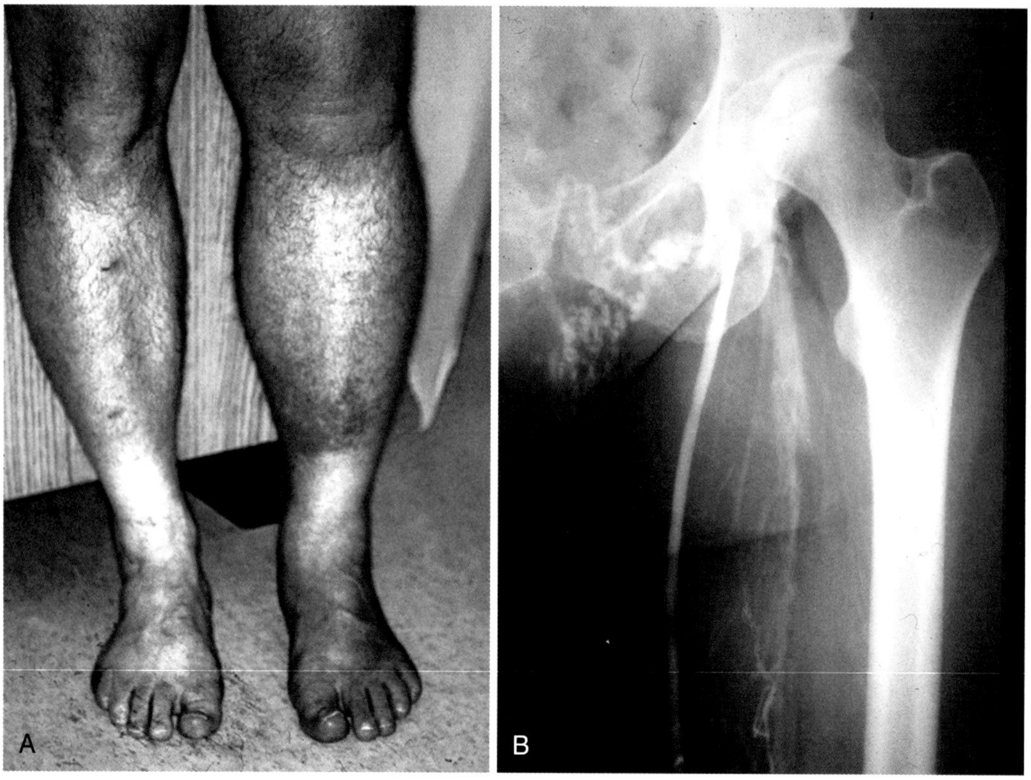

FIG 50.1 (A) Photograph of the lower extremities of a patient suffering iliofemoral deep venous thrombosis 3 months earlier treated with anticoagulation alone. (B) The associated ascending phlebogram demonstrating extensive deep venous obstruction. The saphenous vein is patent, but it too is obstructed at the saphenofemoral junction.

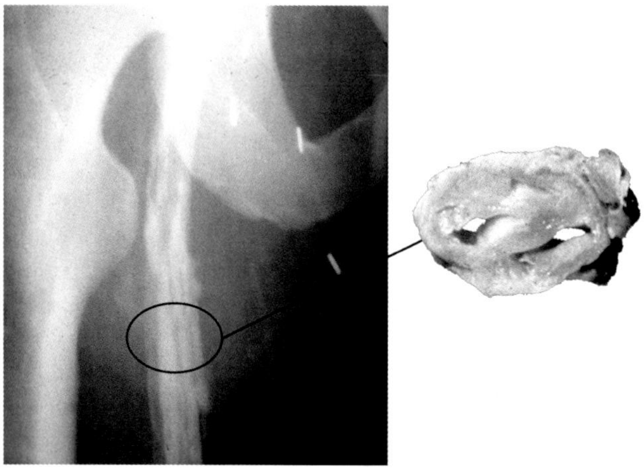

FIG 50.2 Ascending phlebogram of a patient treated for iliofemoral deep venous thrombosis with anticoagulation alone 10 years earlier. A noninvasive vascular laboratory test measuring maximal venous outflow was normal. The ascending phlebogram was read by the radiologist as "tree-barking appearance of chronic venous disease with no evidence of obstruction." The specimen demonstrates a cross-section of the femoral vein just below the profunda femoris vein after the patient had a classic Linton procedure. One can see extensive luminal obstruction with typical recanalization channels.

NATURAL HISTORY STUDIES

Natural history studies of patients with acute DVT treated with anticoagulation alone have revealed a number of important principles. Meissner and colleagues[3] followed patients with acute DVT with sequential venous duplex examinations. Some patients' thrombus was lysed during the first few months of follow-up, whereas in others the thrombus persisted. When thrombus lysed early (within 60 to 90 days), patients were likely to retain normal valve function. However, in patients whose thrombus did not lyse, valve reflux occurred. In longer-term follow-up studies, patients who had persistent thrombus had a significantly higher risk of recurrent DVT.[4]

Acute DVT of the lower extremity includes a spectrum of clinical presentations ranging from asymptomatic isolated calf vein thrombosis to severely symptomatic extensive IFDVT. Cumulative evidence suggests that iliofemoral venous thrombosis is accompanied by more dramatic clinical manifestation, predicts poor immediate and long-term outcomes, and warrants a treatment strategy of thrombus removal. A likely explanation of the underuse of strategies of thrombus removal is the underappreciation of postthrombotic sequelae of extensive proximal venous thrombosis.

Kahn and colleagues[5] performed a prospective analysis of 387 patients with acute DVT. Their intent was to evaluate postthrombotic syndrome following acute DVT. They found that patients with IFDVT had the most severe postthrombotic morbidity (odds ratio [OR] 2.23; $P < .001$). They also found that the patients' clinical condition at 1 month was the best predictor of long-term outcome ($P < .001$).

A number of authors have followed patients with IFDVT who were treated with anticoagulation alone.[6,7] These patients uniformly suffered with chronic venous disease. Within 5 years, 15% developed venous ulceration and up to 40% had venous claudication. The patients' quality of life (QOL) was significantly diminished.

An observation which is often overlooked is that recurrent DVT is more frequent in patients with IFDVT than in patients with femoropopliteal DVT.[8] This is likely due to the large burden of thrombus resulting in postthrombotic obstruction following anticoagulation alone.

VENOUS THROMBECTOMY

The purpose of this short section is not to address operative venous thrombectomy, which is beyond the scope of this chapter. It is to emphasize the principles of restoring patency, normalizing venous pressures, and long-term benefits are well illustrated by the randomized trial performed by Plate and colleagues.[9–11] The Scandinavian investigators randomized patients with IFDVT to venous thrombectomy plus arteriovenous fistula (AVF) followed by anticoagulation or anticoagulation alone. A careful follow-up at 6 months, 5 years, and 10 years demonstrated significant benefits in those patients who underwent venous thrombectomy. Patients randomized to thrombectomy had improved patency, lower venous pressures, less leg swelling, and fewer postthrombotic symptoms compared with anticoagulation alone. These data illustrate the benefit of eliminating obstruction to venous drainage from the leg to the vena cava. The details of contemporary operative venous thrombectomy have been reviewed by Comerota and Gale.[12]

A report by Rodriguez described a novel technique called hybrid open thrombectomy (HOT).[13] The method uses a single surgical access to the common femoral vein to remove thrombus from the iliofemoral venous segment. The same access is used to clear more distal segments, including tibial veins, by means of careful retrograde manipulation with a guidewire followed by balloon catheter thrombectomy. Technical success comparable with pharmacomechanical thrombolysis was achieved in 38 patients.

CATHETER-DIRECTED THROMBOLYSIS

Mechanisms of Fibrinolysis

All drugs currently used for thrombolytic therapy are plasminogen activators. That means that clot dissolution occurs as a result of plasminogen being activated, resulting in the production of plasmin, which is the active clot dissolving enzyme.

Catheter-Directed Thrombolysis

Systemic thrombolytic therapy is an inefficient method of treating acute DVT. A relatively small amount of systemically infused plasminogen activator will contact the thrombus to activate fibrin-bound plasminogen. The results of studies evaluating systemic thrombolytic therapy for acute DVT have been disappointing and generally are associated with higher than acceptable bleeding complications and lower than acceptable success rates.[14] It is understandable that techniques that deliver the plasminogen activator into the thrombus, thereby maximally activating fibrin-bound plasminogen and minimizing the systemic delivery of the plasminogen activator will be associated with greater success rates and fewer bleeding complications.

Numerous reports have demonstrated good outcomes of catheter-directed thrombolysis (CDT) for acute DVT. Most of these reports (≥20 limbs) are listed in Table 50.1, which also includes pharmacomechanical techniques used as adjuncts to CDT. In general, when patients with acute DVT are treated with catheter-based techniques, success rates in the range of 75% to 90% can be anticipated. The rate of bleeding complications ranges from 5% to 11%. Fortunately, serious distant bleeding is uncommon and intracranial bleeding is a rarity. Most bleeding complications are localized to the venous access site, and reports surfacing in the past 7 years generally report bleeding complications as 5% or less. Symptomatic pulmonary embolization during infusion is uncommon and fatal PE a rarity.

The National Venous Registry[15] reported a large cohort of patients treated with lytic therapy for acute DVT. Seventy-one percent of these patients had IFDVT, and 25% had femoropopliteal DVT. It is interesting to note that patients with IFDVT seem to have had better and more durable results than patients with femoropopliteal DVT.

Patients treated in the National Venous Registry were treated with intrathrombus infusion of urokinase via CDT. In the group with acute first-time IFDVT, 65% had complete clot resolution. There was an important correlation ($P < .001$) of thrombosis-free survival with the results of initial therapy. At 1 year, 78% of patients with initially complete clot resolution had patent veins and only 37% of patients who had less than 50% lysis. In the patients with first-time IFDVT who initially had successful thrombolysis, 96% of the veins remained patent at 1 year. Initial lytic success also correlated with valve function at 6 months. Thirty-eight percent of patients with less than 50% thrombolysis had normal valve function, whereas 72% with complete lysis retained normal valve function ($P < .02$).

A cohort-controlled QOL study was performed to assess whether lytic therapy impacted QOL in patients with IFDVT.[16] Patients with IFDVT treated by CDT were compared with a contemporaneous cohort of patients with IFDVT from the same institutions who were treated with anticoagulation alone. All patients treated with anticoagulation alone were candidates for lytic therapy; however, the choice of treatment was determined by physician preference. Patients were evaluated with a validated QOL questionnaire, with patients queried at 16 and 22 months following acute treatment.[17] Ninety-eight patients were evaluated, 68 of whom were treated with CDT and 30 with anticoagulation alone. CDT was associated with better QOL than anticoagulation alone. QOL was directly related to thrombolytic success. Patients who had a successful lytic outcome reported a better Health Utilities Index, improved physical functioning, less stigma of chronic venous disease, less health distress, and fewer postthrombotic symptoms. Not surprisingly, patients in whom CDT failed

TABLE 50.1 Studies of Catheter-Directed Thrombolysis (Drip Technique) and Pharmacomechanical Thrombolysis

			RESULTS			COMPLICATIONS			
						BLEEDING			
Author	Patients (Limbs)	Intervention	Significant/ Complete Resolution (%)	Partial Resolution (%)	No Resolution (%)	Minor (%)	Major (%)	PE	Death From Rx (%)
Semba et al.[57]	21 (27)	CDT with UK, angio/stenting	18 (72)	5 (25)	2 (8)	1 (4)	0 (0)	0	0
Semba et al.[58]	32 (41)	CDT with UK, angio/stenting	21 (32)	9 (28)	2 (6)	0 (0)	0 (0)	0	0
Verhaeghe et al.[59]	24	CDT with rt-PA, stenting	19 (79)	5 (21)	0 (0)	0 (0)	6 (25)	0	0
Bjarnason et al.[60]	77 (87)	CDT with UK, angio/stenting, thrombectomy,	69 (793)	0 (0)	18 (21)	11 (14)	5 (6)	1	0
Mewissen et al.[15]	287 (312)	CDT with UK, stenting, systemic lysis	96 (31)	162 (52)	54 (17)	15 (28)	54 (11)	6	2 (<1)
Comerota and Kagan[61]	54	CDT with UK or rt-PA, thrombectomy	14 (26)	28 (52)	6 (11)	8 (15)	4 (7)	1	0
AbuRahma et al.[62]	51	CDT with UK or rt-PA, stenting	15 (83) 1 (3)	0 0	0 0	3 (17) 3 (9)	2 (11) 2 (6)	0 2 (6)	0 0
Vedantham et al.[23]	20 (28)	CDT with UK, rt-PA, or rPA, thrombectomy, stenting	23 (82)	0	0	0	3 (14)	0	0
Elsharawy et al.[19]	35	CDT with SK, angio/stenting	13 (72) 2 (12)	5 (28) 8 (47)	0 (0) 7 (41)	0 0	0 0	0 0	0 0
Grunwald et al.[63]	74 (82)	CDT with UK, tPA, or rPA, angio/stenting	54 (73)	26 (32)	0	6 (8)	4 (5)	0	0
Laiho et al.[64]	32	CDT with rt-PA or systemic lysis with rt-PA	8 (50) 5 (31)	5 (31) 8 (50)	0 0	4 (25) 6 (38)	2 (13) 1 (6)	2 (13) 5 (31)	0 0
Vedantham et al.[65]	18 (23)	CDT with reteplase + mechanical thrombectomy	7 (31)	12 (52)	4 (17)		1 (6)	0	0
Bush et al.[66]	20 (23)	Pharmacomechanical thrombectomy with reteplase, UK, and rt-PA, angio/stenting	15 (65)	8 (35)	0	2	0	0	0
Sillesen et al.[22]	45	CDT with rt-PA, angio/stenting	42 (93)	0	0	4 (8)	0	1 (2)	0
Jackson et al.[67]	28	CDT with UK or rPA, stenting	5 (18)	20 (72)	0	2 (7)	0	0	0
Ogawa et al.[68]	24	CDT with UK or CDT with UK + IPC	0 (0) 5 (36)	10 (100) 9 (64)	0 0	0 0	0 0	0 0	0 0
Kim et al.[69]	37 (45)	CDT with UK or CDT + PMT	21 (81) 16 (84)	3 (11) 3 (16)	2 (8) 0	1 (4) 0	2 (7) 1 (5)	1 (4) 1 (5)	0 0
Lin et al.[24]	93 (98)	CDT with rPA, rt-PA, or UK, angio/stenting or PMT with rPA, rt-PA, or UK, angio/stenting	32 (70) 39 (75)	14 (30) 13 (25)	5 (11) 4 (8)	2 (4) 2 (4)	1 (2) 0	0 0	0 0
Cynamon et al.[70]	24	Pharmacomechanical thrombectomy, CDT, angio/stenting	12 (50)	12 (50)	0	0	2 (8)	0	0
Protack et al.[71]	69	CDT with UK, tPA, retavase, pulse-spray, mechanical thrombect, stenting, IVC filters	40 (63)	19 (30)	4 (6)	0	0	0	0
Arko et al.[72]	30	Pharmacomechanical thrombectomy with tenecteplase	27 (90)	Not reported		0	0	0	0
Martinez et al.[73]	52	CDT with rt-PA or ISPMT with rt-PA	19 (70) 23 (92)	8 (30) 2 (8)	0 0	6 (27) 5 (19)	1 (4) 1 (4)	0 0	0 0
Parikh et al.[28]	47 (53)	CDT using ultrasound-accelerated catheter with UK, rPA, tPA, and tenecteplase. Adjunctive PTA, stenting, mechanical thrombectomy, AVF	37 (70)	11 (21)	5 (9)	0	2 (4)	0	0

TABLE 50.1 Studies of Catheter-Directed Thrombolysis (Drip Technique) and Pharmacomechanical Thrombolysis—cont'd

						COMPLICATIONS			
			RESULTS			BLEEDING			
Author	**Patients (Limbs)**	**Intervention**	**Significant/ Complete Resolution (%)**	**Partial Resolution (%)**	**No Resolution (%)**	**Minor (%)**	**Major (%)**	**PE**	**Death From Rx (%)**
Rao et al.[74]	43	Pharmacomechanical thrombectomy in pts with contraindication to lysis	95% based on >50% lysis				2 (4)	0	0
Baekgaard et al.[32]	101 (103)	CDT with rt-PA, stenting, stockings, anticoagulation	82% had patent veins with no reflux at 6-year follow-up		8 (8)	5 (5)	1 (1)		0
Gasparis et al.[33]	23	Pharmacomechanical thrombectomy, CDT	14 (61)	9 (39)	0	1	0	0	0
Enden et al.[20]	50	CDT, angio/stenting	24/50 (48)	20/53 (38)	4 (8)	2	1	0	0
Kim et al.[75]	26 (29)	Single-session pharmacomechanical thrombectomy with UK	24 (83)	5 (17)	0	0	0	0	0

AVF, Arteriovenous fistula; *CDT,* catheter-directed thrombolysis; *Hep,* heparin; *IPC,* intermittent pneumatic compression; *IVC,* inferior vena cava; *ISPMT,* isolated segmental pharmacomechanical thrombolysis; *PE,* pulmonary embolism; *PMT,* pharmacomechanical thrombolysis; *PTA,* percutaneous transluminal angioplasty; *rPA,* recombinant plasminogen activator; *rt-PA,* recombinant tissue plasminogen activator; *Rx,* treatment; *SK,* streptokinase; *tPA,* tissue plasminogen activator; *UK,* urokinase.
CDT-Catheter-directed thrombolysis: Drip Technique—no highlight
PMT-Pharmacomechanical thrombolysis—yellow highlight

had outcomes similar to those treated with anticoagulation alone. A subsequent single-center observational study demonstrated that QOL following CDT for IFDVT directly correlated with success of clot lysis.[18]

A small randomized trial performed by Elsharawy and colleagues[19] compared CDT with anticoagulation alone. CDT resulted in significantly better patency and valve function at 6 months. Enden and colleagues[20] reported the results from a randomized trial of CDT and anticoagulation versus anticoagulation alone for IFDVT. Patients treated with CDT had better patency of the iliofemoral system which directly correlated with less postthrombotic morbidity than those treated with anticoagulation.

PATIENT EVALUATION AND TECHNIQUE

Patients with IFDVT have a large thrombus burden and have a significant stimulus to thrombosis, with 40% to 50% having asymptomatic pulmonary emboli. There is value to detecting asymptomatic pulmonary emboli because up to 25% can develop pleuritic chest pain days later, when the infarct reaches the pleural surface of the lung.[21] Clinicians may mistakenly assume that the subsequent pleuritic symptoms are due to a new PE, incorrectly attributing the PE to failure of treatment. A spiral computed tomography (CT) scan of the chest with contrast evaluates the pulmonary vasculature for PE and other thoracic pathology. The CT is then extended to the brain, abdomen, and pelvis to identify the proximal extent of thrombus and to evaluate for intracranial, abdominal, or pelvic pathology. This has been an important addition to the evaluation of these patients because we have found pathology not previously diagnosed with surprising frequency. Renal cell carcinoma, adrenal tumors, retroperitoneal lymphoma, cerebral infarct, pulmonary adenocarcinoma, hepatic metastases, iliac vein aneurysms, vena caval atresia, and asymptomatic abdominal aortic aneurysms have all been identified. Evaluations for a heritable underlying thrombophilia are not performed, although first-degree female relatives of childbearing potential are evaluated for factor V Leiden, prothrombin 20210, and antithrombin deficiency because their management during future pregnancy will be altered if one or more of these tests is positive.

The technique of CDT has evolved. The preferred approach is through an ultrasound-guided popliteal puncture with antegrade passage of an infusion catheter. Patients who have distal popliteal vein and tibial vein thrombosis are also treated with a second catheter passed with ultrasound guidance into the posterior tibial vein at the ankle and advanced to the proximal popliteal vein. Adjunctive mechanical techniques are frequently used to speed clot resolution and shorten the duration of lysis.

The dose and volume of the plasminogen activator have also evolved. Because the activation of fibrin-bound plasminogen is not a dose-dependent phenomenon, its exposure to the plasminogen activator appears to be the most important factor. The volume of lytic solution has increased over the years, with a corresponding decrease in the concentration (dose) of the plasminogen activator. It is now our preference to increase the volume of lytic infusion to 100 mL/h. The larger volume is intended to saturate the thrombus, thereby exposing more fibrin-bound plasminogen to the plasminogen activator. The dose of recombinant tissue plasminogen activator (rt-PA) is generally 1 mg/h. If two catheters are used, the dose is increased to 1.5 to 2 mg/h split between the catheters.

Phlebograms are usually repeated at 12-hour intervals and are used to monitor the success of lysis, reveal the need for additional interventions, and reposition the catheters if necessary. Vena caval filters are not routinely used but are recommended for patients with free-floating thrombus in the vena cava. A retrievable filter can be used in patients for whom only temporary protection is required.

Following successful thrombolysis, the venous system is examined with completion phlebography. If an underlying stenosis exists, which is frequently observed in the left common iliac vein, where it is compressed by the right common iliac artery, the vein is dilated and stented as necessary. It is important to use a stent of adequate diameter (Fig. 50.3). The common iliac vein frequently requires a 14- to 16-mm stent and the external vein a 12- to 14-mm stent. The addition of intravascular ultrasonography has improved the evaluation of iliac compression and the precision of stent deployment. Residual areas of stenosis must be corrected to achieve long-term success; otherwise, the patient faces a high risk of rethrombosis.

PHARMACOMECHANICAL THROMBOLYSIS

Although good results have been achieved with CDT, treatment times can be unacceptably long, and therefore bleeding risk and cost associated with therapy are high. A contemporary report of extensive DVT treated with CDT alone demonstrated a 93% success rate.[22] These patients were generally treated within 7 days of symptom onset. It would be expected that lysis could be achieved efficiently in these patients because they represented a true acute DVT. However, treatment times for CDT alone averaged 71 hours. This duration of infusion is logistically difficult, if not impossible, for many practitioners and many medical centers. The associated cost is high because patients receiving lytic therapy are generally monitored in intensive care units. Therefore techniques to speed lytic success are important for efficient patient care and cost containment.

ENDOVASCULAR MECHANICAL THROMBECTOMY

Mechanical techniques alone or in combination with thrombolysis have been developed to more rapidly clear the venous system. Vedantham and associates[23] evaluated the effectiveness of mechanical thrombectomy alone or in combination with pharmacologic thrombolysis in 28 limbs of patients with acute DVT. They evaluated multiple devices. Venographic scoring was performed at each step of the procedure. Twenty-six percent of the thrombus was removed by mechanical thrombectomy alone, whereas adding a plasminogen activator solution to the mechanical technique (pharmacomechanical) removed 82% of the thrombus. Mechanical thrombectomy (rheolytic technique) alone was highly successful when removing intraprocedural thrombus, which is usually gelatinous and not cross-linked by factor XIII. The average infusion time was approximately 17 hours per limb, and 14% of patients had major bleeding complications.

RHEOLYTIC THROMBECTOMY

Lin and colleagues[24] reported their 8-year experience with pharmacomechanical thrombolysis using a rheolytic thrombectomy catheter. Of their 98 patients, 46 received CDT alone and 52 underwent pharmacomechanical thrombolysis using the AngioJet catheter (Medrad, Minneapolis, MD). Their observations demonstrated that the pharmacomechanical technique was associated with significantly fewer phlebograms, shorter intensive care unit (ICU) stays, shorter hospital stays, and fewer blood transfusions. Bleeding complications were not different between the two groups. A smaller patient group treated by rheolytic thrombectomy was reported by Kasirajan and associates,[25] who demonstrated that mechanical thrombectomy alone was less effective than the combined pharmacomechanical technique.

The efficacy of high-pressure delivery of the plasminogen activator solution into the thrombus was reported by Chang and colleagues.[26] Twelve patients with extensive lower extremity DVT were treated with repeat, high pressure, intermittent infusion of rt-PA. They used the higher-pressure pulse-spray technique. Following the pulse-spray infusion, the catheter was removed and the patient returned to their hospital room. Patients had repeat venograms the following day and additional pulse spray infusion if indicated. Significant or complete lysis was observed in 92% (11/12), with the remaining patient having 50% to 70% lysis.

Bookstein and colleagues[27] reported the benefit of forceful pulse-sprayed plasminogen activator in thrombosed arteries and dialysis access grafts.

This calls attention to the importance and effectiveness of the plasminogen activator penetrating the thrombus and of the plasminogen activator penetrating the thrombus and binding to fibrin-bound plasminogen with subsequent production of intrathrombus plasmin.

ULTRASOUND-ACCELERATED THROMBOLYSIS

Parikh and colleagues[28] reported an early clinical experience with ultrasound-accelerated thrombolysis (USAT) in 53 patients treated for acute DVT with the EKOS EndoWave system (EKOS Corp, Bothell, WA). Both upper and lower extremity DVT patients were included, as well as use of a variety of lytic agents. This makes a comparison with other reports difficult because axillosubclavian DVT responds more quickly than lower extremity venous thrombosis.

Complete lysis (≥90%) was observed in 70% of patients and overall lysis (complete or partial) in 91%. The median infusion time was 22 hours, and 4% of patients had major complications, which were essentially puncture site hematomas. It was the authors' impression that, compared with historical controls, treatment times and dose of lytic agents were reduced with ultrasound-accelerated thrombolysis compared with CDT using the drip technique alone.

Engelberger and his colleagues from Bern, Switzerland performed the "Bernutiful Trial" designed to answer the question, "Does intravascular high frequency, low power ultrasound facilitate resolution of thrombus during catheter-directed thrombolysis?"[29] They randomized 48 patients with acute IFDVT to be treated with conventional CDT using an ultrasound-accelerated thrombolysis catheter without the ultrasound-activated versus standard ultrasound-accelerated CDT. All patients received 20 mg rt-PA infused over 15 hours. The study end point was the amount of thrombolysis at 15 hours assessed by readers blinded to the treatment group. After 15 hours of treatment, there was 54%

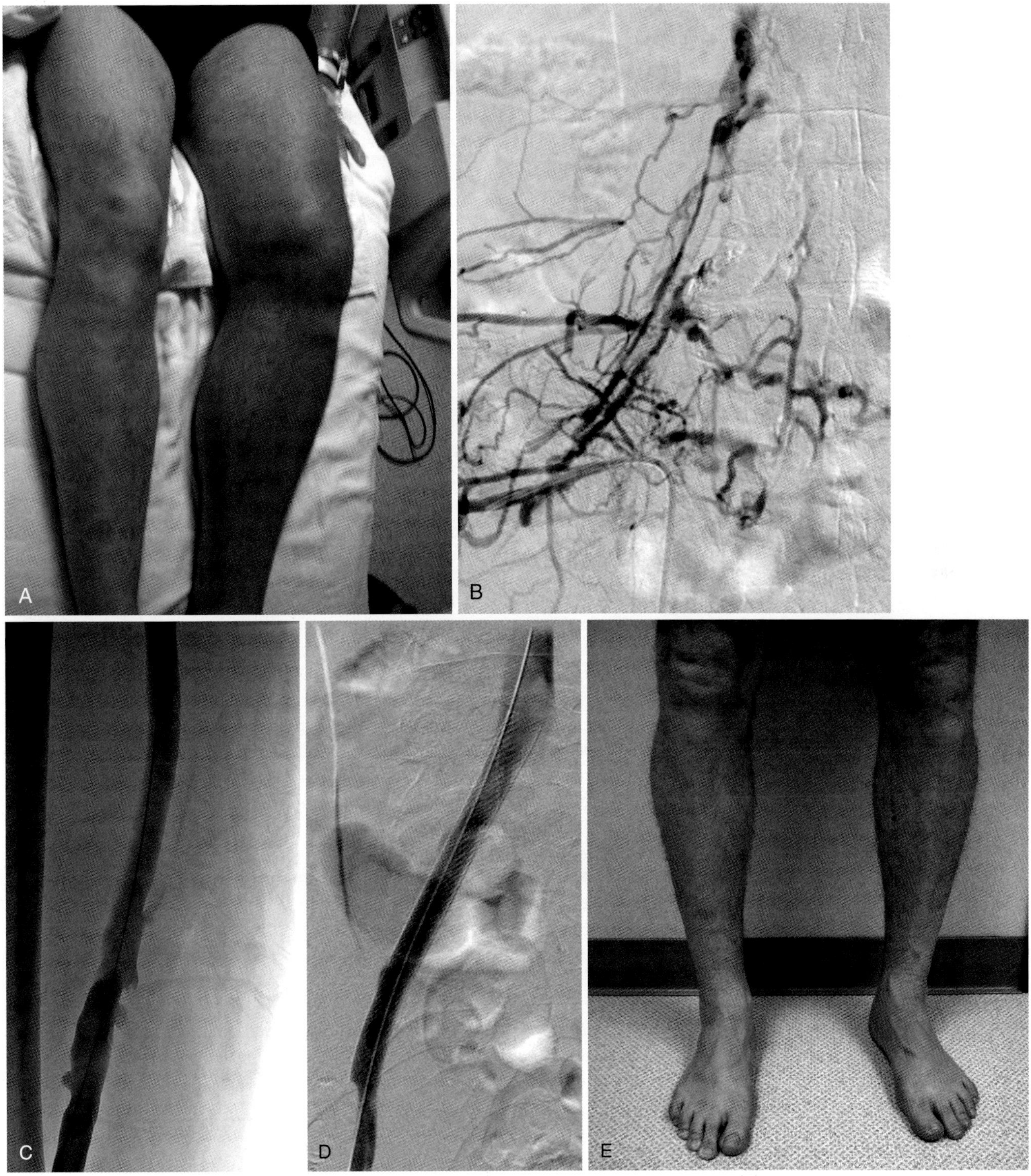

FIG 50.3 (A) Photograph of a patient presenting with phlegmasia cerulea dolens after being treated with Lovenox for 7 days. (B) Ascending phlebogram shows extensive thrombotic obstruction of the iliofemoral venous system. (C) Following pharmacomechanical thrombolysis and CDT, patency and valve function were restored to the patient's femoral vein and (D) iliac venous system. Stenting was required to correct an underlying iliac vein stenosis. (E) Twelve-month follow-up demonstrated a normal physical examination, and noninvasive evaluation demonstrated patent veins with normal valve function.

lysis in the CDT patients and 55% lysis in the ultrasound-accelerated thrombolysis patients. Because the infusion pump used with the EKOS catheter is a low-pressure pump, the lytic agent does not disperse much beyond the catheter, thereby minimizing the potential advantage of the rt-PA contacting the expanded fibrin surface area. If the rt-PA was delivered by an intermittent high-pressure injection pump that dispersed the plasminogen activator into the thrombus with an increased fibrin surface area, there may have been improved results with USAT.

ISOLATED SEGMENTAL PHARMACOMECHANICAL THROMBOLYSIS

The Trellis catheter (Medtronic, Minneapolis, MN) is a double-balloon catheter that is passed through the thrombus with the proximal balloon inflated above the clot and the distal balloon inflated to isolate a segment of the venous system. Between these two balloons, a plasminogen activator is infused and a dispersion wire causes the intraballoon segment of the catheter to assume a spiral configuration. The catheter is then activated and spins at 3500 rpm for 15 to 20 minutes. Liquefied and fragmented thrombus can be aspirated and treatment success evaluated by repeat segmental phlebography. If thrombus is resolved, the catheter is repositioned and additional thrombosed segments treated. If residual thrombus persists, a second treatment is performed or repeat treatment of another appropriate intervention (rheolytic thrombectomy, balloon angioplasty, stenting) is performed.

Martinez and coworkers[30] reviewed 52 consecutive limbs treated for IFDVT, the first 27 with CDT alone and the following 25 with isolated segmental pharmacomechanical thrombolysis (ISPMT) plus CDT when necessary. Thrombus burden and treatment outcomes were quantified. Ninety-three percent of the patients were treated with rt-PA. Venoplasty and stenting were used to correct underlying stenoses, and all received long-term therapeutic anticoagulation. Sixteen of the 27 limbs treated by CDT required adjunctive mechanical techniques to clear the thrombus, such as the AngioJet, ultrasound-accelerated lysis, or pulse-spray techniques, whereas only 7 of the limbs treated with ISPMT had additional mechanical techniques. A larger percentage of the thrombus was removed with ISPMT than with CDT. Complete lysis (≥90%) was achieved in 11% of the limbs of CDT patients as opposed to 28% of the limbs treated by ISPMT ($P = .077$). Treatment time was shorter (23.4 vs. 55.4 hours, $P < .001$) and the rt-PA dose was lower (33.4 vs. 59.3 mg, $P = .009$) with ISPMT. Hospital and ICU length of stay was no different, which was likely due to underlying patient comorbidities. Only 18% of the limbs had complete lysis following the use of the ISPMT catheter alone. Bleeding complications occurred in 5% of patients undergoing CDT alone, as well as 5% of patients treated with ISPMT.

The Trellis catheter was removed from the market for redesign. It is anticipated that an improved version will be released soon.

PHARMACOMECHANICAL TECHNIQUES AND VEIN VALVE FUNCTION

Physicians have been concerned that mechanical techniques added to CDT would adversely affect vein valve function. Vogel and colleagues[31] reported their observations in 69 limbs of 54 patients treated with either CDT alone ($N = 20$) or pharmacomechanical thrombolysis ($N = 49$). There was a tendency toward more complete thrombus resolution with the pharmacomechanical techniques. There was no difference in valve function between the groups; 53% of patients treated with pharmacomechanical thrombolysis had vein valve reflux greater than 1 second versus 65% treated with CDT ($P = .42$). An interesting observation was that of the patients with unilateral IFDVT, 31% had valvular reflux in their contralateral, uninvolved vein. The best predictor of reflux in the treated limb was reflux in the contralateral, uninvolved limb.

Pharmacomechanical thrombolysis does not adversely affect valve function compared with CDT alone.

OUTCOMES OF CATHETER-BASED INTERVENTION FOR ILIOFEMORAL DEEP VENOUS THROMBOSIS

Contemporary results of CDT, using the drip technique alone or by adding PMT, have improved patient outcomes. Baekgaard and colleagues[32] reported 103 patients followed for 6 years after CDT for IFDVT. Eighty-six percent of patients at 6 years had patent veins and normally functioning valves.

Grewal and colleagues[18] performed a QOL evaluation on patients undergoing CDT for IFDVT. The question they posed is whether patient QOL is related to the degree of successful lysis. They found a direct correlation indicating that the better the success of lytic therapy, the better the patient's QOL. In a smaller study, Gasparis and colleagues[33] also found that patients enjoying successful thrombolysis for IFDVT had a good QOL.

Comerota and colleagues[34] reported a direct correlation of postthrombotic morbidity with residual thrombus following CDT. The greater the amount of residual thrombus, the worse the postthrombotic syndrome as measured by the validated Villalta scale. The better the clot resolution, the lower the Villalta scale. Patients who had 90% or more clot resolution essentially had no postthrombotic morbidity.

As mentioned earlier, the large thrombus burden of IFDVT is associated with significantly higher recurrence rates compared with patients with infrainguinal DVT alone.[8] It has been our observation that patients treated with CDT for extensive venous thrombosis had a low incidence of recurrence. This was studied by Aziz and colleagues,[35] who reported that residual thrombus at the end of lysis correlated with recurrence. Patients with more than 50% (mean 65%) residual clot had a significantly higher recurrence rate than patients with less than 50% (mean 16%) thrombus remaining. It appears evident that residual thrombus is in large part responsible for recurrent thrombosis.

OVERVIEW

Extensive DVT is associated with severe postthrombotic morbidity. One can restore venous hemodynamics to near normal or normal with successful thrombus removal. Pharmacomechanical techniques have increased treatment success, decreased treatment time, and reduced dose of plasminogen activator.

Successful thrombus removal improves QOL, reduces or eliminates subsequent postthrombotic morbidity, and appears to reduce the risk of recurrence.

ATTRACT TRIAL

The ATTRACT trial (Acute Venous Thrombosis: Thrombus Removal with Adjunctive Catheter-directed Thrombolysis) is the largest randomized study evaluating a strategy of thrombus removal using catheter-based techniques compared to anticoagulation alone for patients with acute proximal DVT[35a] (Fig. 50.4). This was a National Institutes of Health–funded study.

Among the questions to be answered by the ATTRACT trial are: (1) Is thrombus removal better than anticoagulation alone regarding long-term postthrombotic syndrome? (2) Is there differential benefit in patients with IFDVT versus femoropopliteal DVT? (3) How does treatment affect QOL? (4) Is degree of clot lysis correlated with benefit (postthrombotic morbidity)? (5) How is valvular reflux and residual obstruction correlated with postthrombotic morbidity? (6) Is pharmacomechanical thrombolysis better than CDT with the drip technique alone? (7) Is percutaneous intervention cost effective? Six hundred ninety-two patients with symptomatic proximal DVT were randomized within 56 clinical centers in the United States to standard anticoagulation or catheter directed pharmacomechanical thrombolysis (PCDT). Prior to randomization, patients were stratified by the extent of their thrombosis (femoropopliteal DVT or IFDVT) (Fig. 50.5). The primary efficacy outcome measure was

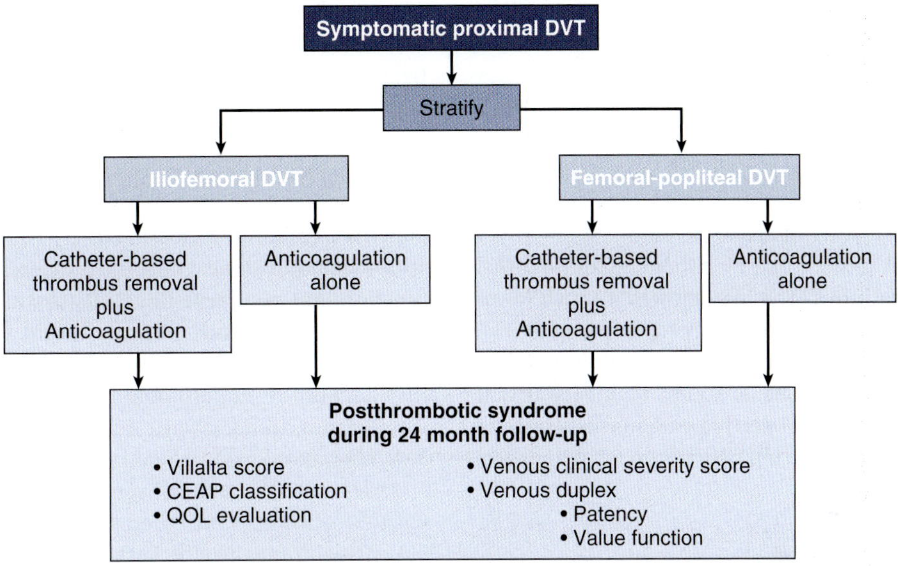

FIG 50.4 Basic outline for the conduct of the ATTRACT trial. *CEAP,* Clinical Etiologic Anatomic Pathophysiologic; *DVT,* deep venous thrombosis; *QOL,* quality of life.

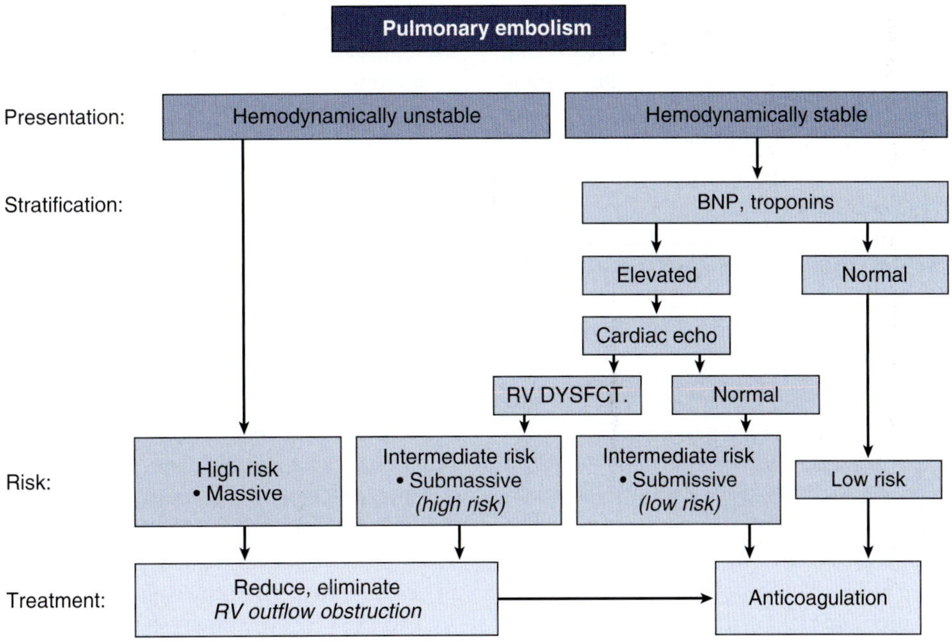

FIG 50.5 An algorithm for the approach to managing patients with symptomatic pulmonary embolism. *BNP,* Beta natriuretic polypeptide; *RV,* right ventricular.

PTS defined by a Villalta Score of >4, and the primary safety outcome measure was major bleeding.

All patients were treated with standard therapeutic anticoagulation and received 30 to 40 mm Hg ankle-gradient compression stockings. During follow-up, patients were assessed for postthrombotic syndrome using the validated Villalta scale, severity of leg pain, QOL, and the Venous Clinical Severity Score. Objective assessment of vein patency and venous valve function were performed with venous duplex examinations.

When evaluating the primary efficacy endpoint—PTS defined by a Villalta Score >4—there was no difference between treatment groups: 47% and 48% in the PCDT and anticoagulation groups, respectively. However, there was more rapid and significant reduction in pain and swelling in patients treated with PCDT and significantly less moderate-to-severe PTS (Villalta Score >9: 18% vs. 24%, $p = 0.035$). In patients presenting with a Villalta score >14, there was a major reduction in moderate to severe PTS compared to those treated with anticoagulation alone.

Major bleeding occurred in 1.7% of the PCDT treated patients and 0.3% of those treated with anticoagulation alone ($p = 0.049$). There were no intracranial bleeds. All but one major bleed occurred in patients over 65 years, and 100% of major bleeds occurred in patients >60 years of age.

The ATTRACT trial showed that all patients with proximal DVT do not benefit from PCDT. It also showed a much lower bleeding complication rate than previously reported for PCDT, although higher than anticoagulation alone, and clustered in older patients. Important additional analyses are underway that will assist physicians on properly selecting patients for strategies of thrombus removal and counseling patients on what to expect from outcomes of treatment.

PULMONARY EMBOLISM: SYSTEMIC THROMBOLYSIS

It would seem that appropriate goals of therapy for the management of patients with acute PE are: (1) restore cardiopulmonary hemodynamics in these patients in whom it is deranged; (2) avoid recurrent PE; and (3) avoid chronic thromboembolic pulmonary hypertension with its associated morbidity and mortality. Chronic thromboembolic pulmonary hypertension is associated with recurrent PE, a younger age of onset, large perfusion defects, and idiopathic PE.[36]

Pulmonary emboli large enough to cause right ventricular dysfunction are associated with a sixfold increase in hospital mortality and a 2.4-fold increase in 1-year mortality.[37]

The National Institutes of Health (NIH)-sponsored trials[38,39] of PE randomized patients to systemic thrombolytic therapy versus anticoagulation alone. The entry criteria included anyone with a documented symptomatic PE. All patients had arteriographically confirmed PE and had arteriographic and lung scan follow-up. The results from the NIH trials demonstrated that lytic therapy rapidly improved arteriogram and lung scan resolution of pulmonary emboli compared with patients treated with anticoagulation alone ($P < .05$). Thrombolytic therapy reduced pulmonary artery pressures and right atrial pressures ($P < .05$). However, bleeding complications were 46% with lytic therapy versus 27% in patients randomized to anticoagulation. There was no difference in mortality between the two groups; however, the design of these trials was not to evaluate mortality as a primary end point.

At 1-year follow-up, patients treated with lytic therapy had normal pulmonary capillary blood volumes and their oxygen diffusing capacity was 93%.[40] Patients treated with anticoagulation alone had a significantly reduced pulmonary capillary blood volume and their oxygen diffusing capacity was only 72% ($P < .05$).

At 7-year follow-up, patients underwent right heart catheterization.[41] There was a significant reduction in pulmonary artery pressures both at rest and at exercise in patients treated with lytic therapy, and pulmonary vascular resistance was significantly lower both at rest and with exercise the lytic therapy group. This resulted in several important clinical benefits: namely, fewer patients developed DVT or recurrent PE who had been treated with lytic therapy and there were significantly fewer patients in the lytic therapy group who suffered with congestive heart failure.

Goldhaber and colleagues[42] performed a randomized trial of patients with acute PE to evaluate early functional benefit; 101 patients were randomized to either rt-PA 100 mg × 2 hours or anticoagulation alone. Outcome measures were right ventricular function and recurrent PE. Patients who were randomized to rt-PA had significantly improved right ventricular function at 24 hours ($P = .005$), their end diastolic area was less ($P = .01$), they had improved pulmonary perfusion ($P = .0001$), and there was a strong trend toward a reduction in recurrent PEs at 14 days ($P = .06$).

Jerjes-Sanchez and collegues[43] designed a study to assess whether thrombolytic therapy would improve survival in patients with massive PE. Patients with massive PE (PE causing hypotension) were randomized to streptokinase plus heparin or heparin alone. The ethics committee terminated the trial after eight patients were randomized. The four patients receiving heparin alone died, whereas four patients receiving streptokinase plus heparin survived. The committee thought it unethical to continue the trial. This trial has been criticized because of the small sample size.

Wang and colleagues[44] studied reduced-dose rt-PA versus standard dose for the management of massive and submassive PE. They reasoned that the standard dose of rt-PA (100 mg) was arbitrarily chosen, although it was found to be effective. Bleeding complications were a recognized side effect.

Two recent trials randomized patients with acute submassive PE to either systemic thrombolysis with anticoagulation plus tenecteplase versus anticoagulation alone. The TOPCOAT trial randomized 83 patients.[45] The primary outcome was adverse events defined as death, shock, intubation, recurrent PE, or poor functional capacity. At 5 days, adverse events were observed in 2.5% of tenecteplase-treated patients versus 7.0% of anticoagulation patients (P = NS). At 90 days, adverse events occurred in 15% of tenecteplase-treated patients compared with 37% of patients treated with anticoagulation alone ($P = .017$).

The PEITHO investigators randomized 1005 patients with submassive PE.[46] Similarly, they used tenecteplase (TNK) and anticoagulation versus anticoagulation alone. They reported their efficacy and safety end points. The primary efficacy end point was death or hemodynamic collapse. The primary safety end point was major bleeding or ischemic/hemorrhagic stroke within 7 days of treatment.

A protocol studying one-half dose rt-PA (50 mg) versus full dose (100 mg) in PE patients was completed. They found that reduction in the right ventricular (RV) to left ventricular (LV) ratio, reduction in the systolic pulmonary artery pressure, decrease in the pulmonary perfusion defect score, and the decrease in pulmonary artery obstruction were no different between doses. There was no difference in mortality or recurrent VTE. However, there was a 47% reduction in bleeding complications ($P = .05$) with lower-dose rt-PA.

There was significant benefit with systemic thrombolysis with tenecteplase. Primary outcome (death/hemodynamic collapse) occurred in 2.6% of tenecteplase-treated patients versus 5.6% in anticoagulation alone patients ($P = .002$). However, the stroke rate of TNK-treated patients was significantly elevated to 2.4% compared with 0.2% in anticoagulation patients ($P = 0.003$), with the majority of the strokes being hemorrhagic (2%). There were also more major extracranial bleeds with tenecteplase 6.3% versus 1.2% ($P < .001$). In both the TOPCOAT and PEITHO trials, patients were anticoagulated during their course of systemic thrombolysis.

PATIENT SELECTION

Observational studies have demonstrated the importance of abnormal cardiopulmonary hemodynamics, abnormalities on echocardiography,[47] and biomarkers indicating ventricular stretch[48] and myocardial damage.[49] Echocardiography has become a helpful tool in the evaluation of patients with PE. Poor prognostic indicators on echocardiography in patients with PE include right ventricular thrombus, right ventricular hypokinesis, right ventricular dilation, pulmonary hypertension, tricuspid insufficiency, ventricular septal deviation, and a patent foramen ovale.

A meta-analysis of right ventricular dysfunction in patients with PE demonstrates a high short-term mortality from PE (12% to 14%) in patients with right ventricular dysfunction compared with less than 1% in patients who have a normally functioning right ventricle.[47] Longer-term observations correlated mortality with right ventricular dysfunction, increased mortality 6- to 13-fold in patients with right ventricular dysfunction versus those with a normally functioning right ventricle. Therefore, based upon the observed natural history of PE patients with reduced right ventricular function, it would appear that this subset of patients should be considered as candidates for thrombolysis.

A systematic review of elevated pro-beta natriuretic polypeptide (BNP) in PE was performed by Klok and colleagues.[48] They found that in patients with an elevated pro-BNP there was a significant increase in right ventricular dysfunction (OR 38.6, $P = .00001$), adverse clinical outcomes (OR 6.8, $P = .00001$), and death (OR 6.5, $P = .002$). Likewise, PE causing pathologic myocardial stretch is associated with increased morbidity and mortality and should be considered for lytic therapy.

Myocardial damage resulting from PE can be measured with troponins. A troponin-1 >.03 μg/L was a significant predictor of mortality.[49] Konstantinides and colleagues[50] showed a linear correlation of increased troponins with death, systemic complications, and recurrent pulmonary emboli. Troponins can be considered another biomarker of hemodynamically significant PE which would benefit from a treatment strategy designed to eliminate the PE causing obstruction to right ventricular outflow.

It is our practice to assess patients with PE clinically; calculate their RV/LV ratio; obtain their biomarkers, pro-BNP, and troponin; and perform an echocardiogram if biomarkers are abnormal. In general, patients who are on the borderline of stable hemodynamics (tachycardia but normal blood pressure) have suboptimal oxygenation, abnormal cardiac echo, and elevated pro-BNPs and troponins, would be those who we would consider treating with thrombolytic therapy, in addition to those with massive PE (Fig. 50.6).

The Seattle II investigators reported the results of 150 patients with acute massive PE ($N = 31$) and submassive PE ($N = 119$) treated with ultrasound-accelerated thrombolysis.[51] All patients had a RV to LV diameter ratio of ≥0.9 on chest computed tomographic angiography (CTA). rt-PA was infused at 1 mg/h per catheter, which was positioned within the embolus. If patients had unilateral catheters, they were treated for 24 hours, if bilateral catheters, treatment was discontinued after 12 hours, therefore achieving a maximal dose of rt-PA of 24 mg.

The efficacy results are detailed in Table 50.2, demonstrating a significant reduction in RV/LV ratio at 48 hours and a significant reduction in the Miller index score and Pulmonary Artery Systolic Pressure (PASP) post treatment.

There was one Global Utilization of Streptokinase and Tissue plasminogen activator for Occluded Coronary Arteries (GUSTO)-defined severe bleed (groin hematoma with hypotension) and 16 defined GUSTO moderate bleeding events (10%).[51a] There was no intracranial hemorrhage.

The American College of Chest Physicians (ACCP) in 2008 recommended that all patients with PE should undergo rapid risk stratification (grade 1C).[52] They further suggested that patients with hemodynamic compromise and no contraindication to lytic therapy receive thrombolytic therapy (grade 1B). They also

TABLE 50.2 Imaging and Hemodynamic Outcomes of the Seattle II Study

Variable	Pretreatment	Posttreatment	*P*-Value
RV/LV ratio	1.55	1.13	<.0001
Miller index score	22.5	15.8	<.0001
PASP (mm Hg)	54.1	36.9	<.0001

PASP, Pulmonary Artery Systolic Pressure; *LV*, left ventricular; RV, right ventricular.

From Piazza G, Hohlfelder B, Jaff MR, et al: A prospective, single-arm, multicenter trial of ultrasound-facilitated, catheter-directed, low-dose fibrinolysis for acute massive and submassive pulmonary embolism: the SEATTLE II Study. *JACC Cardiovasc Interv* 8:1382–1392, 2015.

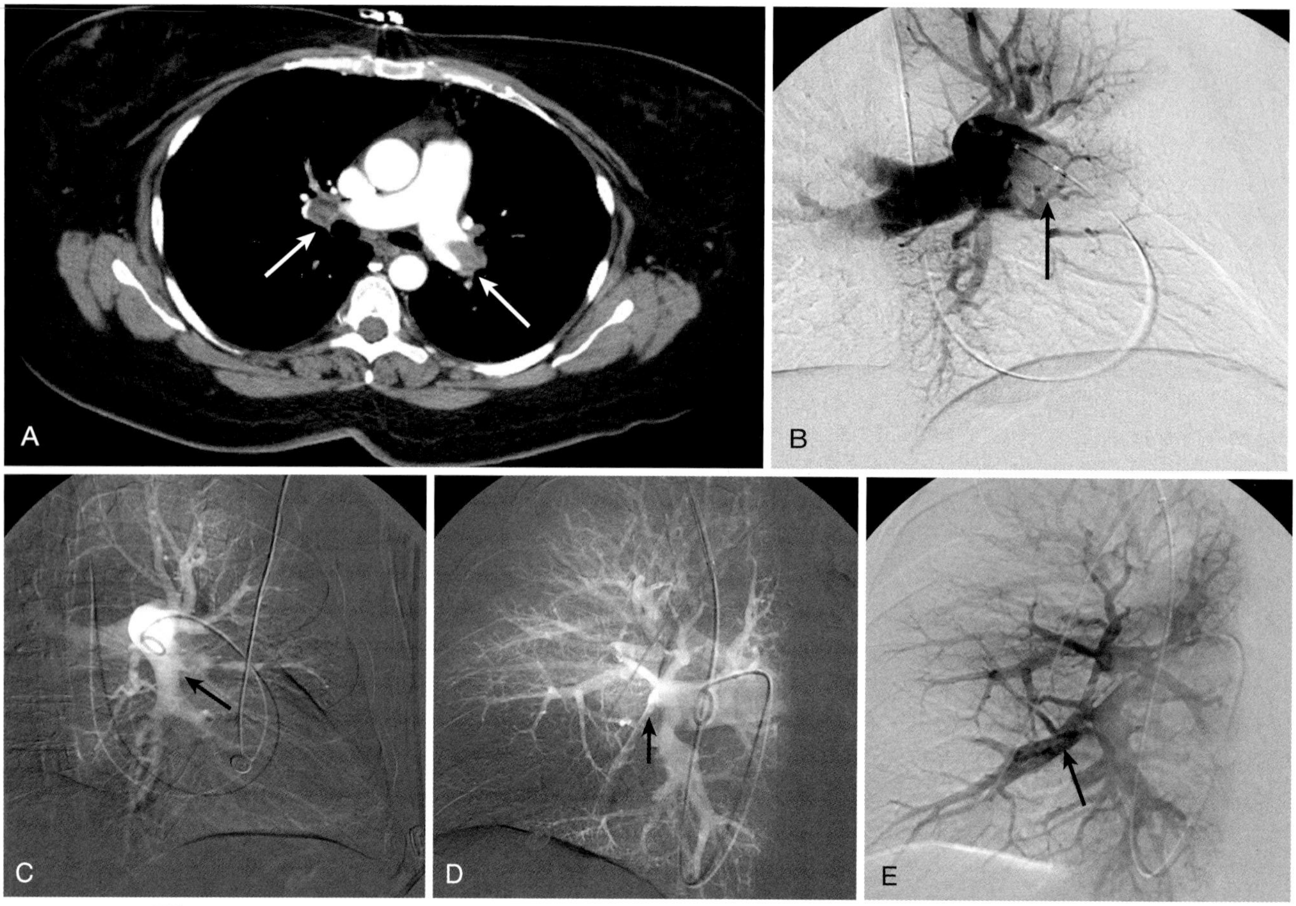

FIG 50.6 (A) Computed tomography scan showing bilateral submassive pulmonary emboli *(arrows)* in a patient with active gastrointestinal bleeding. (B) A direct pharmacomechanical intervention was performed using the AngioJet catheter, showing the large left-sided pulmonary embolism (*arrows;* PE), (C) posttreatment perfusion of the left lung, and (D) obstructing PE of the right lung with (E) posttreatment perfusion. The patient's hemodynamics and oxygenation rapidly stabilized.

suggested that additional selected patients without hypotension at low risk of bleeding receive thrombolytic therapy (grade 2B). They went on to suggest that in compromised patients unable to receive lytic therapy, interventional catheter techniques are recommended (grade 2C). Since the publication of the 2008 guidelines, technology has improved considerably, increasing the success rates of direct catheter-based treatment and reducing the rates of complications.

CATHETER-BASED INTERVENTION FOR PULMONARY EMBOLISM

Catheter-based intervention for large pulmonary emboli is becoming more popular, with observations of rapid improvement following fragmentation and/or dissolution of proximal pulmonary emboli.

Tajima and coauthors[53] reported 25 patients with hemodynamically important pulmonary emboli who were treated with a modified rotating pigtail catheter. After embolic disruption, 13 mg of rt-PA was injected into the affected pulmonary arteries followed by manual clot aspiration. All patients survived, and their clinical status improved. After treatment, arteriography showed improved pulmonary perfusion that resulted in a significant reduction in the Miller score and a 30% decrease in the mean pulmonary artery pressure ($P < .01$).

Zeni and colleagues[54] treated 17 patients with the AngioJet device, 10 of whom also received an infusion of reteplase. Immediate angiographic improvement with relief of symptoms occurred in 16 of 17 patients. Heart block, which is a potential complication of this technique, occurred in one patient in whom the procedure was terminated. Fifteen patients survived the initial hospitalization. Two were lost to follow-up, and the remaining 13 were alive 19 months later, more than would have been expected based upon their natural history if treated with anticoagulation alone.

Fourteen patients with significant pulmonary emboli (10 with massive PE) who were ineligible for systemic thrombolysis or operative embolectomy were treated with rheolytic thrombectomy by Chauhan and Kawamura.[55] Five of the 14 patients also received catheter-based pulse-spray fibrinolytic treatment. One patient died as a result of sustained cardiogenic shock, and posttreatment hemoptysis developed in another. Successful treatment

TABLE 50.3 **Results of Rheolytic Pulmonary Thrombectomy**[51]

Parameter	Pretreatment	Posttreatment	*P*-Value
sBP (mm Hg)	119	145	.02
Heart rate	101	84	.02
sPAP (mm Hg)	54	44	.048
dPAP (mm Hg)	21	16	.02
PVR	758	637	.004
PaO_2/FiO_2	169	325	.001
Miller score	17.9	11.8	.0003

dPAP, Diastolic pulmonary artery pressure; *PVR,* pulmonary vascular resistance; *sBP,* systolic blood pressure; *sPAP,* systolic pulmonary artery pressure.

was observed in 12 of 14 patients (Table 50.3). During a mean follow-up of 9 months, all survivors reported significant improvement in symptoms without recurrent PE. The high-pressure repetitive pulsed infusion in the pulmonary arteries can result in bradycardia arrhythmias and heart block; therefore a transition to other techniques has occurred. Although pure mechanical pulmonary embolic fragmentation is possible in high-risk patients and reduces pulmonary artery pressure, administration of plasminogen activator solution pulsed into the thrombus during fragmentation is likely to result in better short- and long-term benefit. Small doses (5 to 10 mg rt-PA) diluted into relatively large volume and infused into the embolus are unlikely to cause bleeding complications, yet offer the opportunity of clot dissolution after fragmentation as a result of the plasminogen activator penetrating the thrombus and binding to fibrin-bound plasminogen (LYS-plasminogen).

Akin and colleagues[56] reported our initial experience with catheter-based fragmentation and hand-pulsed low-dose thrombolysis in 17 patients, 5 with massive PE and 12 with high-risk submassive PE (see Fig. 50.6). Rapid and significant reduction in pulmonary artery pressures, correction of right ventricular dilation, correction of right ventricular dysfunction, and marked reduction of tricuspid regurgitation was observed. These catheter-based techniques are increasingly being used in high-risk PE patients, with gratifying results. Our approach to patient management is summarized by the algorithm in Fig. 50.5.

SUMMARY

Patients with extensive VTE, namely those with IFDVT and massive or submassive PE, should be considered for strategies of thrombus removal. Thrombolytic therapy delivered by intrathrombus infusion is more effective than systemic infusions by virtue of activation of fibrin-bound plasminogen. Contemporary outcomes of CDT for IFDVT demonstrate a marked reduction in postthrombotic morbidity and preliminary observations that recurrent DVT is reduced.

Patients with PE who are appropriately stratified, such as those with an enlarged right ventricle, abnormal echocardiogram, increased pro-BNP, and increased troponins, also appear to have better short- and long-term outcomes when treated with lytic therapy and catheter-based techniques to disobliterate the large central embolus. Systemic lytic therapy is effective, and lower doses appear to be as effective but safer than large-dose short-term infusion. There is an increased risk of major bleeds and intracranial bleeds, especially in patients older than 70 years.

As technology improves, delivery of plasminogen activators to the clot and the addition of mechanical manipulation of the thrombus speeds resolution. Randomized trials are necessary to establish these treatment modalities with confidence, and whenever possible, patients should be entered into randomized trials. However, absent a randomized trial, patient stratification and good clinical judgment should guide therapy. In patients with central venous or pulmonary obstruction, a strategy of thrombus removal is generally favored.

REVIEW QUESTIONS

1. Which of the following statements regarding iliofemoral DVT is true?
   - **a.** Iliofemoral DVT is associated with the highest risk of postthrombotic morbidity, exceeding the risk imposed by ipsilateral recurrent DVT.
   - **b.** Patients with femoropopliteal DVT have the same resting and hyperemic venous pressures as those with iliofemoral DVT.
   - **c.** Natural history studies show that approximately 40% of patients with iliofemoral DVT suffer serious postthrombotic morbidity.
   - **d.** There are no level 1 data supporting either venous thrombectomy or catheter-directed thrombolysis for the management of patients with iliofemoral DVT.
2. Which of the following statements is true regarding postthrombotic syndrome?
   - **a.** The underlying pathophysiology of the postthrombotic syndrome is ambulatory venous hypertension.
   - **b.** Ambulatory venous hypertension is caused by venous valve reflux, venous luminal obstruction, or both.
   - **c.** The combination of venous valve reflux and luminal obstruction produces the highest ambulatory venous pressure and the most severe postthrombotic syndrome.
   - **d.** All of the above.
3. Which of the following statements regarding postthrombotic syndrome is the most accurate?
   - **a.** Patients with venous obstruction suffer the most severe postthrombotic syndrome.

b. Venous obstruction is reliably identified by noninvasive maximal venous outflow studies.
c. Noninvasive diagnostic tests for venous obstruction are more reliable than those for venous valvular incompetence.
d. Luminal obstruction is reliably diagnosed by ascending phlebography.

4. *Phlegmasia Cerulea Dolens* is a term often used to categorize some patients with acute DVT. Which of the following statements is correct?
   a. It is reserved for patients who have impending venous gangrene.
   b. It is seen only with patients with iliofemoral DVT.
   c. It refers to all patients with a painful, swollen limb having bluish discoloration.
   d. Fasciotomy is the most important step in management following therapeutic anticoagulation.
5. Which of the following statements is most correct in the management of patients with iliofemoral DVT?
   a. Approximately 50% of patients with iliofemoral DVT have asymptomatic PE.
   b. If a patient with DVT is found to have a PE, all patients should have a vena caval filter inserted prior to venous thrombectomy or catheter-directed thrombolysis.
   c. If catheter-directed thrombolysis is chosen to treat the patient, a much higher dose of lytic agent should be infused to dissolve the pulmonary embolus.
   d. Following catheter-directed thrombolysis, a repeat CT scan of the chest should be performed to assess the status of asymptomatic pulmonary embolus.
   e. All of the above
   f. None of the above
6. A 62-year-old gentleman presents with a painful, swollen left leg with bluish discoloration. You are discussing a catheter-based strategy of thrombus removal with the patient. Which of the following pieces of information will you give the patient?
   a. He has a 90% to 100% chance of serious postthrombotic morbidity if treated with anticoagulation alone.
   b. If pharmacomechanical thrombolysis is used instead of a catheter drip technique, treatment times will be shorter, the dose of plasminogen activator will be less, and overall success rate will be improved.
   c. It is important to persist with treatment to remove as much clot as possible because postthrombotic morbidity is related to the amount of residual thrombus at the end of catheter-directed thrombolysis.
   d. The ACCP 12 guidelines do not recommend catheter-directed thrombolysis for iliofemoral DVT.
   e. All of the above
7. Which of the following statements regarding the ATTRACT trial is correct?
   a. It is the largest randomized trial to date addressing catheter-directed thrombolysis versus anticoagulation alone for acute DVT.
   b. It stratifies femoropopliteal DVT versus iliofemoral DVT.
   c. It will evaluate the efficacy of pharmacomechanical techniques versus a catheter-based drip technique alone.
   d. It will answer quality of life and cost effectiveness questions.
   e. All of the above
8. You are called to see a 48-year-old woman in the emergency room who is short of breath, has a PO_2 on room air of 88%, a heart rate of 100, and a blood pressure of 126/70. A CT scan of the chest with contrast demonstrates large bilateral PE. A cardiac echo demonstrates an RV/LV ratio of 1.0. The patient and her family have numerous questions about her acute management and how it relates to her long-term outcome. You tell them the following:
   a. She has a submassive PE and is much more likely to suffer chronic thromboembolic pulmonary hypertension than most patients with PE.
   b. Systemic thrombolysis with rt-PA is associated with more rapid return of normal cardiopulmonary hemodynamics than anticoagulation alone.
   c. Nonrandomized trials have demonstrated significant survival advantage to lytic therapy.
   d. The randomized NIH PE trials have shown significant advantage in restoring normal cardiopulmonary hemodynamics and reduction in congestive heart failure over the long term if lytic therapy was used.
   e. All of the above
9. Which of the following is true regarding risk assessment in patients with pulmonary emboli?
   a. The ACCP 12 recommends that patients with an abnormal echocardiogram undergo thrombolytic therapy.
   b. Troponin elevation reflects excessive myocardial stretch.
   c. Elevated pro-beta natriuretic polypeptide (pro-BNP) in PE patients reflects myocardial damage.
   d. None of the above
   e. All of the above
10. Catheter-based intervention for PE:
    a. Is not recommended
    b. Is associated with cardiac tamponade secondary to ventricular perforation.
    c. Offers no advantage over systemic thrombolysis
    d. None of the above
    e. All of the above
11. Which of the following statement regarding aspirin in the use of patients with venous thromboembolism is correct?
    a. Aspirin should not be used for DVT prophylaxis in any patient.
    b. Randomized trial data demonstrate that aspirin significantly reduces recurrent venous thromboembolism when used following a full course of anticoagulation.
    c. Aspirin augments the inhibition of activated factor Xa.
    d. All of the above
    e. None of the above

References available online at ExpertConsult.com.

CHAPTER 51

Surgical Management of Chronic Venous Obstruction

Peter Gloviczki, Ying Huang

Reconstruction of the occluded iliofemoral vein or the inferior vena cava (IVC) may be required in patients with postthrombotic venous occlusion if they exhibit signs and symptoms of advanced chronic venous insufficiency (CVI). Reconstruction of large veins may also be needed in patients with traumatic or iatrogenic venous injuries or in those who undergo excision of primary or metastatic malignant tumors invading the IVC or the iliac veins. Nonthrombotic iliac vein lesions (NIVLs)—as seen in May-Thurner syndrome, which are caused by occlusion or stenosis of the left common iliac vein due to compression by the overriding right common iliac artery (Fig. 51.1)—can lead to acute deep venous thrombosis (DVT) more frequently than previously thought.[1] Chronic NIVL can be symptomatic in up to one-third of the patients with CVI. The advent and development of intravascular ultrasound (DUS) and high-resolution imaging techniques have helped us to recognize that obstruction of the iliac veins occurs ubiquitously due to both postthrombotic and nonthrombotic lesions.[2]

Endovascular treatment for iliocaval obstruction has progressed rapidly, and venous stenting is currently the primary choice for benign iliac, iliofemoral, or iliocaval venous occlusions in patients who fail conservative compression therapy (see Chapter 52). Further studies on the effectiveness of venous stenting are still needed, since comparative studies are few and the quality of evidence to support the use of deep venous stenting is still weak.[3]

In the last 2 decades, results of open surgical reconstruction have also improved and symptomatic patients who are not candidates or who fail endovascular reconstruction can be treated with venous bypasses to relieve symptomatic venous outflow obstruction.[4] A thorough preoperative evaluation to identify the underlying cause of CVI in these patients is essential.

INCIDENCE AND ETIOLOGY

In most series of patients with CVI, previous DVT is the most common cause of venous outflow obstruction. DVT is very prevalent; Heit and colleagues found that the incidence for DVT ranged from 45 to 117 per 100,000 person-years and that recurrent DVT ranged from 15 to 29 per 100,000 person-years.[5] Postthrombotic syndrome (PTS) develops in 20% to 50% of patients with previous DVT, and about 5% to 10% will have advanced disease, including venous ulcers.[6] There is evidence that PTS develops more frequently in patients who have proximal venous obstruction.[7,8]

Venous outflow obstruction can also be the result of primary venous disease, most frequently of NIVL. May-Thurner syndrome is the most prevalent NIVL, although iliac vein compression has been described in other areas as well, including the right iliac vein. May and Thurner observed secondary changes, such as an intraluminal web or spur, in the proximal left common iliac vein in 22% of 430 autopsies.[9] Kibbe and colleagues found that 24% of asymptomatic patients who underwent computed tomography for other reasons had greater than 50% compression of their left common iliac vein.[10] Among 4026 patients with symptoms of chronic venous disease, iliac vein obstructive lesions were found in 938 limbs of 879 patients; 53% were nonthrombotic, 40% were postthrombotic, and 7% were a combination.[1]

Other less common causes of venous outflow obstruction include retroperitoneal fibrosis; iatrogenic, blunt, or penetrating trauma; placement of an IVC filter; congenital venous anomalies such as deep venous agenesis or hypoplasia; and benign or malignant tumors.

The most frequent primary malignant tumor originating from large veins is venous leiomyosarcoma, and suprarenal involvement occurs in more than 40% of cases; three-fourths of these tumors involve retroperitoneal and abdominal veins. Secondary cancers or sarcomas that involve the IVC are more common than primary venous leiomyosarcoma. Renal cell carcinoma is the most common cancer involving the IVC and requires operative intervention, and the tumor thrombus in some patients may reach all the way into the right atrium, although invasion of the wall of the IVC is rare.[11]

Congenital suprarenal caval occlusion can occur because of webs or caval coarctation that may also develop with associated hepatic vein occlusion (Budd-Chiari syndrome).[12,13]

PATHOPHYSIOLOGY

During the acute phase of DVT, the thrombus in the vein activates the inflammatory cascade, which in turn promotes partial lysis of the thrombus and leads to recanalization (see Chapter 49). However, these processes are also responsible for damage to the vein wall and to the venous valves, leading to chronic obstruction and valvular incompetence. If collateral venous circulation is inadequate, ambulatory venous hypertension develops because of a functional venous outflow obstruction and the incompetence of damaged valves. In the PTS, deep reflux and obstruction of multiple venous segments often coexist.

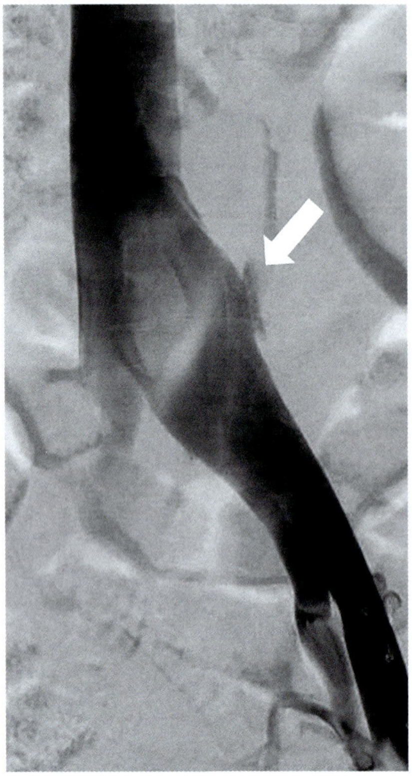

FIG 51.1 Venogram of May-Thurner syndrome with compression of the left common iliac vein by the overriding right common iliac artery *(arrow)*. (Reproduced with permission of the Mayo Foundation.)

In a prospective study of 83 lower extremities with acute DVT in 78 patients, DUS was performed for follow-up study. Strandness and colleagues observed that at a median follow-up of 3 years (range 1 to 6 years), 41% of the limbs had features of the PTS. Additionally, limbs with PTS had over 3 times the odds of having combined reflux and obstruction than did limbs without the PTS (OR 3.5, 95% CI 1.4% to 8.6%).[14] Factors that predispose patients to develop PTS include DVT involvement of the iliac vein, poor resolution of DVT, and recurrent DVT. The lesions can vary from stenosis to chronic total occlusion (CTO).[2]

Nonthrombotic obstructive lesions in the ilieocaval vein segments are due to fibrotic or membranous stenosis that develops where the vein is crossed by arteries or fibrous ligaments. The lesions may be ontogenic or result from traumatic injury from repeated pulsations of the closely related artery. Because a majority of these patients are asymptomatic, Raju suggested the explanation of permissive pathologies—namely, that the venous obstructive lesions were permissive, remaining silent until additional insult such as trauma, cellulitis, or additional pathology such as venous reflux, DVT, or sedentary leg dependency precipitated symptoms.[2]

PRESENTATION

Unilateral limb swelling and pain during and after exercise that is relieved with rest and leg elevation (venous claudication) is the typical presentation of patients with chronic venous obstruction owing to previous DVT, PTS, or obstruction of the common iliac vein (May-Thurner syndrome).[15] Patients with obstruction may also have symptoms similar to those associated with primary valvular incompetence, such as varicose veins, edema, skin changes, or venous ulcers; however, claudication and edema are usually more severe with venous obstruction, and relief with limb elevation is not as pronounced.

TABLE 51.1 Clinical Symptoms in 60 Patients Undergoing Venous Reconstructions for Benign Disease at the Mayo Clinic

Symptom	*n* (%)
Venous edema	56 (94)
Venous claudication	54 (90)
Edema and claudication	50 (84)
Healed ulceration	8 (13)
Active venous ulcers	12 (19)

From Garg N, Gloviczki P, Karimi KM, et al: Factors affecting outcome of open and hybrid reconstructions for nonmalignant obstruction of iliofemoral veins and inferior vena cava. *J Vasc Surg* 53(2):383–393, 2011.

Depending on the extent of the collateral circulation, patients with outflow obstruction will have pain, swelling, and heaviness of the limb, and the most severe forms of venous obstruction can interfere with the viability of the limb. Obstruction alone can also result in skin changes and venous ulcerations. In the Mayo Clinic experience with 64 venous reconstructions performed in 60 patients with benign disease, the mean duration of symptoms was 6 years (Table 51.1).

A collateral vein on the abdominal wall or across the pubic bone can be a sign of venous obstructive disease at the level of the groin or higher in patients with CVI. Kurstjens and colleagues compared 295 patients with a collateral vein on the abdominal wall or pubic bone, visible on physical examination, with a randomly selected control group of 365 patients without a collateral vein. This study found that abdominal wall collaterals have a 93% positive predictive value for deep venous obstruction, with a sensitivity of 68% to predict a high-degree iliac vein obstruction.[16]

CLINICAL EVALUATION

A detailed medical history may establish the diagnosis of primary, secondary, or congenital venous problems. The history should address previous DVT or thrombophlebitis, previous abdominal or pelvic interventions, trauma, tumor or symptoms of malignancy, personal or family history of thrombophilia, medication history (particularly oral contraceptive pills), smoking, obstetric history, and a family history of venous disorders (most patients with varicose veins relate their parents' or grandparents' disease).

An abdominal mass or lymphadenopathy can provide a clue to venous compression and outflow obstruction. Perineal, vulvar, or groin varicosities can be seen in iliac vein obstruction or internal iliac vein or gonadal vein incompetence causing pelvic congestion syndrome. Scrotal varicosities may be a sign of gonadal vein incompetence, left renal vein compression between the superior mesenteric artery and the aorta (Nutcracker syndrome), or occasionally IVC lesions or renal carcinoma.

INVESTIGATIONS

Plethysmography

Air or strain-gauge plethysmography is designed to evaluate the global leg hemodynamics by measuring reflux, obstruction, and calf muscle pump function (see Chapter 14). Venous plethysmography is rarely used today, but it can provide information on venous function in patients with CVI. Plethysmography quantifies venous reflux and obstruction and has been used to monitor venous functional changes and assess the physiologic outcome of surgical treatments.[17,18] These studies can be helpful in patients with suspected outflow obstruction but normal duplex findings, or in those suspected of having venous disease because of calf muscle pump dysfunction but with no reflux or obstruction noted on duplex scanning.

A recent report, however, questions the value of plethysmography in patients with outflow obstruction. Although the positive predictive value was 95%, the sensitivity of air plethysmography (APG) was 35% and the negative predictive value was 30%. Thus APG did not prove useful in identifying chronic deep venous obstruction compared with DUS or magnetic resonance venography (MRV).[19]

Duplex Scanning

Venous DUS should be performed in all patients with symptoms of CVI to help to define the location, cause, and severity of the underlying problem. The test is safe, noninvasive, cost-effective, and reliable and is recommended as the first diagnostic test for all patients with suspected CVD.[20–22] It has a grade 1A level-of-evidence recommendation in the clinical practice guidelines of the Society for Vascular Surgery (SVS), the American Venous Forum (AVF),[22] and of the European Society for Vascular Surgery (ESVS).[23] DUS is also excellent for evaluation of both infrainguinal venous obstruction and valvular incompetence.[24] In the PTS, DUS identifies residual obstruction, persistent occlusion, and valvular incompetence in the affected segments, with greater accuracy in the infrainguinal areas.

The four components that are essential in a complete duplex scanning examination for CVD are visibility, compressibility, venous flow, and augmentation. The typical appearance of a postthrombotic vein during duplex scanning is that of a thickened, hardly compressible vessel with damaged, incompetent valves and variable degrees of venous flow owing to partial recanalization. Asymmetry in flow velocity, lack of respiratory variations in venous flow, and waveform patterns at rest and during flow augmentation in the common femoral veins indicate proximal obstruction. Obesity and bowel gas may prevent good visualization of the iliac veins, vena cava, and common hepatic veins with ultrasound.

Metzger and colleagues studied the sonographic criteria for the diagnosis of iliac venous outflow obstruction by assessing the correlation of DUS with intravascular ultrasound (IVUS) in patients with advanced CVI. DUS had high agreement with IVUS for the detection of obstructions 50% or greater. The velocity ratio equal to or greater than 2.5 was the best criterion for the detection of significant venous outflow obstructions in iliac veins.[25] Monophasic flow of the common femoral vein at rest and continuous flow during the Valsalva maneuver are highly suggestive of iliac vein obstruction.[26]

Computed Tomography and Magnetic Resonance Venography

Early venous disease (C_{1-2}) rarely requires advanced imaging studies in addition to DUS. Computed tomography and magnetic resonance venography have progressed in the last decade and provide excellent three-dimensional imaging of the venous system. Both modalities are suitable for identifying pelvic or iliac venous obstruction in patients with lower limb varicosities when proximal obstruction or iliac vein compression (May-Thurner syndrome) is suspected.[27] Venous phase examination will help to identify any obstructing mass or tumor and provides sufficient information in most patients about venous anatomy, obstruction, or stenosis. The sensitivity of imaging techniques can be increased if diameter measurements of the iliac vein segments are included for comparison with anatomic norms for assessment.[2]

Contrast Venography and Hemodynamic Studies

Diagnostic ascending or descending (or both) contrast venography for CVI is performed only selectively in patients with postthrombotic syndrome and suspected deep venous obstruction. Ascending venography is performed with the patient in a standing position to evaluate patency of the superficial and/or deep venous system. Ascending venography is useful as a map of the deep veins of the limb; it defines the sites of obstruction and images the collateral venous circulation and the patterns of preferential flow. Descending venography is used to study associated venous valve incompetence with Valsalva maneuver and classifies the severity of reflux (grade 1 to 4 : 1 = to upper thigh; 2 = to distal thigh; 3 = popliteal reflux; 4 = reflux to tibials and perforators).[28,29] This test has been much less frequently used in recent years. The relatively low sensitivity of single-plane transfemoral venography can be increased by biplane imaging and by measurement of femoral venous pressure measurements during venography.[2]

Contrast venography is routinely used in CVD before performing endovenous procedures, such as angioplasty or venous stenting, and it also helps in planning open venous reconstructions. A pressure gradient across iliofemoral obstruction of 3 mm Hg at rest in the supine patient or 10 mm Hg after exercise confirms functional venous obstruction. Exercise consists of 10 dorsiflexions of the ankles or 20 isometric contractions of the calf muscle. Arm or foot venous pressure tests and ambulatory venous pressure measurements in a dorsal foot vein are additional tests that can be performed. Detailed descriptions and techniques for these tests are provided in the consensus statement.[30]

Intravascular Ultrasound

Studies have shown that IVUS is useful tool to detect and assess iliofemoral venous occlusive lesions in patients with suspected or confirmed iliac vein obstruction.[2,25–27] IVUS can be used in veins with stenosis without occlusion to assess the venous wall morphology and mural thickness; it can also identify trabeculations and recanalization, frozen valves, and external compression. Some of these lesions, as emphasized by Neglen and Raju,[27] are not seen with conventional contrast venography. IVUS provides measurements in assessing the degree of stenosis and is useful to measure surface area and assist in the selection of stent size. IVUS has also been used as a comparative method to examine the sensitivity of DUS in detecting venous obstructive lesions.[25,26] In addition, IVUS confirms the position of the stent in the venous segment and the resolution of the stenosis.[27]

Laboratory Evaluation

Based on their history, selected patients with recurrent DVT thrombosis at a young age or thrombosis in an unusual site should undergo screening for thrombophilia (a grade 1A level of evidence recommendation by the SVS and AVF).[22]

TREATMENT

Conservative Management

Symptoms of CVI due to venous obstruction should be treated initially with compression therapy and local wound care of venous ulcerations, if any. In addition, lifestyle modifications including weight loss, exercise, and elevation of the legs whenever possible are recommended. The rationale for compression treatment is to compensate for increased ambulatory venous hypertension and to facilitate ulcer healing, maintain the patient's functional mobility, and prevent recurrence (see Chapter 54). Pressures needed to compress the superficial veins in supine patients range from 20 to 25 mm Hg, since pressures of 35 to 40 mm Hg in the upright position have been shown to narrow the superficial veins, and pressures higher than 60 mm Hg are needed to occlude them.[31] Ambulatory compression techniques and devices include elastic compression stockings and multilayer elastic bandages. Pneumatic compression devices, applied primarily at night, are also employed in patients with refractory edema and venous ulcers.[32] Compression garments result in variable degrees of success, dependent on patient compliance, which in a hot climate can be difficult to wear. Patients with persistent disabling symptoms—such as venous claudication, severe swelling, and nonhealing or recurrent ulcers—not responding to conservative treatment should be considered for endovascular or open surgical reconstruction.

Endovascular Treatment

Iliac or iliocaval stenting has become the primary treatment for chronic venous obstructions. Indications, techniques, and results are discussed in detail in Chapter 52.

Hybrid Reconstruction

In patients with obstruction of the central femoral vein (CFV) and proximal venous disease, conventional venous stenting is frequently not possible because of poor inflow. Endovenous recanalization and stent placement, however, can be combined in selected cases with femoral vein endophlebectomy and patch angioplasty using autologous vein or bovine pericardial patch (Fig. 51.2). Balloon angioplasty and stenting is performed before or after completion of the patch angioplasty. Jugular vein access is obtained for retrograde recanalization as an alternative to or in combination with femoral access. The stent is extended across the inguinal ligament distally, frequently into the venous patch.[4] Others have reported good outcomes with the hybrid technique by adding a temporary arteriovenous fistula (AVF).[33-35]

Open Surgical Treatment

Patients who are not candidates for endovascular reconstruction or who fail to endovascular reconstructions can be treated with venous bypasses to relieve symptomatic nonmalignant venous outflow obstruction. Venous reconstruction is also performed in patients who undergo excision of malignant tumors invading the vena cava or iliac veins. Saphenopopliteal or saphenotibial bypass may be used for infrainguinal venous obstruction; whereas femorofemoral, femoroiliac, iliocaval, or femorocaval bypass is used for the treatment of iliofemoral or iliacocaval venous obstruction.

Saphenopopliteal Bypass

First described independently by May and Husni in 1970s,[36] saphenopopliteal bypass (SPB) is indicated for femoral or proximal popliteal vein obstruction. The great saphenous vein (GSV), which most commonly is the major outflow from the leg via collaterals in these patients, is exposed above the knee joint, and a direct anastomosis is performed between the GSV and the popliteal vein (end-to-side) (Fig. 51.3). Alternatively, a free vein conduit can be used if the ipsilateral GSV is not suitable.

In a study of 17 patients undergoing SPB with an average follow-up of 103 months, the primary patency rate was 69%; 82% of the patients had complete or nearly complete resolution of venous claudication, and three out of five chronic ulcerations healed. Of note, three patients in this study had a concomitant AVF created during the bypass procedure to improve venous inflow.[37] A more recent series of 12 patients reported improvement of venous claudication, hyperpigmentation, and pain in 10 patients, with a median follow-up of 60 months.[38]

Crossover Saphenous Vein Transposition (Palma Procedure)

Patients with symptomatic unilateral iliac vein obstruction are candidates for the Palma procedure (Figs. 51.4 and 51.5). With this technique, the contralateral saphenous vein is used for a crossover bypass to decompress venous congestion in the affected limb. The common femoral vein on the affected side is exposed first through a 6- to 8-cm long longitudinal groin incision. The collateral veins should be preserved if possible. The GSV of the contralateral leg is dissected through a 3- to 5-cm incision made in the groin crease, starting just medial to the femoral artery pulse. Tributaries of the saphenous vein are ligated and divided, and the saphenous vein is mobilized for a length of 10 to 12 cm. A short, second upper-thigh incision is made to dissect a 20- to 25-cm long portion of the saphenous vein. The vein is ligated distally and pulled up to the groin incision. Alternatively, endoscopic harvesting of the saphenous vein can be performed.

It is essential to free the saphenofemoral junction completely and dissect at least the anterior wall of the common femoral

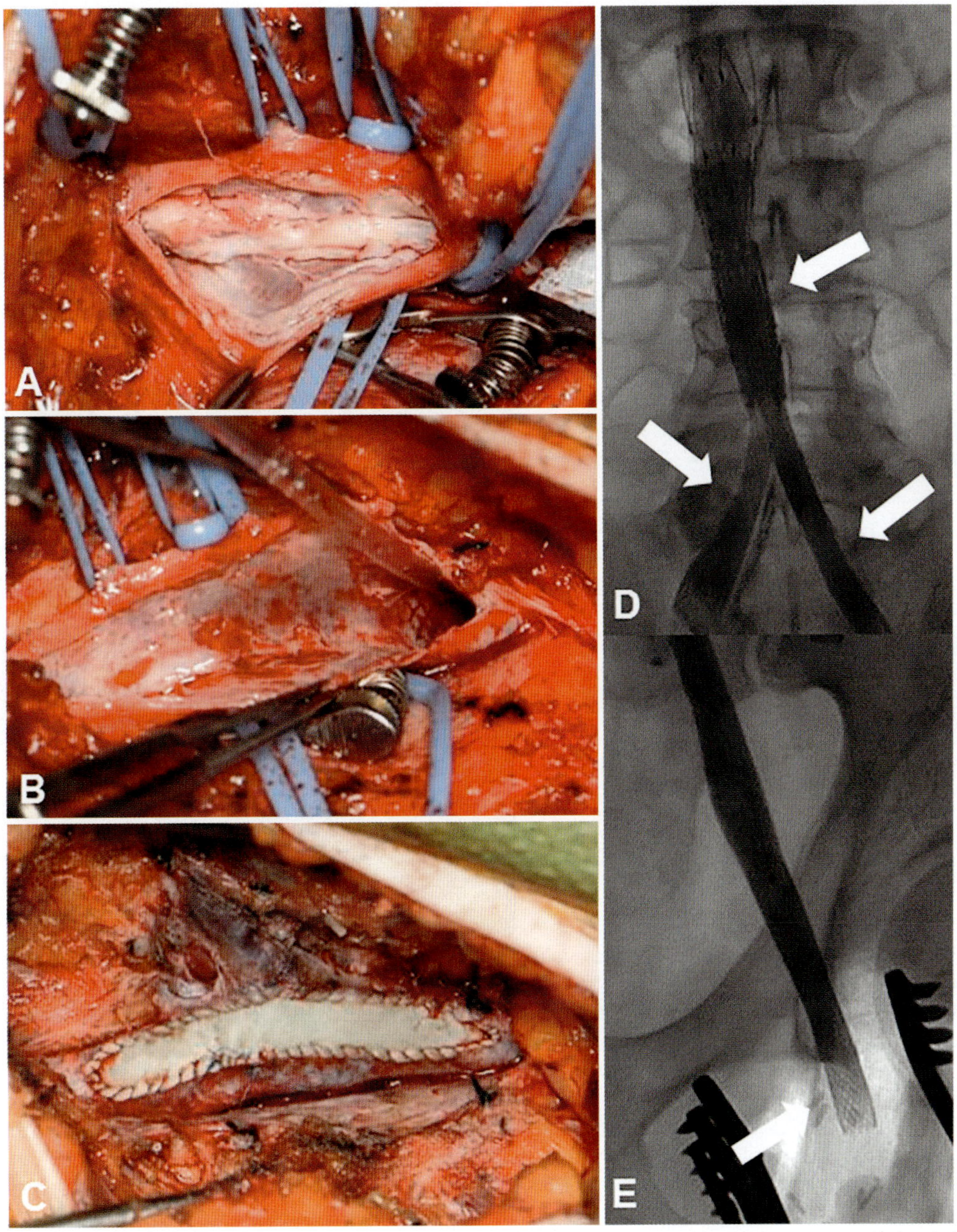

FIG 51.2 Hybrid reconstruction. (A) Hybrid reconstruction with endophlebectomy of the left common femoral vein (CFV). (B) Stenting of the left iliac veins. (C) Bovine pericardial patch closure of the left CFV. (D) Full reconstruction with bilateral iliac vein and inferior vena cava stenting *(arrow)*. (E) Follow-up venogram at 11 months revealing an occluded left femoral venous stent *(arrow)*. ([A–D] From Garg N, Gloviczki P, Karimi KM, et al: Factors affecting outcome of open and hybrid reconstructions for nonmalignant obstruction of iliofemoral veins and inferior vena cava. *J Vasc Surg* 53:383–393, 2011, Fig. 6.)

vein around the saphenous vein so that there is no kink or buckle when the saphenous vein is pulled through the suprapubic tunnel. Before tunneling, a small Satinsky clamp is placed on the common femoral vein to allow distension of the saphenous vein and the saphenofemoral junction under gentle pressure using a heparinized papaverine-saline solution. If there is a kink at the saphenofemoral junction, excision of the saphenous vein with a 2-mm cuff from the common femoral vein and reanastomosis to the femoral vein with running 6/0 polypropylene suture—after turning the junction upward 180 degrees—is a way of solving this problem. The vein is then tunneled subcutaneously in the suprapubic space over to the contralateral side using an aortic clamp to ensure a large tunnel without any extrinsic compression of the graft. The common femoral vein is clamped and opened longitudinally for approximately 2 cm. An end-to-side anastomosis is performed between the saphenous vein and ipsilateral common femoral vein. This anastomosis can be spatulated onto the ipsilateral GSV if the femoral or deep femoral veins

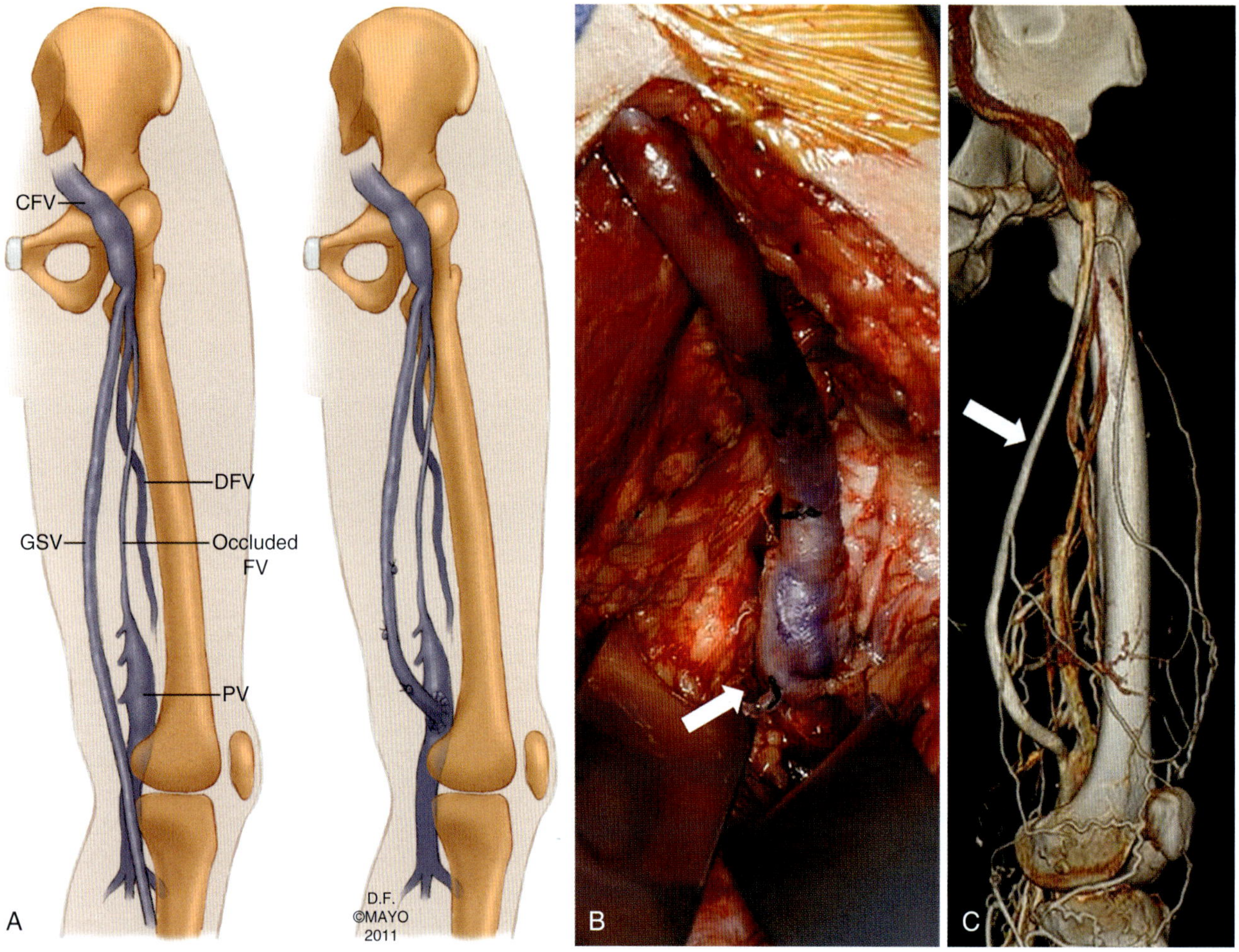

FIG 51.3 (A) Postthrombotic femoral vein *(FV)* obstruction with patent great saphenous vein *(GSV)* is a suitable anatomy for the May-Husni operation (saphenopopliteal transposition). (B) Intraoperative photograph of the saphenopopliteal anastomosis. Completed operation with an end-to-side anastomosis between the GSV and the popliteal vein *(PV)*. (C) A computed tomography venogram at 14 months showing a widely patent popliteosaphenous anastomosis with preferential flow of contrast into the transposed GSV. *DFV,* Deep femoral vein. ([A–C] From Ryer EJ, Misra S, McBane RD, et al: Great saphenous vein transposition to the popliteal vein [the May-Husni procedure]. *J Vasc Surg Venous Lymphat Disord* 1:82–83, 2013, Figures C, B, and cover image. Used with permission of Mayo Foundation for Medical Education and Research. All rights reserved.)

are diseased and the GSV is the predominant outflow in the affected leg. The anastomosis between the saphenous and femoral veins is performed with running 6/0 polypropylene suture. A vein at least 5 mm in diameter is required to provide a high venous flow and correct the poor venous emptying. Saphenous vein grafts in morbidly obese patients have a lower chance of success because of possible external compression of the vein.

Although few large series have been reported, the patency of Palma grafts in nine series ranged between 70% and 83% at 3 to 5 years.[12] Results were better in patients who had no or minimal infrainguinal venous disease and those with May-Thurner syndrome without previous DVT. We observed a 70% primary and a 78% secondary patency at 5 years in 25 Palma vein grafts.[4] Endoscopic vein harvest was associated with decreased primary but not secondary patency rates.

Crossover Femoral Venous Prosthetic Bypass

An externally supported 10- to 12-mm diameter polytetrafluoroethylene (PTFE) graft is used if the GSV is inadequate, less than 5 mm in diameter, or of poor quality. Similar to the autologous femoral suprapubic bypass, the femoral veins are exposed bilaterally, the externally supported PTFE (ePTFE) graft is positioned in the subcutaneous suprapubic tunnel, and an end-to-side anastomosis is performed to the common femoral veins on each side. A distal AVF on the affected side is routinely added to the procedure using a 4- to 5-mm PTFE graft for the fistula between the PTFE graft and the superficial femoral artery. Sottiurai[39] recommended cutting out a small window rather than just making a longitudinal cut in the cross-femoral graft at the hood of the femoral anastomosis to optimize inflow and decrease intimal hyperplasia in the AVF.

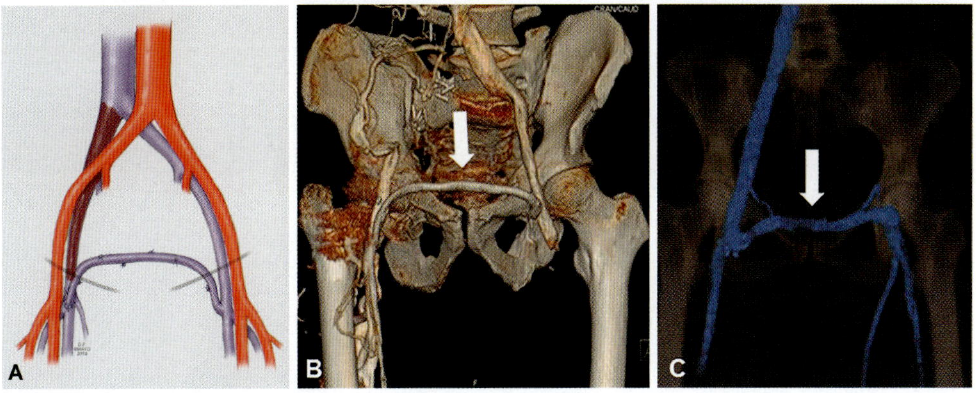

FIG 51.4 Femoral crossover bypass. (A) Artist's drawing of a left saphenous vein transposition to the right femoral vein (Palma procedure) to treat right iliac vein thrombosis. (B) Computed tomographic venogram at 2 months demonstrating patency of the left great saphenous vein (GSV) used to bypass the right iliac vein obstruction due to previous pelvic surgery *(arrow)*. (C) Computed tomographic venogram at 22 years after Palma procedure shows widely patent enlarged GSV graft *(arrow)*. ([A and B] From Garg N, Gloviczki P, Karimi KM, et al: Factors affecting outcome of open and hybrid reconstructions for nonmalignant obstruction of iliofemoral veins and inferior vena cava. *J Vasc Surg* 53:383–393, 2011, Figure 1; [C] From Mendes BC, Gloviczki P, Akhtar N. Patency and clinical success 22 years after the Palma procedure. *J Vasc Surg Venous Lymphat Disord* 4:95–96, 2016, Figure D. Used with permission of Mayo Foundation for Medical Education and Research. All rights reserved.)

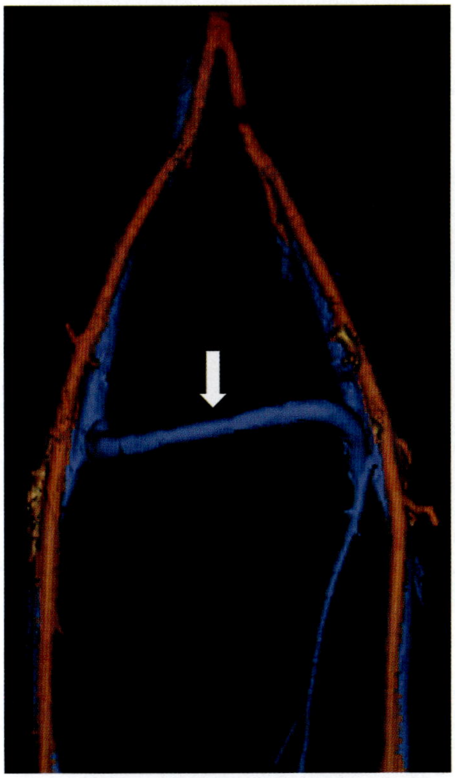

FIG 51.5 Computed tomography venogram of a patent right saphenous transposition to the left femoral vein because of left iliac vein thrombosis *(arrow)*. (From Power AH, Gloviczki P: Left iliac vein occlusion treated with a Palma procedure. *J Vasc Surg Venous Lymphat Disord* 2:204–205, 2014, cover image.)

Variable patency rates of ePTFE grafts in this location have been reported and range between 0% and 100%.[40] Externally reinforced grafts with large diameters and heparin bonding may improve the outcome. In the authors' experience, the secondary patency of these bypasses is only 50%, and preference still should be given to saphenous crossover grafts or in-line PTFE femorocaval reconstruction.

Femorocaval or Complex Bypass

Long bypasses from the femoral vein to the IVC have good results if inflow is adequate. They must be constructed with an arteriovenous fistula to improve chances of long-term patency. Patients with bilateral disease or those with obstruction of the suprarenal or suprahepatic IVC and those who have failed endovascular intervention are evaluated for a complex reconstruction using either a bifurcated or tube graft with a contralateral jump graft.

For in-line reconstruction of iliocaval occlusions, an ePTFE graft with external support is the preferred conduit. Large-diameter (12 mm) grafts are used most frequently; a diameter of 12 to 14 mm is used for iliocaval bypasses and at least 10 mm for femorocaval bypass (Figs. 51.6 and 51.7). The upper portion of the infrarenal IVC at and immediately distal to the renal veins is best approached transperitoneally through a midline incision, reflecting the ascending colon medially and mobilizing the duodenum using the Kocher maneuver. The IVC just above the iliac bifurcation is best approached retroperitoneally through a midline transabdominal or right flank incision. If the occlusion is limited to the right common iliac vein, the same incision is used to expose the external iliac vein for the distal anastomosis. Inflow is obtained from the iliac vein, exposed via a flank incision, or from the femoral vein, through a standard groin incision. The graft is always tunneled under the ureter. To all grafts originating from the femoral vein and to most long iliocaval grafts, an AVF is added at the groin (see Figs. 51.6 and 51.7).

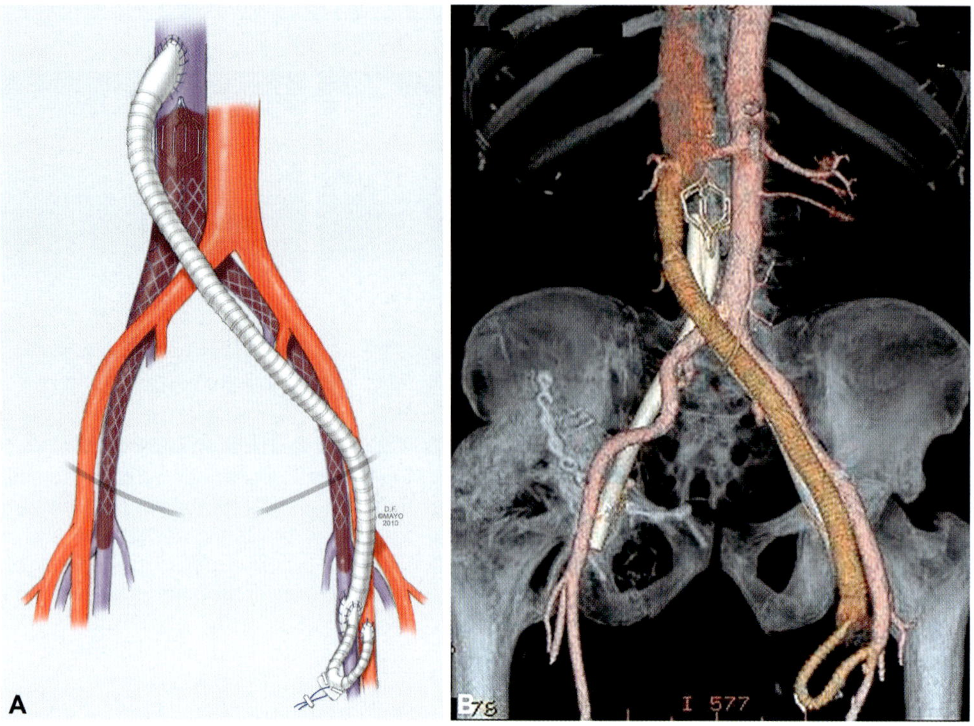

FIG 51.6 Femorocaval or complex bypass. (A) Left femorocaval polytetrafluoroethylene (PTFE) bypass with a left femoral arteriovenous fistula using a 6-mm externally supported PTFE graft. (B) Computed tomographic venogram at 7 months revealing a patent bypass graft. Previous inferior vena cava filter is seen proximal to occluded stents. (From Garg N, Gloviczki P, Karimi KM, et al: Factors affecting outcome of open and hybrid reconstructions for nonmalignant obstruction of iliofemoral veins and inferior vena cava. *J Vasc Surg* 53:383–393, 2011, Figure 4, p 387. Used with permission of Mayo Foundation for Medical Education and Research. All rights reserved.)

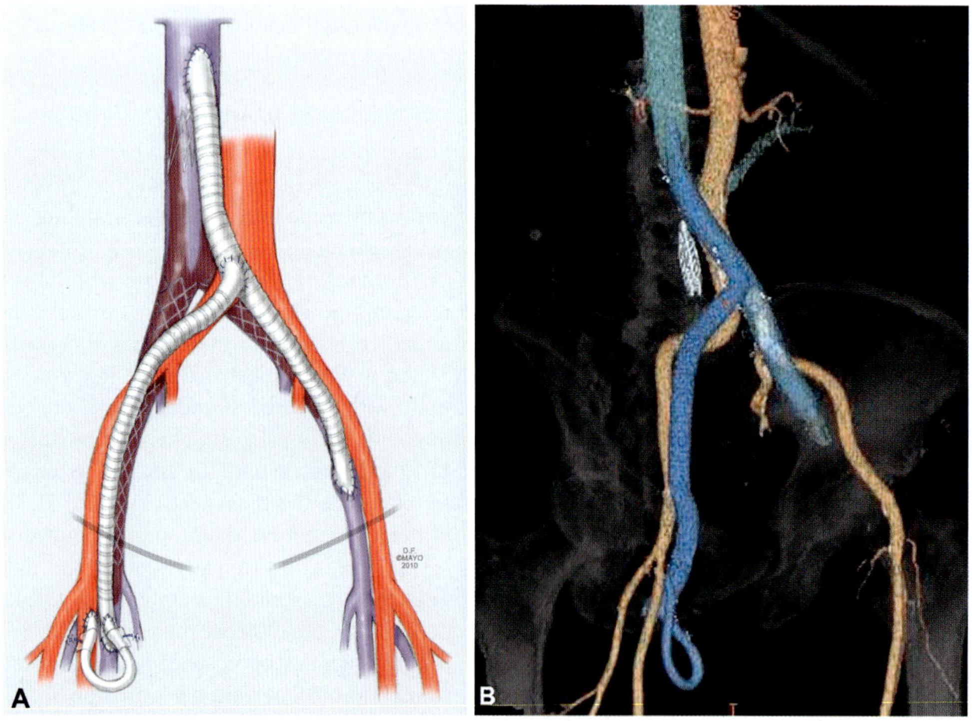

FIG 51.7 (A) Complex venous reconstruction with polytetrafluoroethylene grafts from the right common femoral vein and the left external iliac vein to the inferior vena cava (IVC). Note arteriovenous fistula at the right groin. (B) Computed tomographic venogram done at 2 months revealing patent bypass and previous IVC filter. (From Garg N, Gloviczki P, Karimi KM, et al: Factors affecting outcome of open and hybrid reconstructions for nonmalignant obstruction of iliofemoral veins and inferior vena cava. *J Vasc Surg* 53:383–393, 2011, Figure 5. Used with permission of Mayo Foundation for Medical Education and Research. All rights reserved.)

The use of autologous vein for femoroiliac or femorocaval reconstruction is also an option. Because of its relatively small size, saphenous vein in this location can rarely be used. If a short segment of the common femoral or iliac vein has to be reconstructed, a better size match is a spiral saphenous vein graft prepared using the contralateral saphenous vein. The excised vein is opened longitudinally, the valves are excised, and the graft is wrapped around a 28- or 32-mm argyle chest tube. The edges are approximated with running 6/0 polypropylene sutures or with stainless steel nonpenetrating vascular clips. The internal or external jugular veins are other conduits that can be considered for venous reconstruction. The femoral vein is also an alternative for the reconstruction of abdominal veins, although the morbidity from removing this vein in many of these patients with underlying thrombophilia or postthrombotic syndrome is high and other options are recommended. Cryopreserved saphenous or femoral vein has also been reported for venous reconstruction, but the long-term patency of these grafts for venous replacement is not known.

Experience with femorocaval or iliocaval PTFE bypass grafts for benign disease has been limited. Long-term patency of 77% was reported in one series published by Sottiurai.[39] A 5-year primary and secondary patency of 31% and 57%, respectively, was also observed for femoroinfrahepatic IVC bypasses.[4]

Femoroiliac or Iliocaval Bypass

The iliac vein is exposed via a flank incision, and the femoral vein is exposed through a standard groin incision as detailed previously. In cases with common iliac vein occlusion, infrahepatic vena cava is used as outflow; it is exposed through a midline incision or right flank incision. These short bypasses have a hemodynamic advantage because of their length and high flow. An externally supported 10- to 14-mm PTFE graft is preferred for these bypasses. Among 17 patients who underwent a short bypass, 5-year primary and secondary patency of 63% and 86%, respectively, were observed.[4]

Inferior Cavoatrial Bypass

Patients with symptomatic short membranous occlusion of the IVC or longer congenital or acquired narrowing (caval coarctation) without or with hepatic venous outflow obstruction (Budd-Chiari syndrome) can be treated with cavoatrial bypass when attempts at percutaneous angioplasty or stenting have failed. The largest experience for the treatment of Budd-Chiari syndrome comes from Asian countries, and multiple modalities have been described to treat associated caval occlusion. Some of the preferred techniques include membranectomy, endovenectomy with patch angioplasty, cavocaval bypass, and mesoatrial bypass with or without caval limb.[13,41] Results of these techniques are encouraging, with greater than 85% long-term success in appropriately selected patients. Recent data suggest significantly better outcomes with mesoatrial caval bypass compared with mesocaval bypass,[42] and originating one limb from the superior mesenteric vein has higher patency rates compared with the splenic vein.[43]

The suprahepatic inferior vena cava or right atrium is approached through an anterolateral right thoracotomy. The pericardium is opened anterior to the phrenic nerve. If the membranous occlusion is short and is located to this area, a short PTFE interposition graft can be performed from this exposure. If the occlusion extends distal to the hepatic veins, the abdomen is entered through the same thoracotomy, transecting the diaphragm circumferentially and mobilizing the liver forward and medially. Division of the triangular and the right coronary ligament will help mobilization of the liver. The adrenal gland and the kidney are left in their bed, and dissection is performed more medially. Excellent exposure of the suprarenal IVC can be achieved through this approach. If the distal anastomosis has to be made more distally, a separate right subcostal or midline incision can be performed.

For a cavoatrial bypass, an end-to-side anastomosis to the IVC is performed, and the graft is routed under the liver, parallel to the IVC. The graft is then anastomosed end to side to the suprarenal IVC or the lower portion of the right atrium. Partially occluding clamps are used to perform the anastomosis, and cardiopulmonary bypass is not needed. Traumatic or iatrogenic occlusions can also be managed by this technique. The use of a 16- to 20-mm externally supported PTFE graft is recommended.

The reported success rate with cavoatrial grafts is approximately 77%, with a perioperative mortality of 3% and 2-, 5-, and 10-year patency rates of 86%, 78%, and 57%, respectively.[40,44]

Inferior Vena Cava Reconstruction Following Excision of Malignant Tumors

Primary venous leiomyosarcoma or secondary tumors invading the vena cava are the most frequent indications. Most renal carcinomas that extend into the vena cava do not invade the wall of the vessel, and the tumor thrombus can frequently be removed from the IVC without the need for venous reconstruction. Partial excision of a chronically dilated cava in most of these cases permits resection of up to 50% of the caval circumference with primary closure. Patch angioplasty or graft replacement is necessary when tumor adherence or wall invasion requires greater than 50% partial or circumferential resection of the IVC. An externally supported PTFE graft or patch or bovine pericardial patch are options for reconstruction. Attention must be paid to avoid tumor or air embolization to the right atrium, and extension of the tumor thrombus into right atrium may mandate cardiopulmonary bypass and circulatory arrest to permit its safe removal.

The incision for resection of primary IVC tumors is transperitoneal, usually midline or right subcostal. If circulatory arrest is required, a median sternotomy is also performed. Hepatic tumor resection may require a right thoracolaparotomy. The infrahepatic IVC is exposed as described before. PTFE grafts (14 to 20 mm) with external support provide excellent patency of the reconstructed suprarenal or infrarenal inferior vena cava (Fig. 51.8) because inflow is usually excellent and there is no associated iliofemoral venous thrombosis. Short 10-mm wide externally supported PTFE grafts can also be used to reconstruct the renal veins if nephrectomy for treatment of the tumor does not have to be performed.

A venovenous bypass between the IVC or iliac vein and the axillary or internal jugular vein using a mechanical (Bio-Medicus, Medtronic, Minneapolis, MN) pump is occasionally needed in

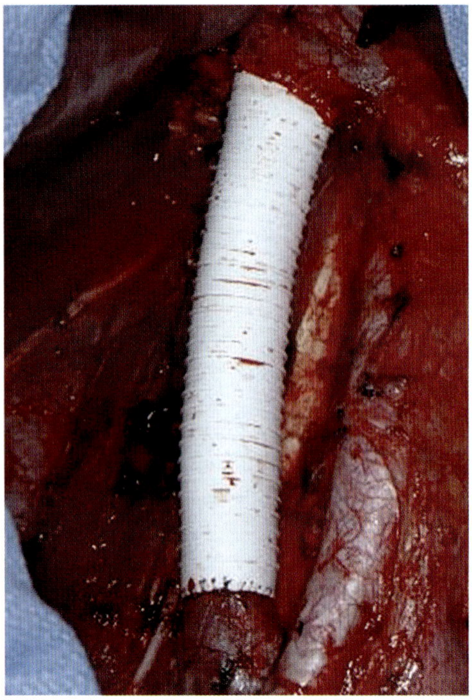

FIG 51.8 Reconstruction of the infrarenal inferior vena cava with externally supported polytetrafluoroethylene interposition graft after excision of a retroperitoneal tumor invading the inferior vena cava. (From Gloviczki P, Kalra M, Duncan AA, et al: Open and hybrid deep vein reconstructions: to do or not to do? *Phlebology* 27[Suppl 1]:103–106, 2012, Figure 1.)

patients with poor cardiac function who cannot maintain a systolic blood pressure greater than 100 mm Hg when both the IVC and the hepatic veins are occluded for an anastomosis. When resection of the retrohepatic suprarenal vena cava has to be performed, the proximal anastomosis is performed first to allow early restoration of hepatic venous outflow. A femoral AVF is usually not required because of the excellent venous inflow.

Perioperative complications are frequent (43%) and operative mortality, because of the associated liver resection, can be high (7%). Graft patency is excellent at 93% at 3 years.[45] Survival in many patients, however, is limited because of recurrent local tumor or distant metastases. Nevertheless, aggressive surgical management may offer the only chance for cure or palliation of symptoms for patients with primary or secondary IVC tumors. Caval reconstruction can result in significant improvement of the quality of life in these patients even if their survival is short owing to the underlying malignant disease.

At the Mayo Clinic, we replace the IVC if it is only partially obstructed and a majority of its circumference requires resection to provide clear tumor margins. We prefer large-diameter, externally supported PTFE grafts (20 mm) and have found their patency rates to be greater than 95% in more than 90 patients who have now been operated on at our institution.[11] The University of California, Los Angeles, group favors smaller-diameter grafts to assure higher blood flow velocities to maintain good long-term patency.[46]

Reconstruction of the Superior Vena Cava

Patients with SVC syndrome with benign disease who have extensive chronic venous thrombosis not anatomically suitable for endovascular treatment and those with less extensive disease who have failed to respond to endovascular therapy are candidates for open surgical reconstruction.[47]

Regarding graft materials, autologous spiral saphenous vein graft (SSVG) has been our favorite graft and it has excellent long-term patency. Short, large-diameter (12 to 14 mm), externally supported PTFE grafts, however, also have very good long-term patency (see Fig. 51.8). Cryopreserved aortoiliac arterial graft or femoral vein are other alternatives, as are grafts prepared from autogenous or bovine pericardium.[47]

The operation is performed through a full or partial median sternotomy. If the internal jugular vein is used for inflow, the midline incision is extended obliquely into the neck along the anterior border of the sternocleidomastoid muscle on the appropriate side. The mediastinum is exposed, and biopsy of the mediastinal mass or resection of the tumor is performed before caval reconstruction.

After biopsy or tumor resection is performed, the pericardial sac is opened to expose the right atrial appendage, which is most frequently used for the central anastomosis. A side-biting Satinsky clamp is placed on the right atrial appendage, which is then opened longitudinally. Some trabecular muscle is excised to improve flow into the heart and an end-to-side anastomosis with the vein graft is performed with a running 5-0 monofilament suture. If it is not involved in the fibrosing process, a patent SVC central to the occlusion can also be used for this purpose. The peripheral anastomosis of the graft is performed with the internal jugular or innominate vein in an end-to-side or preferably an end-to-end fashion.

A single straight graft from the internal jugular or innominate vein to the SVC or right atrial appendage (Fig. 51.9) is our current operative choice for SVC reconstruction. Because collateral circulation in the head and neck is almost always adequate, unilateral reconstruction is sufficient to relieve symptoms in most patients. When only part of the circumference of the SVC is invaded by the tumor, resection plus caval patch angioplasty with a prosthetic patch, bovine pericardium, or autogenous material such as saphenous vein or pericardium is also a good option.[47]

Open surgical treatment of SVC syndrome has excellent long-term results. Outcome depends on the etiology, conduit, and length of the venous reconstruction. Of the autologous graft materials, our experience with SSVGs and femoral vein grafts has been the largest, with reported secondary patency rate of 86% at 5 years and good to excellent clinical results. The 2-year patency rate of ePTFE grafts was approximately 70%.[47]

SPECIAL CONSIDERATIONS

Endophlebectomy

Postthrombotic femoral veins frequently have multiple lumens due to partial recanalization of the thrombus. Excision of the organized and fibrotic thrombus will enlarge the lumen, although the exposed collagen in the media of the vein wall is more thrombogenic than

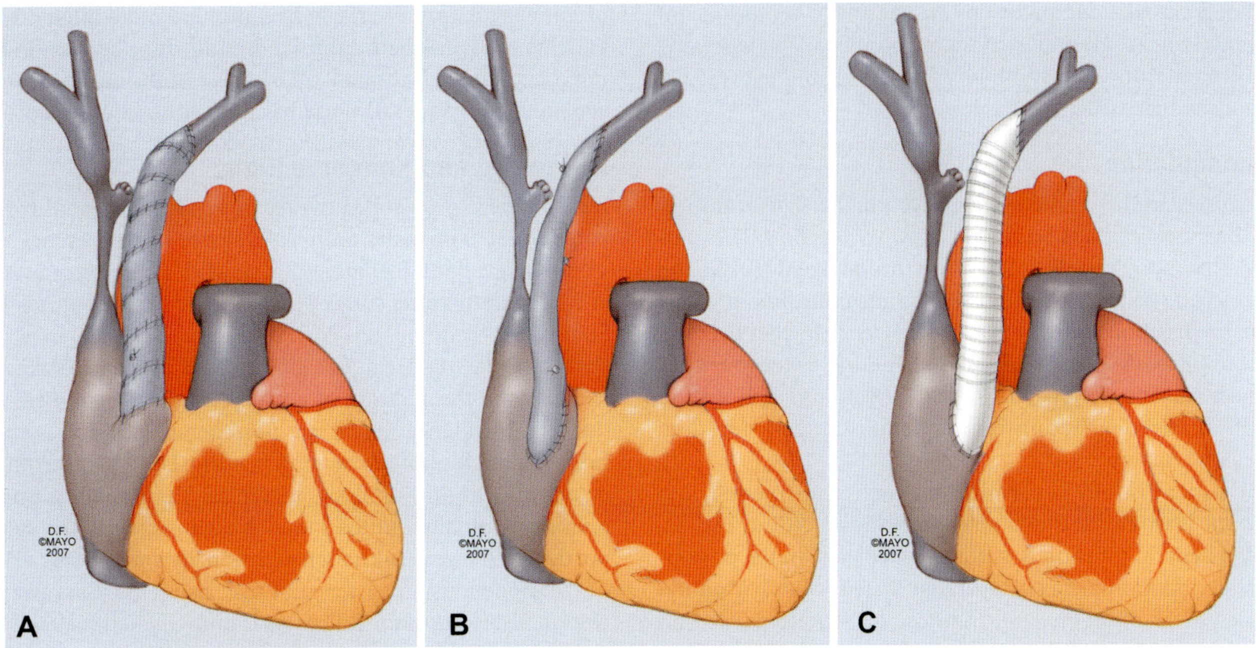

FIG 51.9 Artist's drawings of (A) left innominate vein–right atrial appendage spiral saphenous vein graft. (B) Left innominate vein–right atrial appendage femoral vein graft. (C) Left innominate vein–right atrial appendage externally supported polytetrafluoroethylene graft. (Used with permission of Mayo Foundation for Medical Education and Research. All rights reserved.)

the intact venous wall. Still, careful endophlebectomy will improve inflow; attention, however, must be paid to avoid injury to the thin residual venous wall. In patients who have localized high-grade stenosis of the common femoral vein, this operation alone is sufficient to improve venous outflow. This procedure has also been performed combined with deep venous valve transplantation in patients with PTS. The defect is closed with a patch, using a segment of the saphenous vein or bovine pericardium. The endophlebectomized segment can also be used to improve inflow for iliocaval stenting (see the discussion of hybrid reconstructions, further on, and Fig. 51.2) or for a cross-femoral or femorocaval bypass. An AVF will improve patency rates.

In a series of patients who underwent endophlebectomy, early results showed 77% primary patency of the operated segments at 8 months and a 93% secondary patency rate.[48] Comerota and colleagues reported 20 patients undergoing this procedure had significant improvements in terms of the Venous Clinical Severity Score (VCSS) and the VEINES Quality of Life (VEINES-QOL).[49]

Arteriovenous Fistula

Caval reconstructions or short iliocaval grafts, including prosthetic bypasses, do not need an adjunctive temporary AVF to maintain patency except in cases of poor inflow and distal anastomosis at the level of common femoral vein (see Figs. 51.6 and 51.7). Even in these distal cases, the additional benefit provided by AVF to prevent early thrombosis is questionable.[4]

Yet Kurstjens and colleagues suggest that placement of the AVF in the cranial part of the endophlebectomy during hybrid recanalization may result in a more favorable outcome, although this tendency was not statistically significant. In their single-center retrospective study, hybrid procedures—including recanalization of the occluded caval, iliac, and/or CFV using PTA and stenting followed by the creation of an AVF using a ring-enforced PTFE loop, a straight nonenforced PTFE tube, or a side branch of the GSV to connect the CFA with the CFV—were performed in 65 limbs, 42 cranially, and 23 with caudally placed AVFs in the endophlebectomy area.[50]

Prevention of Complications

Complications associated with open surgical venous reconstruction depend on the magnitude of the underlying disease and patient comorbidities. In general large vein reconstructions for benign disease are performed in good surgical candidates only, with a low risk of systemic complications. Of the local, nonvascular complications, wound infection, hematoma, and lymphatic leaks (fistula, lymphocele) are the most frequent. Atraumatic surgical technique, antibiotic prophylaxis, and standard surgical principles are helpful for prevention. Intraoperative air embolism, especially during caval reconstruction, is a potentially fatal complication and can be prevented by meticulous flushing of the grafts before reestablishment of the circulation and passive Valsalva maneuver (30 mm Hg) in addition to Trendelenburg positioning before release of the proximal clamp.

DVT and PE are serious vascular complications. During a series of 64 procedures performed for nonmalignant disease, there was no mortality and no pulmonary embolism.[4] Although the early graft thrombosis rate was high (20%) and reinterventions were needed, 96% of the patients left the hospital with a patent graft after open surgical bypass. Perioperative anticoagulation with heparin and warfarin, the use of elastic stockings, intermittent pneumatic compression pumps, and early ambulation help to prevent thromboembolic complications, which are fortunately rare. Local vascular complications are specific to venous reconstructions and include graft stenosis or thrombosis, perioperative bleeding, graft infection, and injury to the surrounding vascular and nonvascular structures.

Anticoagulation

Grafts placed in the venous system have a higher rate of thrombosis than arterial grafts because of a low venous flow. The presence of thrombophilic disorders and a thrombogenic surface on any prosthetic graft increase the risk of graft failure. Infrainguinal venous obstruction and valvular incompetence further decrease inflow to the graft; this is a major contributing factor to failure. For these reasons, perioperative anticoagulation is indicated in patients undergoing reconstructive venous surgery for deep venous obstruction.

The patient is fully heparinized during reconstruction, and protamine is avoided at the completion of the procedure. Unfractionated heparin infusion is started immediately in the postoperative period. Complete postoperative systemic heparinization is achieved for 48 hours, and full-dose low-molecular-weight heparin is continued subcutaneously for another 3 to 5 days, given simultaneously with warfarin. The incidence of postoperative bleeding has been between 5% and 10%, mainly as a result of anticoagulation. Warfarin is continued indefinitely in most patients with prosthetic grafts and in all with a known underlying coagulation abnormality. The effect of the new oral anticoagulants in postoperative use has not yet been well studied.

Follow-Up and Reinterventions

DUS on the first postoperative day is performed to confirm graft patency. DUS provides indirect evidence of the patency of an intrathoracic graft; therefore CTV or MRV is also recommended at 3 to 6 months after surgery and anytime that symptoms recur. Stenosis or thrombosis is corrected immediately after recognition. If thrombosis occurs in a graft without fistula, thrombectomy is done with the addition of a fistula. Graft stenosis discovered during surveillance in the late postoperative period is treated first with angioplasty or venous stenting. Late graft thrombosis is treated with thrombolysis, angioplasty, and stenting. Surgical revision is usually limited to patch angioplasty of the stenotic portion of the graft, although occasionally aneurysmal dilation of the saphenous crossover graft may also require surgical correction. On long-term follow-up, approximately half of these patients require some kind of reintervention. More than 60% of the patients had no venous claudication and no or minimal swelling on long-term follow-up.

REVIEW QUESTIONS

1. What is the first line of management of chronic iliac vein obstructions?
   a. Compression therapy and lifestyle changes
   b. Balloon angioplasty
   c. Venous stent placement
   d. Femorocaval bypass
2. A 40-year-old male with history of left iliofemoral deep venous thrombosis and recurrent ulcerations despite compression therapy presents with large lower extremity varicosities and great saphenous vein reflux. No infrainguinal venous obstruction is obvious on duplex scan. What would you recommend?
   a. High ligation and great saphenous vein stripping
   b. Endovenous ablation of the saphenous vein
   c. Endovenous ablation and stab phlebectomies
   d. CT or MR venogram of the abdomen and pelvis
3. What is the minimal diameter of the great saphenous vein that is acceptable for a cross-femoral bypass (Palma procedure)?
   a. 3 mm
   b. 7 mm
   c. 5 mm
   d. 6 mm
4. In which of the following patients is a cross-femoral venous bypass (Palma procedure) ill advised?
   a. Morbidly obese
   b. Hypercoaguable disorder
   c. Recurrent ulceration
   d. Previous failed venous stenting
5. An adjunctive femoral arteriovenous fistula improves the patency of femorocaval prosthetic bypasses.
   a. True
   b. False
6. A Palma procedure using autologous saphenous vein has the best chance of long-term patency in patients with
   a. Isolated unilateral iliac vein obstruction
   b. Multilevel obstruction
   c. Severe infrainguinal obstruction
   d. Failed previous iliac vein stent
7. In patients requiring resection of the inferior vena cava for invasion by a malignant tumor, up to 50% of the circumference of the vena cava can be resected with primary closure.
   a. True
   b. False
8. A femoral arteriovenous fistula is frequently needed in patients who undergo segmental replacement of the inferior vena cava invaded by a malignant tumor.
   a. True
   b. False
9. Postprocedure antiplatelet therapy has been conclusively shown to reduce thrombotic events in venous bypasses.
   a. True
   b. False
10. Patients with prosthetic grafts for venous replacement require lifelong anticoagulation in most cases.
    a. True
    b. False

References available online at ExpertConsult.com.

CHAPTER 52

Endovascular Repair of Chronic Venous Obstruction

Seshadri Raju, Arjun Jayaraj

Percutaneous endovenous stenting has emerged as a powerful technique for treating chronic venous obstructions. Stenosis and chronic total occlusions (CTOs) are amenable to endovascular correction.[1-4] The technique is minimally invasive, safe, and effective and does not preclude open correction in case of failure. Endovenous procedures can be applied in geriatric patients and in those who have significant comorbidities that would otherwise preclude open procedures. Intravascular ultrasound (IVUS) diagnostics have revealed that obstruction is present in a broader spectrum of chronic venous disease (CVD) than previously imagined.[5] Furthermore, stent correction of obstruction alone in combined obstruction-reflux appears to yield good symptom relief even when the reflux component remains uncorrected[6]; this suggests that the pathophysiologic importance of obstruction has been underestimated.[7] These observations point to a broad, dominant role for stent usage in highly symptomatic CVD patients, signifying a major therapeutic paradigm shift in the management of advanced CVD.

PATHOPHYSIOLOGY

Postthrombotic etiology for chronic venous obstruction is well established. With the use of IVUS, it has become clear that nonthrombotic iliac vein lesions (NIVLs) are also a common feature among "primary" CVD patients with advanced symptoms.[5] The lesions occur at arterial crossover points over the vein (Fig. 52.1). Intraluminal webs and strictures are often present and are thought to result from pulsatile trauma in an intimately associated artery.[8] Other less common causes of chronic venous obstruction include tumors, retroperitoneal fibrosis, and radiation injury. Inferior vena cava (IVC) filters are also emerging as a significant cause of iatrogenic iliocaval obstruction; some filters appear to be more prone to this development than others.[9]

Postthrombotic disease often involves multiple venous segments, but symptom production appears to be mainly related to the iliac vein segment because of its poor collateral potential.[10] Natural collateral pathways based on embryology appear to develop rapidly in obstructions of other venous segments, particularly in femoral vein obstructions and to a lesser extent in caval obstructions. These collateral pathways may already exist in putative form, becoming functional when straight-line flow faces higher resistance than in the quiescent collaterals.[11] The process is just the reverse of that seen in venous stenting, when collaterals disappear instantaneously with clearance of obstruction. The profunda femoris vein is an embryologic collateral and often becomes visible on venography within a few hours after the onset of femoral vein thrombosis. Lesions causing CTO of the IVC are sometimes found incidentally in asymptomatic patients.[10] In contrast, pelvic vein collaterals that appear impressive on venography are often functionally inadequate, and such patients continue to be symptomatic.[12] Some postthrombotic iliac vein lesions develop a tough perivenous sheath that restricts the vein and retards collateral development. Such diffuse iliac vein stenosis, first noted by Rokitanski in autopsy studies, appears as a patent but smaller-caliber iliac vein on venography. The reduction in luminal size is clearly evident on IVUS examination but is easily missed on venography (Fig. 52.2). Focal iliac vein lesions may be impervious to routine venography as well.[13] For these reasons a symptomatic iliac vein lesion may remain occult, whereas the more obvious femoral vein occlusions are readily apparent. The latter are seldom the main source of symptoms, however, and a diligent search for the culprit lesion in the iliac veins is in order.

The discovery through IVUS of a high incidence of NIVLs in patients with symptomatic CVD and relief of symptoms with venous stenting has highlighted the pathophysiologic peculiarities of these lesions. First, these lesions are widely prevalent in the asymptomatic population, with a gross prevalence of up to 30% in autopsy studies[14] and up to 66% with more sensitive modern imaging techniques.[15] With IVUS, the lesions are found in greater than 90% of patients with advanced symptoms.[5] These are characteristics of *permissive pathology,* which is widely prevalent in human disease. Patent foramen ovale (PFO), with an incidence of approximately 25% in the asymptomatic general population, becomes symptomatic in a small fraction, with onset of paradoxic embolus. Not surprisingly, PFO is invariably found in patients with paradoxic embolus. Other examples of permissive or secondary pathologies include obesity and diabetes, diabetes and neuropathy, carotid plaque and transient ischemic attack, ureteric reflux and pyelonephritis, *Helicobacter pylori* and peptic ulcer, and acid reflux and asthma. In case of silent iliac vein obstructions, a number of secondary events may trigger the onset of symptoms (Box 52.1). A postthrombotic iliac vein lesion related to a remote thrombotic event can also remain silent for years or decades before symptoms are precipitated by a later trigger event (Fig. 52.3).

A general principle in treating these complex pathologies is to address the permissive pathology first, which usually provides

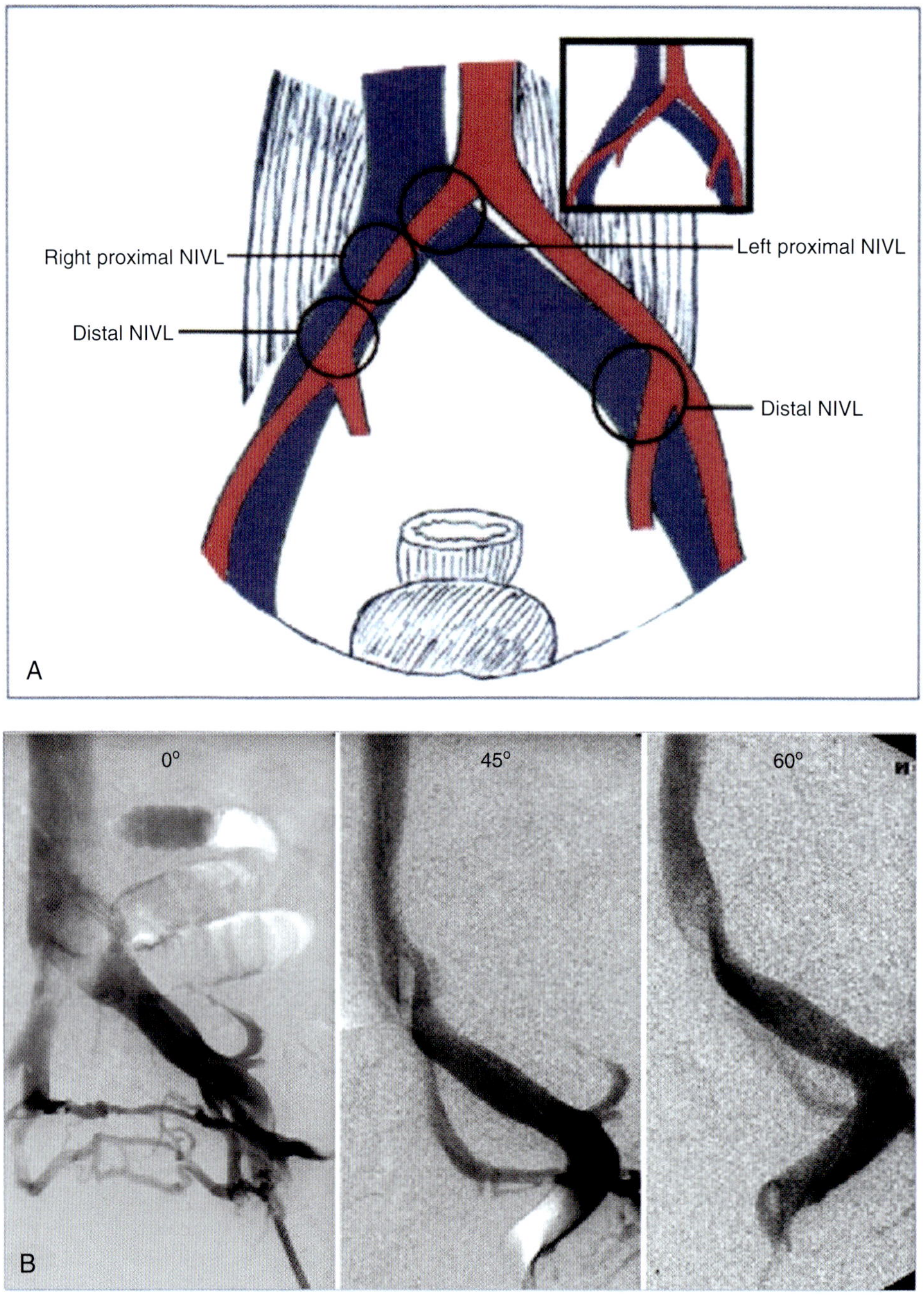

FIG 52.1 (A) The pathologic anatomy of a nonthrombotic iliac vein lesion *(NIVL)*. The classic left-sided proximal lesion is related to abrupt crossing of the left iliac vein by the right iliac artery. Coursing lazily across the vein, the right iliac artery may be related to the proximal or distal NIVL or both. The left hypogastric artery crossing may be related to the left distal NIVL. The hypogastric veins have been omitted to reduce clutter. (B) The proximal NIVL appears as a translucent area on venography in frontal projection. The tight stenosis is clearly visible in 60-degree projection. Collaterals seen in this case are present in only one-third of cases.

definitive cure. The experience with iliac vein obstructions has been similar. In cases of combined obstruction and reflux, iliac vein stenting alone has resulted in effective symptom remission even when associated reflux was quite severe and remained untreated.[6] In an analysis of 528 limbs treated by iliac vein stenting for obstruction, severe reflux (reflux segment score ≥3) was present in 58% and axial reflux in 42% that remained uncorrected. Cumulative ulcer healing and clearance of dermatitis were noted in 54% and 81% of the limbs, respectively, at 5 years. No difference was noted between limbs with severe residual reflux and those with no reflux or less severe reflux. Venous pathologies uniquely respond to partial correction with symptom remission. For example, in combined superficial and deep reflux, the correction of superficial reflux alone may provide symptom relief.

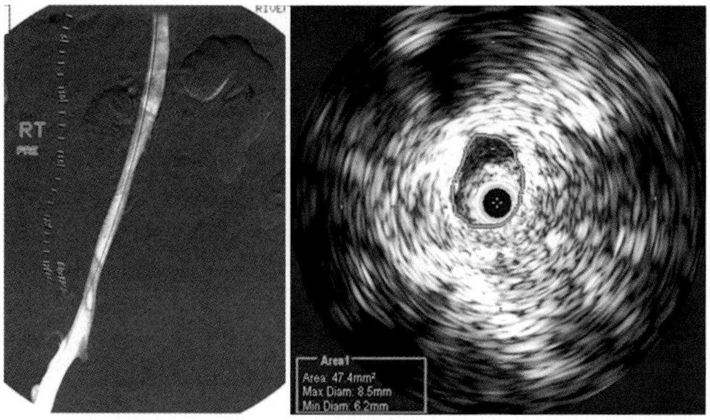

FIG 52.2 Diffuse postthrombotic stenosis may not be recognized on venography *(left)*. It is clearly visible on intravascular ultrasound (IVUS) examination *(right)*. Cross-sectional area by IVUS planimetry measured 47 mm^2 (normal external iliac vein luminal area ≥150 mm^2).

BOX 52.1 Secondary Insults That May Precipitate Symptoms in the Presence of a Silent Iliac Vein Lesion

- Trauma
- Infection (cellulitis)
- Reflux
- Deep venous thrombosis
- Joint surgery
- Orthostasis and poor calf pump (in the elderly)
- Obesity
- Edematogenic medications (many cardiovascular drugs)
- Postmenopausal hormonal changes
- Lymphatic damage and venous disease itself or from cancer, chemotherapy, radiation, or surgery

In axial reflux, the repair of a single valve may suffice.[16] Valve reconstruction of a refluxive valve below an obstructed venous segment has been shown to be effective.[17] With the advent of stent technology, repair of obstruction has become much easier than correction of reflux, which still requires open surgery. The satisfactory therapeutic response to partial pathologic correction means that a stepwise treatment paradigm starting with the simplest and minimally invasive techniques can be pursued; more complex or open treatment modalities can be reserved until later if there is recurrence of symptoms. The satisfactory clinical relief obtained with correction of chronic venous obstruction has suggested that in terms of pathophysiology, obstruction is as important as reflux, which has been the focus for the last 3 centuries.[18] IVUS-proven iliac vein obstruction occurs in isolation without associated reflux in 27% to 36% of CVD patients who present with advanced symptoms.[5,6] Venous ulceration appears to occur most commonly with combined obstruction and reflux, and only rarely with a single pathology of either obstruction or reflux.

There is an intimate relationship between the venous and lymphatic systems in genesis as well as in function. Lymphatic dysfunction can be demonstrated in approximately 30% of

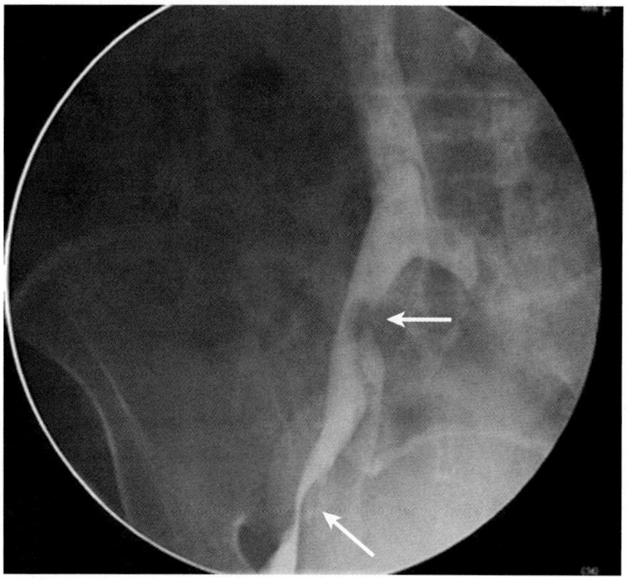

FIG 52.3 The postthrombotic iliac vein lesion shown here is likely a result of deep venous thrombosis related to a motor vehicle crash when the patient was in her twenties. There was onset of leg swelling when the 80-year-old patient suffered a fibular fracture after a fall. Stent placement resolved the swelling.

patients with advanced CVD.[19] Lymphoscintigraphic delay in node visualization appears to be a defect in the precollectors at the microcirculatory level; the form and function of large collector lymphatics are apparently preserved. The precise nature of the damage to the precollectors is unknown but presumably related to the overloaded lymphatic transport imposed by venous dysfunction.

CLINICAL FEATURES

The clinical presentation of chronic venous obstruction is often indistinguishable from that attributed to reflux alone or in combination. Venous obstruction can manifest in the entire spectrum of clinical classes represented in the Clinical Etiology Anatomy Pathophysiology (CEAP) classification. All age groups, both sexes (women more often), and both sides (left more often) are affected. Advanced clinical manifestations of pain, swelling, or skin changes have a high likelihood of being associated with venous obstruction with or without reflux, as already outlined. These clinical features can occur alone or in combination. Some aspects of clinical presentation associated with iliac vein obstruction deserve special commentary.

Limb pain usually has strong orthostatic (standing or seated) features. It is typically diffuse over the limb (differing from pain localized to varices), although pain may be predominant in one region, such as the calf or shin. The character of the pain may vary from "bursting," to "shooting," to "heaviness." In some patients, no overt pain is present, but there is soreness to touch or contact. Restless legs and cramps are common. Pain is relieved by elevation or ambulation, both of which reduce venous pressure. Compression stockings, when properly used, provide relief. Many of these pain-relieving maneuvers have become habitual in long-standing disease, and leading questions are necessary to elicit the information. Many patients routinely sleep with their legs on pillows, for example, and may not offer this information unless specifically asked. Atypical pain presentation is not uncommon, such as pain occurring at night while the patient is recumbent. Patients often get up and "walk off" the nocturnal pain. In some patients, venous limb pain can mimic claudication, with difficulty going long distances or climbing stairs without intermittent rest. A special form of orthostatic venous pain (venous hypertension syndrome) occurs in approximately 10% of patients and is often missed because the limb looks entirely healthy, with no venous signs. Venous pain disproportionate to clinical signs of venous disease is usually due to iliac vein obstruction.

Limb swelling occurs more commonly and more extensively with iliac vein obstruction than with superficial or deep reflux alone. With saphenous reflux, swelling is usually intermittent and confined to the ankles. With extensive deep venous reflux, swelling may advance to involve the leg but is confined to below the knee and is generally only mild to moderate in severity. Massive limb swelling is invariably due to iliac vein obstruction. Recurrent cellulitis of the limb usually indicates the presence of iliac vein obstruction.

Venous dermatitis and ulceration most commonly result from a combination of deep venous reflux and obstruction. However, in a small subset of patients with isolated saphenous reflux, venous dermatitis or ulceration can occur if the saphenous vein is large (often >10 mm). Venous swelling can mimic all the "classic" features of lymphedema, including humping of the dorsum of the foot, squaring of the toes, and Stemmer's sign. A diagnosis of lymphedema should not be made without lymphoscintigraphy. Because of the high prevalence of chronic venous disease and frequently associated lymphatic damage, it is probably the most common cause of secondary lymphedema dwarfing the incidence of primary lymphedema. Therefore, it is worthwhile to do an IVUS examination to rule out iliac vein obstruction in patients presenting with lymphedema.

Iliac vein thrombosis is a special form that can propagate distally, prompted by an underlying NIVL type of lesion.[20] Recurrent venous thrombosis is a recognized cause of symptoms in postthrombotic syndrome.[21] The etiology of iliac vein obstruction (i.e., NIVL vs. postthrombotic) cannot be determined in most cases by clinical features alone except when there is a clear history of prior deep venous thrombosis.

DIAGNOSTIC IMAGING

Standard investigative techniques have poor sensitivity to detect iliac vein obstruction. Routine duplex ultrasound does not provide adequate color-flow images of the iliac vein. The technique described by Labropoulos and colleagues[22] offers better visualization and velocity measurements, but its accuracy has not been determined. The presence of reflux, even severe reflux (multisegmental or axial), does not rule out the presence of iliac vein obstruction or the possibility of symptom remission with stent correction. Absence of reflux or trivial reflux (reflux in only one or two segments, nonaxial reflux, or reflux in a small saphenous vein) in the context of severe symptoms does suggest iliac vein obstruction. It is well established that routine venography in frontal projections, even through the transfemoral route, is approximately only 50% sensitive to iliac vein obstructive lesions.[6] Recent data have demonstrated that the location of the iliocaval bifurcation varies substantially, averaging almost one full vertebral level between IVUS and venography. This review demonstrated that relying on venography alone may result in a missed proximal lesion of the common iliac vein (up to 78% incidence) and potential inadvertent jailing of the contralateral limb (up to 12% of patients). In addition, the anatomic characteristics of venous lesions, including degree and location of maximal disease, were not accurately identified with venography.[23] The accuracy of modern imaging techniques, such as high-resolution computed tomography or magnetic resonance imaging, in detecting iliac vein lesions remains undetermined. No hemodynamic tests have adequate sensitivity to detect iliac vein obstruction. Exercise femoral vein pressures, outflow fraction measurement, and arm/foot pressure measurement can be useful when positive but because of their low sensitivity, they do not rule out obstruction. Using a combination of these techniques and transfemoral venography, it is possible to predict the presence of an iliac vein obstruction with approximately 80% accuracy.[6] Currently, IVUS examination, a morphologic method, remains the most reliable technique in detecting iliac vein obstruction.[24] IVUS is typically performed using a 0.035 probe (Volcano, San Diego, CA) with planimetric evaluation of the luminal areas of the common femoral vein (CFV), external iliac vein (EIV), and common iliac vein (CIV) using 125 mm^2, 150 mm^2, and 200 mm^2 to define normal luminal area cutoffs in the CFV, EIV, and CIV, respectively (Table 52.1). Any decrease in luminal area in a symptomatic patient is considered abnormal, meriting angioplasty and stenting. Because of the high diagnostic yield with this method in symptomatic patients, IVUS remains the preferred diagnostic modality at present. With prior consent, stent correction of the detected stenosis can be performed concurrently.

TABLE 52.1 Luminal Areas and Corresponding Diameter on Intravascular Ultrasound Examination

Vein	Luminal Area (mm^2)	Diameter (mm)
CFV	125	12
EIV	150	14
CIV	200	16
IVC	N/A	17

Because IVC is partially collapsed, only the transverse diameter is used, not the area (N/A).
CFV, Common femoral vein; *CIV*, common iliac vein; *EIV*, external iliac vein; *IVC*, inferior vena cava.

TECHNIQUE OF STENT PLACEMENT

Venous stenting differs from arterial stenting in several respects (Box 52.2), and modification of the endovascular technique learned in arterial practice is essential for symptom relief.

The optimal access point is at the midthigh, where the femoral vein is posterolateral to the artery. The midthigh access offers close proximity to the lesion and antegrade maneuvers while allowing adequate room above the sheath to deploy the stent below the inguinal ligament, if necessary. Access through the internal jugular vein or the popliteal vein is farther removed from the target lesion. In addition, the technique has the disadvantage of requiring prone positioning in an increasingly obese population. Large (10 or 11 French) sheaths are used. Access complications have been rare with the routine use of ultrasound guidance for access and sealant devices.

After an optional on-table venogram (omitted in patients with renal dysfunction), IVUS examination is performed and the presence of an obstructive lesion is confirmed. IVUS planimetry provides accurate measurements of even irregular stenoses, which are common in iliac veins. The luminal area cutoffs for planimetry have already been discussed. The proximal common iliac vein where the artery crosses over is the classic site for nonthrombotic obstruction. Obstructive lesions near the orifice of the hypogastric vein occur frequently[5] but are sometimes impervious to IVUS examination. Gentle balloon dilation of this location is necessary to identify such lesions. Minor lesions are commonly present behind the inguinal ligament. In postthrombotic disease, these compressive points from arterial or ligamentous structures are particularly prone to fibrosis because thrombus resolves poorly at these locations.[20] In severe postthrombotic disease, the entire iliofemoral segment may be involved.

BOX 52.2 Venous Stenting Technique Is Different From Arterial Stenting Technique

- Balloon angioplasty alone does not work because the lesion is fibrous and recoil is the rule.
- Large-caliber stents approximating natural luminal size are necessary to normalize distal venous pressure; patency alone is not enough.
- Stents should be extended into the inferior vena cava, otherwise the choke band at the iliocaval junction will squeeze the stent distally, causing recurrence.
- Venous stents (braided) can be extended across the inguinal ligament without erosion or fracture.
- Iliac veins are intolerant of residual lesions; the result is residual or recurrent symptoms.
- Extensive stenting is often required; veins are very tolerant of metal load (no thrombosis).
- Intravascular ultrasound is mandatory to ensure good results.

Large-caliber 18-mm balloons are commonly used in normal-sized adults for predilation prior to stent placement. Iliac vein obstructions are fibrotic, and recoil is the norm after balloon dilation alone. Stent placement is therefore universally required. Large-caliber 18- to 20-mm Wallstents are deployed under fluoroscopy, with generous overlap between stents to avoid disconnection. The oversizing enables later hyperdilatation in case of stent compression or in-stent restenosis.[25] The preferred upper landing site is the distal vena cava, just above the iliocaval confluence as determined by IVUS.[26] A large-caliber 25- by 50-mm Z stent (Gianturco stent) is used across the iliocaval confluence for additional radial strength. All lesions in symptomatic patients should be corrected in continuity without short skip areas. Currently stents in the majority of patients are extended from the distal inferior cava to the common femoral vein (Fig. 52.4).

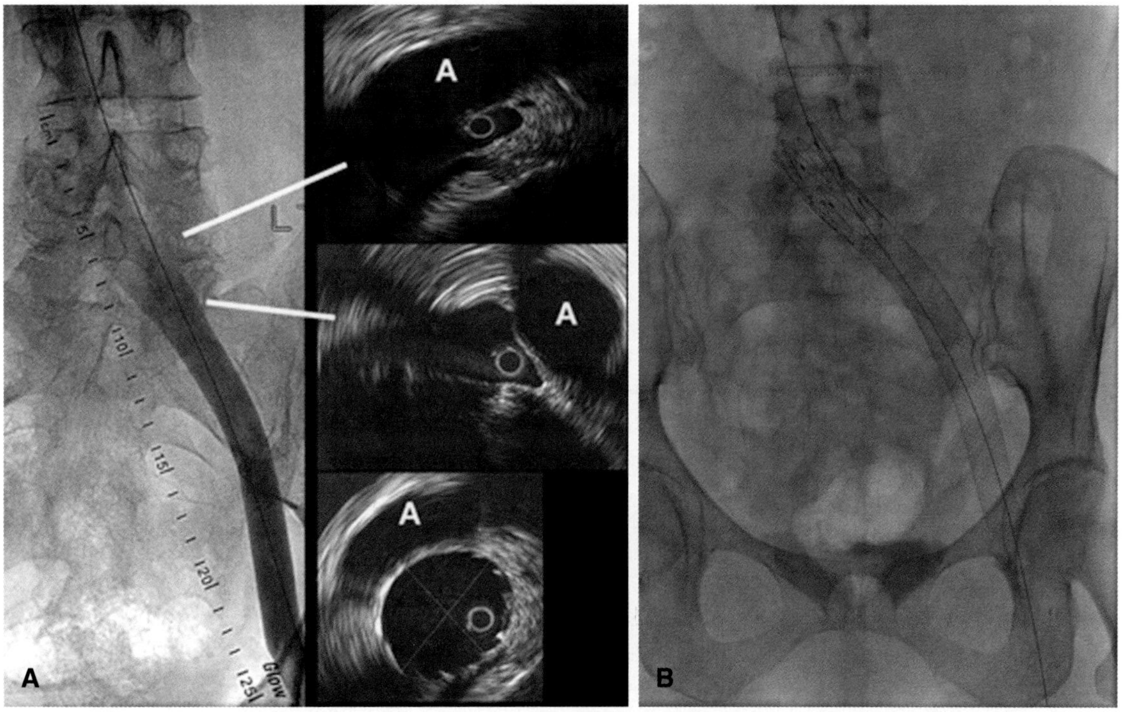

FIG 52.4 (A) The venogram on the left appears grossly normal. Note the absence of collaterals. However, intravascular ultrasound (IVUS) examinations at indicated locations show significant stenosis. The crossing artery is marked *A* in the IVUS images. The IVUS image at the bottom *(right)* shows a normal lumen after stent placement. (B) A stent stack extending from just beyond the iliocaval confluence to the common femoral vein.

Infrainguinal deployment has not resulted in stent fractures, erosions, or stent thrombosis.[27] Metal load from extensive stent stack length does not appear to adversely affect patency.[10] Leaving uncorrected residual lesions has often been responsible for residual or recurrent symptoms.[25] IVUS is used extensively during the procedure to identify lesions, determine optimal landing sites for the stent, and to ensure proper apposition between stent stack members after postdilatation.

BILATERAL STENT PLACEMENT

About 20% of CVD patients in advanced clinical classes have bilateral disease. The limb with more severe symptoms is treated first, using the technique already described (see Fig. 50.4B). Contralateral symptom improvement has been observed after unilateral iliac vein stenting in some cases, presumably because the collateral load is removed. Contralateral limb symptoms may advance over time, however, due to disease progression. In that event, sequential bilateral stenting may be required and can be performed in a similar fashion as the original stent. The second Z stent can, however, be flowered by partially deploying it on the back table, cutting the distal nylon suture and resheathing it. In this manner, the second Z stent can be accommodated in the limited space provided by the vena cava (Fig. 52.5A). If the previous stenting has been carried out using only a Wallstent, a fenestrum can be created using large-caliber balloons and stenting of the fenestrum can be performed using Wallstent and Z stents (see Fig. 52.5B).[28] The technique of double-barreled stents involves a higher risk of complications and reintervention over time. Although the results of the double-barreled technique are initially good, most such cases have failed over time due to compression of one barrel by the other (unpublished data). The ideal treatment of the iliocaval confluence—which overcomes the iliocaval choke-point effect, prevents contralateral jailing, and has a minimal reintervention rate—remains elusive. A vein-specific stent that would address these issues is needed.

INFERIOR VENA CAVA FILTERS

Previously placed IVC filters pose a special technical problem during iliac vein stent placement. Some makes of filters may be associated with stenosis of the vena cava at the implantation site. This can be assessed by IVUS examination during the procedure. If no stenosis is found, the iliac vein stent can be safely placed below the filter. If the filter site is stenotic (>50%), the filter can be removed and the area stented across. If filter retrieval is not possible, then stenting can be performed across the filter after its compaction by repeated balloon dilations[29] (Fig. 52.6). Good long-term results (97% secondary patency) have been noted.[30] Temporary filters that are not retrieved as intended may be associated with a higher incidence of stenosis or thrombosis of the IVC.[31,32]

RECANALIZATION OF ILIOCAVAL CHRONIC TOTAL OCCLUSIONS

Recanalization of iliocaval CTOs involves manipulating a guidewire through the CTO segment.[4] Unlike arterial CTO lesions, postthrombotic venous occlusions do not have solid cores but are traversed by recanalized channels (Fig. 52.7, color insert). Even dense trabeculations can be crossed with patience (80% procedure success). CTO lesions that appear long on venography may be relatively short because of poor contrast opacification of the segment above the lesion. A recanalization attempt is worthwhile despite a daunting venographic appearance. An angled-tip 5 or 6 French catheter with hydrophilic coating is used to direct the guidewire through the CTO segment without

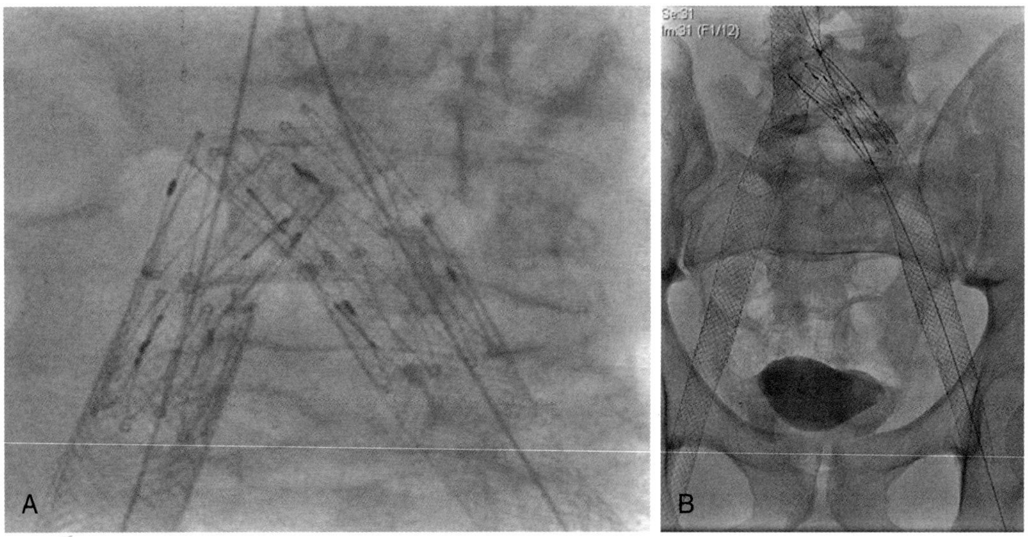

FIG 52.5 (A) Bilateral stenting using the Z-stent technique. (B) Fenestration technique for sequential stenting in patients with a prior isolated contralateral wall stent.

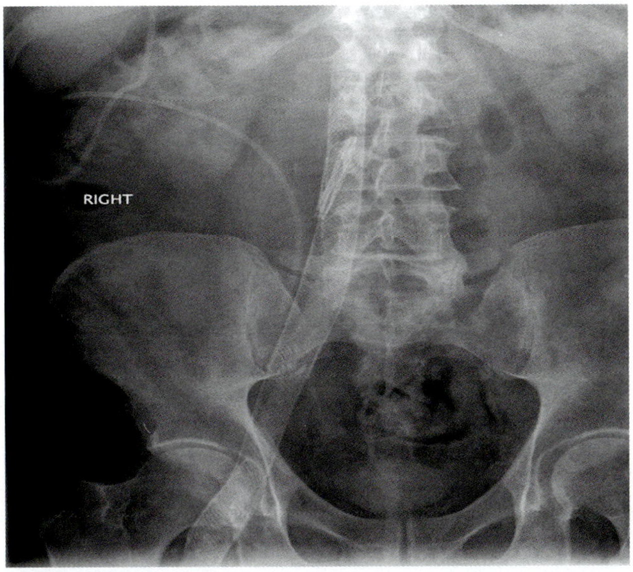

FIG 52.6 Stent across an inferior vena cava filter that was compacted by balloon dilation. Note stent extension below the inguinal ligament. Stent fractures, erosions, or thromboses do not result from stent extension across the groin crease.

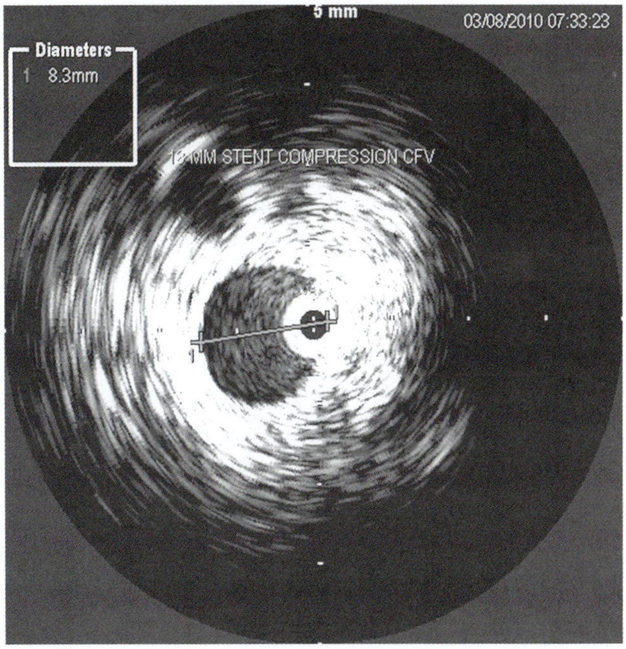

FIG 52.8 Stent compression by perivenous fibrosis is unique to venous stenting. An 18-mm stent has been compressed to 8.3 mm.

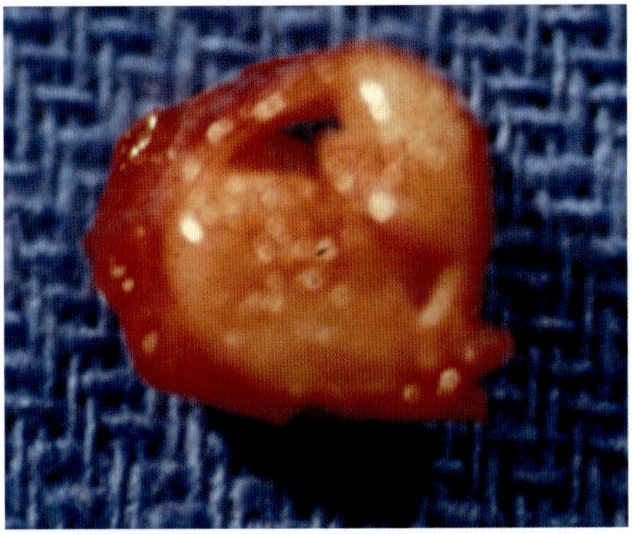

FIG 52.7 Transverse section of a postthrombotic vein. The guidewire is threaded through these small channels in the trabeculated vein during the recanalization procedure.

straying into branches or collaterals. A long 45- to 55-cm sheath is often required to provide additional rigid support for guidewire passage. Perforations that can occur during the maneuvers are innocuous, unlike the case in arterial stenting, because of the low venous pressure and the constraining influence of perivenous fibrosis and fascial sheaths. The guidewire can be withdrawn and the procedure resumed without ill effect. Proper reentry into the vena cava above the obstruction should be confirmed by advancing the guidewire into the right atrium by venography or by IVUS examination. The next step is to enlarge the guidewire tract to normal luminal size for the location. A 7 French hydrophilic-coated sheath with obturator (Shuttle Sheath, Cook Medical, Bloomington, IN) is used first to enlarge the tract and allow easy passage of the balloon catheter. The recanalized channel should be dilated to a size appropriate for the anatomic location, as specified previously; this is essential for adequate peripheral venous decompression. Dilating a CTO fibrous cord to such large sizes may seem hazardous, but it has not proved to be threatening in practice. Oversized 18- to 20-mm stents are placed with generous overlap in the recanalized channel. Stent compression in the dense fibrous channel is a common feature in recanalization procedures (Fig. 52.8). The oversizing allows for hyperdilation should it occur. IVUS again is distinctly superior to venography in confirming luminal adequacy of the stented recanalized channel.

ANTICOAGULATION

Low-molecular-weight heparin at a prophylactic dosage is routinely used immediately before the procedure and for 1 or 2 days thereafter. Intraoperatively, bivalirudin (75 mg) is administered intravenously. Long-term anticoagulation is not necessary for nonthrombotic cases or postthrombotic patients with previous provoked thrombosis. Aspirin (81 mg daily) is used for stent maintenance in these patients. Long-term warfarin anticoagulation is recommended for the following patient groups: those with thrombophilia, recurrent venous thrombosis, unprovoked deep venous thrombosis, and patients who have undergone complex stenting procedures (e.g., IVC recanalizations).

STENT SURVEILLANCE

Stent imaging, using the technique described by Labropoulos and colleagues,[22] has become the standard for monitoring stent patency. Transfemoral venography can be used in selected cases when the duplex ultrasound findings are equivocal. Newer modalities, like B-flow ultrasound, show promise in determining flow patterns and picking up early stent malfunction.

Stent patency is monitored the day after the procedure and at intervals of 2 weeks, 4 weeks, 3 months, 6 months, and yearly thereafter. More frequent monitoring is required in postthrombotic cases,[3] particularly CTO recanalizations, in the first 3 months after the procedure, as stent occlusions occur most often in this subset. Residual or recurrent symptoms are an indication for stent imaging outside the routine intervals.

REINTERVENTIONS

Residual or recurrent symptoms indicate stent malfunction or a missed or de novo lesion.[24] Obstructive lesions that cause residual or recurrent symptoms are due to lesions within the stent stack or in the outflow-inflow tracts immediately adjacent to the stent.

Approximately 25% of stent placements will require reintervention in the succeeding years. The nature of the problem is often evident on duplex imaging or venography. However, discrete focal lesions may be impervious to these techniques. IVUS examination may ultimately be required to identify and correct the problem.

In nonthrombotic cases, the distal NIVL near the hypogastric vein orifice can be missed, even on IVUS examination, and is often the source of symptoms when the original stent placement was confined to the common iliac vein. Less often, a residual uncorrected lesion behind the inguinal ligament is present. Inadequate stent extension into the IVC during the original procedure often leads to local stent migration distally, resulting in recurrent stenosis at the iliocaval junction.

In postthrombotic cases, lesions at the inflow or outflow site to the stent may be the cause of symptoms. Diffuse postthrombotic stenosis of the IVC is easily missed on venography alone unless routine IVUS measurements are taken. A peculiar form of new stenosis that develops late after stenting involves the external iliac vein (i.e., de novo stenosis), the nature of which remains unknown.

Stent malfunction can be divided into two categories, regardless of the original pathology: (1) stent compression by anatomic fibrous bands in nonthrombotic cases and by postthrombotic fibrous tissue in thrombotic cases and (2) in-stent restenosis (Fig. 52.9). The latter appears to have two forms, a soft variety lined by layered thrombus owing to sluggish flow and a hard variety more similar to the one seen in arterial stenting. Both types appear to have an affinity for the external iliac vein. In either cases of in-stent restenosis, associated lesions below or above the stent that might have been contributory should be corrected by stent extensions. Hyperdilation (balloon dilatation with 18- to 24-mm angioplasty balloons, larger than the largest indwelling stent, yield satisfactory results in clearing in-stent restenosis; however, this procedure is much less effective in cases of stent compression.

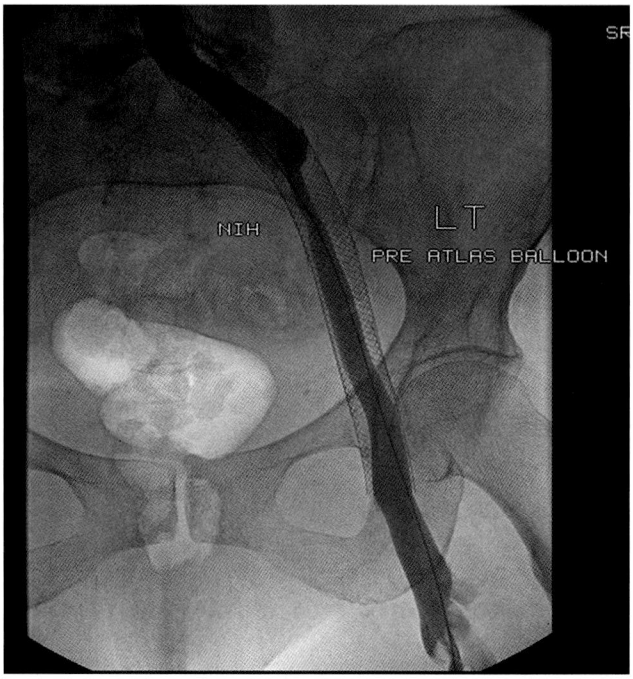

FIG 52.9 In stent restenosis, this pathology seems to have a special affinity for the stented external iliac vein.

MORBIDITY

Percutaneous stent placement is associated with low morbidity and is well tolerated by geriatric patients, even by those with comorbidities that preclude open procedures.[3] There has been one procedure-related mortality in more than 3000 patients treated by stent placement. Lower back pain is a common complaint immediately postprocedure (25% of patents) but is generally easily controlled by nonsteroidal anti-inflammatory drugs and supportive measures on an outpatient basis. The incidence of poststent DVT (<30 days) is 1.5%. The incidence of pulmonary embolism has been 0.02%.

OUTCOMES

Cumulative secondary patency for primary and postthrombotic limbs with a separate curve for CTO recanalizations are shown in Fig. 52.10. Excellent patency is also noted for stenting following the compaction of IVC filters, as noted earlier.[32] Stent thrombosis is an extreme rarity among nonthrombotic limbs after venous stenting, with an observed incidence of 3.5%.[3,33] Stent thrombosis is almost exclusive to postthrombotic limbs, particularly the CTO subset. Among 464 postthrombotic limbs, there were 31 stent thromboses; 7 were reopened by thrombolysis.

Pain relief and improvement in swelling are shown in Fig. 52.11. Nearly two-thirds of patients were completely relieved of pain. Many patients are able to tolerate residual swelling if

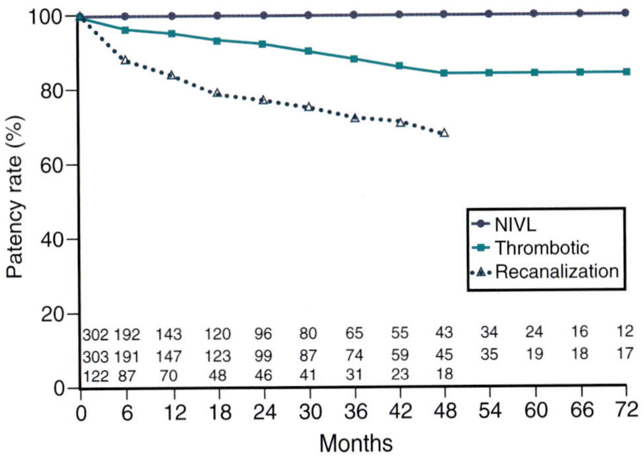

FIG 52.10 Cumulative secondary stent patency rates for nonthrombotic and thrombotic limbs. Patency after chronic total occlusion recanalization is shown separately. Stent thrombosis is extremely rare in nonthrombotic limbs. *NIVL*, Nonthrombotic iliac vein lesion.

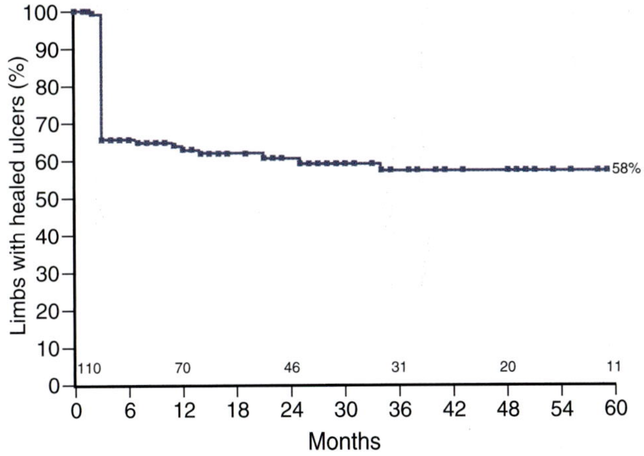

FIG 52.12 Cumulative ulcer healing after iliac vein stent placement. A large number of limbs were censored because of follow-up loss soon after stent placement before the ulcers had a chance to heal. There is little ulcer recurrence after healing, yielding a flat curve.

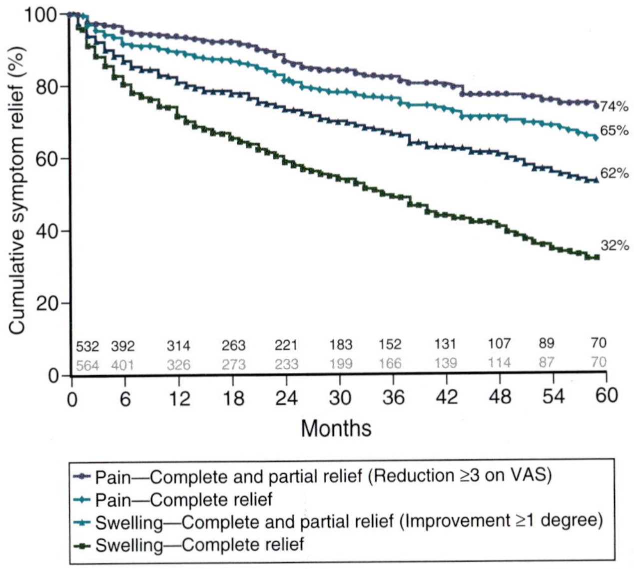

FIG 52.11 Cumulative improvement in pain and swelling after iliac vein stent placement. Partial improvement in pain (≥3/10 visual analogue scale) and partial swelling relief (≥1 grade) are shown separately from complete relief.

the pain component is relieved. Swelling relief is less than pain relief. Approximately one-third of patients were completely relieved of swelling over the long term. Cumulative healing of venous stasis ulcerations is shown in Fig. 52.12. There was cumulative ulcer healing of 58% at 5 years. Quality of life (CIVCQ) showed improvement in every category and in the overall score.[3]

CONCLUSION

Iliac vein stenting has emerged as a powerful minimally invasive technique for the treatment of a wide spectrum of advanced venous disease. The procedure is safe and effective. As a result, it can be applied to a wider spectrum of patients, including those of advanced age and patients with comorbidities, which is not possible with traditional open techniques. Its efficacy even in patients with severe uncorrected reflux has focused new attention on the relative pathophysiologic importance of venous obstruction vis-á-vis reflux in chronic venous disease.

REVIEW QUESTIONS

1. "Primary" NIVL iliac vein obstruction is due to
   - **a.** Prior resolved thrombus
   - **b.** Predominantly ontogenic
   - **c.** Traumatic
   - **d.** Endothelial hypertrophy
   - **e.** Vascularized proliferation
2. Postthrombotic iliac vein lesions are commonly
   - **a.** Focal
   - **b.** Diffuse (Rokitanski type)
   - **c.** Segmental
   - **d.** Poorly collateralized
   - **e.** All of the above
3. With modern imaging, NIVLs are found in:
   - **a.** 20% of the population
   - **b.** 66% of the population
   - **c.** 90% of symptomatic patients
   - **d.** Less than 10% of the population
4. The sensitivity of venography for iliac vein obstruction is
   - **a.** 72%
   - **b.** About 50%
   - **c.** 100% in NIVL
   - **d.** 30%
   - **e.** Increased by reactive hyperemia

5. Iliac vein obstruction without reflux occurs in
   a. 27% to 36% of CVD patients
   b. Very rare
   c. 58% of CVD patients
   d. Postthrombotic disease only
   e. NIVL exclusively
6. The incidence of lymphoscintographic abnormalities in chronic venous diseases is
   a. Less than 5%
   b. Greater than 75%
   c. Extremely rare
   d. About 30%
   e. Unknown
7. The preferred technique of correcting iliac vein obstructions involves the use of
   a. Angioplasty
   b. Large-caliber self-expanding stents
   c. Short dilatable balloon stents
   d. Large-caliber covered stents
   e. 8- to 10-mm stents to restore flow
8. Recanalization of chronic total occlusions is technically achieved by
   a. Subintimal guidewire passage
   b. Subadventitial guidewire passage
   c. Passage through collaterals
   d. Passage through trabeculae
9. A major complication of venous stenting and recanalization procedures is
   a. Hemorrhage
   b. New intimal hyperplasia, higher than in arterial stenting
   c. Stent thrombosis requiring effective anticoagulation
   d. Pulmonary embolism in some 10% of cases
   e. None of the above
10. Venous stenting has been shown to
   a. Heal venous ulcers
   b. Completely relieve venous pain in the majority of patients
   c. Improve leg swelling
   d. All of the above
   e. Only b and c are correct

SELECTED REFERENCES

1. Knipp BS, Ferguson E, Williams DM, et al. Factors associated with outcome after interventional treatment of symptomatic iliac vein compression syndrome. *J Vasc Surg*. 2007;46:743–749.
3. Neglen P, Hollis KC, Olivier J, et al. Stenting of the venous outflow in chronic venous disease: long-term stent-related outcome, clinical, and hemodynamic result. *J Vasc Surg*. 2007;46: 979–990.
4. Raju S, Neglen P. Percutaneous recanalization of total occlusions of the iliac vein. *J Vasc Surg*. 2009;50:360–368.
6. Raju S, Darcey R, Neglen P. Unexpected major role for venous stenting in deep reflux disease. *J Vasc Surg*. 2010;51:401–408, discussion 8.
10. Raju S, Hollis K, Neglen P. Obstructive lesions of the inferior vena cava: clinical features and endovenous treatment. *J Vasc Surg*. 2006;44:820–827.
15. Kibbe MR, Ujiki M, Goodwin AL, et al. Iliac vein compression in an asymptomatic patient population. *J Vasc Surg*. 2004;39: 937–943.
17. Raju S, Hardy JD. Technical options in venous valve reconstruction. *Am J Surg*. 1997;173:301–307.
18. Labropoulos N, Volteas N, Leon M, et al. The role of venous outflow obstruction in patients with chronic venous dysfunction. *Arch Surg*. 1997;132:46–51.
21. Prandoni P, Lensing AW, Prins MR. Long-term outcomes after deep venous thrombosis of the lower extremities. *Vasc Med*. 1998;3:57–60.
26. Neglen P, Berry MA, Raju S. Endovascular surgery in the treatment of chronic primary and post-thrombotic iliac vein obstruction. *Eur J Vasc Endovasc Surg*. 2000;20:560–571.

References available online at ExpertConsult.com.

CHAPTER 53

Etiology and Management of Varicose Veins: Surgery, Endovenous Ablation, and Sclerotherapy

Mark M. Archie, David A. Rigberg

The term *chronic venous insufficiency* (CVI) encompasses a spectrum of symptoms, such as edema, skin changes, or ulceration, which are attributed to functional abnormalities of the venous system and, in turn, venous hypertension.[1] Varicose veins alone are not considered evidence of CVI unless they are associated with other symptoms.[2] CVI is a common problem, affecting more than 2 million patients in the United States. There are 150,000 new cases diagnosed each year, with an estimated cost of half a billion dollars annually for their care.[3,4] In the Edinburgh vein study, more than 1500 patients were screened with a questionnaire, physical examination, and duplex ultrasound.[5] CVI prevalence closely correlated with sex and age, with rates of 21.2% and 12% in men and women greater than 50 years of age, respectively. The most common symptoms of CVI include pain, sensations of heaviness, swelling, aching, restless legs, cramps, itching, tingling, throbbing, and tired legs. Of these symptoms, those significantly correlated with worsening grade of CVI included heaviness, swelling, aching, itching, and ulceration.[2] The Bonn Vein Study examined more than 3000 people from the general population and found signs of CVI, including edema in 13.4%, skin changes in 2.9%, and healed or active ulceration in 0.6% or 0.1%, respectively.[6]

ANATOMY

Standardized nomenclature of lower extremity venous anatomy was published by Caggiati and colleagues in 2002,[7] and this terminology should be adopted to provide uniform description and treatment of CVI. The venous system can be considered as three interconnected groups: (1) superficial veins, which lie above the fascia and drain both the skin and subcutaneous tissue; (2) deep veins, which lie below the fascia and drain the leg musculature; and (3) perforating veins (PVs), which penetrate the fascia and connect the deep and superficial systems. These veins have bicuspid valves that are found at the termination of major tributaries, with increasing numbers found more distally in the venous tree.[8] The superficial veins are usually involved with CVI and include the great and small saphenous veins (SSVs). The great saphenous vein (GSV) drains into the femoral vein at the saphenofemoral junction; a valve lies at this junction in 94% to 100% of individuals, and this is the most common site for clinically significant reflux.[9] The GSV has approximately six valves and branches into an anterior branch and posterior arch below the knee. The SSV runs in the posterior calf and has 7 to 10 valves. Although there is variation in the anatomy, it usually drains into the deep system at the popliteal vein via the saphenopopliteal junction.[9]

There are more than 150 PVs in the lower extremity; however, the four clinically significant groups are found within the foot, medial and lateral leg, and thigh.[10] These perforators may drain directly into the deep venous system or indirectly via venous sinuses of the lower leg. The thigh and calf perforators contain one to three valves and provide a pathway for blood to flow from the superficial to deep venous system. In contrast, PVs in the foot direct blood from the deep to superficial systems.[10] The medial lower leg perforators include the paratibial (or Sherman and Boyd) and posterior tibial (or Cockett) PV. Paratibial PVs direct blood from the posterior arch and GSV to the posterior tibial veins, whereas posterior tibial PVs connect the posterior accessory GSV with the posterior tibial veins. The medial thigh PV includes the inguinal and femoral canal (Dodd) perforators, and these connect the GSV with the superficial femoral vein at the groin or proximal to the knee, respectively.[7]

The deep veins run with their similarly named arterial counterparts and are subfascial structures. The number of valves increases distally down the limb, with one valve at the external iliac–common femoral junction, one valve at the saphenofemoral junction, three valves in the proximal superficial femoral vein, two valves in the distal superficial femoral and popliteal veins, and numerous valves in the anterior and posterior tibial veins, as well as the peroneal veins.[8,10] Venous sinuses are present in the deep compartments of the lower extremity and include both gastrocnemius and soleal sinuses. Although these muscular venous sinuses are valveless, they empty into adjacent valved veins and are the principle collecting system within the calf.[8]

PATHOPHYSIOLOGY

The physiology of venous return is useful in understanding the signs, symptoms, and treatments available for venous disease. Resting venous pressure is a function of capillary inflow, valve function, outflow obstruction, and muscle pump action. Approximately 90% of blood return occurs through the deep venous system via muscular contraction of the foot, calf, and thigh.[11] Under normal conditions, postcapillary venous pressure ranges between 12 and 18 mm Hg. However, in the dependent lower extremity, hydrostatic pressures can range from 30 to 100 mm Hg.[12] Contraction of the calf can generate pressures as high as 250 mm Hg, with a resultant ejection fraction of 65%.[13] Clinically it has been demonstrated that after walking 7 to 12 steps, lower-extremity venous pressure is reduced from 100 mm Hg to a mean of 22 mm Hg.[14] With intermittent muscle pump action (in the presence of competent valves), the deep veins empty, and the resting venous pressure is reduced. During muscular relaxation, venous pressure slowly rises secondary to capillary inflow, as well as emptying from the superficial venous system via perforators. Thus the valves serve to compartmentalize the hydrostatic column of blood and prevent reflux.[15]

Valvular dysfunction reduces venous emptying and contributes to venous hypertension. In addition, in the presence of incompetent perforator valves, increased pressure may be transmitted back to the superficial venous system.[12] Venous hypertension can also lead to dilation of the venous segment below the malfunctioning valve, resulting in subsequent failure of the valve at this level. This simple pathology explains why patients with CVI consistently report that their symptoms are minimized in the morning, prior to getting out of bed. In the supine position the effects of gravity are essentially eliminated from the venous system, thus minimizing pressure gradients across the valves. Large varicosities, which are branches of refluxing veins that have been chronically under high pressure, may all but disappear with leg elevation.

The underlying etiology of venous disorders may be congenital, primary, or secondary. Primary venous disorders pertain to pathology without a precipitating event and involve structural and biochemical changes of the venous wall, whereas secondary disorders occur after an event, such as an acute deep venous thrombosis (DVT). According to the North American subfascial endoscopic perforator surgery (SEPS) registry, CVI results from primary venous disease in 70% of the population and from a postthrombotic state in 30%.[16] The pathogenesis of primary valve dysfunction is not entirely clear; however, connective tissue defects involving both the cellular and extracellular matrix have been identified. Multiple investigators have documented smooth muscle cell proliferation and infiltration, increased numbers of fibroblasts, and atrophied vasa vasora.[17–19] The composition of varicose veins has been found to have reduced total elastin content,[20] variations in both the content and types of collagen, and alterations in the activity of matrix metalloproteinases as well as their tissue inhibitors.[18,21,22] These changes in venous composition are thought to compromise the structural integrity of the vein wall, resulting in venous dilatation and the development of valvular incompetence, with reflux as a consequence.[23]

With secondary venous disorders, a deep venous thrombus can trigger an inflammatory response, thereby contributing to endothelial injury. The direct apposition of thrombus against the vein wall has been shown to activate leukocytes, upregulate activity of matrix metalloproteinases, and promote fibrosis.[24] In addition, recanalization of the vein is often incomplete, with only 55% of patients demonstrating complete resolution of DVT within 6 to 9 months.[25] The resulting hemodynamic abnormality is thus one of both reflux and obstruction.[26]

The interaction of venous anatomy and physiology has yet to completely explain the clinical manifestations of CVI. Venous ulceration is not clearly colocalized with PVs, and single lesions may be associated with multiple levels of valvular incompetence within the superficial, deep, or perforating systems.[27] Despite these minor discrepancies, chronic venous hypertension typically has physical signs concordant with the severity of the underlying disease. Prolonged venous hypertension creates a hydrostatic profile that favors edema formation because of the transudation and exudation of macromolecules and fluid.[28] Hyperpigmentation can result from hemosiderin deposits within dermal macrophages after extravasated red blood cells are broken down.[29] Early signs of advanced disease are corona phlebectatica: numerous, fine intradermal veins overlying the medial or lateral aspects of the foot found in a fan-shaped pattern.[1] With more severe venous disease, fibrosis of the skin and subcutaneous tissue, known as lipodermatosclerosis, results secondary to localized, chronic inflammation.[1] Atrophie blanche is a localized, atrophic, white area of skin surrounded by dilated capillaries or hyperpigmentation, and is also a sign of severe CVI.[1] Venous ulceration is the most advanced form of venous disease and manifests as a full-thickness defect in the skin, with greater than 75% of lesions localized to the medial aspect of the ankle, about the distribution of the posterior arch.[27]

CLASSIFICATION

Given the panoply of signs and symptoms, the classification and treatment of CVI suffered from tremendous heterogeneity. A consensus statement regarding chronic venous disorders was released at the American Venous Forum (AVF) in 1994, which proposed a standardized categorization of chronic venous disorders based on both the clinical classification and severity of disease.[11] The CEAP system was later updated in 2004, with seven categories of clinical manifestations (C), four etiologic categories (E), four categories of anatomic distribution (A), and four basic pathophysiologic categories (P) (Table 53.1).[1] The subgroups that describe the clinical

TABLE 53.1 Classification of Chronic Venous Insufficiency

C-Clinical Class	Characteristics
0	No visible or palpable signs of venous disease
1	Telangiectasias or reticular veins
2	Varicose veins (diameter of 3 mm or more)
3	Edema
4a	Pigmentation or eczema
4b	Lipodermatosclerosis or atrophie blanche
5	Healed venous ulcer
6	Active venous ulcer
A, S	Asymptomatic, symptomatic

The CEAP system considers the clinical class, etiology (congenital, primary, and secondary), anatomy (superficial, perforator, or deep) and pathophysiology (reflux, obstruction, or both). The clinical classes are listed above. Each clinical class is characterized by the presence or absence of symptoms (A or S).

manifestations include: class 0, no visible or palpable signs of venous disease (i.e., symptoms only); class 1, telangiectasias or reticular veins; class 2, varicose veins; class 3, edema; class 4, skin changes due to venous disease; class 5, skin changes with healed ulceration; and class 6, skin changes with active ulceration. The etiologic classification includes congenital, primary, secondary (postthrombotic), or without any venous cause. Anatomic classification includes superficial, perforator, or deep veins, as well as no identifiable venous location. Finally, the basic pathophysiologic classification describes reflux, obstruction, both reflux and obstruction, or no venous pathophysiology identifiable.

In the CEAP revision the following example is offered. A patient has painful swelling of the leg, varicose veins, lipodermatosclerosis, and active ulceration. Duplex scanning shows GSV reflux above and below the knee, incompetent calf perforator veins, and axial reflux in the femoral and popliteal veins. There are no signs of postthrombotic obstruction. Classification according to basic CEAP: C6s, Ep, Aspd, Pr.[1] Of note, physician-derived CEAP scores have been demonstrated to predict both symptom severity and patient-reported quality of life.[30]

DIAGNOSIS

The Society for Vascular Surgery (SVS) and the AVF released practice guidelines for the care of patients with CVI.[31] The workup for CVI starts with a complete history and physical examination. Although there is a fair amount of variation in the presentation of this condition, there are common elements in the history that are of great use in securing the diagnosis. Symptoms include pain, sensations of heaviness, swelling, aching, restless legs, cramps, itching, throbbing, and tired legs.[2] One of the hallmarks of CVI is symptom progression throughout the day, particularly when the patient has been standing for prolonged periods of time. This is true for subjective complaints such as heaviness and fatigue, as well as more objective signs like swelling and engorged varicosities. Many patients, after determining this for themselves, will have learned to elevate their legs or have even started wearing compression stockings. Symptoms that occur during and after exercise and improve with rest and leg elevation may be indicative of venous claudication, which is due to proximal large vein obstruction rather than reflux.[32] The history may also establish whether the etiology is primary, secondary, or congenital. The history of prior DVT, hypercoagulable state, or any other factors that predispose patients to thrombosis (e.g., oral contraceptives, pregnancies, smoking), and family history of CVI or thrombotic disorders should be elicited.

The physical examination is useful not only for arriving at the diagnosis of CVI but also for determining the pattern of disease. Patients should be examined in the standing position, with attention paid to the presence of varicosities, palpable cords, tenderness, thrills, bruits, or pulsatility. The presence of telangiectasia, leg swelling, induration, hyperpigmentation, corona phlebectatica, lipodermatosclerosis, atrophie blanche, or ulceration must be carefully noted.[31] CVI can also coexist with peripheral arterial disease; therefore the pedal pulses must be assessed and documented. The saphenous veins should be examined, and if they can be seen or felt, their size and depth should be noted. For patients with numerous varicosities, a diagram can be drawn or a digital photograph taken. Swelling is best documented by taking measurements of the leg below the knee and at the ankle. The time of day of the measurements should also be recorded because there can be considerable variation, as was previously described. Finally, one must record the presence of any varicosities that have eroded or appear to be on the verge of ulcerating through the skin. If ulceration occurs, bleeding can be impressive, and patients should be instructed on how to dress their leg if this occurs.

The anatomic pattern should be established, with an attempt to determine whether signs are localized to the superficial, deep, or perforator systems; this can be accomplished with duplex ultrasonography.[31] This modality is more accurate than continuous wave Doppler ultrasound because B-mode imaging can help to identify anatomic points of obstruction or turbulence and to determine directionality of flow.[12] The SVS/AVF clinical practice guidelines describe four components of the examination: visibility, compressibility, venous flow, and augmentation.[31] In addition, confirmation of valvular incompetence should be performed in the upright position using one of the following methods. A Valsalva maneuver will increase intraabdominal pressure and should be performed in conjunction with duplex assessment of the common femoral vein or the saphenofemoral junction. Alternatively, manual or cuff compression and release of the limb distal to the point of examination can be performed to evaluate the more distal veins.[31] Many noninvasive vascular laboratories have a protocol for CVI, and the clinician should always specify why the venous examination is being ordered. The study should include all the elements of a DVT study, as well as examination of the great and SSVs. Notation should be made whether reflux occurs spontaneously, and it is useful to document the presence of reflux with the patient in a standing position. The recommended cutoff value for reflux is 1 second in the femoral and popliteal veins, whereas it is 500 ms for the great saphenous, small saphenous, tibial, deep femoral, and PVs.[31] However, many health insurers require greater times; therefore the actual time should be carefully recorded in the study. The sizes of the saphenous veins are also needed, and these structures should be measured at the level of the saphenofemoral junction, the mid thigh and just below the knee (for GSV), and at the popliteal space and ankle (for SSV). These size measurements should also be performed with the patient in a standing position. Larger varicosities should be examined as well, and reflux should be reported if present. As with the saphenous veins, the sizes of the branches need to be recorded in the study. Finally, perforator veins need to be noted in the study. Those with an outward flow of duration greater than 500 ms or a diameter greater than 3.5 mm, which are associated with a healed or open venous ulcer, are considered pathologic, but these perforators should be noted even in the absence of localized disease.[31]

The CEAP system, described earlier, should be used to determine the class, etiology, anatomy, and pathophysiologic classification of CVI.[1] An adjunct evaluative instrument, the revised Venous Clinical Severity Score (VCSS) released by Vasquez and colleagues, should also be incorporated to document the severity of CVI.[33] It generates a score based on (1) patient-reported intensity of pain or other discomfort, (2) severity of varicose veins, (3) severity of lower extremity edema, (4) degree of skin pigmentation, (5) extent of inflammation, (6) distribution of induration, (7) number of active ulcers, and (8) duration of active ulceration.[33] In conjunction, these instruments will provide unambiguous classification and a means of serial assessment for patients with CVI.

TREATMENT

For most patients the diagnosis of CVI is secured with the history, physical examination, and duplex ultrasonography. The initial therapy for the vast majority of patients with mild venous insufficiency is conservative treatment with (1) compression, (2) leg elevation, and (3) nonsteroidal antiinflammatory drugs (NSAIDs). Compression therapy exists in various forms, including elastic stockings, elastic wraps, and pneumatic compression devices, with the more compressive devices used for more advanced disease. While supine, superficial venous pressures range from 20 to 25 mm Hg, whereas, while standing, pressures can be measured as high as 100 mm Hg.[12] In the upright position, applying pressures greater than 60 mm Hg is required to occlude the superficial veins, whereas 35 to 40 mm Hg of pressure has been demonstrated to narrow them.[34] In a study of more than 100 patients, treatment with 30 to 40 mm Hg stockings in patients with CVI, described as CEAP clinical classes 0 to 6, resulted in improvement of pain, edema, skin changes, and overall well-being at 16 months.[35] However, a systematic review of compression stockings for uncomplicated varicose veins found that although compression therapy provided symptomatic relief, there was no evidence for prevention of varicose vein recurrence or cessation of disease progression.[36] The SVS/AVF Guideline Committee currently suggests stockings with an ankle pressure of 20 to 30 mm Hg for treatment of symptomatic varicose veins.[31] With more significant CVI, compression therapy is the standard of care. A systematic review of graded compression for venous ulcers confirmed that this modality improves the healing of ulcers, with greater effectiveness found with higher levels of compression.[37] Most patients with typical CVI symptoms are prescribed stockings of 20 to 30 mm Hg, with different levels of compression available for various indications (Table 53.2). The length of the garment depends on the patient's pattern of disease and the location of tender varicose branches. Typically, a stocking that is knee-high will suffice, and patients will more consistently use garments of this length instead of longer, more restrictive stockings.

As mentioned previously, many patients determine on their own that elevation is beneficial in alleviating their symptoms. As part of their conservative treatment, the physician should encourage the patient to find time to elevate his or her legs at intervals throughout the day. Many patients find that they are able to continue exercise regimens if they elevate their legs for a period of time directly following these activities. For patients with continued aching and pain, NSAIDs can be helpful and are considered an integral part of first-line conservative therapy. Additional adjuvant conservative therapy may consist of weight loss, when appropriate.

TABLE 53.2 Compression Stocking Options

Pressure	Clinical Situation
15–20 mm Hg	Mild edema, mild varicosities, aching legs
20–30 mm Hg	Advanced aching/fatigue, moderate edema, DVT prophylaxis
30–40 mm Hg	Established CVI, advanced edema, post thrombotic state
40–50 mm Hg	Severe edema, open venous ulceration
≥50 mm Hg	Severe edema not responsive to lesser pressures, severe post thrombotic syndrome

Graded compression stockings are available in a range of pressures. Venous indications for the pressures are listed above. They are also available in various lengths, from knee-high up to panty hose. Consideration should be given to the likelihood that the patient will wear the garments; a knee-high stocking is more beneficial if the patient uses it than a more restrictive appliance that is avoided. *DVT,* Deep venous thrombosis; *CVI,* chronic venous insufficiency.

Throughout the course of conservative treatment, the physician must follow the progress of the patient and note any effects of the therapy. The therapy itself can have diagnostic implications. For example, a patient who has no benefit from compressive therapy may have a different etiology for their symptoms. If a patient tries but is unable to tolerate the compression stockings, this must be clearly documented in the medical record. Patients are occasionally wary of reporting a beneficial effect of compression because they may be under the false impression that if their stockings are helpful, they will not receive any further therapy. Although most health insurers require a trial of compression therapy usually in the range of 6 weeks to 6 months, patients will usually qualify for treatment if there is an appropriate definitive therapy available.

Patients with CVI secondary to GSV or SSV incompetence may be treated with open surgery or endovenous ablation. The classic high ligation and stripping of the GSV or SSV involve division of the GSV at the junction with the common femoral vein, along with all its tributaries, and removal with a vein stripping device.[38] The incompetent vein is removed from the circulation so that passive reflux of venous pressure down the leg does not occur. However, with stripping from the groin to the ankle, saphenous nerve injury occasionally occurs, so the technique has been modified to remove the vein from the groin to the knee only.[39] Additional refinements such as microphlebectomy, sclerotherapy, and transilluminated powered phlebectomy (TIPP) for tributary (branch) varicose veins in the calf and thigh have made the procedures for branch removal less invasive.[40,41]

Over the past 15 years, endovenous interventions have replaced open surgical treatment of CVI for the vast majority of patients. These techniques reproduce the effects of high ligation and stripping of the saphenous veins and are done in a minimally invasive fashion. They are now routinely performed in an office setting under local anesthesia. Initial techniques have used thermal energy to ablate the veins, although more recent technology has incorporated the use of mechanicochemical ablation (MOCA) and nonthermal adhesive therapy. Direct thermal injury results in endothelial destruction, denatured collagen in the media, and both fibrotic and thrombotic venous occlusion.[31] The source of heat generation is either a laser fiber (endovenous laser therapy [EVLT]) or a radiofrequency generator (radiofrequency ablation [RFA]). Both of these sources of energy produce high, focused temperatures. As a result, normal body temperature can be maintained within 5 mm of an RFA catheter that is 120°C at its surface or a laser fiber with a temperature of 1000°C. This method prevents extended thermal damage to the vein and surrounding tissues (particularly the skin and adjacent nerves) during treatment.

The principles of therapy are the same for both modalities and for treatment of both the GSV and SSV. Initially, there must be confirmation that the vein is refluxing, enlarged (>4 to 5 mm with patient standing), no greater than 1.5 cm, and not excessively tortuous (which precludes catheter advancement). The vein is accessed under ultrasound guidance via Seldinger technique, usually 5 to 10 cm below the knee, and a sheath is placed in the vein. A laser fiber or RFA catheter is then advanced through the sheath under ultrasound and positioned 2 to 3 cm from either the saphenofemoral or saphenopopliteal junction. This portion of the case is done under great care, as inadvertent placement of the catheter close to the confluence with the deep system may cause damage to the deep veins. The target vein is then surrounded with tumescent anesthetic. This solution is composed of saline, lidocaine, epinephrine, and bicarbonate and accomplishes three goals: (1) anesthesia of the target area, (2) prevention of thermal injury via a heat sink, and (3) compression of the target vein. The GSV is located between layers of fascia, and the fluid can be administered between these layers such that the vein is both surrounded and depressed away from the skin to a minimal depth of 2 cm. The bed is then placed in steep Trendelenburg position to further drain the target vein. Energy is then applied while the physician provides external pressure over the segment of vein being treated. For RFA, segments of 7 cm of vein are treated for approximately 20 seconds, with retraction to the next level every 20 seconds. For the EVLT, there is continuous withdrawal of the catheter at a rate of 1 to 2 mm/s for the first 10 cm and 2 to 3 mm/s for the remaining distance. The process of actual thermal ablation is rapid and on the order of 90 to 120 seconds for both modalities. The sheath and catheter are removed, and the patient's leg is wrapped with an ace bandage for 48 hours. Patients are encouraged to ambulate in the immediate postprocedural time, although also require limb elevation following activity. Strict bed rest is discouraged because it may theoretically lead to thrombotic complications.

Newer endovenous therapies have recently been introduced to address the discomfort associated with the tumescence administration that thermal ablation requires. Their utility below the knee may also be critical in reducing the risk of saphenous nerve injury. The ClariVein occlusion catheter system (Vascular Insights, Madison, CT) uses mechanical injury and sclerosant therapy of the endothelium, thereby avoiding the use of tumescence and tissue injury related to thermal forms of closure. Fig. 53.1 shows the tip of the catheter. Care must be taken to visualize the tip via duplex ultrasonography prior to initiating treatment, because it can be difficult to see and placement too close to the saphenofemoral or saphenopopliteal junctions can lead to thrombus propagation into the deep system. Although not heat related, this thrombus appears very similar to endothermal heat-induced thrombi and appears to behave in the same manner. To date, trials have shown comparable closures of GSV and SSV. Van Eekeren and colleagues evaluated the feasibility, safety, and 1-year follow-up data for MOCA of the GSV. The technical success rate was 99%, with no major complications noted. At 1 year, there was occlusion of the GSV in 88% of patients.[42] The MARADONA trial is a randomized control trial comparing MOCA to RFA and is currently underway. Results will include 1-, 2-, and 5-year data.[43]

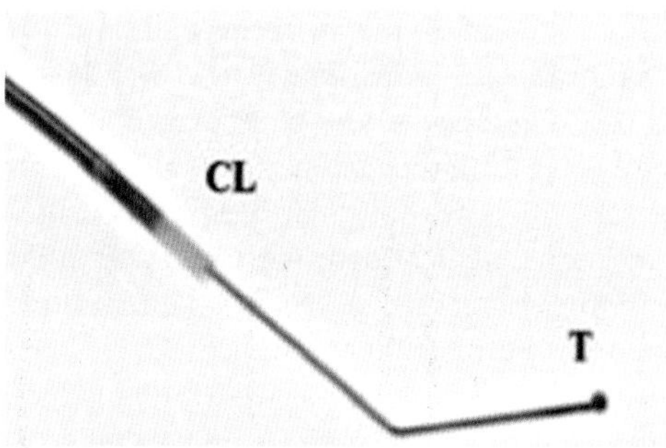

FIG 53.1 Tip of ClariVein catheter.

The other new nonthermal technique for saphenous ablation uses cyanoacrylate adhesives. The VenaSeal closure system (VSCS, Medtronic), which attained US Food and Drug Administration (FDA) approval in February 2015, is adhesive based and avoids the risks of thermal injury and the need for tumescent use. The feasibility and eSCOPE trials for this method also found no need for postoperative compression therapy.[44,45] Early results from the feasibility trial and subsequent follow-up of these patients demonstrated a closure rate of 92% up to 12 months following the procedure. The VeClose trial was a prospective randomized trial comparing RFA to Venaseal. Closure rates at 3 and 6 months were 98.9% and 98.9% for VSCS and 95.4% and 94.3% for RFA, respectively. This was statistically significant in assessing non-inferiority of Venaseal.[46]

Follow-up in most practices includes physical examination of the treated limb and a duplex ultrasound examination of the treated vein up to the saphenofemoral junction within 48 to 72 hours. For the GSV the ideal finding is an occluded GSV with a patent epigastric vein (Fig. 53.2). Complications include bruising and hematoma formation (usually associated with the injection of the tumescent anesthetic), paresthesias secondary to nerve injury, and, rarely, thermal injury to the skin. As stated earlier, a more serious complication of endovenous thermal ablation is extension of a thrombus from the GSV into the deep venous system; this has been reported with an incidence as high as 16% of procedures,[47] although in most series this number is less than 1%. Lawrence and colleagues[48] established a classification system for the level of proximal endovenous closure of the GSV and proposed a standardized treatment algorithm for thrombus extension. Closure levels were graded from levels 1 to 6, based on the extent of thrombus extension into the femoral vein, in proximity to the epigastric vein, as follows (Fig. 53.3): (1) below the epigastric vein, (2) flush with the orifice of the epigastric vein, (3) flush with the saphenofemoral junction, (4) extension into the common femoral vein, (5) past the saphenofemoral junction and adherent to the adjacent wall, and (6) into the common femoral vein—consistent with DVT. Levels 1 and 2 require no treatment; level 3 can be managed at the discretion of the physician with either observation and repeated duplex ultrasound or with low-molecular-weight heparin (LMWH); levels 4 and 5 warrant treatment with LMWH until thrombus retraction is observed; level 6 demands systemic anticoagulation for 3 months. Of the 500 patients studied, 99.6% had successful occlusion of the GSV; however, 2.6% were found to have a thrombus of level 4 or greater. The authors noted that a significantly higher rate of thrombus extension occurred in patients with a history of DVT or with a GSV diameter greater than 8 mm.[48] Although progression to true DVT and even pulmonary embolism have been reported, the thrombus following endovenous ablation is considered an endovenous heat-induced thrombus rather than a DVT because the behavior of this thrombus tends to follow a more self-limited course than does conventional thrombus (Fig. 53.4).

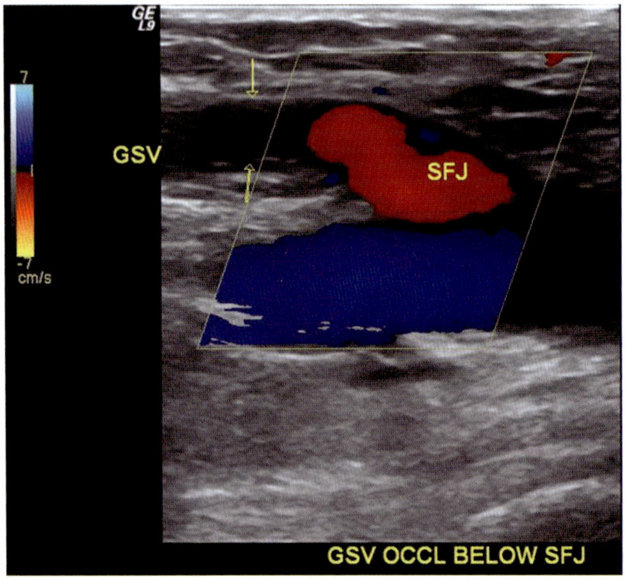

FIG 53.2 An ultrasound image obtained 48 hours after endovenous ablation of the great saphenous vein *(GSV)* is shown. The GSV is occluded, as evidenced by the lack of color flow. The saphenofemoral junction *(SFJ)* is patent, and clearly there is no involvement with the common femoral vein (*blue flow* on scan).

Long-term studies of RFA using first-generation devices have revealed occlusion rates of 87% at 1 and 5 years after the procedure in more than 1200 treated limbs.[49] They identified three types of anatomic failures, including: (1) nonocclusion owing to primary treatment failure, (2) recanalization after an initially successful ablation, and (3) groin reflux involving an accessory vein. In patients with any type of failure, they still reported improvement of pain, fatigue, and edema in 70% to 80% of limbs. This clinical symptom improvement was even greater (85% to 94% of limbs) in patients with anatomic success. The authors noted that catheter pullback speed and body mass index were significant risk factors for anatomic failure, and those with type II or III failures were prone to recurrent varicose veins.[49] A more recent report using a newer device describes occlusion rates of 99.6% at 3 days, 3 months, and 6 months, with sustained improvements in VCSSs.[50] Long-term results of EVLT reveal similar outcomes. In a study of 499 limbs, 98.2% demonstrated immediate successful GSV occlusion, and closure similarly persisted at 2 years (93.4%). Long-term studies using the newer nonthermal devices have yet to be completed, although short-term follow-up studies have shown occlusion rates similar to those of RFA and EVLT.

TREATMENT OF BRANCHES AND PERFORATORS

Many patients with CVI have large, symptomatic varicosities. During a duplex examination, an astute clinician will note that a large varicose vein branching from the saphenous system can

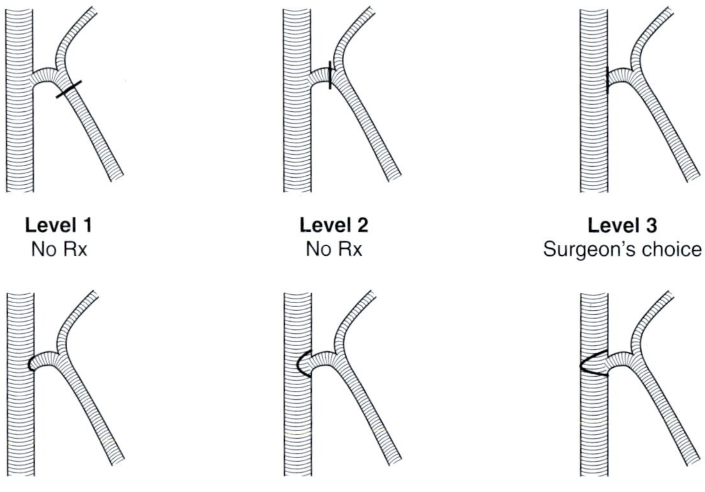

FIG 53.3 Classification of closure level and treatment algorithm. *LMWH,* Low-molecular-weight heparin; *Rx,* prescription.

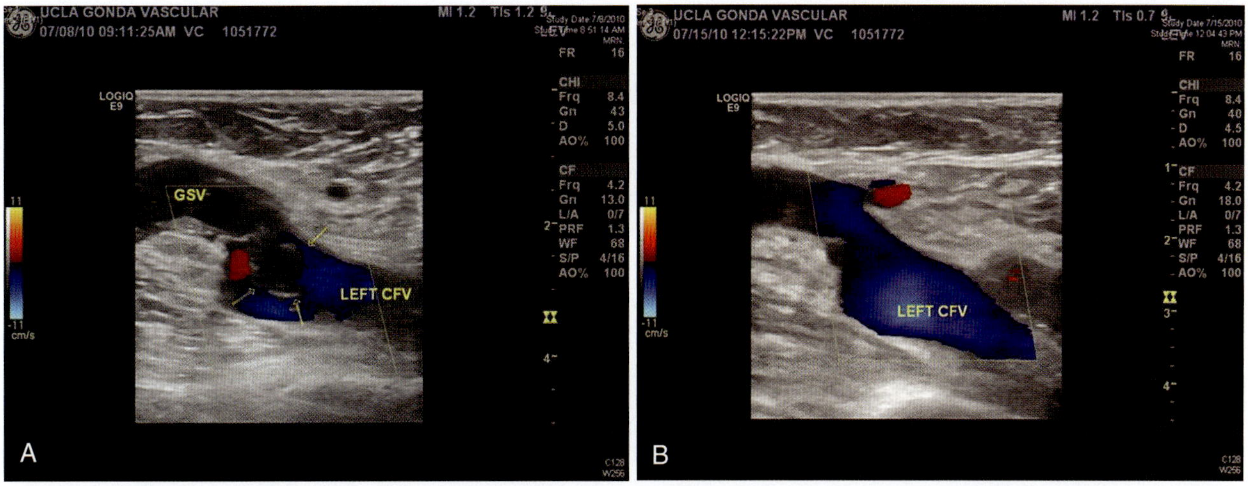

FIG 53.4 (A) Initial scan after radiofrequency ablation demonstrates thrombus extending into the common femoral vein *(CFV)*. This patient was given enoxaparin (Lovenox), and the scan was repeated 1 week later. (B) Note the complete retraction of the thrombus and patency of the epigastric vein on the follow-up scan. Lovenox was stopped after the second scan demonstrated an appropriate level of closure. Of note, most patients with level 4 and 5 closures do not have postprocedure symptoms that differ from patients with closure levels of 3 or less. *GSV*, Great saphenous vein.

essentially siphon off the majority of refluxing flow. In this situation the GSV appears enlarged down the level where the branch joins it. The GSV can all but disappear below this level, whereas the branch, now running superficial to the saphenous fascia, attains a very large size. Phlebectomy is often performed in combination with saphenous vein ablation in order to address both the varicosities and eliminate the etiologic source of reflux. These branches, if straight, can be accessed directly and treated with endovenous ablation. However, these branches are usually tortuous and must be treated using an alternate modality. For larger branches, Muller microstab phlebectomy works well.[51] Tumescent local anesthesia is injected around the veins, 2- to 3-mm incisions are made adjacent to the varicosity, and a hook-shaped instrument is inserted and used to grasp and lift the vein above the level of the skin. The branch is then gently rotated to disrupt attachments to the surrounding tissues, and gentle traction is continued until the vein avulses. Pressure is held over the site for several minutes, and a compression dressing avoids the formation of a hematoma. TIPP is an alternative technique that uses an endoscopic device with a fiberoptic light source and irrigation pump, and an endoscopic tissue dissector. A randomized trial comparing stab phlebectomy and TIPP for local avulsion of varicose veins found that patients who underwent TIPP had significantly fewer incisions; however, they reported increased bruising, prolonged pain at 6 weeks, and reduced early postoperative quality of life.[52] In contemporary venous practice, TIPP has become less commonly used.

Although the pathophysiologic role of incompetent PVs in the development of venous ulceration has been established, the indications for their ablation are unclear. Historically, to ablate these veins, large operations were required to access the subfascial anatomy. Several minimally invasive techniques are now used, including SEPS, percutaneous ablation, RFA, EVLT, and sclerotherapy. SEPS involves balloon dissection and CO_2 insufflation to access the subfascial space. A paratibial fasciotomy is necessary to identify medial PVs, and endoscopic clips or a harmonic scalpel can be used to ligate PVs. The North American SEPS Registry described the results from 17 medical centers in the United States and Canada for patients with CVI. VCSS was significantly improved in most patients, and cumulative ulcer healing was 88% by 1 year and 95% by 2 years.[53] In subgroup analysis, they also examined patients who underwent SEPS without saphenous vein ablation. They still identified significant improvements in clinical scores but also identified significantly reduced cumulative ulcer healing at 1 year (78%) and 2 years (88%). A systematic review of outcomes in patients undergoing treatment for CVI by SEPS (both with and without saphenous vein ablation) similarly described healing of ulcers in 88% of treated limbs, with 13% recurrence at a mean of 21 months. However, the authors qualified their recommendations because of the study's inability to discern the contribution of saphenous vein closure or compression therapy.

More recent data suggest a demonstrable connection between the treatment of incompetent perforator veins and venous ulcer healing. In a study looking at recalcitrant venous ulceration, patients who underwent ablation of their perforator veins had a 90% healing rate, and this was in patients undergoing intensive wound care both before and after their perforator treatment.[54] Additional studies with detailed mapping of the wound healing process have confirmed these findings (Fig. 53.5).[55]

SCLEROTHERAPY

Another alternative for the treatment of both varicose branches and smaller spider and reticular veins is sclerotherapy. In this treatment the vein is injected with a detergent solution (e.g., polidocanol, sodium morrhuate, sodium tetradecyl sulfate [STS]), osmotic sclerosant (e.g., hypertonic saline), or alcohol agent (e.g.,

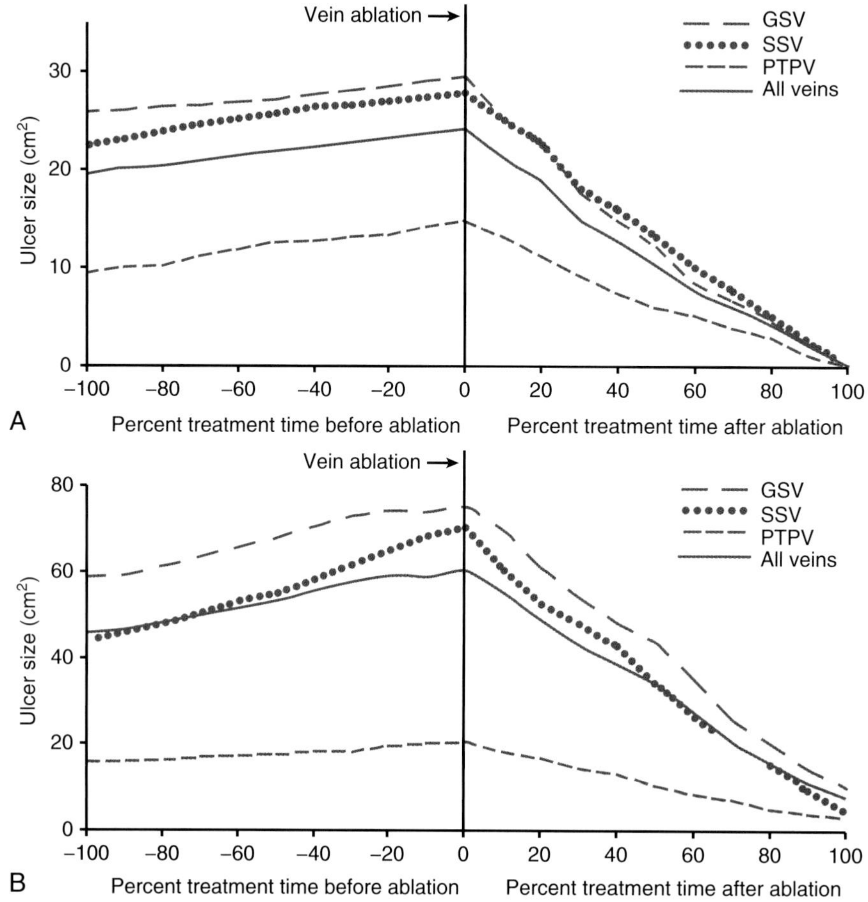

FIG 53.5 (A) The healing rate for venous ulcers that have achieved complete resolution. Ulcer size increased during compression therapy before ablation and decreased after ablation. (B) The healing rate for venous ulcers that have not resolved. These patients started with venous ulcers that were more than twice as large as those that completely healed during the study. As with the healed ulcers, the size increased before ablation, with a similar healing trend seen post ablation. *GSV*, Great saphenous vein; *PTPV*, posterior tibial perforating vein; *SSV*, small saphenous vein.

chromated or nonchromated glycerin). The material damages the endothelium in the target vessel and exposes subendothelial collagen fibers, leading eventually to obliteration.[31] Hypertonic saline is used in a concentration of 23.4% and results in osmotic dehydration of endothelial cells followed by cell death. Polidocanol is the most commonly used agent and is injected in concentrations between 0.6% and 3%, depending on the size of the vein. STS is used in concentrations of 0.125% to 3% in a similar fashion. These agents are injected intraluminally, starting proximally, with a maximum volume of 1 mL per site, and no more than 20 injections per session.[56] A multicenter, randomized trial comparing 0.5% polidocanol and 0.25% STS for the treatment of telangiectasia and reticular veins demonstrated superiority of polidocanol in terms of effectiveness and patient satisfaction.[57] Sclerotherapy has been used primarily for closure of spider veins or telangiectasia, but foam sclerotherapy has been found to be a safe and effective method to treat varicose veins. A ratio of 1 part STS or polidocanol to 4 parts air is mixed, using a three-way stopcock connected to two syringes.[58] The veins are injected starting with the saphenous trunk, followed by varicose and PVs, and a maximum of 20 mL is injected per session. After both liquid and foam sclerotherapy, patients are then instructed to wear 30- to 40-mm Hg graduated compression stockings for 1 to 2 weeks. A multicenter, randomized trial was conducted to compare 3% polidocanol in foam or liquid forms for treatment of primary varicose veins because of an incompetent GSV.[59] They reported elimination of reflux in 69% and 27% of patients who underwent foam or liquid sclerotherapy, respectively. These procedures can also be performed under ultrasound guidance, and there are advocates of using foam sclerotherapy for treatment of everything from the refluxing saphenous veins and their associated branches to perforator veins and spider veins. At this time, insurance coverage varies widely, with many plans denying use of sclerotherapy because of the lack of a randomized prospective trial demonstrating rates of venous closure commiserate with that achieved by endovenous ablation.

CONCLUSIONS

CVI and varicose veins are common conditions with underappreciated clinical sequelae. Newer technologies allow the modern clinician to approach these disorders with an array of minimally invasive therapies that are especially useful in a patient population that is frequently young, working, and active. Developing a practice to care for varicose veins requires the clinician to develop the skills to interpret venous duplex scans, both for diagnosis and during treatment. An understanding of the pathophysiology behind the disorder allows the clinician to appropriately diagnose and treat CVI with techniques that are both acceptable to the patients and successful in correcting the disorder.

REVIEW QUESTIONS

1. Which of the following situations is most closely associated with endovenous heat-induced thrombosis (EHIT)?
   a. History of superficial thrombophlebitis
   b. Reflux in both the superficial and deep systems
   c. Double treatment with laser or radiofrequency catheter along entire length of vein
   d. 18-mm diameter of saphenous vein at level of saphenofemoral junction
   e. Use of oral contraceptive pills
2. Which of the following statements is true?
   a. There is greater anatomic variation at the saphenofemoral junction than the saphenopopliteal junction.
   b. The vein of Giacomini provides a direct connection between the greater saphenous vein and the deep system of the thigh.
   c. There are no valves in the popliteal veins.
   d. Perforator vein flow should be superficial to deep in normal flow conditions.
   e. The posterior and anterior arch veins typically arise above the knee.
3. Which of the following is true regarding the CEAP classification system?
   a. CEAP class 3 represents edema.
   b. CEAP 4b represents eczema
   c. The etiologic classification includes congenital as a criterion.
   d. CEAP class 2 requires varicose veins greater than 2 mm in size.
   e. Patients with healed ulcers are CEAP class 5.
4. Which of the following is a component of treatment for reflux disease?
   a. Leg elevation
   b. Compression stockings
   c. Manual massage of the lower extremities
   d. Nonsteroidal antiinflammatory agents
   e. Endovenous ablation.
5. With regard to endovenous ablation, the role of tumescent anesthesia is:
   a. not needed with EVLT
   b. only needed when treating the entire length of saphenous vein
   c. to deaden sensory nerves running inside the saphenous vein
   d. helpful for draining blood from the saphenous vein
   e. not needed if adequate Trendelenburg position is attained.
6. A postendovenous ablation scan demonstrates a level 2 closure. This patient:
   a. needs a follow-up scan within a week.
   b. needs to start low-molecular-weight heparin and then Coumadin.
   c. should have a hypercoaguable workup initiated.
   d. needs no further treatment.
   e. should be placed on periprocedural Lovenox if the contralateral leg is treated.
7. Which of the following regarding perforator veins is true?
   a. Refluxing perforator veins are a common cause of CEAP class 2 disease.
   b. Treatment always requires open surgical ligation.
   c. Perforator reflux should be dealt with before saphenous reflux.
   d. Foam sclerotherapy is more effective than laser for treating perforator reflux.
   e. Perforator treatment is usually indicated in patients with CEAP 5 or 6 disease.
8. Which of the following is not a consideration when planning endovenous ablation?
   a. Use of compression stockings
   b. Depth of the target vein
   c. Ability of patient to tolerate epinephrine containing tumescence.
   d. Tortuosity of target vein
   e. Age of patient
9. Which of the following has not been reported following endovenous ablation?
   a. Sural nerve injury
   b. Arterial thrombosis
   c. Acute suppurative thrombophlebitis
   d. Pulmonary embolism
   e. Skin burns
10. Which of the below agents is a detergent used for sclerotherapy?
    a. Glycerin
    b. Hypertonic saline
    c. Polidocanol
    d. Doxycycline
    e. Lidocaine

References available online at ExpertConsult.com.

54 CHAPTER

Management of Venous Leg Ulcers

Peter F. Lawrence, Steven M. Farley

A venous leg ulcer is defined as "an open skin lesion of the leg or foot that occurs in an area of venous hypertension." Venous ulcers are one of the most common chronic vascular diseases: they are estimated to have a prevalence in the United States of approximately 1%, and the frequency of venous leg ulcers increases with age.[1] Once a venous ulcer occurs, the average time to healing is 22 months, and approximately 5% of patients who develop a venous ulcer never heal, due to patient factors such as obesity or poor compliance, as well as health care system factors, such as inappropriate management or uncoordinated care. The monthly cost of treatment of a venous ulcer is approximately $2500 until healed.

These staggering statistics indicate that venous ulcers are one of the most common and costly medical conditions in the United States, and the American health care system spends a huge amount of its health care dollars trying to heal venous ulcers. One of the reasons ulcers do not heal is that the recent advances in venous ulcer diagnosis and management have not been disseminated to all health care providers, so many venous ulcer patients are receiving outdated venous ulcer care.

VENOUS ANATOMY AND PHYSIOLOGY RELATED TO VENOUS ULCERS

The physiologic principle central to understanding the etiology of venous ulcers is that they occur only due to "ambulatory superficial venous hypertension." This hypertension can be due to valvular incompetence in the deep, perforator, or superficial system, or from occluded deep veins, and the high pressure in the deep system is transmitted to the superficial system, resulting in localized venous hypertension in the skin and subcutaneous tissue. Clinically, a leg with ambulatory superficial venous hypertension becomes hardened and pigmented and is described as having lipodermatosclerosis. The location of the lipodermatosclerosis is primarily in the "gaiter zone" of the ankle, which is both the most dependent portion of the leg when standing, leading to the highest venous pressures, as well as being closest to the largest cluster of perforator veins that transmit the pressure to the superficial system. Formerly called "Cockett" perforators, these perforator veins are currently identified by the distance from the sole of the foot. To help identify the location of leg perforator veins that may need treatment, Geza and Gloviczki[2] dissected all superficial and perforating veins in the leg and identified the most common locations (Fig. 54.1), including those arising from the posterior arch vein, paratibial perforators, and connecting veins between perforator veins and other tributary veins. They found that very few perforator veins connect to the saphenous veins, which is the reason why stripping or ablation of the saphenous veins does not eliminate incompetent perforator veins that transmit the high venous pressure and cause venous ulcers.

DIAGNOSIS OF VENOUS ULCERS

The combination of physical exam and duplex ultrasound is the best method of diagnosing the presence of venous disease in a patient with a leg ulcer, to determine the extent of venous disease, the need for any further workup, and indications for treatment. The initial evaluation should determine not only if a venous ulcer is present but also if there are other diseases or conditions which coexist, such as diabetes, arterial insufficiency, and infection. In addition, the age of the ulcer, its depth and appearance, and the previous treatments to heal the ulcer, as well as initiating factors, such as trauma, biopsy, or chronic edema, all contribute to understanding how the ulcer developed, how it has been treated, and why it has not healed. A photograph of the ulcer (Fig. 54.2) is useful to document its size and depth as well as the extent of edema and infection; the photo can also be used for planimetry, which is a precise measurement of venous ulcer dimensions.

IMAGING OF VENOUS ULCERS

Duplex ultrasound is the best method for determining whether chronic venous insufficiency is causing a venous leg ulcer. It is a cost-effective, accessible, and accurate diagnostic tool. When further anatomic definition is needed, particularly of the deep veins above the inguinal ligament, computed tomography (CT) venography or magnetic resonance (MR) venography may be used to supplement ultrasound. Intravascular ultrasound (IVUS) is an additional imaging modality used to determine the degree of iliac vein and vena caval stenosis by providing three-dimensional images, but it requires puncture of the femoral vein and therefore is primarily used during venous stenting procedures.

The duplex ultrasound should be done using standardized diagnostic protocols by technologists trained in the appropriate techniques. Ultrasound of the deep, superficial, and perforator veins must be performed to determine the location and extent of venous incompetence. Color Doppler and pulsed wave Doppler

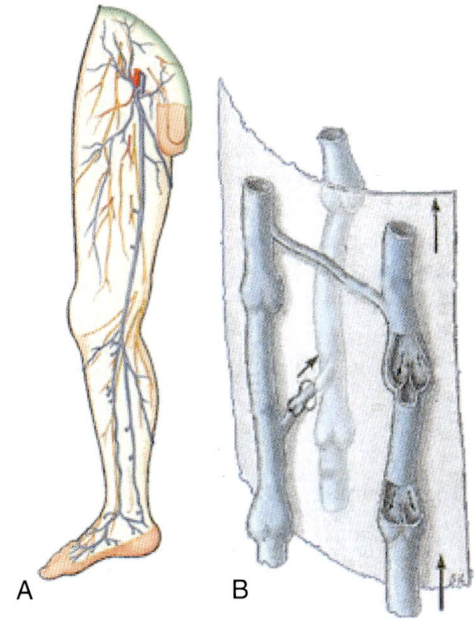

FIG 54.1 (A) Superficial venous anatomy of the leg, showing that the perforator veins arise off of the posterior and anterior arch veins, rather than the saphenous vein. (B) Connections between veins include both superficial veins to other superficial veins and from superficial veins to deep veins.

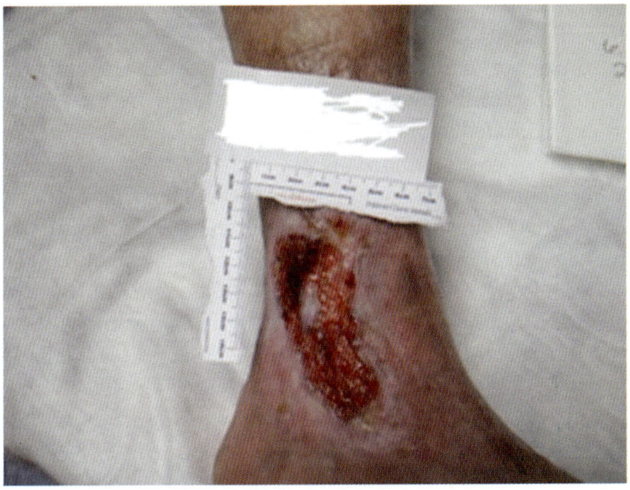

FIG 54.2 A photo of a typical appearing venous ulcer of the ankle can be useful for both initial measurements and determining healing rate.

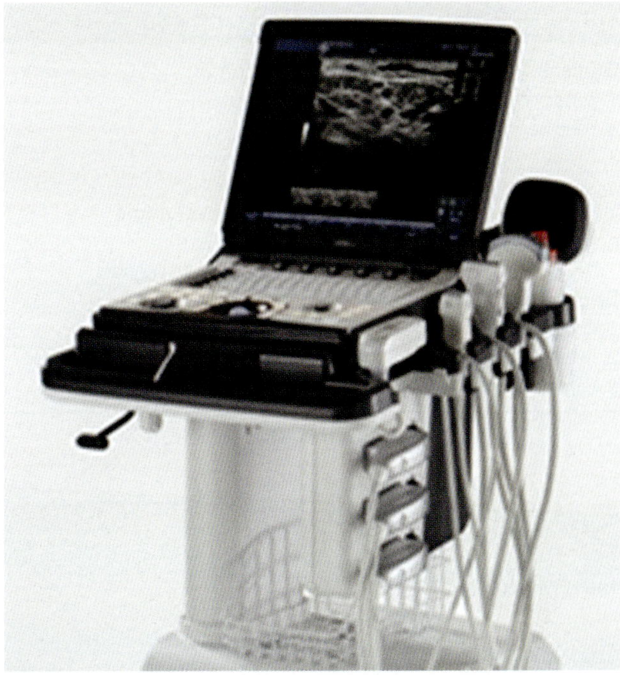

FIG 54.3 Duplex ultrasound equipment for venous disease diagnosis and endovenous procedures include 6 to 12 MHz transducers, which will image most leg veins, whereas 4 MHz transducers are better for iliac and abdominal veins.

BOX 54.1 Duplex Ultrasound Evaluation Assessment of Venous Leg Ulcers

1. Measurement of diameter and duration of reflux of each superficial vein
2. Identification of tributary veins that are adjacent to the venous ulcer
3. Documentation of refluxing perforating veins adjacent to the venous ulcer
4. Determination of deep venous reflux in the common femoral, femoral, and popliteal veins
5. Assessment of signals in the common femoral vein

with a linear 7.5 to 10 MHz transducer can directly visualize flow and venous reflux (Fig. 54.3). The examination must include evaluation of the common femoral vein and other deep veins, saphenous veins, perforator veins, and tributaries (Box 54.1). Indirect evidence of proximal iliac vein or vena cava obstruction can also be assessed by duplex ultrasound of the common femoral vein, where loss of normal respiratory cycling and loss of augmentation with compression occur with proximal venous disease. In this same region the saphenofemoral junction should be assessed for reflux, and, if reflux is present, the great saphenous vein should then be evaluated along its course for patency and duration of reflux, as well as looking for any incompetent accessory, perforator, or tributary veins. When patients have lateral ankle ulcers, the popliteal fossa should also be assessed for small saphenous vein incompetence. After the truncal and deep veins have been evaluated, the calf veins, including the deep and perforator veins, should be evaluated for reflux, as well as any tributary veins near the ulcer. Duplex ultrasound criteria for abnormal veins in patients with venous leg ulcers include incompetence of the deep system (veins with a maximum vein diameter >3.5 mm and reflux >1 second) and superficial and perforator veins incompetence with a vein diameter greater than 3.5 mm and reflux greater than 500 ms.

CLASSIFICATION OF VENOUS ULCERS

The CEAP (Clinical Etiologic Anatomic Pathophysiologic) classification system[3] was developed to standardize venous diagnosis and treatment when caring for patients with venous insufficiency

BOX 54.2 CEAP Classification

Clinical
1. Telangiectasias (spider veins)
2. Varicose veins
3. Edema
4. Lipodermatosclerosis
5. Healed venous ulcer
6. Open venous ulcer

Etiologic
1. Primary
2. Secondary
3. Congenital

Anatomic
1. Superficial
2. Deep
3. Perforator

Pathophysiologic
1. Reflux
2. Obstruction
3. Reflux + obstruction

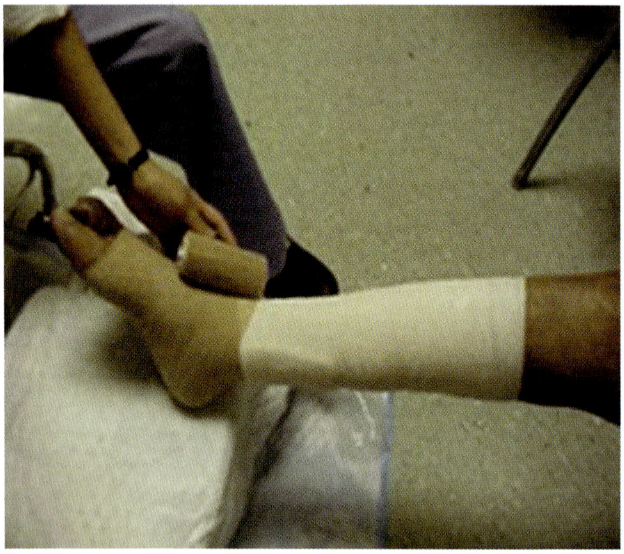

FIG 54.4 Compression of a venous ulcer is the mainstay of therapy and is often used in conjunction with other procedures that eliminate reflux from the deep to the superficial system. Approximately 30 to 40 mm Hg of pressure, uniformly applied, are required to promote wound healing.

(Box 54.2). Venous ulcers are classified as CEAP 6, and once they heal, they are moved to the CEAP 5 classification level. The CEAP clinical classification score can most precisely be defined after imaging of the superficial, deep, and perforator veins of the leg with duplex ultrasound.

TREATMENT

The mainstay of treatment for venous ulcers is compression, which both prevents venous ulcers, facilitates healing, and prevents recurrence (Fig. 54.4). Compression can be provided by medicated short stretch gauze wraps, multilayer semistretch wraps, or compression stockings, measured at a minimum of 30 to 40 mm Hg pressure. There are also reusable inelastic segmental straps that allow patients to apply and adjust them to provide proper pressure. The greatest challenge with compression is patient compliance. In a landmark study,[4] published a number of years ago, but as relevant today as in the past, patients who faithfully used compression had an approximately 80% probability of healing their ulcers and keeping them healed, whereas those who are noncompliant have less than 50% probability of venous ulcers healing and staying healed.

When patients have an open venous ulcer (CEAP 6) in addition to compression, some clinicians use topical agents, such as antibiotics, growth factors, and fluid absorbents, to facilitate healing. Although there are many products available, the one consistently successful treatment of venous wounds has been aggressive débridement, usually with a curette, which stimulates intrinsic growth factors and wound closure. There is also evidence that skin and dermal substitutes facilitate wound closure after the venous hypertension is corrected, but they are costly, often not covered by health plans, and therefore used primarily in patients with recalcitrant wounds that have delayed healing.

TRUNCAL (GREAT SAPHENOUS AND SMALL SAPHENOUS) VEIN ENDOVENOUS TREATMENT

There are both thermal and nonthermal devices available for the treatment of incompetent axial veins, which is the initial step in healing venous ulcers.[5] The truncal vein to be treated, whether it is the great saphenous, small saphenous, a duplicated saphenous vein, or an accessory saphenous vein, is imaged from its junction with the deep venous system to the site distally in the leg where it becomes normal in size and without reflux. The site for access to the vein and sheath placement is selected so that the entire incompetent vein can be treated. Distal incompetent veins, in the region of the ankle, should be treated only if they are located in the region of the ulceration because sensory nerves run alongside the veins in the ankle and calf region.

The vein is accessed and a sheath or catheter placed in the incompetent vein while the patient is in the Trendelenburg position (Fig. 54.5). A catheter is advanced up the vein and parked 2 to 3 cm from the deep venous junction. The vein is then treated and confirmation of its closure and absence of flow within it confirmed with duplex ultrasound. Compression is applied to the path of the vein for several days to reduce the likelihood of painful superficial phlebitis. Successful closure of the vein can be confirmed from days to weeks after treatment.

POTENTIAL COMPLICATIONS FOLLOWING ENDOVENOUS ABLATION

Patients with significant postoperative pain or swelling and those who have high risk factors for deep venous thrombosis (DVT) should undergo duplex ultrasound to assess the site of the endovenous procedure for hematoma or excessive superficial branch or truncal vein thrombus, and to evaluate the deep venous system adjacent to the ablated vein for thrombus and/or extension of superficial thrombus into the deep venous system, called endovenous heat-induced thrombosis (EHIT). Differentiating EHIT from DVT clinically is difficult, unless ultrasound is used to image the site of concern, but there are significant differences between EHIT, DVT, or other causes of persistent pain, such as hematoma or superficial thrombophlebitis, all of which may all

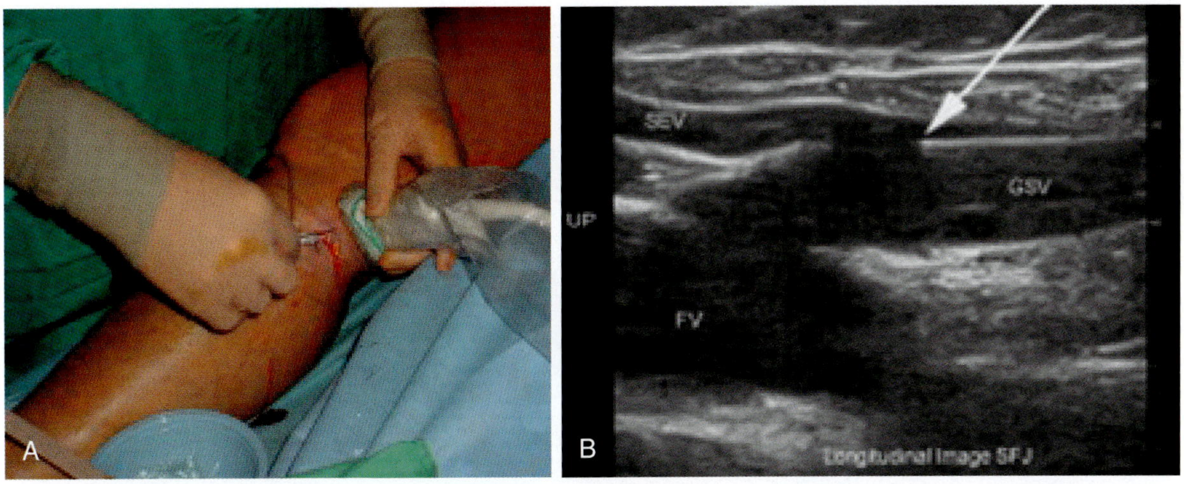

FIG 54.5 (A) Ablation of the saphenous vein is accomplished by placing a guidewire, followed by a sheath, followed by the catheter into the vein. (B) Catheter tip is seen *(arrow)*, properly placed, adjacent to the epigastric vein and 2 cm from the junction with the femoral vein *(FV)*. After tumescence is placed around the saphenous vein, the vein is ablated with heat throughout its course and the catheter is then removed. *GSV,* Great saphenous vein; *SEV,* superficial epigastric vein.

occur. Even though the risk of EHIT is low (<2%), it is a common concern of most treating physicians.

The approach to EHIT has been controversial because some surgeons do not perform routine postprocedure ultrasound to determine if EHIT is present, whereas others perform it routinely. A taskforce of the American Venous Forum is currently developing guidelines for EHIT and to determine when, if ever, EHIT screening is indicated. However, symptomatic patients with leg pain and swelling should be managed like any postoperative patient who has symptoms in a treated leg, with a physical examination, appropriate imaging, and treatment, based on the findings of the ultrasound exam. If a significant portion of the deep venous system is occluded with thrombus, patients should be treated with anticoagulation and followed for extension or retraction of the thrombus. When the thrombus has retracted into the treated vein, anticoagulation can be discontinued. Long-term anticoagulation is not required for EHIT, because the thrombus is not attached to the deep vein wall and therefore that wall does not remain thrombogenic.

ENDOVENOUS PERFORATOR VEIN TREATMENT

Since Linton's original description of the "Linton procedure," it has been known that incompetent perforator veins create ambulatory venous hypertension and prevent wound healing, and that closure of these perforator veins is based on the theory that perforator reflux is the primary problem. Unfortunately, Linton not only ligated perforator veins using a long leg incision, but he also ligated the refluxing femoral vein, which created more venous hypertension. Modifications in the Linton approach have evolved, from long incision that is difficult to heal, to endoscopic perforator vein ligation, to the current approach, in which all incompetent perforator veins are closed with an endovenous approach, using radiofrequency energy, a laser, foam sclerotherapy, or mechanical ablation. The endovenous approach[6] now allows these procedures to be performed in an ambulatory setting, which makes them very appealing to patients and very cost effective.

TECHNIQUE OF PERFORATOR VEIN TREATMENT

The incompetent perforator veins must be identified at the time of the procedure and compared with any prior duplex ultrasound to confirm location. The best system is to measure each incompetent perforator vein from the sole of the foot (e.g., 17-cm perforator) and from a bony landmark, such as the tibia (for medial perforators) or fibula (for lateral perforators). It is not uncommon for patients with venous ulcers to have two or three incompetent perforators, some of which are difficult to identify during the procedure. During the perforator ablation procedure, ultrasound must be used to guide needle or trocar placement into the perforator vein (Fig. 54.6) and during treatment of the vein. Duplex ultrasound can also be used to visualize thermal catheters while treating a perforator vein and to confirm the effect of the catheter and solution at the tip of the catheter during treatment.

The technique of endovenous perforation ablation, whether by sclerotherapy, thermal ablation with laser or radiofrequency energy, or with nonthermal techniques such as glue or foam, depends on the accurate identification of the junction of the perforator vein, before it branches or bifurcates, with the leg fascia. All techniques depend on the identification of this site, followed by placement of a needle within the vein at this level. If the perforator vein is treated below the fascia, there is a risk that a deep vein will thrombose, leading to calf vein thrombosis. In addition, there is a risk of tibial nerve injury because this nerve is adjacent to the deep veins. When the treatment of the perforator vein is performed too far above the fascia, the vein has often already bifurcated or branched, so that the entire field of the perforator vein is not treated and there may be continued

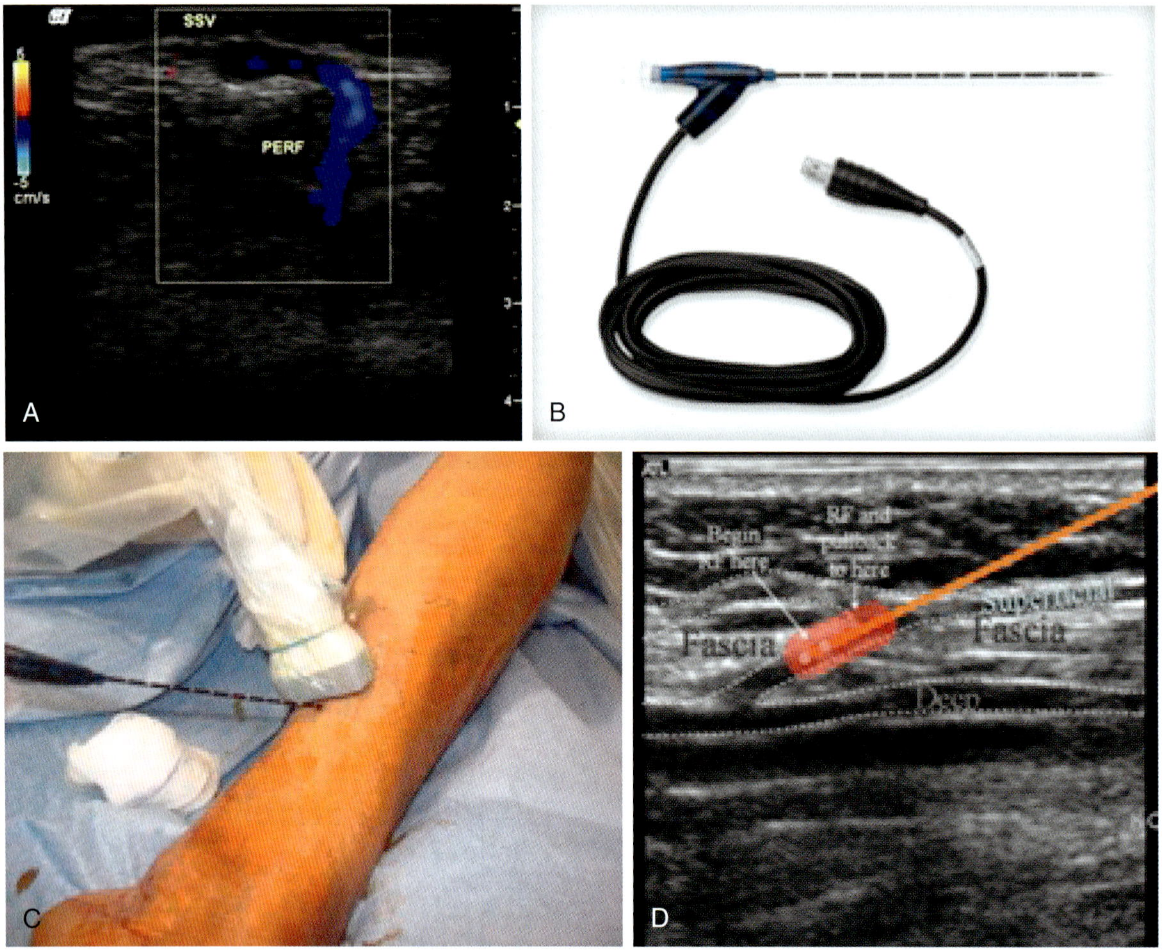

FIG 54.6 (A) A perforator *(PERF)* vein is seen passing through the fascia of the leg. (B) A radiofrequency catheter is used to ablate an incompetent perforator vein. (C) Ultrasound-guided placement of a trocar into a perforator vein. (D) The proper position for the catheter is with the tip at the level of the fascia and in the center of the perforator vein. The *red zone* indicates the area of the perforator vein to be treated, and the *orange line* simulates the catheter. Ablation in each quadrant can now be performed. *RF,* Radiofrequency; *SSV,* small saphenous vein.

reflux into parts of the superficial system. Consequently, precise placement of every treatment device used for disconnecting the deep from the superficial veins requires that the incompetent perforator vein be treated at the level of the fascia. In addition, there is recent interest in filling the remaining incompetent superficial venous plexus directly above the perforator vein and below the venous ulcer with sclerosing solution, and duplex ultrasound can visualize this plexus while foam, glue, or sclerosant fills it. It is important that the solution fills the entire plexus but does not reflux into the deep veins

CONFIRMATION OF SUCCESS FOLLOWING ENDOVENOUS PROCEDURES

Successful endovenous procedures are measured by complete occlusion of the treated vein (Fig. 54.7). If there are persistent ulcers or recurrence of a venous ulcer, this may require a second procedure to close any remaining refluxing veins. If a venous ulcer does not heal, it is important to determine if the vein that was treated has closed and remains closed.

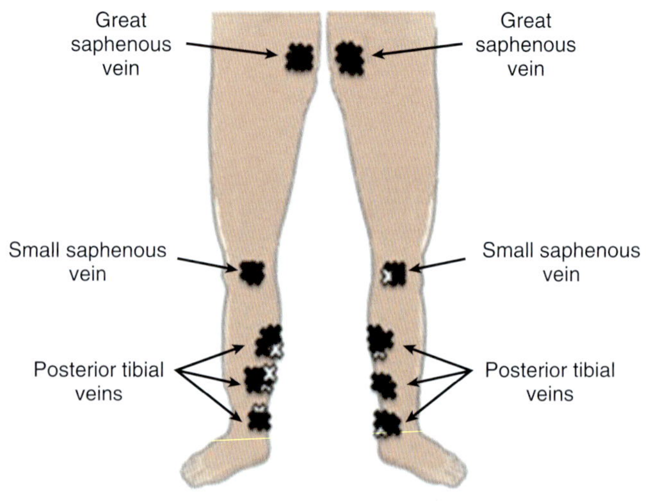

FIG 54.7 The locations of incompetent veins in patients with CEAP 6 nonhealed venous ulcers are shown as *x,* with those successfully closed *blackened* and those unsuccessfully closed shown as *white x. CEAP,* Clinical Etiologic Anatomic Pathophysiologic.

PROXIMAL VENOUS PROCEDURES FOR TREATMENT OF VENOUS ULCERS

The importance of proximal stenotic or occlusive deep venous disease in patients with chronic venous insufficiency, and the need to correct it, has been reported by Raju and colleagues.[7] They have emphasized imaging techniques to identify proximal disease, as well as the method of correcting it, whether due to external compression or postthrombotic disease, with proximal venous balloon angioplasty and stent. They have also emphasized the critical role of proximal venous stenosis or occlusions over infrainguinal reflux in patients with venous insufficiency. Marston[8] looked specifically at venous leg ulcers and found that more than 50% have a greater than 50% iliac stenosis and 25% have greater than a 75% iliac stenosis. DeRubertis and Rollo[9] have reported on a simple algorithm and technique to stent the proximal iliac stenosis or occlusion, whether the etiology is postthrombotic or May-Thurner syndrome. Fig. 54.8 shows the compression of the iliac vein, which can be managed by treating the proximal venous stenosis with a stent.

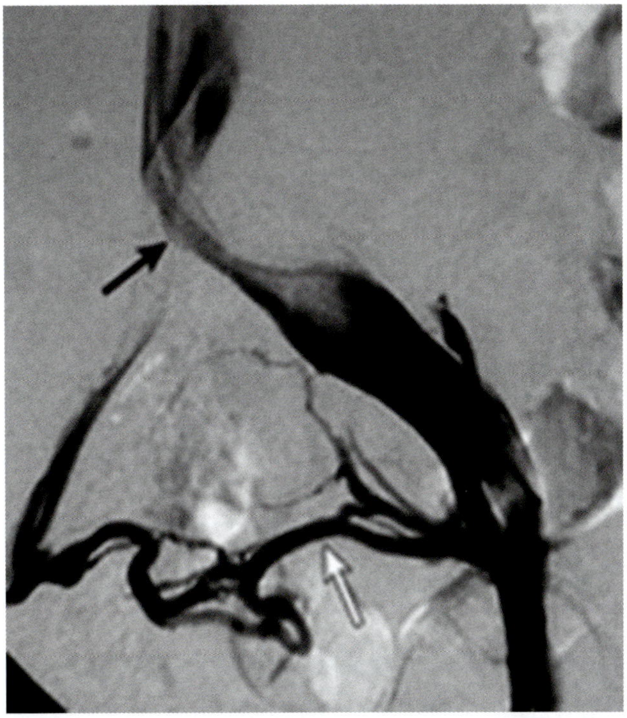

FIG 54.8 The *black arrow* denotes proximal left iliac venous stenosis causing venous hypertension is shown in this venogram of May-Thurner syndrome. The *white arrow* demonstrates large collaterals, which have developed in response to the venous hypertension.

VENOUS BYPASS

Occasionally, proximal iliac occlusions cannot be treated with an endovascular approach, and bypass of the proximal deep venous system is required to eliminate proximal venous hypertension. The practice guidelines of the American Venous Forum/Society for Vascular Surgery[1] suggest that a venous bypass be performed with saphenous vein or polytetrafluoroethylene, from one femoral vein to another, or from the femoral vein to the iliac vein or vena cava, with or without an arteriovenous fistula to improve graft patency.

CONCLUSIONS

The healing of a venous ulcer requires a multipronged approach, with control of swelling using compression, elimination of superficial venous reflux, elimination of perforator reflux, and elimination of proximal deep venous stenosis or occlusion. Compliance by patients is critical, particularly with compression, and most studies that have followed patients closely have emphasized how rarely patients are truly compliant. After the hemodynamics have been corrected, then local wound care is required for skin closure and healing, and after skin healing occurs, the leg must be protected to prevent the recurrence of superficial ambulatory venous hypertension and eventual reulceration. With our current understanding of chronic venous disease, a compliant patient, and facility with the many treatment options currently available, most patients with venous leg ulcers can both heal them and maintain healing.

REVIEW QUESTIONS

1. The cause of venous leg ulcers is:
   - **a.** Trauma to pigmented skin
   - **b.** Deep venous obstruction
   - **c.** Superficial venous insufficiency
   - **d.** Ambulatory superficial venous hypertension
   - **e.** Supine deep venous hypertension
2. The best screening test for patient with a venous ulcer to determine the treatment options is:
   - **a.** Trendelenburg test
   - **b.** Marginal ulcer biopsy
   - **c.** Computed tomography (CT) venogram
   - **d.** Ankle pressure study
   - **e.** Duplex ultrasound
3. The initial treatment of a patient with a venous leg ulcer should be:
   - **a.** local wound care
   - **b.** compression of the leg
   - **c.** ablation of all incompetent veins
   - **d.** stenting of the left iliac vein
   - **e.** antibiotics orally or topically

4. The treatment of iliac venous stenosis or occlusion by stenting should be performed:
   - **a.** Only in patients with femoral vein pressures greater than 30 mm Hg
   - **b.** Only in patients with demonstrated collateral veins
   - **c.** Only in patients with a stenosis demonstrated on IVUS
   - **d.** Only in patients who have had treatment of the incompetent superficial veins
   - **e.** Only in patients with a recalcitrant nonhealing venous ulcer
5. Patients who undergo ablation of an incompetent saphenous vein for a nonhealing venous ulcer will:
   - **a.** Uniformly heal the ulcer
   - **b.** Heal the ulcer if there is no other superficial or deep venous reflux
   - **c.** Heal the ulcer without compression
   - **d.** Rarely heal the ulcer
   - **e.** Heal the ulcer if a compression garment is worn
6. Ablation of an incompetent perforator vein in a patient with a venous ulcer should not be performed with:
   - **a.** A stocking seam incision
   - **b.** Laser
   - **c.** Radiofrequency
   - **d.** Foam sclerotherapy
   - **e.** Mechanicochemical ablation (MOCA)
7. Iliac stenosis in a patient with a venous ulcer is:
   - **a.** Rare
   - **b.** Most commonly due to May-Thurner syndrome
   - **c.** Usually eliminated with stenting
   - **d.** Usually cured with balloon angioplasty
   - **e.** Requires a drug-eluting stent
8. Open surgical bypass for a chronic iliac venous occlusion:
   - **a.** Should never be performed
   - **b.** Is more durable that stenting
   - **c.** Requires a prosthetic bypass graft for long-term patency
   - **d.** Can be performed from the common femoral vein to the vena cava
   - **e.** Requires a permanent AV fistula for long-term patency
9. Healing with compression of a venous ulcer in a compliant patient is:
   - **a.** Approximately 10% long term
   - **b.** Greater than 90% long term
   - **c.** Dependent on the status of reflux in the calf veins
   - **d.** Approximately 70%
   - **e.** Associated with a recurrence rate of greater than 80%
10. The best topical treatment associated with venous ulcer wound healing is:
    - **a.** Antibiotics
    - **b.** Skin substitutes
    - **c.** Electrical stimulation
    - **d.** Balneotherapy
    - **e.** Skin grafting

References available online at ExpertConsult.com.

CHAPTER 55

Portal Hypertension

Rameen S. Moridzadeh, David A. Rigberg, Hugh A. Gelabert

Portal hypertension and variceal hemorrhage are important clinical problems in which vascular surgeons may still have a significant interest and concern. New developments have altered the once-familiar approach to this disease, with endoscopic and endovascular approaches having replaced what was once treated predominantly with open surgical procedures. Orthotopic liver transplantation has also become a vital component in treating this disease in appropriately selected patients.

For a surgeon to have a role in treating these patients, it is important to understand the underlying liver disease, the pathophysiology of portal hypertension, and the alternative management options for variceal hemorrhage and portal hypertension.

DEFINITION

Portal hypertension is a condition in which the normal circulation of blood in the portal venous system is impeded, resulting in an increase in portal venous pressure. Elevation of the portal venous blood pressure results in a series of physiologic alterations, including ascites, hypersplenism, and variceal hemorrhage. Normal portal venous pressure is between 5 and 10 mm Hg. Portal hypertension is present when portal pressure is elevated above 15 mm Hg. Clinically significant portal hypertension exists when the portal pressure is elevated more than 10 mm Hg above systemic pressure in the inferior vena cava (corrected portal pressure).

The natural history of patients with portal hypertension differs, depending on the cause of the condition and the stage of presentation. The patient's ability to withstand the stress of hemorrhage or surgery largely depends on the functional hepatic reserve.

PATHOGENESIS

Physiologically, portal hypertension results from either an increase in the portal blood flow (rare) or an obstruction to the outflow of blood from the portal circulation (common). Obstructions to the portal circulation have been classified anatomically based on their location relative to the hepatic sinusoids. Accordingly, the obstruction may be presinusoidal, sinusoidal, or postsinusoidal. Presinusoidal and postsinusoidal obstructions have been subclassified as intrahepatic or extrahepatic (Box 55.1).

Extrahepatic Presinusoidal Obstruction

Presinusoidal extrahepatic obstruction is most commonly due to thrombosis of the portal vein. Although less common than other forms of obstructive portal hypertension, portal vein thrombosis occurs in a significant number of children and can also occur in adults, although the causes are remarkably different between children and adults.

Portal vein thrombosis in children most commonly occurs as a complication of an infectious process such as omphalitis and appendicitis, while in adults, the most common cause of portal vein thrombosis is a gradual and relentless decrease in the portal blood flow secondary to the high resistance in the hepatic circulation caused by cirrhosis. Other causes in adults include pancreatitis, hypercoagulable states or tumor thrombus, and mechanical obstruction of portal venous flow. The last may be the result of malignant invasion, lymphadenopathy, or caudate lobe compression. Hypercoagulable conditions may result from polycythemia, cancer, or hypovolemia. Sepsis can also lead to portal vein thrombosis by several mechanisms: low-flow states, hypovolemia, and activation of the coagulation system.

Intrahepatic Presinusoidal Obstruction

Most causes of intrahepatic presinusoidal obstructive portal hypertension relate to fibrosis and compression of the portal venules, with subsequent restriction of portal flow. Included among these diseases are congenital hepatic fibrosis, sarcoidosis, chronic arsenic exposure, Wilson disease, hepatoportal sclerosis, primary biliary cirrhosis, schistosomiasis, and myeloproliferative disorders.

Schistosomiasis is the most common cause of portal hypertension in third-world countries. Deposition of ova in the portal vein walls results in a granulomatous inflammatory reaction, which in turn results in fibrosis and portal flow restriction. Hepatic function is preserved in the early stages, but later stages of this disease are characterized by advanced cirrhosis and loss of hepatic function.[1] Myeloproliferative disorders such as myelosclerosis and myeloid leukemia occasionally lead to presinusoidal hypertension by virtue of the deposition of primitive cellular material infiltrating the portal zones.[2] Sarcoidosis causes portal hypertension by two mechanisms: sarcoid granulomas within the portal vein leading to obstruction, and increased portal blood flow.

Hepatic function is usually preserved in the early stages of presinusoidal diseases. In later stages, significant hepatic impairment may result from progressive cirrhosis. Hemodynamic characteristics are similar to those of extrahepatic portal vein obstruction: low hepatic wedge pressure and elevated portal venous pressure.

BOX 55.1 Causes of Portal Hypertension

Presinusoidal

Extrahepatic: portal vein thrombosis
- Omphalitis
- Pancreatitis
- Trauma
- Malignancy
- Polycythemia
- Periportal lymphadenopathy

Intrahepatic
- Biliary atresia
- Schistosomiasis
- Sarcoidosis
- Arsenic toxicity
- Congenital hepatic fibrosis
- Myeloproliferative disorders
- Primary biliary cirrhosis
- Hepatoportal sclerosis

Sinusoidal

Cirrhosis
Toxic hepatitis
Fatty metamorphosis

Postsinusoidal

Intrahepatic
- Cirrhosis
- Postnecrotic
- Portal
- Hemochromatosis

Veno-occlusive disease

Extrahepatic
- Budd-Chiari syndrome
- Hepatic vein webs
- Malignant obstruction
- Oral contraceptives
- Pregnancy
- Plant alkaloids

Cardiac causes
- Congestive heart failure
- Constrictive pericarditis

Increased Blood Flow: Arteriovenous Fistulas

Splenic artery to splenic vein
Hepatic artery to portal vein

Intrahepatic Sinusoidal and Postsinusoidal Obstruction

Sinusoidal portal hypertension may be the sequelae of alcoholic hepatitis, viral hepatitis, or toxic hepatitis. Although pure sinusoidal obstruction is relatively rare, it is frequently part of a combined sinusoidal and postsinusoidal obstructive picture. As such, it is the most common cause of portal hypertension in the United States and is estimated to be the tenth leading cause of death. Postsinusoidal obstruction is seen most commonly in cases of alcoholic liver disease, postnecrotic cirrhosis, or hemochromatosis. As would be expected in these diseases, hepatic function is usually significantly impaired.

Two mechanisms account for the portal hypertension in these patients. First is the mechanical obstruction of the portal blood flow by the regenerating hepatic nodules and cirrhotic bands within the damaged liver. These changes may extend beyond the confines of the hepatic sinusoids, accounting for the presence of presinusoidal, sinusoidal, and postsinusoidal distortion of the hepatic architecture. The second element is an increase in the splanchnic perfusion, in part attributed to the genesis of multiple arteriovenous shunts and collateral channels. One-third of portal blood flow may bypass functional hepatocytes through these channels.[3] The clinical correlate of this increased blood flow is the hyperdynamic state that typifies cirrhosis: elevated cardiac output and a diminished systemic resistance.[4]

The portal hemodynamic characteristics of these diseases usually consist of elevated hepatic wedge pressure along with elevated portal vein pressure. Because most of these diseases directly affect hepatocytes, hepatic function is usually impaired, even in the early stages of disease. These patients frequently have poor hepatic reserve and decompensate with each bleeding episode. Selection and timing of interventions are important aspects of their management.

Extrahepatic Postsinusoidal Obstruction

Postsinusoidal hepatic vein obstruction is usually the result of thrombosis in the hepatic veins. Although the cause of most cases is unknown, a number of associated diseases have been identified. Membranous webs of the hepatic veins, malignancies (hepatomas, renal carcinomas, adrenal carcinomas), trauma, pregnancy, contraceptive use, acute alcoholic hepatitis, veno-occlusive disease, and *Senecio* species (ragwort) toxicity may all result in hepatic vein thrombosis.[5] Constrictive pericarditis and chronic congestive heart failure may also cause postsinusoidal obstruction.

Budd-Chiari syndrome is the result of hepatic venous occlusive disease and is characterized by massive ascites, esophageal varices, variceal hemorrhage, hepatic failure, and death. Chiari disease is due to primary hepatic vein ostial occlusion. The clinical progression after hepatic vein occlusion may be fulminant or gradual. Hepatic failure is the result of chronic congestion and ischemia from impaired hepatic blood flow. The factors that determine the rate of progression are not well understood. Angiography is essential in establishing the diagnosis; it identifies the presence of thrombus and its location.[6,7]

The fulminant course is marked by the rapid development of fatigue, ascites, and jaundice. In addition, elevated liver enzymes and prothrombin time indicate hepatocellular damage. Patients who do not improve with anticoagulation should be considered for either shunting or liver transplantation.

The more gradual presentation may have many similar features, such as ascites and chronic fatigue, but hepatic function is preserved to a greater degree. Hypersplenism and variceal hemorrhage may be more prominent features in these patients.

An initial trial of anticoagulation may allow endogenous fibrinolysis to resolve the venous thrombosis. Patients whose course is gradually progressive and who have intact hepatocellular function should be considered for portal decompression by a portacaval, mesocaval, or mesoatrial shunt. Shunt selection is dependent on the patient's anatomy, as defined by angiography. When Budd-Chiari syndrome leads to the deterioration of hepatic function, as demonstrated by abnormal liver function tests, hepatic transplantation is the procedure of choice.[8]

Arteriovenous Fistulas

Arteriovenous fistulas are a relatively rare cause of portal hypertension. Most fistulas are either traumatic or splenic. Traumatic arteriovenous fistulas may occur as a consequence of transhepatic biliary manipulations or as a result of penetrating trauma. Splenic fistulas may be associated with splenic artery aneurysms, sarcoidosis, Gaucher disease, myeloid metaplasia, or tropical splenomegaly. Women of childbearing age are at the greatest risk. The portal hypertension results initially from increased flow in the portal circulation. At later stages, fibrosis, along with secondary obstruction of the presinusoidal spaces, exacerbates the portal hypertension.

DIAGNOSIS

The diagnosis of portal hypertension rests on demonstrating increased portal venous pressure or anatomic evidence of this increased pressure. In practical terms, the diagnosis of portal hypertension is made by identifying signs of elevated portal venous pressure in a patient with a history that supports these findings.

The signs of elevated portal venous pressure include the presence of esophageal varices, splenomegaly, ascites, or abdominal wall venous collaterals. Ascites, splenomegaly, and abdominal wall collateralization may be apparent on physical examination. Esophagogastric endoscopy is currently considered the most reliable means of identifying gastroesophageal varices.

Signs of underlying hepatic disease include spider angiomas, palmar erythema, gynecomastia, muscle wasting, loss of pubertal hair growth, and testicular atrophy. Encephalopathy, asterixis, fetor hepaticus, and fatigue may also be noted in patients with chronic hepatic insufficiency, but the presence of liver disease is not conclusive evidence that the patient has significant portal hypertension.

Historical support for the diagnosis of portal hypertension includes identification of any of the diseases that are known to lead to portal hypertension (e.g., alcohol ingestion, hepatitis, hepatotoxins). The duration of such problems is also important in substantiating the diagnosis of portal hypertension. Both alcoholic toxicity and viral hepatitis lead to cirrhosis and usually portal hypertension, but the time between the onset of these insults and the development of hypertension may be 10 years or more.

Hemodynamic measurement of the portal circulation is most commonly accomplished by transjugular venous catheterization and measurement of the wedge hepatic vein pressure.[9,10] This technique is able to record the pressure in the hepatic veins and the hepatic sinusoids. Elevation in the wedge pressure reflects elevation in the portal venous pressure. False-negative results may be encountered in patients with presinusoidal obstruction and in cases of catheter malfunction. Normal hepatic venous pressure is essentially the same as the right atrial pressure (0 to 5 mm Hg); portal venous pressure is approximately 2 to 6 mm Hg higher than hepatic venous pressure. A gradient greater than 10 mm Hg is considered abnormal.

The most recent development in assessing the portal circulation is the application of noninvasive ultrasonography. Duplex scanning has been used to establish patency and measure the direction and velocity of portal blood flow. Information gathered from this technique identifies portal vein thrombosis, hepatopetal and hepatofugal flow, and portal hypertension.[9-12] Bolondi and associates[13] documented high sensitivity and specificity with these techniques.

DIAGNOSTIC EVALUATION

Laboratory Testing

The initial step in evaluating most patients is to assess their serum chemistries. Specific attention should be given to testing the liver enzymes (serum glutamic-oxaloacetic transaminase [SGOT], serum glutamic-pyruvic transaminase [SGPT], lactate dehydrogenase [LDH], alkaline phosphatase) and hepatic synthetic function (prothrombin time and serum albumin). Information from these two sets of tests identifies patients who are suffering from acute hepatocellular damage and those who have had sufficient damage to reduce the liver's ability to synthesize essential proteins. This represents two distinct gradations of hepatic dysfunction. The first is indicative of an acute insult; the second represents the degree of hepatic dysfunction. The presence and degree of abnormalities in liver function tests correlate with outcome: the more abnormal the test results, the worse the prognosis.[14,15]

Abnormal liver function tests combined with physical findings and historical data form the basis for classifying patients with portal hypertension. The Child classification or, more recently, the combined Child-Pugh classification predicts the survival in cirrhotic patients who undergo both emergent and elective surgery (Table 55.1).[16]

Additional laboratory investigations should include a determination of serum ammonia and a complete blood count (CBC)—white blood cells (WBCs), red blood cells (RBCs), and platelets. Serum ammonia may be elevated in cases of severe hepatic dysfunction and coma. It correlates loosely with mentation but may also serve as an indicator of a treatable cause of encephalopathy, hyperammonemia.[17]

The CBC detects the presence of anemia and hypersplenism. Anemia in cirrhotic patients can result from a number of causes other than hemorrhage. Chronic malnutrition is a particularly important cause of anemia in these patients. Although splenomegaly is present in virtually all portal hypertensive patients, hypersplenism may not develop until later in the course of the disease. The size of the spleen does not correlate directly with either the degree of portal hypertension or the severity of hypersplenism, but an enlarged spleen is found in virtually all patients with portal hypertension and hypersplenism.[18] Hypersplenism is defined by the degree of splenic sequestration and destruction of platelets and WBCs. This leads to significant depression in the platelet and WBC counts. Platelet counts less than 50,000/mm^3 and WBC counts less than 2000/mm^3 support this diagnosis.

TABLE 55.1 Classification of Portal Hypertension Patients as Prognosticator of Survival

Child Classification

	RISK		
Criteria	**Good**	**Moderate**	**Poor**
Bilirubin (mg/dL)	<2.0	2.0–3.0	>3.0
Albumin (mg/dL)	>3.5	3.0–3.5	<3.0
Ascites	Absent	Easily controlled	Poorly controlled
Encephalopathy	Absent	Minimal	Advanced
Nutrition	Excellent	Good	Poor

Pugh Classification

	POINTS SCORED FOR INCREASING ABNORMALITY[a]		
Criteria	**1**	**2**	**3**
Albumin (mg/dL)	>3.5	2.8–3.5	<2.8
Bilirubin (mg/dL)	1.0–2.0	2.0–3.0	>3.0
Ascites	Absent	Slight	Significant
Encephalopathy	Normal	1 or 2	3 or 4
Prothrombin time (seconds prolonged)	1–4	4–6	>6

[a]5 or 6 points for class A encephalopathy; 7 to 9 points for class B encephalopathy; 10 to 15 points for class C encephalopathy.

Upper Gastrointestinal Endoscopy

Endoscopy plays a pivotal role in the management of portal hypertensive patients. For both diagnostic and therapeutic reasons, endoscopy should be one of the first tests performed. Endoscopy identifies not only the presence of varices but also the source of bleeding in patients with hemorrhage.

The diagnosis of portal hypertension can be established by noting the presence of varices. The size, appearance, and location of the varices may significantly affect the patient's management. Endoscopy also notes the presence of other sources of bleeding in portal hypertensive patients, such as hypertensive gastropathy, gastritis, gastric ulceration, duodenal ulceration, gastric mucosal lacerations (Mallory-Weiss tears), or esophageal ulcerations. Because of the variety of possible bleeding lesions and the significant differences in the management of these lesions, patients admitted for hemorrhage must undergo upper gastrointestinal endoscopy on each admission. As many as 40% to 60% of patients with documented varices have associated gastritis or peptic ulcer disease.[19] In patients with esophageal and gastric varices, the gastric varices have been found to be the site of bleeding in up to 18%.[20]

Liver Biopsy

The role of liver biopsy in the preoperative evaluation of portal hypertensive patients has been a focus of controversy. The goal of liver biopsy in this setting is to identify those patients who have active hepatitis. In alcoholic patients, this is most commonly determined by the presence of Mallory bodies, which signify acute hyaline necrosis. Mallory bodies may also be seen in patients with Wilson disease, cholestasis, and primary biliary cirrhosis. The reason for identifying patients with acute hepatic necrosis is that these patients are thought to be at increased risk of dying during shunt surgery.

The current recommendation is that patients suspected of having acute hepatitis and who are candidates for elective shunt surgery should undergo percutaneous liver biopsy. If Mallory bodies are identified, consideration should be given to postponing the elective operation to give the liver time to recover. This must be carefully balanced against the risk of recurrent hemorrhage and the likelihood of the patient's compliance.

Duplex Ultrasound Scanning

Duplex scanning is finding greater application in the evaluation of portal hypertensive patients. In patients who are being considered for portacaval shunting or hepatic transplantation, the duplex scan is frequently sufficient to document portal vein patency. Duplex scanning determines both the patency of the portal vein and the direction of portal venous blood flow. This is the minimal anatomic information required to proceed with an operation. The combination of color-flow imaging and duplex scanning has improved the accuracy and extended the diagnostic abilities of duplex scanners.[11]

Angiography

Preoperative anatomic definition is essential for optimal surgical management, particularly when peripheral shunts are being considered. Although angiography was previously performed on all patients who are to undergo elective shunting procedures, CT angiography and MR angiography have replaced catheter-based imaging.

Most portal angiography is performed by selective cannulation of the celiac and superior mesenteric arteries, with observation of the venous phase of these angiograms. Additional studies that should be obtained include an injection of the renal veins and a hepatic wedge angiogram with pressure recording. The combination of these studies is commonly referred to as a *liver package*.

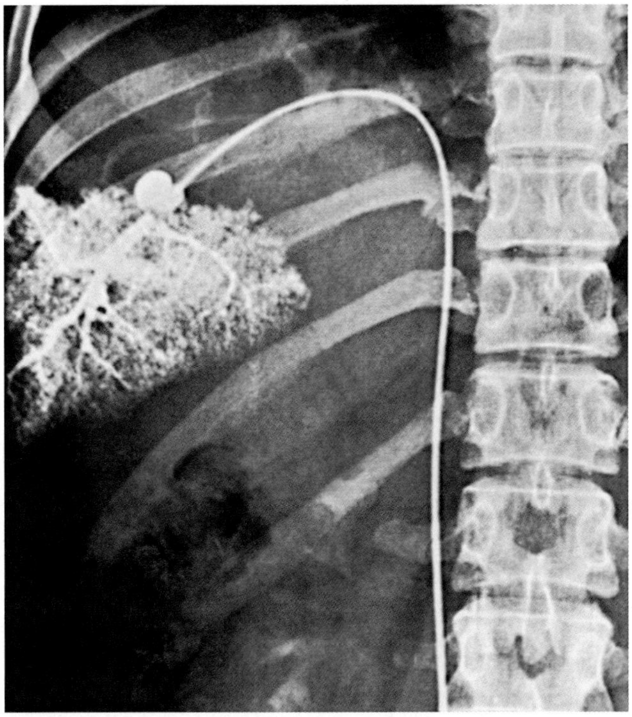

FIG 55.1 Abnormal wedged hepatic venogram demonstrating a coarse, mottled parenchymal pattern consistent with cirrhosis.

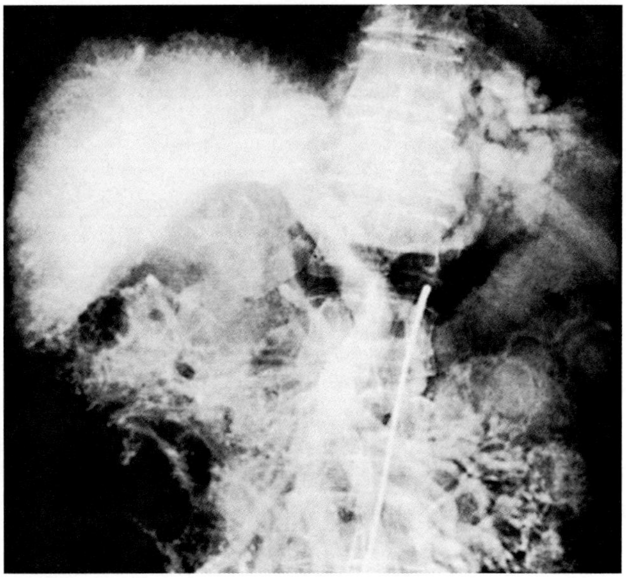

FIG 55.2 Venous phase superior mesenteric angiogram demonstrating superior mesenteric, portal, and dilated coronary veins.

The goal of these studies is to delineate the major portal tributaries—the splenic vein, the superior mesenteric vein (SMV), and the portal vein itself—and their relation to the renal vein. An additional goal of the liver package is to measure the hepatic wedge pressure and visualize the hepatic sinusoidal circulation. These last two elements are helpful in confirming the presence of portal hypertension, estimating the severity of the hypertension, and determining the cause of the elevated pressure. Low hepatic wedge pressure (<10 to 12 mm Hg) in a patient with variceal hemorrhage should prompt a careful search for evidence of portal vein thrombosis.[21] The wedge hepatic vein catheter allows determination of the morphology of the sinusoids and the direction of blood flow (Fig. 55.1). The wedge hepatic venogram in cirrhotic patients demonstrates irregular sinusoids with multiple scattered filling defects. Retrograde portal vein filling indicates hepatofugal flow.[22]

COMPLICATIONS

Esophageal Varices

Esophageal varices develop in approximately 30% of cirrhotic patients. Of those who have upper gastrointestinal bleeding at presentation, approximately 30% bleed from varices. The other 70% bleed from chemical gastritis, hypertensive gastritis, ulceration, erosions, mucosal tears, and neoplastic growth. Of the cirrhotic patients who bleed from esophageal varices, 5% to 15% have massive hemorrhage that is difficult to control. The mortality of these patients—bleeding to death from esophageal varices—is approximately 30% to 50%.

The pathogenesis of esophageal varices centers around the development of collateral circulatory pathways for blood exiting the portal circulation. The impetus for the development of these collaterals is the difference in pressure between the portal system and the systemic venous circulation. Several major collateral networks have been described in cirrhotic patients: the coronary-esophageal veins, the umbilical vein, the hemorrhoidal veins, and the retroperitoneal veins (veins of Retzius). Each of these venous systems may develop into significant collateral networks (Fig. 55.2).

Any blood vessel that is attenuated and distended under supranormal pressures is at risk of disruption and bleeding. The addition of mechanical trauma or chemical irritation may increase the likelihood of bleeding. Consequently, any of the collaterals that develop because of portal hypertension may bleed. Hemorrhoidal vessels, intestinal varices, and stomal varices have all been documented as bleeding sites in cirrhotic patients. The mechanical and chemical irritants that bathe the gastroesophageal region result in esophagitis, attenuation of the mucosal layers, and disruption of the varices. When the increased pressure within the varices is combined with periodic exacerbations of this pressure by activities that increase the intraabdominal and intrathoracic pressure (e.g., coughing, retching), the risk of bleeding from esophageal varices is significantly increased. The elevation of portal pressure results in dilatation of all of these collateral pathways (Fig. 55.3).

Several attempts have been made to predict the risk of hemorrhage from esophageal varices. Determination of the severity of portal hypertension on the basis of corrected sinusoidal pressure has not correlated with subsequent hemorrhage. Factors that predict the risk of bleeding include the size of the varices, the Child class of the patient, and the presence of erosions on the varices (red-dot signs).[23-27]

Encephalopathy

Although not usually a life-threatening complication of portal hypertension, encephalopathy can have a disabling effect on

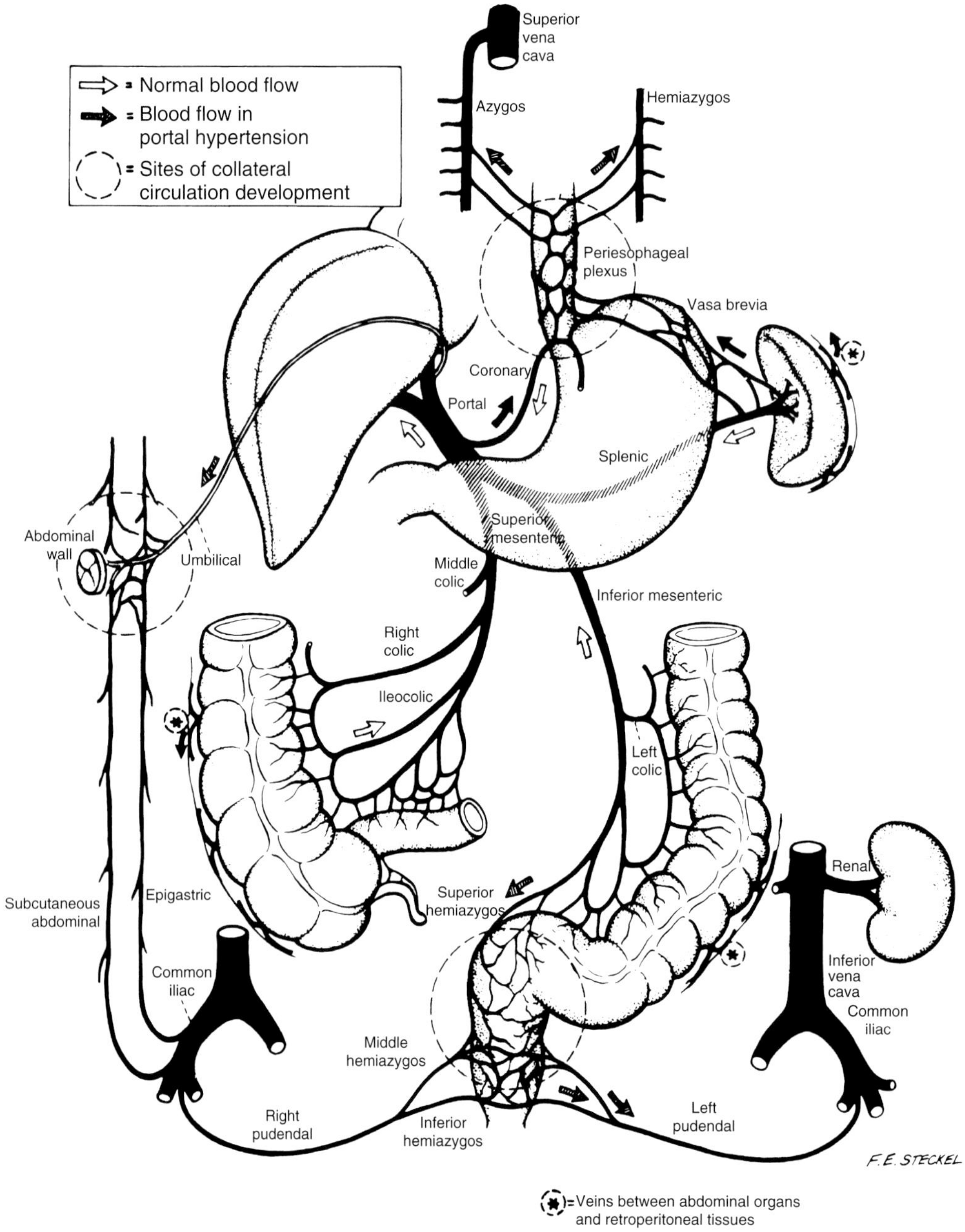

FIG 55.3 Schematic diagram of collateral venous pathways. (From Sedgwick CE, Poulantzas JK: *Portal hypertension*, Boston, 1967, Little Brown.)

patients. The clinical manifestations of encephalopathy cover a spectrum from mild inattention to frank coma. The most commonly used system of staging encephalopathy classifies patients from stage I through stage IV. Progression begins with mild personality alterations and occasionally with asterixis or clonus in stage I. Stage II may be characterized by drowsiness, sometimes with mild confusion. Stage III is typified by stupor and obtundation. Coma is the hallmark of stage IV. Electroencephalography is not specifically diagnostic, but characteristically shows only slow wave activity, primarily in the frontal regions.[28]

The mechanism by which liver failure leads to coma is not clearly understood. Several agents have been postulated as encephalopathic, especially in the presence of a diseased liver. Ammonia, nitrogenous amines, increased false neurotransmitters, decreased true neurotransmitters, and an increased ratio of aromatic to branched chain amino acids are the most likely candidates.

Elevated ammonia levels have several significant repercussions. First, they elevate glucagon levels. This in turn stimulates gluconeogenesis, which produces more ammonia. In addition, gluconeogenesis leads to elevated insulin levels, which promotes catabolism of branched chain amino acids. This ultimately leads to increased levels of straight chain amino acids such as phenylalanine, tyrosine, and methionine. An elevated ratio of straight chain to branched chain amino acids drives neutral amino acids past the blood-brain barrier. The cerebral uptake of these neutral amino acids is possible because ammonia stimulates brain glutamine synthesis, allowing rapid equilibration of brain glutamine for straight chain neutral amino acids. These same neutral amino acids may act as false neurotransmitters and are thought to produce encephalopathy.[29]

The treatment of encephalopathy is based on reduction of ammonia levels and supplementation of branched chain amino acids. Lactulose and neomycin reduce ammonia uptake from the gut by altering the intestinal pH, reducing the number of intestinal bacteria, and reducing intestinal transit of protein. Other agents such as levodopa have been used, with mixed results, in improving encephalopathy.[30]

Ascites

Ascites is a common symptom of portal hypertension. Up to 80% of these patients may have some degree of ascites. The mechanism by which ascites develops is a combination of hemodynamic, physiologic, and metabolic factors. The hemodynamics of the portal circulatory system in the face of cirrhosis is caused primarily by the increased portal venous pressure. In such a state, Starling forces tend to drive fluids out of the vessels and into the interstitial space. Compounding this problem is the low oncotic pressure in many cirrhotic patients due to their hypoalbuminemia. Finally, many patients have a chronically low intravascular volume, which in turn triggers the renal aldosterone-renin-angiotensin system and, perhaps, an additional natriuretic hormone. These changes produce a state in which the patient retains free water and salt, both of which aggravate the ascites. The net effect is the translocation of fluid from the intravascular space to the interstitial space and the abdominal cavity.

The compensatory mechanism that normally counteracts the accumulation of interstitial and peritoneal fluid is primarily the lymphatic system. In a cirrhotic patient, the lymph flow is frequently increased. Ascites accumulates when the ability of the lymphatics to reabsorb this fluid is overwhelmed.

The cornerstone of the management of ascites is the restriction of salt intake and judicious use of diuretics. These measures control the vast majority of ascitic patients. In only 5% of cases is ascites intractable, when other means of addressing ascites are required.

MEDICAL THERAPY

General Medical Care

Medical care starts by evaluating and defining the cause of the liver disease. The first step is to address any factors related to the cause of the liver disease that are amenable to change (e.g., stopping alcohol consumption). The second step is establishing the patient's current state of health and hepatic function: defining the presence of portal hypertension, splenomegaly, ascites, or varices. An assessment of the hepatic disease and the degree of hepatic deterioration helps in predicting the risks of treatment and eventual course of the patient. The next step involves maintenance of nutrition, supplementation of vitamins and minerals, and avoidance of salt (especially in ascitic patients).

Management of Acute Complications

The management of acute complications in portal hypertension patients is a highly specialized field. The most common problem that requires urgent care is hemorrhage. The significance of hemorrhage in these patients is difficult to understate. Hemorrhage may be associated with up to a 70% mortality, depending on the cause and severity of the liver disease and the degree of decompensation of the patient at the time of presentation. Furthermore, the risk of a second hemorrhage within 1 year may be as high as 60%.[16]

The essential steps in caring for a cirrhotic patient with an upper gastrointestinal hemorrhage include establishing peripheral venous access, volume-resuscitating the patient, and determining the source of bleeding. This is best accomplished by upper gastrointestinal endoscopy. As mentioned previously, between 40% and 60% of cirrhotic patients with known varices who have upper gastrointestinal hemorrhage are not bleeding from their varices.[31] If the patient is bleeding from an esophageal varix or hypertensive gastritis, several specific steps are taken promptly. First, the rate of bleeding is assessed. Second, the patient must be adequately resuscitated. Third, the patient must be prepared for a possible therapeutic intervention.

Assessing the rate of bleeding is essential. The assessment is based largely on the progressive change in the patient's vital signs, mentation, and perfusion during the course of resuscitation. A nasogastric tube also provides information about continued bleeding. Emergency endoscopy may provide insight into whether the patient is suffering a massive hemorrhage or is bleeding at a moderate rate. The change in the patient's hematocrit is not necessarily the best indicator of bleeding because there may be a significant lag between the bleeding episode and the subsequent drop in hematocrit.

Patients with relatively minor bleeding episodes frequently stop bleeding spontaneously. The few patients who are actively bleeding at the time of admission almost always respond to an infusion of octreotide. The key to managing these patients is to avoid overloading them with fluid and salts because this may precipitate rebleeding with further decompensation.

Patients with moderate bleeding rates have a reasonable chance of stopping bleeding without surgical intervention. These patients frequently respond to infusions of octreotide, emergency sclerotherapy, or balloon tamponade. Patients who bleed massively may require more advanced intervention, often in addition to octreotide and balloon tamponade. Emergent endoscopy is frequently difficult, due to massive bleeding. Subsequent steps include angiographic embolization, percutaneous attempts to create an intrahepatic shunt (transjugular intrahepatic portosystemic shunt [TIPS]), or emergency surgical shunting.

SPECIFIC MEASURES FOR THE CONTROL OF ACUTE HEMORRHAGE

Protein and Gut Lavage

Hemorrhage into the gastrointestinal tract poses a significant risk of encephalopathy, particularly in patients with bleeding varices. The combination of a large protein load in the intestinal tract and poor hepatic function frequently results in encephalopathy. The intestinal tract must be cleansed of the blood and any other nitrogenous substances by a combination of enemas and oral cathartics or gastric lavage.

The upper gastrointestinal tract should be lavaged with the aid of a large-bore tube (e.g., Ewald tube) to remove the clotted blood from the stomach. The rest of the GI tract is cleansed at the appropriate time by the administration of lactulose and neomycin by mouth. Neomycin and lactulose are given to alter the intestinal absorption of ammonia. Neomycin is a relatively nonabsorbed antibiotic; it destroys urease-producing bacteria and thereby decreases ammonia production. Lactulose is converted by lactase-containing intestinal bacteria into lactic acid and acetic acid, thus decreasing the intraluminal intestinal pH. The lower pH ionizes ammonia into ammonium (NH_4^+), which is less able to diffuse through the colonic mucosa. Lactulose also promotes diarrhea, cleansing the intestine of its contents.[17,32,33]

Vasopressin

Vasopressin (Pitressin) should no longer be considered first-line therapy in the management of active bleeding varices; however, information from its previous use has provided significant insight into the early management of variceal bleeding. The drug is directed at slowing and stopping variceal hemorrhage. It has been recognized since 1917 for its vasoconstrictive effects and its ability to decrease portal pressure.[34] Vasopressin is a naturally occurring nonapeptide that demonstrates general vasoconstrictive effects, with particular efficacy in the splanchnic bed. This splanchnic vasoconstriction leads to decreased portal flow. Vasopressin is also known to diminish cardiac output by an average of 14% and heart rate by 11%. This, in turn, reduces hepatic blood flow by approximately 44% and wedge hepatic vein pressure by 11%. As much as a 23% reduction in the gradient between hepatic venous pressure and wedge hepatic vein pressure has been documented.[35]

A consequence of the vasoconstrictive effects of vasopressin is the potential exacerbation of cardiac ischemia. To counter these ischemic effects, a number of pharmacologic agents have been used in conjunction with vasopressin.[35–37] Isoproterenol, when administered with intravenous vasopressin, results in an equivalent reduction of portal vein pressure but maintenance of cardiac output.[36] Sublingual nitroglycerin plus vasopressin has been shown to reduce the deleterious effects of vasopressin alone while preserving the decrease in portal vein pressure.[35,38] In the course of a controlled trial, Gimson and associates[39] noted that nitroglycerin may reverse some of the cardiac suppressive effects of vasopressin, as well as enhance the portal hypotensive effects.

Intravenous vasopressin should be used before balloon tamponade. It stops variceal bleeding in at least 80% of cases. The initial dose is 0.2 to 0.4 units/min. If bleeding does not cease with the initial dose, the dose may be increased up to 1 unit/min.

Somatostatin and Octreotide

Because of its fewer side effects and equal efficacy compared with vasopressin, octreotide has become the agent of choice in managing acute variceal hemorrhage. Somatostatin is a tetradecapeptide derived from the hypothalamus that has demonstrated an ability to decrease splanchnic blood. Octreotide is a synthetic octapeptide analog of somatostatin. It has a longer half-life than somatostatin (100 minutes vs. 2 to 3 minutes). Both have been demonstrated to be as effective as vasopressin for the control of acute bleeding, with fewer complications.[40] Hemodynamic studies indicate that somatostatin decreases the portal venous pressure gradient.[32,41] Randomized studies have shown equal efficacy between the two, and meta-analysis has demonstrated no survival benefit. Somatostatin has been repeatedly shown to have fewer side effects than vasopressin.[40,42]

Octreotide is effective in reducing and halting variceal hemorrhage in 80% of cases. Intravenous octreotide should be used before, and along with, balloon tamponade. It should be started before endoscopy. The initial dose of octreotide is a bolus infusion of 50 µg. This is followed by an infusion of 50 µg/h. As with vasopressin infusions, the octreotide infusion should be continued over a 3-day period. After this period, the drug should be gradually discontinued.[37]

Data have been mixed regarding somatostatin and related agents, but several studies demonstrated decreased blood loss when these drugs are used. For example, a meta-analysis comprising 12 trials (1452 patients) showed an overall decrease in transfusion requirements of 1 unit of blood per patient,[43] but mortality, rebleeding, and the need for balloon tamponade were not decreased. As the authors concluded, the transfusion requirements are significant, but it is not evident that there is any clinical benefit in saving a single unit of blood.

Terlipressin is a synthetic vasopressin analog that can be given intermittently as an injection, unlike vasopressin, which must be administered as an intravenous drip. In comparison with vasopressin, no significant differences in outcome were shown in a meta-analysis of 20 studies comprising 1609 patients.[44] It is not clear whether this drug will become a front-line treatment agent.

In summary, because these drugs are easy to administer, have relatively safe profiles, and may be effective, many centers use them routinely for bleeding varices. Additional support for their use comes from a recent update of a Cochrane Database review demonstrating that vasoactive drugs appeared to work well when sclerotherapy was not readily available. The therapy was also found to be associated with few risks.[45]

Propranolol

Propranolol, a beta-blocking drug, has been found to be useful in controlling chronic portal hypertension and reducing the risk of recurrent bleeding from esophageal varices. Its action is thought to be mediated on the basis of reduced cardiac output, reduced systemic pressure, and subsequent reduction in portal venous pressure.

Evidence of propranolol's efficacy in the reduction of recurrent bleeding has been mixed. Burroughs and colleagues[46] compared propranolol with placebo and found no significant difference in rebleeding or survival. Fleig and colleagues[47] randomized 70 patients to sclerotherapy or propranolol and found no difference in the rebleeding rate or survival; however, propranolol decreased the size of the varices significantly after 3 months of treatment. In a prospective, controlled, randomized study of 79 patients, Lebrec and associates[48,49] noted that after 3 months, 2.6% of patients maintained on propranolol had recurrent gastrointestinal tract bleeding, compared with 66% maintained on a placebo drug. Similar findings have been reported by others.[50] Poynard and coauthors analyzed 127 patients treated with propranolol and found five factors that were associated with rebleeding: (1) hepatocellular carcinoma, (2) lack of persistent decrease in heart rate, (3) lack of abstinence from alcohol, (4) lack of compliance, and (5) prior history of rebleeding[51] Schepke and associates[52] compared propranolol therapy with band ligation in primary prophylaxis of varices in high-risk patients, noting that there were no differences in bleeding between these treatments. Other data suggest that sclerotherapy is more effective in this regard, reducing the risk of a first variceal bleeding episode to 5% versus a cohort receiving propranolol alone, which had a risk of 20%.[53] More recent data from Sauerbruch and colleagues compared propranolol in combination with isosorbide-5-mononitrate against TIPS in a randomized controlled trial in the prevention of rebleeding for patients with variceal hemorrhage. At 2 years, TIPS had significantly fewer patients with rebleeding than the medical group (7% vs. 26%), although it carried higher adverse event rates (mainly hepatic encephalopathy) and failed to improve survival when compared with medical therapy.[54]

In addition to the mixed evidence for the efficacy of nonselective beta-blockers (NSBB) such as propranolol, the safety of NSBB in advanced cirrhosis has recently been questioned. However, a recent meta-analysis by Bossen and colleagues[55] suggests that NSBB do not increase the risk of mortality in cirrhotic patients with ascites. They examined data from three randomized trials with 1198 patients. After controlling for a number of factors, including age, gender, MELD score, Child-Pugh score, and ascites severity, they found that NSBB users and nonusers had similar cumulative all-cause mortality at 52 weeks (23.2% vs. 25.3%). The authors conclude that their data support current clinical practice, which entails the use of NSBB such as propranolol to prevent rebleeding of varices. They also found that NSBB are safe in patients with ascites, though dose reduction or discontinuation should be considered based on renal function, serum sodium concentration, and systolic blood pressure.

Propranolol has been specifically used as maintenance therapy to decrease the risk of recurrent esophageal variceal bleeding in patients with portal hypertension. Its use in acute bleeding episodes has not been studied.

Carvedilol has been shown to have better efficacy in controlling the hemodynamics of portal hypertension as compared with propranolol. However, trials have failed to consistently demonstrate a benefit in mortality over propranolol. Recently, Aguilar-Olivos and colleagues conducted a meta-analysis of randomized controlled trials comparing carvedilol to propranolol in preventing primary variceal bleeding in cirrhotic patients.[56] Although carvedilol was more effective in reducing the hepatic vein pressure gradient in acute and long-term settings, there was a trend toward more frequent and serious adverse events associated with carvedilol use. For this reason, additional studies with larger series and long-term follow-up are necessary to elucidate the role of carvedilol in this setting.

Antibiotics

Recent advances in our understanding of portal hypertension and its complications have underscored the role of the microbial milieu in the pathogenesis of variceal hemorrhage. In a recent Cochrane review and meta-analysis, Chavez-Tapia and colleagues examined 12 trials (1241 cirrhotic patients) with upper gastrointestinal bleeding, comparing antibiotics against placebo or no antibiotics.[57] Patients with antibiotic therapy not only had reduced duration of hospitalization but also had improved survival and reduced rebleeding events. As such, nearly all modern guidelines recommend some form of antibiotic therapy.

Balloon Tamponade

Balloon tamponade is a technique that uses compression by an intragastric balloon to stem the bleeding of esophageal and gastroesophageal varices. The technique dates to the early 1950s, when Linton, Nachlas, Sengstaken, and Blakemore developed the tubes that now bear their names.

All these tubes work on the same principle—tamponade of varices. The design variations include the presence of one or two balloons for compression of the stomach alone or the esophagus and stomach (Linton-Nachlas vs. Sengstaken tube) and the presence of adjunctive ports for aspiration of the stomach and esophageal secretions (Sengstaken-Blakemore vs. Edlich modification or Minnesota tube).[58,59] The Sengstaken-Blakemore tube is probably used more often because it can compress both esophageal and gastric varices, whereas the Linton-Nachlas tube can compress only gastric varices.

The Sengstaken-Blakemore tube can be passed through either the mouth or the nose. Passage of this tube must be performed carefully and precisely to prevent complications. The manufacturers recommend that the gastric balloon be inflated with a low volume of air (250 mL) and that an abdominal radiograph be taken to ensure that the gastric balloon is on the stomach before full inflation (with 750 mL of air). This should avoid the problem of fully inflating the gastric balloon in the esophagus, which could lead to an esophageal wall tear.

Once the gastric balloon is inflated, it is taped to the facemask of a football helmet with approximately 1 kg of pressure. The gastric and esophageal ports are connected to intermittent low suction. The position of the gastric balloon is checked periodically to ensure that migration into the esophagus has not occurred. If bleeding does not cease with gastric balloon inflation and tension, the esophageal balloon is inflated to 24 to 45 mm Hg pressure. If bleeding ceases with the Sengstaken-Blakemore tube insertion, it is left inflated for 24 hours. After this period, the esophageal balloon should be deflated. Twenty-four hours later, the gastric balloon is deflated. If bleeding does not recur, the tube is deflated and left in place. It should be removed after an additional day.[58] Esophageal variceal tamponade results in the cessation of hemorrhage in 45% to 92% of cases.[60–63] Bleeding recurs shortly after the Sengstaken-Blakemore tube is deflated in 24% to 42% of cases, however, and cannot be controlled in

33% to 37% of cases.[60,61] The incidence of recurrent bleeding after a second period of balloon control is 40%.[62]

This tube has been associated with significant complications: gastroesophageal tears, ulceration, and perforation. Pulmonary complications include aspiration pneumonia and asphyxia from tracheal intubation. Conn and Simpson reported a complication rate of 41% and a mortality rate of 20%,[64] but more commonly, the incidence of major complications is in the range of 4% to 9%.[60–62]

SURGICAL SHUNT CORRECTION

Shunt Nomenclature

The anatomic naming of shunts is based on the elements of the shunt; the principal shunts are portacaval, mesocaval, and splenorenal. The first portion of the name denotes the donor vessel, and the second portion denotes the recipient vessel. A portacaval shunt may be either side-to-side or end-to-side. Similarly, a splenorenal shunt may be either a proximal or a distal splenorenal shunt. The principal advantage of this system is that it allows a clear, descriptive means of labeling an operation.

The taxonomic nomenclature is derived from both physiologic and anatomic considerations. The two principal types are central and remote and selective and nonselective. A central shunt is one constructed in the region of the porta hepatis, or at the center of the portal confluence. Included among these are the various portacaval shunts. The term is used to distinguish shunts that involve the portal vein itself from those that are remote from the portal vein, such as splenorenal and mesocaval shunts. The selectivity of a shunt refers to its effect on the portal venous blood flow. Selective shunts preserve the flow of mesenteric blood through the portal vein to the liver, while decompressing esophageal varices. Nonselective shunts drain all portal blood flow into the vena cava. The selective shunts include the distal splenorenal shunt (DSRS) and the coronary-caval shunts. Nonselective shunts include the end-to-side portacaval shunt, side-to-side portacaval shunt, mesocaval shunt, and proximal splenorenal shunt. Many shunts are also still associated with the names of their proponents. Included are the Warren shunt (DSRS), Linton shunt (proximal splenorenal), Clatworthy shunt (mesocaval shunt using the inferior vena cava [IVC]), Drapanas shunt (mesocaval shunt using a Dacron interposition graft), Inokuchi shunt (coronary-caval), and Sarfeh shunt (portacaval polytetrafluoroethylene [PTFE] interposition graft).

Prophylactic Shunting

Prophylactic shunts do not benefit patients with asymptomatic varices. Although the incidence of variceal hemorrhage is virtually eliminated, these patients tend to suffer from hepatic encephalopathy and die of hepatic failure. Encephalopathy is increased following portacaval shunting, and long-term survival may in fact be decreased by a shunt procedure. Only 30% of patients who have varices lead to bleeding, and the decreased incidence of death from bleeding may be offset by the operative mortality of a shunt procedure, as well as by the effects of subsequent hepatic encephalopathy.

Therapeutic Shunting

The efficacy of portosystemic shunting has been studied with prospective, randomized clinical trials. Four such trials were performed in the United States and France to evaluate the fundamental question of whether therapeutic shunts prolong survival and maintain the quality of life compared with conventional medical therapy.[65–68]

The VA study, begun in 1961, followed the survival of 155 selected patients over a 5.5-year period. Although 78 patients were randomized to the surgical group, only 67 actually received shunts. Operative mortality following therapeutic portacaval shunts was 8%. Recurrence of variceal bleeding was 7% in the surgical group and 65% in the medical group. Encephalopathy occurred with approximately equal frequency in both groups, but was more severe in the shunted group. The long-term survival rate at 5 years was 57% in the shunt group and 36% in the medical group. The increase in long-term survival was not, however, statistically significant.[69]

In the BILG study,[70] patients underwent end-to-side portacaval shunt, side-to-side portacaval shunt, or medical therapy. The long-term survival was better in the shunt group than in the medically treated group, but this difference was not statistically significant. On the basis of both the VA and the BILG studies, Conn concluded that despite the lack of statistical significance, therapeutic portacaval shunts prolong the mean duration of life in cirrhotic patients who have suffered from variceal hemorrhage.[71]

Researchers at the University of Southern California published a 12-year follow-up of a prospective, randomized study comparing end-to-side portacaval shunts with medical therapy. There were 190 episodes of bleeding in the group receiving medical therapy, compared with 11 in the surgical group. Encephalopathy of a moderate to severe degree occurred in 35% of shunt patients. A 5-year life-table analysis revealed a 44% survival rate among patients treated with shunts and a 24% survival rate among those treated medically. This difference was not statistically significant.[72]

Rueff and associates, in a study at the Hôpital Beaujon in Clichy, France, compared therapeutic end-to-side portacaval shunts with medical therapy.[68] The long-term survival was 47% in the shunt group and 56% in the medical group. The diminished long-term survival in the shunt group is unique to this study and may be due to the high operative mortality (19%, compared with 13% for the BILG study and 8% for the VA study). Encephalopathy was equally common in the medical and surgical groups, with an incidence of 40%. As in the other studies, it tended to be more severe and chronic in the shunt group, however. Recurrent bleeding occurred in 8% of the shunt group and in 72% of the medical group.

The most compelling conclusion drawn from these studies is that they failed to demonstrate a survival advantage. Portacaval shunts are clearly superior in preventing recurrent variceal bleeding. Encephalopathy is not more common in patients undergoing portacaval shunting, but it tends to be more severe and chronic than in medically treated patients.

Emergency Portacaval Shunting

Portacaval shunting on an emergency basis is no longer widely performed because of the reported high mortality. Despite this risk, it has proved highly efficacious in its ability to stop bleeding and prevent recurrent bleeding.[73] Orloff and colleagues[74] continued to advocate the portacaval shunt in the acute setting, and they achieved a 4-year actuarial survival of 69%. Interestingly, this same group reported actuarial survivals of 99% at 5 years and 97% at 10 years when all patients (those bleeding acutely and those operated on for recurrent bleeds) were considered.[75] Villeneuve and coworkers also supported the use of this shunt in acutely bleeding patients who have mild to moderate liver disease and in whom other forms of treatment have failed.[76] In general, emergency surgical intervention is performed less frequently as nonsurgical options become more effective.

Common Portosystemic Shunts

Nonselective Shunts

Portacaval shunts. Both end-to-side and side-to-side portacaval shunts are nonselective and cause diversion of portal flow into the systemic circulation. The only specific indication for the portacaval shunt is esophageal variceal hemorrhage. Intractable ascites was once treated with a side-to-side portacaval shunt, but this technique has been discarded in favor of peritoneovenous shunting and TIPS.[77,78]

The question of whether an end-to-side or a side-to-side portacaval shunt is more effective is still debated. An end-to-side portacaval shunt is certainly not indicated in the presence of Budd-Chiari syndrome, because the portal vein serves as a decompressive outflow tract for intrahepatic portal blood. Uncontrolled studies comparing end-to-side with side-to-side shunts indicate that the side-to-side shunt is associated with a lower surgical mortality in patients with poor hepatic function.[79] Others find the side-to-side portacaval shunt to be more technically demanding. Encephalopathy has been shown to be somewhat more common in side-to-side than in end-to-side portacaval shunts.[80] Investigators previously found that in addition to allowing total diversion of portal venous flow, the side-to-side shunt may create a siphon effect, permitting egress of hepatic arterial blood through the portal vein rather than the hepatic vein. This may be an explanation for the increased incidence of encephalopathy with side-to-side portacaval shunts.

End-to-side portacaval shunt. Two approaches have been described: the midline incision and the right subcostal incision. After the abdomen has been entered, the duodenum is mobilized medially to expose the IVC. The dissection is carried up along the IVC to the level of the first hepatic vein under the liver. The portal vein should be exposed by rotating the bile duct and hepatic artery using a vein retractor or peanut sponges. The division of the portal vein should be done after it has been securely clamped (proximally and distally) and the hepatic portion of the vein suture-ligated.

A Satinsky clamp is placed at the appropriate point on the vena cava, and an ellipse of cava is removed to allow anastomosis. Pressure in the portal vein should be measured to document the adequacy of the decompression and to detect any unobserved technical problems. A 50% reduction in portal venous pressure should be expected after the shunt is completed.[81,82]

Arterialization of end-to-side portacaval shunts. In an attempt to reduce the morbidity of end-to-side portacaval shunts, a variety of measures have been used to maintain portal perfusion of the liver. Portal vein arterialization refers to the anastomosis of an arterialized conduit to the hepatic end of the portal vein. Various arteries have been used for this purpose, including the right gastroepiploic artery, splenic artery, and saphenous vein grafts from the hypogastric artery or aorta.

Side-to-side portacaval shunt. The side-to-side portacaval shunt is technically more difficult than the end-to-side shunt. The initial approach is similar to the end-to-side shunt; a longer segment of the vena cava is exposed and circumferentially dissected so that it can be lifted out of its bed. The portal vein must also be exposed for a greater length, because a 4-cm segment is necessary for the anastomosis. Portal pressures are measured before the shunt is performed. After applying the vascular clamps, an elliptic segment measuring approximately 2 cm is excised from the IVC and portal vein directly opposite each other. Again, mesenteric venous pressure measurements should demonstrate a 50% reduction in portal vein pressure.[81]

Portacaval H-graft. An alternative to the side-to-side portacaval shunt is the portacaval H-graft. Technically easier than the side-to-side shunt, the large-diameter (16 to 20 mm) H-graft effectively prevents variceal rebleeding, but encephalopathy occurs frequently. Building on this experience, Sarfeh and colleagues[83] systematically reduced portacaval H-graft diameters and found that an 8-mm PTFE graft combined with portal collateral ablation effectively prevented rebleeding, maintained hepatic perfusion, and reduced encephalopathy. The 5-year cumulative late patency rate was 97%.

Mesocaval shunts. In 1955, Clatworthy and associates devised a portosystemic shunt procedure involving division of the IVC above its bifurcation and anastomosis of the proximal cava to the side of the SMV.[84] The portosystemic shunt procedure has been particularly successful in children with extrahepatic portal vein thrombosis, but in adults, massive lower extremity edema has limited its usefulness. Because of the extensive dissection necessary to expose the vena cava, a number of alternative graft materials have been used, including cadaveric IVC, iliac vein, PTFE, and Dacron, which is currently favored.[85–89]

There has been considerable debate about whether portal perfusion (hepatopetal flow) is maintained by mesocaval shunts. Drapanas and colleagues[90] documented continued hepatopetal flow in 44% of their patients. Others have noted, however, that portal perfusion can persist only if there is partial or total H-graft occlusion.[91] Misinterpretation of angiographic studies may also be attributable to the phenomenon of portal pseudoperfusion, as explained by Fulenwider and coauthors.[92] Overall, H-graft mesocaval shunts are considered nonselective shunts.

Clinical role of mesocaval shunts. The primary application of the interposition H-graft mesocaval shunt is for the urgent control of massive variceal hemorrhage. This graft is technically easier to perform than a portacaval or a selective shunt and is frequently indicated in the emergency management of variceal hemorrhage.[93] In the case of previous surgery in the right upper quadrant, a portacaval shunt of any type is especially challenging and is usually contraindicated. If a selective shunt is contraindicated, a mesocaval shunt may be a good alternative. This is true in patients with significant ascites. Other factors that favor mesocaval shunting include extensive periportal fibrosis, a large overriding caudate lobe, an obliterated portal vein, extreme obesity, and Budd-Chiari syndrome.[94]

Interposition mesocaval H-graft. The operation, as described by Drapanas and coauthors in 1975, remains essentially unchanged to this day.[90] The transverse mesocolon is elevated superiorly, and the small intestine is retracted inferiorly. At the root of the small intestine mesentery, the peritoneum is opened transversely to expose the superior mesenteric vessels. An important goal is to preserve as many branches of the SMV as necessary to preserve intestinal venous flow. After the SMV is isolated, the anterior surface of the vena cava is exposed through the right transverse mesocolon. Only dissection sufficient to permit the use of a Satinsky clamp on the vena cava is required. Once the vena cava is partially isolated, the third and fourth portions of the duodenum must usually be mobilized to allow the duodenum to ride above the graft. Failure to do this may cause obstruction of the occasional low-lying duodenum or occlusion of the interposed graft.

The graft length should be only 3 to 6 cm to minimize kinking of the prosthesis. Anastomosis is performed in the posterior surface of the vein, with a continuous suture of 5-0 polypropylene (Prolene, Ethicon, Sommerville, NJ). With the clamps removed, the graft should distend quickly. In most instances, a palpable thrill should be present. Postshunt pressures are then measured in the SMV; if the shunt is functioning properly, there should be at least a 50% reduction of pressure with the shunt open.

Clinical results. Sarr and colleagues[95] published a series of 33 patients who underwent the mesocaval C-shunt procedure. There was a 24% operative mortality rate (all Child class C nonelective cases), an 8% rebleed rate, and a 46% incidence of encephalopathy. However, there were no graft thromboses.

The average incidence of encephalopathy after a mesocaval graft is approximately 25%.[94,96] The reported incidence of encephalopathy ranges from 9% to 45%.[89,93] Late graft occlusion is caused by excessive layering of thrombus, possibly aggravated by perigraft scarring, leading to kinking and constriction.[91] The incidence of shunt occlusion ranges from 4% to 24%.[90,91,97-101] Rebleeding occurs in approximately 14% of mesocaval shunts (range, 12% to 16%). One-third of these cases may be related to occlusion of the graft.[93] Overall, the mortality is approximately 15%. The cumulative long-term mortality ranges from 28% to 57%. The long-term mortality is probably dependent on the state of liver function rather than the type of shunt.

Mortality related to mesocaval H-shunts is not significantly different from that for other types of shunts and is dependent on the patient's Child classification. Initial hospital mortality is related to the urgency of surgery, significant elevation of SGOT or bilirubin, or the presence of encephalopathy.[91]

Proximal splenorenal shunts. Currently of historical interest only, the nonselective splenorenal shunt, or Linton shunt, was first developed by Blakemore and Lord in 1945 using a Vitallium tube.[102] Linton and coworkers[103] advocated this shunt in the years that followed and considered it the operative procedure of choice for the correction of portal hypertension. Early reports of noncontrolled studies suggested a decreased incidence of encephalopathy with this shunt compared with the portacaval shunt.[104] This finding, however, has not been substantiated. Other investigators failed to demonstrate significant differences between central splenorenal and portacaval shunts in regard to encephalopathy or long-term survival. In fact, some reports noted an increased incidence of thrombosis associated with the central splenorenal shunt.[105]

Splenorenal shunts. Portacaval shunts suffer from two significant problems: progressive hepatic failure and progressive, occasionally disabling, encephalopathy. These problems are thought to be due to the diversion of portal blood from the liver. In an attempt to avoid the complications of total diversion of portal flow, the DSRS, or Warren shunt, was developed in the late 1960s.[106]

This operation is based on the principle of compartmentalization, as discussed by Malt.[1] The portal-azygos system and the portal-splanchnic system can be surgically separated into parallel and independent hemodynamic units. Thus decompression of the portal-azygos system can be accomplished without reducing the portal-splanchnic system perfusion pressure or blood flow.[105] Therefore one should be able to decompress esophageal varices and prevent hemorrhage without diverting the hepatopetal flow of the portal-splanchnic blood. In principle, this is accomplished in two steps: First, by disrupting the coronary vein and right gastroepiploic vein, blood flow into the esophageal variceal system is reduced. Second, by anastomosing the distal splenic to the left renal vein, without performing a splenectomy, blood is able to freely drain from the esophageal varices through the short gastric into the lower-pressure systemic circulation (Fig. 55.4).

The theoretical benefit of the DSRS includes preservation of hepatic perfusion and function, with consequent prolongation

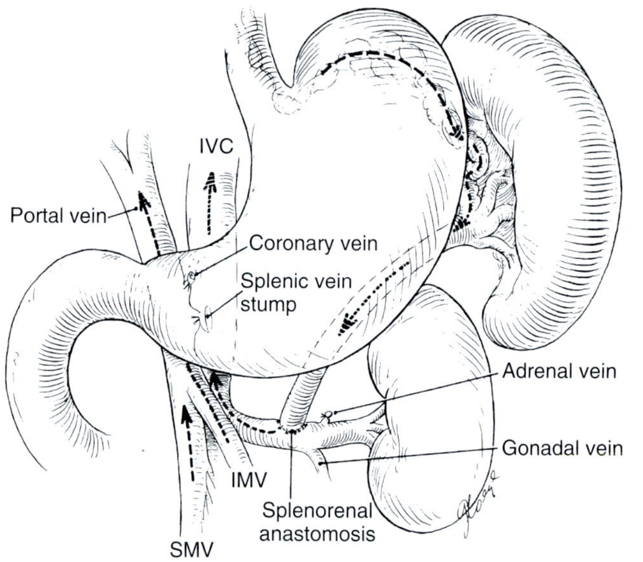

FIG 55.4 Illustration of the selective distal splenorenal shunt. *IMV,* Inferior mesenteric vein; *IVC,* inferior vena cava; *SMV,* superior mesenteric vein.

of survival and lower risk of disabling encephalopathy. The search for evidence of this benefit has led to the creation of several randomized trials. Five trials compared the DSRS and portacaval shunts. Three trials compared the DSRS with best nonsurgical management and sclerotherapy.

Distal splenorenal shunt versus other shunts. The DSRS was compared with the end-to-side portacaval shunt in three randomized studies by Langer and colleagues in Toronto,[107] Resnick and coworkers in the Boston–New Haven trial,[108] and Harley and associates at the University of Southern California Medical Center (Fig. 55.5).[109] Langer's group reported a 14% incidence of postshunt encephalopathy in the selectively shunted patients, but a 50% incidence in the end-to-side portacaval group. There was no difference in long-term survival.[107] Preliminary data from Resnick's group indicated no substantial difference between the two operations in regard to either encephalopathy or long-term survival. It should be noted, however, that the follow-up period was relatively short.[108] Harley and associates randomized 54 patients between the two shunts and failed to demonstrate any superiority of one over the other in regard to encephalopathy or survival. They did, however, experience an unusually high rate of rebleeding with the DSRS (27%).[109]

A study in Atlanta compared the DSRS with nonselective shunts, most commonly interposition mesorenal shunts.[110,111] The operative mortality was similar for the two groups: 12% for the DSRS and 10% for nonselective shunts. Early postoperative angiography demonstrated persistent hepatopetal flow in 88% of the DSRS patients, but in only 5% of the nonselective shunt patients. Corresponding to this were quantitative measurements of hepatic function, maximal rate of urea synthesis, and the Child class, which were similar to preoperative values in the DSRS group but greatly decreased in the nonselective group. The incidence of encephalopathy correlated with preservation of hepatopetal blood flow. Patients with hepatopetal flow suffered no encephalopathy; patients with hepatofugal flow experienced a 45% incidence of encephalopathy. Overall, encephalopathy occurred in 27% of the DSRS group and 52% of the nonselective group ($P < .001$). Recurrent variceal hemorrhage occurred in 4% of selective and 8% of nonselective shunts. Although survival was similar for the two groups, it appears that the quality of survival was improved in the DSRS group.

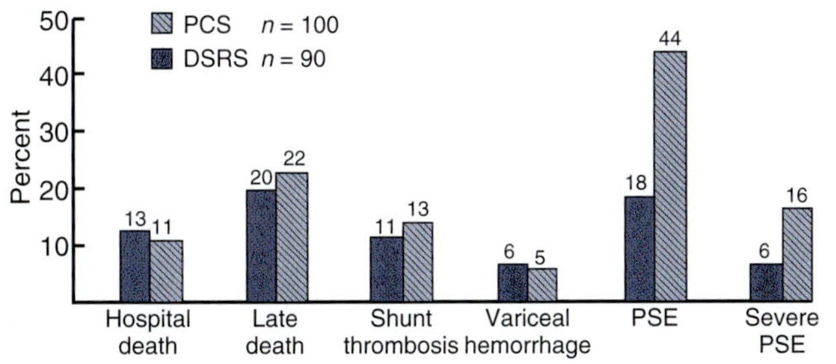

FIG 55.5 Combined experience of the distal splenorenal shunt *(DSRS)* versus the portacaval shunt *(PCS)*. *PSE,* Portosystemic encephalopathy. (Data from randomized trials by Rikkers and colleagues,[116] Langer and colleagues,[113] Reichle and colleagues,[106] and Harley and colleagues[115] and their respective colleagues.)

Zeppa's group[112] demonstrated that the 5-year survival of patients with nonalcoholic cirrhosis after DSRS was 89%, compared with 39% in the alcoholic cirrhotic group. It should be noted that improved survival in nonalcoholic cirrhotic patients was also suggested by another group,[111] but other investigators have contested this point.[19] In addition, a number of other unmatched studies have demonstrated excellent results with the DSRS.[113–111] A combined review of the literature comparing mesocaval H-grafts to DSRSs unequivocally demonstrated the latter to be superior in decreasing the incidence of both encephalopathy and recurrent hemorrhage.[93]

More recently, Henderson and colleagues compared DSRS with TIPS in a prospective randomized trial of 140 patients with Childs-Pugh class A and B cirrhosis refractory to endoscopic and medical therapy for variceal bleeding.[112] They found no statistically significant difference between the two modalities with respect to rebleeding, encephalopathy, need for OLT, or survival. The TIPS group, however, required more frequent reinterventions. Interestingly, quality of life scores were not statistically different between TIPS and DSRS.

Splenopancreatic disconnection. Because of the results of trials indicating that, with the passage of time, the DSRS gradually becomes a nonselective shunt, Warren modified the operation. In 1986, he and his coauthors proposed that the DSRS procedure include complete dissection of the splenic vein and division of the splenocolic ligament (splenopancreatic disconnection).[113] In theory, this should reduce the pancreatic sump or siphon effect—the tendency of pancreatic branches of the splenic vein to progressively enlarge and serve as an outflow collateral for the portal mesenteric circulatory system. This modification was intended to prolong and preserve the selective quality of the DSRS. Clinically, Warren's group found that this modification preserved postoperative portal perfusion in alcoholic cirrhotic patients better than the DSRS alone.[113] It also considerably extended the magnitude of the operation.

Indications for distal splenorenal shunt. The principal indication for a DSRS is to prevent recurrent variceal hemorrhage that is not controllable with sclerotherapy. The specific strengths of the DSRS include its lower incidence of encephalopathy and its anatomic remoteness from the porta hepatis. For these reasons, it is considered the shunt of choice in patients who require elective shunting and have no specific contraindications to the DSRS. The most important of these contraindications is the presence of significant ascites, which in practice means ascites that is difficult to control by the administration of diuretics. In addition, patients should have an adequately sized patent splenic vein. Some authors consider the presence of hepatofugal portal blood flow to be a contraindication to the DSRS. In cases of portal hypertension owing to extrahepatic portal vein thrombosis, the DSRS has been demonstrated to be effective in preventing recurrent hemorrhage.[118] Finally, although the DSRS has been performed as an emergency procedure, it is not widely considered the shunt of choice in these circumstances because of the relative difficulty of the operation.

Results: Patency and portal perfusion. The maintenance of portal perfusion in the early postoperative period has been documented in more than 90% of patients.[104,109,110,121] The principal question regarding this operation, however, is one of durability: how long does the benefit of the DSRS last? It has been shown that the incidence of early partial portal vein thrombosis may be as high as 22%, and that of complete portal vein occlusion at 6%. When followed over a 6-month period, most nonocclusive portal vein thromboses resolve spontaneously.[124] A 10-year follow-up by Warren and coworkers of the DSRS group revealed that 75% had persistent portal perfusion at 10 years.[121] Patients who were demonstrated to have portal perfusion at 3 years maintained this until the conclusion of the study at 7 years.[111,115]

The DSRS has several advantages over other nonselective shunts: it preserves portal flow to the liver, it maintains hepatotropic perfusion, it permits the metabolism of toxic metabolites, and it maintains a high portal perfusion pressure in the intestinal venous bed, decreasing the absorption of toxic substances.[62] It is the best procedure to perform under elective conditions in a patient with hepatopetal flow. Child classes A and B patients under emergent conditions also benefit from selective shunts. It should be noted that the DSRS has not been clearly demonstrated to improve survival by itself, but when used in conjunction with judicious sclerotherapy, it appears to provide the best chance of survival for these patients.

Current Indications for Shunt Procedures

As noted, shunting operations are performed infrequently since the advent and proliferation of TIPS procedures. In a recent report by Orug and coauthors,[125] less than 1% of patients with portal hypertension at their institution over a 9-year period underwent open shunt procedures. In a multicenter study of bleeding varices, 3.3% of patients underwent open procedures.[126] The need for repeated intervention is the primary disadvantage of TIPS compared with open operations, but even this aspect can be improved with the use of covered stents (discussed later). Nonetheless, one of the compelling reasons for choosing an open shunt over a TIPS procedure continues to be the lack of access for follow-up. Wong and coworkers[127] reported on their use of splenorenal shunts in patients with poor access to follow-up care in the South Pacific. They concluded that open procedures can be performed safely and are appropriate when tertiary care centers are not easily available. The other clinical scenario in which open shunts continue to be performed is when other methods fail to control variceal hemorrhage, particularly in Child class A patients. Interestingly, if one considers the available data, open procedures could be recommended in many low-risk Child class A and B patients.[128] A recent meta-analysis examined shunts versus TIPS in the setting of bleeding varices in Child class A and B patients. There were fewer shunt failures and longer survival in the shunted patients than in the TIPS patients.[129] Indeed, in properly selected patients, surgical portocaval shunts may offer not only a small survival benefit but may do so at essentially a very modest increase in cost.[130] However, the trend in clinical practice is clearly otherwise. Finally, the effectiveness of emergency portacaval shunts in the setting of bleeding has recently been reported by Orloff and colleagues.[131] In comparison to sclerotherapy, which achieved long-term control of bleeding in only 20% of patients, emergency shunting was successful in 100% of patients. Patients undergoing the shunting procedures also had increased survival rates up to 15 years out from the initial intervention.[131]

NONSHUNT SURGICAL PROCEDURES

Emergency portosystemic shunting results in an operative mortality of approximately 47%.[15] Furthermore, in the presence of certain clinical laboratory test results, including an SGOT greater than 300 units/L, or the presence of ascites or other determinants of Child class C status (e.g., bilirubin >6 mg/dL, hyaline necrosis, severe muscle wasting), a portosystemic shunt is almost sure to result in death. Because of this, numerous nonshunting surgical procedures have been developed.

Splenectomy

Based on Banti's theory that the diseased spleen caused portal hypertension and ascites, splenectomy was one of the first operations proposed for the treatment of Banti syndrome (splenomegaly, hypersplenism, and ascites, often accompanied by esophageal varices). The use of splenectomy in this setting was largely due to its advocacy by Osler, a great admirer of Banti's work. It was not until 1936, when Rousselot reviewed the experience at Columbia University in New York, that the failings of this operation were noted: a significant incidence of recurrent hemorrhage after splenectomy and the consequent loss of the splenic and portal veins, which would preclude possible shunt surgery.[132] In 1940, Thompson was able to demonstrate statistically that splenectomy was of value only to those patients with isolated splenic vein thrombosis[133]; this continues as an indication for splenectomy and can be performed as either an open or laparoscopic procedure.[134] Finally, in 1945, Pemberton and Kiernan[135] reported a 54% incidence of recurrent variceal hemorrhage with splenectomy alone.

Collateralization

The development of collateral pathways between the portal circulation and the systemic circulation was the goal of several procedures. Omentopexy, introduced by Talma in 1898, produces collateral pathways by suturing the omentum to the peritoneum.[136] Another collateral-promoting operation was the transposition of the spleen into the thorax.[137,138] Like omentopexy, its goal was to allow the development of large venous collateral pathways between the portal venous system and the systemic venous circulation. Unfortunately, these collateral pathways were never able to adequately decompress esophageal varices. Thus the patients were doomed to repeated hemorrhage.

Ablation

Perhaps the most successful devascularization procedure was that developed by Suguira and Futagawa in Japan.[139,140] Because of the significant risk of encephalopathy, shunt procedures were abandoned in favor of an extensive periesophagogastric devascularization accompanied by esophageal transection. The procedure is performed via separate thoracic and abdominal incisions; in poor-risk patients, a two-stage procedure is indicated. The esophagus is devascularized from the gastroesophageal junction to the left inferior pulmonary vein. The vagus nerve is carefully preserved. At the level of the diaphragm, the esophagus is partially transected, leaving only the posterior muscular layer intact. Esophageal varices are occluded, not ligated, by oversewing each with interrupted sutures. The esophageal muscle is closed, but the mucosa is not sutured. The abdominal operation is performed through a separate midline incision and includes splenectomy, devascularization of the abdominal esophagus and proximal stomach, and pyloroplasty and fundoplication.

The early results of this operation, as reported by Suguira and Futagawa,[139] were excellent. The authors reported an overall operative mortality of 4.6%, and the emergency operative mortality was 20%. Varices were eradicated in 97% of patients, and recurrent bleeding occurred in only 2.5%. Their long-term survival was 84%. A follow-up report by the authors on 276 patients indicated equally good survival rates, with excellent control of variceal bleeding and no encephalopathy.[141] In a later report, they analyzed their results according to the patients' Child classification. They found that in class C patients, both operative mortality and long-term survival were discouraging. For classes A and B patients, the results were very good, with combined (A, B, and C) 15-year survival as high as 72%.[142]

Reports by Suguira's group have been confirmed by others in Japan, as well as by selected investigators in the United States.[143] A number of other reports have suggested the use of esophageal transection procedures in the management of selected patients with poor hepatic reserves (Child class C patients). The end-to-end anastomosis (EEA) stapler has made this a relatively simple procedure, but the possibility of esophageal perforation still makes the procedure a risky one. Overall, these studies demonstrate that esophageal transection should be considered a reasonable option in the management of acute hemorrhage in a debilitated patient with both gastric and esophageal varices.[144–148]

TRANSJUGULAR INTRAHEPATIC PORTOSYSTEMIC SHUNT

TIPS has become a mainstay of therapy for controlling variceal hemorrhage and has had a dramatic effect on the performance of operative shunting procedures, despite the fact that TIPS has been used clinically only since 1988. Over the last few years, the indications for TIPS have expanded, although these applications have not always been backed by randomized trials. Recent developments in TIPS research, most notably the use of covered stents, have improved the patency of TIPS and will most likely lead to even more widespread use of this procedure.

Rosch and colleagues demonstrated 30 years ago that intrahepatic portacaval shunts could be created in a minimally invasive fashion.[149] Palmaz and colleagues applied his stent to this type of procedure, leading to prolonged patency of these shunts in animal models.[150] After its initial application in human subjects, there was a rapid expansion in its application, so that a large number of interventionists became skilled in this technique. Most major medical centers now perform TIPS.

TIPS can be performed with conscious sedation and is frequently carried out in interventional suites. Ultrasonography should be done before the procedure to document the patency of the portal vein and assess the need for a peritoneal ascites tap. Most interventionists minimize the amount of ascites before performing TIPS so that the liver is not "floating" in the abdomen. Access is ideally attained via the right internal jugular vein, which provides the most direct route for cannulation of the right hepatic vein branches. Wedged venogram and portal pressures are obtained, and a portal vein branch is then punctured. There are a number of commercially available devices for advancing through the liver parenchyma to the portal vein; the Rosch-Uchida transjugular liver access set (Cook Surgical, Bloomington, IN) is used at our institution. These devices combine a cutting needle with an aspiration port and are usually designed to fit a 10 French sheath. Portal access is confirmed by aspirating blood during needle advancement. A guidewire is advanced so that the hepatic and portal circuits are in continuity. Finally, the track is balloon-dilated and stented. At the end of the procedure, pressure measurements can be repeated to confirm that the portal-systemic gradient is less than 12 mm Hg. A completion venogram must also be obtained to assess stent placement and to ensure that varices are no longer filling.

The best indication for TIPS is for secondary prevention of variceal bleeding, as supported by evidence from 12 randomized controlled trials. A recent meta-analysis by Zheng and colleagues concluded that TIPS reduces risk of rebleeding and death due to rebleeding as compared with endoscopic therapy.[151] The most common causes of death in the TIPS arm was liver failure (10.2% of patients); in the endoscopic arm, variceal bleeding was the most common cause of death (7.9% of patients). Despite the benefits of TIPS, this treatment modality suffers from higher rates of posttreatment hepatic encephalopathy as compared with endoscopic therapy (odds ratio 2.21). More recently, Holster and colleagues conducted a randomized controlled trial comparing TIPS with covered stents versus endoscopic therapy and beta-blocker management in patients with first or second episodes of gastric or esophageal variceal bleeding.[152] None of the TIPS patients experienced variceal rebleeding compared to 29% of the endoscopic treatment patients. Although hepatic encephalopathy was higher in the TIPS group at 1 year, this difference diminished on long-term follow-up (38% vs. 23%, $P = .121$).

TIPS for acute variceal bleeding stops hemorrhage in more than 90% of patients.[153] Nonetheless, it is generally avoided as the initial treatment of acute variceal bleeding, as bleeding is usually readily managed with less invasive measures including medical management and endoscopic variceal ligation.[154] However, a recent randomized controlled trial compared contemporary medical management plus endoscopic therapy to early TIPS (within 72 hours of after diagnostic endoscopy) in Child-Pugh Class B and C patients.[155] Patients with early TIPS had statistically better survival rates (86% vs. 61%) and freedom from rebleeding (97% vs. 50%).

As with rebleeding following other therapies, a significant number of patients (25% to 30%) will have a different, nonvariceal lesion as the hemorrhage source. Confirmation of the source is thus extremely important. When the bleeding is from varices, it is almost invariably associated with improper function of the shunt. As with other vascular conduits, short-term problems are usually technical in nature, whereas those developing later are related to neointima formation. Although TIPS can be revised to control the bleeding, one of the chief criticisms of these shunts is the need for repeated interventions.[156] In fact, the primary patency of TIPS is approximately 40% at 1 year, but secondary patency approaches 90%.[157]

Another application of TIPS has been for the management of refractory ascites. In a randomized study by Rossle and coauthors,[158] TIPS was shown to be more effective than paracentesis in controlling refractory ascites. In a study by Lebrec and coworkers,[159] TIPS was shown to benefit Child class B patients with ascites but was of no help in class C patients, in whom it had little effect on ascites and increased mortality. In a more recent review of randomized trials, Saab and associates,[160] using clinical registries, found that TIPS reduced ascites reaccumulation better than paracentesis at 3- and 12-month follow-up. Encephalopathy was more common in the TIPS group, but all other variables analyzed were equal. Finally, Rosemurgy and colleagues[161] performed a randomized, prospective trial comparing TIPS and peritovenous shunts. They concluded that TIPS was more beneficial in patients unless they had only a very short life expectancy.

D'Amico and colleagues conducted a meta-analysis of randomized controlled trials comparing TIPS to paracentesis for ascites.[162] They identified five trials with a total of 330 patients in their analysis. TIPS had superior outcomes with respect to recurrence of ascites as well as a trend toward improved survival as compared to paracentesis. Consistent with previously published work, this study also found that TIPS was associated with increased rates of hepatic encephalopathy. Despite this drawback, the treatment of refractory ascites with TIPS is supported by some of the best available evidence. In a more recent study, Bureau and colleagues compared TIPS with covered stents to paracentesis in a randomized trial of 62 patients with cirrhosis with a primary endpoint of survival without a liver transplant at 1 year following the procedure.[163] 93% of the TIPS patient met the endpoint as compared to 52% of the paracentesis patients. In addition, patients in the paracentesis group had higher rates of variceal-related bleeding (18% vs. 0%) and spent twice as many days in the hospital.

It is clear that TIPS has replaced open surgical shunt procedures for most Child classes B and C patients. This is underscored by the fact that it is not uncommon for a surgical resident to finish his or her training without performing a single shunting procedure. Interestingly, in the largest prospective trial comparing TIPS and surgical shunts (8-mm prosthetic H grafts), TIPS was found to have higher rates of death, rebleeding, and treatment failure.[164] This trial, as well as an additional 4 years of follow-up, was published by Rosemurgy and colleagues[164] and evaluated 35 patients in each arm, pairing them based on their Child class. A comparison of the rates of posttreatment encephalopathy generally favored surgery as well. These data are in agreement with that in the metaanalysis by Clark, cited in the shunt section of this chapter.

TIPS has been applied in several other clinical situations. One broad category is as a bridge to hepatic transplantation. Theoretically, the procedure leaves the porta hepatis unperturbed and allows for easier subsequent operation. Some have argued that TIPS actually accelerates liver failure in patients awaiting transplantation.[165] However, several studies support the use of TIPS in this setting, particularly as a means for improving patients' general condition, sometimes with decreased blood loss at the time of surgery.[166–170] One technical note of importance is placement of the distal end of the stent well above the IVC so that it does not interfere with the transplant itself or cause damage to the portal vein.

TIPS has also been used with some success in the treatment of Budd-Chiari syndrome. There are several small studies investigating its use in this setting. Perello and coauthors[171] managed 13 such patients with TIPS and found that 11 were doing well after a follow-up of 4 years. Interestingly, many of the patients' TIPS were no longer patent but did not require treatment owing to the absence of signs of portal hypertension. Blum and coauthors[172] reported on 12 Budd-Chiari patients who underwent TIPS.[172] Two of the patients had fulminant hepatic failure and died, but the remaining 10 had resolution of their ascites. In a larger series, Rossle and colleagues reported on 35 patients receiving TIPS for Budd-Chiari syndrome.[173] The cumulative 1- and 5-year survival rates without transplantation in this group were 93% and 74%. The largest series investigating TIPS for Budd-Chiari syndrome examined long-term results in 124 patients with high MELD scores and Rotterdam scores (a well-established index for predicting mortality in patients with Budd-Chiari).[174] The authors concluded that TIPS confers high long-term survival, with OLT-free survival at 5 years improved by 30% compared with that predicted by the Rotterdam score. Taken together, these studies suggest that TIPS will continue to evolve as a treatment for this disease.

One additional application of TIPS has been for hepatorenal syndrome. Brensing and colleagues[175] reported an improvement in renal function in these patients compared with nonshunted patients. Other studies also support the use of TIPS in this setting.[176,177] Recently, Wong and colleagues[178] demonstrated prospectively that TIPS can be used in conjunction with a protocol of midodrine, octreotide, and albumin to improve renal function in type 1 hepatorenal syndrome.

As mentioned previously, some of the main drawbacks of TIPS are the poor primary patency and the need for repeated interventions to maintain the shunt. It has been shown in animal studies that the use of covered stents improves the patency of TIPS, and there are now human data to support this contention. Otal and associates[179] used PTFE-covered nitinol stents in a recent series of 20 patients and reported primary and secondary patency rates of 80% and 100% at 387 days (as opposed to 58% primary patency at 1 year for uncovered stents reported in the literature).[179] Rossi and coworkers[180] reported 1-year primary patency rates of 83.8% with these stent-grafts, and Maleux and associates[181] reported only a single occlusion after 56 TIPS procedures using PTFE-covered stents at a mean follow-up of 246 days (range, 3 to 973 days). A meta-analysis of observational studies (including one randomized controlled trial) comparing PTFE-covered stents versus bare metal stents for use in TIPS demonstrated not only improved patency for the covered stents but also a trend toward increased survival. No concomitant increase in encephalopathy was noted.[182] Perarnau and colleagues recently published the results of the second randomized controlled trial addressing this issue.[183] After randomizing 133 patients to either PTFE-covered stents or bare metal stents, the 2-year rate of shunt dysfunction (defined as portocaval pressure greater than 12 mm Hg or stent lumen stenosis greater than 50%) was 44% for PTFE-covered stents versus 60% for bare metal stents. There was no difference between the two groups with respect to early complications, 2-year survival, or rates of hepatic encephalopathy.

TIPS has also been used successfully in patients who have already undergone orthotopic liver transplantation (OLT). King and coauthors[184] recently reported on a series of OLT patients who went on to develop either variceal bleeding or refractory ascites. The patients with a pre-TIPS model for end-stage liver disease (MELD) score of less than 15 essentially did, as well as a control group (i.e., non-OLT) of patients undergoing TIPS for the same indications. However, with a MELD score greater than 15, patients in the OLT group did poorly.[184]

Despite the wide application of TIPS to a variety of pathologies, several contraindications to TIPS must be considered.[154] Absolute contraindications to TIPS include congestive heart failure or severe tricuspid regurgitation, severe pulmonary hypertension, multiple hepatic cysts (e.g., increased risk of hemorrhage with polycystic kidney disease), uncontrolled systemic infection or sepsis, and unrelieved biliary obstruction. Relative contraindications to TIPS include hepatocellular carcinoma (especially central type), total obstruction of all hepatic veins, portal vein thrombosis (necessitates extensive stenting to prevent shunt failure), and preexisting hepatic encephalopathy (may be exacerbated by TIPS).

ORTHOTOPIC LIVER TRANSPLANTATION

With the advent of liver transplantation as an established modality for patients with end-stage liver failure, the role of nontransplantation procedures (shunt surgery in particular) has been the subject of considerable debate. Currently the best transplant survival rates are generally more favorable than those of Child class C patients after the best care with a combination of sclerotherapy and shunting. This issue has been the subject of two reports from Iwatsuki and colleagues[185,186] at the University of Pittsburgh Liver Transplant Unit. These reports described the survival of 302 patients who had bleeding esophageal varices. According to the authors, these patients were all ranked as Child class C in regard to hepatic function. Their survival was reported in a life-table format as 79% at 1 year, 74% at 2 years, and 71% at 5 years. The authors then compared these results with shunt survival as reported in the medical literature and concluded that in Child class C patients with bleeding varices, liver transplantation should be considered the treatment of choice, assuming that the patients are reasonable transplant candidates.

Our experience at the University of California–Los Angeles has revealed that transplantation affords superior survival to Child class C patients (Table 55.2). In a series of 761 patients operated on between January 1986 and December 1991, 77 underwent portosystemic shunting as their initial procedure, and 684 underwent hepatic transplantation. Of the patients receiving transplants, 86% were Child class C, whereas only 16% of the shunt patients were class C. Despite this, 15% of shunt patients eventually required liver transplantation for progressive hepatic deterioration. Furthermore, the 5-year survival for the shunt group was 64%, in contrast to 73% for the transplant patients. Similar 5-year survival data in excess of 75% were recently published by Roberts and associates,[187] reflecting patients' studies through 1999. These data support the impression that portosystemic shunting is an appropriate therapy for Child classes A and B patients, but that class C patients who are reasonable candidates are best managed by liver transplantation.

TABLE 55.2 Results of Portosystemic Shunting and Liver Transplantation From January 1986 to December 1991[a]

	No. of Patients	Child Class C (%)	5-Year Survival
Portosystemic shunt	77	16	64
Liver transplantation	684	86	73

[a]University of California, Los Angeles, experience. Distal splenorenal shunts constituted 50% of shunt operations; 15% of shunt patients eventually underwent liver transplantation because of deterioration of hepatic function.

Further complicating the issue is the effect of a prior shunt operation on a subsequent transplant operation. It has been reported that patients who must receive a liver transplant after having a portacaval shunt have considerably greater blood loss, longer operative procedures, increased morbidity, and higher mortality.[188] The portacaval shunt is a particularly troublesome procedure to overcome, because the performance of a successful liver transplantation requires dissection through the scarred tissues about the portal structures, disconnection of the shunt, and reconstitution of the normal caval anatomy; only then can the liver transplant operation begin. This is in contrast to peripheral shunt operations, such as the mesocaval shunt or the DSRS. Although these shunts have an effect on the transplantation procedure, they are not as difficult to manage as the central shunts are. In the case of a mesocaval shunt, the shunt must be disconnected or occluded before the transplant operation is completed, or the new liver may be deprived of portal nutrient blood flow. A similar problem can arise with the DSRS, although because of the nature of this shunt, the siphon effect (drainage of portal blood through peripancreatic collaterals into the shunt) is usually relatively minor, and the shunt frequently does not require dismantling.

In any consideration of the role of shunting versus liver transplantation, the essential factors are the underlying cause of the hepatic disease, the current stage of hepatic dysfunction, and the expected progression (the natural and treated history) of the hepatic disease. Assuming that the patient is a reasonable transplant candidate and that the liver disease is approaching the end stage (Child class C), transplantation should be strongly considered. If the patient requires an emergent procedure to control bleeding before undergoing transplantation, all efforts should be made to provide a peripheral shunt. If the patient is not a transplant candidate, treatment should consist of the best

TABLE 55.3 Sclerotherapy Versus Medical Management (Control)

		SCLEROTHERAPY			CONTROL		
Study	**Follow-up (Months)**	**No. of Patients**	**Rebleed (%)**	**Percentage Surviving (Years)**	**No. of Patients**	**Rebleed (%)**	**Percentage Surviving (Years)**
Terblanche and colleagues[198]	60	37	43[a]	45 (5)	38	73	45 (5)
Paquet and Feussner[193]	9–52	93	48	36 (2)	97	54	25 (2)
Westaby and colleagues[197]	3–60	56	55[a]	60 (4)	60	80	31 (4)
Korula and colleagues[200]	3–35	63	44[a]	60 (2)	57	70	56 (2)
Soderlund and Ihre[199]	12–48	57[b]	49 (2)	50[b]	34 (2)		

[a]There was a significant decrease in transfusion requirements in the sclerotherapy group, as well as fewer rebleeding episodes per patient-month if followed up.
[b]Overall recurrent hemorrhage was 3.6 times more frequent in the control group.

therapy available: sclerotherapy supported by either esophageal transection with devascularization or shunting.

VARICEAL SCLEROTHERAPY

Esophageal variceal sclerotherapy was introduced by Crafoord and Frenckner in 1939.[189] These authors reported a single patient who underwent rigid endoscopic sclerotherapy to prevent further variceal bleeding. With the upsurge in the variety of surgical procedures for variceal hemorrhage in the 1940s, however, sclerotherapy was soon forgotten. Once it was recognized that therapeutic portacaval shunts, with their inherent operative mortality and risk of encephalopathy, were not the ultimate surgical procedure, attention was redirected toward less invasive, more direct methods of treatment, and there was renewed interest in sclerotherapy after the results of several controlled trials.

The first major review of sclerotherapy was by Johnston and Rodgers in 1973.[190] In 117 patients, bleeding was initially controlled in 92%, and the hospital mortality per admission was 18%. The average time to recurrence of variceal hemorrhage was 10 months. This group, however, made no attempt to perform sequential variceal sclerotherapy and recommended a shunt for long-term variceal control.

Endoscopy is necessary to confirm the presence of varices and differentiate those that are actively bleeding from those that have ceased to bleed. The use of sclerotherapy to stop acute bleeding at the time of initial endoscopy has been advocated as the treatment of choice.[191,192] Urgent or emergent sclerotherapy is used in many institutions after stabilization with balloon tamponade or after failure of conservative supportive therapy and somatostatin. Several controlled trials have compared sclerotherapy with medical management with the Sengstaken-Blakemore tube in the acute setting.[193–197] Three studies demonstrated a significantly lower early rebleeding rate,[193–195] and all the studies supported the use of sclerotherapy for acute bleeding. Only Paquet and Feussner demonstrated significantly improved overall survival with sclerotherapy.[193]

The ability of sclerotherapy to prevent recurrent variceal hemorrhage and improve long-term survival with extended treatment has been examined in numerous controlled trials (Table 55.3).[196–200] When sclerotherapy was performed to eradicate all varices and compared with conservative medical management, sclerotherapy patients had fewer recurrent bleeds[196,198] and improved long-term survival.[197] Terblanche and colleagues[198] were able to demonstrate complete eradication of varices in 95% of sclerotherapy patients; however, they could not demonstrate a significant difference in survival, and varices recurred in more than 60% of the sclerotherapy patients.[198]

TABLE 55.4 Sclerotherapy Versus Portacaval Shunt in Management of Variceal Hemorrhage

	Sclerotherapy ($n = 32$)	**Shunt ($n = 32$)**	***P* Value**
Rebleed rate (%)	50	19	<.009
Encephalopathy (%)	13	13	NS
Surgery not required	7 (22%)	—	—
Long-term cost	\$23,000	\$28,000	NS
18-Month survival (%)	28	13	NS

NS, Not significant.
Data from Cello J, Grendell J, Crass R, et al: Endoscopic sclerotherapy versus portacaval shunt in patients with severe cirrhosis and variceal hemorrhage. *N Engl J Med* 311:1589–1594, 1984.

Only since 1984 has sclerotherapy been systematically compared with portosystemic shunts in the management of variceal hemorrhage. Cello and associates[201,202] compared the portacaval shunt with sclerotherapy in Child class C patients, showing greater rebleeding, increased rehospitalization, and higher blood transfusion requirements in the sclerotherapy group, with 40% of sclerotherapy patients ultimately requiring surgical therapy. However, they were unable to demonstrate any significant difference in survival (Table 55.4). The authors concluded that in high-risk patients, sclerotherapy and portacaval shunting are equal in the acute setting, but one must consider shunt surgery if varices are not totally obliterated.

The DSRS has been compared with endoscopic sclerotherapy for the long-term management of variceal bleeding in three controlled trials (Table 55.5). Warren and coworkers[203] showed that although early mortality was the same, there was a higher

TABLE 55.5 Sclerotherapy Versus Distal Splenorenal Shunt in Long-Term Management of Variceal Hemorrhage[a]

	Sclerotherapy	DSRS	*P* Value
Warren and Colleagues[203]			
No. of patients	36	35	
Rebleed rate (%)	53	3	<.05
Portal perfusion (%)	95	53	<.05
Patients requiring surgery	10	(28%)	
2-Year survival (%)	84	59	<.01
Rikkers and Colleagues[205]			
No. of patients	30	27	
Rebleed rate (%)	57	19	.003
Encephalopathy (%)	7	16	
2-Year survival (%)	61	65	NS
Teres and Colleagues[204]			
No. of patients	55	57	
Rebleed rate (%)	37.5	14.%	<.02
Encephalopathy (%)	8	24	<.05
2-Year survival (%)	68	71	NS

[a]All controlled trials.
DSRS, Distal splenorenal shunt; *NS,* not significant.

rebleeding rate with sclerotherapy, and one-third of the patients failed treatment and required surgery.[203] Treatment with sclerotherapy resulted in significant improvement in liver function when successful, with less encephalopathy and improved survival when backed up by surgical therapy for patients with uncontrolled bleeding. Therefore the improved survival in the sclerotherapy group actually represents a combination of sclerotherapy and surgical therapy. Teres and colleagues[204] found no difference in early and long-term mortality—nor did Rikkers and coworkers.[205] However, the rebleeding rate was greater in patients who had sclerotherapy, and encephalopathy rates were higher in shunt patients in the study by Teres and colleagues.[204]

In 1989, Burroughs and associates[206] concluded a prospective, randomized study comparing staple transection with sclerotherapy for emergency control of variceal bleeding. They found no difference in overall mortality and improved control of bleeding with esophageal transection compared with a single injection, but there was a similar incidence of hemorrhage after three injection treatments. Teres and colleagues[207] randomized cirrhotic patients with uncontrolled bleeding to portacaval shunt or staple transection in low-risk patients and staple transection or sclerotherapy in high-risk patients. Survival was similar in the two groups. In the low-risk patients, portacaval shunt had a greater hemostatic effect but a greater incidence of encephalopathy. In high-risk patients, sclerotherapy and staple transection had similar rebleeding rates and survival, but fewer complications were observed in the sclerotherapy group. The authors therefore recommended staple transection for low-risk patients and sclerotherapy for the initial management of high-risk patients. Although a consensus has not yet been reached, sclerotherapy may represent an appropriate alternative ablative procedure in selected patients with hepatic dysfunction.[207–214]

More recently, interest has increased in an alternative endoscopic technique, variceal banding. This has the advantage of avoiding the caustic agents required for sclerotherapy. In comparison studies, the rates of efficacy in halting bleeding are similar between the two techniques. There is debate whether the incidence of complications with banding is reduced compared with sclerotherapy. Clearly the same major complications attend both techniques: recurrent bleeding, as well as esophageal ulceration and perforation.[214] Indeed, a multicenter prospective randomized trial compared endoscopic ligation to combination ligation with sclerotherapy.[214] There were more complications in combined therapy group, including deep ulcers (65% vs. 20%) and dysphagia (30% vs. 0%).

Endoscopic variceal sclerotherapy and variceal banding have the distinct advantages of no risk of portal vein thrombosis, good control of variceal hemorrhage, and easy accessibility for repeat sclerotherapy. There is no question that in patients with acute variceal bleeding who have had a prior splenectomy or a portosystemic shunt that has failed, endoscopic therapy is indicated. Because of the high mortality associated with emergency shunting procedures, variceal sclerotherapy in conjunction with octreotide is indicated in the acute management of variceal hemorrhage. Recurrent variceal hemorrhage is likely if follow-up routine sclerotherapy is not performed; therefore sclerotherapy should be considered an adjunctive therapeutic management tool for the acute control of variceal bleeding rather than definitive treatment.

TREATMENT PLAN FOR VARICEAL HEMORRHAGE

When a patient has an upper gastrointestinal tract hemorrhage and the history and physical examination suggest esophageal varices in association with hepatic disease, a preset treatment plan should be followed (Fig. 55.6). It is important to remember that time is of the essence in these patients, and delays to consider, define, and formulate a plan of action may jeopardize the patient's life. The initial care of a bleeding portal hypertensive patient should be as routine as the initial care of a trauma patient, following the *ABC*s. Special variations are implemented because of the underlying hepatic disease and the associated risks.

Initial laboratory studies should include a CBC, electrolytes, blood typing, and crossmatching. In addition, determinants of liver function, including bilirubin, SGOT, LDH, SGPT, prothrombin time, partial thromboplastin time, albumin, total protein, and alkaline phosphatase, should be obtained. Nasogastric tubes must be placed in all patients; if blood is present in the stomach, then gastric lavage and emergency endoscopy are indicated. This allows verification of the source of the hemorrhage and emergent sclerotherapy, if required.

Initial fluid management is crucial. Treatment with fluids and blood products should be directed at maintaining adequate tissue perfusion. Resuscitation should include packed RBCs and fresh frozen plasma, as needed. Cryoprecipitates and calcium may be required in cases of massive bleeding. It is generally

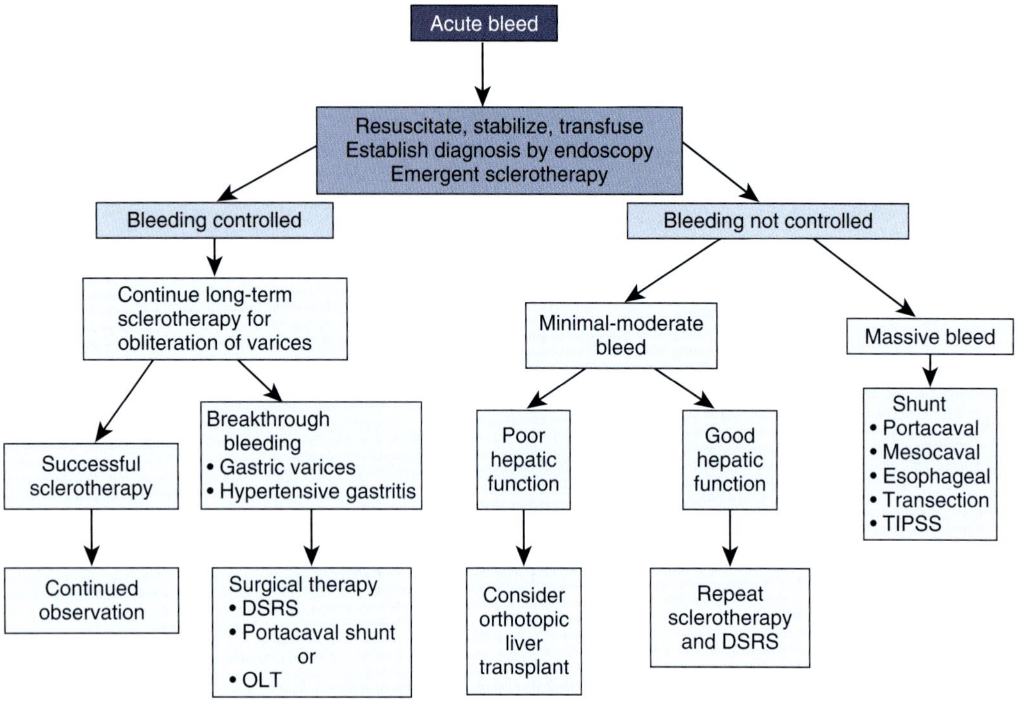

FIG 55.6 Protocol for the management of variceal hemorrhage. *DSRS,* Distal splenorenal shunt; *OLT,* orthotopic liver transplantation; *TIPSS,* transjugular intrahepatic portosystemic stent-shunt.

preferable to resuscitate with a combination of crystalloid and blood components (albumin and packed RBCs) rather than with saline only. Thiamine should be administered to prevent Wernicke encephalopathy. Propranolol or diazepam (Valium) may be required for the symptoms of alcohol withdrawal.

If the bleeding does not stop during resuscitation and transfusion, octreotide should be administered intravenously and repeated sclerotherapy should be performed. Balloon tamponade may be especially helpful at this juncture. If the patient fails to stop bleeding after injections and balloon tamponade, emergent intervention is indicated. Depending on the institution's resources, the patient should be considered for a TIPS, portosystemic shunt, or esophageal transection with devascularization. If the patient is a potential liver transplant candidate, a peripheral shunt (DSRS or mesocaval) should be performed. The choice of TIPS or surgical shunt should probably be based on the local expertise and ability of the managing physicians.

Once bleeding is controlled, patients with relatively good hepatic function (Child class A or B) should undergo long-term sclerotherapy until varices are obliterated. If this is successful, the patient should continue to be observed, and no further intervention need be planned. If the patient has breakthrough bleeding from noncompliance, gastric varices, or hypertensive gastritis and is an appropriate candidate for an elective shunt, a preoperative evaluation should be done (angiography, duplex scan) and a shunt is performed.

Patients with poor hepatic function should be considered for transplantation if they meet the appropriate criteria. While the patient is awaiting orthotopic liver transplantation, a peripheral shunt may be necessary as a bridge. Child class C patients with marked muscle wasting and obvious hyaline necrosis have a prohibitively high operative mortality rate and should undergo endoscopic sclerotherapy followed by transplantation. If this technique is not available, esophageal transection with or without the EEA stapler and ligation of portal-azygos collateral pathways is indicated, although the mortality can be expected to be greater than 60%.

MANAGEMENT OF ASCITES

Ascites predisposes portal hypertensive patients to potentially lethal complications, including renal failure, peritonitis, variceal hemorrhage, pleural effusions with respiratory insufficiency, abdominal wall hernias, anorexia, and generalized malaise. In most patients, ascites can be controlled with a restricted-salt diet and a diuretic regimen. However, a subgroup (5% to 10%) of ascites patients have refractory ascites, and this is associated with increased mortality.[215] Treatment options for these patients include paracentesis, TIPS, peritoneovenous shunting, or OLT. Paracentesis can be an effective strategy, particularly when large volume paracentesis can be tolerated.[216] When this treatment modality is not successful or practical, TIPS may provide an attractive alternative (studies comparing outcomes of TIPS to paracentesis were previously discussed under the TIPS section).[158] A return of ascites should prompt a diagnostic workup for a TIPS stenosis or occlusion.

Although rarely performed, peritoneovenous shunting can also be used for the treatment of ascites. In 1974, LeVeen and colleagues introduced the peritoneovenous shunt.[217] This device consists of a Silastic tube that runs from the peritoneum to the superior vena cava. It is controlled by a one-way valve so that a pressure gradient of 5 cm H_2O suffices to transfer the ascitic fluid from the abdomen to the intravascular space. The Denver shunt, a variation of the LeVeen shunt, incorporates a pump in line with the shunt and is implanted into the subcutaneous tissues in the chest wall. Its proposed benefit is the ability to clear the shunt of debris by using the pump mechanism.[116]

Although promising innovations, both of these shunts are dogged by complications. Early complications include congestive heart failure (from the infusion of ascitic fluid) and disseminated intravascular coagulation (DIC).[218] Coagulation values tend to improve after the first postoperative week, possibly related to diminished ascitic flow into the venous system.[219] If clinically apparent DIC develops, the only definitive treatment is shunt ligation. Because of the host of complications accompanying these shunts, they are rarely performed today.

The final option for the management of refractory ascites is OLT, which is performed as a definitive treatment in this situation. However, data evaluating the role OLT for ascites are actually lacking. Ascites is not considered in the MELD score; therefore it is unclear how patients transplanted in this clinical scenario ultimately do.

SUMMARY

The management of portal hypertension and its sequelae of ascites, encephalopathy, and recurrent variceal hemorrhage continue to be significant challenges to clinicians. Its cause and pathogenesis have been well described. Alcoholic cirrhosis resulting in intrahepatic sinusoidal and postsinusoidal obstruction continues to be the most common cause.

Long-term survival depends on rapid control of hemorrhage and institution of the most appropriate care for the patient according to the nature and severity of the hepatic disease. A patient who has variceal hemorrhage should be resuscitated quickly. Endoscopy should be performed to establish the source of gastrointestinal bleeding, followed by sclerotherapy. Initial management should include intravenous vasopressin followed by balloon tamponade. Angiography or duplex Doppler studies should be performed in patients being considered for shunting. Emergent shunt surgery should be avoided if possible, because the mortality is excessive.

Selective shunt procedures (e.g., DSRS), although they do not extend long-term survival, produce less encephalopathy and stop bleeding. Patients should be considered for elective shunting if they cannot be controlled with sclerotherapy and have relatively good hepatic function (Child class A or B). Child class C patients and "unshuntable" patients are best treated with nonshunt procedures or transplantation. Esophageal variceal sclerotherapy provides effective control of acute variceal hemorrhage; however, if it is unsuccessful after several attempts, a portal-azygos devascularization procedure should be performed. Ultimately, the survival of these patients depends on the degree of hepatic function. Patients with end-stage liver disease should be considered for liver transplantation.

Encephalopathy is a consequence of hepatic failure. It may be ameliorated by a medical regimen of neomycin, lactulose, and a low-protein diet. Ascites can usually be managed with salt restriction and diuretics. In a patient with intractable ascites, a peritoneovenous shunt may provide control, although complications are common.

Determining the best treatment for patients with portal hypertension relies on the recognition that the hepatic disease dictates the progression of liver failure. Depending on the stage of hepatic dysfunction, different options are available. In deciding how best to manage a particular patient, it is necessary to keep in mind that the goal is not merely survival but also quality of life.

REVIEW QUESTIONS

1. A 35-year-old woman with a history of viral hepatitis and cirrhosis, status postcholecystectomy, has a clinical presentation of variceal hemorrhage unresponsive to medical therapy. Which surgical procedure is indicated if sclerotherapy fails?
   a. End-to-side portacaval shunt
   b. Side-to-side portacaval shunt
   c. H-graft mesocaval shunt
   d. EEA abdominal esophageal transection
   e. Distal splenorenal shunt
2. A 10-year-old boy with a history of omphalitis experiences his first episode of variceal hemorrhage. Which is the most appropriate therapy?
   a. Distal splenorenal shunt
   b. Medical regimen
   c. Variceal sclerotherapy
   d. End-to-side portacaval shunt
   e. H-graft mesocaval shunt
3. Specific contraindications to peritoneovenous shunts include all of the following except:
   a. Hepatic necrosis
   b. Bilirubin greater than 6 mg/dL
   c. Hepatorenal syndrome
   d. Infected ascitic fluid
   e. Prothrombin time prolonged more than 4 seconds
4. Which of the following statements about prophylactic portacaval shunts is true?
   a. They prolong longevity
   b. They decrease encephalopathy
   c. They have a greater than 50% recurrent hemorrhage rate
   d. They are associated with a prohibitively high operative mortality
   e. They are not indicated

5. The Budd-Chiari syndrome may be treated by all of the following except:
   a. Anticoagulants
   b. Side-to-side portacaval shunt
   c. End-to-side portacaval shunt
   d. Mesoatrial shunt
   e. Mesocaval shunt
6. Technical considerations in favor of performing a distal splenorenal shunt include which of the following?
   a. Cavernomatous transformation of the splenic vein
   b. Acute hyaline necrosis
   c. Splenic vein greater than 4 mm in diameter
   d. Intractable ascites
   e. Hepatopetal flow
7. Which of the following statements regarding sclerotherapy is false?
   a. Percutaneous transhepatic coronary vein occlusion is associated with a 20% portal vein thrombosis rate.
   b. Sclerotherapy should not be used in the acute setting because of high mortality.
   c. Sodium morrhuate and ethanolamine oleate are appropriate sclerosing agents.
   d. Repeated sclerotherapy is necessary for control of hemorrhage.
   e. Esophageal ulcerations usually resolve spontaneously without sequelae.
8. Which of the following is an advantage of selective shunts?
   a. Continued portal perfusion
   b. Gastric and esophageal varix decompression
   c. No greater incidence of shunt thrombosis than with portacaval shunts
   d. Decreased incidence of encephalopathy
   e. All of the above
9. A 40-year-old man has hematemesis and hypotension. What initial diagnostic measures should be performed after stabilization?
   a. Superior mesenteric arteriography
   b. Splenoportography
   c. Esophagogastroscopy
   d. Celiac angiogram with venous phase
   e. Upper gastrointestinal series
10. What is the most common site of obstruction causing portal hypertension in the Western world?
   a. Portal vein (thrombosis)
   b. Extrahepatic postsinusoidal
   c. Intrahepatic presinusoidal
   d. Intrahepatic sinusoidal and postsinusoidal
   e. Extrahepatic presinusoidal
11. A 40-year-old man with cirrhosis is determined to be Child class A; his bleeding has been controlled with sclerotherapy and vasopressin. What is the most appropriate treatment plan?
   a. Emergency shunt surgery
   b. Warren shunt
   c. Mesocaval shunt
   d. TIPS procedure
   e. Periodic sclerotherapy

References available online at ExpertConsult.com.

CHAPTER 56

Lymphedema

Andrew K. Kurklinsky, Thom W. Rooke

Lymphedema is an important topic for vascular surgeons for three reasons. First, it is very common. There are hundreds of thousands of lymphedema patients in the United States,[1] and hundreds of millions are affected worldwide.[2] Second, even the best surgeons may have patients who develop lymphedema after operations involving the limbs or trunk. Third, lymphedema may be confused with venous disease or other vascular anomalies that are typically referred to vascular surgeons.

PATHOGENESIS

Fluid, proteins, and various soluble substances extravasate from the capillaries into the interstitial space. This fluid is removed through venous capillaries and lymphatic vessels, which provide equilibrium between the amount of fluid released into the interstitium and that removed from it. Fluid transported by the lymphatic vessels carries macromolecules and is rich in protein, increased concentrations of which raise osmotic pressure of the tissues by binding fluid in the interstitium.[3] Once it enters the lymphatic vessel, interstitial fluid is called *lymph fluid*. If the flow of lymphatic fluid through the lymphatic vessels is hindered, it accumulates in the tissues producing edema.

Normal lymphatic vessels exhibit spontaneous regular rhythmic contractions that pump fluid centripetally. This process is independent of hydrostatic pressure, muscle contractions, or external pressure in healthy individuals. These mechanisms become important for maintaining fluid flow when lymphatic vessels are damaged. Various insults may produce a range of lymphatic vessel abnormalities, such as total obstruction of lymphatic trunks in erysipelas or vessel wall changes in staphylococcal dermatitis or after trauma. Progressive stages of lymphedema are marked by increasing abnormalities of the lymphatic vessel contractions leading to stasis and increased tissue pressure.[4]

Lymphedema occurs when interstitial fluid builds up because of lymphatic obstruction or reflux (rarely from extreme overproduction of lymph fluid). Over time, inflammatory alterations in connective tissues are marked by altered cytokine production, accumulation of plasma proteins, and fibrous proliferation with deposition of collagen lead to dermal fibrosis. The brawny or "woody" texture of lymphedema (Fig. 56.1) is thought to be caused by chronic inflammation associated with the excessive interstitial protein trapping that overwhelms intrinsic neutrophil and macrophage proteases.[5] In addition to mechanical obstruction and inflammation, other factors, such as impaired capacity for lymphangiogenesis causing a reduced number of collaterals and lymphovenous communications, may contribute to lymphedema formation in breast cancer–related lymphedema.[6]

CAUSES

Lymphedema may be either primary or secondary, resulting from either the failure of lymphatics to develop normally or the degeneration and loss of lymphatics over time. Primary lymphedema may occur shortly after birth (heritable forms include Milroy disease)[7,8]; around the time of puberty (lymphedema praecox)[8]; or, rarely, during adulthood (lymphedema tarda).[9] Phenotypic characterization of the genetic defects has been possible for some forms of primary lymphedema.[10] More than 30 mutations in vascular endothelial growth factor receptor-3 (VEGFR3 or FLT4) have been identified for Milroy disease. Due to incomplete penetrance, the presence of these mutations results in lymphedema in 64% to 90% of all patients with the genetic defect. In this condition, skin lymphatics are abundant but are nonfunctional.[10] In lymphedema-distichiasis the mutation is in *FOXC2*[11] with penetrance 94% to 100%. A characteristic double row of eyelashes is present at birth, while lymphedema onset is delayed until puberty. Lymphedema-distichiasis may also include another disease variant known as lymphedema-ptosis syndrome.[10] Hypotrichosis-lymphedema-telangiectasia syndrome is due to mutation in *SOX18*.[12] Isolated pubertal-onset primary lymphedema (Meige disease) does not have an identified genetic defect. Many complex syndromes, such as Hennekam; Aagenaes (cholestasis-lymphedema syndrome); microcephaly-chorioretinopathy-lymphedema; Mucke; Noonan; Turner; Prader-Willi; neurofibromatosis type I (von Recklinghausen); lymphedema-hypoparathyroidism; Klippel-Trenaunay-Weber; and yellow nail syndromes include lymphedema as a clinical feature.[10,13,14] Several new genetic mutations responsible for the development of lymphedema have been identified in the last few years.

Secondary lymphedema is much more common than the primary form and may result from anything that leads to the destruction of lymphatic vessels or nodes.[9] In the United States and other developed countries, most cases are secondary to surgical interventions and radiation treatment, which leads to lymphatic sclerosis and is usually related to cancer.[15] Incidence ranges from 9% to 41% after axillary lymph node dissection, although it decreased to 4% to 10% with sentinel node biopsy.[16-18] Other common causes include trauma, invasion of the lymphatic system by tumor, recurrent infections or lymphangitis (usually caused by streptococci or, less often, staphylococci) that obliterate the vessels, and certain parasites. Many other conditions, including autoimmune diseases, pregnancy, illegal drug injections, and factitial injuries, may produce lymphedema.[19-22] Lymphangiodysplastic syndromes are characterized by lymphatic obstruction and loss of lymphatic fluid from "chylous cysts" as a result of lymphangiectasia with formation of "chylomas" and "protein-losing enteropathy" when chyliferous vessels in the enteric villi break into the intestinal lumen. This causes loss of proteins, lipids, and lipoproteins. In some cases, chylous ascites or even "chyloperitoneum" develop, and paracentesis with fluid analysis is important for differential diagnosis. Then, total parenteral nutrition with replacement of medium chain triglycerides is vital until the final diagnosis and surgical plans are made.[23]

Worldwide, filariasis was treated in nearly half a billion people (primarily in tropical countries) in 2009 and thus is the most common cause of lymphedema.[2] The most common filariae are the *Wuchereria bancrofti* and *Brugia* species.[24] Although most of these are tropical organisms, some *Brugia* species are found in North America.

Risk factors for lymphedema development include weight gain and/or obesity, trauma, history of malignancy, family history of lymphedema, and travel to endemic geographic areas.[25]

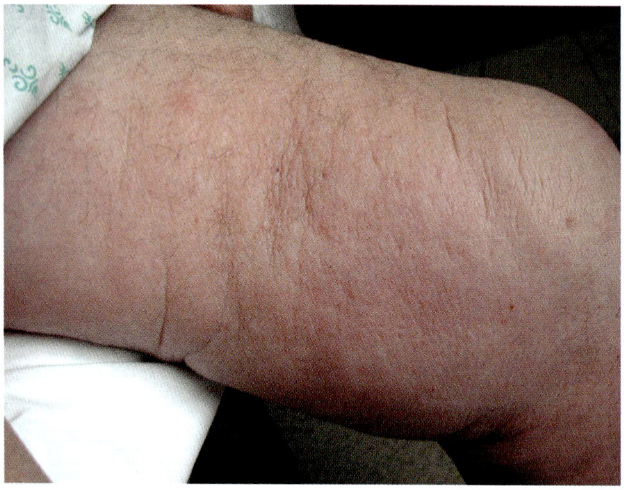

FIG 56.1 Skin changes in lymphedema. Protein accumulation within the interstitial space produces "brawny" induration of the skin. The resulting "orange peel skin" is a common clinical finding in chronic lymphedema.

DIAGNOSIS

Lymphedema is often suspected or diagnosed on clinical grounds. Age, an appropriate history describing the circumstances leading to the onset of edema, and the presence of comorbid conditions help discern primary and secondary lymphedema cases. In some variants of primary lymphedema, family history along with characteristic phenotypical traits may facilitate the diagnosis.[10]

Lymphedema is usually confined to a single upper or lower limb, although the involvement of multiple limbs (including hemihypertrophy) is possible. Local pressure may cause "pitting" indentation of the skin in early lymphedema, but it is less prominent than in venous edema. As tissue induration progresses, the pitting becomes less notable.

Lymphedema is typically worse at the distal end of the extremity. However, swelling may be compartmentalized in some cases (with sparing of the most distal parts of the extremity), thus challenging the simplistic, traditional "stopcock hypothesis" of impeded lymphatic flow.[6] When it affects the lower limb, the feet and toes are rarely spared (Fig. 56.2), unlike in lipedema,

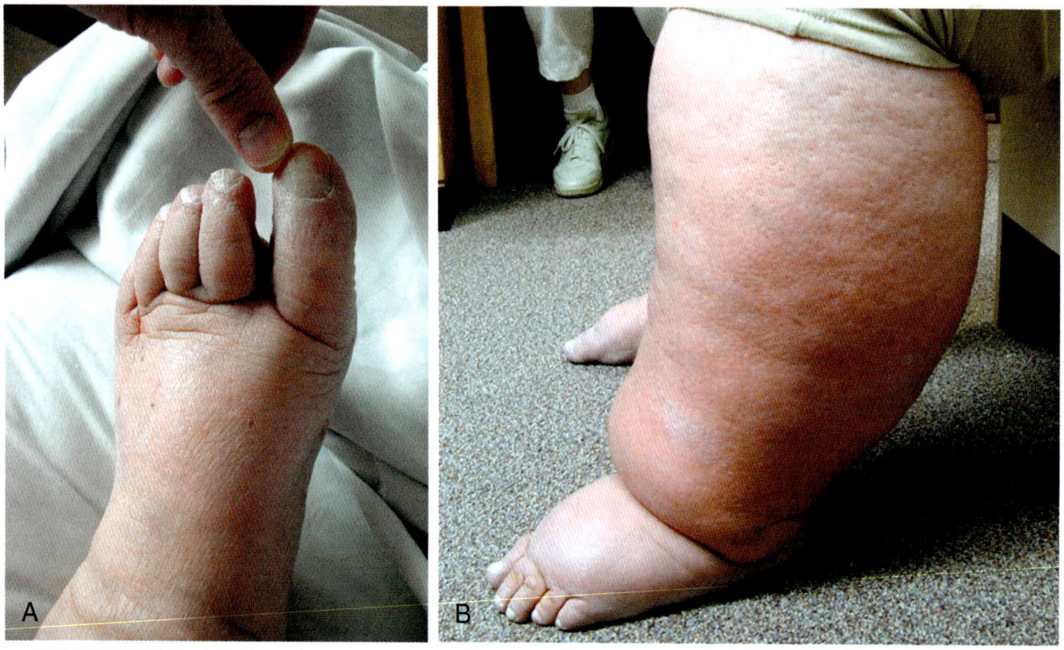

FIG 56.2 Clinical findings in lymphedema. (A) Typical "swollen sausage" appearance of the toes. Lymphedema is usually most severe in the distal limb. (B) When lymphedema involves the leg, the toes and feet are almost always affected.

where feet are characteristically spared.[26] Indeed, chronic toe edema leads to remodeling changes that produce the "squaring" of the toes (or "boxcar" toes) classically seen in lymphedema. *Stemmer sign* is a classic feature of lymphedema and denotes the inability to pinch the skin on the dorsum of the second digit of the foot. Venous prominence and "ski-jump" toenails are found in Milroy disease, a form of primary lymphedema. In lymphedema-distichiasis venous varicosities, ptosis, cleft palate, congenital heart disease, spinal extradural cysts, and other abnormalities are also commonly found.[10] Verrucous or papillomatous skin changes are common; these wartlike lesions may lead to unnecessary biopsies in some cases. In extreme cases, particularly those produced by tropical filariae, the limb may take on a grotesque appearance associated with massive edema, fibrosis, and verrucous changes (Fig. 56.3). This appearance is commonly called *elephantiasis.*

It may be necessary to rule out other problems that can cause or contribute to limb swelling, especially venous occlusion or chronic reflux. This is particularly problematic when limb swelling occurs after an operation such as mastectomy or pelvic surgery (Fig. 56.4), during which lymph nodes and vessels may have been damaged or removed (producing lymphedema) and veins may have been injured or thrombosed (producing venous edema).

In diagnosing lymphedema and assessing response to therapy, both qualitative and quantitative assessments of lymphedema are useful.[16] Volumetric methods assess changes in the size of the extremity and compare them with the contralateral extremity that is unaffected and not at risk for lymphedema. In addition to volume changes, tissue properties are altered by the pathologic process, and a number of methods have been developed for the evaluation of tissue elasticity and electric conductivity.

In practice, the clinical grading of lymphedema (Table 56.1) is commonly used based on the physical condition of the affected tissues.[27,28] Volumetric documentation and bioimpedance technologies improve diagnostic precision and may help detect subclinical disease.[25,29] Many scales exist, so the precision of lymphedema grading depends on the purpose (clinical vs. research) and varies in terms of time and cost.[30] The quantification of lymphedema is clinically meaningful and is commonly performed by simple circumferential measurements at 4 cm intervals using a measuring tape. More sophisticated methods include volumetry, opto-electronic volumetry (perometry),[31] 3D

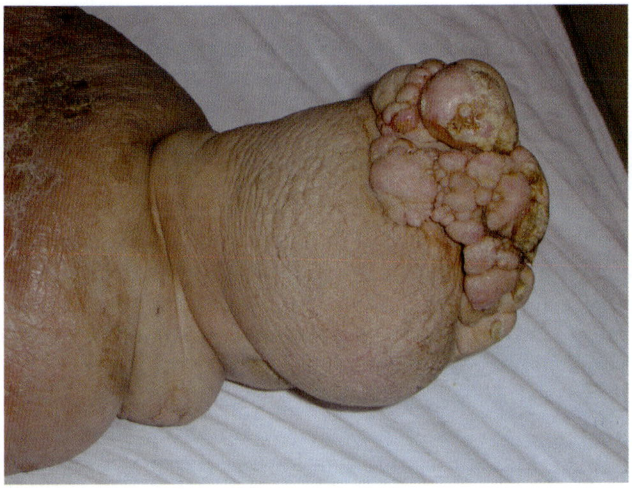

FIG 56.3 End-stage changes in lymphedema. Wartlike (verrucous) skin changes are commonly seen in advanced cases of chronic, long-standing lymphedema.

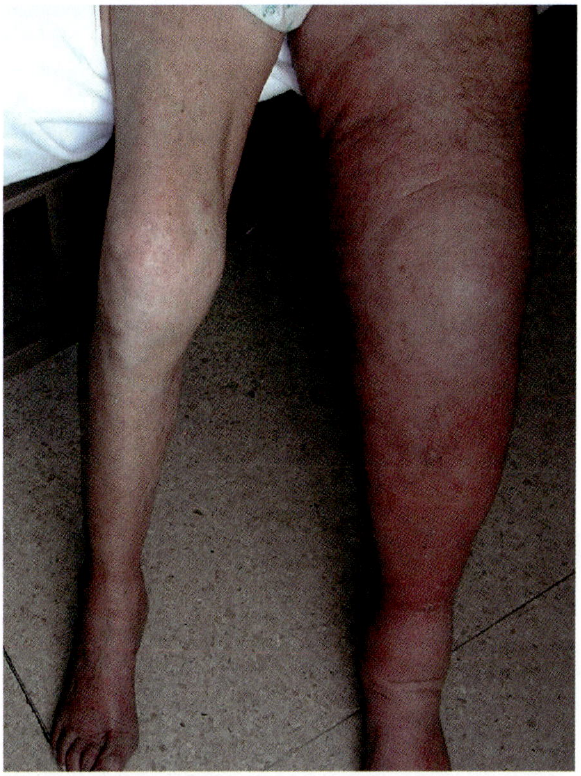

FIG 56.4 Lymphatic versus venous disease. This man developed progressive left leg edema following radical prostatectomy. The question is: Is it due to lymphedema or venous obstruction? In this case, the answer is both. The left limb has a perioperative iliofemoral deep venous thrombosis and secondary lymphedema from surgical disruption of the nodes and lymphatics.

TABLE 56.1 Stages of Lymphedema

	Fibrosis	Pitting	Elevation	Skin
Stage 0 (latent or sub-clinical condition)	None	None	No effect	No change
Stage 1 (early protein rich fluid accumulation)	None or minimal	May be present with pressure	Reduces edema	No change
Stage 2 (initial fibrosis development)	Moderate	May be present	Minimal to no reduction	Early changes
Stage 3 (marked fibrosis)	Substantial	None to minimal	No reduction	Marked trophic changes

stereophotogrammetry,[32] quantitative lymphoscintigraphy,[33] and bioimpedance spectroscopy (BIS).[29] Tonometry measures resistance of tissues to compression.[34] No single standard of lymphedema severity assessment or staging exists, and the choice of specific methods varies among institutions.

The two tests used to assess lymphatic patency are *lymphangiography* and *lymphoscintigraphy*. They provide both anatomical and functional information. Lymphangiography involves the cannulation of a distal lymphatic vessel via a surgical incision.[35] Contrast dye is injected into the cannulated vessel, and x-ray images are obtained. The study provides a detailed view of the lymph vessels and nodes. It is now rarely used, as it is painful, technically difficult to perform, and in some cases may cause sterile lymphangitis and worsen lymphatic obstruction.[36] Lymphoscintigraphy involves the subcutaneous injection of a radiolabeled colloid into the distal extremity.[37] The colloid travels through lymphatic vessels and lymph nodes, and its flow can be assessed using traditional nuclear imaging cameras. In normal subjects, transport to the abdominal level occurs in an hour or less, but when lymphatic obstruction is present, the colloid never ascends the lymphatics and becomes trapped in the interstitial spaces of the distal limb, producing a "dermal back-flow" pattern. Delayed transport or dermal back-flow patterns identify limbs with lymphatic obstruction (Fig. 56.5).[3,38]

Early lymphedema is more amenable to interventions; thus early detection plays an important role. The recently developed methods of BIS and tissue dielectric constant (TDC) determination have similar specificity, albeit TDC may have greater sensitivity, in detection of early and latent lymphedema in cancer patients.[39]

Duplex ultrasound scanning and venography help assess the possible contribution of venous pathology to edema. Cross-sectional imaging with computed tomography (CT) or magnetic resonance imaging (MRI) may also be appropriate to look for enlarged, tumor-filled lymph nodes or other lesions, such as nonmalignant masses and fluid collections, which can produce lymphatic obstruction. In addition, CT may reveal characteristic honeycomb appearances of the tissues. MRI can help differentiate the cutaneous edema of lymphedema from other types of limb swelling, including lipedema and phlebedema.[40-43] Additional methods of assessment include CT lymphography, dual-emission x-ray absorptiometry (DXA), and bi-photonic absorptiometry.[27] Fluorescent microlymphography (FML) utilizes fluorescein isothiocyanate (FITC), a fluorescent tracer attached to dextran molecules, which, upon injection into the interstitial space, are transported in the lymph. After 10 minutes, the spread of the medium from the point of maximum congestion is assessed with fluorescent light microscope and compared with the spread from the symmetrical point of the contralateral extremity. Considerable experience with this method exists at some centers. This test is safer, quicker, and simpler compared with lymphangiography and lymphoscintigraphy, and may gain wider acceptance as a more practicable alternative.[44-46]

In diagnosing protein-losing enteropathy, albumin-labeled (^{99m}Tc) scintigraphy may be used. Several immunohistochemical markers may aid the examination of the lymphatic system.[47,48] However, there is a scarcity of basic research of the lymphatic system, partially due to the lack of animal models.[49-51]

In addition to venous disease, there are other conditions that may mimic the clinical appearance of lymphedema. Myxedema associated with thyroid dysfunction, cardiac or renal failure, hypoproteinemia, and chronic dependency may resemble lymphedema or can aggravate otherwise mild cases of lymphedema. Obesity (including morbid obesity and lipedema) is frequently seen in conjunction with or mistaken for lymphedema.

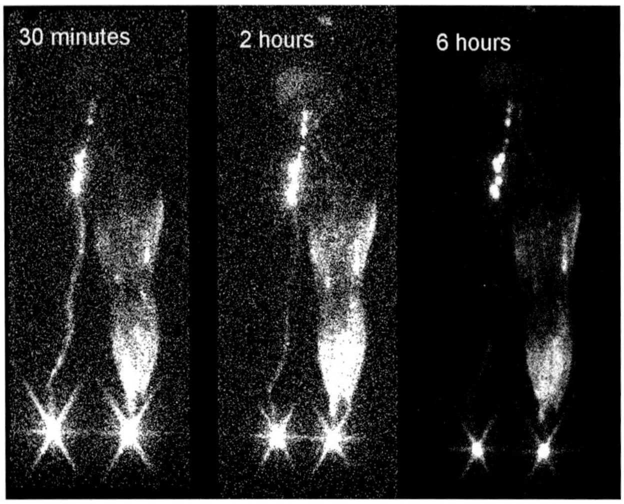

FIG 56.5 Lymphoscintigram (anterior view) in patient with left leg secondary lymphedema obtained 30 minutes, 2 hours, and 6 hours after injection of radionuclide shows significant uptake asymmetry. Isotope quickly reaches ilioinguinal lymph nodes via a single lymphatic channel on the right. Marked dermal backflow is noted on the left without reaching the ilioinguinal lymph nodes. By 6 hours, isotope transit from the injection site is completed on the right; dermal backflow persists on the left.

RATIONALE FOR TREATMENT

Lymphedema is generally an incurable, chronic disease that often requires lifelong care, but is almost never life-threatening.[27] The goals of treatment are to improve limb function, reduce pain, improve cosmesis, and prevent long-term complications. The natural history of the disease is characterized by progression both in terms of the amount of lymphedema and its grades. This progression is slower for primary cases compared with secondary ones, and slower for arms than for legs. In general, secondary lymphedema cases are marked by accelerated fibrosis.[28] Adverse psychological effects of lymphedema can be significant.

The rationale for therapy directed at pain relief, functional improvement, or appearance seems obvious; therapy intended to prevent future complications is less intuitive but often of greater importance. Limbs with lymphedema are at risk for numerous problems, including increased susceptibility to injury and infections, such as cellulitis or lymphangitis (Fig. 56.6; both of which lead to progressive destruction of lymphatics and increasing edema), and tumor formation (particularly angiosarcoma or Stewart-Treves syndrome).[52] It may be difficult to appreciate the importance of lymphedema treatment for the prevention of complications in patients with no limb pain, no

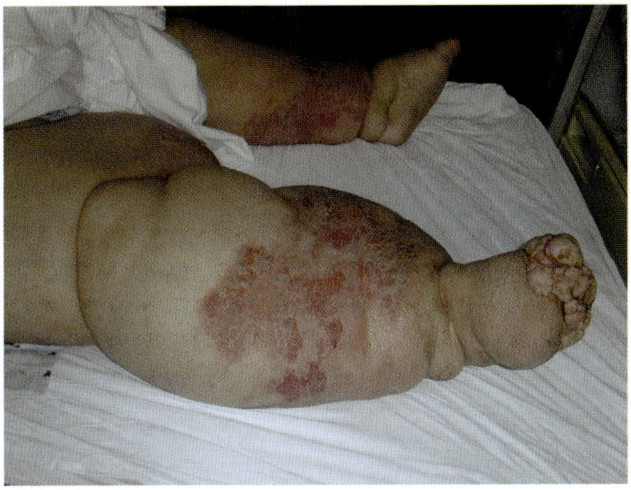

FIG 56.6 Complications of lymphedema. A limb with lymphedema is highly susceptible to cellulitis and other infections. The causative agents are usually streptococci or staphylococci.

functional impairment, and no cosmetic concerns. However, the ensuing complications may be devastating when patients develop cellulitis or lymphangitis that ravages the remaining lymphatics and leaves the limb dysfunctional with severe lymphedema. Even more devastated are patients who develop angiosarcoma, a condition that usually leads to the rapid loss of the limb and life (5-year survival time 10% to 16%; mean survival of 19 to 31 months).[53-55]

It is easy to conclude that a young, healthy patient with severe, disabling, painful, cosmetically disfiguring lymphedema warrants treatment. Other decisions may not be so easy. What about the young woman whose swelling is so mild that she notices it only when she tries to wear tight jeans, or the patient whose lymphedema is caused by the obstruction of lymph nodes due to metastatic cancer, or an elderly patient with significant lymphedema? In these instances, the "cost" of treating lymphedema (given the mild symptoms, bad prognosis, or advanced age) must be weighed against the likely "benefits."

Unfortunately, cost-benefit determinations may be extremely challenging. Cost is determined not only by the dollars spent on therapy but also by less tangible factors such as the time devoted to therapy (which may be substantial), the inconvenience of certain treatment measures (e.g., wearing stockings or wraps all day), and the emotional challenge of having to incorporate regular treatment sessions into one's lifestyle. The benefits of therapy are likewise often subjective. How much better does the patient feel or function after treatment? How much better does he or she look? There is no one right answer, and therefore therapy must be individualized for each patient. Differences in treatment rationale and patient demographics define the variety of institutional practices.

GOALS OF THERAPY

The goals of therapy may seem obvious—to reduce the size of the limb and thus to minimize functional impairment, pain, cosmetic disfigurement, and the chance of long-term complications. However, how much fluid needs to be removed from a lymphedematous limb to achieve these goals, and what degree of reduction is feasible? Is it a rational goal to make the limb as close to perfect as possible? Beyond a certain point, very aggressive treatment compared with less intensive treatment, although producing further limb size reduction, may actually become disadvantageous to the patient by compromising the patient's ability to participate in regular daily activities or to hold down a job. Thus "better" lymphedema therapy may paradoxically decrease the patient's quality of life.

Even in this era of evidence-based medicine, lymphedema treatment remains more art than science. Effective therapy is often a balancing act—the more aggressively the edema is controlled, the more intense (and often lifestyle-altering) the treatment is. The patient and the physician may have vastly different ideas about the ultimate goals of therapy. Realistic outcomes should be communicated to the patient, and the patient's individual preferences and expectations should always be carefully considered.

TREATMENT OPTIONS

There is no universal consensus on the best approach to lymphedema treatment, so protocols vary among institutions. Attempts have been made by the International Society of Lymphology and the International Union of Phlebology to amalgamate the spectrum of these diverse diagnostic and treatment approaches into consensus documents.[56,57]

For resolution of edema, either fluid production and sequestration must be decreased, or fluid removal must be enhanced. Conservative therapy is traditionally the preferred initial approach.[58] However, improving microsurgical techniques may eventually lead to wider and earlier application.[59]

The use of pharmacological methods in lymphedema is very limited. Diuretics are generally not recommended due to the risk of increased fibrosis and worsening fluid accumulation. They may be adjunctive in patients with certain comorbidities (e.g., cardiac or renal failure, prolonged dependency) that aggravate their lymphedema. Benzopyrones (coumarins) are thought to increase proteolysis by macrophages and used to be touted as drugs that can help patients with lymphedema.[60,61] Lack of evidence to support these early claims of beneficial effects[62] and links to hepatotoxicity[63] caused these drugs to fall out of favor. Nutritional supplements have not shown to be effective.[25]

In practical terms, since lymphedema appears to be largely the result of impaired interstitial fluid removal, most treatment modalities aim to enhance fluid drainage. Evacuation of the excessive fluid from the extremities affected by lymphedema can be accomplished by maximizing the evacuation through the remaining lymphatic vessels; alternatively, new conduits for lymphatic outflow can be created to replace defective ones.

The mainstay of conservative therapy is complex decongestive lymphatic therapy (DLT), based on the principles developed by Vodder and Foldi.[58,64] In 1936, Emil Vodder, PhD, a massage practitioner who initially did not realize he was trying to manipulate lymphatic flow, presented his method of light-pressure massage, called manual lymph drainage (MLD), in Paris.[64]

MLD is not only very safe but also has the greatest amount of supportive evidence from a number of trials. It is often combined with other techniques, such as compression bandaging as part of decongestive therapy, and may vary in its effectiveness, depending on the degree of fibrosis. It is more effective in the early stages of lymphedema when collateral lymphatic flow rerouting is more easily achievable and before the more pronounced fat tissue changes and fibrosis develop.[65]

In the 1980s, Foldi incorporated MLD into a multidisciplinary approach of complex decongestive lymphedema therapy.[58,66,67] This approach encompasses several treatment modalities, such as MLD, physical therapy, compression garments, and external sequential pneumatic compression devices (lymphedema pumps). It is geared toward augmenting the contractility of lymphatic vessels and increasing lymphatic flow through cutaneous lymphatics (thus improving lymphatic fluid evacuation from deeper tissues). Randomized controlled studies have been performed, some demonstrating a 40% to 60% decrease in the excess limb volume. However, follow-up is generally limited and the individual results are variable, which may be due to the differences in the stage of the disease.[25] Lymphedema compression pumps[68,69] have been used for decades and evolved over time to include a range of single and multichamber models. Some of the newer pumps encase the trunk and limbs, and are composed of individually inflatable chambers that can be programmed to mimic lymphatic massage. The newest generation of pumps may indeed offer the best of both worlds (Fig. 56.7). The concept of compression therapies to enhance lymphatic flow through existing lymphatic channels as well as to stimulate the formation of new channels is very intuitive. Lymphatic pumps are used for several short sessions a day or for prolonged periods. Normal lymphatic pressures are significantly lower than venous or arterial pressures in the same extremity. However, to stimulate creation of new lymphatic channels in more fibrotic tissues of advanced lymphedema, higher pressures may be needed. The exact pressures, duration, frequency, and other application parameters of the lymphatic compression pumps depend on the lymphedema stage, are not well studied, and will have to be elucidated in current and future clinical trials.[70,71] The applied pressure varies, depending on the model (generally 60 to 100 mm Hg), and concern about potential additional tissue damage, especially with high-pressure systems, may not be a real problem.[72,73] Several clinical trials have demonstrated the efficacy of lymphatic pumps in reducing lymphedema, especially in the early postprocedural period, and the effects seem to be greater in combination with MLD.[74-78]

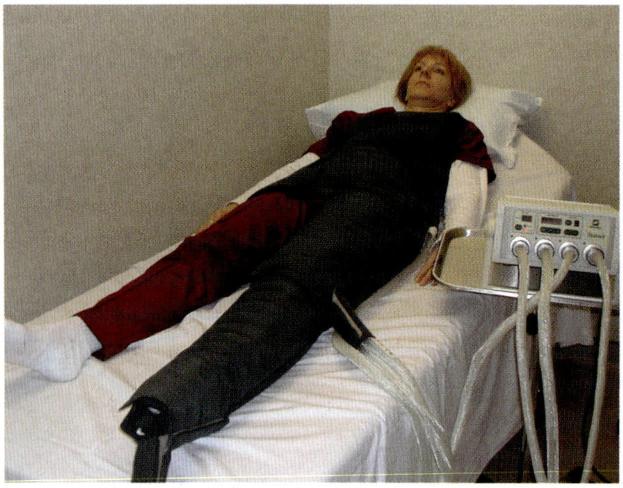

FIG 56.7 Pumps for lymphedema. This pump is coupled to a "body cuff" containing scores of inflatable chambers. By sequentially activating each cell in a predetermined order, the pump can be programmed to simulate lymphatic massage.

Gravity may also be used to improve passive drainage through limb elevation and is helpful, especially in the early stages of lymphedema.[27] A special lymphedema sling[79] or foam wedges can be used for these purposes.

The durations of the intense initial and then maintenance lymphedema treatments are not well established, and symptomatic recurrence may occur within several months of initiating maintenance therapy.[80]

Functional outcomes and quality of life measures are the ultimate end-point metrics of lymphedema therapy. Functional outcomes, such as strength and range of motion, may be improved with physical therapy, and physical activity involving the affected limb should be encouraged. Even regular, progressive exercises appear to be safe and beneficial in patients with secondary lymphedema. Patients should be counseled that obesity is a risk factor of lymphedema, and thus weight optimization may be beneficial.[81,82]

Finally, quality of life measures of therapeutic success are related to functional outcomes, where subjective factors may be definitive but not correlate directly with the volumetric status of the limb. This highlights the need for individualized goals, modes, duration, and intensity of therapy. Several functional assessment scales have been developed for clinical and research use.[65,83]

While surgery is a well-recognized lymphedema risk factor in breast cancer patients, the risk of lymphedema development may be reduced by immediate breast reconstruction. This approach also improves quality of life.[84]

Surgical approaches for the treatment of lymphedema are generally classified into ablative (debulking) and physiological operations that aim to restore lymph flow. Traditionally, the first report of a debulking procedure is attributed to Charles in 1912,[85] although the credit may actually belong to Baldwin in 1910.[86] Charles's procedure underwent modifications by Sistrunk and Thompson.[16,87-90] These interventions are now very rarely used, given the significant associated morbidities. Liposuction is an effective debulking alternative when lymphovenous shunts cannot be created, but it may also disrupt residual lymphatics, resulting in the exacerbation of lymphedema, although clinical reports using lymphoscintigraphy demonstrated that it did not cause the further compromise of lymph kinetics.[91-93]

Physiologic operations are becoming more popular and may be more effective in the earlier stages of lymphedema.[16] They aim to improve the drainage of the trapped lymph into other lymphatic basins or into veins. Omentum flaps have been used in the past in the hope that their rich lymphatics might provide lymphatic shunting.[94] Microvascular lymph node transfer is designed to provide a substrate from which new lymphatic vessels could sprout.[95,96] Surgical techniques of vascularized lymph node transfer (VLNT) are evolving with encouraging results. In VLNT, vascularized tissue and healthy lymph nodes are brought into the sites affected by lymphedema. The resultant formation of the new lymphatic channels is thought to be achieved by a combination of primary pump function of the transferred lymph nodes and by local production of lymphatic growth factors.[97]

Lymphaticolymphatic bypass procedures may be more promising, with initial lymphatic patency demonstrated by lymphoscintigraphy and volume reduction maintained at 3 years after the operation. Interposition grafting has been performed between the proximal and distal lymphatic vessels.[98-102] Preliminary results of lymphaticoventricular bypass are promising in breast cancer patients with upper extremity lymphedema.[16,103] Microvascular surgical techniques continue to improve. However, earlier stages of the disease are most amenable to microsurgical techniques, and in the more advanced stages, the best outcomes are achieved by nonoperative methods. The best results are also achieved in specialized centers. In cases of lymphangiectasia and local lymphorrhea, successful ablation is occasionally performed via CO_2 laser.[23,104,105]

Once a limb has been reduced in volume, its smaller size must be maintained. This maintenance almost always involves elastic compression, sometimes with foam padding underneath the wraps. Both high-stretch and low-stretch wraps have their advocates. Whenever possible, patients are encouraged to use compression stockings. Stockings generally have a superior cosmetic appearance to wraps and can be worn all day without the need for constant rewrapping or readjustment. It is generally recommended that pressures be around 30 to 40 mm Hg, although compression of 50 to 60 mm Hg (or more) may be necessary to adequately control edema. Indeed, physiological studies suggest that the compression bandages may raise lymphatic pressures to 40 to 70 mm Hg and that sequential intermittent pneumatic compression devices may be producing a similar effect. Massage and active foot movements are also effective in the earlier lymphedema stages; these therapies are to no avail in the last stage of lymphedema, when nearly all lymphatic transport has ceased.[4,106] Various nonelastic compression devices with static pressure gradient can also be used for the maintenance of the limb size.[107] Pumps and massage can also be incorporated into a regular maintenance program to keep the limb at a reduced size, and in some cases, a combination of modalities is best. As noted earlier, expensive, highly aggressive, time-consuming programs may not be necessary for every patient. The use of specific treatment modalities and specific protocols depend on the patient's preference, availability of the treatment methods, financial resources afforded, and access to care. In general, the simplest maintenance programs that reasonably control edema are the best. Practitioners must resist the temptation, often encouraged by industry advertising, to prescribe aggressive, expensive, or inconvenient therapies for every lymphedema patient.

In addition to the specific edema reduction measures just described, there are adjuvant therapies that may be useful in selected patients. An appropriate diet, particularly one that helps the patient lose weight and control obesity, can be valuable. Many patients with lymphedema report that their edema worsens with a high salt intake; avoiding salt, therefore, may make the edema easier to manage. Exercise is useful in most patients with lymphedema not only for controlling obesity but also for promoting lymphatic drainage. Concerns exists about safety of weight-lifting exercises in lymphedema patients, although recent studies suggest that graduated weight-lifting exercises are not only safe but may provide additional reduction benefits.[108-110] In patients with recurrent episodes of cellulitis, antibiotics may be useful.[111] It is prudent for lymphedema patients to keep penicillin or a first-generation cephalosporin on hand at home to start therapy at the first sign of cellulitis. If patients have frequent episodes, prophylactic therapy (typically 1 week out of every month) may be useful.[111] In rare cases, chronic antibiotic therapy may be necessary.

Considering the large number of cancer patients diagnosed or at risk for developing lymphedema, the risks associated with manipulations are important. Empirically, the practice of advising patients to avoid blood pressure cuff application or venipuncture in the at-risk extremity may be reasonable, even if anxiety provoking to some patients and without good evidence to support such recommendations. Avoidance of the at-risk limb for venipuncture or blood pressure measurements may be undesirable in some cases (e.g., bilateral breast cancer or otherwise lack of reliable venous access for surgery).[112,113] The newest focus of research in the therapy of lymphedema includes gene therapy, such as use of the adenovirally introduced VEGF in animals.[114,115] The blockade of transforming growth factor (TGF) has been shown recently to promote lymphangiogenesis in animal studies.[116]

REVIEW QUESTIONS

1. Which of the following statements is true?
   a. Lymphedema is rare in the United States.
   b. Lymphedema is extremely common affecting up to 500 million people worldwide.
   c. Modern surgical techniques that are carefully applied completely prevent lymphedema fibrosis.
   d. Lymphedema is always easy to distinguish from other causes of swelling.

2. Which of the following statements about lymphatic vessels is true?
   a. Unlike veins, they do not contain valves.
   b. They are characterized by constant slow flow of the lymphatic fluid.
   c. Lymphedema develops only when lymphatic vessels become obstructed.
   d. The fluid contained within lymphatic vessels is rich in proteins and other macromolecules.

3. What is the correct term for primary lymphedema that develops around the time of puberty?
   a. Lymphedema praecox
   b. Milroy disease
   c. Secondary lymphedema
   d. Lymphedema tarda
4. What is NOT a cause of secondary lymphedema?
   a. Tumor
   b. Trauma
   c. Mutation in the FOXC2 gene
   d. Infection
5. Which of the following is the most common cause of lymphedema worldwide?
   a. Autoimmune disease
   b. Pregnancy
   c. Filarial disease
   d. Cellulitis
6. The clinical features of classic, chronic lymphedema do not include which of the following?
   a. Very soft, easily pitting edema
   b. Verrucous skin changes
   c. Square toes
   d. Swelling of the foot or hand
7. Which of the following modalities may be helpful in counseling families of patients with primary lymphedema?
   a. CT scan
   b. Genetic consultation
   c. Lymphoscintigraphy
   d. MRI
8. Which of the following statements is true of lymphangiography?
   a. It usually gives poor-quality images.
   b. It is technically difficult to perform.
   c. It is less likely to injure the lymphatic vessels than lymphoscintigraphy.
   d. All of the above
9. What is the least common reason for treating lymphedema?
   a. Improve cosmetic appearance
   b. Improve mobility of the limb
   c. Alleviate pain
   d. Prevent the occurrence of future problems
10. What is the conventional initial treatment approach to lymphedema?
   a. Complex DLT
   b. Debulking operation
   c. Liposuction
   d. Coumarin pharmacotherapy

BIBLIOGRAPHY

Campisi C, Witte MH, Fulcheri E, et al. General surgery, translational lymphology and lymphatic surgery. *Int Angiol.* 2011;30:504–521.

Cormier JN, Askew RL, Mungovan KS, et al. Lymphedema beyond breast cancer: a systematic review and meta-analysis of cancer-related secondary lymphedema. *Cancer.* 2010;116: 5138–5149.

European Journal of Lymphology. The diagnosis and treatment of peripheral lymphedema: Consensus document of the International Society of Lymphology. *European Journal of Lymphology and Related Problems.* 2010;21:13–20.

Ezzo J, Manheimer E, McNeely ML, et al. Manual lymphatic drainage for lymphedema following breast cancer treatment. *Cochrane Database Syst Rev.* 2015;(5):CD003475.

International Society of Lymphology. The diagnosis and treatment of peripheral lymphedema: 2013 Consensus Document of the International Society of Lymphology. *Lymphology.* 2013;46:1–11.

Lee BB, Andrade M, Antignani PL, et al. Diagnosis and treatment of primary lymphedema. Consensus document of the International Union of Phlebology (IUP)—2013. *Int Angiol.* 2013;32:541–574.

Northup KA, Witte MH, Witte CL. Syndromic classification of hereditary lymphedema. *Lymphology.* 2003;36:162–189.

Raju A, Chang DW. Vascularized lymph node transfer for treatment of lymphedema: a comprehensive literature review. *Ann Surg.* 2015;261:1013–1023.

Runowicz CD, Leach CR, Henry NL, et al. American Cancer Society/American Society of Clinical Oncology Breast Cancer Survivorship Care Guideline. *J Clin Oncol.* 2016;34:611–635.

World Health Organization. Global programme to eliminate lymphatic filariasis. *Wkly Epidemiol Rec.* 2010;85:365–372.

References available online at ExpertConsult.com.

CHAPTER 57

Hemodialysis and Vascular Access

Richard F. Neville, Ahmed Kayssi

INTRODUCTION

Access to the vascular system in order to perform life-sustaining dialysis in the face of renal failure remains an important and challenging clinical scenario for vascular surgeons. The number of individuals requiring vascular access for hemodialysis continues to rise. Up to 16% of the world's population now suffers from chronic kidney disease (CKD), which is defined according to "the presence or absence of kidney damage and level of kidney function."[1] CKD most commonly occurs secondary to diabetes and hypertension.[2] Many of those patients have advanced cardiovascular disease and live in low- or middle-income countries whose economies are ill equipped to shoulder the considerable financial burden of this vulnerable patient population.[3] In 2008, there were 382,000 patients in the United States with end stage renal disease (ESRD), defined as a progression of CKD requiring the initiation of renal replacement therapy.[1,4] Over 90% of those patients were hemodialysis-dependent. This chapter briefly discusses the history of dialysis access to supply perspective to the problem and then reviews catheter and permanent access in the form of an arteriovenous fistula constructed with an autogenous or prosthetic conduit. This discussion includes a review of configuration, results, and complications associated with the different methods of dialysis access.

HISTORICAL PERSPECTIVE

The earliest recorded attempt at hemodialysis was made in 1913 by Abel, Rowntree, and Turner in Baltimore, Maryland. Abel and colleagues created the first "artificial kidney" while studying the physiologic consequences of partial plasma removal in animals. They developed a method of plasmapheresis, which they called *vividiffusion*, to advance this research.[5] In 1924, Haas, in Germany, was credited with the first human use of hemodialysis to treat a uremic patient.[6] The procedure was short and experimental, lasting about 15 minutes, and his avant-garde research was largely ignored by the medical community of the time. In 1943, Kolff, in Holland, developed the first clinically effective hemodialysis machine.[7] He used cellophane tubing to build a rotating drum artificial kidney. Over the course of World War II, Kolff treated 17 patients, of whom only 1 survived.[8] The subsequent success of early dialysis machines was dulled by their inefficiency, requiring up to 10 hours per session, as well as a lack of reliable vascular access options. Therefore treatment was limited to patients with acute kidney failure who did not require long-term therapy. In 1960, in Seattle, Washington, Dr. Belding Scribner and colleagues, including Wayne Quinton, developed an external arteriovenous (AV) polytetrafluoroethylene (PTFE) shunt that was successfully used to dialyze a machinist,[9] who survived for 11 years after starting treatment. Scribner went on to found the Seattle Artificial Kidney Center, the first outpatient dialysis facility. At around the same time, Shaldon, a British nephrologist, created a homemade indwelling hemodialysis catheters using yellow plastic tubing. These catheters were introduced into the femoral vein using the Seldinger technique.[10] The advent of these indwelling vascular access devices heralded the era of chronic dialysis therapy. The first AV fistula created for dialyzing patients with ESRD was described in 1966 by Brescia and colleagues from the Veterans Administration Hospital in the Bronx, New York.[11] Appel, the group's surgeon, performed a side-to-side anastomosis between the radial artery and the cephalic vein using a continuous silk suture.[12] Of the 14 procedures that were performed, 12 matured without complication. In 1976, Baker and colleagues in Phoenix, Arizona, described the first use of expanded polytetrafluoroethylene (ePTFE) AV grafts for dialysis access.[13] The authors placed 8-mm ePTFE grafts in 72 patients. Their satisfactory short-term results encouraged the further development of prosthetic grafts for patients with ESRD.

Much progress has been made in the management of patients with ESRD since the early days of hemodialysis, including important guidelines from the National Kidney Foundation's Kidney Disease Outcomes Quality Initiative (NKF KDOQI) and the National Vascular Access Improvement Initiative known as the Fistula First Breakthrough Initiative (FFBI).[14] This initiative has led to an increase in the creation of autogenous arteriovenous fistulas and a decrease in the use of chronic central venous catheters. However, the number and complexity of patients with CKD who require dialysis has also grown considerably over the past several decades. The best approach to addressing these challenges is with multidisciplinary teams that include internists, nephrologists, and access surgeons. This approach has been associated with superior clinical outcomes after the initiation of dialysis therapy.[15]

CLINICAL EVALUATION

History

Most patients with CKD have multiple medical comorbidities that place them at a higher perioperative surgical risk, so it is imperative for the surgeon to obtain a careful medical and surgical history that will guide the operative decision-making process. The surgeon should first assess the patient's dominant hand, history of treatment for CKD, and the projected dialysis starting date if the patient still has a functioning kidney. A thorough medical and surgical history should be obtained to determine the patient's other ongoing medical issues, such as diabetes, hypertension, hypercholesterolemia, and smoking status. A complete list of current medications and allergies should also be documented. As with all vascular reconstructions, it is most useful to plan for AV access procedures in terms of inflow, conduit, and outflow.

To evaluate inflow, the surgeon should inquire about any history of prior AV access creation and the artery or arteries that were used. Operative notes should be obtained, if possible, and any postoperative complications documented. Peripheral arterial disease (PAD) of the upper or lower extremities—as manifested by claudication, tissue loss, or rest pain—may need further assessment to ensure the appropriate choice of an artery as an AV access inflow vessel. Outflow should be evaluated by assessing the patient's venous anatomy and risk for central venous stenosis. Patients with a history of neck or chest radiation, upper extremity or chest trauma, pacemakers, defibrillators, and central venous line placements for hemodialysis, chemotherapy, or fluid resuscitation are at a higher risk of central venous stenosis and subsequent AV access failure. Finally, conduit options should be evaluated by determining which veins are available for AV access creation or to serve as potential targets for the venous outflow for an AV graft. Patients with a history of multiple access procedures may have fewer autogenous conduit choices compared with patients presenting for their first AV access procedure. The availability of competent superficial and deep veins in a lower extremity may also allow the surgeon to consider a lower-extremity site for dialysis access.

Physical Examination

The physical examination should evaluate the patient's overall physical status as well as the arterial and venous systems. A careful inspection should look for superficial veins in the upper extremities and surgical scars or skin marks indicative of previous surgical procedures, trauma, or radiation therapy. Evidence of central venous stenosis or occlusion includes uni- or bilateral neck or arm swelling and chest wall telangiectasia.

Vital signs should be obtained and blood pressures measured in both arms. A markedly lower blood pressure in one arm is concerning for proximal arterial disease and should be further investigated. Radial and ulnar pulses as well as femoral, popliteal, and pedal pulses should be palpated and diminished or absent pulses documented.

An Allen test can be performed in each hand to assess whether the palmar circulation is dependent on the radial or ulnar artery. First described in 1929 by Allen in Rochester, Minnesota, the test has since undergone numerous modifications to improve its clinical utility.[16] First, the radial and ulnar arteries are palpated at the proximal skin crease of the wrist and then compressed with three fingertips. With both arteries compressed, the patient is instructed to clench and unclench the hand 10 times, after which the blanched hand is held open without any hyperextension or splaying of the fingers. The ulnar artery is then released and the capillary refill time measured. If the capillary refill time is greater than 6 seconds, the test is considered positive and the patient's palmar circulation deemed to be predominantly dependent on the radial artery.[17] Kohonen and colleagues in Finland reported a sensitivity of 73% and specificity of 97%.[18] Numerous reports, however, have questioned the accuracy and clinical utility of the Allen test for assessing the palmar circulation.[19-21]

Investigations

Bilateral upper extremity vein mapping should be performed in an accredited vascular lab to determine venous patency and diameter.[22] There is currently no consensus on the usefulness of arterial Duplex in the workup of AV access patients who do not demonstrate any clinical signs or symptoms of arterial insufficiency. However, Kim and colleagues in Los Angeles performed arterial Duplex ultrasound examinations on 163 patients undergoing upper extremity AV fistula creation and found that the addition of arterial Duplex to venous mapping resulted in a change in the operative plan in up to 12% of patients in the study, particularly when a radiocephalic fistula had been planned.[23]

Patients with abnormal clinical findings suggestive of central arterial or venous disease should be further evaluated with computed tomography angiography (CTA) or digital subtraction arteriography or venography. The advantage of the last two modalities is that they are both diagnostic and therapeutic, allowing for the angioplasty or stenting of any obstructing arterial or venous lesions.

HEMODIALYSIS CATHETERS

Hemodialysis catheters are commonly inserted in patients with acute kidney failure who require short-term hemodialysis, or as a bridging tool before the patient undergoes an AV fistula or graft procedure or receives a kidney transplantation. Indwelling catheters are also used in patients with no other viable AV access options and in patients with a limited life expectancy.

Limitations of hemodialysis catheters include a higher incidence of thrombotic complications, vascular stenosis, and bacterial infections compared with AV fistulas and grafts.[24] Despite their numerous disadvantages, however, the use of hemodialysis catheters has been increasing. In the United States, the number of patients receiving dialysis through central catheters between 1995 and 2002 increased from 13% to 26%.[25] However, this has also been associated with an increase in the proportion of AV fistulas created and a decline in AV graft procedures.

Hemodialysis catheters can be acute, intended for short-term use, or chronic, in which case a Dacron-cuffed catheter is tunneled under a subcutaneous tissue bridge that anchors the catheter and decreases the incidence of line infections. Most are constructed with polyurethane, silicone, or the copolymer Carbothane, although there is no conclusive evidence that any of those materials is associated with superior clinical outcomes.[26] Catheters may also be coated with antithrombotic or antimicrobial treatments such as antibiotics, silver, or heparin.[27,28] Of those, heparin has demonstrated the best antimicrobial properties by reducing bacterial trapping within fibrin clots and sheaths and decreasing bacterial adhesion on catheter material.[29]

Catheters can have two separate lumens, one for arterial and another for venous flow, or a single double lumen. Two randomized controlled trials comparing the two designs concluded that, although there were no significant differences in infection rates, double-lumen catheters were easier to use.[30,31] Furthermore, although most hemodialysis catheters have a staggered tip design to prevent recirculation, there is no evidence of an advantage for any particular tip design.[31] The most important factor to consider in choosing a catheter should be its long-term function and complication rate.[26]

Acute Catheters

Acute hemodialysis catheters are used primarily in critically ill patients in need of hemodialysis, patients with temporary loss of permanent access as an "in and out" strategy, and, far less frequently, in ambulatory patients being treated at centers that do not use tunneled catheters.[32] Acute catheters are preferentially placed in the internal jugular or common femoral veins. The subclavian vein should be avoided, if possible, to prevent catheter-related stenosis, which would adversely impact future AV fistula or graft patency rates.[33]

The advantage of acute hemodialysis catheters is that they can be inserted at the bedside without requiring an operating room (OR) or fluoroscopic guidance. If possible, the right internal jugular vein should be used preferentially as it is associated with a better hemodynamic profile due to its short and direct path to the right atrium compared with the left internal jugular vein, and is associated with a lower incidence of complications.[34] Furthermore, line insertion should be performed using ultrasound guidance to decrease the risk of procedural complications. Indeed, studies have shown that ultrasound guidance increases the success rate to 95% compared with placement based on anatomic landmarks, and is associated with a lower risk of catheter placement failure, failure to place the catheter on first attempt, arterial punctures, and hematoma formation.[35,36] It is also associated with a significantly decreased time to cannulate the vein and a lower number of attempts per catheter insertion.[36]

For an internal jugular vein placement, the patient's neck is prepped with an antiseptic skin cleansing solution and draped in a sterile fashion. The patient is then placed in the Trendelenburg (head down) position to dilate the neck veins and decrease the risk of accidental air embolization to the brain. An ultrasound probe is used to identify the internal jugular vein, and the skin puncture site is infiltrated with a local anesthetic solution. A blade is used to create an entry incision in the anesthetized skin, and the puncture needle supplied in the hemodialysis catheter kit is flushed with saline solution and used to puncture the vein using ultrasound guidance while maintaining suction using a syringe. Once the vein has been accessed, the Seldinger technique is used to introduce a wire, followed by a dilator; finally the hemodialysis catheter is placed into the vein. Generally a 15-cm catheter is inserted into the right internal jugular vein and a 20-cm catheter into the left internal jugular vein. The catheter should be flushed with heparinized solution and then locked with a cap. An anchoring stitch should be placed at the entry site to tether the catheter to the skin. Finally, an upright chest x-ray confirms adequate catheter placement and rules out any immediate complications such as a pneumothorax. Femoral catheters are placed similarly; however, they are more likely to become infected and occluded due to the groin location. Femoral catheters range from 20 to 24 cm in length.

Chronic Tunneled Catheters

Tunneled hemodialysis catheters are also commonly placed in the internal jugular and femoral veins. The procedure should be done under ultrasound and fluoroscopic guidance. For a tunneled internal jugular vein line, the ipsilateral neck and chest are washed with antiseptic solution before the patient is draped. The neck skin approximately 1 to 2 cm superior to the clavicle is infiltrated with local anesthetic solution, and access to the internal jugular vein is obtained using ultrasound guidance and the Seldinger technique. Unlike the acute catheter technique, however, the vein puncture site is deeper along the course of the vein. Wire access is obtained, but the catheter is not yet introduced into the vein. The chest wall is generously infiltrated with local anesthetic, and an incision is made for the catheter entry site. A subcutaneous tunnel is then fashioned bluntly along the projected course of the catheter, and the catheter is introduced through the chest incision and exteriorized through the previously created neck incision, taking care not to displace the wire that is resting in the jugular vein. The wire is used to place a peel-away sheath into the jugular vein, and this is subsequently used to advance the catheter tip, under fluoroscopic guidance, into the distal superior vena cava or junction with the right atrium. A similar approach is carried out for a tunneled femoral hemodialysis line, although the catheter tip is positioned in the inferior vena cava. Similar to nontunneled catheters, tunneled femoral vein catheters are also more likely to be infected and occluded compared with jugular catheters and should be avoided if possible.[37]

More complex pathways for tunneled hemodialysis catheters include collateral and small veins that develop in the mediastinum and chest wall secondary to chronic jugular vein occlusion, the thyrocervical collaterals, the inferior vena cava via a translumbar approach, and the hepatic vein in patients with infrarenal inferior vena cava occlusion.[38] The advantage of using collateral veins is that they preserve other veins for future use, but they can be technically difficult to access and are associated with significant anatomic variability.[39] The translumbar approach to the inferior vena cava is less technically challenging but is associated with poor patency and is a better bridging modality than a reliable long-term option for hemodialysis.[40] Finally, the transhepatic approach is associated with frequent catheter exchanges, likely because of the dynamic variation in the position of the liver with the respiratory cycle.[41]

Catheter Patency and Function

Hemodialysis catheter malfunction is defined as "failure to attain and maintain an extracorporeal blood flow sufficient to perform hemodialysis without significantly lengthening the hemodialysis treatment."[14] The minimum blood flow to maintain sufficient extracorporeal function is 300 mL/min. Malfunction can be positional, due to kinking or poor positioning, or, more commonly, mechanical, due to thrombosis, fibrin sheaths, and infection.[42]

Shingarev and colleagues examined the natural history of tunneled hemodialysis catheters and reported a median primary patency of 202 days.[43] Of the catheters examined in the study, 69% were still in place at 3 months, 53% at 6 months, and 34% at 12 months. The most common reason for nonelective removal of the catheters was catheter failure in 44% of the cases. The only predictor of catheter malfunction was placement in the left internal jugular vein. The most common strategy to prevent catheter malfunction is to employ "catheter locks" with anticoagulant agents such as heparin, citrate, tissue plasminogen activator (tPA), and oral medications such as warfarin, aspirin, and ticlodipine.[42] None of those strategies, however, has been demonstrated to be clearly superior, and future large studies are needed to adequately determine the best strategy.

Catheters that are not complicated by intraluminal thrombosis usually fail secondary to the development of fibrin sheaths. Such sheaths form at the point of contact between the catheter and vessel wall and may encapsulate the full length of the catheter within 7 days of its insertion.[44] Oliver and colleagues reported a 70% incidence of fibrin sheath obstruction in patients with long-term tunneled hemodialysis catheters with refractory catheter dysfunction.[45] The authors concluded that the disruption of sheaths by angioplasty results in durable patency and modestly improves blood flow and clearance over the duration of catheter use.

ARTERIOVENOUS FISTULAS

AV fistulas are the most durable modes of access for hemodialysis and are associated with the fewest complications (Fig. 57.1). Despite the fact that most patients begin hemodialysis with a catheter, Huber and colleagues demonstrated that access surgeons who adopt an "all autogenous policy" can attain up to a 90% rate for constructing a native AV fistula.[46] The key to successful AV fistula creation is careful patient selection and optimization. Indeed, up to 25% of AV fistulas fail secondary to thrombosis or failure to mature.[47] Preoperative workup should determine whether the patient has adequate arterial inflow, venous outflow, and an adequate vein to act as a conduit.

Configuration of AV Anastomoses

Four possible AV anastomotic configurations have been described: side to side, vein end to arterial side, arterial end to vein side, and end to end. Our group consistently uses the vein end–to–arterial side configuration, which can provide adequate flow while reducing the risk for venous hypertension that has been described with the side-to-side and arterial end–to–vein side configurations.[48] Although the end-to-end anastomosis was common in the past, it should be avoided, especially in elderly and diabetic patients, because it requires severing of the radial artery and is disadvantaged by AV size mismatch.[49] There is no high-quality evidence to suggest that any particular fistula configuration is associated with better clinical outcomes. O'Banion and Moini both reported that a side-to-side anastomoses with

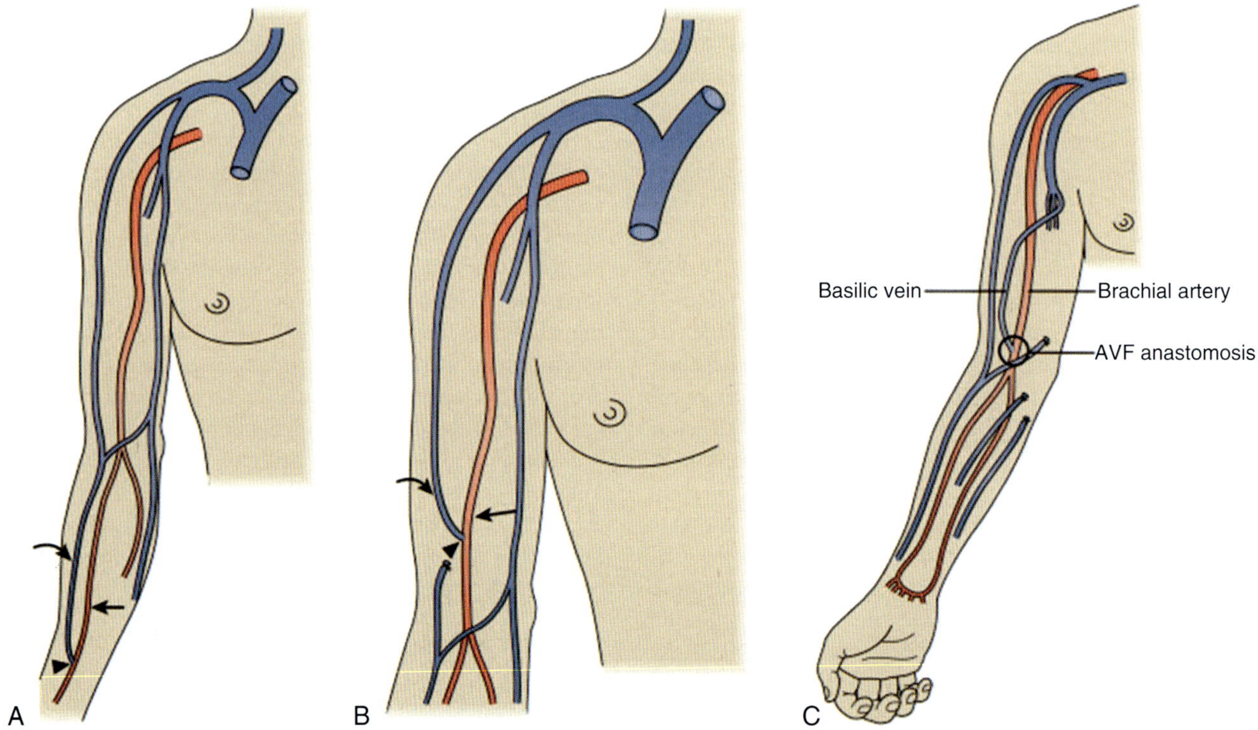

FIG 57.1 Autogenous upper extremity arteriovenous fistula configurations. (A) Radiocephalic, (B) brachiocephalic, and (C) brachiobasilic vein transposition. *AVF,* Arteriovenous fistula. (From Valji K: *The Practice of Interventional Radiology,* Philadelphia, Elsevier, 2012, Fig. 19.1.)

distal cephalic vein ligation was associated with better patency rates compared with vein end–to–arterial side anastomoses, Mozaffar and colleagues performed a small randomized controlled trial that showed no difference in clinical outcomes between patients receiving an end-to-side and a side-to-side AV fistula.[50-52]

Type of Anesthesia

The anesthetic techniques used in AV fistula creation include monitored anesthesia care (MAC), which combines local anesthesia with conscious sedation, as well as regional anesthesia and general anesthesia. The use of MAC is popular because it is quick and easy to administer, allowing for shorter operative times and less hospital resource utilization. However, it is challenging to maintain in long cases and difficult dissections. Furthermore, the administration of large doses of local anesthetic may lead to neurologic and cardiac toxicity and is associated with significant vasoconstriction.[53-55] Conversely, general anesthesia is associated with vasodilation and is commonly used in complex AV fistula procedures where a prolonged procedural time is anticipated.[56] It is also the most commonly used anesthetic option in the United States, as reported by Siracuse and colleagues, who reviewed the National Surgical Quality Improvement Project (NSQIP) data for the years 2007 to 2010 and found that 85% of patients undergoing new upper extremity AV fistula creation received a general anesthetic.[57] However, in addition to the greater operative and recovery room resources required with general anesthesia, it may not be an ideal option in dialysis patients, who carry a greater burden of comorbid disease compared with the general population.

Regional anesthesia has gained favor for AV access surgery. It can be performed preoperatively in a designated "block room," which does not interfere with OR work flow. Regional anesthesia is also associated with vasodilation of the basilic and cephalic veins, making the creation of the AV anastomosis less technically challenging.[58] However, regional anesthetic techniques require more resources than MAC. Ultimately the type of anesthesia used does not seem to affect fistula maturation and complication rates.[59] In the absence of randomized controlled trials comparing local, regional, and general anesthesia, practice continues to be guided by physician and patient preferences and institutional norms rather than high-quality evidence.[60]

Intraoperative Anticoagulation

The use of intraoperative anticoagulation during AV fistula creation is controversial. Patients with ESRD are uremic and have an impaired coagulation system, likely due to the altered metabolic interactions of the components of the coagulation cascade, platelets, and the vessel wall.[61] As such, some have reasoned that intraoperative anticoagulation is superfluous while placing the patient at an increased bleeding risk. In an attempt to address this issue, Smith and colleagues conducted a meta-analysis of four randomized controlled trials, demonstrating that systemic anticoagulation led to a significant improvement in AV fistula patency but a highly significant increase in the risk of bleeding-related complications.[62] Interestingly, the AV access advantage was lost when studies of AV grafts were included in the analysis. In our practice, intraoperative anticoagulation is selectively administered to patients with a prior history of hypercoagulable state and those with intraoperative evidence of small and thus technically challenging arteries or veins. Furthermore, when systematic anticoagulation is not administered, we occasionally flush the arteries with heparinized saline solution prior to clamping.

Femoral Vein Translocation

In patients without a viable upper extremity vein option for AV fistula construction, the femoral vein may be harvested and used as a conduit. The femoral vein is attractive for numerous reasons: its diameter is usually greater than 6 mm and it is more resilient than superficial arm veins, making it more durable and easier to manipulate. However, there are numerous disadvantages with this approach. First, harvesting the femoral vein adds a significant amount of time to the procedure. Second, there is a significant amount of morbidity associated with this procedure, including surgical site infections and venous insufficiency. Third, the use of this vein as a conduit precludes its use in other procedures.[63] Unfortunately its use is also associated with high failure rates and a primary patency of just 20% at 2 years.[64]

Radiocephalic AV Fistula (Brescia-Cimino)

The patient is placed in the supine position with the operative arm extended on a board (Fig. 57.2). If not done preoperatively,

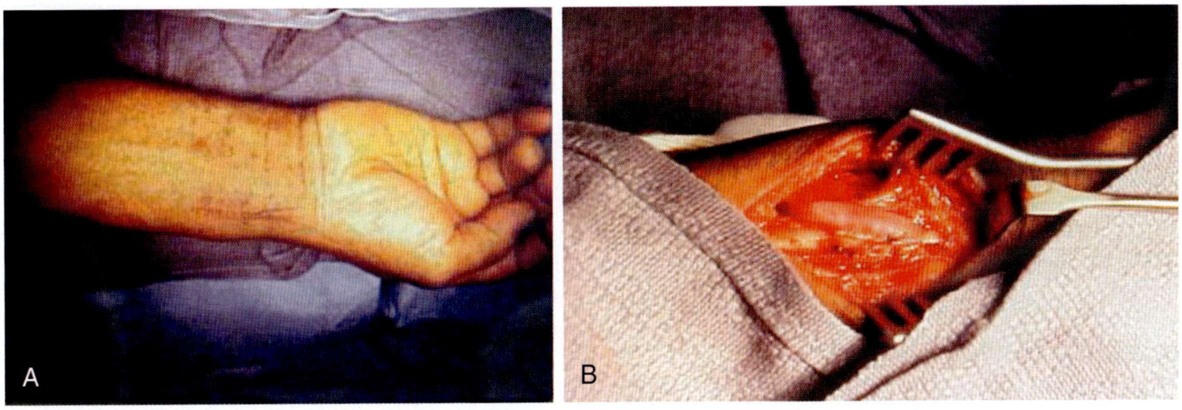

FIG 57.2 Creation of radiocephalic fistula. (A) Right-hand positioning, (B) radiocephalic anastomosis.

a bedside ultrasound can be used to map the course of the cephalic vein to assist with a precise dissection. The arm is then washed circumferentially with antiseptic solution from the shoulder to the fingertips and the arm is free-draped to allow for positional adjustments. If the patient has undergone a regional block, the skin is tested for anesthesia using toothed forceps before an incision is made. Alternatively, if a MAC strategy is pursued, conscious sedation may be administered intravenously followed by local anesthetic that is infiltrated along a line midway between the course of the palpable radial artery and the previously marked cephalic vein at the wrist. We do not routinely administer perioperative antibiotics in AV fistula procedures.

After adequate anesthesia has been established, a no. 15 blade is used to create a 2- to 3-cm incision along the course of the previously infiltrated skin midway between the radial artery and the cephalic vein. The dissection is carried down through subcutaneous tissue and flaps are created both medially and laterally. Separate incisions can be made over the radial artery and cephalic vein if an extensive flap would be required for exposure of both through a single incision. The cephalic vein is exposed laterally and mobilized proximally to enable creation of the anastomosis with minimal tension. The radial artery is then identified medially and proximal and distal control is established with vessel loops without occluding the artery. At this point, heparin is administered intravenously according to the surgeon's preference. The artery is clamped using microvascular clips (preferred) or the previously placed vessel loops, and the vein is transected, spatulated, and gently injected with heparinized saline to hydrostatically dilate the vein prior to the formation of the AV anastomosis. Handling of the vein should be as atraumatic as possible and kept to a minimum. The proximal aspect of the vein, closer to the wrist, is ligated with a silk suture ligature. The vein is superimposed onto the artery and an arteriotomy is created using a no. 11 blade and Potts scissors. The length of the arteriotomy depends on the diameter of the vein and its angle of approach. The arteriotomy should equal the vein diameter if the angle of approach is 90 degrees and be adjusted according to the longitudinal access of the artery for more acute angles.[49,65] A venous end–to–arterial side anastomosis is created using a 6-0 or 7-0 nonabsorbable monofilament suture and the "parachute" technique at the toe and heel of the anastomosis with knot formation at the midportion of the anastomosis on either side. At the completion of the anastomosis, a Doppler ultrasound is used to interrogate the cephalic vein for the characteristic "machinery murmur" humming flow. If the murmur is absent, it may indicate a technical failure due to stenosis, kinking, or torsion, and the anastomosis should be taken down, inspected, and repeated if necessary. After adequate hemodynamic control is obtained, the skin is reapproximated with an absorbable running subcuticular suture. The newly created fistula is again palpated and auscultated with a Doppler to ensure adequate flow and the incision site is covered with sterile gauze dressing, taking care not to apply too much pressure, which would occlude the fistula.

Brachiocephalic Fistula Technique

The approach to a brachiocephalic fistula is the same as for a radiocephalic fistula, as outlined earlier. However, there is no need for free draping of the operative arm. After the vein has been marked, the patient is prepped and draped and adequate anesthesia is confirmed. Using a no. 15 blade, a 3- to 4-cm transverse incision is then created approximately 1 fingerbreadth below the antecubital crease to minimize the occurrence of postoperative wound complications. Proximal and distal flaps are created and the cephalic vein or the median antecubital vein, as deemed appropriate by the surgeon, is identified and mobilized to allow for a tension-free anastomosis. Exposure of the brachial artery requires the incision of the bicipital aponeurosis, which separates the superficial and deep contents of the antecubital fossa. Care should be taken to prevent direct trauma or thermal injury to the median nerve, which runs in close proximity to the brachial artery. Proximal and distal control of the artery is obtained using vessel loops; the patient may receive an intravenous dose of heparin at this point, as per the surgeon's preference. The artery is then clamped with the vessel loops or microvascular clips. The vein is transected, spatulated, and injected with normal saline to dilate it with gentle hydrostatic pressure. Care should be taken to not traumatize the vein. The proximal aspect of the vein is suture-ligated with a monofilament nonabsorbable suture. The vein is then superimposed onto the artery and an arteriotomy is created using a no. 11 blade and Potts scissors. The length of the arteriotomy depends on the diameter of the vein and its angle of approach. A venous end–to–arterial side anastomosis is then created using the "parachute" technique with a 6-0 or 7-0 nonabsorbable monofilament suture. The patency of the fistula is checked by feeling for a thrill or Doppler ultrasound if the thrill is questionable. The anastomosis should be taken down and repeated if there is no evidence of adequate flow in the cephalic vein. After adequate hemostasis is confirmed, the subcutaneous tissue is then reapproximated with a running absorbable suture and the skin is reapproximated with an absorbable subcuticular suture. Adequate flow is then confirmed once more with palpation of a thrill and/or Doppler ultrasound interrogation of the fistula.

Brachiobasilic Vein Transposition Technique

For patients who are not candidates for radio- or brachiocephalic AV fistula creation or if the basilic vein is of markedly better quality than the cephalic system, a brachiobasilic vein transposition can be performed using a single- or two-stage approach (Fig. 57.3). In the single-stage approach, the basilic vein is transected, tunneled laterally, and anastomosed to the brachial artery in a single procedure. The two-stage approach, however, starts by creating a brachiobasilic AV fistula that allows the basilic vein to arterialize and mature. In a second stage, the fistula is taken down and the basilic vein is tunneled laterally and reanastomosed onto the brachial artery. A meta-analysis by Cooper and colleagues found that the two-stage approach is associated with improved 1-year patency and reduced primary failure rates, although the authors cautioned that their findings were limited by the small size, observational design, and inconsistent quality of the included studies.[66]

The single-stage procedure begins with placing the patient in the supine position with the operative arm extended. The entire course of the basilic vein is mapped using ultrasound if

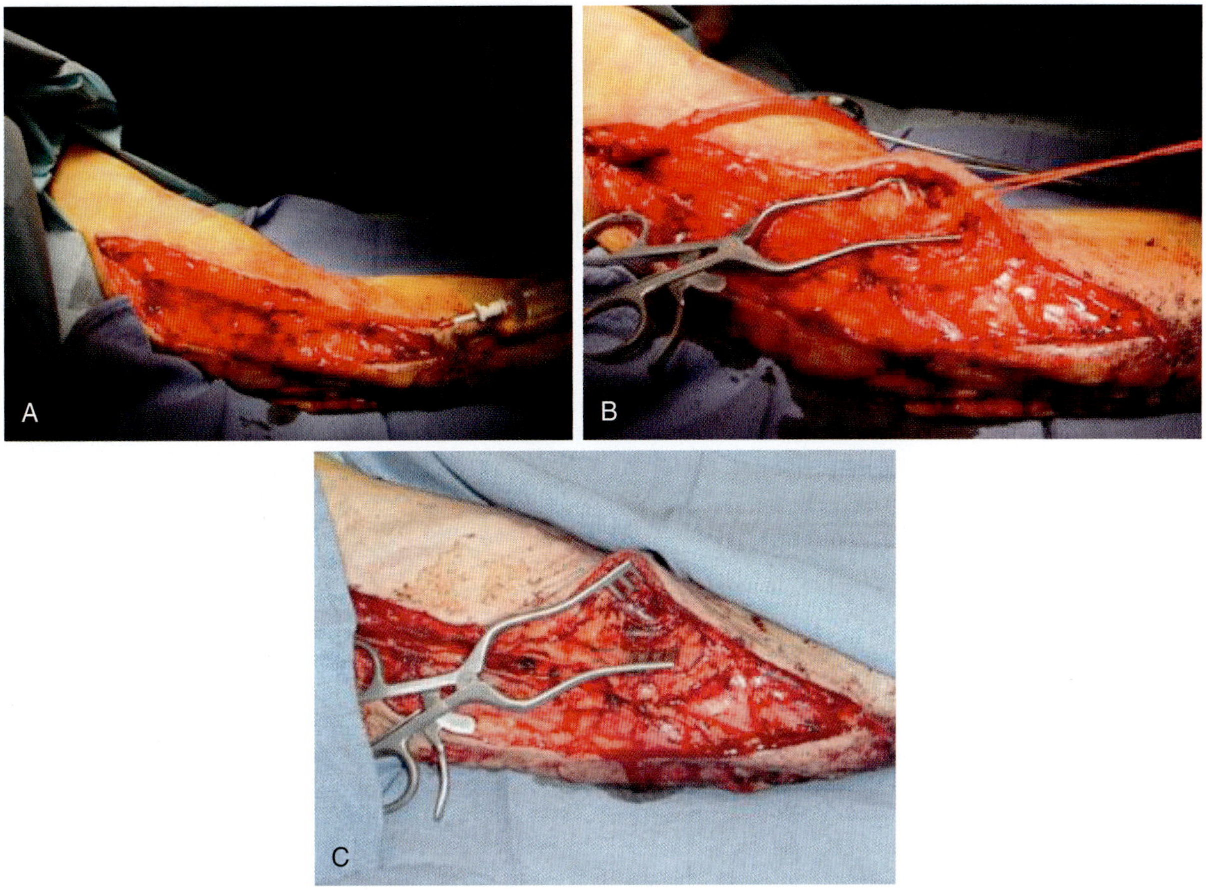

FIG 57.3 Creation of brachiobasilic fistula. (A) Exposure of left basilic vein, (B) anterolateral tunneling of basilic vein, (C) brachiobasilic anastomosis.

needed to facilitate dissection. The extent of dissection needed makes MAC anesthesia difficult and a regional block or general anesthesia is usually preferred. After the patient is prepped and draped as described above, an incision is made along the course of the vein. During the dissection and mobilization of the vein, the medial antecubital cutaneous nerve is commonly encountered and should be preserved to prevent postoperative neurologic deficits that can lead to neuropathy and patient dissatisfaction.[67] The basilic vein should be mobilized from the antecubital fossa to the axilla, and its tributaries should be ligated and transected. The brachial artery should then be exposed through a medial approach, taking care to preserve and avoid injuring the median nerve. The brachial artery is then dissected and controlled with vessel loops both proximally and distally without clamping. The vein should then be harvested as proximally as possible and a curved tunneler or tunneling clamp used to create a lateral pathway for the vein on the outer aspect of the upper arm that can be accessed for dialysis. Again, the vein is flushed with heparinized saline solution with gentle hydrostatic dilation. Therapeutic anticoagulation can then be administered, as per the surgeon's preference, and the artery is clamped with the previously placed vessel loops or vascular clips. The vein is transposed onto the artery using the previously created tunnel. An arteriotomy is made using a no. 11 blade and extended as needed with Potts scissors. A venous end–to–arterial side anastomosis is then created as described earlier with wound closure.

The advantage of the two-stage brachiobasilic AV fistula procedure is that it prevents the patient from undergoing a potentially morbid dissection of the medial arm if the basilic vein fails to sufficiently arterialize after the first stage. The vein also elongates after the first procedure and is easier to handle because of maturation and distention. After stage one as described, the basilic vein's maturation is monitored and a second-stage procedure arranged if and when the basilic vein reaches a reasonable diameter (6 mm). The second-stage procedure is identical to the single-stage procedure already described, although it has been our experience that the arterialized basilic vein is somewhat thicker and easier to handle. Of note, we do not leave drains in either single- or two-stage brachiobasilic vein transposition procedures.

Lower Extremity AV Fistula Technique

Lower extremity AV fistulas are similar to brachiobasilic vein transposition procedures but should be reserved for those patients in whom upper extremity options have been exhausted. The lower extremity fistulas carry a greater morbidity and increased risk of infection and edema. These procedures are performed with a regional block or general anesthesia, depending on the patient's preference and comorbidity. The femoral vein is mobilized distally, from the adductor hiatus, to proximally to its insertion onto the common femoral vein. The vein is divided at the adductor hiatus, tunneled laterally in the thigh, and then anastomosed to the distal superficial femoral artery near the adductor hiatus as a single-stage procedure.[68] An alternate and often preferable option for an autogenous lower extremity AV fistula is a great saphenous vein (GSV) loop graft. The GSV is mobilized from the knee proximally toward the saphenofemoral junction. Careful ligation and division of all GSV tributaries should be performed. The vein is flushed with heparinized saline solution. The vein is then tunneled from medially to laterally in the thigh and anastomosed onto the common femoral artery.[69] The arterial anastomosis is often preferentially performed to the proximal superficial femoral artery to avoid any impact on the origin of the profunda femoris. The major complications associated with lower extremity AV fistulas are infection and distal limb ischemia secondary to steal syndrome.[70]

Postoperative Follow-Up

Most procedures can be performed on an outpatient basis, and the patient is seen 10 to 14 days postoperatively to examine the wound and ensure that the fistula is patent and without other complication. Patients with upper extremity AV fistulas can use a stress ball to encourage hand exercises and expedite the fistula maturation process. Indeed, hand exercises after AV fistula surgery have been associated with enlargement of the arterialized vein, an improved capacity for vasodilatation, and improved fistula maturation.[71] The diameter of the arterialized vein is followed with examination and ultrasounds with the maturation process considered to be ideal when the vein reaches 6 mm in diameter with a minimum flow of 600 mL/min, as per the societal guidelines discussed below. In our experience, this process often requires a minimum of 6 weeks. If veins fail to mature, a fistulogram can be considered to investigate treatable conditions such as inadequate inflow through the artery or, more commonly, central venous outflow disease, which may be amenable to endovascular repair. Sometimes the fistulogram reveals accessory venous branches that diminish the flow within the fistula and are subsequently ligated in the OR, with excellent results.

After patients begin hemodialysis using a newly created AV fistula, they are not routinely followed in a clinic setting but are reassessed on an as-needed basis when requested to do so by the dialysis team. Signs of impending access failure include decreased fistula flow rates, increased venous pressure, as measured by the dialysis machine, and a decreased urea reduction ratio.[72] However, Casey and colleagues found no compelling evidence to support routine surveillance of AV access and concluded that the quality of the current evidence for doing so is very poor.[73]

Outcomes

In order to assess outcomes after AV access creation, it is crucial to be familiar with the concepts of primary patency, assisted primary patency, and secondary patency. According to the Committee on Reporting Standards of the Society for Vascular Surgery, primary patency is defined as "the interval from the time of access placement until any intervention designed to maintain or reestablish patency, access thrombosis, or the time of measurement of patency." Assisted primary patency is defined as "the interval from the time of access placement until access thrombosis or the time of measurement of patency, including intervening manipulations (surgical or endovascular interventions) designed to maintain the functionality of a patent access." Finally, secondary patency is defined as "the interval from the time of access placement until access abandonment, thrombosis, or the time of patency measurement including intervening manipulations (surgical or endovascular interventions) designed to reestablish functionality in thrombosed access."[74]

Despite being the gold standard for hemodialysis access, up to 50% of upper extremity AV fistulas are never used for hemodialysis and 25% fail after 2 years.[75] The outcomes in the lower extremity are no better. However, the 12-month patency rates of femoral vein transposition arteriovenous fistulas are better than those of upper- and midthigh grafts, with weighted mean primary patency rates of 83% versus 48% and 43%, respectively, and weighted mean secondary patency rates of 93% versus 69% and 67%, respectively.[70] Conversely, the cumulative patency rate of saphenous vein transposition fistulas has been reported to be 66% at 2 years and 40% at 3 years.[76]

Several studies have examined the factors that predict outcomes after AV fistula creation. The functional ability of the artery and vein to dilate and achieve a rapid increase in blood flow after surgery may be the most important determinant of AV fistula maturation.[77] Furthermore, accelerated venous neointimal hyperplasia, as a result of the AV fistula configuration or of vascular injury, is another important cause of maturation failure.[78] Factors such as increased age, diabetes, diastolic hypotension, artery and vein diameter, arteriosclerosis, and venous distensibility have all been correlated with AV fistula patency.[79] Gender, however, has not been shown to be a significant predictor.[80] Unfortunately the ability of clinicians to predict AV fistula maturation is still limited. Physical examination and Duplex ultrasound remain the most reliable tools for preoperative assessment.[81]

ARTERIOVENOUS GRAFTS

When autogenous AV fistula options are exhausted, patients should be considered for the creation of an AV graft using a synthetic or biologic conduit (Fig. 57.4). Although AV grafts have numerous disadvantages, including lower patency and a higher complication rate, their main advantages are the wide availability of conduit compared with the limited autogenous vein options and the shorter time to access the graft, as there is no need to wait for a fistula to mature.

Graft Types

The ideal AV graft should be readily available, easy to handle, nonthrombogenic, immunologically inert, resistant to infection and repeated access, able to retain tensile strength, and cost-effective.[82] ePTFE is among the most commonly used prosthetic graft materials due to its durable nature and wide availability. However, there is a 2-week waiting period for the graft to be

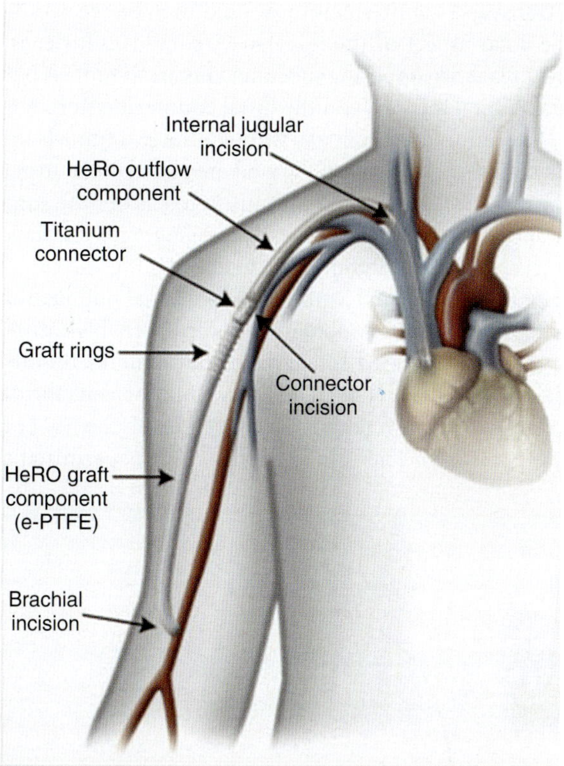

FIG 57.4 HeRO graft catheter. (From *Annals of Vascular Surgery*, Volume 25, Issue 3, April 2011, pages 387–387, Fig. 3.)

incorporated before it can be accessed to minimize the risk of hematoma or seroma formation as well as thrombosis. This may force the placement and use of temporary central lines for those patients with an ongoing hemodialysis requirement. This has given rise to a generation of multilayered and self-sealing "early cannulation" grafts that can be accessed within 72 hours.[83] The main disadvantage of those grafts is that they are more expensive and less readily available compared with ePTFE, with an increased conduit thickness during construction of the anastomosis. Heparin-bonded ePTFE has also been used to decrease prosthetic graft thrombosis by bonding heparin to the inner surface of the conduit, thus reducing platelet deposition and thrombus formation. While demonstrating some benefit in lower extremity bypass, there is questionable benefit at best in the in dialysis access population.[84]

Unfortunately prosthetic grafts have higher rates of thrombosis due to intimal hyperplasia and a relatively high rate of infection. In order to minimize these complications and extend dialysis access performance, biologic alternatives to prosthetic grafts have been attempted, including bovine carotid artery, cryopreserved vein grafts, biosynthetic composite grafts, bovine ureteric grafts, and bovine mesenteric veins.[82,85,86] First studied by Matsuura and colleagues, cryopreserved venous grafts were intended for patients with infected grafts and no autogenous AV access options.[87] The authors reported no infections, a 1-year primary graft patency rate of 49%, and a secondary graft patency rate of 75%. However, other groups have reported a significant incidence of graft infection and rupture with this technique; its use in hemodialysis access creation has consequently been limited.[88] Biosynthetic grafts such as the Omniflow vascular prosthesis (LeMaitre Vascular, Burlington, MA) are biosynthetic composites of polyester mesh and ovine connective tissue components.[89,90] Although the evidence for their use is based on small institutional series, a review by Al Shakarchi and colleagues from the United Kingdom reported a primary patency rate of 60% and a secondary patency rate of 82%, with infection rates ranging between 0% and 6%.[91] Other modern bioprostheses, such as bovine mesenteric veins and ureteric grafts, are prepared using a process of gluteraldehyde cross linking and gamma radiation or detergent processing.[82] They have shown encouraging results compared with ePTFE and a better infection resistance profile, but they are expensive and there have been no large randomized studies to support their use.[92-94] Unfortunately these biologic conduits have not improved on the results of standard prosthetic grafts with a significant incidence of thrombosis and dilation of the conduit.

Lawson and colleagues have reported an initial clinical experience with a bioengineered conduit constructed from banked human vascular smooth muscle cells cultured on a biodegradable polymer.[95] A process of decellularization removes viable tissue elements, leaving an intact conduit with preserved mechanical properties. This trial is the largest reported for a tissue-engineered vascular conduit. These bioengineered conduits demonstrated no dilation and minimal postcannulation bleeding, with a 6-month primary patency of 63% (primary assisted patency 73%, secondary patency 97%). Thrombosis at 12 months resulted in a 28% primary patency (secondary patency 89%). The rate of reintervention was similar to reported rates with ePTFE, including 16 venous anastomotic revisions showing no demonstrable reduction in anastomotic hyperplasia. Although patency rates were acceptable, there was no obvious improvement over prosthetic graft results, and patency was not as good as that with arteriovenous fistula construction. However, the potential benefits and significant scientific efforts surrounding this conduit support further testing and a larger controlled clinical study.

HeRO Graft

Despite the availability of a range of prosthetic and biologic grafts, many patients are ineligible for graft placement because of central venous stenosis or lack of venous outflow. To address this challenge, the Hemodialysis Reliable Outflow (HeRO) graft (Merit Medical Systems, South Jordan, UT) was developed to combine fluoroscopic central venous access with a prosthetic AV graft (see Fig. 57.4).[96] The HeRO graft's placement success rate is greater than 90%, which has allowed patients who would otherwise be dependent on tunneled catheters the opportunity to benefit from an AV graft configuration.[97] A literature review including 400 patients from eight centers showed only 22% 1-year patency with a 6% incidence of arterial steal and 0.13 to 0.7 incidents of bacteremia per 1000 days of use, with the authors calling for randomized trials.[98] Contraindications for HeRO graft placement include a brachial artery diameter smaller than 3 mm, an internal jugular vein that cannot accommodate a 19-Fr sheath, cellulitis or infection at the implantation site, and known or suspected bacterial sepsis or systemic infection.

Forearm Prosthetic Graft Technique

The approach to this procedure is similar to the brachiocephalic AV fistula technique described previously (Fig. 57.5A). The patient is placed in the supine position with the operative arm extended on a board. The arm is then washed circumferentially with antiseptic solution from the shoulder to the wrist and draping is applied, exposing the forearm. After adequate anesthesia is administered, a transverse incision is created using a no. 15 blade approximately 1 fingerbreadth inferior to the antecubital crease. The dissection is carried deep to the subcutaneous fascia and the antecubital or cephalic vein is identified and controlled with vessel loops. The bicipital aponeurosis is then incised and the brachial artery exposed and similarly encircled with vessel loops.

A transverse counterincision should then be created distally on the volar aspect of the forearm. A curved tunneler is then used to create two opposing subcutaneous arced tunnels between the antecubital incision and the distal counterincision. A 6-mm graft is introduced sequentially through the two tunnels to form a loop, such that both ends of the graft are placed at the antecubital incision. A dose of heparin is administered as per the surgeon's preference and the artery is clamped. Using a no. 11 blade and Potts scissors, an arteriotomy is created along the anterior aspect of the brachial artery and a graft end–to–arterial side anastomosis is created using a 6-0 monofilament nonabsorbable suture. The clamp is then migrated to the proximal graft to restore flow within the brachial artery. The antecubital or cephalic vein is then clamped and a venotomy is created using the no. 11 blade and Potts scissors. The vein is flushed with heparinized saline

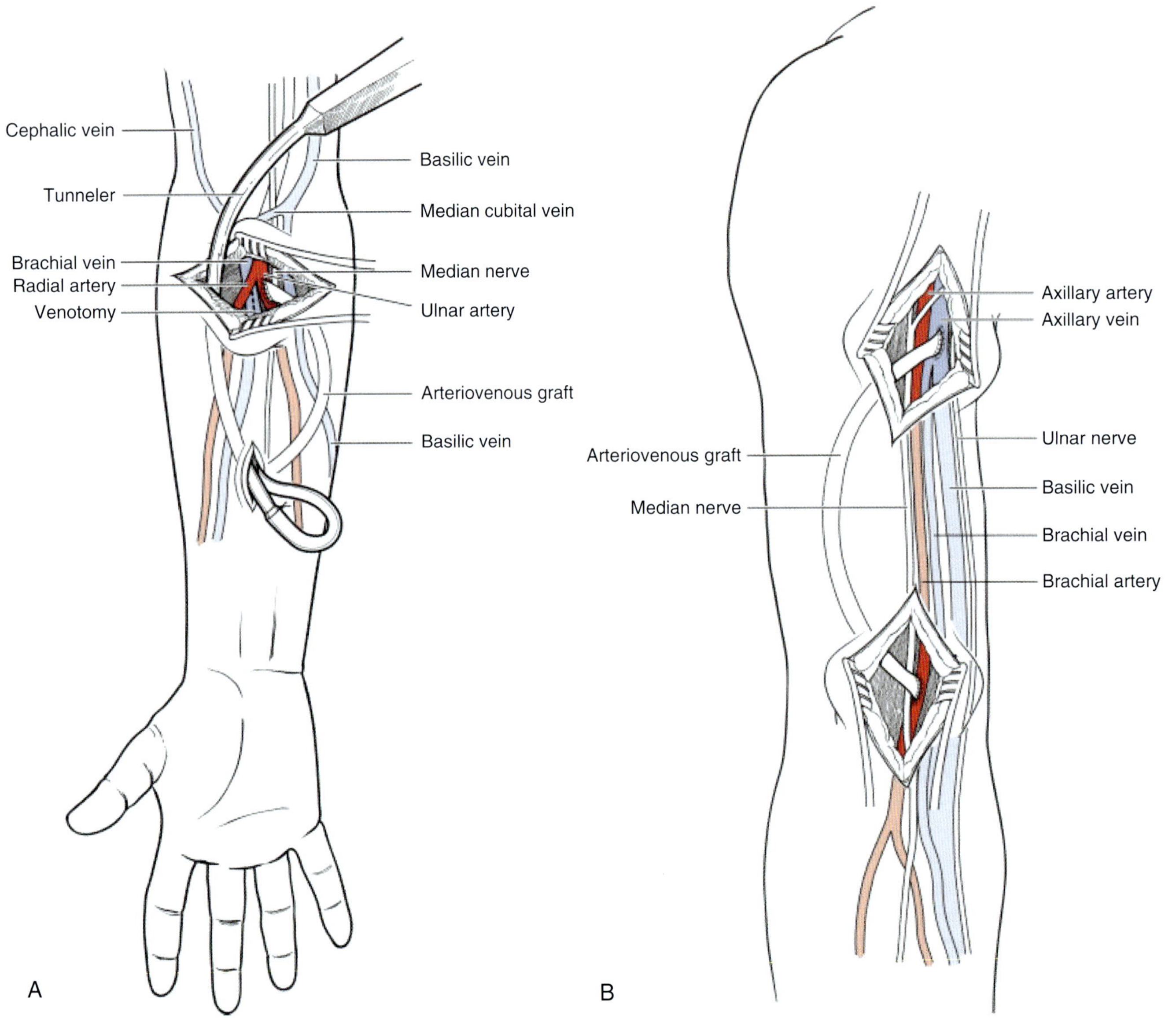

FIG 57.5 Prosthetic vascular access configurations: (A) forearm loop graft, (B) brachial artery–to–axillary vein interposition graft. (From Chaikof EL, Cambria RP: *Atlas of Vascular Surgery and Endovascular Therapy*, Philadelphia, Elsevier, 2014, Figs. 64.3 and 64.4.)

solution. A graft end-to-venous side anastomosis is then similarly created using the 6-0 monofilament suture. The clamp is then released sequentially to "de-air" the graft, and flow is established. In keeping with the preoperative exam, a pulse or Doppler signal is confirmed in the radial artery to ensure adequate distal flow. The antecubital and distal incisions are then closed with a subcuticular absorbable suture.

Upper Arm Prosthetic Graft Technique

For this procedure, we prefer placing the brachial artery inflow distally above the antecubital crease rather than in the axilla because it is easier to expose the artery distally and tunnel the graft laterally than to expose the artery in the axilla and create a loop configuration (see Fig. 57.5B). The patient is placed in the supine position with the operative arm extended at a 90-degree angle on a board. It is easier to perform this procedure under general anesthesia due to the deep dissection that is sometimes required in the axilla. The arm is then washed with antiseptic solution circumferentially from the chest to the wrist and draped.

The procedure starts with exposure of the brachial artery, as previously described. A separate medial incision is created in the upper arm distal to the axilla, and the axillary vein is exposed and encircled with vessel loops. A curved tunneler is then used to create an arced tunnel between the axillary incision and the distal antecubital incision as lateral on the arm as possible to facilitate future hemodialysis access. A 6-mm graft is then introduced through the tunnel. A weight-based dose of heparin is then administered as per the surgeon's preference and the artery is clamped. Similar to the forearm AV graft procedure, the arterial anastomosis is performed and a clamp is migrated to the proximal graft to allow distal flow within the brachial artery but close to the arterial anastomosis so as to prevent thrombus from developing in the graft. The axillary vein is then clamped, with care taken to identify the major axillary vein trunk as the vein exits the axilla to the chest. As the anastomosis is completed, the graft is "forward flushed" to de-air and the axillary vein flushed in a retrograde and prograde manner. The anastomosis is then completed, a thrill is assessed in the axillary vein, and a pulse is palpated in the radial artery to ensure adequate distal flow. The subcutaneous tissue at the axillary incision is reapproximated with a running absorbable suture and the two skin incisions are closed with a running absorbable subcuticular suture.

Lower Extremity Prosthetic Graft Technique

The approach to this procedure will depend on the inflow and outflow vessels chosen for creating the AV graft. Our preference is to use the proximal superficial femoral artery and femoral vein or proximal saphenous vein if it is of reasonable caliber. This avoids a groin incision and preserves the common femoral vessels for any future procedures that may be required while minimizing the chance of lower extremity arterial steal and ischemia.

Lower extremity AV procedures can be performed using a regional block or general anesthesia, as per the patient's and anesthesiologist's preference in communication with the surgeon. The patient is placed in the supine position and the operative side washed with antiseptic solution from the hip to the knee. The patient is then draped and a longitudinal incision or transverse incision can be made in the medial aspect of the midthigh along the course of the sartorius muscle. The sartorius muscle is identified and retracted laterally to expose the superficial femoral artery and femoral or proximal saphenous vein. Both vessels are then encircled with vessel loops and a tunneler is used to create a subcutaneous loop with the help of a counterincision distally, as described in the earlier section titled Forearm Prosthethic Graft Technique. The course of the tunnel should be as anterior and lateral in the thigh as possible; it should be deep to the sartorius muscle laterally and superficial to the muscle medially to prevent graft kinking. A 6-mm graft is then introduced through the tunnel. A weight-based dose of heparin is given to the patient as per the surgeon's preference and the artery is clamped. The arterial and venous anastomoses are performed as previously described.

Postoperative Follow-Up

AV graft procedures can often be performed on an outpatient basis. All patients receiving an AV graft are seen in clinic 10 to 14 days after the procedure to assess the surgical wound and determine the graft's readiness for hemodialysis access. Patients with ePTFE grafts usually begin hemodialysis through their newly created access after a 2-week maturation period, whereas patients receiving an early-cannulation graft are usually accessed within 72 hours. If the patient has a tunneled hemodialysis catheter, it is removed as soon as the AV graft has been confirmed with several successful episodes of AV graft utilization for dialysis. Long-term follow-up is carried out using a similar protocol with AV graft patients as with fistula patients, with clinic visits on an as-needed basis if the hemodialysis team has any concerns, as outlined earlier. If flow rates drop consistently below 600 mL/min while on dialysis, examination with Duplex ultrasound and selective imaging with a fistulagram is indicated.

Patency Outcomes

The cumulative patency rates of all AV grafts have been reported at 59% to 90% at 1 year and 50% to 82% at 2 years, which are inferior to AV fistulas.[99] ePTFE AV grafts, which are the most commonly used prosthetic grafts, are associated with primary 1-year patency rates of 28% and secondary patency rates of 76%, 59%, and 43% at 6, 12, and 24 months, respectively.[82] Although no large prospective studies are available, current evidence suggests that ePTFE and newer, "early access" vascular grafts have similar patency rates and clinical outcomes.[100-104] Furthermore, heparin-bonded PTFE grafts have also been used in dialysis access creation, although there is insufficient evidence to suggest improved patency compared with other prosthetic grafts.[105] Suemitsu and colleagues in Japan investigated the factors predictive of primary patency after forearm AV graft creation and found that radial artery inflow was associated with superior patency compared with the brachial artery (53.8% vs. 24.4%; $P = .03$).[106] HeRO grafts have been associated with similar patency rates compared with other AV grafts but better clinical outcomes compared with tunneled catheters.[107] And although HeRO grafts and thigh grafts have similar secondary patency and infection rates, HeRO grafts have been shown to be more cost-effective as compared with tunneled catheters and thigh grafts.[108,109]

COMPLICATIONS

The most common complications after AV access creation are thrombosis, bleeding, infection, noninfectious fluid collections, pseudoaneurysm formation, venous hypertension, arterial steal syndrome, high-output cardiac failure, and neuropathy (Table 57.1).[110]

Thrombosis

Thrombosis is the most common cause of autogenous and prosthetic AV access failure.[111] Factors that have been associated with thrombosis include the prosthetic graft material, a vein less than 2.5 mm in diameter, or the presence of diabetes mellitus. There is no apparent difference between direct anastomoses and the translocated configuration. Thrombosis of an arteriovenous fistula (AVF) is most often the result of diminished venous outflow because of a poor venous conduit or venous stenosis, either centrally or peripherally. Arteriovenous graft (AVG) thrombosis is most often related to anastomotic stenosis related to myointimal hyperplasia that occurs between the graft and venous outflow. If thrombosis occurs within the initial 30-day postoperative period, a problem with venous outflow should be suspected regardless of whether it is an AVF or AVG. However, a technical error or arterial inflow problem should also be suspected. Early thrombosis can also be due to medical factors such as endothelial injury, stasis of the blood, and hypercoagulability.[112] As previously mentioned, late thrombosis is most often related to venous stenosis with an AVF or anastomotic stenosis with an AVG.

Intervention for a failing or thrombosed access includes both endovascular and open surgical options. Endovascular options for an identified failing access include balloon angioplasty of any stenotic venous segment or anastomosis, with or without stent placement. Several studies have examined the technical factors associated with improved patency of an AV access after endovascular intervention, as the type of balloon and duration of inflation, but none were associated with improved long-term patency.[113] Options for open repair include patch angioplasty of the stenotic anastomosis or venous segment with a vein or other patch. If the access failure is due to stenosis of a venous segment, then resection and placement of an interposition graft might be considered. Alternatively, if there are several stenotic segments within the venous outflow, a composite AVG procedure might be considered.[114]

Management of the thrombosed AV access can be performed with an endovascular or open approach. Although endovascular therapy for a thrombosed autogenous AVF is often not effective or durable unless the vein can be completely cleared of mural thrombus and the underlying etiology of failure effectively treated. Percutaneous chemical, mechanical, and open thrombectomy have unfortunately been associated with poor outcomes and only limited short-term success.[115,116] Furthermore, there is no difference in outcomes between the different interventional modalities with the exception of a possible advantage for the surgical treatment of autogenous AV fistula thrombosis with correction of any underlying abnormality, although high-quality evidence is lacking.[117,118] This underscores the importance of a prompt workup and intervention in a failing AV access before thrombosis occurs.

Bleeding

Bleeding complications associated with AV access can occur intraoperatively with intractable oozing or postoperatively with prolonged bleeding after dialysis access. An underlying etiology in both instances is dysfunctional hemostasis in uremic patients with ESRD, although venous hypertension in the limb may also contribute to prolonged bleeding and should be considered in the differential diagnosis. Bleeding has been classified according to its severity: grade 0 (no bleeding), grade 1 (resolves without treatment), grade 2 (resolves with medical therapy), and grade 3 (requires a surgical intervention).[74]

The management of uremic bleeding aims to correct the underlying coagulopathy and poor platelet function in ESRD. Dialysis improves platelet abnormalities and reduces the risk of hemorrhage but does not entirely eliminate the risk of bleeding.[119] Other strategies include the administration of cryoprecipitate, vasopressin, and erythropoietin. Cryoprecipitate was successfully used by Janson and colleagues in 1980 for the temporary treatment of uremic bleeding.[120] However, subsequent research has shown that there is a variable response to this treatment among some patients, and different doses might be needed.[121] Mannucci and colleagues showed that vasopressin can similarly stem uremic bleeding for a short duration of time.[122] It is associated with fewer potential complications compared with cryoprecipitate, including mild facial swelling, tachycardia, and headache.[123] Finally, the use of erythropoietin to correct anemia in chronically uremic patients has been shown to decrease the risk of bleeding by shortening the bleeding time in these patients.[124,125] Fortunately use of these medical interventions is rarely required.

Infection

Infection is a major source of morbidity and mortality in ESRD patients who are dialysis dependent.[126] Uremic patients are immunocompromised due to the impaired coordination between the different components of the immune system.[127] Furthermore, repeated access places the hemodialysis patient at a higher risk of infection compared with other patients. AV access can be classified according to the following grading system: grade 0 (no infection), grade 1 (resolves with antibiotics treatment), grade 2 (loss of AV access), and grade 3 (loss of limb).[74] Septic episodes can be expected up to 0.15 times per dialysis year, or, 1.5 episodes per 10 years of dialysis. Overall, there is approximately a 20% incidence of some degree of infection associated with prosthetic AVGs and only 5% with AVFs. Additionally, bacterial colonization is present in up to 60% of dialysis patients and 30% of dialysis staff.

The most common organisms in AV access infections are *Staphylococcus aureus* and *Enterococcus*.[110] Patients typically present with clinical signs of cellulitis, induration, purulence, or a draining sinus along the course of the AV access. The treatment of an infected AV access depends on whether it is autogenous or prosthetic, its location, the type of bacteria, and the clinical presentation. A patient presenting with asymptomatic cellulitis

TABLE 57.1 **Grading Severity of Arteriovenous Access Complications**

Complication	Severity
Local Access Complications	
Bleeding	0, None
Early, postoperative	1, Resolves without treatment
Prolonged bleeding from needle puncture sites	2, Medical therapy needed to correct coagulation abnormality 3, Intervention needed
Infection	0, None
Early (<30 days)/late (>30 days)	1, Resolved with antibiotic treatment
Culture: positive/negative	2, Loss of AV access because of ligation, removal, and possible bypass
Site of infection: anastomosis/mid-AV access/runoff vein	3, Loss of limb
Noninfectious fluid collections	0, None
Hematoma	1, Observed, resolved
Seroma	2, Aspirated, surgical drainage
Lymphocoele	3, Loss of AV access
Anastomotic complications	0, None
Hemorrhage: external bleeding/hematoma	1, Observed
Pseudoaneurysm: mechanical/infectious	2, Aspirated, surgical drainage, or correction maintaining AV access functionality
Stenosis with intimal hyperplasia: venous anastomosis	3, Loss of AV access
Mid-AV access/runoff vein complications	0, None
Dilation/aneurysm	1, Observed, no treatment needed
Pseudoaneurysm at needle stick site	2, Local treatment: interventional/surgical revision
Mid-AV access stenosis	3, Loss of AV access
Access thrombosis	0, None
Early (<30 days)/late (>30 days)	1, Clot removal
Cause found (technical, anastomotic intimal hyperplasia, coagulation disorders)	2, Revision with or without clot removal
Cause not found	3, Loss of AV access
AV access malfunction	0, Functional AV access
Insufficient inflow	1, Not corrected
Insufficient runoff	2, Required revision
Inability to puncture: too small/too deep	3, Loss of AV access
Remote Complications	
Steal syndrome	0, None
Healthy vasculature (anastomosis/runoff vessel too large)	1, Mild (cool extremity with few symptoms but demonstrable by flow augmentation with fistula occlusion), no treatment needed
Abnormal vasculature	
Inflow obstruction	
Decreased collateral flow (e.g., occluded ulnar artery with cephaloradial direct access)	2, Moderate (intermittent ischemia only during dialysis/claudication), intervention sometimes needed
Distal arterial occlusive disease	3, Severe (ischemic pain at rest/tissue loss), intervention mandatory
Venous hypertension	0, None
Valvular incompetence with retrograde flow	1, Mild (minimal symptoms/discoloration/minimal extremity swelling), no treatment needed
Central vein thrombosis: axillary/subclavian/internal jugular/ brachiocephalic/superior vena cava	2, Moderate (intermittent discomfort/severe swelling), intervention usually needed
Runoff vein stenosis	3, Severe (persistent discomfort with hyperpigmentation/ persistent swelling, severe or massive/venous ulceration), intervention mandatory
Neuropathy (excluding ischemia/steal)	0, None
Systemic: uremia (β2-microglobin amyloidosis)/diabetes	1, Mild, intermittent sensory changes (pain/paresthesia/numbness with sensory deficit)
Mechanical: entrapment or compartment syndromes (carpal tunnel/ cubital or ulnar nerve compression)	2, Moderate, persistent sensory changes 3, Severe, sensory changes and progressive loss of motor function: movement/strength/ muscle wasting

AV, Arteriovenous.
From Sidawy AN, et al: Recommended standards for reports dealing with arteriovenous hemodialysis accesses. *J Vasc Surg* 35(3):603–610, 2002, Table VI.

overlying an AV fistula would require a different treatment than a patient presenting with a purulent *Pseudomonas* discharge from an infected AV prosthetic graft.

Patients with an infected AV fistula should be treated with a short course of antibiotics and reassessed on a regular basis. If the infection does not subside, an ultrasound should be obtained to rule out a drainable abscess. In certain circumstances, such as infections with antibiotic-resistant bacterial strains or the presence of previously placed stents or other prosthetic materials, a prolonged course of intravenous antibiotics may be necessary. Conversely, the treatment of prosthetic AV graft infections with antibiotics alone is usually not sufficient but can be attempted with only an overlying cellulitic reaction. Any AVG with a fluid collection, drainage, or resulting in sepses requires resection of the infected segment or the entire graft, depending on the extent of the infection and the infectious organism.

Noninfectious Fluid Collections

Fluid collections that sometimes develop around an AV access include hematomas, seromas, and lymphoceles. These collections have also ben classified according to a grading system: grade 0 (no fluid collection), grade 1 (observed and resolved fluid collection), grade 2 (aspirated or surgical drainage of fluid collection), and grade 3 (loss of AV access).[74] Hematomas result from a combination of dysfunctional hemostasis in uremic patients and frequent access of the AV fistula. However, most hematomas are benign and will resolve spontaneously; therefore they and should be observed. An intervention is warranted only if the hematoma becomes symptomatic, either by compressing the AV access or by infection. Evacuation of an asymptomatic hematoma can be associated with an increased risk of infection and should be avoided. Seromas tend to occur around prosthetic rather than autogenous grafts, are infrequent, and are also usually managed conservatively. Fluid collections are more common in the upper arm versus the lower arm and can require graft excision or a bypass procedure of the affected segment.[128] Lymphoceles are collections of fluid that accumulate secondary to disruption of the lymphatic microcirculation around the AV access. Like seromas and hematomas, they are managed nonoperatively, and the majority will reabsorb spontaneously without intervention.

Pseudoaneurysms

Aneurysms and pseudoaneurysms of AV fistulas and grafts have been reported in 5% to 60% of patients with a large variability in the literature likely due to the absence of a standardized definition for this condition.[129] The challenge in defining aneurysms is that both arteries and veins dilate in response to hemodialysis access creation. It is therefore difficult to set a diameter increase threshold beyond which a vessel is deemed to be aneurysmal. To address this issue, Mudoni and colleagues suggested defining AV fistula aneurysms as an "abnormal localized dilatation of the vessel and classify it on the basis of true aneurysm or false (pseudo) aneurysm, location (arterial/venous/graft) and site (anastomotic/puncture site/native vessel and whole outflow vein)."[129] Pseudoaneurysms at the anastomotic site or body of the access conduit are easier to define, being encountered as complications with other vascular bypass procedures.

The treatment of aneurysms is often nonoperative, with intervention reserved for evidence of bleeding, infection, skin breakdown or ulceration, and impending failure due to thrombosis within the aneurysmal segment or largest diameter greater than 2 cm. Treatment options include open and endovascular interventions. Surgical revision of the aneurysmal segment either with aneurysmorrhaphy or resection and bypass with saphenous vein or prosthetic graft is associated with good clinical outcomes (Fig. 57.6).[130,131] Graft extension around a pseudoaneurysm should include exclusion or resection of the aneurysmal sac and maintenance of a segment of the access for active dialysis to avoid the need for a temporary catheter. Endovascular exclusion of the aneurysmal segment using a covered stent can also be performed, but is associated with a higher risk of graft thrombosis and should not be considered a first-line therapy.[132-134]

Venous Hypertension

Patients with ESRD are at a high risk for venous hypertension. Most have a history of central venous access through an acute or tunneled dialysis line. Furthermore, the change in venous hemodynamics after AV access creation increases the risk of central venous stenosis and thrombosis, which results in venous hypertension.

The clinical features of venous hypertension include regional edema, high venous pressures, a strong pulse in the hemodialysis fistula or graft, and prolonged bleeding after dialysis.[110] In approximately 20% of patients, some symptom of venous hypertension will become severe enough for intervention. If intervention is considered, a fistulogram should be obtained to investigate the underlying pathology, which often involves subclavian vein involvement. Angioplasty can be performed to address any significant venous stenosis identified with selective stenting for a suboptimal result or recurrent stenosis. Surgical decompression can also be effectively performed with axillary to internal jugular vein bypass if the jugular vein is found patent on Duplex ultrasound. This remains an option for subclavian lesions that are resistant or recur after endovascular therapy.

Arterial Steal Syndrome

The phenomenon of arterial steal occurs in up to 90% of all AV connections. Ischemia secondary to this steal phenomenon, also known as dialysis access steal syndrome (DASS), occurs in 10% to 20% of patients and can lead to significant patient morbidity and tissue loss if uncorrected.[135] There are three underlying etiologies to explain arterial steal syndrome. First, an arterial lesion, either proximal or distal to the AV anastomosis, may cause decreased blood flow to the hand. Second, true steal can result when excess blood is siphoned through the AV access. This is more apt to occur if the AVF diameter is more than twice that of the arterial inflow. Finally, steal can result from a lack of arterial adaptation or collateral flow after the creation of the AV access.[136] It is important to note that some degree of steal is inevitable with flow diversion and that the majority of patients remain asymptomatic despite abnormal Doppler lab findings. Therefore the management of this condition should be reserved for symptomatic patients. The most important risk factors for steal syndrome are the use of prosthetic conduit, female gender,

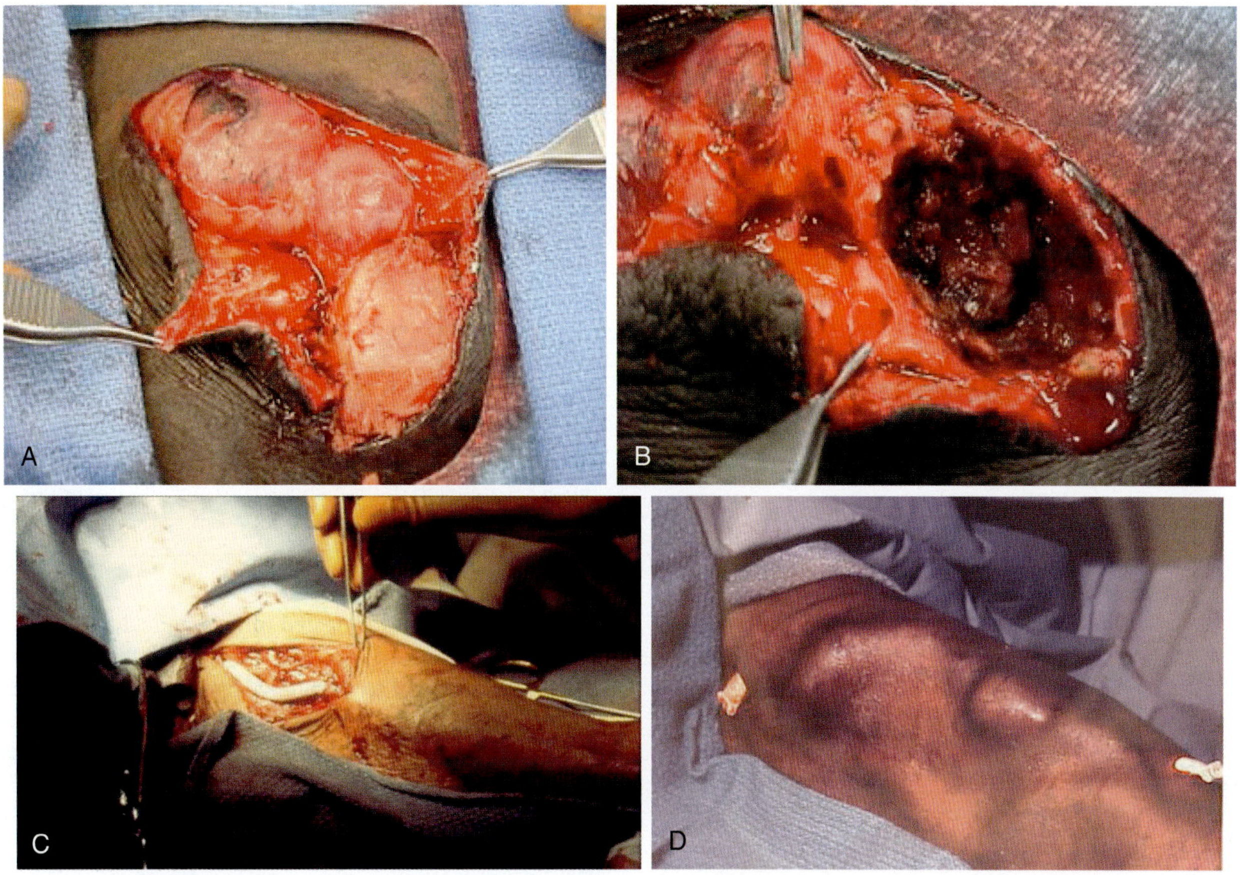

FIG 57.6 Repair of aneurysmal left-arm arteriovenous fistula with evacuation and interposition graft placement or exclusion and lateral bypass graft placement: (A) exposure of aneurysmal cephalic vein segment, (B) evacuation of intraluminal thrombus, (C) placement of prosthetic interposition graft to replace aneurysmal segment, (D) exclusion and lateral prosthetic bypass graft placement around the aneurysmal segment.

diabetes mellitus, and brachial artery origin of the AV access.[110] Steal syndrome can be classified according to a grading system: grade 0 (no evidence of steal), grade 1 (mild steal, manifested by a cool extremity with few symptoms but demonstrable by flow augmentation with fistula occlusion, does not need treatment), grade 2 (moderate steal, intermittent ischemia only during dialysis/claudication, intervention is sometimes needed), and grade 3 (severe steal, ischemic pain at rest/tissue loss, and intervention is mandatory).[74]

Symptoms of arterial steal can vary from distal extremity coolness to tissue loss and permanent neurologic injury. Patients with steal syndrome typically experience transient improvement of their symptoms with compression of the AV access. In addition to a thorough clinical examination documenting the vascular and neurologic status of the affected limb, an objective assessment should also be carried out using noninvasive testing.[22] Although no clear guidelines exist for the definition of upper extremity abnormalities after AV access creation, Tordoir and colleagues have proposed the following thresholds as an indication of significant steal: digital pressures of less than 50 mm Hg, a digital-brachial index of less than 0.6, and a transcutaneous oxygen pressure of less than 20 to 30 mm Hg.[137] Using Doppler flow studies, AV access flow can be further stratified by flow: high flow (>800 mL/min in AV fistulas, >1200 mL/min in AV grafts), normal flow, and low flow (<400 mL/min in AV fistulas, <600 mL/min in AV grafts).[138] Digital plethysmography with and without AVF or AVG compression can be helpful in the clinical diagnosis.

Interventions for steal syndrome are warranted in patients with moderate and severe steal. An arteriogram with fistulogram component is important and may reveal a significant lesion in the arterial inflow or outflow responsive to angioplasty with possible stenting. Such arterial lesions are present in up to 14% of all patients with AV access, and up to 80% of patients with symptomatic steal syndrome.[139,140] After arterial imaging, surgical options include banding, distal revascularization-interval ligation (DRIL), revision using distal inflow (RUDI), proximalization of the arterial inflow (PAI), and ligation of the access. Access ligation is reserved for patients with critical ischemia without the time for appropriate diagnostic and therapeutic procedures (Figs. 57.7 and 57.8).

Banding is the oldest surgical intervention for high-output fistulas and can be performed with nonabsorbable sutures, prosthetic material, or functionally with a tapered interposition graft

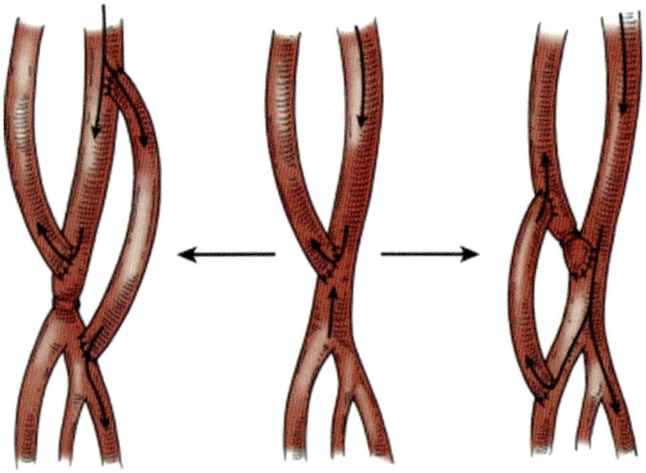

FIG 57.7 DRIL and RUDI procedures for the management of arterial steal syndrome. *AVF,* Arteriovenous fistula; *DRIL,* distal revascularization-interval ligation; *RUDI,* revision using distal inflow. (From *Annals of Vascular Surgery,* Volume 23, Issue 4, July–August 2009, pp. 485–490, Fig. 1.)

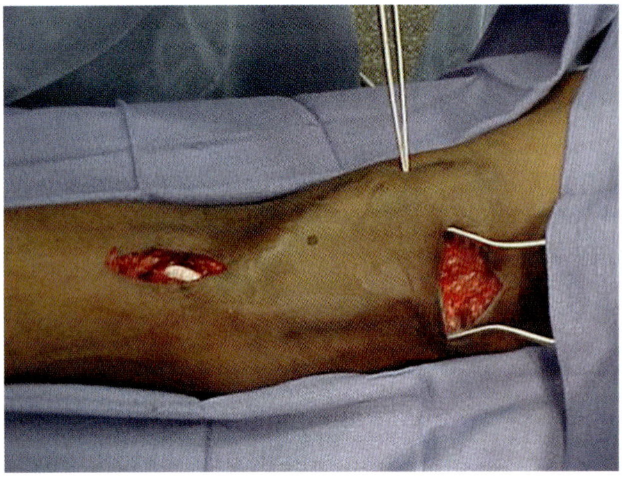

FIG 57.8 Intraoperative view of DRIL procedure for the management of right arm arterial steal syndrome. *DRIL,* Distal revascularization-interval ligation; *RUDI,* revision using distal inflow.

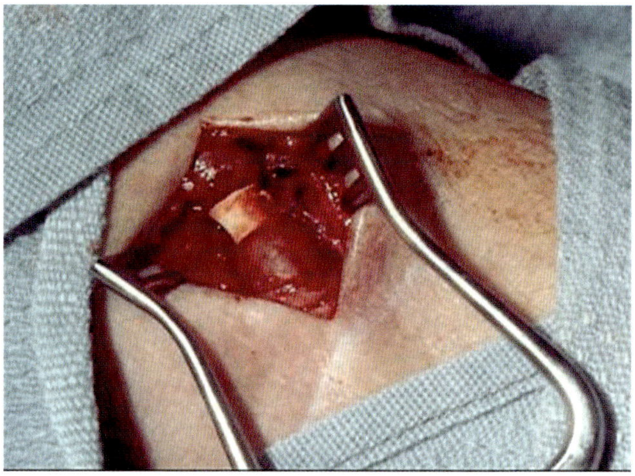

FIG 57.9 Banding of the cephalic vein for the treatment of arterial steal syndrome.

(Fig. 57.9).[141] Although the treatment has excellent outcomes in high output AV fistulas, it is also associated with diminished long-term access patency.[138] More recently, Miller and colleagues described a hybrid approach, aptly named the Minimally Invasive Limited Ligation Endoluminal-Assisted Revision (MILLER) procedure, where banding is performed against a percutaneously placed inflated angioplasty balloon to prevent excessive narrowing of the fistula vein.[142] The authors and others have reported excellent primary and secondary patencies up to 24 months, although this approach has not been examined in multicenter studies.[143,144]

The DRIL and RUDI procedures use a bypass to improve perfusion to the distal arm with interval ligation. In the DRIL procedure, the artery is ligated immediately distal to the origin of the AV fistula and a bypass is constructed to deliver flow from the artery proximal to the site of ligation to an artery at least 5 cm distal to the AV anastomosis.[145] This procedure has been associated with excellent postoperative outcomes, including an 89% to 100% freedom of symptoms and a 73% to 100% patency of the AV fistula and bypass graft.[138] Conversely, the RUDI procedure involves the ligation of the vein immediately distal to the AV anastomosis followed by a reversed saphenous vein bypass from a more distal arterial source to the AV fistula vein distal to the site of ligation.[146] The RUDI procedure is also associated with excellent postoperative outcomes and has similar results as compared with the DRIL procedure.[147-149] The PAI procedure is performed by ligating the vein immediately distal to the AV anastomosis and creating a bypass from the fistula vein to the feeding artery more proximally, usually the brachial artery. A prosthetic graft can be used because the brachial artery is larger more proximally.[150] There is currently insufficient evidence, however, to rigorously compare the PAI procedure with other treatment modalities for steal syndrome.

High-Output Cardiac Failure

Heart failure is common among patients with ESRD, and half of those patients will die from the sequelae of cardiovascular disease.[151] The creation of an AV access tends to exacerbate heart failure due to progressive cardiac dilatation. Conversely, ligation of the AV access has been associated with regression of this dilatation process and subsequent decrease in the incidence of heart failure.[152] Although there are no validated diagnostic parameters for this condition, MacRae and colleagues have noted that published reports have consistently shown that access flow greater than 2 L/min and an access flow to cardiac output ratio greater than 30% to 35% were consistent with high-output heart failure.[152] The treatment of high-output cardiac failure is to decrease the flow through the AV access, either by banding, the RUDI procedure, or distalization of the AV anastomosis.[153-155] In some instances, however, salvage procedures are unsuccessful and the AV access must be ligated.

Neuropathy

Although the most common cause of unilateral neuropathy in hemodialysis patients is ischemia secondary to steal syndrome, other etiologies—such as uremic and diabetic neuropathies and carpal tunnel syndrome—should also be considered.[74] Ischemic monomyelic neuropathy (IMN) is an acute neuropathic condition that may involve a form of steal syndrome; it affects the median nerve fibers of the forearm and hand. First described by Bolton and colleagues in Canada, the term *ischemic monomyelic neuropathy* was coined by Wilburn and colleagues, who defined it as an "ischemic neuropathy produced by the shunting of blood away from, or the acute noncompressive occlusion of, a major proximal limb artery."[156,157] Risk factors for IMN include diabetes, dissection of the brachial artery, female gender, and a history of atherosclerotic disease.[158] Several clinical features are helpful in differentiating IMN from other entities, especially steal syndrome. Steal syndrome onset is usually insidious and can occur after access creation in the wrist, forearm, or upper arm. The tissues affected by steal syndrome are most commonly the skin, followed by muscles and then nerves. The degree of ischemia is severe and diffuse and the radial pulse is usually absent, with a finding of decreased digital pressures. Conversely, the onset of IMN is acute, often presenting in the recovery area postoperatively as pain and sensory loss. The obvious degree of ischemia can be minimal, with a warm hand, palpable radial pulse, good thrill in the fistula, and mildly diminished or normal digital pressures.[159] It can sometimes be difficult to diagnose IMN, however, especially if the AV access creation was performed with a regional block, as postblock neuromuscular deficits can range from weakness, dysesthesia and loss of motor and sensory function.[160] However, IMN is a surgical emergency that warrants immediate return to the OR and ligation of the AV fistula or graft. Delay is associated with progressive and permanent nerve injury. Unfortunately correction of ischemia may not improve the neuropathy, which underscores the importance of a quick intervention in these patients.[161]

SOCIETAL GUIDELINES

Several societal guidelines have been developed to standardize the management of hemodialysis patients and provide evidence-based recommendations for access surgeons. The Society for Vascular Surgery, British Renal Association, Kidney Health Australia, and the Canadian Society of Nephrology have all published guidelines that are freely available.[162-165] The differences between the various guidelines are minor, as they were all based on systematic reviews of the most up-to-date literature when they were compiled. The most widely applied guidelines in the United States are the NKF KDOQI guidelines.[14] Last updated in 2006, the document includes guidelines for patient and type of hemodialysis access selection, postoperative monitoring and surveillance, and the detection and management of access-related complications. It also sets targets for type of access creation and incidence of complications. Although a detailed discussion of the NKF KDOQI guidelines is beyond the scope of this chapter, some important points are highlighted here.

AV fistulas should be placed at least 6 months and grafts 3 to 6 weeks before the anticipated start date of hemodialysis. Long-term catheters should be avoided, and the order of preference for access creation, in descending order, should be a radiocephalic AV fistula, brachiocephalic AV fistula, and a brachiobasilic transposition, followed by forearm and upper arm AV grafts. The rule of sixes should be used to determine whether an AV fistula is likely to be usable: flow greater than 600 mL/min, diameter greater than or equal to 6 mm, and an AV fistula depth of 6 mm or less. Fistulas that fail to mature within 6 weeks should be investigated, and ePTFE grafts should not be cannulated for at least 2 weeks. Centers should aim for an AV fistula placement rate of greater than 65%, with a tunneled catheter rate of less than 10%.

REVIEW QUESTIONS

1. A 58-year-old patient with a previously created left brachiobasilic fistula is referred by his nephrologist because of newly formed pulsatile masses in the left upper arm. The fistula was created 14 months earlier and is functioning well, with adequate flow. Physical examination shows intact skin with a palpable thrill and no evidence of infection or bleeding. The patient has three areas of marked subcutaneous dilatation along the course of the arterialized vein but does not complain of any pain or discomfort. What is your management?
   - **a.** Duplex ultrasound followed by ligation and bypass of the diseased segment using autogenous saphenous vein
   - **b.** Continued dialysis through the fistula using the "buttonhole technique"
   - **c.** Fistulogram and balloon angioplasty of any central venous lesions
   - **d.** Ligation of the fistula and hemodialysis catheter placement

2. A 72-year-old diabetic woman with end-stage renal disease is in the recovery room after creation of a right-upper-extremity loop graft for hemodialysis access. The recovery room nurse calls you to assess the patient because she is complaining of substantial pain. All of the following are risk factors for ischemic monomelic neuropathy except
   - **a.** Diabetes
   - **b.** Old age
   - **c.** Prosthetic graft
   - **d.** Forearm graft

Questions 3 and 4 refer to the same clinical scenario.

3. A 47-year-old smoker develops severe pain and coldness in his left forearm and hand during dialysis via a left brachiocephalic fistula. You examine the patient in your clinic and find that his hand appears warm and well perfused. There is no evidence of tissue loss. His neuromuscular examination is normal. The patient says that the symptoms began 3 weeks earlier and that they occur only during dialysis. According to the Society for Vascular Surgery Reporting Guidelines, what is the grading severity of this patient's steal symptoms?
   a. 0
   b. 1
   c. 2
   d. 3
4. A 47-year-old smoker develops severe pain and coldness in his left forearm and hand during dialysis using a left brachiocephalic fistula. You examine him in your clinic and find that his hand appears warm and well perfused. There is no evidence of tissue loss. His neuromuscular examination is normal. The patient says that the symptoms began 3 weeks earlier and that they occur only during dialysis. What is the best treatment for the management of this condition?
   a. Ligation of the fistula and placement of a dialysis catheter
   b. Distal revascularization with interval ligation (DRIL)
   c. Physiotherapy and short-term follow-up in clinic
   d. Banding of the arteriovenous fistula's venous outflow
5. A 39-year-old male presents to the office from dialysis for evaluation of his right prosthetic brachial-axillary upper arm graft, which is currently being used for dialysis. On physical examination of his right arm, you note a thrill and bruit overlying his graft. There are two separate 5-cm soft pulsatile masses along the length of the graft with mild skin ulcerations overlying the masses but no erythema or edema and palpable radial, ulnar, and brachial artery pulses. What is the likely diagnosis?
   a. Seroma
   b. Abscess
   c. Pseudoaneurysm
   d. True aneurysm
6. A 65-year-old female presents with increasing edema of her left upper extremity approximately 18 months after the creation of a right brachiocephalic upper arm fistula. On physical examination of her right arm, you note a bounding pulse overlying the fistula, moderate edema, and palpable radial, ulnar, and brachial artery pulses. Venography of the right upper extremity shows an 80% subclavian vein stenosis and patent internal jugular and innominate veins with no stenosis. What is the best treatment plan for this patient?
   a. Right subclavian vein balloon angioplasty alone.
   b. Ligation of the fistula and placement of a dialysis catheter
   c. Right subclavian vein balloon angioplasty and stent placement
   d. Right subclavian vein–to–internal jugular vein bypass with autogenous saphenous vein graft

Questions 7 and 8 refer to the same clinical scenario.

7. A 42-year-old male presents with a thrombosed right prosthetic forearm loop arteriovenous graft that was being used for dialysis access until 3 days earlier. The graft was placed a year ago. On physical examination of his right arm, you note that there is no thrill or bruit in the graft and no edema. He has palpable radial, ulnar, and brachial pulses, appears comfortable, and does not complain of pain. What is the most likely reason for the graft thrombosis in this patient?
   a. Graft infection
   b. Central venous stenosis
   c. Stenosis at the graft-arterial anastomosis
   d. Stenosis at the graft-venous anastomosis
8. A 42-year-old-male presents with a thrombosed right prosthetic forearm loop arteriovenous graft; it was being used for dialysis access until 3 days earlier. The graft was placed a year earlier. On physical examination of his right arm, you note that there is no thrill or bruit in the graft and no edema. He has palpable radial, ulnar, and brachial pulses, appears comfortable, and does not complain of pain. What is the optimal next step in the management of this patient?
   a. Admit the patient to hospital, start catheter-directed thrombolysis
   b. Admit the patient to hospital, perform thrombectomy in the operating room
   c. Start the patient on an oral Factor Xa inhibitor, follow up in clinic in 1 week
   d. Admit the patient to hospital, place dialysis catheter

BIBLIOGRAPHY

Berardinelli L. Grafts and graft materials as vascular substitutes for haemodialysis access construction. *Eur J Vasc Endovasc Surg.* 2006;32:203–211.

KDOQI Clinical Practice Guidelines and Clinical Practice Recommendations for 2006 Updates: Hemodialysis Adequacy, Peritoneal Dialysis Adequacy and Vascular Access. *Am J Kidney Dis.* 2006;48(suppl 1):S1–S322.

Konner K. History of vascular access for haemodialysis. *Nephrol Dial Transplant.* 2005;20:2629–2635.

Miles AM. Vascular steal syndrome and ischaemic monomelic neuropathy: two variants of upper limb ischaemia after haemodialysis vascular access surgery. *Nephrol Dial Transplant.* 1999;14:297–300.

Mudoni A, Cornacchiari M, Gallieni M, et al. Aneurysms and pseudoaneurysms in dialysis access. *Clin Kidney J.* 2015;8:363–367.

Padberg FT Jr, Calligaro KD, Sidawy AN. Complications of arteriovenous hemodialysis access: recognition and management. *J Vasc Surg*. 2008;48:S55–S80.

Sidawy AN, Gray R, Besarab A, et al. Recommended standards for reports dealing with arteriovenous hemodialysis accesses. *J Vasc Surg*. 2002;35:603–610.

Sidawy AN, Spergel LM, Besarab A, et al. The Society for Vascular Surgery: clinical practice guidelines for the surgical placement and maintenance of arteriovenous hemodialysis access. *J Vasc Surg*. 2008;48:S2–S25.

Tal MG, Ni N. Selecting optimal hemodialysis catheters: material, design, advanced features, and preferences. *Tech Vasc Interv Radiol*. 2008;11:186–191.

Tordoir JH, Dammers R, van der Sande FM. Upper extremity ischemia and hemodialysis vascular access. *Eur J Vasc Endovasc Surg*. 2004;27:1–5.

References available online at ExpertConsult.com.

58 CHAPTER

Neointimal Hyperplasia

Neel A. Mansukhani, Melina R. Kibbe

Nearly all vascular interventions are prone to the development of neointimal hyperplasia because any manipulation of the arterial wall induces endothelial cell injury. Current enthusiasm for less invasive but more locally injurious percutaneous peripheral vascular therapies increases the importance of developing strategies designed to suppress neointimal hyperplasia after such interventions. Arterial injury initiates a cascade of inflammatory events that ultimately results in neointimal hyperplasia and limits the durability of these vascular interventions. Some vascular interventions are more prone to the development of neointimal hyperplasia; these include prosthetic bypass and arteriovenous grafts.[1] However, percutaneous balloon angioplasty with or without stenting, endovascular atherectomy, vein bypass grafting, and endarterectomy are all susceptible to this process.[2-5] Thus peripheral vascular interventions will remain temporarily effective and palliative rather than durable and potentially curative unless effective treatment of neointimal hyperplasia is achieved.

The classic description of neointimal hyperplasia resulting from the proliferation and migration of vascular smooth muscle cells (VSMCs) from the media to the intima, along with deposition of the extracellular matrix after endothelial cell injury, no longer accurately represents the pathophysiologic changes that occur during this injury process.[6,7] Neointimal hyperplasia results from a complex cascade of inflammatory cellular events that involves all three layers of the arterial wall as well as circulating blood elements.[8] Much has been learned about this process in the past decade that has changed the way neointimal hyperplasia is viewed and has opened up new strategies for therapeutic development. We now recognize that the adventitia as well as resident and circulating stem and progenitor cells play a large role in this process. In addition to the well-described role of cytokines and growth factors that are secreted from platelets and leukocytes at the site of injury, reactive oxygen species (ROS) and adiponectin, an adipokine produced from periadventitial adipose tissue, are intimately involved in the regulation of this process. This chapter summarizes the current concepts regarding the pathology, pathophysiology, and treatment strategies of neointimal hyperplasia.

PATHOLOGY

Neointimal hyperplasia is the abnormal continued proliferation of cells and connective tissue elements that occurs at sites of arterial injury. During the first decade of the 20th century, Carrel and Guthrie[9] noted that "within a few days after the operation, the stitches placed in making the anastomosis became covered with a glistening substance similar in appearance to the normal endothelium." This early description of arterial healing most likely represents the normal response of an artery to injury. Neointimal hyperplasia, in contrast, is the result of an exaggeration of this response through the inability to control or the continued stimulation of this normal regenerative process.

Lesions of neointimal hyperplasia are firm and homogeneous on gross examination. They look smooth, shiny, and subendothelial. These lesions were often referred to as *myointimal hyperplasia,* initially highlighting the thought that the medial VSMC is the origin of the proliferating tissue. However, we now recognize that multiple cell types contribute to the neointimal mass; therefore the term *neointimal hyperplasia* or *intimal hyperplasia* is more commonly used today. Assessment of neointimal lesions using intravascular ultrasound supports the notion that the majority (≈90%) of lesions are homogeneous in appearance. However, with advances in technology, such as intravascular optical coherence tomography, it appears that up to 40% of lesions may be heterogeneous in nature.[10] Pathologic histologic examination of neointimal lesions reveals mainly stellate cells surrounded by a clear fibromyxomatous stroma and connective tissue. These stellate cells contain smooth muscle–like features and stain positively for actin and sulfated glycosaminoglycans.[11,12] They appear to originate from several different sources, including the media, the adventitia (i.e., fibroblasts), the endothelium, and resident and circulating stem cells. Cellular proliferation begins within 24 hours of injury and is one of the hallmarks of neointimal hyperplasia. However, proliferation, migration, phenotypic differentiation, cellular infiltration, and extracellular matrix deposition all occur, resulting in wall thickening that continues to develop over several weeks (Fig. 58.1).[13]

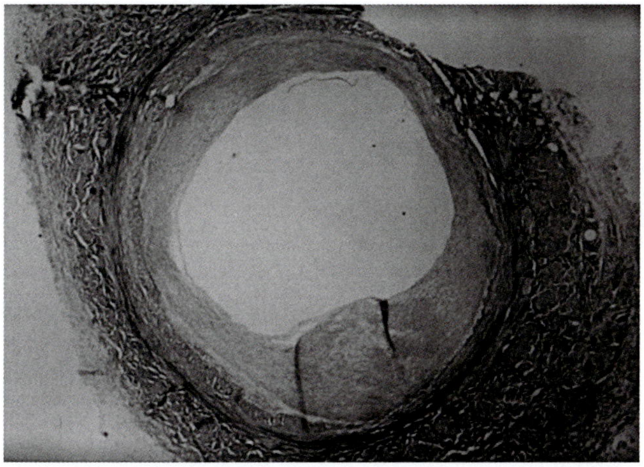

FIG 58.1 Photomicrograph of a failed infrainguinal autogenous vein bypass graft showing a large amount of hyperplastic intimal proliferation (Verhoeff–van Gieson stain; original magnification ×20).

TABLE 58.1 Proliferating Cell Number per Square Millimeter After Arterial Injury

Time Point	Media	Adventitia
Noninjured	0.2	0.1
4 h	42	286
8 h	37	510
12 h	38	531
24 h	369	582
48 h	972	691
72 h	930 (29%)	1164 (53%)
7 days	576 (14%)	1424 (41%)
14 days	420 (13%)	810 (23%)
30 days	22 (0.4%)	75 (2%)

Modified from Couffinhal T, Dufourcq P, Jaspard B, et al: Kinetics of adventitial repair in the rat carotid model. *Coron Artery Dis* 12:635–648, 2001.

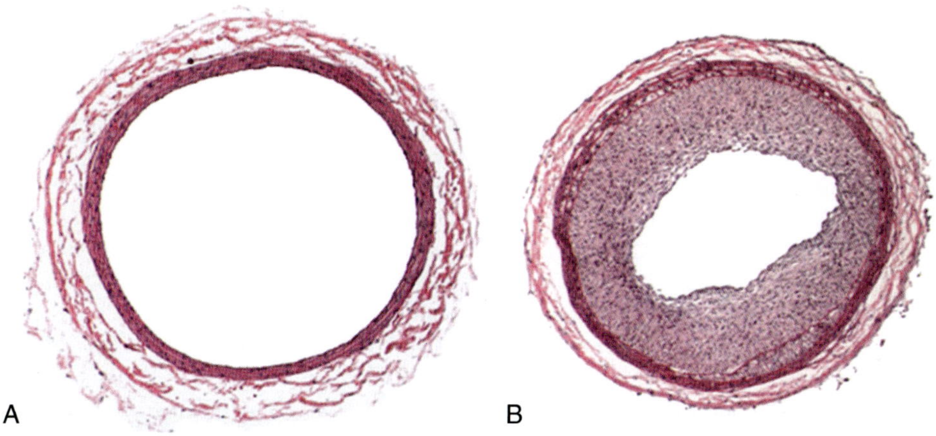

FIG 58.2 (A) Cross section of a rat carotid artery. (B) Cross section of a rat carotid artery 2 weeks after balloon injury.

PATHOPHYSIOLOGY

The classic description of the arterial injury response by both Clowes and Ross involves damage to the vascular endothelium and exposure of the underlying VSMCs to circulating blood elements.[6,7,14-16] Exposure of the subendothelial arterial wall elements triggers the activation of a myriad of cellular and enzymatic events. The underlying internal elastic lamina and VSMCs are exposed to circulating blood elements. Platelets immediately aggregate and adhere to the site of injury.[17] An inflammatory response follows, with the infiltration of neutrophils, macrophages, and leukocytes.[18,19] Twenty-four hours after injury, under the influence of growth factors and cytokines, medial VSMCs convert from a contractile to a synthetic phenotype and begin to proliferate.[20] VSMCs migrate to the neointima, where they continue to proliferate for up to 8 weeks.[6,21,22] Endothelial cells concurrently regenerate through the stimulation of basic fibroblast growth factor (bFGF) within 24 hours after injury; this can continue for 6 to 10 weeks.[23] Finally, transforming growth factor beta (TGF-β) stimulates extracellular matrix deposition.[24,25] The culmination of these events results in the formation of neointimal hyperplasia (Fig. 58.2).

The classic arterial injury response just described does not account for the role of the adventitia. However, the adventitia is now thought to be one of the main driving forces in the development of neointimal hyperplasia. The proliferative response after arterial injury has been characterized in rat and pig arteries.[26,27] The proliferative response in the adventitia, compared with the intima and media, is much greater at almost all time points after arterial injury in both rat and pig animal models. Although 1.5- to 2-fold more proliferation was reported in the adventitia compared with the media in rat carotid arteries (Table 58.1), nearly 7-fold more proliferation was reported in the adventitia than in the media in pig coronary arteries.[26,27] On examination of early time points, proliferation was seen in the adventitia before the media as early as 4 hours after arterial injury (see Table 58.1).

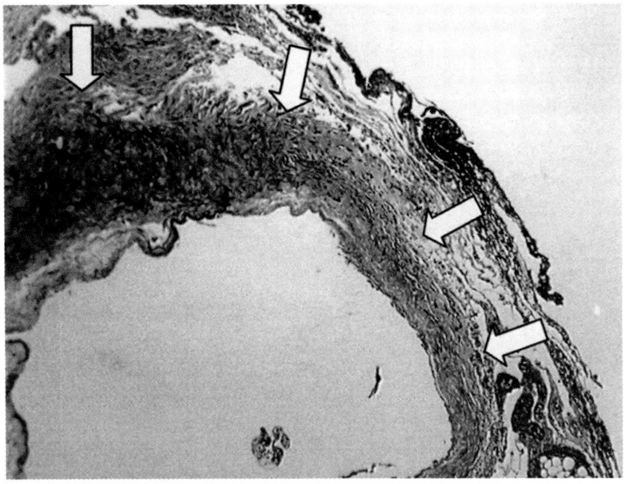

FIG 58.3 Trichrome-elastin stain of a 72-hour-old vein graft. The luminal side is depicted on the bottom edge of this tissue section. There is evidence of endothelial and smooth muscle cell denudation, with adherence of leukocytes and platelets.

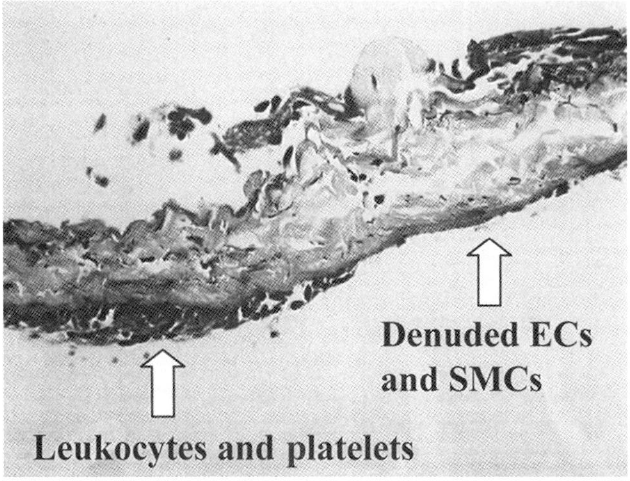

FIG 58.4 Trichrome-elastin stain of a 2-week-old vein graft. *Arrows* denote the region of the external elastic lamina, within which resides the neointima. Many of the nuclei visualized in the neointima proved to be macrophages when stained with ED-2 macrophage stain (not depicted). *ECs,* Endothelial cells; *SMCs,* smooth muscle cells.

The development of neointimal hyperplasia in vein grafts is similar to neointimal hyperplasia after arterial injury but differs in that there are fewer medial cells that respond and there is an additional response to increased wall tension. Prominent features in rodent models of vein grafting include extensive early denudation of the endothelium and smooth muscle cell layers, attachment of leukocytes and platelets to the subendothelial matrix, and elaboration of cytokine and growth factor products by these cells. This results in the activation, migration, and proliferation of vein graft adventitial myofibroblasts to form a neointima.[28-33] Pathologically, the trauma resulting from surgical manipulation and exposure of the vein graft to arterial pressure and flow results in nearly complete denudation of the endothelium and loss of the smooth muscle cell layers within the first 24 hours (Fig. 58.3). Soon after denudation, attachment of leukocytes and platelets occurs. Macrophage infiltration dominates the early inflammatory changes observed with vein graft pathobiology. This prominent inflammatory response peaks during the first 2 weeks of vein graft adaptation, which exceeds the response observed in models of arterial injury (Fig. 58.4). Stark and Hoch elegantly demonstrated that by inhibiting macrophage activity early in this inflammatory process, a significant reduction in neointimal hyperplasia was achieved.[31,32]

Vein graft neointimal changes persist and can progress despite reendothelialization. In contrast, arterial neointimal proliferation tends to halt its progression upon restitution of the endothelial cell layer. The ongoing neointimal thickening associated with vein graft neointimal hyperplasia is believed to be an adaptive response to arterial pressure and flow.[34] Wall thickening is greater in regions of low shear (e.g., at the inner wall of a curve). Neointimal hyperplasia results in wall thickening, which decreases wall stress to more physiologic levels. These hyperplastic changes were first described by Carrel and Guthrie when artery and vein grafts were first examined histologically. They referred to this process as *arterialization.*[9,35] We now known that this arterialization process involved phenotypic transformation of the vein cells to an arterial phenotype, as indicated by the loss of ephrin-B4.[36] Wall thickening can be accentuated at valve cusps, perhaps because of local flow abnormalities; at the anastomoses, where shear and wall tension are greatest; and at sites of clamp injury. Hemodynamically significant lesions caused by intimal hyperplasia usually occur after the first month and are rare after a year. After the first year, vein grafts are prone to develop lesions similar to atherosclerosis.

In addition to the processes just described—which involve platelets, inflammatory cells, VSMCs, adventitial fibroblasts, and the extracellular matrix—there is now an understanding of the contribution of resident and circulating stem cells to the development of neointimal hyperplasia as well as the role of ROS in regulating many of these processes. Several mechanisms are likely responsible for stimulating these responses, including mechanical changes, such as turbulence and compliance mismatch, and complex interactions between these different cells. Thus a complex view has emerged that involves the synergistic action of several biologic pathways. The remainder of this section reviews, separately, the experimental basis for the hypothesized involvement of each of these systems.

Hemodynamic and Mechanical Factors

A wide variety of hemodynamic and mechanical factors—including high- and low-flow velocities, high and low wall shear stress, and mechanical compliance mismatch—have been implicated in the formation of intimal hyperplasia.[37-39] In general, low blood flow velocity tends to favor the development of neointimal hyperplasia. For example, in a canine carotid vein interposition model, segments with low-flow velocities developed significantly thicker intimal layers[40]; however, there are exceptions to this rule. In a high-flow renal artery–to–vena cava anastomosis, significant intimal thickening was documented by electron microscopic examination 3 months after formation.[41] Similar intimal lesions have also been noted in arteriovenous fistulas (AVFs) constructed for hemodialysis access.[42] This may be a result of the compliance mismatch noted between the arterial and venous systems. In a monkey iliac AVF model 6 months after construction, no increase in intimal thickening occurred on the experimental side.[43] In that study, although flow rate and velocity were markedly increased on the side of the AVF, the calculated wall shear stress was equal on both sides. Equality of shear stress, despite a significant difference in flow velocities, was the result of a twofold increase in the diameter of the vessel lumen. The vessel wall regulates its diameter to produce a physiologic level of shear stress at the lumen. The endothelium regulates diameter by producing both vasoconstrictors such as endothelin and vasodilators such as nitric oxide (NO). These factors also affect VSMC proliferation and, when chronically present, induce remodeling of the vessel to maintain the new diameter without vasoactivity.

In other primate studies, arteriovenous flow was shown to inhibit neointimal thickening in highly porous polytetrafluoroethylene (PTFE) grafts.[44] Return to normal flow causes neointimal thickening. In a rodent model of arterial injury, low flow caused increased intimal hyperplasia.[45] These and many other studies demonstrate that intimal hyperplasia is increased by low shear and inhibited by high shear. Postmortem studies have shown that early atherosclerotic lesions occur more commonly in areas of low wall shear stress.[46] As an example, in the carotid artery atherosclerosis starts at the outer wall of the bulb, where shear forces are low and oscillating.[47,48]

Compliance mismatch is also an important hemodynamic factor in the production of anastomotic intimal hyperplasia.[49] Compliance is the percentage of radial change per unit pressure and is a useful index of vessel wall distensibility to a pressure force. Experimental and clinical studies show that conduits with compliance values approaching that of the native artery have better patency. In one study, femoropopliteal autografts made from glutaraldehyde-treated carotid arteries had better patency when fixation produced a more compliant graft.[49,50] However, other studies have shown that the creation of stiffer, less compliant grafts by treating arteries with glutaraldehyde results in markedly diminished patency rates.[49,51] Textile and fabric prostheses are relatively noncompliant; this is another factor that contributes to their lower patency rates due to the aggressive formation of neointimal hyperplasia.

To curb the effect of compliance mismatch, some have suggested imposing a short interposition of autogenous vein between the native artery and prosthetic grafts.[52] These modifications include vein cuffs, vein patches, vein boots, and AVFs at the distal anastomosis (Fig. 58.5).[53] A prospective randomized trial to examine the efficacy of Miller vein cuffs in improving lower extremity PTFE graft patency showed that vein cuffs did not improve patency rates in bypasses to the above-knee popliteal artery.[54] However, cuffed below-knee popliteal artery grafts had a 45% 3-year patency rate versus a 19% patency rate in uncuffed grafts (P = .018).[55] Similarly, the use of vein patches, such as those developed by Taylor and Linton, at the distal anastomosis yields better long-term patency rates versus prosthetic material alone.[56,57] Although there have been no randomized prospective trials to date, retrospective reviews have demonstrated improved patency of vein-patched PTFE versus PTFE alone when used for below-knee bypasses. Taylor and colleagues reported a 5-year primary patency of 54% for 83 infrapopliteal PTFE grafts using his vein patch modification.[56] Although there is no control arm to this study, previously reported patency rates with PTFE alone are significantly worse.[1] A review of 145 patients who had undergone either above- or below-knee bypasses using autologous vein, unmodified PTFE, and Linton patch–modified PTFE found

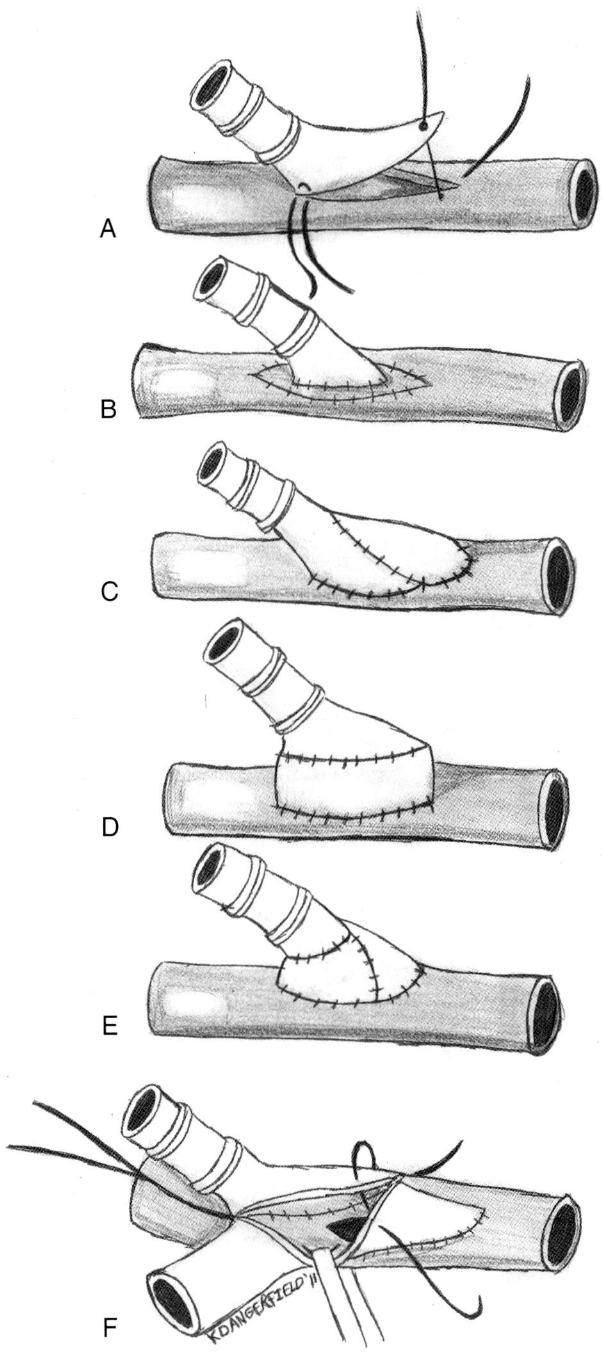

FIG 58.5 Surgical techniques using vein interposition for creation of distal anastomoses. (A) Standard end-to-side anastomosis, (B) Linton patch, (C) Taylor patch, (D) Miller cuff, (E) St. Mary's vein boot, and (F) arteriovenous fistula.

that above-knee bypasses had no statistical difference in 1- and 3-year patency rates between the three groups.[58] However, the cumulative patency rates for 1, 3, and 5 years after below-knee bypasses were 93%, 75%, and 75% for the autologous vein group ($n = 30$); 74%, 52%, and 42% for the unmodified PTFE group ($n = 37$); and 93%, 93%, and 93% for the Linton patch–modified PTFE group ($n = 16$), respectively. They speculated that the improved results over unmodified PTFE bypass grafts were due to improved compliance mismatch between the prosthetic graft and the targeted native artery. The study was limited by the small number of Linton patch–modified PTFE grafts used compared with the autologous vein and PTFE groups. Finally, a retrospective analysis of outcomes of patients with AVF-modified PTFE grafts versus PTFE alone to the infrapopliteal arteries showed that the 2-year patency rates were significantly better for grafts with the AVF modification (23% vs. 5% for the PTFE alone grafts, $P < .05$).[59] The AVF, originally described by Ascer and colleagues to improve bypass graft outflow, is created by first mobilizing an adjacent vein and transecting it.[60] The vein is then anastomosed to the artery in an end-to-side fashion. A venotomy is created near the AVF and the ePTFE is anastomosed, creating the AVF modification at the distal anastomosis (see Fig. 58.5). Despite these surgical improvements, patency rates remain poor, especially when the distal outflow is at or below the level of the popliteal artery, primarily as a result of the formation of neointimal hyperplasia.

Endovascular interventions, similarly, are prone to neointimal hyperplasia. Despite antiplatelet therapy and drug-eluting stents designed to inhibit neointimal hyperplasia, in-stent stenosis exists because stenting alters the circumferential and shear stress on a vessel. In stented rabbit arteries, neointimal hyperplasia occurred most frequently in areas of low shear stress.[61] Stent oversizing worsened neointimal hyperplasia, as was demonstrated in a porcine model with intentionally oversized stents and in human clinical studies examining percutaneous coronary interventions.[62,63] Stenting in geometrically asymmetrical or stenotic arteries further alters shear stress on the endothelium and exacerbates the development of intimal hyperplasia (Fig. 58.6).[64,65]

Platelets

Platelets have long been known to play a central role in the reaction of a vessel wall to injury. Activation of platelets by the injured endothelium is a major factor in the development of intimal hyperplasia. Denudation of the arterial wall exposes the subendothelial matrix, which leads to adherence and subsequent activation of platelets. Platelet adherence requires the interaction of subendothelial collagen, a platelet membrane glycoprotein receptor (GP Ib), plasma von Willebrand factor, and fibronectin. After adherence, platelets undergo a morphologic change, stretching to cover the exposed surface. Activated platelets release adenosine diphosphate and activate the arachidonic acid pathway to release thromboxane A2. Both of these factors lead to platelet aggregation. The luminal surface quickly passivates by adsorption of plasma proteins, limiting the period of platelet aggregation to less than 24 hours. Recruitment of platelets requires the rapid expression of the platelet membrane receptor complexes GP IIb and GP IIIa, both of which promote platelet aggregation through the binding of circulating fibrinogen. Platelet adhesion and granule release also lead to a parallel acceleration of the coagulation cascade. This activation of clotting pathways, combined with high local concentrations of fibrinogen mediated by binding to the GP IIb/IIIa complex, creates a fibrin protein network that further stabilizes the aggregated platelet plug. Once platelet aggregation has been initiated by the pathways mentioned earlier, its continuation is actively inhibited by an intact endothelium. Thus a damaged endothelium not only initiates platelet activation but also impairs its inhibition.

Platelet-derived growth factor (PDGF) is secreted along with other granule constituents, including platelet factor 4, thromboglobulin, and thrombospondin. PDGF is a cationic protein with a molecular weight of 28 to 31 kDa. It comprises two subunits (α and β). Physiologically, PDGF functions as both a chemoattractant and a mitogen for VSMC and fibroblasts. Because it binds with high affinity to VSMC, some have suggested that PDGF may attract the VSMCs from the media into the intima, bind to them, and stimulate their proliferation. Interestingly, evidence has shown that the platelet may not be the only source of this protein. PDGF (α and β subunits) is produced by human umbilical vein and saphenous vein endothelial cells. In fact, a large increase in PDGF production can be measured in injured endothelial cells. Also, both α- and β-subunit messenger RNAs (mRNAs) have been noted in fresh endarterectomy specimens obtained during carotid surgery.[66] VSMCs themselves also produce PDGF-like activity in response to arterial injury, and VSMCs from human atheromas contain mRNAs for the PDGF α subunit.[67] Taken together, these findings may explain how proliferation continues after reendothelialization occurs. PDGF may be released by both platelets and endothelial cells, causing the activation and migration of VSMCs and myofibroblasts, which then secrete additional PDGF, leading to proliferation. Demonstrating the importance of PDGF to the arterial injury response, inhibition of PDGF using antibodies or antisense oligonucleotides in animal models of arterial injury has been shown to inhibit neointimal hyperplasia by 60% to 80%.[68-70] Hence PDGF is a popular focus for the development of targeted therapy and nanotherapeutics designed to inhibit neointimal hyperplasia.[71,72] From our understanding of platelet physiology during arterial injury came the clinical practice of pretreatment with antiplatelet agents prior to endovascular interventions as well as postprocedural antiplatelet therapy.[73] Furthermore, in animal studies, technology is under development to create rouvastatin-loaded stents which accelerate endothelialization, and antiplatelet acetylcalicylic acid–eluting biodegradable stents with the potential to obviate the need for daily oral antiplatelet therapy to inhibit platelet aggregation and neointimal hyperplasia formation following endovascular interventions.[74,75]

Inflammatory Cells

Inflammatory cells are intimately involved in the arterial response to injury. Electron microscopic studies after balloon catheter intimal injury show that leukocytes attach to the deendothelialized surface of an arterial lumen within minutes.[18,19,76] This includes polymorphonuclear neutrophils (PMNs), monocytes, and lymphocytes. In addition to adhering to the damaged endothelium,

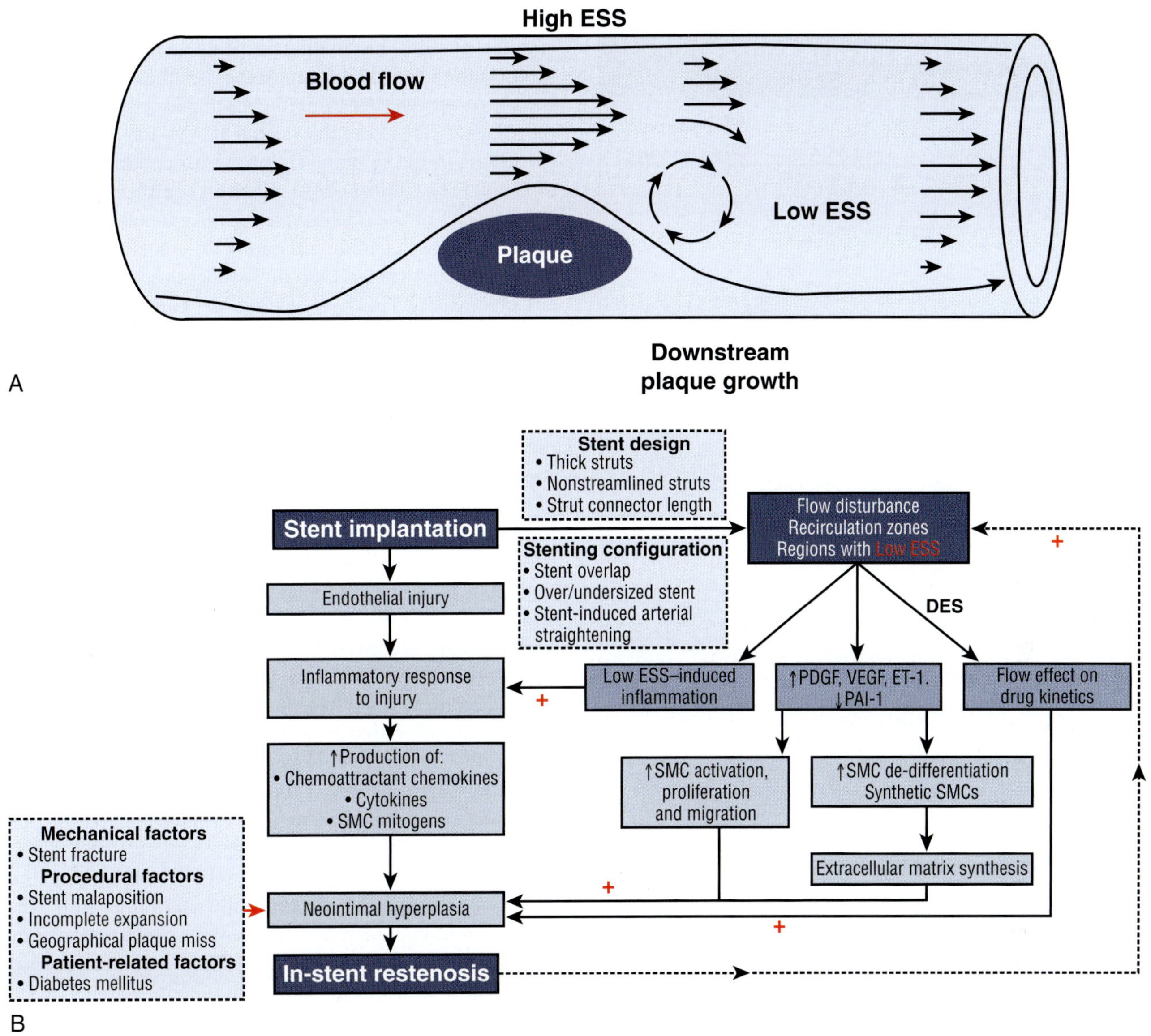

FIG 58.6 Model of low endothelial shear stress *(ESS)* in native atherosclerotic plaque and in stented lesions. (A) Model of blood flow around native atherosclerotic plaque with low ESS due to hemodynamic disturbance downstream from the plaque. (B) Schematic flow model depicting the relationship between low ESS and restenosis. *DES*, Drug-eluting stent; *SMC*, smooth muscle cell. (Modified from Koskinas KC, Chatzizisis YS, Antoniadis AP, Giannoglou GD: Role of endothelial shear stress in stent restenosis and thrombosis: pathophysiologic mechanisms and implications for clinical translation. *J Am Coll Cardiol* 59[15]:1337–1349, 2012, with permission from Elsevier.)

these cells even penetrate it in some instances. These adherent leukocytes are paramount to the secretion of many cytokines and growth factors that influence the subsequent events in neointimal hyperplasia (Table 58.2).[77-79] One model that supports the role of inflammation in the development of neointimal hyperplasia consists of delivering leukocyte-derived myeloperoxidase in the presence of its substrate hydrogen peroxide (H_2O_2). The infusion of myeloperoxidase and H_2O_2 into an isolated rat common carotid artery without mechanical injury elicited the development of neointimal hyperplasia.[80]

In another model, an endotoxin-soaked thread was placed on half of a rat femoral artery to produce an inflammatory response. This technique consistently caused significant leukocyte infiltration, which occurred only on the treated side of the vessel. Histologic examination performed 14 days later revealed nonuniform neointimal lesions in which proliferating VSMCs were located exclusively on the side of the lumen adjacent to the treated half of the arterial wall.[81] These animal models suggested a strong association between inflammation and neointimal hyperplasia.

TABLE 58.2 Cellular Sources of Growth Factors and Cytokines Involved in the Arterial Response to Injury

Growth Factor/Cytokine	Leukocytes	Monocytes/ Macrophages
IGF-1		X
PDGF		X
TGF-α		X
TGF-β	X	X
VEGF	X	X
EGF		X
FGF		X
TNF-α	X	X
IL-1β	X	X
IL-4	X	
IL-6		X
IL-8	X	X
IL-10		X
IL-18	X	X
MCP	X	X
IGF-1		X
PDGF		X

EGF, Epidermal growth factor; *FGF,* fibroblast growth factor; *IGF,* insulin-like growth factor; *IL,* interleukin; *MCP,* macrophage chemoattractant protein; *PDGF,* platelet-derived growth factor; *TGF,* transforming growth factor; *TNF,* tumor necrosis factor; *VEGF,* vascular endothelial growth factor.
Modified from Mitra AK, Del Core MG, Agrawal DK: Cells, cytokines and cellular immunity in the pathogenesis of fibroproliferative vasculopathies. *Can J Physiol Pharmacol* 83:701–715, 2005.

The adhesion of PMNs to the surface of endothelial cells is controlled by several complex glycoproteins located on the surface of both endothelial and white blood cells. Two endothelial cell adhesion molecules involved in neutrophil binding have been well characterized: endothelial leukocyte adhesion molecule-1 (ELAM-1) and intercellular adhesion molecule-1 (ICAM-1). ELAM-1 is either unexpressed or remains intracellular in the inactive endothelial cell. However, after activation by a variety of different cytokines, this adhesion complex is rapidly induced and appears on the membrane surface of the stimulated endothelial cell. ICAM-1 is located in small amounts on the surface of inactive endothelial cells. After activation by either injury or a variety of stimulating agonists, the expression of this binding complex is significantly increased. ICAM-1 is the binding ligand for the CD11a/CD18 receptor on the leukocyte membrane.

Histochemically, the adhesion molecules located in the surface membranes of the white blood cells responsible for leukocyte binding to endothelial cells can be separated into three related heterodimers. Each of these heterodimer protein complexes are composed of an α and a β subunit. The α subunit differs among the three glycoprotein complexes (CD11a, CD11b, or CD11c), whereas the β subunit remains constant (CD18). The CD11a/CD18 complex is found on the surface of all white blood cells and mediates the attachment of unstimulated PMNs to stimulated endothelial cells. This binding probably occurs through an interaction with the ICAM-1 receptor that is expressed on the luminal surface of activated or injured endothelial cells. The binding of the CD11a/CD18 complex to the ICAM-1 receptor may also play a role in the cytokine-induced transendothelial migration of PMNs. The CD11b/CD18 adhesion complex is referred to as either *Mac-1* or the *C3b complement receptor.* This glycoprotein has been implicated in the adhesion of chemotactically stimulated PMNs and controls several cellular functions such as aggregation and cytotoxicity. The third heterodimer complex, CD11c/CD18, exists on both PMNs and monocytes, but its role in binding to endothelial cells remains undetermined.

During inflammatory states, the attachment of PMNs to the involved endothelium is greatly increased, primarily because of the upregulation and enhanced expression of the binding glycoproteins described earlier. A variety of substances are capable of stimulating this enhanced PMN adherence. Interleukin (IL)-1, tumor necrosis factor (TNF)-α, lymphotoxin, and bacterial endotoxins (lipopolysaccharide) all increase the production of both ELAM-1 and ICAM-1 on the surface of affected endothelial cells. In addition, PMN activation can be stimulated by several substances that are released secondary to inflammation. Examples include the complement factors C5a and C3b, which stimulate PMN chemotaxis and phagocytosis, respectively. Likewise, PMN adhesion and chemotaxis can also be stimulated by IL-1, xanthine oxidase, PDGF, and the lipid mediators leukotriene B and platelet-activating factor. Finally, TNF-α is an important mediator of PMN phagocytosis and can lead to the increased release of lysosomal enzymes.

After activation and adhesion to the damaged vessel lumen, leukocytes migrate into the arterial wall. In one study, 42 days after a denuding injury, leukocytes were shown to penetrate the arterial media and were seen deep within the hyperplastic lesions.[82] VSMCs and macrophages elaborate potent chemotactic factors for leukocytes, which could sustain continued leukocyte recruitment.[83] Supporting this notion, serum containing medium that was conditioned from VSMCs stimulated leukocyte migration. Other chemotactic agents for leukocytes include PDGF and, in some reports, factors released by fibroblasts. VSMCs removed from atherosclerotic plaques expressed ICAM-1, suggesting a possible connection between these medial cells and leukocyte recruitment and activation.

The mechanism by which leukocytes may initiate the formation of intimal hyperplasia after penetrating the injured arterial wall remains unknown. After a denuding endothelial injury and the deposition of inflammatory cells, a variety of inflammatory products may be involved. These include chemotactic factors, growth factors, complement components, and enzymes. One of the most studied substances is monocyte- and macrophage-derived growth factor (MDGF). MDGF is a well-known stimulator of VSMC and fibroblast proliferation. This growth factor is similar and may be identical to PDGF. Thus the stimulation of VSMC proliferation is one mechanism by which inflammatory cells may contribute to the formation of neointimal hyperplasia. A second possibility involves the production of lysosomal degradation enzymes. Activated leukocytes secrete several potent proteases capable of degrading collagen, basement membranes, and other important extracellular structural proteins. One example of a PMN-derived enzyme that has been implicated in peri-inflammatory extracellular damage is myeloperoxidase. Liberation of these destructive enzymes into the wall of an injured vessel may weaken the extracellular matrix. This "loosening" of the vessel wall may facilitate the migration of VSMCs from the medial layer toward the lumen. Finally, leukocytes may act directly at sites of vessel injury to extend endothelial injury. PMNs can produce oxygen-free radicals through the action of the nicotinamide adenine dinucleotide phosphate (NADPH) oxidase system present on their membranes. The toxic substances elaborated by these activated PMNs—including superoxide anion, hydrogen peroxide, and hydroxyl radicals—can damage endothelial cells and alter capillary permeability. With PMN activation, marginally injured endothelial cells bordering a lesion may be destroyed, increasing the magnitude of the damage to the vessel wall. This further exposure of the subendothelial layer allows more platelet cell adherence, aggregation, and activation as well as the recruitment of more leukocyte mediators and thus the stimulation of a continued cycle of inflammatory injury.

In addition to luminal entry, the adventitia has been recognized as an important site of inflammation after arterial injury (Fig. 58.7). The accumulation of B cells, T cells, and macrophages in the adventitia has been documented in numerous studies.[84-87] Okamoto and colleagues[88] characterized macrophage localization to the adventitia after porcine coronary artery angioplasty and identified which receptors are important to macrophage recruitment. Macrophages present in the adventitia were significantly increased at day 1 after injury, peaked at day 3, and then slowly decreased back to baseline at day 14. Interestingly, the number of adventitial macrophages was larger than the number found in either the media or the intima. In addition, macrophage accumulation preceded cell proliferation by 48 to 72 hours. Remarkably, they also found that macrophages had a nearly 20-fold greater presence than neutrophils. Early and sustained expression of E-selectin, P-selectin, and VCAM-1 by the vasa vasorum indicated that these receptors were important in allowing the macrophages to localize to the adventitia. Macrophages have also been noted to phenotypically differentiate into myofibroblasts after arterial injury and contribute to the development of neointimal hyperplasia.[89] Bayes-Genis and coworkers demonstrated that 14 days after arterial injury to the pig coronary artery, 42% of the neointimal cells expressed the macrophage-specific antigen SWC3, and 9% of the cells coexpressed SWC3 and alpha smooth muscle actin (αSMA).[89] Finally, macrophage localization and activation has been found to rely on angiotensin II (Ang II)–induced upregulation of CCL2 and IL-6. Tieu and associates were recently able to quantify the degree to which Ang II increases the macrophage population in the adventitia and found a 5.3-fold increase in populations of mice treated with Ang II.[90] They also documented the important role that CCL2 plays in Ang II–induced macrophage localization, because the absence of CCR2, a CCL2 receptor, in $CCR2^{-/-}$ mice significantly attenuated the accumulation of adventitial macrophages. The cytokine IL-6 was shown to be important to the activity of Ang II because the adventitia in $IL\text{-}6^{-/-}$ mice did not show the same propensity to recruit macrophages as it did in the $IL\text{-}6^{+/+}$ mice after Ang II stimulation. IL-6 has also been implicated in the recruitment of bone marrow–derived endothelial progenitor cells (EPCs) for reendothelialization after vascular injury.[91]

Gregory and colleagues utilized all-trans retinoic acid delivered via a polydiolcitrate perivascular membrane to the adventitia after carotid artery balloon injury in rats. All-trans retinoic acid and polydiolcitrate are thought to exert their effects by an antiinflammatory mechanism. Compared with untreated controls in this study, treatment with locally delivered periadventitial all-trans retinoic acid by a polydiolcitrate membrane reduced neointimal hyperplasia by 50% as measured by the intima/media area ratio ($P < .001$).[92] In a study by Akagi and coauthors, specialized pro-resolving lipid inflammatory mediators derived from omega-3 fatty acids were used to attenuate the formation of neointimal

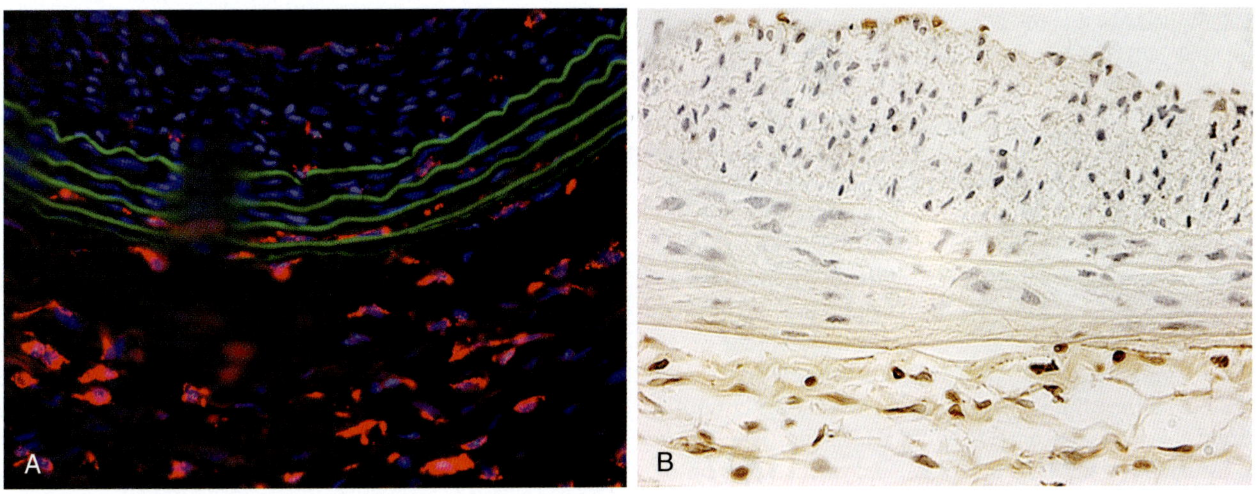

FIG 58.7 Arterial cross sections of immunohistochemical staining for (A) monocytes/macrophages *(red staining)* and (B) lymphocytes *(brown staining)* 2 weeks after arterial balloon injury in the rat carotid artery. Note that the majority of infiltrates are found in the adventitia.

hyperplasia in the mouse carotid artery ligation model. With systemic treatment of the inflammatory mediators resolving D2 and maresin 1, development of neointimal hyperplasia was reduced by 62% and 67% compared with untreated controls.[93] Liu and colleagues targeted the inflammatory cascade in their study using endosomal vesicles derived from adipose mesenchymal stem cells (MSCs). These anuclear endosomal vesicles contained several proteins, mRNAs, microRNAs, organelles, and lipids. In both in vitro and in vivo models, endosomal vesicles derived from adipose MSCs inhibited macrophage migration, proliferation, migration of VSMCs, and intimal hyperplasia as measured by intimal thickness compared with controls ($P < .05$).[94] These data further confirm the inflammatory nature of neointimal hyperplasia and validate the inflammatory cascade as a treatment target.

Growth Factors

The stimulation of cellular proliferation is the final common pathway of all postulated mechanisms leading to the development of intimal hyperplasia. There is now enough evidence that the vascular wall is a complex integrated organ, complete with its own endogenous local autocrine system. By this view, neointimal hyperplasia is postulated to result from an imbalance of these local hormonal systems. This could be caused by an excess of stimulatory molecules or from the absence or reduction of inhibitory hormones, or both mechanisms may synergistically contribute to the development of neointimal hyperplasia.

PDGF and MDGF are both examples of growth factors believed to be involved in the formation of hyperplastic neointimal lesions; each has been reviewed in detail earlier. bFGF, a smooth muscle cell mitogen that is not secreted, is released from damaged VSMCs and acts in an autocrine fashion to stimulate the proliferation of adjacent, viable cells. This mitogen is largely responsible for the proliferative response after balloon injury.[6] Denudation of endothelium with a fine wire that does not damage the underlying media results in much less VSMC activation.[95] Lindner and associates observed that administration of bFGF after an injury increased VSMC proliferation from 11.5% to 54.8%.[20] Their finding of an equivalent increase in proliferation after wire loop injury demonstrates that bFGF can act as a mitogen for undamaged medial cells. bFGF administered to normal, nondenuded arteries has no effect on VSMC growth. bFGF is also a potent stimulator of endothelial cells and, accordingly, stimulates angiogenesis. After arterial injury, bFGF is important for stimulating endothelial cell growth to completely cover injured regions that would normally remain denuded. Cuevas and colleagues demonstrated that the direct local infusion of bFGF into either normal adventitia or injured media results in proliferation of both vasa vasorum and VSMCs.[96] More recently, Syndecan-4 (Syn4) has been identified as a key coreceptor in the regulation of the bFGF pathway and migration of VSMCs. Using the femoral artery wire injury model of neointimal hyperplasia in Syn4 knockout mice, Ikesue and colleagues noted less neointimal formation after injury due to regulation of VSMC proliferation and vascular progenitor cell mobilization.[97]

TGF-β is classically known for its role in stimulating the deposition of extracellular matrix. It is now understood to have a role in negatively regulating endothelial cell activation, VSMC migration, and macrophage and lymphocyte accumulation.[98] Early studies demonstrated that TGF-β was expressed after arterial injury.[25] Furthermore, application of TGF-β to the arterial wall using gene therapy or intraluminal delivery stimulated the development of neointimal hyperplasia.[24,99,100] Inhibition of TGF-β using antibodies inhibited neointimal hyperplasia.[101-103] These early studies focused on the stimulation of procollagen and fibronectin. Identification of SMAD3 as a downstream target of TGF-β has revealed more precisely the role of TGF-β in neointimal hyperplasia. SMAD3 knockout mice exhibited significantly more neointimal hyperplasia after injury compared with wild-type controls. Specifically, they exhibited more cellular proliferation, and bone marrow transplantation studies revealed that the neointima that developed in SMAD3 knockout mice was derived from resident cells, not circulating cells.[104]

In the mouse aortic allograft model, Sun and colleagues tested the effect of an oral TGF-β inhibitor, which functions by deactivating SMAD3, on intimal hyperplasia. They noted up to a 48% reduction in intimal hyperplasia in the oral TGF-β inhibitor group compared with the control group 8 weeks after aortic transplantation.[105] Subsequently, following carotid angioplasty in the rat, Shi and colleagues revealed that the TGF-β/SMAD3 system led to SMC secretion of VEGF. After angioplasty, VEGF functions as an inhibitor of VSMC apoptosis, contrary to its effects in vitro; and the survival of VSMCs after angioplasty contributes to the formation of intimal hyperplasia.[106] DiRenzo further revealed that the TGF-β/SMAD3 pathway upregulates the proliferation of VSMCs and therefore intimal hyperplasia by upregulating the Wnt/β-catenin pathway in cultured aortic SMCs.[107]

Coagulation and Fibrinolytic Pathways

Products of coagulation pathways participate in the development of neointimal hyperplasia in complex and diverse ways. Formation of a fibrin matrix in an area of endothelial damage helps stabilize the aggregating platelet plug. Many substances released by organizing thrombus can affect VSMC growth and migration. Among thrombin's many actions, it is a VSMC mitogen. The locally active vascular fibrinolytic system allows VSMCs to detach from the surrounding matrix and migrate to the intima. Several molecules participate in this activity, including plasmin, the active end product of the tissue plasminogen-plasmin system. Other important components of this system include the precursor plasminogen and its main endogenous activators: urokinase plasminogen activator (u-PA) and tissue plasminogen activator (t-PA). The catalytic action of these proteases is inhibited in vivo by the plasmin inhibitors α_2-antiplasmin, α_2-macroglobulin, and a group of related plasminogen activator inhibitory proteins.

Several studies link plasmin to VSMC migration. First, circulating plasminogen is a relatively large protein that is normally prevented from entering the medial layer by an intact endothelium. However, after endothelial damage, this protein diffuses readily.[108] Once present in the extracellular medial layer, plasminogen converted into plasmin directly degrades several matrix proteins and activates other collagenases.[109] VSMCs express plasminogen activator activity in tissue culture and are a likely source of this enzyme locally in the vessel wall.[110,111] In an in vivo model of arterial repair, Clowes and associates demonstrated that VSMC contain increased levels of both urokinase plasminogen activator (u-PA) and tissue type PA (t-PA). These plasminogen activators act synergistically; their secretion depends on the functional state of the VSMCs. During cellular proliferation, u-PA is the major product, whereas during migration, t-PA expression predominates. These experimental observations suggest that injury to the endothelium allows the local penetration of plasminogen and chemotactic substances elaborated from activated platelets and leukocytes into the arterial wall. The conversion of extracellular plasminogen into plasmin by VSMCs degrades the structural matrix proteins. This process may be enhanced by the presence of leukocyte-derived enzymes. Activation of VSMCs by the elaborated growth and chemotactic factors initiates migration of these cells through the weakened arterial wall. The direction of migration is determined automatically by the gradient of plasminogen and mitogenic activity, which is highest adjacent to the endothelial defect.[28] Fu and colleagues have suggested the tissue factor pathway inhibitor as a potential gene therapy for atherosclerosis and neointimal hyperplasia. In their viral gene transfer study they noted that the proliferation of VSMCs was markedly decreased in in vitro mouse VSMCs infected with adenovirus containing the recombinant tissue factor plasminogen inhibitor gene.[112] In related work, Chen and colleagues noted the inhibition of neointimal hyperplasia after mouse femoral artery wire injury in a transgenic mouse that expressed a membrane-tethered tissue factor pathway inhibitor. Later, Chen and colleagues further developed this finding in a mouse aortic interposition model in the same genetic background. After aortic transplantation, transgenic mice expressing TFPI developed a quiescent endothelium instead of progressive neointimal hyperplasia as seen in wild-type mice.[113,114]

Nitric Oxide

NO is a small gaseous molecule normally produced in endothelial cells that serves to protect the vascular health of the vessel wall. NO was originally described as endothelium-derived relaxing factor by Furchgott and Zawadzki[115] in 1980. It is a small diffusible molecule with a very short half-life that is produced from L-arginine by one of three different enzymes—endothelial nitric oxide synthase (eNOS), neuronal nitric oxide synthase (nNOS), or inducible nitric oxide synthase (iNOS). Although these isoforms share a number of similarities, they are also clearly distinct. They all require the cofactors NADPH, FAD, FMN, heme, and tetrahydrobiopterin to catalyze the reaction.[116] In general, however, eNOS and nNOS are constitutively expressed enzymes and NO production is regulated predominantly by intracellular Ca^{2+} fluxes that permit calmodulin binding, which activates the enzymes.[116] In contrast, iNOS is transcriptionally regulated and is not normally produced by most cells.

NO possess many different vasoprotective properties that serve to protect the artery against the development of neointimal hyperplasia. NO inhibits platelet aggregation, inhibits leukocyte chemotaxis and adherence, inhibits the proliferation and migration of VSMCs and adventitial fibroblasts, stimulates VSMC apoptosis, inhibits endothelial cell apoptosis, and stimulates

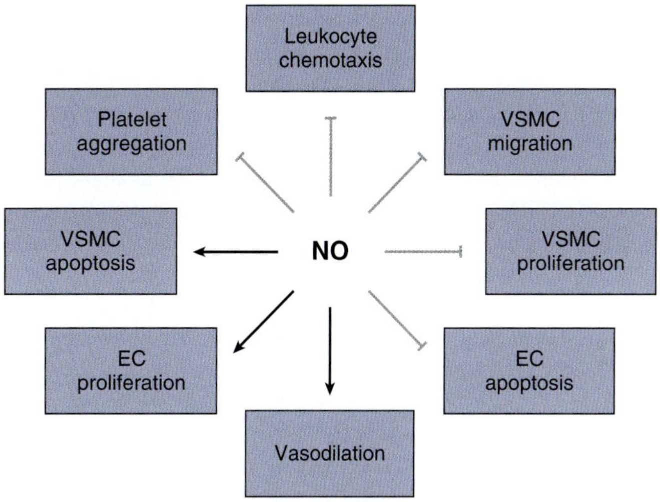

FIG 58.8 Schematic of the vasoprotective effects of nitric oxide. *EC,* Endothelial cell; *VSMC,* vascular smooth muscle cell.

endothelial cell growth (Fig. 58.8).[117-124] NO is also a potent vasodilator. By stimulating soluble guanylate cyclase and leading to the increased release of cyclic guanosine monophosphate, NO regulates basal vasomotor tone.[125,126] All of these properties of NO serve to maintain vascular homeostasis by affecting all the key components of the injury response.

Endothelial cell injury results in loss of NO, given that endothelial cells are the main source of constitutive NO production. This loss of NO after vascular injury is pivotal to the development of neointimal hyperplasia. Rudic and coworkers studied eNOS knockout mice and found that these mice developed significantly more neointima after carotid artery ligation than did their wild-type partners.[127] Fischer and associates used a different approach. They performed the balloon injury to the rat carotid artery, but in some animals they administered a NO synthase inhibitor, N-nitro-l-arginine, in the drinking water. Two weeks after injury, the animals exposed to the NO synthase inhibitor developed 30% more neointimal hyperplasia.[128] Mayr and coworkers evaluated the effect of iNOS deletion on vein graft intimal hyperplasia. They found that autologous vein grafts implanted into the carotid artery of iNOS knockout mice developed twofold more vein graft intimal hyperplasia compared with the wild-type controls.[129]

NO is also an important regulator of progenitor cell involvement in the development of neointimal hyperplasia after arterial injury (see Stem and Progenitor Cells section). Using an animal model of hind-limb ischemia, Aicher and colleagues originally described that eNOS knockout mice had impaired endothelial progenitor cell (EPC) mobilization.[130] Shortly thereafter, Iwakura and coworkers, and later Wegiel and coworkers, demonstrated impaired recruitment of EPCs in eNOS-deficient mice after arterial injury, which was associated with impaired reendothelialization and greater neointimal hyperplasia.[131,132] Using a mouse vein-graft model, Mayr and coworkers demonstrated impaired regeneration of endothelial cells in the vein graft of iNOS knockout versus wild-type mice.[129] They also showed that the iNOS knockout mice expressed less VEGF and had fewer microvessels in the adventitia compared with the wild-type controls, suggesting that the vasa vasorum in the adventitia may be important to the development of intimal hyperplasia in vein grafts. Zhang and colleagues evaluated the contribution of $Sca1^+$ progenitor cells in eNOS knockout mice using the carotid artery ligation model. They reported increased expression of stromal cell–derived factor-1α (SDF-1α), a chemokine known to regulate hematopoietic progenitor cell mobilization, increased circulating $Sca1^+$ cells, and increased $Sca1^+$ cells in the adventitia 1 week after carotid artery ligation in eNOS knockout versus wild-type control mice.[133] These data correlated with increased adventitial proliferation and neointimal hyperplasia. Together, these studies demonstrate a role for NO in regulating progenitor cell recruitment after arterial injury, but the effects may differ according to the progenitor cell type and the injury model being used.

Solidifying the role of NO in the arterial injury response, many investigators have shown that supplementation of NO at the site of injury prevents the development of neointimal hyperplasia. These NO-based approaches have included systemic delivery of L-arginine or NO donors, inhalational NO, local application of NO donors or NO-releasing polymers/gels, NO-releasing prosthetic materials, and gene therapy of one of the NOS enzymes.[134-149] Demonstrating the potency of NO, simple periadventitial application of the diazeniumdiolate NO donor PROLI/NO, a short-acting NO donor, inhibited the development of neointimal hyperplasia by 91% when applied to the carotid artery after balloon injury (Fig. 58.9).[143] In addition, it appears that these effects are mostly caused by NO and less by its metabolites nitrite or nitrate.[150] Although NO demonstrated potent inhibitory effects on cellular proliferation and inflammation, nitrite and nitrate inhibited inflammation only in a normoxic animal model of neointimal hyperplasia.

Recent advances in nanotechnology have allowed for some interesting therapeutic advances with resect to NO-based therapies. Systemic administration of NO causes hypotension and is limited due to its short half-life. Thus, to overcome these challenges, Kapadia and collaborators develop a therapy that delivers NO locally at the site of injury. Using a nanofiber gel–based platform and the NO donor PROLI/NO, they were able to deliver NO directly to areas of vascular injury in the rat model of carotid artery balloon angioplasty, in which treatment with PROLI/NO nanofiber gel reduced neointimal hyperplasia by 77% as measured by the intima/media area ratio compared with controls ($P < .05$).[151] This study validated NO as a feasible treatment strategy to mitigate the formation of neointima after open vascular interventions. Havelka and colleagues extended the utility of NO to endovascular interventions. They performed rat carotid artery balloon injury and delivered NO either via a permeable balloon catheter or periadventitially in the form of a powder at the time of injury. Both periadventitial and endoluminal NO at the time of arterial injury reduced neointimal hyperplasia formation (55% and 65%, respectively) compared with untreated controls ($P < .001$).[152] Further developing NO treatment technology, Bahnson and colleagues developed a targeted therapy. Using a similar nanofiber platform as employed in the study by Kapadia and a different NO donor strategy with S-nitrosothiols (SNOs), they developed a targeted therapy for intimal hyperplasia designed to be delivered systemically, bringing NO directly to sites of intimal hyperplasia. In vitro, targeted NO-releasing nanofibers inhibited VSMC proliferation; after rat carotid artery balloon injury, treatment with the targeted nanofibers reduced neointimal hyperplasia by 46% compared with untargeted nanofiber controls ($P < .05$); this inhibition was durable out to 8 weeks.[153] Finally, in ex vivo human saphenous vein samples, Wong and colleagues demonstrated release of NO and inhibition of neointimal hyperplasia after stimulation of Eph-B4 with its natural ligand.[154] These studies serve as a foundation for future strategies to mitigate neointimal hyperplasia after vascular surgery.

Reactive Oxygen Species

ROS are recognized as important contributors to the pathophysiology of neointimal hyperplasia. The precursor for all ROS

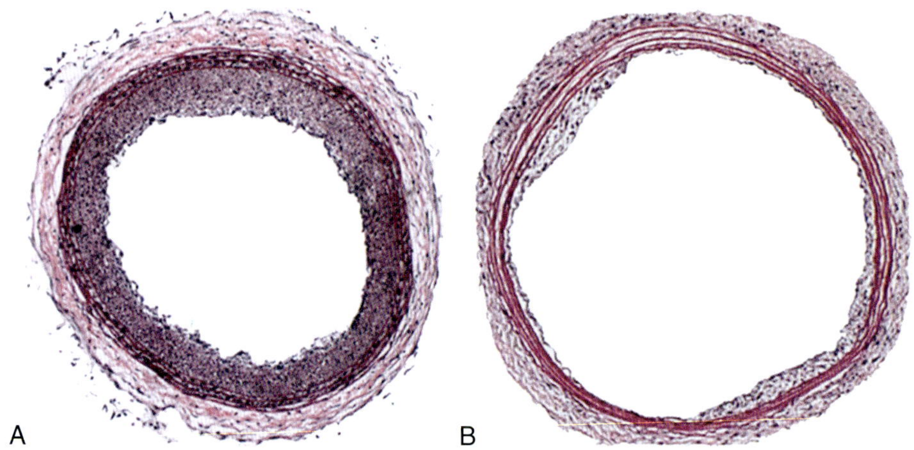

FIG 58.9 The nitric oxide donor PROLI/NO applied to the periadventitial surface of the rat carotid artery after balloon injury inhibits the development of neointimal hyperplasia at 2 weeks. (A) Rat carotid artery cross section after balloon injury; (B) rat carotid artery cross section after balloon injury and application of PROLI/NO.

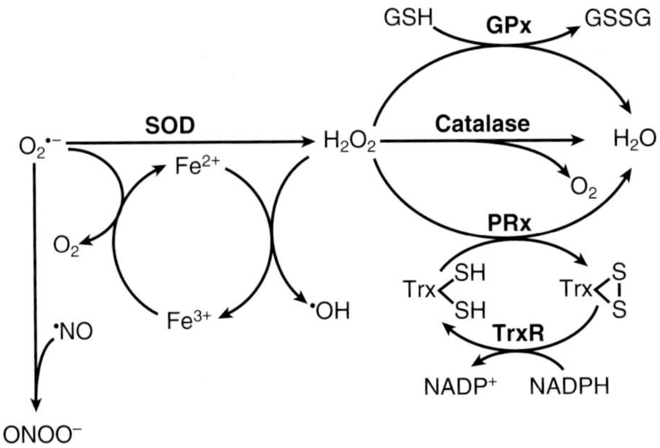

FIG 58.10 Schematic of superoxide ($O_2^{\bullet-}$) metabolism. *GSH,* Gluthathione; *GSSG,* oxidized glutathione; *GPx,* glutathione peroxidase; *Fe^{2+},* iron II; *Fe^{3+},* iron III; *H_2O,* water; *H_2O_2,* hydrogen peroxide; *NADP+,* dihydrophyrimidine dehydrogenase; *NADPH,* nicotinamide adenine dinucleotide phosphate; *NO,* nitric oxide; *O_2,* oxygen; *$ONOO^-$,* peroxynitrite; *PRx,* peroxiredoxin; *SOD,* superoxide dismutase; *Trx,* thioredoxin; *TrxR,* thioredoxin reductase.

is $O_2^{\bullet-}$, which can be produced from NADPH oxidase (NOX), the mitochondrial respiratory chain, lipoxygenases, xanthine oxidase, cytochrome p450, and uncoupled eNOS.[155] However, in the vasculature, $O_2^{\bullet-}$ is produced mainly by the stimulation of the NOX enzymes.[156,157] Seven different homologs of the NOX family exist, but only four have been identified in the vasculature: NOX1, NOX2, NOX 4, and NOX5. Once $O_2^{\bullet-}$ is formed, it is rapidly dismutated by superoxide dismutase (SOD) to H_2O_2, which in turn is metabolized by catalase, peroxiredoxin, or glutathione peroxidase to oxygen and water (Fig. 58.10). $O_2^{\bullet-}$ can also react with NO to form peroxynitrite ($ONOO^-$), or it can react with iron to form hydroxyl radical (•OH). Both superoxide and H_2O_2 have been shown to be involved in the regulation of endothelial cell function, VSMC apoptosis, VSMC and fibroblast migration, VSMC and fibroblast proliferation, and inflammation after arterial injury.[155,158-165] However, the more direct role of oxidative stress has been shown through the use of animal models of arterial injury and bypass grafting.

Several animal models have demonstrated a more direct role for ROS after vascular injury. One of the first suggestions of the importance of ROS to the arterial injury response was a study by Laurindo and colleagues in 1991 showing that the infusion of SOD inhibited neointimal growth after balloon angioplasty in dogs.[166] Subsequently Nunes and coworkers demonstrated that high levels of superoxide were detectable after balloon injury in pigs, even 14 days after injury, and that the administration of vitamins C and E affected vascular remodeling in association with reducing superoxide production.[167,168] Azevedo and associates characterized the oxidative stress after balloon injury in rabbits. They reported a marked increase (100-fold induction) in superoxide production immediately after injury, with a slow decline to baseline levels 4 weeks after injury. This increase in superoxide levels correlated with cellular proliferation and a decrease in the glutathione/oxidized glutathione ratio, a marker of reduced/oxidized glutathione.[169] Similarly, Souza and coworkers characterized oxidative stress after injury in a balloon injury model in rabbits, with comparable results, and suggested that the redox imbalance is likely caused by NOX.[170] Shi and coauthors showed that balloon injury of porcine coronary arteries resulted in an increased production of O_2^- and specifically an increased expression of the NOX subunits p47phox and p67phox in the adventitial fibroblasts, but not in the media.[171] Dourron and coauthors more directly demonstrated the importance of ROS production in the development of neointimal hyperplasia. They delivered an adenoviral vector carrying a NOX inhibitor periadventitially to rat common carotid arteries after balloon catheter injury. The NOX inhibitor resulted in a significant reduction of distention-induced ROS production. Furthermore, subsequent analysis of the intima-to-media area ratio showed significant attenuation in neointimal development in the group in which NOX had been inhibited compared with controls.[172] Other investigators have found reduced ROS after arterial injury with different antioxidants. NOX inhibitors, genetic NOX deletions, or xanthine oxidase inhibitors have been shown to decrease the formation of neointimal hyperplasia.[172-177] Investigators have also overexpressed SOD using adenoviral-mediated delivery of SOD or treatment with a SOD mimetic to attenuate the formation of neointimal hyperplasia.[178-180] Thus oxidative stress is intimately involved in regulating the arterial response to injury.

Given the importance of the NOX enzymes to the vasculature and the arterial injury response, special mention of each family member is warranted.[156] NOX1 is expressed in endothelial cells, VSMCs, and adventitial fibroblasts. NOX2 is found in cells throughout the arterial wall except in VSMCs from large arteries. NOX4 is present in all three cell types and is much more abundant than the other NOX enzymes. NOX5 is present in at least endothelial cells and VSMCs, but because it is not present in rodents, less is known about it. With respect to function, NOX1 appears to stimulate the proliferation and inflammation of VSMCs and is upregulated after vascular injury; lack of NOX1 in knockout mice is associated with less neointimal hyperplasia.[173] NOX2 may have more of a role in affecting blood pressure, inflammation, and atherosclerosis. The unique feature of NOX4 is that it is thought to be responsible for basal superoxide production. However, recent reports have suggested that NOX4 is distinct from the other NOX enzymes in that it produces mainly basal H_2O_2, not basal superoxide, and that the other enzymes produce superoxide that is then converted to H_2O_2.[181,182] Haurani and colleagues discovered something unexpected when myofibroblasts were transfected with NOX4/p22. Initially, they hypothesized that overexpression of NOX4/p22 would increase Ang II-induced production of H_2O_2. Interestingly, their data showed the opposite.[160] Transfection and overexpression of NOX4/p22 led to a reduction in the migratory capacity of myofibroblasts after treatment with Ang II compared with empty-vector transfection (46% decrease vs. 192% increase, respectively). The hypothesis postulated by the authors to explain these data included the unique ability of H_2O_2 to downregulate NOX4. They postulated that elevated levels of exogenous NOX4 exert negative feedback on endogenous NOX4 mRNA, or that the protein produced by the NOX4 mRNA has a negative feedback effect on the mRNA itself. Thus each of the NOX isoforms is intimately involved in regulating some aspect of the arterial injury response.

Stem and Progenitor Cells

Human stem cell research with respect to the vasculature has really expanded in this past decade. With the description of the EPCs, the appreciation of the multipotency of the vascular pericyte, and the discovery of the resident adventitial stem cells, a more detailed look into the world of the vascular stem cell has commenced. The first vessel wall resident cell to be identified as possessing progenitor cell properties was the pericyte.[183] Pericytes, which incompletely surround the endothelial cells of the microvasculature and share the same basement membrane and numerous junctions with endothelial cells, have traditionally been described and characterized by their supportive role. These cells play an important role in the development of capillaries through the regulation of the surrounding endothelial cells. However, pericytes can differentiate into multiple different cell types—adipocytes, chondrocytes, osteoblasts, VSMCs, macrophages, and fibroblasts—depending on the stimuli.[184-187] With this pluripotent ability, pericytes serve as a reservoir of precursor cells, giving rise to cells of multiple different lineages. In coculture experiments, Bagley and colleagues show endothelial cells and pericytes in close association with each other spontaneously forming capillary-like networks. This suggests that pericytes are involved in guiding endothelial cells and other precursor cells to sites of vascular injury.[188]

Progenitor cells are not limited to the pericytes within the vascular wall. In fact, the vascular wall, specifically the adventitia, is an active site of recruitment of circulating stem and progenitor cells. Hematopoietic stem cells (HSCs), MSCs, and EPCs all contribute to the formation of the neointima after arterial injury, expanding our understanding of what occurs in the arterial wall after injury.[189-192] Sata and colleagues and Han and colleagues were the first investigators to independently demonstrate, using bone marrow–irradiated mice transplanted with labeled or sex-specific bone marrow, that bone marrow–derived cells constituted approximately 50% to 60% of the neointima after injury.[189,193] Some cells stained positive for CD31 and others stained positive for αSMA. Wang and coauthors studied the response to injury in mice deficient in stem cell factor (SCF) or c-Kit, both important molecules for stem cell signaling. A near-complete lack of neointima in these mice after arterial injury compared with wild-type controls confirmed the importance of stem cells to the formation of the neointima.[194] Further studies by Tanaka and coauthors demonstrated that the degree of incorporation of bone marrow–derived cells into the neointima was dependent on the type of injury model used, with the wire-mediated injury resulting in the largest percentage of bone marrow–derived cells in the neointima.[195] Stem and progenitor cells are mobilized and recruited to the site of arterial injury and undergo phenotypic differentiation to endothelial cells or VSMCs. Boyd and colleagues showed that differentiation of human embryonic stem cells to VSMCs occurs upon stimulation with TGF-β.[196] However, much remains unknown about the forces regulating these processes and the multipotency and differentiation capabilities of VSMC.

Tigerstedt and coworkers characterized the involvement of precursor cells in the arterial injury response. After rat arterial injury, there was a fivefold increase in adventitial cells preceding the formation of the neointima. This was accompanied by a fourfold increase in the adventitial microvasculature, which peaked at day 14. The cytoskeletal marker vimentin—which stains VSMCs, fibroblasts, and myofibroblasts—stained mostly positive in the adventitia at days 3 to 4; thereafter, the staining declined in the adventitia and shifted to the neointima. Flk-1 staining, a stem cell marker, was noted in the first cells that localized to the neointima and adventitia. By day 14, all layers of the vascular wall expressed flk-1, with the greatest intensity seen in the neointima. These findings support the assertion that cells in the adventitia are activated or recruited very early in the injury response and contribute to neointima formation. To further characterize the adventitial cell types contributing to neointima formation, outgrowth assays were performed from aortic explants. Cells from these outgrowth assays coexpressed markers of multiple cell lineages including VSMCs, endothelial cells, and myofibroblasts; a high percentage of these cells was also positive for the stem cell markers flk-1, Sca1, and CD34.[197] These data suggest that stem and progenitor cells contribute significantly to the development of neointimal hyperplasia after arterial injury.

An interesting study by Shoji and associates described a mechanism by which human MSCs block macrophage involvement with neointimal hyperplasia. Human MSCs were injected into the left ventricle of rats immediately and also 6 days and 13 days after ligation of the left common carotid artery. The ligated arteries were then harvested at 7, 14, and 28 days after ligation. Assessment of the human MSCs incorporation into the resulting neointimal lesion revealed an absence of transplanted stem cells despite a significant reduction in the size of the neointima. Monocyte recruitment into the neointima decreased by 30% ($P < .05$). In addition, human MSC–treated rats exhibited 44% less monocyte chemoattractant protein-1 (MCP-1), a protein responsible for the mobilization and targeting of monocytes ($P < .05$).[198] The authors argue that human MSCs, although not incorporated into neointimal lesions, exert vasoprotective properties by limiting the activation of circulating monocytes after vascular injury. In a similar but contradicting study, Zhao and coauthors suggest that MMP-14 releases activated TGF-β, which then recruits MSCs from the periphery, and that, in turn, MSCs differentiate into neointimal cells at sites of arterial injury.[199] There is still much to be learned regarding their exact roles and relationships, but these studies highlight the complex relationship between growth factors and progenitor cells in the response to arterial injury and formation of neointimal hyperplasia.

The adventitia is also home to resident adult pluripotent cells, including Sca1+ cells, CD34+ cells, and pericytes. Passman and coworkers found that Sca1$^+$ cells, which are integral to the developing artery, are present in adult arteries in the adventitia, near the media/adventitia interface. In an effort to determine how the adventitial Sca1$^+$ cells are targeted to and maintained within the adventitia, they identified a layer of sonic hedgehog protein (Shh) located between the media and the adventitia.[200] Shh is important in the retention of other progenitor cell populations in areas such as the skin, nervous system, and lymphoid tissue.[201-203] Shh knockout mice also have significantly fewer adventitial Sca1+ cells compared with wild-type mice. In a quiescent state, adventitial Sca1 cells do not express VSMCs or endothelial cell markers in vivo. However, these cells can readily differentiate into VSMCs or endothelial cells in vitro depending on the stimulus.[200,204] For example, Hu and coworkers demonstrated the presence of progenitor cells within the adventitia of the aortic root in an atherosclerotic mouse model, the apolipoprotein E knockout mice. These cells were found to express a number of markers characteristic of progenitor cells, including stem cell antigen–1 (Sca-1), c-Kit, and CD34. Similar cells were notably absent from the media and intima. Sca-1–positive cells carrying the *LacZ* gene were then transferred to the adventitia of vein grafts in these atherosclerotic mice. *LacZ*-positive cells were subsequently found to populate the intimal atherosclerotic lesions of the vein grafts.[204] This study has far-reaching implications and suggests that resident adventitial stem cells may play an important role in the development of neointimal hyperplasia, however, to date there have been no identified cell-specific conditional lineage of the Sca-1+ stem cell populations.[205]

Zengin and coauthors identified the presence of resident adventitial CD34+ cells in the walls of adult human arteries. These cells were located in the same zone as the Sca1+ cells described earlier, at the media/adventitia interface, and demonstrated the potential to differentiate into endothelial cells and contribute to the vasa vasorum.[206] Subsequently Wu and colleagues identified CD34+ resident progenitor cells in the adventitia of young and old female rats. They noted less cells of this phenotype in older rats and induced differentiation of CD34+ progenitor cells into VSMCs with exposure to estrogen. This study further supports the many roles of resident progenitor/stem cells in the adventita and has implications for the mechanism of estrogen protection against cardiovascular disease in females.[207]

Finally, the CD44+ multipotent resident adventitial stem cells were identified by Klein and colleagues in the vasculogenic zone of the adventitia, where other progenitor cells have been identified. These cells were able to differentiate into not only VSCMs but also pericytes.[208] In a follow-up study, this group also identified the Hox genes as epigenetic regulators of CD44+ differentiation in the vascular wall, implying a role for CD44+ resident adventitial MSCs in the formation of angiogenesis, tumor vascularization, and neointimal hyperplasia.[209]

Adiponectin and Periadventitial Adipose Tissue

Adiponectin is a small 30-kDa protein produced by periadventitial adipose tissue. It belongs to a class of compounds called adipokines and can be found systemically in the plasma in concentrations between 3 and 30 μg/mL.[210,211] In general, adipokines increase as a person's adiposity increases (i.e., obese individuals produce more adipokines). Interestingly, this is not the case with adiponectin. In fact, the level of adiponectin is inversely related to the amount of adipose tissue in a person.[212] Low levels of adiponectin have been linked to the development and progression of obesity-related diseases, including type 2 diabetes and hypertension.[213-216] In addition, adiponectin levels have been linked to the severity of peripheral artery disease. Higher levels of adiponectin are associated with better ankle-brachial indices and improved symptom-free walking distances.[217] In addition, adiponectin levels found in perivascular adipose tissue were negatively correlated with the severity of both coronary and aortic atherosclerosis.[218] Given its relationship with arterial disease, adiponectin has recently garnered more attention as to the role it plays in the vasculature.

Adiponectin has already been shown to have numerous beneficial effects on the endothelium. It stimulates endothelial cell proliferation and inhibits endothelial cell apoptosis (programmed cell death), both of which are important in attenuating the progression of arterial disease.[219,220] Repair of damaged endothelium involves the recruitment and differentiation of circulating EPCs. Shibata and coauthors showed that adiponectin influences the degree to which EPCs are used: adiponectin knockout mice show attenuated activity of EPCs, whereas adenovirus-mediated adiponectin overexpression restored the activity level of EPCs.[221] In addition, adiponectin has been shown to be a chemoattractant for EPCs to the endothelium and to induce EPCs to differentiate. NO, which exhibits numerous vasoprotective properties, has also been shown to be regulated in part by adiponectin. Adiponectin modulates the production of NO by upregulating the phosphorylation and thus activation of eNOS.[220,222,223] Thus, adiponectin has been shown to be a protector of the vascular endothelium: it increases endothelial cell proliferation and migration, increases the activation and chemotaxis of EPCs, and increases the local concentration of NO.

Further supporting the vasoprotective role of adiponectin, Takaoka and coworkers demonstrated that adiponectin produced by periadventitial adipose tissue, and not systemic adiponectin, is an important regulator of neointimal hyperplasia. First, the ability of periadventitial adipose tissue to inhibit the formation of neointima was established. Wild-type mice underwent femoral artery injury after removal of the periadventitial adipose tissue. Neointimal hyperplasia was markedly increased in the wild-type mice after the removal of adipose tissue. This effect was attenuated if subcutaneous adipose tissue was transplanted back to the adventitia of the injured artery, demonstrating that local adipose tissue inhibits neointimal hyperplasia. Second, Takaoka and coauthors demonstrated that this protective effect was, in fact, caused by locally produced adiponectin. They did so by studying neointimal hyperplasia in the setting of adiponectin knockout mice. At 4 weeks after femoral artery injury, wild-type mice showed significantly less neointimal hyperplasia than the adiponectin knockout mice. Perivascular application of an adiponectin donor (i.e., adiponectin gel) caused a significant reduction in the development of neointimal hyperplasia compared with adiponectin delivered subcutaneously and in adiponectin knockout mice.[224] Together, these data demonstrate the important role of adiponectin in limiting the formation of neointimal hyperplasia after arterial injury.

In a subsequent study, Takaoka and colleagues demonstrated a 66% decrease in adiponectin expression in periadventitial adipose tissue 24 hours after balloon injury of rat iliac arteries ($P < .05$). This was accompanied by an increase in proinflammatory adipocytokines: a 2-fold increase in TNF-α, a 2-fold increase in MCP-1, and a 10-fold increase in IL-6 ($P < .05$). TNF-α appeared to be the driving force behind the subsequent increases in MCP-1 and IL-6, because these increases were attenuated in TNF-α knockout mice. Further investigation demonstrated that TNF-α acted on adiponectin levels through MCP-1 because postinjury decreases in adiponectin were attenuated in MCP-1 knockout mice. Immunofluorescent staining revealed that the ultimate source of postinjury TNF-α was from infiltrating periadventitial macrophages, with a minority of TNF-α derived from the adipocytes themselves. Neointimal hyperplasia development was reduced in TNF-α knockout mice. Neointimal severity was then restored by supplying the TNF-α knockout mice with a periadventitial infusion of TNF-α, elegantly confirming the importance of TNF-α to neointimal growth.[225]

In a model of rabbit carotid interposition with autologous vein graft, Morisaki and colleagues treated rabbits with oral pioglitazone for 4 weeks. In their study they saw a twofold increase in circulating adiponectin levels, over a twofold decrease in VSMC proliferation, over a twofold increase in VSMC apoptosis, and ultimately decreased formation of neointimal hyperplasia in interposition vein grafts at 28 days postsurgery as measured by the intima/media index (1.16 control, 0.652 pioglitazone treatment, $P < .01$).[226] Most recently, Bahnson and coauthors further demonstrated the implications of periadventitial fat on the development and treatment of neointimal hyperplasia. Using the rat carotid artery balloon injury model, rats in which the periadventitial adipose tissue was stripped at the time of injury developed 27% more neointimal hyperplasia compared with rats that retained intact periadventital adipose tissue ($P < .0001$). Using the NO donor PROLI/NO, they treated rats after carotid artery balloon injury and compared neointimal hyperplasia in rats with periadventitial adipose tissue intact with rats in which periadventitial adipose tissue was stripped at the time of carotid artery injury. Compared with intact rats, rats stripped of periadventitial adipose tissue had a 35% greater decrease in intimal area when treated with NO.[227] Thus regulation of the arterial injury response extends into the periadventitial tissue, creating a proinflammatory milieu that promotes the growth of the neointima.

Vasa Vasorum

The vasa vasorum consists of a network of microvascular channels that supply oxygen and nutrients to the vessel wall. These conduits consist of a lumen lined by endothelial cells surrounded by smooth muscle cells. This architecture allows its caliber to be modified by vasodilatory compounds. In addition to delivering nutrients, the vasa vasorum can act as a port of entry for different circulating cell types into the adventitia. Monocytes, progenitor cells, and cytokines can take advantage of the branching vasa vasorum to enter the adventitia and participate in the reaction to arterial injury.

Arterial injury alters the adventitial density of the vasa vasorum. Kwon and coauthors were among the first to describe the neovascularization that occurs in the adventitia after balloon angioplasty. To induce arterial injury and neointima formation, they used a porcine model of coronary artery balloon angioplasty. After 28 days, the animals were sacrificed and the arteries were perfused with a radiopaque liquid polymer, MV-122. Microscopic three-dimensional computed tomography reconstruction was then used to image the arteries. The authors found that the density of the vasa vasorum per square millimeter increased by 66% in the vessel wall of injured arteries versus in uninjured controls ($P < .01$), but the overall percentage of vessel wall composed of vasa vasorum decreased by 30% after injury ($P = .018$). There was a strong, direct relationship between the number of vasa vasorum and intimal thickness, but it was unclear from this study whether increased vasa vasorum number was a cause or effect of the thickness of the neointima.[228] A well-developed vasa vasorum network present soon after injury can promote neointimal growth by serving as a better route through which monocytes and other inflammatory cells invade the vascular wall. However, an increase in vasa vasorum density after injury could reduce adventitial hypoxia, a potent inducer of neointimal hyperplasia. Supporting the latter is a study by Mayr and associates of vein graft intimal hyperplasia in iNOS knockout versus wild-type mice. Although they found that iNOS knockout mice developed greater vein graft intimal hyperplasia, they also noted that the iNOS knockout mice exhibited a lower density of vasa vasorum, as indicated by CD31 staining, in the adventitia compared with the wild-type mice.[129] In a rabbit double arterial injury model, Ye and colleagues confirmed a proportional increase in vasa vasorum and intimal hyperplasia. Furthermore, they identified a decreased density of vasa vasorum after injury compared with control.[229] From these data it appears that injury increases vasa vasorum arborization in the vessel wall; however, the effect this has on neointimal hyperplasia may be due to ischemia, as evidenced by a decreased density of vasa vasorum.

The transcription factor nuclear factor-κB (NF-κB) is known to be important to the development of neointimal hyperplasia early after arterial injury, because inhibition of NF-κB attenuates neointimal growth.[230-234] A recent study by Damrauer and colleagues sought to identify the role of NF-κB in vasa vasorum neovascularization after arterial injury. Irradiated rats underwent bone marrow transplant with cells ubiquitously expressing green fluorescent protein (GFP). Neointimal hyperplasia was then induced by performing balloon injury of the common carotid artery, after which the rats were transfected with A20, a compound known to inhibit NF-κB. There was a significant reduction in CD31 expression, an endothelial cell marker, in arteries transfected with A20 versus arteries transfected with an empty vector. The endothelial cells present in the adventitia sometimes expressed GFP, indicating that some were derived from the bone marrow. Importantly, although the presence of endothelial cells was reduced in the adventitia, the rate of reendothelialization of the vessel lumen, necessary for arterial recovery from injury, actually accelerated. The endothelial cells repopulating the endothelium were GFP-negative, indicating that they did not originate in the bone marrow.[235] The authors were able to conclude that inhibition of NF-κB affected the layers of the vessel wall differently, with the adventitia exhibiting a marked reduction in neovascularity and the endothelium exhibiting an increase in the rate of reendothelialization. In a similar study, Wihastuti and colleagues used the antioxidant mangosteen pericarp ethanolic extract (MPEE), a known NF-κB inhibitor. Rats were fed a hypercholesterolemic diet with MPEE for 3 months, and treated mice had significantly decreased vasa vasorum angiogenesis compared with controls ($P < .05$).[236]

The studies by Damrauer and Wihastuti may be explained in part by an inability of the adventitia to recruit circulating endothelial cell precursors, which may serve as the building blocks for vasa vasorum angiogenesis. Nieves Torres and colleagues cultured endothelial cells isolated from porcine blood (blood outgrowth endothelial cells, BOECs) and cocultured them with fibroblasts under hypoxic conditions to determine if BOECs reduced conversion of fibroblasts to myofibroblasts. They concluded that contact with BOECs caused reduced conversion of fibroblasts to myofibroblasts, reduced migration, but did not change proliferation.[237] This represents a possible explanation for the adaptive role of the vasa vasorum in arterial injury and a possible future treatment strategy for neointimal hyperplasia.

A study by Misra and coworkers investigated the influence of hypoxia on murine adventitial fibroblasts in vitro. Mouse fibroblasts were grown under hypoxic conditions (3% O_2) or normoxic conditions (20% O_2) for 24, 48, and 72 hours. These investigators found that hypoxic conditions cause acceleration in fibroblast differentiation into myofibroblasts, as evidenced by an increase in the expression of αSMA, a myofibroblast marker. Cell lysates were then collected and the proteins concentrated by immunoprecipitation. Western blot analysis was then performed to assess the level of expression for hypoxia-induced factor 1α (HIF-1α) and matrix metalloproteinase 2 (MMP-2). HIF-1α is a transcription factor upregulated under hypoxic conditions and affects the expression of many genes. One such gene is for MMP-2, an enzyme that degrades the extracellular matrix and eases the migration of myofibroblasts from the adventitia to the media. Misra and coworkers showed that hypoxia leads to an increase in HIF-1α and MMP-2 at 24, 48, and 72 hours. They concluded that hypoxia acts as a driving force behind neointimal growth by stimulating fibroblast differentiation, increasing HIF-1α levels, and increasing the expression of MMP-2.[238] This study implies that adventitial hypoxia is optimal for neointimal growth.

CONCLUSION

It is apparent that the arterial injury response represents a complex interplay of events that culminates in the formation of neointimal hyperplasia. It can no longer be viewed as a simple proliferative response of the medial VSMCs to the intima under the stimulation of growth factors and cytokines released from platelets and leukocytes. Instead, all three layers of the arterial wall are involved, with the adventitia playing a much more important role than was appreciated originally, given that the adventitia is the portal of entry for many cells through the vasa vasorum, contains adiponectin, and prominently expresses NOX4. The cell types involved in the arterial injury response include both resident and circulating cells, and these include platelets, leukocytes, endothelial cells, VSMCs, adventitial fibroblasts, as well as stem and progenitor cells. Finally, ROS have also been shown to play a prominent role. By gaining a better understanding of the pathophysiology of neointimal hyperplasia, targeted therapies can be developed to prevent restenosis after vascular interventions.

REVIEW QUESTIONS

1. The origin of the proliferating cells found in neointimal hyperplastic lesions includes all of the following except:
   a. Adventitial fibroblasts
   b. Macrophages
   c. Progenitor cells
   d. Vascular smooth muscle cells
   e. All of the above
2. Which hemodynamic force has been implicated as a contributing factor in the development of intimal hyperplasia?
   a. Vessel wall compliance
   b. High shear stress
   c. Flow velocity
   d. Low shear stress
   e. All of the above
3. Which surface membrane receptor regulates vascular smooth muscle cells' accumulation of low-density lipoprotein (LDL)?
   a. Glycoprotein receptor Ib
   b. High-affinity LDL receptor
   c. Glycoprotein receptor IIb/IIIa
   d. Low-affinity LDL receptor
   e. High-affinity high-density lipoprotein receptor
4. Platelet aggregation is stimulated by which of the following?
   a. Adenosine triphosphate
   b. Platelet-derived growth factor
   c. Adenosine diphosphate
   d. LDL
   e. Prostacyclin
5. Angiotensin-converting enzyme is located primarily on the membrane surface of which of the following?
   a. Platelets
   b. Neutrophils
   c. Fibroblasts
   d. Vascular endothelial cells
   e. Macrophages
6. Nitric oxide is constitutively expressed in the vasculature in which cell type?
   a. Platelets
   b. Neutrophils
   c. Endothelial cells
   d. Vascular smooth muscle cells
   e. Adventitial fibroblasts
7. Which of the following NOX enzymes directly produces hydrogen peroxide?
   a. NOX1
   b. NOX2
   c. NOX3
   d. NOX4
   e. NOX5

8. Which of the following has been shown to be a resident progenitor cell in the arterial wall, just external to the external elastic lamina?
   a. Pericytes
   b. Sca1+ cells
   c. flk+ cells
   d. CD34+ cells
   e. CD31+ cells
9. In the vasculature, adiponectin stimulates:
   a. Platelet aggregation
   b. Leukocyte chemotaxis
   c. Endothelial cell proliferation
   d. Vascular smooth muscle cell proliferation
   e. Adventitial fibroblast proliferation
10. Arterial injury has been shown to alter which characteristic of the vasa vasorum?
   a. Absolute number of the vasa vasorum
   b. Density of the vasa vasorum
   c. Percentage of the vessel wall consisting of the vasa vasorum
   d. a and b
   e. a, b, and c

References available online at ExpertConsult.com.

CHAPTER 59

Prosthetic Graft Infection

Mimmie Kwong, John George Carson, Christopher J. Abularrage, Julie Ann Freischlag

The development of prosthetic biomaterial devices has made it possible to treat conditions that otherwise would have resulted in significant morbidity and mortality. Examples of such clinical conditions include but are not limited to aortic aneurysms, hemodialysis access in patients in whom autologous fistulas are not possible, and infrainguinal bypass for limb ischemia. The advent of prosthetic conduits has also resulted in the problem of prosthetic graft infection. The morbidity associated with infected prosthetic vascular grafts is considerable and can be catastrophic, resulting in limb loss, sepsis, and death. This chapter examines the causes, diagnosis, and management of prosthetic graft infection.

INCIDENCE

Prosthetic graft infection is relatively uncommon, with a reported incidence ranging from 1% to 6%.[1-4] Graft infections are influenced by the implant site, the indications for operation, and the host's defense status as manifested by comorbid disease.[5,6] Szilagyi and colleagues'[1] analysis of 2145 patients undergoing a variety of vascular reconstructions—including aortofemoral, aortoiliac, and femoropopliteal reconstructions—revealed an overall graft infection rate of 1.5%. A prospective multicenter Canadian study of repair of unruptured abdominal aortic aneurysms revealed a graft infection rate of 0.2%.[7] A prosthetic graft inserted in the femoropopliteal or femorotibial position has a higher rate of infection, ranging up to 18% in some reports.[8] It has been theorized that the true percentages of prosthetic graft infection may be higher than reported due to the wide range in the time course of presentation, when many affected patients are lost to follow-up.

In recent years, there has been a sharp rise in the use of endovascular interventions for aneurysmal and occlusive vascular disease. Although it is relatively early, reports of infections in endovascular prosthesis are increasing. Extrapolating from the data regarding aortic aneurysm repair, endograft infections occur in around 1%.[9]

CLASSIFICATION

Prosthetic graft infections can be classified in one of three ways:

1. Timing: Early (<4 months after initial implantation) or late (>4 months after initial implantation)
2. Depth of wound infection (Szilagi classification)[1]:
   - Szilagyi grade I: Infection confined to the dermis
   - Szilagyi grade II: Infection involving the subcutaneous tissue but not the graft
   - Szilagyi grade III: Arterial graft involvement
3. Site and extent of graft involvement (modified Bunt classification)[10]:
   - P0: Infection of intracavitary graft (intrathoracic or intra-abdominal)
   - P1: Infection of extracavitary graft (neck, extremities, subcutaneous tissue of the trunk)
   - P2: Infection of extracavitary component of graft with intracavitary origin
   - P3: Infection of prosthetic patch
   - Graft—enteric erosion
   - Graft—enteric fistula
   - Aortic stump sepsis after excision of infected aortic graft

MICROBIOLOGY

The cause of vascular graft infections can be determined by examining the microorganisms recovered from infected grafts. Although any microorganism can potentially cause a graft infection, *Staphylococcus aureus* is the most prevalent bacterium.[1,2,4] However, over the last 2 decades, *Staphylococcus epidermidis* has increasingly been identified as the responsible pathogen for a significant proportion of graft infections, predominantly the late-appearing indolent type.[11,12]

Early-appearing graft infections are more often associated with organisms of higher virulence, including *S. aureus*. Coagulase-positive strains elaborate toxins that result in a vigorous host inflammatory response, including systemic signs such as fever, leukocytosis, hypotension, and bacteremia with positive blood cultures as well as severe symptoms such as abdominal pain or distension and cellulitis or drainage over the graft. Late-appearing graft infections are caused by less virulent gram-positive bacteria such as *S. epidermidis*. This organism is indolent and normally harbored in natural skin. It has the ability to adhere to prosthetic material and to secrete a glycocalyx biofilm that insulates the organism from white blood cells (WBCs). Over time, this biofilm induces an inflammatory response that results in perigraft inflammation, which is observed clinically as perigraft fluid, although severe systemic responses are rare. This innocuous presentation has led many to view *S. epidermidis* infections as inflammatory allergic reactions rather than bacterial graft infections.[13] Additionally, *S. epidermidis* is not easily cultured or isolated, and ultrasonication is often required to physically separate *S. epidermidis* from the graft surface in order to culture it.[14]

Other microorganisms such as fungi and gram-negative bacteria can also cause graft infections. Gram-negative bacteria such as *Pseudomonas* species, *Escherichia coli, Serratia, Enterobacter* species, and *Proteus* species are highly virulent and result in dramatic clinical manifestations, such as anastomotic disruption and frank hemorrhage.[15] These organisms induce a substantial host inflammatory response with secretion of potent tissue proteases, which account for the tissue destruction leading to artery-graft dehiscence. Severely immunosuppressed patients are also vulnerable to fungal (*Candida* and *Aspergillus* species) graft infections, an otherwise rare clinical entity in the general population.

CAUSE AND PATHOPHYSIOLOGY

The fundamental question concerning the cause of prosthetic graft infections is when exposure to the infection-causing microorganisms occurred. The three major potential mechanisms that can result in prosthetic graft colonization and subsequent infection are

1. Intraoperative contamination
2. Hematogenous spread of bacteria
3. Direct contamination of graft by infection emanating from the skin, soft tissue, gastrointestinal tract, or genitourinary tract

Although all these factors can result in a graft infection, the third mechanism is the least common.

Intraoperative Contamination

The patient's bacteria are the most common source of bacterial contamination resulting in infection of the surgical site. The resident microflora, usually referred to as the *indigenous microflora,* consists of a complex mixture of microbial species ranging from nonpathogenic saprophytes to pathogens. Endogenous bacteria are a more important source of surgical site infection than exogenous bacteria.

The patient's endogenous flora from a site close to the prosthetic bed—especially from a colonized site, such as the skin or gut—is a common source of graft infection. Most of the intertriginous areas of the body, such as the axillae, groin, and interdigital spaces of the foot, contain large numbers of eccrine sweat glands and harbor large bacterial populations. Indeed, prosthetic grafts placed in the groin have a well-characterized propensity to develop *S. aureus* infection.[16-18] *S. aureus* bacteria from the groin area may contaminate the wound, resulting in a wound infection, or contaminate the graft surface if it is inadvertently dragged across the skin, resulting in a graft infection. The lymphatics in the groin may be contaminated at the time of surgery, especially if the patient has an open infected wound in an extremity, and these lymphatics can be a source of intraoperative graft infection.

Bacteria can be present in diseased vessels or in the thrombus lining an aortic aneurysm.[19] One prospective study demonstrated that among patients undergoing peripheral vascular bypass surgery, 41% had positive arterial tissue cultures, 68% of which were coagulase-negative *Staphylococcus*[20]; but subsequent graft infections were not reported. Therefore, although the positive cultures are intriguing, their significance is unclear. Interestingly, in another study, the aneurysm contents of 216 patients were cultured. Positive cultures were found in 55 patients (25.5%). However, after 3 years of follow-up, only four graft infections occurred (1.9%); among these, only two grew the same organism as the original cultures.[21]

Hematogenous Spread

Seeding of an indwelling prosthesis by hematogenous spread of bacteria is an important mode of prosthetic graft infection, although the frequency with which this occurs is unknown. In experimental animals, infusion of 10 million organisms of *S. aureus* immediately after implantation of a prosthetic aortic graft resulted in a 100% incidence of graft infection.[22,23] Later studies demonstrated an inverse relationship between the incidence of graft infection and time after implantation, suggesting that graft incorporation and the development of a pseudointima may provide some protection.[24,25] Vulnerability to infection from bacteremia has been documented at even 1 year after implantation, with 30% of aortic grafts becoming infected after a single bacterial infusion at that time.[20] The anatomic difference between the infected and uninfected grafts was the absence or presence of a complete neointimal lining. Systemic and local antibiotics significantly reduced the incidence of graft infection.[26-28] The significance of remote infection is unclear, but it has been theorized that transient bacteremia associated with, for example, dental procedures or colonoscopy may account for very late infections.

Direct Contamination

Any direct exposure of the graft to bacterial sources can result in graft infection. Failure of the skin incision to heal after an operation can result in direct bacterial contamination and places the underlying graft at significant risk of subsequent infection. Moreover, hematomas and lymphoceles near or around the graft not only inhibit graft incorporation, thus increasing the duration of susceptibility to infection, but serve as niduses for bacterial growth, which may directly contaminate the adjacent graft. Finally, contamination of prosthetic grafts can occur from contact with adjacent bacteria-containing organs. For this reason, it is prudent to avoid any operation on the gastrointestinal tract at the time of insertion of an aortic prosthetic graft. Rarely, injury to bowel can occur during the placement of an aortic graft. Care must be exercised in tunneling graft limbs cautiously to avoid injury to the bowel, as these injuries can go unrecognized and lead to severe sepsis, peritonitis, and devastating graft infections (Fig. 59.1A and B). Should bowel injury with entry into the bowel lumen and spillage of bowel contents occur while a prosthetic aortic graft is being placed, the procedure should be aborted if possible. Of note, one important means of contamination from adjacent organs is the formation of an aortoenteric fistula or

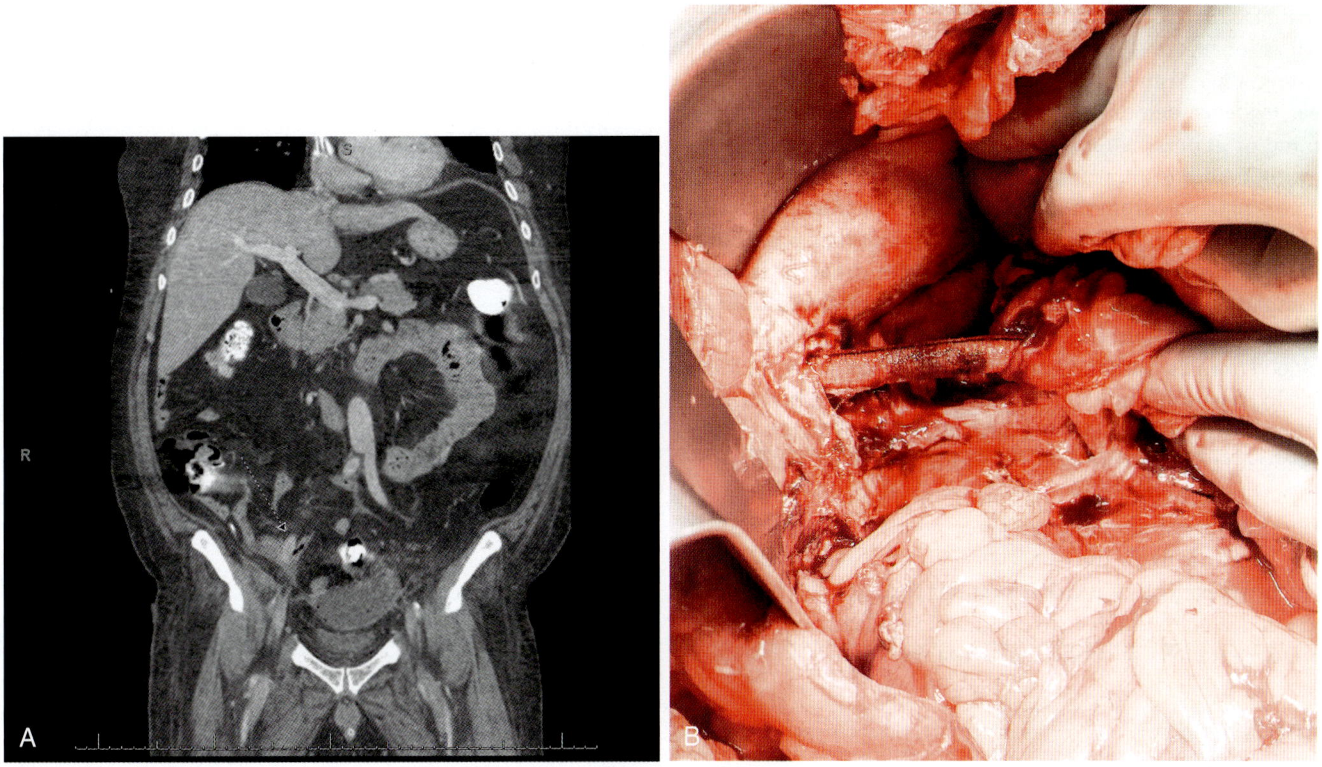

FIG 59.1 (A) Preoperative computed tomographic scan of patient presenting with infected aortic graft showing one limb of the aortobifemoral graft impaled through the terminal ileum *(arrow)*. This type of injury can occur during tunneling of the graft limb. (B) Intraoperative image of prosthetic aortobifemoral graft limb that has pierced through the terminal ileum.

erosion (AEF or AEE). With an incidence of 0.4% to 1.6% with open repair and likely less with endovascular repair, AEFs/AEEs are rare.[29-31] Although the pathogenesis of an AEF/AEE remains unknown, pulsatility of the aorta against the bowel and adhesions between the inflamed aortic graft and adjacent bowel have been postulated as a possible etiology of AEFs and AEEs.[32,33]

PREVENTION

The best way to avoid graft infection is to prevent it in the operating room and during the postoperative period. It has been shown that the cutaneous microflora of patients who are hospitalized for any length of time undergo change.[34] It is unclear whether this is caused by the underlying illness or the use of antibiotics. Thus the preoperative stay, if any, should be as short as possible to avoid colonization by resistant bacteria. Prophylactic antibiotics have been shown to decrease the incidence of graft infections.[27,28] Most authors recommend the administration of a first-generation cephalosporin approximately 30 to 60 minutes before incision, with continuation of the scheduled antibiotic dosing for the first 24 hours after surgery.[28,35,36] If the operation lasts for an unusually long time, additional doses should be administered to maintain adequate circulating levels. Although bacteremia is noted in 4% to 8% of angiographic procedures, it is usually asymptomatic. Antibiotic prophylaxis is not routinely recommended in endovascular procedures except for patients at high risk (e.g., repeated intervention within 7 days, prolonged indwelling arterial sheaths, prolonged duration of procedure) and for interventions where aortic or peripheral endograft placement is planned.[37] There is no evidence to support the continuation of prophylactic antibiotics until indwelling lines, such as central venous or urinary bladder catheters, are removed.[28] Indeed, the prolonged use of postoperative antibiotics may even be detrimental in some patients, leading to antibiotic-associated colitis or the development of other resistant infectious organisms.

The use of antibiotic-impregnated or soaked grafts has been proposed as a potential method to reduce the risk of prosthetic graft infection. In particular, rifampin, which has a higher affinity for collagen and gelatin coatings of grafts as compared with other antibiotics, has been the most extensively studied.[38] However, randomized controlled trials have shown mixed results, with lower short-term infection rates in patients treated with antibiotic-impregnated grafts. This is attributable largely to infection reduction in patients in whom a groin incision was made, although no benefit has been demonstrated in long-term follow-up.[39,40] The latter finding may be due to the development of bacterial resistance to rifampin or gradual loss of the rifampin coat over time.

Finally, meticulous surgical technique is vital in preventing wound and graft infections. The graft must be handled carefully, with minimal if any contact with the patient's skin, even after skin has been prepped prior to the start of surgery. With no strong evidence favoring iodophors versus chlorhexidine preparations, the decision regarding skin prep should be driven by patient factors, costs, and potential side effects.[41] Adhesive drapes, such as Ioban, are commonly used to aid in preventing contact between the prosthetic graft and the skin, although there is no clear evidence demonstrating a reduction in the incidence of wound or graft infection with the use of adhesive drapes with or without iodine impregnation. However, if the adhesive plastic drape is separated from the skin during the operation, the infection rate increases.[42,43] Simultaneous gastrointestinal procedures should be avoided to prevent intraoperative contamination; if an unplanned enterotomy occurs, graft implantation should be postponed if possible. Irrigation should also be used to remove all blood from the peritoneal cavity, because blood acts as medium for bacterial proliferation. If irrigation of a wound is performed, every effort should be made to evacuate the fluid. Wounds should be closed in layers, with efforts to minimize dead space using the least amount of suture material. Incisions should be covered with clean dressings, although there are new data suggesting some benefit with the use of negative-pressure wound dressings in high-risk patients or incision locations (e.g., groin),[44] However, these data remain inconclusive, with other studies failing to show a significant effect of specialized dressings.[45,46]

DIAGNOSIS

Graft infections can result in limb loss, systemic sepsis, and sometimes death, even in the setting of correct diagnosis and treatment. Therefore prompt diagnosis is essential to avoid or minimize complications. The consequences of a missed diagnosis in this setting can be catastrophic. Clinicians should maintain a high index of suspicion for graft involvement in any patient with a prosthetic graft presenting with local or systemic signs of infection, and every attempt should be made to confirm or exclude the diagnosis by either imaging or operative exploration.

Clinical Presentation

The clinical presentation of graft infection is influenced by the anatomic location of the graft and the time of presentation. Infection of an infrainguinal graft frequently appears as cellulitis, soft tissue infection, drainage tract, or pseudoaneurysm. Conversely, an intraabdominal graft infection may appear as systemic sepsis or as an ileus or abdominal distension with or without tenderness. Occasionally an aortic graft infection can result in an aortoenteric fistula, the first sign of which is a herald gastrointestinal bleed. A patient with upper gastrointestinal bleeding and an aortic graft must be presumed to have an aortoenteric fistula until proved otherwise (Fig. 59.2).

Early graft infections, usually caused by virulent organisms such as *S. aureus*, can manifest with pain, erythema, induration, or purulent drainage from the graft site. Patients may have signs of systemic sepsis (tachycardia, tachypnea, hypotension, and fever) or infective endocarditis (splinter hemorrhages, septic emboli, etc.) with positive blood cultures. A late graft infection, usually caused by indolent organisms such as *S. epidermidis*, often appears as a healing complication such as a seroma or pseudoaneurysm or as late graft thrombosis with no anatomic reason. Systemic signs of illness, such as fever, are often not present.

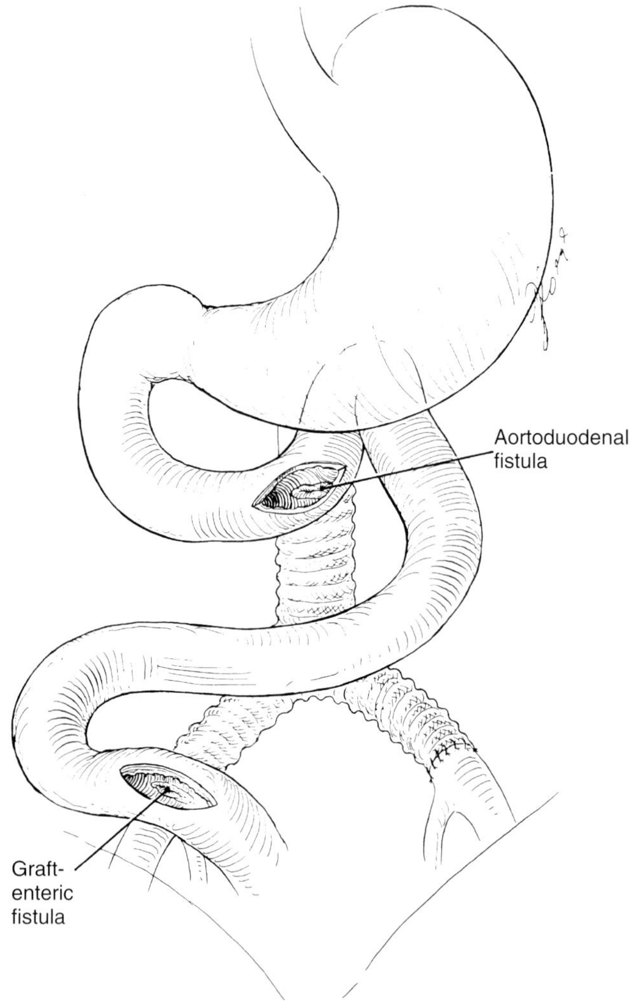

FIG 59.2 A communication may develop between the bowel lumen and the graft. Hemorrhage may be due to a direct communication between the aorta and the bowel (aortoenteric fistula) or from vessels in the bowel wall that have been eroded by the prosthetic graft (enteroparaprosthetic fistula).

Laboratory Studies

A leukocytosis with a left shift and an elevated erythrocyte sedimentation rate (ESR) often accompany prosthetic graft infections, particularly early infections, but their lack of specificity limits their diagnostic utility. Late-appearing infections with *S. epidermidis* may present with no laboratory abnormalities or mild leukocytosis and an elevated ESR without a significant left shift. Blood cultures may be positive with more virulent infections but they may also often be negative, particularly with indolent infections.

Imaging

Imaging plays an important role in the diagnosis of prosthetic graft infection. The particular imaging modality used depends on the site being investigated and the information desired. Computed tomography (CT), angiography, ultrasonography, nuclear medicine, and magnetic resonance imaging (MRI) constitute the diagnostic armamentarium for the evaluation of potential graft infection.

Ultrasonography

A duplex ultrasound scan is an excellent initial test for the identification of graft infections in the upper and lower extremities. Perigraft fluid and anastomotic pseudoaneurysms can be diagnosed by ultrasound, and these aberrancies can be distinguished from more benign findings such as hematomas or seromas. Ultrasonography can also be useful in determining the patency of a prosthetic bypass, since an infection can often result in thrombosis. Ultrasonography is quick, portable, and noninvasive. The accuracy of the test depends on the technician's expertise, but in skilled hands it is informative and reliable. The role of duplex ultrasound in the diagnosis of cavitary graft infections is more limited due to the difficulty of penetrating through bowel gas (in the case of intraabdominal grafts) and or bone/lung (in the case of intrathoracic grafts) (Fig. 59.3C).

Computed Tomography

A CT scan with contrast is a sensitive test for the diagnosis of graft infections and can be reliably obtained within a reasonable time at most hospitals. Perigraft fluid collections, perigraft gas, anastomotic aneurysms, adjacent bone osteomyelitis, and distortion of normal tissue planes are all findings suggestive of graft infection and are all well visualized by a contrast-enhanced CT scan (see Fig. 59.3A and B). Although perigraft gas and fluid can be normal findings immediately after surgery, the presence of these findings more than 6 to 8 weeks after implantation is abnormal and concerning for graft infection. In one study examining the natural history of periprosthetic air after abdominal aortic surgery, 26 consecutive patients undergoing elective aortic aneurysm repair had CT scans performed at 3, 7, and 52 days postoperatively. Perigraft air was seen in 65% of patients in the

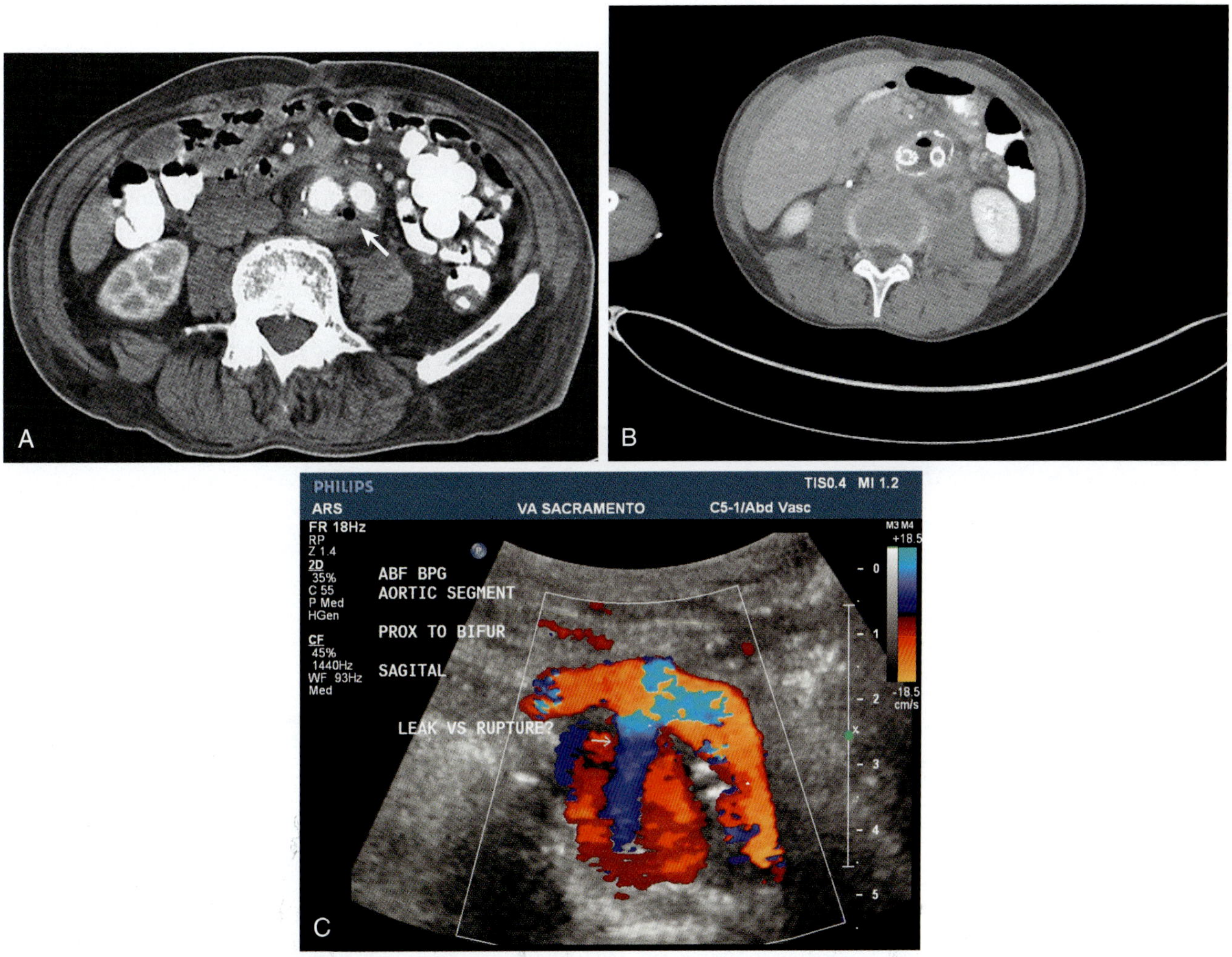

FIG 59.3 (A) Postoperative computed tomographic scan of a patient who underwent abdominal aortic aneurysm repair showing air within the aneurysm sac *(arrow)*, consistent with graft infection. (B) Postoperative computed tomographic scan of a patient who underwent surgery for an abdominal aortic aneurysm with a stent-graft repair showing air within the aneurysm sac, consistent with graft infection. (C) Duplex scan of a cryopreserved aorta with a pseudoaneurysm. ([A] From Abularrage CJ, Deaton DH: Vascular surgery. In Ho VB, Reddy GP, editors: *Cardiovascular imaging*, Philadelphia, 2011, Elsevier.)

first week following operation. All patients with periprosthetic air had spontaneous resolution by a mean of 52 days postoperatively (range, 21 to 85 days).[47]

CT-guided aspiration of perigraft fluid is a means of verifying graft infection in cases where the diagnosis is less certain; it can provide material for Gram stain and culture and direct medical therapy. However, aspiration can also result in contamination of a previously sterile field and thus be the inciting event resulting in a graft infection. Furthermore, ambiguous cases are rare, and suspicious CT findings in a patient more than 6 to 8 weeks postprocedure in the appropriate clinical setting should prompt timely graft excision and reconstruction with the rare exception of a patient too frail to undergo a major operation.

Magnetic Resonance Imaging

MRI is a useful modality for identifying perigraft fluid because of its ability to distinguish fluid from tissue, using differences in signal intensity between T1- and T2-weighted images. The efficacy of MRI was highlighted in one study in which patients suspected of having an aortic graft infections underwent preoperative MRI. MRI was positive in 14 of 16 patients studied, who were ultimately found intraoperatively to have an aortic graft infection. Comparatively, CT was positive in only 5 of 12 patients.[48] Indeed, MRI may be particularly useful during the early postoperative period, where the role of CT imaging is limited, as grafts undergoing incorporation only show mild enhancement on T2-weighted images, whereas infected perigraft tissue demonstrates significantly increased signal intensity.[49] However, due multiple factors—including limited availability, high operative costs, and the time-consuming nature of the test—MRI is not routinely used for the diagnosis of prosthetic graft infections.

Angiography

Angiography is useful in delineating extraluminal from intraluminal blood flow and thus can help in identifying the location of graft pseudoaneurysms (Fig. 59.4). However, the presence of a pseudoaneurysm is neither sensitive for nor specific to a graft infection. Furthermore, angiography is unable to assess for extraluminal gas or fluid collections. Therefore the role of angiography in the diagnosis of prosthetic graft infections is limited.

White Blood Cell Scanning

^{111}In-labeled WBC scanning has high positive and negative predictive values for graft infection.[50] Compared with ^{67}Ga-labeled scans, ^{111}In-labeled leukocyte scanning is more reliable, with less nonspecific bowel uptake, resulting in a high target-to-background ratio and better results.[51] In one study, 10 of 10 patients with positive scans were confirmed to have graft infections at the time of surgery. Conversely, of the 15 patients in this study with negative scans, only 1 proved to be a false-negative (patient with a quiescent aortoduodenal fistula) (see Fig. 59.4B).[52]

Gastrointestinal Endoscopy

Endoscopy is a vital diagnostic tool in the evaluation of upper gastrointestinal tract bleeding.[53] A patient with an aortic prosthesis and upper gastrointestinal bleeding should be suspected of having an aortoenteric fistula or erosion until proved otherwise. The initial test for this diagnosis is upper gastrointestinal endoscopy, which should be performed expeditiously once the diagnosis of aortoenteric fistula has been considered. The endoscopic examination should be done thoroughly, with adequate visualization of the third and fourth portions of the duodenum,

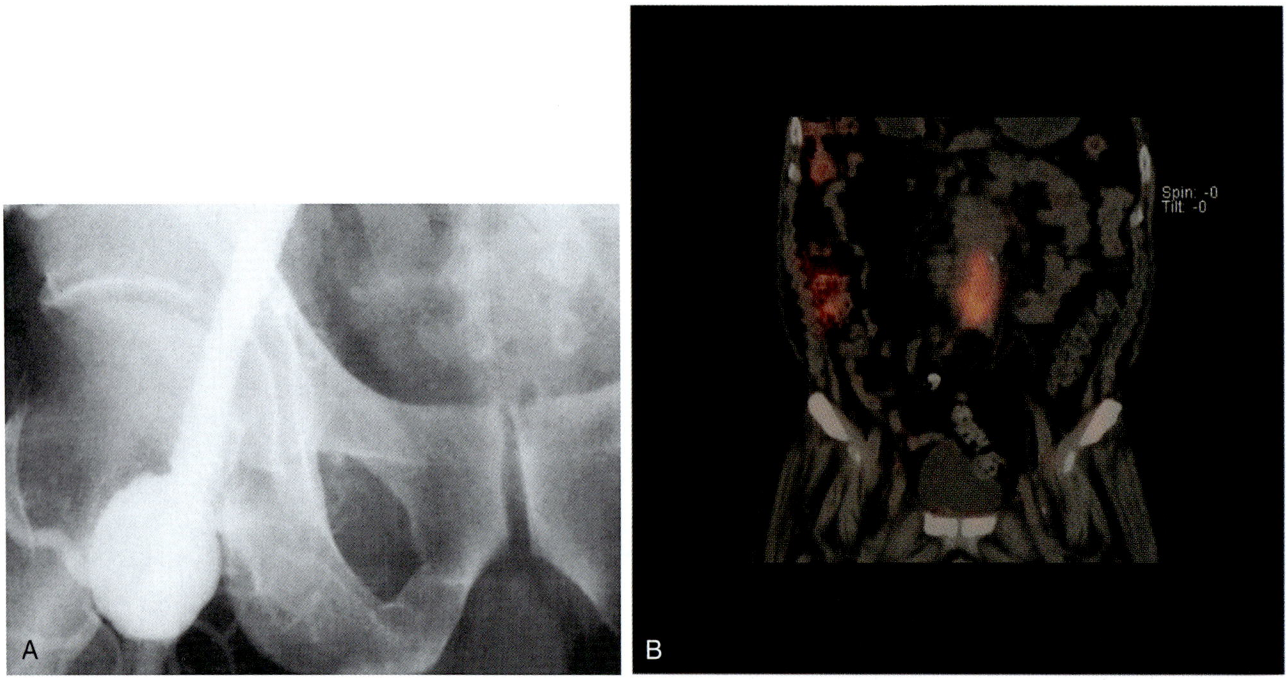

FIG 59.4 (A) Graft infection was first manifested by the development of a false aneurysm. (B) ^{111}In-labeled white blood cell scan with activity noted around the aortic graft, consistent with graft infection.

and carefully, as the endoscope can inadvertently dislodge any clot that has formed over ulcer or erosion and caused bleeding. The finding of an ulcer or an erosion with adherent blood clot in the duodenum can be pathognomonic for an AEF/AEE. If endoscopy does not reveal any pathology—such as bleeding varices, gastritis, or a stomach or duodenal ulcer—an aortoenteric fistula may still be present though not seen.

MANAGEMENT OF GRAFT INFECTION: GENERAL PRINCIPLES

Preoperative Preparation

Any unstable patient, such as a patient in hemorrhagic shock from an anastomotic rupture or a one with massive gastrointestinal hemorrhage from an aortoenteric fistula, should be managed according to the standard principles of resuscitation. In these categories of patients, there may not be much time for preoperative planning, diagnosis, or adjuvant therapy.

In a stable patient where there is adequate time for investigation and planning, the appropriate diagnostic tests should be ordered and the patient's medical condition optimized in advance of a potentially extensive operation. Imaging studies—including CT, MRI, tagged WBC scans, angiography, and duplex ultrasound—should be ordered to confirm the diagnosis, determine the extent of involvement, and evaluate possible options for autogenous extraanatomic or in situ reconstruction. The patient's cardiac and pulmonary status, including fluid resuscitation, should be evaluated and optimized. Parenteral nutrition should be initiated in severely malnourished patients.[54] Broad-spectrum empiric antibiotic coverage should be initiated to contain the graft infection and prevent progression to sepsis. Good glycemic control is required, as hyperglycemia can cause suppression of neutrophil function, thus worsening infection. Finally, a detailed discussion with the patient and family must be held to ensure their understanding that treatment may involve a very demanding operation, both physiologically and psychologically.

Antibiotic Therapy

Preoperative administration of culture-specific antibiotics is ideal. If the infecting organism is not known, broad-spectrum antibiotics, in doses adequate to reach minimal inhibitory concentrations should be administered. Subsequent therapy with antibiotics should be tailored to culture results once available. After source control with surgical resection, the appropriate duration of antibiotic therapy is debated, with most using at least 2 weeks of systemic antibiotic therapy, as patients treated with at least 6 weeks of parenteral antibiotics had significantly better outcomes than those treated for 2 weeks or less.[55] Interestingly, some case series have shown positive outcomes with long-term use of antibiotics for suppressive therapy in patients for whom surgery was not an option and the infected graft or device had to be left in situ.[56,57]

More recently, antibiotic-loaded beads have been used in conjunction with serial irrigation and debridement in an effort to sterilize groin wounds and preserve infected lower extremity grafts.[58] The beads are left in place or changed during debridement until the intraoperative wound cultures have no bacterial growth, at which time soft tissue or muscle flap coverage is obtained. In vitro and animal studies have shown a benefit to the inhibition of bacterial activity and reduction of biofilm production with use of antibiotic-impregnated beads.[59,60] In one promising study, after an average of 2.5 antibiotic bead replacements, sterile wounds were achieved in 90% of patients with a 2-year recurrent graft infection and mortality rate of 11%.[61] A more recent study demonstrated similar wound sterilization (87%) with less bead replacements (average 1.4), but recurrent infection occurred in 19% of patients, with the vast majority recurring early in the postoperative course, and 19% of patients experiencing limb loss.[62]

Revascularization

Removal of an infected graft usually mandates a revascularization procedure. For infected prosthetic grafts used in arteriovenous access, excision may be performed without immediate placement of a new access. Moreover, in thrombosed grafts or in bypass grafts placed for claudication, excision without revascularization may be considered. However, without the reestablishment of blood flow, removal of a patent but infected graft placed for critical limb ischemia may result in recurrent ischemia and subsequent tissue loss. Removal of an infected aortic graft without revascularization is associated with a 33% to 36% risk of limb loss.[63] As a result, use of this technique has become increasingly rare.[64]

Studies have shown that, for aortic graft infections, staged operations, with initial revascularization followed by graft excision in 1 to 2 days, are associated with significantly less morbidity and mortality. In one study, the perioperative mortality rate for an aortic graft infection was 71% if graft excision preceded extraanatomic bypass and 26% if bypass preceded graft excision.[65] Many reasons for this have been theorized, including decreased physiologic stress as demonstrated by decreased metabolic derangements in the patient undergoing a staged approach.[55] Another reason may be that performing the revascularization before the graft excision obviates the need for systemic heparinization and minimizes extremity ischemic time, enabling a more thorough and radical debridement. For extracavitary graft infections, revascularization is recommended to avoid extremity ischemia, which can result in major amputation.[66]

The ideal conduit for revascularization is autogenous vein, endarterectomized artery, or cryopreserved allograft, as they all trigger a reduced host inflammatory response, have lower rates of reinfection, and obviate the need for extraanatomic bypass. If a prosthetic conduit is chosen for an extraanatomic bypass, polytetrafluoroethylene (PTFE) is preferable to Dacron. In vitro studies have found that PTFE is more resistant to bacterial colonization than are other prosthetic conduits.[67] This has been validated clinically in a retrospective analysis that revealed a lower infection rate for PTFE compared with Dacron.[68] Indeed, some studies have suggested that, in selected patients, grafts infected with low-virulence *S. epidermidis* can be safely treated with an in situ PTFE prosthetic graft.[69,70]

Graft Excision

Open excision remains the gold standard for treatment of an infected prosthetic graft. Suture line involvement in the infectious process is an absolute indication for removal of the entire infected graft, since equivocation on the decision for an infected anastomosis can risk eventual rupture and hemorrhage. However, many authorities have begun to advocate conservative treatment in selected cases, such as infections with less virulent organisms, the involvement of inguinal or infrainguinal grafts, or in those cases where patients may not tolerate a complete excision.[69,71,72] The process of graft preservation consists of drainage, debridement, and systemic and local antibiotic coverage for the management of perigraft infection. Calligaro and colleagues have shown that partial or complete graft preservation has been successful in the treatment of extracavitary graft infections, with a hospital mortality rate of only 8.5% and a limb preservation rate of 87%.[73] Similarly, they have shown efficacy of conservative management in intraabdominal graft infections, with seven of nine patients surviving hospitalization and no recurrent infection at long-term follow-up at a mean of 7.6 years.[74] Patients must be carefully selected for graft preservation; the graft anastomosis cannot be involved with infection, and the patient should not demonstrate any uncontrolled arterial bleeding or systemic signs of sepsis, which would warrant immediate graft excision.

Should graft preservation be attempted, one must also consider using tissue coverage after debridement. Tissue coverage of the debrided area can be achieved with a rotational flap or a free flap.[75] Among patients treated with muscle flap coverage of their infected graft site, poor prognostic indicators of graft preservation have included exposure of the arterial anastomosis, infection occurring more than 1 month postoperatively, methicillin-resistant bacteria, and *Pseudomonas* species infection.

More recently, vacuum-assisted closure (VAC) therapy has been advocated in the treatment of groin and lower extremity bypass infections. Some studies have shown success in achieving tissue coverage over exposed grafts without muscle flap coverage, with complete healing in up to 100% of patients treated and no short-term mortality or limb amputation.[76,77] However, other studies have shown high complication rates with this strategy, with a 29% mortality rate and 33% amputation rate among patient with synthetic grafts treated with debridement and wound VAC therapy alone.[78]

Aortoenteric fistulas, particularly aortoduodenal fistulas, have traditionally required complete excision of the graft, closure of the intestinal wall defect, and placement of an extraanatomic bypass (Fig. 59.5A and B). The sequence of these procedures can be important. In an actively bleeding patient or one in whom the diagnosis has been made at celiotomy, graft excision should precede extraanatomic bypass. It is often difficult to determine whether a patient needs a remote bypass in such a setting; therefore the safest approach is to perform immediate revascularization in the majority of cases. Some studies have also looked at in situ replacement of the infected graft rather than extraanatomic bypass, with good outcomes. One study showed a 90% survival for the operation with no cases of limb loss and 83% of surviving patients experiencing no issues after a mean of 5.2 years' follow-up.[79]

Some have suggested a role for endovascular repair, with case studies reporting good short-term outcomes with endovascular stent placement in the treatment of an AEF/AEE, whereas others have noted increased complications, primarily due to reinfection.[80,81] In one case series, seven patients who were deemed too high risk for excision underwent conservative management with endovascular intervention. One of seven died of fungal septicemia, and one of seven required laparotomy for persistent sepsis. Three of seven patients died after their acute illness of unrelated causes. Three of seven patients were alive at long-term follow-up at a mean of 3 years without evidence of recurrent infection or bleed. These data suggest that endovascular treatment may be

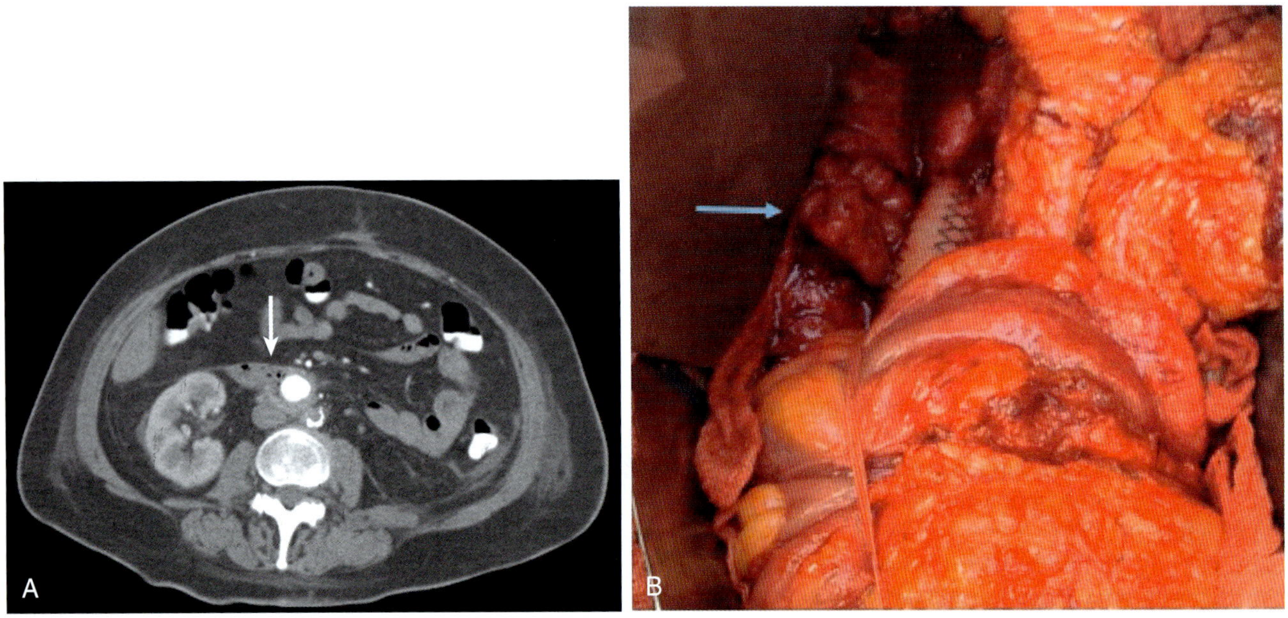

FIG 59.5 (A) Aortoenteric fistula *(arrow)* resulting from erosion of the proximal anastomosis into the duodenum. (B) Duodenum separated from the graft *(blue arrow)* resulting from erosion of the proximal graft anastomosis into the duodenum.

an alternative in high-risk patients.[82] However, a recent large systematic literature review revealed a 44% rate of recurrent hemorrhage or infection among 41 patient studied, with the preoperative diagnosis of sepsis as a strong predictor of poor outcome. These findings prompted the authors to conclude that, among patients with evidence of severe infection, endovascular repair should be considered only as a bridge to more definitive excision.[83]

Debridement

Blowout and late hemorrhage from the proximal aortic stump may occur in some patients after successful excision of the graft. This is most likely due to residual infection in the bed of the graft in the perigraft and para-aortic tissues. The perigraft debridement must therefore be generous enough to ensure eradication of all infected tissue. The aorta must then be oversewn in two layers, if possible, using polypropylene sutures.

TREATMENT OF SPECIFIC GRAFT SITE INFECTIONS

Aortic Grafts

When one is faced with an aortic graft infection, some fundamental points must be addressed. First, one has to determine whether the aortic graft was performed for aneurysmal or occlusive disease. If the graft was placed for aneurysmal disease, it will be an end-to-end anastomosis; if the graft was placed for occlusive disease, the configuration of the anastomosis may be end to end or end to side. The distal implantation site has to be addressed as well; if the graft extends down to the femoral vessels, revascularization will be a bit more involved than if the distal anastomosis is to the iliac arteries.

Aortoiliac and Aortic Interposition Grafts

Aortoiliac graft infections have traditionally been treated by preliminary axillobifemoral bypass through uninfected tissue planes followed by aortic graft excision (Fig. 59.6). The inflow anastomosis is created at the proximal axillary artery. The distal anastomoses can be constructed at both common femoral arteries because the distal limbs of the infected aortic graft are confined to the abdomen. This operation can be followed immediately by graft excision or, alternatively, graft excision can be performed 1 to 2 days later. This staged approach is associated with significantly less morbidity than the traditional simultaneous procedure (see section Revascularization).

For aortic graft excision, celiotomy is performed, and the aortic graft is isolated through the retroperitoneum. Although systemic heparin is indicated for the axillofemoral bypass, the advantage of the staged operation is that no anticoagulation is necessary during the aortic graft excision. If the procedures are done consecutively, the heparin should be reversed before the aortic graft is approached. Careful dissection in the abdomen is performed, and the graft is separated from adherent bowel and viscera. Once the entire graft has been exposed, proximal control is obtained at the supraceliac aorta. The iliac arteries distal to the anastomoses are similarly isolated and control is obtained. The entire graft is then excised, and the aorta is debrided back

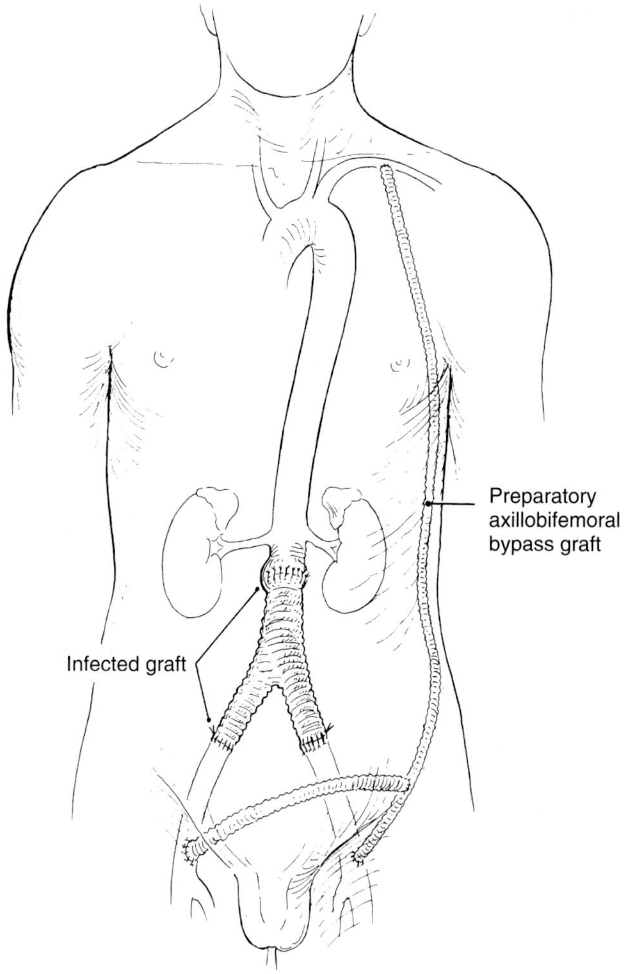

FIG 59.6 Before removing an infected intraabdominal prosthetic graft, perfusion of the lower extremities is established by an axillobifemoral bypass graft. This technique provides uninterrupted perfusion of the lower limbs and reduces the morbidity associated with ischemic changes occurring when reconstitution of flow is delayed until after the aortic graft has been removed.

to normal, healthy-appearing tissue. The aortic stump is then closed with locking monofilament polypropylene sutures. The iliac arteries are similarly closed. Perigraft tissue that may be infected is carefully but completely debrided. Closed suction drains may be placed. Care is taken to avoid injury to the ureters, and placement of ureteral stents prior to the procedure is often helpful. If debridement is necessary above the renal arteries, it should be performed without compromise and the renal arteries then revascularized by antegrade bypasses from branches of the celiac axis. Perfusion of the pelvic circulation is maintained by retrograde flow from the axillofemoral bypass through the external and internal iliac arteries. If the distal anastomoses are to the external iliac arteries and require excision, perfusion to at least one internal iliac artery should be maintained by means of a bypass.

Axillobifemoral bypass has long been considered an imperfect solution to aortic graft infection.[84,85] It is associated with high perioperative mortality rates, with a 30-day mortality as high as

27%, although this has dropped to 11% in more recently published data. Long-term survival is poor, with only 56% to 78% survival at long-term follow-up reported in recent studies.[86-88] Of particular concern is the risk of blowout of the remaining aortic stump, which is often a fatal event. Reported incidence rates have been noted to be as high as 30% for aortic stump blowout after excision and extraanatomic bypass, although more recent data suggest that these events have become rarer, with rates closer to 3%.[87,89] Moreover, primary patency of the axillofemoral graft is low, with a 5-year patency of 40% to 73%,[90,91] although these rates may see improvement with increasing use of ringed grafts (9% occlusion vs. 22%).[68] Recent publications have called into question whether axillobifemoral bypass grafting should remain the gold standard for the treatment of infected aortic grafts. One systematic review of 37 clinical studies showed a high mean rate of conduit failure and early and late mortality in extraanatomic bypass as compared with other treatment modalities, including in situ replacement with rifampin-bonded PTFE, cryopreserved allograft, and autogenous vein. Reinfection rates were higher for extraanatomic bypass as compared with cryopreserved and autogenous in situ conduits, and amputation rates were higher for extraanatomic bypass as compared with rifampin-bonded PTFE and cryopreserved in situ conduits. When all negative outcomes were combined, *any* one of the in situ reconstructions was favored over extraanatomic bypass.[92]

One alternative to prosthetic revascularization has been autogenous reconstruction with femoral vein as the conduit, the neoaortoiliac system (NAIS).[93,94] The femoral vein is a large-caliber vein that can be used to reconstruct the aortoiliac or aortofemoral system in a variety of configurations. The advantage of this approach is that the reconstruction is completely autogenous, thereby avoiding the need for extraanatomic bypass. Thirty-day mortality rates are reported to be low at less than 10%, and 5-year mortality rates are noted to be similar to extraanatomic bypass at 30% to 50%. Patency rates are high, with less than 4% early thrombosis and 62% to 91% primary patency at 5 years.[94,95] The disadvantage of this approach lies in the long operative time and concern for venous morbidity, particularly the risk of compartment syndrome. In one study, 12% of patients who underwent placement of the NAIS required fasciotomy and 15% developed chronic venous insufficiency (CVI).[94] However, in other studies, rates for fasciotomy were as low as 0% to 4%, with similar rates of CVI at 11% to 15%.[95,96]

Another alternative approach for in situ reconstruction is the use of cryopreserved arterial homograft. Animal studies have suggested reduced rates of reinfection with cryopreserved allografts.[97] Clinical studies have verified this, with reinfection rates of 0% to 5%.[98,99] Studies have reported 30-day mortality rates of 13% to 28% and reintervention rates of 5% to 6% within 1 year.[98-101] However, superior outcomes have been noted at more experienced centers. In one study of 57 in situ revascularizations of the abdominal aorta using cryopreserved arterial homograft, 30-day mortality was found to be 9%, with the majority of deaths caused by sepsis-related multiorgan system failure.[102] The 3-year freedom from revascularization and postoperative survival rates were 89% and 81%, respectively. The authors concluded that cryopreserved arterial homografts decreased the risk of recurrent infection, early thrombosis, late graft failure, and amputation compared with extraanatomic bypass using prosthetic conduits. One disadvantage of cryopreserved arterial homografts is that they are prone to long-term degeneration because of an immune response or imperfections in the cryopreservation method.[103,104] Thus continued surveillance for anastomotic breakdown is necessary. Postoperative immunosuppression following implantation of cryopreserved arterial homograft may theoretically decrease the risk of degeneration; however, the risks of immunosuppression in the setting of infection must be weighed in this clinical scenario.

Next, placement of in situ rifampin-soaked prosthetic grafts with omental coverage and antibiotic suppression has been advocated for the treatment of aortic graft infection. Studies have revealed a 30-day mortality of 7% to 21% and a 1-year survival of 64% to 100% associated with this technique.[105-107] One recent study reported a 9% 30-day mortality and a 1- and 5-year survival of 85% and 59%, respectively, when patients with aortoenteric fistulas were treated with in situ rifampin-soaked graft replacement. Moreover, despite concern for a high risk of reinfection, graft reinfection occurred in only 4% of patients.[108]

A prospective randomized trial in the United Kingdom attempted to define the role of the rifampin-bonded prosthesis in extraanatomic bypass grafts by studying whether they resulted in a decreased risk of graft infection compared with controls. A total of 257 patients were randomized at 14 vascular centers to either rifampin-bonded grafts or regular collagen-impregnated grafts. There was no significant difference in the incidence of graft infection on early follow-up (1 month).[109] The 2-year follow-up of these patients revealed an infection rate of 4.5%, with six infections in the rifampin-bonded group, four infections in the nonbonded group, and no significant difference in the rate of graft infection or mortality between the two groups. The authors concluded that, despite studies on almost 3000 patients, there was no convincing evidence that rifampin bonding decreases the incidence of prosthetic extraanatomic graft infection.[110] This finding is in contradistinction to the treatment of aortic graft infections with in-line rifampin-soaked grafts.

Also of some concern with use of rifampin-bonded grafts is the efficacy of this method in the face of rising antibiotic resistance. Although rifampin enjoys broad activity against many organisms, including *Streptococcus* and *Staphylococcus* species, animal and clinical studies have suggested possible limitations in the use of rifampin-bonded grafts against methicillin-resistant *S. aureus* (MRSA).[105,111] Moreover, reinfections among patients treated with rifampin-bonded grafts have been noted to occur with organisms resistant to rifampin.[107]

Finally, silver-coated prosthetic conduits represent another option for the treatment of infected aortic grafts. The silver is thought to inhibit bacterial colony formation on the prosthetic graft. One recent study compared silver-coated grafts with arterial homografts with and without immunosuppression. Postoperative morbidity and mortality were 7% and 11% in the silver-coated group, 16% and 8% in the arterial homograft with immunosuppression group, and 35% and 23% in the arterial homograft without immunosuppression group. There was a statistically significant difference in morbidity between the silver-coated and arterial homograft without immunosuppression groups; however, there were no statistically significant differences between the three groups in terms of mortality.[112] Another study comparing silver-coated Dacron grafts with cryopreserved arterial homografts without immunosuppression showed similar perioperative mortalities of 18% and 14%, respectively, and similar 2-year survival rates of 73% and 82%, respectively, although 2 of 11 patients treated with the silver-coated grafts experienced reinfection.[113] The authors concluded that silver-coated grafts could be considered as an alternative to cryopreserved arterial homograft, given their comparable outcomes, lower cost, and greater availability.

One recent systematic review questioned whether extraanatomic bypass and subsequent graft excision should remain the standard treatment of aortic graft infection. The study compiled 37 clinical studies and compared amputation, conduit failure, reinfection, and early and late mortality between extraanatomic bypass and in-line rifampin-bonded prosthetic, cryopreserved allografts, and autogenous venous reconstruction. Autogenous venous reconstructions were associated with the lowest infection rates, followed by cryopreserved allografts. Rifampin-bonded prosthetic grafts were associated with the fewest amputations, conduit failures, and early mortalities. However, late mortality was lowest in the autogenous vein and cryopreserved allograft groups. When examining combined outcomes, extraanatomic bypass was associated with statistically inferior outcomes compared to each of the other groups. The authors concluded that selection of the appropriate revascularization technique depends on the patient; whereas autogenous venous reconstruction may be better for younger, healthier patients who might enjoy the longer patency rates, whereas extraanatomic bypass may be better for older, sicker patients in whom step-wise intervention may result in less stress and for whom long-term patency may not be as important. Selection will also depend on the extent of the infection, with infections with more resistant organisms being less amenable to revascularization with grafts such as rifampin or silver-bonded Dacron.[92]

Aortobifemoral Grafts

Although the treatment principles for aortofemoral graft infections are fundamentally the same as those stated previously, the issue of revascularization is more troublesome. The distal femoral anastomoses of an aortobifemoral graft may preclude the attachment of distal limbs of an extraanatomic bypass to the common femoral artery. Therefore, if a prosthetic bypass via an extraanatomic route is to be used, the distal anastomosis of the extraanatomic bypass must be at the profunda femoris artery, the superficial femoral artery, or the popliteal artery. If the graft was performed for occlusive disease in an end-to-side fashion, it may be possible to excise the graft and repair the aortotomy primarily, relying on flow through the native vessels to the lower extremities. Although the native vessels in these cases are undoubtedly diseased, there may be adequate flow to avoid the need for immediate revascularization. In this situation, the neoaortoiliac system, with the femoral vein as the conduit and its associated decreased risk of reinfection, represents an attractive option for reconstruction in an infected field.

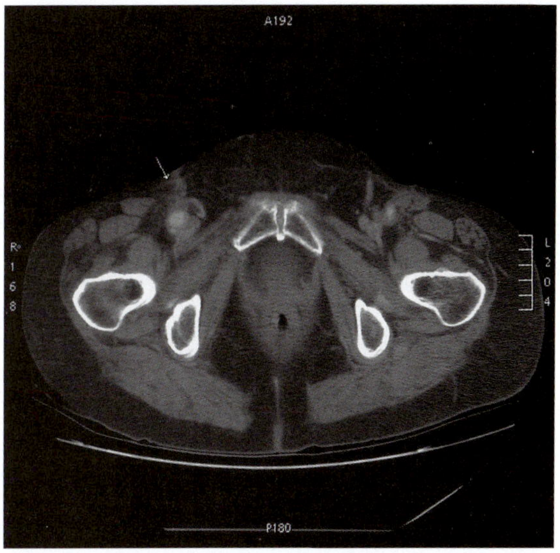

FIG 59.7 Computed tomography (CT) scan of a patient with an aortobifemoral bypass graft and chronic occlusion of the right limb of the bypass. The patient had one episode of pulsatile right groin bleeding. CT scan showed perigraft stranding in the right groin and edema tracking to the skin, suggestive of graft infection *(arrow)*.

If the graft infection is localized to the groin and the proximal and distal anastomoses are not involved, graft preservation can also be attempted (Fig. 59.7; see section Graft Excision). This is done by drainage of the abscess, aggressive debridement of the infected perigraft tissues, possibly with multiple repeated operations, and adequate coverage of the graft with healthy tissue. The use of muscle flaps in the treatment algorithm of infected graft preservation not only provides coverage in the presence of a large soft tissue defect but can also provide better-vascularized tissue to transport antibiotic therapy. Although the majority of muscle flaps—including rectus femoris, rectus abdominis, and gracilis rotational flaps—are usually performed by plastic surgeons, the sartorius muscle flap is a common flap that can be performed by vascular surgeons. This flap is based on segmental vessels that feed the muscle from the medial side. The muscle is divided from its attachment to the iliac spine, mobilized laterally, and then rotated medially onto the graft.

Patients selected for graft preservation must meet all the previously mentioned criteria. Contraindications to graft preservation techniques include graft occlusion, arterial hemorrhage, and the presence of sepsis or infection with a virulent organism, particularly *Pseudomonas aeruginosa*.

If the femoral anastomosis is involved with the infection, that graft limb should be excised. The limb can be approached by means of an ipsilateral retroperitoneal exposure (Fig. 59.8). Proximal control can be obtained at that level and the graft limb can be excised. If the proximal (aortic) anastomosis is involved, the entire graft must be excised according to the principles elucidated earlier. Next, the groin is exposed and the graft-artery anastomosis is excised, the native artery is debrided, and the femoral arteriotomy is then closed with patch angioplasty, preferably with autologous tissue. If a portion of the common femoral

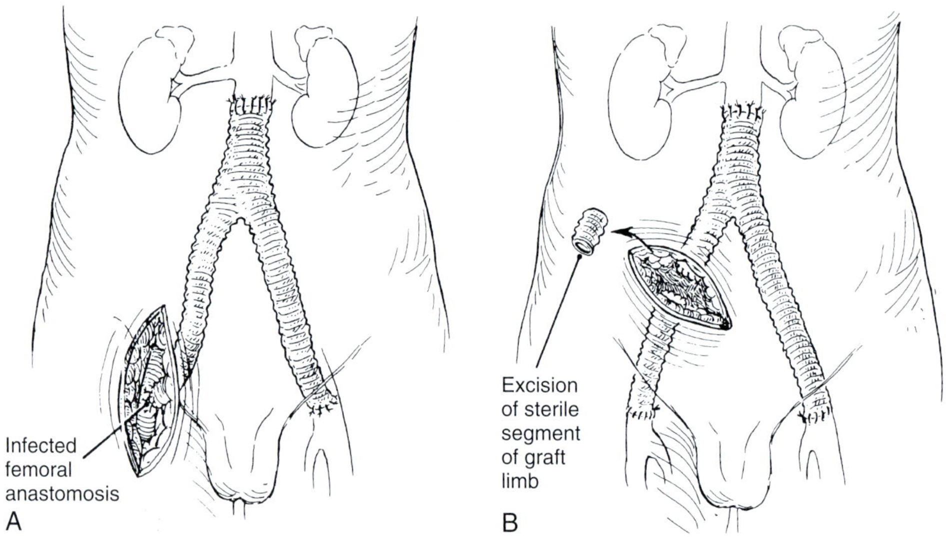

FIG 59.8 Through a retroperitoneal approach, the sterility of the proximal portion of the graft limb is determined. (A) The sterile graft above is isolated from the area of infection at the groin by excision of a segment of graft and obliteration of the communicating tissue planes between the two areas. (B) The distal portion of the graft limb is then removed from below after the clean procedure has been performed in the retroperitoneal space and the wound has been closed.

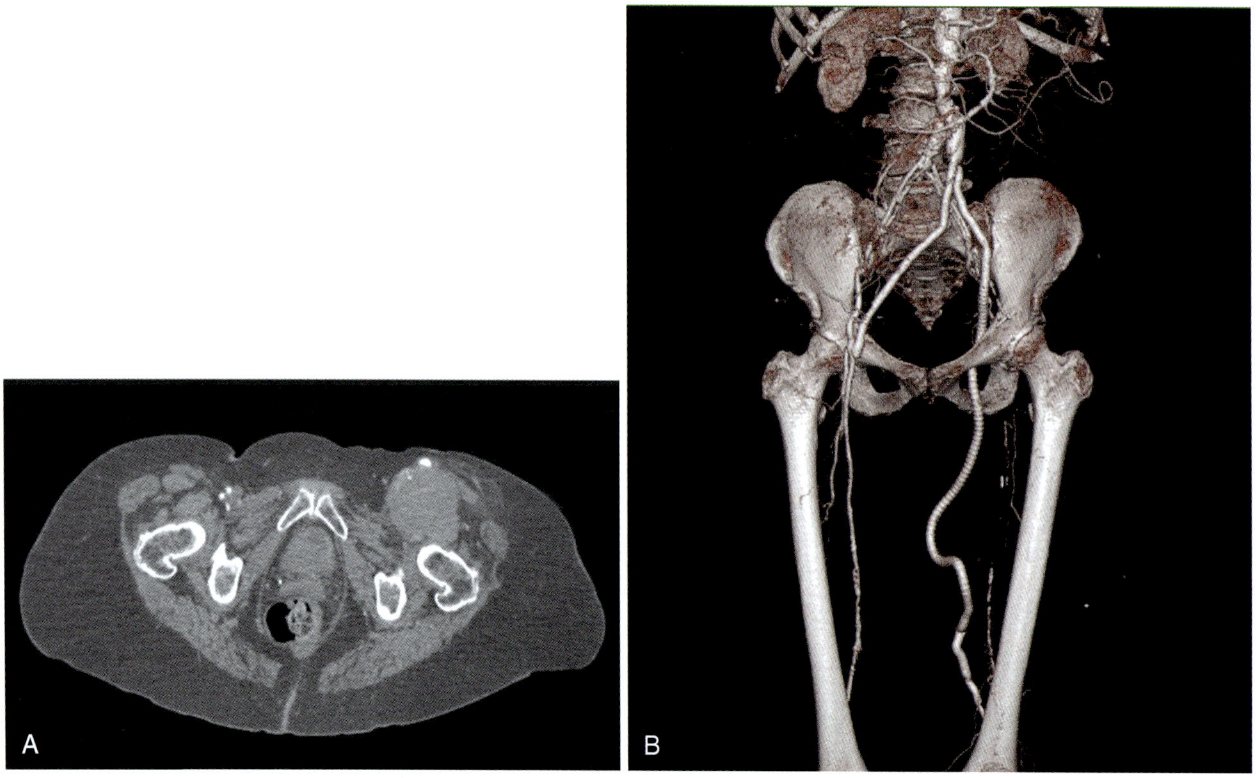

FIG 59.9 (A) Left femoral pseudoaneurysm *(arrow)* due to late graft infection and anastomotic rupture in a patient who previously had an aortobifemoral bypass and left femoropopliteal bypass for rest pain. At the time of surgery, the left limb of the aortobifemoral graft was approached from a retroperitoneal incision and found to be well incorporated. (B) Therefore an obturator bypass was performed from the left limb of the aortobifemoral bypass to the distal aspect of the previous femoropopliteal bypass with immediate excision of the infected segments.

artery at that level must be debrided or excised, an attempt should be made to perform an end-to-end anastomosis of the superficial femoral artery to the deep femoral artery to maintain retrograde perfusion of the pelvis. An extraanatomic bypass can then be fashioned, depending on the need for revascularization of the involved limb. The choice of the vessel for distal bypass depends on the condition of the native vasculature. If only the unilateral limb is excised, the limb can be revascularized by a bypass tunneled via a retropubic route or through the obturator canal or by a femorofemoral bypass tunneled via a medial route (Fig. 59.9). The bypass conduit has to be routed through clean, uninfected tissue (Fig. 59.10). If the entire graft must be excised,

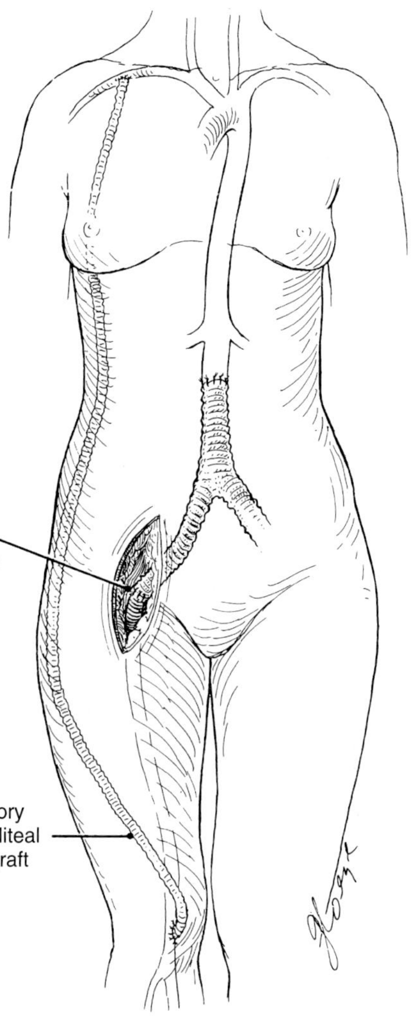

FIG 59.10 Perfusion of an ischemic extremity in the presence of sepsis in the ipsilateral groin is achieved with an axillopopliteal bypass graft. Care is taken to bring the graft wide of the groin through unaffected tissue planes.

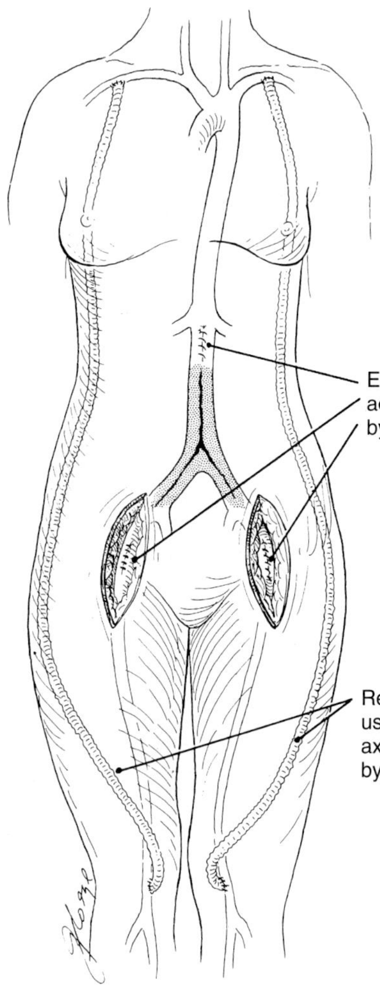

FIG 59.11 Ischemia of the lower extremities caused by a return to dependence on the native circulation after the removal of an infected aortic graft. This can be successfully managed by bilateral axillopopliteal bypass grafts.

as would be the case with proximal anastomosis involvement, an extraanatomic bypass originating from the axillary artery can be anastomosed to the deep femoral artery, the superficial femoral artery, or the popliteal artery (Fig. 59.11); alternatively, an in situ replacement (such autogenous vein or cryopreserved arterial allograft, as discussed earlier) can be considered.

Femoropopliteal Bypass Grafts

An infected femoropopliteal bypass graft should be excised in its entirety (Fig. 59.12), although partial or complete graft salvage can be attempted in selected cases (see section Graft Excision). The same principles as with aortic, aortobi-iliac, and aortobifemoral grafts apply, including radical debridement of infected tissue, debridement of the artery to healthy viable tissue, and closure of the artery with monofilament nonabsorbable suture. The viability of the limb determines the need for immediate versus delayed revascularization. Should immediate revascularization be needed, it is ideally performed with autogenous vein, and only if the anastomosis is not done in an infected area.

For anastomoses performed in infected fields, use of cryopreserved cadaver vein graft or cadaver arterial graft can be considered. The advantage of the cadaver artery or vein is its ease of handling, its resistance to infection, and appropriate size matching to the artery. Its principal disadvantages are the significant cost and the poor medium- and long-term patency rates. One study with 17 patients who received a cryopreserved artery bypass for revascularization in infected lower extremity bypass showed good short-term outcomes with no perioperative mortality or limb loss but poor primary patency (68% at 18 months) and risk of aneurysmal degeneration and rupture (2 of the 17 patients studied).[114] Another, larger study with 27 patients showed a 2.6% 30-day mortality and a 2.6% amputation rate, with 7% 1-year procedure-related mortality.[115] Cryopreserved vein in this setting has also been studied, but results were poor, with a 20% occlusion rate at a mean follow-up of 9.5 months.[116] This is in line with studies on cryopreserved vein for infrainguinal bypass, which showed primary patency rates of 83% at 1 month, 50% at 6 months, 30% at 12 months, and 18% at 24 months.[117] Revascularization should be performed with adherence to the same

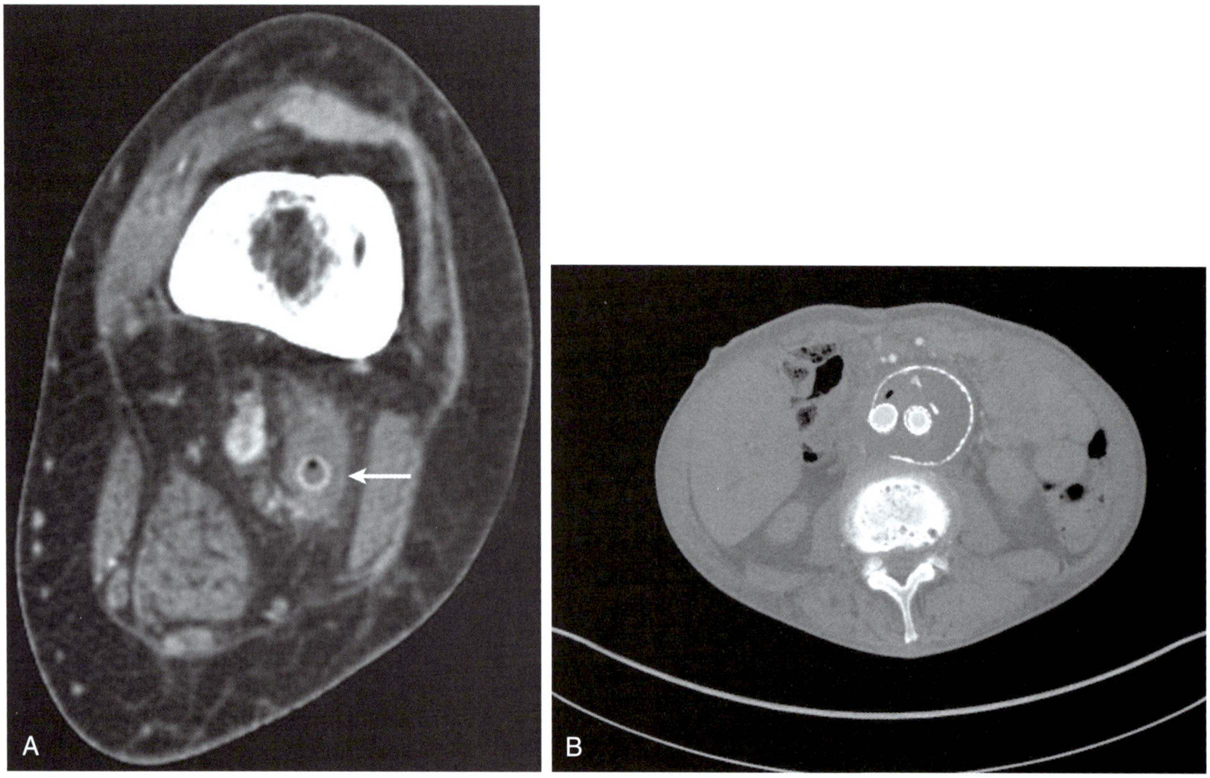

FIG 59.12 (A) Axial image from computed tomographic angiography shows a thrombosed lower extremity bypass with intraluminal air and surrounding fluid collection *(arrow)* consistent with graft infection. (B) Axial image from computed tomographic angiography shows air within a previously treated aortic aneurysm sac. (From Abularrage CJ, Deaton DH: Vascular surgery. In Ho VB, Reddy GP, editors: *Cardiovascular imaging,* Philadelphia, 2011, Elsevier.)

principles outlined earlier, with the route of the graft through clean, uninfected tissue.

Endovascular Stent-Grafts

The overall incidence of aortic endograft infection is thought to be less than 1%.[118] The diagnosis can also be uncertain, especially soon after graft insertion, as there is a well-described post-implantation inflammatory profile of fever and leukocytosis. One early study of 12 patients who underwent endovascular repair with Dacron-covered stent-grafts showed that the majority of patients developed a fever (body temperature >101.4°F [38.5°C]), leukocytosis, and CT evidence of perigraft air. All patients became afebrile with resolution of their leukocytosis, and none had any evidence of graft infection on follow-up.[119] Approximately one-third of patients present with acute sepsis, one-third with chronic or low-grade sepsis, and one-third with aortoenteric fistulas (see Fig. 59.12B).[120]

The cause of endograft infection is similar to that of open grafts. Graft infection can occur at the time of implantation, as a consequence of hematogenous seeding, or through direct contamination from adjacent infection. The last mechanism is especially important because approximately 11% of patients will require secondary interventions to maintain aneurysm occlusion.[121] As a result, not only are preoperative antibiotics indicated at the time of initial endograft implantation, but they are also indicated when performing percutaneous procedures for reintervention.

One of the largest studies to examine aortic endograft infections found 12 infections in 1431 procedures (incidence of <1%); 42% of patients presented within 3 months of their procedure, with no significant difference among patients who underwent endovascular aortic repair (EVAR) versus thoracic endovascular aortic repair (TEVAR). Endograft infections were more common after an emergency procedure (0.56% vs. 2.79%) and were more likely due to *Staphylococcus* or *Streptococcus* infections. Over the study period, 3 of the 12 patients died, corresponding to a mortality rate of 25%, with no significant difference in mortality between those treated with excision versus those treated with medical therapy alone. Although the study was limited by a small sample size, the authors concluded that the lack of significant difference in mortality might suggest a role for nonoperative management of infected endografts after EVAR or TEVAR.[122]

Operative mortality of infected endograft excision is substantial, with studies reporting a perioperative mortality of 19% to 28%, likely, at least in part, due endografts often being performed in patients at high risk for open repair,[123,124] though more recent studies have noted lower perioperative mortality rates of 11%.[125] Surgical treatment is similar to open graft infection, with excision and extraanatomic or in situ reconstruction. One review suggested a lower mortality with in situ reconstruction (5.8%) versus extraanatomic bypass (16%).[126] Antibiotic therapy without graft excision can be performed in high-risk patients who have a good initial response to parenteral antibiotics but is associated with a higher mortality rate (36.4% vs. 16% in one review).[126,127] A more recent review suggests there may be a lower perioperative mortality of 21% with non-operative management, though long-term mortality remains high at 45%. Mortality is the highest in those presenting with an aortoenteric fistula and lowest among those that received some intervention (such as drainage, surgical debridement, sac irrigation, and/or omentoplasty).[128]

CONCLUSIONS

The underwhelming success of traditional modes of managing graft infections has spurred experimentation with alternative methods, such as selective graft preservation, antibiotic- and silver-bonded grafts, and the use of autogenous vein or cryopreserved allograft for reconstruction in situ. Although evolution in the management of graft infection is ongoing and encouraging, the most fruitful endeavor may be an enhanced understanding of the pathophysiologic factors that predispose certain patients to develop graft infection. The interaction of a foreign body with the host and the subsequent response of the host determine the clinical outcome. With a better understanding of this interaction and the disparate responses of different hosts, more successful attempts at immunomodulation may reduce the incidence of graft infection and its considerable morbidity and mortality.

REVIEW QUESTIONS

1. Which of the following organisms is most likely to cause graft anastomotic disruption and hemorrhage?
   - **a.** *Staphylococcus epidermidis*
   - **b.** *Pseudomonas* species
   - **c.** *Candida* species
   - **d.** All of the above
2. Which of the following statements regarding perigraft air or fluid in the setting of a prosthetic graft is not true?
   - **a.** Perigraft air 3 months after placement of the graft should raise concern of a graft infection.
   - **b.** Ultrasonography or CT is an acceptable imaging technique for the diagnosis of perigraft fluid.
   - **c.** Graft infections manifesting as perigraft fluid can be appropriately treated by percutaneous drainage of the fluid and long-term antibiotics.
   - **d.** The great majority of patients have complete resolution of perigraft air by approximately 8 to 12 weeks following implantation.
3. Which of the following statements regarding *Staphylococcus epidermidis* graft infections is true?
   - **a.** *S. epidermidis* infections manifest most commonly with sepsis and hemorrhage.
   - **b.** Revascularization for *S. epidermidis* graft infections may be performed with in-line PTFE grafts.
   - **c.** Routine Gram stain and culture of the graft are usually adequate for establishing the diagnosis.
   - **d.** Extended (>24 hours) perioperative coverage with antibiotics is more effective at preventing graft infections compared with a single preoperative dose.
4. The options for reconstruction of an infected aortofemoral bypass graft include all of the following except:
   - **a.** Axillobifemoral bypass
   - **b.** Autogenous reconstruction with superficial femoral vein
   - **c.** Cryopreserved allograft
   - **d.** Collagen-impregnated Dacron graft
5. Which of the following statements regarding prosthetic graft infection is true?
   - **a.** Grafts involving the femoral artery have a higher rate of infection than grafts anastomosed to the iliac arteries.
   - **b.** An emergency operation (e.g., for a ruptured abdominal aortic aneurysm) carries an equivalent rate of infection as an elective operation.
   - **c.** The surgeon is the principal and most likely source of the organism infecting the prosthesis.
   - **d.** The mortality of an operation to treat prosthetic aortic graft infection approaches 75% to 80%.
6. Examples of extraanatomic bypass include all of the following except:
   - **a.** Obturator bypass
   - **b.** Axillopopliteal bypass
   - **c.** Femorofemoral bypass
   - **d.** Neoaortoiliac system involving the superficial femoral vein
7. Which of the following is not a clinical presentation of graft infection?
   - **a.** Pseudoaneurysm
   - **b.** Recurrent graft thrombosis
   - **c.** Hemorrhage
   - **d.** Malaise, fever, weight loss
   - **e.** Neointimal hyperplasia at the proximal anastomosis

References available online at ExpertConsult.com.

60 CHAPTER

Noninfectious Complications in Vascular Surgery

Glenn C. Hunter, Juan Carlos Jimenez

With an increasing number of endovascular interventions replacing open vascular reconstruction, the management of open surgical complications may become less familiar to surgeons currently finishing training. Complications after aortoiliac and peripheral arterial reconstruction often develop and progress rapidly to produce disastrous consequences, including major organ failure or loss of limb or life.

These complications may be the result of technical errors, the extent of the pathologic process, or one or more frequently associated diseases. A timeworn surgical principle applies, especially to vascular surgery: "A complication not anticipated is sure to be experienced." There are currently fewer and more complex open operative procedures being performed by surgeons who lack the suitable training to undertake these operations. Since the introduction of endovascular aneurysm repair (EVAR), the number of patients undergoing open aneurysm repair (OAR) requiring suprarenal clamp placement and adjunctive renal and/or visceral grafts has increased from 6% to 44% and 12% to 44% respectively. Patients undergoing OAR also have a higher incidence of renal vein division (4% to 11% vs. 18%), iliac artery aneurysms (25% vs. 42%), and occlusive disease (12% vs. 20%). Adjunctive renal and/or visceral grafts were required in only 1.9% of patients with infrarenal clamp placement. Although OAR with suprarenal clamp placement can be performed with relatively low mortality rates in major academic centers (0.8% to 6.1%), early recognition and treatment of complications is essential if mortality rates are to be maintained in this range in the future.[1-4] Additionally, with EVAR becoming the standard of care for aortic aneurysm management, vascular surgeons must become familiar with open conversion in the setting of endograft explant and possible suprarenal clamping.

The primary problems reviewed in this chapter are perioperative bleeding, thrombosis, acute renal injury and failure, spinal cord ischemia, operative embolization, iatrogenic ureteric injury and obstruction, bowel obstruction and intraabdominal compartment syndrome (ICS), chylous ascites, graft deterioration, anastomotic false aneurysms, incisional hernias, and postoperative lower extremity lymphoceles and edema.

AORTOILIAC SURGERY

Complications of aortoiliac arterial reconstruction are similar regardless of whether the procedure is for abdominal aortic aneurysmal or occlusive disease. A recent comparison of aortofemoral bypass to alternative inflow procedures in the veteran population demonstrated a trend toward higher mortality at 30 days postoperatively (2.7% vs. 0.53%. $P = 0.6$). Aortofemoral bypass also had higher rates of pneumonia, deep vein thrombosis, pulmonary embolus, postoperative transfusion, and urinary tract infection.[5]

Perioperative Bleeding

Operative Bleeding

Operative bleeding may occur during dissection of the major vessels from failure to secure hemostasis or from difficulties encountered while sewing in the graft. Venous tears are the most common cause of intraoperative bleeding and usually result from injury to unrecognized venous anomalies and during mobilization of the aorta and iliac arteries from the inferior vena cava (IVC) and iliac veins. The inferior mesenteric, left renal, adrenal, gonadal, and lumbar veins are all at risk of injury during dissection or retractor placement to expose the infrarenal aorta when undertaking aortic bypass procedures for occlusive or aneurysmal disease (Fig. 60.1).[6] A thorough understanding of the anatomy, and familiarity with the characteristics of major venous anomalies and careful operative dissection, are essential to avoid this complication.[7] Venous anomalies can involve the infrarenal, renal, or suprarenal segments of the IVC. Infrarenal segment anomalies include agenesis of the IVC, a left-sided IVC (0.2% to 0.5%), and duplicate IVCs (1% to 3%). Either of these anomalies may be associated with a right or, rarely, left retrocaval ureter. When present, the proximal ureter is dorsal to the IVC and, inferiorly, runs between the vena cava and the aorta. In rare instances, a double right vena cava has been observed. Anomalies of the renal segment of the IVC include a retroaortic renal vein (1.7% to 3.4%; Fig. 60.2) and circumaortic venous rings (Fig. 60.3), in which the retroaortic segment is located in a more caudal position relative to the preaortic segment. Anomalies of the suprarenal segment of the IVC are extremely rare and associated with either azygos or hemiazygos continuation and absence of the hepatic venous segment.[8]

The distal IVC and iliac veins are most vulnerable at the level of the posterolateral aspect of the aortic bifurcation in the area of tight adherence of the aorta and common iliac artery to the adjacent wall of the vena cava and right iliac vein. Complete separation of these structures by circumferential dissection is generally unnecessary, because temporary occlusion can usually be achieved by clamp control more distally or with intraluminal

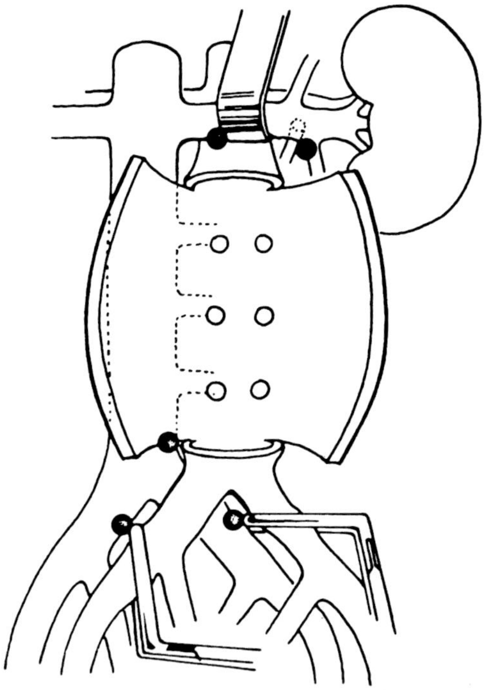

FIG 60.1 Sites of venous injury. (From Downs A: Problems in resection of aortoiliac and femoral aneurysms. In Bernhard VM, Towne JB, editors: *Complications in vascular surgery*, New York, 1980, Grune and Stratton, p 68.)

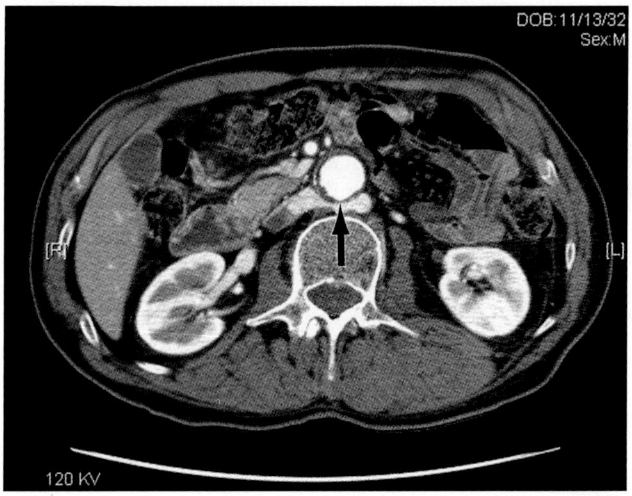

FIG 60.2 Computed tomography scan demonstrating a retroaortic left renal vein *(arrow)* in a patient with an abdominal aortic aneurysm.

balloon occlusion catheters. If the IVC or one of the iliac veins is inadvertently lacerated, bleeding should be controlled by gentle finger pressure or sponge stick tamponade, and the venous laceration closed with interrupted pledgeted Prolene sutures. Application of clamps is hazardous and may enlarge the rent in the vein.

The left renal vein should be routinely identified early during dissection of the aorta above an aneurysm or proximal to the area of major aortic occlusive disease. The caudal border of the

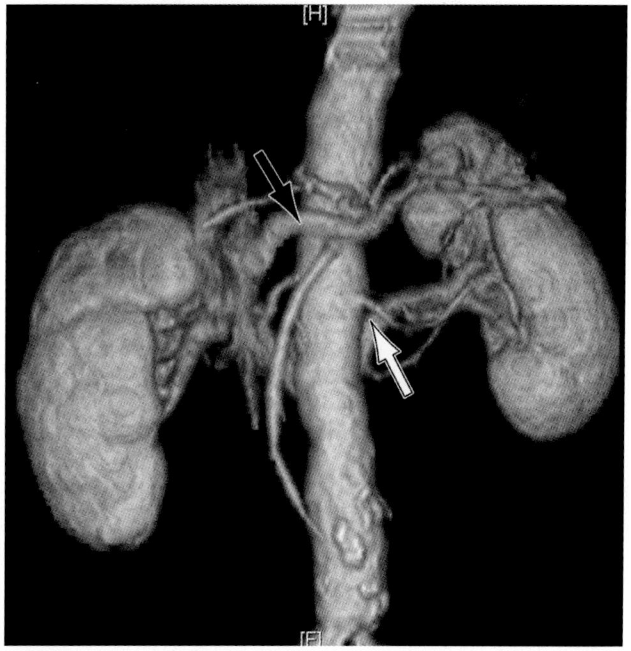

FIG 60.3 Magnetic resonance imaging reconstruction of a circumaortic renal vein *(black arrow)*. Note the caudal position of the posterior branch *(white arrow)*.

left renal vein should be clearly defined so that this structure can be easily retracted cephalad. Division of its adrenal, gonadal, or lumbar branches enhances its mobility and improves exposure. Careful consideration should be given to ligation of these branches if division of the renal vein is contemplated to improve exposure in patients with large or inflammatory aneurysms. Failure to find the left renal vein in its usual position suggests its aberrant location behind the aorta (see Figs. 60.2 and 60.3), where it may be readily injured during circumferential dissection of the infrarenal aorta preparatory to application of an occluding clamp.[6,7,9,10]

An arteriovenous fistula (AVF) involving the aorta or iliac arteries is an uncommon complication of spontaneous aneurysm rupture into an adjacent vein (about 80% of cases) or of penetrating injury to these major vessels (20%). Aortocaval fistula (ACF) has also been reported after EVAR.[11,12] The incidence of this complication is quite low; it occurs in less than 1% of all aneurysms and in 3% to 4% of ruptured aneurysms.[13-16] The presence of an ACF should be suspected when there is a continuous bruit over the aneurysm associated with the sudden onset of abdominal pain, lower extremity venous hypertension, oliguria, hematuria, and congestive heart failure. If suspected, the diagnosis of an ACF or iliac arteriovenous (AV) fistula can be confirmed by color Doppler imaging, computed tomography (CT) scanning, magnetic resonance imaging (MRI), or digital subtraction angiography (DSA). Before the routine use of preoperative imaging studies to evaluate patients with abdominal aortic aneurysms (AAA), the presence of an ACF or ilioiliac AV fistula remained undetected in 25% to 44% of patients undergoing open AAA repair. The patient with an ACF should be rapidly medically optimized before being taken to the operating room. Cardiac catheterization is rarely necessary except in cases of diagnostic uncertainty. The initial medical management should include admission to the intensive care unit (ICU), placement of hemodynamic monitoring lines and catheters, and the use of angiotensin-converting enzyme (ACE) inhibitors and diuretics. Sufficient blood and blood products should be available because intraoperative bleeding may be profuse. The fistula may sometimes be unsuspected intraoperatively because of its small size or its being obscured by the laminated thrombus within the aneurysm, with it becoming apparent only when sudden massive venous hemorrhage occurs within the lumen of the aorta during evacuation of the laminated thrombus from the aneurysmal sac.[17] In all patients undergoing AAA repair without preoperative imaging studies, it is wise to palpate the IVC for the presence of a thrill, indicating an ACF, before opening the aneurysm sac to evacuate the laminated thrombus. If a fistula is suspected, the inferior vena cava should be occluded with a sponge stick or a clamp adjacent to the neck of the aneurysm before the aneurysm is occluded and opened, to prevent embolism of clot or air to the lungs.[14] No attempt should be made to separate the aneurysm wall from the IVC at the fistula site.

Occlusion of the fistulous defect by direct finger pressure over the fistula, followed by proximal and distal caval compression with sponge sticks or insertion of balloon occlusion catheters, are among the maneuvers used to control the venous bleeding so that the defect can be visualized and closed with Prolene pledget sutures (92%) or patch angioplasty (8%) from within the aortic sac (Fig. 60.4).[18,19] Intraoperative bleeding from iliac AVFs is often more difficult to control because of their location deep within the pelvis, the size of the defect, and the intimate relationship between the vein and artery. Elective balloon catheter occlusion or placement of a covered stent to occlude the defect in the femoral vein before entering the aneurysm may control venous bleeding and permit closure of the defect without massive blood loss. Autotransfusion is a useful adjunct in the management of ACF and iliac fistulas.[13] Surgical treatment of ACF includes intraaneurysmal closure of the defect and reconstruction of the aorta with a tube or a bifurcated graft. Although endovascular repair with an aortic stent-graft may be the optimal method of treating ACF and iliac AVFs with suitable anatomy, rupture of an enlarged aneurysm sac into the IVC after EVAR is a recognized cause of ACF. Open repair, relining the endoprosthesis, and percutaneous closure of the defect with an Amplatzar ventricular septal defect (VSD) muscle plug are among the therapeutic options available for treating patients with ACF after EVAR.[20-22] Prophylactic placement of an IVC filter is rarely necessary. Complications of surgical repair, including excessive intraoperative blood loss, myocardial infarction, respiratory failure, stroke, colonic ischemia, paraparesis, and renal failure, occur in 39% of patients. Mortality rates, ranging from an average of 34% (6% to 71%) have declined to 12% in the most recent report by Davidovic and coworkers.[18] Myocardial infarction and multiple-system organ failure remain the major cause of mortality. Long-term survival after repair is greater than 90%.[19]

Arterial bleeding usually arises from the lumbar, anomalous renal, inferior mesenteric arteries, or posterior aortic wall during circumferential dissection or after the aneurysmal sac has been opened.[23-25] Lumbar vessel injury can be avoided in aneurysm surgery by limiting the dissection to the anterior surface of the aorta and by suture ligation of the lumbar orifices from within the aneurysmal sac after the aneurysm has been opened and the thrombus evacuated.[16] Precaval location of the right renal artery (5%) and multiple renal arteries (30% to 40%) should be identified. The inferior mesenteric artery should also be suture-ligated from the interior or close to the wall of the aneurysm (if there is pulsatile backflow) to avoid injury to mesenteric collaterals. The posterior aortic wall is often heavily calcified or attenuated in patients with AAA. Calcified plaque at the site of the proposed anastomosis may require an endarterectomy, which further attenuates the aortic wall. The preemptive use of a Teflon buttress will reduce the risk of bleeding from tears at the anastomotic suture line from the placement of sutures in a fragile aortic wall. When anastomotic bleeding is encountered, the aorta should be clamped briefly while additional sutures, frequently with PTFE pledgets, are placed to control the bleeding and avoid further tears in the aortic wall. In patients with unfavorable aortic tissues, the use of biological tissue glues may sometimes be helpful. These agents are not a substitute for careful hemostasis, however, and their use is associated with more frequent reoperation for bleeding and the potential for infection.[26,27] Reinforcement of the aortic anastomosis with a cuff of graft material is another option.

Continued intraoperative bleeding may result from failure to reverse or discontinue anticoagulants or platelet inhibitors preoperatively or the administration of too large a dose of heparin. The massive blood transfusion requirements during repair of thoracoabdominal or ruptured abdominal aneurysms result in the dilution of coagulation factors and platelets. In patients undergoing repair of pararenal aneurysms or the need for supraceliac clamping to facilitate repair, unrecognized fibrinolysis may be the cause of continued bleeding. Only rarely is the bleeding caused by an unrecognized congenital coagulation factor deficiency. The cause of the coagulopathy is often difficult to determine intraoperatively. Because of the higher mortality rates associated with increased intraoperative blood loss and the delay in obtaining the results of laboratory studies, it is recommended that blood, fresh frozen plasma (FFP), and platelets be administered concomitantly to improve the survival rate of these patients. If supraceliac clamping is anticipated or repair of a thoracoabdominal aneurysm is being undertaken, the transfusion of FFP should be started before clamp placement. Antifibrinolytic agents such as aminocaproic acid (Amicar) or tranexamic acid should be considered if activation of the fibrinolytic pathway is suspected. It should be noted, however, that there are no prospective data available for the clinical use of these agents in vascular surgery patients.[28,29]

Postoperative Bleeding

Bleeding in the immediate postoperative period usually comes from suture lines, inadequately ligated lumbar vessels, or the inferior mesenteric vein. This is manifested by a continuing need for blood replacement and the development of a retroperitoneal hematoma. This can be identified by palpating the flank—usually the left—which loses its normal soft concavity and becomes distended and tense. When aortic or iliac suture line bleeding is rapid, shock is more obvious, and the patient complains of

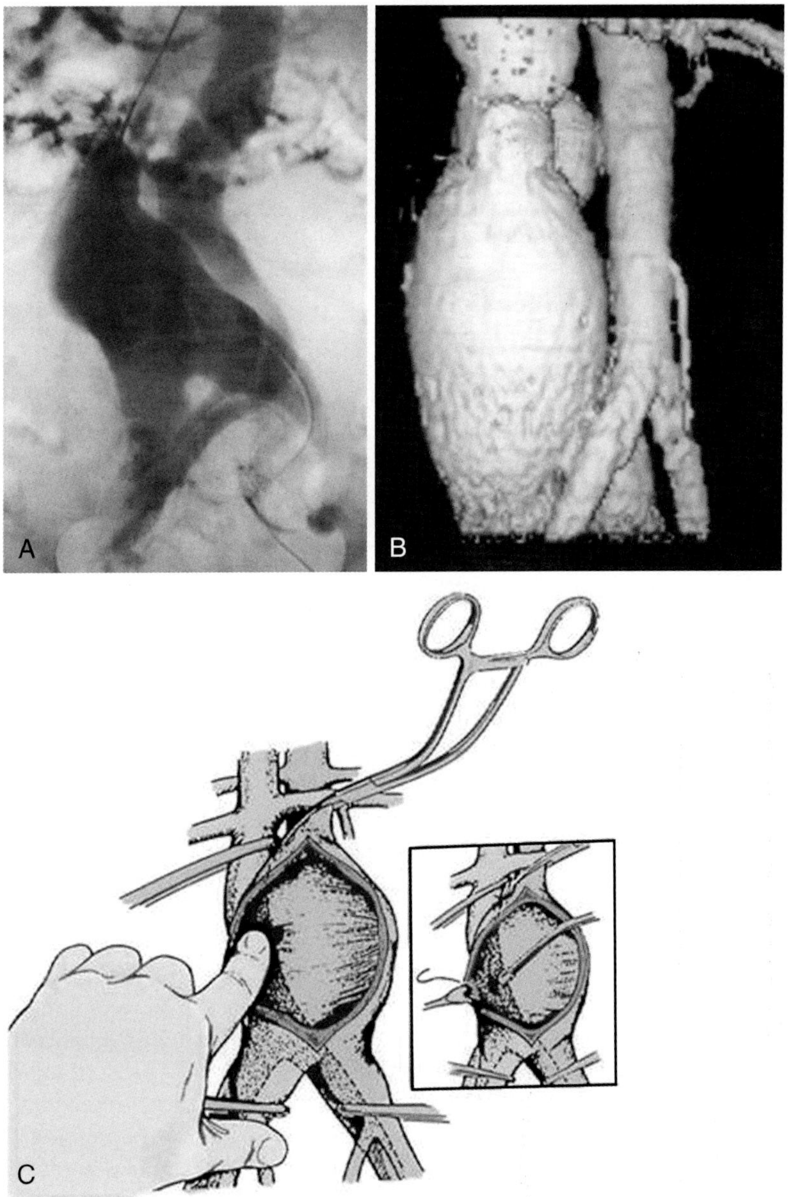

FIG 60.4 (A) Abdominal angiogram showing filling of the vena cava from an aortic aneurysm. (B) Magnetic resonance angiogram showing a traumatic aortocaval fistula. (C) The fistula orifice is exposed through the aneurysm and controlled by simple digital occlusion of the hole into the inferior vena cava. The fistula is closed with interrupted Prolene pledgetted sutures from within the aneurysmal sac. A clear and unencumbered field is provided by rapid aspiration and autotransfusion of blood pouring into the aneurysmal sac from the cava.

severe backache similar to the pain of a ruptured aortic aneurysm. Postoperative hemorrhage is treated by immediate return to the operating room for identification and control of the bleeding site under fully monitored general anesthesia. The surgeon should search for the potential bleeding site when blood volume and pressure are at the patient's normal level before closing the retroperitoneum over the aortoiliac reconstruction.

Prevention of this complication requires thorough inspection of the intraabdominal anastomoses and the periaortic area, with special attention given to the orifices of the lumbar or anomalous renal vessels, the inferior mesenteric artery, and the ligated or oversewn stumps of the aorta or iliac vessels.

Hypothermia and acidosis are correctable causes of persistent coagulopathy and postoperative bleeding. Prevention of hypothermia by using heating blankets, increasing room temperature, and infusing adequate volumes of warm blood and fluids to optimize cardiac output are essential. A recent study by Samoila and colleagues reviewed the effects of hypothermia on outcomes following both open and endovascular aneurysm repair. They reviewed eight studies involving 765 patients. Normothermic patients had a shorter length of hospital stay in the intensive care unit. Hypothermia was associated with higher rates of organ dysfunction, higher in-hospital mortality, and prolonged hospital stay.[30]

An activated clotting time (ACT) is done and specimens sent for a platelet count, fibrinogen, prothrombin time (PT), and partial thromboplastin time (PTT); these tests may not be helpful in the acute setting. Fibrinogen is the first clotting factor to fall in this situation and should be replaced. A platelet count of 100,000 or greater should not negate the need for platelet infusion because the platelets may not be functional. Congenital coagulation factor deficiency is rare and can usually be ascertained by careful preoperative history and evaluation.[31] Preliminary screening studies do not reliably identify the need to search for precise factor deficiencies and direct their replacement before and during surgery. Intraoperative monitoring of the ACT before and after heparin administration is the most effective means of identifying variations in the individual response to intraoperatively administered unfractionated heparin and to determine the adequacy of its reversal before closing the abdomen.[31] Proper management of bleeding caused by congenital or acquired deficiencies requires repeated monitoring of pertinent coagulation parameters during and immediately after the operative procedure.

The rising number of cardiac and peripheral percutaneous and endovascular interventions being performed has resulted in antiplatelet agents being administered to increasing numbers of patients. It is not uncommon for patients undergoing coronary or peripheral vessel angioplasty or stenting to receive a combination of drugs, including aspirin; clopidogrel; heparin; glycoprotein (GP) IIb/IIIa inhibitors such as abciximab, eptifibatide, and tirofiban; and direct thrombin inhibitors such as bivalirudin. Emergency surgical procedures to control bleeding from retroperitoneal hemorrhage or expanding groin hematomas from cannulation sites can be associated with significant perioperative blood loss into the thigh or retroperitoneum.[32-35]

Although thromboelastography may be a useful adjuvant to therapy, it is not universally available. Discontinuation of the antiplatelet agent or anticoagulant therapy and delay of surgery when feasible is sometimes the preferred option. However, should emergency intervention be required, red blood cells, FFP, fibrinogen concentrate, and platelets should be infused. Cryoprecipitate and specific factor replacement should be reserved for patients with specific coagulation factor defects.

Initially approved for treating patients with hemophilia who had antibody inactivating factors V111 and 1X, recombinant activated factor V11 (rFV11a) is used extensively in patients with massive bleeding from surgery or trauma and may be beneficial in patients undergoing ruptured AAA (rAAA) repair. Recombinant activated factor V11a binds locally to the tissue factor at the site of vessel injury, generating small amounts of thrombin sufficient to activate platelets. The activated platelet surface membranes form a template on which rFV11a directly or indirectly mediates further activation of the coagulation pathway, ultimately generating more thrombin and the conversion of fibrinogen to fibrin. Recombinant factor V11a also stabilizes clot by activation of a thrombin-mediated fibrinolysis inhibitor. Clinical studies in patients undergoing prostatectomy, liver transplantation, noncoronary cardiac surgery, and trauma have shown that rFV11a minimizes operative blood loss and reduces transfusion requirements. A major concern with the use of this agent is the risk of thrombosis. The incidence is believed to be low because of the dilution of coagulation factors in patients from massive blood loss.[36,37] One recent study analyzing outcomes following AAA repair and the use of rFVII demonstrated a lower mortality in patients who responded to treatment, however the rate of thromboembolic adverse events was 14%.[38]

It is estimated that there are approximately 2.5 million patients on long-term vitamin K therapy and 40% of the US population over 40 years of age is on antiplatelet therapy. The need for temporary interruption of these therapies for surgical and other invasive procedures is therefore not infrequent.[39] In a recent study, approximately 15% of patients on long-term vitamin K therapy required a major surgical procedure within a 4-year follow-up period.[40] Recommendations for the discontinuation of vitamin K and antiplatelet agents preoperatively or preprocedurally must be balanced with the risk of thrombotic occlusion of recently placed stents or stent-grafts, the type of surgery including the risk of hemorrhagic complications, and the pharmacodynamic/kinetic profile of the therapy used to reverse the vitamin K therapy.

Neilipovitz and colleagues, using decision analysis, showed that the continued use of aspirin in vascular surgery patients reduces perioperative mortality, despite a 2.5% increase in hemorrhagic complications.[35] A more recent study by Khashram and colleagues demonstrated that the perioperative use of aspirin was a significant predictor of improved survival following aortic aneurysm repair.[41] The antiplatelet effects of clopidogrel persist for 7 to 10 days, so this drug should be discontinued 1 week before surgery. These recommendations are based on observations from case studies of patients undergoing coronary artery bypass grafting who received aspirin and clopidogrel or aspirin and placebo.[42] Patients receiving both drugs had a higher rate of major postoperative bleeding (9.6% vs. 6.3%), reoperation (9.8% vs. 1.6%), and blood transfusion (3.0 units vs. 1.6 units) compared with patients receiving aspirin and placebo. The effects of GP IIb/IIIa inhibitors on platelets are quite variable. The antiplatelet effects of eptifibatide are usually abated within 8 hours of cessation of therapy in patients with normal renal function. Abciximab has a biological half-life of 8 hours, but its effects on the surface of circulating platelets can be detected for up to 2 weeks after discontinuing the drug.[32]

The risk of hemorrhage and thromboembolism varies with the international normalized ratio (INR) in patients on vitamin K therapy. With INR ratios between 2 and 3, the relative risk of hemorrhagic events is 2.7 compared with 21.8 at INR ratios between 3 and 5. The risk of thromboembolism increases significantly with low INR; compared with INR ratios between 2 and 3, the relative risk of thromboembolism associated with INR below 2 was 3.5; within the range of 2 to 3, there is still a higher risk of thromboembolic than hemorrhagic events (2.6%/year vs. 1.4%/year). Patients with mechanical heart valves or chronic atrial fibrillation and those at high risk of recurrent deep vein thrombosis who are on long-term vitamin K therapy should have the vitamin K agonist reversed and receive bridging low-molecular-weight heparin (LMWH). Therapeutic options for acute reversal of vitamin K agonists include vitamin K, FFP, prothrombin complex concentrate (PCC), and, possibly, rFVIIa. PCC is obtained from plasma; 60 mL of PCC is equivalent to 1500 mL of FFP, reducing volume requirements.[43]

Thrombosis

Graft thrombosis in the early postoperative period is almost invariably caused by technical problems (Fig. 60.5) that usually occur at the distal anastomoses.[44-46] These include an elevated intimal flap, narrowing of the artery at the anastomotic suture line, failure to remove a clot adherent to the inner wall of the graft before completion of the anastomosis, twisting or kinking in the retroperitoneal tunnel, compression of the femoral limb of the graft by the inguinal ligament, unrecognized inflow disease, or inadequate runoff secondary to unappreciated iliac, deep femoral, superficial femoral, or infrapopliteal disease. Rarely, thrombosis after aortofemoral bypass or aneurysm replacement is caused by hypercoagulability from inadequate doses or resistance to heparin, antithrombin III deficiency, protein C or S deficiency, a mutation in factor V Leiden or prothrombin genes, homocysteinemia, anticardiolipin antibodies, heparin-induced thrombocytopenia (HIT) and thrombosis, or stasis caused by reduced cardiac output.[47-50]

The adequacy of pulsatile blood flow through the graft or endarterectomy should be evaluated in the operating room before the incisions are closed, by palpation of the graft and the arteries immediately distal to the anastomoses and by direct inspection of the pedal circulation beneath the drapes and palpation of distal pulses. If necessary, noninvasive measurements such as Doppler flow or pulse-volume recording tracings can be obtained intraoperatively.[44,45,51-53] Intraoperative completion angiograms or color-flow Doppler imaging should be obtained in all patients who have had extensive reconstructive procedures of the common femoral, superficial femoral, or deep femoral arteries to ensure the adequacy of the repair. Noninvasive studies should be performed routinely in the recovery room when pulses cannot be felt distal to the repair or when the anticipated improvement in circulation has not occurred. Objective information obtained from these easily performed studies is particularly valuable in the immediate postoperative period, when patients are frequently hypothermic and peripherally vasoconstricted. Detection of unsatisfactory graft function mandates immediate direct evaluation of the involved anastomoses before wound closure or prompt return to the operating room if graft flow subsequently deteriorates.

An ACT should be obtained and additional systemic heparin given as necessary. This is especially important if protamine has

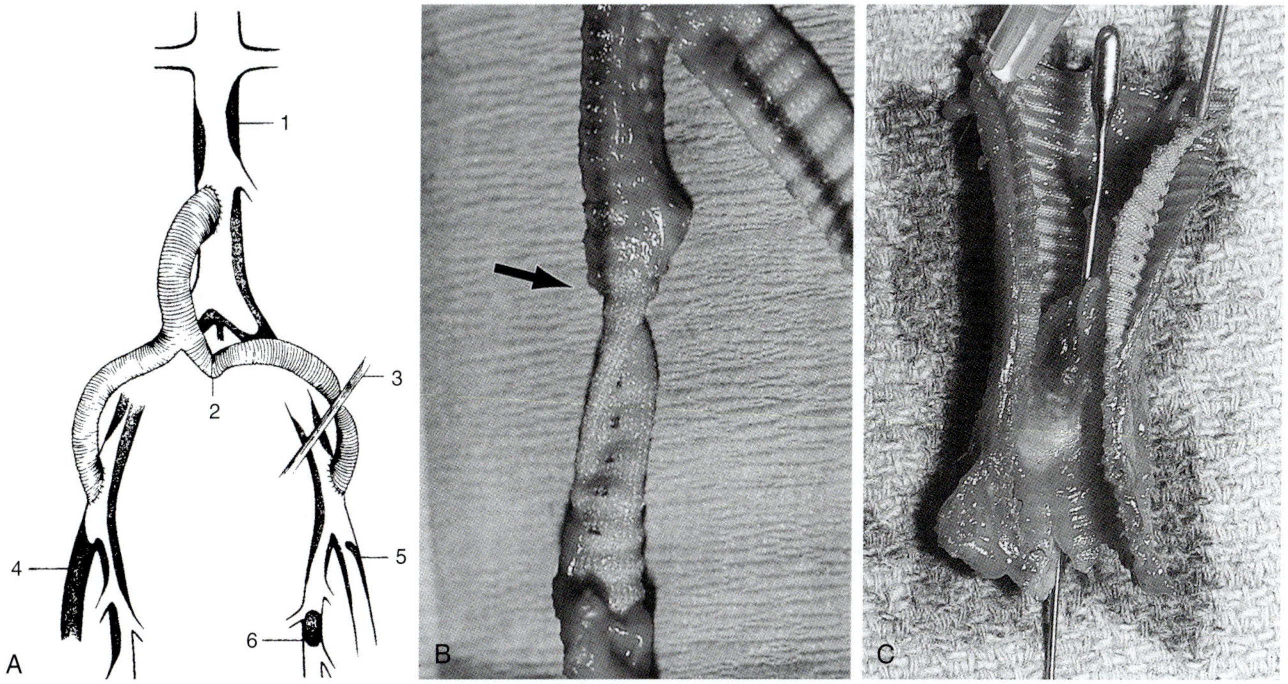

FIG 60.5 (A) Aortic and mechanical factors that may cause early thrombosis of aortofemoral graft: *(1)* aortic anastomosis distal to obstructing atherosclerosis at the infrarenal level; *(2)* kinking of the graft limb caused by placement of the proximal anastomosis low on the aorta, with an overly long aortic graft segment; *(3)* compression by the inguinal ligament; *(4)* inadequate runoff caused by occlusion of the superficial femoral artery and severe stenosis of the deep femoral artery; *(5)* elevation of the distal intima; *(6)* peripheral embolization or thrombosis. (B) Operative picture demonstrating a twist in the right limb *(arrow)* of an aortobifemoral graft. (C) Fibrointimal ingrowth resulting in occlusion of the limb of a bifurcation graft. ([A] From Bernhard VM: The failed arterial graft: lost pulses and gangrene. In Condon RE, DeCosse JJ, editors: *Surgical care*, Philadelphia, 1980, Lea and Febiger, p 155.)

been given at the initial operation. Treatment of immediate postreconstructive thrombosis consists of thorough inspection of the intraluminal aspect of the involved anastomosis. This is best accomplished through an incision in the distal end of the graft or by takedown of the anastomosis to directly view the intima and the runoff vessels adjacent to the arteriotomy. Effective revision may require stabilization of an elevated plaque, extension of an iliac limb to the common femoral artery, or patch angioplasty of a deep or proximal superficial femoral stenosis. Complementary bypass from the femoral to the popliteal or infrapopliteal vessels is only infrequently required when runoff through the deep femoral artery is inadequate.[54,55] The lie of the graft should always be inspected throughout its length to ensure that there is no kinking, twisting, or external compression within the retroperitoneal tunnel.

Prevention of early graft thrombosis depends on an accurate evaluation of the distal runoff bed by preoperative noninvasive hemodynamic testing and imaging; computed tomography angiography (CTA), magnetic resonance angiography (MRA), or DSA. The iliac artery, rather than the femoral, should be palpated throughout its length before the selection of this vessel as the site for distal anastomosis. The orifices of the runoff vessels should be inspected and calibrated with dilators. Special attention should be given to the deep femoral orifice, which often requires endarterectomy or extension of the graft over its orifice when the distal anastomosis is performed at the common femoral level. Tacking sutures may be required to prevent distal intimal dissection. Finally, technical perfection in the performance of anastomoses is mandatory to avoid narrowing of the runoff vessels.

The widespread use of unfractionated heparin and LMWH has resulted in an increased frequency of HIT, reported to occur in 5% of patients receiving unfractionated heparin and in 0.5% receiving LMWH. The heparin/platelet factor 4 (PF4) complex generates predominantly IgG and to a lesser extent IgM antibodies, which activate prothrombotic platelet microparticles, resulting in platelet consumption, increased thrombin generation, and the risk of venous and arterial thrombosis. A milder form of HIT that is neither immune-mediated nor prothrombotic occurs more often in patients receiving heparin. Heparin-induced thrombocytopenia with thrombosis (HITT) should be suspected when the platelet count decreases by more than 50% from baseline or drops to 150,000 or less in patients receiving heparin therapy. Thromboembolic complications usually become evident between 5 and 14 days after heparin therapy and can involve the deep veins of the lower extremity, the pulmonary arteries, and major cerebral veins. Arterial thrombotic complications may involve the lower extremities and the coronary, mesenteric, renal, or cerebral arteries. When HITT is encountered intraoperatively, the surgeon has to act without confirmatory tests. If HITT is suspected because of the presence of "white clots" or unexplained intraoperative thrombosis, blood should be drawn immediately for diagnostic confirmation and a specimen of the thrombus sent to the laboratory for a touch prep to confirm the predominance of platelets in the clot. The administration of all unfractionated heparin should be discontinued and the ACT normalized with protamine if heparin has been administered recently.[56-58]

Laboratory confirmation of HITT using the PF4/polyanion immunoassay is specific if strongly positive but has low specificity (as a result of IgM, IgG, and nonspecific antibodies) if the enzyme-linked immunosorbent assay is weakly positive. The platelet serotonin release assay is more specific if there is greater than 80% serotonin release. The principles of treatment include discontinuation of all heparin, and administration of direct thrombin inhibitors such as argatroban, lepirudin, or bivalirudin to maintain the PTT between 1.5 times and 3.0 times baseline. Prophylactic platelet transfusions should be avoided. Because warfarin may predispose to microvascular thrombosis in patients with acute HITT receiving direct thrombin inhibitors, it should be reversed with vitamin K if a dose has already been given and should be reintroduced only when the platelet count is greater than 150×10^4/L.

Thrombosis caused by the progression of downstream atherosclerosis or anastomotic intimal hyperplasia (AIH) is the most frequent late complication of aortoiliac and aortofemoral procedures.[59,60] The impaired outflow through the external iliac artery or the branches of the common femoral usually manifests as unilateral limb ischemia (Fig. 60.6).[61-67] Anastomotic intimal hyperplasia causes stenosis, usually at the graft-artery interface of the distal anastomosis: occlusion occurs when flow diminishes sufficiently to result in stasis thrombosis.[66] The majority of patients initially treated with aortofemoral bypass have stenosis/occlusion of the superficial femoral artery at the time of the primary procedure. Therefore, an adequate lumen at the origin of the deep femoral artery is the most significant factor in ensuring long-term patency of these grafts.[52,60,62,65,67] Underestimating the severity of outflow disease at the time of primary reconstruction is an important cofactor in progressive atherosclerosis that increases susceptibility to late graft limb occlusion.[68] Despite an adequate primary procedure, progression of femoral or infrapopliteal atherosclerotic disease is more likely to occur in patients with continued exposure to atherogenic risk factors, particularly patients who continue to smoke.[61,68] Impaired inflow is the second most common cause of late postrevascularization thrombosis. Although it is four to nine times less frequent than impaired outflow, it is the most common cause of simultaneous bilateral postreconstructive lower limb ischemia after aortoiliac or femoral surgery.[60,63,68] The most common mechanism is obstruction from progressive infrarenal aortic atherosclerosis proximal to the site of previous repair (see Fig. 60.5A). This is usually the consequence of placing the proximal anastomosis too low on the aorta (i.e., at or below the inferior mesenteric artery; see Fig. 60.6A). The area between this site and the renal arteries is an active site of progressive atherosclerosis.[52] Likewise, after aortoiliac endarterectomy, late occlusion is more likely if the proximal infrarenal aorta is not included in the endarterectomy.[69] The use of an end-to-end rather than an end-to-side aortic anastomosis may be associated with fewer thrombotic failures, although this has not been clearly defined. Superior hemodynamic flow characteristics, the absence of competitive flow, less chance of embolization from the host aorta, and less angulation of the limbs as they arise from the body graft have been cited as the advantages of the end-to-end aortic anastomosis.[52,69]

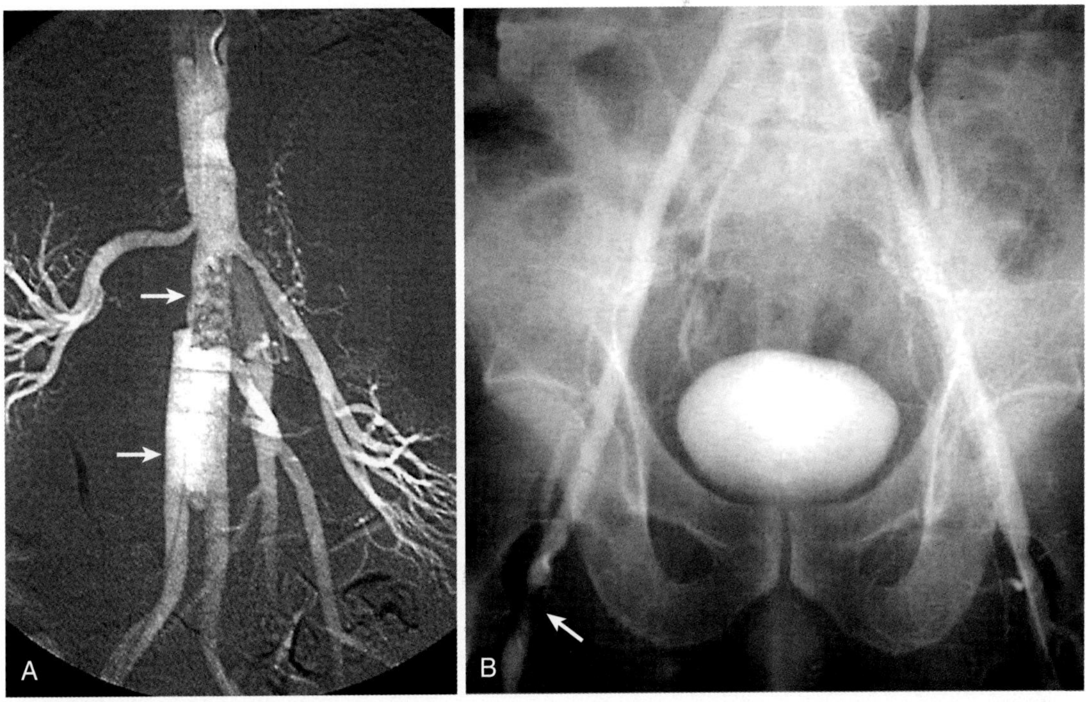

FIG 60.6 (A) Digital subtraction angiogram demonstrating progression of atherosclerosis above an aortofemoral graft *(upper arrow)*. The graft is placed well below the renal arteries and the body of the graft is too long *(lower arrow)*. (B) High-grade stenosis caused by intimal hyperplasia at the distal limb of an aortofemoral graft *(arrow)*.

Angulation of the graft limb at the bifurcation may produce kinking because of failure to pull the graft limb out to full length before the distal anastomoses are performed or excessive length of the graft body, resulting in too wide a bifurcation angle (see Fig. 60.5B). Inadequate retroperitoneal tunneling of the graft limbs may promote thrombosis as a consequence of extrinsic compression from the mesentery of the sigmoid colon or the recurrent portion of the inguinal ligament (see Fig. 60.5C).[68]

Less frequent causes of late thrombosis of aortoiliac and femoral reconstructions include accumulation of mural thrombus and false aneurysms. Mural thrombus develops when the graft diameter is significantly larger than the outflow artery. The flow pattern of the larger graft adjusts itself to the smaller outflow artery, leaving a peripheral layer of slowly moving blood that clots to form the mural thrombus. The normal, smooth, firmly adherent fibrous neointima becomes lined with a thick, gelatinous, loosely adherent mural thrombus that reduces the functioning lumen to the diameter of the outflow vessel. Fragmentation with distal embolization or progressive narrowing of the graft lumen with secondary acute thrombotic occlusion may then occur.[66] Anastomotic false aneurysms, although relatively rare causes of late limb ischemia, may also produce peripheral embolization or thrombosis of the aneurysm and the adjacent vessel lumen.[68] Finally, aortoiliac and femoral reconstructions can progress suddenly to thrombosis from percutaneous catheter interventions, cardiac embolization, or decreased cardiac output secondary to myocardial infarction or congestive heart failure. Rarely, no apparent cause for late thrombosis can be identified, implicating thrombogenicity of the graft surface or degeneration and disruption of the neointima.

The diagnosis of late thrombosis is suggested by the sudden or progressive recurrence of symptoms, a decrease or loss of previously present distal pulses, and a concomitant reduction in ankle pressure indices, Doppler flow, or pulse-volume recording waveforms. The degree of ischemia after thrombosis of a reconstruction is usually more severe than before the primary revascularization procedure.[60,63] The frequency of late thrombosis increases from 5% to 10% in the first 5 years to 20% to 30% at 10 years.[52,67,70-72] Therefore, routine and long-term follow-up of these patients at regular intervals is required to monitor the adequacy of graft function. If significant stenosis can be demonstrated before complete thrombosis, surgical correction is simplified. When either abrupt or gradual change is apparent, prompt imaging studies should be performed to determine the status of the graft, the anastomoses, the inflow, and the runoff bed.[51,73]

The severity of recurrent ischemia may range from minimal to severe claudication to rest pain to gangrene, depending on the extent of compensating collaterals and the vigor of the patient's normal activity. Imaging studies are required to determine whether further surgery is feasible and to guide the surgeon in the selection of the most appropriate reoperative or interventional procedure, considering the patient's age, health status, and level of activity.[61,68]

Correction of late thrombosis requires preoperative delineation of the underlying anatomical problem, followed by appropriate corrective maneuvers.[68,74] The occlusion of one limb of an aortoiliac bifurcation graft is usually caused by overlooked or progressing disease in the external iliac and femoral arteries. Thrombolytic therapy may be useful in delineating the artery involved by the progression of atherosclerosis. Balloon catheter angioplasty with stenting is not usually indicated because of the extent of the disease or location beneath the inguinal ligament. One reliable solution consists of retroperitoneal exposure of the occluded limb, balloon catheter thrombectomy, and graft extension to the femoral level. Femorofemoral bypass is an alternative if the donor iliofemoral inflow is satisfactory, especially in a high-risk patient. Axillofemoral bypass may be required if neither of the preceding methods is feasible.[7,54]

The most commonly encountered situation is a thrombosed aortofemoral graft limb with impaired outflow. Inflow can usually be restored by the use of catheter-based thrombolysis, or surgical or percutaneous graft thrombectomy using a balloon thromboembolectomy catheter or mechanical thrombectomy device with or without regional lytic agents (Fig. 60.7).[74] A thromboendarterectomy stripper or adherent clot catheter is often required to complete the extraction of adherent clots and old pseudointima. The Fogarty occlusion catheter is passed through the ring of the stripper into the patent aortic portion of the graft, and its balloon is fully inflated and pulled down to occlude the proximal end of the limb to control bleeding and prevent crossover embolization. The stripper is passed back and forth and rotated around the catheter within the occluded graft limb up to the distended balloon to scrape thrombus from the graft wall. Thereafter, the balloon is deflated just enough to permit its tight withdrawal through the graft limb along with the stripper and detached thrombus (see Fig. 60.7). Use of the Fogarty adherent clot catheter obviates the need for the thromboendarterectomy stripper. The patient is systemically heparinized (100 to 125 units/kg) during all these maneuvers.

Thrombectomy is usually combined with a profundoplasty of varying extent to provide outflow. However, femoropopliteal or femorodistal bypass may be required, depending on the extent and location of outflow disease (Fig. 60.8).[54,55,74,75] If an occluded graft limb cannot be reopened by thrombectomy, a femorofemoral graft can be inserted. Replacement of the graft limb is another alternative but is technically more difficult. Endovascular options include thrombus removal by catheter aspiration, thrombus dissolution with hydrodynamic catheters such as the Cordis Hydrolyser, the BSIC Oasis, and Angiojet systems. These mechanical therapeutic modalities are often combined with the use of thrombolytic agents.[76] Percutaneous thrombectomy is more frequently used to treat lower extremity graft or native arterial occlusions. The use of these mechanical and aspiration thrombectomy catheters to treat aortofemoral limb occlusion is limited to small series and isolated case reports.[77]

If an entire bifurcated graft is thrombosed, a problem at the proximal anastomosis such as low placement of the graft with progression or unrecognized proximal disease, kinking, or anastomotic aneurysm, or cardiac embolization is a likely cause. Imaging with CTA, MRA, or DSA is required to identify proximal progression of disease. If no proximal problem can be demonstrated, thrombectomy with a balloon or an adherent clot catheter can be attempted but is usually not successful. The alternatives are to replace the original prosthesis or insert an axillobifemoral bypass. The latter procedure is less technically

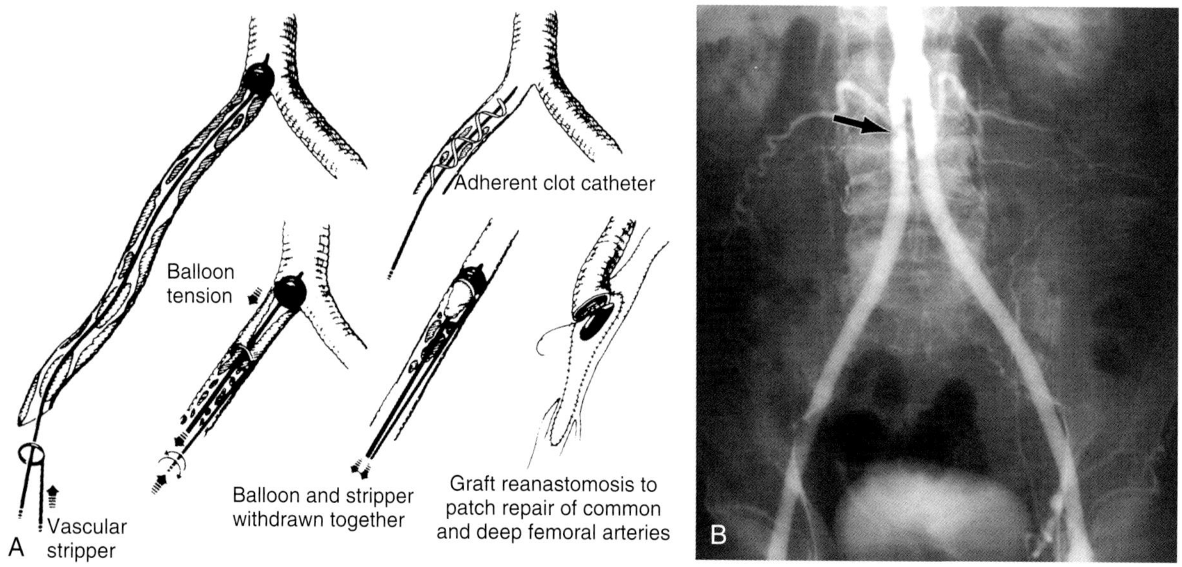

FIG 60.7 (A) A ring endarterectomy stripper is used in conjunction with a balloon catheter or adherent clot catheter to remove thrombus and pseudointima adherent to the wall of an occluded limb of an aortofemoral graft. The cleared graft limb is then sutured to the common or deep femoral outflow after patch angioplasty. (B) Intraoperative arteriogram demonstrating residual thrombus *(arrow)* in the proximal right limb of an aortobifemoral graft after attempted thrombectomy. ([A] From Bernhard VM: Late vascular graft thrombosis. In Bernhard VM, Towne JB, editors: *Complications in vascular surgery*, ed 2, New York, 1985, Grune and Stratton, p 193.)

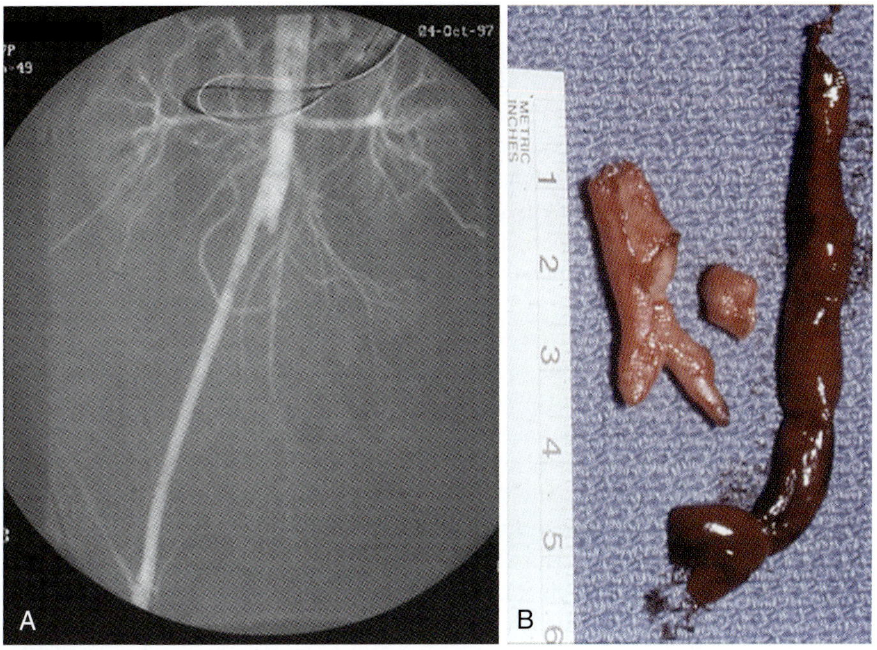

FIG 60.8 (A) Angiogram of the occluded limb of an aortofemoral graft. (B) The operative specimen demonstrating the thrombus and plaque removed from the proximal superficial femoral and profunda femoris arteries.

demanding and less hazardous and is the reoperation of choice in a physiologically compromised patient.[74] When groin scarring is especially intense, bypass to the mid-deep femoral artery simplifies the outflow repair of the reoperative procedure by avoiding a tedious and hazardous dissection in the area of a previous femoral anastomosis.[78]

Endovascular treatment of this complication may be feasible in selected patients by establishing inflow with covered stents or stent grafts after dissolution or removal of the thrombus. An aggressive attitude toward reoperation after thrombotic failure of aortoiliac reconstruction is warranted, especially if the patient will derive sustained benefit from long-term patency and improved limb function.[74] Operative morbidity and mortality rates are low. Reoperative mortality rates of 3% and cumulative 3-year patency rates of 68% to 75% have been reported.[60,74] Judicious use of extraabdominal approaches has contributed significantly to reduced reoperative morbidity and mortality.[68]

Lytic Therapy for Graft Thrombosis

Although thrombectomy has been the treatment of choice in the management of occluded aortofemoral and femoropopliteal bypass grafts, incomplete removal of thrombotic material and the difficulties associated with reoperation have led to the evaluation of direct intraarterial infusion of thrombolytic agents, either preoperatively or intraoperatively, for the management of this problem.[79] The potential benefits of lytic therapy include delineation of the cause of the graft thrombosis (most commonly distal occlusion caused by intimal hyperplasia or progression of disease) and, as a consequence, shorter operation time, reduced blood loss, ease of extracting any residual thrombus, and reduced wound complication rate. Potential disadvantages and complications of thrombolytic therapy include the need for monitoring in an intensive care unit, delay in surgical intervention, and risk of bleeding or renal impairment from the contrast load required for frequent angiographic evaluation. Further, mechanical thrombectomy for aortofemoral graft limb occlusion is at least as effective as clot lysis and adds little to the operative procedure required to restore outflow.

Kuhn and colleagues,[80] in a series of 129 patients with acute and subacute occlusions of native arteries (77) and bypass grafts (55), reported recanalization with r-tPA thrombolysis in 73.6% of cases. There was no statistically significant difference in primary therapeutic success rates between native arteries and bypass grafts. The morbidity rate was 31% (minor complications, 20.2%; major complications, 10.9%), and the mortality rate was 2.3%. Twenty-seven patients required radiologic and surgical interventions within 12 months, with a limb salvage rate after primary successful recanalization of 89.5%.[80] Successful lysis, which does not appear to be affected by the duration and cause of the graft thrombosis, can be achieved in 50% to 90% of occluded prosthetic graft limbs, 50% to 77% of saphenous veins, and 38% to 71% of prosthetic grafts.[81-86] Despite successful clot lysis, however, a recent study by Schrijver and colleagues suggested that long-term amputation-free survival at 1 and 5 years is still lower than expected (76% and 65% for native arteries and 78% and 51% for bypass grafts).[87]

The thrombolytic agents used clinically are recombinant thrombolytic peptides represented by recombinant tissue plasminogen activator (r-tPA), which enzymatically breaks down cross-linked fibrin strands within the thrombus by converting plasminogen to plasmin. The three recombinant thrombolytic peptides that are clinically relevant are alteplase (r-tPA), reteplase (r-PA), and tenecteplase (TNK). r-PA and TNK have been structurally modified from native r-tPA to increase their half-life and fibrin specificity. TNK possesses a longer half-life, improved fibrin specificity, and increased resistance to plasminogen activator inhibitor and has been shown to have a better safety profile compared with t-PA in patients with acute myocardial infarction (MI). A metaanalysis of studies comparing thrombolysis with surgical intervention concluded that catheter-directed peripheral intraarterial thrombolysis (PIAT) resulted in higher limb salvage rates and lower mortality rates than surgical intervention. Limb salvage rates at 30 days in patients receiving PIAT were 93% compared with 85.5% with surgery. These higher limb salvage rates were maintained at 6- to 12-month follow-up (89% vs. 73%). Mortality at 30 days was 4% for PIAT compared with 15% for surgical patients. This trend in mortality rates was maintained at 6- to 12-month follow-up (8% vs. 29%), respectively.[88-90]

Infusion of the thrombolytic agents is usually accomplished by a multi–side-hole catheter or an infusion wire placed so that it covers the extent of the thrombus. There are multiple dosage regimens advocated for the use of these agents. Usually a loading dose followed by a continuous infusion is given: t-PA at 0.25 to 10 mg/hour, r-PA at 0.25 to 1 units/hour, and TNK at 0.25 to 0.5 mg/hour. Heparin in a dose of 300 to 500 units/hour is usually administered through the access sheath to prevent pericatheter thrombosis.[91-95]

Patients are monitored carefully in the ICU for evidence of bleeding. Blood is drawn for hemoglobin, hematocrit, platelet count, fibrinogen, PT, and activated PTT (aPTT) every 6 hours. After successful lysis, the underlying lesion is treated with catheter-based techniques or surgery. Long-term anticoagulation with warfarin is usually indicated.

Bleeding, the major complication of lytic therapy, occurs after 7% to 48% of infusions.[84,96] The most common sources of bleeding are angiography or venous puncture sites, the interstices of prosthetic grafts, and systemic bleeding at remote sites. Central nervous system bleeding is the most lethal complication. Bleeding from a groin arterial puncture site may also result in femoral pseudoaneurysm or retroperitoneal hematoma, which may compress the femoral nerve within the iliac fascia or in the thigh. The resulting femoral neuralgia, reported to occur in up to 30% of patients, may persist for as long as 1 year.[97,98] Rarely, a femoral nerve palsy develops in patients; this may be extremely debilitating, especially in patients with claudication or amputation of the contralateral limb. There is some evidence that the risk of bleeding may be higher with t-PA than with r-PA or TNK.

The most important determinant of the long-term success of lytic therapy is the presence of a lesion correctable by surgical revision or balloon catheter dilatation.[99] Such lesions responsible for the occlusion can be identified in approximately 21% to 30% of patients with 86% to 89% patency at 1 year compared with 37% of a similar number of grafts without correctable lesions.[99]

The results of three prospective studies comparing the efficacy of intraarterial thrombolysis and surgery in patients with lower limb ischemia reported successful catheter placement in 72%, clot dissolution in greater than 70%, and limb salvage at 1 year in greater than 80%.[80,100-102] In a study of 114 patients with acute lower limb ischemia of less than 7 days' duration who were randomized to thrombolytic therapy or surgery, Ouriel and colleagues achieved clot dissolution in 70% and observed equivalent limb salvage rates (82%) and improved patient survival (82% vs. 58%) in the patients receiving thrombolytic therapy at 1 year.[100] They attributed the improved survival in the thrombolytic group to the more frequent occurrence of cardiopulmonary complications in the patients undergoing surgery. In a subsequent study, Ouriel and associates randomized 213 patients with acute limb ischemia of less than 14 days' duration to recombinant urokinase or surgery.[101] Clot lysis was achieved in a similar number of patients (71%) but there was no difference in mortality rate (14% vs. 16%) or amputation-free survival rate (75% vs. 65%) between the two groups at 1 year. In the Surgery versus Thrombolysis for Ischemia of the Lower Extremity (STILE) trial,[102] the efficacy of rt-PA and urokinase was compared with that of surgery in 393 patients with limb ischemia of less than 6 months' duration. Failure of catheter placement occurred in 28% of patients. Patients with ischemia of less than 14 days' duration receiving lytic therapy had lower amputation rates than did surgical patients, whereas patients with ischemic symptoms of more than 14 days' duration fared better with surgery. The results of these studies suggest that in selected patients, thrombolytic therapy may be a useful adjunct or alternative to surgical therapy. However, long-term patency rates of 28% to 37% of thrombolysed grafts are clearly inferior to those obtained with surgery.[99,103] Thrombolytic therapy may be extremely valuable in patients with limb-threatening ischemia secondary to thrombosed popliteal aneurysm. Thrombolysis may improve the chances of achieving long-term patency and limb salvage.[104]

Reteplase differs from alteplase both in its structure and biochemical composition and in its lower affinity for thrombin. McNamara reported a 34% incidence of bleeding in a series of 40 patients treated with t-PA compared with 3% among those receiving r-PA at doses of 2 to 8 mg/hour.[105] Even reducing the dosage of t-PA to 0.5 to 1 mg/hour was still associated with a 25% incidence of bleeding requiring transfusion.

In all cases, the risks and benefits of the use of lytic therapy in the treatment of patients with graft limb occlusions must be evaluated carefully.

The relatively low incidence of complications, improved technique of administration, and efficacy of thrombolytic agents have reduced the need for urgent surgical thrombectomy in patients with noncritical limb ischemia. Successful lytic therapy readily identifies the cause of the graft limb occlusion and may allow a less extensive repair. In addition, lytic therapy may reduce the risk of wound and graft complications and reduce the incidence of reperfusion edema and compartment syndrome associated with extensive redo procedures.

Mechanical Thrombectomy

Mechanical thrombectomy devices that theoretically permit rapid revascularization of an ischemic extremity using minimally invasive techniques are gaining in popularity. The use of mechanical energy to cause fragmentation, dissolution, and aspiration of thrombus is appealing. These devices can be classified broadly into (1) aspiration thrombectomy catheters that remove the thrombus by steady manual suction through a large-lumen aspiration catheter; (2) pull-back thrombectomy catheters that withdraw the thrombus with a balloon catheter or basket into a trapping device, allowing the clot to be removed; (3) recirculation thrombectomy devices that ablate the thrombus by hydrodynamic vortices, which pulverize the thrombus into microscopic fragments; (4) nonrecirculation thrombectomy devices, which macerate the thrombus mechanically into fragments that are larger than those produced by recirculation catheters; and (5) energy-assisted devices that use ultrasound, laser, or radiofrequency to lyse the thrombus or enhance the effects of pharmacologic agents.[106] Several of these devices are currently being evaluated clinically, with complete angiographic success reported in approximately 50% of patients and partial success in an additional 27%.[107] Concomitant lytic therapy or balloon angioplasty is often a necessary adjunct. The most extensively studied device is the AngioJet rheolytic thrombectomy system, which is approved for peripheral arterial and coronary applications.[108] Chief limitations of the current devices include catheter size and working length, the possibility of fluid overload, hemolysis, and cost effectiveness. The major treatment limitation of these devices is their lack of efficacy against organized thrombotic or embolic material.[76,77,109]

Atheroembolism

Preoperative Embolism

Atherothrombotic debris is present to varying degrees in most atherosclerotic arteries but especially in the distal aorta. Protruding atheromas of the aortic arch and descending aorta have assumed increasing importance as potential sites for embolization during catheter manipulation in the aorta for cardiac catheterization, carotid stenting placement of thoracic endografts, or bypass surgery.[110] Embolization may also occur spontaneously or with the use of anticoagulants and thrombolytic therapy.[111] Readily detectable by transesophageal echocardiography, lesions greater than 0.5 cm are most likely to be associated with embolic events.[112,113] Evidence of spontaneous embolization has also been demonstrated at autopsy studies, but the incidence appears to be low (0.3% to 0.7%).[114,115] The effects of spontaneous embolization may be exacerbated by dislodgement of atheromatous debris during intraoperative manipulations.

Intraoperative Embolism

Variable amounts of atherothrombotic material may be dislodged and carried to a downstream territory as a consequence of manipulation during arterial dissection and clamp placement.[36,94,95] After cardiac operative procedures, 66% of emboli lodge in the gastrointestinal (GI) tract and 48% lodge in the kidneys. Visceral embolization occurs in 40.9% of patients undergoing aortic reconstruction with the "shaggy" aorta syndrome.[116] Embolization may also occur on reestablishment of circulation as a result of the accumulation of fresh thrombus in the temporarily static column of blood above or below the clamps if it is not carefully evacuated before circulation is restored. In the immediate postoperative period, atheroembolism should be suspected if the blotchy areas of discoloration of the skin of the abdominal wall and extremities and toes and impaired renal function do not improve with warming and optimization of cardiac output. A nonspecific systemic response characterized by fever, eosinophilia, elevated erythrocyte sedimentation rate (ESR), and highly specific C-reactive protein (hsCRP) may accompany an embolic episode.

Larger emboli lodging in major vessels can usually be retrieved with a balloon thrombectomy catheter. Smaller embolic particles that cannot be retrieved will be flushed into end arteries of the feet or toes, leading to the "trash foot" syndrome.[6,51,113,117] The end result is the appearance of patchy areas of painful skin gangrene at these sites (Fig. 60.9). This may be a minor and self-limited problem, or it may produce extensive gangrene of all the digits and the forefoot, leg, buttocks, and rarely the abdominal wall.

Prevention is key because it is frequently difficult or impossible to treat this complication. Careful review of preoperative imaging studies will determine the site of clamp placement. A variety of technical maneuvers has been used to prevent or minimize operative embolization.[6] Unnecessary and overly vigorous handling of vessels before the application of clamps should be avoided. Effective preclamping heparinization, monitored by intraoperative measurement of the ACT, reduces stasis thrombus formation above the proximal clamp and in the sluggish circulation distally. In patients with suspected or demonstrable atheromatous debris within the aorta on CT scans, the distal clamps should be applied to the common femoral or iliac arteries before proximal occlusion to avoid downstream displacement of debris when the aortic clamp is placed. The proximal clamp may need to be placed at the level of the diaphragm if the pararenal segment

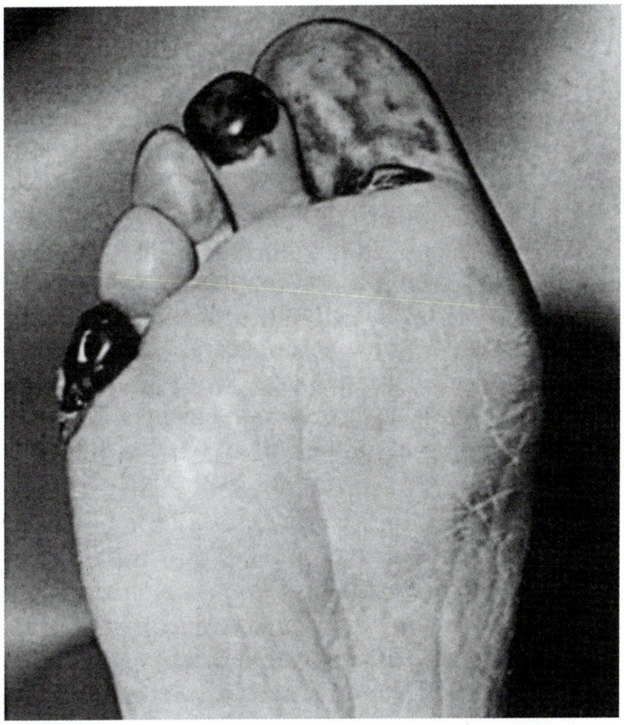

FIG 60.9 Atheroembolic ischemic lesions of the toes. (From Eastcott HHG: Complication of aortoiliac reconstruction for occlusive disease. In Bernhard VM, Towne JB, editors: *Complications in vascular surgery*, New York, 1980, Grune and Stratton, p 59.)

of the aorta appears to be involved. The lumen of the aortic prosthesis should be thoroughly aspirated to remove blood and debris after testing the proximal suture line, and efforts should be made to prevent the accumulation of blood within the prosthesis while distal iliac or femoral anastomoses are being performed. Vigorous antegrade flushing of the proximal vessel and retrograde flushing from the distal arteries as the last few stitches are being placed in an anastomosis, before the restoration of circulation, is the most reliable maneuver to ensure that retained debris and clot are effectively removed.[117]

Treatment depends on the severity of embolization. Minor patchy areas of cyanosis or necrosis can be observed, with spontaneous recovery anticipated. More extensive involvement with threatened viability of the distal foot requires attempted removal of embolic material with small Fogarty balloon catheters passed into the distal vessels through the patent popliteal artery. Distal intraarterial infusion of r-tPA may be applicable in selected patients. Occasionally, when there is severe ischemia of a single or multiple digits, lumbar sympathectomy or amputation may be necessary. Low-dose corticosteroids may offer short-term benefit in patients with acute or subacute renal failure with systemic symptoms but have no favorable effect on long-term renal outcome.[118,119] Statins, which stabilize atherosclerotic plaques and potentially improve outcomes, should be offered to all patients. Whether intensive lipid-lowering statin therapy for 3 to 6 months before surgery in patients at known risk of embolization will prove beneficial is presently unknown.[120]

Declamping Hypotension

A sudden decrease in blood pressure should be anticipated after removal of the aortic clamp to restore flow to one or both extremities after aortoiliac reconstruction.[121-124] The cause is hypovolemia resulting from incompletely replaced blood loss and fluid sequestration during surgery, compounded by a variable degree of preoperative dehydration that is usually present.[125] Contributing factors are peripheral vasodilatation secondary to limb ischemia during the period of aortic occlusion and a decrease in cardiac output caused by a sudden return of acidic blood and other vasoactive metabolites to the central circulation on restoration of limb perfusion. The major consequences are significant reduction in coronary perfusion, which may promote myocardial injury, especially in patients with significant coronary artery disease, and temporary renal ischemia, which may contribute to renal failure. Prevention is preferable to treatment after a hypotensive insult has already occurred and depends on adequate hydration and effective restoration of intravascular volume during the procedure, and especially before clamp release.[123-125] Effective volume replacement requires careful monitoring of blood loss and accurate estimation of the extracellular fluid shifts caused by sequestration and loss from evaporation. The extent of intravascular depletion is directly related to the duration of intraperitoneal and retroperitoneal exposure during surgery.

The most reliable guide to ensuring adequate volume replacement without circulatory overload is the use of a Swan-Ganz catheter to monitor left-heart filling pressures and myocardial performance.[125] Cooperation between the surgeon and the anesthesiologist is essential during the critical moments before clamp release. Left atrial filling pressures should be optimized before release of the clamps. The arterial pressure must be continuously observed while blood flow is slowly restored to the extremities by gradual release of the clamps until full flow can be tolerated without hypotension. Finally, when a bifurcated graft is inserted, it is best to complete the anastomosis to one limb and restore its circulation immediately so that lower body perfusion can be resumed with the least amount of delay; this avoids washout acidosis and reduces declamping hypotension.

Acute Renal Failure

Renal impairment in patients undergoing abdominal aortic surgery is an important cause of morbidity and mortality and can range in severity from acute renal injury (ARI) to acute renal failure (ARF). Acute renal injury, manifested by the occurrence of albuminuria (93%) and proteinuria (22%) in patients undergoing aortic surgery, is the mildest form of impairment. Albuminuria usually occurs before cross-clamping and peaks between 0 and 6 hours after declamping. Acute renal dysfunction according to the RIFLE criteria (risk, injury, failure, loss of renal function, and end-stage renal disease), defined as an increase in serum creatinine (sCR) of 50% from baseline or oliguria of less than 0.5 mL/kg per hour for 6 hours, may progress to acute renal failure, which manifests as a 200% increase in sCR and oliguria of less than 0.5 mL/kg per hour for 24 hours or anuria.[126]

The reported incidence of ARF after elective aortic aneurysmectomy is 1% to 8%, with a mortality rate of 40%. However, if the aneurysmectomy is emergent, the reported incidence of ARF is 8% to 46%, with a mortality of 57% to 95%.[127,128] A more recent study by Siracuse and colleagues reported the incidence of acute renal failure following open repair of ruptured AAA to be 17.3%.[129] The major cause of ARI is reduced renal perfusion resulting from decreased cardiac output, decreased blood volume, and dehydration. A contributing factor is renal cortical vasospasm produced by infrarenal application of the aortic clamp, which stimulates the renin-angiotensin mechanism.[130,131] Other promoting factors include: underlying renal artery stenosis; suprarenal aortic cross-clamping (which totally eliminates renal perfusion); ischemia reperfusion injury; ligation of the left renal vein; intraoperative embolization; older age; hypertension; and drugs such as diuretics, β-blockers, calcium antagonists, nephrotoxic antibiotics, nonsteroidal antiinflammatory drugs, cyclooxygenase 2, and angiotensin-converting enzyme inhibitors.[132] Cholesterol embolization to the kidneys may originate from debris and clot accumulating proximal to the aortic clamp or from manipulation of the juxtarenal aorta.[128,133] Preoperative contrast (CTA, DSA) and endovascular catheter manipulations may produce a mild to moderate degree of renal dysfunction, which can be compounded by blood loss, hypotension, and dehydration during the operative procedure. Renal artery obstruction may be produced by displacement of large atherosclerotic plaques, thrombus, or dissection at the orifices of the renal arteries when an aortic clamp is applied. Myoglobinemia can occur after restoration of circulation to limbs that have been severely ischemic for an extended period. Finally intraabdominal hypertension resulting in ICS, especially in patients with ruptured aneurysms, must be considered.

Although the consequences of ischemic injury to the kidney are complex, injury to the tubules, especially the S3 segment of the proximal tubule and the thick ascending limb of the loop of Henle, is central to the development of oliguria.[134] Obstruction of the tubular lumen by cellular debris and casts results in a reduction of the ultrafiltration pressure and sequestration of tubular fluid within obstructed tubules, in addition to back-leakage of fluid into the interstitium.[135]

The critical issue in ARF is prevention, which is related primarily to the maintenance of an effective circulating blood volume and adequate hydration in the immediate perioperative period.[128,136] It is essential that the patient be well hydrated and have a good urinary output at the commencement of surgery. Any significant extracellular fluid volume deficits should be restored the evening before surgery, especially if CTA, DSA, or mechanical bowel preparation has recently been performed. The sCR level should be measured after procedures requiring contrast administration, and if a decrease in renal function is identified, surgery should be delayed, if possible. Central filling pressures should be monitored perioperatively to ensure that volume replacement is optimal in relation to cardiac output and myocardial performance.[125] It is appropriate to give mannitol and commence an infusion of renal-dose dopamine (2 to 3 μg/kg) just before cross-clamping the aorta to promote an osmotic diuresis and reduce the effects of renal cortical vasospasm.[130] Bicarbonate is given to alkalinize the urine if there is any question of significant contrast-related nephrotoxicity or myoglobin washout from renewed perfusion of limbs that have undergone prolonged ischemia. Renal insufficiency is a significant complication of surgical procedures requiring cross-clamping of the thoracic or suprarenal aorta. Currently, a number of therapeutic maneuvers including preoperative statins, *N*-acetylcysteine, heme-oxygenase, ischemic preconditioning, fluid loading, renal cooling, calcium-channel blockers, atrial natriuretic peptide, endothelin antagonist, and fenoldopam are being evaluated in cardiac patients to determine their efficacy in reducing the incidence of ARF. The data regarding renal protection in vascular surgery patients are conflicting and have been extrapolated primarily from patients undergoing cardiac surgery procedures.[137-143]

During dissection required to gain proximal control of large infrarenal or juxtarenal aneurysms, the left renal vein and its branches are vulnerable to injury. Access to this portion of the aorta is facilitated by division of the left renal vein close to its origin from the IVC, thus preserving the tributaries and reducing renal venous congestion if the vein cannot be re-approximated at the completion of the aortic anastomosis.[144] In the past, this maneuver was viewed as one of little long-term consequence. However, Huber and coworkers[145] and Abu Rahma and associates[146] demonstrated increased sCR concentrations in patients who had renal vein ligation. Whether the renal dysfunction after renal vein ligation is solely a consequence of the resultant increased venous pressure or develops from a combination of venous hypertension and transient ischemia from intraoperative suprarenal clamp placement, which is required more frequently than with infrarenal clamp placement (11% vs. 18%), is not yet clear. Nonetheless, it is prudent to repair the renal vein if there is congestion of the left kidney and reanastomosis can be accomplished without undue tension or prolongation of the procedure.[1,144,147,148]

Renal arteries should be dissected free and temporarily clamped in patients with aortic occlusion and thrombus that extends up to the renal orifices. The quality of the renal pulses must be evaluated and the blood flow assessed by Doppler color-flow imaging after restoration of circulation through the aorta in any patient who has had significant juxtarenal aortic manipulation.

Postoperatively, the continued retroperitoneal and intraperitoneal sequestration of extracellular fluid requires replacement with lactated Ringer solution, within the limits imposed by left-heart filling pressures, to ensure adequate renal output.[24] Volume replacement should be reduced after the second postoperative day to prevent fluid overload from the mobilization of large volumes of sequestered extravascular fluid. The urinary output is monitored continuously and should be maintained at or above 0.5 mL/kg per hour. The specific gravity is determined frequently, and the blood urea nitrogen and sCR are measured daily for 2 or 3 days to determine the quality of renal function. Diuretics should not be given until intravascular volume has been fully restored. A rise in sCR, the standard marker used to detect ARF, does not allow for the early diagnosis of ARI because of a lack of specificity for ARI; poor correlation with glomerular filtration rate; and the influence of age, sex, body mass index, hydration, and nutrition. Several biomarkers are currently being investigated in patients undergoing cardiac surgery to improve the detection of early renal dysfunction. Cystatin C, kidney injury molecule-1 (KIM-1), *N*-acetyl β-D-glucosaminidase (NAG), and neutrophil gelatinase–associated lipocalin (NGAL) are among the early detectable biomarkers in the serum and urine of patients with ARI. However, correlation of individual markers with glomerular filtration rate is variable, and a combination of markers may be required to improve the sensitivity of these molecules in the early diagnosis of ARI.[126,149] At the onset of ARF, urinary specific gravity increases (>1.015) and sodium and urea decrease. Once tubular necrosis occurs, the urine becomes isosthenuric; the urinary sodium, fractional excretion of sodium, and urea increase to greater than 20 mml/L, greater than 1%, and greater than 35%, respectively; and the ratio of blood urea nitrogen (BUN)-to-creatinine ratio falls from 20:1 to 10:1.[134] If ARF is diagnosed, fluid replacement should be restricted to maintain central filling pressure in the normal range. Dialysis is used aggressively to control excess volume and relieve azotemia and hyperkalemia.[128,150] Intravenous hyperalimentation or parenteral nutrition should be instituted early in the clinical course of patients with ARF to minimize protein catabolism.[151]

Renal artery stenosis or impaired renal function is frequently present in patients undergoing aortic reconstruction for occlusive and aneurysmal disease. The liberal use of CTA, MRA, and DSA before surgery is recommended to identify renal anomalies, renal artery stenoses, or suprarenal extension of an aneurysm so that appropriate alterations in operative management can be planned. Often, renal revascularization can be accomplished by balloon angioplasty and stenting, along with operative or endovascular correction of the aortic disease. In this setting, patients often have impaired renal function, and the large volume of contrast agents used for imaging studies or intervention may result in additional nephrotoxicity. The preoperative administration of *N*-acetylcysteine has been shown to reduce contrast-related ARF from 12% to 2% to 4%.[152,153] A cautionary note regarding the use of *N*-acetylcysteine in the immediate perioperative period: Wijeysundera and coworkers have shown that its use is associated with greater transfusion requirements in patients undergoing cardiac surgery procedures.[139] Additional maneuvers to reduce the risk of renal ischemia include the use of temporary renal perfusion with cold lactated Ringer solution containing heparin, mannitol, and methylprednisolone.[128] Postoperatively, a renal perfusion scan or aortography should be performed immediately if total renal shutdown occurs because this suggests a renal artery occlusion. This requires immediate reoperation to restore kidney circulation. The use of statins in the early postoperative period has been shown to lower the incidence of AKI in cardiac surgery patients. Welten and associates, in a study of 2170 patients undergoing lower extremity bypass or abdominal aortic surgery, demonstrated that early statin use increased the odds of recovery if renal function deteriorated postoperatively.[154,155] In addition, statin use was also associated with improved long-term survival irrespective of changes in renal function.

Intestinal Ischemia

Intestinal ischemia may complicate aortic bypass or endarterectomy for occlusive disease, but the majority of cases involve the colon and follow aneurysmectomy.[156,157] Almost all reported instances of intestinal ischemia following aortic surgery are a result of arterial obstruction or hypotension; venous ischemia is extremely rare.[158] Small bowel ischemia occurs in 0.15% of cases.[156] The clinical presentation of ischemic colitis occurs in 0.2% to 10% of aortic procedures and most commonly involves the rectosigmoid area.[156] Data from the Swedish Vascular Registry showed a frequency of transmural colon necrosis of 7.3% and 2.8% in patients undergoing repair of ruptured AAA with and without preoperative hypotension; 23% of deaths were associated with colonic ischemia. The overall mortality rate for patients with colon ischemia is approximately 50% and approaches 90% for transmural colon involvement.[159,160]

The cause of bowel ischemia is interruption of the primary or collateral arteries to the bowel wall or operative atheroembolization.[156,157] Two sets of vessels are critical to colon perfusion: (1) the inferior mesenteric artery and its left colic branch, which connect with the superior mesenteric artery through the arc of Riolan and, to a lesser extent, the marginal artery of Drummond, and (2) the superior rectal branch of the inferior mesenteric artery, which connects with the middle and inferior rectal branches of the hypogastric vessels, thus connecting the visceral and systemic circulations.[161] The former connection is referred to as the "meandering mesenteric artery," especially when it becomes enlarged as a collateral to compensate for superior or inferior mesenteric artery obstruction.[162] This vessel is present in approximately two-thirds of healthy people and can be seen on angiography in 27% to 35% of patients who have aneurysmal or occlusive disease.[163] Areas of deficiency in this normal anatomic relationship are at Griffith's point at the splenic flexure and in the collateral vessels of the rectosigmoid (Fig. 60.10).

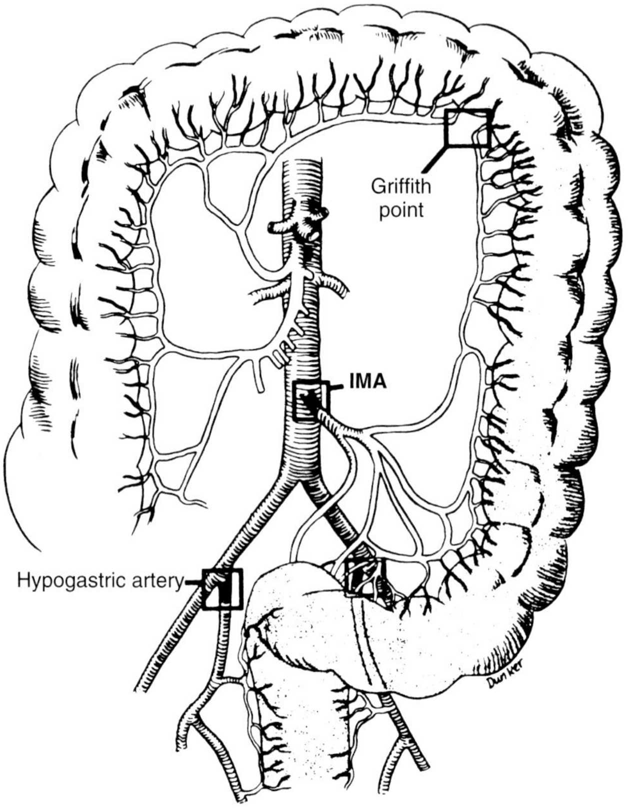

FIG 60.10 Lack of marginal artery continuity at the splenic flexure (Griffith point), with inferior mesenteric artery *(IMA)* and hypogastric artery occlusions predisposing to left colon ischemia. (From Ernst CB: Colon ischemia following abdominal aortic reconstruction. In Bernhard VM, Towne JB, editors: *Complications in vascular surgery*, New York, 1980, Grune and Stratton, p 383.)

Obstruction of the primary arteries supplying the viscera makes viability of the bowel dependent on this collateral circulation. Occlusion of the orifice of the inferior mesenteric artery is frequently associated with aneurysmal disease and obstructive aortic atherosclerosis, thus placing the burden of bowel circulation on collaterals from the superior mesenteric artery and the hypogastric vessels. Severe obstruction or occlusion of the superior mesenteric artery is compensated for by branches from the celiac artery and retrograde flow from the inferior mesenteric artery through the left colic and middle colic arteries. Hypogastric obstruction requires collateral flow from branches of the inferior mesenteric artery. When this source is also impaired, colon circulation must depend on more tenuous connections between the arch of Riolan and the marginal artery and the distal branches of the hypogastric, which in turn take their blood supply from the parietal circulation.

A critical loss of blood flow to an intestinal tract that is dependent on this extensive collateral network may occur if a patent inferior mesenteric artery is ligated during aortic surgery. Collateral flow may be further compromised by ligating the inferior mesenteric artery peripherally rather than flush with the aortic wall because this may occlude the connection between the left colic and superior rectal arteries. Failure to ensure perfusion

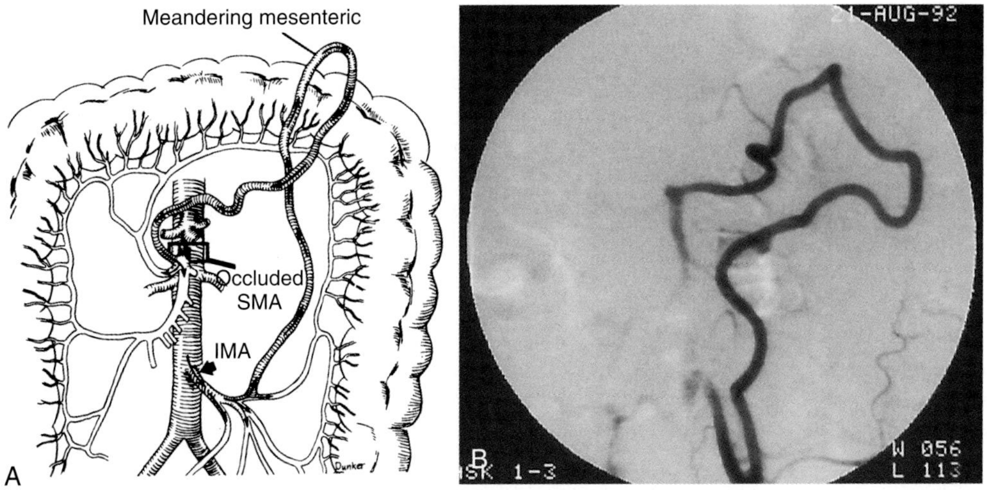

FIG 60.11 (A) When the superior mesenteric artery *(SMA)* is occluded, meandering mesenteric blood flow is from the inferior mesenteric artery *(IMA)* to the SMA. Meandering mesenteric sacrifice under these conditions predisposes to small bowel and colon ischemia. (B) Selective visceral angiogram demonstrating a meandering mesenteric artery. ([A] From Ernst CB: Colon ischemia following abdominal aortic reconstruction. In Bernhard VM, Towne JB, editors: *Complications in vascular surgery,* New York, 1980, Grune and Stratton, p 385.)

through at least one hypogastric may promote colon ischemia if this is the primary supply in the absence of the inferior mesenteric artery or effective collateral flow from the meandering artery. Loss of the inferior mesenteric artery or the meandering artery produces right colon and small bowel ischemia when these viscera depend on retrograde flow because of superior mesenteric arterial occlusion (Fig. 60.11). The large hematoma associated with a ruptured aneurysm may compress significant collateral vessels, which may explain the high incidence of colon ischemia in this circumstance.[156] Furthermore, angiography is almost never available before repair of a ruptured aneurysm, and the surgeon has no precise information regarding intestinal circulation to allow the design of an operative procedure that will conserve or augment colon perfusion. Prolonged hypotension and the use of vasopressors may exacerbate the effects of preexisting occlusive disease. Recently, Djavani and coworkers demonstrated a correlation between ICS and colonic hypoperfusion in patients with ruptured AAA.[164] A relatively unrecognized cause of mesenteric ischemia is cardiopulmonary bypass. Abdominal complications after coronary artery bypass occur in less than 1% of patients. Acute mesenteric ischemia accounts for 10% to 67% of these complications, with mortality rates of 70% to 100%.[165] Preexisting visceral occlusive disease, cardiac or aortic arch embolization, use of an intraaortic balloon, postoperative renal failure, female gender, duration of cardiopulmonary bypass, and cross-clamp times are important contributing factors.[166]

Depending on the severity of ischemia and the thickness of the bowel wall involved, three forms of ischemic colitis are recognized. Type I is mucosal ischemia, which is transient and mild. Type II, with mucosal and muscularis involvement, reflects more severe ischemia that may result in healing with fibrosis, scarring, and stricture. Type III is transmural ischemia, which produces irreparable damage with gangrene and bowel perforation.[167]

The clinical manifestations of intestinal ischemia immediately after aortic surgery are often masked by incisional discomfort and other problems that may explain abdominal pain, tenderness, fever, an elevated white blood cell count, and fluid sequestration. Findings that suggest the presence of intestinal ischemia and progressing infarction of the colon include progressive distention, sepsis, increasing peritoneal signs, and unexplained metabolic acidosis. The most common clinical presentation is diarrhea—either brown liquid or bloody—which occurs in 65% to 76% of patients with intestinal ischemia.[161,168] Although the onset may occur as long as 14 days after operation, diarrhea usually appears within 24 to 48 hours after surgery.[161] Bloody diarrhea has been reported to be a more ominous prognostic sign than nonbloody diarrhea; however, some investigators have noted no correlation between the extent of ischemic injury and the presence of bloody diarrhea.[169]

Postoperative *Clostridium difficile* colitis may mimic ischemic colitis. Therefore, in critically ill patients who develop fever, abdominal distension, diarrhea, and leukocytosis after emergency aortic procedures, stool specimens for culture and for *C. difficile* toxin should be obtained and endoscopic evaluation of the colon performed. Real-time polymerase chain reaction (PCR) assay to detect the *C. difficile* gene toxin confirms the diagnosis more rapidly than stool culture. Appropriate oral antibiotic therapy (metronidazole or vancomycin) should be instituted if the diagnosis of *C. difficile* is confirmed.[170,171]

Because of the high mortality rate associated with transmural colonic ischemia (80% to 100%), early diagnosis is the key to effective management. The diagnosis depends on a high index of suspicion and the prompt performance of endoscopy with the flexible sigmoidoscope or colonoscope.[170] In a prospective study of 100 patients undergoing aortic reconstructive procedures, Zelenock and associates[172] observed a 3% incidence of endoscopic colonic ischemia. Adjunctive procedures were used in 12% of these patients, compared with 4% in earlier studies from their institution. Sigmoid colon pH monitoring begun before surgery and continued postoperatively has been used with some success by Björck and Hedberg to identify patients at risk for ischemic colitis.[173] They found that a sigmoid colon pH below 6.86 for 9 to 12 hours had a sensitivity of 100% and a specificity of 97% for predicting ischemic colitis. When sigmoid colon acidosis below 7.10 pH was reversed within 2 hours, no major complications developed, but when it was prolonged, 8 of 10 patients developed major complications. Further evaluation of sigmoid colon pH monitoring appears warranted before its widespread application. The occurrence of ischemic colitis without left colon involvement is rare enough that endoscopy to 40 cm is usually sufficient to establish the diagnosis.[156] Once ischemic colitis is detected, endoscopy should be terminated to avoid perforation. Mild changes of ischemic colitis consist of submucosal hemorrhage and edema that is usually circumferential. Pseudomembranes, erosions, and ulcers indicate more advanced ischemia. A yellowish-green, necrotic, noncontractile surface indicates gangrene.[161] Repeated endoscopy, every other day by the same individual, is required to document resolution or progression of the process. In a recent report, Acosta and colleagues demonstrated elevated D-dimer concentrations in patients with acute mesenteric ischemia.[174] This elevation was especially helpful in female patients with atrial fibrillation. Wider application of this test to other causes of acute mesenteric ischemia awaits validation.

Patients under observation for intestinal ischemia are managed by frequent reexamination; serial endoscopy; sigmoid colon and gastric intramucosal pH monitoring; monitoring of blood gases and serum lactate levels, white blood cells and D-dimers, urine output, and fluid requirements; institution of broad-spectrum antibiotic coverage; and bowel rest with nasogastric suction. Intramucosal pH measurements are not readily available and serial endoscopy may result in bowel perforation. Plain radiographs may demonstrate a nonspecific ileus, dilated loops of bowel, or thumb printing; intramural or portal vein gas are rarely seen and usually indicate late-stage disease. Computed tomography scans may show vascular occlusion, intramural gas, free air or intraperitoneal fluid, and infarcts in the kidneys, liver, and spleen (Fig. 60.12). CTA is also helpful in diagnosing nonocclusive mesenteric ischemia. If the colon appears distended, either clinically or radiographically, it should be decompressed by the gentle insertion of a rectal tube because increased intraluminal pressure may further compromise colon blood flow.[161,173] If sustained IAH is present (intraabdominal pressure >20 mm Hg), the patient should be treated with muscle relaxants or abdominal decompression. Optimum fluid management remains controversial. Balogh and colleagues compared two different fluid regimes in trauma patients (500 mL and 600 mL/minute per m^2) and concluded that overaggressive resuscitation doubled the risk of IAH, ICS, organ dysfunction, and death. Although no similar studies have been done in patients with ruptured AAA, there is some evidence that resuscitation with large volumes of isotonic crystalloids increases the risk of complications.

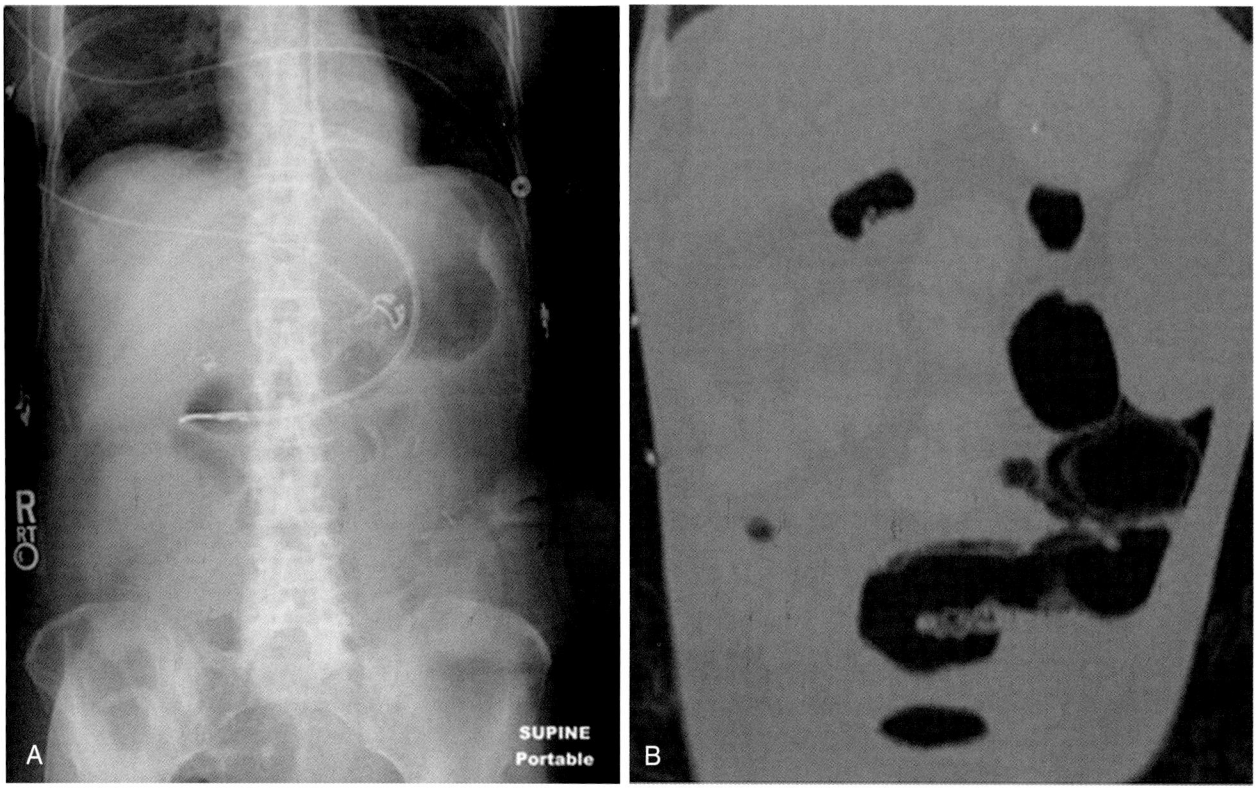

FIG 60.12 (A) Plain abdominal radiograph showing air in the wall of the colon. (B) Computed tomography scan showing dilatation of the sigmoid colon and edema of the bowel wall, which is characteristic of colonic ischemia.

Improvement of the patient, as evidenced by diminishing diarrhea, improvement in vital signs, clinical examination, laboratory values, and resolution of the ischemia documented by endoscopy, permits continuation of nonoperative management.[156] Reversible ischemic lesions should improve within 7 to 10 days.[167,175] Continuing clinical evidence of ischemia beyond 2 weeks requires operative intervention because this usually reflects a walled-off perforation with local peritonitis.[161] Finally, progression of intestinal ischemia during the period of observation, identified by deteriorating clinical signs and symptoms, requires prompt celiotomy. Surgery for transmural ischemic colitis requires resection of nonviable bowel, end-colostomy, and formation of a Hartmann pouch or resection of the rectum, if involved.[176]

Prevention of intestinal ischemia depends on an appreciation of the potential for this complication and the institution of appropriate steps to either avoid injury to the collateral circulation of the colon or augment circulation to the bowel as part of the aortic reconstructive procedure.[177] Spiral CTA or MRA is frequently used preoperatively to evaluate the abdominal aorta and its visceral branches. This technique permits multiple views of complex aortic lesions, reflects the true diameter of aortic aneurysms, and may alleviate the need for angiography.[178,179] Identification of a patent inferior mesenteric artery with retrograde flow through a large meandering artery that is functioning as a collateral pathway for an obstructed superior mesenteric artery requires preservation of flow through the inferior mesenteric; this orifice is spared by constructing an end-to-side aortic anastomosis or by reimplanting the inferior mesenteric onto the side of an aortic graft using a variation of the Carrel patch technique.[156]

Bypass to the superior mesenteric artery should also be considered.[177] A large, meandering artery with flow from the superior mesenteric toward the sigmoid and rectum in the presence of inferior mesenteric artery occlusion is strong evidence of adequate collateral supply to the bowel.[162] Ischemic colitis is unlikely under these circumstances if this collateral is not impaired by surgery. The status of the hypogastric vessels should be identified on the aortogram or other imaging study so that arterial reconstruction can be designed to maintain flow through at least one of these arteries by direct revascularization or by retrograde perfusion from a femoral anastomosis, especially if a patent inferior mesenteric artery must be ligated.[175]

Measurement of the inferior mesenteric artery backpressure during aortic reconstruction may be a useful guide to the need for restoration of flow to the inferior mesenteric artery.[175] A mean pressure greater than 40 mm Hg and an inferior mesenteric artery–systemic pressure ratio greater than 0.4 indicate satisfactory collateral circulation without the need for mesenteric arterial repair.

Intraoperative duplex ultrasonography in patients undergoing visceral artery repair allows prompt correction of underlying technical defects.[180]

Thorough mechanical preparation of the bowel before aortic surgery reduces the fecal burden to which the potentially ischemic bowel is exposed.[156] During aortic surgery, every effort should be made to prevent injury to the mesenteric vessels. Undue traction on the left colon mesentery should be avoided. When inferior mesenteric ligation is required, this should be carried out by suture ligature within the aortic lumen or immediately adjacent to the aortic wall to avoid injury to its ascending and descending branches.[156] Finally, the presence of Doppler flow signals over the base of the bowel mesentery and the serosal surface of the colon suggests that adequate collateral circulation is present.[168] Absence of a flow signal after reconstruction suggests the need to restore perfusion through the inferior mesenteric artery or through some other major collateral vessel. The association of severe visceral and aortic occlusive disease in younger female patients is accompanied by high mortality and morbidity rates. The severe weight loss resulting from celiac and superior mesenteric artery occlusive lesions makes complete revascularization a hazardous undertaking. In these individuals, a combination of endovascular treatment of the visceral occlusive disease before aortic revascularization may decrease the early morbidity and mortality rates, and improve long-term survival.[181]

Gastrointestinal Complications

Gastrointestinal complications occur in 6% to 21% of patients undergoing elective procedures and in 27% of those undergoing emergent aortic procedures. This complication is associated with a prolonged ICU stay and increased mortality (48%) from multisystem organ failure. Paralytic ileus, mechanical small bowel and duodenal obstruction, acute pancreatitis, upper GI bleeding, *C. difficile* enterocolitis, acute cholecystitis, chylous ascites, colonic and rectal ischemia, and liver failure are among the GI complications described. This discussion will be limited to paralytic ileus and mechanical small bowel and duodenal obstruction, the most common problems encountered. The increase in intraoperative blood loss and postoperative fluid requirements associated with these complications accounts for the prolonged requirement for mechanical ventilation and the occurrence of renal failure. Intraoperative hypotension, gastric hyperacidity, visceral embolization, hematoma, sac seroma, superior mesenteric artery syndrome, bowel wall edema, adhesions, and a compromised collateral blood supply are among the etiologic factors contributing to the development of GI complications after aortic surgery. Paralytic ileus is the most common cause of delayed return of small bowel function after abdominal aortic procedures. Small bowel obstruction (SBO) is reported to occur in approximately 2.9% of patients undergoing aortic reconstruction for AAA ($n = 818$) or occlusive ($n = 657$) disease within 4 to 28 (mean, 6) days postoperatively. The incidence of SBO after aortic surgery is much lower than the 9.5% reported after nonvascular abdominal operations, although almost 50% of the patients reported by Ellozy had undergone a previous abdominal operation. Duodenal obstruction after AAA repair is rare, with only 16 cases reported in the English literature. The presentation is often delayed, with symptoms occurring 8 to 60 days (mean, 13.3) postoperatively. Surgeons must maintain a high level of suspicion to anticipate possible GI complications. Symptoms include increased nasogastric tube output, nausea, bilious vomiting, abdominal pain, distension, hematemesis, hematochezia, diarrhea, fever, leukocytosis, and a decrease in hematocrit level. Diagnostic tests should include plain abdominal and chest radiographs; CT scanning; upper GI endoscopy; and laboratory monitoring of hemoglobin, hematocrit, white blood cells, amylase and lipase, BUN, sCR, and electrolytes. Early postoperative SBO requiring surgical intervention carries significant morbidity, including abdominal and wound sepsis, fistula formation, wound disruption, and persistent obstruction. Therefore, a 1- to 2-week trial of conservative therapy in these patients is reasonable. Patients with obstruction lasting longer than 2 weeks almost always require operative relief of the obstruction.

Fluid and electrolytes should be replaced, a nasogastric tube reinserted, and nutrition provided. In the series reported by Siporin and colleagues, 18 of 44 (41%) patients with SBO required reoperation (lysis of adhesions, 18; bowel resection, 2) within 6 to 30 days (mean, 14.2) of the initial aortic procedure, whereas only 13% of the nonvascular patients required reexploration: one required small-bowel resection.[182-187] Conservative treatment with nasogastric decompression is recommended in all patients initially in the absence of bowel ischemia or perforation. Operative relief of the obstruction is indicated in patients with obstruction lasting longer than 2 weeks or if complications ensue. The mortality rate ranges from 0% to 5%. There were no bowel infarctions, small bowel fistulas, or late graft infections in the aortic patients undergoing laparotomy for bowel obstruction.

Abdominal Compartment Syndrome

ICS is defined as an increase in intraabdominal pressure (IAP) greater than atmospheric pressure (IAP >20 mm Hg or bladder pressure >30 mm Hg) with the new onset of organ dysfunction. In vascular patients, ICS is most commonly encountered with intraperitoneal or contained retroperitoneal AAA rupture after open surgery or EVAR. In a recent analysis of 73 patients undergoing both open repair and EVAR for ruptured AAA, the incidence of ICS was 29%. Mortality was higher in patients who developed ICS (62% vs. 33%, $P = .022$). The morbidity of ICS following EVAR for rAAA was especially pronounced (83% vs. 17%, $P = .05$).[188]

Sometimes ICS may occur after mesenteric revascularization for ischemic bowel or massive retroperitoneal bleeding in patients on anticoagulants. The increase in intraabdominal pressure is exacerbated by massive fluid resuscitation and positive end-expiratory pressure ventilation (PEEP). Physiologically, an increase in IAP causes elevation of the diaphragm, resulting in a decrease in lung capacity and compliance and respiratory compromise. The associated decrease in venous return, compounded by hypotension, reduces cardiac output and increases peripheral resistance, resulting in impaired renal, hepatic, and mesenteric perfusion; an increase in bacterial translocation from the gut; and raised intracranial pressure, which, if uncorrected, results in the increased morbidity and mortality in these patients. Ischemia of the abdominal wall results in edema and decreased compliance, further exacerbating the effects of ICS. Direct measurement of IAP is possible but increases the risk of infection. The indirect method requires emptying the bladder and instilling 50 to 150 mL of saline; the drainage tubing is clamped and a needle attached to the pressure transducer is inserted above the clamp and the pressure determined. If the bladder pressure exceeds 20 mm Hg, the pressure should be monitored hourly. A bladder pressure of greater than 30 mm Hg is diagnostic of ICS.

In patients at high risk for postoperative ICS, leaving an open abdomen (OA) at the completion of the initial surgery should be considered. Several options including suture or sequential towel clip closure of the skin; use of a Bogota bag silo; fascial interposition of an absorbable, biological, or nonabsorbable mesh; and use of a vacuum pack or wound vac dressing are available to manage the OA. A short course of a neuromuscular blocking agent may decrease fascial edge retraction and be a useful adjunct to negative pressure devices and conservative measures. Neuromuscular blockade decreases IAP; however, once the paralysis wears off, the IAP returns to baseline levels. Once ICS is diagnosed, decompressive laparotomy and creation of an OA as outlined above is undertaken. Patients with an acute increase in IAP (25 mm Hg) without acute organ dysfunction should also be considered for prophylactic decompressive laparotomy. Postoperatively, efforts should be focused on correcting the oxygen and energy debt, hypothermia, and coagulopathy. As the visceral edema resolves, the abdomen is closed either primarily or with biological or nonabsorbable mesh. The survival of patients with ruptured AAA treated with OA and delayed fascial closure is 50% compared with 27% when the fascia is closed primarily.[164,189,190] Djavani and associates reported 0% mortality and 0% left colon ischemia in patients with rAAA and normal IAPs compared with 22% and 44%, respectively, when the IAP was greater than 21 mm Hg.[164] Patients reoperated for ICS had a mortality rate of 84%.[191]

Abdominal Wall Hernias

The relationship between AAA and abdominal wall hernias (AWHs) is well recognized. However, the prevalence of AAA in patients undergoing inguinal hernia repair remains controversial. In a study of men older than 55 years of age undergoing inguinal hernia repair, Antoniou and colleagues[192] detected AAA in 8.1% in the hernia group and 3.9% in controls. In subjects with aortic diameters greater than 4.0 cm, the prevalence was 5.1% in the hernia group compared with 1.5% in those without inguinal hernias. In contrast, Andersen and Shiralkar detected only two AAAs (3%) in a prospective evaluation of 70 men older than 65 years undergoing inguinal hernia repair.[193] Midline, paramedian, oblique, and transverse incisions are commonly used to expose the abdominal aorta.[194-198] Although transverse incisions are associated with the lowest complication rate, their use is often limited to patients with pulmonary insufficiency. Despite the reported benefits of oblique incisions, a significant number of complications, including long-lasting wound pain and bulging in 11% to 23% of patients and incisional hernias in 7%, have been reported.[197,199] Presumably, the diffuse bulging is caused by muscle atrophy resulting from a combination of factors, including division of the intercostal nerves, incision-related muscular injury, and reduced blood supply. Gardner and colleagues were able to decrease the incidence of bulging from 11% to 0.03% by preserving the 11th intercostal nerve.[200]

The incidence of midline ventral hernias ranges from 10% to 37% and is more common in patients undergoing aortic repair of AAA than those having surgery for occlusive disease. Takagi and associates reported a threefold increased risk in both inguinal and incisional hernias in patients with AAA compared with those with occlusive disease.[199,201,202] CT scans and MRI are used with increasing frequency to diagnose the discontinuity of the fascial layers with protrusion of the abdominal viscera because clinical examination may underestimate the prevalence of incisional hernias. The prevalence of incisional hernia detected by CT was 22% at 24 months compared with 8% detected clinically.[203] Two distinct types of defects can be identified. Focal periumbilical defects are almost invariably the result of poor technique. The diffuse bulging associated with lateral retraction of the recti is far more commonly observed in patients with incisional hernias after undergoing aortic aneurysmal resection than aortofemoral bypass for occlusive disease (Fig. 60.13). Several studies have found no difference in the incidence of the usual risk factors—age, chronic obstructive pulmonary disease, diabetes, smoking, wound infection, length of ICU stay, and amount of blood transfused—between patients who developed incisional hernias and those who did not.

Mass suturing of the musculoaponeurotic layers of the abdominal wall using monofilament or braided suture is the most frequently used technique to close midline incisions. A meta-analysis of the method of abdominal wound closure after AAA repair concluded that the ideal suture for abdominal fascia closure was a running nonabsorbable monofilament suture. Also, a suture length–to–wound length ratio greater than 4 reduces the incidence of incision lesions.[204,205] It cannot be overemphasized that careful suture technique with placement of bites 2 cm from the edge and 1 cm apart is essential if this complication is to be prevented. The prophylactic placement of a polypropylene mesh has been shown by Bevis and coauthors to reduce the incidence of incisional hernias without increasing the rate of complications in patients undergoing elective AAA repair.[206] Whether these data can be verified in larger series and the prophylactic use of mesh proves cost effective remain to be determined.

Primary repair using monofilament nonabsorbable suture is appropriate for closure of small periumbilical defects. Surgical or laparoscopic repair using prosthetic mesh is usually necessary to repair large defects in the upper abdomen.[207,208] The incidence of seromas and recurrence rates remain high. The relationship among AWH, AAA, and circulating proteases and their inhibitors is currently being investigated.

Chylous Ascites

Chylous ascites, issuing from a damaged cisterna chyli and its tributaries at the root of the mesentery, is a rare complication of aortic reconstruction and performance of a Warren shunt.[209] In a review of the literature, Pabst and coauthors found that approximately 75% of cases occurred after AAA resection, 19% after aortic reconstruction for occlusive disease, and the remaining 7% after resection of infected aortic grafts.[210] Interruption of the lymphatics and chylous ascites are not invariably related because the lymphatics are often interrupted during aortic operations without apparent sequelae.[209,211] Patients with chylous ascites typically present within 2 or 3 weeks of aortic repair with anorexia and progressive abdominal distension. Chylous ascites can result in nutritional imbalance, immunologic deficit, and respiratory dysfunction. Ascites is usually evident on physical examination and can be confirmed by abdominal radiography, ultrasonography, or CT scanning. Abdominal paracentesis reveals a milky fluid, with a high lymphocyte count and lipid content, which is bacteriologically sterile. The ascitic fluid is usually contained within the abdomen. Leakage of ascites to the outside through a defect in the incision increases the fluid and protein loss and heightens the risk of infection. Such a leak should be repaired surgically or laparoscopically under sterile conditions and prophylactic antibiotic coverage. Methods used to identify the site of the leak include lymphoscintigraphy, lymphangiography, direct

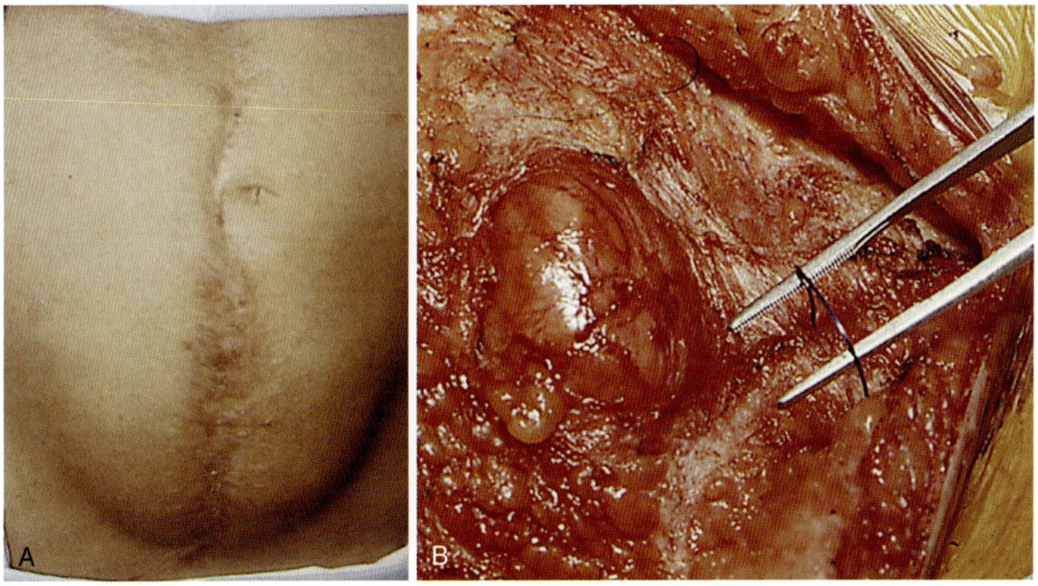

FIG 60.13 (A) Photograph demonstrating a large abdominal incisional hernia in a patient after repair of an abdominal aortic aneurysm. (B) Operative photograph demonstrating the intact sutures adjacent to the fascial defect.

opacification of the thoracic duct with oral fat emulsion observed by CT, and injection of Evans blue dye. The reliability of these tests in identifying the location of the leak or fistula remains unestablished.[212]

The management of chylous ascites includes abdominal paracentesis, a low-fat diet rich in medium-chain triglycerides, and total parenteral nutrition. However, repeated paracentesis may result in the loss of large amounts of protein and lipid that cannot quickly be replaced. An additional risk is that of line-related sepsis. In patients who do not respond to repeated paracentesis, a peritoneal venous shunt, in addition to diet control or total parenteral nutrition, may relieve the ascites. Whether the use of octreotide or fibrin glue accelerates the resolution of ascites remains unclear.[213] Surgical or laparoscopic ligation may be necessary in resistant cases.[209,210] Recurrence of ascites after surgical repair is rare.[214]

Spinal Cord Ischemia

Spinal cord ischemia occurs most frequently during repair of thoracic and thoracoabdominal aneurysms but is sometimes encountered during resection of AAA and, rarely, after aortoiliac bypass for ischemia.[132,215,216] The overall incidence of this complication has been reported as 0.26% after open AAA repair, 0.21% after endovascular aneurysm repair, and is 10-fold higher after rAAA repair than after elective aneurysm resection.[216-218] In a review of a series of more than 100 patients undergoing open repair for rAAA, Peppelenbosch and coauthors found an incidence of spinal cord ischemia of 1.2% (0% to 2.8%), with a mortality rate of 46.9% (35.6% to 65.2%).[219] The incidence of spinal cord ischemia after thoracic aortic reconstruction is in the range of 1% to 10%, depending on the extent of the lesion repaired. Patients undergoing thoracic endovascular aortic aneurysm repair (TEVAR) after prior AAA repair have a 12.5% risk of spinal cord ischemia compared with 1.7% for those without prior AAA repair.[220]

The upper level of the neurologic deficit was found to be T10 to L2 in 39 of 44 patients (88.6%) reviewed at the Henry Ford Hospital.[217] Postoperative mortality was directly related to the severity of paraplegia. When the neurologic deficit was complete initially, involving both sensory and motor function, 76% of the patients died; there were only two complete neurologic recoveries and one partial recovery. By contrast, when the initial deficit was only partial motor or sensory loss, 24% died and some degree of recovery was noted in all but one patient.[216,221,222]

In the report of spinal cord ischemia by Peppelenbosch and colleagues, 72.7% of the patients presented with hemodynamic shock and 38.2% required suprarenal clamp placement during rAAA repair; 42% of the patients had complete infarction of the spinal cord, 33% had anterior spinal artery syndrome, and the remaining 21% had varying degrees of cord involvement. The diagnosis was often delayed and made within 3.2 ± 5.2 days after surgery.

The major cause of spinal cord ischemia is interruption of flow through the great radicular artery of Adamkiewicz, which is the major source of supply to the anterior spinal artery at the lower end of the cord.[215,223] The great radicular artery is a major branch of the posterior division of one of the intercostal vessels, arising between T8 and L1. On occasion, it may originate from a lumbar branch of the infrarenal aorta. The anterior spinal artery itself is long and has rather poor collateral contributions from the posterior spinal arteries or from the radicular arteries derived from more proximal intercostal vessels. Because the spinal cord is only tenuously supplied in its lower portion by vessels other than the great radicular artery, embolization or injury to this vessel during aortic reconstruction may lead to some degree of cord infarction. The effectiveness of collateral pathways may be further compromised by hypotension, especially in patients with ruptured aneurysms; prolonged clamp placement; ligation or occlusion of the hypogastric, lumbar, or sacral arteries; and retrograde dissection from the aortic anastomosis occluding intercostal arteries. The placement of a high aortic clamp for temporary control of a ruptured aneurysm, however, does not clearly correlate with the incidence or severity of spinal cord ischemia.[216]

Noninvasive CTA and MRA are the most frequently used imaging modalities to visualize the artery of Adamkiewicz in patients with thoracoabdominal aneurysms. MRA has detection rates of 67% to 100% compared with 18% to 100% with CTA.[224-226] The very low incidence of spinal cord ischemia after operations of the infrarenal aorta and the frequent use of CTA and MRA in the evaluation of patients with AAA render angiographic visualization impractical and potentially dangerous.[146,223-225] Moreover, the occurrence of this complication remains unpredictable and may not be preventable in association with infrarenal aortic reconstruction. Monitoring of somatosensory evoked potentials during thoracic surgery has been shown to correlate with cord ischemia.[227] These abnormal findings have been reversed by temporary shunting and implantation of intercostal vessels into the thoracic aortic graft. Practical application of this technique to abdominal aortic surgery is undergoing continued investigation.[227-230]

Perioperative lumbar drainage decreases cerebrospinal fluid (CSF) pressure, increases perfusion pressure to the spinal cord, and may reduce the risk of postoperative paraplegia. A recent review by Tshomba and colleagues reported a significant decrease in spinal cord ischemia after performing CSF drainage in patients prior to type IV thoracoabdominal aortic aneurysm (TAAA) repair from 11.4% to 2.4%.[231] A recent position paper from the European Association for Cardio-Thoracic Surgery recommended preoperative CSF drainage for all patients undergoing open thoracic or thoracoabdominal aneurysm repair and recommended that it continue for 48 hours postoperatively. They also recommended that the perioperative mean arterial pressure be maintained at 80 mm Hg or higher and hemoglobin levels greater than 10 mg/dL.[232]

It is prudent to avoid prolonged high aortic clamping unless absolutely necessary, to maintain cord perfusion pressure by avoiding systemic hypotension, and to prevent stasis thrombosis in collateral vessels by effective heparinization. Suturing a patch of posterior aortic wall with its intercostal vessel orifices into a window cut out of the graft has been recommended for thoracoabdominal aneurysms.[132] Finally, it is important to ensure pelvic perfusion through one or both hypogastric arteries to maximize collateral contribution to the spinal cord (Fig. 60.14).[233]

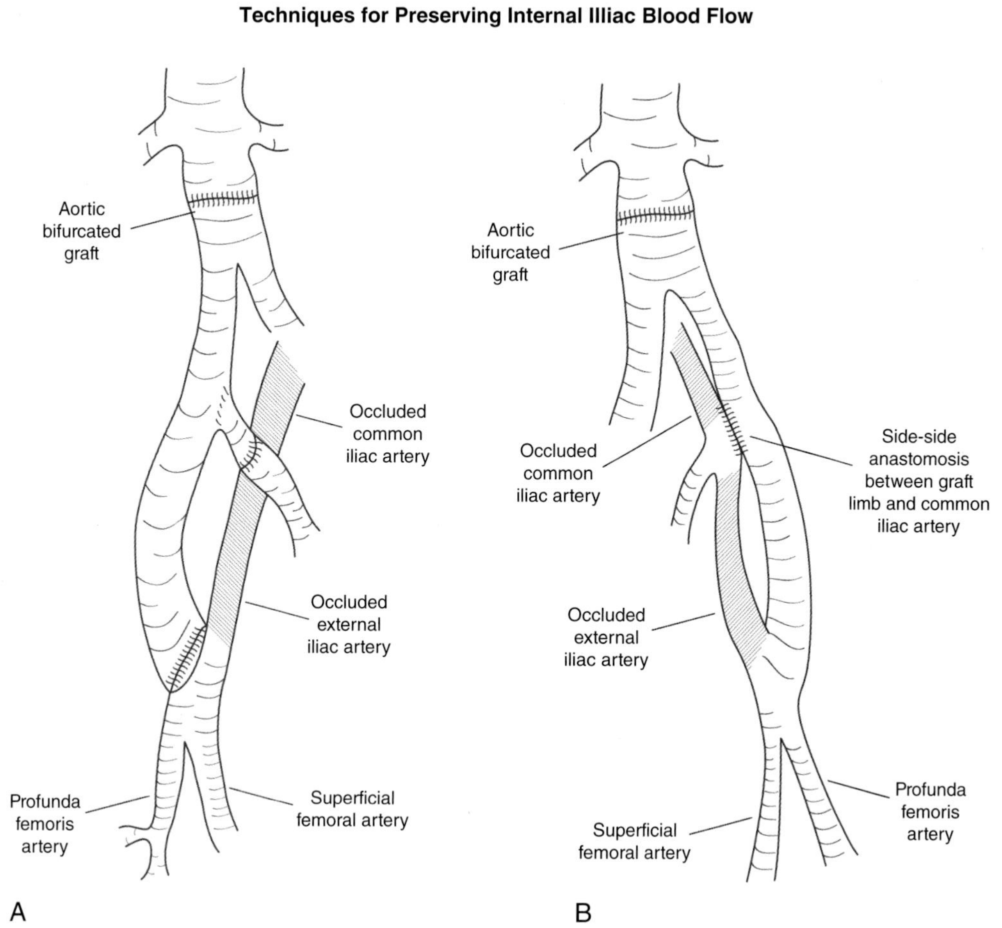

FIG 60.14 Techniques for internal iliac revascularization in patients with external and common iliac occlusion. (A) Interposition graft. (B) Endarterectomy and side-side anastomosis.

The diagnosis of spinal cord ischemia is made clinically and can be confirmed by CT and MRI.

When ischemic injury to the spinal cord is clinically evident postoperatively, treatment is supportive.[216] Immediate placement of a spinal drain is indicated if not already present. Several drugs, including steroids, rosuvastatin, cilostozol, angiotensin ll receptor blockade, and oxygen-free radical scavengers, are being investigated to limit the extent of, or prevent neurologic damage after, aneurysm repair.[234-237]

Ureteral Injury and Obstruction

The ureters are immediately adjacent to the operative field and may be easily injured during dissection and aortoiliac repair.[238] This is especially important in patients with large iliac and hypogastric aneurysms or when there is increased adherence to vascular structures in the presence of an "inflammatory" aneurysm or retroperitoneal fibrosis.[239] Nachbur and associates, in a study of 220 patients with asymptomatic aneurysms evaluated with CT scanning, observed 20 cases of ureteral obstruction.[240] In eight patients, ureteral obstruction was associated with inflammatory aneurysms; in the remaining 12, it was associated with abdominal aortic, common iliac, and hypogastric atherosclerotic aneurysms. Thorough knowledge of the anatomic relationships of the ureters at the level of the iliac bifurcation is essential. Sometimes, multiple ureters may be present or they may be in an aberrant position, owing to congenital anomalies. Although intravenous pyelography and sonography have been used as first-line studies, contrast-enhanced CT and MRI are the most reliable diagnostic modalities. A preoperative contrast-enhanced CT scan is especially indicated in reoperative aortoiliac surgery to identify postoperative changes in the ureteral anatomy or demonstrate possible injury incurred during the initial surgery.

Direct injury to the ureter can best be avoided by keeping the dissection close to the iliac artery at the point where the ureter normally crosses the common iliac bifurcation in transit to the bladder. This is especially important during the blind development of the retroperitoneal tunnel for aortofemoral bypass. The ureter should be elevated away from the iliac vessels so that the graft will lie dorsal to it. Inadvertent passage of the graft ventral to the ureter may cause it to be compressed between the graft limb and the underlying iliac artery, producing hydroureter and hydronephrosis. The incidence of ureteral obstruction after aortic grafting in one prospective study was 2%.[241] However, the ureter may be entrapped in perigraft scarring, even if it is placed in its proper position ventral to the prosthesis.[238]

Both ureters should be demonstrated before closing the retroperitoneum. The right ureter must be carefully protected during retroperitoneal closure because this structure can easily be caught up in the suture line. Iatrogenic ureteral injuries sustained during placement or revision of a vascular graft should be repaired primarily. Although renal salvage is possible when the diagnosis is delayed, nephrectomy is often necessary if there has been extensive contamination of the graft.[242] Sometimes, an intraoperative ureteral injury is overlooked, and the diagnosis is delayed for days or weeks. Once recognized, placement of a percutaneous nephrostomy tube may be associated with a shorter hospital stay and lower infection rate than with open repair.[243,244]

Ureteral obstruction was present in 57% of patients with idiopathic retroperitoneal fibrosis (IRF) reported by Kermani and coauthors.[245] Retroperitoneal fibrosis may be idiopathic (2/3) or secondary (1/3) to drugs (e.g., alkaloids, dopamine agonists, β-blockers, hydralazine, and analgesics); malignancy (carcinoma of the prostate, colon, or breast; lymphoma, carcinoids); infection; renal trauma; hemorrhage; and radiation or chemotherapy. Retroperitoneal fibrosis with encasement of the ureters also accompanies inflammatory aortic aneurysms.[245-247] The fibrotic encasement of IRF is usually concentrated at the aortic bifurcation. Ureteric obstruction may also occur after open or endovascular AAA repair and is the most common cause of hydronephrosis after aortic surgery. Postoperative hydronephrosis can be categorized as early (occurring within 6 months) or late (after 6 months). Temporary asymptomatic hydronephrosis can be detected on CT scans in 12% to 30% of patients, and mild to moderate permanent ureteral dilatation is seen in 2% to 14% of patients undergoing aortic surgery. The fibrosis is usually secondary to bleeding; excessive dissection, ligation, or devascularization of the ureter; or pseudoaneurysm formation. Ureteral obstruction is believed to be more common when the limb of the graft is tunneled anterior to the ureter. However, hydronephrosis secondary to anterior graft placement occurs in only 30% of cases. The majority of patients have a clinical presentation within 1 year of the procedure, but delayed presentation up to 14 years has been reported. Approximately 30% of patients manifest with symptoms, including pain, recurrent bouts of urinary tract infection, azotemia, or hematuria.[248-250]

Wright and associates reported a 35-year experience with 58 ureteral complications in 50 patients undergoing aortoiliac reconstructions.[251] Two of the six patients with ureteral obstruction treated before, or in conjunction with, repair of the aneurysm developed graft complications (one graft limb thrombosis and one graft infection). The remaining 44 patients had 46 complications, including hydronephrosis (42), ureteral leaks (3), and ureteral necrosis (1). Twenty-four patients had 36 graft complications, including anastomotic aneurysm (19), graft limb thrombosis (8), graft infection (6), and aortoenteric fistula (3). Twenty-nine of the 44 patients underwent graft or ureteral operations, or both, with a mortality rate of 21%.

The status of the ureters should be carefully evaluated in patients with inflammatory aortic aneurysms with retroperitoneal fibrosis. Hydronephrosis recognized preoperatively should be treated with ureteral stent placement to decompress the obstruction and facilitate ureteral identification during repair. In a systematic review of open surgical repair (OSR) versus EVAR of inflammatory AAA, Paravastu and colleagues[252] reported regression of the periaortic fibrosis in 73% of the OSR patients compared with 65% in the EVAR group. Forty-five patients undergoing OSR and 29 undergoing EVAR had preoperative ureteric obstruction, which regressed postoperatively in 69% and 38% of patients, respectively. Inflammation progressed in 1% and 4%, respectively. The authors suggest that OSR may be the preferred treatment in patients with hydronephrosis. Postoperative hydronephrosis detected by ultrasonography or CT can initially be followed expectantly because it often resolves on its own. Only 12 of the 58 patients reported by Wright and coworkers required surgical intervention for progressive hydronephrosis.[251] The selective use of balloon dilatation, stents, and antibiotics in conjunction with operative repair is essential if the high incidence of graft complications is to be reduced (Fig. 60.15).

Impotence

The loss of ability to achieve or maintain an erection adequate for satisfactory coitus may be a result of psychogenic or vasculogenic causes. Current evidence suggests that up to 80% of cases have organic causes,[6] which are subdivided into vasculogenic, neurogenic, and hormonal etiologies. Vasculogenic etiologies represent the largest group, with arterial or inflow disorders being the most common.[253]

Eighty percent of patients who have aortoiliac occlusive disease have significant erectile dysfunction (ED).[254] Among the contributing factors are age, hypertension, diabetes, smoking, alcohol abuse, lipid disorders, heart disease, β-blockers, ACE inhibitors, and urologic and liver disease. Medications account for up to 25% of cases. In a survey of sexual function after elective open (EO), ruptured open (RO), and endovascular AAA repair, the prevalence of ED was 27% (EO), 63% (EVAR), and 45% (RO) preoperatively, and postoperatively was 58%,76%, and 67%, respectively.[255,256] Approximately 25% of patients will have iatrogenic ED if appropriate technical modifications are not used. Therefore, careful evaluation of penile erectile function by history, noninvasive techniques, and angiography should be included in the preoperative evaluation before elective aortic surgery.[257,258] This will determine whether there is normal sexual function that should be preserved or whether there is already an established pattern of impotence that might be relieved by altering pelvic blood flow. This information provides valuable insights into the possible psychogenic and cultural factors contributing to an existing problem and gives the surgeon an estimate of the importance of sexual function to the patient. Such preoperative information may alter the type of aortic operation planned.

Preoperative evaluation of erectile function includes nocturnal tumescence studies. The absence of tumescence during an adequate sleep study is strong evidence of organic impotence. Documentation of normal erections during rapid eye movement sleep establishes the psychogenic basis of the patient's ED. Unfortunately, the failure to achieve erection is often qualitative rather than complete, making tumescence studies less discriminating between organic and psychogenic impotence.[254,258]

If organic impotence is suspected, the next step is noninvasive vascular testing. At present, the most reliable measurement is the penile systolic pressure and the penile-brachial index (PBI).[254] Kempczinski and Birinyi found that age had a deleterious effect on the PBI independent of sexual potency.[254] Patients younger

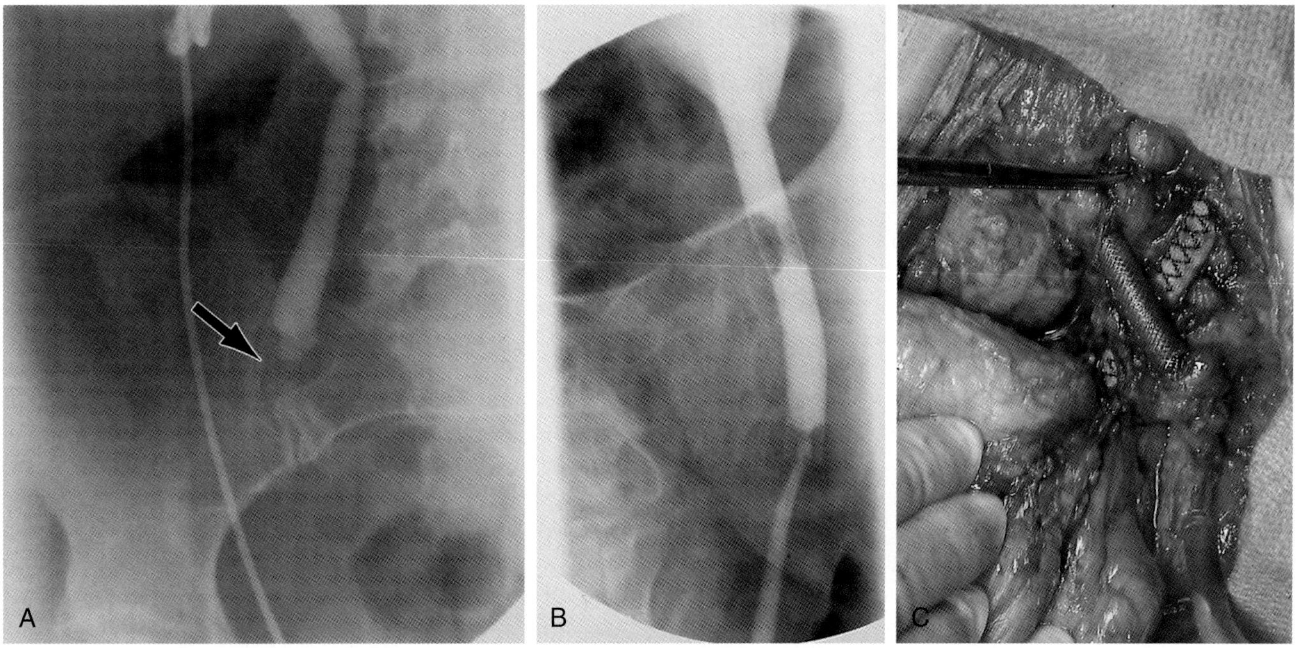

FIG 60.15 (A) A stricture is present in the distal ureter as it crosses over the limb of an aortofemoral graft *(arrow)*. (B) After dilatation of the stricture, a stent was placed. (C) Erosion of the ureter by the stent resulted in a 3-cm defect in the ureter and exposure of the limb of the graft.

than 40 years had a mean PBI of 0.99 compared with a PBI of 0.74 for equally potent men older than 40. This difference was statistically significant. By contrast, impotent men older than 40 had a mean PBI of 0.58, also a statistically significant difference. Despite the significant differences in PBI measurements in these three groups, there is poor correlation between PBI and the degree of ED.[258,259] Although a low PBI is not sufficient to establish the diagnosis of vasculogenic impotence, the finding of a PBI greater than 0.8 confirms the adequacy of penile blood flow and suggests that a vasculogenic cause is extremely unlikely.[254]

Neurogenic impotence is commonly a result of neuropathy secondary to diabetes mellitus, or it may follow autonomic nerve injury from genitourinary or abdominopelvic surgery. This diagnosis is often one of exclusion, but abnormal pudendal nerve velocity studies (sacral latency testing) and abnormal cystometrography (the anatomic pathways in micturition and erection being similar) can implicate this cause.[254,260]

The diagnosis of endocrinologic impotence requires measurement of thyroid function and serum levels of testosterone and other associated hormones. Finally, a thorough medication history is required.[260]

Preoperative angiography is useful in identifying the patency of the hypogastric vessels and their contribution to pelvic perfusion. Unfortunately, angiographic findings correlate poorly with the patient's erectile function.[254] Selective injections to identify the flow through the pudendal vessels into the penis may be required to more accurately assess patients with primarily vasculogenic impotence.[254]

Although the findings on preoperative angiograms correlate poorly with erectile function, preservation of adequate perfusion into at least one hypogastric artery appears to be a vital component in minimizing iatrogenic impotence.[254] When possible, direct antegrade perfusion of the internal iliac artery should be ensured. This may require thromboendarterectomy of the hypogastric orifice. Sometimes angioplasty, stenting, or operative endarterectomy of the orifices of one or both hypogastric arteries will improve erectile function. If both external iliac arteries are occluded or stenotic, and bypass into the common femoral arteries is anticipated precluding retrograde iliac flow, the proximal aortic anastomosis should be constructed end to side when feasible to preserve pelvic blood flow. When proximal aortic disease is extensive (requiring an end-to-end proximal anastomosis) and impaired penile perfusion has been diagnosed by preoperative, noninvasive testing, it may be necessary to reimplant the hypogastric artery into one limb of an aortobifemoral graft or add a jump graft to one hypogastric artery to improve pelvic inflow (see Fig. 60.14).[254,260] Finally, careful flushing of the graft in both directions before completion of the final suture line is important to prevent embolization of small particles into the pelvic arteries. DePalma and colleagues[261] reported spontaneous erectile function in 58% of patients with impotence undergoing aortoiliac reconstruction compared with 27% after microvascular procedures.

Retrograde Ejaculation

Ejaculatory dysfunction is not uncommon after aortic surgery. Earlier series reported an incidence of 30% to 75%, but in more contemporary series, the incidence ranges from 3% to 9%.[262,263] This lower incidence is clearly the result of both an increased awareness of the anatomy controlling ejaculation and improved surgical technique. Emission and closure of the bladder neck to ensure antegrade ejaculation are dependent on innervation by postganglionic fibers of the lumbar sympathetic nerves arising from T11 to L3. The loss of one or both functions as a result of dissection in the region of the aortic bifurcation results in dry ejaculation.[264,265]

Careful preservation of the sympathetic-parasympathetic plexus overlying the aorta and its bifurcation and maintenance of blood flow through the hypogastric and pudendal arteries are the important factors in preventing retrograde ejaculation and impotence in men undergoing elective aortic surgery.[257,263,266] Dissection should be carried down to the aortic wall on its right anterolateral surface and the paraaortic structures gently retracted to the left to avoid trauma to the nerves contained within these tissues (Fig. 60.16). During aneurysm resection, the inferior mesenteric artery should not be dissected free but should be controlled by suture ligature from inside the aorta after the aneurysm has been opened to avoid disruption of nerve fibers at the junction of the inferior mesenteric artery with the aorta (see Fig. 60.16). There should be minimal division of the longitudinal periaortic tissues to the left of the infrarenal aorta, and the nerve plexuses that cross the left common iliac artery should be spared.[254,266] The limbs of bifurcated grafts should be routed within the lumens of the common iliac arteries in patients undergoing aneurysm resection to avoid external dissection and minimize injury to perivascular nerve fibers.

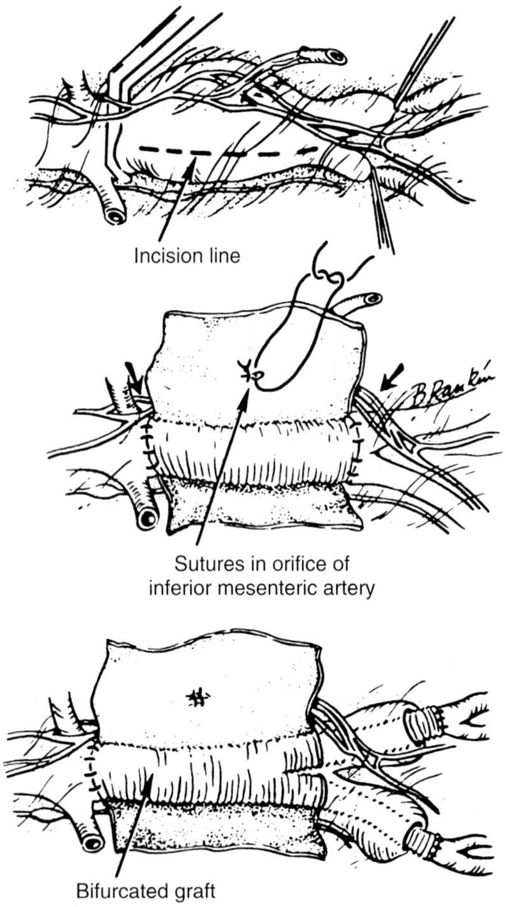

FIG 60.16 Approaches to abdominal aortic and aortoiliac aneurysm. The sac is left intact and sutured over an inlay graft. (From DePalma RG: Impotence as a complication of aortic reconstruction. In Bernhard VM, Towne JB, editors: *Complications in vascular surgery*, New York, 1980, Grune and Stratton, p 437.)

Anastomotic False Aneurysm

False aneurysms can develop at any anastomotic site. They are almost invariably associated with prosthetic rather than autogenous tissue suture lines.[267-273] The most common sites of occurrence are femoral anastomoses after placement of aortofemoral bypass grafts.[268,270,273] Femoral anastomotic aneurysms (FAAs) develop in approximately 3% of all femoral anastomoses and in 6% to 8.7% of patients undergoing aortofemoral bypass. In 3.4% of patients, FAAs may be bilateral or recurrent; aortic anastomotic aneurysms occur in 2.9% of patients.[267,270,272,274] Pathologically, there is a partial separation of the graft from the arterial wall. The perianastomotic fibrous tissue prevents immediate hemorrhage and forms a capsule around the hematoma that gradually expands, owing to the pressure transmitted from the arterial lumen. The fibrous capsule may rupture, with rapid, painful enlargement of the mass, or it may erode the overlying skin to produce infection and external hemorrhage. In the abdomen, false aneurysms are prone to erode into adjacent bowel, forming aortoenteric fistulas.[273,275,276] Because blood flow within the pseudoaneurysm is static, its lumen becomes partially filled with thrombus, which may embolize.[267,273] The luminal distortion produced by the pseudoaneurysm and its thrombus may also cause occlusion of a graft limb.[273]

In the immediate postoperative period, the integrity of all vascular anastomoses is entirely dependent on suture material alone. With time, a prosthesis-artery junction is maintained by the integrity of the suture material and also by external fibrous bonding caused by scarring.[277] The important factors involved in the development of an anastomotic false aneurysm include arterial wall weakness,[272] endarterectomy at the anastomotic site,[278] compliance mismatch between the graft and host artery,[279,280] dilatation of the graft material,[276,281] prosthetic deterioration or an actual flaw in the graft material,[282] increased tension at the anastomotic site because of insufficient length of the prosthesis,[282] uneven tension on the anastomosis as a result of beveling of the end of the graft,[277] and deterioration of suture material, which is extremely rare.[283]

Pseudoaneurysm is occasionally caused by underlying infection, although this is seldom identified.[270,273] When infection is the causative factor, a purulent perigraft exudate is usually, but not always, present. The lack of incorporation of the graft into the surrounding tissue may be the only sign of an infection. Therefore, during repair of any pseudoaneurysm, its wall and contents should be routinely cultured by aerobic and anaerobic techniques.

Recognition is usually quite simple at groin anastomoses, where a large, pulsatile, and sometimes tender mass becomes apparent to both the patient and the examining physician. In a series of a 142 FAAs (76% for A-I occlusive disease, 24% for AAA) reported by Demarche and associates, the presenting features included a painless pulsatile mass (64%), acute leg ischemia (19%), a painful pulsatile mass (8%), hemorrhage (7%), pseudo-postphlebitic edema (0.01%), and microemboli of the toes (0.01%).[284] Skourtis and coauthors reported 11 cases of rupture and 4 cases with thromboembolic complications in their series of 49 cases.[285] False aneurysms developing in the retroperitoneum at an aortic or iliac anastomosis rarely become palpable and go unnoticed until rupture produces pain and shock or erosion occurs in an adjacent loop of bowel, with gastrointestinal hemorrhage.[286] Sometimes, false aneurysms are identified during routine CT scanning or angiography for some other vascular or unrelated problem. Ultrasonography, CTA, and MRA are reliable methods for evaluating grafts and anastomoses for dilatation and pseudoaneurysm formation and the presence of infection.[287] Angiography is seldom indicated except to delineate the distal runoff vessels.[286] If fluid is detected surrounding the graft, it should be aspirated under sterile conditions and sent for culture.

Retroperitoneal false aneurysms should be repaired as soon as they are identified to avoid rupture or bowel erosion.[271,275,286] Unfortunately, these complications are frequently the first indication that a false aneurysm is present. When there is no evidence of infection, the suture line defect can be dissected free and repaired either directly or by the interposition of fresh graft material. Endovascular treatment of thoracic, paraanastomotic aortic, iliac, and femoral pseudoaneurysms is an attractive alternative to surgery in patients with favorable anatomy.[288-290] Lagana and colleagues were able to treat 30 false aneurysms, 13 at the aortic anastomosis and 17 at the distal iliac anastomosis of patients who underwent previous aortoiliac reconstructive surgery with endovascular techniques with primary and secondary success rates of 81% and 91%, respectively at 1 year.[291] In general, FAAs should be repaired as soon as they are identified. However, false aneurysms that are small (<2.5 cm), stable, and asymptomatic may be observed first, especially if the patient is at increased risk for reoperation.[270,272,273] If surgery is delayed, reexamination at frequent intervals is mandatory so that repair can be carried out when expansion is evident but before complications develop.

When infection or visceral erosion has taken place, the graft must be removed entirely, the aorta and iliac vessels closed, and the extremities revascularized. Management of this problem is discussed in detail elsewhere in this text.

Surgical repair of an FAA is usually performed through the site of the original incision. Dissection is carried down to the graft wall proximally so that it can be controlled with a circumferential tape. Further dissection is then carried distally along the graft to define the anastomosis, the aneurysmal bulge, and the branches of the common femoral artery. It is usually difficult and tedious to dissect out the major branches of the artery at the anastomotic site. When extensive scarring is encountered, further dissection may be abandoned, and the patient is given intravenous heparin. The graft is then clamped and disconnected from the aneurysm, and branch control is achieved by the insertion of balloon occlusion catheters into the lumens of the major branches.[271] The anastomotic site is surveyed carefully to identify the cause of the pseudoaneurysm. The distal frayed end of the graft at the anastomosis is resected, and the edges of the artery are trimmed back to healthy tissue. To avoid tension at the new anastomosis, a short piece of new graft material is usually required to connect the proximal end of the old prosthesis with the freshened arterial orifice. The diameter of the interposed graft segment generally should not exceed 8 mm, to more closely approximate the size of the outflow tract rather than the larger inflow prosthetic limb.[281] Unless retrograde flow up the external iliac artery must be preserved, it is best to convert the femoral anastomosis from end to side to end to end.[271] Before repairing the anastomosis, the orifices of the superficial and deep femoral arteries should be inspected so that significant stenoses can be repaired by endarterectomy or patch angioplasty to ensure adequate runoff. Madiba and coworkers[292] treated 25 femoral anastomotic aneurysms with an interposition graft (15), resuture (6), tube graft, (1), crossover graft (1), graft-popliteal bypass (1), and ligation (1). There were no deaths or recurrences in the 49-month follow-up period. Wound infection occurred in two patients and occlusion of the opposite limb occurred in one. Endovascular repair of FAA is also an option in selected patients.[293] In a review by Demarche and colleagues, overall mortality for repair of FAA was 2.7% and 20% in patients with infected FAA. Results are distinctly better if this lesion is repaired electively rather than emergently.[272,273] Emergent procedures are associated with increased mortality (46.6%), whereas elective operation resulted in high patency rates and no mortality.[285]

Recurrent Anastomotic Aneurysm

Repair of FAAs remains durable in approximately 80% of patients; however, recurrent FAAs develop in a small percentage of patients. The recurrence rate of anastomotic femoral false aneurysms after initial repair has been reported to range between 5.7% and 19%.[277,281,294] Factors predisposing to recurrent FAA include graft dilatation, local wound complications, cigarette smoking, and previous repair of an FAA in a woman.[281,294] Although there appears to be an inverse relationship between atherosclerotic heart disease and recurrent FAA, the significance of this observation is difficult to explain. Furthermore, factors that have been implicated in the development of primary FAAs (e.g., hypertension, smoking, diabetes, suture material, type of graft, performance of an endarterectomy) have not been related to the development of recurrent FAAs. Recurrent FAAs are subject to the same complications as primary FAAs, including rupture, thrombosis, and peripheral embolization.

Repair is indicated in good-risk patients with recurrent FAAs larger than 2 cm. For those smaller than 2 cm, management includes careful follow-up, especially if coexisting medical problems make surgical intervention risky. The principles of repair are similar to those for primary FAAs and include careful dissection of the distal outflow vessels, use of graft material approximately the size of the outflow vessel, and conversion from end-to-side to end-to-end anastomosis.[281,294]

Infrainguinal Arterial Reconstruction

Femoropopliteal and femoroinfrapopliteal bypasses are the most commonly performed procedures for revascularization of the lower extremity below the inguinal ligament. Specific problems related to endarterectomy of the superficial femoral, popliteal, or deep femoral arteries are reviewed in the discussion of these procedures. The basic principles of infrainguinal bypass are similar to those for aortoiliac reconstruction, with the following significant differences: the vessels involved are smaller, and the length of the bypass conduit is greater, with a consequent increase in the incidence of early and late thrombosis; vein grafts rather than prostheses are used for the majority of procedures; and there is a tendency for less severe systemic complications because of the more peripheral and less traumatic nature of the operative procedure.

Bleeding

Major blood loss or hemorrhage is not a frequent complication during this surgery but may become a problem in the immediate postoperative period. Ali and coauthors[295] reported a 3% incidence of hemorrhage associated with femoropopliteal vein grafts within 1 hour to 180 days after the procedure. The most common sources are the anastomoses, insecure ligatures on branches of a vein graft, laceration of the vein wall by instruments in the in situ technique, blind disruption of small vessels encountered during blunt dissection of thigh and leg tunnels, inadequate hemostasis during dissection of the major vessels, incomplete reversal of heparin anticoagulation, and oozing from antiplatelet medication.[296] In the immediate postoperative period, bleeding usually appears as wound swelling of the extremity, and the severity of hypotension, if present, mirrors the extent and rapidity of hemorrhage. Prompt return to the operating room is required to control the source of bleeding and to evacuate the hematoma, which may interfere with healing and promote infection. Wound hemorrhage that occurs after 48 to 72 hours is frequently caused by uncontrolled infection or poor healing at anastomosis sites.[296] However, hemorrhage may occur later in the immediate postoperative period in patients who have been maintained on anticoagulants or in whom fibrinolytic agents have been infused for graft thrombosis within 10 days to 2 weeks of surgery.[297] The management of bleeding after lower extremity bypass requires treatment of the underlying cause and replacement of blood and coagulation factors and the restoration of platelet function. In patients undergoing infrainguinal revascularization, intraoperative blood transfusion is associated with a higher risk of mortality and pulmonary and infectious complications.[298] Long-term graft patency has been shown to be significantly reduced in patients in whom wound hemorrhage develops in the immediate postoperative period.[296]

Thrombosis

The most common significant complication of infrainguinal bypass or endarterectomy is thrombosis of the reconstruction. In the early postoperative period (±30 days), thrombosis is usually related to technical factors (Fig. 60.17).[51,73,299,300] The most common of these is imprecise construction of the anastomotic suture line, resulting in stenosis or elevation of a distal intimal flap that obstructs flow; this is especially important at a distal anastomosis to a small-caliber tibial or peroneal vessel. A prosthetic or reversed saphenous vein graft may become twisted when drawn through

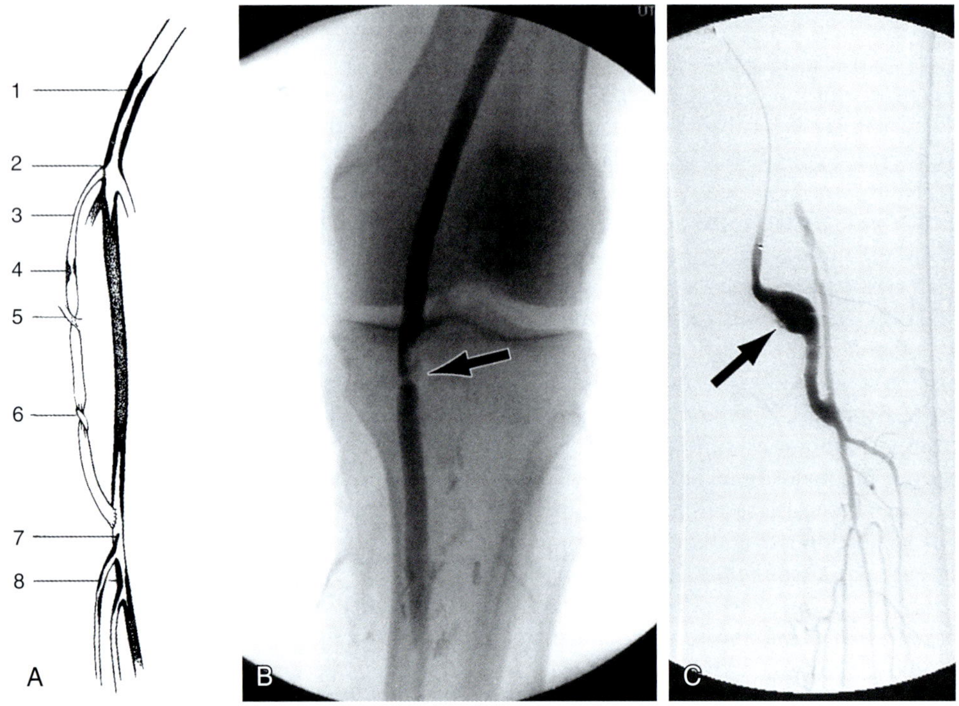

FIG 60.17 (A) Mechanical factors underlying early thrombosis of femoropopliteal and femorotibial grafts: *(1)* Stenosis of iliac inflow; *(2)* stenosis of proximal anastomosis produced by suturing a small vein to a thick-walled femoral artery; *(3)* proximal vein graft <4 mm in diameter; *(4)* recanalized saphenous phlebitis; *(5)* external compression tissue bands in tunnel; *(6)* graft twist; *(7)* elevation of distal intima; *(8)* inadequate runoff. (B) Stenosis and platelet deposition *(arrow)* in a below-knee saphenous vein graft. (C) Aneurysmal dilatation *(arrow)* of a saphenous vein graft proximal to a stenosis in a patient with distal embolization. ([A] From Bernhard VM: The failed arterial graft: lost pulses and gangrene. In Condon RE, DeCosse JJ, editors: *Surgical care*, Philadelphia, 1980, Lea and Febiger, p 156.)

the thigh tunnel. Kinking or entrapment may occur because of compression by nerve trunks or other tissues crossing the tunnel, or by tracking the graft inappropriately in relation to the adductor muscles of the thigh or the medial head of the gastrocnemius. Vein graft stenosis may be produced by a branch ligature placed too close to the main saphenous trunk. For reversed saphenous vein grafts, factors leading to early thrombosis are vein diameter less than 3.5 to 4 mm, thick-walled vein, marked varicosities, and evidence of previous phlebitis.[301,302] In the in situ saphenous vein bypass, technical factors causing early thrombosis are platelet deposition at sites of endothelial damage from improper intraluminal instrumentation, missed valves or incomplete cusp lysis, diversion of flow by significant fistulas, venospasm, and torsion or kinking of the proximal or distal-free segments of the vein. Atherosclerotic disease in the inflow or outflow arteries that was inadequately evaluated before surgery is another significant cause of graft thrombosis. Other technical errors include inadequate heparinization, improper flushing of the arterial system before restoration of graft flow, and clamp injury to the inflow or outflow vessels or the bypass conduit.[73,303] Nonmechanical causes of early thrombosis are decreased cardiac output, arterial vasospasm, and hypercoagulability.[73,304]

Thrombosis that occurs from 1 month to 1 year after implantation is most frequently caused by degenerative changes in the graft itself or at an anastomosis.[299,300,305,306] In reversed saphenous vein bypass, thrombosis is usually caused by fibrosis of a valve or fibrotic changes in the vein graft wall as a result of injury during harvest and preparation before insertion.[73,300,301] These intrinsic vein graft defects are more common in the narrow proximal portion of reversed vein grafts.[300] In in situ saphenous vein bypass grafts, stenoses of the conduit have been reported at the mobilized upper or lower ends of the graft caused by fibrous dysplastic lesions and in the midportion as the result of thickening around a valve cusp.[307] For all types of arterial bypasses, intimal hyperplasia at or just beyond the distal anastomosis may be produced by turbulent flow secondary to alteration of the arterial stream at the junction of graft and artery,[66,308-310] a compliance mismatch,[279,311] and the interplay of platelets and other blood factors at anastomoses.[312] Intimal hyperplasia may also be a consequence of clamp injury to the graft or artery incurred at the time of surgery.[300]

Thrombosis occurring after 1 to 2 years is most frequently caused by progressive atherosclerosis in the arteries proximal or distal to the arterial repair.[300,301,305,313,314] Arterialized venous conduits in an atherosclerotic patient tend to become atherosclerotic themselves[314]; this appears to apply only to reversed, not in situ, vein bypass grafts.[307,315] Giswold and coworkers showed that continued smoking, hemodialysis, hypercoagulable states, and early duplex surveillance failure are independent factors associated with vein graft occlusion.[314] Pedal bypass for previous graft occlusion was also independently predictive of poor graft patency at 1 year.[316]

There is a higher incidence of thrombosis when prosthetic conduits are used, especially when they are carried below the knee to the distal popliteal or infrapopliteal vessels.[254,302,317-320] Thrombosis after vein grafting appears to level off between 1 and 2 years, whereas it is progressive in prosthetic grafts.[300,318] The specific causes of prosthetic thrombosis are the absence of a true intima, with its antithrombotic characteristics; the tendency to develop progressive intimal hyperplasia, usually at the distal anastomosis because of the complex interactions between the more rigid prosthetic graft and the arterial wall; and the greater likelihood of kinking of prosthetic materials as they cross the knee joint. Thrombosis may also occur as a consequence of false aneurysm formation, which is more frequent with prostheses than with vein grafts. Hooded grafts, vein cuffs, and patches have been used at the distal anastomoses of prosthetic grafts to improve their patency. Patency rates range from 37% to 57% for below-knee prosthetic grafts.[321-324]

Heparin-bonded Dacron and heparin-bonded PTFE grafts have been used to reduce the incidence of prosthetic graft thrombosis. In a prospective, randomized comparison of heparin-bonded Dacron (HBD) with standard PTFE (predominantly above knee) bypasses, Devine and colleagues reported primary and secondary patency rates of 46% and 47% for HBD compared with 35% and 36% for PTFE, respectively, at 5 years.[325] In a prospective comparison of Propaten (heparin-bonded PTFE, or HBPTFE) with standard PTFE grafts for femoropopliteal bypass, the investigators observed a 37% reduction in the overall risk of primary graft failure with HBPTFE. Primary and secondary patency rates were 86.4% and 88% and 79.9% and 81% for HBPTFE grafts and PTFE grafts, respectively, at 1 year.[326] In a multicenter comparison of saphenous vein (SV) and HBPTFE grafts in the treatment of critical limb ischemia in diabetics, Dorigo and colleagues[327] reported primary, assisted primary, and secondary patency rates at 48 months of 63.5%, 69%, and 69.6% for SV compared with 46.3%, 47.3%, and 57.5% for HBPTFE, respectively. Limb salvage and amputation-free survival rates for SV and HBPTFE were 75.4% and 82.4% and 59.9% and 64.4%, respectively. Thrombosis in a bypass graft may involve only the graft itself, without loss of flow in the segments of the vessel proximal and distal to the points of anastomosis. Under these circumstances, the leg will return to its previous degree of ischemia, assuming there has been no significant change in the inflow or outflow vessels and collateral pathways. If thrombosis extends beyond the anastomosis into the popliteal and infrapopliteal arteries, however, ischemia will invariably be more severe, and the limb may become acutely nonviable unless circulation can be restored.[51]

When a reversed vein graft becomes thrombosed in the immediate postoperative period, the intima and muscularis suffer prolonged anoxic injury because of a loss of nutritive blood flow from the lumen, in addition to the absence of normal graft wall perfusion through the vasa vasorum, which was disrupted during vein graft harvest.[305] The vein thus becomes a less satisfactory conduit, even though flow can be restored within a few hours. This is reflected in the reduced long-term patency of vein grafts that have undergone thrombosis and initially successful thrombectomy.[300,308]

In the case of late or neglected thrombosis of a vein conduit, either reversed or in situ, the vein tends to undergo irreversible changes. The vein wall becomes thick and edematous, and the lumen becomes stringlike. Thrombus usually cannot be removed by any means, and dilatation of the vein by a balloon catheter may result in splitting of the wall.[307]

In the immediate postoperative period, hypothermia and peripheral vasospasm may make clinical evaluation unreliable. However, noninvasive tests permit the identification of thrombosis at the earliest possible moment.[53,328,329] Therefore, the quality of graft flow and overall limb circulation should be evaluated by noninvasive hemodynamic techniques, and by clinical observation intraoperatively, immediately after completion of the reconstruction, and at frequent intervals in the early postoperative period.[72,330] Doppler waveform analysis, duplex imaging, ankle pressure indices, and pulse-volume recordings provide reliable objective information. Surgical reintervention should be carried out immediately in the event of obstructed graft flow to limit propagation of thrombus into distal vessels and minimize the period of ischemia in the limb and the wall of a vein graft.

Beyond the immediate postoperative period, patients with infrainguinal arterial reconstruction, especially with vein grafts, should continue to be examined at regular intervals at least every 3 to 4 months for 12 to 18 months and every 6 months thereafter. A history of worsening claudication, the recognition of reduced distal pulses, and the development of new bruits over the graft or its anastomoses are important findings that should be documented at each visit. In addition, noninvasive hemodynamic tests, including duplex scanning, should be performed; they provide quantitative and objective information and can identify impending thrombosis in the absence of symptoms or clinical findings.[328,330-332] Any evidence of decreasing graft function signals the need for prompt angiography to identify the problem before thrombosis occurs.

Correction of abnormalities within the graft or in the vessels adjacent to a failing graft should be carried out as soon as reduced perfusion has been identified.[328] When possible, intervention should occur before thrombosis has taken place or in the early postthrombotic period, when mechanical obliteration or lytic therapy is most effective. Delay of an aggressive surgical approach may be required in patients who are poor operative risks. Anticoagulants may prevent thrombosis in the presence of progressing stenosis if surgery must be delayed. However, once occlusion has occurred, the longer the thrombus has been present, the less effective recanalization attempts will be.

Areas of isolated stenosis within the graft, at an anastomosis, or in the inflow or outflow arteries can be successfully managed by percutaneous balloon angioplasty.[297] These fibrous vein graft lesions are often difficult to dilate and may require the use of cutting balloons and high-pressure balloons often inflated from 10 to 20 atm. Primary, primary assisted, and secondary patency rates of 38%, 58%, and 84%, respectively, at 24 months after balloon angioplasty have recently been reported by Eisenberg and colleagues.[333] If this technique is not satisfactory, a direct surgical approach at the site of the stenosis is indicated.[51,300] Vein patch angioplasty can usually be accomplished with relative ease to relieve stenosis of the graft itself or at an anastomosis (see Fig. 60.17). If the proximal segment of a reversed saphenous vein graft is too narrow, it can be widened (Fig. 60.18). Progressive disease in the inflow vessels requires a jump graft from the lower end of the original graft to a patent distal popliteal or infrapopliteal artery to bypass the obstruction.[300]

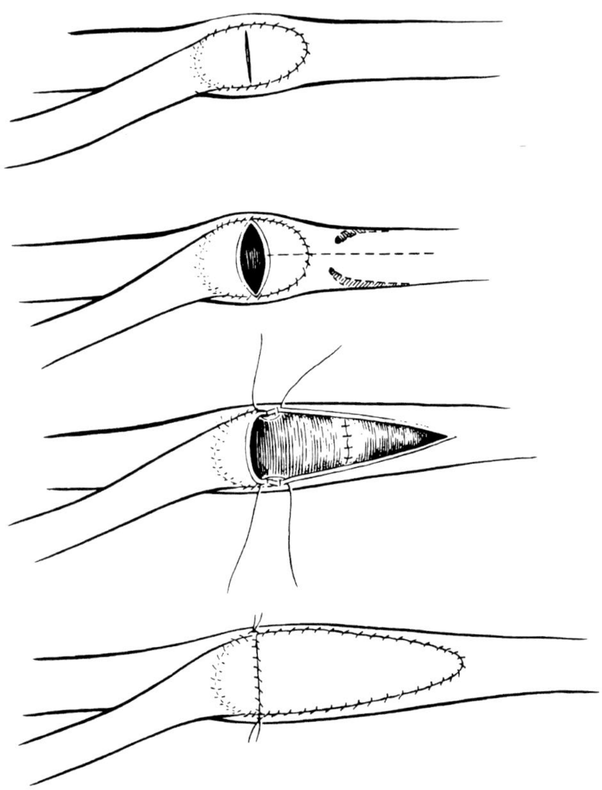

FIG 60.18 Technical sequence for inspection and repair of distal anastomosis of femoropopliteal or femorotibial graft. (A) Transverse incision in a wide "cobra head" overlying the distal anastomosis facilitates thrombus extraction, visualization of the internal aspect of the suture line, and close without stenosis. (B and C) When the distal intima is elevated, the arteriotomy is extended beyond the areas of injury, redundant intima is removed, and the cut edge is secured with tracking sutures. (D) Closure of the defect with a vein patch. (From Bernhard VM: The failed arterial graft: lost pulses and gangrene. In Condon RE, DeCosse JJ, editors: *Surgical care*, Philadelphia, 1980, Lea and Febiger, p 160.)

When thrombosis has already occurred and is recent, the graft lumen may be restored by mechanical extraction of the thrombus with a balloon thromboembolectomy catheter or mechanical devices such as the AngioJet device; prosthetic grafts are more amenable to this procedure than are vein grafts.[51,300,334] Thrombectomy of a fresh reversed saphenous vein graft usually requires exposure of both anastomoses. A transverse incision is made at the distal, wider end of the graft so the thrombus at that level can be removed and the internal aspect of the distal anastomosis viewed directly (Fig. 60.19). A second incision over the proximal anastomotic vein hood or partial takedown of the proximal suture line is required for passage of balloon thromboembolectomy catheters and for vigorous forward flushing because retrograde manipulations will be impeded by valves (Fig. 60.20). Prosthetic graft declotting can sometimes be accomplished through a single distal graft opening if the thrombosis is recent. The thoroughness of thrombus removal is determined by the vigor of flow through the graft from the proximal to the distal end, which also suggests that there is no inflow obstruction. Operative angiography

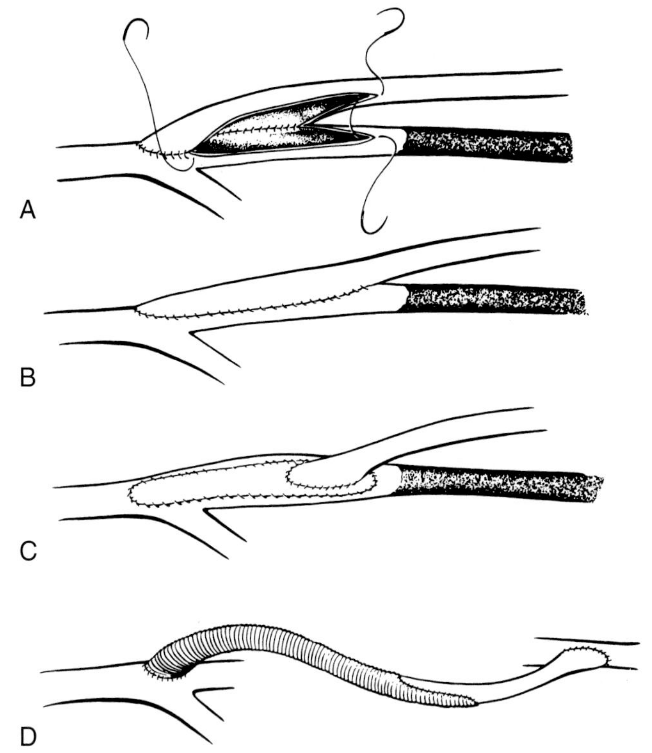

FIG 60.19 Techniques for revision of the femoral anastomosis to avoid stenosis caused by a narrow vein and thick arterial intima. (A) The proximal superficial femoral artery is incised to match the long incision in the vein graft; the vein graft incision is carried distally until the vein diameter is at least 4 mm. (B) Completion of anastomosis. (C) Alternative technique using a vein patch to increase the diameter of the artery; the vein graft is then anastomosed to the patch. (D) Composite vein–Dacron graft is another solution when the available saphenous vein is too short. (From Bernhard VM: The failed arterial graft: lost pulses and gangrene. In Condon RE, DeCosse JJ, editors: *Surgical care*, Philadelphia, 1980, Lea and Febiger, p 165.)

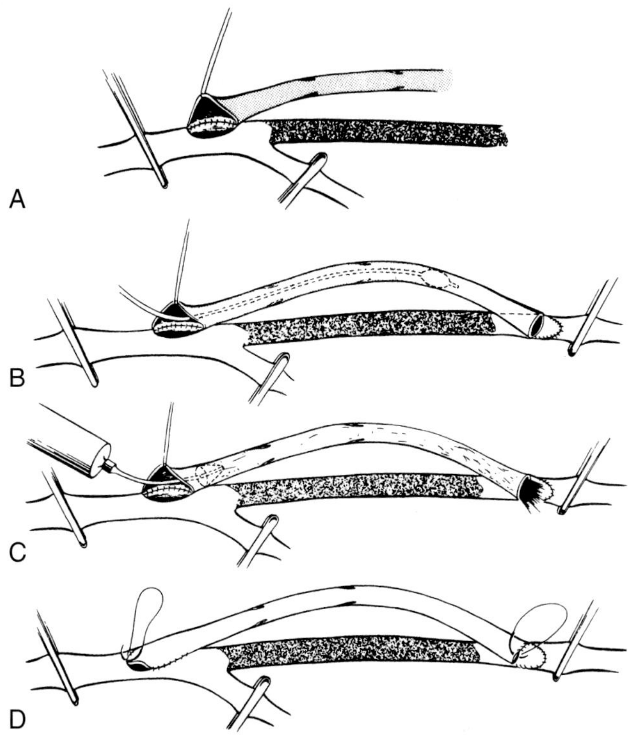

FIG 60.20 Partial detachment of the proximal anastomosis and graft thrombectomy. (A) Partial takedown of the proximal suture line. (B) Passage of a Fogarty catheter to the distal end of the graft and retrograde extraction of clot. (C) Vigorous flushing of the thrombectomized graft with heparinized Ringer lactate solution. (D) Resuture of the proximal anastomosis and distal transverse venotomy. (From Bernhard VM: The failed arterial graft: lost pulses and gangrene. In Condon RE, DeCosse JJ, editors: *Surgical care*, Philadelphia, 1980, Lea and Febiger, p 161.)

under fluoroscopic guidance is required after declotting of either venous or prosthetic grafts to confirm the thrombus has been extracted completely, to view both anastomoses, to evaluate the entire length of the intervening graft to identify areas of stenosis that need to be repaired, and to reevaluate the inflow and the runoff bed.[335]

The direct intraarterial infusion of thrombolytic agents is an alternative to balloon catheter thrombectomy in a patient who has no sensory or motor deficits and no signs of impending muscle necrosis.[84,297,307,336,337] Thrombolytic therapy has been successfully applied to vein grafts, prostheses, and endarterectomized segments at all levels of the lower extremity arterial system. The endothelial lining of vein grafts and of small runoff vessels is spared the trauma of mechanical thrombectomy, which may be an important factor in restored vein graft function long term. Although effective lysis can be accomplished several weeks after an occlusion has occurred,[79,338] best results with this form of therapy are usually achieved within hours or days of thrombosis.[339] The technique of percutaneous intraarterial thrombolytic therapy is discussed elsewhere in this book.

As soon as the clot has been effectively cleared from the graft by lytic therapy, angiographic investigation of the entire length of the graft, both anastomoses, the inflow, and the runoff bed is required to identify the cause of graft failure, which must be corrected to avoid reocclusion. In the interim between lytic recanalization and correction of the causes of graft thrombosis, patients must be effectively anticoagulated to forestall rethrombosis.[79] It is important to recognize that although lytic recanalization of occluded grafts can be achieved, thrombolytic therapy alone suffices in only a minority of patients. Graft stenoses or deterioration of inflow or runoff vessels must be identified and corrected to achieve long-term patency and limb salvage.[84,328,338,340]

Several reports indicate that intraoperative fibrinolytic therapy is an effective adjunct to catheter or mechanical thrombectomy in select cases when residual clot in the distal artery threatens the success of thrombectomy.[341-343] The use of intraoperative fibrinolytic agents has not been associated with significant bleeding complications.[341,342]

Graft thrombosis that is old or that cannot be reopened by mechanical or lytic therapy requires a secondary bypass procedure if the limb is in jeopardy or if claudication is truly incapacitating. Autogenous vein is preferable to prosthetic material, especially for bypasses to the infrapopliteal arteries. When the saphenous vein is not available for reoperation, lesser saphenous and arm veins, when available, are preferable to prosthetic conduits. The long-term results with prosthetic material are poor when used for secondary bypass, whereas arm veins have been shown to have long-term patency rates nearly equal to those of saphenous vein.[344]

It is important to emphasize the need to search for nonmechanical reasons for decreased graft flow, such as diminished cardiac output or hypercoagulability, especially when no other causes of thrombosis can be identified. Curi and associates[345] reported a 13% incidence of diverse hypercoagulable states in this patient population. Failure to identify and correct the reason for graft occlusion usually suggests a poor prognosis, because the underlying cause has not been removed.[75] However, thrombosis in PTFE grafts may occur for no apparent reason other than presumed platelet adherence to a relatively thrombogenic surface. For this reason, antiplatelet therapy in the immediate postoperative period is indicated.[312,346] Long-term anticoagulation with warfarin sodium should be considered in patients who have recurrent thrombosis for no apparent reason.

Reoperation to maintain extremity circulation is worthwhile because prolonged limb salvage can be achieved in 40% to 60% of patients undergoing four or more reoperative procedures.[300] The best results after reoperation for failure of an infrainguinal reconstruction are achieved in patients who require only a vein patch to relieve a stenosis that is repaired before thrombosis takes place.[300,330] For example, Whittemore and associates achieved a 19% 5-year patency rate after thrombectomy and patch angioplasty of thrombosed femoropopliteal vein grafts, a 36% 5-year patency rate after secondary autogenous vein bypass, and an overall 50% long-term limb salvage rate.[300] However, vein patch angioplasty of a stenotic graft or anastomotic lesion before thrombosis occurred yielded an 86% 5-year patency rate. For 72 early and late occlusions of PTFE femoropopliteal grafts that placed the limb in jeopardy, Veith and colleagues reported a 5-year graft patency rate of 37% and a 5-year limb salvage rate of 56% in patients undergoing reoperation.[347] PTFE femoropopliteal bypasses appear to be unusual in that thrombectomy alone, even when delayed up to 30 days after thrombosis, can sometimes restore long-term patency. The success rate for reoperation for thrombosis of PTFE grafts to infrapopliteal arteries is considerably lower than that for femoropopliteal bypasses. Brumberg and colleagues in a study of 131 infrainguinal prosthetic bypasses (44 above the knee, 27 distal popliteal, and 59 tibial/pedal) reported that treatment with warfarin sodium was associated with a patency rate of 89% in patients with an INR in the therapeutic range compared with 55% in patients who were subtherapeutic or nonanticoagulated. Warfarin in the therapeutic range augmented the patency of low-flow grafts, which occluded more frequently than higher-flow grafts (46% vs. 13%).[348]

Wound Complications

Major wound complications after lower extremity bypass grafting to the tibial or pedal vessels are not often reported but may jeopardize the success of these procedures. The reported incidence of significant wound complications after autogenous and prosthetic infrainguinal bypass grafting ranges from 7.5% to 34%.[349-352] In a prospective study of 77 inguinal incisions, Kent and coworkers reported a 10% incidence of wound complications; however, complications occurred in 44% of 79 distal (popliteal or tibial) incisions.[353] More recently, Turtiainen and colleagues[349] reported a 34% incidence of surgical wound complications and 27% incidence of surgical wound infections in patients undergoing aortoiliac and infrainguinal revascularization. Independent predictors for wound infection were infrainguinal surgery, obesity, and an angiography injection site within the operative area. Predisposing factors include age, female gender, obesity, diabetes mellitus, renal failure, anemia, postoperative anticoagulation, steroid therapy, ipsilateral limb ulceration or infection, and severity of ischemia. Technical factors, including the length and placement of the incision, prolonged retraction, location of the distal anastomosis, and technique of wound closure, may all influence the ultimate healing of these incisions.[350-354] In a recent analysis of 9932 patients undergoing lower extremity revascularization, O'Hare and colleagues found no significant differences in wound complications or return to the operating room for graft-related complications between patients with renal insufficiency and those without.[355] The amputation rate at 1 year, however, was significantly higher (29% vs. 10%) in patients on dialysis than in those with normal renal function.[356] The use of a continuous incision increases the risk of wound hematoma or seroma and, if it is not positioned directly over the saphenous vein, elevation of a large posterior flap, which is likely to become devascularized. The two parallel incisions required to mobilize the artery and vein for in situ grafting to the dorsalis pedis artery risk necrosis of the intervening skin bridge. Wound complications range from erythema, hematoma/hemorrhage, and superficial necrosis of the margins, to infection of the deeper layers with exposure of the graft. Gram-positive cocci and mixed bacterial flora are frequently cultured from these wounds.[350-353] In a report by Turtiainen and colleagues, staphylococcal species were cultured from 66% of the infected wounds and in 29%, cultures were negative.

Several steps help to prevent wound complications after infrainguinal bypass procedures. Preoperative mapping of the course of the saphenous vein with duplex ultrasound minimizes the likelihood of creating a large posterior flap. The use of skip incisions and leaving skin bridges may be of value in some patients. Isolation of necrotic or ulcerative skin lesions of the foot before preparation of the skin limits contamination of the operative field. In patients undergoing in situ vein bypasses, valve incision with the LeMaitre valvulotome and detection of side branches with Doppler ultrasound, angiography, or angioscopic guidance (when available) and ligation of side branches through small incisions, may obviate the need for long continuous incisions and, as a consequence, reduce the incidence of wound complications.[357-359] A metaanalysis of 4953 patients showed a significant reduction in wound infections from 13% in open vein harvest (OVH) to 3% with endoscopic saphenous vein harvest (EVH).[360] The severity of postoperative pain, extremity edema, and hospital length of stay is also reduced. Suture repair of side branch avulsions was required 3 to 5 times more often with EVH than with OVH. There is also some concern that the use of CO_2 insufflation pressures greater than the central venous pressure may result in severe hypercapnia, subclinical

(10.2%) or massive (0.22%) CO_2 embolization and the formation of microthrombi in the collapsed saphenous vein caused by the pressurized tunnel. Damage to the endothelial lining evidenced by reduced calcium mobilization, nitric oxide production, and esterase activity has also recently been demonstrated with EVH.[361,362] A comparison of the 1753 subjects who had EVH with 1247 subjects who had OVH in the Prevent IV trial showed that patients with EVH had higher rates of vein-graft failure (46.7% vs. 38%) at 12 and 18 months. Patients were not randomized based on harvest technique and no details of the harvest technique are provided.[363] Compared with open surgery, endoscopic saphenous vein harvest has been shown by Illig and colleagues to be associated with fewer overall wound complications (34% vs. 20%), as well as fewer class II and class III wound complications.[364] Review of the currently available data and analysis of our own cases has led to limiting the use of EVH for infrainguinal bypass in patients who have increased risk factors for wound complications: morbid obesity, poorly controlled diabetes, and renal failure and transplant. If a continuous incision is used, careful placement of the incision, meticulous hemostasis, and careful skin closure also reduce the incidence of wound complications. Once a wound complication has occurred, however, the treatment should be tailored to the severity of infection. Wound erythema with minimal necrosis of the wound margins usually responds to appropriate antibiotics and local wound care. More extensive wound infection and necrosis require extensive débridement and, often, skin grafting, muscle transfers, or myocutaneous-free flaps. Rarely, an exposed vein graft ruptures, requiring removal of the graft and placement of a new conduit routed through uninvolved sites. If this is not feasible, amputation may be necessary.

GRAFT SURVEILLANCE

Vein Grafts

When implanted in the arterial system, vein grafts undergo a series of morphologic adaptive changes that include thickening of the wall, anastomotic intimal hyperplasia, valvular stenosis, dilatation, aneurysm formation, and atherosclerosis as a response to arterial blood pressure.[314] The saphenous vein may be used in situ or reversed when used for infrainguinal bypass procedures. The merits of one technique over another remain a topic of considerable debate. Proponents of the in situ technique emphasize the theoretical benefits of better endothelial preservation and compliance characteristics, but there is limited objective evidence to support this assumption. In actuality, the in situ technique may entail more manipulation and damage to the intima from the use of valvulotomes.

Graft failure within the first 30 days is usually a result of fibrin platelet thrombus, retained valves, twists, unrecognized AVFs, or technical problems with the anastomoses; this occurs in up to 3% to 10% of grafts.[365,366] Careful intraoperative assessment of the entire length of the graft with Doppler spectral analysis or angiography is essential if these early complications and subsequent stenosis are to be avoided.[358,359] An unsuspected technical problem (e.g., stenosis, stricture, platelet thrombus, tunneling error) may produce thrombosis or be the source of a subsequent graft stenosis. Platelet thrombi occur at the sites of valve incision or splits in the intima along the length of the vein. Exploration of these sites, with careful removal of any thrombotic material and repair by patch angioplasty or replacement of the damaged vein segment, is often necessary.

Intraoperative duplex scanning of infrainguinal vein bypass grafts has been shown to identify problems that require revision in 10% to 27% of procedures (arm or spliced vein, 27%; in situ saphenous vein, 16%, nonreversed saphenous vein, 13%; reversed saphenous vein, 10%).[367] Bush and coworkers reported a 10% incidence of competent valves in the presence of "normal" operative angiograms.[368] Controversy remains regarding the efficacy of duplex ultrasound surveillance after infrainguinal vein bypass. The 2007 Inter-Society Consensus for the Management of Peripheral Arterial Disease document (TASC II) recommended a clinical surveillance program consisting of an interview for new symptoms of limb ischemia; limb examination with palpation of the proximal graft and outflow vessel pulses; and measurement of resting and, if possible, postexercise ankle-brachial indices (ABIs). Testing is begun in the immediate postoperative period and repeated at 6-month intervals for at least 2 years.[369]

Duplex imaging of the bypass was not recommended on the basis of a European multicenter, randomized, controlled clinic trial (Vein Graft Surveillance Trial [VGST]) that found no clinical benefit for routine duplex testing after femoral-distal vein bypass grafting; at 18 months, graft patency, amputation rate, and quality of life assessment were similar. Davies and coauthors[370] found no differences in primary, primary assisted, and secondary patency rates between clinical (69%, 76%, and 80%) and duplex (67%, 76%, and 79%) surveillance of vein grafts despite a higher incidence of stenosis in the clinical group (19% vs. 12%). The authors conclude that intensive surveillance did not show any additional benefit in terms of limb salvage but did incur additional cost.[370] The optimal surveillance program to detect bypasses at risk for imminent occlusion continue to evolve but should include both a clinical assessment for new or changes in limb ischemic symptoms, measurement of ankle and/or toe systolic pressures, and duplex ultrasound imaging of the bypass graft. The majority of lesions detected by duplex surveillance by Tinder and Bandyk[367] were asymptomatic, progressed in severity on subsequent scans, and amenable to treatment with endovascular techniques. The finding of low graft flow during intraoperative assessment or at a scheduled surveillance study predicts failure, and if associated with an occlusive lesion, a graft revision can prolong patency. The frequency of testing to detect the failing bypass should be individualized to the patient, the type of arterial bypass, and the results of prior duplex imaging. A peak systolic velocity 300 cm/s and peak systolic velocity ratio across the stenosis greater than 3.5 correlates with greater than 70% stenosis and is an indication for repair. Recently Shrikhande and colleagues questioned the validity of the aforementioned criteria for tibial bypasses and suggested a velocity ratio of greater than 2.0 as indicative of a greater than 70% stenosis. However, tibial graft stenoses accounted for only a small number of the lesions evaluated and validation of these findings await the results of studies with larger numbers of patients undergoing tibial bypasses. Johnson and coauthors,[371] using intraoperative duplex scanning, detected lesions requiring revision in 15% (96/626) of infrainguinal bypasses. The lesions detected included 82 vein/anastomotic stenoses, 17 vein segments with platelet thrombus, and 5 low-flow grafts. The revision rate was highest for arm and lesser saphenous vein bypass grafts (27%) compared with reversed saphenous vein bypass grafts (10%); nonreversed translocated saphenous vein (13%) and in situ saphenous vein bypass grafts (16%).[371] A normal initial intraoperative imaging scan, or one performed after revision, was associated with a thrombosis rate of 0.2% at 30 days, whereas 21% of bypass grafts with a residual or unrepaired stenosis by duplex or low flow required a corrective procedure for thrombosis. Ferris and associates[372] found that despite normal completion angiography, early graft velocity abnormalities could be detected in 26% of 224 grafts. Fifty-two percent of these lesions required correction, 38% resolved, and the remaining lesions were revised at a later date. When conducted appropriately, a graft surveillance program should reduce the incidence of unexpected graft failure to less than 3% per year.[367]

Beyond the initial postoperative period, approximately one-third of infrainguinal vein grafts develop stenoses that may predispose to thrombosis. Reoperation to correct such defects before graft occlusion permits salvage of the grafts and prevents recurrent ischemia. Unfortunately, between 20% and 40% of grafts occlude without warning or with recently recorded normal ankle pressure indexes.[373] Because of these grafts' propensity to fail, every attempt should be made to detect obstructive changes within the graft, at anastomoses, or in the inflow or runoff vessels before occlusion occurs.

A hemodynamically significant graft stenosis can be detected during carefully executed duplex scanning of the graft. The exact criteria mandating graft revision to prevent graft thrombosis remain controversial. Our observations suggest that when the peak systolic velocity progresses to 350 cm/s or more, or the velocity ratio is 3.5 or more, the graft is at significant risk of failure.[374] These threshold criteria may seem high compared with other published criteria, and larger surveillance studies are necessary to resolve this remaining controversy. Other important parameters are a decreased graft velocity of less than 45 cm/s and a fall in the ABI of greater than 0.15 (Fig. 60.21).[374] The former is particularly suggestive of a more proximal lesion, whereas the latter, if isolated, may be indicative of an outflow lesion or a missed graft stenosis on duplex scan. Nonetheless, these abnormal values warrant immediate attention, which may consist of closer follow-up, further evaluation, or immediate intervention, as dictated by the information obtained. After revision or an initial bypass procedure, the patient is seen every month for 1 year and every 6 months thereafter.[373,375]

The majority of vein-graft stenotic lesions respond to endovascular interventions. Use of a cutting balloon in conjunction with a high-pressure balloon may be necessary to achieve optimal results. Repeat interventions are not infrequent and are associated with excellent technical success rates. However, primary and secondary patency rates of 33% ± 7% and 63% ± 7% at 2 years suggest that surgical repair should be considered after early endovascular failure. Surgical repair with patch angioplasty or replacement of a segment of vein offers good long-term results.[376]

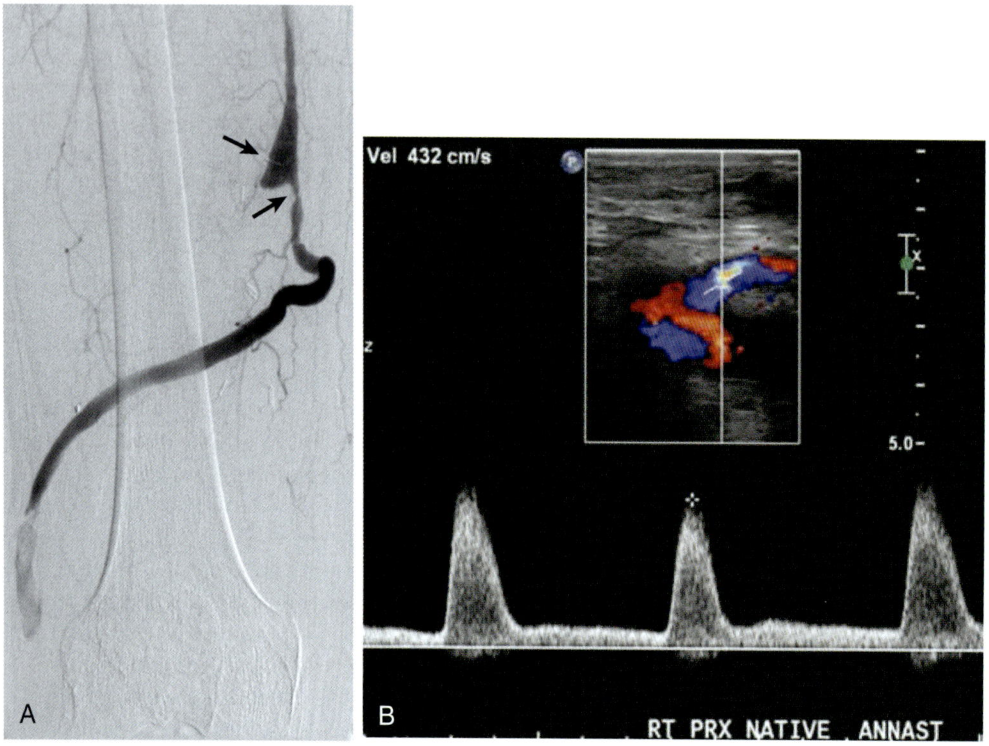

FIG 60.21 Vein graft stenosis. (A) Digital subtraction angiogram demonstrating a high-grade proximal stenosis of an arm vein femoropopliteal graft. (B) Duplex scan demonstrating increased velocities at the origin of the graft.

Functional failure of patent infrainguinal bypass grafts manifested by extension of necrosis or failure to control infective processes in the foot occurs in 2% to 4% of cases for reversed vein grafts, up to 7.5% for in situ vein grafts, and 8.1% to 9.5% for PTFE grafts.[377-379] Amputation may be required unless graft extension to an additional tibial or pedal vessel is possible. An alternative may be microvascular free flap transfer of healthy muscle to cover a persistent defect that usually involves exposed tendons, bones, or joints. Simons and colleagues, in an analysis of lower extremity bypasses for critical limb ischemia from the Vascular Study Group of Northern New England database, reported that 10% of patients with patent grafts met the criteria for the composite end points of clinical failure: tissue loss and rest pain (7.4%) and major amputation (2.7%) at 1 year.

Dialysis-dependent renal failure and the preoperative inability to ambulate independently were the significant predictors of clinical failure on multivariate analysis.

Graft Dilatation

With the increased life expectancy of patients undergoing aortofemoral and femoropopliteal bypass grafting, continued surveillance to detect deterioration in the graft material or complications resulting from the implantation of prosthetic devices is becoming more important. Although florid rupture of Dacron grafts and dilatation of PTFE grafts have been nearly eliminated by improvements in manufacturing techniques of the former and by increasing the wall thickness of or applying an external wrap around the latter, deterioration in prosthetic grafts still occurs.

Dacron Grafts

The true incidence of dilatation is unknown because patients with apparently well-functioning grafts, as evidenced by palpable distal pulses or normal ankle pressure indexes on follow-up examinations, are seldom evaluated unless a problem such as an anastomotic aneurysm or acute occlusion of a graft limb supervenes. Textile grafts initially dilate approximately 15% to 20% after implantation. This is believed to be caused by yarn slippage and is accompanied by a small decrease in tensile strength, which then stabilizes but may continue throughout the life of the graft. Three factors are believed to contribute to dilatation of Dacron grafts: (1) a flattening of the crimp when the graft is subjected to arterial pressure; (2) an increase in diameter and a decrease in length caused by rearrangement of the textile structure (i.e., the lighter the graft fiber, the greater the porosity and the more likely it is to dilate); and (3) an increase in diameter and length because of deformation of the graft material.[276,380-383] Dilatation is more likely to occur in knitted rather than woven grafts.[382] Berman and coworkers reported mean dilatation of 49.2% ± 4% for knitted Dacron prostheses, 28.5% ± 3% for woven Dacron grafts, and 20.6% ± 1.9% for PTFE grafts from their preimplantation diameter using CT (Fig. 60.22).[383] Although prosthetic rupture and anastomotic aneurysm formation have been reported in patients with dilated grafts, the natural history of such grafts left in place is presently unknown, although Stollwerck and colleagues reported no complications in their series of dilated Dacron grafts that were followed for up to 6 years.[276,281,384-387]

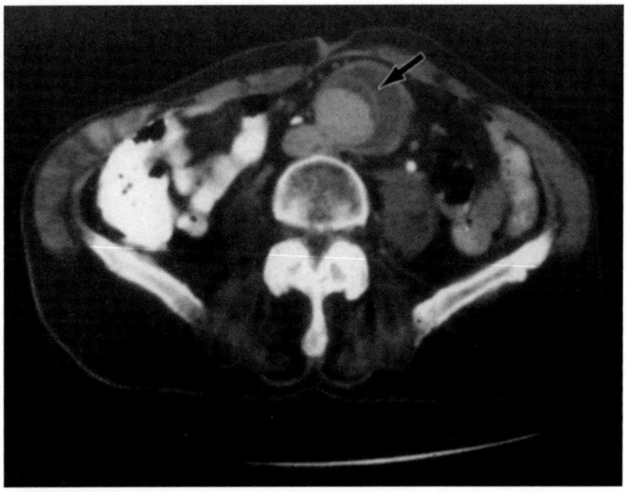

FIG 60.22 Abdominal computed tomography scan demonstrating a dilated graft *(arrow)* and the surrounding thrombus from an aortic anastomotic aneurysm. (From Hunter GC, Bull DA: The healing characteristics, durability, and long-term complications of vascular prostheses. In Bernhard VM, Towne TB, editors: *Complications in vascular surgery*, St Louis, 1991, Quality Medical Publishing, p 65.)

Nevertheless, removal of a grossly dilated graft or lining it with an endograft may be prudent in asymptomatic low-risk patients. In practice, dilated segments of grafts associated with anastomotic aneurysms are replaced. Care should be taken to use a graft corresponding to the diameter of the outflow vessel, and no attempt should be made to match the diameter of the interposition graft to that of the dilated implanted graft.

Umbilical Vein

Umbilical vein has been used as a substitute for saphenous vein, with a 5-year patency rate of approximately 45%.[388] Dardik and colleagues,[389,390] in a series of 756 glutaraldehyde-stabilized umbilical vein grafts (UVGs) implanted over a 7-year period, identified aneurysmal change in 7 grafts (1%) in the entire series. The incidence of such aneurysms increased over time, from 1.2% at 4 to 6 years to 7.7% at 6 to 8 years. In a recent report of 211 consecutive femoropopliteal bypass operations with human umbilical vein (HUV; 65 above knee and 146 below knee), Neufang and colleagues[391] reported primary, primary assisted, and secondary patency rates of 54%, 63%, and 76%, respectively, after 5 years; limb salvage was achieved in 92%. There were no significant differences in patency between above- and below-knee anastomoses. Segmental aneurysmal degeneration occurred in six grafts (0.03%), with operative reintervention in three cases.[391] In an evaluation of 283 grafts implanted over a 10-year period, Dardik and colleagues reported no aneurysms. Neufang and colleagues more recently reported a 7% incidence of aneurysmal dilatation of HUV grafts patent beyond 3 years; 3.5% required repair.[391,392] Because of the small but definite risk of continued deterioration of these grafts, it is recommended that HUV grafts be monitored with noninvasive surveillance and an angiogram performed if dilatation is detected.[389,390]

Polytetrafluoroethylene

PTFE grafts do not dilate significantly over time and are only infrequently associated with anastomotic pseudoaneurysms. In a study of 99 consecutive patients undergoing open surgical treatment of AAA with tube grafts, Stollwerck and colleagues observed dilatation of the midgraft segment of 1% ± 5% (ePTFE/Gore), 10% ± 9% (polyester/Braun), and 7% ± 8% (polyester/Vascutek) at discharge, which increased to 19% ± 21% (ePTFE/Gore), 33% ± 22% (polyester/Braun), and 23% ± 19% (polyester/Vascutek) after 6 years. Graft patency was 100% and no graft-related failures or ruptures occurred.[387] Because of its resistance to dilatation, PTFE remains the material of choice for open and endovascular repair of anastomotic aneurysms and possibly for aortofemoral bypass.[393,394]

Edema

Some degree of lower extremity edema accompanies the majority of successful infrainguinal arterial reconstructions and saphenous vein harvesting for coronary artery bypass grafting (CABG). The incidence of unilateral limb swelling ranges from 70% to 100% after femoropopliteal bypass grafting and from 8.9% to 41% after CABG. At 3 months, 56% of patients with leg swelling after CABG had improved: in 23%, swelling persisted beyond 2 years.[395] Endoscopic vein harvest is associated with a lower incidence of edema than occurs with the minimally invasive or OVH method (12% vs. 28% at 7 days, 6% vs. 19% at 3 months).[75,396] Although the most important factor in the development of edema appears to be lymphatic interruption at the inguinal, thigh, and popliteal areas during the lower extremity arterial reconstruction, the high incidence seen in cardiac patients suggests that other etiologic factors may be operative. Microcirculatory derangements that exist in the ischemic limb, such as loss of arteriolar autoregulation, loss of the orthostatic vasoconstrictor reflex, capillary recruitment, and focal capillary endothelial injury, all seem to contribute to this lymph-related edema by increasing the net flux of interstitial fluid into the lymphatic system, accounting for the 32% increase in limb volume compared with the non-operated leg reported by Haaverstad and coworkers.[397] Venous thrombosis has been shown to be an infrequent cause of postreconstruction edema (Fig. 60.23).[398-401]

The severity of the edema increases in relation to the severity of prebypass ischemia. It is less frequent after aortoiliofemoral reconstruction, presumably because there is less limb lymphatic disruption.[358]

Technical modifications to minimize inguinal and popliteal lymphatic injury during infrainguinal arterial reconstruction may reduce the incidence of postoperative edema.[402] Endoscopic vein harvest, use of a transverse versus vertical incision, and single-layer wound closure are among the technical factors associated with less edema.[403] Edema after lower extremity bypass procedures can be reduced by the use of elastic support stockings (18 mm Hg), bed rest, elevation, and diuretics. Intermittent compression has not been shown to be effective in controlling edema.[404] Fortunately, in most instances, postreconstructive edema is self-limited and improves or disappears during the first few postoperative months. However, the swelling may persist in approximately 10% of patients for up to 1 year.[75]

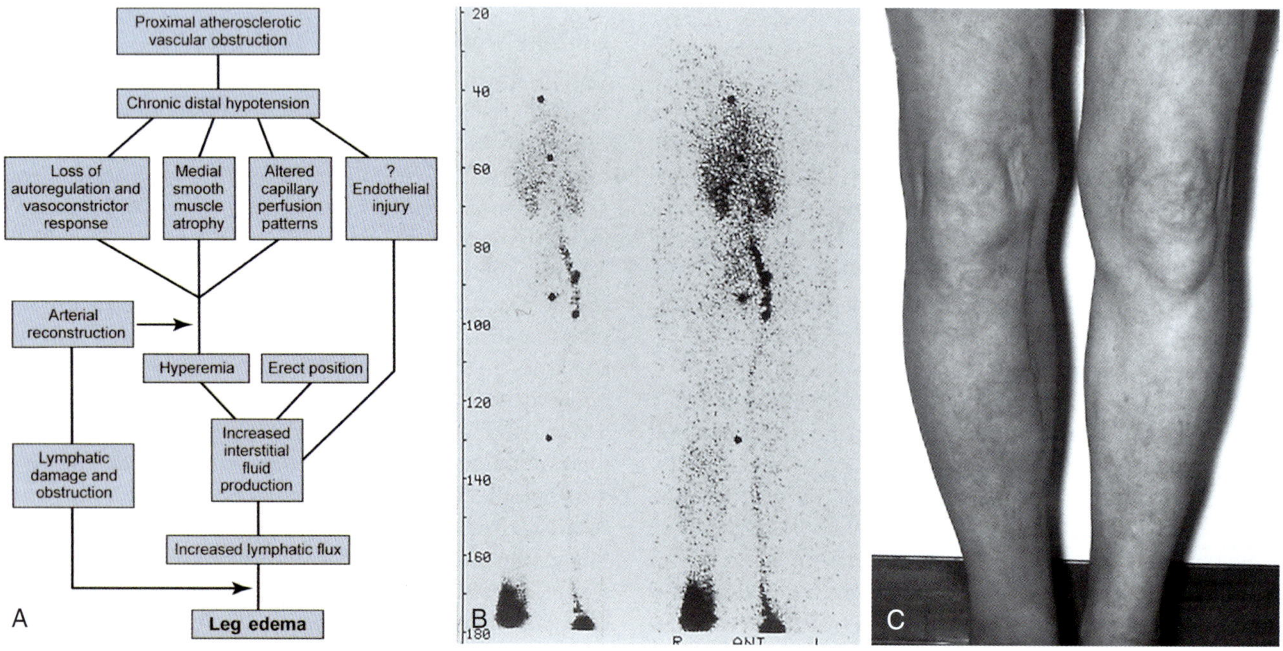

FIG 60.23 (A) Schematic overview of the factors involved in postoperative lower extremity edema after femorodistal reconstruction. (B) Lymphoscintigram showing decreased uptake of the radionuclide tracer in the swollen right lower extremity. (C) Patient after femoropopliteal bypass grafting. ([A] From Schubart PJ, Porter JM: Leg edema after femorodistal bypass. In Bergan JJ, Yao JST, editors: *Reoperative arterial surgery*, New York, 1986, Grune and Stratton, p 328.)

Lymphoceles and Lymph Leaks

The accumulation of lymph after groin surgery usually appears as an asymptomatic mass without evidence of overlying inflammation. The incidence of lymphoceles and lymphocutaneous fistulas was 1.2% per incision in a retrospective study reported by Tyndall and colleagues.[405] The highest incidence was seen after aortofemoral bypass (8.1%) for aneurysmal disease and isolated femoral procedures (5.3%) in previously operated groins, with the lowest frequency seen after femoropopliteal/tibial bypasses (0.5%). The diagnosis of a groin lymphocele is confirmed clinically and with duplex scanning. Aspiration of the fluid under sterile conditions should only be considered if there is suspicion of infection. If the lymphocele is small and located some distance from the incision, it can be followed expectantly. Should the lymphocele fail to resolve spontaneously, increase in size, communicate with the incision, or begin to leak, it should be explored and treated as in patients with lymph leaks.

Drainage of lymphatic fluid from the groin incision is a relatively infrequent complication of arterial reconstruction. In the series reported by Kent and associates,[353] a seroma/lymph leak occurred in 4% of the patients with groin incisions who were evaluated prospectively. The leak appears as a persistent, clear, watery drainage through the wound after the first few postoperative days or as the onset of drainage when the patient resumes ambulation.[75] The frequent presence of bacteria in the lymphatic channels draining ulcerative or gangrenous lesions of the extremity may lead to graft infection and anastomotic disruption. Lymphatic leakage results from transected and unligated lymphatic channels and lymph nodes in the groin wound. Possible contributing factors include poor wound edge and tissue layer approximation and subcutaneous fat necrosis.[75] Suture ligation of the veins and subcutaneous tissues rather than dissection with diathermy cautery during exposure of the femoral vessels is thought to reduce the risk of this complication. Nonoperative treatment of lymphorrhea includes bed rest and leg elevation to reduce lymph flow while allowing the lymphatics to heal. Wound care must be meticulous, and systemic prophylactic antibiotics should be administered to reduce the risk of secondary infection.[75] If the wound continues to drain for more than 2 to 3 days, the patient should be returned to the operating room and the wound explored. Manual massage of the thigh, the preoperative injection of isosulfan blue dye, or lipiodol or radiolabeled isotopes into the foot several hours before surgery are useful adjuncts in identifying and potentially sealing the leak site.[406,407] The divided lymphatic channels are suture-ligated and the wound is closed in layers over suction drainage, with care being taken to separate the drain from the prosthesis. This technique controls wound drainage and decreases the risk of secondary infection of the lymphatic cavity.[408,409] The reported experience with early wound reexploration suggests shortened hospitalization and a reduction in the incidence of graft infection. There have been anecdotal reports of the successful use of negative pressure suction devices such as wound vacs to control lymph leaks from groin wounds. Whether the routine application of fibrin glue to the femoral lymphatics before wound closure provides an added advantage remains unanswered. Several authors have advocated the use of vacuum-assisted closure for treating lymphatic complications following peripheral vascular surgery and have reported good results.[410,411]

REVIEW QUESTIONS

1. Venous bleeding is the more commonly encountered source of intraoperative bleeding because:
   - **a.** Duplication of the inferior vena cava is present in 1% to 3% of patients.
   - **b.** Veins are often adherent to adjacent arteries.
   - **c.** Venous pressure is lower than arterial pressure.
   - **d.** Circumferential mobilization is always necessary to obtain proximal and distal control.
2. Which of the following statements regarding aortocaval arteriovenous fistulas are true?
   - **a.** Common presenting symptoms include hematuria, pedal edema and congestive heart failure, and abdominal murmur.
   - **b.** They occur in 10% of patients with ruptured aneurysms.
   - **c.** Complete mobilization from the aorta is always required.
   - **d.** Cardiac catheterization is always performed because of congestive heart failure.
3. A 75-year-old patient presents with recurrent left lower extremity claudication and an absent left femoral pulse 5 years after undergoing an aortobifemoral bypass. The most likely cause of the aortic graft limb occlusion is:
   - **a.** Presence of a hypercoagulable state.
   - **b.** Progression of atherosclerosis at the proximal anastomosis.
   - **c.** Angulation of the graft or compression by the inguinal ligament.
   - **d.** Fibrointimal hyperplasia or atherosclerosis obstructing the profunda femoris artery.
4. Which of the statements are true regarding acute renal failure after infrarenal aortic repair?
   - **a.** Prompt intraoperative volume replacement with fluid and blood is not beneficial.
   - **b.** The mortality rate ranges from 57% to 95%.
   - **c.** Intraoperative embolization and infrarenal clamping are the only causative factors.
   - **d.** Biomarkers are routinely used to distinguish between acute renal injury and acute renal failure.

5. Which of the following statements about postoperative intestinal ischemia are true?
   a. Clinical signs and symptoms: plain abdominal radiographs and CT scans have improved diagnostic accuracy.
   b. Ligation of the inferior mesenteric artery (IMA) should always be done some distance from the aortic wall.
   c. An elevated serum lactate and normal D-dimer are diagnostic of mesenteric ischemia in the postoperative period.
   d. An IMA backpressure of 20 mm Hg and an index of 0.20 confirm the adequacy of flow through the IMA.
6. Twenty-four hours after repair of an abdominal aortic aneurysm, an 80-year-old patient demonstrates low blood pressure, decreasing urine output, increasing ventilatory pressures, and mental confusion. You suspect intraabdominal compartment syndrome. Which of the following interventions may be the most beneficial?
   a. Increase the fluid infusion rate and add vasopressors to improve the blood pressure.
   b. Increase positive end-expiratory pressure ventilation (PEEP) to improve the oxygenation.
   c. Monitor intraabdominal pressure and open the abdomen if the bladder pressure exceeds 30 mm Hg.
   d. Consult the gastroenterologist to perform immediate endoscopy.
7. Which of the following statements about spinal cord ischemia after infrarenal aortic repair are true?
   a. Interruption of the blood supply to the spinal cord between T-7 and L-3 is the usual cause.
   b. The mortality rate is decreased if the patient is paraplegic from the onset.
   c. Abnormalities during monitoring of spinal cord evoked potentials are diagnostic.
   d. Spinal cord ischemia occurs in 0.23% of patients undergoing infrarenal aortic repair.
8. Two weeks after repair of an abdominal aortic aneurysm, a 65-year-old patient presents with complaints of malaise, loss of appetite, increasing abdominal girth, and extremity edema. Which of the following studies would be most appropriate to confirm the diagnosis?
   a. Obtain an immediate CT scan of the abdomen.
   b. Maintain the patient on a high-protein, high-fat diet.
   c. Obtain abdominal paracentesis and biochemical analysis of fluid.
   d. Obtain a cardiology consult, give Lasix, replace potassium, and infuse albumin.
9. Which of the following statements regarding lower extremity edema after femoropopliteal bypass or saphenous vein harvest are true?
   a. It is always associated with venous thrombosis.
   b. Ankle edema after saphenous vein harvest in patients undergoing coronary artery bypass is rare.
   c. It occurs in 70% to 100% of patients after femoropopliteal bypass.
   d. It is unrelated to the severity of preexisting limb ischemia.
10. A patient presents with clear fluid draining from the left groin 10 days after an iliofemoral bypass. All of the following statements regarding lymphatic groin leak are true except:
   a. It is more common after femoropopliteal than aortic reconstructions.
   b. It may be preventable by careful ligation of lymphatic channels in the groin, application of fibrin glue, and multilayered wound closure.
   c. Apply a wound vac device.
   d. Admit to the hospital for bed rest, culture of the fluid, and empiric antibiotic therapy.

References available online at ExpertConsult.com.

CHAPTER 61

Management of Complications After Endovascular Abdominal Aortic Aneurysm Repair

Margaret W. Arnold, Daniel Silverberg, Sharif H. Ellozy

Endovascular abdominal aortic aneurysm repair (EVAR) for abdominal aortic aneurysms (AAAs) has gained wide acceptance since it was first reported in 1991.[1] Randomized controlled trials have shown decreased short-term morbidity and mortality when compared with open controls.[2,3] Increasing clinical experience coupled with refinements in device design, such as the development of lower-profile delivery systems and improvements in preoperative imaging for procedure planning and device sizing, have reduced the complications associated with EVAR. However, as with any therapy, the potential for complications exists. This chapter reviews the common short- and long-term complications of EVAR as well as their prevention and management options.

It is useful to classify complications of stent grafting according to their temporal occurrence. Early complications may be related to difficulty with percutaneous access, the passage of the device, failure at a seal zone, or accidental coverage of a side branch, such as the renal artery. Late complications are most often related to endoleaks but can include other entities such as limb occlusion, degeneration of the proximal neck, device fatigue, graft infection, and rupture.

EARLY COMPLICATIONS

Access

In order for EVAR to be considered as an option for a patient, the access vessels (the femoral and iliac arteries) must be fully evaluated and deemed to be of adequate caliber and acceptable tortuosity to accommodate the device and the delivery system. Challenges related to the access vessels can result in significant perioperative morbidity and potential mortality.[4,5]

As device delivery profiles have decreased in size, fully percutaneous endovascular aneurysm repair (P-EVAR) has gained popularity as a technique. Most authors report using percutaneous closure with larger-profile devices up to 24-French sheaths. A recent review of the Targeted Vascular data set from the American College of Surgeons National Surgical Quality Improvement Program database comparing P-EVAR with traditional cutdown demonstrated shorter operative time, shorter length of stay, and fewer wound complications associated with P-EVAR. On multivariate analysis, the only predictor of percutaneous access failure was performance of any concomitant procedure.[6]

Major complications of the percutaneous approach stem from failure to adequately close the femoral arteriotomy. These complications include retroperitoneal hemorrhage and femoral artery pseudoaneurysm formation. In most cases, the failure is noted immediately and the femoral artery is repaired by open technique. One study examined 279 femoral arteries that were accessed percutaneously with an immediate failure rate of 6%.[7] The midterm follow-up data on this group showed 3 of 156 (1.9%) having late complications, including one femoral artery dissection and two pseudoaneurysms.[8]

Relative contraindications to percutaneous repair, which may be associated with a higher rate of complication, include circumferential or anterior calcifications of the femoral arteries, small access-vessel size, severe groin scarring, a high femoral bifurcation above the inguinal ligament, and large groin pannus.[9] A high puncture site can be associated with hemorrhage on mobilization, whereas a low puncture site can be associated with vessel occlusion. Ultrasound guidance can be a useful adjunctive technique to find the optimal puncture site and avoid potential complications.

Iliac Artery Complications

Iliac artery rupture during passage of the device can lead to significant blood loss; if not controlled expeditiously, it can be potentially lethal. Fortunately, with the quality of current computed tomography (CT) imaging, it is possible to anticipate the majority of access problems. Technologic improvements including smaller sizes and hydrophilic coating make endografting accessible to more patients. However, although the delivery profile of abdominal aortic endografts has been decreasing in size, the smallest endograft approved by the US Food and Drug Administration still requires a 14 French sheath. Typically the size requirements range from 18 to 25 French. As such, depending on the device, the iliac arteries should have a minimal luminal diameter of 7 to 9 mm. Apart from vessel diameter, other anatomic factors must be considered, such as the extent of calcification as well as tortuosity and the presence of previous stents (Fig. 61.1). In general, if only one of these factors is marginal, transfemoral delivery can be attempted. However, if more than one factor is marginal, an alternative access such as an iliac conduit should be considered.

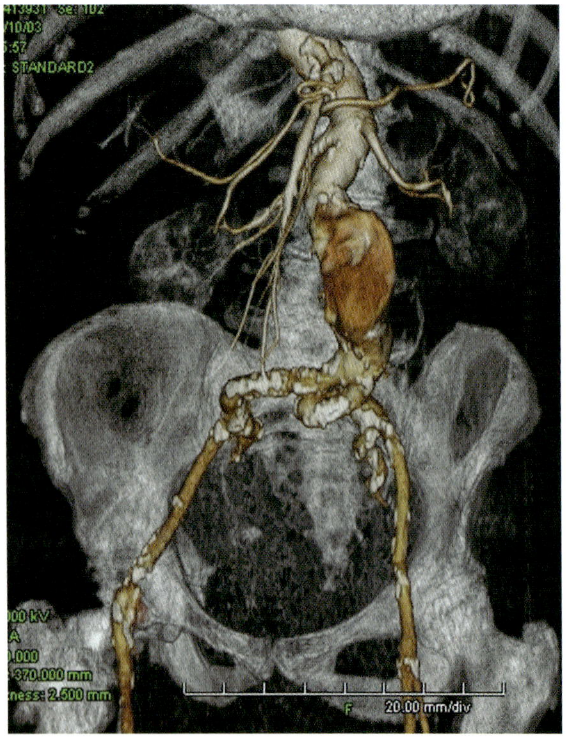

FIG 61.1 Challenging iliac access vessels. Note the calcification and severe tortuosity. (From Moore WS, Ahn SS: *Endovascular surgery*, ed 4, Philadelphia, 2011, Saunders.)

Two classes of conduits have been described: open and endovascular. Open conduits are typically performed through a retroperitoneal incision. It is the authors' preference to construct this conduit under combined spinal-epidural anesthesia. A 10-mm crimped Dacron graft is sewn in an end-to-side fashion to the distal common iliac artery and the graft is clamped distally. The graft can then be punctured and used analogously to a native vessel to allow for delivery of the device. After delivery, the graft can simply be ligated, or it can be tunneled down to the groin and anastomosed to the femoral artery to treat any significant iliac occlusive disease. An open conduit also maintains perfusion to the ipsilateral internal iliac artery (Fig. 61.2).

Endoluminal conduits consist of either a commercially available self-expanding stent-graft deployed in the iliac artery prior to delivery of the aortic stent graft[10] or a balloon-expandable stent sewn to a thin-walled 8-mm polytetrafluoroethylene (PTFE) graft delivered through an open femoral arteriotomy. The PTFE graft is predilated at the tip to an appropriate diameter to match the diameter of the common iliac artery at the seal zone. The graft is sewn to an appropriately sized balloon-expandable metal stent and then crimped onto a balloon sized for the iliac seal zone (Fig. 61.3A and B). The balloon, stent, and PTFE graft are then back-loaded into a sheath (typically 16 to 18 French), and an angioplasty balloon (typically 6 mm by 2 cm) is used to form a tapered tip for the delivery system. The commercially available conduit is simpler to use, but the "homemade" conduit allows

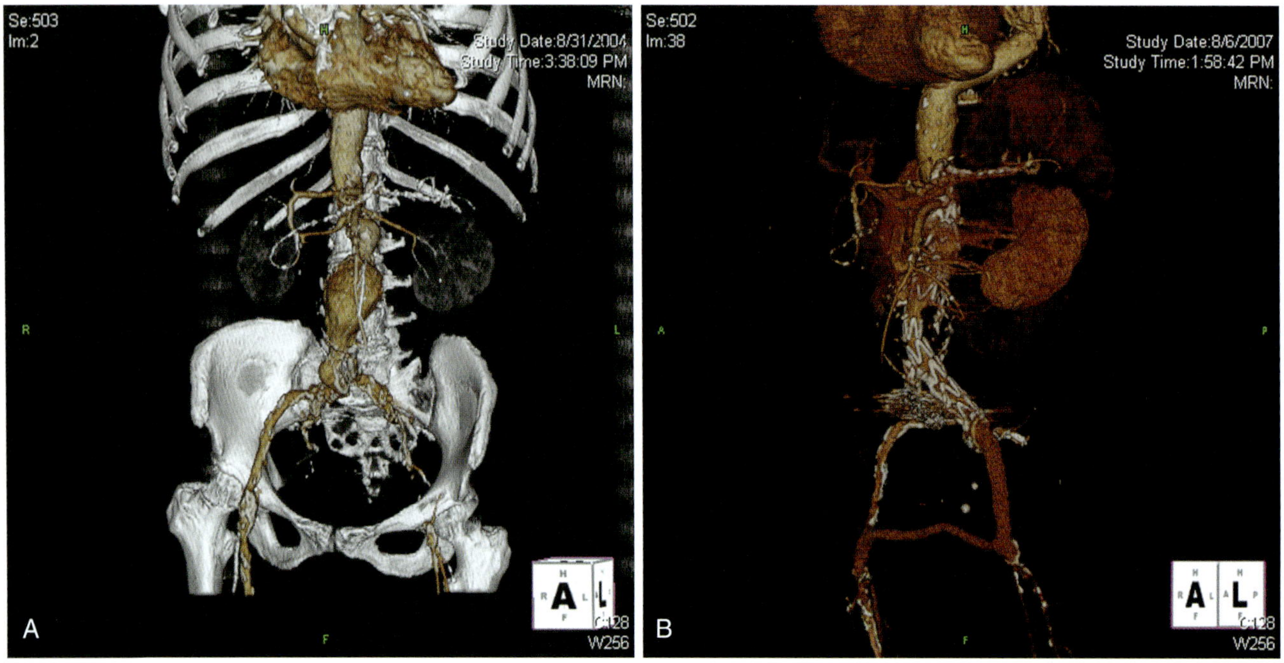

FIG 61.2 Open iliac conduit. (A) Preoperative computed tomography (CT) angiogram demonstrating occlusion of the left external iliac artery, with tortuosity, stenosis, and calcification seen on the right. (B) Follow-up CT angiogram after repair with an aorto-uniiliac device delivered via a left common iliac conduit. The conduit was then anastomosed to the left common femoral artery and a femorofemoral bypass was performed. (From Moore WS, Ahn SS: *Endovascular surgery*, ed 4, Philadelphia, 2011, Saunders).

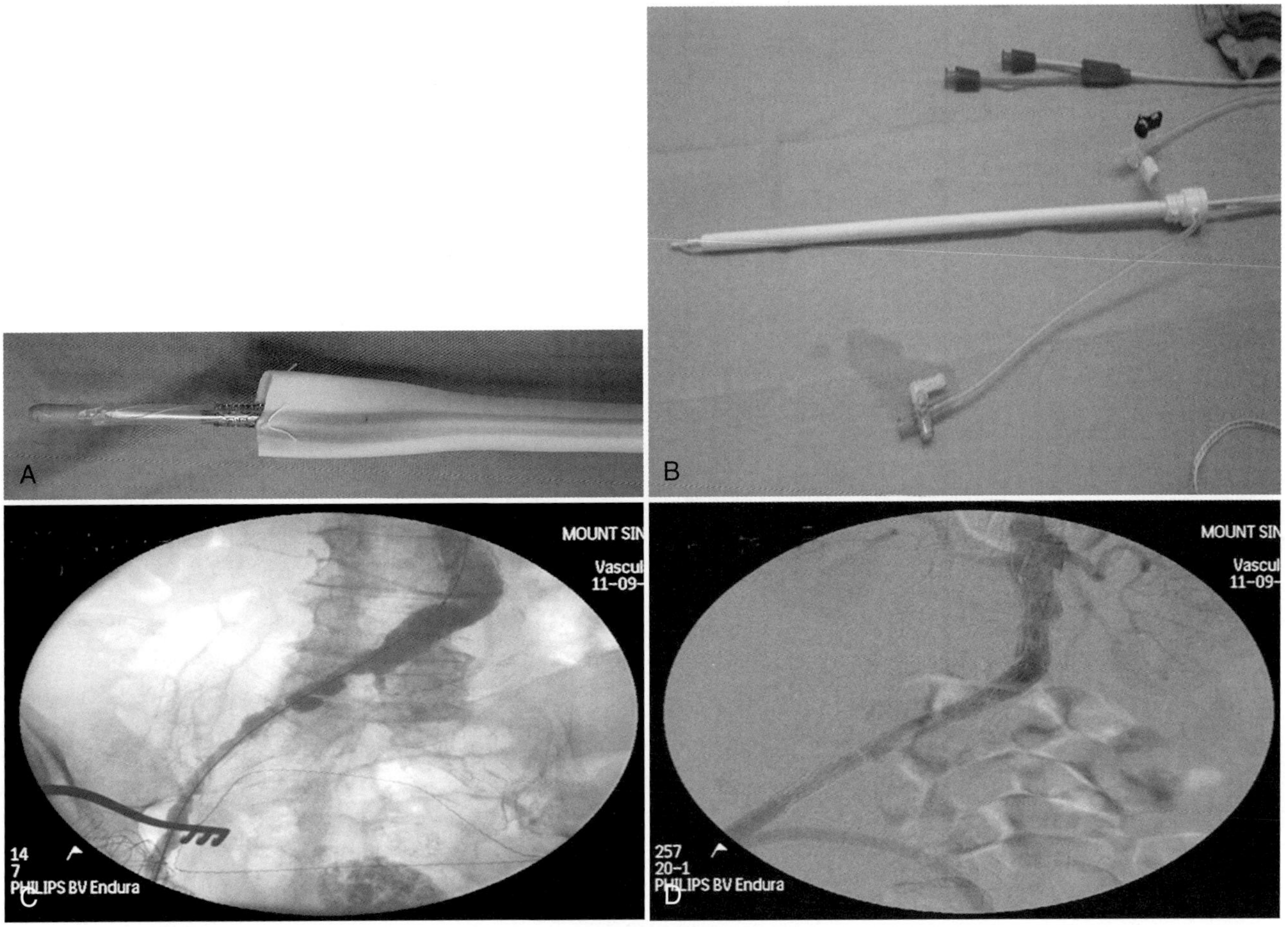

FIG 61.3 Endoluminal conduit. (A) Balloon-expandable stent sewn to an expanded polytetrafluoroethylene graft. (B) Endoluminal conduit in its delivery sheath. (C) Predeployment angiogram demonstrating occlusion of the left common iliac and right internal iliac arteries with a stenosed and calcified right iliac system. (D) Completion angiogram after delivery of an aorto-uniiliac device through the endoluminal conduit. (From Moore WS, Ahn SS: *Endovascular surgery*, ed 4, Philadelphia, 2011, Saunders.)

for surgical reconstruction of a diseased common femoral artery. Either type of endoluminal conduit can be placed using only local anesthesia if necessary. The endoluminal conduit is delivered transfemorally after judicious predilatation of the iliac arteries. Once the stent is in the common iliac artery, the sheath is withdrawn, the stent is expanded, and the iliac artery is dilated throughout its entire length down to the groin. At this point the endoluminal conduit can be accessed in a fashion similar to a native vessel to allow for delivery of the device (see Fig. 61.3C and D). Upon completion of the procedure, the PTFE graft is anastomosed to the femoral artery. The benefit of an endoluminal conduit is that it obviates a retroperitoneal incision in a patient with a hostile abdomen. In addition, in patients with circumferential iliac calcification, the conduit does not have to be sutured to the artery. Disadvantages include the fact that the ipsilateral internal iliac artery must typically be covered. This may result in a higher risk of spinal cord injury in patients with extensive thoracic or thoracoabdominal aneurysms.

Despite adequate planning, access vessel rupture can occur (Fig. 61.4). Two conditions are necessary to allow for a safe outcome. First, prompt recognition of the rupture is mandatory. Any unexplained hypotension noted intraoperatively should be investigated with a retrograde injection of contrast through the iliac artery. Second, it is absolutely essential to maintain wire access. This allows for placement of a compliant balloon for aortic occlusion to control hemorrhage. The compliant balloon can be inflated in the common iliac artery just proximal to the site of rupture to allow for continued perfusion of the contralateral iliac artery. At this point, a decision can be made as to how to repair the iliac rupture. If the device has already been delivered, an extension limb or a commercially available stent graft can be deployed over the site of rupture. There are several types available (Viabahn, VBX, Fluency and Atrium) and the delivery systems range in size from 6 to 12 French. If the rupture is not amenable to repair with a stent-graft, then a retroperitoneal incision can be made in a controlled fashion and either direct repair of the artery or placement of an open iliac conduit can be performed at this time.

A small-caliber calcified distal aorta may present access problems as well, especially when a bifurcated device is planned. A

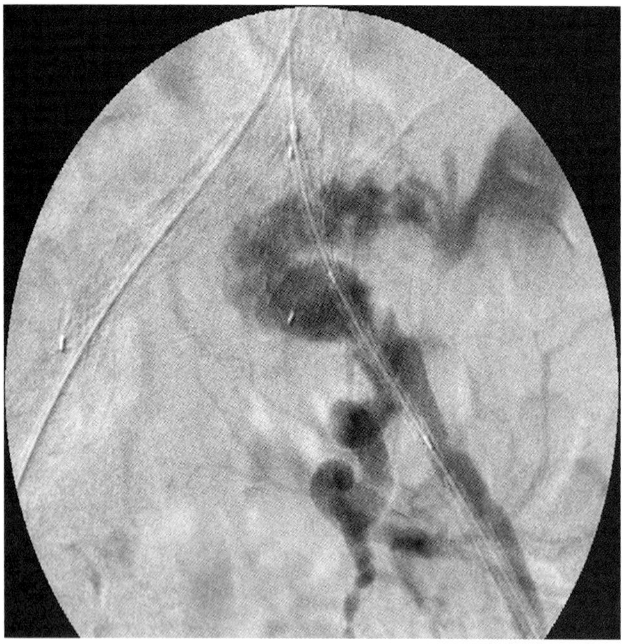

FIG 61.4 Retroperitoneal rupture after dilatation of the left iliac limb. (From Moore WS, Ahn SS: *Endovascular surgery*, ed 4, Philadelphia, 2011, Saunders.)

narrow lumen in the distal aorta might not allow full deployment of the main device, making access of the contralateral gate difficult. If possible, partial deployment of the device with constraint of the iliac limb can be performed. Then, after cannulation of the contralateral gate, the device can be fully deployed. This will hopefully prevent jailing out the contralateral gate. Once the aneurysm is excluded, judicious postdilatation of the iliac limbs should be performed to eliminate any stenoses. An alternative strategy is to use an aorto-uniiliac device.

Acute Neck Complications

Although access vessel issues are responsible for the majority of acute complications, the long-term success of EVAR is ultimately dependent on the seal zone at the proximal neck. A recent study by AbuRahma and colleagues[11] found that aortic neck length of less than 10 mm correlated with an increased rate of both early and late type I endoleaks. In addition to length, three other anatomic characteristics of the proximal neck determine suitability: angulation, shape, and the extent of mural thrombus (Fig. 61.5). In general, long, straight necks with minimal thrombus are ideal. Preoperative assessment with three-dimensional CT angiography is essential in assessing these characteristics. Centerline reformatted images can provide an accurate assessment of neck length, shaded surface reconstructions can give an accurate view of the angulation and shape of the neck, and orthogonal reconstructions allow for accurate diameter measurements and assessment of the extent of mural thrombus. If one anatomic factor is unfavorable, one can consider attempting EVAR. However, if multiple factors are unfavorable, the likelihood of long-term failure increases significantly.[12]

The choice of device may contribute to the success or failure of the proximal seal zone. Advances in device design such as suprarenal fixation, increased graft flexibility, and an increased range of sizes have allowed endografts to be used in a broader range of patients. However, there are no definitive data proving superiority of any one graft over another.[13] The clinician should base his or her choice of device on several factors, such as diameter, conformability, trackability, and precision of deployment. In addition, the importance of operator familiarity with the device cannot be overemphasized.

Accurate sizing and placement of the device is essential. Angiography from multiple projections should be performed to identify the true origin of the lowest renal artery. Three-dimensional reconstruction technology can allow for optimal determination of gantry angulation prior to the procedure. The entire length of suitable neck should be used to allow for durable fixation of the stent-graft. If a proximal type I endoleak is present after placement of the main device, several maneuvers may be helpful. It is the authors' practice to complete deployment of the contralateral limb before addressing the proximal leak. This provides additional column strength to the device before any salvage maneuvers are undertaken. At this point, the cause of the endoleak must be determined. If the device is too low, then placement of a proximal extension cuff is generally the first step. Occasionally the device abuts the lowest renal artery but does not cover the entire length of neck on the opposite wall due to poor device apposition from neck angulation. In this case, a second cuff may be helpful, as it may position itself in a different fashion once the main body is in place (Fig. 61.6).

If a proximal endoleak persists despite coverage of the entire available neck, then the mechanism of the endoleak must be determined. Occasionally the device may be correctly sized and positioned but fails to seal because of conformability issues. Should this be the case, a large balloon-expandable stent may help seal the endoleak. Care should be taken when inflating the stent so as not to overdilate the aortic neck (Fig. 61.7). It should be noted that the durability of a balloon-expandable stent deployed inside a commercially approved device has not been rigorously studied.

Accidental coverage of a renal artery can be a challenging complication. Other authors have described pulling the devices downward using either an aortic occlusion balloon or a wire and a catheter pulled over the device bifurcation and grasped from both femoral arteries.[14] These maneuvers can be challenging to perform with any amount of control, particularly if the device has active fixation. Should there be any residual renal lumen, it is the preference of the authors to simply stent the renal arteries to maintain patency. As with most endovascular interventions, the key is to establish wire access. Brachial access can be particularly helpful because the stent grafts cover the inferior aspect of the renal ostium. Low-profile systems are preferable (Fig. 61.8). Long-term salvage of renal function after accidental renal artery coverage is possible.[15,16]

In addition, other authors describe using the "snorkel" or "chimney" technique as a means to prevent occlusion of the renal artery during endograft deployment. In this method, a brachial approach is used to deploy a stent in the renal artery prior to endograft placement. The stent ends up running parallel to the endograft to provide inflow to the renal artery (Fig. 61.9).[17]

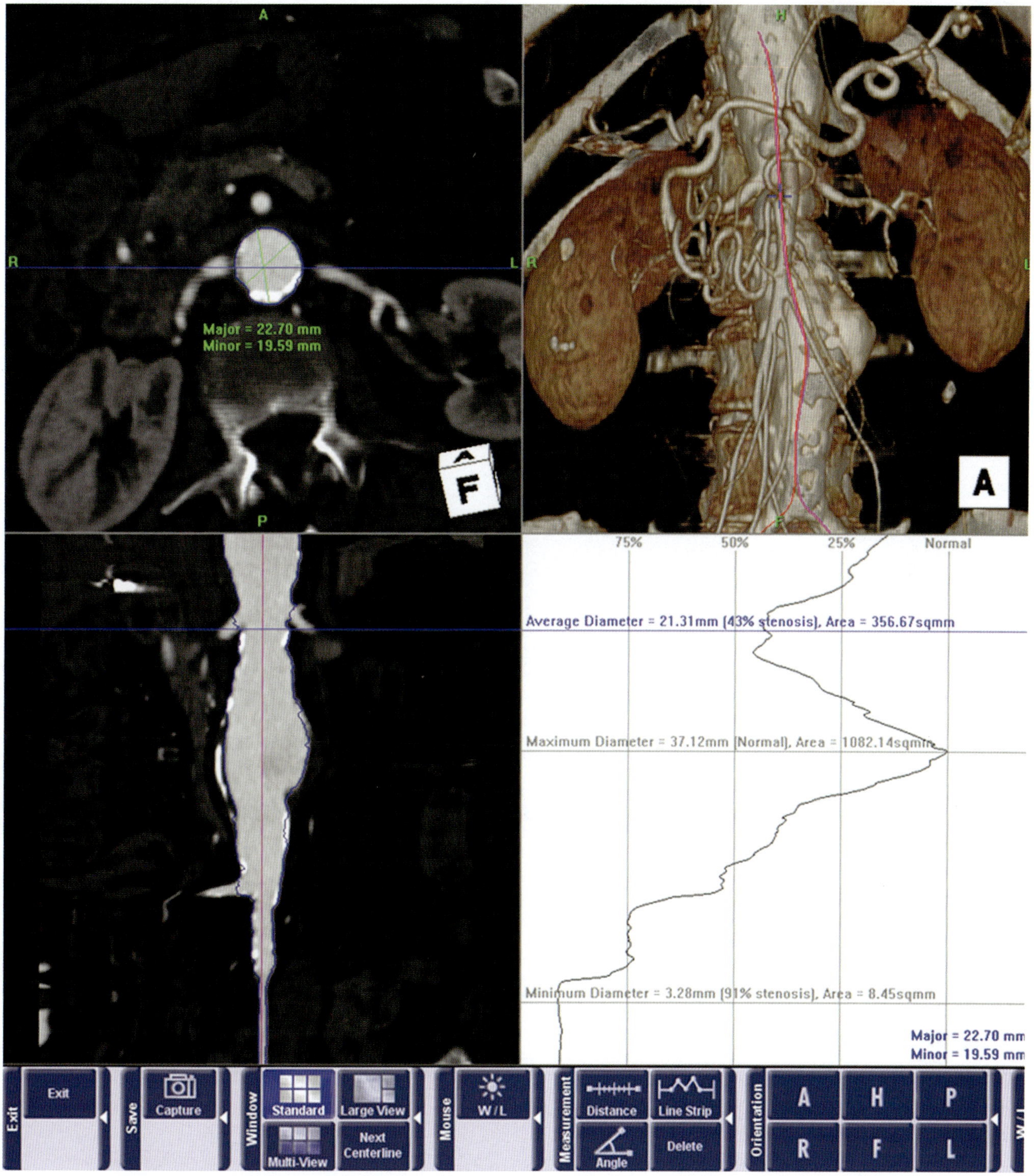

FIG 61.5 Three-dimensional computed tomographic reconstruction showing orthogonal, shaded surface and stretched views of the abdominal aorta. (From Moore WS, Ahn SS: *Endovascular surgery*, ed 4, Philadelphia, 2011, Saunders.)

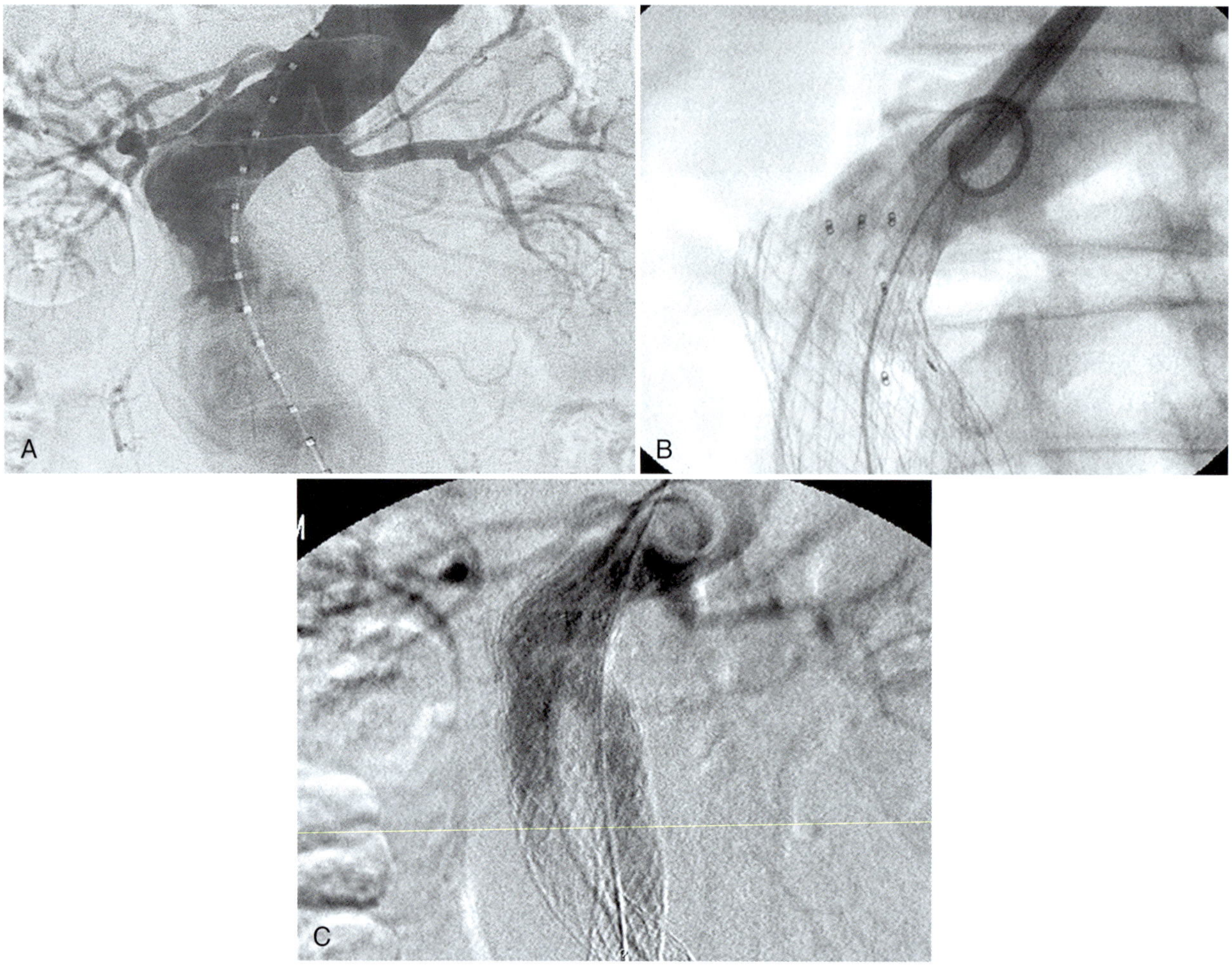

FIG 61.6 (A) Angled neck. (B) Deployment of the main body. The graft is low on the greater curve despite being just below the left renal on the lesser curve. This is primarily due to the stiffness of the device, which prevents it from conforming to the neck angulation. (C) Deployment of a proximal cuff allows for better coverage on the greater curve. (From Moore WS, Ahn SS: *Endovascular surgery*, ed 4, Philadelphia, 2011, Saunders.)

This maneuver requires a skilled practitioner but has been shown to have good results in small series.[18,19]

LATE COMPLICATIONS

Endoleak

Endoleaks are defined as any persistent perfusion seen inside the aneurysm sac. They are classified by their point of origin (Table 61.1). The incidence of endoleak has been reported to be from 15% to 50%.[20-22] The majority of these endoleaks are type II, resulting from retrograde filling of the sac via patent side branches. In the absence of sac enlargement, most clinicians believe that these endoleaks are benign and do not warrant intervention. Type I or III endoleaks, however, are believed to convey systemic pressure to the aneurysm sac. Patients with type I or III endoleaks are believed to be at risk of rupture, and the presence of one of these endoleaks mandates correction. Any patient with an enlarging sac and a persistent type II endoleak should be investigated further because of the possibility that this could represent an unappreciated type I endoleak.

TABLE 61.1 Endoleak Classification

Endoleak Type	Point of Origin
I	Proximal or distal seal zone
II	Patent aortic side branch (inferior mesenteric artery or lumbar arteries)
III	Failure of device integrity (fabric tear or junctional leak)
IV	Graft porosity at the initial implantation
V	Endotension (enlarging sac with no demonstrable endoleak)

Accurate characterization of an endoleak is the key to its management. CT angiography is the most common form of surveillance after EVAR, and it is highly sensitive for the presence of an endoleak. However, CT angiography is a static study and does not demonstrate the direction of flow. This is of clinical significance because type I endoleaks often show flow in patent aortic side branches. The flow is antegrade, in contrast to the

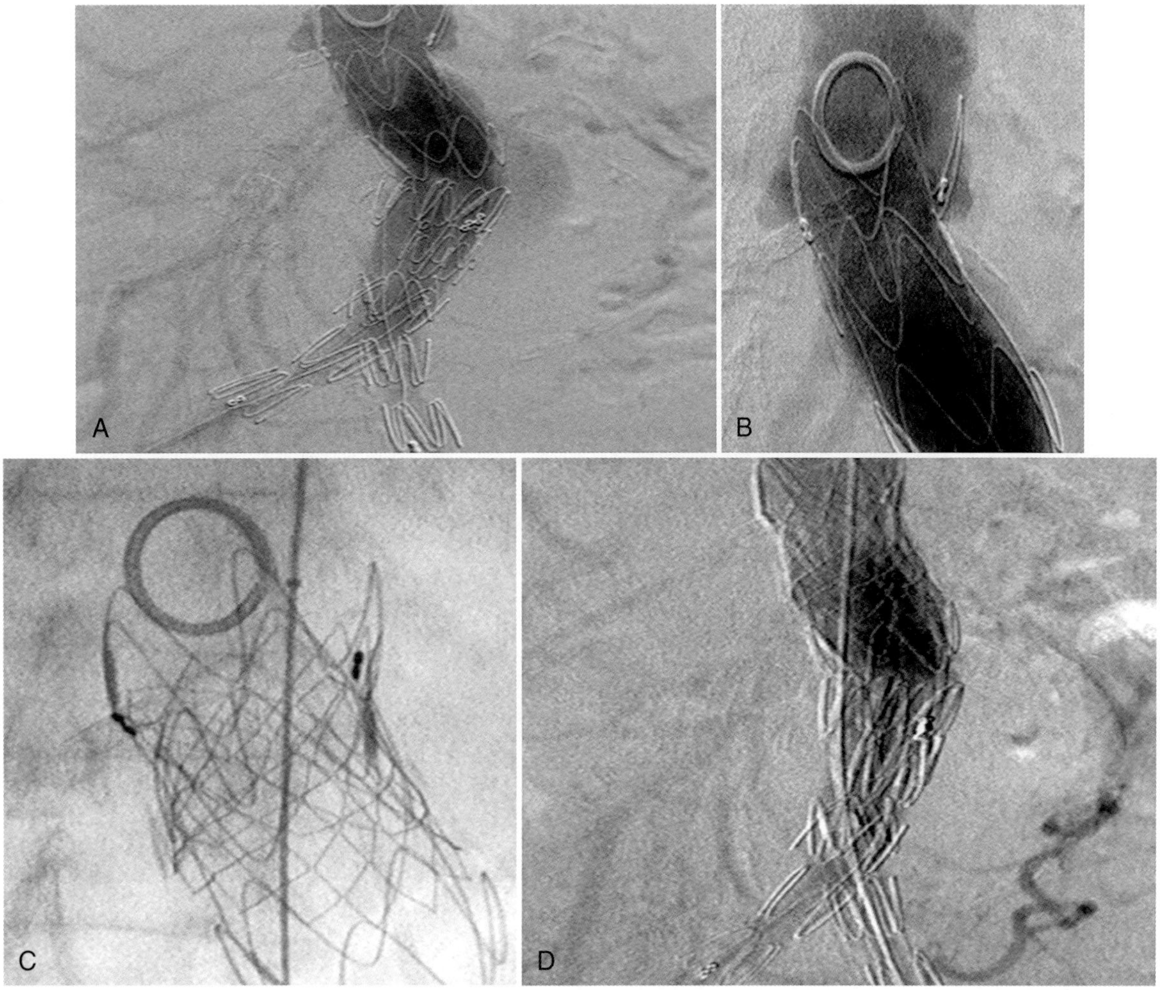

FIG 61.7 Neck irregularity treated with a large balloon expandable stent. (A) Proximal type I endoleak noted despite adequate position and sizing of the graft. (B) Poor apposition of the graft against the aortic wall calcification. Note the calcification in the wall. (C) Improved device apposition against the wall after stent placement. (D) Resolution of the proximal type I endoleak. (From Moore WS, Ahn SS: *Endovascular surgery*, ed 4, Philadelphia, 2011, Saunders.)

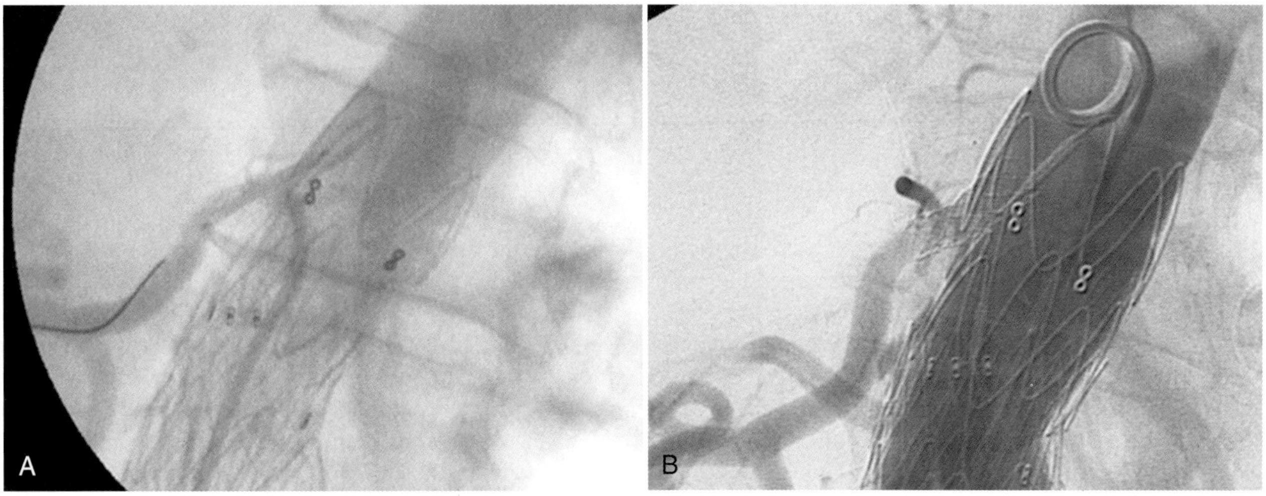

FIG 61.8 (A) Significant of a single renal artery by stent-graft fabric. Renal wire access has been obtained using a brachial approach. (B) Completion angiography after stent deployment demonstrates a widely patent renal artery. (From Moore WS, Ahn SS: *Endovascular surgery*, ed 4, Philadelphia, 2011, Saunders.)

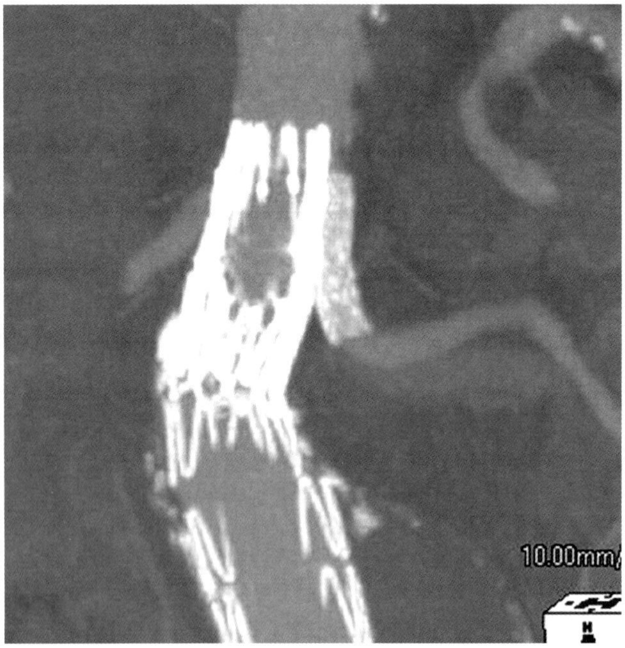

FIG 61.9 Left renal artery "snorkel" stent running parallel to the main body component of an aortic stent graft. (From Hiramoto JS, Chang CK, Reilly LM, et al: Outcome of renal stenting for renal artery coverage during endovascular aortic aneurysm repair. *J Vasc Surg* 49:1100–1106, 2009.)

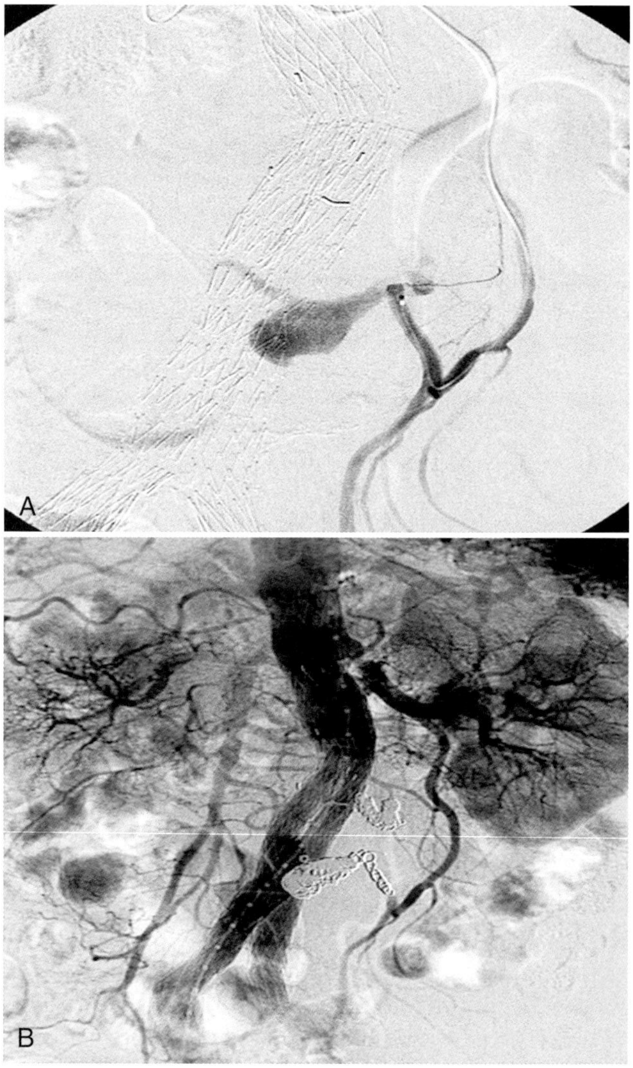

FIG 61.10 (A) Type II endoleak through a patent inferior mesenteric artery. The microcatheter was advanced into the sac through the superior mesenteric artery via the arc of Riolan. (B) Completion angiogram after embolization of the sac with microcoils demonstrates no further endoleak. (From Moore WS, Ahn SS: *Endovascular surgery*, ed 4, Philadelphia, 2011, Saunders.)

retrograde flow seen in type II endoleaks. As such, CT angiography might not always differentiate between type I and II endoleaks. A dynamic study, such as conventional angiography or time-resolved magnetic resonance angiography, is needed to tell the direction of flow in the endoleak.

Conventional angiography can be both diagnostic and therapeutic in the management of endoleaks. Flush aortography, selective injection of the superior mesenteric and both internal iliac arteries, and interrogation of the seal zones may be needed to define the nature of the endoleak. The type of treatment depends entirely on the character of the endoleak. Should the sac enlargement be due to a type II endoleak, embolization at the time of angiography can be performed. Access to the sac can be gained typically in one of three ways: (1) transarterially, via a microcatheter through the superior mesenteric artery and the marginal artery into the inferior mesenteric artery or through the hypogastric artery into a lumbar artery; (2) via direct translumbar puncture of the sac; or (3) through a transcaval approach. Each of these methods has its advantages, but it should be kept in mind that a translumbar or transcaval puncture cannot definitively define the origin of an endoleak, as these methods will only demonstrate the outflow from the sac. Therefore a transfemoral angiogram must be performed first for diagnostic purposes. Once a catheter has been introduced into the aneurysm sac, a variety of embolic agents, such as coils or glue, can be used (Fig. 61.10). Retrospective data suggest that translumber or transcaval embolization may result in higher rates of clinical success than transarterial embolization; however, there is significant heterogeneity in reported outcomes.[23]

Delayed failure of the proximal seal zone is perhaps the most challenging complication of endovascular stent-grafting. If the endoleak is demonstrated to be a proximal type I endoleak, then the determination needs to be made as to whether this can be salvaged with another endovascular device or whether the patient will require open conversion. The same anatomic criteria for endovascular suitability exist for a revision as they do for a primary repair: length, shape, angulation, and presence of thrombus in the neck. Review of the original, pretreatment images can be useful in determining further therapy. If the original device was undersized or misdeployed, then repeat endovascular repair may be feasible. However, if the original films demonstrate circumferential thrombus in the neck or if the device failed despite adequate sizing and deployment, endovascular revision is likely to fail. In addition, the presence of a device in the aneurysm

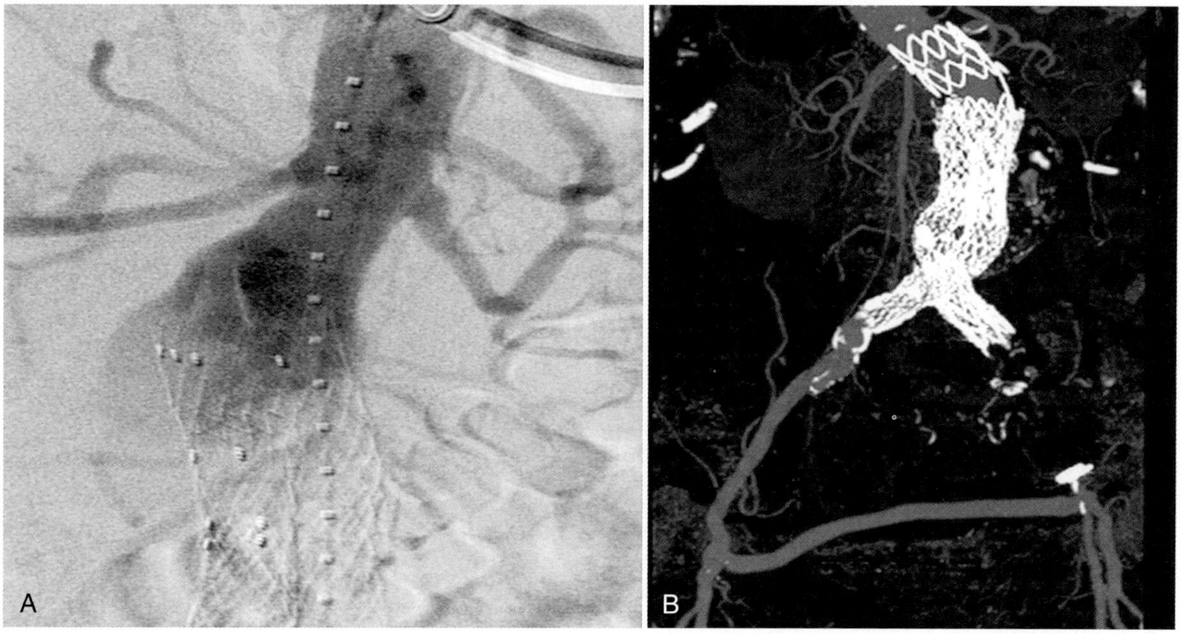

FIG 61.11 (A) Delayed proximal type I endoleak. Note that the device is sitting in the aneurysm sac. (B) Computed tomographic reconstruction after conversion to an aorto-uniiliac device with a femorofemoral bypass. (From Moore WS, Ahn SS: *Endovascular surgery*, ed 4, Philadelphia, 2011, Saunders.)

may complicate access issues, as it can make passage of a secondary device more difficult. Two approaches have typically been used for endovascular salvage: placement of a proximal cuff or conversion to an aorto-uni-iliac device with a femorofemoral bypass. Although the placement of a cuff is simpler, it relies on a seal between the old device and the new device for long-term fixation. This seal may be difficult to achieve if there is significant angulation in the neck. The aorto-uniiliac repair is more labor-intensive because the goal is to reline the entire aorta from the renal arteries to the iliac seal zone; it also requires creation of a femorofemoral bypass (Fig. 61.11). However, it does not depend on the integrity of the old device or on a seal between the old and the new device. In the authors' experience, aorto-uniiliac repairs seemed to be more durable.[24] The use of a device with a suprarenal stent should be considered when revising proximal failures. The advent of branched and fenestrated devices as well as the off-label use of chimney and snorkel grafts may be of use in salvaging proximal type I endoleaks.

Distal type I endoleaks can easily be treated with internal iliac artery embolization and extension of the limb to the external iliac artery. This can usually be performed percutaneously. Currently available iliac branch devices may allow for the preservation of hypogastric flow in anatomically appropriate cases.

Type III endoleaks can often be salvaged endovascularly by relining the stent-graft because the seal zones are still intact. Although rare, fatigue and junctional failures can be seen with all devices (Fig. 61.12).[25] It is essential to characterize the site of failure in order to correct it. If the endoleak is junctional, then simply placing a limb to bridge the leak typically solves the problem. If, however, the problem with device integrity is in the body of the graft, then the entire device must be excluded. This

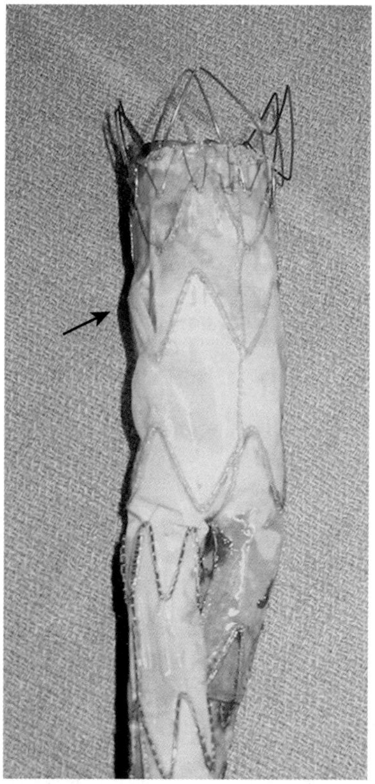

FIG 61.12 Fabric tear noted at explant *(arrow)*. (From Moore WS, Ahn SS: *Endovascular surgery*, ed 4, Philadelphia, 2011, Saunders.)

usually requires an aorto-uniiliac device with a femorofemoral bypass because a second bifurcated device cannot be placed inside the first.

Branched or Fenestrated Endografts

The use of branched or fenestrated endografts has allowed practitioners to offer EVAR to more patients, but it has also resulted in an increased source of endoleaks and a greater need for secondary procedures.[26] One study followed 107 patients who underwent either fenestrated or branched endografting or both from 2001 to 2010. The investigators found that 26.2% of these patients developed complications requiring 34 secondary procedures (six repeated interventions). The complications included limb-graft stenoses or thromboses, in-stent visceral vessel stenoses or occlusions, as well as type I and III endoleaks.[26] In addition, a retrospective review from a multicenter group in France reported reinterventions in 12 of 134 patients who had undergone fenestrated endografting.[27] This is comparable to the complication rate seen in the pivotal trial for the Zenith fenestrated endovascular graft, with a 22% secondary intervention rate. The majority of interventions (11 of 15) were for renal artery stenosis or occlusion.[28]

Limb Occlusion

Iliac limb occlusion after endovascular stent-graft placement reportedly occurs in 3% to 7% of patients. The risk factors for limb occlusion include extension of the limb to the external iliac artery, extensive calcification, the use of unsupported graft limbs, kinking of the graft limbs, and small-caliber vessels.[29-31] The clinical presentation can vary from an incidental finding on surveillance CT to an acutely ischemic, threatened limb, depending on the collateral circulation. Important collaterals around the area of occlusion include the internal iliac artery and the profunda femoris (Fig. 61.13).

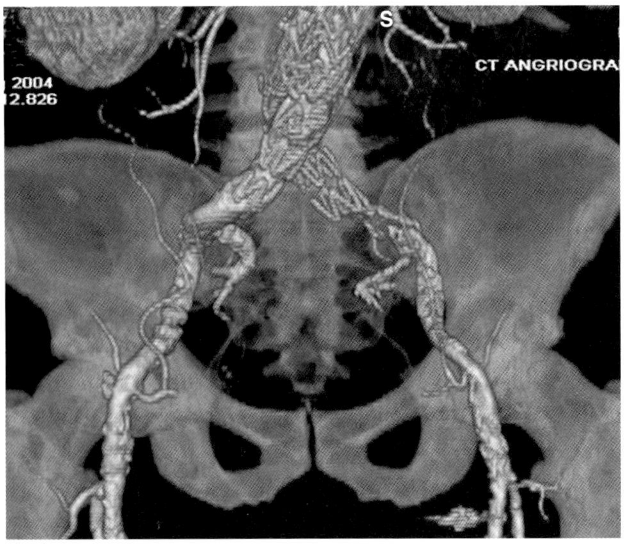

FIG 61.13 Occlusion of the left iliac limb with reconstitution at the level of the iliac bifurcation via pelvic collaterals. (From Moore WS, Ahn SS: *Endovascular surgery*, ed 4, Philadelphia, 2011, Saunders.)

The management of an iliac limb occlusion depends on the acuity of the ischemia and the underlying anatomic defect. Certain authors have described endovascular approaches to limb occlusion. Catheter-directed thrombolysis and thrombectomy will reveal any contributing stenosis. This can then be managed with angioplasty and stenting.[29] This strategy offers the potential benefit of a completely percutaneous approach. However, in the acutely ischemic patient, it may take several hours to restore perfusion. An additional concern is that it may be difficult to correct the anatomic cause of the occlusion. An alternative approach, generally favored by the authors, is to simply perform a femorofemoral bypass. This avoids the risks of thrombolysis and allows for rapid restoration of perfusion. Long-term patency of the femorofemoral bypass in this setting is very good.[32]

Graft Infection

Endovascular stent-graft infection is a rare but potentially lethal complication. It can arise in the setting of an aortoenteric fistula or come about because of contamination of the graft. Graft infection may be suspected if air is seen in the aneurysm sac on CT more than 1 month out from the initial implantation or if the patient develops inflammatory findings around the aneurysm with systemic signs of infection. When feasible, the treatment of choice is graft excision with either in situ or extraanatomic bypass and debridement of all infected tissue (Fig. 61.14).

Open Conversion

Under certain circumstances, an endovascular repair must be converted to an open repair to prevent severe patient morbidity or mortality. A recent systematic review found that of the 14,289 AAA patients who underwent endovascular repair, 279 (1.9%) required late conversion, with a mortality rate of 10%.[33] The authors found that the most frequent cause of late open conversion was persistent aneurysm expansion with or without diagnosed endoleak, migration, or stent-graft disconnection.[32] Open conversion after failed endovascular repair can be facilitated with several techniques. Positioning of the proximal clamp is determined by the presence or absence of suprarenal stents. If there are bare stents across the renal arteries, an initial supraceliac clamp can be placed until the device is out; then the clamp can be moved into the infrarenal position. Balloon occlusion catheters, deployed either transfemorally or transbrachially, can be helpful in patients with challenging anatomy. Some authors have even described deploying the catheters directly through the indwelling stent-graft. Care should be taken in removing the device to prevent damage to the aorta at the pararenal segment. If the suprarenal stents are embedded in the wall of the aorta, a sterile wire cutter can be used to leave the wires in situ. Distally, the iliac arteries and the device limbs can be clamped directly. Vascular clamps with Fogarty inserts can facilitate occlusion of the stent-graft limbs. If the distal seal is intact, the iliac limbs do not have to be removed. The limbs can be transected, and an end-to-end anastomosis can be fashioned to the limbs using the native iliac as an external pledget. Despite the increased complexity of repair in the setting of a failed stent-graft, some authors have reported good long-term outcomes.[34]

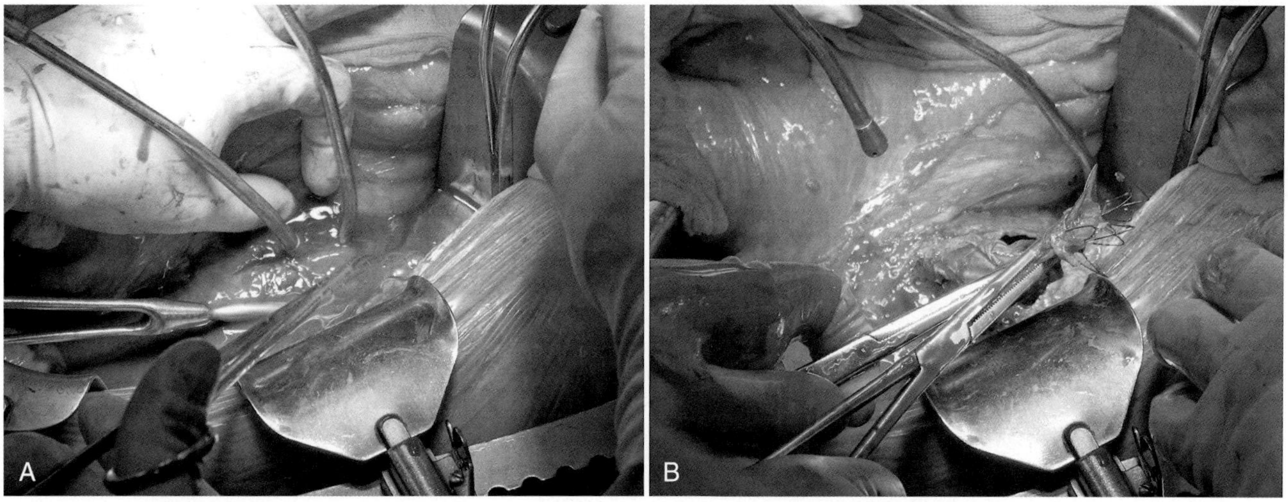

FIG 61.14 Stent-graft infection. (A) Grossly infected sac contents. (B) Removal of the stent-graft. (From Moore WS, Ahn SS: *Endovascular surgery*, ed 4, Philadelphia, 2011, Saunders.)

CONCLUSIONS

The key to managing complications in EVAR is anticipation and case selection. The most serious acute complications are related to access vessels, and these are typically predictable. The liberal use of conduits in challenging cases allows for safe endovascular repair. Close surveillance after repair, with the use of dynamic imaging in equivocal cases, allows for early identification and safe treatment of late complications. Precise imaging is key in determining whether endovascular revision of failed stent-grafts is possible. Should the patient need open conversion, balloon occlusion catheters, Fogarty vascular clamps, and sterile wire cutters can significantly simplify the operation.

BIBLIOGRAPHY

Baril DT, Silverberg D, Ellozy SH, et al. Endovascular stent-graft repair of failed endovascular abdominal aortic aneurysm repair. *Ann Vasc Surg*. 2008;22(1):30–36.

Buck DB, Karthaus EG, Soden PA, et al. Percutaneous versus femoral cutdown access for endovascular aneurysm repair. *J Vasc Surg*. 2015;62:16–21.

Greenhalgh RM, Brown LC, Kwong GP, et al. Comparison of endovascular aneurysm repair with open repair in patients with abdominal aortic aneurysm (EVAR trial 1) 30-day operative mortality results: randomised controlled trial. *Lancet*. 2004; 364(9437):843–848.

Jimenez JC, Moore WS, Quinones-Baldrich WJ. Acute and chronic open conversion after endovascular aortic aneurysm repair: a 14-year review. *J Vasc Surg*. 2007;46(4):642–647.

Moulakakis KG, Dalainas I, Mylonas S, et al. Conversion to open repair after endografting for abdominal aortic aneurysm: a review of causes, incidence, results, and surgical techniques. *J Endovasc Ther*. 2010;17:694–702.

Oderich GS, Greenberg RK, Farber M, et al. Results of the United States multicenter prospective study evaluating the Zenith fenestrated endovascular graft for treatment of juxtarenal abdominal aortic aneurysms. *J Vasc Surg*. 2014;60:1420–1428.

Parodi JC, Palmaz JC, Barone HD. Transfemoral intraluminal graft implantation for abdominal aortic aneurysms. *Ann Vasc Surg*. 1991;5(6):491–499.

Prinssen M, Verhoeven EL, Buth J, et al. A randomized trial comparing conventional and endovascular repair of abdominal aortic aneurysms. *N Engl J Med*. 2004;351(16):1607–1618.

Sidloff DA, Stather PW, Choke E, et al. Type II endoleak after endovascular aneurysm repair. *Br J Surg*. 2013;100:1262–1270.

Silverberg D, Baril DT, Ellozy SH, et al. An 8-year experience with type II endoleaks: natural history suggests selective intervention is a safe approach. *J Vasc Surg*. 2006;44(3):453–459.

References available online at expertconsult.com.

62 CHAPTER

Diabetic Foot Complications: A Primer for Vascular Surgeons

Neal R. Barshes, Joseph L. Mills

Diabetic foot complications are common, costly, and impactful.[1] The experience of many diabetic programs has demonstrated that multidisciplinary or interdisciplinary management of patients with diabetic foot ulcers (DFUs) can significantly reduce complications and produce outstanding outcomes[2-4]; participation in these groups may be one of the most beneficial roles a vascular surgeon may play. Vascular surgeons should therefore have a fundamental understanding of the spectrum of diabetic foot complications and their management.

PATHOGENESIS AND PRESENTATION OF DIABETIC FOOT ULCERS AND INFECTIONS

The development of a foot ulcer—defined as a full-thickness epithelial defect on the foot (skin distal to the malleoli) lasting more than 14 days—is usually the initial complication that develops in the diabetic foot. A multitude of risk factors may predispose to the development of a foot ulcer, but sensory neuropathy is the most significant single factor. Changes in the morphology of the foot may also lead to an abnormal or uneven distribution of pressure across various areas of the foot during walking. This abnormal distribution of pressure may lead to repetitive trauma during walking and may ultimately lead to full-thickness ulceration. Although this ulcer would generally be very painful in persons with normal sensation, it often goes unnoticed in patients with sensory neuropathy; this has been termed "loss of protective sensation" (often abbreviated in medical literature as LOPS).

Once established, foot ulcers act as the portal of entry for bacterial infection of the foot. Among those with a foot ulcer, the incidence of foot infection is also twofold higher among those with peripheral arterial disease (PAD) compared with those without PAD.[5] The incidence of foot infection is associated with foot ulcers that have been present for more than 30 days and recurrent foot ulcers, as well as penetrating trauma to the foot.[5] In addition, the combination of foot infection and PAD triples the amputation risk in patients with diabetes.[6]

Like ulcers, gangrenous digits can also pose a risk for foot infection. Gangrene of an entire digit occurs when oxygen and nutrient supply becomes insufficient to maintain soft tissue viability. Inflammation from local trauma or an infected ulcer may change the balance between supply and demand sufficiently to result in digit gangrene. Systemic illness (including volume overload from kidney failure or severe heart failure; hypotension requiring vasopressor support) and some tumors (via paraneoplastic syndromes) can rarely also cause digit gangrene. In most patients, foot ulcers and digit gangrene should *not* be ascribed to embolization of more proximal atherosclerotic lesions or to microvascular occlusive disease because these are phenomena not thought to be involved in the pathogenesis of diabetic foot complications.[7] Similar to a foot ulcer with overlying eschar or acellular debris, the interface between viable and nonviable tissue may serve as a portal of entry for bacterial inoculation in the remainder of the foot.

Infection in the diabetic foot often has a more subtle presentation than does infection in other areas or infection in patients without diabetes. Typically, diabetic foot infections may present with erythema, swelling, and often with fluctuance. Purulent drainage is a more specific sign of infection, but serous discharge should also be viewed as suspicious for infection. Foul odor can sometimes be caused simply by necrotic tissue on the surface of the wound but should also be considered a sign of possible infection. The presence of unilateral edema in the affected foot or calf should signal the presence of an underlying foot infection, even if the appearance of the ulcer and skin immediately surrounding it is unremarkable.

Systemic symptoms and signs also help to identify infection. As with infections in other areas, such systemic signs may include fever, tachycardia, and evidence of inadequate end-organ perfusion (tachypnea, mental status changes, oliguria). However, similar to local signs of infection, only subtle symptoms or signs may be present, including malaise, anorexia, nausea, fatigue, or a degree of hyperglycemia that is unusual for a particular patient. Patients with a foot ulcer and systemic signs of infection should be assumed to have a foot infection, unless another plausible cause of infection can be clearly identified.

Infections may affect virtually any of the structures in the foot. Cellulitis and abscesses are particularly common. Diabetic foot osteomyelitis complicates approximately 20% to 30% of foot ulcers,[8,9] and the risk of osteomyelitis appears to be directly correlated with the duration of a foot ulcer as well as the depth.[8] Other things being equal, foot ulcers complicated by osteomyelitis have twofold to threefold higher rate of leg amputation than those with only soft tissue infection.[9,10]

The organisms involved in both soft tissue infections and osteomyelitis are similar; approximately one-third of foot infections are monomicrobial, whereas the remainder are polymicrobial, with two to five organisms commonly found. Approximately 60% of isolates are gram-positive aerobic bacteria, 20% are gram-negative aerobic bacteria, and 15% are anaerobic bacteria.[11] *Staphylococcus aureus* is the most common species of organism isolated in most series, with methicillin-resistant and methicillin-sensitive strains (MRSA and MSSA, respectively) being found in a near equal distribution.[11] Compared with MSSA osteomyelitis, MRSA osteomyelitis has been associated with a higher fever, more pronounced leukocytosis, fetid odor, a higher prevalence of cutaneous necrosis, as well as a higher incidence of radiographic evidence of bony changes suggestive of osteomyelitis. Patients with MRSA osteomyelitis also have longer hospital stays and slower healing times.[12] However, MRSA osteomyelitis is not associated with higher rates of treatment failure or leg amputation, when compared with MSSA infections.[11,12]

In contrast to MRSA, two gram-negative aerobic bacteria—*Escherichia coli* and *Pseudomonas aeruginosa*—have been associated with higher rates of treatment failure and leg amputation compared with other organisms.[9,11] These organisms are not as common in North America (generally <5% to 10% of isolates) compared with other areas in the world but still should be treated aggressively with surgery and appropriate isolate-specific antimicrobial therapy when found.

Fungal isolates are rare, not often found as the sole isolate, and are generally considered a contaminant or colonizing organism rather than a pathogen. Anaerobic bacteria generally comprise only 10% to 20% of isolates in series that use conventional techniques for cultures of operative specimens. However, one study that used 16s rRNA to identify organisms at a higher sensitivity found anaerobes in 87% of bone specimens.[13] The role of anaerobes in foot osteomyelitis will need to be clarified with further study.

ROLE OF THE SURGEON IN THE EARLY MANAGEMENT OF DIABETIC FOOT INFECTIONS

The surgeon must play a critical role in the early treatment of foot infections: identification and operative drainage of foot infection. Specifically, the surgeon should be available to rapidly evaluate for the signs of infection. Aside from cellulitis or osteomyelitis without associated soft tissue infection, the surgeon should have a low threshold to operate on a patient with a suspected diabetic foot infection. Surgeons from all of the appropriate specialties, including vascular, general, orthopedic, podiatric, and plastic surgeons, should be sufficiently trained to be capable of evaluating and treating deep soft tissue infections.

It has been recognized since at least 1931 that foot infections usually track along longitudinally oriented soft tissue structures (including tendon sheaths, the plantar aponeurosis, and fascial planes separating the compartments of the foot); therefore transectioning the forefoot transversely to treat infection using partial foot amputations is not be the most effective means of draining these longitudinally oriented infections. Rather, amputation should initially be limited to only obvious areas of irreversible necrosis. Probing with a metal instrument and incising along the identified sinus tract will help to establish drainage of abscess tracts. Drains can be placed through these tracts and eventually be used to facilitate opening them along their entire length (Fig. 62.1).

Deep soft tissue infection must be drained aggressively. Even with an initial aggressive approach, the need for reoperation at 24 to 72 hours is frequent and should not be viewed as signaling a poor prognosis. When performed comprehensively, operative drainage is very effective at controlling a septic diabetic foot. Severity of infection should only be the indication for a major amputation in rare situations. In addition to operative drainage of any suppurative infection, broad-spectrum antibiotics should be initiated and continued until culture results are obtained from surgery. They can help to tailor an isolate-specific antibiotic

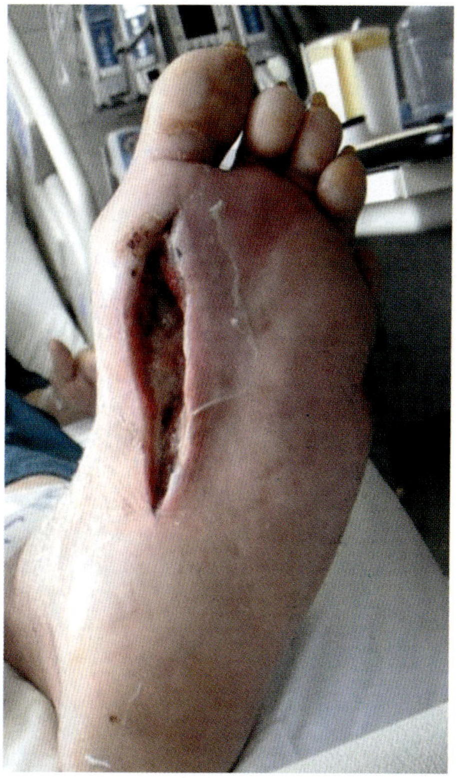

FIG 62.1 A longitudinal incision on the plantar aspect of the forefoot to drain an abscess tracking through the medial compartment of the foot.

regimen. All organisms identified from a deep operative culture (including *Staphylococcus epidermidis* and other organisms not typically considered pathogenic) should be covered by this therapeutic antibiotic regimen. Societal guidelines have recommended up to 1 to 2 weeks of antibiotics for soft tissue infections or osteomyelitis that has been resected to a negative margin, 6 weeks for osteomyelitis with grossly normal but histologically positive margins, and more than 3 months for osteomyelitis treated nonsurgically or with residual dead or grossly infected bone.[14]

The surgical drainage of deep soft tissue infection should not be postponed by studies to assess arterial blood flow. Such evaluations should generally be done after drainage, although it may be reasonable to combine surgical drainage for focal and more limited infections and angiography with possible endovascular intervention in centers with the available resources and expertise to offer this approach.

OPERATIVE TREATMENT OF DEEP SOFT TISSUE INFECTIONS OF THE FOOT

Surgical drainage of a foot infection is a skill with which all surgeons should be well versed. Effectively draining deep soft tissue infections while minimizing further soft tissue destruction is critical to the success of the subsequent foot reconstruction process.

An ankle block is always sufficient for anesthesia, even if edema is present at the level of the ankle. The surface of the foot should be sterilized with an iodine-based two-step solution. The foot and ankle should be draped.

1. If obviously gangrenous tissue such as a necrotic toe or eschar is present, this should be resected. The underlying wound or amputation base should be used to probe for a sinus tract extending from the area of gangrenous tissue.
2. Alternatively, if no gangrenous tissue is present, a hemostat or other pointed metal instruments should be used to probe the instigating ulcer. The tip of the instrument should be used to find any sinus tracts. These sinus tracts often follow anatomic structures, including flexor tendons or the plantar aponeurosis, although sometimes an abscess will track from the plantar aspect of the foot around the metatarsal head and toward the dorsum of the foot.
3. After the presence and location of any existing sinus tracts is known, an incision extending from the edge of the ulcer may be used for cavities that are not very extensive. A counterincision with placement of a Penrose drain should be used for sinus tracts that are lengthier. If necrotic soft tissue or obviously necrotic bone is seen along the sinus tract, an incision should be used to provide adequate drainage and resection of obviously necrotic tissue. However, a definitive resection to clean bone margins is not needed at this initial operation because the focus should be on draining deep soft tissue infection. Resection of bone to grossly normal margin can be done after the soft tissue infection is controlled or resolved, with delayed primary closure of soft tissue and/or skin over the remaining bone.
4. Deep fluid or necrotic tissue should be sent for Gram stain and culture in a sterile container. A small volume of sterile saline may be added if the specimen will not be immediately processed. Swabs should not be used because the yield is significantly lower than with a tissue specimen.
5. Any existing abscess cavity or sinus tract should be copiously irrigated with sterile saline solution. An antibiotic does not need to be added to the solution.

Postoperative care should focus on pain control and empiric antibiotics until causative organisms are identified from culture.

ROLE OF THE VASCULAR SURGEON

There are several reasons why vascular surgeons should be involved early in the care of patients with foot infections and nonhealing foot ulcers. First and foremost is the task of ensuring or establishing arterial blood flow to the foot that is sufficient for wound healing. Contrary to what many clinicians believe, the accurate identification of PAD in patients with diabetes is subtle and often requires more than a physical examination. Palpating for pedal pulses in patients with diabetes has a sensitivity of approximately 50% and low levels of interrater reliability. Other physical findings, including temperature, hair loss, and atrophic skin, have even lower diagnostic accuracy.[15] Therefore uniformly obtaining noninvasive testing, especially toe pressure or skin perfusion pressure measurements, is the most effective strategy for identifying significant PAD, although it is reasonable to proceed directly to angiography if palpable pedal pulses are not appreciated.[16] With 1-year major amputation rates of 30% to 40% among patients with nonhealing foot ulcers and significant PAD that do not undergo revascularization,[17,18] clinicians should use screening strategies that maximize the likelihood of identifying PAD prior to confirmation with an angiogram. The Society for Vascular Surgery Threatened Limb Classification system[19] can help surgeons to weigh the relative importance of revascularization in the setting of ischemic, infected wounds of various severities. Once identified, vascular surgeons should use patient-specific factors (including but not limited to arterial anatomy) to determine the feasibility of and preference for various revascularization options.

In addition, the vascular surgeon should be in frequent communication with the patient and with the surgeon who is assuming responsibility for reconstruction of the foot, discussing the overall prognosis of the patient's limb and how various outcomes may influence mobility and social functioning. The authors feel that the potential benefits of attempting even aggressive limb preservation in functional individuals generally outweigh the potential risks, but each case needs careful evaluation. The combination of suboptimal options for revascularization (e.g., inadequate autologous vein conduit, limited pedal outflow) and suboptimal options for reconstruction (e.g., extensive midfoot osteomyelitis associated with Charcot deformity) may favor palliative wound care[20] or even primary amputation instead of limb preservation attempts, especially in those with both low functional status and multiple comorbidities. Systemic comorbidities alone should rarely represent a contraindication to revascularization because leg amputation does not decrease operative mortality when compared with limb salvage attempts.[21] Vascular surgeons may also evaluate patients with large but uninfected wounds that would benefit from surgical reconstruction. Such wounds include midfoot ulcers associated with Charcot neuroarthropathy; extensive forefoot necrosis or defects requiring soft tissue reconstruction for closure of a partial foot amputation (transmetatarsal, Lisfranc, or other amputation); or heel wounds in patients with ambulatory function. In these situations, a foot surgeon's early input is needed to help the vascular surgeon determine whether revascularization and reconstruction efforts have a realistic chance of success.

There are some clinical circumstances in which limb preservation efforts would be of little or no value to a patient. The most obvious is a limb with little or no function, as a result of stroke, in a patient with a major residual neurologic deficit, spinal cord injury, or fixed joint contractures. The other situation would be foot wounds that cannot be healed or closed in ways that would provide meaningful functional benefit to a patient. For many centers, this might include partial foot amputations proximal to the Lisfranc (tarsometatarsal) joint because the function following such proximal amputations (including Chopart, Syme, and Pirigoff amputations) is no better than a transtibial amputation. These proximal foot amputations are often associated with difficulties in prosthesis fitting that exceed that of a transtibial amputation, but local experience and expertise may also allow these to be feasible options.

EARLY AND LATE FOLLOW-UP AFTER REVASCULARIZATION AND/OR RECONSTRUCTION

As already mentioned, foot infections are extremely rare in patients who do not have an ulcer or have not had recent penetrating trauma to the foot.[5] For this reason, early follow-up should focus on healing any surgical incisions on the leg and working to heal the foot wound that led to revascularization. Results from several series have suggested that expediting the wound-healing process, including using delayed primary closure of foot wounds, may reduce the need for additional foot surgery to treat infection and may reduce the incidence of leg amputation.[11,22-24] However, new or recurrent foot ulcers do occur in late follow-up,[25] and it is important to ensure that patients regularly see providers (including an internal medicine physician, a family practitioner, an endocrinologist, a vascular surgeon, or a podiatrist) who can either manage a recurrent foot ulcer or reliably refer the patient to a provider or team that has expertise in diabetic foot infections and ischemic limbs. The vascular surgeon should routinely perform a clinical evaluation and surveillance ultrasound evaluation of infrainguinal bypass vein grafts and prosthetic bypass grafts as well, but the exact role of "surveillance" after endovascular intervention is not clear at this time.[26]

REVIEW QUESTIONS

1. Which of the following is the most common result of testing for microbial organisms in foot infections using conventional culture techniques?
   a. Monomicrobial with a predominance of gram-positive organisms
   b. Monomicrobial with a predominance of gram-negative organisms
   c. Polymicrobial with a predominance of gram-positive organisms
   d. Polymicrobial with a predominance of gram-negative organisms
2. Which organisms have been associated with higher rates of major (above-ankle) amputations?
   a. Methicillin-resistant *Staphylococcus aureus* (MRSA) and *Escherichia coli*
   b. MRSA and *Pseudomonas aeruginosa*
   c. *E. coli* and *P. aeruginosa*
   d. *P. aeruginosa* and anaerobes
   e. *P. aeruginosa* and *Candida* fungal species
3. When might a primary major (above-ankle) amputation be appropriate?
   a. An 82-year-old man with osteomyelitis of two or more metatarsal bones
   b. A 68-year-old woman with a severe soft tissue infection of the forefoot, a leukocytosis of 15,000/μL, and hemoglobin A1C of 12%.
   c. A 52-year-old man with Charcot arthropathy and a midfoot ulcer.
   d. A 62-year-old man who is a bedbound nursing home resident since a major stroke 2 years ago and presents with a 4-cm necrotic patch of skin on the heel.

References available online at ExpertConsult.com.

63 CHAPTER

The Wound Care Center and Limb Salvage

Peter F. Lawrence, Steven M. Farley

Knowledge about the management of wounds is a distinct subspecialty requiring knowledge of both normal and nonhealing wound physiology, products to accelerate wound healing, and new therapies for the treatment of recalcitrant wounds. Many subspecialties—such as vascular surgery, plastic surgery, podiatry, and primary care—share a role in managing wounds in the community. Current literature and research regarding wound healing is often published outside of traditional surgical or medical journals, so that many vascular surgeons are not familiar with up-to-date best practices.

In many institutions, surgeons and particularly vascular surgeons are the primary consultants for the management of wounds, as few other physicians train in the evaluation and treatment of wounds. Classifying wounds as arterial, venous, mixed/arterial venous, neuropathic, or vasculitic requires thoughtful evaluation of the wounds but also the patient in total.

One of the most common clinical presentations for patients with peripheral arterial disease (PAD) is a nonhealing ischemic wound. Although revascularization may be required for limb salvage, the meticulous management of the primary wound before and after surgery is critical to the success of limb salvage as well as the time that it will take for a patient to return to function. Wound care after revascularization may be required for months or even years, and a nonhealing wound can lead to limb loss, even if revascularization has been successful.

Patients with PAD who have limb-threatening ischemia often have diabetes. Lower extremity ulcers are not only common in diabetics but they may also develop during the course of treatment. Diabetic wounds require specific management and are often managed by the vascular surgeon.

In the process of limb salvage, vascular surgeons create surgical wounds in ischemic limbs by harvesting vein conduit and exposing distal vessels. These newly created wounds occasionally result in graft exposure or infection or delay the return to normal activity. Knowledge about the methods of minimizing the risk of creating wounds in ischemic limbs and their management is the province of vascular surgery.

NORMAL WOUND HEALING

Wound healing involves a well-organized, multifaceted series of events beginning after the actual event of wounding and ends with the formation of mature scar tissue (Fig. 63.1). The acute wound is caused by external trauma; in normal healing, the acute injury heals by progressing through orderly phases in a predictable time frame. Chronic wounds, however, do not follow this predictable course of events and should be viewed differently from acute wounds undergoing normal healing. For chronic wounds, health care providers are now beginning to comprehend the complex cellular and biological abnormalities in nonhealing wounds.

Much of the latest research on wound healing involves investigation of the effects of various cytokines, growth factors, proteinases, and their regulators and how they control the process of wound healing (Fig. 63.2). To understand the effect of these substances on the chronic wound, the normal healing process of the acute wound must be understood. In acute wounds, the healing process begins with tissue injury and progresses predictably through the four phases of wound healing: hemostasis, inflammation, proliferation, and remodeling.

Acute Wounds

Hemostasis

At the time of the initial injury, platelet activation and vasoconstriction occur after injury to the endothelium. Platelet aggregation, vasoconstriction, and clot formation begin the process of hemostasis. A number of soluble mediators are released by the platelets, including platelet-derived growth factor (PDGF), insulin-derived growth factor 1 (IGF-1), epidermal growth factor (EGF), fibroblast growth factor (FGF), and transforming growth factor-β (TGF-β). These mediators are responsible for initiating the healing process. Growth factors stimulate the proliferation of wound cells, act as chemotactant agents, and regulate the differentiated functions of wound cells.[1] Neutrophils and macrophages are recruited to the injured site, attracted by the chemotactant release by the platelets.

Inflammation

Aggregated platelets begin to degranulate and mediators are released that help form the fibrin clot. Initially in the inflammatory phase, there is significant vasodilation, increased capillary permeability, complement activation, and migration of polymorphonuclear neutrophils (PMNs) and macrophages to the site of the wound. The antimicrobial defense and removal of devitalized tissue is initiated by the macrophages and PMNs. As they engulf and destroy bacteria, proteases are released, including elastase and collagenase, which begin the degradation process of the damaged extracellular matrix (ECM) components.

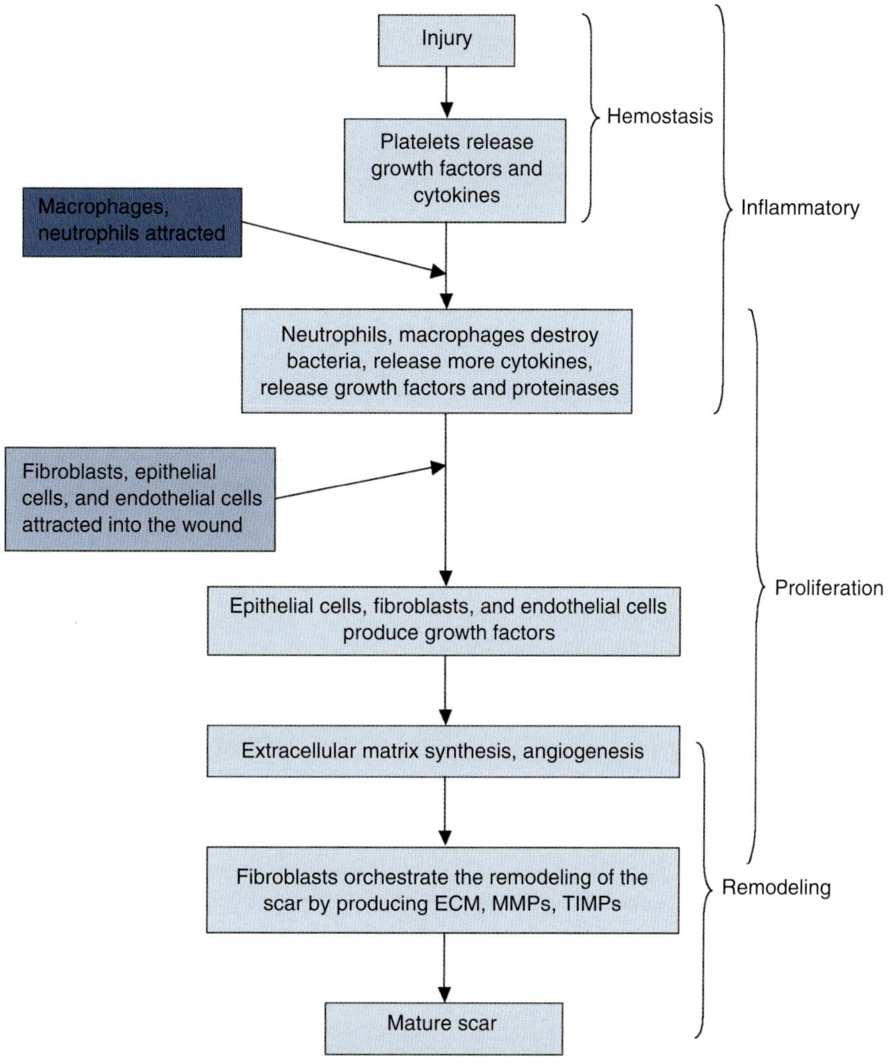

FIG 63.1 The normal process of wound healing is complex and involves a series of phases that overlap. *ECM*, Extracellular matrix; *MMPs*, matrix metalloproteinases; *TIMP*, tissue inhibitor of metalloproteinases.

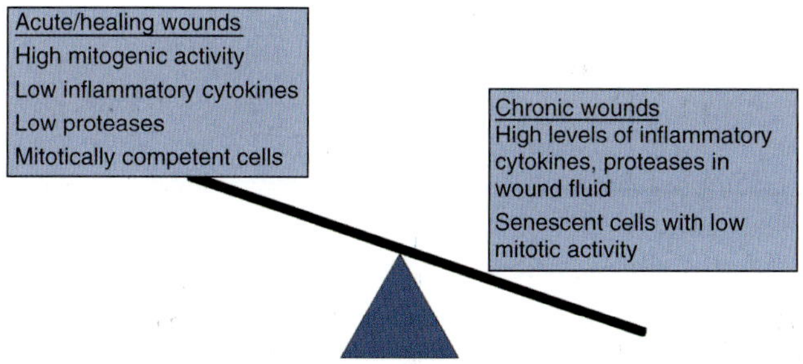

FIG 63.2 Balance of healing and nonhealing factors in wounds. (Modified from Schulz GS, Sibbald G, Falanga V, et al: Wound bed preparation: a systemic approach to wound management. *Wound Rep Reg* 11:1-28, 2003.)

Along with their role in defense and debridement, macrophages and neutrophils induce the formation of granulation tissue by secreting growth factors that stimulate fibroblast proliferation (PDGF), collagen synthesis (TGF-β), and the formation of new blood vessels (FGF). The cytokine IL-β stimulates the proliferation of fibroblasts, and TNF-α and IL-1β stimulate fibroblasts to synthesize matrix metalloproteinases (MMPs).

Proliferation

The proliferative phase begins as the number of inflammatory cells in the wound bed decreases. The synthesis of growth factors continues in the wound bed but is populated by the fibroblasts, endothelial cells, and keratinocytes. Keratinocytes synthesize TGF-β, TGF-α, and IL-1. Fibroblasts secrete IGF-1, bFGF, TGF-β, PDGF, keratinocyte growth factor, and connective tissue factor. Endothelial cells produce b-FGF, PDGF, and vascular endothelial growth factor. The process of cell migration and proliferation continues as the processes of new capillary formation and synthesis of ECM components are begun.

Fibrin and fibronectin form a provisional wound bed matrix. New collagen and elastin and proteoglycan molecules that form the initial scar are synthesized by fibroblasts. Proteases have an essential role at this point. No integration of the newly formed matrix with the dermal matrix can occur until the damaged proteins in the existing matrix are removed. Neutrophils, macrophages, fibroblasts, epithelial cells, and endothelial cells secrete proteases. Key proteases include collagenases, gelatinases, and stromelysins, which are all members of the matrix MMP superfamily, and neutrophil elastase, a serine protease.

In the wound bed, cell proliferation and the formation of new ECM is continuing and sustained by a dramatic increase in the vascularity of the wound bed. The epidermal layer is reformed by the proliferation and migration of epithelial cells across the highly vascularized ECM.

Remodeling

Once the initial scar is formed, the synthesis of ECM continues for several weeks. The newly healed red, raised scar changes over the course of weeks to months to a scar that is less red and may be barely visible. At the cellular and molecular level, the breakdown of the ECM components reaches a balance with the process of synthesis of ECM, allowing remodeling to occur. The increased concentration of fibroblasts and capillaries present in the early phase of healing declines, primarily through apoptosis. In the final remodeling phase, tensile strength reaches a maximum of 80% of the initial strength, as cross-linking of collagen fibrils plateaus.

Chronic Wounds

In contrast to the acute wound, the chronic wound does not heal in a predictable fashion. Lazarus and colleagues[2] define the chronic wound as one in which the normal process of healing has been disrupted at one or more points in the phases of hemostasis, inflammation, proliferation, and remodeling. Chronic ulcers are characterized by defective remodeling of the ECM, a failure to epithelialize, and prolonged inflammation.[3-5] In the chronic wound, fibroblasts do not readily respond to growth factors such as PDGF-β and TGF-β; this failure to respond is hypothesized to be due to a form of cellular senescence. Hyperproliferation at the wound margin interferes with normal cellular migration across the wound bed, probably because of inhibition of apoptosis within the fibroblasts and keratinocytes.[6,7]

The phases of wound healing are replete with factors that have played important roles in the progression of wound healing; therefore any alteration in one or more of these components may interfere with the progression of healing. Growth factors such as PDGF, EGF, bFGF, and TGF-β are present in the chronic wound, but the levels remain constant rather than displaying the variation seen in normal acute wound healing. The proinflammatory cytokines—such as IL-1, IL-6, and TNF-α—remain elevated in chronic wounds compared with the normal, acute wound, where a dramatic decrease is seen during healing, because there is a reduction in the inflammatory state.[8]

Several studies have shown that chronic wounds stall in the inflammatory phase of the wound healing process.[9-11] This phase is most often associated with an increased amount of exudate, postulated to be from infection, heavy colonization, or from reaction to increased necrotic tissue in the wound bed. The amount and character of fluid produced by the chronic wound can severely impede and even reverse the healing process.[12-15]

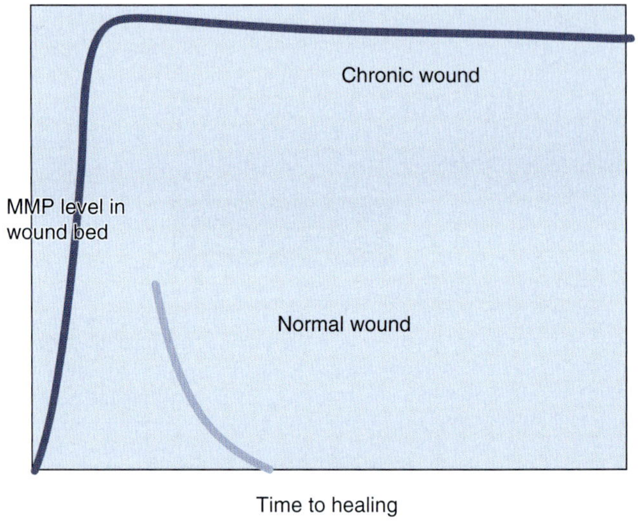

FIG 63.3 Matrix metalloprotein *(MMP)* levels in wound fluid remain high in patients with chronic nonhealing wounds, whereas they recede in the normal wound.

Studies investigating chronic wound effluents have provided increasing evidence that the cellular and molecular environments are substantially altered in chronic wounds. Bucalo and colleagues[16] collected exudate from venous ulcers and examined the effects of chronic wound fluid on the proliferation of dermal fibroblasts, microvascular endothelial cells, and keratinocytes in culture. This study found that wound fluid is not only cytotoxic, but that it inhibited or failed to stimulate the proliferation of dermal fibroblasts, endothelial cells, and keratinocytes. Fluid from acute wounds, in contrast, has been found to stimulate fibroblast proliferation.[17] Proteases in chronic wound fluid have also been shown to degrade growth factors such as PDGF and TGF-1.[18,19]

MMPs are a necessary component of the wound healing process and have an important role in cell migration and modification of the ECM. If the regulation of these protease molecules is disrupted, excessive MMP production may lead to degradation of the ECM, preventing cellular migration and attachment and ultimately causing tissue destruction.[20] It has been shown that MMP activity is significantly elevated in a high percentage of chronic wounds when compared with acute wounds, suggesting dysregulation in chronic wounds (Fig. 63.3). The activity of these proteases decreases consistently in patients whose ulcers progress from a nonhealing to a healing phase.[21]

The chronic wound can also be heavily colonized or infected by bacteria that can substantially increase the amount of exudate. Thus a copious amount of exudate produced by the chronic wound, whatever its cause, can be a barrier to healing.[15,16,22,23]

ASSESSMENT OF WOUND HEALING CAPABILITY

Chronic wounds are the result of altered cellular and molecular processes. Hence wound management must focus on both the wound and the patient as a whole. The goal of wound management is to attain a healthy, well-vascularized granulating wound bed. For this to happen, factors that can impede healing must be addressed. The way in which chronic wounds are viewed and managed should be based on a model that is both different from the acute wound paradigm and representative of the complex nature of nonhealing wounds.[24]

Wound bed preparation has become part of the standard nomenclature in wound healing. The concept of wound bed preparation is the management of a wound in order to accelerate endogenous healing or to facilitate the effectiveness of other therapeutic measures. The main barriers to healing in a chronic wound are necrotic tissue, high bioburden, increased exudate, and altered composition of exudate. The goal of wound bed preparation is to remove or reduce these barriers to healing by using ongoing debridement, reduction of bacterial burden in the wound bed, and management of exudate.

Patient Assessment

Identification of patient factors that would act as an impediment to healing is an essential component of the healing paradigm. The presence of diabetes, renal disease, heart disease, or liver disease can have detrimental effects on wound healing. Autoimmune diseases such as scleroderma, rheumatoid arthritis, vasculitis, or lupus erythematosus will deter wound healing. Systemic steroids, immunosuppressant medications, and nonsteroidal antiinflammatory drugs will also interfere with the healing wound.

The nutritional status of the patient is an overlooked factor in wound healing. Protein-calorie malnutrition can have devastating effects on the integrity of the body and on any wounds the patient might have. Protein-calorie malnutrition is defined as insufficient intake of both protein and calories. In protein-calorie malnutrition, morbidity and mortality increase as a result of the proportionate decline in body weight.[25] A decrease in lean body mass of greater than 10% is associated with compromised wound healing despite therapeutic interventions. Once depletion of lean body mass reaches 30%, the wound becomes a secondary issue as the body seeks to restore and replenish lost muscle.[26] Correction of any nutritional deficit should begin at the first visit and be maintained throughout the wound healing process. Assessment of dietary intake, including vitamin supplementation, is a necessary part of any wound healing assessment. Appetite stimulants, such as megestrol (Megace), may be helpful. If assessment shows moderate to severe protein-calorie malnutrition, supplementation with oxandrolone has been shown to be beneficial to facilitate restoration of lean muscle mass.[27]

Assessment of Wound Characteristics

Accurate classification of the etiology of the wound is the basic starting point for proper wound care. For example, improper classification of active pyoderma gangrenosum may result in improper debridement or compression of ischemic wounds. Basic history taking is critical: How long has the wound been present, how did it start, what has been the progression, and how much pain exists? What aggravates or relieves the pain? What are the associated diseases, such as peripheral arterial or coronary artery disease, type 1 or 2 diabetes, or rheumatoid arthritis?

TABLE 63.1 Documentation of Wound Characteristics

Category	Observation to Be Documented
Wound size	Length, width, depth, area, volume Undermining presence, location, measurement
Appearance	Granulation tissue; slough, necrotic, eschar; friability
Exudate	Amount, color, type (serous, serosanguineous, sanguineous, purulent), odor
Wound edge	Presence of maceration, advancing epithelium, erythema, even, rolled, ragged

Assessment of the wound includes the location, size, depth, and color of the wound bed (Table 63.1). A cotton swab has been shown to accurately gauge the depth and involvement of deep structures. The depth of a wound can be used to predict the likelihood of healing without extensive debridement of tendon or bone. The most common classification system of diabetic lower extremity wounds is the Wagner system, which grades the depth from superficial skin involvement to a deeper level, involving tendon and bone.

These variables should be photographed, measured, and recorded. The amount and type of exudate should also be assessed. Associated signs—such as callus surrounding the ulcer, skin changes in the gaiter (ankle) distribution, peripheral neuropathy, and ischemic (trophic) changes—should also be noted and recorded.

Diagnostic Studies for the Nonhealing Wound

Three questions must be answered through diagnostic studies. First, what is the depth of the wound? Depth determines treatment, because involvement of deep structures such as tendon or bone reduces the likelihood of healing without removal of the deep tissue and increases the risk of an ascending infection along tendon sheaths. Subfascial infection is particularly worrisome in diabetic patients, who have reduced sensation of the foot and a reduced ability to fight infection. The simplest test of depth is to probe the wound to determine whether tendon or bone is involved. This inexpensive and simple method has been shown to be as reliable as more expensive tests in determining the presence of osteomyelitis. Other tests such as plain radiographs and bone scans have less sensitivity and specificity than a magnetic resonance imaging (MRI) scan (Fig. 63.4). All these tests have false negatives and positives, so that surgical debridement may be required to determine the presence of deep infection and osteomyelitis by bone biopsy and culture.

Second, is the wound infected? The differentiation between colonization, cellulitis, abscess, and osteomyelitis is critical for optimal wound management. The degree of bacterial involvement is difficult to quantify and requires clinical acumen. Quantitative cultures are often difficult to obtain and have more use in research than in daily clinical decision making.

Wounds are not sterile and colonization is normal. A wound culture will have multiple skin organisms and there may be no clinical signs of infection, such as erythema, swelling, and pain. Clinically significant bacterial involvement is seen with cellulitis,

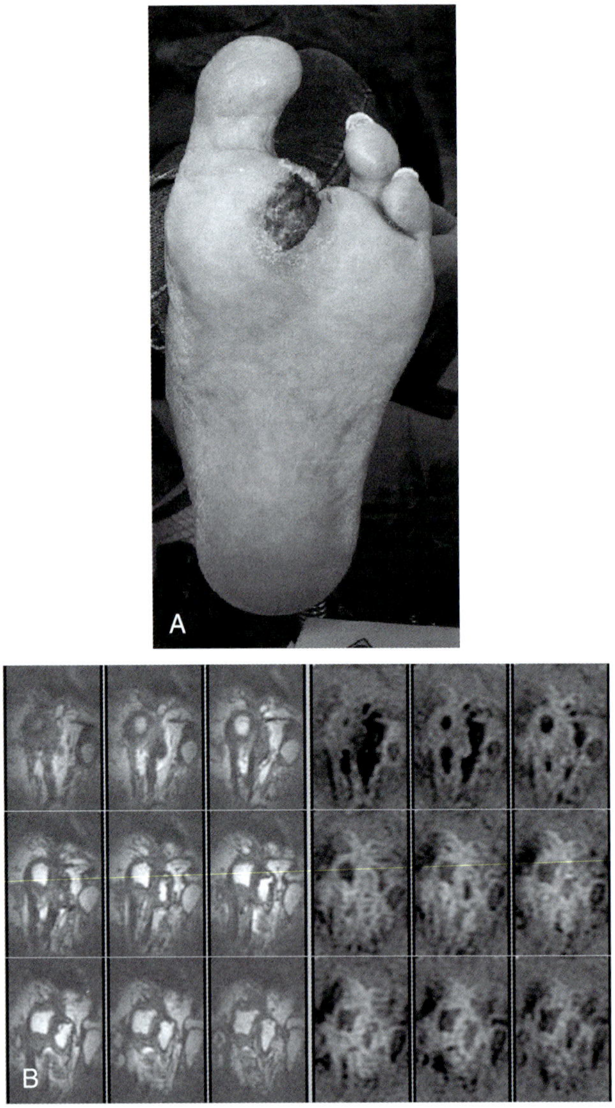

FIG 63.4 (A) A foot with a superficial ulcer needs further diagnostic studies to determine its depth. (B) Magnetic resonance imaging scan of the foot can show the depth of the wound and evidence of osteomyelitis when it is not clinically apparent.

increasing wound pain, wound enlargement, and increasing tissue necrosis. Plain film of the bone in a patient with osteomyelitis becomes positive in the late stages, long after osteomyelitis is established, whereas MRI scan has been shown to be reliable for determining osteomyelitis and detecting early signs, such as changes in marrow intensity, periosteal reaction, and cortical erosion.

Third, is the limb ischemic and does it have adequate blood flow to heal the wound? Adequate tissue oxygenation must be present for wound healing. Oxygen is available bound to hemoglobin and dissolved in plasma. In chronic wounds, plasma-dissolved oxygen can be adequate for wound healing assuming that perfusion of the tissue is satisfactory.

Assessment of the large vessel vascular supply is a critical component of the examination. A palpable pulse indicates a blood pressure of greater than 80 mm Hg in the foot and 70 mm Hg in the hand.[28] If a pulse is not easily palpable, use of a vascular laboratory examination is essential. Doppler waveforms and ankle-brachial index (ABI) as well as plethysmography (Fig. 63.5) can be used with transcutaneous pressure of oxygen ($TcPO_2$) and skin perfusion pressure to determine the adequacy of blood supply. In patients with falsely elevated "stiff" arteries (high ABI with poor Doppler signals), pulse volume recordings, Doppler waveforms, and toe pressures are more reliable.

Normal acute wounds usually have oxygen tensions ($TcPO_2$) of 60 to 90 mm Hg, whereas chronic nonhealing wounds are most often associated with varying degrees of hypoxia because of low oxygen tension and poor blood perfusion. A tissue oxygen tension of greater than 40 mm Hg is adequate for wound healing. Tissue oxygen levels of less than 20 mm Hg in the wound bed are usually associated with failure to heal. When there is inadequate blood flow or perfusion pressure for wound healing, treatment must be directed at increasing the perfusion by revascularization.

TREATMENT OF NONHEALING WOUNDS

Elimination of Edema

Edema reduces microvascular blood flow and the clearance of bacteria and protein from the wound. It eliminates or reduces the likelihood of healing, and other management is often futile until edema is eliminated. The most challenging wounds are those with edema and ischemia, because patients with limb ischemia often place the limb in a dependent position to relieve ischemic rest pain. Prolonged dependency increases the limb edema and reduces perfusion; this paradoxically leads to a further need for dependency. In ischemic limbs, the best way of reducing edema is to elevate the limb above the level of the heart. Compression using sequential devices (e.g., Lymphopress, wraps [Unna boot or Profore], or support hose at 20 to 40 mm Hg pressure) should be limited to patients with a documented normal ABI of greater than 0.80 (Fig. 63.6).

Debridement

The presence of necrotic tissue in a wound is the most obvious marker of a chronic wound. Reestablishing the balance of cytokines, proteases, and growth factors should be the focus of wound treatment. Efficient removal of devitalized tissue (necrotic burden) is an essential step in chronic wound management. The underlying pathogenic abnormalities in chronic wounds cause a continual buildup of necrotic tissue, and regular debridement is necessary to reduce the necrotic burden and achieve healthy granulation tissue. The debridement of devitalized tissue reduces tissue damage and destruction, removes bioburden, and exposes dead space that can harbor bacteria. Debridement can be accomplished in several different ways (Table 63.2); the method chosen should be dictated by the condition of the wound and the skill of the practitioner as well as the patient's situation.

Autolytic Debridement

Autolytic debridement uses the body's own natural enzymes to dissolve necrotic tissue within the wound and occurs spontaneously to some extent in all wounds. The macrophages and endogenous proteolytic enzymes liquefy and spontaneously separate

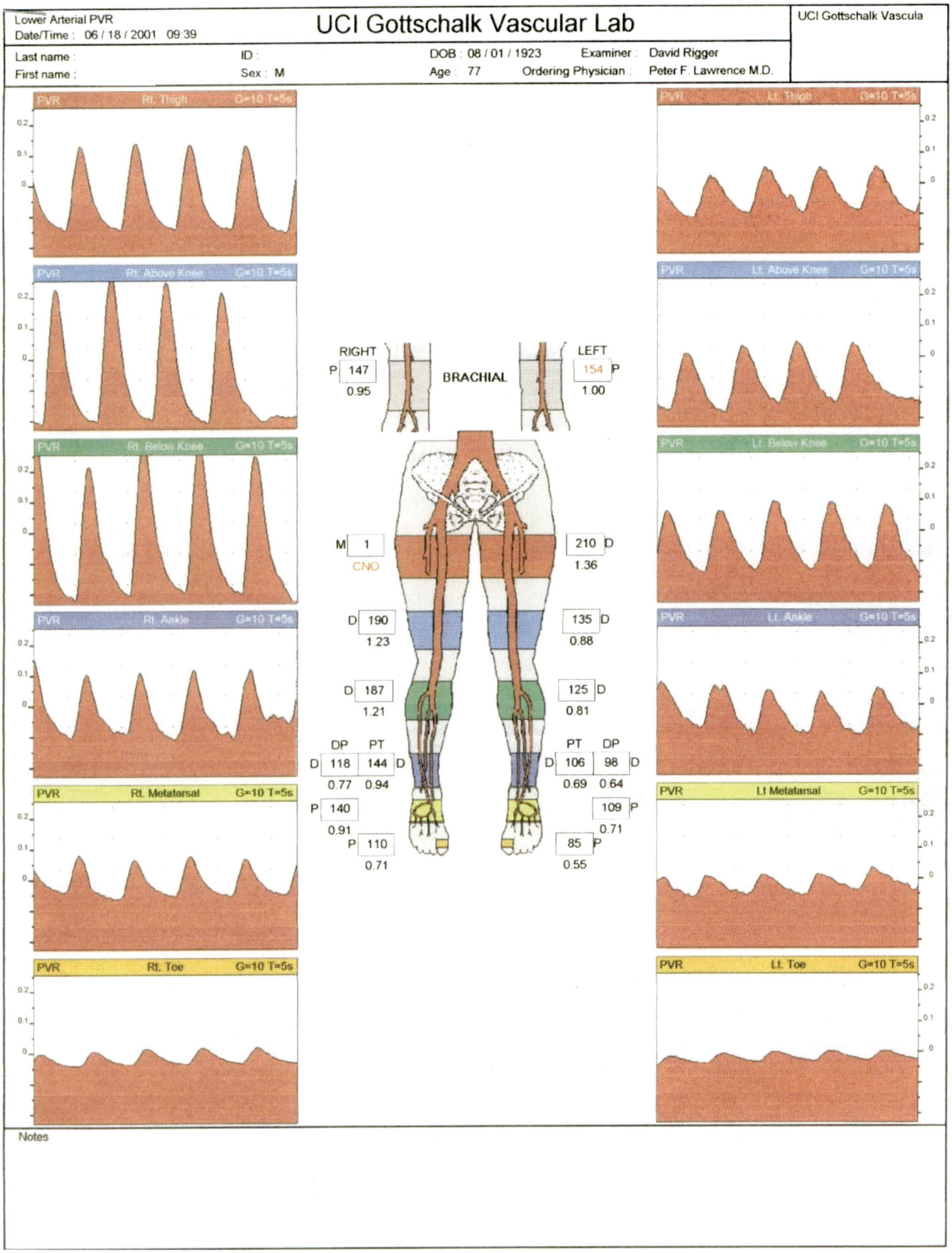

FIG 63.5 Physiologic studies of the lower limb are useful to determine the likelihood of wound healing. An ankle-brachial index (ABI) greater than 0.6 and biphasic or triphasic Doppler waveforms suggest a high likelihood of healing, whereas an ABI less than 0.4 and monophasic waveforms make the likelihood of healing low.

necrotic tissue and eschar from healthy tissue. Autolytic debridement is most effective in a moist wound environment. Dressings most commonly used for this method include hydrogels and hydrocolloids, both of which can produce a more effective environment for the destruction and phagocytosis of the necrotic tissue. Dressings that are occlusive or semiocclusive facilitate contact between the necrotic tissue and the enzymes within the wound. This method of debridement is selective, with little discomfort, but it is often slow. If there is no improvement in the wound bed within 72 hours, another method of debridement should be used. This method is inappropriate for a wound that has a significant amount of necrotic debris or is heavily infected.

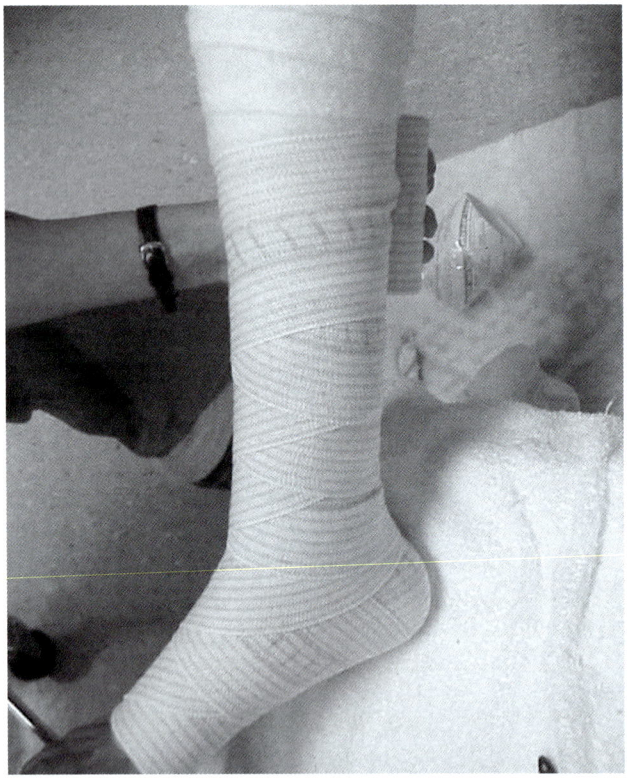

FIG 63.6 If there is adequate perfusion, compression with a multilayered wrap is useful to reduce edema. With an ankle-brachial index greater than 0.8 or an ankle pressure greater than 80 mm Hg, the use of three- or four-layer wraps is recommended because they create 30 to 40 mm Hg of pressure.

Enzymatic Debridement

Enzymatic debridement uses the application of topical agents to the surface of the wound, which chemically disrupts or digests devitalized extracellular proteins present in wound. There are two main preparations used in enzymatic debridement: collagenase (Santyl) and papain urea (Accuzyme). Collagenase is a partially purified preparation of collagenase derived from *Clostridium histolyticum*. It has been shown to have specificity for collagen types I and II. It cleaves glycine in endogenous collagen and digests collagen but is not active against keratin, fat, or fibrin. Papain urea is composed of papain (from papaya fruit) mixed with a chemical agent, urea. Papain digests necrotic tissue by liquefaction of fibrinous debris but is inactive against collagen. Urea is an activator of the papain. Urea also digests nonviable protein, making it more susceptible to proteolysis. Studies have demonstrated that the combination of papain and urea is approximately twofold more effective than the enzyme alone.

Alvarez and colleagues showed that the papain urea product achieved a better wound response than did collagenase, but there was no significant difference in wound closure between the two groups.[29] Some patients complain of burning when the papain urea is applied, which may limit its use in some patients.

Mechanical Debridement

Mechanical debridement is a nonselective method of removing necrotic tissue from the wound using mechanical force. This method can damage healthy tissue in the wound bed and at the margins of the wound, and it can be extremely painful for the patient. Wet-to-dry dressings are the simplest method of mechanical debridement but require frequent dressing changes; therefore they result in increased costs because of increased nursing time. Wet-to-dry debridement involves covering a wound with saline-moistened gauze and allowing it to dry. It is then removed along with the necrotic tissue that has adhered to the dressing. This method is nonselective and painful because it lifts away viable tissue as well. Strings from the gauze can be left behind in the

TABLE 63.2 Selecting Methods of Wound Debridement

	DEBRIDEMENT METHOD			
Characteristic	**Autolytic**	**Surgical**	**Enzymatic**	**Mechanical**
Rapidity of debridement action	4	1	2	3
Tissue specificity	3	2	1	4
Exudate	1	4	2	3
Infection	3	1	4	2
Cost	4	1	3	2
1	4	2	3	

1, Most appropriate; *2,* appropriate; *3,* somewhat appropriate; *4,* least appropriate.

Modified from Sibbald RG, Williamson D, Orsted HL, et al: Preparing the wound bed—debridement, bacterial balance, and moisture balance. *Ostomy Wound Manage* 46(11):14–22, 24–28, 30–35, 2000.

wound bed, creating a further inflammatory reaction to the presence of a foreign body. Wet-to-wet dressings maintain a moistened dressing until removal and accomplish the same results with less destruction of viable tissue.

Pressurized irrigation involves the application of streams of water at a high or low pressure to wash away bacteria, foreign matter, and necrotic tissue from the wound, but bacteria may be driven even further into soft tissue with this technique.

Biosurgical Debridement

Biosurgical debridement involves the use of maggots to remove nonviable tissue from a wound bed. This technique uses sterile maggots applied to the wound bed and covered with a dressing. The maggots then digest necrotic material from the wound bed without damaging the healthy tissue. Maggots also demonstrate the ability to consume bacteria, thus decreasing the patient's risk of developing infection. The precise mechanism by which the maggots debride the wound and promote healing is not clear. It is speculated that the pH of the wound is changed by the maggots, increasing the bacteriostatic effect. It is thought the maggots also secrete proteolytic enzymes that enhance protein degradation. Despite their effectiveness and encouraging reports on wound healing, some patients complain of increased pain with maggot therapy, and some patients are uncomfortable with the idea of maggots on their wounds.

Sharp Debridement

Surgical (or sharp) debridement is the fastest way to remove devitalized tissue. Removing dead tissue decreases bacterial burden in the wound bed. Use of the scalpel to remove senescent cells converts a chronic wound into an acute wound within a chronic wound and has been shown to increase the healing rate of diabetic neurotrophic foot ulcers.[30] The major problem with this form of debridement is that both viable and nonviable tissue may be removed. This method can also be painful, but the use of topical or local anesthetic (eutectic mixture of local anesthetics [EMLA] cream) can alleviate the discomfort.

TREATMENT OF INFECTION

The presence of bacteria in the wound bed can be categorized as contamination, colonization, critical colonization, or infection. Contamination is the presence of nonreproducing bacteria in the wound bed; they do not interfere with healing. Colonization is the presence of reproducing bacteria in the wound bed; they are adherent to the surface of the wound but do not impede wound repair. Critical colonization is a step between colonization and infection; replicating bacteria are present in the wound and interfere with wound healing but do not show the typical signs of infection. Treatment is necessary to rid the wound of the bioburden. The infected wound will show the signs of delayed healing as well as increased pain, an increased amount of exudate, and a change in the color of the wound bed to friable, red granulation tissue or the absence of granulation tissue, along with odor and purulence. Treatment strategies include sustained-release silver dressings or slow-release iodine formulations such as cadexomer iodine, along with systemic antibiotics.

Chronic wounds are usually colonized with at least three species of microorganisms.[31] The concentration of bacteria necessary to impede the healing of open wounds is controversial; however, 1×10^5 organisms per gram of tissue have historically been associated with impaired healing.[32,33] The type and pathogenicity of the organisms in a wound bed may be a better predictor of the risk of infection than simply the number. Some combinations of bacteria act synergistically to enhance the virulence of a previously benign organism.[33]

Another important factor in infections is the biofilm on some bacteria, which can contribute to delayed healing. Biofilm occurs as some bacteria proliferate; they form microcolonies that become attached to the wound bed, secreting a glyocalyx sheath of biofilm that protects the microorganisms from systemic antimicrobial agents.[34]

Treatment of an infected wound should begin without delay. Antibiotics are useful to prevent the spread of infection in the soft tissue beyond the wound, but repeated use of antibiotics in patients with chronic wounds can lead to the development of resistant organisms. Therefore systemic antibiotics should be used judiciously and should be avoided unless infection is established.[35] The use of antiseptic agents is useful in the treatment of the infected wound and may be essential.[36] Topical cadexomer iodine and nanocrystalline silver target the bacteria at the cell membrane, cytoplasmic organelle, and nucleic acid level; this combination of actions means that development of resistant bacteria is improbable. Cadexomer iodine is a formulation of cadexomer beads that absorb a significant amount of exudate while slowly releasing iodine into the tissues in a concentration low enough to be bactericidal but not cytotoxic. Cadexomer iodine has been shown to be effective against *Staphylococcus aureus*, methicillin-resistant *S. aureus,* and vancomycin-resistant enterococci.[37,38] Nanocrystalline silver dressings provide an antibacterial dressing that has been shown to be effective in partial- and full-thickness wounds. The silver is slowly released into the wound bed and maintains an effective antimicrobial barrier for up to 7 days. Nanocrystalline silver is effective against a number of pathogens, including methicillin-resistant *S. aureus* and vancomycin-resistant enterococci.

MANAGEMENT OF THE EXUDATE

Patients, primary care providers, and the general public commonly promote the "drying" of a chronic wound. Common quotes include "let it dry" or "leave it in the sun" or "wounds like fresh air." However, the wound-healing community has long recognized that wounds heal faster in a closed, moist environment. Eagelstein and colleagues[39] showed that experimentally induced wounds healed 40% faster in a closed, moist environment compared with wounds left exposed to the air.[39] A moist environment has also been shown to facilitate epithelial migration, maintain optimal temperature, decrease pain, and provide a better cosmetic result; however, excess exudate in a chronic wound has an adverse effect on wound healing.[40] The buildup of wound fluid must be managed to minimize the negative biochemical factors. On the other hand, excessive desiccation slows the migration of epidermal cells and limits epidermal regeneration.[41] Therefore the choice of dressings must be made with the goal of controlling exudate while maintaining optimal moisture in the wound bed.

DRESSING THE NONHEALING WOUND

All wound dressings are designed with a specific purpose in mind; many serve more than one purpose. The wound, the patient, and their multiple needs must be considered in choosing a dressing (Box 63.1). Optimal wound care decision making focuses on the need for moist dressings, which will maintain the healing environment at the optimum moisture. The Agency for Health Care Policy and Research published guidelines in 1994 for the selection of dressings (Table 63.3).

Hydrogels provide a high level of moisture (70% to 90% water), which is contained in insoluble polymers.[42] Hydrogels are the best choice for dry, sloughy wounds with minimal to moderate levels of exudate. Gels must be reapplied every 24 to 72 hours because they are not antibacterial; they are nonadherent and soothing. Wound gels facilitate autolytic debridement.

Hydrocolloids provide an occlusive dressing for the wound bed, forming a matrix gel on contact with the wound exudate. Hydrocolloids are suited to autolytic debridement for mild to moderately exudative wounds, but care should be taken to avoid maceration of the healthy epidermis. Mild antibacterial activity is present within hydrocolloids because of the lowered pH. Occlusion is achieved with foam or a film-sheet backing with adhesive, which can cause an allergic reaction in some patients.[43,44]

Film dressings are ideal at the later stage of wound healing, when there is no significant exudate. The dressings are permeable to water and oxygen while maintaining impermeability to bacteria and water. Foam dressings are appropriate for moderately to heavily exudative wounds. Foams come in many forms and sizes. All provide thermal insulation, high absorbency, and a moist environment. Most have a polyurethane backing to prevent excess fluid loss. Hydrofibers are considered in the category with foam dressings, although visually they are quite different. Hydrofibers are highly absorbent and have good tensile strength. Both foams and hydrofibers can be worn for up to 1 week, are easy to cut to the size and shape of the wound, and do not shed fibers in the wound bed.[45]

Alginates are best used on heavily exudative wounds. They form a gel upon contact with the exudate, promoting a moist wound healing and autolytic debridement. They are made from brown seaweed. After debridement, they donate calcium to the wound bed, facilitating hemostasis. Silicone dressings are among the first products that were engineered specifically for painless removal of the dressing from the wound. Silicone dressings have a hydrophobic soft silicone layer that prevents the dressing from adhering to the wound surface. They maintain contact with the wound bed, allowing exudate to pass through and be absorbed while also allowing antimicrobials or biologically active properties of other dressings to interact with the wound bed.

BOX 63.1 Principles for Wound Dressings

Wound dressing should

- Debride necrotic tissue
- Identify and eradicate infection, reduce wound contamination
- Obliterate dead space
- Absorb excess drainage
- Maintain moist wound environment while keeping periwound skin protected
- Provide thermal insulation
- Protect the wound from bacteria and trauma
- Promote wound healing

GROWTH FACTORS

Research on wound healing has focused on the development, use, and effect of various cytokines and growth factors on the wound bed. The only growth factor approved by the US Food and Drug Administration (FDA) and readily available is PDGF, in the form of becaplermin (Regranex), approved for use in neuropathic ulcers. In 1995, Steed[46] reported that becaplermin gel improved healing rates in diabetic foot ulcers in 48% of patients, as opposed to 25% in the control group. Other studies have not shown similar results in the treatment of neuropathic foot ulcers, but the dose of 100 μg/g facilitated 50% complete closure within the prescribed time, compared with 35% in the placebo group.[47] Studies examining becaplermin for use in other types of ulceration, such as pressure ulcers, have not met with the same degree of success.[48] Recently platelet-rich plasma (PRP) has been used in orthopedic, maxillofacial, and plastic surgery. PRP is an autologous concentration of human platelets in a

TABLE 63.3 Selection of Dressings for Chronic Wounds

	APPEARANCE OF WOUND BED				
Dressing	**Eschar**	**Slough-Dry**	**Slough-Moist**	**Pink/Red, Wet**	**Pink, Healthy Granulation, Epithelialization**
Hydrogels	++	+++			+++
Hydrocolloids	+	++	++		++
Film dressings			++		++
Calcium alginate			+	++	
Foam			++	++	
Enzymes	+++	+++			+
Antimicrobial (silver, cadexomer iodine)			+++	+++	

+, mild efficacy for listed wound type; ++, medium efficacy for listed wound type; +++, large efficacy for listed wound type.

small volume. Because it is a concentration of platelets, it is also a concentration of seven fundamental protein growth factors proved to be actively secreted by platelets to initiate all wound healing. These growth factors include the three isomers of PDGF (PDGF-αα, PDGF-ββ, and PDGF-αβ), two of the numerous transforming growth factors-β (TGF-β1 and TGF-β2), vascular endothelial factor, and epithelial growth factor.[49] PRP, because it is suspended in a small amount of plasma, also contains fibrin and fibronectin, which are cellular adhesion molecules. It is known that degranulation of the platelet with the release of growth factors initiates and facilitates the healing cascade. The active secretion of these growth factors is initiated by the clotting of blood and begins within 10 minutes. More than 95% of the growth factors are secreted within 1 hour; therefore the PRP must be developed in the anticoagulated state and should be used within 1 hour.

The literature has been mixed about the results of PRP. In maxillofacial, orthopedic and cosmetic surgery, it has been associated with positive results.[50] After the initial use of PRP-related growth factors, the platelets synthesize and secrete additional growth factors for the remaining 7 days of their life span.[51-58] Recently PRP has been used to promote wound healing. Knighton and colleagues[59] evaluated the use of PRP in patients with wounds of various etiologies; wounds healed in 15% of controls and 81% of patients treated with platelet concentrate. Patients who had failed to heal in the control arm were then treated with PRP, and all patients had epithelialization in an average of 7.1 weeks.[59] Currently there are two office devices that are used to develop PRP and have been cleared by the FDA: the Smart PreP (Harvest Technologies, Plymouth, MA) and the Platelet Concentration Collection System (Implant Innovations, West Palm Beach, FL).

TISSUE TRANSFER

Autologous tissue transfer has been used for many years to cover tissue defects; however, the use of autologous tissue creates another tissue defect at the donor site, requires anesthesia, and creates additional pain. Tissue substitutes arose from the need to treat large burns with insufficient donor skin for grafting.[60] This work has extended to wound care, and now there are several choices of skin substitutes. The purpose of a skin substitute is to provide a temporary dressing that is biologically active and accelerates skin tissue regeneration and wound healing by stimulating recipient wound bed growth factors and skin cells.[61] Significant progress has been made in progressing from a simple synthetic material to products that have increasing structural and biochemical complexity. Many skin substitutes now closely approximate the biochemical and cellular composition and behavior of the dermal and epidermal structures. Numerous products have entered the wound care space in a wide variety of constructs, including placental, neonatal, and xenogenic sources.

Commercially bioengineered skin consists of sheets of biomaterial matrix containing allogeneic cells, which are typically derived from neonatal foreskin, a convenient tissue source with the added advantages of having a higher content of putative keratinocyte stem cells, vigorous cell growth and metabolic activity, and minimal antigenicity.[62,63] The skin substitutes approved for use in vascular and diabetic ulcers include Dermagraft (Smith and Nephew, Largo, FL), a cryopreserved human fibroblast-derived dermal substitute approved for treatment of diabetic foot ulcers of greater than 6 weeks' duration. Fibroblasts are isolated from neonatal tissue and then cultured on a bioabsorbable polyglactin mesh for 3 weeks. During incubation, the cells secrete matrix proteins, including human dermal collagen and soluble factors to create a human protein-containing three-dimensional matrix that can be used as a dermal replacement.[64,65] Marston reported an increase in complete healing with Dermagraft (30% vs. 18%).[66] Another study examining Dermagraft in diabetic foot wounds of long duration showed increased healing at week 12 (71% vs. 14%) compared with saline-soaked gauze–treated control group.[67] The product must remain frozen prior to use and requires thawing and rinsing prior to placement.

Apligraf (Organogenesis Inc., Canton, MA) is a bilayered, living skin construct developed to provide multiple functions, similar to human skin (Fig. 63.7). These functions include providing a barrier against mechanical damage and infection, producing structural and regulatory substances (e.g., growth factors or cytokines), and interacting with the underlying tissue to promote more effective wound repair.[68] Apligraf assimilates allogeneic cultured human skin cells from neonatal foreskin in a full-thickness skin construct that contains both epidermal and dermal layers. The well-differentiated epidermal layer is formed of living human keratinocytes; the dermal layer is formed of living human fibroblasts that are dispersed in a type I bovine-derived collagen matrix.[69,70] Apligraf is approved for use in venous ulcers and diabetic foot ulcers.[71] The pivotal Apligraft (Organogenesis

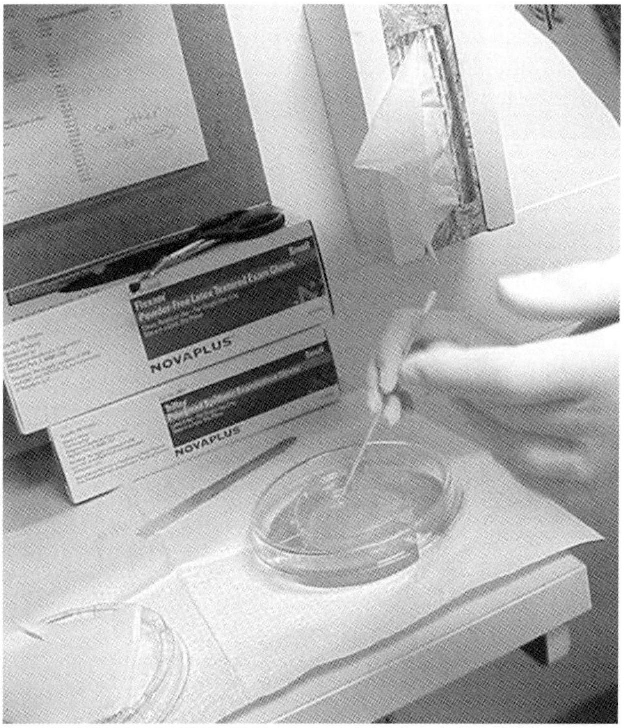

FIG 63.7 Apligraft is a skin and dermal substitute that can be useful in the coverage of chronic wounds once adequate perfusion has been restored.

Inc.) study provided to the FDA for approval in diabetic foot ulcers was done by Veves and colleagues.[72] This multicenter trial of the healing rates of neuropathic, diabetic, and plantar foot ulcers showed a 56% complete wound closure at 12 weeks, compared with 38% in the control patients.[72]

Hyperbaric Oxygen Therapy

Oxygen makes up 21% of the earth's atmosphere. When administered at higher concentrations, oxygen is technically an inhaled drug. The hyperbaric chamber is a delivery system that can deliver oxygen in superphysiologic concentrations, well beyond what is possible at normobaric pressures (Fig. 63.8). Unquestioned absolute indications for hyperbaric treatment are decompression illness, crush injuries, gas embolism, carbon monoxide poisoning, and cyanide toxicity.

Controversy surrounds the benefit of the temporary delivery of high concentrations of oxygen to wound beds. Hyperbaric therapy is expensive and time-consuming; it should be seen as an advanced therapy for problem wounds. Considering these factors and the historical and current unscientific use of hyperbaric oxygen for a host of medical problems including dementia and multiple sclerosis, there is still skepticism surrounding hyperbaric oxygen therapy (HBOT).

Patients with problem wounds make up a majority of those who undergo modern HBOT. More specifically, approximately 80% of patients undergoing HBOT receive treatment for wounds—40% radiation-associated and another 40% diabetes-associated. In other wounds, modern hyperbaric centers mainly treat wounds and are available for occasional emergency indications. Contraindications to HBOT include untreated pneumothorax and ongoing treatment with several chemotherapies, such as bleomycin or doxorubicin (Adriamycin). Relative contraindications include severe chronic obstructive pulmonary disease with air trapping, poorly compensated congestive heart failure, history of claustrophobia, seizure disorders, history of ear surgery, or retinal surgery.

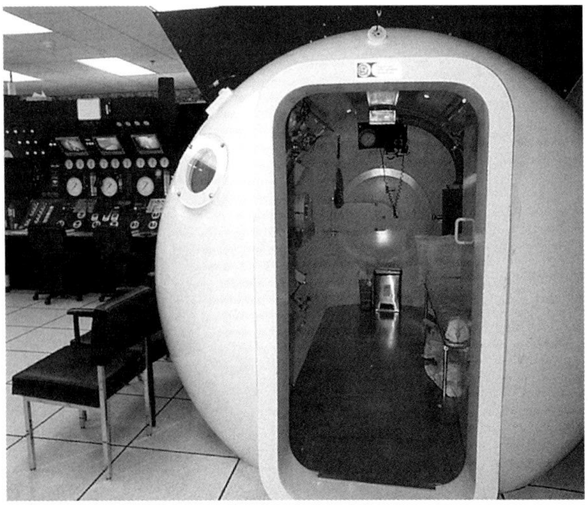

FIG 63.8 A hyperbaric chamber can improve healing in chronic wounds that show a low $TcPO_2$; this increases to greater than 30 mm Hg when 100% oxygen is given to the patient.

Central to the evaluation of patients with chronic wounds is tissue oxygenation. Using transcutaneous oxygen sensors, the partial pressure of oxygen at the skin can be measured. To achieve meaningful results, $TcPO_2$ testing must be done by a certified technologist under controlled conditions. In general a $TcPO_2$ of greater than 40 mm Hg is associated with wound healing. Patients with a $TcPO_2$ of less than 40 mm Hg are given a normobaric 100% oxygen challenge. An increase in 50% or a $TcPO_2$ greater than 100 mm Hg represents a positive oxygen response and identifies patients who can benefit from hyperbaric oxygen. Currently HBOT is approved by the Centers for Medicare and Medicaid Services (CMS) for wound treatment in patients with chronic refractory osteomyelitis, failing or threatened free tissue grafts, diabetic foot wounds involving deep space infection (Wagner stage III or IV), and radiation-associated wounds.

Vacuum-Assisted Closure

Vacuum-assisted closure (VAC) relies on negative pressure or a vacuum to promote wound healing; it has gained increased acceptance in the management of a wound with a heavy exudate and edema that cannot be controlled by conventional methods of wound care. Use of the VAC requires adequate limb perfusion (ABI > 0.6) and absence of osteomyelitis and active infection. A portable device is available that can create negative pressure and collect drainage from the wound while also reducing edema. During therapy, negative pressure facilitates contraction of the wound. Large wounds often contract dramatically in size in a relatively short time. The positive experience of physicians and nurses with the VAC has led to its increasing use for large wounds in swollen limbs with adequate perfusion.

New Therapies for Nonhealing Wounds

Some wounds remain recalcitrant despite the established wound care approaches already discussed. Oral or intravenous steroids are often used for vasculitic ulcers that do not respond to conventional treatment, and occasionally colectomy is required to heal pyoderma gangrenosum in a patient with ulcerative colitis. Currently there are nonapproved options for the nonhealing wound, including use of the Art Assist, a pneumatic leg compression device used for to treat intermittent claudication that augments limb blood flow, intravenous PGE or PGI2 prostaglandin infusion, and oral sildenafil (Viagra). Although none of these therapies have been demonstrated by level 1 evidence to close wounds, they are occasionally used when the only alternative is an amputation or a wound that remains open and dysvascular for a prolonged time.

ORGANIZATION OF A WOUND CARE PROGRAM

A critical component of optimal wound care is an integrated program in which continuity can be provided from the hospital to the ambulatory clinic to home health care. Nurses, physicians, access to all subspecialties, and a facility with equipment and dressings are necessary for optimal wound care and a successful wound care program.

Personnel

The key component of a successful wound care program is personnel. Because wound problems often need treatment more than once a week, a typical physician's office is unable to provide the environment for an excellent wound care program. Nurses and physicians with expertise in wound management must be available every day to heal recalcitrant wounds, and they must be available for consultation with home health and visiting nurse services.

The core of most wound care programs is a complement of nurses with training in wound care. Their expertise must include the ability to assess changes in the status of the wound, training to mechanically debride the wound, and knowledge of optimal dressings for different clinical situations. Nurses provide continuity of care for most patients who have wounds, because physicians often rotate coverage of wound centers and are not available daily. This applies particularly to vascular surgeons, who may be in the operating room for an entire day and thus unavailable to patients on some days of the week.

Specialists who have expertise in the management of patients with dysvascular or nonhealing wounds are an important component of all wound care centers. Plastic surgery, orthopedic surgery, podiatry, endocrinology (diabetes), nephrology, infectious disease, rheumatology, and cardiology are the specialties are most often asked to provide help with the management of this group of patients, who have many risk factors and comorbidities.

Facility

The optimal wound center has dedicated rooms used to treat patients with wounds. These rooms are designed for patients who are often not ambulatory and have special needs. Rooms dedicated for wound care need ready access to a variety of debriding instruments, wound care products, and dressings and have increasingly become hospital-based outpatient clinics. For patient ease, diagnostic facilities—such as plain radiography, foot MRI, and computed tomography (CT)—are optimally located close to the wound care center. A treatment room for the debridement of wounds is also useful. The most expensive capital expense for wound care, hyperbaric therapy, is not necessarily needed within the center because a small percentage of wound care patients need hyperbaric therapy; nevertheless it should be readily accessible. Other capital equipment that is often useful includes a multichamber mechanical compression device (e.g., Lympha Press [Mego Afek, Kibbutz Afek, Israel]) and a platelet concentrator for PRP.

REVASCULARIZATION IN PATIENTS WITH NONHEALING WOUNDS

Dysvascular patients with nonhealing wounds present a unique challenge to the vascular surgeon because the process of revascularization, which is often necessary, is frequently associated with the creation of another wound, exposure to cardiovascular risk, prolonged hospitalization, and further protein-calorie depletion. To determine the need for revascularization, a systematic approach must be taken to this complex group of patients. Several questions should be asked to determine the best approach for dysvascular patients with nonhealing wounds:

First, how ischemic is the limb? Patients with mild or moderate ischemia but without rest pain, dependent rubor, or infection may be treated less urgently than those with more advanced ischemia. In addition, the method of revascularization does not require the same degree of durability as in a patient who would need revascularization for limb ischemia, even if the nonhealing wound were not present.

Second, what is the level of the disease? Patients with proximal PAD of the iliac arteries are much more easily treated with revascularization procedures than those with distal, infrapopliteal disease. In addition, distal revascularization procedures are often less durable and require an incision in the ischemic limb for either conduit harvest or exposure of the vessels.

Third, what conduit is available? For a distal bypass in an ischemic limb that requires long-term patency, the ideal conduit is autogenous vein. Patients who do not have conduit because of prior harvesting, small size, or prior thrombosis have more limited options.

And last, will the patient have a functional limb if the ulcer is healed with revascularization? For the limb to be functional, the patient must have the motivation and strength, adequate plantar skin, and biomechanics to walk. If it is unlikely that the patient will use a revascularized limb, the risks and complexity of the procedure must be weighed against the patient's desire for a cosmetic, nonfunctional limb.

Options for Revascularization

Nonrevascularization

In the presence of mild ischemia, a trial of optimal wound care is a reasonable approach in some patients. Traumatic toe and pressure wounds, particularly in diabetics, that are superficial and not associated with severe preexisting ischemia may heal with relief of pressure, optimal wound care, and patience. Although these wounds might not heal at the rate seen in patients without ischemia, if there is otherwise no indication for revascularization, then a trial of wound care may be the best option. Veith and colleagues[73] showed that a significant number of mildly dysvascular patients healed ulcers without revascularization using a program of bed rest and wound care.

Angioplasty

Angioplasty is an attractive option for a patient with a dysvascular, nonhealing wound because it rarely causes additional tissue trauma, which occurs with surgical vessel exposure and vein harvest. Angioplasty alone can often improve perfusion enough to heal a wound. Proximal lesions (iliac and aortic) are optimal for angioplasty and stenting. As the hemodynamically significant disease occurs more distally, the durability of angioplasty and stenting is reduced, although recent reports have shown excellent early patency and results comparable to those of bypass.[74] In the superficial femoral artery, the type of lesion (TASC A, B, or C, which is a classification system[75] for the length, extent, and degree of calcification of the lesions) determines the likelihood of initial and long-term success. For infrapopliteal disease, Chandra and colleagues[76] recommend angioplasty as the optimal procedure to improve blood flow and heal ischemic ulcers in limbs that do not otherwise require revascularization.

Bypass

Bypass is the standard treatment for patients with limb ischemia and a nonhealing wound. Although an extensive discussion of the alternative techniques and conduits is beyond the scope of this chapter, certain principles should be applied in deciding on a revascularization procedure.

First, limit distal incisions. Kalra and colleagues[77] advise surgeons to limit distal incisions by harvesting more proximal veins and tunneling them distally and to avoid foot and ankle incisions in dysvascular limbs (Fig. 63.9). In situ bypasses should be performed with a closed technique if technically feasible. The LeMaitre valvulotome as well as other commercially available valvulotomes perform the valvulotomy without an incision to expose the vein. Treiman and colleagues[78] have reported on the management of wound complications in a small series of patients who developed incision complications after distal bypass, as well as alternatives designed to maintain patency of the exposed graft.

Second, use tissue transfer procedures. The patient with advanced ischemia who needs both limb revascularization and closure of a large wound can often have both accomplished with a flow-through flap using the radial artery or other arterial conduits.[79] This procedure provides a conduit for revascularization with an elliptical flap of attached, vascularized tissue (Fig. 63.10). The radial artery usually matches the size of the distal foot vessel and is optimal for this procedure. If a long conduit is needed for the proximal anastomosis, then saphenous vein can be spliced to the radial artery, although the proximal radial artery anastomosis can usually be placed in a proximal tibial or peroneal artery. Vascularized skin and subcutaneous tissue can then be used to cover large ulcers and skin defects. Other flaps, which can be anastomosed to a vein conduit, can even provide fascia to reconstruct the Achilles tendon if needed.

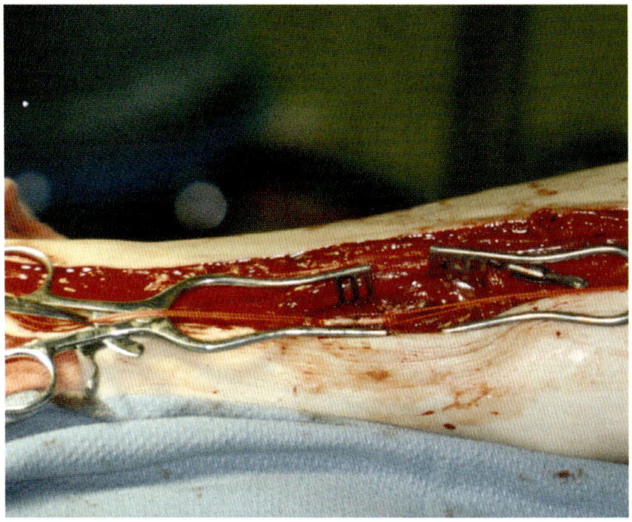

FIG 63.9 Incisions that are made in the distal part of an ischemic limb are at significant risk for wound complications of infection or dehiscence. An alternative is to harvest a more proximal vein and tunnel it distally.

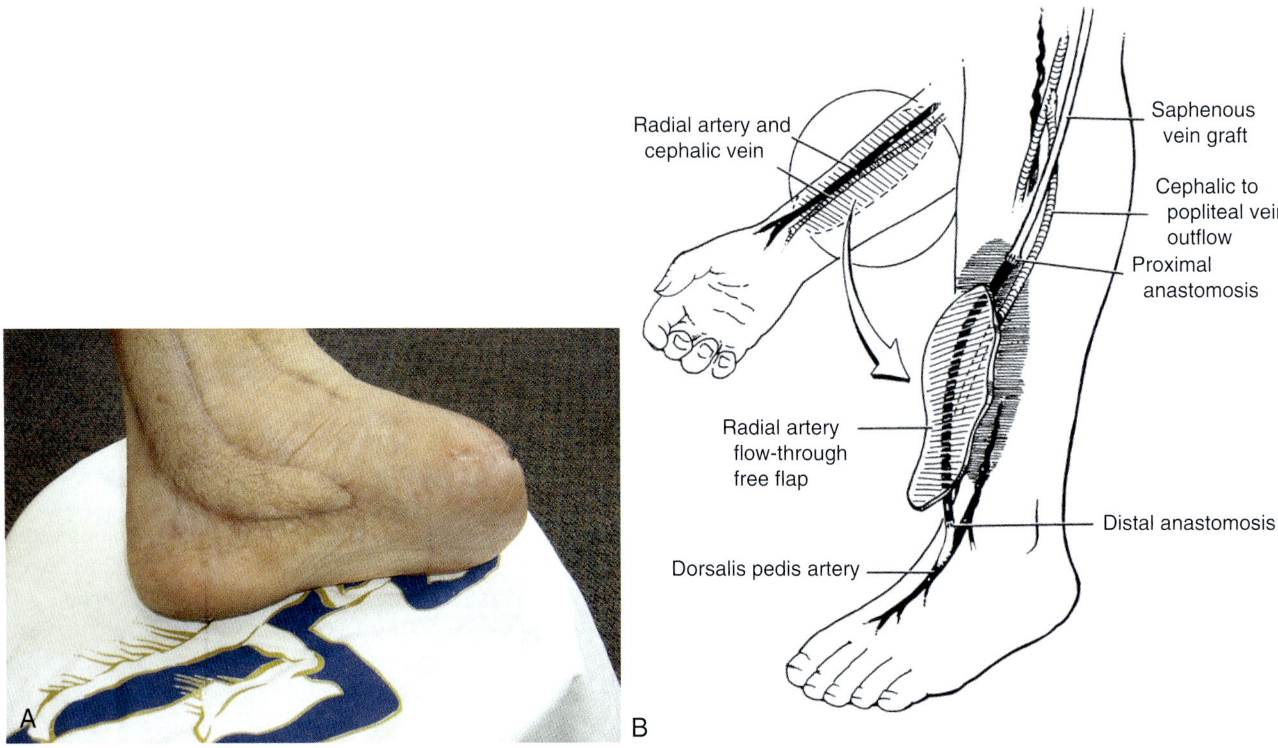

FIG 63.10 (A) The photograph depicts the final clinical result after transmetatarsal amputation and successful flow-through. (B) Anatomic representation of a donor radial flow-through flap and surgical anastomosis with the midposterior tibial artery to the inframaleolar posterior tibial artery.

Third, use prosthetic or cryopreserved conduit for ulcer healing. If a dysvascular, nonhealing wound cannot be healed with wound care or angioplasty, then a conduit with good short-term patency but poor long-term patency can be used to temporarily provide an increased blood supply to the healing wound.[80,81] This alternative should be used only if the rest of the limb does not need long-term revascularization. These grafts often require anticoagulation to maintain patency, and they are at increased risk for graft infection.

CONCLUSION

Wound care and revascularization in the dysvascular patient are inextricably intertwined if limb salvage is to occur. Vascular surgeons are the common link in diagnosing, treating, and coordinating care. To achieve an optimal patient outcome, vascular surgeons must be familiar with the principles of wound healing, the alternatives for wound bed preparation, and the techniques for revascularization in the ischemic limb.

REVIEW QUESTIONS

1. What defines a wound as chronic?
2. What does proper documentation of wound characteristics include?
3. What are the basics in the treatment of nonhealing wounds?
4. How is a chronic wound defined as infected versus colonized?
5. True or false: Hyperbaric oxygen has a broad role in managing chronic wounds.
6. True or false: Wound healing is promoted by creating a dry environment rather than a moist one.
7. True or false: The management of chronic wounds requires a significant infrastructure including nursing, home health, and multiple specialists including podiatry, plastic surgery, vascular surgery, and endocrinology.
8. Diagnostic studies used to evaluate patients with chronic wounds include
   - **a.** Ankle brachial index
   - **b.** Venous insufficiency studies
   - **c.** X-ray
   - **d.** $TcPO_2$
   - **e.** MRI
   - **f.** All of the above
9. True or false: Tissue transfer is widely available, can heal most wounds, and is low in cost.
10. Current indications for hyperbaric oxygen therapy for chronic wounds include
    - **a.** Refractory osteomyelitis
    - **b.** Diabetic foot ulcer
    - **c.** Radiation-associated wounds
    - **d.** Failing skin flaps or threatened skin grafts
    - **e.** All of the above

References available online at ExpertConsult.com.

64 CHAPTER

Lower Extremity Amputation

Juan Carlos Jimenez

OVERVIEW AND HISTORICAL PERSPECTIVE

Amputation is thought to be one of the oldest surgical procedures.[1] The earliest artificial limb dates from the Samnite wars of 300 BC. Until the time of Ambroise Paré (1510–1590), the techniques for amputation surgery and amputation level selection were extremely crude. Paré improved the surgical technique of amputation through the use of vascular ligatures and developed guidelines for the selection of appropriate levels of amputation. Because many of his original drawings and descriptions are not greatly different from today's surgical and prosthetic practices, he is considered the originator of the modern principles of amputation surgery. Paré's work was expanded by Dominique Jean Larrey (1776–1842) during the Napoleonic wars. Larrey advocated early amputation for traumatic limb injuries and was instrumental in the acceptance of both complete stump debridement and the modern surgical technique whereby bone is buried deep in the amputation stump, rather than the previous method of suturing skin tightly over the bone. Larrey was also involved in developing methods of early mobilization of war amputees.[2]

The idea of immediate or rapid fitting of an artificial leg after lower extremity amputation is relatively recent. Credit for the concept of rapid fit is generally given to Berlemont,[3] based on his work with patients who experienced delayed healing after lower extremity amputation; the concept of immediate postsurgical prosthetic fitting was developed by Weiss.[4] In the late 1960s, Burgess and colleagues noted accelerated rehabilitation, increased acceptance of a prosthesis, and less psychological trauma associated with loss of a limb when a prosthesis was applied immediately after lower extremity amputation.[5] Other advances in lower extremity amputation include the development of new techniques for amputation level selection, extension of the frontiers for limb salvage, and fabrication of prosthetic limbs that incorporate new designs and materials as well as energy storage.

Despite the long and colorful history of amputation surgery, most surgeons considered amputation a surgical defeat and an uninteresting and unrewarding surgical procedure. In many surgical institutions, amputation surgery was traditionally passed down to the youngest and least experienced member of the surgical team, who often operated without senior supervision. A report from the European surgical literature suggests that amputation failure is statistically linked to the lack of amputation experience of the surgeon.[6]

There has been a resurgence of interest in amputation surgery and rehabilitation. It is my view that amputation surgery is not a failure; it is clearly a reconstructive surgical technique. In addition, rehabilitation must be provided to patients following amputation surgery.

Historically, amputations were performed by orthopedic rather than general surgeons. However, two thirds of all lower extremity amputations are necessitated by complications of peripheral vascular disease or diabetes mellitus, so it is not surprising that the majority of lower extremity amputations are now performed by general and vascular surgeons. Unfortunately, most general surgical training programs fail to provide education in prosthetics, prosthetic design, biomechanics, and rehabilitation. The qualifications of the surgeon performing the amputation are not nearly as important as his or her interest in providing postoperative rehabilitation for the newly amputated patient.

This chapter reviews important features of lower extremity amputation surgery and amputation rehabilitation and includes detailed subsections on patient evaluation and preparation for amputation; amputation level selection; indications, surgical techniques, and prosthetic requirements for each level of amputation; surgical morbidity and mortality; common principles of lower extremity prosthetics; techniques of postsurgical rehabilitation; and future trends.

PATIENT EVALUATION AND PREPARATION FOR AMPUTATION

A review of the literature suggests that the mortality rates for below-knee and above-knee amputation are 4% to 16% and 12% to 40%, respectively.[7–12] It has been estimated that two thirds of patients undergoing lower extremity amputation have diabetes mellitus and that one half to two thirds have symptoms of cardiorespiratory disease.[7,9,13] A review of the causes of late mortality following successful amputation surgery discloses that two thirds of patients die of cardiovascular disease, approximately half of whom die from myocardial infarction.[7,14]

There are between 30,000 and 50,000 new lower extremity amputations performed in the United States each year.[7,9] At present, it is unclear whether the increase in distal revascularization has decreased the number of amputations. It is clear that diabetes-related amputation rates exhibit high regional variation, even after adjustment for age, sex, and race.[15] The indications for lower extremity amputation are listed in Table 64.1. For

TABLE 64.1 Indications for Lower Extremity Amputation

Indication	Percentage (Range)
Complications of diabetes mellitus	60–80
Nondiabetic infection with ischemia	15–25
Ischemia without infection	5–10
Chronic osteomyelitis	3–5
Trauma	2–5
Miscellaneous (neuroma, frostbite, tumor, pain, nonhealing)	5–10

Data from references 7, 9, 13, 14, 20.

patients with diabetes mellitus, it has been estimated that the risk of losing the second leg in the 5 years after amputation of the first leg ranges from 15% to 33% (3% to 7% per year)[16–18]; however, one third to one half of amputees with diabetes mellitus die of complications of diabetes or cardiorespiratory disease before undergoing amputation of the second extremity.[16,18,19]

In view of the mean age of patients undergoing lower extremity amputation (62 years),[7,8,13,14,20] the incidence of associated diseases, and the morbid and nonmorbid complications associated with surgery, the importance of a careful preoperative physical examination cannot be overstated. The physical examination should include a search for physical signs and symptoms suggestive of cardiorespiratory disease. Documentation of all pulses, as well as a careful assessment of the presence or absence of physical findings suggestive of extremity ischemia (pain, paresthesias, elevation pallor, rubor, alteration of sensory or motor function), should be performed. The extent and depth of infection or gangrene should be noted. The presence of malnutrition or systemic diseases, such as diabetes mellitus, collagen-vascular diseases, and immunodeficiency syndromes, or the systemic administration of antiinflammatory drugs, such as steroids, should be noted because their presence may have a major influence on the preoperative preparation and timing of lower extremity amputation, as well as postsurgical recovery. All diabetic patients should be carefully screened for silent but significant coronary artery disease. A paper by Pinzur and colleagues reinforced the concept that multidisciplinary presurgical evaluation helps in amputation level selection and prosthetic limb fitting and improves patient rehabilitation.[21]

The presence of lower extremity infection in a diabetic patient requires special mention. Historically, most studies have suggested that the primary organisms were *Staphylococcus aureus* and enteric gram-negative bacilli. More recent information, however, suggests that 60% of lower extremity infections in patients with diabetes mellitus involve both obligate and facultative anaerobic organisms.[22] Fierer and associates also pointed out that patients with mixed infections required more operations than those with simple staphylococcal infections and that their surgical wounds tended to heal more slowly.[22] I therefore recommend that antibiotic coverage for diabetics with lower extremity infections include drugs that provide broad-spectrum bactericidal aerobic and anaerobic coverage. A note of caution: there have been increasing reports of methicillin-resistant *S. aureus* infections, especially in patients with wound complications after vascular surgery.[23]

In the absence of acute arterial embolization, diabetes mellitus, immunodeficiency syndromes, collagen-vascular diseases, or drugs that inhibit the immune system, it is unusual to see tissue loss with or without infection in patients without multilevel vascular occlusive disease. Chronic single-level arterial obstruction is not usually associated with limb loss. As a general guideline, chronic occlusion of the superficial femoral artery does not cause limb loss without outflow (tibial trifurcation) or inflow (iliofemoral or deep femoral) occlusive disease.

The aims of amputation are to remove gangrenous tissues, relieve pain, obtain primary healing of the most distal amputation possible, and obtain maximal rehabilitation after amputation. For purposes of further discussion, the indications and management of patients undergoing amputation are divided into three general categories: (1) acute ischemia, (2) progressive chronic ischemia, and (3) ischemia complicated by infection.

Acute Ischemia

The choice of amputation for the management of acute ischemia in a patient whose arterial tree is considered unreconstructible or in a patient who presents late in the course of acute ischemia, such that arterial reconstruction may be contraindicated, is a decision that taxes the judgment of even the most experienced surgeon.[24] In addition, urgent or emergent amputation following acute arterial occlusion is generally associated with the greatest risk of morbidity and mortality in the entire field of amputation surgery. The degree of urgency for amputation in the face of acute arterial ischemia is governed by multiple factors that include, but are not limited to, the extent of extremity ischemia, especially the muscle mass; the pain the patient is experiencing from the ischemic tissues; and the presence of signs of systemic toxicity resulting from products of necrotic muscle or bacteria reaching the general circulatory system. If the affected ischemic area is small (e.g., the toes or forefoot), the pain is relatively moderate, and there are no signs of supervening infection or systemic toxicity, amputation can and should be postponed as long as possible to allow maximum development of collateral circulation. Delay of amputation in such a case improves the likelihood that a more distal limited amputation will heal. Mild to moderate pain can be controlled with narcotics. Adjunctive therapy, including systemic heparin, low-molecular-weight dextran, or fibrinolytic agents (urokinase, tissue plasminogen activator, tenecteplase, or reteplase) may be valuable in preventing progression of thrombus within capillary beds during the period of reduced blood flow, thus maintaining the viability of marginally ischemic tissues while collateral channels are beginning to enlarge. The presence of severe pain, extensive muscle necrosis, or systemic toxicity may require more emergent amputation with less patient preparation preoperatively. If muscle necrosis is extensive, the need for urgent or emergent amputation is critical because of the risk of renal damage secondary to circulating myoglobin. In addition to renal dysfunction, necrotic muscle tissue may cause cardiovascular or respiratory compromise, adding to the need for emergent amputation. The presence of systemic toxicity, especially a necrotizing infection, often necessitates emergent amputation. For those patients with significant medical comorbidities or systemic toxicity, cryologic or physiologic amputation allows extended time for patient preparation for surgery and decreases mortality.[25]

Several features of patient evaluation and clinical progression are helpful in this decision-making process. The first consideration is the extent of nonviable skin. Although discoloration or gangrene is readily apparent, hyposensitive areas due to severe skin ischemia do not allow adequate healing and may not be so easily identified. Except in patients with diabetic neuropathy, sensation to pinprick and light touch is a useful discriminant. If there is diminished sensation below the knee, for example, the chances of performing a successful below-knee amputation are small, and morbidity may be avoided by proceeding expeditiously to an above-knee amputation. The presence of significant calf muscle swelling or muscle rigidity is an ominous sign suggestive of myonecrosis. Careful monitoring of calf circumference, skin sensation, urine color and output, and signs of systemic toxicity such as lethargy, confusion, or hallucinations must be done on an hourly basis. The presence of systemic toxicity or significant changes in the physical examination indicate the need for immediate amputation or physiologic amputation.[25] Similarly, the presence of myoglobinuria or cardiovascular instability represents an indication for immediate amputation. It is generally impossible to obtain rapid myoglobin determinations in serum or urine, but the presence of a urinary heme-positive dipstick in the absence of red blood cells under microscopic examination or pink serum (hemoglobin) is consistent with a diagnosis of myoglobinuria. In addition, the presence of markedly elevated creatine phosphokinase or lactate dehydrogenase isoenzymes in the serum is suggestive of myonecrosis in the absence of trauma, myocardial infarction, or recent surgery. If continued observation is elected, prophylaxis against renal damage from myoglobin pigment is recommended and includes maintenance of a diuresis in the range of 75 to 100 mL/hour by the administration of osmotic diuretics such as mannitol and fluids. In addition, the urine should be maintained at an alkaline pH, because myoglobin precipitates in the renal tubules at a pH less than 7. Usually, a mixture of mannitol and sodium bicarbonate in a balanced salt solution can be used to titrate urine output and pH. Finally, the presence of infection in the ischemic extremity is an ominous complication requiring careful consideration. The presence of such an infection in a diabetic patient is even more ominous because of the sometimes rapid progression of seemingly innocuous infections. Any evidence of systemic toxicity or progressive infection is an indication for immediate surgical debridement, which may take the form of a debriding amputation or a physiologic amputation followed by a formal surgical amputation later.

As long as there is continued improvement in collateral blood supply to an acutely ischemic extremity and there is no sign of systemic or renal toxicity, observation may be continued. As soon as circulatory improvement ceases or signs of toxicity develop, amputation should be performed promptly. An alternative to amputation in an unstable or high-risk patient is physiologic amputation, as previously discussed.

Evaluation for potential vascular reconstruction in a patient with a clear-cut demarcation of a nonviable area of a lower extremity after a period of observation for acute ischemia is not likely to be beneficial; however, if there is a question of marginal tissue viability above an area that is believed to be nonviable and the questionable tissue might permit a lower amputation level, evaluation for vascular reconstruction may be beneficial.[26] For example, the presence of a nonviable forefoot and a marginal lower extremity between the knee and ankle may be an indication for evaluation for vascular reconstruction in an attempt to perform a below-knee rather than an above-knee amputation.

Progressive Chronic Ischemia

A patient with progressive chronic ischemia who ultimately presents for amputation has experienced one or more of the following problems: rest pain, nonhealing skin lesion or ulceration, gangrene, or gangrene with superimposed infection. Gangrene complicated by infection is a special problem and is discussed in a separate section.

From the patient's point of view, ischemic rest pain is one of the most compelling indications for amputation. Characteristically, the patient seeks relief by sitting up and allowing his or her legs to hang over the side of the bed or by ambulation. The dependent position provides relief of ischemic rest pain because gravity favors improved collateral blood flow, which augments arterial perfusion pressure. In its more severe forms, ischemic rest pain forms part of a vicious circle. As the patient more frequently uses dependency to achieve pain relief, the extremity becomes edematous and lymphatic return decreases, which eventually results in more ischemia. The end result of this vicious circle is a massively swollen, very painful ischemic extremity. Mild to moderate rest pain can often be successfully managed with narcotics. There have been reports that early mild rest pain may be relieved by sympathectomy. If there are no signs of systemic toxicity or supervening infection, and if mild ischemic rest pain can be controlled with medication, a patient can be followed and amputation postponed.

Another manifestation of chronic ischemia is the presence of ischemic skin ulcerations or nonhealing skin lesions on the lower extremity. Unfortunately, many of these skin ulcers occur in hospitalized patients as a result of abrasion of the foot or pressure necrosis (due to poor foot protection in the hospital bed). In a diabetic patient, ulceration usually occurs at pressure points, and the patient is often unaware of the problem because of diabetic neuropathy. Patients without peripheral neuropathy are very much aware of these ischemic ulcers because they are typically extremely painful. Besides obvious areas of pressure necrosis, such as the heel and the lateral and medial malleoli, other common points of ulceration include the bony prominences over the metatarsal heads and midphalangeal joints or between the toes.

Fortunately, most patients with chronic progressive ischemia come to medical attention before the presence of frank tissue loss. Even patients with tissue loss usually present early with involvement of one or more toes or, in more severe cases, the entire forefoot. Under these circumstances, there is usually ample opportunity to fully prepare and evaluate the patient for lower extremity amputation or arterial reconstruction if possible. Preoperative evaluation and management should include proper medical attention to all associated diseases and a careful evaluation for potential critical organ dysfunction, especially the heart, lungs, and kidneys.

All patients with chronic ischemia should undergo consideration for vascular reconstruction for limb salvage. Angiographic evaluation from the infrarenal abdominal aorta down to and including the pedal arches is mandatory. In general, the surgeon should ensure good inflow to the level of the deep femoral artery. Reconstruction distal to the level of the deep femoral artery should be done only if chances for success are reasonably high and if a successful procedure would obviate the need for a major amputation. There is continuing controversy over the effect of prior revascularization on amputation level.[27–35] In my opinion, revascularization should always be attempted unless contraindicated by the patient's medical condition. If vascular reconstruction is brought below the knee, the incision required for approaching the distal popliteal artery and tibial trifurcation vessels should be planned along the lines of the posterior skin flap that might be required for a subsequent below-knee amputation. Techniques for selecting an amputation level are discussed later. However, one of the interesting spinoffs from studies of amputation level selection is the identification of patients who are unable to heal a low-level amputation and in whom the chance for rehabilitation at a high level of amputation is unlikely. When such objective information is available, attempts at proximal or extended distal extremity bypass to salvage a knee joint, for example, may be indicated to keep a patient ambulatory.[26,28,29]

Gangrene Complicated by Infection

The presence of dry gangrene is not an emergent surgical problem or necessarily the hallmark of an ominous clinical situation. Dry gangrene, limited to the toes, for example, may be treated conservatively and requires little, if any, surgical or ancillary medical support; however, infection complicating dry gangrene (i.e., wet gangrene), especially in a diabetic patient, is a limb- and life-threatening emergency. Control of sepsis can sometimes be achieved with antibiotic therapy plus limited debridement and drainage, or it may require radical excision and debridement; antibiotic therapy alone is seldom adequate treatment for gangrene complicated by infection. Failure to institute prompt therapy, especially in diabetic patients, results in rapid ascension of the infectious process, the loss of potentially salvageable tissue, and a large increase in patient mortality. As noted earlier, in patients with systemic toxicity, cryoamputation before definitive surgical amputation helps decrease mortality.

The first step in the management of infected or wet gangrene is identification of the infecting organisms. Usually, the urgency of the clinical situation does not allow the identification of specific organisms by culture, although culture should be obtained and submitted for both anaerobic and aerobic organisms. It has been my practice to assume that gangrene complicated by infection includes a mixture of aerobic and anaerobic organisms; therefore broad-spectrum bactericidal antibiotic coverage is used.[22]

Once antibiotic therapy has been started, the patient's status must be monitored carefully, including pulse rate, white blood cell count, blood pressure, temperature, extent of infection, severity of pain, and diffuse signs of systemic toxicity such as lethargy, hallucinations, and general mental status. In a diabetic patient, serum glucose and insulin requirements are additional useful monitoring parameters. If a prompt response to antibiotic therapy is noted, therapy should be continued for maximum effect and a definitive amputation then performed. If the patient does not respond promptly to antibiotic management or if undrained purulent material was initially evident, debridement of gangrenous tissue and establishment of drainage should be employed as an early adjunct to antibiotic therapy.

If the gangrenous infection extensively involves the foot and contaminates tendon and tissue spaces, especially in a diabetic patient, radical debridement should be performed. One of the better methods to obtain radical debridement and establish open drainage is a guillotine amputation of the foot carried out at the level of the malleoli (Fig. 64.1). Guillotine amputation eliminates the septic focus and allows drainage of contaminated lymphatics and tissue spaces in the lower leg. The presence of cellulitis and lymphangitis at the level of ankle guillotine is not a contraindication to this type of debridement technique. After performance of a guillotine-type amputation for debridement, systemic antibiotics are continued until the definitive amputation is performed, usually 3 to 5 days later. Definitive amputation is performed after ascertaining that the infection has been controlled and the patient's preoperative status has been optimized.

The incidence of stump infection in patients who present with a septic foot is decreased if a preparatory ankle guillotine amputation is performed before definitive amputation. In my experience, such a two-stage surgical approach decreased the stump infection rate from 22% to 3% ($P = .01$).[36] This approach

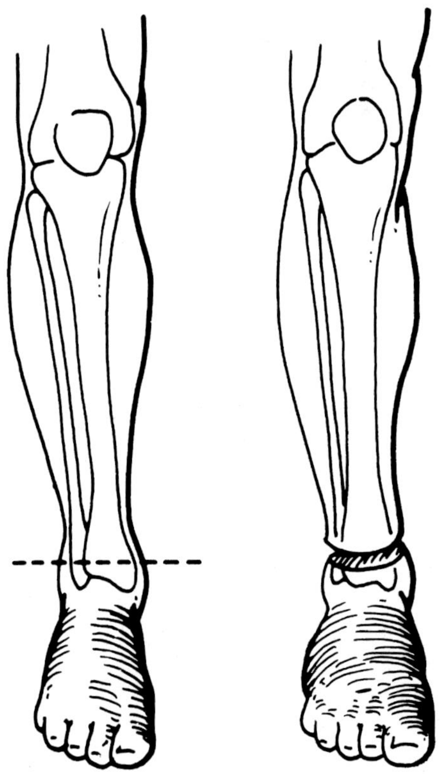

FIG 64.1 Schematic representation of an open ankle guillotine, or preparatory, amputation in a patient with a septic foot.

was reaffirmed in a prospective, randomized study by Fischer and colleagues,[37] in which the incidence of stump infection was decreased from 21% (one stage) to 0% (two stage) ($P = .05$).

Amputation for Trauma

Patients undergoing traumatic lower extremity amputation tend to be young and in good medical health, so patient evaluation and preparation for amputation are easier than that described for geriatric patients with peripheral vascular disease and diabetes. As a general principle, formal traumatic amputation is performed to achieve healing at the lowest amputation level possible, and amputation level selection is usually predetermined by the injury. Adequate debridement of dead tissue is mandatory. The presence of a large amount of marginally viable tissue or potentially infected tissue may be an indication for debridement and open amputation followed at a later date by formal amputation with skin closure. A special effort should be made to rule out proximal bony or ligamentous injuries. Careful attention must be paid to other potentially life- or limb-threatening injuries, and management of such injuries must be handled in an appropriate sequence to achieve the best overall result for the patient. The use of a proximal extremity tourniquet for control of bleeding is optional but should be discouraged in a dysvascular patient. The use of drains after traumatic amputation is controversial, although there is some evidence that drainage results in a more rapid resolution of postamputation stump edema. If drains are used, they should be the closed-system type (not open Penrose drains).

DETERMINATION OF AMPUTATION LEVEL

The objective of preoperative amputation level selection is to determine the most distal amputation site that will heal. The general requirements are as follows: (1) the amputation must remove all necrotic, painful, or infected tissue; (2) the amputation stump must be able to be fitted with a functional and easily applied prosthesis; and (3) the blood supply at the level of the proposed amputation must be sufficient to allow primary skin healing. Appropriate selection of the amputation level is critical. If the surgeon elects too proximal an amputation, such as a midthigh amputation, the patient may be deprived of the opportunity for ambulation and rehabilitation, although the amputation might heal without difficulty. If a distal amputation site is selected and the blood supply is inadequate for amputation healing, further surgery will be required for amputation at a higher level. This latter approach may result in increased morbidity and mortality and may ultimately result in rehabilitation failure.

The inherent advantages of a below-knee amputation as opposed to an above-knee amputation should be obvious. It is easier to ambulate on a below-knee prosthesis; this is extremely important, especially in geriatric patients. In general, a unilateral below-knee amputee requires a 10% to 40% increase in energy expenditure for ambulation compared with the energy required for walking with an intact extremity. In contrast, a unilateral above-knee amputee (using a prosthesis with a locked or unlocked knee) requires approximately a 50% to 70% increase in energy expenditure. Crutch walking without a lower extremity prosthesis uses approximately 60% more energy, whereas wheelchair use necessitates only a small increase in energy expenditure (9%). Patients with severe coronary artery disease or severe chronic obstructive pulmonary disease may be physically unable to provide the additional energy required for ambulation on an above-knee compared with a below-knee prosthesis.

It is usually possible for the surgeon to decide on an amputation level that will remove necrotic, painful, or infected tissue as well as to plan an amputation stump that can be fitted with a prosthesis. However, the decision regarding the adequacy of blood supply at the proposed amputation level is one of the most difficult problems facing the amputation surgeon.

The earliest attempts at amputation level selection used the presence of pulses in the affected extremity, skin temperature, correlation of arteriographic findings, and "clinical judgment." It has been well documented that none of these selection techniques has a consistent enough correlation with amputation healing to provide a sound basis for clinical decision making. In a study by Robbs and Ray, the morbidity, mortality, and rates of healing of lower limb amputations in 214 patients, wherein the amputation level was determined by nonobjective criteria, were retrospectively analyzed.[38] Six of 67 (8.9%) primary above-knee amputations and 37 of 147 (25%) primary below-knee amputations had to be revised to a higher level. The authors concluded "that flap viability could not be predicted by the extent of ischemic lesion in relation to the ankle joint, the popliteal pulse status, or lower limb angiography."[38] In a 1992 study comparing clinical parameters and skin perfusion pressure for amputation level selection, Dwars and coworkers noted that the presence of palpable pulses immediately above the selected level correlated well with primary healing.[39] However, the absence of palpable pulses and angiographic patency scores were of no clinical value in amputation level selection. Golbranson and colleagues presented promising data on improved methods of skin temperature measurement that had a high degree of accuracy (90%) for selecting below- versus above-knee amputation levels.[40] In addition, Spence and Walker demonstrated a clear correlation between three different temperature isotherms (1.8°C separation) and isotopically derived skin blood flow ($P < .001$).[41] Stoner and associates reported that when the ratio of temperatures at the posterior and anterior incision sites (Burgess posterior flap below-knee amputation) was greater than 0.98, healing was improved.[42] In a study comparing several modalities for amputation level selection, Wagner and colleagues noted (for above- and below-knee amputations) that the average skin temperature at the amputation site was higher (34.3°C) in patients who healed primarily compared with those who required operative stump revision (33.3°C) ($P = .001$).[43] One physical finding that has some value in differentiating proposed amputation levels is the presence of dependent rubor. Skin that develops dependent rubor is clearly ischemic and thus, like gangrenous tissue, is an absolute contraindication to amputation at that level; however, the absence of dependent rubor does not necessarily ensure healing ability. Early workers in the field of amputation surgery solved the problem of level selection by performing above-knee amputations on almost all patients. In the 1960s, Lim and coworkers demonstrated that 83% of all patients requiring a lower extremity amputation would heal following a below-knee amputation.[44]

However, using empirical below-knee amputation selection may be detrimental to some patients who might have healed following a more distal amputation, such as a transmetatarsal or Syme amputation. In addition, identifying the 20% to 30% of patients in whom a below-knee amputation is doomed to failure would be advantageous so that either a knee disarticulation or an above-knee amputation could be performed primarily, saving the patient additional surgical procedures.

The need for more sensitive and objective methods for the preoperative selection of amputation level led to the development of numerous noninvasive techniques, including Doppler ankle and calf systolic blood pressure determinations, with or without pulse-volume recordings[45–52]; xenon 133 (^{133}Xe) skin blood flow studies[53–59]; digital or transmetatarsal photoplethysmographic pressures[50]; transcutaneous oxygen determination[11,59–68]; skin fluorescence after intravenous fluorescein dye[69–72]; laser Doppler skin blood flow measurements[55,73] (F.A. Matsen, personal communication, 1978); pertechnetate skin blood pressure studies[74,75]; and photoelectrically measured skin color changes.[76]

An overview of the various criteria for predicting the healing of digit and forefoot amputations is shown in Table 64.2. Totals from Table 64.2 suggest that preoperative selection techniques correctly predicted primary healing in 174 of 189 toe and forefoot amputations (97%). Similar data for below-knee amputation levels are summarized in Table 64.3. Excluding empirical below-knee selection, the tests listed in Table 64.3 correctly

TABLE 64.2 Selection Criteria for Toe and Forefoot Amputation

Criterion	Reference	Amputation Level	Number of Healing Patients (%)
Doppler Ankle Systolic Pressure			
70 mm Hg	45	Forefoot	38/44 (86)
116 mm Hg	50	Digit/forefoot	25/27 (93)
35 mm Hg	51	Digit	44/46 (96)
Fiberoptic fluorometry DFI >44	72	Foot/forefoot	18/20 (90)
Photoplethysmographic digit or TMA pressure 20 mm Hg	50	Digit	20/20 (100)
Xenon skin clearance >2.6 mL/100 g tissue/min	57	Digit/forefoot	25/28 (89)
Transcutaneous Po_2 >20 mm Hg	65	Forefoot	4/4 (100)
Total			174/189 (92)

DFI, Dye fluorescence index; *TMA*, transmetatarsal-ankle.

TABLE 64.3 Selection Criteria for Below-Knee Amputation

Criterion	Reference	Number of Healing Patients (%)
Doppler systolic ankle pressure 30 mm Hg + calf pressure 65 mm Hg + pulsatile PVR	49	27/27 (100)
Doppler systolic calf pressure 70 mm Hg	46	32/32 (100)
Doppler systolic thigh pressure 80 mm Hg or calf pressure 50 mm Hg	52	36/36 (100)
Empirical below-knee	44	38/46 (83)
Fiber-optic fluorometry DFI >44	72	12/12 (100)
Fluorescein dye	70	24/30 (80)
^{99m}Tc-pertechnetate skin blood pressure	86	24/26 (92)
Laser-Doppler velocimetry >20 mV	78	25/26 (96)
Photoelectric skin pressure 20–100 mm Hg	76, 87	60/71 (85)
Transcutaneous Po_2 >10 mm Hg or >10 mm Hg increase on 100% O_2	62, 80	76/80 (95)
>35 mm Hg	60, 64, 67	51/51 (100)
>20 mm Hg	65	16/16 (100)
>0 to <40 mm Hg	60	17/19 (89)
0 mm Hg	60	0/3 (0)[a]
Index >0.59	64	17/17 (100)
Index >0.20	77	33/34 (97)
Xenon skin clearance = 3.1 mL blood flow/100 g tissue/min	54	23/26 (88)
>2.6 mL blood flow/100 g tissue/min	57	35/36 (97)
Epicutaneous >0.9 mL/100 g tissue/min	53, 56	14/15 (93)
Total		560/603 (93)

[a]Excluded from total.
DFI, Dye fluorescence index; *PVR*, pulse-volume recording.

predicted primary healing of below-knee amputations in 560 of 603 elective amputations (93%). Clearly, objective amputation level selection can not only predict potential healing of a more distal level of amputation but also accurately assess the likelihood of healing of a below-knee compared with an above-knee amputation. It is my opinion that elective lower extremity amputation should not be performed without some type of preoperative testing to ensure primary healing of the most distal amputation possible.

The techniques for the use of ankle, calf, and popliteal Doppler systolic blood pressure determinations have been well described[45–49,51,52] and are not covered in this chapter. Similarly, use of the photoplethysmograph for determining digital and transmetatarsal blood pressures has been well described by Schwartz and coworkers[50] and is not presented here. The potential advantages of both the Doppler instrument and the photoplethysmograph are that they are relatively simple, inexpensive, and totally noninvasive. The problem with these instruments is that the presence of a blood pressure less than a predetermined level does not necessarily guarantee failure of amputation healing at that level (negative predictive value). This problem was nicely summarized by Verta and colleagues, who noted that "for forefoot amputation a high Doppler ankle pressure did not guarantee successful healing and a low ankle pressure did not contraindicate primary healing."[51] In an effort to increase the accuracy of Doppler ankle pressures, both Gibbons and coworkers[48] and Raines and associates[49] suggested the ancillary use of pulse-volume recordings. Although Raines's group reported 100% successful healing in 27 below-knee amputations in which the Doppler systolic ankle pressure was greater than 30 mm Hg, calf pressure was greater than 65 mm Hg, and there was a pulsatile pulse-volume recording in the foot, Gibbons's group was unable to duplicate these results and concluded, "we find no consistent criteria which are more accurate and reliable than clinical judgment and no ankle pressure above which primary healing was guaranteed." Gibbons and coworkers also noted decreased accuracy in amputation level prediction using pulse-volume recording and Doppler ankle systolic pressures in patients with diabetes mellitus. The problem with diabetic patients (falsely high systolic pressure measurements) is likely due to medical calcinosis of their vessels. Wagner and colleagues reported that Doppler pressures at the thigh, popliteal, midcalf, or ankle level were unreliable in predicting healing of a below-knee amputation.[43]

Theoretically, the measurement of skin fluorescence with a Wood's ultraviolet lamp after intravenous injection of fluorescein dye (Funduscein) should be a reliable test for amputation level selection. Although this technique is somewhat more invasive than Doppler ankle systolic pressure measurements or pulse-volume recordings, it is less complicated and less invasive than ^{133}Xe skin blood flow or pertechnetate skin perfusion measurements. The commercial availability of two new types of fluorometers (Fiberoptic Perfusion Fluorometer, Diversatronics, Broomall, PA; Fluoroscan, V. Elings, PhD, University of California, Santa Barbara), which can provide objective numeric readings quickly and in the absence of a Wood's lamp, may further enhance the use of this technique.[69,71,72] Development of a computerized video camera system to analyze skin perfusion after oral ingestion of fluorescein obviates the risk of intravenous injection and allows easy data manipulation for limb mapping. Such a system has been under study at Maricopa Medical Center in Phoenix, Arizona. McFarland and Lawrence reported an accuracy rate of 80% for skin fluorescence, compared with 47% for Doppler popliteal systolic blood pressure (50 mm Hg) for the prediction of healing of a below-knee amputation (see Table 64.3).[70] In addition, when skin fluorescence and Doppler pressure did not agree on the level of amputation, fluorescein always predicted a more distal level. Silverman and associates, in 1985, reported their data on fiberoptic fluorometry for amputation level selection at the below-knee, below-ankle, and above-knee levels in dysvascular limbs.[72] The overall success rate was 92% (36 of 39), and individual rates were 18 of 20 below-ankle (90%), 12 of 12 below-knee (100%), and 6 of 7 above-knee (86%) amputations. Discriminate analysis demonstrated an optimal reference point between healing and nonhealing amputations, and a dye fluorescence index of greater than 44 had 93% accuracy. Two later studies, however, did not demonstrate such promising results.[77,78] In a blinded, prospective review of 56 patients undergoing below-knee amputation, objective measurement of fluorescein perfusion did not correlate with amputation healing.[79] In a study comparing multiple methods of amputation level selection, Wagner and colleagues found that qualitative skin fluorescence was not as successful as cutaneous oxygen measurement.[43]

Promising work with a modified Clark-type oxygen electrode (with a heating element and thermostat for temperature control; Transoxode, Hellige-Orager, FRG; US manufacturer, Litton Industries [Woodland Hills, CA]) for amputation level selection has been reported by several groups.[60,62,64,65,67,80] Franzeck and colleagues reported that the mean transcutaneous partial pressure of oxygen (Po_2) values of patients who healed primarily compared with those who failed to heal were 36.5 ± 17.5 mm Hg and less than 0.3 mm Hg, respectively.[62] However, in those patients with a transcutaneous Po_2 less than 10 mm Hg, six of nine failed to heal, and three of nine healed primarily. In a study on below-knee amputations, Burgess and coworkers found that 15 of 15 amputations healed primarily if the transcutaneous Po_2 was greater than 40 mm Hg, 17 of 19 healed if the transcutaneous Po_2 was greater than 0 mm Hg but less than 40 mm Hg, and none of the three amputations with a Po_2 of 0 mm Hg healed.[60] Katsamouris and coworkers reported that 17 of 17 lower extremity amputations healed if the Po_2 was greater than 38 mm Hg or if the Po_2 index (chest wall control site) was greater than 0.59.[64] Ratliff and colleagues noted that 18 below-knee amputations healed if the Po_2 was greater than 35 mm Hg, while 10 of 15 failed if the Po_2 was less than 35 mm Hg.[67] Kram and associates noted success in 33 of 34 (97%) below-knee amputations with multisensor transcutaneous oxygen mapping when the critical Po_2 index was greater than 0.20.[77] In addition, all six patients with an index less than 0.20 failed to heal. All investigators have reported some amputations that healed in patients with low Po_2 values. A partial explanation for this observation might be the nonlinear relationship between Po_2 and cutaneous blood flow. In a careful study, Matsen and coworkers reported that Po_2 measurements are most dependent on arteriovenous gradients and cutaneous vascular resistance.[66] Techniques to improve the accuracy of transcutaneous Po_2 probes include local heating (to 44°C, which minimizes local vascular resistance and makes Po_2 more linear with respect to cutaneous blood flow), measurements before and after oxygen administration, oxygen isobar extremity mapping, and transcutaneous oxygen recovery half-time.[81] Oishi and associates noted—in a study comparing skin temperature, Doppler pressure, and transcutaneous oxygen—that after the inhalation of oxygen, if the Po_2 increased 10 mm Hg or more, the Po_2 predicted amputation healing with a sensitivity of 98%.[82] In another study, the authors prospectively compared the following tests for their accuracy in amputation level selection: transcutaneous oxygen, transcutaneous carbon dioxide, ratio of transcutaneous oxygen to transcutaneous carbon dioxide, foot-to-chest transcutaneous oxygen, intradermal ^{133}Xe, ankle-brachial index, and absolute popliteal artery pressure.[65] All metabolic parameters had a high degree of statistical accuracy in predicting amputation healing, whereas none of the other tests had statistical reliability. All amputations—transmetatarsal, below-knee, and above-knee—healed primarily if the transcutaneous Po_2 level was greater than 20 mm Hg, and there was a 0% incidence of false-positive and false-negative studies. Most authors of transcutaneous oxygen testing studies suggest using a cutoff point of 35 to 40 mm Hg. I have used 20 mm Hg with excellent results. Recent data reconfirm the accuracy of a threshold of 20 mm Hg, especially in distal limb amputations.[68] Also of importance is the observation that amputation site healing is not affected by the presence of diabetes mellitus, nor are the test results for any of the metabolic parameters. Similar data have been reported by Bacharach and colleagues, who stated that 51 of 52 limbs (98%) healed (primary and delayed) with a Po_2 greater than or equal to 40 mm Hg, whereas a Po_2 of less than 20 mm Hg was associated with universal failure.[83] In that study, Po_2 measurements during limb elevation improved the predictability of outcome for patients with supine Po_2 values greater than 20 mm Hg but less than 40 mm Hg.

Theoretically, laser-Doppler velocimetry should be an ideal tool for skin blood flow determination; it is noninvasive and "measures" capillary blood flow (good correlation between laser-Doppler blood flow measurements using microspheres, electromagnetic flow probes, and ^{133}Xe clearance).[84] However, data by Holloway and Burgess,[54] Holloway and Watkins,[55] Holloway,[84] and Matsen (personal communication, 1978) suggest that although there is a linear relationship among techniques, there is a fair amount of variance. These groups noted that the use of local skin heating may enhance the accuracy of the laser-Doppler and make it a more valuable adjunct for amputation level selection.[84] Holloway and Burgess reported their experience with laser-Doppler velocimetry in 20 lower extremity amputations at the foot, forefoot, below-knee, and above-knee levels, and the accuracy rates were as follows: foot and forefoot, two of six (33%); below-knee, eight of eight (100%); and above-knee, six of six (100%).[73]

Malone and coworkers'[57] and Moore's[58] greatest postsurgical experience was with the use of ^{133}Xe skin clearance for amputation level selection. These techniques have been well described by Moore,[58] Daly and Henry,[85] and Malone and associates.[57] One of the major difficulties with the application of ^{133}Xe skin clearance for amputation level selection is its reproducibility by other investigators. In an earlier publication, Holloway and Burgess were unable to document a clear-cut end point above which all amputations healed.[54] In contrast, Silberstein and colleagues reported that 38 of 39 patients (11 above-knee amputations, 18 below-knee or transmetatarsal amputations, and 9 no amputation) healed when ^{133}Xe skin blood flow was greater than 2.4 mL/100 g tissue per minute; when flow was less than 2.4 mL/100 g tissue per minute, only four of seven patients healed.[59] One significant advantage of ^{133}Xe clearance techniques that may offset both of these problems, if its ultimate reliability is demonstrated in other centers, is its potential ability to predict healing at all levels of lower extremity amputation.[57]

A final problem with the intradermal use of ^{133}Xe for skin blood flow measurements is that the manufacturer no longer supplies ^{133}Xe. The product must be made by nuclear medicine departments. This limitation may further preclude widespread use of the intradermal ^{133}Xe technique. Finally, despite past publications and excellent results,[57,58,85] I no longer use ^{133}Xe skin clearance for amputation level selection. In part, this change was made because of the enumerated difficulties; however, the major reason for this change was a study wherein ^{133}Xe was not found to be statistically reliable as a selection method for amputation level.[65] (As noted previously, transcutaneous oxygen is very reliable.)

Using the disappearance of intradermal technetium 99m pertechnetate, ^{131}I-sodium, ^{131}I-antipyrine, or ^{133}Xe in the presence of external pressure, Holstein[74] and Holstein and Lassen[86] reported amputation level selection data comparable to data reported by Moore, Daly, Henry, Malone, and others. Because ^{133}Xe is trapped in subcutaneous fat, there are solid theoretical reasons to use an isotope other than ^{133}Xe. Holstein and associates found no significant difference among ^{131}I-sodium, ^{131}I-antipyrine, and ^{99m}Tc-pertechnetate for the measurement of skin perfusion pressure.[75]

Stockel and coworkers[76] and Ovesen and Stockel[87] reported preliminary data on the use of a photodetector and plethysmography (Medimatic, Copenhagen) for amputation level selection; these findings correlate well with the ^{133}Xe skin perfusion pressure techniques of Holstein and colleagues.[74,75] This technique uses a blood pressure cuff placed over a photoelectric detector, which is connected to a plethysmograph, to measure the minimal external pressure required to prevent skin reddening after blanching. To date, 66 of 71 (93%) below-knee amputations healed with skin pressures between 20 and 100 mm Hg. In 1992, Dwars and associates reported that skin perfusion pressure measurements were of excellent predictive value for the healing of lower extremity amputations (positive predictive value, 89%; negative predictive value, 99%).[39]

In summary, it is my opinion that elective lower extremity amputation should not be performed in the absence of objective testing to determine the most distal amputation that will heal primarily, yet allow the removal of infected, painful, or ischemic tissue. A variety of techniques are available, and the technique chosen depends on the available equipment, the amputation level under consideration, and the current accuracy rates for the reported techniques. However, in my opinion, the most reliable, easiest to use, and best overall technique for prospective amputation level selection is transcutaneous oxygen testing.

LOWER EXTREMITY AMPUTATION LEVELS

This section discusses only those amputation levels that are relevant to patients with peripheral vascular disease or diabetes mellitus. Amputation levels that are less desirable from the standpoint of healing or rehabilitation or those that present specific prosthetic fitting problems are omitted. In my experience and that of others, Chopart, Lisfranc, and Boyd forefoot amputations have been fraught with controversy because of healing problems, prosthetic fitting problems, and equinus deformities.[88] Because these amputation levels are occasionally used by vascular surgeons, they are reviewed here only briefly.

Toe Amputation

Toe amputation is the most frequently performed peripheral amputation. It is especially common in patients with diabetes mellitus, who are prone to lesions (ulceration, osteomyelitis, gangrene) that necessitate amputation.

Patients who present with dry gangrene allow the surgeon a choice between direct surgical intervention and autoamputation. In the absence of supervening infection or pain, expectant management permits epithelialization to take place under the dry gangrenous eschar. As soon as epithelialization is complete, the toe will drop off, leaving a cleanly healed stump. Autoamputation is preferable to direct surgical intervention because it obviates the need for healing after amputation and probably results in a more distal site of healing than would be achieved with surgical intervention. However, this process often requires months before it is complete.

Indications

Gangrene, infection, neuropathic ulceration, or osteomyelitis should be confined to the midphalanx or distal phalanx. There must be no dependent rubor, and venous filling time should be less than 20 to 25 seconds. Sizer and Wheelock demonstrated that the presence of pedal pulses, even in patients with diabetes, is associated with a very high rate of healing after toe amputation (98%).[89]

Contraindications

Cellulitis proximal to the area of proposed toe excision, the presence of dependent rubor, forefoot infection, and involvement of the metatarsophalangeal joint or (distal) metatarsal head all represent specific contraindications to toe amputation.

Surgical Technique

A single toe should never be amputated by disarticulation but should be transected through the proximal phalanx, leaving a small button of bone to protect the metatarsal head. Skin flaps can be of any design, as long as they obey basic surgical principles and have an adequate base for the length of flap. The flaps can be fish-mouth, plantar base, dorsal base, side to side, or any variation or combination; however, they must be long enough to close without tension. The most commonly used incision is circular (Fig. 64.2). Amputation through the metatarsophalangeal joint or an interphalangeal joint should be avoided because of the avascular nature of cartilage and the likelihood of supervening infection or failure to heal.

Careful atraumatic edge-to-edge skin closure without the use of forceps maximizes the chances of primary healing. Suture material that produces minimal reaction when left in place for long periods should be used, such as monofilament wire or plastic. A soft postoperative dressing that provides gentle wound compression should be applied.

Chronic osteomyelitis of the great toe without gangrene in a diabetic patient presents a difficult surgical problem. Because complete healing is not common, and total resection of the great toe results in some imbalance in walking (which can be accommodated with proper shoe orthotics), debridement and resection of the infected phalanges through a medial or lateral incision, leaving a soft tissue toe remnant in place, are probably best from a functional standpoint.

Advantages and Disadvantages

The primary advantage of toe amputation is the lack of requirement for prosthetic rehabilitation and the fact that minimal tissue is excised.

Except for the risk of nonhealing or secondary infection and stump breakdown, requiring a higher level of amputation, there are no disadvantages to this level of amputation.

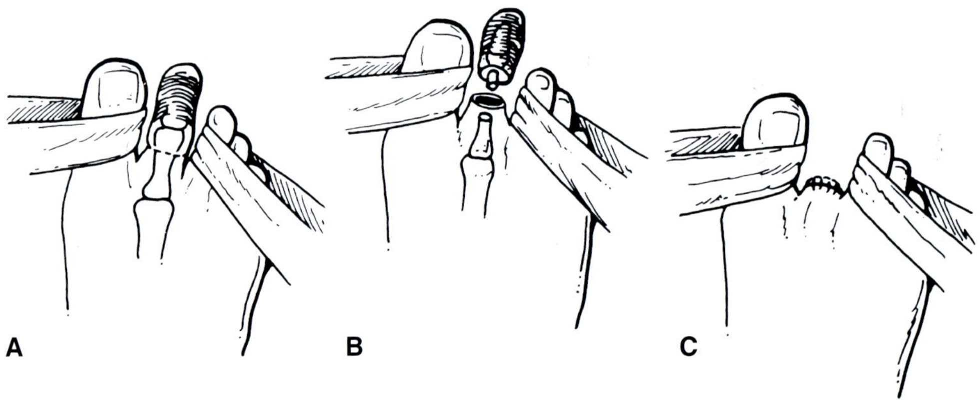

FIG 64.2 Single-toe amputation using a circular incision and transverse wound closure. (A) Circular incision for toe amputation. (B) Disarticulation of interphalangeal joint. (C) Wound closure.

Rehabilitation Potential

Rehabilitation potential is 100%. However, the performance of a toe amputation in a patient with peripheral vascular disease, especially with concomitant diabetes, is an ominous sign with regard to long-term prognosis. Little and coworkers found that by 3.5 years after toe amputation, almost three fourths of their patients required a more proximal major amputation.[90]

Ray Amputation

Indications

If the gangrenous skin or infectious process approaches the metatarsophalanged crease or includes the (distal) metatarsal head, this precludes a toe amputation. A conservative partial distal forefoot amputation can still be performed by extending the toe amputation to include the distal metatarsal shaft and head.

Contraindications

Gangrene, infection, cellulitis, and dependent rubor involving skin proximal to the metatarsophalangeal crease are contraindications to ray amputation. In addition, involvement of multiple toes is a relative contraindication, because a transmetatarsal amputation would be a more suitable surgical procedure. Ray amputation for gangrene or infection of the great toe also is a relative contraindication, because removal of the first metatarsal head leads to unstable weight bearing and difficulties with ambulation; however, with proper shoe orthotics, ray amputation of the first or great toe results in excellent foot salvage and provides patients with a stable gait pattern.

Surgical Technique

The incision begins vertically on the dorsum of the foot, bifurcates laterally and medially to encircle the toe, meets on the plantar aspect of the foot, and extends for a variable distance on the plantar aspect of the foot. The plantar incision is extended proximally as needed to allow removal of the toe and distal metatarsal head. Care should be taken not to injure the digital arteries or nerves adjacent to the metatarsal bone and not to enter into the deep tension or joint spaces of the medial and lateral toes. The distal metatarsal shaft is divided at its neck, and soft tissues are removed by sharp dissection. The surgical specimen consists of the toe, metatarsophalangeal joint, and distal portion of the metatarsal shaft and head. If possible, the surgical specimen should be removed in continuity. The metatarsal shaft must be transected in an area of normal bone. "Soft bone" suggests osteomyelitis, especially in diabetic patients, and mandates higher (i.e., more proximal) bone division.

I recommend that the surgical wound be generously irrigated with an antibiotic solution (the content of which is based on preoperative cultures, if available). Once again, attention is paid to meticulous hemostasis and atraumatic deep tissue and skin closure. Interrupted monofilament sutures that achieve edge-to-edge skin coaptation (without the use of forceps) should be placed (Fig. 64.3). The postoperative dressing can be either a soft dressing with an outer elastic wrap (which allows compression of the forefoot and removes tension from the suture line) or a combination of a soft dressing with foot and lower leg plaster cast (which provides maximum skin and wound protection). In the event that adequate hemostasis cannot be obtained, the use of a drain is suggested. In the presence of infection in either the metatarsophalangeal joint or skin flaps, consideration should be given to leaving the wound open and doing a delayed primary closure or allowing secondary healing.

Advantages and Disadvantages

This relatively conservative amputation results in minimal cosmetic deformity and maximum (100%) rehabilitation potential. There are no prosthetics required; however, ray resection of the first metatarsal head causes some walking imbalance, and the foot should be fitted with a specially constructed shoe to minimize foot trauma and improve ambulatory balance.

There are no disadvantages, except for the risk of hematoma formation, nonhealing, secondary infection, or chronic osteomyelitis of the remaining metatarsal shaft.

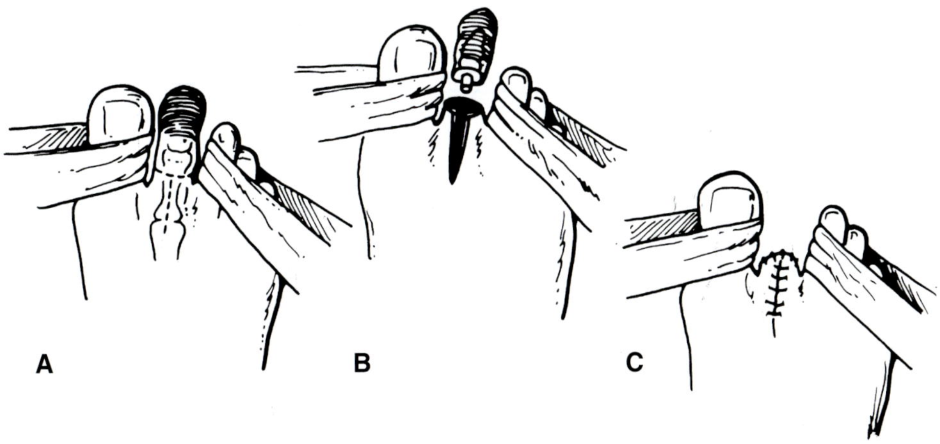

FIG 64.3 Single-digit ray amputation of the foot. The dorsal and plantar incisions are closed in their original direction; the toe incision can be closed either vertically or transversely. (A) Incision encircles the toe and extends onto the dorsum. (B) Disarticulation of the joint. (C) Wound closure.

Transmetatarsal Amputation

Indications

The indication for transmetatarsal amputation is gangrene or infection involving several toes or the great toe (on the same foot). This amputation may also be used if the gangrenous or infectious process extends a small distance on the dorsal skin past the metatarsophalangeal crease (but not up to the distal third or midthird junction of the forefoot), provided that the plantar skin is uncompromised.

Contraindications

Deep forefoot infection, cellulitis, lymphangitis, or dependent rubor involving the dorsal forefoot proximal to the metatarsophalangeal crease all represent contraindications to amputation at this level. In addition, gangrenous changes on the plantar skin of the foot, even those extending only a small distance past the metatarsophalangeal crease, is a specific contraindication to amputation at this level. Foot pulses are not necessary for healing, and venous refill should probably be less than 25 seconds.

Surgical Technique

An excellent description of the technique for transmetatarsal amputation was presented by McKittrick and associates in 1949.[91] A skin incision is designed that uses a total plantar flap. A slightly curved dorsal incision is carried from side to side of the foot at the level of the midmetatarsal shafts. The incision extends to the base of the toes medially and laterally in the midplane axis of the foot and then across the plantar surface at the metatarsophalangeal crease. It is important to place the dorsal skin incision slightly distal to the anticipated line of bone division. The dorsal skin incision is carried down to the metatarsal bones, and each metatarsal shaft is transected with an air-driven oscillating saw approximately 4 mm to 1 cm proximal to the skin incision (Fig. 64.4).

The plantar tissues in the distal forefoot are separated from the metatarsal shafts with a scalpel. The tissues of the plantar flap are thinned sharply, excising exposed tendons and leaving the underlying musculature attached to the skin flap. The plantar flap is then rotated dorsally for closure. Further tailoring or thinning of the plantar flap may be necessary to achieve good skin coaptation.

The importance of attention to absolute hemostasis cannot be overemphasized. A simple closure is performed, consisting of a deep layer of absorbable interrupted sutures and skin closure with a monofilament suture using a vertical mattress technique. Once again, careful approximation of skin edges is important, and I recommend not using forceps on the skin.

If adequate hemostasis cannot be readily achieved, use of a closed drainage system is suggested. Bone wax should not be used to control bleeding from the metatarsal shafts; the use of electrocautery to achieve hemostasis is preferable.

A well-padded short leg plaster cast is the best postoperative dressing because it controls edema and prevents stump trauma. I do not advise early ambulation after transmetatarsal amputation because of problems with flap necrosis and stump healing. If wound healing is satisfactory at the first cast change (7 to 10 days after surgery), a rubber heel may be incorporated into the second cast for ambulation. Subsequent casts are changed when they become loose, generally every 7 to 14 days, and a rigid dressing is used until the transmetatarsal flap is well healed, usually 3 to 4 weeks after surgery.

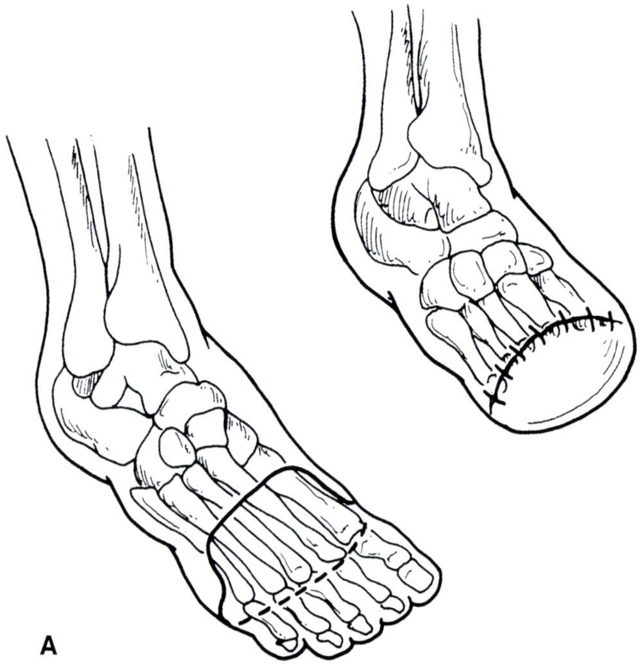

A

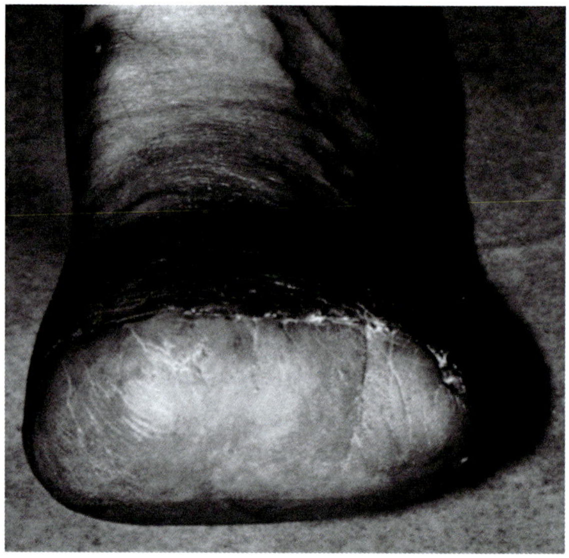

B

FIG 64.4 (A) Planned transmetatarsal plantar-based skin flap and appearance of the completed closure. (B) Healed right transmetatarsal amputation treated with immediate postsurgical prosthetic fitting, 1 month after amputation.

Advantages and Disadvantages

Transmetatarsal amputation provides an excellent result compared with more proximal foot or lower extremity amputation. Disability is minimal, and the prosthetic requirements are relatively simple.

The primary disadvantages of a transmetatarsal amputation are the risks of nonhealing, infection, and hematoma formation and the necessity for a secondary higher-level amputation.

Prosthetic Requirements and Rehabilitation Potential

To achieve maximum ambulation potential, some minor prosthetic modification should be considered. A shoe that incorporates a steel shank in the sole allows normal toe-off during ambulation. The spring steel shank reproduces the action of the longitudinal arch of the foot during ambulation. A custom-molded foam pad or lamb's wool can be used to fill the toe portion of the shoe. An alternative approach is to use a custom-molded shoe with a roller-shaped sole to provide toe-off motion during walking.

There are relatively few, if any, limitations in rehabilitation for a transmetatarsal amputation. With proper shoe modification, there should be no discernible physical disability for a transmetatarsal amputee during ambulation. It is important, however, that the shoe or other prosthetic device be properly constructed to avoid stump ulceration and breakdown. There are increased numbers of anecdotal reports combining guillotine forefoot amputation with secondary distal split-thickness skin graft to achieve successful healing at this amputation level. Although this latter technique allows the salvage of more proximal transmetatarsal amputations, I do not favor its use because of frequent problems with distal stump (skin graft) breakdown in active patients.

Lisfranc and Chopart Amputations

Indications

Some reports have called attention to foot-sparing amputations when a transmetatarsal amputation is precluded because of the extent of ischemia or infection.[92–95] The Lisfranc amputation is a tarsometatarsal joint amputation, and the Chopart amputation is a midtarsal joint amputation. I agree with Chang and coworkers[95] that both of these midforefoot amputations are easier to perform than a Syme amputation and may improve long-term ambulation.[96]

Contraindications

Both Lisfranc and Chopart amputations result in the development of equinovarus deformity and require lengthening of the Achilles tendon to achieve maximum rehabilitation potential.[93,94] In addition, Hirsch and colleagues documented force plate data showing that an abnormal pattern characterized by reduced stance duration and deficient forward propulsion on the amputated side was greater in a Chopart's prosthesis than in a transmetatarsal prosthesis.[96] That study also documented stump problems as the principal difficulty with Chopart amputations over time.

Surgical Technique

Both Lisfranc (tarsometatarsal joint) and Chopart (midtarsal joint) amputations are well described in articles by Sanders[94] and Chang and coworkers,[95] to which interested readers are referred.

Prosthetic Requirements and Rehabilitation Potential

I agree with a modified version of the conclusion reached by Chang and coworkers that ischemic foot necrosis extending beyond the limits of conventional transmetatarsal amputation does not necessarily require a major limb amputation.[95] With improvements in patient selection and surgical technique, Lisfranc and Chopart amputations are viable options when attempting to salvage mid- to hindfoot structures. From a prosthetic standpoint, fitting of these more distal and conservative amputation levels should emphasize unloading the distal part of the stump and smoothing out the impulsive force peak on the stump in late stance to minimize pain, decrease stump breakdown, and enhance ambulation capacity.[96]

Syme Amputation

Syme first described this amputation in 1843.[97] Then, as now, there were arguments over its merit. Harris (in Toronto) has championed Syme amputation and has written several excellent articles concerning its development and the surgical technique necessary for successful results.[98,99] I believe that the Syme amputation is the most technically demanding lower extremity amputation, and attention to surgical detail is crucial for its success.

Indications

If the gangrenous or infectious process precludes transmetatarsal amputation, the next level to be considered is an ankle disarticulation, or Syme amputation.

Contraindications

If the gangrenous or infectious process involves the heel, if there are open lesions on the heel or about the ankle, if there is cellulitis or lymphangitis ascending up the distal leg, or if dependent rubor is present at the heel, Syme amputation is contraindicated. The presence of a neuropathic foot in a diabetic patient, when there is absence of heel sensation, is also a relative contraindication to Syme amputation. A high rate of primary healing demands the use of objective, noninvasive amputation level selection techniques before surgery and preservation of the posterior tibial artery (if patent).

Surgical Technique

The skin incision is placed to construct a posterior flap using the heel pad. The dorsal incision extends across the ankle from the tip of the medial malleolus to the tip of the lateral malleolus. The plantar incision begins at a 90-degree angle from the dorsal incision and progresses around the plantar aspect of the foot distal to the heel pad (Fig. 64.5). The dorsal incision is deepened through subcutaneous tissues and carried down to bone without dissection in the tissue planes. The anterior tendons (tibialis anterior, extensor hallucis longus, and extensor digitorum longus) are pulled down into the wound, transected, and allowed to retract. The anterior tibial artery is identified, clamped, divided, and suture-ligated. The incision is then deepened, and the capsule of the tibial-talar joint is opened. The tibialis posterior tendon is divided, and the foot is forced into plantar flexion to provide

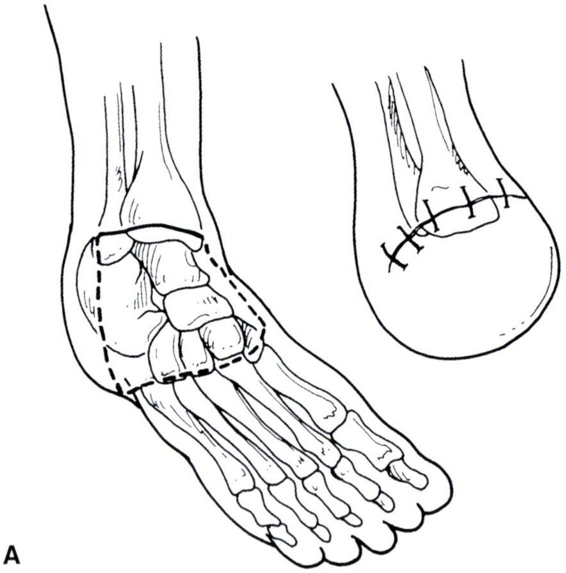

A

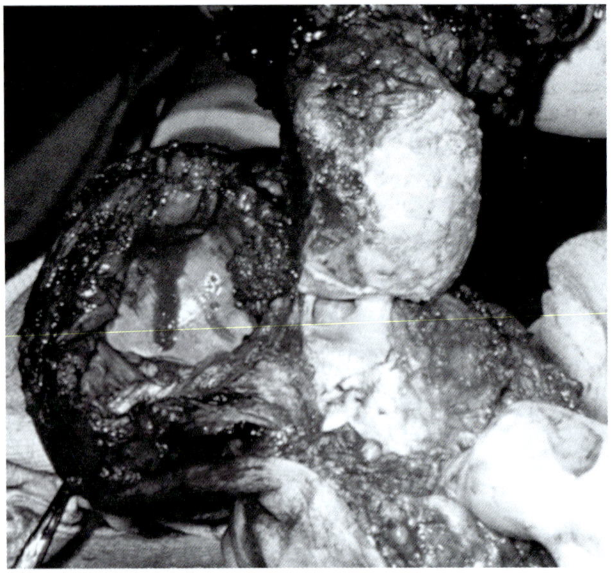

B

FIG 64.5 (A) Syme amputation, with a posterior heel-based skin flap, performed with the one-stage surgical technique. (B) Intraoperative photograph of a Syme amputation showing the Achilles attachment of the calcaneus *(midsuperior portion of picture)*, the tibial plateau, and the heel flap *(lower left corner)*.

increased visualization of the tibial-talar joint. Great care should be taken during medial dissection to preserve the posterior tibial artery. The joint is further dislocated by incising the posterior capsule. The peroneus brevis and tertius tendons are transected. The plantar aspect of the incision is deepened through all layers of the sole of the foot down to the neck of the calcaneus. The calcaneus is then carefully and sharply dissected from the heel pad. Dissection of the calcaneus is the most difficult part of the operation, and great care is needed to maintain the dissection on the bony surface of the calcaneus to prevent damage to the soft tissues of the heel, injury to the posterior tibial artery, and buttonholing of the posterior skin as the Achilles tendon is transected. Performance of Syme amputation by the one-stage and two-stage techniques is identical up to this point.

If the surgeon chooses the one-stage technique, the lateral and medial malleoli are transected flush with the articular surface of the tibial-talar joint with an air-driven reciprocating saw. Once again, the importance of hemostasis cannot be overemphasized. If adequate hemostasis cannot be achieved, a closed drainage system should be incorporated. Even in dry surgical wounds, the use of a drain is advocated by some authors.[88,98,99] I prefer to irrigate the surgical wound with copious amounts of antibiotic solution before closure. The heel pad is rotated anteriorly and sutured to the proximal dorsal skin edge with a single layer of interrupted vertical mattress sutures. Once again, atraumatic placement of skin sutures is mandatory, and forceps should not be used on the skin edges.

If the two-stage technique is selected,[88] the lateral and medial malleoli are not transected. A drain is placed, and the wound is closed as previously described. Approximately 6 weeks after performance of the first stage, the patient is returned to surgery for the second stage (which can be done under local anesthesia). Medial and lateral incisions are made over the dog ears on the amputation stump, and the incisions are carried down to bone with sharp dissection. The malleoli are removed flush with the ankle joint. The tibial articular cartilage is not disturbed. The distal tibia and fibula are exposed subperiosteally approximately 6 cm above the ankle joint, and the tibial and fibular flares are removed with an osteotome and a smooth rongeur. This last procedure produces a relatively square stump that simplifies postoperative prosthetic fitting and improves cosmesis. If the heel pad is loose after removal of the malleoli, it can be secured to the tibia and fibula through drill holes in the bones.

The postoperative dressing for a Syme amputation stump (for both one- and two-stage procedures) is extremely important; it is critical to maintain correct alignment of the heel pad over the end of the tibia and fibula during healing. Either a soft compression dressing or a rigid plaster cast can be used as a postoperative dressing; however, most authors prefer the application of a short leg plaster cast. If a cast is used, great care must be taken to avoid injury to the medial and lateral skin flaps (dog ears). Weight bearing should not occur during the early phases of healing of a Syme amputation because of the risks of nonhealing and flap necrosis. When the first cast is removed, usually 7 to 10 days after surgery, a second cast that incorporates a walking heel can be applied if healing is satisfactory. I prefer to keep Syme amputation patients nonambulatory for 3 weeks after amputation to allow good heel pad fixation and healing. After ambulation begins, the patients are kept in a short leg walking cast for an additional 3 to 4 weeks before construction of a temporary removable prosthesis.

Advantages and Disadvantages

The Syme amputation stump is extremely durable because it is end-weight bearing. It involves minimal disability from the standpoint of walking. Performance of a one-stage Syme amputation results in a somewhat bulbous distal stump compared with a two-stage Syme amputation. For cosmetic reasons, a two-stage procedure is probably preferable in female patients, although I generally do not perform Syme amputations in young female patients because of concerns about cosmesis. Clinical evaluation by patients, prosthetists, and surgeons has consistently shown that the Syme amputation is superior to amputation levels above the ankle. Oxygen uptake, gait velocity, cadence, and stride length are significantly better in patients with Syme amputations than in those with higher-level amputations.[100]

Delayed healing or healing complications due to hematoma formation or infection are not uncommon. Careful preoperative amputation level selection helps ensure primary healing of a Syme amputation. Failure to heal almost always results in performance of a more proximal amputation. Long-term follow-up of my diabetic patients with normal or "almost normal" sensation in whom a Syme level was chosen demonstrates a high incidence of revision to the below-knee level because of problems resulting from a progressive insensate Syme stump (i.e., progressive neuropathy). Other authors have not reported similar problems.

Prosthetic Requirements and Rehabilitation Potential

Ambulation in the home can be achieved without the application of a prosthetic appliance; however, ambulation outside the home requires some type of prosthetic device. The usual cosmetic prosthesis consists of a foot and a plastic shell that incorporates the lower leg. A typical prosthesis for a patient with a one-stage Syme amputation is shown in Fig. 64.6. Ambulation in the home or for limited distances can be achieved with the application of a simple strap on a cup slipper with a built-up heel.

A patient with a successful Syme amputation and an appropriately fitted prosthesis can expect a minimal degree of disability. Energy consumption compared with that of a nonamputee is, at most, 10% above normal. Many patients with Syme amputations continue to be employed, including some who perform heavy manual labor. The salvage of a Syme amputation, especially in patients who are likely to become bilateral amputees, may be the ultimate difference between continued ambulation and nonambulation.

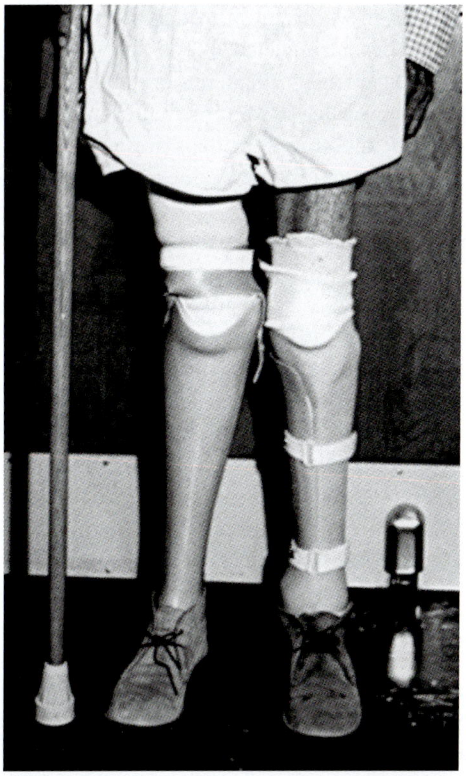

FIG 64.6 Bilateral lower extremity amputee with a right below-knee amputation and a left Syme amputation. The Syme prosthesis is a standard medial window design for a one-stage Syme amputation. Note the bulbous distal ankle on the Syme prosthesis *(left leg)*, compared with the cosmetic ankle on the below-knee prosthesis *(right leg)*.

Below-Knee Amputation

Indications

Below-knee amputation is the most common amputation level selected for the management of lower extremity gangrene, infection, or ischemia with nonhealing lesions that preclude more distal amputations. When the blood supply is inadequate for healing at more distal levels, amputation at the below-knee level can be expected to provide adequate blood supply for healing in the majority of cases. In fact, as previously noted, 83% of all patients undergoing lower extremity amputation can expect healing of a below-knee amputation (see Table 64.3).[44] With objective amputation level selection, primary healing rates in excess of 94% can be expected.

Contraindications

A below-knee amputation is contraindicated if the gangrenous or infectious process involves skin on the anterior portion of the lower extremity within 4 to 5 cm of the tibial tuberosity or skin that would be used to construct the posterior flap. A flexion contracture of the knee greater than 20 degrees also represents a contraindication to below-knee amputation. Great caution should be used when attempting below-knee amputation in patients with an occluded deep femoral artery (the superficial femoral is almost always occluded) in the absence of objective amputation level selection data that suggest that the amputation will heal. Finally, a patient with stroke or neurologic dysfunction on the side of proposed amputation, in whom muscle spasticity or rigidity is marked, should not have a below-knee amputation because spastic muscles will force the knee into flexion and ultimately result in amputation failure.

Surgical Technique

Two significant advances in amputation technique have contributed to better results after below-knee amputation: use of a long posterior flap, and application of a rigid dressing in the immediate postoperative period. There is considerable clinical and theoretical information available to support the use of a long posterior flap. The gastrocnemius and soleus muscles and the overlying posterior calf skin derive their major blood supply through the sural arteries, which originate proximal to the knee joint. Blood flow is maintained to this area in many patients, particularly diabetic patients, in whom flow through the popliteal artery and its major branches is restricted. Blood supply via the anterior tibial artery and geniculate collaterals to the skin and soft tissues of the anterior lower leg is so poor that even if equal anterior and posterior below-knee skin flaps are used, there is a high incidence of rehabilitation failure due to wound necrosis of the anterior skin flap.

The operation can be performed under general or spinal anesthesia, with the patient in the supine position on the operating table. If there are open infected lesions on the foot, a plastic bag or plastic adherent drape can be placed over the open infected portion of the extremity to isolate it. As mentioned previously, in a patient with a septic foot, a preparatory ankle guillotine amputation followed by a delayed primary below-knee amputation results in a higher rate of healing and fewer stump infections than the performance of a one-stage primary below-knee amputation.[36,37] An alternative to the two-stage approach (one-stage technique with delayed primary closure) that works well for diabetic patients, except those with Wagner grade 5 foot infection, was reported by Kernek and Rozzi.[101]

I prefer to use a long posterior flap and no anterior flap for reasons previously stated; however, there is at least one prospective, randomized study comparing a sagittal technique and long posterior musculocutaneous flaps that found no significant difference with respect to healing, limb fitting, ambulation, and ultimate rehabilitation.[102] Another report of sagittal incisions for below-knee amputation pointed out the utility of this type of incision in patients in whom a long posterior flap may be contraindicated because of infection or skin necrosis.[103] A report by Ruckley and coworkers noted that for below-knee amputations in patients with end-stage peripheral vascular disease, the skew flap is an excellent alternative to the long posterior flap.[104] The techniques for construction of a long posterior flap in below-knee amputation have been well documented in many previous publications[10,105–107]; however, the salient features of the amputation are outlined here.

For a standard below-knee amputation, I select a point of bone division approximately a handbreadth, including the thumb, below the tibial tuberosity. When there is concern that the posterior flap may impinge on distal infection or ischemia, a palm breadth (minus the thumb) can be used for the point of division below the tibial tuberosity. The absolute minimum length for a below-knee amputation is three fingerbreadths (7 to 8 cm) below the tibial tuberosity. The skin incision should be approximately 1 cm distal to the intended point of bone division. The transverse diameter of the midshaft calf at the level of the anterior incision, plus 1 inch, represents the approximate length of the posterior skin flap. It is usually my preference to outline the flap with a marking pencil before making a skin incision. The anterior skin incision represents the anterior half of the circumference of the extremity. The skin incision then abruptly turns distally with gentle curves and proceeds down the medial and lateral aspects of the extremity, in the midplane axis of the leg, to the point of the distal extent of the posterior skin flap. The two lateral incisions are then connected posteriorly. My preference is then to incise the flap through skin and fascia in all areas before muscle transection. Use of a proximal tourniquet for hemostatic control is optional in patients undergoing traumatic below-knee amputation but is relatively contraindicated in patients undergoing elective below-knee amputation for ischemia. Use of electrocautery is preferred for division of all muscles. The anterior tibial muscle is divided at the level of bone division, and the anterior tibial neurovascular bundle is identified, clamped, divided, and suture-ligated. Electrocautery is used to incise the tibial periosteum circumferentially, and a periosteal elevator is used to mobilize the periosteum of the tibia proximal to the point of proposed bone division. The tibia is then divided with an air-driven reciprocating saw. Using electrocautery, the fibula is isolated at the level of the transected tibia and divided approximately 0.25 inch proximal to the tibia, using the saw. Following division of the fibula and tibia, proximal traction is placed on the transected tibia (use of a bone hook is easiest), and the lower extremity is bent at 90 degrees and retracted distally. The posterior tibial artery and vein and the common peroneal artery and vein are identified, clamped, transected, and individually suture-ligated. The posterior tibial nerve is identified, pulled into the wound, ligated, transected, and allowed to retract out of the area of surgical incision. The posterior calf muscle musculature is transected, leaving the gastrocnemius muscle as part of the posterior skin flap. The surgical specimen is then divided at the same point as the posterior flap skin incision, which permits removal of the surgical specimen. Care should be taken not to thin the posterior flap so much that there is inadequate coverage for the tibia when the flap is closed. The saw is used to bevel the tibia at a 45- to 60-degree angle, and the bony edges are filed smooth. Care is also taken to ensure that the distal ends of the fibula are smooth (Fig. 64.7).

The wound is copiously irrigated with an antibiotic solution. Once again, the importance of meticulous hemostasis cannot be stressed enough. Generally, drains are not necessary in below-knee amputations for peripheral vascular disease; however, drains are frequently used in below-knee amputations performed for trauma or other reasons. If a drain is required, I prefer a closed suction drain, which is brought through a separate stab wound in the lateral aspect of the lower leg. The sural nerve (posterior flap) is identified, pulled down, ligated, transected, and allowed to retract back from the edge of the flap. The flap is rotated anteriorly, and the muscle fascia of the posterior flap is approximated to the anterior fascia with interrupted absorbable sutures. The skin is carefully approximated with interrupted vertical mattress sutures using a monofilament plastic or metal suture. I avoid the use of tissue forceps and believe that closure of the below-knee stump, especially in patients with peripheral vascular disease, should be performed with the care of a plastic surgical procedure. Tailoring the corner of the skin flap may be required to prevent excessive dog ears.

The use of a rigid plaster of Paris dressing incorporating the knee is ideal, regardless of whether an immediate postoperative prosthesis will be used. A rigid dressing controls edema, promotes healing, and protects the stump during the postoperative period. In addition, a rigid dressing prevents flexion contracture. Application of an immediate postoperative prosthesis as part of the rigid dressing is described in detail later.

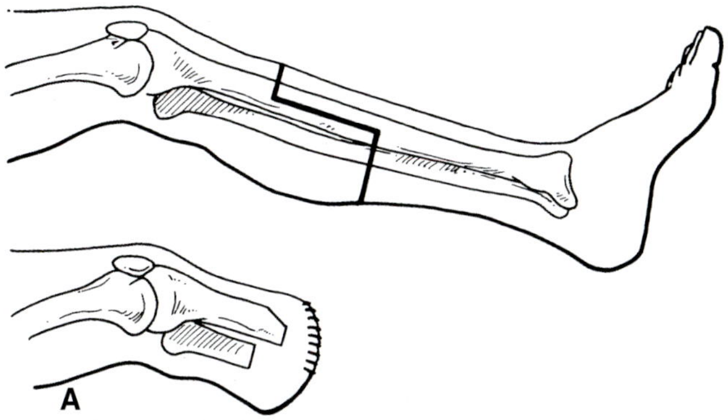

A

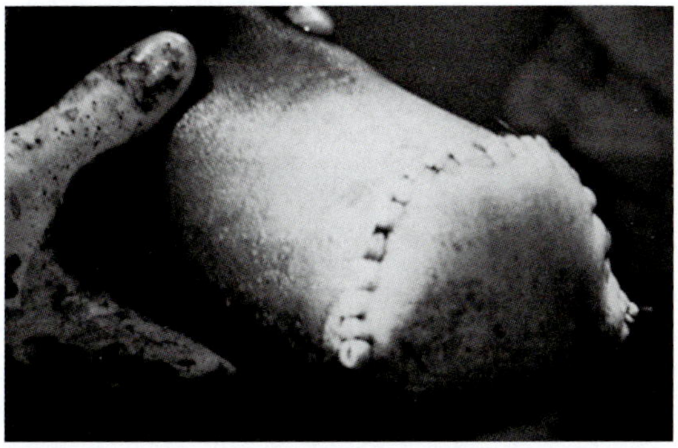

B

FIG 64.7 (A) Standard posterior flap below-knee amputation. Note the beveled tibia and the proximal shortening of the fibula compared with the tibia. (B) Intraoperative photograph showing a below-knee amputation. Note the skin coaptation with interrupted sutures and the minimal dog ears.

Advantages and Disadvantages

The below-knee amputation is an extremely durable amputation. The likelihood of primary healing is very good, and the ability to rehabilitate a patient with a below-knee prosthesis is excellent. In a report by Kim and coworkers in 1976, 90% of their patients with unilateral below-knee amputations were able to ambulate.[108] Roon and colleagues achieved a 100% ambulation rate with unilateral below-knee amputations and a 93% ambulation rate in patients with bilateral below-knee amputations.[14] In addition, 91% of the patients reported by Roon's group were still ambulatory an average of 44 months following amputation.[14]

In the absence of the ability to perform a more distal amputation, there are no specific disadvantages of a below-knee amputation.

Prosthetic Requirements and Rehabilitation Potential

A below-knee prosthesis is required for ambulation at this level of amputation. A variety of prostheses are available, but all generally involve total stump contact (with or without a prosthesis liner) with weight bearing on the patellar tendon and tibial-fibular condyles. Newer types of below-knee prostheses incorporate total contact and total weight-bearing designs. The prosthesis can be suspended with a variety of techniques, including a thigh lacer with external joints, Silastic sleeve suspension, standard patellar tendon-bearing (PTB) strap, supracondylar medial clip, suction, and self-suspension secondary to muscle control. These prostheses can incorporate a variety of feet, some of which have flexion and extension motion or "ankle rotation" (with weight loading) or energy storage (Seattle Foot [Model & Instrument Works, Inc., Seattle]; Flex-Foot [Össur, Scheck & Siress, Gakbrook Terrace, IL]). The energy requirement for a unilateral below-knee amputee is increased approximately 40% to 60% compared with normal (energy consumption with an energy-storing leg has not yet been reported).

It has been my experience, as well as that of others, that any patient (regardless of age) who was ambulatory before below-knee amputation and who undergoes amputation within 30 days of hospital entrance can ambulate successfully on a below-knee prosthesis. In fact, most patients who require bilateral below-knee amputations can ambulate successfully, as shown by Roon and associates.[14] The importance of aggressive rehabilitation after unilateral below-knee amputation in patients who are at high risk for bilateral lower extremity amputation was stressed in a report by Inderbitzi and coworkers.[109] Delay in rehabilitation resulted in a high rate of nonambulatory patients after the second amputation. The time required for gait training for a unilateral below-knee amputee is approximately 2 to 3 weeks, and most patients develop a very good gait pattern. There are some physical limitations for geriatric below-knee amputees; however, young below-knee amputees are able to negotiate ladders, stairs, and other obstacles with minimal difficulty.

Knee Disarticulation

Indications

The indications for knee disarticulation amputation are limited, and it is performed primarily on young, active males for whom the advantages of strength and serviceability outweigh prosthetic cosmesis. Disarticulation amputation of the knee is the second most technically difficult lower extremity amputation following Syme amputation. Successful performance of a knee disarticulation amputation with a high degree of primary healing usually requires some type of objective technique of preoperative amputation level selection. Knee disarticulation is indicated primarily when the gangrenous process, infection, trauma, tumor, or orthopedic disability encroaches too close to the anterior and posterior (or sagittal) limits of a below-knee amputation flap or has resulted in an unsalvageable knee joint. Another potential indication for knee disarticulation is a patient who has had either acute or chronic failure of a below-knee amputation in whom skin flaps at the knee are viable enough to consider knee disarticulation. In general, British surgeons have been more enamored of knee disarticulation than their American colleagues. Interest in this level of amputation has arisen as a result of advances in cosmetic prosthetic components and prosthetic fitting techniques. Moreover, in a study of 169 unilateral lower extremity amputees, Houghton and coworkers found that rehabilitation results were better for through-knee amputation (62%) than for above-knee (33%) ($P < .02$) or Gritti-Stokes (44%) amputation.[110]

Contraindications

Contraindications to knee disarticulation are inadequate blood flow to the skin in the region or ulceration, gangrene, or infection involving tissues about the knee joint or the joint space.

Surgical Technique

There are two excellent reviews of the surgical techniques of disarticulation of the knee[111,112]; therefore they are described only briefly here. I prefer the knee disarticulation technique described by Burgess,[111] owing to failure with other types of knee disarticulation amputation and success using the modified Burgess technique.

Anesthetic management of knee disarticulation is best handled with either spinal or general anesthesia, with the patient in the prone position. The operation can be performed, but is more difficult, with the patient in the supine position. At the discretion of the surgeon, a gown or pack can be placed beneath the thigh to hyperextend the hip joint and provide an easier working surface on the anterior portion of the knee and lower leg. The leg is held in a flexed position. Depending on the availability of suitable skin, a classic long anterior, equal flap, or sagittal flap–type incision can be used (Fig. 64.8). A marking pencil should be used to outline the skin flaps before making the skin incision. Construction of the knee disarticulation skin flaps is crucial to avoid tension on the skin suture line when the amputation stump is closed. Dissection is first carried anteriorly down to the insertion of the patellar tendon on the tibia. The tendon is severed at its insertion and sharply dissected proximally. Deep dissection on the medial side of the knee results in exposure of the hamstring muscles. The tendons are sectioned and allowed to retract. The deep fascia is reflected with the overlying tendon and skin flap. On the lateral side of the knee, the tendon of the biceps femoris muscle and iliotibial band are sectioned low. The knee joint is entered anteriorly, the knee is flexed, and the cruciate ligaments are transected at their tibial insertion. The posterior knee capsule structures are divided, and the individual members of the popliteal vascular sheath are clamped, transected, and suture-ligated. The tibial and peroneal nerves are identified, retracted under moderate tension, ligated, sectioned with a sharp knife, and allowed to retract into the proximal amputation stump. The patella is removed subperiosteally, and the fascial defect in the patellar tendon is closed with interrupted sutures.

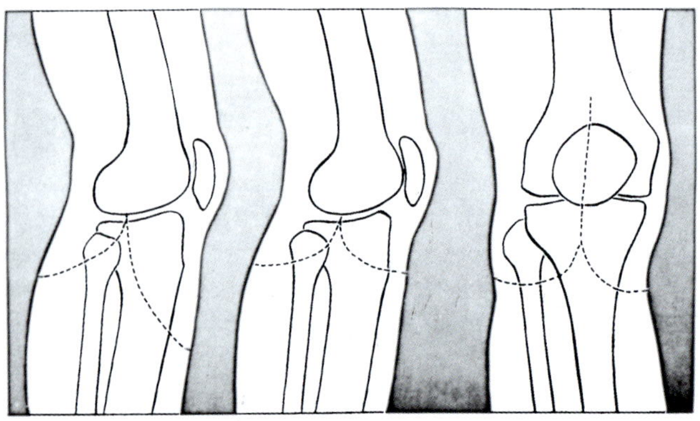

FIG 64.8 The three types of skin incisions commonly used for knee disarticulation amputation. (From Burgess EM: Disarticulation of the knee: a modified technique. *Arch Surg* 117:1251, 1977.)

The femoral condyles are now transected transversely, approximately 1.5 cm above the level of the knee joint (Fig. 64.9). Sharp distal femoral margins are carefully contoured. The patellar tendon is pulled down into the intracondylar notch under moderate tension and sewn to the stump of the crus ligaments. The semitendinosus and biceps tendons are likewise pulled into the notch, tailored, and sewn to the stump of the patellar tendon and cruciate ligaments. This approximation of the tendons and ligaments allows muscle stability. The superficial skin fascia is approximated with interrupted absorbable sutures, and the skin is meticulously closed using a vertical mattress technique with monofilament metal or plastic sutures, without the use of forceps. Alternatively, skin staples may be used. The use of a through-and-through or a suction drain is optional and is left to the discretion of the surgeon. A rigid dressing, with or without the incorporation of an immediate postoperative prosthesis, should be applied.

Advantages and Disadvantages

The advantages of a knee disarticulation amputation include excellent durability and end–weight-bearing capacity; retention of a long, powerful, muscle-stabilized femoral lever arm; improved proprioception; and a limb-socket interface with improved prosthetic suspension and rotational control (compared with an above-knee amputation). This amputation level is almost as good as a below-knee amputation and is therefore a tremendous benefit to the patient in comparison to the next higher level, the above-knee amputation.

The absence of a knee joint and increased energy expenditure make this amputation level less advantageous than a below-knee amputation.

Prosthetic Requirements and Rehabilitation Potential

Historically, knee disarticulation amputations were not well liked in the prosthetic community because of cosmetic and knee-thigh length problems resulting from existing prosthetic components (nonequal knee centers); however, the availability of lightweight polycentric hydraulic knee joints and endoskeletal systems has helped solve these problems. The usual knee disarticulation socket incorporates some type of medial window to allow the bulbous stump to pass through the smaller lower thigh portion of the socket.

Knee disarticulation amputation is probably most useful in young, active patients without peripheral vascular disease. However, this amputation is also an excellent choice for geriatric patients. Patient performance is better than that with a mid- to high above-knee amputation, although not nearly as good as that with a standard below-knee amputation. There are some physical limitations resulting from the absence of a knee joint, specifically involving climbing stairs and ladders and physical tasks that require rotational or flexion-extension knee motions.

Above-Knee Amputation

Indications

The indications for an amputation at the above-knee level are inadequate blood flow for healing at a more distal level, a disabled patient who is not expected to walk again, profound

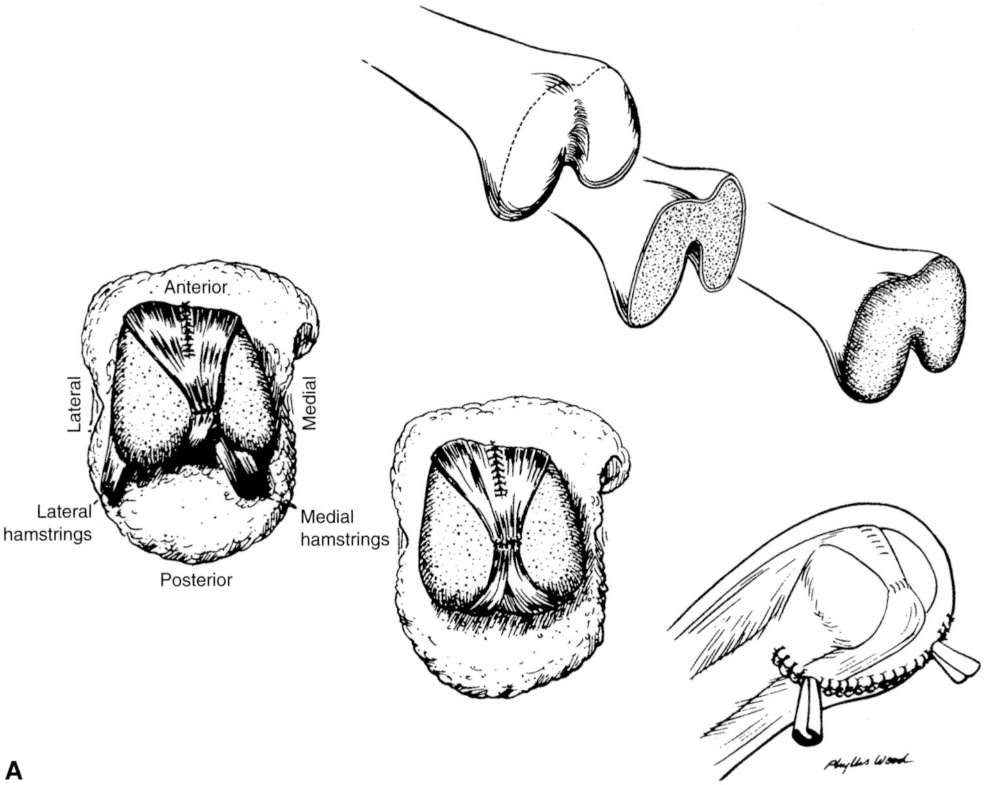

A

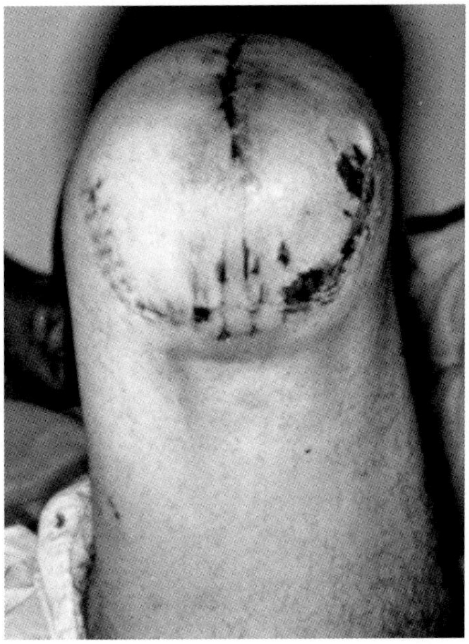

B

FIG 64.9 (A) The femur is transected 1.5 cm above the condylar ends, the patellar tendon is sewn to the cruciate ligaments, the hamstring tendons are sutured to the cruciate-patellar ligaments, and the wound is closed over a drain. (B) Anterior flap knee disarticulation amputation at the first postoperative cast change (7 to 10 days) with the patient in the supine position (in this case, the patella was removed transcutaneously). (From Burgess EM: Disarticulation of the knee: a modified technique. *Arch Surg* 117:1253, 1977.)

life-threatening infection with questionable viability of the lower extremity, and extensive infection or gangrene that would preclude a knee disarticulation or below-knee amputation. Historically, above-knee amputation has been the operation of choice for many surgeons because greater than 90% primary healing can be anticipated, regardless of the vascular status of the patient.

Contraindications

Extension of the infectious or gangrenous process to the level of the proposed above-knee amputation is the most common contraindication. Severe necrotizing lower extremity infection is a relative contraindication unless a high above-knee amputation is performed.

Surgical Technique

There are three basic levels for the above-knee amputation (Fig. 64.10). In general, the longer the above-knee amputation stump, the more likely the patient is to ambulate, so the stump should be as long as possible. If an amputation is being performed to control sepsis or toxicity, a midthigh or high-thigh amputation provides more assurance of healing and control of systemic toxicity, although the chances of rehabilitation are less.

Either a circular or a sagittal-type incision can be used. I prefer a circular (or fish-mouth) incision appropriate for the level of anticipated bone division. A circumferential line of incision is drawn with a marking pen 2 to 3 cm below the level of the proposed bone transection. The incision is then carried down through skin and fascia. The skin and fascia are retracted superiorly to allow more proximal muscle division. I prefer to use electrocautery for muscle division. The femoral artery and vein are identified, clamped, divided, and suture-ligated in the subsartorial canal. All the muscles of the anterior, medial, and lateral thigh are transected. The muscle mass is then retracted proximally, the proposed line of bone transection is exposed, and the periosteum is cut using electrocautery. An air-driven reciprocating saw is then used to transect the femur. The posterior muscles are transected using electrocautery. The sciatic nerve is identified, pulled down into the wound, ligated, transected, and allowed to retract into the proximal amputation stump. The rough edges of the femur are filed smooth. The amputation stump should be irrigated with an antibiotic solution, especially if the amputation is being performed for infection. The soft tissues and skin are drawn distally to ensure adequate soft tissue coverage for the femur. If soft tissue coverage is adequate, the wound is closed in two layers. The fascia is closed with an interrupted absorbable suture, and the skin is closed with interrupted vertical mattress sutures of plastic or metal monofilament. Good skin coaptation is important, and the use of forceps on the skin should be avoided. If the soft tissue coverage for the bone is inadequate, the femur is shortened as required to allow adequate soft tissue coverage without tension on the skin suture line (Fig. 64.11). If the amputation is being performed for infection, especially a necrotizing infection, the wound should be left open. If a fish-mouth incision is used, the apex of the "angle of the mouth" approximates the point of bony division. Closure, although spatially different, encompasses the careful atraumatic technique described previously.

A rigid dressing can be applied and is advantageous for control of stump edema, but it is much more cumbersome and less valuable than a rigid dressing used at lower amputation levels. I prefer to use a soft dressing suspended with a Silesian type of elastic bandage or a modified waist suspension belt.[113] After the wound has healed satisfactorily (1 to 2 weeks after surgery), a temporary removable prosthesis can be provided if appropriate.

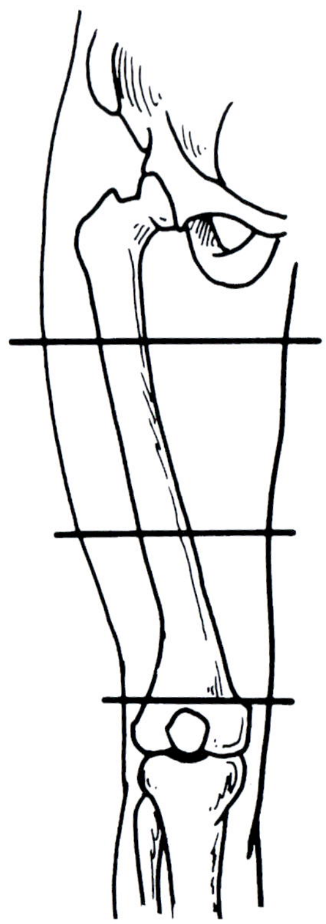

FIG 64.10 The three common levels of above-knee amputation.

Advantages and Disadvantages

The primary advantage of an above-knee amputation is the very high likelihood of primary healing. Prosthetic rehabilitation is very difficult at this level of amputation. Whereas 80% to 90% of all patients with unilateral or bilateral below-knee amputations can be expected to ambulate, only 40% to 50% of unilateral above-knee amputees can be expected to do so. It has been my experience that less than 10% of bilateral lower extremity amputees, when one side is an above-knee amputation, will successfully ambulate.

Prosthetic Requirements and Rehabilitation Potential

A variety of prostheses are available for above-knee amputees. Newer prosthetic devices incorporate contoured axially aligned sockets, ultralightweight materials, endoskeletal design, hydraulic-assisted knee joints, ankle rotators and motion feet, and energy storage. There is a direct correlation between successful ambulation at this level of amputation and the weight of the prosthesis because of the energy expenditure required for walking. Compared with normal, the energy expenditure of an above-knee amputee is increased 80% to 120%.

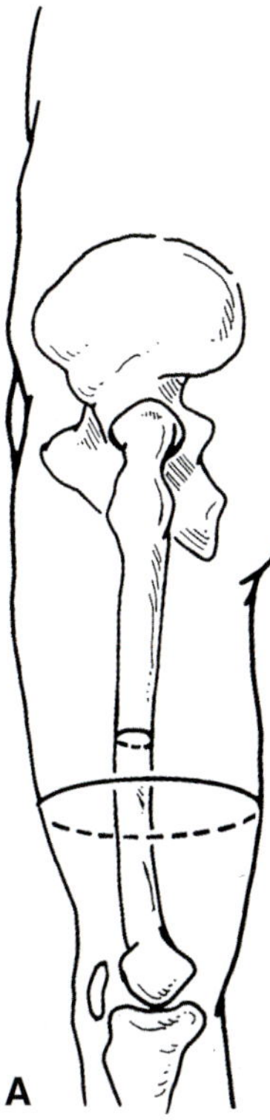

A

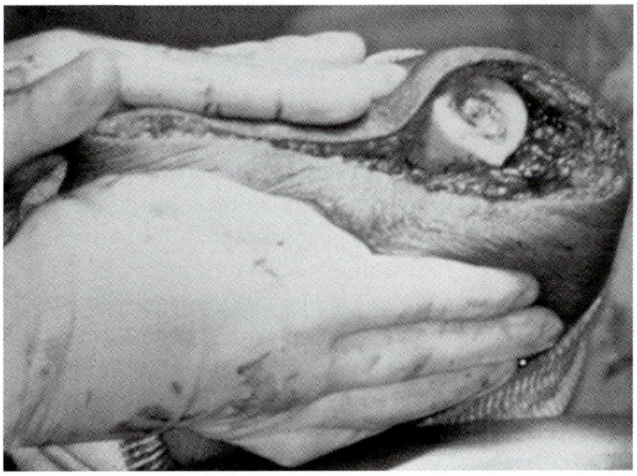

B

FIG 64.11 (A) Standard circular incision technique for above-knee amputation. Sagittal flaps can be used if appropriate. The key to closure is adequate femur shortening to avoid later bone protrusion through the distal end of the stump. (B) Intraoperative photograph of an above-knee amputation stump demonstrates why skin and soft tissue length for bone coverage should be checked before closure. Proximal femur shortening was required to decrease wound tension.

As noted, the rehabilitation potential for a unilateral above-knee amputee is only fair and averages 10% to 50%.

Hip Disarticulation Amputation

In general, hip disarticulation amputation is not an operation that general or vascular surgeons usually perform, because almost all patients will heal after a high above-knee amputation.

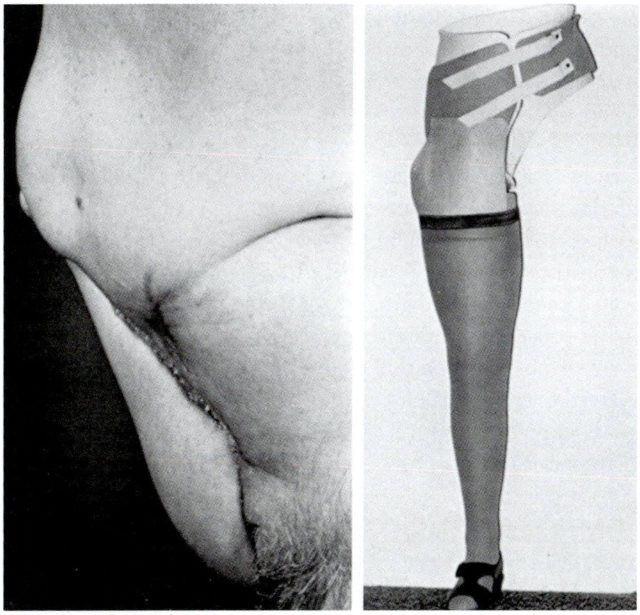

A B

FIG 64.12 (A) Photograph of a left hip disarticulation stump 6 months after amputation. The operation was performed with a posterior gluteal flap technique. (B) Ultralightweight (4.5 pounds) left hip disarticulation prosthesis based on an Aqualite plastic endoskeletal system with cosmetic cover (US Manufacturing Co., Pasadena, CA) and a Scotchcast Canadian-type socket (bucket).

Indications

The indications for hip disarticulation are inadequate blood flow (usually in patients with occlusion of both the deep and superficial femoral arteries) for healing of a more distal amputation, a life-threatening infection or extensive gangrene that precludes amputation at a lower level, trauma, tumor, and failed hip reconstruction.[114] Wound complications occur frequently, and their incidence is increased for urgent or emergent operations and in patients with prior above-knee amputations.[115] In addition, both limb ischemia and infection increase the mortality rate.

Contraindications

In my experience, infection that precludes hip disarticulation amputation is almost uniformly fatal. There are no contraindications to this level of amputation, except infection and gangrene (or tumor) that extends above the level of the proposed amputation.

Surgical Technique

Because this procedure is performed only occasionally by general and vascular surgeons, and because there are excellent articles describing this operation,[114–118] the surgical technique is not presented here. Based on a limited experience, I favor a posterior flap technique (Fig. 64.12A).

Advantages and Disadvantages

In the absence of healing at an above-knee level, there is a higher likelihood of primary healing.

Prosthetic rehabilitation at this level of lower extremity amputation is uncommon (<10%), even with unilateral amputation in geriatric patients.

Prosthetic Requirements

Various types of prostheses have been described and created for hip disarticulation amputees. Most of them entail a pelvic bucket (Canadian-type) prosthesis (see Fig. 64.12B) and are endoskeletal in construction (to save weight); few involve the use of sophisticated knee joints, ankle joints, or motion feet. A full discussion of the prosthetic requirements for this level of amputation is beyond the scope of this chapter, and interested readers are referred to appropriate references.[114–117] Compared with normal, the energy expenditure of a hip disarticulation amputee is increased 1.5 to 2.5 times.

COMPLICATIONS OF LOWER EXTREMITY AMPUTATION

Historically, postoperative morbidity and mortality following major lower extremity amputation were common, and the incidence of fatal complications was high enough to engender considerable debate about the optimal preoperative, operative, and postoperative management. In general, however, the morbidity and mortality following a major lower extremity amputation have decreased with time.[119–121]

The major postoperative complications following lower extremity amputation and their frequency of occurrence are listed in Table 64.4. Each of these complications is addressed separately in the following paragraphs.

Early Postoperative Complications

Pain

The literature suggests that the incidence of disabling stump pain and phantom limb pain following major lower extremity amputation ranges from 5% to 30%.[122–127] In a retrospective random survey of 5000 Veterans Administration (VA) amputees, Sherman and coworkers noted that 85% of the respondents reported significant phantom limb pain.[128,129] Their explanation for the high incidence of pain was based in part on the fact that most reports, especially those citing pain treatment modalities, have inadequate posttreatment follow-up. In addition, Sherman and coworkers suggested that most amputees quickly learn that physicians are not interested in pain problems and therefore fail to give accurate responses when questioned, often to protect their credibility and relationship with their physician (thereby guaranteeing long-term care). Of more concern was the fact that statistical analysis of 42 of the most common treatment modalities for phantom limb pain, including drug therapy, local injections, and surgery, showed that no treatment provided satisfactory results.[128,129] At most, 8.4% of survey respondents were helped to any real extent. In my experience, based on an amputation program that uses immediate postsurgical prosthetic fitting and aggressive postamputation rehabilitation, the incidence of disabling pain problems following major lower extremity amputation is less than 5%. I have no objective explanation for the difference between reports in the surgical literature and my personal experience, but I believe that rapid rehabilitation and the use of rigid dressings, with or without a pylon, have a positive impact in decreasing postamputation pain problems.

In my personal experience, the perioperative administration of gabapentin (Neurontin) in dogs, ranging from 100 to 300 mg orally twice a day, seems to be associated with less postoperative pain and phantom pain.

TABLE 64.4 Postoperative Complications

Complication	Incidence (%)	References
Stump pain/phantom pain	5–80	9, 14, 20, 122–129
Death	0–35	7, 9, 20, 100, 119, 120, 130, 131
Pulmonary complications	8	14
Stump infection	12–28	120, 131
Nonhealing stump	3–28	9, 14, 20, 119, 120, 130
Pulmonary embolus	4–38	7, 14
Deep venous thrombosis	1–3	9, 14, 20
Flexion contracture	1–3	9, 14, 20, 57
Renal insufficiency	1–3	9, 14, 20

Death

The incidence of death following major lower extremity amputation ranges from 0% to 35%.[7,9,17,20,119,120,130,131] Although the postoperative death rate has decreased each decade since the 1950s, an overall death rate of 6% to10% is still the average for centers treating large numbers of amputees.[9,14,20] As might be expected, the postoperative death rate for above-knee amputation (20% to 40%) exceeds that for below-knee amputation (3% to 10%).[9,14,20,100,119,120,131] Two thirds of all postoperative deaths are due to cardiovascular complications, including myocardial infarction, stroke, congestive heart failure, and visceral ischemia, with approximately one third to one half of these deaths due to myocardial infarction alone. Death after lower extremity amputation is related to patient age. In my experience and that of others, the mortality increases for patients older than 75 years.[132]

Nonhealing

Nonhealing of an amputation stump represents a major complication because it almost always results in amputation at a higher level. Nonhealing results from inadequate blood supply at the level selected for amputation, rough or traumatic intraoperative handling of marginally vascularized tissue, or stump hematoma with or without secondary infection. The incidence of nonhealing after major lower extremity amputation ranges from 3% to 28%.[9,14,20,119,120,130,133] In other words, the primary healing rate after major lower extremity amputation ranges from 63% to 97%. Because the literature suggests an overall healing rate of 97% for digit and forefoot amputations (see Table 64.2) and 94% for below-knee amputations (see Table 64.3) when objective techniques of amputation level selection are used, it can be inferred that failure to heal is directly related to the method used for amputation level selection. In a modern amputation program using objective amputation level selection techniques, the rate of nonhealing should be no higher than 4% to 8%. In my last 250 consecutive lower extremity amputations, there has been one failure (0.8%) due to nonhealing from ischemia (transcutaneous Po_2 >20 mm Hg).

The literature is somewhat controversial on healing differences between patients with and without diabetes mellitus. However, it has been my experience, as well as that of others, that there is no significant difference in the healing rates of major lower extremity amputations between diabetic and nondiabetic patients.[9,20,54,57,60,65,76,134] The rate of infectious stump complications might be slightly higher in diabetics; however, this has not been my experience.

In a review of 59 consecutive lower extremity amputations in diabetics, Bailey and associates noted that the preoperative hemoglobin level was statistically significantly lower in patients whose amputations healed primarily.[135] Eighteen amputations done in patients with a preoperative hemoglobin value of less than 12 g/dL healed primarily, whereas all 30 amputations in patients with a hemoglobin level greater than 13 g/dL failed to heal.

It seems reasonable to consider isovolemic hemodilution in patients with marginally viable skin or borderline values as measured by amputation level selection methods. In a study of skin flap survival, Gatti and colleagues suggested that isovolemic hemodilution might be a valuable technique for the salvage of marginally ischemic tissues.[136]

Stump Infection

The incidence of infection in an amputation stump ranges from 12% to 28%.[9,18,20,57,120] As might be expected, the incidence of postoperative stump infection is directly related to the reason for performing the amputation. The incidence of this complication can be reduced by appropriate management of preexisting infections, including the use of perioperative antibiotic therapy, as well as wide debridement or drainage of infection before definitive amputation. Reviews by McIntyre and coworkers[36] and Fischer and colleagues[37] noted a statistically significant decrease in the rate of stump infection in patients undergoing definitive below-knee amputation for a septic foot in whom prior ankle guillotine amputation was performed to control infection. The incidence of below-knee stump infection in patients managed with a one-stage surgical procedure was 22% and 21% in these reports, respectively, whereas the incidence in patients who had undergone preparatory guillotine ankle amputation was 3% and 0%, respectively ($P < .05$). My most recent incidence of stump infection is 3% (4 of 134), and most of these infections represent aggressive closure of contaminated wounds or amputations in limbs with distal ipsilateral septic foci.

I recommend the use of prophylactic antibiotics in all patients undergoing lower extremity amputation, even in the absence of established limb infection. It has been my practice to treat patients with preoperative infections with broad-spectrum antibiotics that provide bactericidal aerobic and anaerobic coverage. The necessity for aerobic and anaerobic coverage is especially important in diabetic patients, in whom the incidence of mixed facultative and obligate anaerobic infections may be as high as 60%.[22]

Once an infection is established in an amputation stump, the wound must be opened widely to provide adequate drainage. In general, this means that the amputation will have to be revised to a higher level; for example, a stump infection in a below-knee amputation usually results in an above-knee amputation. The importance of this complication is emphasized by the fact that for a geriatric patient, conversion from a below-knee to an above-knee amputation is often the difference between successful ambulation and the inability to walk.

Stump hematoma after lower extremity amputation is a catastrophic complication, especially when the amputation has been performed for distal extremity infection. Although the correlation between stump hematoma and stump infection is not 1 : 1, it is high enough to make the avoidance of stump hematoma highly desirable. The importance of meticulous hemostasis after amputation cannot be emphasized enough. If an amputation is not dry, the wound should be closed with drains (closed drainage system, not Penrose drains), although several studies have suggested that the use of drains increases the risk of infection.[137]

Pulmonary Embolism and Deep Venous Thrombosis

The incidence of pulmonary embolism and deep venous thrombosis following major lower extremity amputation is 1% to 3%[7,14] and 4% to 38%,[9,14] respectively. The postoperative lower extremity amputee is at high risk for venous thromboembolic complications. Usually, these patients have had a prolonged period of hospitalization and bed rest before amputation. In addition, many have undergone prior attempts at vascular surgical reconstruction that may have injured the deep veins in the leg and prolonged preamputation immobilization. The amputation itself involves division of veins, which may result in stagnation and thrombosis in these vein segments postoperatively. When an active rehabilitation program is not begun on the first day after amputation surgery, this additional period of inactivity or immobilization may further predispose the patient to venous thromboembolic complications. The morbidity and mortality from venous thromboembolic complications may be significant, and impairment of blood oxygenation may further compromise the healing of ischemic tissues.

For patients undergoing elective major lower extremity amputation in whom major risk factors for venous thromboembolic complications exist, appropriate prophylaxis for pulmonary embolism should be instituted. Because there is a slight increase in stump hematoma formation, the use of a closed suction drainage system in these patients is advisable. Probably the most important factor in preventing thromboembolic complications is to not allow patients to become bedridden either preoperatively or postoperatively. A patient being prepared for lower extremity amputation should be undergoing preoperative physical therapy for range of motion and strengthening of the contralateral leg and upper extremities. A postoperative amputee, even if an immediate postoperative prosthesis is not used, should be receiving physical therapy for similar body conditioning. Attention should be paid to the nonamputated extremity, and the use of thromboembolic elastic stockings is recommended during the perioperative period. A final factor that must be considered is the patient's state of hydration, both preoperatively and postoperatively. This is especially important in patients who have undergone prior attempts at vascular reconstruction or angiography.

Pulmonary Complications

The incidence of pulmonary complications, including pneumonia, atelectasis, and sepsis, has been estimated at 8% in patients undergoing major lower extremity amputation.[14] These complications are significantly higher in patients undergoing above-knee amputation, as noted by Huston and colleagues,[7] in whom the incidence of pneumonia and sepsis ranged from 8% to 60%. The same conditions of bed rest, inactivity, dehabilitation, and dehydration that predispose to thromboembolic complications also predispose to atelectasis and pneumonia. Next to myocardial infarction, pulmonary complications are probably the biggest problem with geriatric patients undergoing lower extremity amputation. Attention to good pulmonary toilet, increased muscular activity, and active exercise (physical therapy) are all valuable adjuncts to preoperative and perioperative care.

Flexion Contractures

Flexion contractures of the knee or hip joint can occur quite rapidly following major lower extremity amputation, especially in geriatric patients. In my experience, the incidence of such postoperative flexion contractures has been 1% to 3%.[9,14,20,57]

Irreversible flexion contracture prohibits the successful fitting of a prosthesis and, subsequently, patient ambulation. Such a problem may also necessitate amputation at a higher level. The use of a rigid postoperative dressing, with or without an immediate postoperative pylon, helps decrease the incidence of this complication. In patients who are not receiving immediate postoperative prosthetic (IPOP) treatment, physical therapy directed toward range of motion and muscle strengthening should be instituted preoperatively if possible and as soon as possible after amputation.

Renal Insufficiency

Renal insufficiency represents a low-frequency complication following major lower extremity amputation, with an incidence of 1% to 3%.[9,57] This complication is, for the most part, avoidable if proper attention is paid to adequate preoperative and postoperative hydration. In addition, in patients requiring prolonged antibiotic therapy for perioperative infection, attention must be paid to antibiotic dosage to avoid renal insufficiency as a complication of antibiotic therapy.

Long-Term Complications

Stump Revision

There is little information available in the literature regarding the frequency of stump revision in patients who have been discharged from the hospital following lower extremity amputation. In an early report by Malone and associates, there was a 97% rate of primary healing after lower extremity amputation, and 88% of the amputees were followed for up to 18 months after surgery, with no stump revision.[20] The incidence of prosthesis use in those patients was 100%. Similar information was reported by Roon and coworkers, who noted that 91% of their patients were ambulatory on their prostheses 44 months following amputation.[14] I believe that the frequency of stump revision is probably related to amputation level selection method, quality of prosthesis fit, and careful postoperative follow-up. My current incidence of late stump revision is 2.3% (10 of 450).

Death

Approximately one third of all lower extremity amputees die within 5 years of their amputation, and two thirds of these deaths are due to cardiovascular causes.[120] Roon and coworkers reported a 45% overall 5-year survival following lower extremity amputation, compared with an expected 85% 5-year survival for the age-adjusted normal population.[14] More striking, however, was their analysis of the projected 5-year survival following lower extremity amputation for diabetic and nondiabetic amputees. They reported a 75% 5-year survival for nondiabetics, compared with only 39% for patients with diabetes mellitus (Fig. 64.13). Analysis of the cause of death disclosed that more than one third of deaths were due to myocardial infarction, and two thirds were due to cardiovascular causes.[14]

There are good multivariate data showing that in dialyzed diabetic patients, apolipoprotein A-I, fibrinogen, age, and stroke are independent predictors of both cardiac and noncardiac death.[138] In addition, in type 1 diabetic patients, in spite of intensified insulin therapy, nephropathy is the strongest predictor of mortality and end-stage complications, including amputation.[139]

Contralateral Limb Loss

Estimates of the rate of contralateral limb loss range from 15% to 33% in the 5 years following major lower extremity amputation.[16–18] In all probability, however, diabetic amputees are likely to die before contralateral limb loss.[14,120] Because of the risk of contralateral limb loss, significant attention should be paid to examination of the contralateral limb as well as patient education in prophylactic skin and foot care. Patient instructions

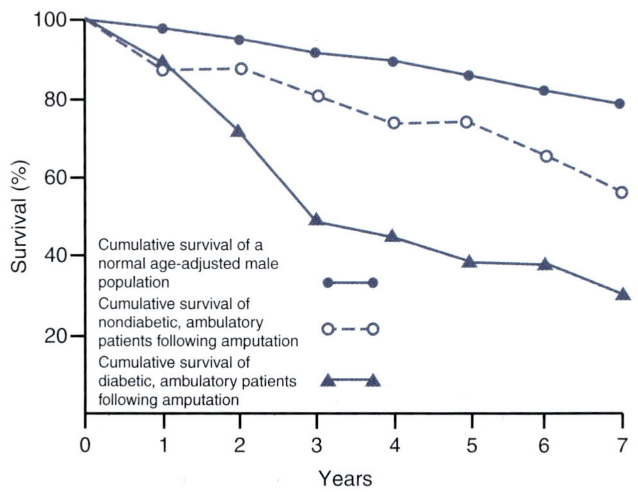

FIG 64.13 Life-table representation of survival after lower extremity amputation for both diabetic and nondiabetic amputees compared with the age-adjusted normal population. (From Roon AJ, Moore WS, Goldstone J: Below knee amputation: a modern approach. *Am J Surg* 134:153–158, 1977.)

BOX 64.1 Patient Instruction Sheet for Care of the Diabetic Foot

1. Inspect your feet daily for blisters, cuts, scratches, and areas of possible infection. Do not miss looking between your toes. A mirror can help you see the bottom of your feet or between the toes. If it is not possible for you to inspect your feet yourself, seek the help of a family member or friend.
2. Wash your feet and toes daily, and dry very carefully, especially between the toes. It is also important to dry carefully after showering or swimming.
3. Avoid extreme temperatures for your feet. Test bath water with your hand to ensure that it is not too hot, and be extremely careful of hot pavement or concrete during the summer.
4. If your feet feel cold at night, wear socks. Do not apply hot water bottles or heating pads.
5. Do not use chemical agents to remove corns or calluses.
6. Inspect your shoes daily for foreign objects, nail points, torn linings, or other problems that might damage your feet.
7. Wear properly fitting stockings, and try to avoid stockings with seams and stockings that are mended. It is important to change stockings daily.
8. All shoes should be comfortable and loose fitting at the time of purchase. Do not depend on shoes to stretch or break in. Try to avoid shoes that are pointed or apply pressure on the toes.
9. Do not wear shoes without stockings.
10. Do not wear sandals with thongs between the toes. Never walk barefoot, especially on hot surfaces. Be extremely careful of walking barefoot at home owing to danger from pins, tacks, or other items dropped on the floor.
11. Toenails should be cut straight across, and if there is a question, please consult your physician or podiatrist.
12. Do not cut corns or calluses yourself; seek counseling from your physician or podiatrist. See your physician or podiatrist regularly, and be sure that your feet are examined on each visit.
13. If your vision is impaired or you have other difficulties with examining your feet, have a family member or friend inspect your feet, trim nails, and otherwise ensure adequate foot care.
14. Be sure to tell your podiatrist or physician that you are diabetic.
15. Do not smoke.
16. Remember that even minor infections can cause significant problems in diabetics, and a physician or podiatrist should be consulted when infection occurs.

for diabetic foot care that are used at the Tucson VA Medical Center and Maricopa Medical Center (Phoenix, AZ) are shown in Box 64.1.

A randomized, prospective educational study at the Tucson VA Medical Center found that an audiovisual education program decreased the incidence of subsequent amputation significantly (at 1 year) among diabetics who presented with foot ulcers, infection, prior amputation, or high-risk lesions.[16] In that study, 203 patients were randomized into two groups: education and no education. There were no significant differences in medical management or clinical risk factors between the two groups. There was no significant difference in the incidence of infection; however, the rate of ulceration and amputation was three times higher in the no-education subgroup (ulceration: 26 of 177 vs. 8 of 177, $P = .005$; amputation: 21 of 177 vs. 7 of 177, $P = .025$), demonstrating that a simple education program significantly reduced the incidence of ulcer and amputation in diabetic patients. Other studies have documented the importance of diabetes education, protective footwear, and preventive foot care.[140–143]

Lehto and associates clearly demonstrated that there is a dose-response relationship between plasma glucose or hemoglobin A_1 and the risk of amputation.[141] Similar data have been published by Muhlhauser and colleagues, showing that the end-stage complications of blindness, amputation, and dialysis were statistically linked to the level of glycosylated hemoglobin.[139] Flores Rivera documented an increased risk for amputation in diabetic patients with cholesterol levels greater than 450 mg.[140] Muhlhauser and colleagues linked serum cholesterol levels to the combined end points of blindness, amputation, or dialysis.[139] Clearly, good blood glucose control should decrease the incidence of amputation in diabetics. However, the benefit, if any, of cholesterol-lowering drugs in decreasing the risk of amputation in both diabetic and nondiabetic patients is not known.

Prosthetic Considerations Following Major Lower Extremity Amputation

In general, as the level of amputation moves proximally up the lower extremity and the age of the patient increases, the success rates for rehabilitation decline and the length of time required to achieve ambulation increases.[17,144–150] Before discussing specific prosthetic considerations, a review of some of the problems associated with rehabilitation of geriatric amputees is worthwhile.

Rehabilitation of Elderly Amputees

In the mid to late 1960s, the literature was replete with reports on the problems encountered in rehabilitating geriatric amputees. Many of these reports have been forgotten, but the information they presented is still valid. Among the most important work of that period was the project of Mazet and associates involving a 10-year follow-up of 1770 geriatric patients from the VA and county hospitals in Los Angeles.[17] Among their findings was the fact that 60% of patients who were given prosthetic limbs discarded them within 6 months. Thirteen years later, Jamieson and Hill, in a review of amputation for peripheral vascular disease, reported that more than half the patients fitted with artificial legs never used them effectively.[151] In addition, they reported that if the rehabilitation process was delayed for 2 or more months after amputation, the likelihood of ultimate ambulation was very poor. In a more recent review of rehabilitation following lower extremity amputation, Kerstein and colleagues noted that it required an average of 27 weeks (189 days) to achieve the maximum benefits of rehabilitation, and it was approximately 6 months before a successfully rehabilitated amputee was returned to society.[152] In an earlier article analyzing the influence of age on rehabilitation, Kerstein and coauthors found that many patients older than 65 required a year to achieve maximum benefit from the rehabilitation process.[146] Malone and coworkers analyzed contemporary series on below-knee amputation in patients treated with conventional rehabilitation techniques and found that the average rate of rehabilitation was 64% and the average time from operation to rehabilitation (ambulation) was 133 days (Table 64.5).[9] In a later review, Malone and coworkers noted that the rehabilitation times for patients treated with conventional

TABLE 64.5 Overview of Postsurgical and Rehabilitation Outcome in Several Series[a]

	Amputations (N)	Primary Healing (%)	Eventual Healing (%)	Mortality Rate (%)	Rehabilitation With Prosthesis (%)	Average Time From Operation to Authors Rehabilitation (Days)
Warren and Kihn	121	48.8	66.9	4.1	69.4	180–270
Chilvers et al.	53	50.0	67.9	7.5	60.4	—
Robinson	47	77.0	88.0	17.0	83.0	—
Bradham and Smoak	84	85.7	—	—	—[b]	—
Block and Whitehouse	43	88.0	95.0	0.0[c]	53.5	120–180
Cranley et al.	101	76.0	86.0	7.0	73.3	—
Lim et al.	55	53.0	83.0	16.0	51.0	70
Ecker and Jacobs	69	77.0	85.0	8.7	52.2	201
Wray et al.	174	92.0	—	3.5	70.0	49–77
Nagrendran et al.	174	80.5	91.4	—	—	—
Berardi and Keonin	44	—	61.4	4.5	29.5	111
Averaged totals	965	74.9	82.0	6.7	63.8	133

[a]Series reporting results with conventional techniques of rehabilitation after below-knee amputation. Note that the overall rehabilitation rate was 64% and the average time to achieve ambulation was 133 days.
[b]Authors commented that very few patients attained ambulation; however, no numbers were given.
[c]Two patients died before discharge and were not included as postoperative deaths.
From Malone JM, Moore WS, Goldstone J, Malone SJ: Therapeutic and economic impact of a modern amputation program. *Ann Surg* 189:801, 1979.

TABLE 64.6 Comparison of Rehabilitation Time With Conventional and Accelerated Techniques[a]

Level of Amputation	Group 1 (Days)		Group 2 (Days)		
	Range	Mean	Range	Mean	P Value
Transmetatarsal	20–60	47.0	10–24	18.4	NS
Syme	—	—	15–17	23.0	—
Below-knee	60–330	132.0	18–140	32.5	.0001
Knee disarticulation	—	—	15–140	60.7	—
Above-knee	360	—	27–30	28.5	NS
Hip disarticulation	—	—	35	—	—
Overall	20–360	128.4	10–140	30.8	.0001

[a]Rehabilitation time following lower extremity amputation for patients treated with conventional surgical and prosthetic techniques (group 1, 128 days) and accelerated techniques incorporating immediate postoperative prostheses (group 2, 31 days) ($P < .001$).
NS, Not significant.
From Malone SM, Moore WS, Leal JM, Childers SJ: Rehabilitation for lower extremity amputation. *Arch Surg* 116:97, 1981.

techniques versus accelerated rehabilitation techniques (including amputation level selection and immediate postoperative prosthesis) were 128 and 31 days, respectively (Table 64.6).[20] The same review pointed out that the success rate for ambulation after amputation with conventional rehabilitation techniques was 70%, whereas it was 100% for amputees treated with accelerated rehabilitation techniques. In addition, it has been my experience that if a geriatric patient is nonambulatory for either a month before or a month after amputation (i.e., rehabilitation is delayed), the likelihood for rehabilitation is significantly less than if the patient remains ambulatory during the perioperative period.

Part of the problem with rehabilitation of geriatric amputees is their decreased cardiorespiratory reserve and the increased energy expenditure required after lower extremity amputation, especially at more proximal amputation levels. These problems are complicated by the fact that individual surgeons probably see too few amputees to treat them with maximum efficiency, and the few patients they do see place a large burden on beds, resources, and physician time.

In a review of the energy cost of walking for amputees, Waters and colleagues found that in both unilateral traumatic and vascular amputees, performance was directly related to the level of amputation.[149] Walking velocity, cadence, and stride length were all decreased in amputation patients compared with control groups. In a detailed analysis of velocity of ambulation, rate of oxygen uptake, respiratory quotient, and heart rate, these authors concluded that amputees adjust their gait velocity to keep their

TABLE 64.7 Energy Expenditure (Compared With Controls) After Lower Extremity Amputation[a]

Level of Amputation	Increase in Energy Expenditure (%)
Unilateral below-knee	9–25
Bilateral below-knee	41
Unilateral above-knee	25–100
Bilateral above-knee	280

[a]As measured by oxygen utilization per minute[149,153,155] or indirect calorimetry.[154] Energy expenditure was measured at comfortable walking speeds that averaged 22% of normal.

rate of energy expenditure within normal limits. The approximate energy expenditures (compared with those of controls) after lower extremity amputation are shown in Table 64.7.[149,153–155] Note that the energy expenditures for both unilateral and bilateral below-knee amputees are less than those for unilateral above-knee amputees. This clearly demonstrates the importance of the knee joint in terms of energy used for ambulation. The additional effort of walking with an above-knee prosthesis is accomplished by the use of small muscles, which are poorly designed for locomotion.[155]

Decreased physical strength due to age, decreased cardiorespiratory reserve due to the ravages of cardiovascular or pulmonary disease, and increased energy expenditures for ambulation after lower extremity amputation all have an additive effect that complicates the rehabilitation of geriatric amputees. It is in this setting that the salvage of the most distal amputation that will heal may mean the difference between ambulation and independence and nonambulation and dependence for an elderly amputee. These factors also explain the higher likelihood of ambulation for a young high-level amputee compared with an elderly high-level or bilateral amputee. In their evaluation of 113 amputations in 103 patients, most of whom underwent amputation for peripheral vascular disease, diabetes, or both (mean age, 61 years), Roon and coworkers found the following rates of successful rehabilitation: 100% for unilateral below-knee amputation, 93% for bilateral below-knee amputation, 17% for a combination of above-knee and below-knee amputation, and 0% for bilateral above-knee amputation.[14]

Postoperative Prosthetic Techniques

After major lower extremity amputation, the surgeon has three choices for prosthetic management: soft dressings or conventional technique, constant environmental treatment (CET) (which at this point is probably of historical interest only), and rigid dressings with or without a postoperative prosthesis. In addition, the surgeon may choose delayed (conventional), rapid, or immediate postoperative rehabilitation.

Conventional Stump Wrap (Soft Dressing)

The historical standard, and a technique that is still used in many institutions, is the application of a soft postoperative dressing. Cotton gauze or fluffs are used to pad the amputation stump, and the stump is wrapped with elastic bandages (Fig. 64.14).

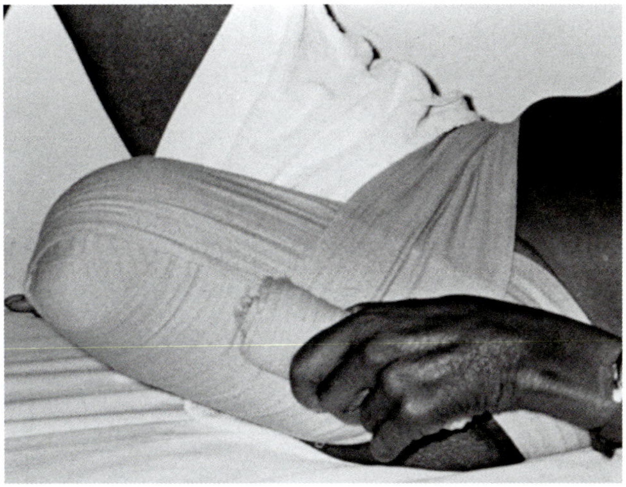

FIG 64.14 Standard, conventional soft dressing and stump wrap being applied by a patient to his right above-knee amputation.

The advantage of this technique is that it does not require a prosthetist to be present in the operating room or at the time of dressing changes. The disadvantages are that it does not readily control stump edema, the dressings are difficult to maintain in place (especially for high-level amputees), there is minimal stump protection from postoperative trauma, the dressing does not prevent knee flexion contracture, and ambulation may be delayed as a result of the prolonged time required for stump maturity (6 months).

Except for the above-knee and hip disarticulation amputation levels, where it is technically difficult to maintain a rigid dressing in good stump contact, there are no valid reasons to continue the use of this postoperative dressing technique.

Constant Environmental Treatment Unit

Developed and used almost exclusively in Great Britain, the CET unit consists of a control console containing a multistage centrifugal air compressor. The air passes through pressure control valves, a pressure cycle timing device, a bacteriologic filter, and a thermostatically controlled heating element that controls heat and relative humidity. The dressing on the patient consists of a transparent flexible polyvinyl bag. The bag is not in direct contact with the residual limb, except on the resting surface. A pleated air seal is incorporated into the proximal end of the bag to maintain a pressure seal. A sterile CET bag is placed over the amputation stump in the operating room. The amputation stump is, in essence, "enclosed" in a sterile environment with cyclic pressure (which controls stump edema) and airflow set to the desired temperature and humidity (Fig. 64.15).

The CET unit was designed for use in a setting in which a prosthetist is not immediately available or one in which the surgeon wants to be able to control stump edema yet have easy access to examine the surgical wound. The system incorporates a long flexible hose so that the patient can undergo rehabilitation training at the bedside. Indications for use of the CET unit are relatively limited; it is probably best used on patients in whom there is some risk of stump infection and in whom the ability to observe the wound without dressing changes is desirable.

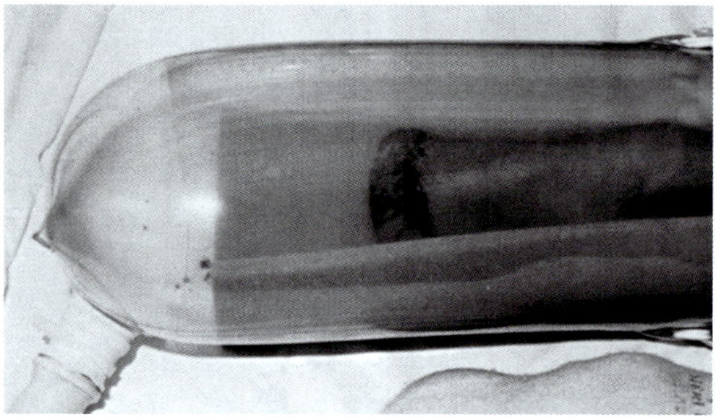

FIG 64.15 Clear polyvinyl controlled environment treatment bag has been placed over a left below-knee amputation. Note the air supply hose at the distal end of the bag.

TABLE 64.8 Overview of Immediate Prosthesis Data: San Francisco and Tucson Veterans Administration Hospitals and Maricopa Medical Center

Stump healing	138/153 (90%)
Rehabilitation time	15–32 days
Rate of rehabilitation	155/175 (88%)
Unilateral below-knee	128/129 (99%)
Bilateral below-knee	17/19 (89%)
Bilateral above- and below-knee or above- and above-knee	6/23 (26%)
Unilateral above-knee	4/4 (100%)

Data from references 9, 14, 20.

Because of its limited application, high cost, and poor patient acceptance due to noise, the CET unit, although successful, has seen limited use in the United States.[156]

Rapid and Immediate Postoperative Prostheses

The application of an immediate postoperative prosthesis has received considerable attention, support, credit, and discredit in the recent past. Proponents of the technique have waxed eloquently on the benefits to the patient, while opponents of the technique have cautioned about the potential detriment to the amputation stump from the casting technique.

Berlemont is generally credited with the early work that led to the establishment of the technique, based on his application of temporary prostheses in patients with delayed (secondary) amputation stump healing.[3] Weiss of Poland is credited with adapting this technique for stumps undergoing primary healing (i.e., immediate postoperative prosthesis). The latter technique proved highly successful, and Weiss reported his initial results at the Sixth International Prosthetic Course in Copenhagen in July 1963. This early presentation and a subsequent publication in 1966 came to the attention of surgeons worldwide.[4] The Prosthetic and Sensory Aids Service of the VA was especially interested in this technique for the management of veteran amputees and was instrumental in bringing this procedure to the US surgical theater. Working with the VA, Burgess, an orthopedic surgeon in Seattle, refined and developed the IPOP technique for the US surgical field.[5,134,157–159] Burgess and his team performed most of the early work in the United States, and he was instrumental in training other investigators in the use of this technique. In the late 1960s and early 1970s, there were multiple reports extolling the virtues and possible pitfalls of the IPOP technique (also called IPPF, IPOP fitting).

Initially, there was general agreement that the IPOP technique was ideally suited for nondiabetic, nondysvascular amputees. Subsequent reports in the literature, however, have shown that, if properly used, the technique may be ideal for geriatric dysvascular amputees because of its ability to shorten hospitalization time and increase rates of rehabilitation.[9,14,20]

In general, proponents of the technique note that its benefits include an increased rate of healing, decreased hospitalization time, decreased rehabilitation time, decreased psychological trauma to the patient, control of stump edema, protection from stump trauma in the early postoperative period, and perhaps an increased rate of rehabilitation.[9,14,20,88,160–163] The paper most commonly cited against the use of the IPOP technique is that by Cohen and colleagues.[164] Using conventional surgical and prosthetic techniques, they were able to achieve 97% stump healing, whereas only two of nine (22%) amputation stumps treated with the IPOP technique healed. They noted no rehabilitation advantage to the IPOP technique and recommended caution in its application. The experience of Cohen and colleagues has not been matched by other reports in the literature. Some reports noted no change in the rate of wound healing,[160] but in general, most papers found no deleterious effects from the use of a rigid postoperative dressing (with or without a prosthesis), decreased hospitalization time, and decreased rehabilitation time.[9,14,20,160,162,163] Importantly, Cohen and colleagues suggested that their problems with the IPOP technique might be with the plaster technique itself or in the application of the technique. A review of their paper shows that four patients sustained what are described as second-degree blisters, which almost certainly indicate problems with plaster fabrication and application rather than problems with the IPOP technique itself. In my own experience with 600 consecutive major lower extremity amputations during the past 12 years, there has been only one stump problem related to the use of an immediate postoperative prosthesis, and that problem was caused by improper application of an immediate postoperative cast.

An overview of data on the use of the IPOP technique reported from the San Francisco VA Hospital, the Tucson VA Hospital, and Maricopa Medical Center by Roon and colleagues[14] and Malone and associates[9,20] is given in Table 64.8. A 1992 paper by Folsum and coworkers documented the overall rate of rehabilitation at 80% and the interval from amputation to ambulation at 15.2 days and 9.3 days for below-knee and above-knee amputees, respectively.[165] Information not tabulated in Table 64.8 suggests that the patient's ambulatory status before surgery is one of the most important predeterminants of postoperative ambulation. Essentially, 100% of patients undergoing unilateral major lower extremity amputation who ambulated before surgery were successfully rehabilitated after amputation, whereas less than 15% of the patients who were nonambulatory before amputation surgery were successfully rehabilitated.[9,14,20]

The advantages of immediate or early postoperative prostheses can be divided into two categories: those derived from the rigid dressing and those derived from early weight bearing and ambulation. The advantages of the rigid dressing include edema control, stump immobilization, perhaps improved healing, prevention of joint flexion contracture, and protection of the stump from external trauma. There may be no difference between soft and rigid dressings with respect to the time required to reach eventual stump maturity (6 months), although postoperative stump edema resolves much more quickly with a rigid dressing. The advantages of immediate or early ambulation include decreased hospital stay, less time from surgery to ambulation, increased rates of rehabilitation compared with patients managed in a more conventional manner, reduction in morbid and nonmorbid complications of amputation, and improvement in the patient's psychological outlook after amputation.[9,14,20,123]

In summary, there is general agreement on both the benefits and the pitfalls of the IPOP technique. I agree with Friedmann's conclusions: "immediate postoperative prosthetic fitting should be confined to large centers with medical and prosthetic facilities available on short notice."[80] In other circumstances, he advocated the use of conventional amputation rehabilitation techniques but specified that such management should include modern postoperative methods, including the early use of temporary prostheses for evaluation and training. The best solution to the problem of choosing a postoperative prosthetic technique would be the routine use of a rigid dressing and the application or use of a temporary prosthesis when the surgeon thinks that adequate wound healing has occurred (usually 1 to 2 weeks after amputation), thereby avoiding some of the potential hazards of immediate ambulation.[166–168]

Another variant of a postoperative rigid dressing that allows early ambulation is the air splint.[145,169] This device may be a practical alternative for a surgeon who wants to achieve early postoperative ambulation but does not have access to a prosthetist skilled in the application of immediate postoperative prostheses or temporary removable prostheses.

Techniques of Immediate Postoperative Prosthetic Application

IPOP use has been described for all levels of major lower extremity amputation—from the transmetatarsal through the high above-knee amputation; however, it is best suited to below-knee amputation. Specific technical details regarding the application of immediate postoperative prostheses can be found elsewhere and are only briefly outlined here.[107]

Transmetatarsal and Syme Amputations

A rigid cast with felt padding for bony prominence relief is used as the first dressing for these distal levels of lower extremity amputation; however, ambulation is not allowed until adequate primary healing has been obtained (3 weeks). Early ambulation for transmetatarsal and Syme amputation patients results in a higher incidence of wound complications. With Syme amputation, it is extremely important that the posterior heel flap be held in good approximation and alignment by the cast and that great care be taken to pad the distal stump and dog ears, as well as the bony prominences. If a two-stage surgical approach for Syme amputation is used,[88] it is probably best to avoid weight bearing until completion of the second stage of the surgical procedure (6 to 8 weeks). Both transmetatarsal and Syme's amputees will ultimately ambulate well, and a short delay in the ambulation process has essentially no impact on their overall rehabilitation. Avoidance of stump trauma to ensure primary wound healing during the early postoperative period is of paramount importance, and rehabilitation efforts can be confined to range of motion and strengthening of the opposite leg and upper extremities during the early postoperative period.

Below-Knee Amputation

Following completion of the amputation, a thin sheet of fine mesh material (Owen's silk) is moistened in antibiotic solution or saline and applied over the suture line, with care taken to avoid wrinkling (Fig. 64.16). Next, lamb's wool or polyurethane foam is placed over the end of the stump to provide stump compression and padding (Fig. 64.17). A Spandex stump sock is then carefully rolled over the stump, with care taken to avoid displacement of the distal stump padding (Fig. 64.18). Relief pads made from nonporous foam are fashioned and glued to the stump sock with Dow-Corning medical adhesive. These pads can be obtained precut or can be hand-fashioned in the operating room. They are placed to pad the bony prominences, specifically including the fibular head, tibial condyles, and patella. Care is taken to leave a relief area between the medial and lateral tibial pads (Fig. 64.19). Next, elastic plaster is used to form the inner layer of the immediate postoperative prosthesis. It is important that an assistant maintain traction on the stump sock during plaster application. Care is taken to maintain compression from posterior to anterior (direction of the posterior skin flap) and

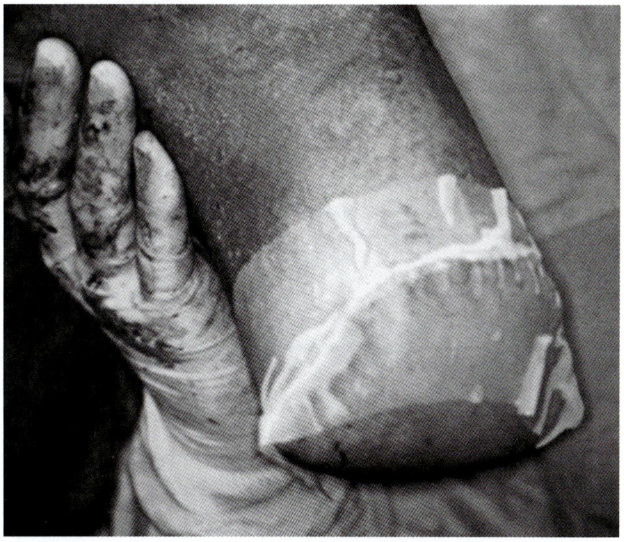

FIG 64.16 A single sheet of moistened Owen's silk is placed over the suture line on the below-knee amputation stump. Care is taken to avoid wrinkling of the silk material.

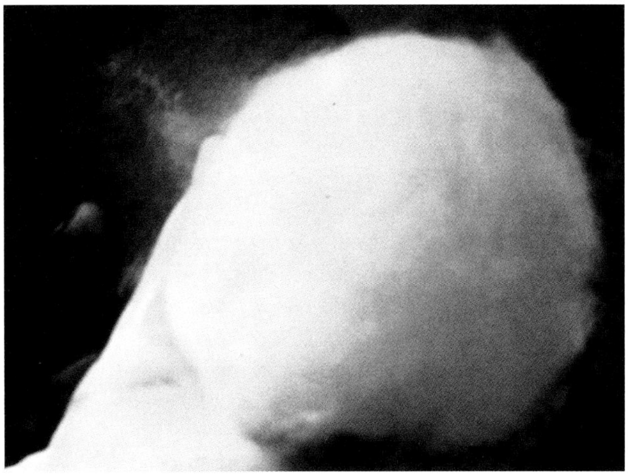

FIG 64.17 Lamb's wool, Dacron, or prefabricated polyurethane foam can be placed over Owen's silk to provide distal stump padding. Care is taken to place padding material both above and below skin dog ears, if they exist.

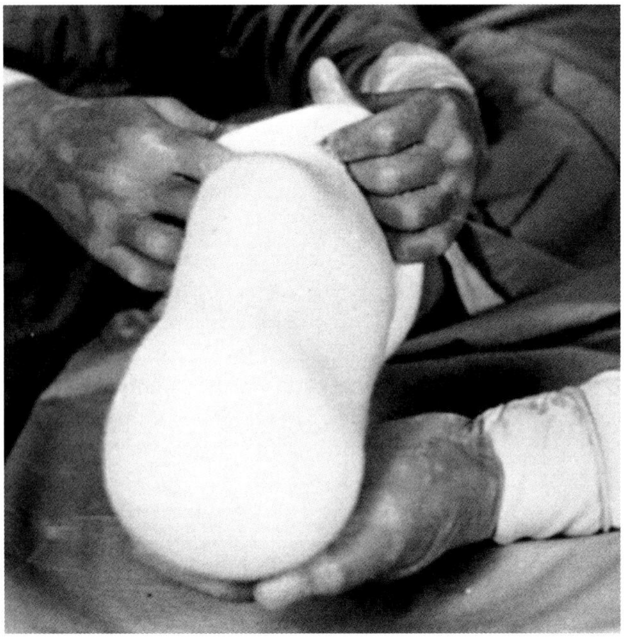

FIG 64.18 Spandex stump sock is carefully pulled over the distal end of a below-knee stump and rolled proximally up the leg. Care is taken not to displace the distal end stump padding during application of the sock. Until the postoperative cast is dry, an assistant must maintain traction on the stump sock.

to grade compression from the distal end of the stump to the more proximal thigh (Fig. 64.20). The suspension assembly of the immediate postoperative pylon is then contoured to the inner cast after the cast has dried (Fig. 64.21). The pylon can be attached and static alignment achieved before incorporating the suspension assembly into the cast. The pylon is removed, and the suspension assembly is secured to the inner cast using fiberglass casting tape. The use of lightweight casting tape decreases the weight of the immediate postoperative prosthesis and significantly increases its durability.[167] A completed immediate postoperative

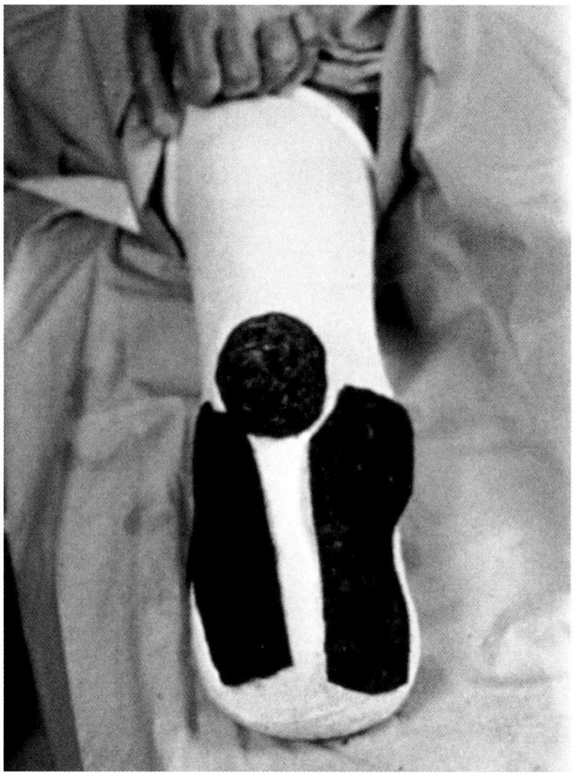

FIG 64.19 Felt relief pads are measured, trimmed, and glued to the Spandex stump sock over the bony prominences of the knee and lower leg. Care is taken to leave a relief area between the medial and lateral tibial pads.

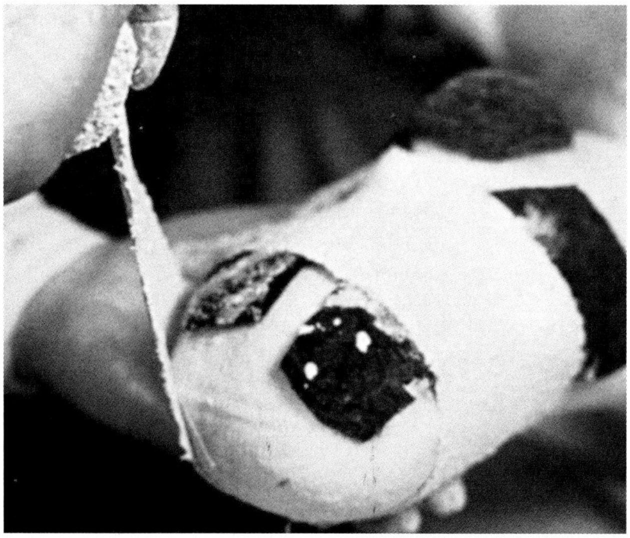

FIG 64.20 The inner layer of the postoperative rigid cast is made using elastic plaster, which provides good control of stump compression. Compression should be from posterior to anterior, in the direction of the posterior flap, and distal to proximal so that the compression decreases as the cast moves higher on the upper leg.

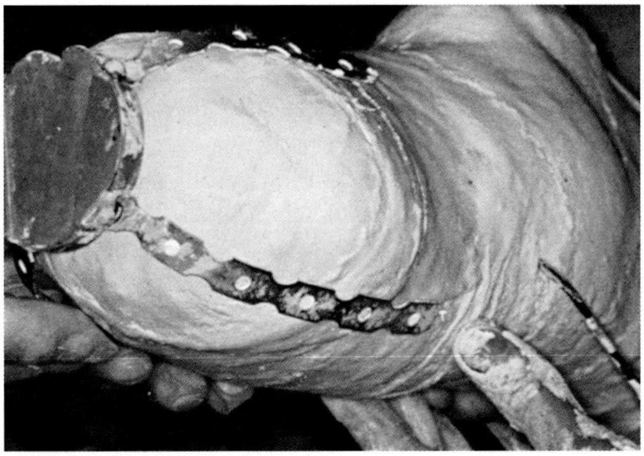

FIG 64.21 The metal arms of the immediate postoperative prosthetic bucket are molded to the contours of the inner plaster shell after the cast has dried.

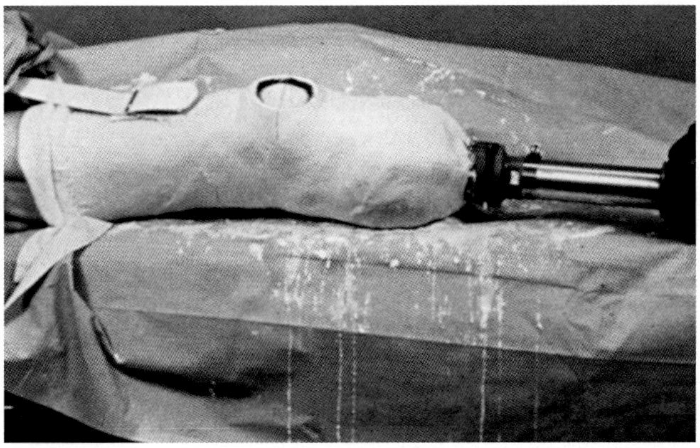

FIG 64.22 Intraoperative photograph of a completed immediate postoperative below-knee prosthesis with pylon, foot, and waist suspension belt. Note that a relief window has been placed over the area of the patella.

prosthesis, waist suspension belt, pylon, and foot are shown in Fig. 64.22. If a drain is employed, the drain should be brought out proximally (and laterally) through a separate hole made in the cast during the fabrication process. The drain should not be secured to the skin, so that it can be pulled out through the cast when appropriate.

Most surgical pain is gone within 36 to 48 hours after surgery. Significant pain more than 48 hours after surgery is an indication that the cast is too tight or that there is a wound complication. In this case, the cast should be removed, the wound inspected, and the cast reapplied if appropriate. Almost all patients comment that their postoperative stump pain diminishes if the heel of the prosthesis is weight-loaded (when they are in the supine position), and this test can be used as a further check for stump swelling and prosthesis fit. One of the most important principles in the postoperative management of these patients is that if there is any question about prosthesis fit or healing of the surgical wound, the prosthesis should be removed, the wound inspected by the surgeon and the prosthetist, and the cast reapplied at the discretion of the surgeon.

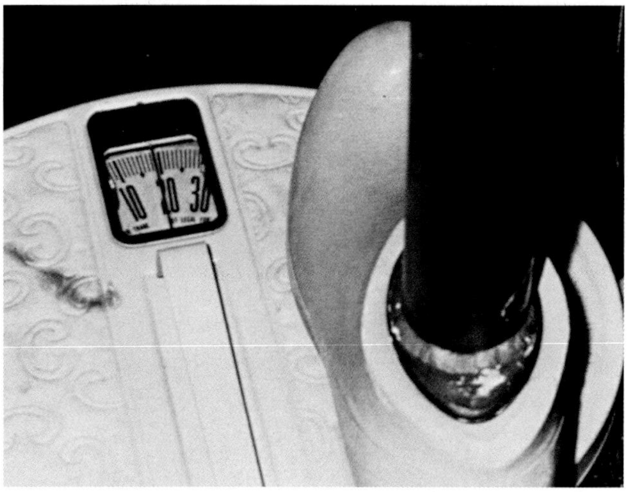

FIG 64.23 To control the amount of postoperative weight bearing by patients, a bathroom scale is used to teach them to distribute their body weight. During the first week after surgery, weight bearing is limited to 10 to 15 pounds. After the second cast change, weight bearing is limited to 50% of total body weight.

On the first postoperative morning, the patient is helped into a standing position at the bedside and instructed in techniques of touchdown weight bearing. At this time, the prosthetist completes the initial static alignment. On the second postoperative morning, the patient goes to the physical therapy department, where he or she is taught touchdown weight bearing using the bathroom scale technique (Fig. 64.23). An alternative to the scale technique is the load cell, which is a pressure-sensing device built into the prosthetic pylon.[170] During the first 7 to 10 days after surgery, the patient ambulates using parallel bars with a maximum of 10 to 15 pounds touchdown weight bearing (10% of body weight). After application of the second postoperative prosthesis, the patient increases weight bearing to approximately 50% of total body weight. At the end of 14 to 21 days, on removal of the second postoperative prosthesis, a decision is made to place the patient either in a third postoperative prosthesis (if there is a question of wound healing) or in a removable temporary prosthesis (if the wound appears to be healing satisfactorily).[167,168] At this time, the patient begins full weight bearing. By approximately 30 to 35 days after amputation surgery, most patients have achieved either independent ambulation or ambulation with some type of ancillary walking aid (cane, walker). If a patient lives close to the hospital and is able to come to daily physical therapy training as an outpatient, he or she may be discharged from the hospital shortly after receiving the second postoperative prosthesis (5 to 10 days); however, if the patient lives a great distance from the hospital, discharge is usually delayed until the surgeon, prosthetist, and therapist are happy with the rehabilitation process (4 to 5 weeks). This approach may have to be modified under the economic restraints that surround current medical care. Reasonable alternatives include transfer to a rehabilitation unit or service or early discharge with outpatient care. In either case, careful follow-up by the surgeon, prosthetist, and therapist is mandatory, especially in patients undergoing early ambulation and rehabilitation.

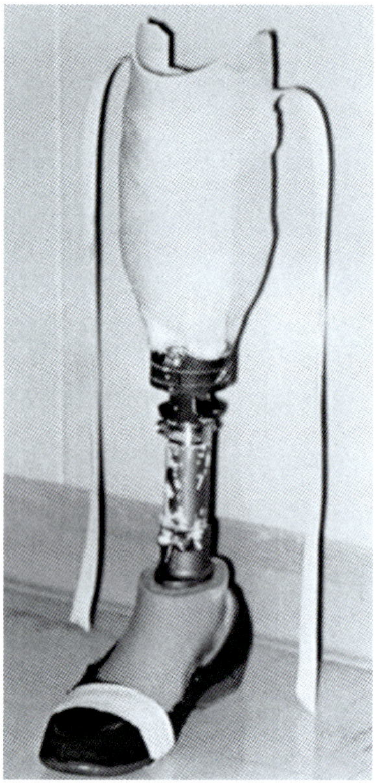

FIG 64.24 Standard removable lightweight below-knee temporary or intermediate prosthesis, prescribed after removal of the last immediate postoperative prosthesis. This particular prosthesis is constructed with 3M Scotchcast (3M, St. Paul, MN). Fabrication with Scotchcast allows construction of a lightweight, cool, yet durable prosthesis.

It can be anticipated that between discharge from the hospital and construction of the first permanent prosthesis (on average, 6 months after amputation), approximately three to six changes in the socket of the temporary prosthesis will be required as a result of progressive stump shrinkage. A typical lightweight, removable, temporary below-knee prosthesis is shown in Fig. 64.24. The same pylon and foot can be used throughout all intermediate (temporary) cast changes, so that the only new requirement is the socket and realignment of the prosthesis. Prosthetic fit is maintained with stump socks, and the primary indication for change of the temporary prosthesis is when the patient has reached a total of 15-ply stockings to maintain a good prosthetic fit. Obviously, great care is taken to educate the patient about the use of the prosthesis and stump care to avoid any problems due to poor prosthetic fit.

Knee Disarticulation Amputation

The techniques for the application of an immediate postoperative prosthesis for knee disarticulation amputation are essentially the same as those for below-knee amputation. Because of the bulbous distal end of the knee disarticulation stump, the immediate postoperative prosthesis for this amputation level is self-suspending. Great care should be taken during cast fabrication to contour the femoral flares and to bring the proximal end of the cast to at least the upper third of the thigh to minimize distal end-weight bearing. My preference is to incorporate a polypropylene quadrilateral above-knee brim into the knee disarticulation cast to provide ischial weight bearing. The stump should be well padded, because there is more stump weight bearing with this level of amputation than with a below-knee amputation. At the discretion of the surgeon and prosthetist, polycentric hydraulic knee units can be incorporated into the initial immediate postoperative prosthesis or at any time during postoperative follow-up. The schedule for cast changes, the rehabilitation techniques, and the use of temporary prostheses are approximately the same as those for below-knee amputation.

Above-Knee Amputation

IPOP techniques for above-knee amputation require more attention to detail to maintain adequate suspension and socket fit. Although techniques using a modified Silesian suspension (contralateral hip sling) or waist suspension belt are simple to implement,[113] I believe that the difficulties of using immediate postoperative prostheses at the above-knee level are not offset by any significant improvement in the overall rehabilitation process. Thus, I use immediate postoperative prostheses at this amputation level only for young amputees. For dysvascular amputees, a temporary above-knee prosthesis is prescribed when primary wound healing has been achieved (2 to 3 weeks). During the postoperative period, the above-knee amputee goes to rehabilitation daily to achieve upper extremity strengthening and balance and to practice ambulation with parallel bars or other walking aids. Once a temporary prosthesis has been constructed, the schedule for prosthesis modification and the rehabilitation techniques are similar to those for below-knee or knee disarticulation amputation.

Overview of Prostheses and Prosthetic Techniques

There is no one type of standard prosthetic prescription for all levels of lower extremity amputation, and knowledge of available components is crucial in determining the proper prescription for each amputee based on his or her activities and lifestyle. A more complete discussion of prosthetic components is beyond the scope of this chapter; however, interested surgeons are referred to their local prosthetists or prosthetic facilities with whom they should be working.

IPOP techniques do not work in all clinical settings. The success of the technique is based on the experience and dedication of the team, and there is no question that if the immediate postoperative prosthesis is improperly applied, significant damage to the amputation stump can occur. In the absence of an experienced prosthetist and physical therapist, I suggest that a rigid postoperative dressing be applied; then, when primary stump healing has occurred, an appropriate temporary prosthesis can be prescribed and the rehabilitation process initiated. A delay of 1 to 2 weeks in the rehabilitation process is meaningless in the overall context of amputee rehabilitation; however, it has been my experience that if the rehabilitation process is delayed for a month or more, the ultimate success of rehabilitation, especially for geriatric high-level amputees, is severely compromised. It is therefore logical and reasonable to provide a temporary prosthesis sometime between wound healing (7 to 10 days after surgery) and 1 month after surgery. Using this "between" approach (i.e., a rigid dressing with early prosthetic application), maximum rehabilitation results can be achieved even in the absence of a formal rehabilitation team.

Prosthetic Components

For a surgeon who performs only an occasional amputation, the number and types of prostheses and prosthetic components for lower extremity amputees can be bewildering. Therefore, a general overview of prosthetic components and specific combinations of components for certain levels of lower extremity amputation may be of value.

Transmetatarsal Amputation

In general, there is minimal, if any, prosthetic requirement for a transmetatarsal amputation. A steel shank placed in the sole of the shoe allows near-normal toe-off, and the void spot in the shoe can be filled with cotton, lamb's wool, or a soft foam material. The other option is construction of a specially designed shoe molded to the patient's foot in which toe-off is built into the shoe during construction.

Syme Amputation

Depending on whether Syme amputation has been performed with a one- or two-stage surgical procedure, the cosmetic quality of the prosthesis will be different (two-stage is more cosmetic). In general, this is an end–weight-bearing stump, and a prosthetic foot is attached to the leg shaft portion of the prosthesis. Because of the bulbous nature of the stump, a medial window has to be cut into the prosthesis to allow the stump to pass through the narrow midportion of the prosthesis. These prostheses are usually built with a nonmotion solid ankle-cushion heel (SACH) foot (Scheck & Siress). The presence of a particularly bulbous distal end precludes a cosmetic prosthesis, and this type of amputation may be contraindicated for cosmetic reasons alone.

Below-Knee Amputation

In general, the below-knee prosthesis consists of a prosthetic socket that is attached to a pylon or ankle block (endoskeletal system) and a foot. The prosthetic shell can be composed of plastic laminate, wood, or one of the newer, lightweight, rolled fiberglass materials such as 3M Scotchcast (3M, St. Paul, MN). The socket may use no liner (skin-socket interface) or may use a liner composed of lightweight plastic such as P-Lite, silicone gel bonded between two sheets of soft leather, or stump socks. The prosthesis can be suspended in a variety of ways, the most common of which is a standard PTB strap, supracondylar clip, Silastic sleeve suspension, suction, or thigh lacer with external hinges (Fig. 64.25). Self-suspending prostheses or physiologic suspension (the prosthesis is held in place by changes in muscle shape and contour with contraction) may be used in young, active amputees. In a young, highly active amputee, an ankle-rotating unit may be placed between the prosthesis and the foot. The feet currently in use include the SACH foot, which is a nonmotion foot; the stationary attachment flexible endoskeletal (SAFE) foot (Scheck & Siress); or the Geisinger 5-Way foot (Danville, PA). The last two feet incorporate flexion, extension, and internal and external rotation when the foot is stressed under weight. The drawback to both of these motion feet is increased weight and perhaps decreased life expectancy compared with the SACH foot. The most popular motion foot, the Seattle foot, overcomes the drawbacks of the previously mentioned motion feet and has a cosmetic design that incorporates toes. A hydraulic ankle unit has recently been developed, but the unit is quite heavy, and there are still problems with oil leakage. New energy-storing feet (energy is "stored" by deformation of carbon-plastic composites and "released" on toe-off), such as the Seattle-Boeing-Burgess Foot and the Flex-Foot (Scheck & Siress), offer significant improvements in gait and activity levels (such as running), especially for young, active amputees. The combination of a motion foot and a lightweight prosthesis provides a very high degree of function for active amputees.

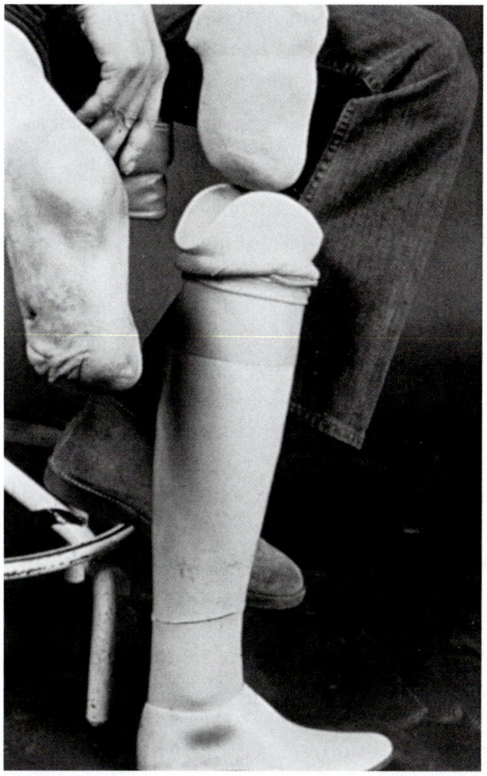

FIG 64.25 This below-knee prosthesis is an ultra-lightweight patellar tendon weight-bearing-type prosthesis using a Silastic sleeve for suspension, a Silastic gel insert, and a stationary attachment flexible endoskeletal motion-type foot. This is an ideal prosthesis for a young, active amputee.

Knee Disarticulation

Historically, knee disarticulation amputations were a prosthetic nightmare because the knee centers (thigh-knee length) could not be matched; however, the availability of polycentric knee joints has allowed construction of a cosmetic knee disarticulation prosthesis. In general, this prosthesis is similar to the Syme-type prosthesis, in that the distal bony end of the stump is passed through the proximal portion of the prosthesis via a window cut in the medial portion of the prosthesis. The prosthetic shell can be constructed of plastic or wood. In general, the prosthetic shell extends from the end of the stump up to the ischium to provide both distal end and ischial weight bearing. Most knee disarticulation prostheses incorporate some type of hydraulic knee unit for both cosmetic and functional reasons. The lower part of the leg can be constructed of solid wood, plastic laminate, or a metal or plastic endoskeletal system for connection to the ankle block and foot. Ankle rotators and energy-storing motion or nonmotion feet can be used at the discretion of the prosthetist and surgeon.

Above-Knee Amputation

The above-knee prosthesis can be constructed of plastic or wood. Suspension techniques include an external hip joint with belt, shoulder suspension, or suction socket suspension. This is not an end–weight-bearing prosthesis, and all the weight is borne by the proximal socket quadrilateral brim design (the soft tissues of the thigh and ischium). Newer prosthetic designs for above-knee sockets include the contoured adducted trochanteric–controlled alignment method (CAT-CAM) design (which holds the stump laterally and medially, providing rigid support for the femur, in contrast to the quadrilateral socket, which holds the stump anteriorly and posteriorly, with poor femur support) and a variety of new flexible socket and strut designs (outer rigid strut attached to the knee joint with a soft flexible inner socket). These new designs significantly enhance function for above-knee amputees. A hydraulic, passive, or manual lock knee joint can be incorporated, based on the individual patient's needs. The lower part of the prosthesis is constructed as outlined in the section on knee disarticulation prostheses.

Hip Disarticulation

In general, hip disarticulation prostheses are built along the lines of the Canadian system, which incorporates a pelvic bucket, an endoskeletal upper and lower leg, simple spring-assisted hip and knee joints, and a nonmotion foot.

AMPUTATION REHABILITATION TEAM

It is exceedingly difficult to achieve consistently reliable rehabilitation results in the absence of a formal, centralized, dedicated rehabilitation team that includes active participation by a prosthetist and members of the physical medicine and therapy departments. Just as some surgical procedures are confined to regional centers because of the cost and necessity of skilled labor, it is my belief that, ideally, amputation rehabilitation should be a centralized resource in a community or group of communities to achieve the best results. My concept of the structure of the amputation rehabilitation team is shown in Fig. 64.26. Note that the center of the rehabilitation team is the patient and that other members of the team interface with the patient through or with an amputation coordinator. This coordinator can be a physical therapist, occupational therapist, nurse, or layperson. In my opinion, this person is key to maintaining coordination and especially long-term follow-up among members of the team. It has been my experience that one break in this rehabilitation circle results in at least a 50% failure rate in amputee rehabilitation. This fact (i.e., a break in the rehabilitation circle) may

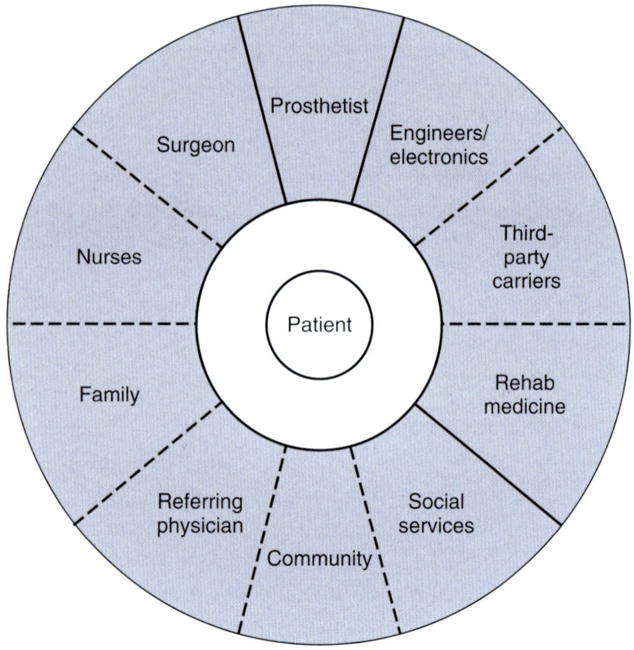

FIG 64.26 The rehabilitation team required for successful amputation rehabilitation. Notice that the patient is at the center, and the surgeon is only one of many coequal team members.

explain why the average rate of rehabilitation after lower extremity amputation is 60% or less.

There are five primary areas of concern in successful amputee rehabilitation: (1) coordination of care, (2) education of patient and family, (3) directed access to community resources, (4) discharge planning, and (5) centralized follow-up. In essence, the coordination of health care and mobilization of resources are under the direct control of the physician; however, once surgery is completed, this task is best organized by the amputation program coordinator. Discharge planning for the patient should start, if possible, before amputation. Education of the patient and family and evaluation of the financial and social resources available to the patient should also begin before amputation or as soon as possible after amputation. Centralized follow-up is important only if the team is interested in evaluating specific treatment techniques or prosthetic components. However, long-term follow-up is mandatory if reliable information on rehabilitation and postoperative complications is to be obtained.

The role of the physician is that of team director and provider of health care. The enthusiasm and interest of the physician will be reflected by all other members of the health care team. In the absence of an interested physician, rehabilitation failures will be common.

It is my belief that the prosthetist should be seen as coequal to the physician in the amputation rehabilitation process. From a practical standpoint, most patients rely more on the prosthetist than on the physician (in the absence of medical problems) once the acute phase of rehabilitation is completed.

The therapist is in the unique position of being able to make or break all the efforts of the surgeon and prosthetist. Only if the rehabilitation process runs smoothly and if attention is paid to small details during the rehabilitation process will the patient successfully regain ambulation. The greatest surgery in the world or the best limb in the world can meet defeat at the hands of an unskilled therapist. The therapist is the third coequal on the rehabilitation team, along with the physician and prosthetist.

Finally, the patient is the most important member of the rehabilitation team. The team can provide the patient with tools and techniques for rehabilitation, but it cannot provide the patient with motivation. It is of the utmost importance that the patient be taught to take primary control of the rehabilitation process. Included in this education are care of the amputation stump, care of the nonamputated leg, and care of the prosthesis. Failure of the patient to take an active role in the rehabilitation process will doom it to failure.[171]

One of the areas in which we as physicians and rehabilitation team members fail our patients is postdischarge follow-up and home care. An excellent review article on this topic appeared in the February 1979 issue of the Orthopedic Nurses Association Journal. All interested rehabilitation physicians and team members are advised to review this information and pass it on to their patients.[121]

I am now in a solo private practice without a dedicated amputation team. Although three experienced prosthetists, all of whom are well acquainted with immediate postoperative prosthesis fitting, are nearby, the lack of trained therapists and capitated-directed patient care contracts makes accelerated rehabilitation difficult if not impossible. Objective amputation level selection (transcutaneous oxygen testing), early if not IPOP filling, utilization of rehabilitation facilities after discharge, education of therapists, and persistence usually lead to a successful outcome. However, the rehabilitation results, especially in elderly or frail patients, are not as good as those documented in this chapter using a dedicated amputation team or center of care model.

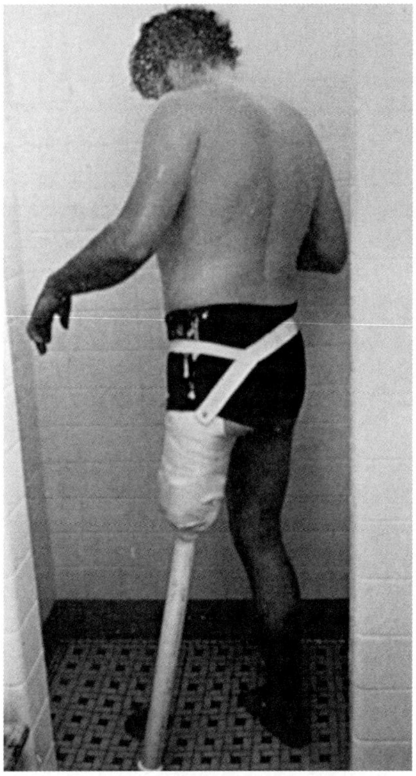

FIG 64.27 Patients with lower extremity amputations usually sit on a stool when taking a shower. The above-knee amputee shown here is wearing an Aqualite shower prosthesis (US Manufacturing Co., Pasadena, CA).

WHAT IS NEW IN AMPUTATION SURGERY?

Instrumentation

As noted earlier, many new instruments are currently undergoing evaluation for amputation level selection. In addition, many of these instruments are being evaluated for their role in arterial insufficiency. Early information is available, but the definitive role for these instruments is undecided. Perhaps more promising than any specific instruments for amputation level selection is the availability of computer software and microprocessors to integrate results from several different types of noninvasive techniques, resulting, in essence, in the era of the "limb viability laboratory." It can be anticipated that multi-instrument testing will result in greater accuracy than single-instrument evaluation. In addition, many of these instruments will find use in the evaluation of limb ischemia, especially in the perioperative period.

Prosthetics

Three current areas of prosthetic development show promise: the emergence of ultralightweight and throwaway or temporary or intermediate prostheses (Fig. 64.27); the design and development of energy-absorbing and energy-returning prosthetic components (designed to return energy on toe-off), as exemplified by the Seattle-Boeing-Burgess foot and the Flex-Foot; and new fabrication techniques such as flexible sockets (ISNY socket [New York University Medical Center, Prosthetics and Orthotics, New York]), flexible suction sockets (Iceross sockets, Össur, Reykjauk, Iceland), and nonquadrilateral or medial-lateral–contoured above-knee sockets. The use of new plastics, fiberglass casting tapes, and carbon fiber polymers is allowing the construction of ultralight-weight yet rugged, durable prostheses. These prostheses have obvious value for geriatric amputees in terms of energy-saving characteristics, especially for high-level amputees, but they also have value for young, active amputees engaging in sports or water-related activities. Lightweight prostheses constructed with these new materials are often easier to fabricate than standard plastic laminate prostheses. Artificial limbs constructed with fiberglass casting tapes, such as 3M Scotchcast, allow a decrease in skin temperature at the socket-skin interface because of the porous nature of the casting material. Preliminary work by my group demonstrated a 5°C to 7°C drop in skin temperature with 3M Scotchcast PTB below-knee prostheses compared with standard plastic laminate PTB below-knee prostheses. The importance of decreased skin temperature is unknown with respect to stump durability, but there is no question that these prostheses result in improved patient comfort in hot, humid climates.

Increasing numbers of studies are now being done with young, active amputees to improve their performance abilities in activities such as running, jumping, and other sports functions.[172] Projects such as this point toward future improvements in prosthetic devices and toward future research efforts, perhaps leading to greater efficiency with which amputees conduct their physical activities.

Surgery

A number of articles in the surgical literature describe arterial reconstruction with free tissue transfer to save limb length,[173,174] myofasciocutaneous flaps to improve stump healing and prosthesis utilization,[175] and foot salvage and avoidance of major lower limb amputations in diabetic patients.[176] In 45 patients with gangrenous lesions of the foot or lower leg due to severe diabetic arterial disease resulting in extensive soft tissue defects with exposed bones or tendons, Vermassen and van Landuyt reported excellent clinical results with arterial reconstruction and combined free tissue transfer.[173] The combined survival and limb salvage rate was 84% after 1 year, 77% after 2 years, and 65% after 3 years. The articles cited are only a small fraction of the published literature, and interested readers can find many more publications using PubMed and doing Internet searches on amputation and skin flaps. The combination of distal vascular reconstruction and free flap utilization, rotational flaps, and other techniques for closure of soft tissue defects of the extremities all offer exciting opportunities for extended limb salvage and avoidance of major limb amputation, especially in patients with diabetes.

NEW CONCEPTS IN LOWER LIMB AMPUTATION

Inflammatory Markers

Recently, inflammatory markers have been studied in order to assist with prediction of amputation levels in patients with lower limb osteomyelitis. Procalcitonin is a hormone precursor released by the follicular cells of the thyroid which is specific for bacterial infection. It is released in response to bacterial toxis by polymorphonuclear cells when infection is present. Reiner and colleagues reviewed procalcitonin levels in 156 consecutive patients and demonstrated higher levels in patients requiring above and/or below knee amputations. They concluded that procalcitonin may be used as a marker to predict amputation level in patients with osteomyelitis.[177]

Saskin and colleagues examined levels of C-reactive protein and mean platelet volume in patients with acute arterial occlusions at their facility. A total of 123 patients underwent thromboembolectomy due to acute embolism in their series. The authors demonstrated that higher levels of C-reactive protein and mean platelet volume were detected as independent risk factors for early extremity amputation after regression analysis.[178]

OUTCOMES FOLLOWING AMPUTATION FOR COMBAT-RELATED INJURY

Recent studies have focused on functional and mental health outcomes following combat-related trauma in military personnel. Ladlow and colleagues recently examined 100 procedures at a UK military complex trauma rehabilitation center. Outcome measures included: mobility and activities of daily living scores, depression, mental health assessments, and pain scores. The authors demonstrated that the unilateral amputation group demonstrated a significant functional advantage over patients who underwent limb salvage procedures and bilateral amputations. They also noted that patients who elected for delayed amputation following limb salvage achieved improved outcomes compared with the limb salvage and immediate amputation groups.[179]

A study by Doukas and colleagues evaluated 324 service members deployed to Afghanistan or Iraq who sustained lower-limb injury or limb salvage. Clinical instruments were used to measure depression, posttraumatic stress disorder, chronic pain, and engagement in sports and leisure activities. Subjects who underwent amputation had better scores in all Short Musculoskeletal Function Assessment (SMFA) measures than patients who had undergone limb salvage. Both groups were equal with regard to depression, chronic pain, and work/school status. The authors did warn that caution is needed when interpreting these results due to possible selection bias.[180]

ACKNOWLEDGMENT

Thanks to James M. Malone, MD, for his work on a previous edition of this chapter.

REVIEW QUESTIONS

1. What is the best overall approach to postamputation prosthetic care and rehabilitation?
   - **a.** Conventional soft dressings
   - **b.** Rigid dressings
   - **c.** Immediate postoperative prosthetics
   - **d.** Rigid dressings with early ambulation
   - **e.** Soft dressings with early ambulation
2. The advantages of a rigid dressing (without an attached prosthesis) after major lower extremity amputation include all of the following except
   - **a.** Control of stump edema
   - **b.** Protection of the wound from trauma
   - **c.** Stump immobilization
   - **d.** Prevention of joint flexion contracture
   - **e.** Accelerated stump maturity
3. Which of the following statements about amputees or amputation rehabilitation is false?
   - **a.** The risk of contralateral limb loss in the 5 years following major lower extremity amputation is greater than 25%
   - **b.** The 5-year life expectancy for patients with diabetes after major lower extremity amputation is less than 50%
   - **c.** Above-knee amputations should be performed in all geriatric patients because of their poor prognosis for successful rehabilitation
   - **d.** When noninvasive amputation level selection techniques are used, primary healing can be expected in more than 90% of all below-knee amputations
   - **e.** None of the above

4. Which of the following statements about amputation surgery or amputees is true?
   a. Clinical judgment is the best technique for amputation level selection
   b. There is no benefit to the patient in performing a knee disarticulation amputation
   c. Amputees reduce their walking speed to control energy expenditure
   d. The successful rehabilitation of bilateral above-knee amputees is common
   e. None of the above
5. Which of the following therapeutic maneuvers is often successful for the treatment of phantom pain?
   a. Surgical stump revision
   b. Psychotherapy
   c. Narcotics
   d. Physical therapy
   e. None of the above
6. Amputation level selection techniques such as transcutaneous oxygen measurement can also be used in which of the following situations?
   a. Intraoperatively
   b. Postoperatively
   c. To evaluate or quantitate the degree of ischemia
   d. All of the above
7. Which statement about major lower extremity amputation is false?
   a. Eighty percent of all patients with a below-knee amputation will heal
   b. Two thirds of patients undergoing amputation surgery have cardiovascular disease
   c. The best amputation level selection technique is a combination of clinical judgment and preoperative arteriography
   d. It takes at least twice as much energy for an above-knee amputee to walk as for a below-knee amputee
   e. Any patient ambulating before amputation can ambulate after amputation, irrespective of age
8. What is the most common cause of major lower extremity amputation?
   a. Failed vascular reconstruction
   b. Trauma
   c. Ischemia
   d. Tumor
   e. Complications of diabetes mellitus
9. Which of the following statements about major lower extremity amputation is false?
   a. Most amputations are caused by complications of peripheral vascular disease or diabetes mellitus
   b. The average rate of ambulation after major lower extremity amputation is 60%
   c. Occlusion of the superficial femoral artery is the most common arterial lesion that leads to below-knee amputation
   d. Patients, especially those with diabetes mellitus, who have undergone successful amputation have a decreased life expectancy
   e. There is no difference in healing between patients with diabetes and those without diabetes
10. Which of the following statements is true?
    a. Amputation surgery is reconstructive surgery
    b. Amputation surgery may be preferable to extended distal bypass or multiple revisions of below-knee distal bypass if good rehabilitation treatment is available
    c. Patient education and foot care of the nonamputated extremity are important
    d. Optimal results after lower extremity amputation require amputation level selection techniques and early or rapid postamputation rehabilitation
    e. All of the above

BIBLIOGRAPHY

Bowker JH, San Giovanni TP, Pinzur MS. North American experience with knee disarticulation with use of a posterior myofasciocutaneous flap: Healing rate and functional results in seventy-seven patients. *J Bone Joint Surg Am.* 2000;82:1571–1574.

Burgess EM, Romano RL. The management of lower extremity amputees using immediate postsurgical prostheses. *Clin Orthop.* 1968;57:137–156.

Chang BB, Bock DE, Jacobs RL, et al. Increased limb salvage by the use of unconventional foot amputations. *J Vasc Surg.* 1994;19: 341–348.

Early JS. Transmetatarsal and midfoot amputations. *Clin Orthop.* 1999;361:85–90.

Flores Rivera AR. Risk factors for amputation in diabetic patients: a case-control study. *Arch Med Res.* 1998;29:179–184.

Hirsch G, McBride ME, Murray DD, et al. Chopart prosthesis and semirigid orthosis in traumatic forefoot amputations: Comparative gait analysis. *Am J Phys Med Rehabil.* 1996;75: 283–291.

Koch M, Kutkuhn B, Grabensee B, et al. Apolipoprotein A, fibrinogen, age, and history of stroke are predictors of death in dialysed diabetic patients: a prospective study in 412 subjects. *Nephrol Dial Transplant.* 1997;12:2603–2611.

Lehto S, Ronnemaa T, Pyorala K, et al. Risk factors predicting lower extremity amputations in patients with NIDDM. *Diabetes Care.* 1996;19:607–612.

Lutz BS, Siemers F, Shen ZL, et al. Free flap to the arteria peronea magna for lower limb salvage. *Plast Reconstr Surg.* 2000;105: 684–687.

Malone JM. Revascularization versus amputation. In: Rutherford R, ed. *Vascular Surgery.* 5th ed. Philadelphia: WB Saunders; 2000: 2255–2266.

Misuri A, Lucertini G, Nanni A, et al. Predictive value of transcutaneous oximetry for selection of amputation level. *J Cardiovasc Surg (Torino).* 2000;41:83–87.

Moore JC, Jolly GP. Soft tissue considerations in partial foot amputations. *Clin Podiatr Med Surg*. 2000;17:631–648.

Muhlhauser I, Overmann H, Bender R, et al. Predictors of mortality and end-stage diabetic complications in patients with type 1 diabetes mellitus on intensified insulin therapy. *Diabet Med*. 2000;17:727–734.

Naylor AR, Hayes PD, Darke S. A prospective audit of complex wound and graft infections in Great Britain and Ireland: the emergence of MRSA. *Eur J Vasc Surg*. 2001;21:289–294.

Reyzelman AM, Hadi S, Armstrong DG. Limb salvage with Chopart's amputation and tendon balancing. *J Am Podiatr Med Assoc*. 1999; 89:100–103.

Sanders LJ. Transmetatarsal and midfoot amputations. *Clin Podiatr Med Surg*. 1997;14:741–762.

Tepel M, van der Giet M, Schwarzfeld C, et al. Prevention of radiographic-contrast-agent-induced reductions in renal function by acetylcysteine. *N Engl J Med*. 2000;343:210–212.

Vermassen FE, van Landuyt K. Combined vascular reconstruction and free flap transfer in diabetic arterial disease. *Diabetes Metab Res Rev*. 2000;16(suppl 1):S33–S36.

Wrobel JS, Mayfield JA, Reiber GE. Geographic variation of lower-extremity major amputation in individuals with and without diabetes in the Medicare population. *Diabetes Care*. 2001;24:860–864.

References available online at ExpertConsult.com.

CHAPTER 65

Anterior Spine Exposure: Operative Techniques for the Vascular Surgeon

Palma M. Shaw, William J. Quiñones-Baldrich

INTRODUCTION

The optimal approach to thoracic, lumbar, and sacral spine exposure depends upon the pathology to be addressed, the level or levels being treated, the patient's other comorbid factors, and the experience of the operator and other team members conducting the procedure. Newer approaches to manage degenerative spondylosis, neural decompression, metastatic and primary tumors of the spine, traumatic fractures, osteomyelitis, and congenital anomalies can be more directly managed via an anterior approach to the spine. The responsibility to safely expose the required levels is that of the access surgeon who most often is a vascular surgeon. Thoracic spine exposure may involve a thoracic surgeon and cervical exposure is most often managed by the spine surgeons. Wide exposure may be necessary requiring mobilization of the thoracic or abdominal aorta, vena cava, iliac artery, or veins. In an effort to minimize complications, preoperative considerations, including the presence of atherosclerosis, history of venous thrombosis, reoperative surgery, obesity, and other co-morbid factors, should be included in the planned approach. Communication between the spine specialist and the access surgeon is essential. Familiarity with the various instrumentations is important so that the access provided is adequate for the particular intervention planned. Although slight anterolateral exposure of the intervertebral disc is adequate for some fusions, true anterior exposure is required for disc replacement and fusions with a cage. Major vascular complications can be avoided with meticulous technique and adjunctive use of specialized retractors, which can optimize exposure while minimizing dissection. Noted complications associated with the anterior approach include vascular injury, thromboembolism, injury to the sympathetic nerve plexus resulting in retrograde ejaculation, lymph leak (lymphocele), ureter or bowel injury, ileus, and infection.[1] The incidence of reported vascular injury ranges from under 1% to 24% and almost double that in redo exposures where hardware removal is required.[2-5] This chapter will present the technique for anterior spine exposure of the more common levels and the principles involved in planning exposure of the spine for instrumentation. Potential complications and their management will be discussed.

PATIENT PLACEMENT

The patient is placed supine on the operating fluoroscopy table. It is imperative that the patient be straight and not rotated. An inflatable airbag behind the lumbar spine can be helpful at times by opening the disc space but should not be routinely inflated. Overinflation can lead to stretching of the vascular structures making them more difficult to mobilize. We prefer to stand on the patient's left side because visualization during exposure of the spine will initially be at an angle from left to right. The fluoroscopy unit is cephalad to the surgeons allowing its intermittent use (Fig. 65.1). An oxygen monitor sensor placed in the left first toe is very useful to monitor return of circulation to the left lower extremity after completion of the procedure (Fig. 65.2). The pulses are examined for comparison at the end of the procedure.

INCISION

Incision placement is a very critical component of anterior spine exposure. It must take into account the angle of the intervertebral disc space so that the spine surgeon has visualization of the posterior part of the space, which helps avoid injuring the dura. This will allow thorough discectomy, which is an essential component of the intervention. The level L5 to S1 is particularly critical because the incision is often several centimeters below the location of the disc space (Fig. 65.3). Nevertheless, the space angle should be taken into consideration for any level. Although the anterior and lateral plain x-ray can be used together with skin landmarks (Fig. 65.4), lateral fluoroscopy with the use of a radiopaque marker gives the most precise location for the incision (Fig. 65.5).

For single-level exposure, a transverse incision is preferred. For multiple levels, an up-and-down longitudinal incision is necessary (see Fig. 65.3). Generous separation of the subcutaneous tissue medial, superior, lateral, and inferior to the incision allows the skin incision to remain relatively small because it permits movement as necessary. The anterior rectus sheath is then incised in an oblique manner. We prefer to curve the distal medial aspect of the anterior rectus sheath incision across the midline. This releases tension of the linea alba to allow for true anterior exposure. In all instances, the exposure of the posterior rectus sheath, particularly for multiple levels, should be medial to the rectus belly to avoid rectus denervation. The inferior epigastric vessels are carefully preserved. When the exposure is below the semilunar line, the fibers of the transversalis can be bluntly separated laterally to enter the retroperitoneal space. This is most often the case for exposure of the L5 to S1 level (Fig. 65.6). For levels requiring entrance above the semilunar line, the posterior

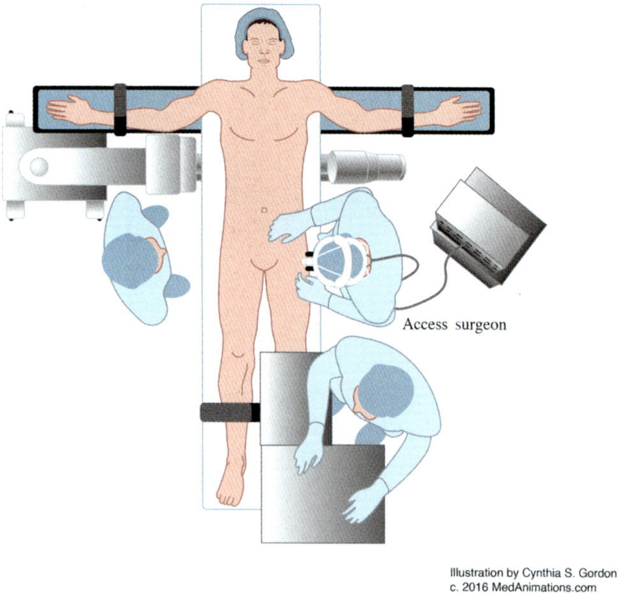

FIG 65.1 Operating room positioning of fluoroscopy equipment and surgeon for spine exposure.

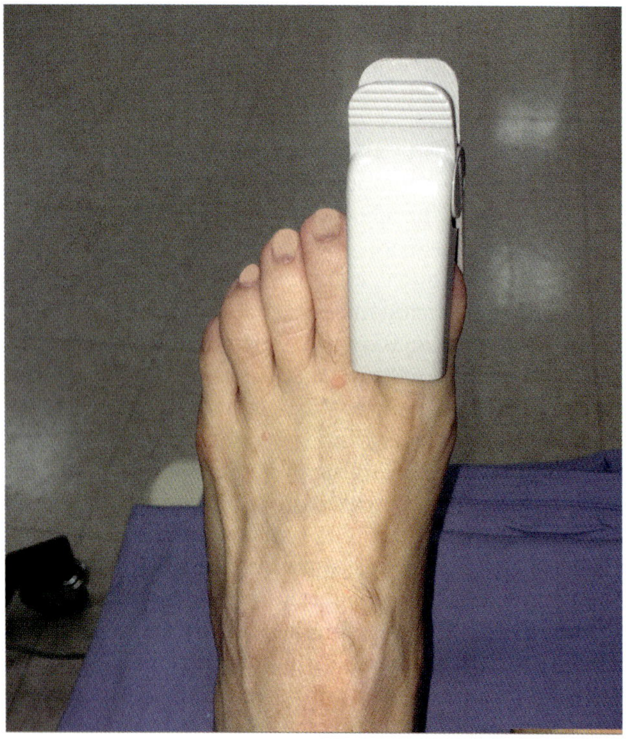

FIG 65.2 Oxygen monitor sensor placed in the left first toe.

rectus sheath is incised and the peritoneum separated to start entering the retroperitoneal space. The more medial the incision on the posterior rectus sheath, the thinner the peritoneum and the greater likelihood of entering the intraperitoneal space. It is therefore best to keep the incision of the posterior rectus sheath at least 2 to 3 cm from the midline. The peritoneum is then separated from the abdominal wall making sure that as the dissection deepens, it stays anterior to the psoas muscle (Fig. 65.7).

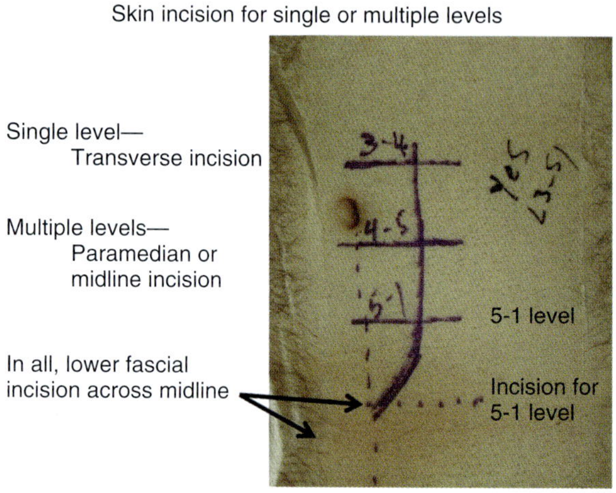

FIG 65.3 Skin incision for single or multiple levels.

Care should be taken to avoid injury to the genitofemoral and the ilioinguinal nerve. The ureter should stay attached to the peritoneum and is retracted medially together with it. Further dissection will depend on the desired level to be exposed. Use of a table-attached retractor is highly recommended (Fig. 65.8).

The access surgeon should remain attentive during the instrumentation by the spine team and re-place the position of the retractors if they are disturbed. This is critical to avoid injury to the surrounding mobilized structures during the actual instrumentation of the spine.

EXPOSURE OF L5 TO S1

Once the peritoneum has been separated from the abdominal wall, the iliac vessels are seen and for the level L5 to S1 are left in place and the exposure most often carried between the right and left iliac vessels. Further separation of the peritoneum is carried out below the aortic and caval bifurcation. Following the proper tissue plane, the iliac vein is separated from the peritoneum and the middle sacral vessels exposed. Use of the cautery in this area should be limited to avoid injury to the sympathetic nerves. The middle sacral vessels are ligated and divided allowing further mobilization of the iliac vein and aortic bifurcation. Smaller venous tributaries can be cauterized with bipolar forceps. The left common iliac vein is then separated from the anterior longitudinal ligament and the right common iliac vein mobilized laterally, which most often can be done with blunt dissection. Use of a peanut dissector is very useful in these maneuvers. A reversed lip retractor is then placed and engaged in the vertebral body retracting all the structures to the right side. Additional superior inferior and left retractors then complete the exposure. A needle is placed in the center of the disc space and its location examined with fluoroscopy to assure proper identification of the correct level and the exact center of the disc space.

On occasion, the L5 to S1 disc space will be higher than usual, in which case, the exposure is similar to the L4 to L5 (see later). We have seen instances where the level is right behind the caval bifurcation making it hazardous to expose. In such a case, aborting the procedure may be the better option.

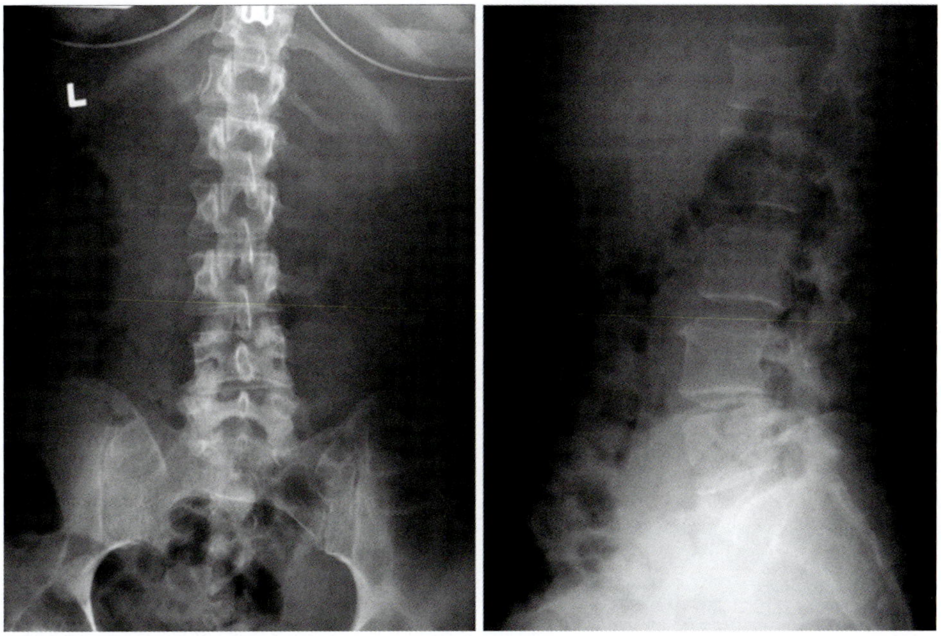

FIG 65.4 Anterior and lateral plain x-ray. Note the angle of the disc spaces, which will dictate the location of the skin incision.

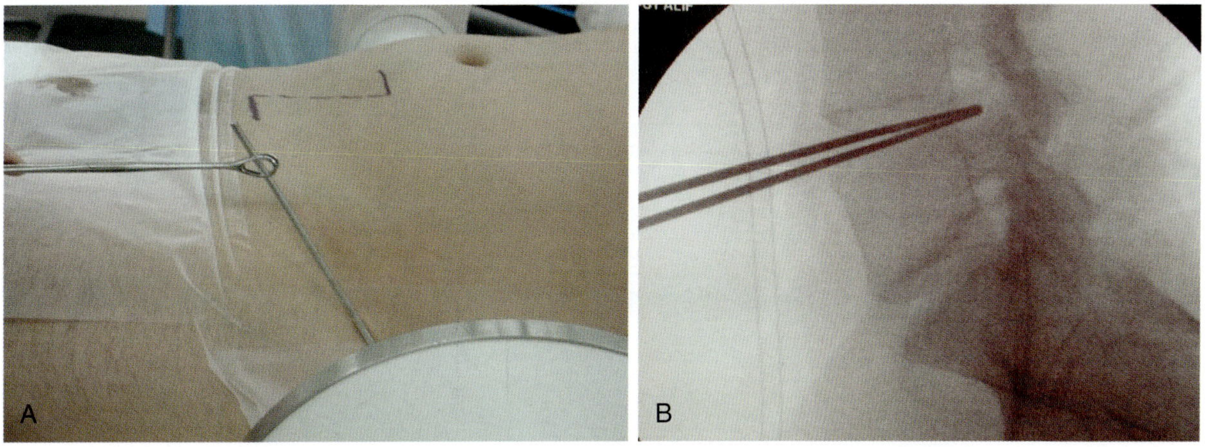

FIG 65.5 (A) Skin landmarks. (B) Lateral fluoroscopy with the use of a radiopaque marker to determine location of the skin incision to account for the angle of the disc space.

Upon completion of the instrumentation, the integrity of the iliac vessels is examined, the femoral pulse documented, and the oxygen saturation by the pulse oximeter in the left foot noted. The peritoneum is allowed to return to its anatomic position. In this particular level, there is usually no posterior sheath to close. The anterior rectus sheath is closed with a 0 absorbable suture in a running fashion. The fascia of Scarpa is closed with a 2-0 absorbable suture and the skin with a subcuticular stitch.

EXPOSURE OF L4 TO L5

The incision is placed according to lateral fluoroscopy taking into account the angle of the intervertebral disc space. Most often for the L4 to L5 disc space, the posterior rectus sheath needs to be incised from above to below the semilunar line. It is best to start the separation of the peritoneum laterally and superiorly and then continue down and medially. Otherwise the initial steps of this exposure are similar to the L5 to S1 approach. The main difference is that the L4 to L5 level is best exposed by retracting the common and external iliac artery and vein medially (see Fig. 65.8). It is best to keep the artery and vein together without separating them from each other. Once the psoas muscle is exposed, the proper tissue plane of the common and external iliac artery is followed mostly with blunt dissection. The common iliac artery from its origin down to the external iliac is fully mobilized. Small tributaries from the external and common iliac artery should be cauterized using bipolar forceps. The common iliac vein is then identified posteromedial to the artery. As the

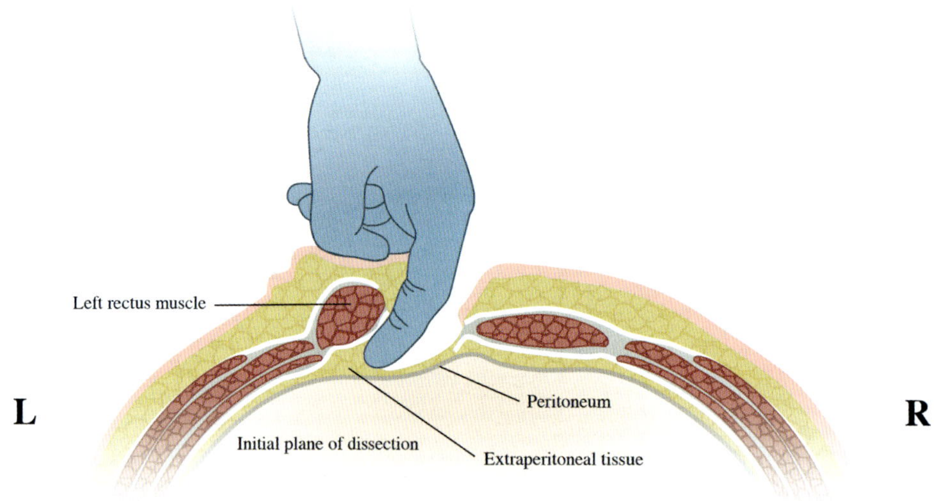

FIG 65.6 Fibers of the transversalis can be bluntly separated laterally to enter the retroperitoneal space. (Illustration by Cynthia S. Gordon. © 2016 MedAnimations.com)

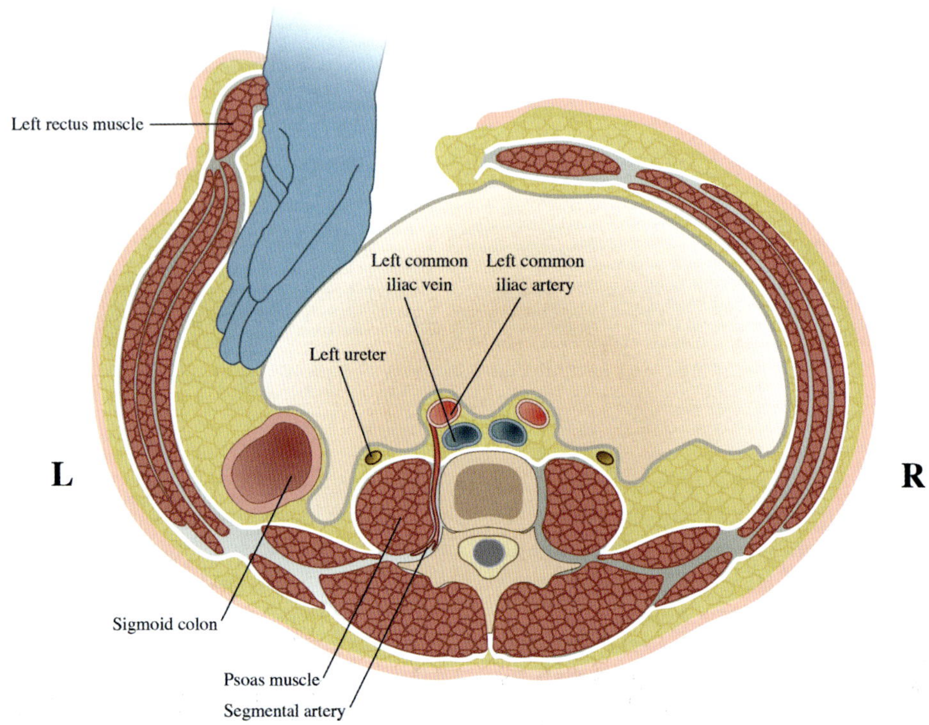

FIG 65.7 Separation of the peritoneum from the abdominal wall making sure that it stays anterior to the psoas muscle. (Illustration by Cynthia S. Gordon. © 2016 MedAnimations.com)

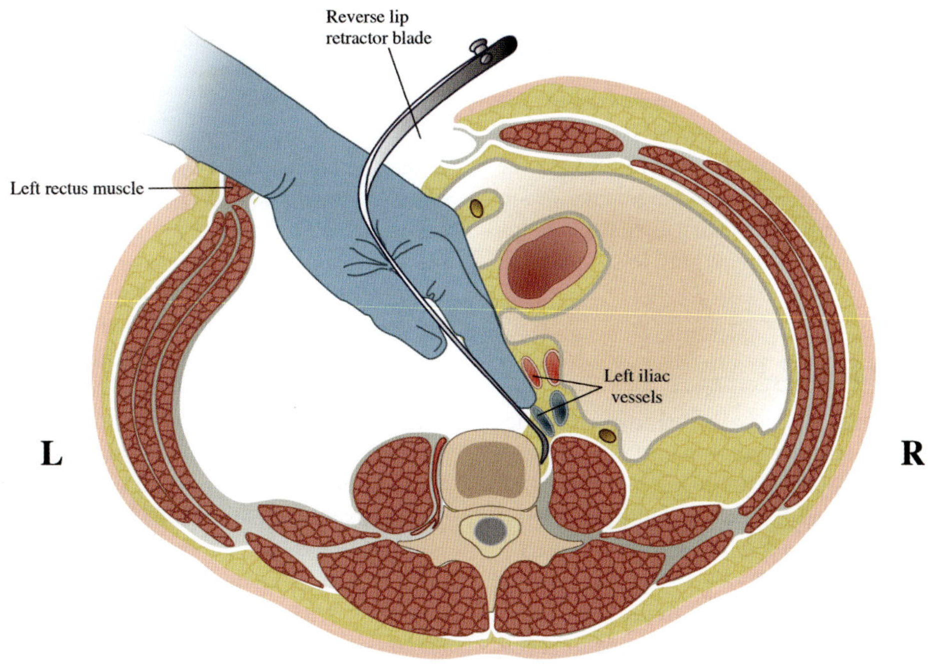

FIG 65.8 Table-attached reverse lip retractor (Brau blades) placed to the right of the vertebral body to retract vascular structures, ureter, and peritoneum. (Illustration by Cynthia S. Gordon. © 2016 MedAnimations.com)

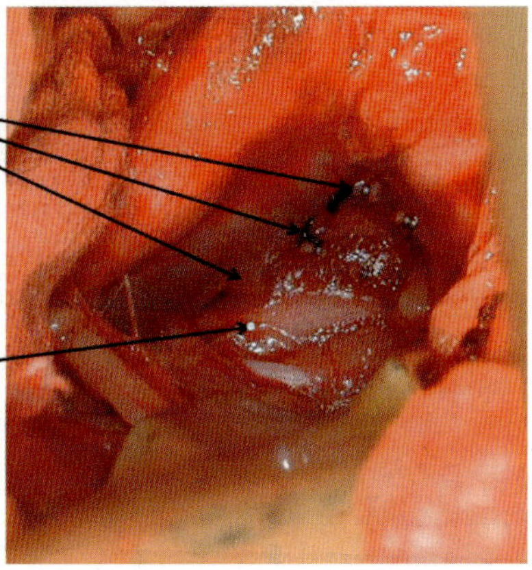

FIG 65.9 Iliolumbar vein. Note the proximity of the obturator nerve.

proper tissue plane is followed, one will encounter the iliolumbar vein (Fig. 65.9). This is a critical step in exposure of this level. In at least 20% of the instances, the iliolumbar vein can be multiple or bifurcates early. With very careful dissection this vein is encircled and must be ligated and divided. The obturator nerve can be in close proximity and its injury should be avoided during iliolumbar vein ligation (see Fig. 65.9). More proximally, one or two lumbar arteries and veins need to be ligated and divided to move the aorta medially. Care should be taken to avoid tearing these segmental vessels because they often retract and make control of bleeding difficult. It is best to identify them. Most of this exposure can be done bluntly with a peanut dissector. Once the spine is identified, sharp incision of the tissue in front of it allows for easy blunt exposure. A reversed lip retractor is then placed to the right side of the intervertebral disc space and the structures retracted to the right (see Fig. 65.8). Superior inferior and left-sided retractors then complete the exposure. Similar to the L5 to S1 exposure, placing a needle in the center of the disc and examination under fluoroscopy is a critical step to assure identification of the correct level.

During instrumentation, the arterial circulation to the left lower extremity is often compromised due to retraction of the left iliac vessels. If the instrumentation is taking longer than 45 minutes, temporary release and reexposure of the level is recommended. Upon completion of the instrumentation, the integrity of the iliac vessels is assured, the left femoral pulse examined, and return of oxygen tension to preoperative levels documented. Wound closure includes reapproximation of the posterior rectus sheath up to the semilunar line. The remainder is the same as the L5 to S1 level.

EXPOSURE OF L4 TO S1

Exposure of the L4 to S1 level requires a longitudinal incision, with our preference being a paramedian angled medially in its lower portion (see Fig. 65.3). Generous mobilization of the subcutaneous tissue from the anterior rectus sheath improves the ease with which the skin can be retracted medially for anterior exposure. The anterior and posterior rectus sheaths are incised in a manner similar to the L4 to L5 exposure. Exposure then proceeds as if each level were to be exposed individually. The L5 to S1 level is exposed between the iliac vessels and the L4 to L5 level exposed by retracting the iliac vessels and aorta to the right. Again, ligation of the iliolumbar vein and segmental vessels is critical. The level that is instrumented first is the spine surgeon's choice. We complete the exposure of both levels and then proceed accordingly.

EXPOSURE OF LEVELS L2, L3

Exposure of these higher levels is rarely performed as a single-level exposure. They require a larger incision and care must be taken particularly at the L2 level to avoid injury to the renal vessels. The left crus of the diaphragm will require division. If full anterior exposure of the L2 level is required, it may be necessary to mobilize the left kidney to allow for safe retraction of the aorta. Segmental vessels are ligated and divided, usually at least one above and one below the level of the exposure. Multilevel exposure from the L2 down is similar to the lower levels.

EXPOSURE OF L1 AND THORACIC LEVELS

Anterior exposure of L1 and thoracic levels is seldom required because lateral or anterolateral access is usually sufficient. At the L1 level, division of the crus of the diaphragm is necessary. At these higher levels, care should be taken not to injure the lymphatic system (cisterna), which usually lies to the right of the vertebral body. Exposure of these levels is usually anterolateral, which requires less mobilization of the surrounding structures. In that instance, it is best to place the patient in a semilateral decubitus or lateral position.

Exposure of the lower thoracic levels may require a combination of a thoracotomy and a retroperitoneal incision. It is important to keep in mind that as the levels proceed cephalad, the size of the vertebral body decreases. Single lung ventilation may be helpful to obtain better exposure. Although levels below T5 can be exposed through a left thoracotomy, levels above that are best exposed through a right thoracotomy. In both instances, particularly on the right, care should be taken to avoid venous bleeding from the azygous or semi-azygos systems.

COMPLICATIONS

The approach of anterior spine exposure has the potential risk of major vascular injury and urogenital complications. These are uncommon and in most cases preventable with proper technique and attention to detail. Major arterial or venous complications occur in 2% of cases, and may vary from those requiring simple suture repair, to bleeding control, to major vascular injuries requiring vascular reconstruction to resolve limb ischemia. Minor vascular injuries are more often venous and most commonly resolve with temporary compression, with or without hemostatic agents, or are easily repaired. These are more common when the exposure is at L4 to L5 and are lowest when L5 to S1 alone are exposed.[6] There is an increased incidence of vascular injury and blood loss in reoperated fields (13.8%) for anterior exposure, previous spinal surgery, or presence of tumor. In one study, the most frequently injured vessel was the left common iliac vein, which accounted for more than 50% of the cases.[2] Brau and colleagues conducted a large study of more than 1300 anterior lumbar procedures and reviewed the type and incidence of vascular injury. They found an incidence of left iliac artery thrombosis (0.45%), and major vein lacerations (1.4%) with a relatively low incidence of vascular injury (1.9%). It was concluded that this type of exposure is safe with respect to vascular injury; however, the importance of careful monitoring of the pulses and O_2 saturation of the left great toe and early intervention when there was a suspicion of injury was emphasized.[7]

Several techniques can help avoid complications. Ligation of the iliolumbar vein or veins to facilitate mobilization of the left common iliac vein toward the right while exposing L4 to L5 will avoid tearing the vein and significant blood loss. Thrombosis of the left iliac artery can be decreased by extending the mobilization of the artery as close to the femoral artery as possible, allowing for less stretch on the artery. Early detection of arterial injury and interruption of blood flow to the extremity can be facilitated with pulse oximetry. This provides a baseline at the beginning of the case and can be monitored throughout. If there is suspicion of thrombosis, this can be addressed through an iliac arteriotomy before the incision is closed, or through a femoral approach if detected after wound closure.[7]

Although rare, urogenital complications of an anterior approach to the lumbosacral spine may present as impotence or sterility in males and needs to be discussed with the patient prior to the procedure as a potential complication.[8-11] It may present postoperatively as failure of normal penile erection or failure of normal ejaculation. Anatomically, the innervation of the urogenital system is via the superior hypogastric plexus (sympathetic), pelvic splanchnic (parasympathetic), and pudendal (somatic) nerves. The sympathetic nerve supply continues from the thoracolumbar sympathetics and along the anterolateral aspects of the lumbar vertebral bodies. At the level of the third and fourth lumbar vertebrae, these join the inferior mesenteric ganglion and almost 80% of these branches occur on the left side of the aorta. These fibers are then referred to as the superior hypogastric plexus because they course distally across the left common iliac artery and vein and cross the pelvic brim to reach the bladder, vas deferens, and seminal vesicles. The sympathetic nervous system has a direct effect upon normal ejaculation and its superior gastric plexus is the most at risk during this approach.[12] Parasympathetic innervation of the urogenital system is derived from the second, third, and fourth sacral segments.[13] These course well below the pelvic brim and course along the side of the rectum as the pelvic splanchnic nerve. Avoidance of dissection below the pelvic brim can prevent parasympathetic (pelvic splanchnic nerve) or pudendal nerve injury.[12] One study focused specifically on the incidence of retrograde ejaculation after anterior lumbar interbody fusion at a single level (L4 to L5 or L5 to S1) found an increased rate of occurrence of postoperative permanent retrograde ejaculation with a transperitoneal approach (10%) versus a retroperitoneal approach (0.86%).[14]

Lymphocele is a rare postoperative complication described in case reports. The differential diagnosis includes abscess, ureteral injury with urinoma, pancreatic injury with pseudocyst formation, and spinal fluid leak with pseudomeningocele.[15] The patient may present with abdominal pain, urinary urgency, or incontinence up to 4 to 6 weeks after surgery. Aspiration of the fluid collection can help with the diagnosis. This has been treated with multiple aspirations,[16] adjunctive sclerosis with povidone iodine,[17] and laparoscopic marsupialization or surgery.[15] Ureteral injury deserves mention given the proximity of the ureter to the surgical site; this is rare and consideration should be given when a patient presents with left flank pain and is found to have a perinephric fluid collection. Ureteral injury or compression can be confirmed with retrograde pyelogram.[18]

CONCLUSION

Anterior exposure of the spine is most often used for intervertebral disc fusion or replacement. The procedure is often conducted as a two-surgeon team approach, which most often includes a vascular surgeon. Understanding the procedure and potential complications can help minimize vascular complications throughout the procedure. Communication between the spine specialist and the surgeon is essential. The approach has been refined, as has the instrumentation to reduce vascular, neurologic, and urologic complications. Early recognition is important and techniques have been discussed to help identify them. Vascular surgeons are well suited to facilitate the approach and address complications when they occur.

REVIEW QUESTIONS

1. Which option is one of the most important advancements in anterior spine surgery?
   - **a.** Minimally invasive approaches for spine fractures
   - **b.** Nerve monitoring to note changes with iliac artery compression
   - **c.** Specialized retractors facilitating better exposure
   - **d.** Spine surgeons routinely performing spine exposure as a single surgeon approach
2. Of the following, which has the highest complication rate of anterior spine surgery?
   - **a.** Major arterial injury
   - **b.** Minor vascular injuries, mostly venous
   - **c.** Lymphocele
   - **d.** Ureteral injury
3. Which of these techniques can best help localize the operative site?
   - **a.** Palpation of the vertebral process over the skin and marking prior to incision
   - **b.** Anteroposterior (AP) and lateral plain x-ray
   - **c.** Palpation of the vertebral body once it has been exposed
   - **d.** Lateral fluoroscopy with a radiopaque marker
4. To facilitate the approach, which of the following is true?
   - **a.** Exposure of the posterior rectus sheath, particularly for multiple levels, should be lateral to the rectus belly.
   - **b.** For multiple levels, an up-and-down longitudinal incision is necessary.
   - **c.** Making the incision on the posterior rectus sheath more medial will lessen the likelihood of entering the intraperitoneal space?
   - **d.** Displacement of the retractors is unusual and can be easily replaced by the spine surgeon with impunity.
5. For L5 to S1 exposure, complications can be minimized by avoiding which technique?
   - **a.** Ligation of iliolumbar vessels and avoidance of cautery
   - **b.** Focused cauterization of bleeders
   - **c.** Use of blunt peanut dissection
   - **d.** Palpation of the iliac artery pulse and documentation of the oxygen saturation by the pulse oximeter in the left foot
6. For L4 to L5 disc space exposure, which of the following is true:
   - **a.** Dissection usually only requires mobilization of a portion of the common iliac artery.
   - **b.** It is best exposed by retracting the common and external iliac artery and vein laterally.
   - **c.** The pudendal nerve can be in close proximity and its injury should be avoided during iliolumbar vein ligation.
   - **d.** The posterior rectus sheath needs to be incised from above to below the semilunar line.
7. Exposure of higher vertebral levels, L2 to L3, would likely require which of the following?
   - **a.** Ligation of the segmental vessels only at the operative level
   - **b.** Division of the left crus of the diaphragm
   - **c.** Single-level exposure
   - **d.** Avoidance of mobilization of the left kidney
8. For exposures of the lower thoracic levels, which of the following is not true?
   - **a.** Levels above T5 are best exposed through a left thoracotomy.
   - **b.** May require a combination of a thoracotomy and a retroperitoneal incision.
   - **c.** Care should be taken to avoid venous bleeding from the azygous or semi-azygos systems.
   - **d.** Single lung ventilation may be helpful to obtain better exposure.

9. Which statement describes vascular injury after anterior spine exposure?
   a. It is unavoidable and should be discussed with the patient prior to the procedure.
   b. The common iliac artery is the most commonly injured vessel.
   c. It is more common when the exposure is at L4 to L5 and is lowest when L5 to S1 alone are exposed.
   d. The incidence of vascular injury is similar in virgin and reoperative fields.

10. The sympathetic nerve supply continues from the thoracolumbar sympathetics and along the anterolateral aspects of the lumbar vertebral bodies. Injury to this during anterior spine exposure causes which of the following?
    a. Lack of penile erection by dysregulation of the venous plexus at the base of the penis
    b. Problems with normal ejaculation
    c. Damage to the pudendal nerves, which control the external urethral sphincter and the muscles of the pelvic floor
    d. An incidence of retrograde ejaculation in men after anterior lumbosacral spinal surgery of 10% to 20%

References available online at expertconsult.com.

CHAPTER 66

Carotid Sinus Stimulation: Background, Technique, and Future Directions

Jeffrey B. Edwards, Karl A. Illig, John D. Bisognano

Hypertension affects more than 65 million people in the United States and is one of the most important risk factors for stroke, heart attack, vascular disease, and death. Cardiovascular risk is estimated to double with each 20 mm Hg increment above 115 mm Hg of systolic blood pressure (SBP).[1,2] Unfortunately, and despite intensive public health efforts and generally effective pharmacologic therapy, control remains poor,[3] in part because adding more antihypertensive medications after a certain point causes increased side effects while efficacy plateaus (Fig. 66.1). In addition, even optimally treated patients who demonstrate perfect compliance can remain significantly hypertensive. A reasonable estimate of those with truly resistant hypertension is 3 to 4 million Americans, and an additional 25 million escape treatment altogether (Fig. 66.2).

One of the major physiologic systems affecting blood pressure (BP) is the carotid sinus baroreflex arc. Increased pressure causes the cells at the sinus to stretch, which directly causes increased glossopharyngeal afferent activity (Fig. 66.3) and leads to three downstream effects: cardiac inhibition (decreased stroke volume and heart rate), vascular smooth muscle inhibition (vasorelaxation), and increased renal sodium and water excretion (Fig. 66.4).[4] This system is responsible for the acute hypotension and bradycardia sometimes seen after carotid stenting or endarterectomy because the sinus is stretched by outward radial force from stent placement or removal of the plaque.

HISTORY

The history of device-based therapy for hypertension has been summarized recently.[5] As early as 1958, it was reported that electrical stimulation of the carotid sinus nerve in normotensive dogs produced an acute decrease in BP,[6] and similar findings were reported in several animal models of hypertension shortly thereafter.[7] Following the original animal model report, it was demonstrated that direct electrical stimulation of the carotid sinus in humans (undergoing neck dissection for cancer) had the same results.[8]

These findings led to more thorough investigation in humans. A single case was reported in 1966 of a 40-year-old man with a BP of 260/165 mm Hg despite four medications. Bilateral stimulation (2.5 V) produced a sustained drop in pressure to 150/90 mm Hg. The device consisted of electrodes at the sinuses connected to a generator placed beneath the pectoralis muscle. The leads were subcutaneously tunneled, and the generator could be turned on or off by placing a magnet over the device, but no further modification could be performed.[9] The first series was reported in 1967 by Seymour Schwartz; he described a mean decrease in BP of 48 mm Hg in eight patients, six of whom reduced their BP medications.[10] Further clinical benefit was demonstrated by at least one other group around this time.[11] Unfortunately this treatment came at the wrong time. Most setups at this time required external power sources and communication and were therefore bulky and impractical for long-term use. In addition, pharmacologic therapy dramatically improved in this era, making the problem less acute. As a result, this concept was essentially forgotten for the remainder of the century.

This phenomenon was reevaluated largely through a large body of work by Thomas Lohmeier, a physiologist at the University of Mississippi. In a large series of animal experiments,[4,12] he was able to reconfirm that this effect was real and reproducible, was effective in normotensive as well as hypertensive (sodium-loaded and obesity models) canines, and, most importantly, was sustainable (Fig. 66.5). This work led to the formation of a company (CVRx, Inc., Minneapolis, MN) whose sole aim was to resurrect this concept using 21st-century technology. A number of trials have demonstrated the efficacy of carotid sinus stimulation in both hypertension and in heart failure,[13] and a second-generation, low-profile device (Barostim *neo*, CVRx, Inc.) has been approved for use in Europe.

Hypertension

Proof-of-concept for antihypertensive therapy via carotid sinus stimulation was demonstrated in 2003 by the BaroReflex Activating System Study (BRASS), in which 11 patients in Switzerland undergoing carotid endarterectomy were tested by direct carotid sinus stimulation. A mean drop in SBP of 18 mm Hg was observed at a maximum of 4.4 V,[14] demonstrating that this effect was reproducible in relatively normotensive humans and that clinically feasible levels of current delivered unilaterally via a small metal electrode could lower BP.

Device-Based Therapy in Hypertension Trial

The Device-Based Therapy in Hypertension Trial (DEBuT-HT) was the initial controlled feasibility trial of the commercially available, clinically practical device. Patients with resistant hypertension (SBP >160 mm Hg despite three medications, one of which included a diuretic) underwent bilateral carotid sinus exposure and lead placement. Electrodes were tunneled subcutaneously

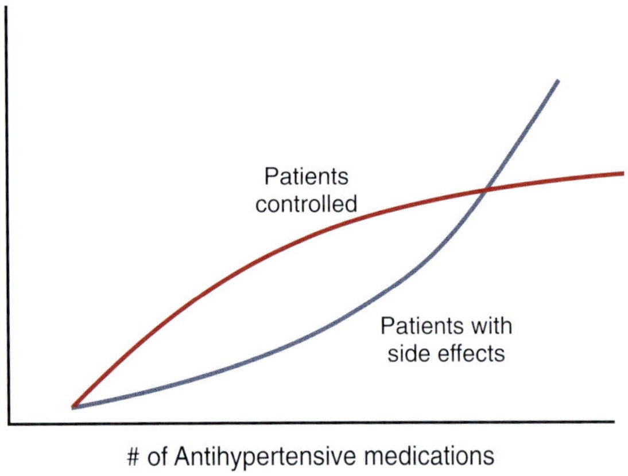

FIG 66.1 Graph illustrating the relationship between increasing numbers of antihypertensive medications (*x* axis) and effects. As the number of medications increases, there is a plateau effect for efficacy but an increase in side effects. (Courtesy CVRx, Inc., Minneapolis, Minnesota.)

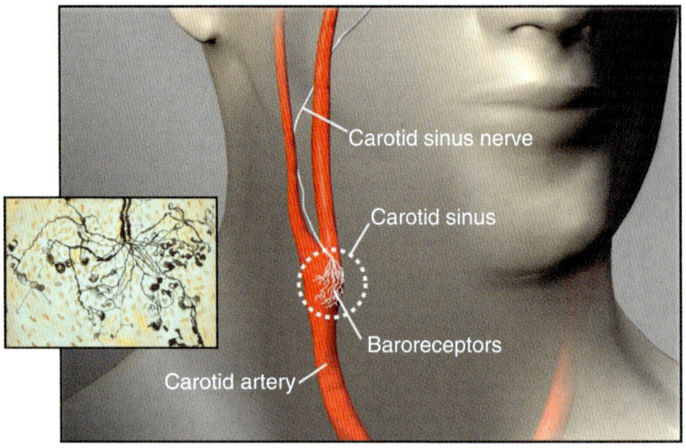

FIG 66.3 Simplified illustration of the carotid sinus baroreceptor arc in humans. The baroreceptors *(inset)* at the carotid sinus sense stretch and increase glossopharyngeal nerve activity via the carotid sinus nerve (nerve of Herring). (Courtesy CVRx, Inc., Minneapolis, Minnesota.)

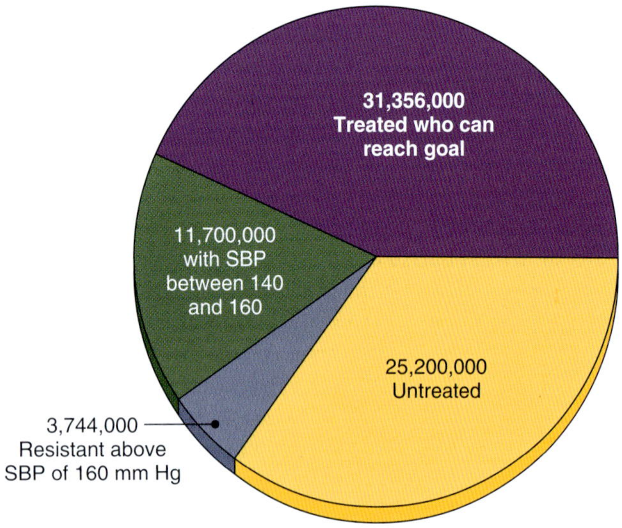

FIG 66.2 Proportions and numbers of Americans in various stages and categories of treatment for hypertension. *SBP,* Systolic blood pressure. (Courtesy CVRx, Inc., Minneapolis, Minnesota. Derived from Cushman WC, Ford CE, Cutler JA, et al: Success and predictors of blood pressure control in diverse North American settings: the Antihypertensive and Lipid-Lowering treatment to prevent Heart Attack Trial [ALLHAT]. *J Clin Hypertension* 4:393–404, 2002; and Hajjar I, Kotchen TA: Trends in prevalence, awareness, treatment, and control of hypertension in the United States, 1988-2000. *J Am Med Assoc* 290:199–206, 2003.)

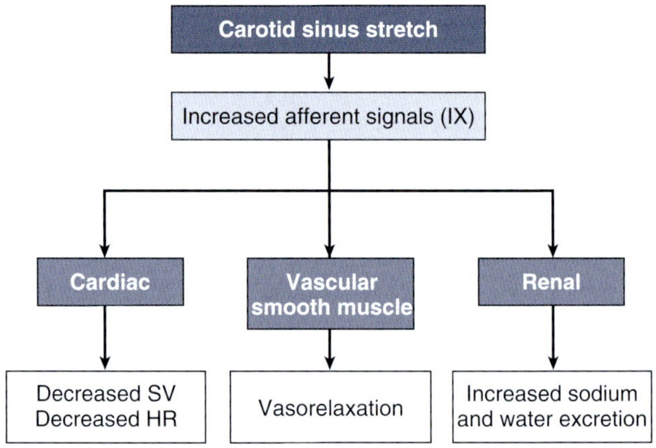

FIG 66.4 Schematic diagram of the effects of the baroreflex receptor arc. *HR,* Heart rate; *SV,* stroke volume. (Modified from Illig KA, Bisognano J: *Carotid Stimulation for Hypertension,* Shelton, CT, 2010, People's Medical Publishing House.)

and attached to a pulse generator implanted in the chest wall (Fig. 66.6). A total of 45 patients were enrolled in this trial, which was performed in Europe starting in 2006. Results on 18 patients after 4 years of therapy were presented in 2010 at the 20th annual meeting of the European Society of Hypertension in Oslo, Norway, and published in abstract form.[15] BP response was sustained, and mean reductions were impressive: 53 ± 9 mm Hg in SBP, 30 ± 6 mm Hg in diastolic pressure, and 5 ± 2 beats per minute in heart rate (Fig. 66.7). Encouragingly, patients were able to decrease their antihypertensive medications

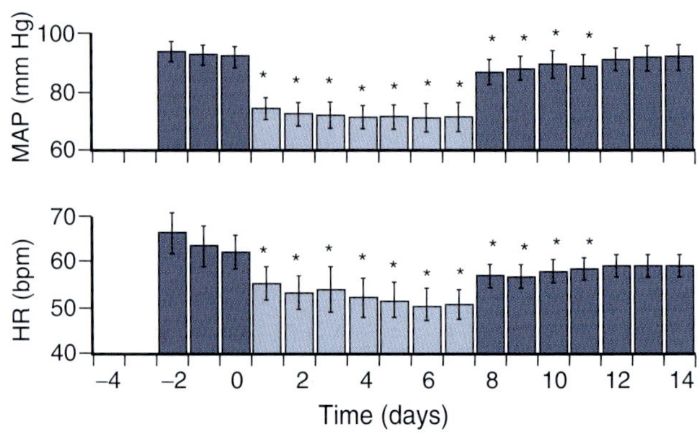

FIG 66.5 Sustained (>7 days) blood pressure and heart rate response to carotid sinus stimulation in normal canines. *Gray shaded bars* denote stimulation; an *asterisk* denotes a significant drop. *HR,* Heart rate; *MAP,* mean arterial pressure. (From Lohmeier TE, Irwin ED, Rossing MA, et al: Prolonged activation of the baroreflex produces sustained hypotension. *Hypertension* 43:306–311, 2004.)

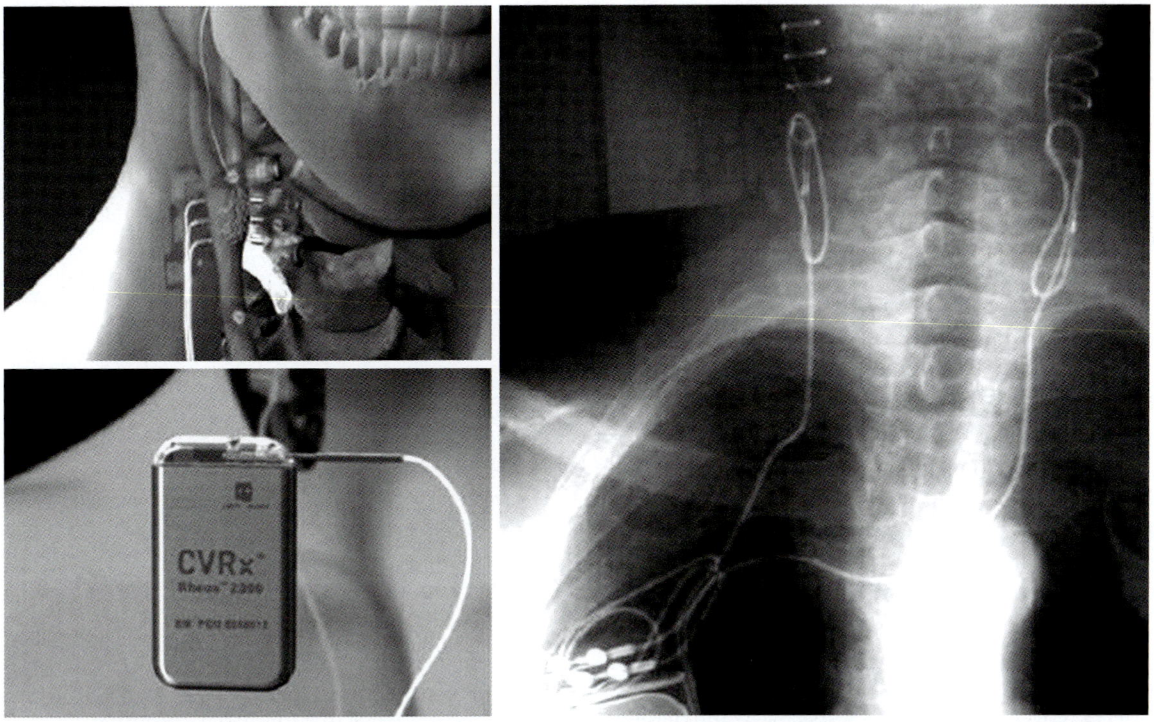

FIG 66.6 Illustration of the original Rheos System implantation for the DEBuT-HT study. *Upper left,* Leads are wrapped around the carotid sinus bilaterally. *Lower left,* Pulse generator (before implantation) and electrode. *Right,* Plain radiograph of patient following implantation. Current practice is to bring the contralateral lead across the neck rather than the chest to allow for future sternotomy. (Courtesy CVRx, Inc., Minneapolis, Minnesota. From Illig KA, Bisognano J: *Carotid Stimulation for Hypertension*, Shelton, CT, 2010, People's Medical Publishing House, pp 25-34.)

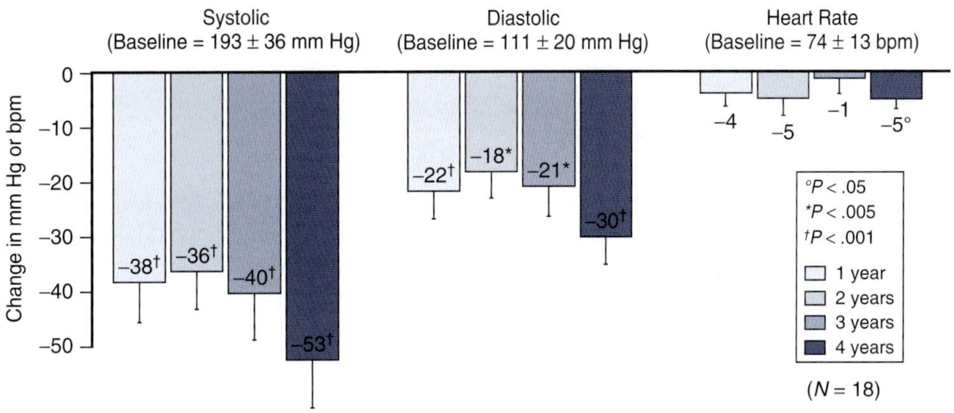

FIG 66.7 Graphic results for 18 of 45 patients enrolled in the Device-Based Therapy in Hypertension Trial study who reached 4 years of stimulation. These results are achieved in the context of a decrease in medication. (Modified from Kroon A, Schmidli J, Scheffers I, et al: Chronically implanted system: 4-year data of Rheos DEBuT-HT study in patients with resistant hypertension. *J Hypertension* 28:278, 2010.)

by approximately one-third (5 ± 1.3 medications at onset to 3.4 ± 1 medications at 4 years).

Rheos Feasibility

Formal testing of the Rheos System (CVRx, Inc.) began in 2006. A total of 16 patients (10 in the United States) were implanted in the phase II feasibility trial. The trial was primarily focused on safety and feasibility, which were both shown to be acceptable.[12] Results were generally combined with those from the DEBuT-HT and the Rheos Pivotal Trial as appropriate; however, after 12 months of therapy, mean systolic ambulatory pressures fell from 171 to 157 mm Hg, and patients spent 20% more time with SBPs less than 140 mm Hg.[16] No injury to or midterm abnormalities of the carotid arteries were identified.[17]

Rheos Pivotal Trial

The Rheos Pivotal Trial was a phase III prospective randomized trial approved by the US Food and Drug Administration (FDA) and designed to prove efficacy in a blinded, randomized, controlled fashion. The device itself, implantation technique, and trial eligibility (SBP > 160 mm Hg despite three medications, one being a diuretic) were the same as for the DEBuT-HT and the Rheos Feasibility Trial. Patients underwent implantation, and the device was turned off for 4 weeks to allow healing. Next, patients were randomized in a 2:1 ratio (study sites and investigators were blinded) to "on" or "off" for the next 6 months, then all patients were "on" for months 7 to 12. The major study endpoints were differences in BP after the 6-month randomization period between those receiving therapy and those whose devices were off, an improvement in BP at 12 months in patients whose devices had been off, and an overall improvement at 12 months versus enrollment baseline in the entire cohort.[18]

Enrollment was completed in late 2009, with 322 patients treated (55 rolled in, 265 randomized). Unblinding occurred in late 2010, and the results have recently been published.[19] Initially "on" and "off" groups were similar at baseline, having mean SBPs of 179 ± 22 and 176 ± 22 mm Hg, respectively, and diastolic BPs greater than 100 mm Hg despite taking an average of 5.2 ± 2 medications. After initial discussions with the FDA, endpoints had been decided to be the percentage of patients achieving a response of 10 mm Hg or greater rather than the absolute BP response. After the first 6 months, 54% of the "on" group showed such a response; however, 46% of the "off" group did as well, illustrating the interaction of the Hawthorne effect combined with a fairly small goal. This difference, at 7.7%, fell below the a priori target of a 20% response rate; however, after 12 months of therapy (all patients being "on" for at least 6 months), sustained improvement was seen in 88% of patients, well above the a priori target of 65% ($P < .001$). Six months of device therapy led to a 40% reduction in hypertensive crises and a 23% reduction in overall hypertension-associated adverse events ($P < .001$). Implantation and therapy were well tolerated, with a 4.4% permanent nerve injury (much of it from peri-incisional numbness) being the most significant complication. Long-term device-related adverse events, at 13%, fell below the a priori target of 28% ($P < .001$). The absolute mean decreases in SBP were 16 ± 29 mm Hg and 9 ± 29 mm Hg in the "on" and "off" groups, respectively. At the 12-month time point, mean decreases in SBP were 25 ± 32 mm Hg and 25 ± 31 mm Hg for those receiving 12 months and 6 months of total therapy, respectively, demonstrating a sustained effect (Fig. 66.8).[19]

Narrowly interpreted in light of a priori agreed-upon categorical endpoints (the percentage of patients who achieved a drop in SBP of ≥10 mm Hg), the goal of a 20% improvement was not seen. However, 80% of patients as a whole responded, 54% met this goal, and mean BP fell by 35 mm Hg; the outcome was negative because more patients in the "off" group did better than expected under care by the "hypertension professionals" involved in this study. As such, the FDA recommended that the study should continue to follow all patients until they had received at least 12 months of therapy and that all consenting patients

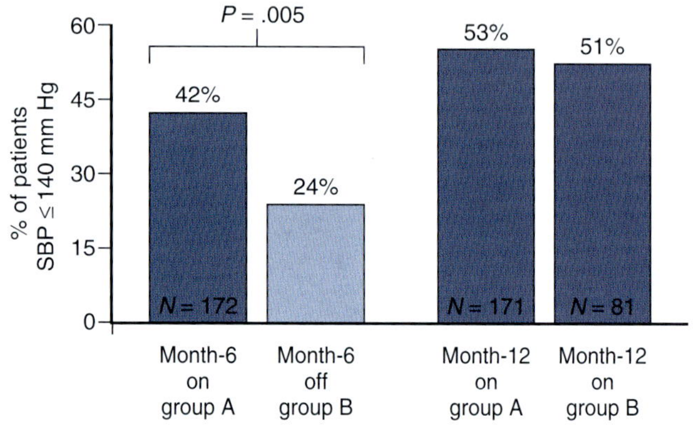

FIG 66.8 Percentage of patients in the Rheos Pivotal Trial whose systolic blood pressure *(SBP)* is less than 140 mm Hg. *Left,* 172 patients *(shaded column)* undergoing stimulation (group A) versus 81 *(white column)* without activation (group B) after 6 months. *Right,* All patients at 12 months. (Modified from Bisognano J, Sica D, Nadim M, et al: Results from the Rheos pivotal trial. *Oral presentation,* Sixtieth Annual American College of Cardiology Annual Meeting, New Orleans, 2011.)

should receive active therapy after 12 months until battery depletion. Of the initial 322 patients, 276 implanted with the Rheos device consented to participate. At an average follow-up date of 28 ± 9 months (maximum 53 months), 88% of patients were clinically significant responders (20 mm Hg drop in SBP or at goal). Characteristics of these patients did not differ from the cohort as a whole, and the number of prescribed medications fell significantly from 5.3 ± 1.9 to 4.7 ± 2.1 antihypertensive agents over the 12-month period. A small cohort (73 patients), initially classified as nonresponders, were reclassified after titration to settings previously prohibited according to the study protocol.[20]

Barostim *neo* Trial

As described earlier, the first-generation Rheos system failed to meet certain trial endpoints and device design required a complex implantation procedure with bilateral carotid exposure. In 2012, initial results for a second-generation device were released (Barostim *neo*, CVRx, Inc.). This nonrandomized open-label verification study enrolled 30 patients at seven centers. The device placement procedure was adapted from the first-generation technique (detailed later) with the following changes: (1) lead implantation required unilateral carotid sinus exposure and (2) carotid sinus exposure did not require exposure of the external carotid artery because the smaller lead was sutured directly to the carotid sinus. Baroreflex activation therapy (BAT) was initiated 2 weeks after implant, and parameters (pulse amplitude, width, and frequency) were individually titrated over the first several months. Although a consistent medical regimen was encouraged, physicians were permitted to make changes when medically indicated.[21]

Thirty patients underwent implantation between February and June 2011, the population being evenly divided between male and female patients with similar comorbidities and on an average of 6.1 ± 2.7 antihypertensive medications. The implant procedure took an average of 107 ± 28 minutes. At 6 months, patients achieved an average SBP reduction of 26.1 ± 3.3 mm Hg, and 43% of patients achieved an average SBP of equal to or less than 140 mm Hg (up from 0% at baseline). There was a 10% perioperative complication rate, including a self-inflicted wound complication, device pocket hematoma, and intermittent pain at device site (which persisted beyond 30 days of follow-up).[21]

This trial demonstrated efficacy for a lower-profile device with an acceptable safety profile and decreased implantation time (107 minutes versus 197 minutes) compared with the Rheos device.[19,21] Six patients in this study had undergone previous unsuccessful renal nerve ablation, which demonstrated the ability of BAT to provide BP reductions despite complete renal denervation. Long-term follow-up on 17 patients treated with unilateral BAT using the second-generation device demonstrated continued efficacy at 12 months of follow-up. Furthermore, there was no attenuation of the mean BP response to deactivation/reactivation of the device after 1 year of follow-up, indicating a sustained antihypertensive effect.[22]

Heart Failure

Multiple ongoing studies have suggested an unexpected benefit of this therapy in patients with heart failure, both with preserved and reduced ejection fraction.[13,23,24] Echocardiograms were obtained in a subgroup of patients within the Pivotal Trial, which showed in aggregate multiple beneficial effects on cardiac function after chronic therapy, including a significant reduction in left ventricular mass and improved diastolic function (Fig. 66.9).[19,25] The Health Outcomes Prospective Evaluation for Heart Failure with Ejection Fraction greater than 40% (HOPE 4HF) is an ongoing prospective randomized trial exploring the effect of BAT to treat diastolic heart failure. The theoretical benefit of carotid sinus stimulation in heart failure with reduced ejection fraction (HFrEF) is in line with current guideline-directed medical therapy (GDMT), which aims to decrease sympathetic activation via reeducation of adrenergic influences. This has been demonstrated in a proof-of-concept study published in 2014. Eleven patients with New York Heart Association (NYHA) class III HF, EF less than 40% and optimized medical therapy who were ineligible for cardiac resynchronization therapy were treated with the second-generation Barostim *neo* device for 6 months. Patients exhibited a significant decrease in muscle sympathetic nerve activity, increased distance in the 6-minute hall walk (6MHW) of 50 m, and improvements in NYHA class, quality of life, and EF.[26]

BEAT-HF Trial

The BEAT-HF Trial is an open-label randomized controlled trial evaluating the safety and efficacy of the *neo* (CVRx, Inc.) device for the treatment of chronic HFrEF. Patients were randomized to either GDMT or BAT and were eligible for participation if they had NYHA class III chronic HF, left ventricular ejection fraction (LVEF) equal to or less than 35% with HR 60 to 100 beats per minute, SBP above 100, estimated glomerular filtration rate (eGFR) above 30 mL/min per 1.73 m^2, and clearance to undergo surgery as judged by surgeon and cardiologist. Ninety-three percent of these patients had existing cardiac rhythm management devices in place, and preoperative evaluation had determined that the BAT device could be safely implanted without impeding existing cardiac devices.[13]

One-hundred forty-six patients were randomized (70 control, 76 intervention) and treated with 97.2% event-free rate from major adverse neurologic and cardiovascular events (cardiovascular-related death, stroke, cardiac arrest, acute myocardial infarction, acute decompensated HF, hypertensive crisis, severe complications of HF treatment, systemic and pulmonary thromboembolism, infection requiring explantation of device, permanent cranial nerve injury). After 6 months of follow-up, statistically significant differences were demonstrated in NYHA functional class (≥1 class improvement, 55% versus 24%), quality-of-life score (19.5-point difference), increase in 6MHW (increase of 58 m),

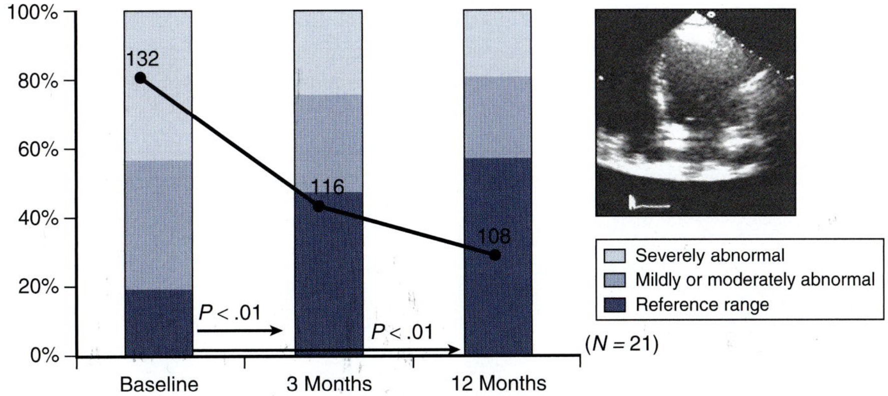

FIG 66.9 Reduction in left ventricular mass index (LVMI) in 21 patients undergoing carotid sinus baroreflex stimulation. LVMI fell from 139 g/m^2 baseline to 114 g/m^2 after 12 months of therapy. The proportion of patients with normal function rose from 19% to 58%, and those with severely abnormal function fell from 42% to 19%. (From Bisognano JD, de Leeuw P, Bach DS, et al: Improved cardiac structure and diastolic flow velocities in early-stage heart failure with chronic treatment using an implantable device: results from European and United States trials of the Rheos system. *J Am Coll Cardiol* 53:A188, 2009.)

each favoring the treatment group. Decreased HF hospitalization was demonstrated in the treatment group while it remained stable in the control group; however, this did not reach statistical significance in a between-group comparison. Interestingly, there was a significant downward trend in SBP in the control group, while SBP increased in the treatment group.[13]

Pitfalls

At least two major pitfalls exist in the minds of surgeons. First is frustration with not being able to reduce the BP to any arbitrary level, as might seem theoretically feasible. The obvious answer is that not all patients are the same and many different interrelated systems work together to regulate BP (and the Rheos system targets only one of them). In fact, it is probably possible to lower pressure to any degree, but at the cost of increasing voltage. This means not only a short battery life but also results in extraneous stimulation (motor as well as sensory) of tissues in the vicinity of the electrodes. As such, this was seen with dose-titration of the second-generation unilateral BAT device.[27] It should be noted that the "average" BP response in a drug that gains FDA approval for hypertension is in the range of 7 to 10 mm Hg; therefore SBP reductions of 35 mm Hg at 1 year and 50 mm Hg at 4 years in the Rheos and DEBuT-HT trials, respectively, are reassuring.

The second issue is that of sustainability and habituation. It is clear from the data, however, that habituation does not occur, at least to 4 years of therapy with the Rheos device and at least 12 months with the *neo* device. The obvious inference is that the habituation seen after carotid endarterectomy occurs at the level of the glossopharyngeal nerve's response to stretch; the nerve will stop firing after 1 day or so. However, the response of the brain and body to glossopharyngeal nerve activity evidently does not habituate (see Fig. 66.3). As a result, if it is possible to artificially produce continuous nerve activity by means of electrical stimulation, the efferent effects will continue.

Surgical Technique

Given current technology, the most critical step in implanting this device is to ensure that it is placed so that electrical stimulation is applied to the most sensitive portion of the carotid sinus—a "sweet spot" that is surprisingly difficult to localize. In practice, this entails 20 to 40 minutes of mapping, providing stimulation at various points (often a few millimeters apart) and noting BP response over the following 1 to 3 minutes. This effect is strongly blunted by most inhalation anesthetics; therefore proper anesthesia technique (in these severely hypertensive patients) is critical.

A detailed anesthetic protocol can be found elsewhere.[12] In brief, anesthetic management is divided into three stages, the middle of which is essentially intravenous general anesthesia alone.

Stage one consists of typical intravenous induction followed by maintenance of anesthesia with inhalation agents. This stage is performed only during the beginning of the procedure itself and is helpful for smooth induction and initial cutaneous stimulation in these very hypertensive patients. Once the skin incision has been made and cutaneous stimulation is complete, stage two begins. At this point all inhalation anesthetics other than nitrous oxide are stopped and general anesthesia is maintained using intravenous agents. These agents are primarily titrated to lack of movement and vital signs, but maintaining bispectral index (BIS) monitor levels between 40 and 60 has been found to allow anesthesia, analgesia, and amnesia while maintaining carotid sinus reactivity. The carotids are usually exposed by 15 to 20 minutes after skin incision, and this timing is usually long enough to allow inhalation agents to wash out of the system. The optimal situation at this point is a relatively high (approximately 150 mm Hg) stable BP, allowing room for electrical stimulation to cause a decrease but ensuring that the electrical stimulation is the only variable being applied. Finally, stage three applies to the phase after mapping is completed. Tunneling and pocket formation are noxious stimuli and baroreflex sensitivity is not as critical; therefore conventional inhalation anesthesia is resumed until the patient wakes.

Formerly, Rheos implantation required bilateral exposure with full circumferential carotid sinus exposure and mapping, but hardware and implantation techniques have evolved significantly and final technique will depend upon the devices finally approved. The device currently being used in heart failure trials (Neo, Fig. 66.10) is much smaller, unipolar, and attached to the anterior surface of the bifurcation only, without the need for circumferential exposure for wrapping.

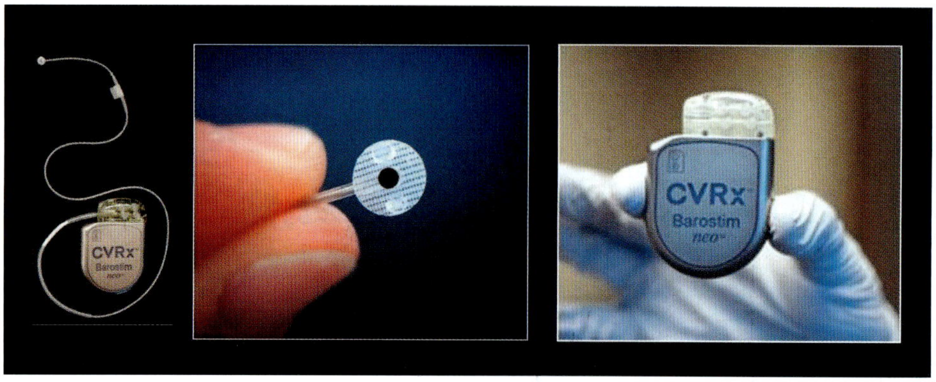

FIG 66.10 The next-generation Neo Barostim system. *Left*, entire system. *Middle*, unipolar lead for sinus stimulation. *Right*, the stimulator itself (about two-thirds as large as the original stimulator). (Courtesy CVRx, Inc., Minneapolis, Minnesota.)

After anesthesia is induced (with further management as detailed previously), the patient is positioned with the back elevated approximately 30 degrees and a towel roll placed vertically on the upper back. The head is extended in midline position, and a Mayo stand is placed symmetrically over the head to about the level of the nose to allow draping without dislodging the endotracheal tube (general anesthesia is still required by protocol for mapping purposes). The entire neck to above the jaw line, including earlobes, as well as the chest, especially the right side, is prepared with Betadine and sterilely draped. Iodoform drapes are used to achieve a thorough seal around all towel edges because a prosthetic implant is to be placed.

The bifurcation is localized by ultrasound and exposed per routine. It is important not to use lidocaine anywhere near the carotid sinus to preserve reactivity for mapping. When dissection is complete, the carotid stimulation electrode is placed on the carotid bifurcation. The lead is then attached to the pulse generator, and testing is commenced at an amplitude of 6 mA, a pulse width of 125 μs, and a frequency of 80 pps. When the "sweet spot" is found, BP response will be obvious, although this might take 60 to 180 seconds. The basic plan is to locate the site at which electrical stimulation produces the greatest and most reliable decline in BP. If only a small response is seen, pressure must reequilibrate before the next spot is tested; this process can take 5 minutes or slightly longer. One useful technique is known as *trolling*; once the best spot in a macroscopic sense is found, the current is left on and the lead is shifted slightly to determine whether any additional benefit can be obtained. A detailed systematic approach to mapping is provided in the manufacturer's instructions for use (IFU). When the site of optimal stimulation is found, the stimulator is sutured to the carotid adventitia with 6-0 Prolene in a circumferential, interrupted fashion. It is important to ensure perfect apposition between the electrodes and the wall of the carotid sinus for best electrical contact. A strain relief loop is created in the lead wire and secured by securing the additional suture tab to the common carotid adventitia.

The implantable pulse generator (IPG) should be placed on the same side as the electrode unless prior device implantation precludes this. Leads should be tunneled deep to the sternocleidomastoid muscle through a subcutaneous or subfascian tunnel, and passage of the lead wire through this may be aided with the use of a red rubber catheter. The IPG is best tolerated if placed subfascially and well secured to the pectoralis major with permanent sutures; enough dissection and loose area should be created medially to allow the leads to exit straight out from the IPG and thus avoid kinking.

WHAT COMES NEXT?

At this point the original technology is close to 10 years old. Rapid advances can be expected in all phases of this system, including smaller generators with more efficient batteries, better recipes for stimulation, less invasive implant strategies, and perhaps internal feedback (e.g., more current is delivered when pressure is high, and less when it is low). The first generation of patients have received bilateral implants while under general anesthesia; however, unilateral stimulation is now being used, appears to be effective, and could probably be performed using local anesthesia once trials are more mature. First-in-man results of a nitinol self-expanding rectangular cuboid implant (MobiusHD, Vascular Dynamics, Mountain View, CA) were released during an oral presentation at the Vascular InterVentional Advances (VIVA) meeting in 2015. This device is designed to increase carotid sinus arterial wall strain without affecting pulsatility or laminar flow, and 17 of 20 patients have had a reduction of SBP of more than 10 mm Hg, although 3 of these patients have had serious adverse events including hypotension and closure device failure.[28] Clinical trials with this device are currently enrolling in the United States and Europe.

In addition to heart failure,[13,25] several other applications of this technology come to mind. Permanent or temporary use of this device can ensure dramatic BP response in the short term and thus could conceivably be used in emergency situations when BP control is needed (e.g., preeclampsia or acute aortic dissection). In addition, survival after medically treated type B aortic dissection is highly dependent on long-term BP control. The Rheos device could be used in this situation to ensure control in patients who will not comply with medication as well as those who will but are resistant to it.

SUMMARY

To date, more than 400 patients worldwide have undergone implantation of the Rheos carotid stimulator system, with acceptably low morbidity and mortality, and the second-generation device has received Conformité Européene (CE) approval for use in hypertension and heart failure in Europe. In the cohort of patients treated longest (4 years), sustained reductions in SBP of approximately 50 mm Hg have been documented. The US Barostim *neo* Hypertension Pivotal Trial is under way currently, with a goal of enrolling 310 patients; approval for use of the system in the United States will be contingent on these results. Both theory and early empiric results are exciting; this technology may represent a significant advance in the care of this difficult group of patients.

REVIEW QUESTIONS

1. For each 20-mm increase in systolic blood pressure over 115, cardiac risk
   a. increases by 10%
   b. increases by 25%
   c. increases by 100% (doubles)
   d. increases by 200% (triples)
2. Truly resistant hypertension is estimated to occur in
   a. no one
   b. thousands of Americans
   c. several million Americans
   d. essentially every patient with hypertension

3. Stimulation of the glossopharyngeal nerve is caused by
   a. carotid sinus stretch
   b. tachycardia
   c. tumors
   d. dehydration
4. Continuous electrical stimulation of the glossopharyngeal nerve in dogs produces hypotension that can be maintained for
   a. only a few seconds
   b. less than an hour
   c. 12 to 18 hours
   d. at least a week
5. Electrical stimulation of the carotid baroreflex is accomplished by stimulation of the
   a. internal carotid artery
   b. carotid sinus
   c. external carotid artery
   d. glossopharyngeal nerve itself
6. Side effects of carotid sinus stimulation could theoretically include
   a. bradycardia
   b. tachypnea
   c. hypertension
   d. jaw claudication
7. Baroreflex stimulation has also been shown to be associated with
   a. preeclampsia in vulnerable subjects
   b. mitral regurgitation
   c. renal hyperplasia
   d. reduction in ventricular mass
8. Baroreflex stimulation has been shown to lower systolic blood pressure by
   a. only 1 to 3 mm
   b. 5 to 10 mm
   c. 30 to 50 mm
   d. 50 to 100 mm
9. In America, baroreflex stimulation is currently (early 2018)
   a. usable only within a clinical trial
   b. usable only for heart failure
   c. useful only in animal models
   d. approved for use in patients with severe hypertension
10. Voltage needed to see a meaningful blood pressure drop is on the order of
    a. a few millivolts
    b. 1 to 6 V
    c. 30 V (low wattage)
    d. 30 V (high wattage)

References available online at ExpertConsult.com.

CHAPTER 67

Building an Outpatient Interventional Suite

Krishna Mohan Jain, John S. Munn, Mark C. Rummel, Daniel J. Johnston, Chris Longton

The United States has the most advanced health technology in the world. At the same time, we have one of the most inefficient health care delivery systems. Most of the technology-driven care is concentrated in hospitals, which are inherently inefficient. In the world of vascular disease management, increasing numbers of patients benefit from endovascular techniques. Most patients are discharged after only a few hours of observation. Therefore almost all patients could be treated in an outpatient setting.[1] This avoids the expensive hospital environment, while still benefiting from the most advanced vascular treatment available.[2] This chapter will describe the process by which an outpatient interventional suite can be built and run ethically and successfully. In the literature, this suite is also referred to as office-based lab or office endovascular suite.

RATIONALE TO BUILD A CENTER

There are many reasons why vascular surgeons should embark on building an outpatient center.

- Schedule: If you own the center, you can control your schedule, reduce cancellations, and decrease turnover time.
- Improve care: If the procedure needs to be done in an expedited manner, it can be done in the office without going through the hospital operating room hierarchy. You control the procedures performed, ensuring patients the most up-to-date technology and techniques. The staff in the center is familiar with the devices and the procedure being conducted, resulting in less likelihood of a complication.
- Improve patient satisfaction[3]: Patients who come to your office are already comfortable with the environment and your office staff. They are much less stressed to come to a known place and meeting familiar people rather than strangers. They do not have to stop at several desks before entering the endovascular suite. Patients can be provided with same-day service.
- Improve revenue: When the procedures are done in the office, the practice collects the technical component, as well as the professional component, as a single payment.

After a decision has been made to explore the possibility of expanding your practice to include an office-based endovascular lab, a specific process needs to be followed. Office-based endovascular laboratories should be located adjacent to the office where the patients are seen. Office-based endovascular labs are not considered to be ambulatory surgery centers, and therefore the rules for operation and billing are different. An office-based lab is regulated by state rules.

STEPS TO SUCCESSFULLY ESTABLISH AN OUTPATIENT ENDOVASCULAR CENTER

Business Plan

The group planning to open an office-based lab in all likelihood already has an existing practice that performs endovascular procedures. Most of the outpatient procedures performed in the hospital could be done in the office. However, we do not recommend discharging patients from the hospital to have a procedure done in the office. A pro forma accounting statement describing "typical financial activities" needs to be created based on last year's outpatient procedures performed in the practice. Projections of growth need to be realistic. While creating the pro forma, one needs to calculate revenue, capital expense, cost of disposables, labor cost, cost of space, and loan expense. For example, the cost structure will change if the building is leased compared with being owned by the practice.

Agreement Among Physicians

Like any other business, all physician employees in the group need to be in agreement that starting an office-based lab is the right decision for the practice. All the cases that can be safely done in the office need to be done in the office. If one partner does not do a particular endovascular procedure, then that case should be transferred to another partner. The compensation formula for physicians may need to be adjusted depending on the practice dynamics. If everyone is not in agreement at the initiation of the outpatient laboratory, the practice should anticipate conflict in the future.

Regulations

The deficit reduction act of 2005 permitted Medicare to pay for endovascular procedures done in the office setting. This was expanded in 2008 to include intervention in peripheral arteries. To qualify for these payments, the procedures should be carried out in the office where the patients are normally seen for established visits. There are no other Medicare rules governing the conduct of these procedures in the office setting. Different states have different rules and laws that govern the conduct of these procedures.[4] Ambulatory surgery centers have their own set of rules that do not apply to office-based endovascular labs. As a result, the procedures done in the office are paid in a global manner that includes both technical and professional components. After the Centers for Medicare and Medicaid Services (CMS) started paying for these services, other insurance companies adjusted their fee structure and also started to pay for these services.

Financing

Various arrangements can be made for financing the center. If the practice is mature, money could be borrowed to build out the center in an existing space or a new space and to buy capital equipment. Cash flow from the existing practice can be used to buy the disposables and pay the salaries of new employees needed for the center. In a less established practice the group could borrow money for the building, lease the equipment, and get disposables on a contingency basis. Another option is to create a separate leasing company to acquire the capital equipment and lease it back to the practice. Cash flow could start as early as 2 weeks after performing the first procedure.

Location

The lab needs to be established in the same physical location where the patients are seen, to qualify as an office-based lab. If the current space is not sufficient to build the center, a separate center can be created, as long as the space is also used for patient care. If building a brand-new space for the office and lab, geographic location should be carefully chosen. Because most labs provide care to a hemodialysis-dependent population, it is important to have the office in close proximity to outpatient dialysis units. Close proximity to a hospital where physicians have operating access and easy access for emergency vehicles is essential in case of an emergency, so a quick transfer can be made. Proximity to a blood analysis lab also helps in case blood needs to be urgently tested prior to procedures.

Building

In addition to the existing facility used for seeing patients, the new endovascular lab space should have an interventional suite, procedure room, preoperative/postoperative area, decontamination room, supply storage area, drug storage area, and office for the laboratory manger. The interventional suite should be lead lined. Although not currently mandated by all states, lead lining the room during the initial build will prevent future remodeling costs if state law changes. With increasing awareness of radiation injury, the laws are likely to change. In addition to the lead-lined interventional suite, a procedure room may be needed to manage patients with superficial venous insufficiency. The interventional suite should be larger than the procedure room. The larger suite should be able to accommodate a C-arm, radiolucent table, intravascular ultrasound (IVUS) machine, supplies, and other equipment needed during the procedure. A preoperative and postprocedure area are also required; however, the same space can be used for both. Depending upon patient volume, the center will need between three and eight bays for patients. This area should be clearly visible to the supervising nurse and other personnel in charge of patient care. The scheduling, coding, and billing is usually done by existing employees so new construction is often not required.

Equipment

The office-based lab is not the interventional suite one is used to in the hospital. It is neither a hybrid suite, a room in the catheterization lab, or interventional radiology lab; it is specifically designed to safely and effectively accomplish the procedures performed by the outpatient endovascular center. The equipment needed is specific to the procedures being conducted. The largest piece of equipment in the suite is the x-ray system. There is a debate between buying a fixed room x-ray system versus a portable C-arm x-ray system. A fixed system is obviously more powerful, could be helpful for obese patients, and have additional features not present in the portable C-arm. However, the fixed system is less versatile compared with a portable C-arm when doing dialysis cases. C-arms have become quite advanced and now provide almost equal-quality imaging when compared with the fixed system. In our outpatient endovascular center, we have not felt the need for a fixed system after performing successfully more than 10,000 cases with a portable C-arm. If one is contemplating coronary angiography or placement of pacemakers/defibrillators, then a fixed system has definite advantages. Fixed systems may also be helpful in renal, mesenteric, and carotid artery procedures. One disadvantage of portable C-arms is the greater radiation exposure risk; therefore appropriate precautions should be taken. In terms of cost, a fixed system is more expensive than a C-arm. Purchasing a new machine is recommended rather than buying a refurbished system because it is very expensive to have a system down for any period of time. The cost of lost business and inability to provide care in a timely manner can be very detrimental to the success of the lab.

The second biggest item in the suite is the radiolucent table. The table should be movable and operator controlled. Side tilt is almost never required in cases being done in the office. Weight limit of the table is important because you may be doing procedures on patients up to 400 lb. Even if the operator is not doing peripheral revascularization procedures in very obese patients, some of the patients on dialysis may fall in that category and the vascular procedures needed for their dialysis can be taken care of in the office.

An IVUS is a required piece of equipment if venous angioplasty and stenting are planned.[5] It can also be beneficial for certain peripheral arterial cases. A power injector is also required for arterial cases. Use of the ultrasound machine for percutaneous access of arteries and veins helps to avoid many complications associated with catheterization.[6] In addition, venous ablation procedures cannot be done without an ultrasound machine. Ultrasound guidance during arterial catheterization diminishes the entry site complications. If a tibial approach is used for arterial revascularization, based on our experience a hockey stick probe is recommended. Other equipment needed can be found in Box 67.1.

Supplies and Medications

The biggest running cost to the center is the disposable supplies and medications, listed in Boxes 67.2 and 67.3. The physicians

BOX 67.1 Equipment for the Endovascular Suite

Equipment for the Endovascular Suite

In the Lab

C-arm/fixed overhead x-ray system
Radiolucent table
Power injector
CO_2 injector
Ultrasound machine
Intravascular ultrasound
Monitoring equipment
Overhead surgical light
Surgical instruments
Arm board
Portable oxygen tanks
Suction machine
Procedure table for instruments

Preoperative and Postoperative Area

Wheel chair
Reclining chair
Beds/stretcher
AED
Monitors
Crash cart

Miscellaneous

Furniture
Computers
Blanket warmer
Autoclave
Emergency battery backup
Lead aprons hats and glasses
PAC image storing
Emergency generator
Storage racks
Data collection software
EHR

AED, Automated external defibrillator; *HER*, electronic health record; *PAC*, picture archiving and communication.

in the group should collaborate and decide what supplies they need. To simplify purchasing and get the best prices, the majority of supplies should come from one vendor; however, some companies will have proprietary products, necessitating specific vendors. The center should provide at the very least the same care that the physicians provide at the hospital. If a patient needs a drug-eluting balloon or a drug-eluting stent, then one should use it despite the fact that they are more expensive and there is no additional reimbursement from insurance companies. There are various atherectomy devices, and the group should decide which devices they will use and stick to that decision unless the data indicate otherwise.

Work Flow

Patients undergoing procedures in the lab will originate from the office. There needs to be a seamless flow of patients between the office and the lab. After a decision has been made to do a procedure on the patient, the procedure needs to be scheduled. The office scheduler who normally schedules cases in the hospital is best suited to schedule cases in the office lab as well, avoiding overlaps and confusion. Patients should be given lab slips for blood work, including partial thromboplastin time (PTT), prothrombin time (PT), blood urea nitrogen (BUN), creatinine, and glomerular filtration rate (GFR), if not being treated for hemodialysis access–related issues. If the lab values are abnormal, these should be addressed prior to performing any outpatient endovascular procedures. Patients who have a GFR of less than 60 should follow a hydration protocol. The patient should be called a day before the procedure to be reminded of the procedure

BOX 67.2 Supplies

Supplies

Preparation for Procedure

Surgical packs
Lead apron
Lead-lined and sterile gloves
Booties, lead-lined hats, and regular hats

Arterial and Venous Procedures

Vascular access kit
Catheter and wires
Sheaths
Support catheters
Crossing devices
Angioplasty balloons
Stents (bare metal and covered)
Atherectomy device
Inflation device
Intravenous ultrasound catheter
Closure device
Snare

Dialysis-Related Procedures

Dialysis permanent and temporary catheters
Over-the-wire Fogarty catheter

Other Procedures

Ports
Stents
Intracaval filters
Filter retrievable kits

BOX 67.3 Medications

Contrast solution
CO_2 cartridge
Intravenous fluid
Fentanyl
Versed
Heparin
Protamine sulfate
Local anesthetic agent
Other drugs if anesthesiology is providing sedation
Local hemostatic agents

and to answer any questions the patient may have. On the day of the procedure, the patient should arrive early enough for proper preparation. If the preoperative area and the postoperative area are the same, the flow of cases needs to be monitored to make sure every patient has a place to recover, depending on the case. Patients should be appropriately prepared; consent taken and the site of procedure should be marked. Before starting the procedure, the appropriate site should be identified with the team. After the procedure, the patient should be followed as per the policies and procedures of the lab. In the postoperative area, patient care needs to be supervised by a registered nurse. At the time of discharge, the patient should be given appropriate instructions about the site of intervention, postprocedure medications to be taken, postprocedure blood work to be done, and complications to look for. A postprocedure follow-up appointment should also be scheduled. After any arterial procedure, the patient should be watched overnight by a responsible adult at home. Following discharge, the office staff should call the patient on the following day.

Training of Surgeons

For the success of the lab, it is crucial that the surgeon's mindset be changed regarding safety and unnecessary wastefulness. Although the basic procedure technique will not change from the hospital interventional suite to the office suite, conduct of the procedure needs to change. A surgeon is typically used to having various disposable items open in the room prior to entering; however, during the procedure, many items that are opened are never used. This contributes to a tremendous amount of waste in a hospital system. In the office-based lab, there should be a zero-waste policy. The same practice should prevail in the hospital, but the surgeon does not control that environment. The procedure should start with basic drapes and be followed by the access kit. After that, each item should be opened only when requested by the surgeon. This is a radical shift from the way one is used to working in the hospital. Another area of caution is aggressiveness during the procedure; there is no back up in the office. If the need to do an open procedure arises, the patient needs to be transferred to the hospital. Do not "push the envelope." Safety is paramount. Finally, surgeons should be certified in advanced cardiac life support (ACLS).

Training of Staff

In the office-based lab, staff needs to be cross-trained for maximum efficiency. The medical assistant who checks in the patient can also get the patient ready for the procedure and monitor the patient in the postoperative period (under the supervision of a registered nurse). In the procedure room a surgical technician, who is usually hired from the hospital, needs to learn the efficiency in the new setting. The technician helps to prepare the patient ready for the procedure, assists with the procedure and with cleaning the room after the procedure, to expedite turnover for a new patient. In most states, there is no requirement to have a registered radiology technician to operate the C-arm. A medical assistant can be trained to run the C-arm, clean the room, and be in charge of the supplies. If anesthesia service is not being used for conscious sedation, a registered nurse needs to monitor the patient and keep appropriate records. There is no need for a circulating nurse. However, all nurses need to be ACLS certified.

Types of Procedures

Every procedure one does in the hospital can be done in the outpatient endovascular laboratory,[3,7] with the exception of carotid stenting and endovascular repair of abdominal aortic aneurysm. The possible procedures are listed in Table 67.1.

Although the procedures listed in the table can be performed in the office-based lab, there are some contraindications, which can be absolute or relative. Absolute contraindications are need for long observation period post procedure, need for general anesthesia, multiple comorbidities requiring hospital admission, and severe allergy to contrast agent. Relative contraindications are sleep apnea, weight greater than 400 lb, and low tolerance to pain if conscious sedation is not available.

TABLE 67.1 Possible Outpatient Endovascular Laboratory Procedures

Dialysis Related	Arterial	Venous	Miscellaneous
Insertion of catheter	Aortogram and run off	Venogram	Carotid angiogram
Removal of catheter	Angioplasty of lower extremity arteries	Venogram, angioplasty, stent	Insertion of port
Fistulogram	Angioplasty and stent	Insertion of intracaval filter	Uterine embolization
Fistulogram angioplasty	Atherectomy, angioplasty and stent	Removal of intracaval filter	PICC line
Fistulogram coiling	Renal artery angioplasty	Embolization	Central venous lines
Fistulogram, angioplasty and stent	Renal artery angioplasty, stent	Thrombolysis	
Thrombectomy of clotted access	Mesenteric artery angioplasty and stent		
Central venous stenosis Angioplasty	Subclavian artery angioplasty		
Central venous stenosis Angioplasty and stent	Subclavian artery angioplasty, stent		
	Upper extremity artery angioplasty		
	Upper extremity angioplasty, stent		

PICC, Peripherally inserted central venous lines.

Dialysis Related

Office labs were initially opened to take care of endovascular needs of dialysis patients. As such, many of the procedures listed in Table 67.1 apply to this group of patients and can be easily done in the office lab. There should be clear-cut clinical indications to perform dialysis access–related procedures. The common indications for doing these procedures are: (1) decreased flow, (2) increased bleeding after needle removal, (3) decreased urea clearance, (4) increased venous pressure, (5) ultrasound finding of hemodynamically significant stenosis, (6) increased circulation time, and (7) inability to access the fistula.[8] Percutaneous mechanical and chemical thrombectomy can be performed. Invariably the stenosis causing the thrombosis needs to corrected by angioplasty or angioplasty and stenting.[9]

Arterial

With the advent of computed tomography (CT) angiography, there is a decreasing need for diagnostic arteriography. If indicated, the aortogram and extremity arteriography can be performed using a retrograde Seldinger technique or via brachial or radial approach. If the patient's GFR is less than 60, appropriate protocols should be used for hydration. With moderate to severe renal insufficiency, CO_2 angiography[10] should be considered for arteriography below the diaphragm. Most of the time the arteriogram is performed with intent to treat. If needed, a tibial approach[11,12] can be used to cross the lesions in the superficial femoral artery or tibial arteries. Patients who have hostile groin or are morbidly obese can also benefit from a radial or tibial approach. Because there are no reported differences in the complication rates if a closure device is used, the use of a device depends on physician preference.[13,14] However, use of these devices may decrease the postprocedure observation period. Above all, the center should offer optimal therapy. Drug-eluting balloons and stents are more expensive than other devices but should be used if indicated.[15-17] There are various atherectomy devices[18,19] with inherent benefits and indications.[19,20] The center should not stock all the devices, so an educated decision must be made about which devices to stock. Limiting the number of devices helps to run a cost-efficient center. IVUS can also be beneficial in selected cases to size the stent and identify intimal flaps that may need to be treated. Carotid angiograms can be performed in the office, but any subsequent intervention is not reimbursable from insurance companies.

Venous

Superficial venous insufficiency can be managed in the outpatient vascular lab. To provide comprehensive venous care, ablation of superficial veins, microphlebectomy, sclerotherapy, and use of new evolving therapies should be offered. A subset of patients will need further management of venous disease and will benefit from the endovascular lab. With the advent of IVUS, management of May-Thurner syndrome has become significantly easier.[21] IVUS is rapidly replacing ascending venography in diagnosing iliac vein stenosis.[5] Conservative treatment should be the first line of therapy, and if that fails, further evaluation using IVUS should be carried out. In cases of iliac vein stenosis, venous angioplasty is not sufficient and a stent is always required. Currently there is no US Food and Drug Administration (FDA)-approved venous stent; however, there are at least two venous stents in clinical trials. The stents required are usually 14 to 28 mm in size. The only stent that is large enough to be usable in the iliac vein is the Wall stent (Boston Scientific, Marlborough, MA). This requires larger balloons that are not usually kept in the lab for arterial procedures. Recently published studies show the benefits of venous stents in managing venous stenosis as a result of external compression or internal obstruction due to previous thrombosis.[22,23]

Most of the time, intracaval filters are placed in the hospital setting; however, sometimes a filter may be required prior to a procedure. The filter can be inserted in the office[24] the day before the main procedure in the hospital. With the advent of retrievable filters, there is a need for a close follow-up of patients who have these filters. The retrievable filter should be removed[25] in a timely manner when clinically indicated. It is easier to remove these in the office rather than requiring the patient to go through the hospital system. The patient does not need to come off anticoagulants for the procedure. Thrombolysis of iliac vein thrombosis can be carried out in the office under appropriate circumstances.[26] Management of pelvic congestion syndrome includes embolization of incompetent veins in the pelvis, which can be easily done in the office setting.

Miscellaneous

Ports for chemotherapy can be placed in the office setting, as long as the patient is not on Coumadin or another anticoagulant, and their platelet count is adequate. The port can be inserted on the day of request if chemotherapy needs to be started quickly. Uterine embolization for fibroids is not a traditional procedure done by the vascular surgeons. However, if the surgeon has special interest in developing expertise in this area, the procedure can be done in the office lab. Central venous lines and peripherally inserted central venous lines can be placed in the office if needed.

Policies and Procedures

No lab should operate without written policies and procedures. These documents guide the operator, physicians, and staff about the conduct of each procedure. The equipment needed, supplies required, conduct of the procedure, and preoperative and postoperative care needs should all be defined in detail. There should be policies to manage complications and transfer of the patient to a hospital in case of an emergency. These documents are always required if the lab wants to get certified by choice or based on state regulation. These documents should be updated as needed.

Billing and Coding

Most surgeons' offices have experience coding and billing for professional services. Many offices use outside billing services. The staff responsible for coding and charging for services will need to be trained on the technical components of the new procedures performed in the endovascular lab. Even if an outside billing service is used, the practice should make sure that the billing process meets federal guidelines. CMS periodically updates the coding of various procedures, thus the staff responsible for coding will need to stay current with these regulations and apply the changes in a timely manner. Periodic internal and external audits should be carried out to make sure that coding is compliant with CMS rules. Penalties for underbilling and overbilling are severe. If preauthorization is required for the procedure, it should be obtained prior to the procedure. If this is not done, you will have a very angry patient or a financial loss to the practice. Account receivables should be managed appropriately. The longer a bill is outstanding, the less chance it will get paid.

Anesthesia

Most procedures are carried out using mild to moderate conscious sedation and local anesthesia. Patients needing intubation should have the procedure performed in the hospital. If an anesthesiologist is not involved in the care of the patient, all physicians and nurses should be ACLS certified. A crash cart should be properly supplied and periodically checked for expired medications. In some states, such as New York,[4] anesthesia personnel are required in the procedure room if moderate to severe sedation is used. Some of the accrediting bodies may also have this requirement. As progressively more complicated procedures are being performed in the office, it is desirable to have anesthesia personnel manage pain, monitor hemodynamic parameters, and keep appropriate records. Some patients who have poor pain tolerance will agree to have the procedure done in the office if they are provided with anesthesia service in the office.

Marketing

Every practice has its own marketing plan. Typically, a practice planning to open an endovascular lab in the office is already successful and has developed a system to continuously recruit new patients to the practice. A great part of the marketing is free. Marketing starts with the surgeon. The way the surgeon presents himself or herself to patients through both attire and communication is essential. Effective communication with patients and their families, staff, and employees in the hospital is crucial to building an image of the practice. The staff is equally important for creating a positive image of the practice. Staff should dress appropriately and be trained to courteously deal with patients. The office environment should be pleasant and inviting for patients, which will help to develop confidence in the practice. Physicians should participate in local medical and specialty societies to build a network. Personal contact between the surgeon and referring physicians is essential in building a long-lasting relationship. Referring physicians include primary care doctors, internists, gynecologists, orthopedic surgeons, neurosurgeons, cardiologists, nephrologists, podiatrists, and radiologists.

There are various mediums to advertise for the new services that you will provide through your office-based endovascular suite. The following avenues can be used for marketing.

1. Print media: Creating a newsletter and periodically sending it to your referring physicians has minimal cost and a big return. An interview about a new procedure with a local newspaper is free and can be helpful. The return on investment in advertising in the print media is decreasing rapidly because most people are shifting away from printed newspapers and magazines.
2. Audiovisual: Periodic interviews with a local radio station or television station can be beneficial. These media outlets are looking to get the latest information to their consumers. Advertising on radio is cheaper than television. These advertisements can be effective but require repetition for consumers to remember the content.
3. Digital: A well-constructed website is a requirement for the practice to succeed. The content on the website needs to be accurate, and the information should be updated to stay current.
4. Billboards: These can be expensive, and it is not clear if they really increase business. Most of the referrals will come from other physicians, who will likely not be swayed by a billboard.
5. Social media: The impact of social media on a vascular surgery practice is unclear. In a venous practice, it may be very helpful.

Research

Research can be a part of your marketing effort. You should collect data on your procedures. The data should be analyzed and shared with your colleagues. This builds confidence in your referring physicians about your ability and competency. An increasing number of patients are interested in the success rate of your procedures, not the success rate of the procedures in general.

Quality Control

Surgeons are used to working in hospitals, where data are collected and analyzed in various quality assurance programs and shared with the surgeons. In the new environment, that responsibility now lies with the owner surgeons of the office-based labs. This requires (1) an appropriate system to store images, (2) electronic health records, (3) management of complications, (4) short- and long-term outcomes, and (5) participation in a regional and/or national registry.[27] Above all, the quality will determine the success of your endovascular lab. Thus it is of utmost importance to track your outcomes and keep referring physicians and patients aware of your results.

Picture Archiving and Communication System

Images from the procedure need to be stored in an easily accessible system. It is both a medical and legal requirement. Many patients will come back for a repeat procedure. The images from previous procedures should be available when planning further treatment. Some of the patients may come to a hospital for further treatment and images should be accessible remotely to plan treatment.

Electronic Health Record

A comprehensive electronic health record (EHR) dedicated to running a vascular practice is critical to run the center efficiently. Because the office-based lab is an extension of the office, the EHR should be seamless between the office and the lab. The data will consist of administrative and clinic records in text and image form. The EHR should be able to manage office notes, images, procedure notes, billing data, medications, and inventory and be able to transfer data into a registry. The data should be in a format that can be used for various analyses. Under the present law, future payments to the practice will depend on quality matrix. The need for an EHR dedicated to the vascular practice cannot be overemphasized.

Management of Complications

Hospitals have a built-in system to manage complications, with many support services available to take care of any complication that arises. However, in the office setting, there are limited resources. This should not deter physicians from providing safe care in the office lab.[3,14] Advance planning is crucial to ensure that patients receive the best care possible, and should a problem occur, an established protocol will help to provide a quick response to an emergency. Physicians should only perform cases in the office that they are comfortable doing. Some patients should not have procedures done in the office. There should be proper protocols for managing any complication, resuscitation, and transfer to a hospital. The patients should be transferred to a hospital where the vascular surgeon has privileges. If the procedure is being performed by a physician who is not a surgeon, the operator should have an understanding with a local vascular surgeon who will manage any complications. A written transfer agreement is not required. When office-based procedures are performed under the right conditions, the results can match or surpass results achieved in the hospital. The complication rates from three published studies of procedures performed in office-based labs are listed in Table 67.2.

There are various complications that should be anticipated in an office-based lab. Complications related to access site include active bleeding, hematoma, pseudoaneurysm, vessel occlusion, embolism, and infection. Complications related to the target site include rupture, dissection, occlusion, and thromboembolism. Device-related complications include broken or retained wire, catheter embolization, and stent migration. Covered stent migration can have disastrous effects. Anesthesia and cardiac complications include hypoxia, myocardial infarction, and cardiac arrhythmia. Other complications such as syncope, seizure, and renal failure should also be planned for.[3,14]

Follow-Up

The patient should be seen within a few days post procedure and then continue to have long-term follow-up for patency and clinical improvement. This should include modification of risk factors. Patients should have an open procedure when indicated. All data should be entered in the EHR and a registry, if available, and analyzed periodically. Repeat procedures should not be performed without clinical indication.

Participation in a Registry

The Medicare access and chip reauthorization act of 2015 (MACRA) mandated payment to physicians should be based on quality measures rather than fee for service. To be able to show quality of care, it is imperative that physician participate in a regional and/or national registry.[27] Physicians should look at the data periodically and continue to improve based on the collective experience of registry participants. This is the only way to compare one's data to peers. Although it will increase the cost of practicing medicine, the downside of not participating is significant. This could result in as much as 9% reduction in payment from CMS.

Radiation Safety

It is important to reduce the radiation exposure of the patient, surgeon, and the personnel in the endovascular suite. Radiation safety begins with the construction of the interventional suite. The walls, ceiling, and floor must provide radiation barriers for anyone outside of the room. The builder or architect can work with a radiation safety physicist to use appropriate materials. Lead-lined doors, frames, and leaded glass may be required.

Within the suite, medical personnel require personal protective equipment. Appropriate lead aprons typically offering 0.5 mm of lead equivalent are required to be worn by personnel in the room. Additional aprons should be available because students, vendors, translators, and other individuals may be required in the suite. Aprons need to be tested regularly. No formal criteria have been devised for office labs with respect to when aprons should be tested or what criteria would be used for rejection of an apron. Typically, access centers would follow the hospital policies, which in turn are based on The Joint Commission (TJC) recommendations. Typically, an annual fluoroscopic examination of the apron can be done to look for any breach.

Most x-ray scattering occurs at the level of the patient and table.[28] Additional barriers such as table-mounted screens and suspended leaded glass windows may be beneficial.[29] Lead-lined eyeglasses and gloves are also available. C-arm certification is typically required on an annual basis. State inspections may occur at random intervals. Radiation dosimeter badges need to be monitored on a regular basis. Several different firms offer this service, and they are easily found online.

The physician is ultimately responsible for minimizing radiation exposure.[30] Techniques should be in accordance with the "as low as reasonably achievable" (ALARA) guidelines.

TABLE 67.2 Complication Rates

	Procedures	Diagnostic angiogram (%)	Arterial intervention (%)	Fistula-related procedure (%)	Venous (%)	Catheter (%)	Whole group (%)	Hospital transfer (%)	Emergency operation (%)
Jain et al.	6458	1	2.7	0.5	2.2	0.3	0.8	0.4	0.15
Lin et al.	5123	3	1.5	1.1	1	0.7	1.4	0.64	0.13
Oskui et al.	500	1.8	1.35	1.9	N/A	N/A	N/A	N/A	N/A

Minimization of x-ray exposure includes increasing one's distance from the x-ray tube and table. Decreased use of magnification or digital subtraction views help to reduce exposure. The pulse rate and collimation settings should be adjusted appropriately. An organized plan prior to commencing the procedure helps to minimize fluoroscopic time. Scatter tends to be less with anteroposterior (AP) projections as opposed to oblique or lateral images.[28,31] Access to the room should be limited.

Conflict With Hospital

If everyone in health care business believes in providing optimal care to the patients, then there is no conflict with the hospitals. Technically all the services being provided by the office-based lab are available in the hospital system. However, the efficiency and the patient satisfaction that is achieved in the office cannot be duplicated in the hospital. This is especially true in taking care of dialysis-dependent patients. If the hospitals are really concerned about the loss of revenue, they could explore the possibility of partnering with physicians. Due to increased efficiency of the office-based lab, the overall number of patients treated increases. Over the past 9 years, the number of cases we have treated in the hospital has remained steady.

Accreditation

There is currently no federal law mandating certification of an endovascular office-based lab by an accrediting agency. However, some states require the lab to be certified. Certifying bodies include the Joint Commission on Accreditation of Healthcare Organizations (JACHO), Accreditation Association Ambulatory Health Care (AAAHC), and the American Association for Accreditation of Ambulatory Surgery Facilities (AAAASF). Currently there is no certifying body that looks at coding compliance, appropriateness of the procedure, and outcomes for endovascular office-based labs. A relevant certification process should look at these elements of the lab, in addition to the factors already being assessed by the currently available certifying bodies. It is the responsibility of the owners of the lab to make sure care is being provided in an environmentally safe office with proper policies and procedures. There is some controversy in the field as to whether certification will improve the quality of care provided by office-based endovascular labs.[3,14] Certification is an added expense that may not increase safety or improve quality. After an accrediting organization is created to meet the specific need of the endovascular lab, it may be desirable to get certified by this body.

Patient Satisfaction

To have excellent patient satisfaction, both the physicians and support staff need to work in concert. Every positive experience the patient has in the office results in a satisfied patient. Every aspect of care, including the phone communication with front desk staff, medical personnel, billing staff, preoperative and postoperative experience, interaction with the physician, and success of the procedure, will factor into the satisfaction of the patient. Communication is the key to having satisfied patients.[2,3] Patients should be adequately educated preprocedure and have a follow-up call after the procedure. Written material given to the patient before the procedure and access to the practice website with enough information about the procedure is very helpful. It is not necessary to have a patient satisfaction survey done by an outside company. The practice can build its own small survey that can be conducted by the office. The two main elements of the survey are: (1) was the patient satisfied by the care? and (2) will the patient come back to the office in the future if another procedure is needed? Under MACRA, patient satisfaction will be one of the elements taken into consideration for the procedure payment.

Office-based endovascular suites have proven to be successful enterprises for both physicians and patients alike. Endovascular procedures performed in this setting have been proven safe, and the ease and success of these procedures has resulted in excellent patient satisfaction. Physicians also benefit by increasing their control over the care they provide, more flexible schedules, and increased financial rewards. Financial challenges will occur as the health care models evolve. However, it is easier to respond to these changes when decision making is in the hands of a few physician owners of the labs rather than hospital bureaucracy.

ACKNOWLEDGMENT

We greatly appreciate and thank Dr. Laura Bauler in helping us with the preparation of this chapter.

REVIEW QUESTIONS

True or False

1. Certificate of need is not required to open an office endovascular suite
   True
   False
2. Carotids stenting can be done in the office lab
   a. True
   b. False
3. All states require lead lining the room if C-arm is used
   a. True
   b. False
4. Anesthesia personnel is required for all procedures
   a. True
   b. False
5. Intravascular ultrasound is a reimbursable procedure
   a. True
   b. False
6. Fistulogram on regular intervals is not permissible under CMS guidelines
   a. True
   b. False

7. With the future payment system, being a part of a registry will facilitate payment
   a. True
   b. False
8. Billing for procedures done in the office is the same as billing for procedures done in an ambulatory surgery center
   a. True
   b. False
9. CMS does not require accreditation of the lab
   a. True
   b. False
10. Intracaval filters cannot be removed in the lab.
   a. True
   b. False

BIBLIOGRAPHY

Akopian G, Katz SG. Peripheral angioplasty with same-day discharge in patients with intermittent claudication. *J Vasc Surg*. 2006;44(1): 115–118. doi:10.1016/j.jvs.2006.03.025.

Cronenwett JL, Kraiss LW, Cambria RP. The Society for Vascular Surgery Vascular Quality Initiative. *J Vasc Surg*. 2012;55(5): 1529–1537. doi:10.1016/j.jvs.2012.03.016.

Fujihara M, Kawasaki D, Shintani Y, et al. Endovascular therapy by CO2 angiography to prevent contrast-induced nephropathy in patients with chronic kidney disease: a prospective multicenter trial of CO2 angiography registry. *Catheter Cardiovasc Interv*. 2015;85(5):870–877. doi:10.1002/ccd.25722.

Jain KM, Munn J, Rummel M, et al. Future of vascular surgery is in the office. *J Vasc Surg*. 2010;51(2):509–513, discussion 513–514. doi:10.1016/j.jvs.2009.09.056.

Jain K, Munn J, Rummel MC, et al. Office-based endovascular suite is safe for most procedures. *J Vasc Surg*. 2014;59(1):186–191. doi:10.1016/j.jvs.2013.07.008.

Jain K, Munn J, Rummel M, et al. VS6. Percutaneous Thrombectomy of a Dialysis Graft in the Office Setting. *J Vasc Surg*. 2012;55(6): 28S. doi:10.1016/j.jvs.2012.03.092.

Ketteler ER, Brown KR. Radiation exposure in endovascular procedures. *J Vasc Surg*. 2011;53(1 suppl):35S–38S. doi:10.1016/j.jvs.2010.05.141.

Lin PH, Yang K-H, Kollmeyer KR, et al. Treatment outcomes and lessons learned from 5134 cases of outpatient office-based endovascular procedures in a vascular surgical practice. *Vascular*. July 2016;doi:10.1177/1708538116657506.

Lo RC, Fokkema MTM, Curran T, et al. Routine use of ultrasound-guided access reduces access site-related complications after lower extremity percutaneous revascularization. *J Vasc Surg*. 2015;61(2): 405–412. doi:10.1016/j.jvs.2014.07.099.

Neglén P, Hollis KC, Olivier J, et al. Stenting of the venous outflow in chronic venous disease: long-term stent-related outcome, clinical, and hemodynamic result. *J Vasc Surg*. 2007;46(5):979–990. doi:10.1016/j.jvs.2007.06.046.

References available online at ExpertConsult.com.

CHAPTER 3

1. b
2. b
3. c
4. b
5. d
6. d
7. c
8. a, d, e
9. b, c
10. a

CHAPTER 4

1. b
2. c
3. c
4. b
5. b
6. d
7. c
8. b
9. c
10. c

CHAPTER 5

1. b
2. d
3. a
4. e
5. c
6. a
7. b
8. e
9. c
10. d

CHAPTER 6

1. d
2. b
3. d
4. a
5. c
6. c
7. c
8. a
9. b
10. e

CHAPTER 7

1. a
2. b
3. a
4. e
5. b
6. e
7. c
8. c
9. b
10. d
11. c

CHAPTER 8

1. a
2. e
3. e
4. a
5. e
6. c
7. d
8. a
9. e
10. d

CHAPTER 9

1. a
2. c
3. a
4. b
5. d
6. c
7. d
8. c
9. b
10. a

CHAPTER 10

1. b
2. False
3. e
4. a
5. d
6. d
7. b
8. c
9. True
10. c

CHAPTER 11

1. True
2. c
3. a
4. e
5. True
6. a
7. False
8. f
9. f
10. e

CHAPTER 13

1. b
2. d
3. c
4. a
5. e
6. b
7. False
8. a
9. a
10. c

CHAPTER 14

1. a
2. c
3. c
4. d
5. c
6. b
7. c
8. a
9. a
10. c

CHAPTER 15

1. False
2. d
3. d
4. a, b, c, d
5. b
6. a, c
7. False
8. True
9. d
10. d

CHAPTER 16

1. c
2. a
3. c
4. True
5. False
6. False
7. b

CHAPTER 17

1. b
2. d
3. d
4. d
5. a
6. b
7. d
8. c
9. c
10. a

CHAPTER 18

1. d
2. c
3. a
4. e
5. b

CHAPTER 19

1. e
2. e
3. b
4. c
5. b
6. b
7. e
8. a
9. a
10. d

CHAPTER 20

1. c
2. b
3. d

CHAPTER 21

1. d
2. d
3. b
4. a
5. b
6. a
7. a
8. d
9. d
10. a

CHAPTER 22

1. a
2. d
3. c
4. d
5. d
6. c
7. d
8. e
9. a
10. e

CHAPTER 23

1. b
2. c
3. d
4. c
5. d
6. d
7. c
8. d
9. c
10. c

CHAPTER 24

1. b
2. a, b, c
3. d
4. e
5. b
6. a
7. a
8. b, c
9. a, b, c
10. c

CHAPTER 25

1. c
2. b
3. c
4. b
5. d
6. b
7. b
8. b
9. d
10. a

CHAPTER 26

1. c
2. a
3. d
4. a
5. d
6. c
7. d

CHAPTER 27

1. a
2. b
3. e
4. e

CHAPTER 28

1. True
2. b
3. False
4. False
5. True
6. False
7. b
8. False
9. True
10. False

CHAPTER 29

1. e
2. c
3. e
4. a
5. b
6. d
7. a
8. e
9. e
10. d

CHAPTER 30

1. a
2. d
3. a
4. d
5. b
6. b
7. c
8. b
9. a
10. b

CHAPTER 31

1. b
2. e
3. b
4. d

5. b
6. d
7. e

CHAPTER 32

1. c
2. c
3. b
4. c
5. b
6. c
7. d
8. a
9. d
10. d

CHAPTER 33

1. c
2. a, b, c
3. a, b
4. e
5. d
6. c
7. c
8. a, b, d
9. e
10. d

CHAPTER 34

1. d
2. d
3. a
4. d
5. b
6. a
7. e
8. b
9. a
10. a

CHAPTER 35

1. d
2. c
3. e
4. b
5. c
6. d
7. a
8. e
9. c
10. a

CHAPTER 36

1. c
2. e
3. a
4. a
5. c
6. a
7. c
8. b
9. a
10. c

CHAPTER 37

1. The indications for TEVAR are the same as for open repair and typically include aneurysms greater than 5.5 to 6 cm in diameter, although saccular and symptomatic aneurysms are often repaired at a smaller size. It is also suggested that aneurysms with a rapid growth rate (more than 1 cm per year, or 0.5 cm in 6 months) should be considered for early intervention.
2. About 10% to 20% is the ideal amount to oversize the aortic diameter at the seal zones, which should be no less than 20 mm long. Grafts that are oversized can lead to folding and gutter formation. Grafts that are undersized tend to migrate and have persistent endoleaks.
3. Each zone is divided by a tangential line along the distal side of each great vessel; zone 0 involves the origin of the innominate artery, zone 1 the origin of the left common carotid artery (LCCA), zone 2 the origin of the left subclavian artery (LSCA), zone 3 the proximal descending thoracic aorta down to the T4 vertebral body, and zone 4 the remainder of descending thoracic aorta. The location of the proximal landing zone depends on the aneurysm's morphology; however; the ideal location in terms of anatomic accommodation of the graft is in zones 3 and 4.
4. Current Society for Vascular Surgery (SVS) guidelines recommend routine preoperative revascularization in elective TEVAR with expectant management in emergency situations. Absolute contraindications of LSCA coverage include a dominant left vertebral artery, left internal mammary to coronary artery bypass, left-arm hemodialysis access, aberrant right SCA, anomalous origin of the left SCA from the aortic arch, hypoplastic right vertebral artery, termination of the left vertebral artery in the posterior inferior cerebellar artery and/or occluded internal iliac arteries. In addition, extended thoracic aortic coverage combined with prior abdominal aortic repair should be considered as posing a higher risk for spinal cord ischemia (SCI), and LSCA revascularization should be performed.
5. After careful interrogation of the gastroduodenal and pancreaticoduodenal arcades and verifying their patency, the celiac access may be covered to assure for a good 20-mm distal seal zone.

6. Data from the three FDA trials showed a cumulative advantage over open repair, with a rate of 6% (vs. 10% in open TAA repair). Several factors have been linked to an increased risk of SCI after TEVAR: concomitant or previous open infrarenal aortic replacement, lack of spinal drainage, extensive thoracic aortic coverage (especially T9 to T12), renal insufficiency, intraoperative hypotension (systolic blood pressure <80 mm Hg), emergency surgery, and coverage of the hypogastric artery or the LSA or both.
7. The stroke rates associated with TAA range from 4% to 8% and are believed to occur primarily because of instrumentation of the aortic arch, causing embolization and occasionally coverage of a critical source of blood to the brain.
8. The published data show the perioperative mortality risk to be 2% (vs. 6% in open repair). The EUROSTAR registry reports a higher but still favorable mortality rate of 5.3%, likely because the patients in the study were deemed not eligible for open repair due to comorbidities and thus represented a sicker cohort.

CHAPTER 38

1. c
2. a
3. b
4. b
5. c
6. b
7. b
8. c
9. c
10. c

CHAPTER 40

1. c
2. e
3. b
4. e
5. b
6. d
7. c
8. d
9. a
10. e

CHAPTER 41

1. e
2. d
3. a
4. a
5. b
6. e
7. b
8. a
9. d
10. a

CHAPTER 42

1. a
2. b
3. True
4. d
5. True
6. False
7. b
8. c
9. False
10. True

CHAPTER 43

1. True
2. False. It depends on the degree of containment of the rupture.
3. False. Only when the rupture is confirmed should a long incision be made.
4. True
5. False. Only by isolating the aorta can clamp control be achieved.
6. True
7. False
8. True
9. True. But only with supraceliac clamp control.
10. d

CHAPTER 44

1. b
2. c
3. a
4. b
5. a, b
6. b
7. b
8. b
9. b
10. b

CHAPTER 45

1. c
2. e
3. e
4. d
5. e
6. c

CHAPTER 46

1. a
2. d
3. a
4. b
5. c

6. c
7. c
8. b
9. c
10. c

CHAPTER 47

1. b
2. c
3. c
4. c
5. a
6. c
7. a
8. a
9. d
10. c

CHAPTER 48

1. d
2. d
3. c
4. a
5. b
6. c
7. b

CHAPTER 49

1. c
2. b
3. a
4. d
5. b
6. d
7. d
8. c
9. c
10. b

CHAPTER 50

1. a
2. d
3. a
4. c
5. f
6. e
7. e
8. e
9. d
10. d
11. b

CHAPTER 51

1. a
2. d
3. c
4. a
5. a
6. a
7. a
8. b
9. b
10. a

CHAPTER 52

1. c
2. e
3. b
4. b
5. a
6. d
7. b
8. d
9. e
10. d

CHAPTER 53

1. d
2. d
3. a
4. c
5. d
6. d
7. e
8. e
9. b
10. c

CHAPTER 54

1. d
2. e
3. b
4. e
5. b
6. a
7. c
8. d
9. d
10. b

CHAPTER 55

1. c
2. b
3. c

4. e
5. c
6. e
7. b
8. e
9. c
10. d
11. e

CHAPTER 56

1. b
2. d
3. a
4. c
5. c
6. a
7. b
8. b
9. c
10. a

CHAPTER 57

1. a
2. d
3. c
4. b
5. c
6. a
7. d
8. a

CHAPTER 58

1. e
2. e
3. b
4. c
5. d
6. c
7. d
8. b
9. c
10. e

CHAPTER 59

1. b
2. c
3. b
4. d
5. a
6. d
7. e

CHAPTER 60

1. b
2. a
3. d
4. b
5. a
6. c
7. d
8. c
9. c
10. a

CHAPTER 62

1. c. Approximately two-thirds of foot infections are polymicrobial, with gram-positive aerobes comprising approximately 60% of isolates. Gram-negative organisms typically comprise 20% of isolates. An analysis using 16s rRNA identified anaerobes in 87% of bone specimens, but conventional culture results generally identify anaerobic bacteria in 10% to 20% of cases.
2. c. Previous studies have identified *E. coli* and *P. aeruginosa* as being associated with a higher rate of major (above-ankle) amputations. MRSA has not been associated with higher rates of amputation.
3. d. Limb preservation efforts will provide no meaningful benefit to patients who have essentially no limb function. Aggressive surgical drainage of infection and antibiotic therapy should be used as the first line strategy to obtain source control in most situations. Osteomyelitis should be treated with antibiotics, possibly in combination with surgical resection of bone. Charcot arthropathy can provide challenges (especially to offloading attempts) but should not exclude patients from being candidates for limb preservation efforts.

CHAPTER 63

1. Wound healing that does not occur in a predictable fashion. The normal processes of healing involving hemostasis, inflammation, proliferation, and remodeling are interrupted.
2. Precise description of wound size, appearance, exudate, and the wound edges.
3. Elimination of edema through leg elevation and compression, debridement of nonviable tissue, treatment of infection, management of the exudate, and dressing the wound.
4. Wounds can be categorized as contaminated, colonized, or infected. Wound infection is often a clinical finding, including increasing pain, exudate, odor, and wound changes. Wound infection is defined by 1 × 105 organisms per gram.
5. False
6. False
7. True
8. f
9. False
10. e

CHAPTER 64

1. d
2. e
3. c
4. c
5. e
6. d
7. c
8. e
9. c
10. e

CHAPTER 65

1. c
2. b
3. d
4. b
5. b
6. d
7. b
8. a
9. c
10. b

CHAPTER 66

1. c
2. c
3. a
4. d
5. b
6. a
7. d
8. c
9. a
10. b

CHAPTER 67

1. True
2. False
3. False
4. False
5. True
6. True
7. True
8. False
9. True
10. False

INDEX

Page numbers followed by "*f*" indicate figures, "*t*" indicate tables, and "*b*" indicate boxes.

G